Burger's Medicinal Chemistry

Fourth Edition

Part II

BURGER'S MEDICINAL CHEMISTRY

Fourth Edition

Part II

Edited by

MANFRED E. WOLFF

Department of Pharmaceutical Chemistry
School of Pharmacy
University of California
San Francisco, California

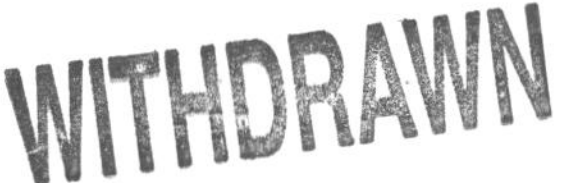

A WILEY-INTERSCIENCE PUBLICATION

JOHN WILEY & SONS, New York · Chichester · Brisbane · Toronto

Notice Concerning Trademark or Patent Rights.
The listing or discussion in this book of any drug in respect to which patent or trademark rights may exist shall not be deemed, and is not intended as a grant of, or authority to exercise, or an infringement of, any right or privilege protected by such patent or trademark.

Library of Congress Cataloging in Publication Data

Burger, Alfred, 1905– ed.
Burger's Medicinal chemistry.

"A Wiley-Interscience publication."
Bibliography: p.
Includes index.

1. Chemistry, Pharmaceutical. 2. Chemotherapy.
I. Wolff, Manfred E. II. Title. III. Title:
Medicinal chemistry. [DNLM: 1. Chemistry, Pharmaceutical. QV744.3 B954]
RS403.B8 1979 615′.7 78-10791
ISBN 0-471-01571-7

Printed in the United States of America

10 9 8 7 6 5 4 3 2 1

Preface

Reading every word in these books, which an editor must do, has given me enormous pride in being a medicinal chemist. It has given me an equally strong confidence that we are only at the beginning of our greatest accomplishments. Nowhere is the rhythm of history and its meaning for the future plainer than in the field of chemotherapy described in this volume.

Antimicrobial sulfonamides, the subject of the initial chapter, began to be developed in the late thirties. The striking progress made at that time came only after 40 to 50 years had passed since the conceptualization of chemotherapy and the development of the aromatic arsenicals. We are now at a similar point relative to a later period of theorizing in medicinal chemistry: these volumes are being published about four decades after the enunciation of the theory of metabolite antagonism by Woods and Fildes. Thus historical precedent and present evidence both suggest that the time for new wide advances is at hand.

The past four decades have been well used by medicinal chemists to build the infrastructure necessary to solve the many problems outlined by the authors of the later chapters of these volumes. An enhanced understanding of the biochemistry of disease, the mechanism of drug action, and the course of drug metabolism has given us a far more accurate view of our science. These basic phenomena have been stressed in each chapter. In such important areas as the antimalarials and other antiparasitic agents covered in Chapters 18 through 21, we may hope that the progress which has been made will result in reducing the huge incidence of these diseases. The same is true for the antiviral and antineoplastic substances covered in Chapters 23 to 25. The hormonal drugs described in Chapters 26–31 include mature fields as well as areas that promise to expand explosively. The use of recombinant DNA techniques for the production of peptide and protein hormones and drugs may well revolutionize drug development in this domain. Chapters 32 to 35 discuss vital areas that are still almost in their infancy but about which a growing body of knowledge is developing; some did not even merit separate chapters at the time of the Third Edition. By contrast, some older declining areas have been dropped from these pages to conserve space.

In this edition of *Burger's Medicinal Chemistry*, Alfred Burger's plan of grouping broad therapeutic classes into contiguous chapters has been retained. This volume deals with most of the chemotherapeutic and endocrine drug classes, although scheduling difficulties resulted in the displacement of a few chapters to Part III. Many of the authors are new to these volumes but all are authorities in their fields. They have invested massive amounts of time and effort in attempting to distill these complex fields into a concise presentation. Errors in a work of this scope are inevitable and we will be grateful to be informed of omissions or mistakes.

MANFRED E. WOLFF

San Francisco, California
January 1979

Contents

CHAPTER THIRTEEN

Sulfonamides and Sulfones

NITYA ANAND

Central Drug Research Institute
Chattar Manzil Palace
Lucknow-226001, India

CONTENTS

1 INTRODUCTION

The development of sulfonamides is one of the most fascinating and informative chapters in medicinal chemistry, highlighting the roles of skillful planning and serendipity in drug research. The discovery of the antibacterial activity of sulfonamides in the early 1930s was the beginning of the present era of chemotherapy. The subsequent recognition of a relationship between the chemical structure of these compounds and their pharmacological response brought into sharp focus the potential power of molecular modification in drug design. The standardization of a suitable method for estimation of sulfonamides in body fluids and tissues added a new dimension—that of pharmacokinetic studies—to drug research. Careful observation of side effects in pharmacological and clinical studies on the early sulfonamides revealed new and unanticipated activities; the sucessful exploitation of these leads opened up such new areas in chemotherapy as oral antidiabetics, carbonic anhydrase inhibitors, and diuretics, and emphasized the importance of side effects of drugs as a source of new leads in drug design. The elucidation of the relationship between sulfonamides and *p*-aminobenzoic acid provided the long sought-after mechanistic basis for a rational approach to chemotherapy. All these studies had a strong impact on thinking in medicinal chemistry and influenced much of the later work in drug research in general and chemotherapy in particular. The rapidity with which new developments took place from 1935 to 1940—from the discovery of the antibacterial activity of sulfonamides to the enunciation of the theory of antimetabolites by Fildes—indicates that the time was just ripe for major developments and needed only a catalyst, which was provided by this discovery.

Interest in sulfonamides has continued unabated. About 30 sulfonamides are now used in clinical practice. They vary widely in their absorption, distribution, and excretion patterns. Some remain largely unabsorbed after oral administration and are useful for gastrointestinal tract infections. Another group characterized by high solubility, quick absorption, and rapid excretion, mainly in the unaltered form, is widely used in urinary tract infections. Yet another group is absorbed rapidly but excreted slowly, resulting in maintenance of adequate levels in the blood for long periods; these sulfonamides require less frequent administration and are particularly useful for chronic conditions and for prophylaxis. The wide difference in the absorption and excretion properties of different sulfonamides has greatly increased their value in therapeutics. This, coupled with their ease of administration, wide spectrum of antimicrobial activity, noninterference with the host-defense mechanism, and relative freedom from the problem of superinfection, is responsible for their extensive use in clinical practice even four decades after their discovery. The use of sulfonamides and sulfones now extends from the treatment of acute and chronic gram-positive and gram-negative bacterial infections, including leprosy, through trachoma, lymphogranuloma venereum, malaria, nocardiosis, coccidiosis, to toxoplasmosis.

2 DEVELOPMENT OF SULFONAMIDES AND SULFONES

2.1 Historical Background

The story of sulfonamides goes back to the early years of this century when Hörlein, Dressel, and Kethe of I. G. Farbenindustrie (1) found that introduction of a sulfamyl group imparted fastness to acid wool dyes, thus indicating affinity for protein molecules. However none of these sulfonamides was investigated for antibacterial activity. The interest in dyes as possible antimicrobials, stimulated by Ehrlich's studies on the relationship between selective staining by dyes and their antiprotozoal activity, led to the testing of azo dyes for antibacterial activity, and some of them indeed showed such activity. In an attempt to improve the bactericidal properties of quinine derivatives, Heidelberger and Jacobs (2) prepared dyes based on dihydrocupreine, which included *p*-aminobenzenesulfonamido-hydrocupreine (13.**1**).

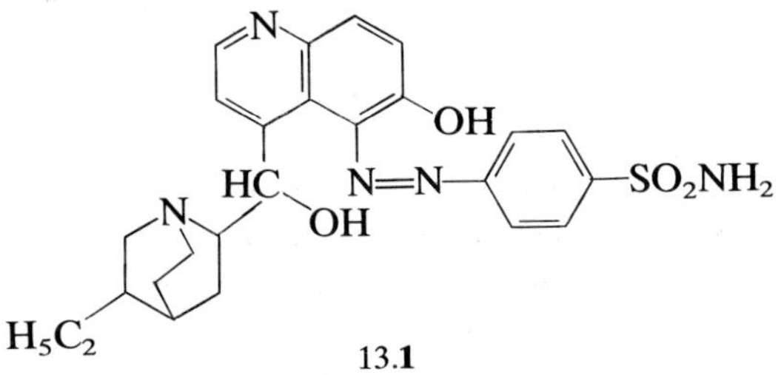

13.**1**

Although the latter was reported to have bactericidal activity, it did not arouse much interest because the activity, having been tested *in vitro,* was found to be low, and no further work was published on these compounds. The work of Mietzch and Klarer of I. G. Farbenindustrie on azo dyes, a continuation of Ehrlich's interest in dyes, led to the development of compounds having high bactericidal activity *in vivo,* but this activity had poor carryover to tests *in vivo.* The lack of correlation between tests *in vitro* and *in vivo* prompted Domagk to take up bactericidal screening *in vitro* in mice in place of *in vitro* testing, a very fortunate decision, since otherwise the fate of sulfonamides might have been different. With the hope of imparting to azo dyes the property of specific binding to bacterial proteins, comparable to the binding to wool proteins, Mietzch and Klarer (3) synthesized a group of such dyes containing a sulfonamide radical, which included prontosil (13.**2**).

13.**2**

Domagk (4) discovered in 1932 that prontosil protected mice against streptococcal infections and rabbits against staphylococcal infections, but had no effect on pneumococcal infections and was without action *in vitro* on bacteria; these epoch-making results were published in 1935. Foerster (5) reported the first clinical success with prontosil in a case of staphylococcal septicemia in 1933.

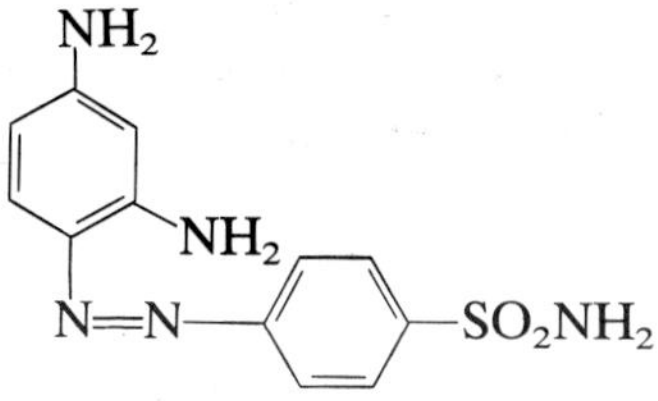

These studies aroused worldwide interest, and further developments took place at a very fast rate. One of the earliest systematic investigations was by Trefouël, Trefouël, Nitti, and Bovet (6), working at the Pasteur Institute in Paris. Under a program of structural modification of this class of compounds, they prepared a series of azo dyes by coupling diazotized sulfanilamide with phenols, with and without amino or alkyl groups. They observed that variations in the structure of the phenolic moiety had very little effect on *in vitro* antibacterial activity, whereas even small changes in the sulfanilamide component abolished the activity. These observations pointed to the sulfonamide group as the active structural unit and led to the conclusion that metabolic cleavage of the azo linkage generates *p*-aminobenzenesulfonamide (sulfanilamide, 13.**3**), which

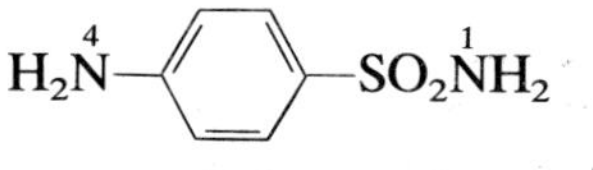

13.**3**

may be responsible for the antibacterial activity. They suggested that prontosil was converted in animals to sulfanilamide and showed that sulfanilamide was as effective as the parent dyestuff in protecting mice infected with streptococci. They also showed that sulfanilamide exerted a bacteriostatic effect *in vitro* on susceptible organisms. Soon after, Colebrook and Kenny (7) observed that although prontosil was inactive *in vitro*, the blood of patients treated with it had bacteriostatic activity. They also reported the dramatic cure of 64 cases of puerperal sepsis by prontosil, while Buttle, Gray, and Stephenson (8) showed that sulfanilamide could cure streptococcal and meningococcal infections in mice. Fuller's (9) demonstration of the presence of sulfanilamide in the blood and its isolation from urine of patients (and mice) under treatment with prontosil firmly established that prontosil is reduced in the body to form sulfanilamide, a compound synthesized as early as 1909 by Gelmo (10). Fuller concluded that the therapeutic action of prontosil was very likely due to its reduction to sulfanilamide. The era of modern chemotherapy had begun. Though Ehrlich's concept of a relationship between the affinity of dyes for a parasite and their antimicrobial activity, which focused attention on sulfonamides, was found to be irrelevant to the activity of the latter sulfonamides proved to be the "magic bullet" of Ehrlich.

These discoveries had a tremendous impact. Sulfanilamide, being easy to prepare, cheap, and not covered by patents, became available for widespread use and brought a new hope for the treatment of microbial infections. Recognizing the potentiality of sulfonamides, almost all the major research organizations the world over initiated research programs for the synthesis and study of analogs and derivatives of sulfanilamide, particularly with a view to improve its antimicrobial spectrum, therapeutic ratio, and pharmacokinetic properties. New sulfonamides were introduced in quick succession till about 1945 when, with the introduction of penicillin, interest gradually shifted to antibiotics. After about a decade, problems encountered with antibiotics, such as emergence of resistant strains, superinfection, and allergic reactions, brought a revival of interest in sulfonamides. The knowledge obtained during this period about the selectivity of action of sulfonamides on the parasite, the relationship between their solubility and toxicity, and their pharmacokinetics, gave a new direction to further developments in this field. New sulfonamides with modified properties began to appear. Thus there are two distinct phases in the development of sulfonamides, the old (pre-1945) and the new (post-1957).

Some of the other developments that had far-reaching effects on future progress not only in the field of sulfonamides but on chemotherapy and drug research in general may be mentioned. The standardization by Bratton and Marshall (11, 12) of a simple method for the assay of sulfonamides in body fluids and tissues permitted precise determination of the absorption, distribution, and excretion of these drugs, thus provided a rational basis for calculating proper dosage requirements. Pharmacokinetic studies thus became an integral part of drug development programs. Wood's (13) observation of the competitive reversal of the action of sulfanilamide by *p*-aminobenzoic acid (PAB) was the first definite demonstration of metabolite antagonism as a mechanism of drug action. This led Fildes (14) to propose his classical theory of antimetabolites, which has been the basis of numerous and intensive studies in chemotherapy and pharmacology. The observation of certain clinical side effects in the early sulfonamides and the success in dissociating these effects from antimicrobial activity by structural modification (*loc. cit.*), resulted in a proper appreciation of the role of side effects of drugs as an important source of leads for drug design (15).

2.2 Nomenclature and Classification

The general term "sulfonamides" has been used for derivatives of *p*-aminobenzenesulfonamide (sulfanilamide), whereas specific compounds are described as N^1- or N^4-substituted sulfanilamides (13.**3**), depending on whether the substitution is on the amido or aromatic amino group, respectively. Most of the sulfonamides used currently are N^1-derivatives. Similarly, the term "sulfone" is used for all derivatives of 4,4′-diaminodiphenylsulfone, whereas specific compounds are described as substituted diaminodiphenylsulfones.

The generic name of a sulfonamide is built up by adding the prefix "sulfa-" to an abbreviated form of the chemical name of the N^1-residue. This is done in two ways: either the amido nitrogen is taken as a part of the "sulfa" residue, as in the case of N^1-heterocyclic sulfonamides, e.g., sulfapyridine (13.**11**), or the amido nitrogen is taken as a part of the N^1-residue as in sulfaguanidine (13.**10**).

Sulfonamides have been classified in many different ways and the one based on absorption and half-life (the time needed for the concentration of the drug in the blood to be reduced to one-half) appears to be the most logical and clinically relevant (Table 13.2). Sulfonamides that have a half-life of less than 10 hr are termed short-acting; between 10 and 24 hr are considered to be medium-acting, and longer than 24 hr are long-acting. "Long-acting" denotes slow excretion and/or reabsorption of the drug into the system from the excretory route and is to be differentiated from the depot form. In the latter case, the drug is formulated in such a way that it is stored in the body in a form in which the total quantity is not available all at once, but is gradually released, e.g., 4.4′-diacetamidodiphenylsulfone (13.**34**) (*loc. cit.*).

2.3 Older Sulfonamides

In an effort to improve on the efficacy of sulfanilamide, more than 5000 derivatives and analogs were investigated in the first phase of research in this field. This work has been described in 1948 in a most exhaustive and thought-provoking monograph by Northey (16), which may be consulted for details of the work of this period. The analogs studied included position isomers, compounds having substituents on the functional groups, isosteres, and ring annellates of the benzene ring. It was realized quite early that the *p*-aminobenzenesulfonyl unit is inviolate for maintaining the activity; therefore almost all the emphasis was laid on preparing N^1-substituted derivatives. The activity shown by some N^4-derivatives was found to be due either to regeneration of the free aromatic amino group or to a mechanism other than antagonism of PAB.

Variation of the N^1-substituent gave a variety of compounds having antimicrobial activity, all acting by PAB antagonism, and most of the sulfonamides used in clinical practice today are N^1-substituted derivatives. For the sake of clarity, these developments are discussed according to the type of N^1-substitution.

2.3.1 N^1-ALKYL, -ARYLAKYL, -CYCLOALKYL, AND CARBOARYL DERIVATIVES. Introduction of these substituents in general leads to lowering or loss of activity, and none of these derivatives is used clinically.

2.3.2 N^1-ACYL DERIVATIVES. N^1Acyl substitution leads to compounds with enhanced biological activity and useful physical properties. Several clinically useful compounds belong to this group. These derivatives are strong acids and form highly soluble neutral sodium salts, giving nonirritant solutions. Such salts are useful for local treatment where the high alkalinity of the sodium salts of other sulfa drugs would be unacceptable. The most important member of this group, widely used in ophthalmic practice, is sulfacetamide (13.**4**) (17, 18), which is more active than sulfanilamide and is as active as sulfadiazine against some organisms *in vivo.* It is quickly absorbed and rapidly excreted without danger of crystallization in the kidney.

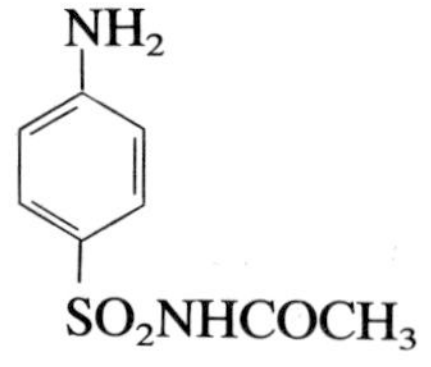

NH_2–C_6H_4–$SO_2NHCOCH_3$

13.**4**

N^1-Aryl-sulfanilamides, though active, do not show any advantage over sulfacetamide or other commonly used sulfonamides (19).

In contrast to sulfacetamide, N^1-higher acyl derivatives are deacylated very substantially in the body and are not clinically useful. N^1-Acetyl derivatives of N^1-heterocyclic sulfanilamides are inactive *in vitro* but have the advantage of being tasteless as compared to the bitter taste of the parent compound; these are quantitatively deacetylated in the intestine and find use in liquid medications (20, 21).

N^4-Carboxyacyl derivatives of sulfacetamide such as N^4-phthalyl- and N^4-succinyl-sulfacetamides (13.**5** and 13.**6**) (22) and of certain N^1-heterocyclic sulfonamides, such as N^4-phthalyl- and succinylsulfathiazoles (13.**7** and 13.**8**) (23), form highly soluble neutral sodium salts and were developed for parenteral administration. Because of rapid excretion, however, adequate blood levels are not built up. These compounds are inactive *in vitro* and remain practically unabsorbed after oral administration, but they undergo gradual intestinal deacetylation to release the active compound. These compounds have found extensive use in intestinal infections. Since they are very poorly absorbed and rapidly excreted, large doses can be administered orally without danger of toxic effects. It is supposed that because of their high solubility under alkaline conditions, they mix well with the intestinal contents and undergo slow hydrolysis, giving a relatively high local concentration of the parent sulfonamide as the effective agent. Because much of the parent sulfonamide would be released low in the intestine where absorption is poor, the drug would not appear in the blood in toxic concentration. It has been suggested that this may be the main reason for their effectiveness. Since these derivatives produce mainly local changes in the bacterial flora, they are extensively used for presurgical sterilization of the gut and for certain intestinal infections; phthalylsulfathiazole is the agent of choice. The concept of the advantage of local action for intestinal infections is, however, questioned by some.

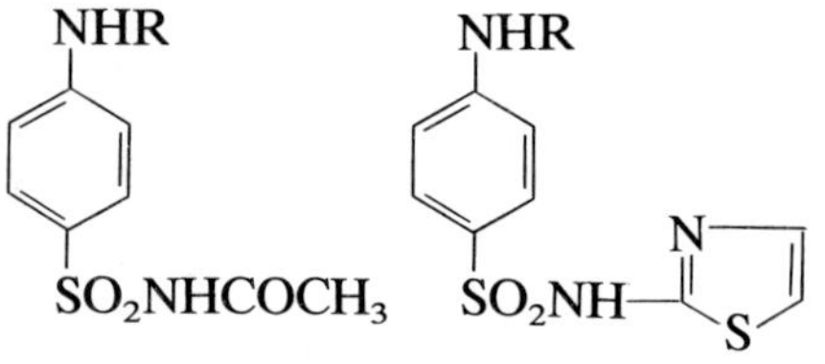

Among the N^1-carbonic acid derivatives, sulfacarbamide (13.**9**) (24, 25) and sulfaguanidine (13.**10**) (26) are of interest.

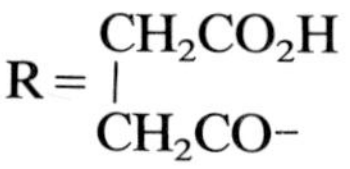

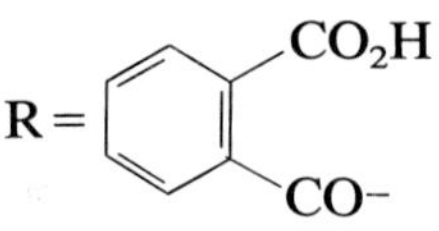

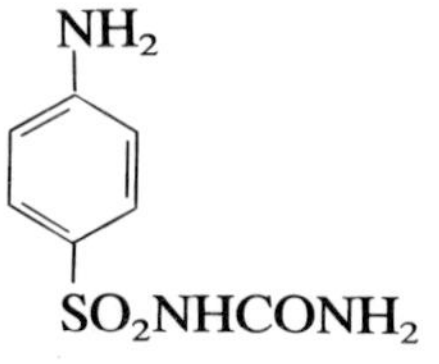

NHR–C_6H_4–$SO_2NHCOCH_3$ NHR–C_6H_4–SO_2NH–(2-thiazolyl)

13.**5** $R = CH_2CO_2H$ / CH_2CO– 13.**7**

13.**6** $R = C_6H_4(CO_2H)(CO$–$)$ 13.**8**

NH_2–C_6H_4–$SO_2NHCONH_2$ NH_2–C_6H_4–$SO_2NHC(=NH)NH_2$

13.**9** 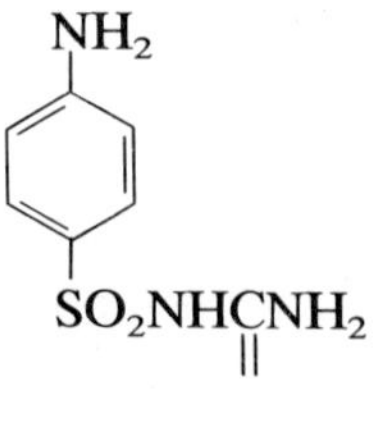 13.**10**

Sulfacarbamide, though not highly active *in vivo* on account of its quick absorption and rapid excretion, finds limited use in pyelitis and urinary tract infections. Sulfaguanidine is more active than sulfanilamide *in vitro*. It is now realized that it is not as poorly absorbed from the gastrointestinal tract as was considered earlier and can cause toxicity when used at a high dose.

2.3.3 N^1-HETEROAROMATIC SULFANILAMIDES. Of the therapeutically used sulfonamides, the more important ones belong to this class. By varying the N^1-heterocyclic residue, it has been possible to greatly enlarge the usefulness of sulfonamides by widening their antimicrobial spectrum, increasing the inhibition index, and modifying their pharmacokinetic properties.

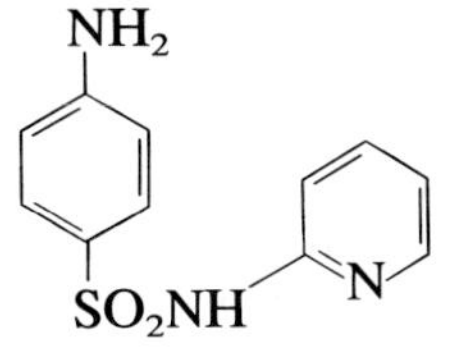

13.**11**

Sulfapyridine (May and Baker 693, 13.**11**) (27), reported in 1938, was one of the earliest of the new sulfonamides to be used in clinical practice for the treatment of pneumonia and remained the drug of choice until it was replaced by sulfathiazole (13.**16**). Apart from sulfapyridine, all the other clinically used N^1-heterocyclic sulfonamides possessing six-membered heterocyclic ring have more than one hetero atom. Diazines (pyrimidines, pyridazines, and pyrazines) have shown the best activity; of these, the derivatives of pyrimidine have received the maximum attention and have provided a large number of clinically useful drugs (28). A sulfonamide linkage at either the 2- or the 4-position gives active compounds. Sulfadiazine (13.**12**) (29) was the first of these derivatives to be introduced and it has retained preeminence among sulfonamides

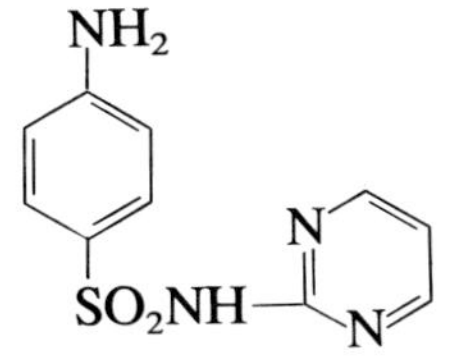

13.**12**

ever since, because of its broad antibacterial spectrum, high *in vivo* activity, low toxicity, and (subsequently discovered) long duration of action. In much of the later work sulfadiazine has been used as a standard for comparison of activity. Two methylated derivatives of sulfadiazine, sulfamerazine (13.**13**) (29–33) and sulfamethazine (13.**14**) (29–33) were soon introduced in therapeutics. Sulfamerazine

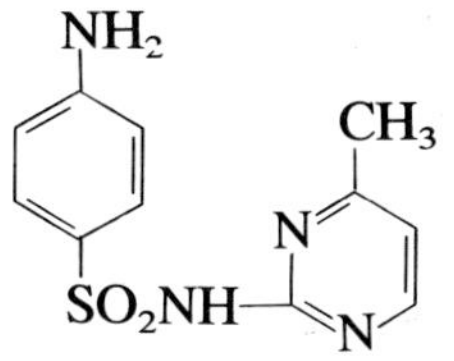

13.**13**

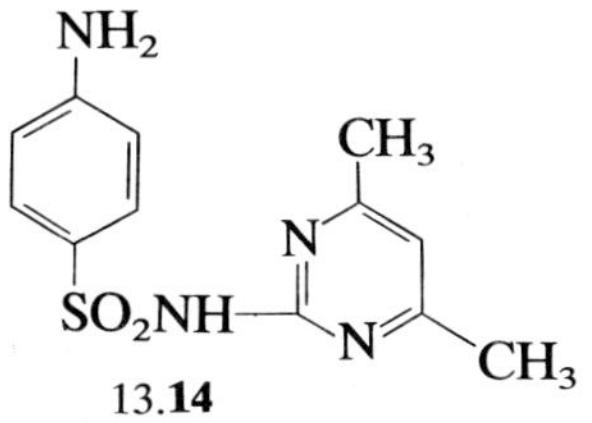

13.**14**

shows greater solubility in water at pH 7.0, and it is more quickly absorbed and more slowly excreted than sulfadiazine. Sulfamethazine is even more soluble than sulfamerazine at pH 5.5; though less active *in vitro* and *in vivo* than sulfadiazine and sulfamerazine, this property gives it a greater tolerance and clinical advantage over the other two. Since these quantitative differences in the properties of the three pyrimidine derivatives seem to complement one another, they have been used in combination as a "triple sulfa." This made it possible to (*a*) lower the dose of each individual component, thus reducing the toxicity of each and lowering significantly the tendency to crystalluria (a major toxicity hazard of earlier sulfonamides), thereby improving the tolerance and activity; (*b*) maintain higher concentrations in plasma and tissue over a long period. The use of combination sulfas was a significant development in this field (34, 35).

Among the 4-sulfapyrimidine derivatives, sulfisomidine (13.**15**) was shown to possess useful activity (36). Its main advantages are high solubility and low tendency to crystalluria, which gives it better tolerance than other pyrimidine derivitives. A useful "disulfa" combination is sulfisomidine and sulfadiazine.

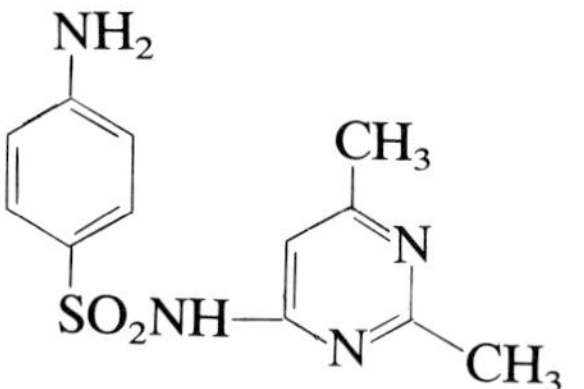

13.**15**

Clinically used sulfas containing five-membered heterocycles have two or more hetero atoms in the ring. The more active compounds belong to the thiazole, oxazole, isoxazole, 1,3,4-thiadiazole, and pyrazole groups. Azoles having an NH in the ring have little activity, but *N*-aryl and *N*-alkyl substituted componds are active, and some of them have been found to be of clinical interest. The corresponding hetero- or benzo- annellates are less active. Most of the clinically used five-membered heterocyclic compounds (except sulfaphenazole) possess one or two CH_3 groups, which must increase their hydrophobicity, and impart favorable properties for binding to protein and perhaps to folate enzyme. The position of substituents in the hetero ring also has a significant effect on the activity pattern of these compounds. Sulfathiazole (13,**16**) (37), the first member of this group to be introduced in clinical practice, replaced sulfapyridine because of its wider antibacterial spectrum and higher therapeutic index. Substitution of the thiazole ring by alkyl groups did not improve the activity, but a 4-phenyl residue enhanced both the activity and the toxicity. An additional nitrogen atom in the ring at position 3, to give 1,3,4-sulfathiadiazole, did not enhance the activity; however a methyl substituent in the 5-position gave sulfamethizole (13.**17**), which has an increased antibacterial activity (38, 39), high solubility, quick absorption, and rapid excretion. Sulfamethizole had, in addition, hypoglycemic activity (*loc. cit.*), which was increased when the methyl group was replaced by an ethyl or an isopropyl group. Another sulfonamide introduced during this period was sulfisoxazole (13.**18**); though less active than sulfadiazine, it is better tolerated because of its high solubility and rapid excretion. Its significant activity against *Proteus vulgaris* and *Escherichia coli* makes it useful in urinary tract infections (40, 41).

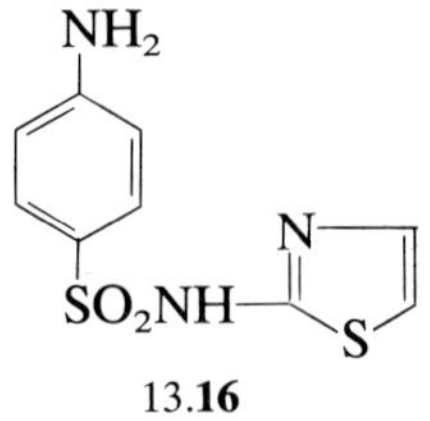

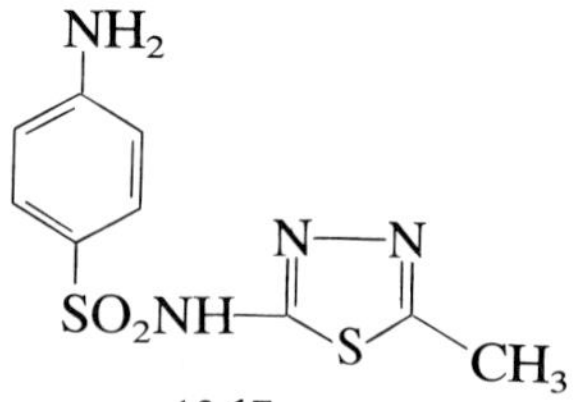

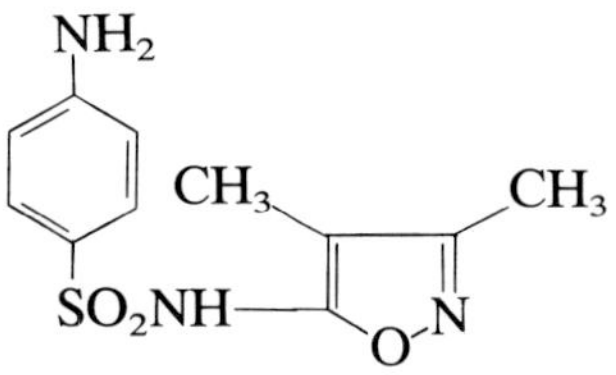

13.**16**

13.**17**

13.**18**

2.3.4 4-SUBSTITUTED DERIVATIVES. The only compound of any importance in this group is 4-aminomethylbenzenesulfanilamide (homosulfanilamide, 13.**19**) (42). Among other organisms, it is active against

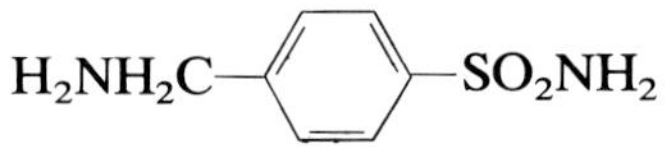

H_2NH_2C—C_6H_4—SO_2NH_2

13.**19**

anaerobic bacteria, therefore finds use for topical application in infected wounds and gas gangrene. It does not act through the PAB mechanism and can be used against organisms resistant to other sulfonamides.

2.4 Newer Sulfonamides

A major advance in sulfonamide therapy came with the proper appreciation of the role of pharmacokinetic studies in determining the dosage schedule of these drugs. It was realized that some of the "older" sulfonamides such as sulfadiazine and sulfamerazine had a long half-life (17 and 24 hr, respectively) and required less frequent administration than normally was prescribed. In fact, a mixture of sulfamerazine and sulfaproxyline was one of the earliest long-acting sulfonamides to be used; it was administered three times a day. The era of newer long-acting sulfonamides started in 1956 with the introduction of sulfamethoxypyridazine (13.**20**) (44), having a half-life of 37 hr, the longest known at that time, which had to be administered only once a day (45). Sulfachlorpyridazine (13.**21**) (46), a related sulfonamide and an intermediate in the synthesis of 13.**20**, was, however, found to have a half-life of about

13.**20** R = OCH_3
13.**21** R = Cl

7 hr and is useful for urinary tract infections. In 1959 sulfadimethoxine (13.**22**) was introduced with a half-life of approximately 40 hr (28, 47, 48). The related 4-sulfonamidopyrimidine, sulfamethoxine (13.**23**) (49, 50), having the two methoxyl radicals in 5,6-positions, has by far the longest half-life—about 150 hr—and would need administration once a week. Sulfamethyldiazine (13.**24**) (51) and sulfamethoxydiazine (13.**25**) (51), each having a half-life of 36 hr, and sulfamethoxypyrazine (13.**26**) (52), with a half-life of 65 hr, were the other long-acting sulfonamides introduced during this period.

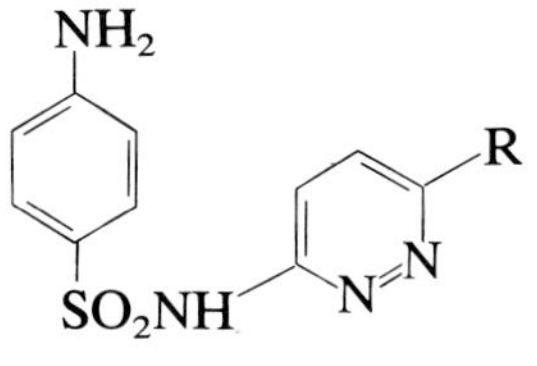

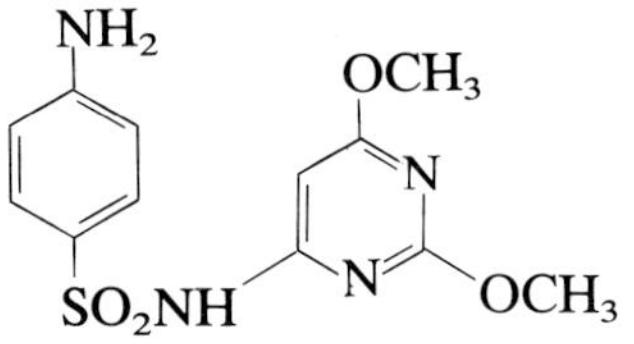

13.**22**

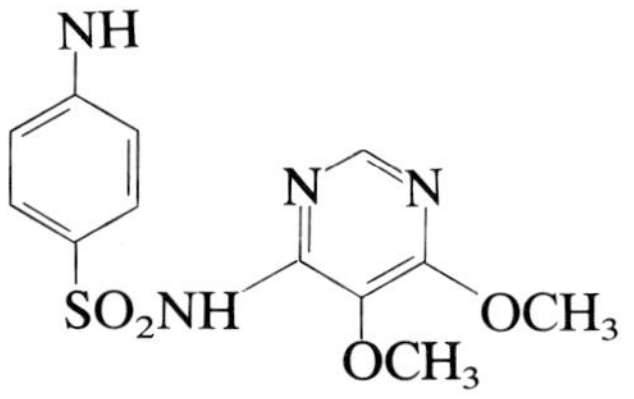

13.**23**

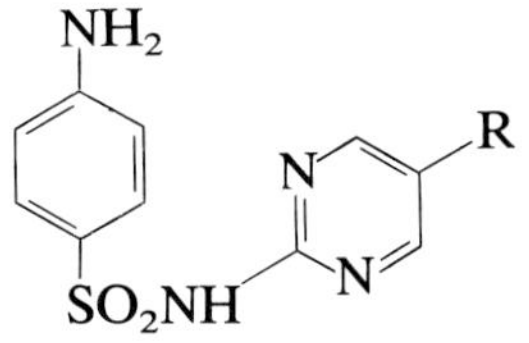

13.**24** R = CH_3
13.**25** R = OCH_3

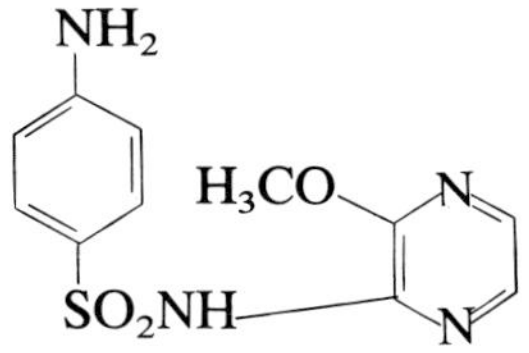

13.**26**

Sulfaphenazole (13.**27**) (53), sulfamethoxazole (13.**28**) (54), and sulfamoxol (13.**29**) (55), the other sulfonamides put into clinical practice during this period, are relatively shorter acting, having a half-life of about 11 hr each.

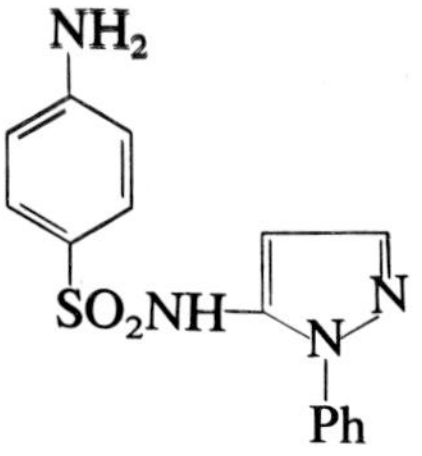

13.**27**

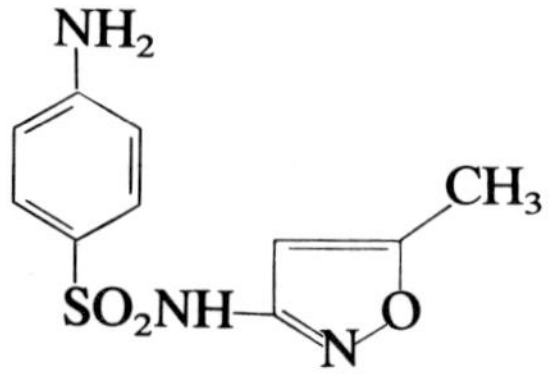

13.**28**

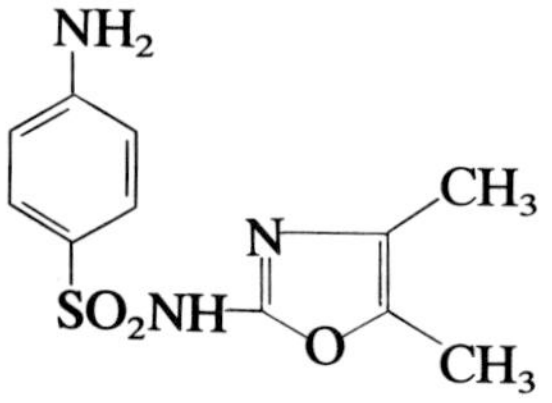

13.**29**

A new broad spectrum sulfonamide, sulfaclomide (13.**30**) (56), has been reported recently. It is relatively nontoxic and gives higher serum levels than other sulfonamides, and patients do not need extra fluid intake or alkalization. Sulfa-1-ethylcytosine (13.**21**) (57) has been reported to be 3–10 times more potent *in vivo* than sulfisoxazole and sulfisomidine. Highly soluble, rapidly absorbed, and excreted almost unchanged, it should find use in urinary tract infections.

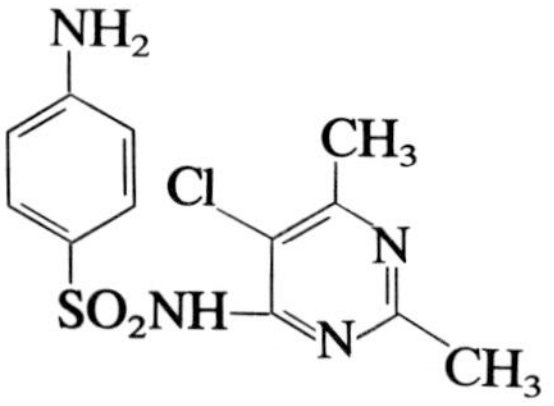

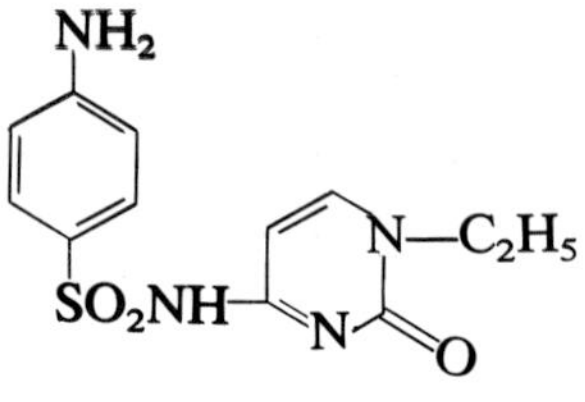

13.**30**

13.**31**

2.5 Sulfones

The demonstration that experimental tuberculosis could be controlled by 4,4′-diaminodiphenylsulfone (dapsone, 13.**32**) (58) and disodium 4,4′-diaminodiphenylsulfone-*N*-*N*′-didextrose sulfonate (promin, 13.**33**) (59), was a major advance in the chemotherapy of mycobacterial infections. Although dapsone and promin proved disappointing in the therapy of human tuberculosis, the interest aroused in

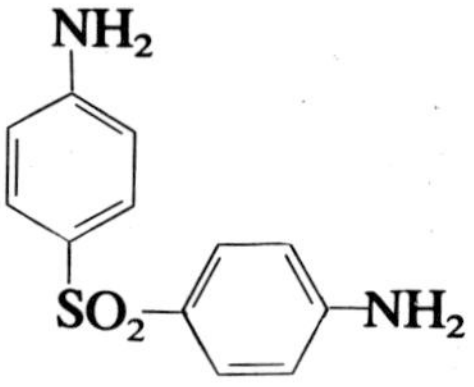

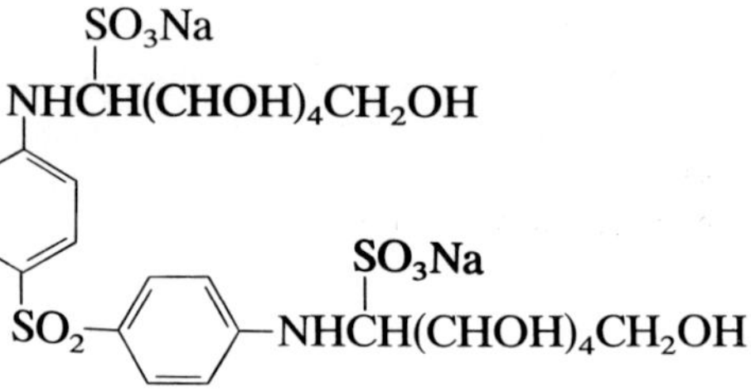

13.**32**

13.**33**

the possibility of treatment of mycobacterial infections with sulfones led to the demonstration of the favorable effect of promin in rat leprosy (60). This was soon followed by the successful treatment of leprosy patients, first with promin, later with dapsone itself. Since then dapsone has remained the drug of choice for the treatment of human leprosy (61). It has now been shown that *Mycobacterium leprae* is unusually sensitive to dapsone (62) and that its growth can be inhibited by a very low concentration of the latter. A successful clinical trial with a weekly dose of dapsone as low as 1–5 mg has been reported (63).

A number of long-acting sulfonamides such as sulfamethoxine have also been found useful in the treatment of leprosy (64, 65).

An important advance in the use of sulfones took place with the demonstration that *N,N′*-diacyl derivatives and certain Schiff bases of dapsone have a repository effect and release dapsone slowly; *N,N′*-diacetamidodiphenylsulfone (acedapsone, 13.**34**) and the Schiff base DSBA (13.**35**)

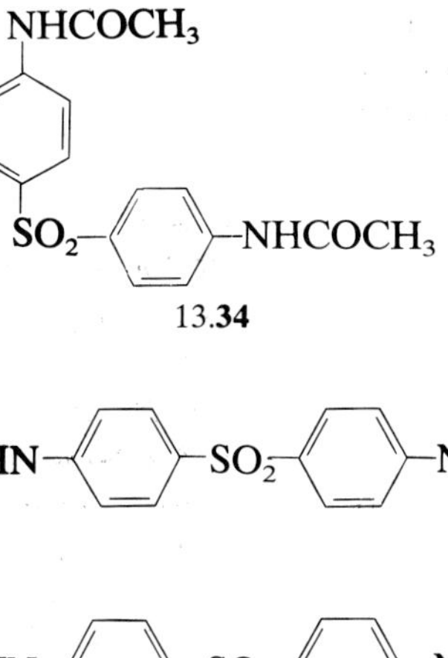

$NHCOCH_3$, SO_2, $NHCOCH_3$

13.**34**

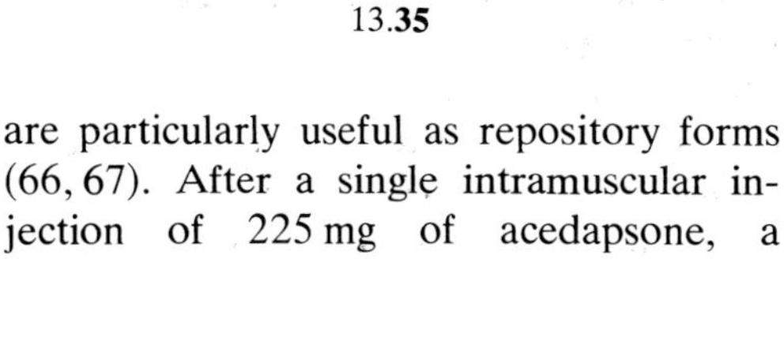

CH_3COHN, SO_2, $N{=}CH$

CH_3COHN, SO_2, $N{=}CH$

13.**35**

are particularly useful as repository forms (66, 67). After a single intramuscular injection of 225 mg of acedapsone, a therapeutic level of dapsone (20–25 ng/ml) is maintained in the blood for as long as 68–80 days. This drug could occupy an important place in the prophylaxis and treatment of leprosy.

A number of mono-*N*-alkylsulfones (68–70) have been prepared, but most of these compounds have been tested against *M. tuberculosis* only, for lack of a suitable rapid method of screening for antileprosy activity. Some of the lower alkyl derivatives, though less active than dapsone *in vitro* against *Mycobacterium* species 707 (71) (a correlation has been reported between MIC against this species and *M. leprae* infection in mouse footpads, 72), were found to be somewhat more active in experimental tuberculosis (73, 74). 4-Ethylamino-4,4′-diaminodiphenylsulfone was also successully tested in leprosy patients and showed a lower incidence of side reactions, but its overall advantage over dapsone was only marginal (75). A number of nuclear substituted derivatives of monoalkyl sulfones carrying a methoxy or hydroxy radical in 2- or 3-position of one or both rings have also been synthesized (76–78) and found to be less active than dapsone in experimental tuberculosis (79).

Compounds in which one benzene ring has been replaced by a 2- or 4-pyridyl, 2- or 5-thiazolyl, or 8-quinolyl residue, preferably carrying an amino group, possess significant activity, but replacement of both benzene rings by these heterocycles leads to inactive compounds. None of these monoheterocyclic sulfones, however, offers any marked advantage over dapsone. As in the case of sulfonamides, the *p*-aminophenylsulfonyl unit seems to be essential for the activity of sulfones.

4.4′-Diaminodiphenylsulfoxide (13.**36**) showed significant antileprosy activity in

H_2N, SO, NH_2

13.**36**

clinical trial but was found to be more toxic than dapsone (80, 81). The activity may be due to its oxidation *in vivo* to dapsone, as both the sulfoxide and its *N*-methyl derivative have been shown to undergo such oxidation (82, 83). 4,4′-Diaminodiphenylsulfide also showed antituberculosis activity in experimental tuberculosis of mice, but was inactive *in vitro* (84). The activity appears to be due to the oxidation of sulfide to sulfone; sulfide is oxidized *in vivo* to the sulfoxide and sulfone (85).

2.6 Antimicrobial Spectrum

Following the initial dramatic results obtained with sulfonamides in the treatment of streptococcal infections, studies with these drugs were extended to other bacteria, viruses, protozoa, and fungi. It was found that many gram-positive and gram-negative cocci and bacilli, mycobacteria, some large viruses, protozoa, and fungi are susceptible to the action of sulfonamides and sulfones. In almost all cases their action is related to PAB antagonism.

The sulfonamides and sulfones have a relatively broad antibacterial spectrum. Individual sulfonamides do differ in their antibacterial spectrum, but these differences are more quantitative than qualitative. The organisms most susceptible to sulfonamides include pneumococci, streptococci, meningococci, staphylococci, some coliform bacteria and shigellae, and lepra bacilli to sulfones (Table 13.1). The main limitation of sulfonamides is their weak activity against bacteria responsible for typhoid fever, diphtheria, and subacute bacterial endocarditis.

Little notice was taken of the antimalarial activity of sulfonamides and sulfones which had been reported as early as 1937 (86, 87), until Archibald and Ross (88), investigating the cause of the lower prevalance of malaria in leprosy patients, showed that dapsone could clear the blood of trophozoites of both *Plasmodium falciparum* and *P. malariae*, though somewhat more slowly than chloroquine. It was soon found that dapsone potentiated the action of pyrimethamine. A combination of the two drugs markedly delayed the development of resistance (89–91), and certain lines of *P. berghei*, *P. cynomolgi*, and *P. gallinaceum* made resistant to either of the drugs were still susceptible to the combination (92, 93). A further advance in therapy took place with the demonstration of the repository effect of *N,N′*-diformyl- and -diacetyl derivatives of dapsone; in the host they are slowly hydrolyzed to release dapsone (94, 95). In the rhesus monkey an intramuscular dose of 50 mg/kg of acedapsone prevented patent *P. cynomolgi* infection for an average of 158 days and suppressed the parasitemia for several weeks longer (96, 97). Human malaria parasites vary greatly in their sensitivity to sulfones; *P. falciparum* is very sensitive, but *P. vivax* is not. A number of long-acting sulfonamides such as sulformethoxine and sulfamethoxypyrazine have been found to possess high antimalarial activity, and their effect is also potentiated by pyrimethamine (98). The action of sulfones and sulfonamides appears to be mainly against the blood forms, and they lack appreciable activity against tissue stages.

The observation of the activity of sulfonamides and sulfones against experimental toxoplasmosis (99, 100) and the synergization of this action by pyrimethamine (101, 102) has led to the wide use of this combination in human toxoplasmosis (103).

Sulfonamides have been shown to be effective against *Eimeria* infection in chickens (104–106) and are now commonly used, alone or preferably in combination with pyrimethamine, for the treatment of coccidiosis (107).

McCallum and Findlay (108) showed that the "large virus" of *Lymphogranuloma venereum* in mice was susceptible to sulfonamides. Later, other Chlamydiae were

Table 13.1 Sensitivity of Microorganisms to Sulfonamides and Sulfones

Gram-Positive, Acid Fast	Gram-Negative	Others
	Highly Sensitive	
Bacillus anthracis (some strains)	*Calymmatobacterium granulomatis*	*Chlamydia trachomatis*
Corynebacterium diphtheriae (some strains)	*Hemophilus ducreyi*	*Lymphogranuloma venereum* virus
Mycobacterium leprae	*H. influenzae*	*Trachoma* viruses
Staphylococcus aureus	*Neisseria gonorrheae*	*Plasmodium falciparum*
Streptococcus pneumoniae	*N. meningitidis*	*P. malariae*
S. pyogenes (group A)	*Pasteurella pestis*	*Toxoplasma*
	Proteus mirabilis	*Coccidia*
	Shigella flexneri	*Actinomyces bovis*
	S. sonnei	*Nocardia asteroides*
	Vibrio cholerae	
	Weakly Susceptible	
Clostridium welchii	*Aerobacter aerogenes*	*Plasmodium vivax*
Streptococcus viridans	*Brucella abortus*	
	Escherichia coli	
	Klebsiella pneumoniae	
	Proteus vulgaris	
	Pseudomonas aeruginosa	
	Salmonella	

also found to be inhibited by sulfonamides, which led to the successful clinical trial of these drugs in the treatment of trachoma (109).

Sulfonamides were also found to have marked activity *in vitro* against *Nocardia asteroides* and are largely used for the treatment of systemic nocardiosis (110, 111).

Table 13.1 gives broadly the range of antimicrobial activity of sulfonamides and sulfones (112).

2.7 Side Effects of Sulfonamides as Leads for New Drugs in Other Areas

The action of sulfonamides is not restricted to antimicrobial activity; they have other weak to strong effects (side effects), unrelated to their antimicrobial activity. Some of these side effects have provided useful leads for developing drugs in several areas (15, 113).

2.7.1 CARBONIC ANHYDRASE INHIBITORS. The clinical acidosis and alkaline urine observed following sulfanilamide administration (114), its carbonic anhydrase inhibiting activity (115), together with the demonstration of high concentration of carbonic anhydrase in the kidney (116), established the causal relationship between the enzyme inhibition and basic physiological changes and suggested that sulfonamides may have a potential as diuretics. Schwartz (117) showed that sulfanilamide did indeed have diuretic action. Further studies led to the synthesis of highly specific carbonic anhydrase inhibitors, including acetazolamide (13.**37**). These were among the earliest

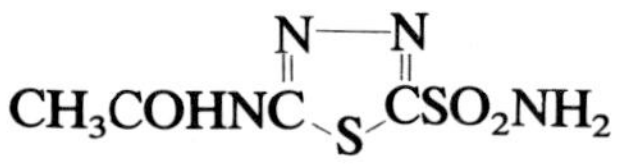

CH_3COHNC–CSO_2NH_2 (N—N, S ring)

13.**37**

nonmercurial diuretics. This was the beginning of the era of modern diuretics. Although carbonic anhydrase inhibitors as diuretics have been replaced by saluretics, they find use for treatment of glaucoma.

2.7.2 SALURETICS. While pursuing the lead provided by sulfonamides having carbonic anhydrase inhibiting activity, it was learned that the introduction of an additional sulfamyl group in the *m*-position led to compounds that, although having diuretic action, had low carbonic anhydrase inhibiting activity and caused increased renal excretion of Na^+ and Cl^- ions in almost equimolar proportions. Ring closure of one of these sulfonamide residues to a thiadiazine ring as in hydrochlorthiazide (13.**38**) (118) yielded more potent diuretics. Replacement of one sulfamyl group by a carboxyl group led to the high ceiling saluretics such as furosemide (13.**39**) (119).

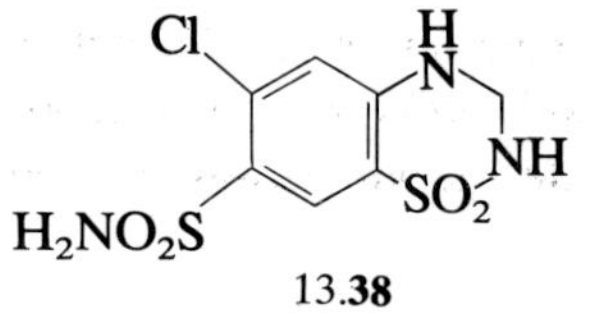

13.**38**

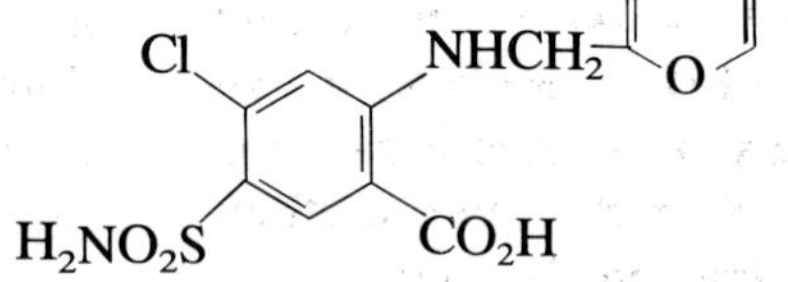

13.**39**

These diuretics have a distinct action on renal tubular function and at maximum dose cause about 3 times as much excretion of sodium chloride as the thiazides. These two classes of diuretics seem to have different modes of action, since even after blocking the renal action of hydrochlorothiazide by a specific antagonist EX4877 the effect of furosemide was retained (120).

2.7.3 INSULIN-RELEASING SULFONAMIDES. That a sulfonamide (13.**40**) could induce hypoglycemia as a side effect was observed in 1942 by Janbon et al. (121); two patients

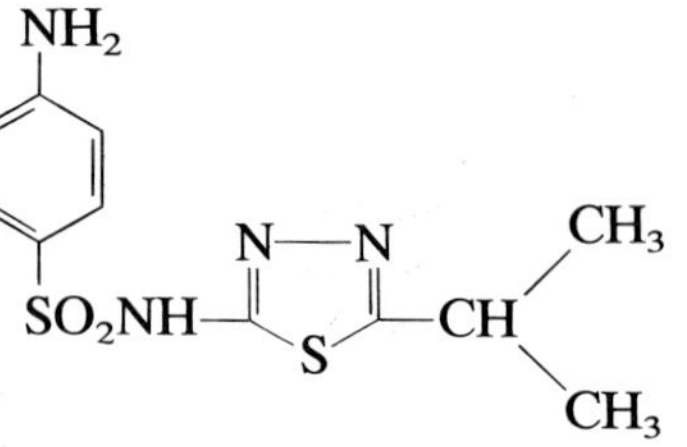

13.**40**

under treatment for typhoid died of hypoglycemic shock. Loubatieres (122), as a result of extensive studies in experimental animals, showed that the compound exerted its hypoglycemic effect by stimulation of the pancreas to secrete insulin. This led to a search for oral hypoglycemic agents among sulfonamides, and it was found that a variety of aromatic sulfonylureas and thioureas could reduce blood sugar in animals and humans with potential insulin stores. The search culminated in the introduction into clinical practice in 1955 of carbutamide (13.**41**), which possesses

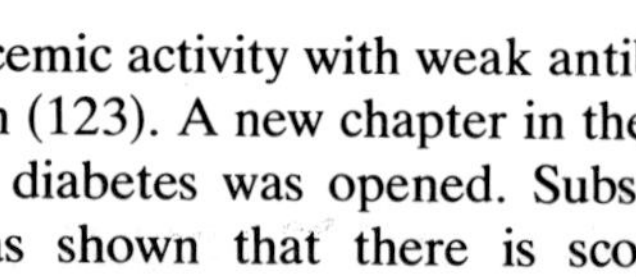

13.**41**

hypoglycemic activity with weak antibacterial action (123). A new chapter in the treatment of diabetes was opened. Subsequent work has shown that there is scope for considerable flexibility in the *p*-substituent; a striking change in activity is brought out by replacing the *p*-amino group by a *p*-acylaminoalkyl moiety as in glybenclamide (13.**42**).

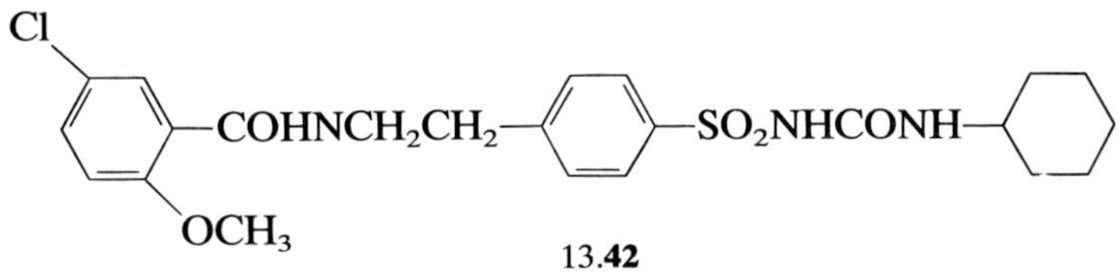

$$\text{Cl},\text{OCH}_3\text{-C}_6\text{H}_3\text{-COHNCH}_2\text{CH}_2\text{-C}_6\text{H}_4\text{-SO}_2\text{NHCONH-C}_6\text{H}_{11}$$

13.**42**

2.7.4 ANTITHYROID AGENTS. Mackenzie et al. (124) observed goiter-inducing action of sulfaguanidine in rats under treatment for experimental intestinal infection in 1942. These results, together with reports of incidence of goiter in factory workers engaged in sulfonamide production, and the chance observation of antithyroid activity of phenylthiourea, set off the research that resulted in the development of the presently used antithyroid agents. It was, however, realized quite early that a sulfonamide group was not essential for antithyroid activity.

2.7.5 TUBULAR TRANSPORT INHIBITORS. The development of probenecid (13.**43**), the first synthetic drug for the control of uric acid excretion, was a result of the observation that some sulfonamides, particularly sulfamyl derivatives of PAB, had a penicillin-sparing effect by decreasing its renal clearance (125). Probenecid has found use both for the treatment of gout and also in prolonging the half-life of penicillin in the body.

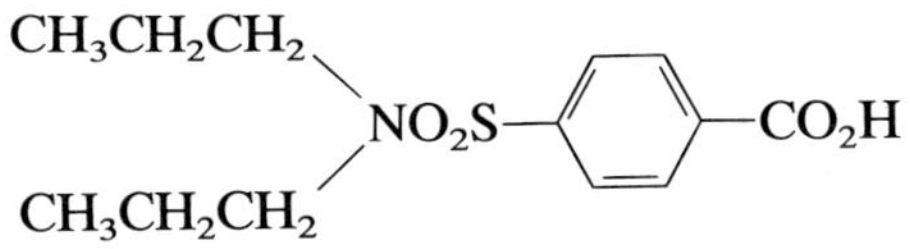

$$(\text{CH}_3\text{CH}_2\text{CH}_2)_2\text{NO}_2\text{S-C}_6\text{H}_4\text{-CO}_2\text{H}$$

13.**43**

3 ACTION OF SULFONAMIDES AND SULFONES

Sulfonamides do have other actions (*vide supra*) apart from their antimicrobial activity. This present discussion, however, is restricted to their antimicrobial action.

3.1 Mode of Action

Sulfonamides are one of the few groups of drugs whose mechanism of antimicrobial action is now known at the enzyme level. Their action is characterized by a competitive antagonism of certain essential factors vital to the metabolism of microorganisms. Evidence for this antagonism started coming soon after the discovery of sulfonamides. It was found that substances antagonizing their action are present in peptones (126), various body tissues and fluids, especially after autolysis or acid hydrolysis (127), pus (128), bacteria (129, 130), and yeast extract (13, 131). Woods (13) obtained evidence that PAB is the probable antagonistic agent in yeast extract and showed that synthetic PAB could completely reverse the bacteriostatic activity of sulfanilamide against various bacteria *in vitro* (31). Selbie (132) and Findlay (133) soon after found that PAB could antagonize the action of sulfonamides *in vivo* as well. Rubbo and Gillespie (134) isolated PAB as its benzoyl derivative, and Kuhn and Schwartz (135) obtained it as the methyl ester from yeast extract. Blanchard (136), McIllwain (137), and Rubbo et al. (138) finally isolated PAB itself from these sources. This led Woods (13) to suggest that because of its similarity of structure with PAB, sulfanilamide interfered with the utilization of PAB by the enzyme systems necessary for the growth of bacteria. Based on these observations, a more general and clear enunciation of the theory of metabolite antagonism to explain the action of chemotherapeutic agents was given by Fildes in 1940 (14) in his now famous paper entitled "A Rational Approach to Research in Chemotherapy".

Further studies showed that the inhibition of growth by sulfonamides in simple media can be reversed not only competitively by PAB, but also noncompetitively by a number of compounds not structurally related to PAB, such as 1-methionine, 1-serine, glycine, adenine, guanine, and thymine (139, 140). The relationship of sulfonamides to purines was uncovered by the finding that sulfonamide-inhibited cultures accumulated 4-amino-5-imidazolecarboxamide ribotide (141), a compound later shown by Shive et al. (142) and Gots (143) to be a precursor of purine biosynthesis.

With the concurrent knowledge gained in the field of bacterial physiology and metabolism, these isolated facts could be gradually fitted into a pattern. The determination of the structure of folic acid by Angier et al. (144) and Mowat et al. (145) revealed that PAB was an integral part of the structure. Following this, Tschesche (146) made the suggestion that folic acid is formed by the condensation of PAB or *p*-aminobenzoylglutamic acid (PABG) with a pteridine and that sulfonamides compete in this condensation. Soon the structure of the active coenzyme form of folic acid, leucoverin (folinic acid, citrovorum factor), was established, and its involvement in biosynthetic steps where 1-carbon units are added was elucidated (147, 148). The amino acids, purines, and pyrimidines that are able to replace or spare PAB are precisely those whose the formation requires 1-carbon addition as catalyzed by folic acid.

Direct evidence of inhibition of folic acid synthesis by sulfonamides was soon obtained by studies on bacterial cultures. It was already known that a number of organisms could use PAB and folic acid as alternative essential growth factors (149). Lampen and Jones (150, 151) found that the growth of some strains of *Streptococcus fecalis, Lactobacillus arabinosus,* and *L. plantarum* in media containing PAB was inhibited competitively by sulfonamides, whereas folic acid caused a noncompetitive type of reversal of this inhibition, suggestive of its being a product of the inhibited reaction. Inhibition of folic acid synthesis by sulfonamides was demonstrated by Miller (152) and Miller et al. (153) in growing cultures of *E. coli* and by Lascelles and Woods (154) in cultures of *Staphylococcus aureus*, a PAB-requiring mutant of *E. coli* and its parent wild strain. Nimmo-Smith et al. (155) showed a similar inhibition of folic acid synthesis by sulfonamides and its competitive reversal by PAB in nongrowing suspensions of *L. plantarum.*

The demonstration of the enzymic synthesis of dihydropteroate and dihydrofolate (Fig. 13.1) in cell-free extracts by Shiota (156), Shiota and Disraely (157), and Shiota et al. (158), using enzymes mainly from *L. plantarum* and *Veillonella* and with an enzyme system from *E. coli* by Brown et al. (159) and Brown and Weisman (160), set the stage for examining the action of sulfonamides at the enzyme level. Brown (161) demonstrated that the synthesis of dihydropteroate from PAB is sensitive to inhibition by a number of sulfonamides. Brown (161) in the *E. coli* system and Shiota et al. (158) in the *Veillonella* system found that the relation between a sulfonamide and PAB remained strictly competitive as long as the two compounds were added simultaneously or PAB was added first. If the enzyme and sulfonamide are preincubated with a low concentration of pteridine, the subsequent addition of PAB fails to reverse the inhibition. If, however, a high pteridine concentration is used, preincubation results in a much lesser degree of inhibition. Brown showed that the enzyme was not irreversibly inactivated. These results were explained by assuming that the sulfonamide reacts enzymatically with the pteridine substrate during preincubation and were suggestive of its incorporation. Thus when

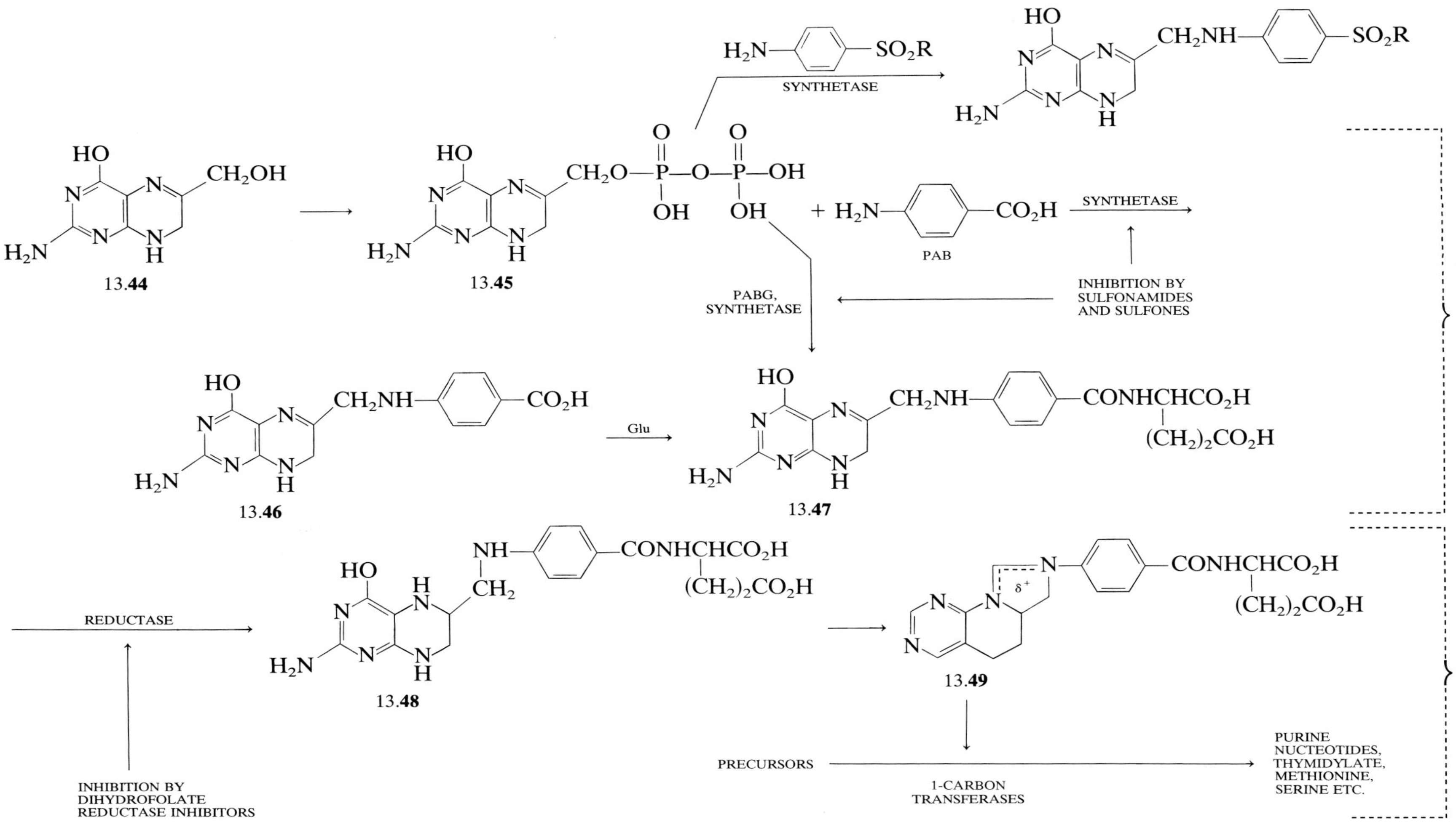

13.**44**

13.**45**

SYNTHETASE

PAB

INHIBITION BY SULFONAMIDES AND SULFONES

PABG, SYNTHETASE

13.**46**

Glu

13.**47**

MICROORGANISMS ONLY

REDUCTASE

INHIBITION BY DIHYDROFOLATE REDUCTASE INHIBITORS

13.**48**

13.**49**

PRECURSORS

1-CARBON TRANSFERASES

PURINE NUCTEOTIDES, THYMIDYLATE, METHIONINE, SERINE ETC.

MICROORGANISMS AND MAN

Fig. 13.1 Sulfonamides, sulfones, and folic acid biosynthesis.

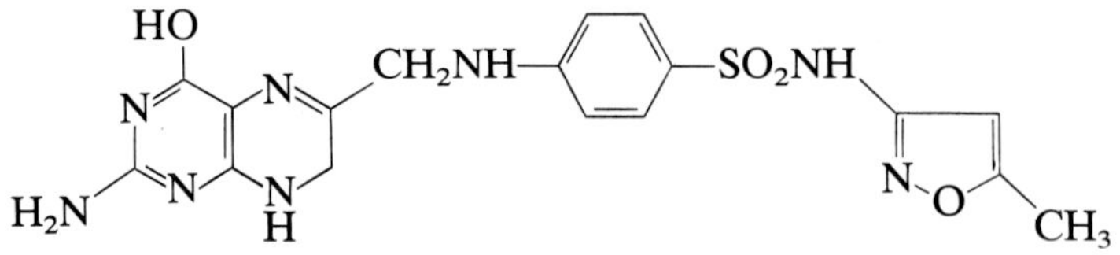

13.**50**

PAB is added after preincubation with sulfonamide at a low concentration of pteridine, very little pteridine remains, but at a high pteridine concentration there is very little inhibitor left. Bock et al. (162) have recently reported similar results using sulfathiazole and sulfamethoxazole. Using ^{35}S-labeled sulfanilic acid in this enzyme system, Brown (160, 161) obtained evidence of incorporation. Though the nature of the resultant product was not elucidated, it was suggested that it may be a sulfanilic acid analog of dihydropteroate (13.**46**, Fig. 13.1) or the fully aromatic form. Bock et al., using ^{35}S-labeled sulfamethoxazole, have confirmed this incorporation by isolating the product formed with partially purified folate-synthesizing enzyme system and in growing cultures of *E. coli*, and identifying the product as N^1-3-(5-methylisoxazolyl)-N^4-(7,8-dihydro-6-pterinylmethyl) sulfanilamide (13.**50**). Metabolic incorporation of antimetabolites is not unknown.

Brown (161) observed that the enzymic synthesis was much more sensitive to inhibition by sulfonamides than bacterial growth, suggestive of impeded permeability of the intact organisms to sulfonamides as compared to PAB. The more potent inhibitors of folate biosynthesis were, in general, better growth inhibitors also. Hotchkiss and Evans (163) have suggested that differences in the response of various organisms to sulfonamides may be due to quantitative differences in the ability of individual isoenzymes to produce folic acid from PAB in the presence of sulfonamides.

Richey and Brown (164) have purified this enzyme from *E. coli*, virtually free from pyrophosphatase, and have proposed that it may be called dihydropteroate synthetase (H_2-pteroate synthetase). This enzyme can also use PABG as the substrate to form dihydrofolate (13.**46**, Fig. 13.1) directly, though PAB is used more efficiently. On the basis of the nonadditive and competitive utilization of these two substrates, it appears that H_2-pteroate synthetase is one single enzyme that can utilize either PAB or PABG (165, 166), and it has been suggested (165) that the enzyme may be allosteric. Recently Toth-Martinez et al. (167) have proposed a multiple enzyme complex for the biosynthesis of folates. They have suggested that the complex, among others, is composed of a glutamate pickup protein, reversibly attached to a PAB pickup protein, which in association with a dihydropteridine pickup protein functions as the enzyme H_2-pteroate synthetase. There is, however, little evidence in the literature that PABG is the natural substrate for this enzyme, except in *M. tuberculosis*, which forms dihydropteroic acid (13.**45**, Fig. 13.1) starting from PABG (163). Brown (161), Shiota et al. (158), and Ortiz and Hotchkiss (168) have shown that the utilization of both the substrates, PAB and PABG, is competitively inhibited by sulfonamides.

Based on consideration of the formal electronic charges on sulfanilamide (169) and PAB (170) determined by the Hückel molecular orbital approach, Moriguchi and Wada (171) have proposed that there are two binding sites on the enzyme, located 6.7–7 Å apart, one being specific for the 4-NH_2 group and the other nonspecific where the acidic group of PAB or sulfonamide binds. Shafter et al. (172), on the basis of X-ray crystallographic data and study of molecular models, noted certain structural similarities between N'-substituted sulfanilamides and *p*-aminobenzoic acid glutamate and have suggested that the N'-substituent may be competing for a site on the enzyme surface reserved for the glutamate residue, either by directly influencing the linking of aminobenzoic acid–glutamate with the pteridine or by the coupling of glutamate to the dihydropteroic acid.

The mechanism of action of dapsone (and other sulfones) is similar to that of sulfonamides, since the action is antagonized by PAB in mycobacteria (173, 174) as in other bacteria (175). The action of diaminodiphenylsulfoxide is similarly antagonized *in vivo* by PAB (175). The action of dapsone (93) against *P. gallinaceum*, like that of sulfonamides (176, 177) against malarial parasites, is inhibited competitively by PAB and noncompetitively by folic acid. Cenedella and Jarrell (178) have suggested a new mechanism for the antimalarial action of dapsone involving inhibition of glucose utilization by the intraerythrocytic parasite; this inhibition was shown to be antagonized by raising the glucose concentration of the medium.

Similarly, in the case of chlamydia it has been shown that the sulfonamide-sensitive members of this group, such as trachoma-inclusion conjunctivitis viruses, have a folic acid metabolism similar to that of bacteria, and that the action of sulfonamides is competitively antagonized by PAB (179–181).

Thus sulfonamides and sulfones, by competing for the enzyme site for PAB, inhibit the biosynthesis of dihydrofolate and thereby of tetrahydrofolate, which is involved in 1-carbon transfer processes. This would prevent or slow down the formation of a number of raw materials of protein, DNA, and RNA biosynthesis, thereby affecting a number of synthetic processes of the organism concurrently. Sulfonamides inhibit only growing organisms, and the bacteriostasis of the latter is preceded by a lag phase. The lag phase can now be explained as being due to stored PAB/folic acid, and its duration is dependent on the quantity stored.

Selectivity of Action. The presence of the folate-synthesizing system has been demonstrated in a number of bacteria (158, 161, 166, 168, 182), protozoa (183–185), yeasts (186), and plants (187–189), and this serves to explain the broad spectrum of action of sulfonamides. However since higher organisms (e.g., mammals) do not possess this biosystem and require preformed folic acid, they are unaffected by sulfonamides. This selectivity of action for the parasite makes sulfonamides "ideal" chemotherapeutic agents. It is not clearly understood how, in spite of the presence of folic acid in blood and tissues, sulfonamides exert their bacteriostatic action. Perhaps folic acid in animal tissues normally occurs linked to polyglutamate conjugates or to proteins and cannot be used in this form by bacteria. Moreover, the concentrations of PAB and other products of the action of folic acid coenzymes, which are able to reverse the action of sulfonamides, may be too low in tissues to prevent the action of sulfonamides when used in adequate dosage.

3.2 Synergism with Dihydrofolate Reductase Inhibitors

In any attempt to synergize the action of sulfonamides and to avoid the development of resistance to them, the most logical approach is to combine them with agents that block the same metabolic pathway as that blocked by sulfonamides, but at different sites. The elucidation of the folic acid pathway and the demonstration of its inhibition by both sulfonamides and "antifolics" provided this possibility (190).

Greenberg (191) and Greenberg and Richesan (192, 193) reported that antifolics, aryloxypyrimidines, and diaminopteridines potentiate the action of sulfonamides in experimental *P. gallinaceum* infection. Since then combinations of pyrimethamine (13.**51**) and sulfonamides has been used for the treatment of plasmodial, toxoplasmal, and coccidial infections, and of trimethoprim (13.**52**) and sulfonamides

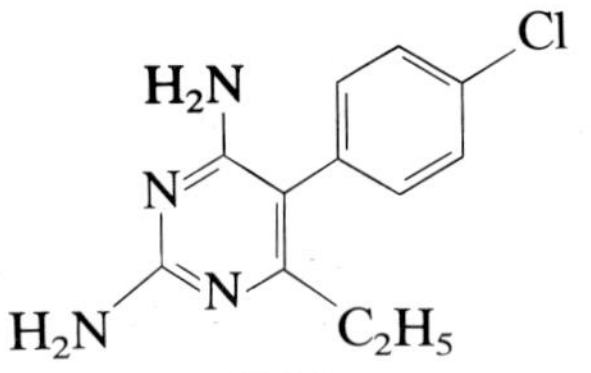

13.**51**

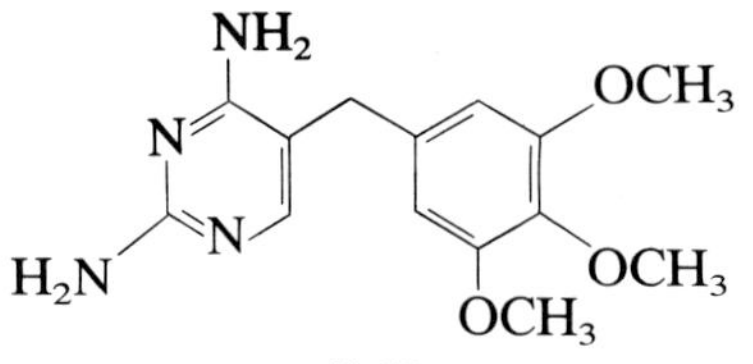

13.**52**

for a number of bacterial infections. This synergism is now recognized as being of general occurrence, and therapy with a combination of dihydrofolate reductase inhibitors and sulfonamides has added a new dimension to treatment with these agents (194). This synergism is clearly a consequence of the sequential arrangement of the twin loci of inhibition (Fig. 13.1). Factors that contribute to the usefulness of such combinations include severalfold increase in chemotherapeutic index, better tolerance of the drugs, ability to delay development of resistance, and ability to produce cures where the curative effects of the individual drugs are minimal (190).

The choice of the combination is based on the best pharmacokinetic fit (195) (trimethoprim plus sulfamethoxazole, both having a half-life of about 11 hr, is a commonly used combination), observed synergism in *in vitro* studies, and the inhibitory index of the antifolate for the particular organism, which is related to the binding to isolated dihydrofolate reductase. Dihydrofolate reductases from various sources differ strikingly in their binding ability to various inhibitors; pyrimethamine is bound much more strongly to the enzyme from plasmodia than from bacteria, and the converse is true for trimethoprim (196). This explains the choice of trimethoprim for bacterial infections and of pyrimethamine for antimalarial chemotherapy.

3.3 Drug Resistance

Emergence of drug-resistant strains of parasites is one of the principal limitations of sulfonamides. Resistant strains develop by random mutation and selection or by transfer of resistance factors. The development of resistance is considered to arise because of over production of PAB (197, 198) or altered permeability of the organisms to sulfonamides (199), or, altered sensitivity of H_2-pteroate synthetase–enzyme from resistant cells can bind PAB more tightly and sulfanilamide less tightly than the corresponding enzyme from the sensitive cells (200–202). It has been shown that several naturally resistant *E. coli* strains contain the sulfonamide resistant enzyme in addition to the sensitive enzyme; the two enzymes differ in their physical characters and stability (202). Different sulfonamides show cross-resistance, but there is no cross-resistance to other antibacterials. In the case of plasmodia a by-pass mechanism (i.e., ability to use preformed folic acid) also seems to be operative. Bishop (203, 204) has described strains resistant to sulfonamide and also to pyrimethamine that presumably can utilize the reduced forms of folic acid available in the host erythrocytes.

One of the important aspects of drug resistance in sulfonamides to come to light during the last decade is the transfer of this resistance from resistant to susceptible strains of different species of Enterobacteriaceae. It was noticed that multiple drug resistance involving streptomycin, chloramphenicol, tetracyclin, and sulfonamides could be transferred between *Shigella* and *E. coli* in mixed cultivation (205). Subsequent studies have established that the transfer of resistant factors (R-factors) is carried out through cell-to-cell contact (conjugation) by autonomously replicating extrachromosomal genetic particles, termed plasmids. This transfer can take place *in vitro* as well as in the alimentary tract. Drug resistance acquired in this manner can be transferred to other sensitive strains indefinitely.

It has been proposed that the R-factors consist of reversible covalently -linked units that separately harbor either transfer (RTF) or resistance functions (R-determinants) (206), and the two may be transferred together or independently (207, 208). Wise and Abou-Donia (202) have shown that in *E. coli* R-plasmid transmitted resistance is the most common mechanism of sulfonamide resistance.

4 STRUCTURE AND BIOLOGICAL ACTIVITY

4.1 Structure-Action Relationships

Although the story of sulfonamides started with the discovery of their antimicrobial action, subsequent work has established their usefulness as carbonic anhydrase inhibitors, diuretics (saluretics), and antidiabetics (insulin-releasers). Compounds with each type of action possess certain specific structural features in common, and it is intended to bring out the broad relationship between structure and action of these four classes without going into details of structure-activity relationship within a group, for which reviews of the particular fields may be consulted. Modification that do not alter these essential features only modulate the activity quantitatively by affecting the physicochemical properties of the compounds.

Antimicrobial sulfonamides and sulfones are characterized by their ability to interfere with the biosynthesis of folic acid by competing with PAB for 7,8-dihydro-6-hydroxymethylpterin at the active site of dihydropteroate synthetase. Northey (16, p. 427), on the basis of the biological activity data of more than 5000 compounds, arrived at the following generalizations:

1. The amino and sulfonyl radicals on the benzene ring should be in 1,4-disposition for activity; the amino group may be unsubstituted or may have a substituent that is removed readily *in vivo*.
2. Replacement of the benzene ring by other ring systems, or the introduction of additional substituents on it, decreases or abolishes the activity.
3. Exchange of the SO_2NH by $SO_2C_6H_4$-(-*p*-NH_2), SOC_6H_4(-*p*-NH_2), $CONH_2$, CONHR, COC_6H_4R retains the activity, though reduced in most cases.
4. N^1-Monosubstitution results in more active compounds, and the activity increases with heteroaromatic substituents; N^1-disubstitution in general leads to inactive compounds.

Subsequent work on structural modification of sulfanilamide, reviewed comprehensively by Shepherd (211), has largely confirmed these generalizations.

A considerable amount of information is now available about the action of carbonic anhydrase inhibitors at the active site of the

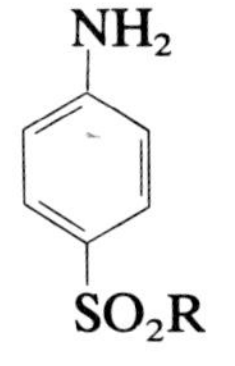

NH_2

SO_2R

R = NHR′, OH, Ph(NH_2-p)

13.**53**

enzyme (212). The minimal structural requirement for this action appears to be an aryl SO_2NH_2 group (13.**54**), in which aryl

Aryl—SO_2NH_2

13.**54**

can be a carboaryl or a heteroaryl residue with preferably 1,4-disposition of the sulfamyl and the ester or amide substituents; particularly high activity is associated with heterocyclic structures (213). Large substituents on the aryl residue lower the activity.

Antidiabetic sulfonamides are characterized by their physiological action on animals and humans whose pancreas contains cells capable of producing insulin. The structural requirement of this class of compounds is shown in 13.**55**, in which X may

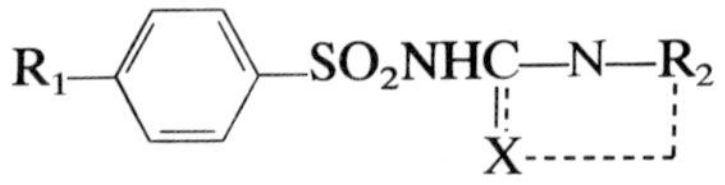

R_1—C$_6$H$_4$—$SO_2NHC(=X)$—N—R_2

13.**55**

be an O, S, or N atom, incorporated into a heteroaromatic structure such as thiadiazole or pyrimidine, or in an acyclic structure such as urea or thiourea. In the case of ureas, the N^2 should carry as substituent a chain of at least two carbon atoms (214).

In sulfonamides possessing saluretic activity, two distinct classes, having separate structural requirements, can be differentiated—the hydrochlorthiazide type (13.**56**)

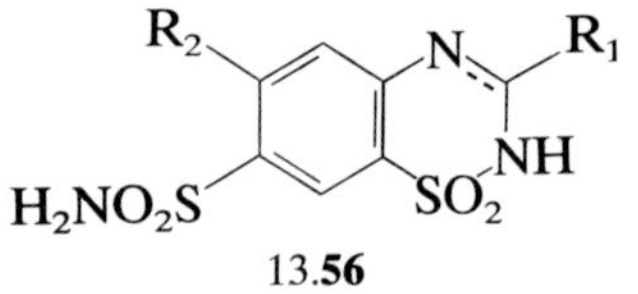

R_2, R_1, N, NH, H_2NO_2S, SO_2

13.**56**

and the high ceiling type such as furosemide and bumetamide, represented by the structure 13.**57**. The main structural requirement is the presence of 1,3-disulfamyl (13.**56**) or 1-sulfamyl-3-carboxy

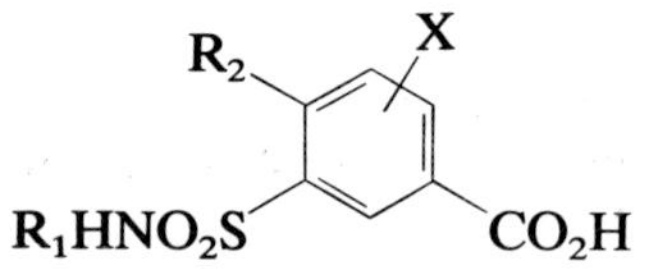

R_2, X, R_1HNO_2S, CO_2H

13.**57**

groups (13.**57**) on a benzene ring. In the former type R_2 is an electronegative group such as chloro, trifluoromethyl, or substituted amino, whereas in high ceiling saluretics R_2 is Cl, Ph, or PhZ, where Z may be O, S, CO or NH, and the substituent X can be at position 2 or 3 and is normally an NHR, OR, or SR (118, 215, 216).

4.2 Physicochemical Properties and Chemotherapeutic Activity

This discussion is restricted to sulfonamides whose antimicrobial activity is antagonized by PAB. Studies to find a correlation between physicochemical properties and bacteriostatic activity of sulfonamides have been pursued almost since their discovery. The parameters that attracted the attention of investigators quite early were the amino and sulfonamido groups in the molecule and several groups of workers almost simultaneously noted the relationship between bacteriostatic activity and degree of ionization of sulfonamides. The primary amino group in sulfonamides apparently plays a vital part in producing bacteriostasis, since any substituent on it causes complete loss of activity. Seydel et al. (220, 221), from a study of the infrared (IR) spectrum and activity of a number of sulfonamides, concluded that the amount of negative charge on the aromatic amino is significant for the activity. However variation in activity within a series of compounds cannot be attributed to a change in ionic strength, since all the active sulfonamides (and sulfones) have a basic dissociation constant of about 2, which is close to that of PAB. Foernzler and Martin (169), by the linear combination of atomic orbitals–molecular orbital (LCAO–MO) method, computed the electronic characteristics of a series of 50 sulfonamide drugs and found that the electronic charge on the *p*-amino group did not vary with a change in the N^1-substituent. Thus attention has been focused mainly on the acidic dissociation constant, which varies widely from about 3 to 11. Fox and Rose (222) noted that sulfathiazole and sulfadiazine were about 600 times as active as sulfanilamide, against a variety of microorganisms, and that approximately 600 times as much PAB was required to antagonize their action as to antagonize sulfanilamide; however the same amount of PAB was required to antagonize the minimum inhibitory concentration (MIC) of each drug. This suggested that the active species in both cases was similar, and that the increase in bacteriostatic activity was due to the presence of a larger proportion of the drug in an active (ionized) form. They found that the concentration of the ionized form of each drug at the minimum effective concentration was of the same order. Thus if only the ionized fraction at pH 7 was considered instead of the total concentration, the PAB/drug ratio was reduced to 1:1.6–6.4. They also observed that with a tenfold increase in ionization of sulfanilamide on altering the pH from 6.8 to 7.8, there was an eightfold increase in bacteriostatic activity. On the basis of these observations, Fox and Rose suggested that only the ionized fraction of the MIC is responsible for the antibacterial action. Schmelkes et al. (223) also noted the effect of pH of the culture medium on the MIC of sulfonamides and suggested that the active agent in a sulfonamide solution is an anionic species.

Bell and Roblin (224), in an extensive study of the relationship between the pK_a of a series of sulfonamides and their *in vitro* antibacterial activity against *E. coli*, found that the plot of log 1/MIC against pK_a was a parabolic curve and that the highest points of this curve lay between pK_a 6 and 7.4; the maximal activity was thus observed in compounds whose pK_a approximated the physiological pH. Since the pK_a values are related to the nature of the N^1-substituent, the investigators emphasized the value of this relationship for predicting the MIC of new sulfonamides. The pK_a of most of the active sulfonamides discovered since then, and particularly of the long-acting ones, falls in this range (Table 13.2). Bell and Roblin correlated Woods and Fildes's hypothesis regarding the structural similarity of a metabolite and its antagonist with the observed facts of ionization. They emphasized the need of polarization of the sulfonyl group of active sulfonamides, so as to resemble as closely as possible the geometrical and electronic characteristics of the *p*-aminobenzoate ion, and postulated that "the more negative the SO_2 group of N^1-substituted sulfanilamides, the more bacteriostatic the compound will be." The acid dissociation constants were considered to be an indirect measure of the negative character of the SO_2 group. The hypothesis of Bell and Roblin stated that the unionized molecules had a bacteriostatic activity too, though weaker than that of the ionized form. Furthermore it was supposed that increasing the acidity of a compound decreased the negativity of the SO_2 group, thus reducing the bacteriostatic activity of the charged and uncharged molecules.

Cowles (225) and Brueckner (226), in a study of the effect of pH of the medium on the antibacterial activity of sulfonamide, found that the activity increased with increase in pH of the medium only up to the point at which the ionization of the drug was about 50%, then decreased. Brueckner assumed different intra- and extracellular pH values to explain the observed effects. Cowles suggested that the sulfonamides penetrate the bacterial cell in the unionized form, but once inside the cell, the bacteriostatic action is due to the ionized form. Hence for maximum activity, the compound should have a pK_a that gives the proper balance between the intrinsic activity and penetration—the half-dissociated state appeared to present the best compromise between transport and activity. This provided an alternative explanation for the parabolic relationship observed by Bell and Roblin between pK_a and MIC.

The activity of sulfaguanidine, the sulfones and the ring N-methyl sulfanilamide-heterocycles appears to be inconsistent with the ionization theory. This inconsistency is resolved by considering the availability of an electron pair, regardless of the anionic charge, in response to the electrophilic center of the enzyme, as of critical importance. Sulfaguanidine has been shown by IR and nuclear magnetic resonance (NMR) spectroscopy to prefer the tautomeric structure $H_2NC_6H_4SO_2N{=}C(NH_2)_2$, represented as the resonance hybrid 13.**58** (227, 228). A lower energy for this structure would be expected in view of the greater stability of symmetrical resonance forms of guanidines in general. The active N^1-heterocyclic sulfanilamides are capable of amido-imido tautomerism and do, in fact, exist substantially in the imido form (228–233). It has been shown, for example, that in aqueous solution sulfapyridine mainly exists as 13.**59** and its anionic form H_2NC_6-$H_4SO_2NC_5H_5N$, their ratio depending on the pH of the solution. The ring N-methyl derivatives (13.**60**) increase the electron density at the sulfonamide group by resonance. The activity of sulfones may be explained similarly when related to the resonance form having a high electron availability at the position para to the amino group of the aminophenyl residue.

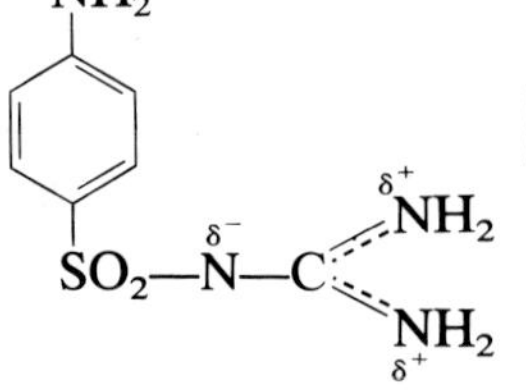

NH_2–C_6H_4–SO_2–$\overset{\delta^-}{N}$–C($\overset{\delta^+}{NH_2}$)($\overset{\delta^+}{NH_2}$)

13.**58**

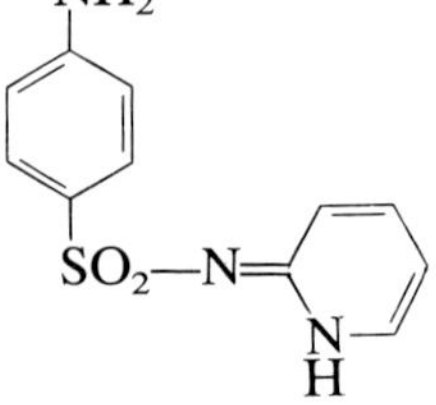

NH_2–C_6H_4–SO_2–N=C_5H_4NH

13.**59**

NH_2–C_6H_4–SO_2–$\overset{\delta^-}{N}$–(pyrimidine ring, δ^+, N–CH_3)

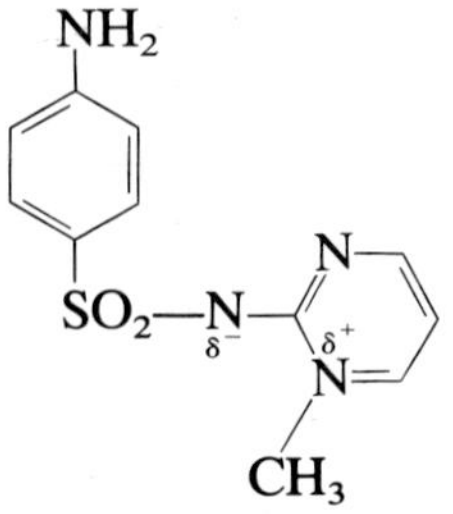

13.**60**

Seydel (234) and Cammarata and Allen (235) have cited examples of active sulfonamides whose pK_a values lie outside the optimal limits given by Bell and Roblin. It has been suggested this may be partly due to the difficulties in titration of weakly soluble compounds. Seydel et al. (220, 221, 236) and Cammarata and Allen (235) also showed that if a small homologous series is used, a linear relationship of the pK_a to the MIC is obtained.

The functional relationship between acid dissociation constant and the activity of sulfonamides has not been questioned since the investigations just cited. This, however, does not mean that the ions of different sulfonamides are equally active; other factors involved can also explain the differences in activity of different sulfonamides, such as affinity for the enzyme. The pK_a is related to solubility, distribution and partition coefficients, permeability of membranes, protein binding, tubular secretion, and reabsorption in the kidneys.

In subsequent studies on correlation of physicochemical properties with activity, additional parameters have been included such as Hammett sigma values and other electronic data for net charge calculated by molecular orbital methods, spectral characteristics, and hydrophobicity constant π.

Bell and Roblin laid emphasis on the polarizability of the SO_2 group and related the negative charge of this group to the MIC. Seydel et al. (221), using IR spectroscopy, and Schnaare and Martin (237) and Foernzler and Martin (169), who calculated the electron density of the oxygen atom of the SO_2 group using LCAO-MO method, could not find any evidence for this correlation. They have, therefore, attached greater importance to the electronic charge on 1-NH. Rastelli et al. (238), however, in a recent study of the correlation of electron indices using the symmetrical stretching mode of the sulfonyl group as determined by IR and Raman spectra, and MIC, have found a direct relationship between the S—O bond polarity and MIC, thus supporting the conclusions of Bell and Roblin. These contradictory results may be due to different conditions used for spectral determination and variability of the antibacterial activity data.

Foernzler and Martin (169) found that the electron densities of the 4–NH_2, S, and O atoms of a large number of N^1-substituted sulfonamides are essentially constant, whereas those for 1-NH vary. They found a correlation between pK_a, electron density, and MIC against *E. coli* of N^1-aryl sulfonamides; this relationship was more significant when the compounds were classified into smaller groups depending on the nature of the N^1-substituent. Seydel and his associates have confined their studies to sulfanilides and N^1-(3-pyridyl)-sulfanilamides. They have extrapolated the electron density on the 1-NH group from a study of IR and NMR data and Hammett sigma values of the parent anilines and have correlated the data with the MIC against *E. coli.* Anilines were used for studying the IR spectra because they could be dissolved in nonpolar solvents, thus giving more valid data; this was not possible with sulfanilamides because of low solubility in such solvents. Seydel (239, 240) and Garrett et al. (241) found an approximately linear relationship between bacteriostatic activity, Hammett sigma value, and electron density of the N^1-nitrogen of a group of *m*- and *p*-substituted sulfanilides and emphasized the possibility of predicting the *in vitro* antibacterial activity of sulfanilamides by use of this relationship. Later, Seydel (242) included in this study 3-sulfapyridines, carried out regression analysis of the data, and obtained a very acceptable correlation coefficient.

Fujita and Hansch (244), in a multiparameter, linear free energy approach, correlated the pK_a, hydrophobicity constant, and Hammett sigma values of a series of sulfanilides and N^1-benzoyl and N^1-heterocyclic sulfanilamides with their MIC data against gram-positive and gram-negative organisms and their protein binding capacity and, by regression analysis, devised suitable equations for this correlation. In the case of sulfanilides they devised separate equations for the meta- and para-substituted compounds; the correlation for the para-substituted compounds was rather poor. The hydrophobicity of the compounds was found to play a definite role in the activity. It was shown that keeping the lipophilicity of the substituents unchanged, the logarithmic plot of activity against the dissociation constant gives two straight lines with opposite slopes, the point of intersection of which corresponds to the maximal activity for a series of sulfanilamides. They suggested the optimal values of the dissociation constant and the hydrophobicity for maximum activity against the organisms studied.

Yamazaki et al. (245), in a study of the relationship between antibacterial activity and pK_a of 14 N^1-heterocyclic sulfanilamides, considered separately the activities of the compounds in terms of the concentrations of their ionized and un-ionized forms and their total concentration in the culture medium. They found that whereas the relationship between pK_a and activity is parabolic when total concentration is considered, it is linear for ionized and un-ionized states giving two lines having opposite slopes and intersecting each other, the point of intersection corresponding to the pH of the culture medium. They found the pK_a for optimal activity to be between 6.61 and 7.4.

In these studies it was noticed that some of the sulfonamides had lower antibacterial activity than expected, possibly because of their poor permeation. To define the role of permeability in the antibacterial activity of sulfonamides, Miller et al. (243) extended this investigation to a cell-free folate synthesizing system and correlated the inhibitory activity of these compounds on this enzyme system and on the intact organisms to their pK_a, Hammett sigma, chemical shift, and π values. The rate-determining steps for sulfonamide action in the cell-free system and a whole cell system were found to have similar substituent dependencies. From a comparison of the linear free energy relationships obtained in the two systems, they suggested that the observed parabolic dependence of the antibacterial activity indicates that it is not the extracellular ionic concentration that governs the potency of the sulfonamides but rather the intracellular ionic concentration, which, in turn, is limited by the permeation of un-ionized compounds, thus supporting Cowles and Brueckner's postulates (*loc. cit.*). They concluded that the lipophilic factors are not important in the cell-free system or for *in vitro* antibacterial activity when permeability is not limited by ionization.

Thus intensive work in this field over the last two and a half decades has fully justified the earlier view of the predominant role of ionization in the antibacterial activity of sulfonamides.

4.2.1 WATER SOLUBILITY. The clinically used sulfonamides, being weak acids, are, in general, soluble in basic aqueous solutions. As the pH is lowered, the solubility of these N^1-substituted sulfonamides decreases, usually reaching a minimum in the pH range of 3–5. This minimum corresponds to the solubility of the molecular species in water (Table 13.2). With a further decrease in pH, corresponding to that of a moderately strong acid, the sulfa drugs dissolve as cations.

The solubility of sulfonamides is of clinical and toxicological significance because damage to kidneys is caused by crystallization of sulfonamides or their N^4-acetyl derivatives. Their solubility in the pH range of human urine (i.e., pH 5.5–6.5) is, therefore, of practical interest. One of the significant advances in the first phase of sulfonamide research was the development of compounds with greater water solubility, such as sulfisoxazole, which helped to overcome the problem of crystallization in the kidney of earlier sulfonamides. However apart from the solubility of the parent compounds, the solubility of their N^4-acetyl derivatives, which are the main metabolic products, is of great importance because these are generally less soluble than the parent compounds. For example, sulfathiazole, which itself is unlikely to be precipitated, is metabolized to its N^4-acetyl derivative, which has a solubility that is likely to lead to its crystallization in the kidney. The solubility of sulfonamides and their principal metabolites in aqueous media, particularly in buffered solutions and body fluids, therefore, has been the subject of many studies aimed at enhancing our understanding of their behavior in clinical situations (16, p. 458; 217, 246).

4.2.2 LIPID SOLUBILITY. An important factor in the chemotherapeutic activity of sulfonamides and their *in vivo* transport is the lipid solubility of the undissociated molecule. The partition coefficients measured in solvents of different dielectric constants have been used to determine the lipid solubility and hydrophobicity constant (217, 241). Recently (247) chromatographic Rm values in a number of thin layer chromatography systems have also been used as an expression of the lipophilic character of sulfonamides and found to correspond well with the Hansch values in an isobutyl alcohol–water system.

Table 13.2 gives the percentage of various sulfonamides passing from aqueous solution into ethylene chloride as determined by Rieder (217). Lipid solubility of different sulfonamides varies over a considerable range. These differences unquestionably influence their pharmacokinetics and antibacterial activity. It has been noted by Rieder (217) that long-acting sulfonamides with a high tubular reabsorption are generally distinguished by a high degree of lipid solubility. The antibacterial activity and half-life are also related to lipid solubility. Although a precise relationship between these factors has not been established, it has been shown in general, that as the lipid solubility increases, so does the half-life and *in vitro* activity against *E. coli* (218).

4.3 Protein Binding

A particularly important role in the action of sulfonamides is played by their binding to proteins. Protein binding, in general, inactivates sulfonamide drugs (the bound drug is chemotherapeutically inactive) and reduces their metabolism by the liver. The binding is reversible; thus the active free form is liberated gradually as its level in the blood is gradually lowered. The sulfonamide concentration in other body fluids, too, is dependent on its protein binding. Thus the unbound fraction of the drug in the plasma seems to be significant for activity, toxicity, and metabolism, whereas protein binding appears to modulate the availability of the drug and its half-life. The manner and extent of binding of sulfonamide has been the subject of many studies (217, 248–250), and the important characteristics of this binding are now reasonably clear. The binding affinity of different sulfonamides varies widely with their structure (Table 13.2) as also with the animal species and the physiological status of the animal (217, 251). In plasma the drug binds predominantly to the albumin fraction. The binding is weak (4–5 Kcal) and is easily reversible by dilution. It appears to be predominantly hydrophobic, with ionic binding relatively less significant (250, 244). Therefore the structural features that favor binding are the same as those that increase lipophilicity, such as the presence of alkyl, alkoxy, or aryl groups (217, 248, 252). N^4-Acetyl derivatives are more strongly bound than the parent drugs. Introduction of hydroxyl or amino groups decreases protein binding, and glucuronidation almost abolishes it. Seydel (253), in a study of the effect of the nature and position of substituents on protein binding and lipid solubility, has shown that among isomers, ortho-substituted compounds have the lowest protein binding. This would indicate that steric factors have a role in protein binding and that N^1-nitrogen atom of the sulfonamide is involved. The binding seems to take place with the basic centers of the arginine, lysine, and histidine in the proteins (217). The locus of binding of several sulfonamides to serum albumin has been shown by high resolution NMR spectral studies to involve more the benzene ring than the heterocycle (254).

There have been attempts to establish correlations between physicochemical properties of sulfonamides, their protein binding, and their biological activity. Martin (255) established a functional relationship between excretion and distribution and binding to albumin, and Krüger-Thiemer et al. (249) have derived a mathematical relationship. Moriguchi et al. (256), observed a parabolic relationship between protein binding and *in vitro* bacteriostatic activity in a series of sulfonamides, and suggested that too strong an affinity between sulfonamides and proteins would prevent them from reaching their site of action in bacteria; with too low an affinity, they would not be able to bind effectively with enzyme proteins to cause bacteriostasis, assuming that affinity for enzyme proteins is paralleled by affinity to bacterial proteins.

Table 13.2 Characteristics of Commonly Used Sulfonamides and Sulfones[a]

Generic Name	R	Common Proprietary Names	*In vitro* activity[b] against *E. coli*, μmol./liter	Water Solubility[c] mg/100 ml at 25°C	pK_a	Lipo-solu-bility[d] %	Protein Binding at 1.0 μmol./ml, % bound	Plasma "Half-life hr" (man)	% N^4-Meta-bolite in Urine[e] (man)
1	2	3	4	5	6	7	8	9	10
		H_2N–C₆H₄–SO_2NHR							
		Poorly Absorbed, Locally Acting							
1. Phthalylsulfacetamide[f]	—$COCH_3$	Enterosulfon Thalisul Thalamyd		Very sparingly soluble	Acid				
2. Phthalylsulfathiazole[f]	N, S	Thalazole Sulfthaladine		Insoluble	Acid				
3. Succinylsulfathiazole[g]	N, S	Sulfasuxidine Thiacyl		20	Acid				
4. Sulfaguanidine	C(=NH)NH_2	Guanicil Resulfon	4[h]	100	Base			5	
		Well Absorbed, Rapidly Excreted							
5. Sulfamethizole Sulfamethylthiadiazole	N—N, S, CH_3	Methisul Lucosil Ultrasul		25 (pH 6.5)	5.5		22	2.5	6
6. Sulfacarbamide Sulfanilylurea	—$CONH_2$	Euvernil	32.2	811 (370)	5.5		95	2.5	
7. Sulfathiazole	N, S	Cibazole Thiazamide	1.6	60 (pH 6)	7.25	15.3	68	4	30 (40)

8.	Sulfisoxazole Sulfanilylurea	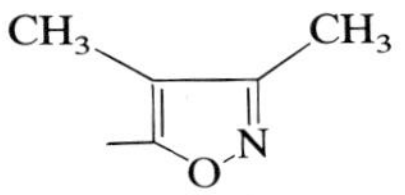 CH_3, CH_3, O, N	Gantrisin Urosulfin	2.15	350 (pH 6)	5.0	4.8	76.5	6.0	16 (30)
9.	Sulfamethazine Sulfadimidine	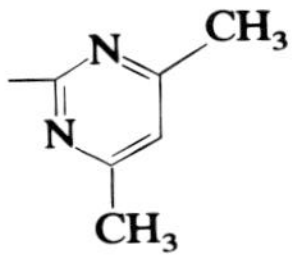 N, N, CH_3, CH_3	Diazil	1.7	150 (29°)	7.4	82.6	66	7	60
10.	Sulfisomidine	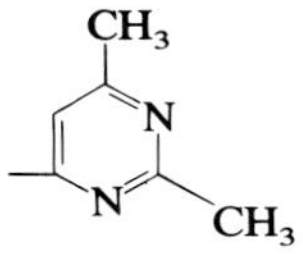 CH_3, N, N, CH_3	Elkosin Aristamid	1.5	300 (30°)	7.4	19.0	67	7.5	4
11.	Sulfacetamide	$—COCH_3$	Albucid	2.3	670	5.4	2.0	9.5	7	5
12.	Sulfachloropyridazine	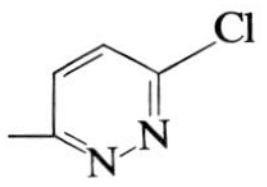 Cl, N, N	Sonilyn		90[i] (pH 5.5)	6.1	14.8	80.5	8.0	
13.	Sulfapyridine	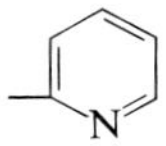 N	Eubasin Dagenan	4.8	30	8.4	14	70	9	30
14.	Sulfanilamide	H	Prontalbin	128	750	10.5	71	9	9	

Readily Absorbed, Medium Rate of Excretion

15.	Sulfaphenazole	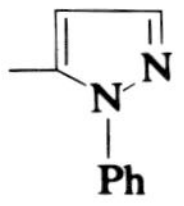 N, N, Ph	Orisul	1.0	150	6.09	69	87.5	10	20 (80)

Table 13.2 (*Continued*)

Generic Name 1	R 2	Common Proprietary Names 3	*In vitro* activity[b] against *E. coli*, μmol./liter 4	Water Solubility[c] mg/100 ml at 25°C 5	pK_a 6	Lipo-solu-bility[d] % 7	Protein Binding at 1.0 μmol./ml, % bound 8	Plasma "Half-life hr" (man) 9	% N^4-Meta-bolite in Urine[e] (man) 10
16. Sulfamethoxazole	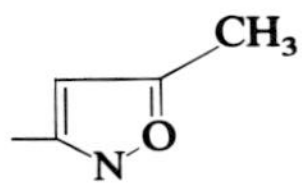 CH_3, N, O	Ganthanol	0.8	Sparingly soluble	6.0	20.5	60	11	60 (14)
17. Sulfamoxol Sulfadimethyloxazole	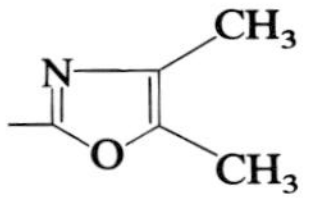 CH_3, N, O, CH_3	Sulfuno	4.0	Soluble	7.4	41.4	76.5	11	
18. Sulfadiazine	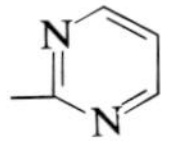 N, N	Debenal Pyrimal	0.9	8	6.52	26.4	37.8	17	25
Readily Absorbed, Slowly Excreted									
19. Sulfamerazine	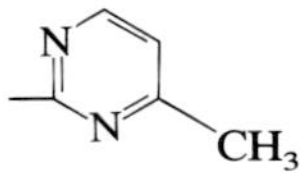 N, N, CH_3	Debenal M Pyrimal M	0.95	16 (37°)	6.98	62.0	56.8	24	50[c], ii
20. Sulfamethyldiazine	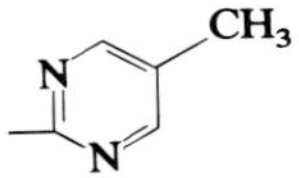 CH_3, N, N	Pallidin	1.0	40 (pH 5.5)	6.7	69.6	74.0	35	
21. Sulfamethoxydiazine Sulfamonomethazine	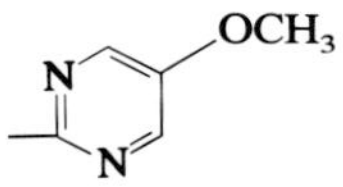 OCH_3, N, N	Sulfameter Durenat	2.0	Very sparingly soluble	7.0	64.0	74.2	37	20[c], ii (30)
22. Sulfamethoxypyridazine	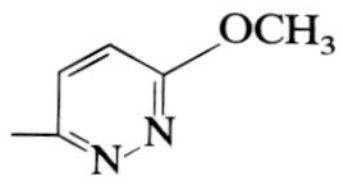 OCH_3, N, N	Lederkyn Kynex	1.0	147 (pH 6.5) (37°)	7.2	70.4	77	37	50 (15)

23. Sulfadimethoxine	OCH_3; N; N; OCH_3	Madribon	0.7	29.5 (pH 6.7) (37°)	6.1	78.7	92.3	40	15 (70)
24. Sulfamethoxypyrazine Sulfametopyrazine	H_3CO; N; N	Sulfalene Kelfizina	1.85	Very sparingly soluble	6.1		65	65	65
25. Sulformethoxine	H_3CO; OCH_3; N; N	Sulfadoxine Fanasil	0.8	—	6.1	5	95	150	60[c], ii (10)
		RHN–◯–SO_2–◯–**NHR**							
26. Diaminodiphenylsulfone	H	Dapsone Avlosulphon	44	14	pK_b 13		50[c], ii	20	
27. Diacetamidodiphenylsulfone	$COCH_3$	Acedapsone		0.3				43 days i.m.	

[a] Unless otherwise stated, the data are from Rieder (217).
[b] From Struller (218).
[c] From (i) *The Merck Index*, M. Windholz, Ed., Merck & Co., N.J., 1976; (ii) Martindale, *The Extra Pharmacopoea*, 26th ed., N. W. Blacow, Ed., Pharmaceutical Press, London, 1972.
[d] Determined by partition between ethylene dichloride and sodium phosphate buffer (217).
[e] From Williams and Park (219).
[f] *N*[4]-Phthallyl.
[g] *N*[4]-Succinyl.
[h] Unpublished results from Dr. O. P. Srivastava, Central Drug Research Institute, Lucknow, India.
[i] Estimated from L. Neipp and R. L. Mayer, *Ann. N.Y. Acad. Sci.* **69,** 448 (1957).

In a multiparameter study of a series of N^1-heterocyclic sulfonamides, Fujita and Hansch (244) considered that in the free state sulfonamides exist as two different species, neutral and ionized, whereas in the bound state they exist only in one form. They developed suitable equations by regression analysis and showed that for a series of sulfonamides of closely related structure, whose pK_a does not vary appreciably, the binding is governed mainly by the hydrophobicity of the N^1-substituent, which supports the earlier results of Scholtan (248).

The implications of protein binding for chemotherapeutic activity are not yet fully understood. The factors favoring protein binding are also those that would favor transport across all membranes, tubular reabsorption, and increased binding to enzyme proteins. N^4-Acetyl derivatives are more strongly bound to proteins and yet are better excreted. No universally applicable relationship has been found between half-life of sulfonamides and protein binding. Strongly bound drugs, such as the long-acting sulfonamides, do not necessarily require a high dosage. However it has been established in general that protein binding modulates bioavailability and prolongs the half-life of drugs.

4.4 Pharmacokinetics and Metabolism

The sulfonamide drugs vary widely in their pharmacokinetic properties (Table 13.2). Some of them having additional acidic or basic groups are not absorbed from the gastrointestinal tract, after oral administration, leading to a high local concentration of the drug in that area; they are, therefore, used for enteric infections. A majority of the sulfonamides, however, are well absorbed, mainly from the small intestine, slightly from the large intestine, and insignificantly from the stomach. Absorption occurs via the un-ionized form, in proportion to its lipid solubility. In rate and extent of absorption, most sulfonamides behave similarly within the pK_a range 4.5–10.5. After absorption they are fairly evenly distributed in all the body tissues. Those that are highly soluble do not, in general, attain a high tissue concentration, show no tendency to crystallize in the kidney, are more readily excreted, and are useful in treating genitourinary infections. The relatively less soluble ones build up high levels in blood, tissues, and extravascular fluids and are useful for treating systemic infections. This wide range of solubilities and pharmacokinetic characteristics of sulfonamides permits their access to almost any site in the body, thus adding greatly to their usefulness as chemotherapeutic agents. The free, non-protein-bound drugs and their metabolic products are ultrafiltered in the glomeruli, then partly reabsorbed. Tubular secretion also plays an important role in the excretion of sulfonamides and their metabolites. The structural features of the compounds have a marked effect on these processes and determine the rate of excretion. The renal clearance rates of the metabolites are generally higher than are those of the parent drugs.

Metabolism of sulfonamides takes place primarily in the liver and involves mainly N^4-acetylation, to a lesser extent N^1-glucuronidation and to a very small degree, C-hydroxylation of phenyl and heterocyclic rings and of alkyl substituents, and O- and ring N-dealkylation. Variation of the substituents markedly influences the metabolic fate of the sulfonamides (Table 13.2); the metabolism also differs markedly in different animal species (219, 257–261). Some of the sulfonamides, such as sulfisomidine, are excreted almost unchanged; in most of them N^4-acetylation occurs to a substantial degree, but some of the newer sulfonamides, such as sulfadimethoxine and sulfaphenazole, are excreted mainly as the glucuronide. The metabolites in human urine of seven of the commonly used sulfonamides given in Fig. 13.2 reveal the

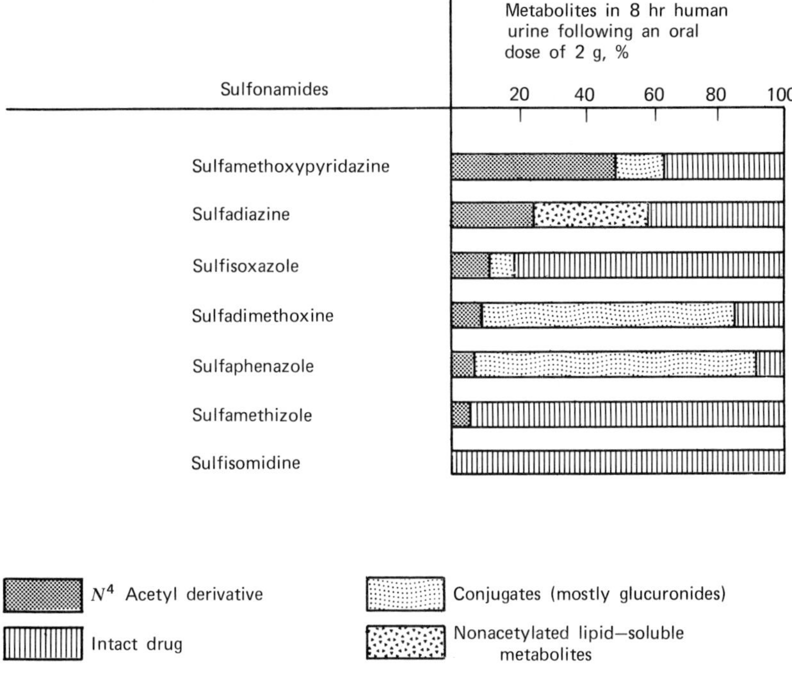

Fig. 13.2

wide variation in the metabolic patterns of sulfonamides (262).

Fujita (263) has performed regression analysis on the rates of metabolism and renal excretion of sulfonamides in terms of their substituent constants. Equations showing the best correlation indicate that the most important factor governing the rate-determining step of the hepatic acetylation is the hydrophobicity of the drug and that pK_a does not play a significant role. The excretion phenomenon seems to be more complex and would have to take into consideration additional parameters to give an acceptable correlation.

4.4.1 SULFONES. Dapsone is well-absorbed after oral administration, and is evenly distributed in almost all the body tissues. It is excreted mainly through the kidneys. Less than 5% is excreted unchanged, very little *N*-acetylation takes place, and most of it is present as the mono-*N*-glucuronide (83, 264, 265). Dapsone has a half-life of about 20 hr. Acedapsone following intramuscular injection is very slowly absorbed and deacetylated. It has a half-life of about 42.6 days. It has been shown that there are marked species differences in the metabolism of dapsone; man is a relatively slow acetylator as compared to rhesus monkey (266, 267). Similarly, mice deacetylate acedapsone efficiently, but rats do not (268).

4.4.2 HALF-LIFE. The half-life of sulfonamides is of great importance because the dosage regimen must be related to it. Dose schedule is a function of the molar activity and pharmacokinetic parameters. Krüger-Thiemer and his associates developed a mathematical model for the relationship between these parameters and evolved a computer program for calculating them (269, 270).

The half-lives of different sulfonamides in clinical use vary widely, from 2.5 to 150 hr (Table 13.2) and also show marked differences in different animal species. Rieder (217) correlated the pK_a, liposolubility, surface activity, and protein binding of a group of 21 sulfonamides with their half-life in man. He found that long-acting sulfonamides were, in general, more lipid-soluble than were the short-acting compounds, but no clear-cut relationship could be established; factors such as tubular secretion and tubular reabsorption seem to be involved. In 2-sulfapyrimidines, a 4-CH_3 group increases the half-life, 4,6-$(CH_3)_2$ reduces it to less than one-half, the corresponding methoxy derivatives have a much longer half-life, and both 5-CH_3 and 5-OCH_3 prolong the half-life to the same extent. Similarly, in 4-sulfapyrimidines, the 2,6-$(CH_3)_2$ derivative is short acting, 2,6-$(OCH_3)_2$ is long acting and the isomeric 5,6-$(OCH_3)_2$ is the most persistent sulfonamide known. Sulfamethoxypyridazine has a half-life about twice as long as that of sulfapyrazine. Thus although no clear-cut pattern of relationship between structure and half-life is discernible, the methoxy group seems to prolong half-life.

5 PRESENT STATUS IN THERAPEUTICS

Sulfonamide drugs now available provide a broad range of pharmacokinetic properties and antimicrobial spectra. Even four decades after their introduction, sulfonamides have an established place in therapeutics. Combination therapy with dihydrofolate reductase inhibitors has greatly increased their usefulness. Clinical indications for sulfonamide therapy have been carefully assessed, and the relative merits of different sulfonamides are reasonably well known (45, 271, 272). In assessing the overall clinical usefulness of a sulfonamide apart from its antimicrobial activity, such other factors as solubility, protein binding, half-life, and metabolism are taken into consideration—thus the best sulfonamide is the one that combines the optimum values of most of these properties.

5.1 Targets of Therapy

Sulfonamides had their spectacular beginning in the treatment of bacterial septicemias. Although they have now been replaced to a large extent by antibiotics, they are recommended for the prophylaxis of rheumatic fever, for meningococcal meningitis when the organisms are sensitive to them, and in *Hemophilus influenzae* meningitis as an adjunct to streptomycin therapy. They are largely used in the control of bacillary dysentery, particularly that caused by *Shigella*. The sulfonamides alone or in combination with trimethoprim occupy an important place in the treatment of urinary tract infections; short-acting soluble drugs, which have a quick throughput, are preferred for this treatment. The combination of sulfamethoxazole with trimethoprim has emerged as a useful treatment for salmonellosis and chronic bronchitis. Sulfonamides remain the drugs of choice in the treatment of chancroid, lymphogranuloma venereum, trachoma, inclusion conjunctivitis, and nocardiosis. Combined with pyrimethamine, they are recommended for toxoplasmosis and chloroquine-resistant falciparum malaria. Salicylazosulfapyridine has been found to be effective in the treatment of ulcerative colitis; combined with steroids, it is considered to be the treatment of choice for chronic, intermittent ulcerative rectocolitis.

Dapsone remains the drug of choice for all forms of leprosy. The possibility of the use of acedapsone as a repository drug is likely to further enhance the usefulness of sulfones in the treatment of leprosy and in malaria.

5.2 Adverse reactions

Crystalluria was one of the earliest serious toxic reactions observed with sulfonamides.

This is a much less perilous problem now than it was years ago, mostly because of the discovery of agents that are highly soluble at the pH of urine, the development of long-acting sulfas that build up adequate blood levels at a dose low enough not to cause crystallization, and the discovery of compounds that are excreted chiefly as highly soluble glucuronides.

Blood dyscrasias are quite uncommon, but when they do occur they may be so serious that drug administration must be stopped immediately. Both topical and systemic administration of sulfonamides can lead to hypersensitivity reactions, such as urticaria, exfoliative dermatitis, photosensitization, erythema nodosum, and in its most severe form, erythema multiforme-exudativum (Stevens-Johnson syndrome). The latter condition is a particularly serious hazard of long-acting sulfonamides.

REFERENCES

1. Hörlein, Dressel, and Kothe quoted by F. Mietzsch, *Chem. Ber.*, **71A,** 15 (1938).
2. M. Heidelberger and W. A. Jacobs, *J. Am. Chem. Soc.*, **41,** 2131 (1919).
3. F. Mietzsch and J. Klarer, German Patent 607,537 (1935); through *Chem. Abstr.*, **29,** 4135 (1935).
4. G. Domagk, *Deut. Med. Wochenschr.*, **61,** 250 (1935)
5. Foerster, *Zbl. Haut-u Geschlechtskr*, **45,** 549 (1933).
6. J. Trefouël, Mme J. Trefouël, F. Nitti, and D. Bovet, *C. R. Soc. Biol.*, **120,** 756 (1935).
7. L. Colebrook and M. Kenny, *Lancet*, **1,** 1279 (1936).
8. G. A. H. Buttle, W. H. Grey, and D. Stephenson, *Lancet*, **1,** 1286 (1936).
9. A. T. Fuller, *Lancet*, **1,** 194 (1937).
10. P. Gelmo, *J. Prakt. Chem.*, **77,** 369 (1908); through *Chem. Abstr.*, **2,** 2551 (1908).
11. E. K. Marshall, Jr., *J. Biol. Chem.*, **122,** 263 (1937).
12. A. C. Bratton and E. K. Marshall, Jr., *J. Biol. Chem.*, **128,** 537 (1939).
13. D. D. Woods, *Br. J. Exp. Pathol.*, **21,** 74 (1940).
14. P. Fildes, *Lancet*, **1,** 955 (1940).
15. M. Tischler, "Molecular Modification in Modern Drug Research," in *Molecular Modification in Drug Design*, Advances in Chemistry Series 45, American Chemical Society, Washington, D.C., 1964, p. 1.
16. E. H. Northey, *The Sulfonamides and Allied Compounds*, American Chemical Society Monograph Series, Reinhold, New York, 1948.
17. M. L. Crossley, E. H. Northey, and M. E. Hultquist, *J. Am. Chem. Soc.*, **61,** 2950 (1939).
18. M. Dohrn and P. Diedrich, *Münch. Med. Wochenschr.*, **85,** 2017 (1938); US Patent 2,411,495 (1946).
19. R. Pulver and H. Martin, *Arch. Exp. Pathol. Pharmacol.*, **201,** 491 (1943).
20. R. E. Flake, J. Griffin, E. Townsend, and E. M. Yow, *J. Lab. Clin. Med.*, **44,** 582 (1954).
21. D. M. Murphy and R. G. Shepherd, US Patent 2,833,761 (1958); *Chem. Abstr.*, **52,** 20,216f (1958).
22. U. P. Basu, *J. Indian Chem. Soc.*, **26,** 130 (1949).
23. M. L. Morre and C. S. Miller, *J. Am. Chem. Soc.*, **64,** 1572 (1942); US Patent 2,324,013–4 (1943).
24. P. S. Winnek, G. W. Anderson, H. W. Marson, H. E. Faith, and R. O. Roblin, Jr., *J. Am. Chem. Soc.*, **64,** 1682 (1942).
25. F. Kurzer, *Chem. Rev.*, **50,** 1 (1952).
26. L. C. Leitch, B. E. Baker, and L. Brickman, *Can. J. Res.*, **23B,** 139 (1945).
27. L. E. H. Whitby, *Lancet*, **2,** 1210 (1938).
28. E. Boehni, B. Fust, J. Rieder, K. Schaerer, and L. Havas, *Chemotherapy*, **14,** 195 (1969); through *Chem. Abstr.*, **71,** 79662q (1969).
29. R. O. Roblin, Jr., J. H. Williams, P. S. Winnek, and J. P. English, *J. Am. Chem. Soc.*, **62,** 2002 (1940).
30. W. T. Caldwell and H. B. Kime, *J. Am. Chem. Soc.*, **62,** 2365 (1940).
31. W. T. Caldwell, E. C. Kornfeld, and C. K. Donnell, *J. Am. Chem. Soc.*, **63,** 2188 (1941).
32. J. M. Sprague, L. W. Kissinger, and R. M. Lincoln, *J. Am. Chem. Soc.*, **63,** 3028 (1941).
33. R. O. Roblin, P. S. Winnek, and J. P. English, *J. Am. Chem. Soc.*, **64,** 567 (1942).
34. D. Lehr, *Proc. Soc. Exp. Biol. Med.*, **58,** 11 (1945); D. Lehr, R. Terranova, S. Blumenfeld, and M. L. Goldfarb, *Postgrad. Med.*, **13,** 231 (1953).
35. E. M. Yow, *Ann. Intern. Med.*, **43,** 323 (1955).

36. T. Matsukawa, B. Ohta, and K. Shirakawa, *J. Pharm. Soc., Japan*, **70,** 283 (1950); through *Chem. Abstr.*, **45,** 2894 (1951).
37. R. J. Fosbinder and L. A. Walter, *J. Am. Chem. Soc.*, **61,** 2032 (1939).
38. J. Vonkennel, J. Kimmig, and B. Korth, *Z. Klin. Med.*, **138,** 695 (1940); *Klin. Wochenschr.*, **20,** 2 (1941).
39. J. P. Bourque and J. Joyal, *Can. Med. Assoc. J.*, **68,** 337 (1953).
40. G. W. Anderson, H. E. Faith, H. W. Marson, P. S. Winnek, and R. O. Roblin, Jr, *J. Am. Chem. Soc.*, **64,** 2902 (1942).
41. E. M. Yow, *Am. Pract. Digest Treat.*, **4,** 521 (1953).
42. E. Miller, J. M. Sprague, L. W. Kissinger, and L. F. McBurney, *J. Am. Chem. Soc.*, **62,** 2099 (1940).
43. A. Wacker and S. Krischfeld, *Arzneim.-Forsch.*, **10,** 206 (1960).
44. R. L. Nichols, W. F. Jones, Jr., and M. Finland, *Proc. Soc. Exp. Biol. Med.*, **92,** 637 (1956).
45. L. Weinstein, M. A. Madoff, and C. M. Samet, *New Engl. J. Med.*, **263,** 793, 842, 900 (1960).
46. M. M. Lester and J. P. English, US Patent 2,790,798 (1957); *Chem. Abstr.*, **51,** 15610 (1957).
47. W. Klötzer anu H. Bretschneider, *Monatsh. Chem.*, **87,** 136 (1956); H. Bretschneider, W. Klötzer, and G. Spiteller, *Monatsh. Chem.*, **92,** 128 (1961).
48. B. Fust and E. Böhni, in "Antibiotic Medicine in Clinical Therapy," Suppl. 1, Vol. 6. p. 3 (1959).
49. G. Hitzenberger and K. H. Spitzky, *Med. Klin.* (Munich), **57,** 310 (1962); *Chem. Abstr.*, **57,** 5274 (1962).
50. M. Reber, G. Rutishauser, and H. Tholen, in "Clearance-Untersuchungen am Menschen mit Sulfamethoxazol und Sulforthodimothoxin," 3rd International Congress on Chemotherapy, Stuttgart 1963, Vol. 1, H. P. Kuemmerle and R. Prezoiosi Eds., Thieme, Stuttgart, 1964, p. 648.
51. H. Horstmann, T. Knott, W. Scholtan, E. Schraufstatter, A. Walter, and U. Wörffel, *Arzneim.-Forsch.*, **11,** 682 (1961).
52. B. Camerino and G. Palamidessi, *Gazz. Chim. Ital.*, **90,** 1815 (1960).
53. J. Tripod, L. Neipp, W. Padowtz, and W. Sackmann, *Antibiot. Chemother.*, **8,** 17 (1960).
54. B. Fust and E. Böhni, *Schweiz. Med. Wochenschr.*, **92,** 1599 (1962).
55. R. Deininger and H. Gutbrod, *Arzneim.-Forsch.*, **10,** 612 (1960).
56. A. Eichhorn, *Zh. Pharm. Pharmakother. Laboratorinmsdiagn.*, **109,** 145 (1970); from *Ann. Rept. Med. Chem.*, 109 (1970).
57. L. Doub, U. Krolls, J. M. Vandenbelt, and M. W. Fisher, *J. Med. Chem.*, **13,** 242 (1970).
58. N. Rist, *Nature*, **146,** 838 (1940).
59. W. H. Feldman, H. C. Hinshaw, and H. E. Moses, *Am. Rev. Tuberc.*, **45,** 303 (1942).
60. E. V. Cowdry and C. Ruangsiri, *Arch. Pathol.*, **32,** 632 (1941).
61. S. G. Browne, *Advan. Pharmacol. Chemother.*, **7,** 211 (1969).
62. C. C. Shepard, D. H. McRae, and J. A. Habas, *Proc. Soc. Exp. Biol. Med.*, **122,** 893 (1966).
63. S. G. Browne, *Int. J. Lepr.*, **37,** 296 (1969).
64. J. Languillon, *Med. Trop.*, **24,** 522 (1964).
65. J. Schneider and J. Languillon, Abstracts, 8th International Congress on Leprology, Rio de Janeiro, 1963, p. 36 (1964).
66. E. F. Elslager, *Progr. Drug Res.*, **18,** 99 (1974).
67. M. I. Smith, E. L. Jackson, and H. Bauer, *Ann. N.Y. Acad. Sci.*, **52,** 704 (1949–1950).
68. B. R. Baker, M. V. Querry, and A. F. Kadish, *J. Org. Chem.*, **15,** 402 (1950).
69. N. Anand, G. N. Vyas, and M. L. Dhar, *J. Sci. Ind. Res.* (India), **12B,** 353 (1953).
70. N. Anand, P. S. Wadia, and M. L. Dhar, *J. Sci. Ind. Res.* (India), **13B,** 260 (1954).
71. N. E. Morrison, *Int. J. Lepr.*, **39,** 34 (1971).
72. W. J. Colwell, G. Chan, V. H. Brown, J. I. DeGraw, J. H. Peters, and N. E. Morrison, *J. Med. Chem.*, **17,** 142 (1974).
73. S. K. Gupta and R. N. Chakravarti, *Brit. J. Pharmacol.*, **10,** 113 (1955); S. K. Gupta, R. N. Chakravarti, and B. Mukerji, *Arch. Int. Pharmacodyn.* **107,** 281 (1956).
74. S. K. Gupta and I. S. Mathur, *J. Sci. Ind. Res.* (India), **16C,** 192 (1957).
75. P. J. Chandy, Mission to the Lepers, Leprosy Home, Faizabad, India, personal communication.
76. W. H. Linnell and J. B. Stenlake, *J. Pharm. Pharmacol.*, **2,** 937 (1950).
77. E. D. Amstutz, *J. Am. Chem. Soc.*, **72,** 3420 (1950).
78. G. N. Vyas, N. Anand, and M. L. Dhar, *J. Sci. Ind. Res.* (India), **13B,** 270 (1954); **14C,** 218 (1955).
79. S. K. Gupta and I. S. Mathur, *Arch. Int. Pharmacodyn.*, **64,** 354 (1958).
80. Ng. Ph. Buu-Hoi, *Int. J. Lepr.* **22,** 16 (1954).

81. S. G. Browne and T. F. Davey, *Lepr. Rev.*, **32,** 194 (1961).

82. M. C. Khosla, P. S. Wadia, N. Anand, and M. L. Dhar, *J. Sci. Ind. Res.* (India), **14C,** 152 (1955).

83. G. A. Ellard, *Brit. J. Pharmacol.*, **26,** 212 (1966).

84. S. K. Gupta, I. S. Mathur, and B. Mukerji, *J. Sci. Ind. Res.* (India), **18C,** 1 (1959).

85. M. C. Khosla, J. D. Kohli, and N. Anand, *J. Sci. Ind. Res.* (India), **18C,** 51 (1959).

86. R. A. Hill and H. M. Goodwin, Jr., *5th Med. J. Nashville*, **30,** 1170 (1937); quoted by W. H. G. Richards, *Advan. Pharmacol. Chemother.*, **8,** 121 (1970).

87. L. T. Coggeshall, J. Maier, and C. A. Best, *J. Am. Med. Assoc.*, **117,** 1077 (1941).

88. H. M. Archibald and C. M. Ross, *J. Trop. Med. Hyg.*, **63,** 25 (1960).

89. S. P. Ramakrishnan, P. C. Basu, H. Singh, and N. Singh, *Bull. W. H. O.*, **27,** 213 (1962).

90. S. P. Ramakrishnan, P. C. Basu, H. Singh, and B. L. Wattal, *Indian J. Malariol.*, **17,** 141 (1963).

91. P. C. Basu, N. N. Singh, and N. Singh, *Bull. W. H. O.*, **31,** 699 (1964).

92. P. E. Thompson, A. Bayles, B. Olszewski, and J. A. Waitz, *Am. J. Trop. Med. Hyg.*, **14,** 198 (1965).

93. A. Bishop, *Parasitology*, **53,** 10p (1963).

94. E. F. Elslager, *Progr. Drug Res.*, **13,** 170 (1969).

95. A. J. Glazko, W. A. Dill, R. G. Montalbo, and E. L. Holmes, *Am. J. Trop. Med. Hyg.*, **17,** 465 (1968).

96. P. E. Thompson, B. Olszewski, and J. A. Waitz, *Am. J. Trop. Med Hyg.*, **14,** 343 (1965).

97. E. F. Elslager, Z. B. Gavrilis, A. A. Phillips, and D. F. Worth, *J. Med. Chem.*, **12,** 357 (1969).

98. W. Peters, *Advanc. Parasitol*, **12,** 69 (1974).

99. A. B. Sabin and J. Warren, *J. Bacteriol.*, **41,** M50, 80 (1941).

100. E. Biocca, *Arq. Biol.* (São Paulo), **7,** 27 (1943).

101. D. E. Eyles, *Ann. N.Y. Acad. Sci.*, **64,** 252 (1956–1957).

102. D. E. Eyles and N. Coleman, *Antibiot. Chemother.*, **5,** 529 (1955).

103. A. Werner, *Bol. Chil. Parasitol.*, **25,** 65 (1970).

104. P. P. Levine, *Cornell Vet.*, **29,** 309 (1939).

105. P. P. Levine, *J. Parasitol.*, **26,** 233 (1940).

106. L. P. Joyner, S. F. M. Davies, and S. B. Kendall, "Chemotherapy of Coccidiosis" in *Experimental Chemotherapy*, R. J. Schnitzer and F. Hawking, Eds., Academic Press, New York, 1963, p. 445.

107, S. B. Kendall and L. P. Joyner, *Vet. Record*, **70,** 632 (1958).

108. F. O. McCallum and G. M. Findlay, *Lancet*, **2,** 136 (1938).

109. W. G. Forster and J. R. McGibony, *Am. J. Ophthalmol.*, **27C,** 1107 (1944).

110. R. E. Strauss, A. M. Kligman, and D. M. Pillsbury, *Am. Rev. Tuberc.*, **63,** 441 (1951).

111. R. G. Connar, T. B. Ferguson, W. C. Sealy, and N. F. Conant, *J. Thorac. Surg.*, **22,** 424 (1951).

112. L. Weinstein, "Antimicrobial Agents," in *The Pharmacological Basis of Therapeutics*, 5th ed. L. S. Goodman and A. Gilman, Eds., Macmillan, New York, 1975, p. 1096.

113. T. H. Maren, *Ann. Rev. Pharmacol. Toxicol.*, **16,** 309 (1976).

114. H. Southworth, *Proc. Soc. Exp. Biol. Med.*, **36,** 58 (1937).

115. T. Mann and D. Keilin, *Nature*, **146,** 164 (1940).

116. H. W. Davenport and A. E. Wilhelmi, *Proc. Soc. Exp. Biol. Med.*, **48,** 53 (1941).

117. W. B. Schwartz, *New Engl. J. Med.*, **240,** 173 (1949).

118. K. H. Beyer and J. E. Baer, *Pharmacol. Rev.*, **13,** 517 (1961).

119. P. W. Feit, O. B. T. Nielson, and H. Bruun, *J. Med. Chem.*, **15,** 437 (1972).

120. A. Small and E. J. Cafruny, *J. Pharmacol. exp. Ther.*, **156,** 616 (1967).

121. M. Janbon, J. Chaptal, A. Vedel, and J. Schaap, *Montpellier Med.*, **21–22,** 441 (1942).

122. A. Loubatieres, *Ann. N.Y. Acad. Sci.*, **71,** 4 (1957–1958).

123. H. Franke and J. Fuchs, *Deut. Med. Wochenschr*, 1449 (1955).

124. J. B. MacKenzie, C. G. MacKenzie, and E. V. McCollum, *Science*, **94,** 518 (1941).

125. K. H. Beyer, H. F. Russo, E. K. Tillson, A. K. Miller, W. F. Verwey, and S. R. Gass, *Am. J. Physiol.*, **166,** 625 (1951).

126. J. S. Lockwood, *J. Am. Med. Assoc.*, **111,** 2259 (1938).

127. C. M. MacLeod, *J. Exp. Med.*, **72,** 217 (1940).

128. D. A. Boroff, A. Cooper, and J. G. M. Bullowa, *J. Immunol.*, **43,** 341 (1942).

129. T. C. Stamp, *Lancet*, **2,** 10 (1939).

130. H. N. Green, *Brit. J. Exp. Pathol.*, **21,** 38 (1940).

131. S. Ratner, M. Blanchard, A. F. Coburn, and D. E. Green, *J. Biol. Chem.*, **155,** 689 (1944).

132. F. R. Selbie, *Brit. J. Exp. Pathol.*, **21,** 90 (1940).

133. G. M. Findlay, *Brit. J. Exp. Pathol.*, **21,** 356 (1940).

134. S. D. Rubbo and J. M. Gillepsie, *Nature*, **146,** 838 (1940).

135. R. Kuhn and K. Schwarz, *Berichte* **74B,** 1617 (1941); *Chem. Abstr.*, **37,** 357 (1943).
136. K. C. Blanchard, *J. Biol. Chem.*, **140,** 919 (1941).
137. H. McIllwain, *Brit. J. Exp. Pathol.* **23,** 265 (1942).
138. S. D. Rubbo, M. Maxwell, R. A. Fairbridge, and J. M. Gillespie, *Aust. J. Exp. Biol. Med. Sci.*, **19,** 185 (1941).
139. E. A. Bliss and P. H. Long, *Bull. John Hopkins Hosp.*, **69,** 14 (1941).
140. E. E. Snell and H. K. Mitchell, *Arch. Biochem.*, **1,** 93 (1943).
141. M. R. Stetten and C. L. Fox, Jr., *J. Biol. Chem.*, **161,** 333 (1945).
142. W. Shive, W. W. Ackermann, M. Gordon, M. E. Getzendaner, and R. E. Eakin, *J. Am. Chem. Soc.*, **69,** 725 (1947).
143. J. S. Gots, *Nature*, **172,** 256 (1953).
144. R. B. Angier, J. H. Boothe, B. L. Hutchings, J. H. Mowat, J. Semb, E. L. R. Stokstad, Y. Subba Row, C. W. Waller, D. B. Cosulich, M. J. Fahrenbach, M. E. Hultquist, E. Kuh, E. H. Northey, D. R. Seeger, J. P. Sickless, and J. M. Smith, Jr., *Science*, **103,** 667 (1946).
145. J. H. Mowat, J. H. Boothe, B. L. Hutchings, E. L. R. Stokstad, C. W. Waller, R. B. Angier, J. Semb, D. B. Cosulich, and Y. Subba Row, *Ann. N.Y. Acad. Sci.*, **48,** 279 (1946–1947).
146. R. Tschesche, *Z. Naturforsch.*, **26b,** 10 (1947).
147. A. D. Welch and C. A. Nichol, *Ann. Rev. Biochem.*, **21,** 633 (1952).
148. M. Friedkin, *Ann. Rev. Biochem.*, **32,** 185 (1963).
149. D. D. Woods, "Relation of *p*-aminobenzoic Acid in Micro-organisms," in *Chemistry and Biology of Pteridines* (Ciba Foundation Symposium), Little Brown, Boston, 1954, p. 220.
150. J. O. Lampen and M. J. Jones, *J. Biol. Chem.*, **166,** 435 (1946).
151. J. O. Lampen and M. J. Jones, *J. Biol. Chem.*, **170,** 133 (1947).
152. A. K. Miller, *Proc. Soc. Exp. Biol. Med.*, **57,** 151 (1944).
153. A. K. Miller, P. Bruno, and R. M. Berglund, *J. Bacteriol.*, **54,** G20, 9 (1947).
154. J. Lascelles and D. D. Woods, *Brit. J. Exp. Pathol.*, **33,** 288 (1952).
155. R. H. Nimmo-Smith, J. Lascelles, and D. D. Woods, *Brit. J. Exp. Pathol.*, **29,** 264 (1948).
156. T. Shiota, *Arch. Biochem. Biophys.*, **80,** 155 (1959).
157. T. Shiota and M. M. Disraely, *Biochim. Biophys. Acta*, **52,** 467 (1961).
158. T. Shiota, M. N. Disraely, and M. P. McCann, *J. Biol. Chem.*, **239,** 2259 (1964).
159. G. M. Brown, R. A. Weisman, and D. A. Molnar, *J. Biol. Chem.*, **236,** 2534 (1961).
160. R. Weisman and G. M. Brown, *J. Biol. Chem.*, **239,** 326 (1964).
161. G. M. Brown, *J. Biol. Chem.*, **237,** 536 (1962).
162. L. Bock, G. H. Miller, K. J. Schaper, and J. K. Seydel, *J. Med. Chem.*, **17,** 23 (1974).
163. R. D. Hotchkiss and A. H. Evans, *Fed. Proc.*, **19,** 912 (1960).
164. D. P. Richey and G. M. Brown, *J. Biol. Chem.*, **244,** 1582 (1969).
165 T. Shiota, C. M. Baugh, R. Jackson, and R. Dillard, *Biochemistry*, **8,** 5022 (1969).
166. P. J. Ortiz, *Biochemistry*, **9,** 355 (1970).
167. B. L. Toth-Martinez, S. Papp, Z. Dinya, and F. J. Hernadi, *Biosystems*, **7,** 172 (1975); from H. H. W. Thijssen, *J. Med. Chem.*, **20,** 233 (1977).
168. P. J. Ortiz and R. D. Hotchkiss, *Biochemistry*, **5,** 67 (1966).
169. E. C. Foernzler and A. N. Martin, *J. Pharm. Sci.*, **56,** 608 (1967).
170. B. Pullman and A. Pullman, *Quantum Biochemistry*, Wiley-Interscience, New York, 1963, p. 108.
171. I. Moriguchi and S. Wada, *Chem. Pharm. Bull.* (Tokyo), **16,** 734 (1968).
172. E. Shefter, Z. F. Chmielewicz, J. F. Blount, T. F. Brennan, B. F. Sackman and P. Sackman, *J. Pharm. Sci.*, **61,** 872 (1972).
173. R. Donovick, A. Bayan, and D. Hamre, *Am. Rev. Tuberc.*, **66,** 219 (1952).
174. G. Brownlee, A. F. Green, and M. Woodbine, *Brit. J. Pharmacol.*, **3,** 15 (1948).
175. C. Levaditi, *C. R. Soc. Biol.*, **135,** 1109 (1941); *Chem. Abstr.*, **38,** 5961 (1944).
176. J. Maier and E. Riley, *Proc. Soc. Exp. Biol. Med.*, **50,** 152 (1942).
177. A. O. Seeler, O. Graessle, and E. D. Dusenbery, *J. Bacteriol.*, **45,** 205 (1943).
178. R. J. Cenedella and J. J. Jarrell, *Am. J. Trop. Med. Hyg.*, **19,** 592 (1970).
179. H. R. Morgan, *J. Exp. Med.*, **88,** 285 (1948).
180. J. W. Moulder, *The Biochemistry of Intracellular Parasitism*, University of Chicago Press, Chicago, 1962, p. 105.
181. L. M. Kurnosova and M. M. Lenkevich, *Acta Virol.*, **8,** 350 (1964).
182. L. P. Jones and F. D. Williams, *Can. J. Microbiol.*, **14,** 933 (1968).

183. R. Ferone, *J. Protozool.*, **20,** 459 (1973).

184. R. D. Walter and E. Konigk, *Hoppe-Seyler's Z. Physiol. Chem.*, **355,** 431 (1974); from H. H. W. Thijssen, *J. Med. Chem.* **20,** 233 (1977).

185. J. L. McCullough and T. H. Maren, *Mol. Pharmacol.*, **10,** 140 (1974).

186. L. Jaenicke and P. H. C. Chan, *Angew. Chem.*, **72,** 752 (1960).

187. H. Mitsuda and Y. Suzuki, *J. Vitaminol.* (Kyoto), **14,** 106 (1968).

188. K. Iwai and O. Okinaka, *J. Vitaminol.* (Kyoto), **14,** 170 (1968).

189. O. Okinaka and K. Iwai, *Anal. Biochem.*, **31,** 174 (1969).

190. G. H. Hitchings and J. J. Burchall, *Adv. Enzymol.*, **27,** 417 (1965).

191. J. Greenberg, *J. Pharmacol. Exp. Ther.*, **97,** 484 (1949).

192. J. Greenberg and E. M. Richeson, *J. Pharmacol. Exp. Ther.*, **99,** 444 (1950).

193. J. Greenberg and E. M. Richeson, *Proc. Soc. Exp. Biol. Med.*, **77,** 174 (1951).

194. L. P. Garrod, D. G. James, and A. A. G. Lewis, *Postgrad. Med. J.* (Suppl.) **45,** 1 (1969).

195. J. K. Seydel and E. Wempe, *Chemotherapy*, **21,** 131 (1975).

196. S. R. M. Bushby and G. H. Hitchings, *Brit. J. Pharmacol. Chemother.*, **33,** 72 (1968).

197. M. Landy, N. W. Larkun, E. J. Oswald, and F. Streightoff, *Science*, **97,** 265 (1943).

198. P. J. White and D. D. Woods, *J. Gen. Microbiol.*, **40,** 243 (1965).

199. M. L. Pato and G. M. Brown, *Arch. Biochem. Biophys.*, **103,** 443 (1963).

200. B. Wolf and R. D. Hotchkiss, *Biochemistry*, **2,** 145 (1963).

201. R. Ho and L. Cormen, *Antimicrob. Agents Chemother.*, **5,** 388 (1974).

202. E. M. Wise, Jr., and M. M. Abou-Donia, *Proc. Nat. Acad. Sci. US.*, **72,** 2621 (1975).

203. A. Bishop, *Biol. Rev.*, **34,** 445 (1959).

204. A. Bishop, in *Drug, Parasites and Hosts*, L. G. Goodwin and R. N. Nimmo-Smith, Eds., Little Brown, Boston, 1962, p. 98.

205. T. Watanabe, *Bacteriol. Rev.*, **27,** 87 (1963).

206. T. Watanabe and T. Fukasawa, *J. Bacteriol.*, **82,** 202 (1961).

207. E. S. Anderson, in *Ecology and Epidemiology of Transferable Drug Resistance, Bacterial Episomes and Plasmids* (Ciba Foundation Symposium) G. W. W. Wolstenholme and M. O'Connor, Eds., Churchill, London, 1969, p.102.

208. S. N. Cohen and C. A. Miller, *Proc. Nat. Acad. Sci., US*, **67,** 510 (1970a); *J. Mol. Biol.*, **50,** 671 (1970b).

209. N. E. Morrison, *Int. J. Lepr.* **36,** Abs. No. 199, 652 (1968).

210. J. M. H. Pearson, J. H. S. Pettit, and R. J. W. Rees, *Int. J. Lepr.*, **36,** 171 (1968).

211. R. G. Shepherd, "Sulfanilamides and Other *p*-Aminobenzoic Acid Antagonists," in *Medicinal Chemistry*, 3rd ed. A. Burger, Ed., Wiley-Interscience, New York, 1970, p. 255.

212. J. D. Coleman, *Ann. Rev. Pharmacol.*, **15,** 221 (1975).

213. T. H. Maren, *Physiol. Rev.*, **47,** 595 (1967).

214. A. Loubatieres, in *Oral Hypoglycemic Agents*, G. D. Campbell, Ed., Academic Press, New York, 1969, p. 1.

215. J. M. Sprague, in *Topics in Medicinal Chemistry*, Vol. 2, J. L. Robinowitz and R. M. Meyerson, Eds., Wiley-Interscience, New York, 1968, p. 1.

216. O. B. T. Nielsen, H. Bruun, C. Bretting, and P. W. Feit, *J. Med. Chem.*, **18,** 41 (1975).

217. J. Rieder, *Arzneim.-Forsch.*, **13,** 81, 89, 95 (1963).

218. T. Struller, "Progress in Sulfonamide Research," in *Progress in Drug Research*, Vol. 12, E. Jucker, Ed., 1968, p.389.

219. R. T. Williams and D. V. Parke, *Ann. Rev. Pharmacol.*, **4,** 85 (1964).

220. J. K. Seydel and E. Wempe, *Arzneim.-Forsch.*, **14,** 705 (1964).

221. J. K. Seydel, E. Krüger-Thiemer, and E. Wempe, *Z. Naturforsch.*, **15b,** 620 (1960).

222. C. L. Fox, Jr. and H. M. Rose, *Proc. Soc. Exp. Biol. Med.* **50,** 142 (1942).

223. F. C. Schmelkes, O. Wyss, H. C. Marks, B. J. Ludwig, and F. B. Stranskov, *Proc. Soc. Exp. Biol. Med.*, **50,** 145 (1942).

224. P. H. Bell and R. O. Roblin, Jr., *J. Am. Chem. Soc.*, **64,** 2905 (1942).

225. P. B. Cowles, *Yale J. Biol. Med.*, **14,** 599 (1942).

226. A. H. Brueckner, *Yale J. Biol. Med.*, **15,** 813 (1943).

227. G. Schwenker, *Arch. Pharm.* (Weinheim), **295,** 753 (1962).

228. A. Rastelli, P. G. DeBenedetti, A. Albasini, and P. G. Pecorari, *J. Chem. Soc., Perkin Trans.*, **2,** 522 (1975).

229. R. G. Shepherd, A. C. Bratton, and K. C. Blanchard, *J. Am. Chem. Soc.*, **64,** 2532 (1942).

230. R. G. Shepherd and J. P. English, *J. Org. Chem.*, **12,** 446 (1947).

231. T. A. Mastrukova, Y. N. Sheinker, I. K. Kuznetsova, and M. I. Kabachnik, *Tetrahedron*, **19,** 357 (1963).
232. T. Uno, K. Machida, K. Hanai, M. Ueda, and S. Sasaki, *Chem. Pharm. Bull.* (Tokyo), **11,** 704 (1963).
233. T. Uno, K. Machida, and K. Hanai, *Chem. Pharm. Bull.* (Tokyo), **14,** 756 (1966).
234. J. K. Seydel, *J. Pharm. Sci.*, **57,** 1455 (1967).
235. A. Cammarata and R. C. Allen, *J. Pharm. Sci.*, **56,** 640 (1967).
236. J. K. Seydel, *Arzneim.-Forsch.*, **16,** 1447 (1966).
237. R. S. Schnaare and A. N. Martin, *J. Pharm. Sci.*, **54,** 1707 (1965).
238. A. Rastelli, P. G. DeBenedetti, G. G. Battistuzzi, and A. Albasini, *J. Med. Chem.*, **18,** 963 (1975).
239. J. K. Seydel, *Mol. Pharmacol.*, **2,** 259 (1966).
240. J. K. Seydel, "Molecular Basis for the Action of Chemotherapeutic Drugs, Structure-Activity Studies on Sulfonamides," in *Physico-Chemical Aspects of Drug Action*, E. J. Ariens, Ed., Pergamon Press, New York, 1968, p. 169.
241. E. R. Garrett, J. B. Mielck, J. K. Seydel, and H. J. Kessler, *J. Med. Chem.*, **12,** 740 (1969).
242. J. K. Seydel, *J. Med. Chem.*, **14,** 724 (1971).
243. G. H. Miller, P. H. Doukas, and J. K. Seydel, *J. Med. Chem.*, **15,** 700 (1972).
244. T. Fujita and C. Hansch, *J. Med. Chem.*, **10,** 991 (1967).
245. M. Yamazaki, N. Kakeya, T. Morishita, A. Kamada, and A. Aoki, *Chem. Pharm. Bull.* (Tokyo), **18,** 702 (1970).
246. D. Lehr, *Ann. N.Y. Acad. Sci.*, **69,** 417 (1957).
247. G. L. Biagi, A. M. Barbaro, M. C. Guerra, G. C. Forti, and M. E. Fracasso, *J. Med. Chem.*, **17,** 28 (1974).
248. W. Scholtan, *Arzneim.-Forsch.*, **14,** 348 (1964); **18,** 505 (1968).
249. E. Krüger-Thiemer, W. Diller, and P. Bünger, in *Antimicrob. Agents Chemother.*, 183 (1965).
250. K. Irmscher, D. Gabe, K. Jahnke, and W. Scholtan, *Arzneim.-Forsch*, **16,** 1019 (1966).
251. W. Scholtan, *Chemotherapia*, **6,** 180 (1963).
252. J. A. Shannon, *Ann. N.Y. Acad. Sci.*, **44,** 455 (1943).
253. J. K. Seydel, "Physicochemical Approaches to the Rational Development of New Drugs," in *Drug Design*, Vol. 1, E. J. Ariens, Ed., Academic Press, New York, 1971, p. 343.
254. O. Jardetzky and N. G. Wade-Jardetzky, *Mol. Pharmacol.*, **1,** 214 (1965).
255. B. K. Martin, *Nature*, **207,** 274 (1965).
256. I. Moriguchi, S. Wada, and T. Nishizawa, *Chem. Pharm. Bull.* (Tokyo), **16,** 601 (1968).
257. H. Nogami, A. Hasegawa, M. Hanano, and K. Imaoka, *Yakugaku Zassi*, **88,** 893 (1968).
258. M. Yamazaki, M. Aoki, and A. Kamada, *Chem. Pharm. Bull.* (Tokyo), **16,** 707 (1968).
259. K. Kakemi, T. Arita, and T. Koizumi, *Arch. Pract. Pharm.*, **25,** 22 (1965).
260. T. Koizumi, T. Arita, and K. Kakemi, *Chem. Pharm. Bull.* (Tokyo), **12,** 428 (1964).
261. R. H. Adamson, J. W. Bridges, M. R. Kibby, S. R. Walker, and R. T. Williams, *Biochem. J.* **118,** 41 (1970).
262. G. Zbinden, "Molecular Modification in the Development of Newer Anti-Infective Agents: The Sulfa Drugs," in *Molecular Modification in Drug Design*, R. F. Gould, Ed., American Chemical Society, Washington, D.C., 1964, p. 25.
263. T. Fujita, "Substituent-Effect Analyses of the Rates of Metabolism and Excretion of Sulfonamide Drugs," in *Biological Correlations—The Hansch Approach*, R. F. Gould, Ed., American Chemical Society, Washington, D.C., 1972, p. 80.
264. S. R. M. Bushby and A. J. Woiwood, *Am. Rev. Tuberc. Pulmo. Dis.* **72,** 123 (1955).
265. S. R. M. Bushby and A. J. Woiwood, *Biochem. J.*, **63,** 406 (1956).
266. H. B. Hucker, *Ann. Rev. Pharmacol.*, **10,** 99 (1970).
267. G. R. Gordon, J. H. Peters, R. Gelber, and L. Levy, *Proc. West. Pharmacol. Soc.*, **13,** 17 (1970).
268. P. E. Thompson, *Int. J. Lepr.*, **35,** 605 (1967).
269. E. Krüger-Thiemer, *Arzneim.-Forsch.*, **16,** 1431 (1966).
270. E. Krüger-Thiemer and P. Bünger, *Arzneim.-Forsch.*, **11,** 867 (1961).
271. L. P. Garrod, D. G. James, and A. A. G. Lewis, *Postgrad. Med. J.* (Suppl.), **45,** 1 (1969).
272. FDA Drug Efficacy Reports, through *J. Am. Pharm. Assoc.*, **NS9,** 535 (1969).

CHAPTER FOURTEEN

Synthetic Antibacterial Agents

RONALD E. BAMBURY

T. R. Evans Research Laboratories
Diamond Shamrock Corporation
Painesville Ohio 44077, USA

CONTENTS

1 INTRODUCTION

The synthetic antibacterial agents are comprised of two major classes of compounds: those effective systematically and those used topically.

The systemically active antibacterials have been divided into three groups, two of which, the sulfonamides and the antimycobacterial agents, are treated in Chapters 13 and 17, respectively. The remaining compounds, principally agents for the treatment of urinary tract infections, are discussed in this chapter.

Antibacterial agents that are employed nonsystemically are commonly termed antiseptics, disinfectants, or preservatives depending on how they are employed. Since there is a considerable degree of overlap in usage among these three groups, this chapter adopts the more convenient method of classifying them, i.e., according to structural types.

The main emphasis is on antiseptics and on disinfectants that have medically related uses, such as skin disinfection, surgical instrument sterilization, and hospital sanitation. Industrial biocides, which are not discussed because they are not used medically, include agents used as slimicides, textile preservatives, cutting oil treatments, paper mill water treatments, and paint preservatives.

Although reports of new compounds possessing antibacterial properties continually appear, especially in the patent literature, only a tiny fraction of these compounds ever reach clinical importance. Consequently, only the compounds and related analogs that have demonstrated clinical utility or compounds of theoretical interest are discussed.

An effort has been made to describe the mode of action on a molecular level for the compounds where it has been determined. Thorough studies have been carried out only for a few agents, however, and it is possible that in some cases investigators observed such secondary effects of cell death as disruption and claimed these as the primary effect of the agent.

2 HISTORICAL (1–3)

The attempts of man to control the effects of microorganisms on his food, his animals, and his person predate recorded history. The skill of the ancient Egyptians in embalming with various herbs, spices, oils, and vegetable gums attests to the success that was achieved in arresting decay without knowing its cause. The drying, salting, and pickling of foodstuffs for preservation was well known before the theory of spontaneous generation was laid to rest. For a further discussion, see Chapter 1.

3 TOPICAL SYNTHETIC ANTIBACTERIALS

The antiseptics and disinfectants are a large, diverse group of chemical compounds that play an important role in the maintenance of human and animal health. Although they are often improperly utilized and overrated in their effectiveness by both lay and medical personnel, they are invaluable when properly employed (4). Many of the older agents have not been subjected to rigorous clinical evaluation, and their use continues despite the availability of superior agents. The hexachlorophene tragedy has shown that extensive toxicological studies are just as important for topical agents as for systemics, and older agents should be employed with due care.

Antiseptics and disinfectants are the subject of an extensive review edited by Lawrence and Block (5).

3.1 Terminology

There are several terms used in conjunction with topical antibacterial agents. Some of these terms have rather strict definitions when used by the US Food and Drug Administration (FDA) or the US Department of Agriculture (USDA). These agencies have jurisdiction over the interstate sale of antibacterial agents used in human and veterinary applications and on inanimate materials. The terms have similar and often overlapping meanings, thus are used rather loosely in everyday language, often with confusing results.

An *antiseptic* is a substance that renders microorganisms innocuous by killing them or preventing their growth. The term is used particularly for preparations applied to living tissue. Antiseptics are found in products such as mouthwashes, douches, soaps, and preparations for minor wounds and burns.

An agent that is used on inanimate objects to kill vegetative bacteria, but not necessarily spores, is termed a *disinfectant.* Disinfectants are commonly found in industrial and household cleaners. To be considered a *sterilizer,* a substance must destroy all forms of life, including spores, viruses, and fungi. Complete sterilization is usually accomplished by a physical process such as treatment with steam under high pressure, but certain organic compounds can be used for the purpose under the proper conditions. "Antiseptic", and "sterilizer" are the basic terms used in describing topically effective antibacterials. It should be recognized, however, that a given agent can fall into all three categories depending on the situation in which it is employed.

Sanitizers are disinfectants that reduce the microbial population to a safe level according to public health requirements. The term most commonly describes products used in dairies, food processing plants, restaurants, or other public facilities where unchecked microbial growth could present a public health hazard.

Compounds that prevent the biological destruction of materials are termed *preservatives.* These agents are found in a wide variety of products including foods, cosmetics, pharmaceuticals, seeds, and industrial products.

The suffix *-cide* widely used in words describing antibacterial agents to denote destruction of the organisms indicated in the prefix. Thus a *biocide* is a substance that destroys all living organisms; *germicides* or *bactericides* are products for killing microorganisms. Other commonly used designations with narrower scope are *sporicide, fungicide, virucide,* and *amebicide.* Another suffix, *-stat* or *-static,* is employed for agents that prevent the increase in numbers of microorganisms without necessarily destroying them. *Bacteriostatic* is often used to describe antiseptic products.

A comprehensive review of the terms used in the field of antiseptics and disinfectants can be found in the monograph edited by Lawrence and Block (5).

3.2 Evaluation of Antimicrobial Activity

Testing of substances for antimicrobial activity began even before it was established that microorganisms were responsible for disease, but rational evaluation of antibacterial effects came into being only with the establishment of the germ theory of disease. Koch, Delepine, and others (6) set forth the early principles for testing of disinfectant properties. The credit for recognizing the need for a standard, reproducible method for the evaluation and comparison of disinfectants and for devising such a method belongs to Rideal and Walker (7). Although their original procedure, now termed the phenol coefficient test, has been subjected to numerous revisions, the fundamental principles are the same, and it is still one of the basic tests for evaluating disinfectants. Their method rests on the simultaneous evaluation of the effect of the test substance and a standard pure chemical, phenol, against the same bacterial culture. A complete description of the test which is currently accepted by the USDA is published by the Association of Official Analytical Chemists (AOAC) (8).

The phenol coefficient test is a tube dilution method in which the highest dilution of disinfectant that will kill the test organism in 10 min but not in 5 min is compared to the dilution of phenol necessary to achieve the same result. Dividing the dilution determined for the new disinfectant by that found for phenol yields the numerical phenol coefficient. Thus in the early stages of the development of the method, a compound with a coefficient of 5 was claimed to be 5 times as effective as phenol. This is clearly misleading and has validity only when applied to phenols, not to other types of disinfectants. Bacteria used in the determination of phenol coefficients are *Staphylococcus aureus*, *Salmonella typhi*, and *Pseudomonas aeruginosa*.

Formerly the phenol coefficient was multiplied by 20 to arrive at a practical dilution factor for a given disinfectant. Thus an agent with a coefficient of 100 would be diluted 1:2000 when put to use. It was felt this yielded a solution equivalent in potency to a 5% phenol solution and provided an adequate margin of safety for overcoming environmental factors that might interfere with the effectiveness of the agent. As it became apparent that this assumption was not valid for all classes of disinfectants, the phenol coefficient became less important, and the USDA now requires more than a phenol coefficient as evidence of efficacy for product registration.

Recognizing the need for a reliable test procedure more closely correlated with the conditions under which disinfectants are used, Stuart and co-workers (9) proposed the *use dilution* method. In this method, which has been adopted by the AOAC, a bacterial suspension is applied to stainless steel cylinders, which are dried and exposed to different dilutions of the disinfectant. Incubation of the cylinders in new media, with precautions to avoid carryover of disinfectant, is used to determine the minimum disinfectant dilution. This procedure has been found to be a more reliable method of judging the effectiveness of disinfectants and determining the safe dilution for use in practical situations. The method is used with *Salmonella chloleraesius*, *Staphylococcus aureus*, and *Pseudomonas aeruginosa*.

Other, more specific, official tests are published for evaluating disinfectants to be used as swimming pool disinfectants, tuberculocides, germicidal sprays, detergent sanitizers, and laundry additives. Special tests are also available for chlorine-releasing agents or chlorine equivalents, sporicides, and fungicides.

Observing that disinfectants must usually function in the presence of organic material that can inactivate them, Miner, Whitmore, and McBee (10) proposed a standard test that attempts to take this factor into account. The test is designed to determine the ability of a disinfectant to kill a fixed number of bacteria in a standard time period in the presence of varying amounts of sterile yeast as the organic contaminant. In the study, several classes of disinfectants were examined at their recommended use levels, and it was found that formaldehyde and glutaraldehyde were 15–100 times more resistant to organic inactivation than representative phenolic, quaternary ammonium, or iodophoric agents.

Antiseptics, because they are used on

living tissue, must be considered to be drugs, which in the United States, places them under the regulatory control of the FDA. The FDA recognizes no standard or official methods of evaluation of antiseptics, and each proposed agent must be shown to meet the criteria of safety and effectiveness by tests relevant to its ultimate use.

Many antiseptic agents are intended for use in products that claim to reduce the microbial flora of the skin. Price (11) devised a test, later modified by Cade (12), that attempted to ascertain the effectiveness of agents intended for this purpose. The test involves making initial bacterial counts of wash water from several successive hand washings under standardized conditions. These counts are then compared with those obtained under the same conditions with the antiseptic agent, giving a measure of the advantage of the antiseptic over plain washing. This test is particularly relevant to products intended for use as surgical scrubs; where maximum reduction in bacteria is the objective. More recently developed procedures for ascertaining the efficacy of antiseptic surgical scrubs have been described by Peterson (13) and Ulrich (14).

The evaluation of antiseptics and disinfectants is complex and difficult to standardize, and has not always been adequate. The most reliable tests are those in which an agent is evaluated under conditions closely resembling those of its intended use. Detailed discussions of the testing of antiseptics, disinfectants, sanitizers, and other topical agents are available (6, 15).

3.3 Halogens and Halophors

The recorded use of halogens as antiseptics dates back to 1839, when iodine was used in the treatment of battle wounds by a French surgeon. Elemental chlorine has been used since the start of the twentieth century for purifying drinking water supplies, and calcium and sodium hypochlorites are widely employed in household and industrial sanitizers.

3.3.1 CHLOROPHORS. The organic "chlorine-releasing" compounds, or chlorophors, were first used as antiseptics during World War I. This group of compounds consists of *N*-chloramine derivatives that release hypochlorous acid on hydrolysis. These compounds were used originally to replace inorganic hypochlorites as treatments for wounds because they were less irritating, longer acting, and slower to be inactivated by organic material. Today they serve mainly as disinfectants, sanitizers, and drinking water treatments, having been replaced in topical applications by other more effective, less irritating antiseptics.

The *N*-chloramines can be segregated into three groups: (1) sulfonamides, (2) cyclic imides, and (3) amidines. The sulfonamide derivatives (16, 17) include chloramine *T* (14.**1**), dichloramine *T* (14.**2**) and halazone (14.**3**). Chloramine *T* was the first chlorophor to be used as an antiseptic (16), and halazone was used extensively during World War II for water purification (18).

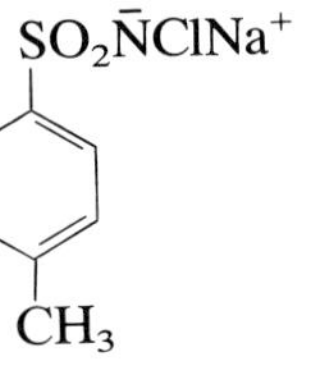

$SO_2\bar{N}ClNa^+$ / CH_3

14.**1**

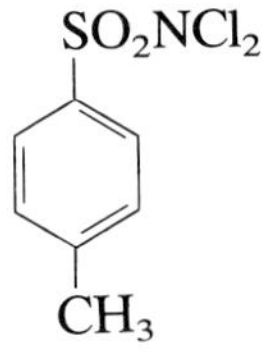

SO_2NCl_2 / CH_3

14.**2**

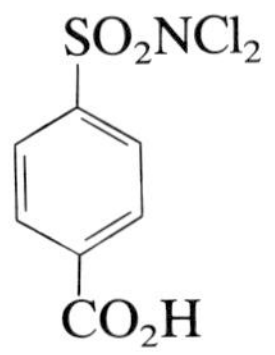

SO_2NCl_2 / CO_2H

14.**3**

Cyclic imide halophors are used in industrial sanitizers, laundry products, and dishwashing compounds, and for water purification (18, 19). They include *N*-chlorosuccinimide, halane (14.**4**), dichloroisocyanurate (14.**5**), and trichloroisocyanurate (14.**6**).

Chloroazodin (14.**7**) is a chlorinated

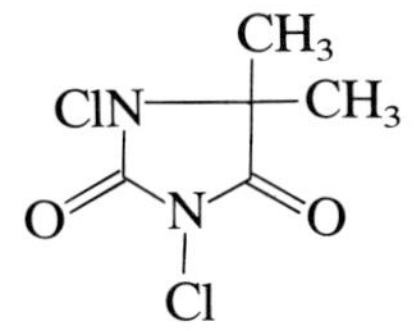

14.**4**

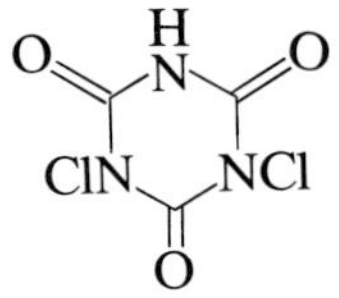

14.**5**

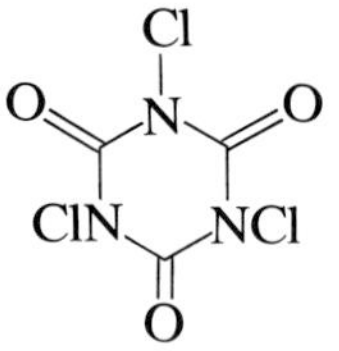

14.**6**

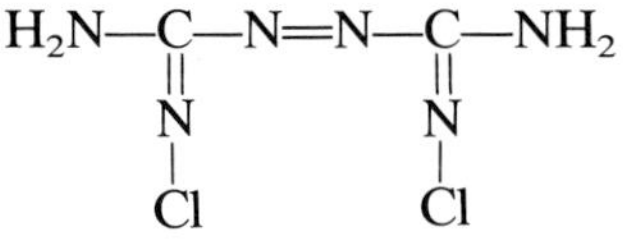

H_2N—C(=N—Cl)—N=N—C(=N—Cl)—NH_2

14.**7**

azoformamidine, once widely used for the treatment of infected wounds and other antiseptic applications (20).

The mode of bactericidal action of *N*-chloramines at the cellular level is not known, although destructive changes in cell wall permeability are a strong possibility (21). Inhibition of key enzymatic reactions and oxidation of sulfhydryl groups have also been suggested as modes of action (22).

The bactericidal activity of *N*-chloramines is dependent on temperature, initial concentration, presence of contaminants, and pH. The pH and organic contaminants are the most important factors. The pH should be in the weakly acid to neutral range, and organic contamination should be kept to a minimum for maximum antibacterial effectiveness of *N*-chloramines.

Early workers felt that the bactericidal action of the *N*-chloramines was due solely to hydrolysis, which formed hypochlorous acid as the killing agent (23). More recently in an extended study of *N*-chloro-α-amino acids and related *N*-chloro derivatives, Bodor and co-workers (24) examined the relationship between the antimicrobial activity of *N*-chloramines and the polarization of the nitrogen–chlorine bond. Their basic assumption was that the bactericidal action of the *N*-chloramines was a manifestation of the direct transfer of positive chlorine to an appropriate receptor in the cell. These studies led them to the synthesis of a class of low chlorine potential (25), "soft" antimicrobial agents. These *N*-chloramines are nontoxic, possess relatively high hydrolytic stability, and are not readily deactivated by the presence of denaturing agents. It was also noted that an increased rate of transfer of positive halogen from an *N*-chloramine to a nitrogen acceptor correlated inversely with antibacterial effectiveness in the presence of horse serum (26). The conclusions drawn from these studies were as follows:

1. Compounds with chlorine potentials between 7 and 8.5 are effective bactericidal agents.
2. The rate at which chlorine is transferred from an *N*-chloro compound to a nitrogen-containing receptor should be considered along with the chlorine potential of the molecules in estimating the bactericidal activity of the compound in solutions containing proteins and other organic material.

Bodor and co-workers considered that 3-chloro-4,4-dimethyl-2-oxazolidinone (14.**8**)

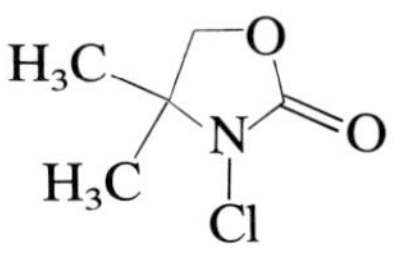

14.**8**

was the best of their synthetic *N*-chloramines, since it possessed effective bactericidal potency and kinetics and was relatively hydrolytically stable. In addition, it retained bactericidal action in the presence of horse serum, and its metabolic and hydrolytic decomposition led to relatively nontoxic materials.

3.3.2 IODOPHORS. Molecular iodine remains one of the most useful antiseptics available. It is highly effective and economical, and has low tissue toxicity at the normal use level. Its main uses are skin disinfection and treatment of wounds and abrasions, and it is probably the most effective agent for this purpose when employed as a tincture.

Iodoform, which was formerly used extensively for treatment of open wounds, owes its germicidal activity to the gradual release of iodine *in situ.* This early iodophor is now no longer in general use, having been supplanted by more effective agents. Other iodophors include various proprietary compositions recommended as sanitizers and disinfectants. They are generally composed of a polyether complex of iodine and a detergent (27).

Povidone-iodine (14.**9**), a complex of iodine and polyvinylpyrrolidinone, is a

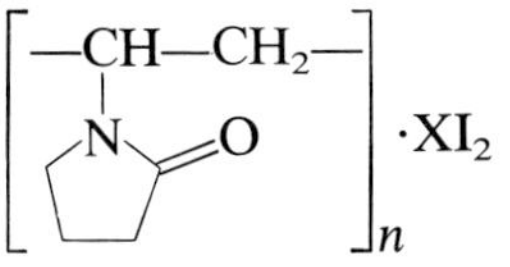

$$\left[\begin{array}{c}-\mathrm{CH}-\mathrm{CH_2}- \\ | \\ \text{N-pyrrolidinone} \end{array}\right]_n \cdot \mathrm{XI_2}$$

14.**9**

widely used, water-soluble iodophor. It is nonstinging and has a rapid, persistent antibacterial action. The major recommended applications include treatment of minor wounds and abrasions, preoperative skin disinfection, and surgical scrub use. The therapeutic uses, toxicity, and history of this product have been detailed by Shelanski and Shelanski (28).

The efficacy of five commonly employed iodophors in relation to that of iodine was investigated by King and Price (29). They found that 1% iodine in 70% alcohol was markedly superior as a skin disinfectant to the iodophors.

3.4 Phenols

Phenols constitute one of the oldest and most widely used classes of antimicrobial agents. The dramatic demonstration by Lister in 1867 of the germicidal effectiveness of phenol and its subsequent use in the struggle to achieve sterile conditions in the operating room represent important milestones of medicinal history. Phenol itself is no longer an important disinfectant, but it is still the standard against which other antibacterials are measured in the AOAC phenol coefficient and use dilution methods.

The antibacterial mode of action of phenolic compounds has been the subject of many investigations. In high concentrations they act as gross cellular poisons, rapidly penetrating the cell wall, denaturing the cellular constituents, and rupturing the cell wall. In concentrations that are not sufficient for protein denaturation it has been observed that amino acids, cations, and other metabolites leak out of bacterial cells (30–32). This alteration of cellular permeability is generally accepted as the major antimicrobial effect of the phenols, but binding to essential protein constituents of bacteria, such as enzymes, has also been implicated (33). Considering the large variation in structure and broad range of antibacterial action of the phenols, it is probable that no single mode of action is responsible for the activity of the group.

3.4.1 SUBSTITUTED PHENOLS. Shortly after the introduction of phenol as a disinfectant, the cresylic acids, a crude mixture of *m* and *p*-cresols, obtained from coal tar, became available for similar uses. The cresylic acids and cresol preparations containing various soaps as solubilizing agents are not used medicinally to any extent today but are widely employed as environmental disinfectants.

A study of the structure-activity relationships of a group of alkylated phenols was described by Coulthard, Marshall, and Pyman (34) in 1930. They found that the antibacterial potency of alkyl phenols increased with increasing size of the alkyl group. This finding was in agreement with later work (35, 36) indicating that the potency of phenol derivatives was correlated with lipid solubility. The sole phenol possessing only alkyl groups that is of any medicinal importance today, besides the cresols, is 2-*n*-amyl-5-methylphenol. It is used as an antiseptic in mouthwashes, gargles, and lozenges for treatment of minor mouth and throat infections.

The potentiation of the antibacterial action of phenols by halogenation was discovered in the early 1900s (37, 38). The most intensive investigations of the structure-activity relationships of the halogenated alkylphenols were reported by Klarmann and co-workers (39–41). Their findings indicated the following:

1. Substitution of halogens para to the hydroxy group generally gave higher potency that ortho-substitution.
2. The introduction of alkyl or aromatic groups usually increased the potency of halophenols, and straight chain alkyl groups were more effective than branched chains groups with an equal number of carbons.
3. The *o*-alkyl-*p*-halophenols were more effective than the *p*-alkyl-*o*-halophenols.
4. With certain homologs a point is reached at which further increase in molecular weight leads to a decrease in activity toward some organisms, while a rapid increase is observed for others. The effect has been termed "quasi-specificity".

In addition to increased antibacterial effectiveness, increasing molecular weight is usually accompanied by decreased mammalian toxicity in the alkyl halophenols.

The most widely used and effective substituted phenols are chlorophene (14.**10**) and *o*-phenylphenol (14.**11**).

Chlorophene is effective against a broad spectrum of pathogenic gram-negative and

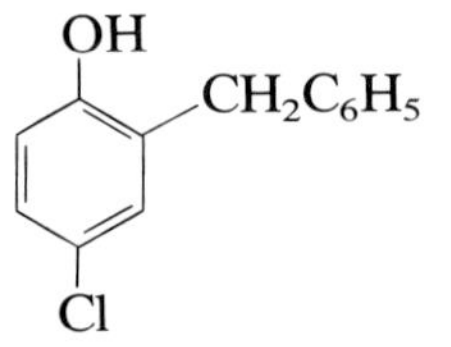

OH, $CH_2C_6H_5$, Cl

14.**10**

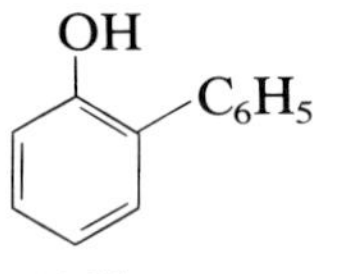

OH, C_6H_5

14.**11**

gram-positive bacteria and has also been found to be effective against certain viruses, fungi, and protozoa. Proprietary preparations containing chlorophene are recommended for environmental disinfection in hospitals, dairies, barns, poultry houses, and rest rooms.

The halogenated xylenols and cresols are used in applications similar to those of chlorophene and in addition are found in antiseptic creams mouthwashes, and gargles. Chlorothymol is also used as a topical antiseptic but is very irritating to mucous membranes.

Although simple brominated phenols have been shown to be antibacterial agents (41, 42), they have not found much commercial application, probably because of their inherent higher cost.

Other substituted phenols formerly used as antibacterials include the nitrophenols, aminophenols, naphthols, and bromonaphthols. These agents have been supplanted by more effective, less toxic materials.

3.4.2 BISPHENOLS. The bisphenols include antibacterial compounds comprised of two phenolic substituents connected by a linking group or bond. Research in this area began with the early observations by Beckhold and Ehrlich of the antibacterial action of substituted diphenols (37). Other studies of bisphenols containing sulfur (43), alkyl (44), and oxygen (45) bridges were reported in the early 1930s.

Studies of the halogenated bisphenols that eventually led to the discovery of 2,2′-methylenebis-3,4,6-trichlorophenol (hexachlorophene, 14.**12**) and 2,2′-methylenebis-4-chlorophenol (dichlorophene, 14.**13**)

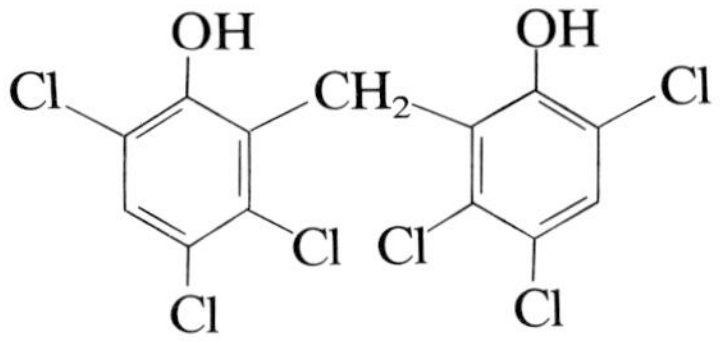

14.**12**

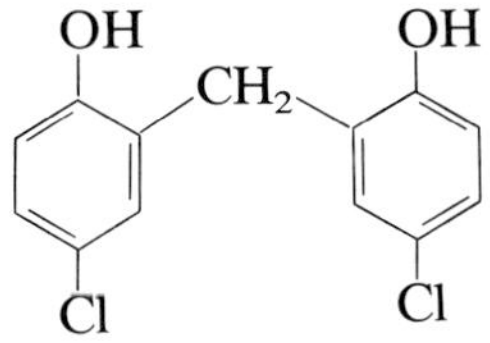

14.**13**

began in 1937 (46). Although it exhibits good antibacterial activity, dichlorophene has been used largely for mildew-proofing. Hexachlorophene, first synthesized by Gump in 1941 (47), was found to possess good antiseptic properties and became one of the most widely used antiseptics in history. At its peak use, it was a standard ingredient in such proprietary items as bath soaps, shampoos, cosmetics, dusting powders, acne preparations, and deodorants. The actual utility of hexachlorophene in many of these products was questionable.

Although only weakly active against gram-negative bacteria, hexachlorophene was an effective agent in reducing skin bacterial counts when used repetitively as a surgical scrub (48, 49). In the late 1950's severe episodes of virulent staphylococcal infections occurred in hospital nurseries throughout the world. One of the more successful efforts to combat this problem was the routine bathing of infants with a 3% hexachlorophene solution.

Early studies of the toxicity of hexachlorophene indicated that it was very toxic when administered to dogs intravenously (50) and moderately toxic to mice (LD_{50}, 80 mg/kg) by the oral route (51). The first indications of systemic toxicity from a normal, topical application of hexachlorophene were described by Larsen in 1960 (52). His descriptions of convulsions in burn patients treated with 3% hexachlorophene led to further work on the dermal absorption and toxicity in rats (53) and monkeys (54). These and other studies correlating the topical application of hexachlorophene, and neurological abnormalities prompted the FDA to publish a regulatory proposal limiting over-the-counter products to concentrations of less than 0.75%. Products containing higher concentrations of hexachlorophene would be required to bear the Rx label and cautionary warnings. This proposal was under review when it was discovered in France that more than 30 infants had died from accidental exposure to baby powder containing 6% hexachlorophene. It was also at this time that Alvord presented to the FDA his study of infant brain sections, which correlated spongiform changes in the brain stem with prior bathing with a 3% hexachlorophene product (55). The receipt of these data prompted the FDA to ban the use of hexachlorophene from all over-the-counter drug and cosmetic products, except at preservative levels. All other products were required to bear an Rx label, as well as warnings concerning absorption and potential neurotoxicity.

An in-depth review of the use of hexachlorophene in the prevention of sepsis in hospital nurseries has been published by Kensit (56). Other reviews of the use of hexachlorophene and its potential for toxicity are available (57–59).

Bithionol (14.**14**) is another chlorinated bisphenol that formerly was widely used in soaps and cosmetics (60). It has an antibacterial spectrum (61) similar to that of hexachlorophene and has also been used as

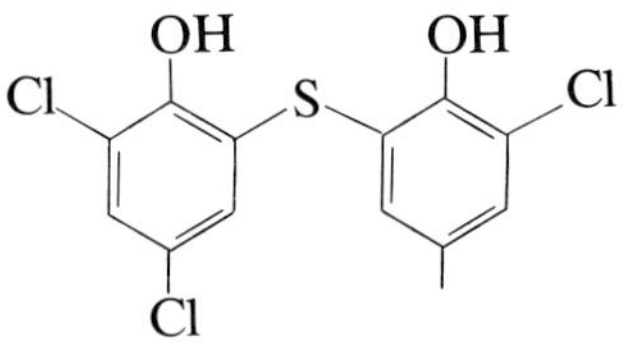

14.**14**

an anthelmintic (62, 63). The FDA withdrew bithionol from the topical over-the-counter market in 1967 because of evidence of contact photodermatitis (64, 65).

Several investigators have studied the mode of action of bisphenols and have attributed their bactericidal effects to chelation of iron (66), interference with dehydrogenase and cytochrome systems (67, 68), and interference with cell membrane function (69). An in-depth study of a nonhalogenated bisphenol (14.**15**) revealed

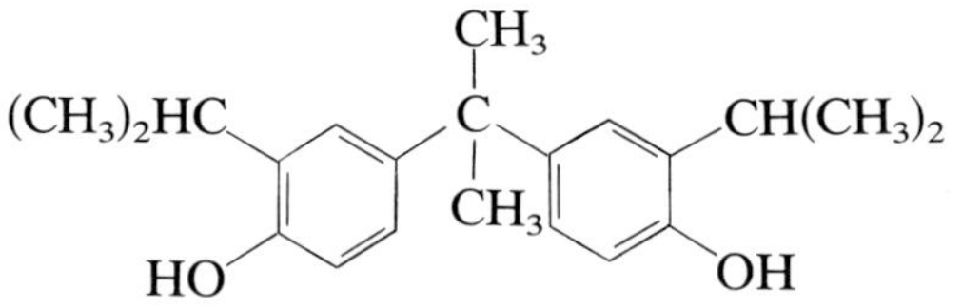

14.**15**

that it was a potent inhibitor of D-glutamyl ligase in *Bacillus subtilis.* This enzyme catalyzes the incorporation of D-glutamic acid into uridine 5′-diphosphomuramyl-L-alanine, which is an essential component of the bacterial cell wall. The compound also had an inhibiting effect on protein synthesis but did not affect DNA or RNA synthesis (70).

3.4.3 SALICYLANILIDES. The antifungal properties of salicylanilide were described in 1936 by Fargher, who recommended its use as a textile preservative (71). Structure-activity studies on halogenated salicylanilides were carried out by Bindler (72), Taborsky (73, 74), and Stecker (75). These investigations showed that optimal antibacterial activity was attained when both rings were halogenated and when a halogen was para to the phenolic hydroxyl group. Their work led to the commercial development of dibromsalan (14.**17**), tribromsalan (14.**16**), metabromsalan (14.**18**), and fluorosalan (14.**19**) as antiseptics and disinfectants. These compounds were once widely used alone and in combination in toilet soaps, detergents, laundry softeners, and

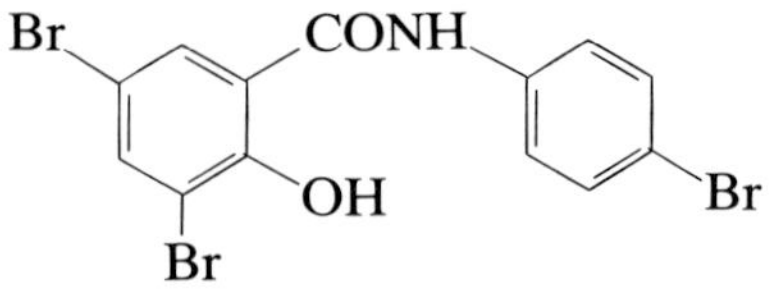

14.**16**

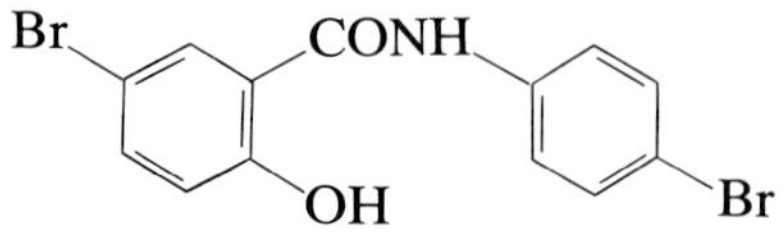

14.**17**

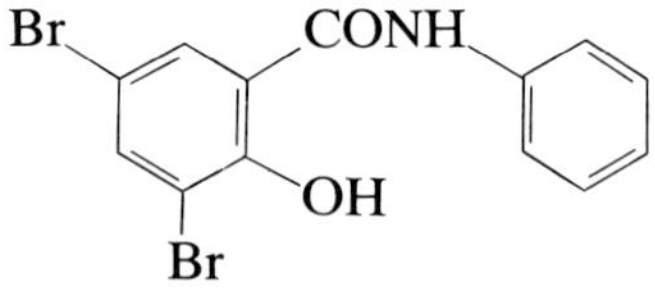

14.**18**

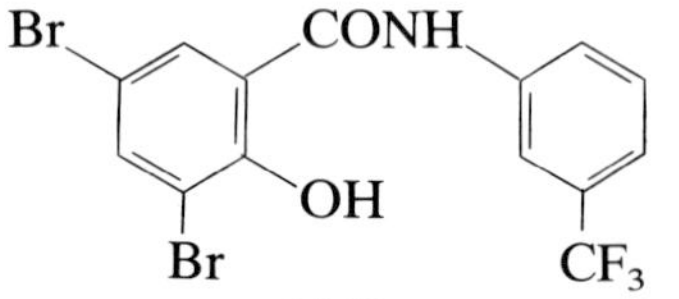

14.**19**

cosmetics. Their use now has been severely restricted by the FDA because of their propensity to induce photosensitization and cross-sensitization to other topical agents (76).

3.4.4 HYDROXYBENZOIC ACIDS. The alkyl esters of *p*-hydroxybenzoic acid (parabens) are used as preservatives in a great number of pharmaceutical, cosmetic, and industrial products. They are bacteriostatic and fungistatic at very low concentrations (77, 78) and exhibit low toxicity, although cases of contact dermatitis have been observed (79).

Benzyl paraben has the best antiseptic properties, and the butyl ester is the best antifungal. A combination of methyl-, butyl-, and ethylparaben has been used in medicaments for pharyngitis. The relationship between physicochemical properties and antimicrobial action of the parabens has been reviewed by Buechi et al (80).

Biphenamine (14.**20**), a substituted 2-hydroxybenzoic acid, was used as an antibacterial in shampoo, but it has recently been withdrawn by order of the FDA (81).

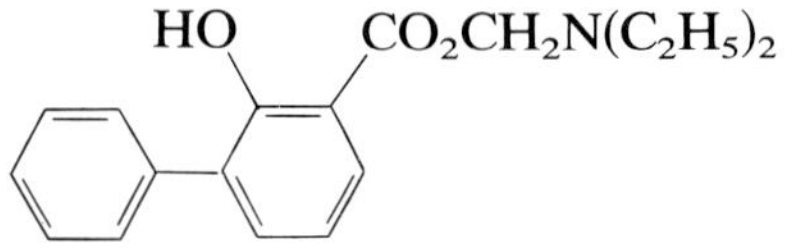

HO $CO_2CH_2N(C_2H_5)_2$

14.**20**

3.4.5 POLYHYDRIC PHENOLS. Resorcinol and its alkyl derivatives were studied by Johnson and co-workers, who first evaluated the antimicrobial activity of this group (82). In general, the level of antibacterial activity increased with the increasing chain length of the alkyl substituent up to a length of six carbons for gram-negative bacteria and nine carbons for gram-positive bacteria. It was also shown that as long as one hydroxyl group remained unsubstituted, the alkyl substituent could be on oxygen or on a nuclear carbon, and the same level of antibacterial activity was maintained (83). Catechol and hydroquinone derivatives have also been evaluated for antimicrobial effects, but they are generally inferior to the resorcinol series.

Resorcinol is still employed in the treatment of ringworm, eczema, psoriasis, and other cutaneous problems, but it is not widely used for its antibacterial properties. Hexylresorcinol is commonly employed as an antiseptic in mouthwashes and other oral preparations. It can be irritating to tissues in high concentrations, and allergic reactions have occurred (84).

3.4.6 HYDROXYQUINOLINES. The uses of 8-hydroxyquinolines in medicine and agriculture have been under investigation since before 1900. The antibacterial and antifungal properties of the 8-quinolinols have been attributed to their ability, unique among the isomeric quinolinols, to chelate biochemically important metals (85, 86). The antibacterial spectrum of 8-quinolinol (oxine, chinosol) is quite broad (87), and it is used in a variety of disinfectant and antiseptic preparations.

Attempts to improve on the antibacterial activity of chinosol led to the discovery of the halogenated 8-quinolinols, which also display broad spectrum antibacterial and antifungal activity. Singly and as mixtures (chinosols) they are used in the same manner as chinosol (88). One of the halogenated 8-quinolinols, 5-chloro-7-iodo-8-hydroxyquinoline (14.**21**) (clioquinol, chinoform), has also been found to be useful in the treatment of amebic dysentery.

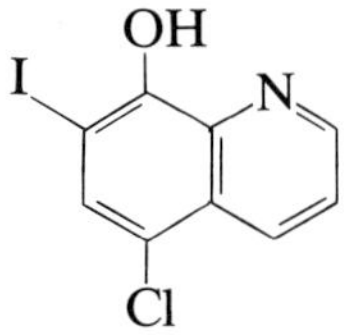

OH I N Cl

14.**21**

Because of its wide spectrum of activity, chinoform became widely used as a preventive and treatment for traveler's diarrhea. The scientific evidence for this use is rather sparse and has come under criticism (89, 90). Chinoform has been associated with an epidemic of subacute myelooptic neuropathy in Japan. Other cases of neurological toxicity have been linked to the use of chinoform, with the result that the drug is no longer available for oral use in Japan and the United States (91).

The 5-nitro derivative of 8-quinolinol has been suggested as a treatment for urinary tract infections (92); since it induces neurological lesions in laboratory animals, however, it does not appear that it will be a useful drug (93).

3.5 Alcohols

Ethyl and isopropyl alcohol are the only alcohols used routinely today as antiseptics and disinfectants. However phenethyl alcohol, benzyl alcohol, 2,4-dichlorobenzyl alcohol, and trichlorobutanol are used as preservatives in many medicinal preparations.

Tanner and Wilson (94) have carried out structure-activity studies with the straight chain alcohols from methyl to undecyl. Using an *in vitro* agar cup–plate method, they found that the size of the zone of inhibition increased from ethyl to amyl alcohol, then gradually decreased with increasing chain length. Methyl alcohol was devoid of activity in this test. A study of branched chain alcohols indicated the following general order of activity: normal-primary>iso-primary>normal-secondary>tertiary (95). Ethyl and isopropyl alcohol possess activity against the vegetative forms of a broad range of bacteria, but they are not sporocidal (96, 97).

The bactericidal activities of ethyl and isopropyl alcohol are essentially equivalent. They are most effective as 60–90% aqueous solutions, and their main uses are in skin and thermometer disinfection. Because of their volatility, they have no residual activity (98). The mode of action of ethyl and isopropyl alcohol at their normal use concentrations is generally regarded to be gross protein denaturation. At lower concentrations, there is some evidence suggesting that interference with metabolism can also play a part (99).

Phenethyl alcohol, benzyl alcohol, and trichlorobutanol have served for some time as preservatives in opthalmic preparations. Phenethyl and benzyl alcohol are no longer recommended for this use because of their slow antibacterial action (100). The mode of action of phenethyl alcohol at the molecular level has received some attention. It has been found to inhibit RNA synthesis, DNA repair, and in particular, may be involved with the synthesis of messenger-RNA (mRNA) (101–103).

3.6 Aldehydes

Formaldehyde has been shown to be active against bacteria, fungi, and viruses and has been used in the past as a gaseous disinfectant or fumigant (104). Because of its slow rate of antibacterial action, poor penetrability, and tendency to polymerize, however, it is not often used for this purpose. In the gaseous state and in aqueous solution, formaldehyde is highly irritating to skin and mucous membranes and is not suitable for antiseptic use. Its main use as disinfectant is as an aqueous or alcoholic solution for the sterilization of surgical instruments and gloves. Studies of the mode of action of formaldehyde have suggested that it may act through nonspecific alkylation of cell constitutents (105).

Polynoxylin is a urea-formaldehyde polymer with a wide antibacterial spectrum (106). Its bactericidal action is presumably due to the slow release of formaldehyde. Polynoxylin is used in creams and powders for the treatment of minor skin infections.

Glutaraldehyde is widely employed in hospitals for disinfection of equipment that cannot be heat sterilized. A 2% aqueous solution has a moderately rapid bactericidal action for a broad spectrum of common pathogenic bacteria and spores (107). The mode of action of glutaraldehyde has been ascribed to a denaturing effect on the outer cell layers, rendering them impermeable (108, 109).

The use of aldehydes as disinfectants has been reviewed by Boucher (110).

3.7. Quaternary Ammonium Compounds

The first record of the preparation of a quaternary ammonium derivative evaluated for antiseptic properties was that of Einhorn and Göttler in 1908 (111). Domagk, however is considered to have successfully introduced quaternary ammonium derivatives (quats) as useful antiseptics and disinfectants (112).

The quats have a broad spectrum of antibacterial activity but are usually more effective against gram-positive than gram-negative bacteria. This difference has been attributed to the higher content of phospholipids in cell wall of gram-negative bacteria (113). Important bacteria that are resistant to quats include *Mycobacterium tuberculosis* and several strains of *Pseudomonas aeruginosa* (114, 115). The development of bacterial resistance to quats has also been demonstrated (116). The quats have not shown sporicidal activity.

Quats are widely used as sanitizers in dairy and food industries because they are generally more effective in the presence of organic contamination than are many other germicides (118, 119). They are used as general environmental sanitizers and for washing clothing, diapers, and eating utensils. The medically related uses include disinfection of skin and mucous membranes and sterilization of surgical instruments. An alcohol solution of a quat has been recommended for the final sterilization step in the hexachlorophene-soap surgical scrub procedure, since the effect of hexachlorophene is mainly bacteriostatic (120). They have also been found to be useful as preservatives in ophthalmic preparations (121).

Since the beginning of the use of quats, it has been known that their antibacterial action may be destroyed by anionic soaps (112). The anionic portion of the soap reacts with the cation of the quat to produce a biologically inert insoluble salt. To achieve effective antibacterial activity when using quats, care must be taken to remove all soap residue from areas to be treated. The calcium, magnesium, and ferric ions found in hard water are also known to interfere with the action of quats (122). Walter has pointed out that cotton, cellulose sponge, cork, rubber, and other materials selectively absorb quats from aqueous solutions (123). This effect must be taken into account when these materials come in contact with solutions used for sterilization, and the quat must be replenished periodically to maintain efficacy.

In the concentrations (1:1000–1:5000) normally employed for use on skin and mucous membranes, quats are quite nontoxic, although they have been shown to cause occasional allergic responses (124). When taken orally in high concentrations, they cause muscle depolarization and can lead to death from respiratory paralysis if large enough quantities are ingested. The fatal dose for humans has been estimated at 1 to 3 g (125).

Early studies on the mode of action of quats by Hotchkiss (126) demonstrated that nitrogen- and phosphorus-containing materials were released into the surrounding medium when bacteria were treated with germicidal concentrations. Examination by light microscopy revealed that no detectable lysis of the cells or morphological change had occurred during the treatment. Other studies have confirmed this release of cellular constituents by bacteria on exposure to quats, and the antibacterial activity has been linked with this effect (127, 128). Evidence has been presented that low concentrations (100 μg/ml) of quats can cause cytological damage that was related to cell death (129). High levels of quats were shown to strip off cell envelopes. A study of the effect of benzalkonium chloride on resistant *P. aeruginosa* using electron microscopy revealed that the quat caused a stripping away of the outer membrane of the bacteria. However this effect occurred with both resistant and susceptible strains, suggesting that the site of resistance to the quat was internal to the outer membrane (130).

Blois and Swarbrick (131) have studied the interaction of quats with model membrane systems using monolayers of gliadin to represent the gram-negative wall. From these studies they concluded that with gram-positive bacteria the quat first associates with cell wall protein, then penetrates, and finally disrupts the cell membrane. With gram-negative bacteria the phospholipids in the outer envelope hinder penetration and afford the organism a degree of protection.

Efforts have been made to relate critical

micelle concentrations and thermodynamic properties of quats to their antibacterial activity (132, 133). Although correlations were found, the studies did not shed light on the mode of action of the quats under study.

The mechanism of antibacterial action on a molecular level is still not well defined for quaternary ammonium compounds, but cell membranes and closely associated structures are likely targets.

A large number of quats have been synthesized and tested for antimicrobial properties. The structure of the majority of these compounds consists of a positively charged head and a hydrophobic tail. The positively charged head is a tetracovalent nitrogen atom, which may either be tetraalkyl substituted or a monoalkyl substituted nitrogen that is part of a heterocyclic ring. Where the hydrophobic tail is a straight chain alkyl moiety and the head is a benzyldimethylamino group, it has been demonstrated that the number of carbon atoms required for activity ranges from 8 to 18, with 14 being optimum (134).

Only a few quats are medically important in the United States. The most widely used are cetylpyridinium chloride (14.**22**), benzethonium chloride (14.**23**), cetrimonium

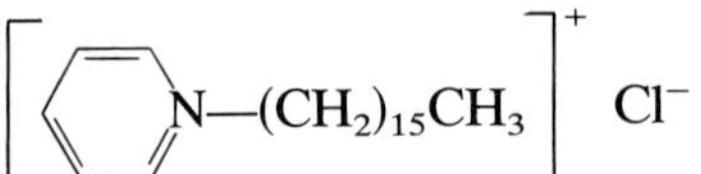

$$\left[C_5H_5N\text{—}(CH_2)_{15}CH_3 \right]^+ \; Cl^-$$

14.**22**

bromide (14.**24**), benzalkonium chloride (R = a mixture of C_8–C_{18} alkyls) (14.**25**), domiphen bromide (14.**26**), and octaphonium chloride (14.**27**). The structure of dequalinium chloride (14.**28**) does not

$$\left[(CH_3)_3N\text{—}(CH_2)_{15}CH_3 \right]^+ \; Br^-$$

14.**24**

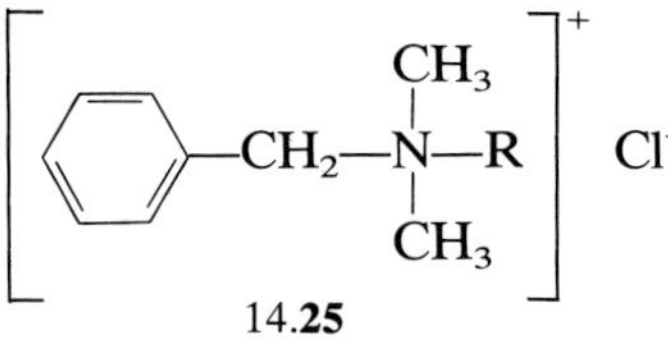

$$\left[C_6H_5\text{—}CH_2\text{—}N(CH_3)_2\text{—}R \right]^+ \; Cl^-$$

14.**25**

$$\left[C_6H_5\text{—}OCH_2CH_2\text{—}N(CH_3)_2\text{—}(CH_2)_{11}CH_3 \right]^+ \; Br^-$$

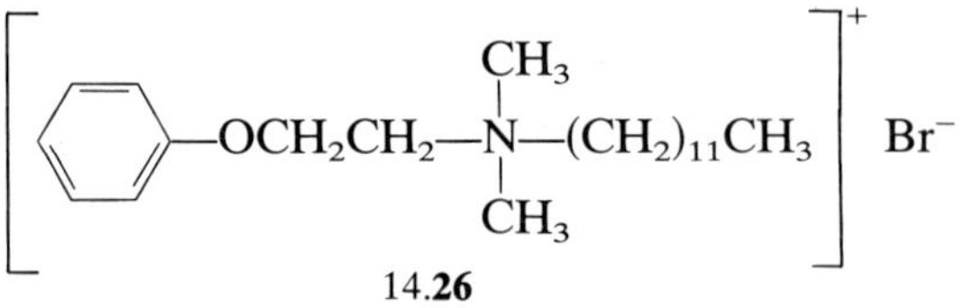

14.**26**

conform to the pattern of the other quats in that it contains two positively charged groups separated by a hydrophobic alkyl chain (135). The main use of this compound is as an oral antiseptic. Studies on the mode of action suggest that its antibacterial action may be due to its effect on components in the cytoplasm containing nucleic acids (136).

Quaternary nitrogen antiseptics and disinfectants have been reviewed by Lawrence (137).

3.8 Dyes

Antimicrobial activity was first ascribed to a dye, crystal violet, by Churchman in 1912 (138, 139). In describing the inhibitory effect of the dye on bacteria, he originated the term "bacteriostasis". There are three main groups of medically important antimicrobial dyes: triphenylmethanes, aminoacridines, and azo compounds.

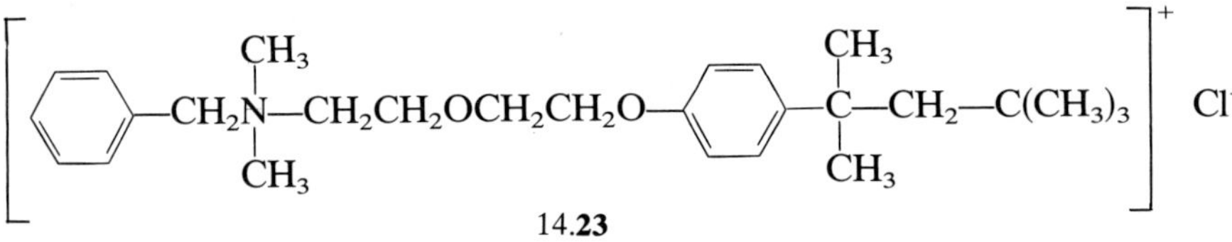

$$\left[C_6H_5\text{—}CH_2N(CH_3)_2\text{—}CH_2CH_2OCH_2CH_2O\text{—}C_6H_4\text{—}C(CH_3)_2\text{—}CH_2\text{—}C(CH_3)_3 \right]^+ \; Cl^-$$

14.**23**

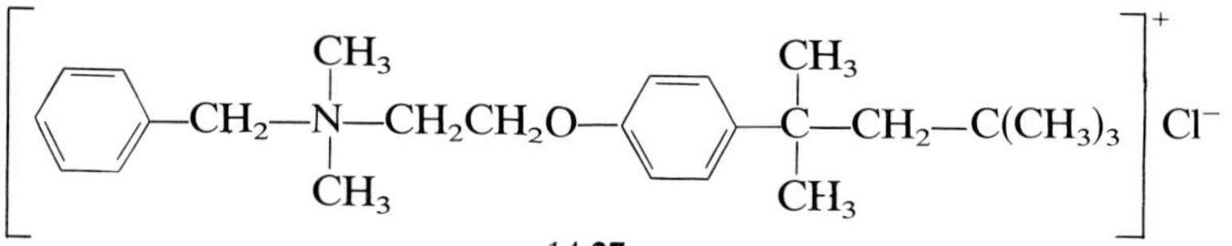

$$\left[C_6H_5-CH_2-\overset{CH_3}{\underset{CH_3}{N}}-CH_2CH_2O-C_6H_4-\overset{CH_3}{\underset{CH_3}{C}}-CH_2-C(CH_3)_3 \right]^+ Cl^-$$

14.**27**

$$\left[H_2N-(\text{quinolinyl, } CH_3)N-(CH_2)_{10}-N(\text{quinolinyl, } CH_3)-NH_2 \right]^{2+} 2Cl^-$$

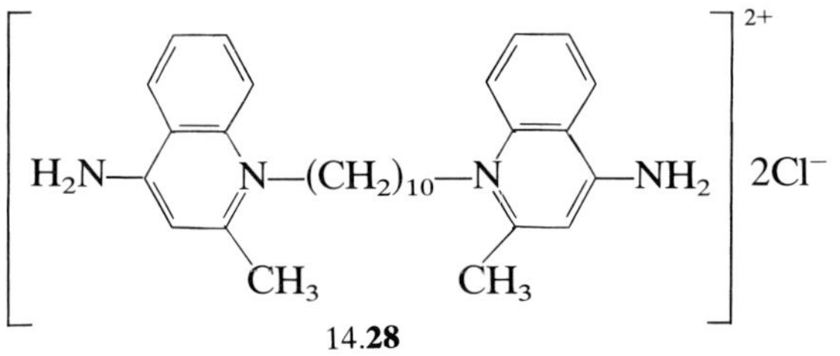

14.**28**

3.8.1 TRIPHENYLMETHANE DYES. The *p*-dialkylamino-substituted triphenylmethane or roseaniline dyes are becoming less important antibacterials as nonstaining, broad spectrum compounds are developed. Roseaniline dyes that are still of some importance as antibacterials include gentian violet (crystal violet, 14.**29**), brilliant green (malachite green, 14.**30**), and fuchsine (roseaniline, 14.**31**).

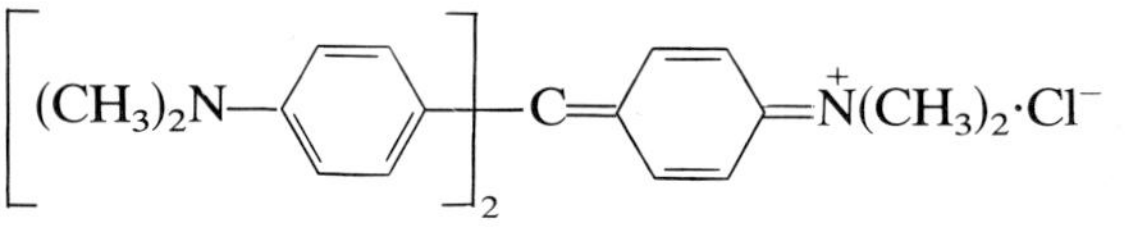

$$\left[(CH_3)_2N-C_6H_4- \right]_2 C=C_6H_4=\overset{+}{N}(CH_3)_2\cdot Cl^-$$

14.**29**

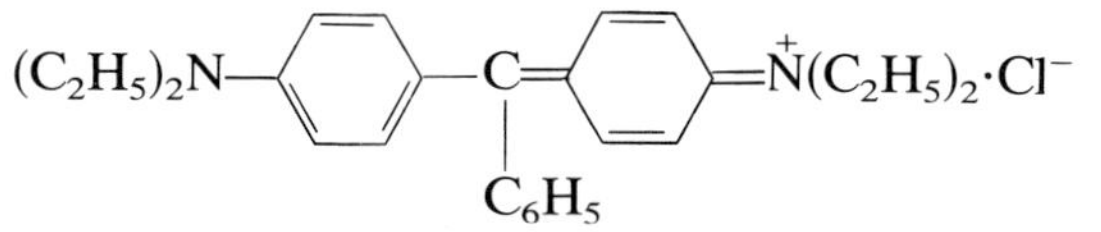

$$(C_2H_5)_2N-C_6H_4-\underset{C_6H_5}{C}=C_6H_4=\overset{+}{N}(C_2H_5)_2\cdot Cl^-$$

14.**30**

$$\left[H_2N-C_6H_4- \right]_2 C=C_6H_4=\overset{+}{N}H_2\cdot Cl^-$$

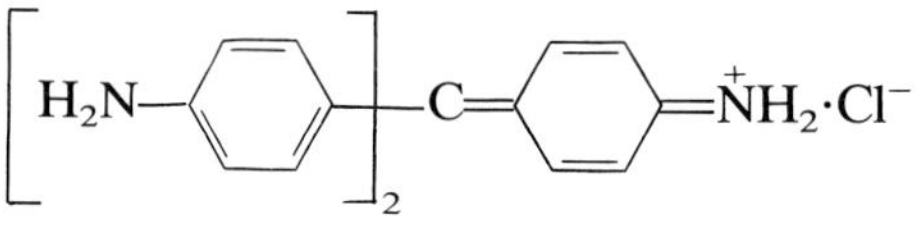

14.**31**

Gentian violet is used more extensively than the other dyes in the United States. It has been used as a topical antibacterial, as an anthelmintic, and as an antifungal agent, but its major medicinal uses at present are for treatment of topical fungal infections and as an antifungal feed additive for poultry (140).

Structure-activity studies on triphenylmethane dyes have been carried out by Fischer and Muñoz (141). They found that triphenylmethanes were more active than diphenylmethanes and that dialkylamino substitution on two or three of the rings was necessary for optimal activity.

Early work by Stearn and Stearn (142) on the mode of action of these dyes attributed their bacteriostatic activity to the formation of complexes with amphoteric substituents of the cells, which blocked biological processes. Other workers have correlated the degree of ionization of the dyes (143) and the pH of the medium (144) with antibacterial activity. More recent work suggests that intercalation of the dye with double helical DNA and subsequent accelerated ribosmal breakdown is involved (145, 146). The poor activity of the dyes against gram-negative bacteria is probably due to the inability of the dye to penetrate the outer envelope of the cell wall (147).

3.8.2 AMINOACRIDINES. Ehrlich introduced the acridine dyes as medicinal agents for the treatment of trypanosamiasis. In 1913 Browning described the antibacterial properties of these dyes, which led to their eventual clinical use (148).

Acriflavin (a mixture of 1 part proflavin and 2 parts 3,6-diamino-10-methyl-acridinium chloride, 14.**32**), Proflavin (14.**33**),

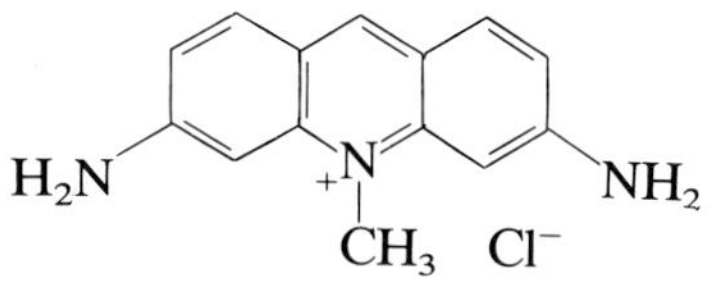

$$H_2N-(\text{acridinium, } \overset{+}{N}-CH_3)-NH_2 \quad Cl^-$$

14.**32**

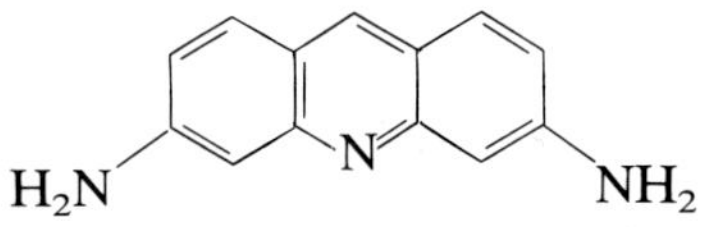

14.**33**

Ethacridine (14.**34**), Aminacrine (14.**35**), and Aminacrine hexylresorcinate (acrisorcin) are the medically important acridines. These agents are employed for the topical treatment of minor fungal and bacterial infections. They have a broad spectrum of activity and are not readily inactivated by serum.

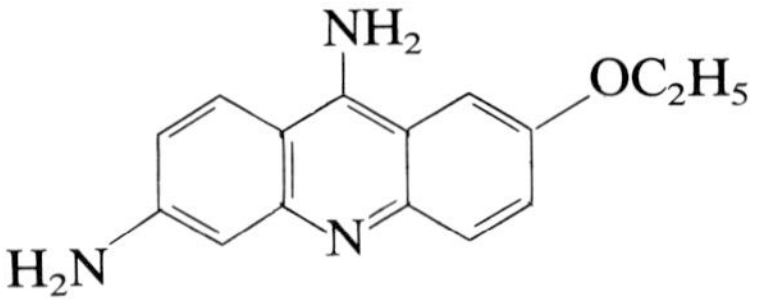

14.**34**

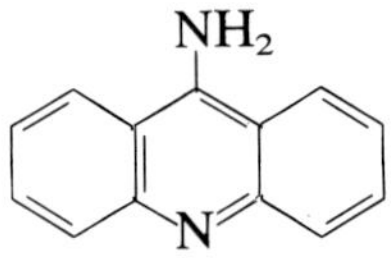

14.**35**

Albert found a direct correlation between the degree of ionization in a group of aminoacridines and their antimicrobial activity (149). In another study of structure-activity relationships of 5,6-acridine derivatives, a regression analysis was used to show an approximately linear relationship between theoretical electronic properties derived using Hückel molecular orbital calculations and antibacterial activity (150).

The mode of action of the acridines on a molecular level is undoubtedly related to their ability to combine with nucleic acids. An important histological stain for DNA and RNA is based on this property. The intercalation of aminoacridines with DNA and their role in the induction of mutations have been reviewed (151–153). These dyes inhibit DNA synthesis and DNA-dependent RNA synthesis and cause "frameshift" mutations in protein synthesis (153). Judging from the recent literature, the importance of the aminoacridines as probes for the study of DNA has probably exceeded their importance as antibacterial agents.

3.8.3 AZO DYES. Scarlet red (14.**36**) and diacetazotol (dimazon, 14.**37**) have been

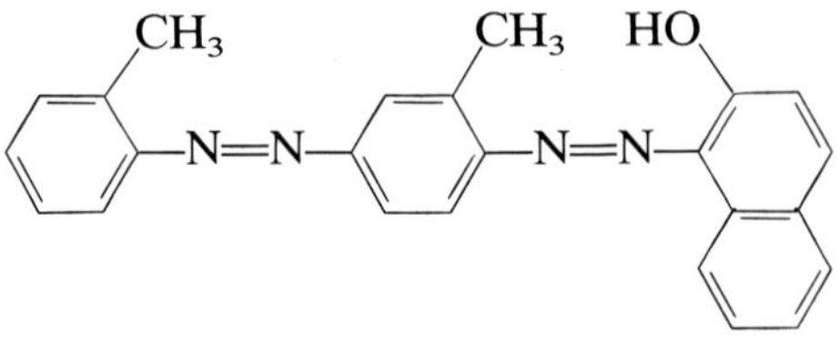

14.**36**

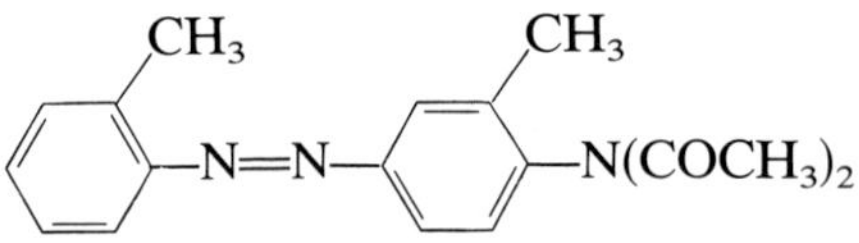

14.**37**

employed in ointments and powders for the treatment of burns, wounds, and chronic ulcers. The antibacterial profile of these drugs is not well documented, and their continued use as antibacterials is probably not warranted.

Although phenazopyridine (14.**38**) was formerly used as a urinary antiseptic, its

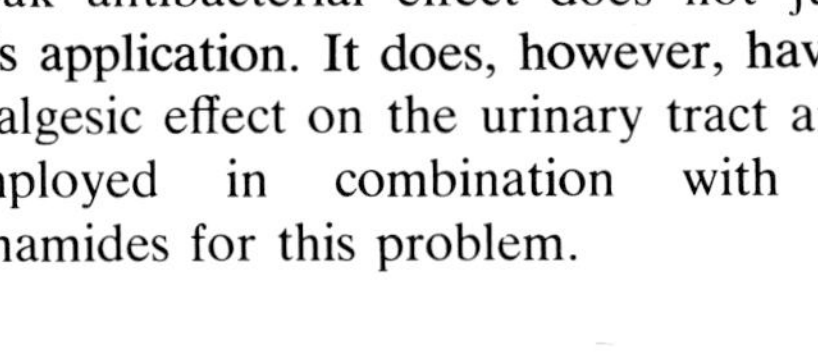

14.**38**

weak antibacterial effect does not justify this application. It does, however, have an analgesic effect on the urinary tract and is employed in combination with sulfonamides for this problem.

3.9 Ureas, Amidines, and Biguanides

The antibacterial properties of urea were noted as early as 1906 (154). Urea, urethane, and substituted carbamates, and their antimicrobial effects have been reviewed by Weinstein and McDonald (155). Early investigations into the antibacterial properties of amidines include the work of Fuller (156), Kohn (157), Thrower (158), and Elson (159). The biguanides were first investigated in 1946 for their antimalarial properties (160), and in 1954 Davies and co-workers described the antimicrobial effects of a number of bisbiguanides (161).

3.9.1 UREAS. In a study of more than 200 urea derivatives Beaver, Roman, and Stoffel (162) identified the very potent antibacterial activity of the diarylureas (carbanilides). The best activity resided with derivatives halogenated in the 3,3′- and 4,4′-positions, with other subsitution patterns greatly decreasing activity. Thioureas were also found to be active, but at lower levels. The compound chosen for commercial development from the group was the 3,4,4′-trichloro derivative, triclocarban (14.**39**). The major uses of this compound

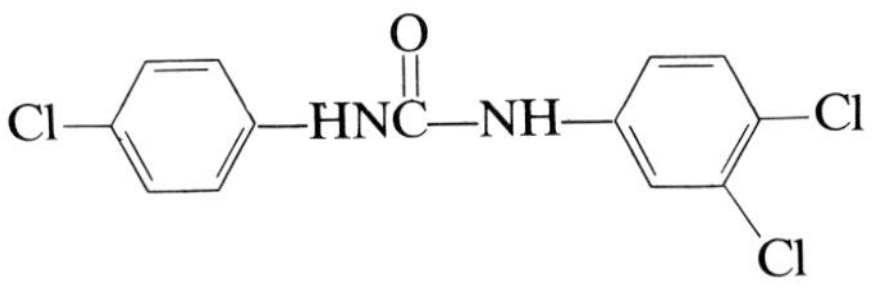

Cl–C₆H₄–HNC(=O)–NH–C₆H₃(Cl)–Cl

14.**39**

include incorporation in deodorants, laundry detergents, toilet soaps, and medicated cosmetics. Triclocarban is active *in vitro* against gram-positive bacteria and certain fungi, less so against gram-negative bacteria. In a Cade serial wash basin study (12), triclocarban exhibited good initial degerming effects and low residual bacterial counts and appeared to be effective for use in surgical scrubs (163).

The toxicity of triclocarban is low, and few cases of irritation, photosensitivity, or primary sensitivity have been reported (164). However reports of methemoglobinemia in infants have been associated with its topical use (165, 166). Further studies of this problem led to the discovery that in diapers, triclocarban breaks down to aniline derivatives, which were implicated as the causative agents of the methemoglobinemia outbreaks in neonates (167). This finding is in accord with recent studies indicating very low levels of cutaneous absorbtion from topical applications of triclocarban (168).

Cloflucarban (14.**40**) is a close analog of triclocarban having similar antibacterial

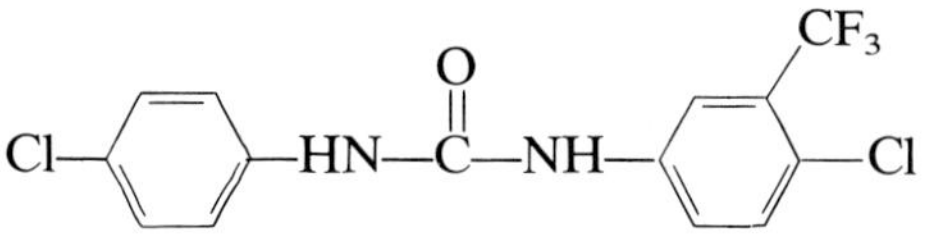

$Cl-C_6H_4-HN-C(=O)-NH-C_6H_3(CF_3)-Cl$

14.**40**

properties and commercial utility (169). Although the antibacterial mode of action of the diarylureas has been the subject of some speculation (162, 170), it has not actually been determined. Alteration of cell membrane permeability has been most recently implicated (171, 172).

3.9.2 AMIDINES. Interest in the chemotherapeutic effects of amidines was first centered on their use in the treatment of trypanosomiasis. It was in a program of synthesis directed toward the preparation of analogs of synthalin (decamethylene diquanidine), a trypanocidal agent, that propamidine (14.**41**) was first prepared (173). The antibacterial properties of aliphatic amidines were first described by Fuller

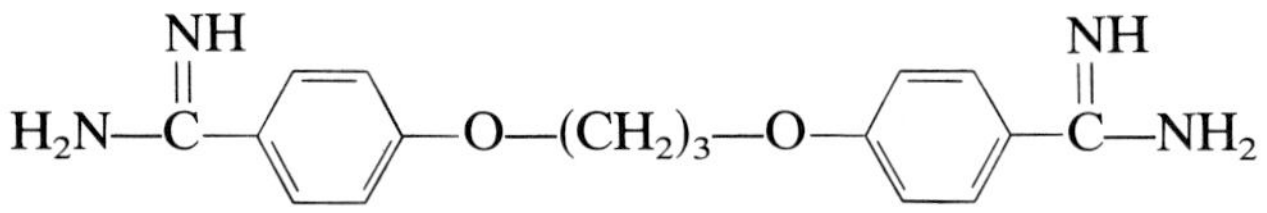

$H_2N-C(=NH)-C_6H_4-O-(CH_2)_3-O-C_6H_4-C(=NH)-NH_2$

14.**41**

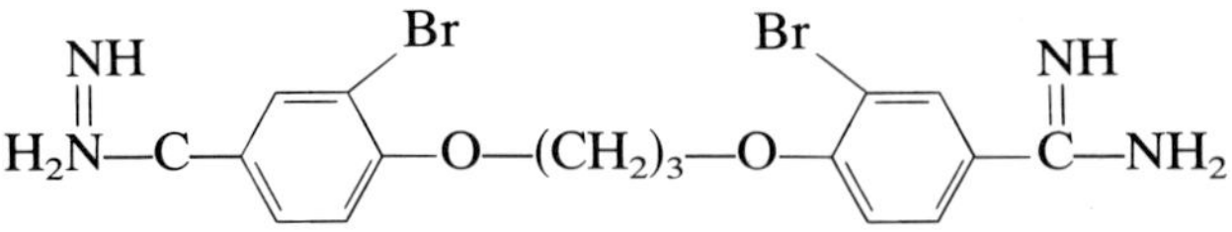

$$H_2N{-}\overset{\overset{\displaystyle NH}{\|}}{C}{-}C_6H_3(Br){-}O{-}(CH_2)_3{-}O{-}C_6H_3(Br){-}\overset{\overset{\displaystyle NH}{\|}}{C}{-}NH_2$$

14.**42**

(156). Thrower and Valentine described the antibacterial properties and clinical utility of propamidine in 1943 (158). Dibromopropamidine (14.**42**) was described by Berg and Newberry (174) in 1949.

Propamidine and dibromopropamidine have essentially the same antibacterial spectrum, with the latter exhibiting somewhat higher potency. The compounds are active against gram-positive bacteria and some fungi but are not effective against gram-negative bacteria or spores (175, 176). The compounds are employed as salts, most commonly as the isethionates (2-hydroxyethansulfonates), in a variety of topical ointments and creams for minor burns, cuts, abrasions, and oral infections. They have also been employed in the treatment of bacterial conjunctivitis.

In spite of several studies on activity of propamidines and related diamidines, there is no clear-cut explanation for their mode of antibacterial action (171–179).

The propamidines have been reviewed by Hugo (180).

3.9.3 BIGUANIDES. Interest in the chemotherapeutic properties of biguanides stemmed from the original observations by Curd and Rose of their antimalarial activity (160). Pursuing these investigations, Rose and Swain (181) synthesized a series of biguanides having the structure 14.**43**. They found that antibacterial activity was much reduced when the biguanide functions were replaced by guanidines or when only one biguanide group was present. The optimum chain length for the central methylene portion was 5–8 carbons, and insertion of aromatic groups or ether linkages in this portion of the molecule did not improve activity. The preferred terminal groups, R and R′, were found to be aromatic as opposed to mono- or dialkyl. Substitution of the aromatic groups with hydroxylic functions such as hydroxyl or carboxyl led to greatly diminished activity. The optimum substituent on the aromatic nucleus was found to be *p*-chloro, which gave the preferred compound of the group, 1,6-di-(4′-chlorophenyldiguanidino)hexane (14.**44**, chlorhexidine). Davies has reported on the biological activity of this series (161).

Chlorhexidine inhibits a broad range of gram-negative and gram-positive bacteria, but is not effective against acid-fast bacteria, spores, or viruses (182). Its activity is not diminished by moderate levels of cationic or neutral detergents or serum but anionic detergents, phosphates, carbonates, and silicates can precipitate it from solution. The compound is usually supplied as a gluconate, acetate, or hydrochloride salt.

Chlorhexidine is one of the most widely used topical antiseptics, especially in the British Commonwealth. Preoperative skin disinfection, surgical scrubs, mouthwash, bladder irrigation, wound irrigation, prevention of mastitis in dairy cattle, general sanitization, and treatment of burns are among the many areas in which chlorhexidine has been useful. An interesting potential application still being investigated is the use of chlorhexidine in oral hygiene for the prevention of bacterial plaque on teeth,

$$RNH{-}\overset{\overset{\displaystyle NH}{\|}}{C}{-}NH{-}\overset{\overset{\displaystyle NH}{\|}}{C}{-}NH{-}(CH_2)_x{-}NH{-}\overset{\overset{\displaystyle NH}{\|}}{C}{-}NH{-}\overset{\overset{\displaystyle NH}{\|}}{C}{-}NHR'$$

14.**43**

Cl—C_6H_4—NH—C(=NH)—NH—C(=NH)—NH—$(CH_2)_6$—NH—C(=NH)—NH—C(=NH)—NH—C_6H_4—Cl

14.**44**

reduction of caries, and reduction of gingivitis (183–185).

Chlorhexidine has been found to possess a very low order of toxicity for animals. It is quite nontoxic to unbroken skin, denuded tissue, and mucous membranes at antibacterially effective concentrations (161, 186, 187). Long-term feeding studies in rats gave no indication of carcinogenicity, teratogenicity, fertility impairment, or other overt effects (188). Absorption studies using radiolabeled material indicated that chlorhexidine was almost unabsorbed when given orally or applied to the skin (189, 190).

Studies of the antibacterial mode of action were initiated by Hugo and Longworth (191), who observed adsorption to the bacterial cell surface followed by a rapid loss of cytoplasmic constituents. Chlorhexidine has been shown to inhibit the activity of membrane-bound ATPase (192) and also to inhibit RNA and protein synthesis (193). From these and many other studies, Hugo (194) has concluded that chlorhexidine exerts a range of effects on the cytoplasmic membrane, from inhibition of biochemical function at low concentrations, to structural damage at the minimum inhibitory concentration. Higher concentrations (50 μg/ml) result in lysis, and further increases cause general precipitation of cell contents.

Picloxydine (14.**45**) (195) and alexidine (14.**46**) (196) are biguanides that have antibacterial properties and uses similar to chlorhexidine but have not enjoyed the commercial success of the latter.

3.10 Heavy Metal Compounds

Preparations containing heavy metal compounds have been used for hundreds of years in attempts to control the consequences of bacterial disease. The first compounds used were inorganic salts and oxides of dubious efficacy. The first effective organic metal derivative was atoxyl, an aromatic arsenic compound used by Thomas (197) in the treatment of trypanosomiasis. Another aromatic arsenic derivative, arsphenamine (Salvarsan) was introduced by Ehrlich in 1910 for the treatment of syphilis. This compound was the first truly effective systemic, organic antibacterial agent and is one of the great milestones in the history of chemotherapy.

Organic derivatives of bismuth and antimony, once used in the treatment of bacterial disease, are now employed only to treat protozoal infections. Organic tin compounds have been suggested for use as disinfectants (198).

Silver and mercury remain the only heavy metals used extensively in the treatment or prevention of microbial disease.

3.10.1 MERCURY COMPOUNDS. The organic mercurial antiseptics possess a carbon–mercury bond and are generally more effective antibacterially and are less easily inactivated than are inorganic mercury salts. They are bacteriostatic, and because of the reversibility of their effect on bacteria and lack of sporicidal activity, some doubt has been raised regarding their suitability as antiseptics (199). However there

Cl—C_6H_4—NH—C(=NH)—NH—C(=NH)—N(piperazine)N—C(=NH)—NH—C(=NH)—NH—C_6H_4—Cl

14.**45**

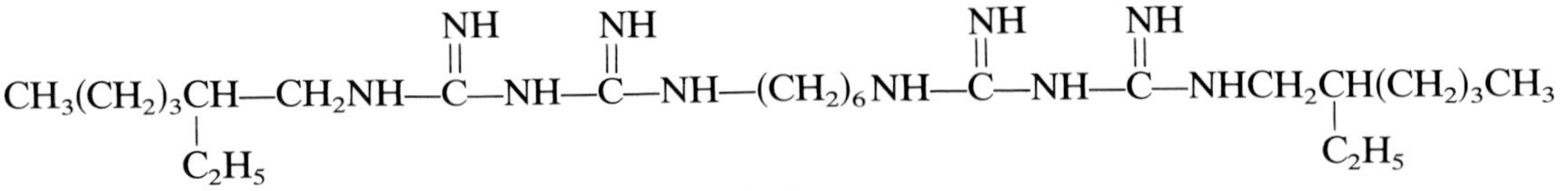

$$CH_3(CH_2)_3CH(C_2H_5)-CH_2NH-C(=NH)-NH-C(=NH)-NH-(CH_2)_6NH-C(=NH)-NH-C(=NH)-NHCH_2CH(C_2H_5)(CH_2)_3CH_3$$

14.**46**

does seem to be ample evidence of effectiveness of these compounds under actual conditions of use as antiseptics (200–202).

The mechanism of action of the organic mercurials is thought to involve the reversible formation of mercaptides with sulfhydryl groups of cellular enzymes (203–205). This theory is in accord with the observed reversal of the bacteriostatic effect of these compounds by ammonium sulfide and 2-mercaptoethanol.

At the levels used in antiseptic preparations, the mercurials have not shown significant toxicity, although sensitization has occurred (206).

Merbromin (14.**47**), (mercurochrome) was the first of the organic mercurials to be introduced an an antiseptic (207). Meralein (14.**48**), a closely related analog (208), was introduced somewhat later. Three phenyl mercury derivatives have achieved importance as antiseptics: nitromersol (14.**49**)

14.**47**

14.**48**

14.**49**

(209), hydrargyraphen (14.**50**) (210), and the acetate, nitrate, and borate salts of phenylmercury.

Two mercaptides of ethyl mercury are also used as antiseptics, thiomersol (merthiolate, 14.**51**) (211) and thiomerfonate (14.**52**) (212).

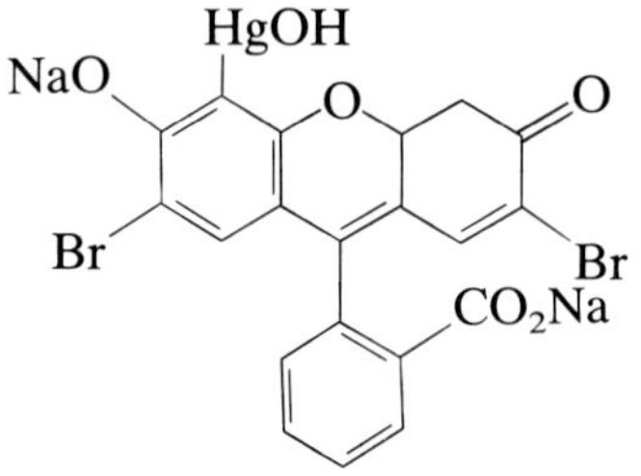

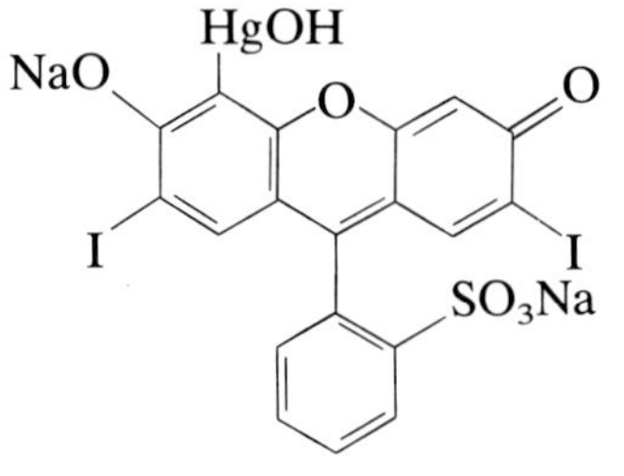

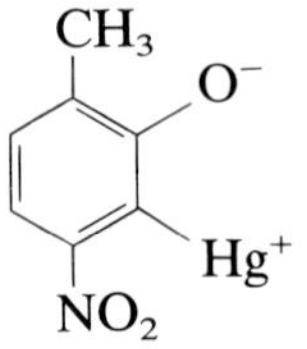

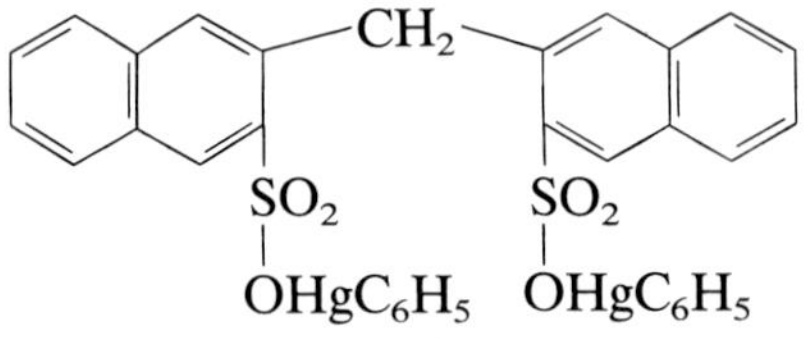

14.**50**

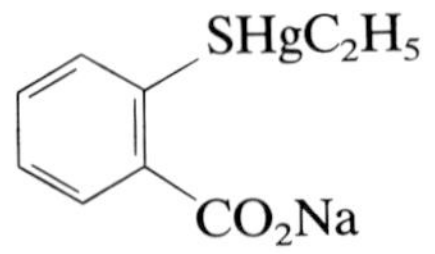

14.**51**

$C_2H_5HgS-C_6H_4-SO_3Na$

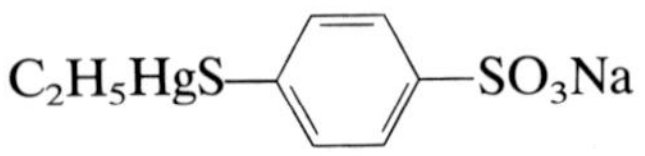

14.**52**

The introduction of topical antibacterials that are bactericidal and sporicidal has resulted in the decline of the use of organic mercurials.

3.10.2 SILVER COMPOUNDS. Credé introduced the use of silver nitrate solution for the prevention of ophthalmia neonatorum in 1884, and this treatment is still routinely employed for the prevention of gonococcal infections in the eyes of newborns. Inorganic salts of silver have been employed for a long time in various preparations for the treatment and preventation of infection, but the only antibacterial agents of importance today that can be considered to be organic compounds of silver are silver protein and silver sulfadizine. These agents are not true organometallics, since they do not contain a silver-carbon bond.

The mode of antibacterial action of silver compounds has long been ascribed to nonspecific binding of silver ions with bacterial protein, but more recent investigations have implicated interference with DNA replication (213, 214) and indirect effects on DNA synthesis by action on the cell membrane (215).

Silver protein, a colloidal preparation of silver combined with protein, was once used as a topical agent for treatment of conjunctivitis and nose and throat infections, and for prevention of gonorrhea. The use of this preparation is no longer recommended because of the availability of more effective, less toxic agents.

A recent prophylactic treatment for severe burns involves the use of silver sulfadizine cream (14.**53**). This compound,

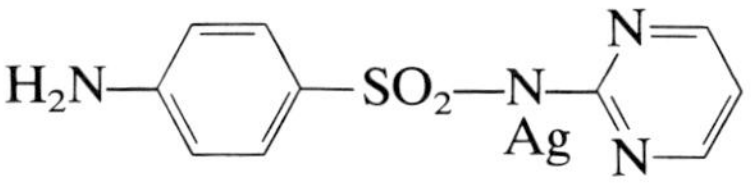

$H_2N-C_6H_4-SO_2-N(Ag)-C_4H_3N_2$ (pyrimidin-2-yl)

14.**53**

first recommended by Fox (216), was approved for use in the United States in 1973. The main topical treatments available for the prevention of infection in severely burned patients at that time were silver nitrate solution, mafenide cream (a sulfonamide), and a gentamicin ointment. Each of these treatments has its disadvantages, and silver sulfadiazine seems to combine the effectiveness of the silver nitrate and sulfonamide treatments without the staining, poor penetration, and potential electrolyte imbalance of the former, and the pain on application, acidosis, and sensitivity problems of the latter. It is effective against *Pseudomonas aeruginosa* and *Staphylococcus aureus*, common invaders of burned tissue, and resistance does not often develop. The use of silver sulfadizine in burn therapy has been reviewed by Moncrief (217) and Fox (218).

3.11 Gaseous Chemosterilants

As medicine and technology have increased in complexity, there has been increased need for effective methods of sterilization that do not depend on heat. Delicate electronic and laboratory equipment, medical devices, biologicals, and numerous other materials unable to withstand autoclaving require alternate means of sterilization.

Attempts at gaseous sterilization began with the fumigation of sickrooms with chlorine or sulfur dioxide at the turn of the century. The first relatively effective gaseous chemosterilant was formaldehyde vapor, which, despite its drawbacks, was the best agent available for several years (see Section 3.6).

Ethylene oxide has supplanted formaldehyde as the agent of choice for gaseous sterilization. Although its antibacterial properties had been described as early as 1929 (219), its commercial use did not begin until the 1940s. Ethylene oxide is highly biocidal against all bacteria, spores, viruses, and fungi; it is not corrosive, and it easily penetrates porous materials (219). Some of the drawbacks associated with ethylene oxide include its toxicity, relatively slow action, and flammability. the latter problem is overcome commercially by supplying ethylene oxide as a 10% mixture in carbon dioxide, which is not flammable when mixed with air (220). The optimum relative humidity for sterilization is approximately 30%, and the rate of sterilization is directly proportional to the temperature and concentration of ethylene oxide (221).

Ethylene oxide is very susceptible to nucleophilic ring opening by attack on carbon, and it is generally accepted that this reaction is the ultimate mechanism of sterilization. It can irreversibly alkylate any of the free amino, carboxyl, mercapto or hydroxyl groups of an organism, giving hydroxyethyl derivatives that block normal metabolic processes (222). Sterilization with ethylene oxide has been reviewed by Ernst (223).

Another alkylating agent that has been used for sterilization is β-propiolactone (224). The mode of action is similar to ethylene oxide, i.e., nonspecific alkylation of essential metabolites. This compound has not achieved the success of ethylene oxide, mainly because of its toxicity and problems encountered in handling. It is still used in certain situations where no other agent is suitable (225).

Other agents that have been considered for use as sterilants include propylene oxide, chlorpicrin, epichlorohydrin, aziridine, glycidaldehyde, and peracetic acid. Reviews on gaseous chemosterilants have been written by Hoffman (226) and Phillips (227).

3.12 Miscellaneous

The biocidal effects of α-halo-α-nitro compounds were first described by Hodge

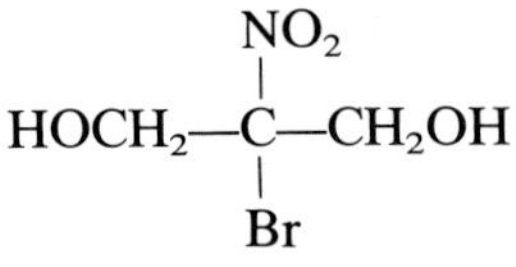

$$HOCH_2—C(NO_2)(Br)—CH_2OH$$

14.**54**

(228), who was investigating the antifungal properties of a series of aralkyl compounds. Further studies of this type of compound led to the synthesis of bronopol (14.**54**) by Spooner and co-workers (229). Bronopol has relatively low toxicity, is nonirritating, and has been used as a preservative in pharmaceutical and cosmetic preparations (230). A broad spectrum of organisms is inhibited by bronopol, including species of *Pseudomonas* and several fungi. The antimicrobial effects of bronopol are inhibited by mercapto compounds such as cysteine, which has led to the hypothesis that its antimicrobial mode of action involves the oxidation of sensitive thiol groups to disulfides (231).

Hexidine (14.**55**) has been employed in an antitricomonal, antibacterial vaginal cream (232).

Quindecamine (14.**56**) was first synthesized in an attempt to find new trypanocidal agents (233). It has been employed as a topical antifungal and antibacterial agent (234).

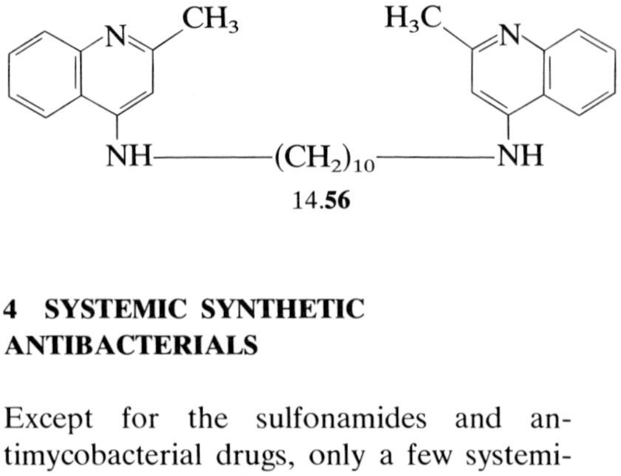

CH_3, H_3C, N, N, NH—$(CH_2)_{10}$—NH

14.**56**

4 SYSTEMIC SYNTHETIC ANTIBACTERIALS

Except for the sulfonamides and antimycobacterial drugs, only a few systemically active synthetic antibacterials are commercially important today. The multitude of highly effective, relatively nontoxic antibiotics (Chapters 15 and 16) available for the treatment of bacterial infections have provided stiff competition for the medicinal chemist attempting to synthesize new antibacterial agents.

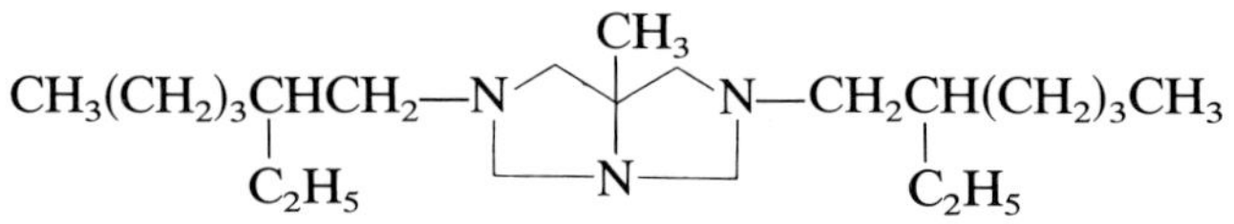

$CH_3(CH_2)_3CH(C_2H_5)CH_2—N$ … CH_3 … $N—CH_2CH(C_2H_5)(CH_2)_3CH_3$, N

14.**55**

Nearly all the synthetic, systemic antibacterials of importance fall into the category of urinary tract antiseptics. They achieve antibacterially effective concentration only in the urine; thus although they are administered orally, they are often termed antiseptics because of their localized action.

4.1 Nitroheterocycles

The first of the chemotherapeutic nitroheterocycles, nitrofurazone, was introduced to human medicine during World War II for the topical treatment of burns and wounds. Other nitroheterocycles gained importance later because of their antiprotozoal activity, especially nitrothiazoles and nitroimidazoles. In the 1960s reports began to appear describing interesting antibacterial activity for a number of new nitroheterocycles. Unfortunately, virtually none of these very promising drug candidates reached the market after toxicological studies revealed mutagenic or carcinogenic liability. Since the mutagenic and antibacterial modes of action are intimately related at the molecular level, it does not seem likely that an important new nonmutagenic antibacterial nitroheterocycle will be found.

4.1.1 NITROFURANS. Dodd and Stillman first described the antibacterial properties of nitrofurazone (14.**57**) in 1944 (235).

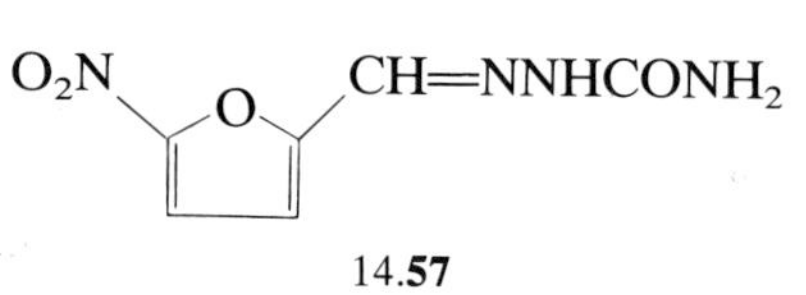

O_2N–(furan)–CH=NNHCONH$_2$

14.**57**

This compound remains on the market today for topical antibacterial therapy of burns, skin grafts, urethritis, and vulvovaginitis.

Nitrofurazone shows broad spectrum antibacterial activity against most important pathogens except *Pseudomonas* species. The activity is not seriously affected by the presence of blood or serum, which is not true of many topical agents (236). Nitrofurazone is well tolerated as a topical agent, with skin reactions reported in only approximately 1% of patients. However the compound has been shown to be mutagenic (237) and carcinogenic when fed to rats (238).

Since the introduction of nitrofurazone, thousands of nitrofurans have been synthesized and examined for antibacterial activity. Of these, only two, nitrofurazone and nitrofurantoin (14.**58**), are on the market in the United States for human use. Nitrofurantoin is active against most gram-positive and gram-negative pathogenic organisms *in vitro* at a range of 5–10 μg/ml, however certain strains of *Klebsiella*, *Aerobacter*, *Proteus*, and *Pseudomonas* are resistant (239). Asnis (240) has shown that bacterial resistance to nitrofurans can develop in the laboratory, however this does not seem to be a serious problem under clinical conditions. Upon oral administration, nitrofurantoin is rapidly absorbed from the gastrointestinal tract; but because of its rapid clearance, antibacterial concentrations are not achieved in the plasma. The concentration of the drug accumulating in the urine is approximately 0.2 mg/ml with an average dose (241). This highly antibacterial level has led to the use of the drug as a treatment and preventive for urinary tract infections. Three other nitrofurans, furazolidone (14.**59**), nihydrazone (14.**60**), and furaltadone (14.**61**) are used as feed additives for animals.

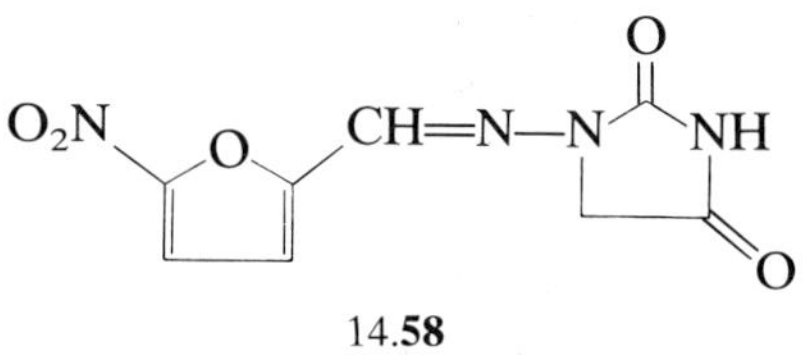

O_2N–(furan)–CH=N–N(hydantoin: C=O, NH, C=O)

14.**58**

O_2N–(furan)–CH=N–N(oxazolidinone: C=O, O)

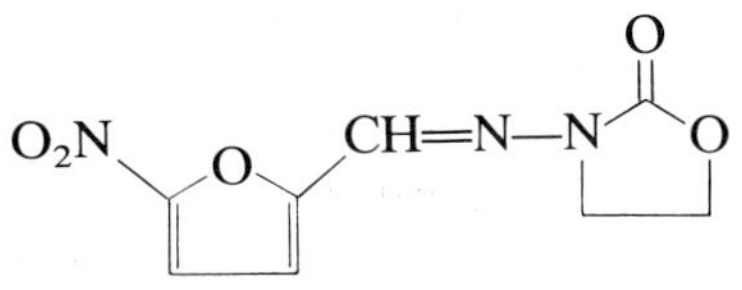

14.**59**

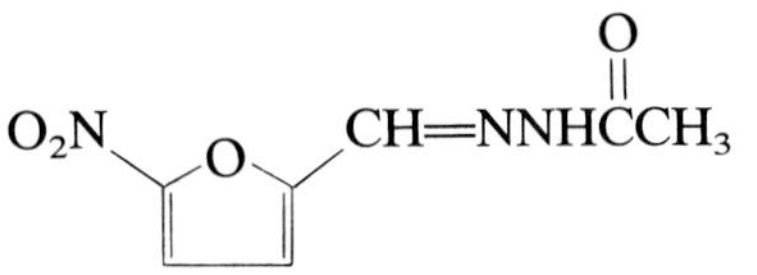

O_2N–(furan)–CH=NNHC(=O)CH_3

14.**60**

O_2N–(furan)–CH=N–N(oxazolidinone)–CH_2–N(morpholine)O

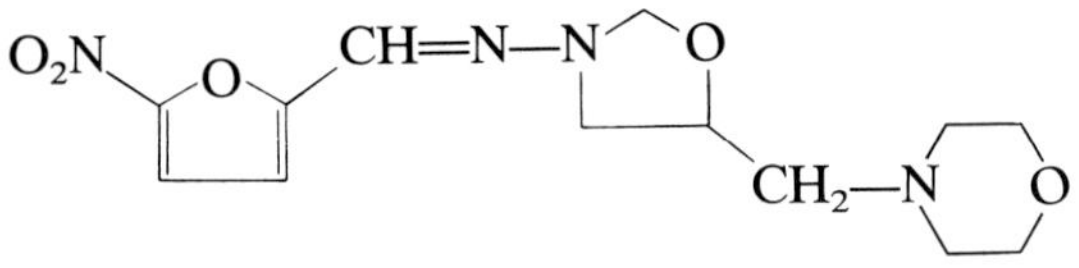

14.**61**

The usual first step in the metabolism of the nitrofuran ring in animals takes place at the cytoplasmic membrane and involves the reduction of the nitro group to a hydroxylamine (242). In the next step further reduction to the amine occurs, followed by ring opening and fragmentation to yield normal cellular constituents (243). Buzard has postulated that nitrofurans are converted to β-ketoglutaramic and ketoglutaric acids, which then enter metabolic pools (244). Hydrolysis can also occur at the azomethine linkage of nitrofuran derivatives, followed by oxidation to give 5-nitrofuroic acid, which has been found in the urine of experimental animals (245). The acute oral LD_{50} of nitrofurantoin in mice was found to be 895 mg/kg (246).

Side effects encountered with the use of nitrofurantoin include, most frequently, nausea and vomiting (247). Less commonly encountered are various allergic responses. The most serious side effect appears to be peripheral neuropathy, which is quite rare and usually occurs only in patients with impaired kidney function (248, 249). A similar but more frequently encountered liability of furaltadone led to its removal from the market after it had enjoyed a period of use as a treatment for systemic staphylococcal infections.

In the animal health area furazolidone (14.**59**) is used as a feed additive in swine for the prevention and treatment of bacterial enteritis and in poultry for the improvement of growth, feed efficiency, and treatment and prevention of bacterial and protozoal infections. Nihydrazone (14.**60**) and nitrofurazone (14.**57**) have similar uses, especially in the prevention of coccidiosis in poultry. Furaltadone (14.**61**) has been used as a mastitis treatment in cows and for enteric infections in cattle and poultry. Currently the FDA is proposing the withdrawal of all the nitrofurans from the animal health market because of their mutagenic and carcinogenic liability (250, 251).

The problems of the oncogenic potential of the nitrofurans began to surface when Morris and co-workers (238) reported on the carcinogenic activity of five nitrofurans in rats orally treated with the drugs at a level of 0.1–0.3% in the diet. The mutagenic behavior of nitrofurazone on *E. coli* was demonstrated by Zampieri and Greenberg (252). These initial reports prompted a considerable amount of investigation of the mutagenic and carcinogenic effects of nitrofurans, as well as the biochemical mechanism of these effects. A review that summarizes the mutagenicity and carcinogenicity of more than 50 nitrofurans has been prepared by Tazima, Kada, and Murakami (253). The studies in this area have shown that the nitro group at position 5 is essential for the mutagenic activity and that reduction to an activated intermediate is the likely first step in the production of the mutagen (254). This theory is supported by the observation that bacterial mutants with decreased levels of nitroreductase are resistant to the mutagenic effects (255). McCalla (254) has described two types of damage to DNA by nitrofurans and has correlated the damage with the potency of the compounds as mutagens and carcinogens. Nitrofurantoin, though exhibiting mutagenic properties, has not proved to be carcinogenic in animal feeding experiments (253).

The study of the mode of antibacterial action of nitrofurans began with the observation of Cramer and Dodd that nitrofurazone increased the lag phase of bacterial growth (256). Later studies focused on enzyme inhibition (257, 258) and the reduction of nitrofurans to active metabolites (259). More recently Herrlich and Schweiger (260) have ascribed the antibacterial effects to inhibition of the synthesis of inducible enzymes by blockage of the initiation of translation. They also attribute the activity to nitrofuran-induced lesions in DNA and the inhibition of the enzymatic repair of these lesions.

The main structural feature for antibacterial activity in the nitrofurans is the absolute requirement for the nitro group at the 5 position. Since the preparation of compounds substituted at the 3- and 4-positions of 5-nitrofurans is synthetically and economically unattractive, few compounds have been prepared with substituents at these positions. The substituents at the 2-position have been varied over an extremely broad range, which can be placed into three general categories for the most active compounds: (1) azomethine (—CH=N—), (2) vinyl (—CH=CH—), and (3) heterocyclic groups.

Nitrofurans that have received some recent attention but have not achieved clinical importance in the United States include nifuratrone (14.**62**) (261), nifurthiazole (14.**64**) (262), nifurpirinol (14.**63**) (263), and nifuraldezone (14.**65**) (264).

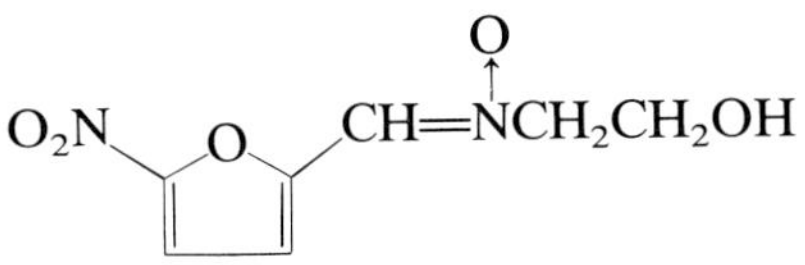

O_2N–(furan)–CH=N(→O)CH_2CH_2OH

14.**62**

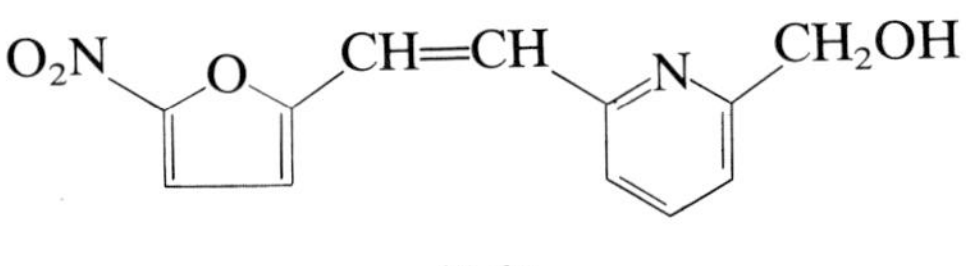

O_2N–(furan)–CH=CH–(pyridine)–CH_2OH

14.**63**

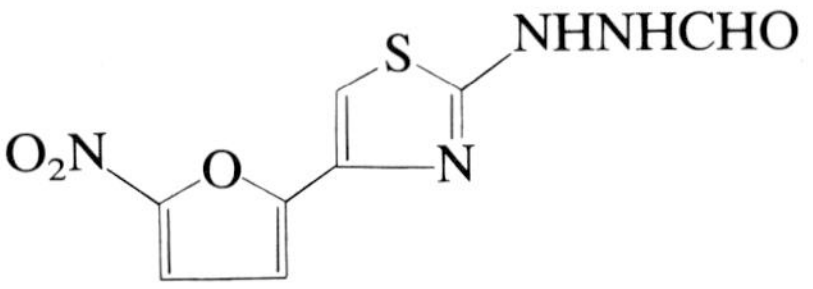

O_2N–(furan)–(thiazole)–NHNHCHO

14.**64**

O_2N–(furan)–CH=NNHCOCONH$_2$

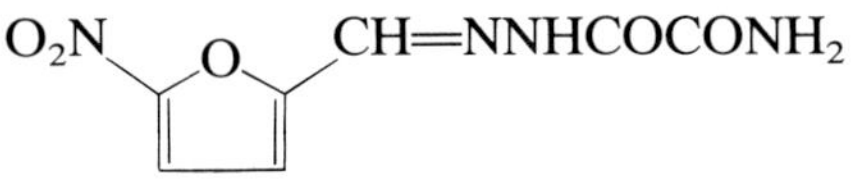

14.**65**

The nitrofurans have been reviewed by Paul and Paul (265), Miura and Reckendorf (266), and Foster and Russell (267).

4.1.2 OTHER NITROHETEROCYCLES. Nitroheterocyclic compounds, with the exception of the nitrofurans, were first developed as antiprotozoal agents. Investigations of their antibacterial activity have shown that they also have potential as antibacterial agents, particularly against gram-negative organisms (268).

Nitroimidazoles for which antimicrobial activity has been reported include an aminothiadiazole derivative (14.**66**) (269), metronidazole (14.**67**) (270), ronidazole (14.**68**) (270), a nitrone (14.**70**) (272), and a 2-nitro derivative (14.**69**) (273).

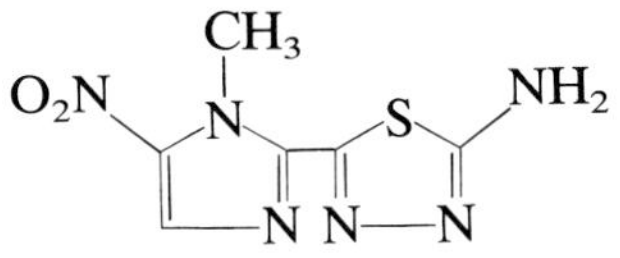

O_2N–(N-CH_3 imidazole)–(thiadiazole)–NH_2

14.**66**

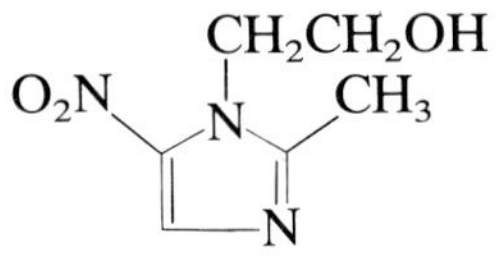

O_2N–(N-CH_2CH_2OH imidazole)–CH_3

14.**67**

O_2N–(N-CH_3 imidazole)–CH_2OCNH_2 (C=O)

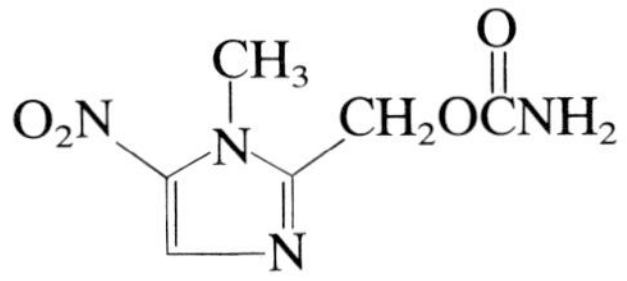

14.**68**

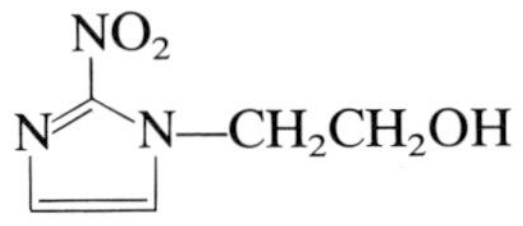

NO_2
N—CH_2CH_2OH

14.**69**

O_2N ... CH_3 ... CH=N(→O)—$CH_2CH_2OC_2H_5$

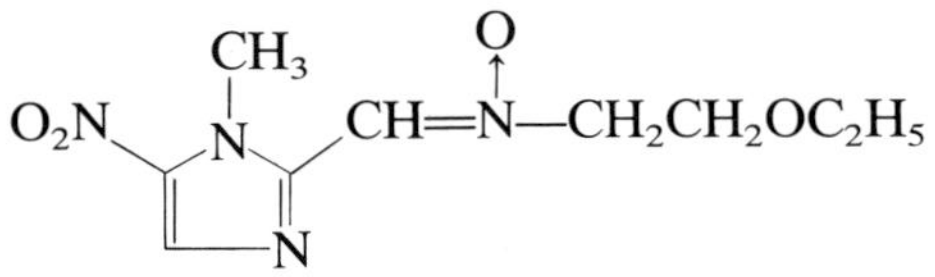

14.**70**

Other nitroheterocyclics for which antibacterial activity has been described include nitropyrroles (274), nitrothiazoles (275), nitrothiadiazoles (276), nitrobenzofurans (277), and nitrothiophenes (278, 279). None of these nitroheterocyclic derivatives have achieved clinical importance as antimicrobials in the United States. It is quite likely, considering the mutagenic problems associated with the nitro group, that many of these compounds failed to pass long-term toxicity evaluations.

The chemotherapeutic properties of monocyclic heterocycles with five-membered rings have been reviewed by Grunberg and Titsworth (280).

4.2 Quinolone Antibacterial Agents

4.2.1 NALIDIXIC ACID. Nalidixic acid (14.**71**) was first described by Lesher and co-workers (281) in 1962. The compound was the most active of a group of substituted 1,8-naphthyridines and was approved in the United States as a treatment for

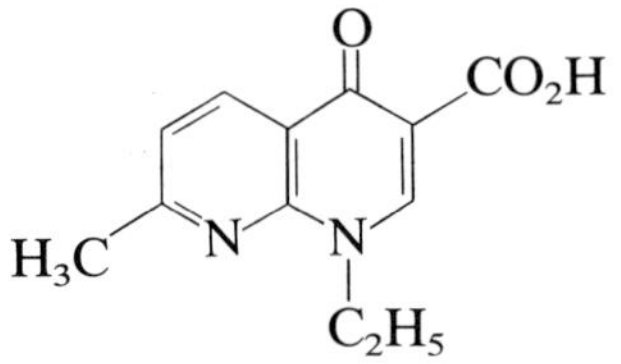

O
CO_2H
H_3C N N
C_2H_5

14.**71**

Table 14.1 *In Vitro* Antibacterial Activity (288)

Organism (number of strains)	Minimum Inhibitory Concentration, μg/ml
Escherichia coli (8)	3.0–7.5
Klebsiella pneumoniae (1)	2.0
Proteus mirabilis (2)	2.5–7.5
Proteus vulgaris (2)	7.5–10.0
Salmonella enteriditis (2)	2.5–10.0
Shigella spp. (3)	2.5–5.0
Staphylococcus aureus (2)	25–50
Streptococcus fecalis (1)	500.0

urinary tract infections in 1964. Antibacterial studies have indicated that nalidixic acid is particularly active against gram-negative organisms. Table 14.1 gives a profile of the *in vitro* activity. Brumfitt and Pursell (282) studied the sensitivity of several strains of bacteria commonly associated with urinary tract infections and found that 99% of strains of *B. coli*, 98% of *P. mirabilis*, 92% of *Klebsiella* and *Enterobacter*, and 80% of other coliform species were sensitive to the drug.

Nalidixic acid is well absorbed orally, and plasma levels of 20–40 μg/ml are readily achieved with a 1 g dose (283, 284). The drug is 93% protein bound and does not appreciably cross the blood-brain barrier (285, 286). Although the plasma levels achieved are well above those that are bactericidal for sensitive organisms, nalidixic acid has not been useful in treating systemic infections. Zinsser (285) found that only half of systemic infections due to a highly sensitive *E. coli* strain could be controlled with intravenous nalidixic acid. It has been recommended, however, for the treatment of *E. coli* enteritis in calves (286).

Hydroxylation at the 7-methyl group of nalidixic acid gives rise to compound 14.**72**, which represents 30% of the biologically active drug in the serum and 85% in the

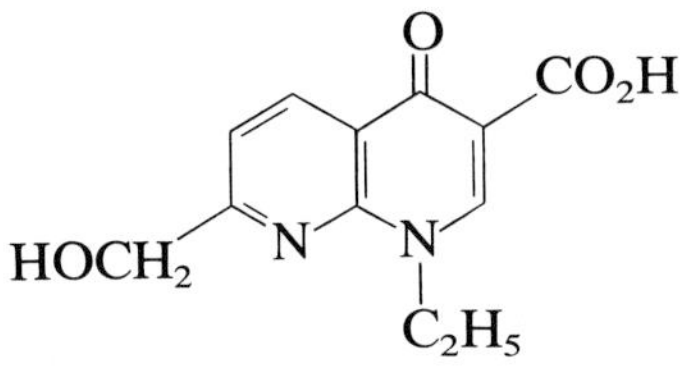

14.72

urine. The antibacterial spectrum of the hydroxylated form is essentially the same as the parent drug (288). The major pathway of excretion is the urine, with the parent drug, the hydroxylated form, and glucuronides of both comprising the important excretion products. Although the glucuronides are inactive, peak urine levels of active drug after a 1 g dose average 150–200 μg/ml, 3–4 hr after administration, with a half-life of 6 hr (283).

The oral LD_{50} in mice for nalidixic acid is reported as 3300 mg/kg and intravenously as 176 mg/kg. Monkeys readily tolerate oral doses up to 500–900 mg/kg. In chronic administration to rats and monkeys, no toxicological evidence of DNA synthesis inhibition could be detected over a period of 1 yr (289).

Nalidixic acid is generally well tolerated. A low incidence of adverse effects is reported, including gastrointestinal disturbances, rashes, urticaria, pruritis, and photosensitivity. Reversible central nervous system disorders, including drowsiness, headache, weakness, vertigo, and visual disturbances have also occurred (290).

The mode of action of nalidixic acid has been the subject of a number of investigations and has been reviewed by Goss and Cook (289) and Bauernfeind (291). Microscopic examination of *E. coli* cultures grown in the presence of nalidixic acid revealed the presence of abnormal, elongated forms. The bactericidal action was found to be correlated with growth in the cultures and further investigation indicated a deficiency in DNA synthesis (292, 293). These initial observations have been confirmed, and it has been suggested that nalidixic acid binds with and inactivates an essential component in the DNA replication complex in susceptible organisms (289, 291, 294).

The emergence of bacterial resistance during therapy with nalidixic acid has been observed (282). Resistance arises in approximately 25% of the cases and usually within 48 hr of the start of therapy. This problem appears to be the most serious drawback in the clinical utility of nalidixic acid.

4.2.2 OXOLINIC ACID. Kaminsky and Meltzer first reported the synthesis of oxolinic acid (14.**73**) in 1968 (295), and the

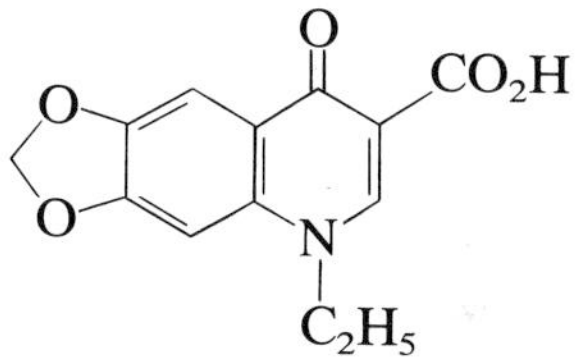

14.**73**

drug was approved in the United States for the treatment of urinary tract infections in 1975. The antibacterial spectrum of the compound is similar to that of nalidixic acid, but the potency is reported to be 2–4 times as great, especially *in vivo* (296). Oxolinic acid is readily absorbed when given orally, and peak levels of activity in the urine are reached within 4 hr. The major metabolites are the glucuronides of the dihydroxy compound 14.**74**, the

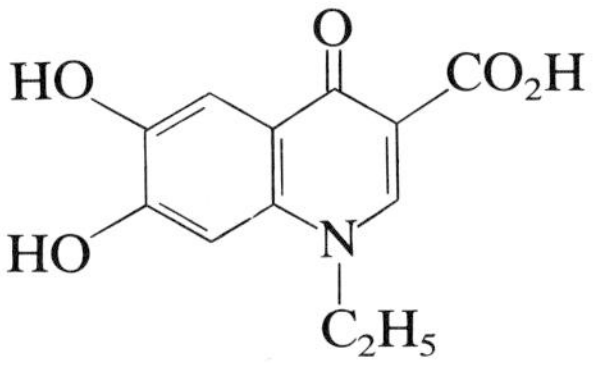

14.**74**

monohydroxy compounds 14.**75**, 14.**76**, and the glucuronide of oxolinic acid (297, 298). The drug is usually well tolerated and has side effects similar to those reported for nalidixic acid. There is some

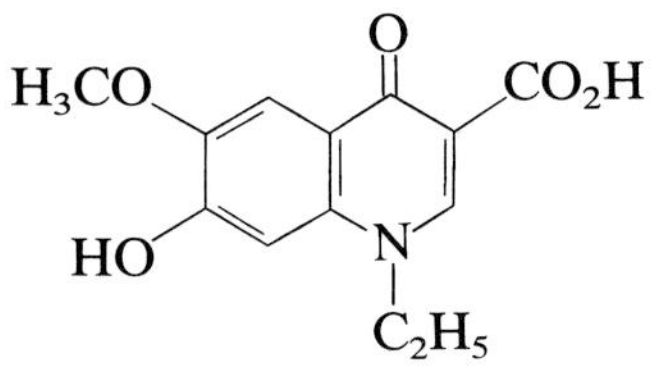

14.**75**

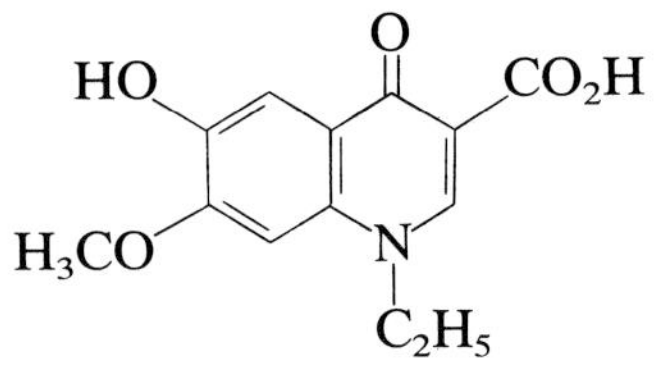

14.**76**

indication that oxolinic acid produces a higher incidence of central nervous system side effects than does nalidixic acid (299).

The emergence of bacterial resistance during treatment with oxolinic acid has been observed, as well as cross-resistance with nalidixic acid (299). Studies of the mode of action of oxolinic acid have indicated that it is identical with that of nalidixic acid in inhibiting ATP-dependent DNA synthesis (300, 301).

4.2.3 OTHER 4-QUINOLONE-3-CARBOXYLATES. The disclosure of nalidixic and oxolinic acids as effective antibacterial agents led to the synthesis of many analogs. Piromidic acid (14.**77**) and its metabolite, hydroxypiromidic acid (14.**78**)

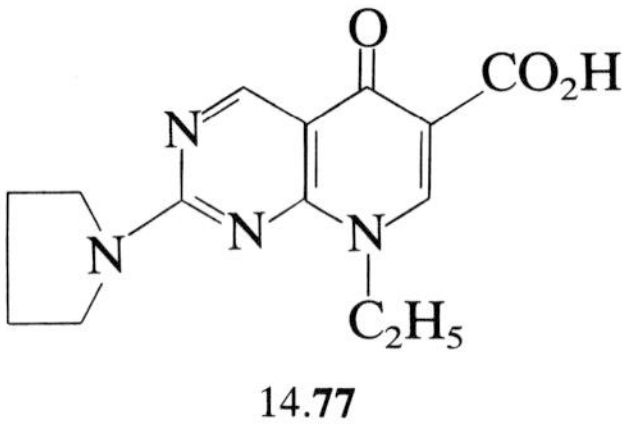

14.**77**

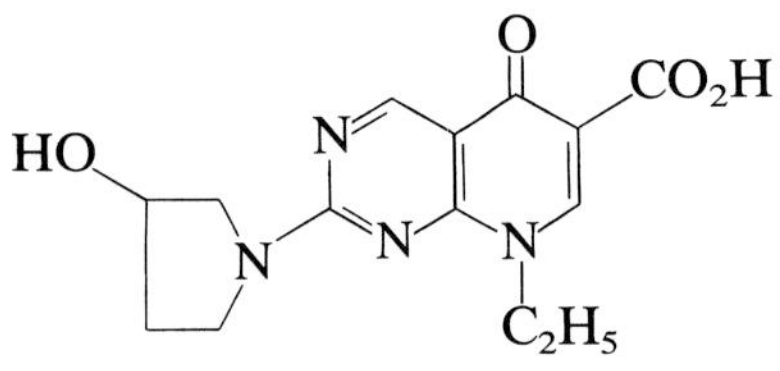

14.**78**

were described as having antibacterial activity comparable to that of nalidixic acid (302). These compounds were found to be inhibitors of DNA synthesis (303), and they exhibited cross-resistance with nalidixic acid (304). They appear to have no clinically significant advantages over nalidixic and oxolinic acids. Another closely related analog, which may have a clinical advantage over nalidixic acid, is pipemidic acid (14.**79**). This drug has been

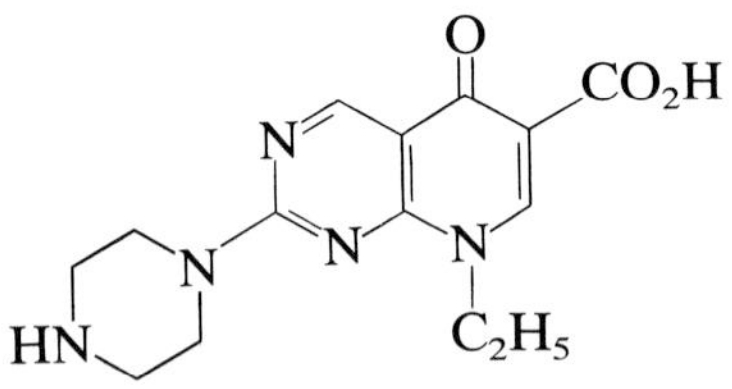

14.**79**

shown to be orally effective in the treatment of systemic *Pseudomonas aeruginosa* infections in mice, in addition to controlling the bacteria normally susceptible to nalidixic acid (305, 306). Since only a very few drugs are available for the effective treatment of *Pseudomonas* infections, pipemidic acid could prove to be a valuable new antibacterial agent.

4.2.4 STRUCTURE-ACTIVITY RELATIONSHIPS (281, 295, 302, 305). A study of the patent literature reveals that hundreds of analogs of nalidixic acid have been prepared, and claims to their efficacy as antibacterial agents have been made. There is also a group of structurally related anticoccidial agents possessing a 6,7-dialkoxy-4-oxo-1,4-dihydroquinoline-3-carboxylate structure that could be included in a structure-activity analysis of this group of compounds (307). An exhaustive analysis of these compounds is beyond the scope of this chapter, but certain structural requirements for antibacterial activity can be summarized. Referring to generic structure

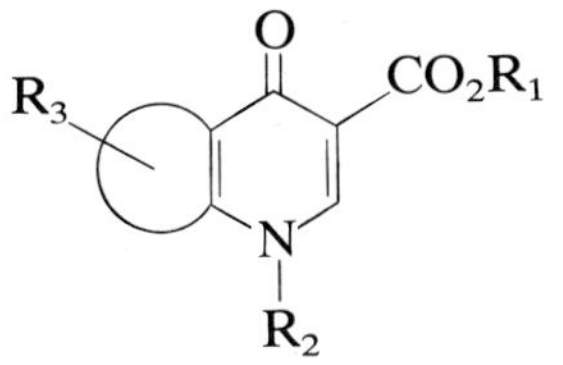

14.80

14.80, the necessary features are as follows:

1. A trisubstituted nitrogen hetero atom at position 1.
2. The 4-oxo group.
3. The carboxyl function at position 3.
4. A second ring attached to the pyridone ring at positions 5 and 6.

The optimum substituent at position 1 appears to be the ethyl group; replacement by methyl or larger alkyl groups usually results in decreased activity. A vinyl or an unsubstituted benzyl can replace R_2 in some cases without loss of activity. Esters and amides of the carboxyl group may show activity but probably need to be enzymatically hydrolyzed to the free acid before they can exert their effects. Although wide variation is possible in the nature of the second ring attached at positions 5 and 6, the effects of variations here are not predictable. Each system has its own peculiarities in regard to substituent(s) R_3, depending on the number and position of hetero atoms in the ring. Active compounds have been reported in which the substituent R_3 consists of a third benzenoid or heterocyclic ring (308). A heterocyclic nitrogen can also be present at position 2 according to a report by Holmes et al. (309). Compounds in which the alkyl group at position 1 has been replaced by an alkoxy group have also shown activity (310).

4.3 Quinoxaline- and Phenazine-di-*N*-Oxides

4.3.1 IODININ. Clemo and McIlwain first isolated iodinin (14.**81**), a violet pigment

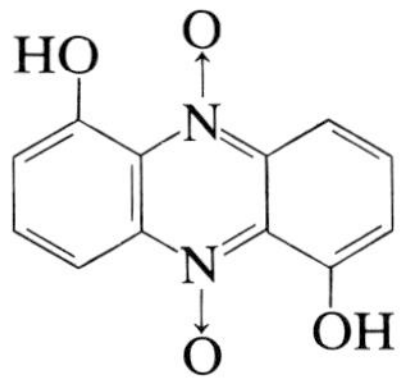

14.81

produced by *Chromobacterium iodinum*, and ascribed a dihydroxyphenazine-di-*N*-oxide structure to the compound (311). Confirmation of the structure by synthesis was made by Clemo and Daglish in 1950 (312). The antibacterial properties of iodinin were described in 1941 by McIlwain, who also showed that the activity was antagonized by naphthaquinone and anthraquinone derivatives (313, 314).

A considerable amount of research has been carried out on iodinin and related phenazine-di-*N*-oxides. They have been found to exhibit antitumor, antiphage, and antifungal activity, in addition to the originally observed antibacterial effects (315). None of the phenazine-di-*N*-oxide derivatives, however, are currently in use clinically.

4.3.2 QUINOXALINE-DI-*N*-OXIDES. The antagonist relationship between the phenazine-di-*N*-oxides and naphthaquinones noted by McIlwain prompted him to prepare a series of quinoxaline-di-*N*-oxide derivatives (14.**82**), hoping that a similar antagonism

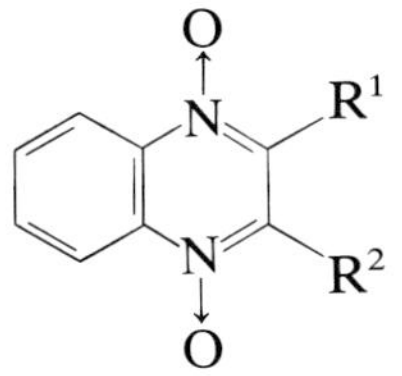

$R^1, R^2 = H$
$R^1 = H, R^2 = CH_3$
$R^1 = CH_3, R^2 = C_5H_{11}$
$R^1, R^2 = —(CH_2)_4—$

14.82

might be observed between these compounds and phthiocol or other compounds related to vitamin K (314). Growth inhibition of *Streptococcus hemolyticus* and *Corynebacterium diphtheriae* was displayed by all the derivatives, but they were not as active as iodinin. McIlwain also found that the *N*-oxide groups were necessary for activity, since the reduced compounds were inactive. Further studies on the antibacterial properties of quinoxaline-di-*N*-oxide derivatives indicated activity against *Mycobacterium tuberculosis*, *Salmonella typhosa*, *S. schottmuelleri*, and *Pseudomonas aeruginosa* (315, 316).

Francis and co-workers noted that 2,3-dimethylquinoxaline-1,4-dioxide appeared to be less active *in vitro* than would have been expected from its *in vivo* activity against experimental infections in mice (317). Speculating that this might be a case of active metabolite formation, they studied the metabolism of the compound and learned that it was converted to the hydroxymethyl methyl derivative 14.**83**. This metabolite was considerably more active *in vitro* than was the parent compound. In further metabolic studies two additional urinary metabolites (14.**84**, 14.**85**) were identified, and the bishydroxymethyl compound exhibited greater *in vitro* and *in vivo* antibacterial activity than 14.**83**, but about the same toxicity. The carboxylic acid metabolite 14.**85** was not active. Although this evidence confirms the *in vivo* formation of active metabolites from 2,3-dimethylquinoxaline-1,4-dioxide, another explanation for the discrepancy between the *in vitro* and *in vivo* activity with two other quinoxaline 1,4-dioxides (14.**86** and 14.**87**) has been postulated. Hennesy and Edwards (318) noted that 14.**87** had weak antimicrobial activity *in vitro* while displaying good *in vivo* activity, particularly against gram-negative organisms. However when 14.**87** was tested *in vitro* under anaerobic conditions, ten- to hundredfold enhancement of activity was found. The same type of enhancement of *in vitro* activity under anaerobic conditions was noted for 14.**86** (319). These authors suggested that anaerobic or semianaerobic *in vitro* testing conditions more closely resembled the *in vivo* environment, which accounted for the seeming discrepancy between the original *in vitro* and *in vivo* experiments.

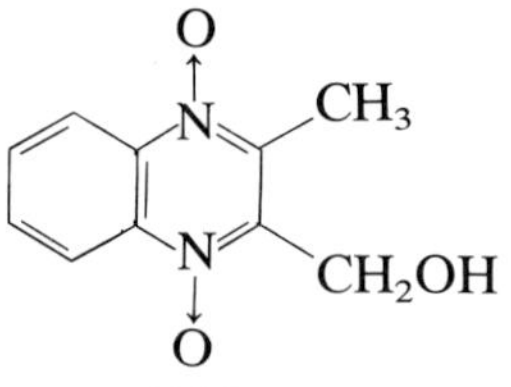

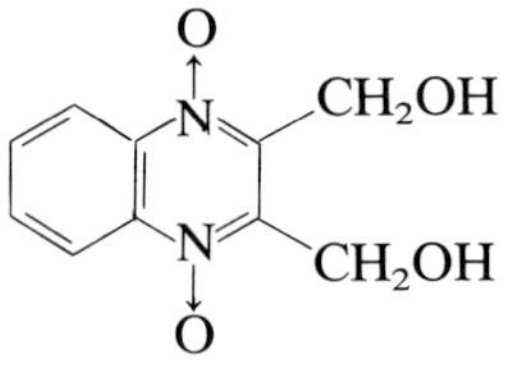

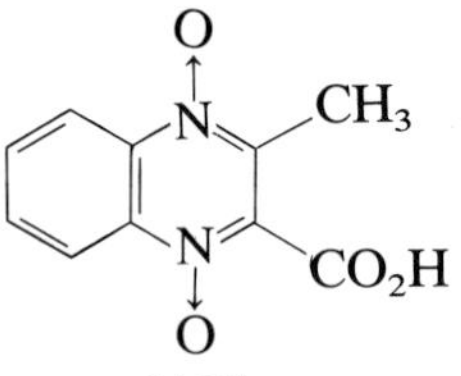

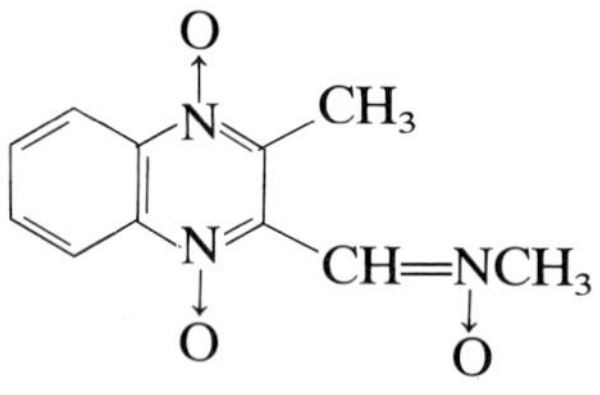

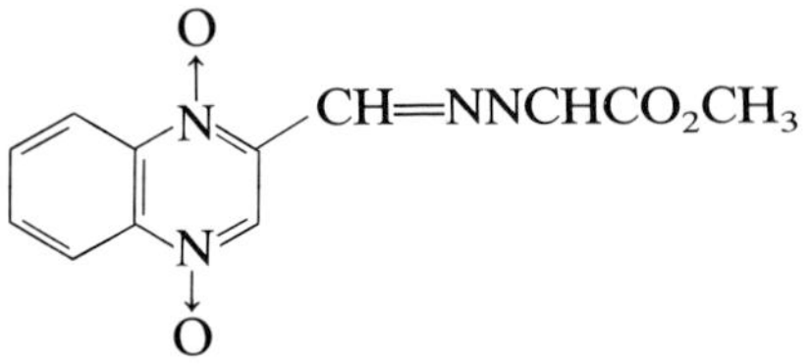

O, N, CH_3, N, CH_2OH, O

14.**83**

O, N, CH_2OH, N, CH_2OH, O

14.**84**

O, N, CH_3, N, CO_2H, O

14.**85**

O, N, CH_3, N, $CH{=}NCH_3$, O, O

14.**86**

O, N, $CH{=}NNCHCO_2CH_3$, N, O

14.**87**

Although a great number of quinoxaline-di-*N*-oxides, phenazine-di-*N*-oxides, and other related heterocyclic-*N*-oxides have been claimed as antibacterial agents in the patent literature, none have reached importance in human medicine. However Carbadox (14.**87**) was approved in 1972 in the United States as a swine feed additive for increased weight gain and improvement of feed efficiency. It is also recommended for the treatment of dysentery and bacterial enteritis.

Except for the early work of McIlwain (314) suggesting a possible relationship to the K vitamins, nothing has been reported on the mode of action of the phenazine and quinoxaline-di-*N*-oxides.

4.4 Cotrimoxazole

Trimethoprim (14.**88**) was first described by Roth and coworkers (322) as the most

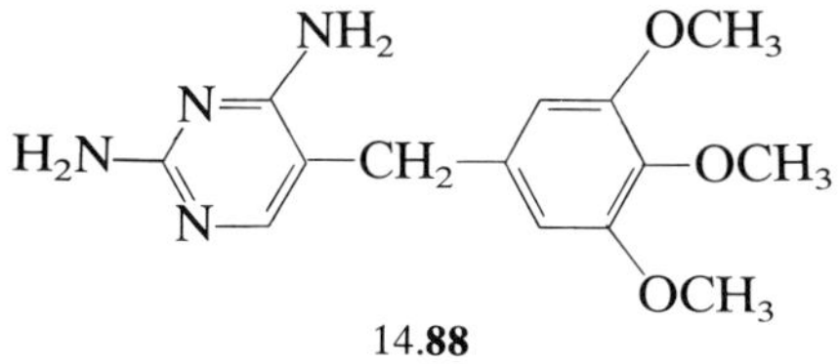

14.**88**

promising antibacterial agent of a group of 5-benzyl-2,4-diaminopyrimidines. This work was an outgrowth of a search initiated by Hitchings (323, 324) for new inhibitors of dihydrofolate reductase as potential antimalarials.

Trimethoprim exhibits high activity against a broad spectrum of gram-positive and gram-negative organisms but is not active against *P. aeruginosa*. Development of resistance by *E. coli* and *S. aureus* has been demonstrated in the laboratory (325), and resistant bacteria have been isolated from patients receiving the drug (326). However resistance does not appear to be a serious problem clinically except in patients with recurrent *E. coli* infections (327). Resistance factors for trimethoprim from the W plasmid group have been found in *E. coli* and other enteric organisms (328, 329).

Trimethoprim is not usually used alone, but is employed in combination with a sulfa drug, sulfamethoxazole (14.**89**). (The sulfa drugs are fully discussed in Chapter 13.)

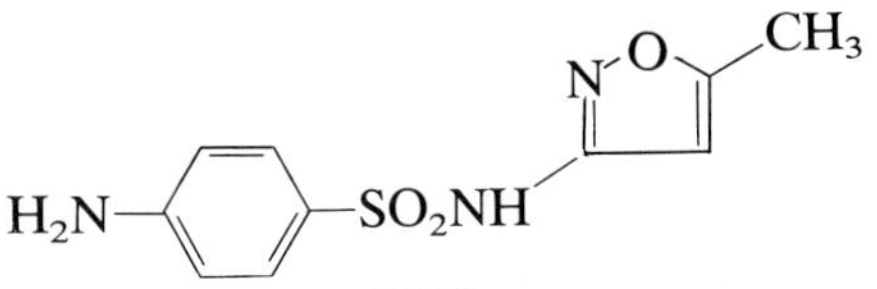

14.**89**

This combination, called cotrimoxazole, has essentially the same antibacterial spectrum as trimethoprim, but resistance is not encountered as often because of the synergistic effects of the combination.

Cotrimoxazole is used principally in the treatment of urinary tract infections. Other uses include treatment of gonorrhea (330), chest infections due to pneumococci and *Hemophilus influenzae* (331), and enteric *Salmonella* infections (typhoid, paratyphoid, carriers) (332). Cotrimoxazole is rapidly absorbed from the gastrointestinal tract. The usual dose of 400 mg of sulfamethoxazole and 80 mg of trimethoprim, 3 times daily, gives a steady state plasma concentration averaging 20 and 1 μg/ml, respectively. The main route of excretion of the components is by way of the urine, with 60% of administered trimethoprim and 50% of the sulfamethoxazole eliminated in 24 hr (333, 334).

In mice the acute LD_{50}'s are greater than 2000 mg/kg orally and 200 mg/kg intravenously. High doses of cotrimoxazole fed to pregnant rats at the eight or ninth day of pregnancy caused the death of most fetuses; and when given on the tenth through twelfth days, a high incidence of fetal malformations was observed (335).

The major side effects observed with the drug are related to folate metabolism and include megaloblastosis, leukopenia, and thrombocytopenia. These side effects are observed only in patients with impaired folate metabolism and do not present a problem in normal individuals (336). Skin rashes and sulfonamide hypersensitivity have also been reported (337). Upon prolonged administration of cotrimoxazole, Whitman (338) observed changes in folate metabolism in man after 7–10 days. The clinical significance of the changes was not apparent.

The mode of action of trimethoprim involves the inhibition of the conversion of dihydrofolate to tetrahydrofolate by dihydrofolate reductase. Enzyme binding studies by Burchall and Hitchings (339) carried out on a number of benzyl diaminopyrimidines showed that trimethoprim was bound to dihydrofolate reductase from *E. coli* 5.2×10^4 times more strongly than to the same enzyme derived from rat liver. Other binding and inhibition studies have confirmed the high specificity of trimethoprim for bacterial as opposed to mammalian dihydrofolate reductase (340). The strong specificity is responsible for the high bacterial and low mammalian toxicity of the drug.

The mode of action of sulfonamides involves the inhibition of the synthesis of dihydrofolate by competitive inhibition with *p*-aminobenzoic acid and is described in Chapter 13.

Cotrimoxazole has been described as a *synergistic* combination of antibacterial agents. The synergistic or potentiating effect of dihydrofolate inhibitors on the antibacterial activity of sulfonamides was first reported by Hitchings and Bushby (341). According to Potter (342) the synergistic effect is due to the "sequential inhibition" of enzymes on the same metabolic pathway. This explanation has been accepted for some time as the basis of the well-documented synergism between trimethoprim and sulfamethoxazole (343). Webb (344), however, has indicated that sequential blockade of linear reactions by multiple inhibitors is theoretically incapable of producing an effect greater than that of a single inhibitor alone. This has been confirmed experimentally by Rubin (345). The concept above is also not a satisfactory explanation of why potentiation still occurs in sulfonamide-resistant organisms (345). Poe (347) has proposed an alternate explanation for the observed synergy based on his observations that in addition to being a competitor for *p*-aminobenzoic acid, sulfamethoxazole is a moderately potent inhibitor of bacterial dihydrofolate reductase. Poe ascribes the observed synergistic effect to the simultaneous binding and inhibition of the sulfa and trimethoprim to the same enzyme. This theory appears more fully to explain the observed data concerning this synergistic combination.

Reviews on cotrimoxazole have been written by Burchall (348), and a supplement to the *Journal of Infectious Diseases* has been devoted to the subject (349).

Another synergistic combination of a sulfonamide and a dihydrofolate reductase inhibitor is used in veterinary medicine. Sulfadimethoxine (14.**90**) and ormetoprim (14.**91**) are recommended for the preven-

H_2N–C_6H_4–SO_2NH–(pyrimidine with two OCH_3)

14.**90**

(H_2N, NH_2 pyrimidine)–CH_2–(C_6H_2 with two OCH_3 and H_3C)

14.**91**

tion of coccidiosis, infectious coryza, colibacillosis, and fowl cholera in chickens and turkeys (350).

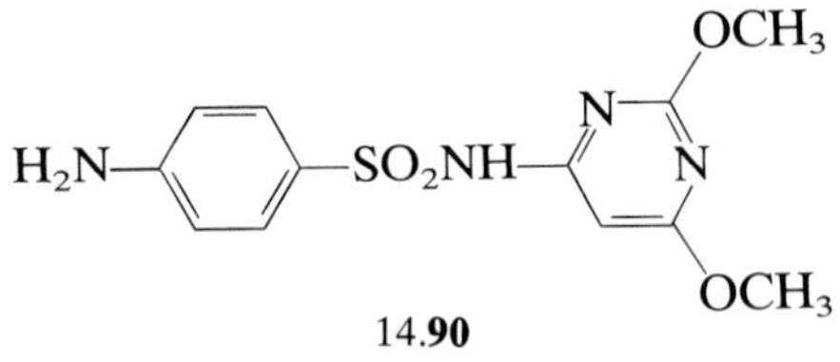

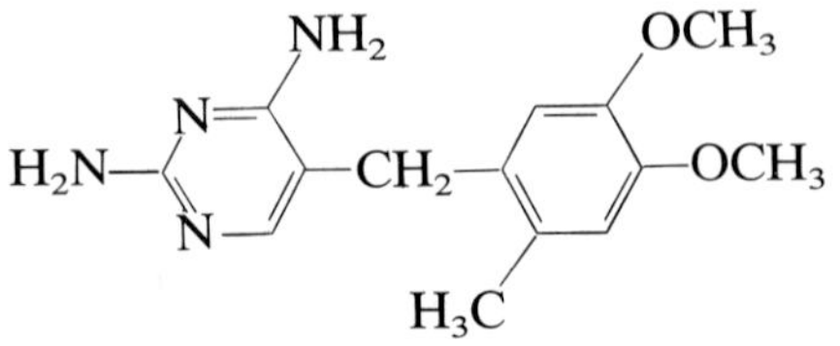

4.5 Methenamine

Hexamethylene tetramine (methenamine, 14.**92**) has been used for some time as a urinary tract antiseptic. Its broad spectrum

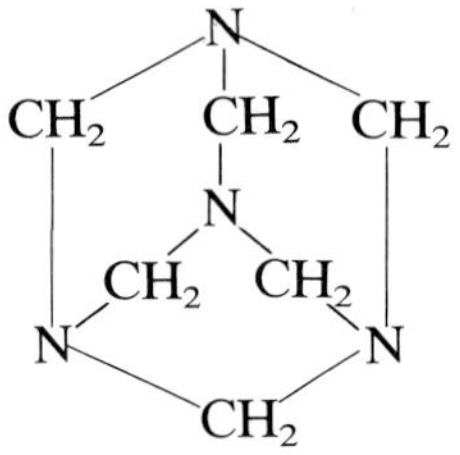

14.**92**

antibacterial action depends on the release of formaldehyde by the hydrolysis of the compound in the urine at an acidic pH. It is generally prescribed as the mandelate or hippurate salt, which helps to maintain acidity of the urine. The compound is not a treatment of choice for acute bacterial urinary tract infections but is sometimes used in long-term suppressive therapy (351, 352).

4.6 Miscellaneous

A unique, fixed-ratio combination antimicrobial drug comprised of α-deutero-3-fluoro-D-alanine (14.**93**) and the 2,4-pentanedione enamine of cycloserine (14.**94**) has recently been described (353–356).

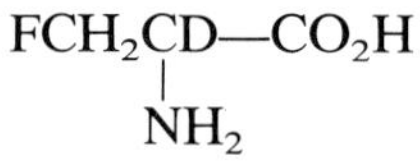

$FCH_2CD(NH_2)—CO_2H$

14.**93**

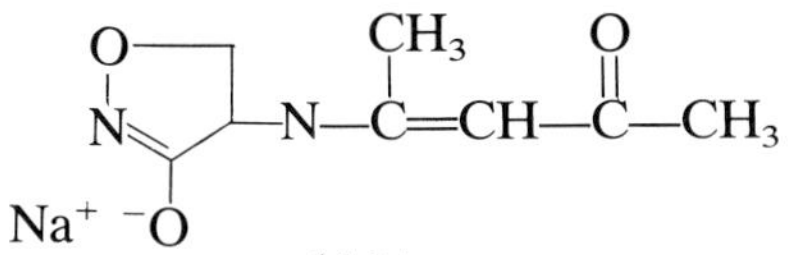

14.**94**

The antibacterial properties of D-fluoroalanine have been described by Kollonitch (357), and the mode of action has been shown to be inhibition of incorporation of D-alanine into the bacterial cell wall by inactivation of alanine racemase. The utility of D-fluoroalanine was limited, however, by the loss of antibacterial activity at drug levels 2–3 times the minimum inhibitory concentration. The D-fluoroalanine apparently becomes a substrate instead of an inhibitor at these concentrations and is incorporated into the cell wall peptidoglycan.

It was discovered that when cycloserine was used at subinhibitory concentrations together with D-fluoroalanine, reversal of antimicrobial activity did not occur. Cycloserine is known to be an inhibitor of alanine racemase and D-alanyl-D-alanine synthetase. It also prevents the incorporation of D-fluoroalanine into the bacterial peptidoglycan, accounting for the inhibition of the reversal of antimicrobial action.

To further improve the activity of the D-fluoroalanine, a derivative was sought that would enhance the metabolic stability of the compound. Since one of the major steps in its metabolism is oxidation by D-aminoacid oxidase, it was postulated that oxidation could be retarded without loss of antibacterial activity by using an α-deutero analog. The α-deutero analog was, indeed, found to be equivalent in antibacterial activity and was also metabolized 2–3 times more slowly both *in vitro* and *in vivo* because of the kinetic isotope effect on the enzymatic oxidation.

A problem encountered with the use of cycloserine in combination was its instability to acid and base and its tendency to dimerize in solution and on storage. The pentanedione enamine derivative did not have these liabilities and was found to release cycloserine, *in vivo*, at a concentration sufficient to prevent reversal of the antibacterial activity of D-fluoroalanine.

This combination drug was reported to be effective, both orally and parenterally, against a broad range of bacterial infections in mice, including *Pseudomonas*, *Serratia*, and gram-negative anaerobes.

Although this drug has not yet achieved clinical importance, it represents an interesting departure from the empirical methods often used in the past to discover new synthetic antimicrobial agents. This attempt to interfere in a highly specific manner, at the molecular level, with a metabolic process common to bacteria but not to mammals, is an excellent example of the biochemically oriented approach to new antimicrobial agents.

REFERENCES

1. P. E. Baldry, *The Battle Against Bacteria*, Cambridge University Press, Cambridge, 1965.
2. Robert Reid, *Microbes and Men*, Saturday Review Press, New York, 1974.
3. S. S. Block, Historical Review, in *Disinfection, Sterilization and Preservation*, S. S. Block and C. A. Lawrence, Eds., Lea and Febiger, Philadelphia, 1968, pp. 3–8.
4. R. E. Dixon, R. A. Kaslow, D. C. Mackel, C. C. Fulkerson, and G. F. Mallison, *J. Am. Med. Assoc.*, **236,** 2415 (1976).
5. *Disinfection, Sterilization and Preservation*, C. A. Lawrence and S. S. Block, Eds., Lea and Febiger, Philadelphia, 1968.
6. G. K. Bass and L. S. Stuart, in *Disinfection, Sterilization and Preservation*, C. A. Lawrence and S. S. Block, Eds., Lea and Febiger, Philadelphia, 1968, Ch. 9.
7. S. Rideal and J. T. A. Walker, *J. Roy. Sanit. Inst.*, **24,** 424 (1903).
8. W. Horwitz, Ed., *Official Methods of Analysis of the Association of Official Analytical Chemists*, Association of Official Analytical Chemists, Washington, D.C., 1975, Ch. 4.
9. L. S. Stuart, L. F. Ortenzio, and J. L. Friedl, *J. Assoc. Off. Agr. Chemists*, **36,** 466 (1953).
10. N. A. Miner, E. Whitmore, and M. L. McBee, *Dev. Ind. Microbiol.*, **16,** 23–30 (1974).
11. P. B. Price, *J. Infect. Dis.*, **63,** 301 (1938).
12. A. R. Cade, *J. Soc. Cosmet. Chem.*, **2,** 281 (1951).
13. A. F. Peterson, *J. Assoc. Cosmet. Chem.* **14,** 125 (1973).
14. A. G. Schenkel, *J. Assoc. Cosmet. Chem.*, **14,** 131 (1973).
15. D. F. Spooner and G. Sykes, in *Methods in Microbiology*, Vol. 7B, J. R. Norris and D. W. Ribbons, Eds., Academic Press, New York, 1972, Ch. 4.
16. H. D. Dakin, J. B. Cohen, and J. Kenyon, *Brit. Med. J.*, **1,** 160 (1916).
17. P. N. Leech, *J. Am. Pharm. Assoc.*, **12,** 592 (1923).
18. G. F. Reddish and A. W. Pauley, *Bull. Nat. Formul. Comm.*, **13,** 11 (1945).
19. J. S. Thompson, *Soap Chem. Spec.*, **40,** 122 (1964).
20. A. F. Guiteras and F. C. Schmelkes, *J. Biol. Chem.*, **107,** 235 (1934).
21. L. Frieberg, *Acta Pathol. Microbiol. Scand.*, **40,** 67 (1957).
22. W. E. Knox, P. K. Stumpf, and D. E. Green, *J. Bacteriol.*, **55,** 451 (1948).
23. C. K. Johns, *Ind. Eng. Chem.*, **26,** 787 (1934).
24. M. Kosugi, J. J. Kaminski, S. H. Selk, I. H. Pitman, N. Bodor, and T. Higuchi, *J. Pharm. Sci.*, **65,** 1743 (1976).
25. I. Pitman, H. Dawn, T. Higuchi, and A. Hussain, *J. Chem. Soc.*, *B.* 626 (1969).
26. J. Kaminski, N. Bodor, and T. Higuchi, *J. Pharm. Sci.*, **65,** 1733 (1976).
27. L. Gershenfeld, in *Disinfection, Sterilization and Preservation*, C. A. Lawrence and S. S. Block, Eds., Lea and Febiger, Philadelphia, 1968, Ch. 22.
28. H. A. Schelanski and M. V. Shelanski, *J. Int. Coll. Surg.*, **25,** 727 (1956).
29. T. C. King and P. B. Price, *Surg. Gynec, Obstet.*, **116,** 361 (1963).
30. D. A. Haydon, *Proc. Roy. Soc.* (London), *Ser. B.*, **145,** 383 (1956).
31. M. C. Allwood, W. B. Hugo, *J. Appl. Bacteriol.*, **1971,** 369.
32. H. L. Josevick and P. Gerhardt, *Bacteriol. Proc.*, **1960,** 100.
33. J. E. Starr and J. Judis, *J. Pharm. Sci.*, **57,** 768 (1968).
34. C. E. Coulthard, J. Marshall, and F. L. Pyman, *J. Chem. Soc.*, 280 (1930).
35. E. M. Richardson and E. E. Reid, *J. Am. Chem. Soc.*, **62,** 413 (1940).
36. A. H. Fogg and R. M. Lodge, *Trans. Faraday Soc.*, **41,** 359 (1945).
37. H. Beckhold and P. Erlich, *Z. Physiol. Chem.*, **47,** 173 (1906).
38. H. Beckhold, *Münch. Med. Wochenschr.*, **61,** 1924 (1914).
39. E. G. Klarmann, L. W. Gates, V. A. Shternov, and P. H. Cox, *J. Am. Chem. Soc.*, **54,** 3315 (1932).
40. E. G. Klarmann, V. A. Shternov, and L. W. Gates, *J. Am. Chem. Soc.*, **55,** 2576 (1933).

41. E. G. Klarmann, L. W. Gates, V. A. Shternov, and P. H. Cox, *J. Am. Chem. Soc.*, **55,** 4657 (1933).
42. N. J. DeSouza, A. N. Kothare, and V. V. Nadkarny, *J. Med. Chem.*, **9,** 618 (1966).
43. F. Dunning, B. Dunning, Jr., and W. E. Drake, *J. Am. Chem. Soc.*, **53,** 3466 (1931).
44. W. C. Harden and E. E. Reid, *J. Am. Chem. Soc.*, **54,** 4325 (1932).
45. F. Muth and G. Wesenberg, German Patent 628,792.
46. W. C. Harden and J. H. Brewer, *J. Am. Chem. Soc.*, **59,** 2379 (1937).
47. W. S. Gump, US Patent 2,250,408 (1941).
48. P. B. Price, *Ann. N.Y. Acad. Sci.*, **53,** 76 (1950).
49. R. B. Kundsin and C. W. Walter, *Arch. Surg.*, **107,** 75 (1973).
50. P. B. Price and A. Bonnet, *Surgery*, **24,** 542 (1948).
51. H. J. Florestano, *J. Pharmacol. Exp. Ther.*, **96,** 238 (1949).
52. D. E. Larsen, *Hospitals*, **42,** 63 (1968).
53. T. B. Gaines, R. D. Kimbrough, and R. E. Linder, *Toxicol. Appl. Pharmacol.*, **25,** 332 (1973).
54. U.S. Food and Drug Administration, *Hexachlorophene and Newborns*, bulletin, December 1971.
55. R. M. Shuman, R. W. Leech, and E. C. Alvord, Jr., *Morbid. Mortal.*, **22,** 93 (1973).
56. J. G. Kensit, *J. Antimicrob. Chemother.*, **1,** 263 (1975).
57. P. M. Catalano, *Arch. Dermatol.*, **111,** 250 (1975).
58. R. D. Kimbrough, *J. Clin. Pharmacol.*, **13,** 439 (1973).
59. A. Davies, *Rep. Progr. Appl. Chem.*, **58,** 491 (1973).
60. S. H. Hopper and K. M. Wood, *J. Am. Pharm. Assoc., Sci. Ed.*, **47,** 317 (1958).
61. R. S. Shumard, D. J. Beaver, and M. C. Hunter, *Soap Sanit. Chem.*, **29,** 34 (1953).
62. W. L. G. Ashton, *Brit. Med. J.*, **1970,** 500.
63. *Trop. Dis. Bull.*, **65,** 288 (1968).
64. O. F. Jillson and R. D. Baughman, *Arch. Dermatol.*, **88,** 409 (1963).
65. S. E. O'Quinn, B. C. Kennedy, and K. H. Isbell, *J. Am. Med. Assoc.*, **199,** 89 (1967).
66. J. B. Adams and M. Hobbs, *J. Pharm. Pharmacol.*, **10,** 507 (1958).
67. B. S. Gould, N. A. Frigerio, and W. B. Lebowitz, *Arch. Biochem. Biophys.*, **56,** 476 (1955).
68. B. S. Gould, M. A. Bosniak, S. Neidleman, and S. Gatt, *Arch. Biochem. Biophys.*, **44,** 284 (1953).
69. A. G. Norman, *Antibiot. Chemother.*, **10,** 675 (1960).
70. I. R. Shimi, S. Shoukry, and Z. Zaki, *Antimicrob. Agents Chemother.*, **9,** 580 (1976).
71. R. G. Fargher, L. O. Galloway, and M. E. Robert, *J. Text. Inst.*, **21,** 245 (1935).
72. J. Bindler, U.S. Patent 2,703,332 (1955).
73. R. C. Taborsky, G. D. Darker, and S. Kaye, *J. Am. Pharm. Assoc. Sci. Ed.*, **48,** 503 (1959).
74. R. C. Taborsky and R. J. Starkey, *J. Am. Pharm., Sci. Ed.*, **51,** 1152 (1962).
75. H. C. Stecker, U.S. Patent 3,041,236 (1962).
76. *Fed. Reg.*, **30 Oct. 1975,** 40 (210), 50527–31.
77. T. R. Aalto, M. C. Firman, and N. E. Rigleo, *J. Am. Pharm. Assoc., Sci. Ed.*, **42,** 449 (1953).
78. H. Sokol, *Drug Stand.*, **20,** 89 (1952).
79. W. F. Schorr, *J. Am. Med. Assoc.*, **204,** 107 (1968).
80. J. Buechi, J. B. Hansen, and S. A. Tammilehto, *Pharm. Acta Helv.*, **1971,** 602.
81. J. W. Burks, M. Schreiber, and C. L. Carpenter, *South. Med. J.*, **55,** 632 (1962).
82. T. B. Johnson and F. W. Lane, *J. Am. Chem. Soc.*, **43,** 348 (1921).
83. E. G. Klarman, L. W. Gates, and V. A. Shternov, *J. Am. Chem. Soc.*, **53,** 3397 (1931).
84. K. Brehm, *Fette, Seifen, Anstrichm.*, **75,** 443 (1973); through *Chem. Abstr.*, **79,** 143010v (1973).
85. W. F. van Ottigen, *Therapeutic Agents of the Quinoline Group*, Chemical Catalog Co., New York, 1933, p. 33.
86. G. R. Pettit and A. K. Das Gupta, *Chem. Ind.* (London), 1016 (1962).
87. K. A. Oster and M. J. Golden, *J. Am. Pharm. Assoc.* (*Sci. ed.*), **37,** 283 (1947).
88. K. Sigg, *Schweiz. Med. Wochenschr.*, **77,** 123 (1947).
89. M. G. Schultz, *J. Am. Med. Assoc.*, **220,** 273 (1972).
90. Anon., *Lancet*, **1968(1),** 679.
91. M. Dunne, M. Flood, and A. Herxheimer, *J. Antimicrob. Chemother.*, **2,** 21 (1976).
92. O. Uhlir, J. Hnatek, and M. Hatala, *Proceedings of the Seventh International Congress* on *Advances in Antimicrobial Antineoplastic Chemotherapy, 1971*, Vol. 1, Pt. 2, E. M. Hejzlar, Ed., University Park Press, Baltimore, 1972, p. 1353.
93. O. Angelova, N. Tyutyulkova, and R. Vasilev, in ref. 92, p. 507.

94. F. W. Tanner and F. L. Wilson, *Proc. Soc. Exp. Biol. Med.*, **52,** 138 (1943).
95. F. W. Tilley and J. M. Schaffer, *J. Bacteriol.*, **12,** 303 (1926).
96. M. Heuzenroder and K. D. Johnson, *Aust. J. Pharm.*, **40,** 944 (1958).
97. C. E. Coulthard and G. Sykes, *Pharm. J.*, **137,** 79 (1936).
98. V. Groupé, C. G. Engle, P. E. Gaffney, and R. A. Manaker, *Appl. Microbiol.*, **3,** 333 (1955).
99. S. Dayley, E. A. Dawes, and G. A. Morrison, *J. Bacteriol.*, **60,** 369 (1950).
100. W. Mullen, W. Shepherd, and J. Labovitz, *Ther. Rev.*, **17,** 475 (1973).
101. C. Prevost and V. Moses, *J. Bacteriol.*, **91,** 1446 (1966).
102. H. S. Rosenkranz, H. S. Carr, and H. M. Rose, *J. Bacteriol.*, **89,** 1370 (1965).
103. C. K. K. Nair, D. S. Pradham, and A. Sreenivasan, *J. Bacteriol.*, **121,** 392 (1975).
104. G. Nordgren, *Acta Pathol. Microbiol. Scand.* (Suppl.), **40,** 1 (1939).
105. C. R. Phillips, *Bacteriol. Rev.*, **16,** 135 (1952).
106. H. Brodhage and A. R. Stofer, *Antibiot. Chemother.*, **11,** 205 (1961).
107. R. W. Snyder and E. L. Cheatle, *Am. J. Hosp. Pharm.*, **22,** 321 (1965).
108. S. Thomas and A. D. Russell, *J. Appl. Bacteriol.*, **37,** 83 (1974).
109. P. V. McGucken and W. Woodside, *J. Appl. Bacteriol.*, **36,** 419 (1973).
110. R. M. G. Boucher, *Can. J. Pharm. Sci.*, **10,** 1 (1975).
111. A. Einhorn and M. Göttler, *Justus Liebigs Ann. Chem.*, **343,** 207 (1908).
112. G. Domagk, *Deut. Med. Wochenschr.*, **61,** 829 (1935).
113. R. Gilby and A. V. Few, *J. Gen. Microbiol.*, **23,** 19 (1960).
114. C. R. Smith, H. Nishihar, F. Golden, A. Hoyt, C. O. Goss, and M. Kloetzel, *US Pub. Health Rept.*, **65,** 1588 (1950).
115. K. Anderson, S. Lillie, and D. Crompton, *Pharm. J.*, **192,** 593 (1964).
116. C. E. Chaplin, *J. Bacteriol.*, **63,** 453 (1952).
117. D. R. MacGregor and P. R. Elliker, *Can. J. Microbiol.*, **4,** 499 (1958).
118. C. K. Johns, *Can. Food Ind.*, **19,** 24 (1948).
119. G. Schneider, *Z. Immunitatsforsch.*, **85,** 194 (1935).
120. C. A. Lawrence, *J. Soc. Cosmet. Chem.*, **3,** 123 (1952).
121. C. A. Lawrence, in *Disinfection, Sterilization and Preservation*, C. A. Lawrence and S. S. Block, Eds., Lea and Febiger, Philadelphia, 1968, Ch. 26, p. 444.
122. W. S. Mueller and D. B. Seeley, *Soap Sanit. Chem.*, **27,** 131 (1951).
123. C. W. Walter, *J. Am. Med. Assoc.*, **179,** 386 (1962).
124. J. K. Morgan, *Brit. J. Clin. Pract.*, **22,** 261 (1968).
125. J. M. Arena, *J. Am. Med. Assoc.*, **190,** 56 (1964).
126. R. D. Hotchkiss, *Ann. N.Y. Acad. Sci.*, **46,** 479 (1946).
127. M. R. J. Salton, *J. Gen. Microbiol.*, **5,** 391 (1951).
128. E. F. Gale and E. S. Taylor, *Nature*, **157,** 549 (1946).
129. M. R. J. Salton, R. W. Horne, and V. E. Cosslett, *J. Gen. Microbiol.*, **5,** 391 (1951).
130. R. M. E. Richards and R. H. Cavill, *J. Pharm. Sci.*, **65,** 76 (1976).
131. D. W. Blois and J. Swarbrick, *J. Pharm. Sci.*, **61,** 393 (1972).
132. N. D. Weiner, F. Hart, and G. Zografi, *J. Pharm. Pharmacol.*, **17,** 350 (1965).
133. H. H. Laycock and B. A. Mulley, *J. Pharm. Pharmacol.*, **22** (Suppl.), 157S (1970).
134. R. A. Cutler, E. B. Cimijotti, T. J. Oklowich, and W. F. Wetterau, *Soap Chem. Spec.*, **43,** 74 (1967).
135. M. H. Babs, O. J. Collier, W. C. Austin, M. D. Potter, and E. P. Taylor, *J. Pharm. Pharmacol.*, **10,** 110 (1956).
136. W. B. Hugo and M. Frier, *Appl. Microbiol.*, **17,** 118 (1969).
137. C. A. Lawrence, in *Cationic Surfactants*, E. Jungermann, Ed., Dekker, New York, 1970, p. 491.
138. J. W. Churchman, *J. Exp. Med.*, **16,** 221 (1912).
139. J. W. Churchman, *J. Am. Med. Assoc.*, **85,** 1849 (1925).
140. T. C. Chen and E. J. Day, *Poult. Sci.*, **53,** 1791 (1974).
141. E. Fischer and R. Muñoz, *J. Bacteriol.*, **53,** 381 (1947).
142. E. W. Stearn and A. E. Stearn, *J. Bacteriol.*, **11,** 345 (1926).
143. A. Albert, S. D. Rubbo, R. Goldacre, M. Davey, and J. Stone, *Brit. J. Exp. Pathol.*, **26,** 60 (1945).
144. E. Adams, *J. Pharm. Pharmacol.*, **19,** 821 (1967).

145. A. D. Wolfe, R. G. Allison, and F. E. Hahn, *Biochemistry*, **11,** 1569 (1972).

146. N. E. Sharpless, C. L. Greenblatt, and W. H. Jennings, *Trans. N.Y. Acad. Sci.*, **35,** 187 (1973).

147. P. Gustafsson, K. Nordstrom, and S. Normak, *J. Bacteriol.*, **116,** 893 (1973).

148. C. H. Browning and W. Gilmour, *J. Pathol. Bacteriol.*, **18,** 144 (1913).

149. A. Albert, *Selective Toxicity*, Wiley, New York, 1968.

150. B. Tinland, C. Decoret, and R. Bodin, *Farmaco, Ed. Sci.*, **27,** 1024 (1972).

151. M. J. Waring, *Nature*, **219,** 1320 (1968).

152. M. Steinert, *Advan. Cytopharmacol.*, **1,** 229 (1971).

153. T. J. Franklin and G. A. Snow, *Biochemistry of Antimicrobial Action*, Wiley, New York, 1975, p. 84.

154. D. C. Schroder, *Chem. Rev.*, **55,** 186 (1952).

155. L. Weinstein and A. McDonald, *Science*, **101,** 44 (1944).

156. A. T. Fuller, *Biochem. J.*, **36,** 547 (1942).

157. F. Kohn, M. H. Hall, and C. D. Cross, *Lancet*, **2,** 140 (1943).

158. W. R. Thrower and F. C. Valentine, *Lancet*, **1,** 133 (1943).

159. W. O. Elson, *J. Infect. Dis.*, **76,** 193 (1945).

160. F. H. S. Curd and F. L. Rose, *J. Chem. Soc.*, 729 (1946).

161. G. E. Davies, J. Francis, A. R. Martin, F. L. Rose, and G. Swain, *Brit. J. Pharmacol.*, **9,** 192 (1954).

162. D. J. Beaver, D. P. Roman, and P. J. Stoffel, *J. Am. Chem. Soc.*, **79,** 1236 (1957).

163. Monsanto Bulletin No. FC-4A, January 1963, through Ref. 5, p. 463.

164. R. E. Gosselin, H. C. Hodge, R. P. Smith, and M. N. Gleason, *Clinical Toxicology of Commercial Products*, 4th ed., Williams and Wilkins, Baltimore, Md., 1976, Section II, p. 184.

165. P. G. Quie, R. O. Fisch, and R. Raile, *Lancet*, **82,** 428 (1962).

166. R. O. Fisch et al., *J. Am. Med. Assoc.*, **185,** 124 (1963).

167. Ref. 5, p. 464.

168. J. G. Block, D. Hawes, and T. Rutherford, *Toxicology*, **3,** 253 (1975).

169. W. E. Frick and W. Stammbach, US Patent 3,214,468 (1965).

170. R. S. Baichwal, R. M. Baxter, S. I. Kandel, and G. C. Walker, *Can. J. Biochem. Physiol.*, **38,** 245 (1960).

171. W. A. Hamilton, *J. Gen. Microbiol.*, **50,** 441 (1968).

172. W. A. Hamilton, *Membranes: Struct. Funct., Fed. Eur. Biochem. Soc., Met.*, 6th **1969,** 71; *Chem. Abstr.*, **74,** 95906g (1971).

173. J. N. Ashley, J. J. Barker, A. J. Ewins, G. Newberry, and A. D. H. Self, *J. Chem. Soc.*, 103 (1942).

174. S. S. Berg and G. Newberry, *J. Chem. Soc.*, 642 (1949).

175. R. Wien, J. Harrison, and W. A. Freeman, *Brit. J. Pharmacol.*, **3,** 211 (1948).

176. R. Wien, J. Harrison, and W. A. Freeman, *Lancet*, 711 (1948).

177. W. Woodside, *Microbios*, **8,** 23 (1973).

178. D. R. Makulu and T. P. Woolkes, *J. Nat. Cancer Inst.*, **54,** 305 (1975).

179. M. J. Pine, *Biochem. Pharmacol.*, **17,** 75 (1968).

180. W. B. Hugo, in *Inhibition and Destruction of the Microbial Cell*, W. B. Hugo, Ed., Academic Press, New York, 1971, Ch. 3d.

181. F. L. Rose and G. Swain, *J. Chem. Soc.*, 4422 (1956).

182. R. Hall, *Process Biochem.*, **2,** 24 (1967).

183. A. Davies, *Rep. Progr. Appl. Chem.*, **58,** 494 (1973).

184. R. P. Quintana, *Advan. Chem. Ser.*, **145,** 290 (1975).

185. P. Gjermo, *J. Clin. Periodontol.*, **1,** 143 (1974).

186. R. C. Buckle and C. E. Seabridge, *Lancet*, 193 (1963).

187. J. S. Cason and E. J. L. Lowbury, *Lancet*, 501 (1960).

188. M. J. Winrow, *J. Periodont. Res.*, Suppl., **12,** 45 (1973).

189. B. Magnusson and G. Heyden. *J. Periodont. Res.* Suppl., **12,** 49 (1973).

190. D. E. Case, J. McAinsh, A. Rushton, and M. J. Winrow, in *Chemotherapy*, J. D. Williams and A. M. Geddes, Eds., Plenum Press, New York, 1976, p. 367.

191. W. B. Hugo and A. R. Longworth, *J. Pharm. Pharmacol.*, **16,** 655 (1964).

192. F. M. Harold, J. R. Baarda, C. Baron, and A. Abrams, *Biochim. Biophys. Acta*, **183,** 129 (1969).

193. W. B. Hugo and D. C. Daltrey, *Microbios*, **11,** 119 (1974).

194. W. B. Hugo and D. C. Daltrey, *Microbios*, **11,** 131 (1974).

195. J. W. James, J. A. Baker, and L. F. Wiggins, *J. Med. Chem.*, **11,** 942 (1968).
196. T. F. McNamara, M. I. Steinbach, and B. S. Schwartz, *J. Soc. Cosmet. Chem.*, **16,** 499 (1965).
197. H. W. Thomas, *Brit. Med. J.*, **1,** 1140 (1905).
198. L. Chalmers, *Manuf. Chem. Aerosol News*, **38,** 37 (1967).
199. H. E. Morton, L. L. North, and F. B. Engley, Jr. *J. Am. Med. Assoc.*, **136,** 37 (1948).
200. H. M. Powell, *J. Am. Med. Assoc.*, **137,** 862 (1948).
201. H. W. Cromwell, *J. Am. Med. Assoc.*, **140,** 401 (1949).
202. J. H. Brewer and C. B. McLaughlin, *J. Am. Med. Assoc.*, **146,** 729 (1951).
203. H. Meyer, *Pharm. Zentralhalle*, **103,** 571 (1964).
204. J. A. de Lonreiro and E. Lito, *J. Hyg.*, **44,** 463 (1946).
205. E. S. G. Barton and T. P. Singer, *J. Biol. Chem.*, **157,** 221 (1945).
206. K. P. Mathews, *Am. J. Med.*, **44,** 310 (1968).
207. H. H. Young, E. C. White, and E. O. Swartz, *J. Am. Med. Assoc.*, **73,** 1483 (1919).
208. F. Dunning and L. H. Farinholt, *J. Am. Chem. Soc.*, **51,** 804 (1929).
209. G. W. Raiziss, M. Severac, and J. C. Moetsch, *J. Am. Chem. Soc.*, **94,** 1199 (1930).
210. A. A. Goldberg, *Manuf. Chem.*, **22,** 182 (1951).
211. W. A. Jamieson and H. M. Powell, *Am. J. Hyg.*, **14,** 218 (1931).
212. J. H. Waldo, *J. Am. Chem. Soc.*, **53,** 992 (1931).
213. M. Wysor and R. E. Zollinhofer, *Pathol. Microbiol.*, **38,** 296 (1972).
214. S. M. Modak and C. L. Fox, *Biochem. Pharmacol.*, **22,** 2391 (1973).
215. H. S. Rosenkranz and H. S. Carr, *Antimicrob. Agents Chemother.*, **2,** 367 (1972).
216. C. L. Fox, *Arch. Surg.*, **96,** 184 (1968).
217. J. A. Moncrief, *Clin. Plast. Surg.*, **1,** 563 (1974).
218. C. L. Fox, *Pahlvai Med. J.*, **8,** 45 (1977).
219. C. R. Phillips and S. Kaye, *Am. J. Hyg.*, **50,** 270 (1949).
220. G. W. Jones and R. E. Kennedy, *Ind. Eng. Chem.*, **22,** 146 (1930).
221. S. Kaye and C. R. Phillips, *Am. J. Hyg.*, **50,** 296 (1949).
222. C. R. Phillips, *Bacteriol. Rev.*, **16,** 135 (1952).
223. R. R. Ernst, *Dev. Biol. Stand.*, **23,** 40 (1974).
224. R. K. Hoffman and B. Warshawsky, *Appl. Microbiol.*, **6,** 358 (1958).
225. G. A. LoGrippo, *Angiol.*, **12,** 80 (1961).
226. R. K. Hoffman, in *Inhibition and Destruction of the Microbial Cell*, W. B. Hugo, Ed., Academic Press, New York, 1971, Ch. 4.
227. C. R. Phillips, in *Disinfection, Sterilization and Preservation*, C. A. Lawrence and S. S. Block, Eds., Lea and Febiger, Philadelphia, 1968, p. 669.
228. E. B. Hodge, J. R. Dawkins, and E. Kropp, *J. Am. Pharm. Assoc., Sci. Ed.*, **43,** 501 (1954).
229. N. G. Clark, B. Croshaw, B. E. Leggetter, and D. F. Spooner, *J. Med. Chem.*, **17,** 977 (1974).
230. G. Sykes and R. Smart, *Am. Perfum. Cosmet.*, **84,** 45 (1969).
231. R. J. Stretton and T. W. Manson, *J. Appl. Bacteriol.*, **36,** 61 (1973).
232. F. H. McMillan, German Patent 1,209,249; through *Chem. Abstr.*, **64,** 14039f.
233. W. C. Austin, M. D. Potter, and E. P. Taylor, *J. Chem. Soc.*, **1958,** 1489.
234. A. Doppstadt, H. C. Stark, H. G. Stoll, and H. K. Grubmeuller, *Arzneim.-Forsch.*, **19,** 1764 (1969).
235. M. C. Dodd, W. B. Stillman, M. Roys, and C. Crosby, *J. Pharmacol. Exp. Ther.*, **82,** 11 (1944).
236. D. L. Cramer and M. C. Dodd, *J. Bacteriol.*, **51,** 293 (1946).
237. D. R. McAlla and D. Vautsinos, *Mutat. Res.*, **26,** 3 (1974).
238. J. E. Morris, J. M. Price, J. J. Lalich, and R. J. Stein, *Cancer Res.*, **29,** 2145 (1969).
239. F. Legler, *Arzneim.-Forsch.*, **12,** 890 (1962).
240. R. E. Asnis, *J. Biol. Chem.*, **213,** 75 (1952).
241. J. Sachs, T. Geer, P. Noell, and C. M. Kunin, *New Engl. J. Med.*, **278,** 1032, (1968).
242. A. H. Beckett and A. E. Robinson, *J. Med. Pharm. Chem.*, **1,** 135 (1959).
243. D. M. Tennent and W. H. Ray, *Fed. Proc. Fed. Am. Soc. Exp. Biol.*, **22,** 367 (1963).
244. J. A. Buzard, *Sci. Sect. Am. Pharm. Assoc.*, 1962; through *Chem. Abstr.*, **60,** 6079g (1964).
245. J. Olivard, S. Valenti, and J. A. Buzard, *J. Med. Pharm. Chem.*, **5,** 524 (1962).
246. S. Toyoshima, K. Shimada, and S. Tanaka, *J. Pharm. Soc. Japan*, **84,** 187 (1964).
247. I. M. Thompson and A. D. Amar, *J. Urol.*, **82,** 387 (1959).
248. J. F. Toole and M. L. Parrish, *Neurology*, **23,** 554 (1973).
249. J. H. Felts, D. M. Hayes, J. A. Gergen, and J. F. Toole, *Am. J. Med.*, **51,** 331 (1971).
250. *Food, Drug Cosmet. Law Rep.*, **711,** Pt. II, August 25, 1976.

251. *Fed. Reg.*, **41,** No. 160, 34884 (1976).
252. A. Zampieri and J. Greenberg, *Biochem. Biophys. Res. Commun.*, **14,** 172 (1964).
253. Y. Tazima, T. Kada, and A. Murakami, *Mutat. Res.*, **32,** 55 (1975).
254. D. R. McCalla and D. Voutsinos, *Mutat. Res.*, **26,** 3 (1974).
255. D. R. McCalla, A. Reuvers, and C. Kaiser, *J. Bacteriol.*, **104,** 1126 (1970).
256. D. L. Cramer and M. C. Dodd, *J. Bacteriol.*, **51,** 293 (1946).
257. M. F. Paul, H. E. Paul, F. Kopko, M. J. Bryson, and C. M. Harrington, *J. Biol. Chem.*, **206,** 491 (1952).
258. T. Suzuki and C. Nishimura. *J. Pharm. Soc. Japan*, **76,** 1013 (1956).
259. R. E. Asnis, *Arch. Biochem. Biophys.*, **66,** 208 (1957).
260. P. Herrlich and M. Schweiger, *Proc. Nat. Acad. Sci. US*, **73,** 3386 (1976).
261. H.K. Kim, R. E. Bambury, and H. K. Yaktin, *J. Med. Chem.*, **14,** 301 (1971).
262. W. R. Sherman and D. E. Dickson, *J. Org. Chem.*, **27,** 1351 (1962).
263. A. Fujito, M. Nakata, S. Minami, and H. Takamatsu, *J. Pharm. Soc. Japan*, **86,** 1014 (1966).
264. W. Stillman and A. Scott, US Patent 2,416,238 (1947).
265. H. E. Paul and M. F. Paul, in *Experimental Chemotherapy*, Vol. 2, R. J. Schnitzer and F. Hawking, Eds., Academic Press, New York, 1964, p. 307.
266. K. Miura and H. K. Reckendorf, in *Progress in Medicinal Chemistry*, Vol. 5, G. P. Ellis and G. B. West, Eds., Butterworths, London, 1967, p. 320.
267. J. H. S. Foster and A. D. Russell, in *Inhibition and Destruction of the Microbial Cell*, W. G. Hugo, Ed., Academic Press, New York, 1971, p. 201.
268. R. Wise, J. M. Andrews, and K. M. Bedford, *Chemotherapy*, **23,** 19 (1977).
269. G. Asato and G. Berkelhammer, *Science*, **162,** 1146 (1968).
270. D. Edwards, M. Dye, and H. Carne, *J. Gen. Microbiol.*, **76,** 135 (1973).
271. A. K. Miller, *Appl. Microbiol.*, **22,** 480 (1971).
272. R. E. Bambury, C. M. Lutz, L. F. Miller, H. K. Kim, and H. W. Ritter, *J. Med. Chem.*, **16,** 566 (1973).
273. H. N. Prince, E. Grunberg, E. Titsworth, and W. F. DeLorenzo, *Appl. Microbiol.*, **18,** 728 (1969).
274. W. T. Colwell, J. H. Lange, and D. W. Henry, *J. Med. Chem.*, **11,** 282 (1967).
275. K. C. Watson, *J. Med. Microbiol.*, **3,** 363 (1970).
276. J. Hiendel, E. Schroeder, and H. W. Kelm, *Eur. J. Med. Chem.- Chim. Ther.*, **10,** 121 (1975).
277. L. J. Powers *J. Med. Chem.*, **19,** 57 (1976).
278. P. M. Theus and W. Weuffen, *Arch. Pharm.*, **300,** 629 (1967).
279. R. J. Alimo and H. E. Russell, *J. Med. Chem.*, **15,** 335 (1972).
280. E. Grunberg and E. Titsworth, *Ann. Rev. Microbiol.*, **27,** 317 (1973).
281. G. Y. Lesher, E. J. Froelich, M. D. Gruett, J. H. Bailey, and R. P. Brundage, *J. Med. Pharm. Chem.*, **5,** 1063 (1962).
282. W. Brumfitt and R. Pursell, *Postgrad. Med. J.*, **47,** (Suppl.), 16 (1971).
283. G. A. Portmann, E. W. McChesney, H. Stander, and W. E. Moore, *J. Pharm. Sci.*, **55,** 72 (1966).
284. L. P. Garrod, H. P. Lambert, and F. O'Grady, "Nalidixic Acid", in *Antibiotics and Chemotherapy*, 4th ed., Churchill Livingstone, Edinburgh and London, 1973, p. 38.
285. H. H. Zinsser, *Med. Clin. N. Am.*, **54,** 1347 (1970).
286. I. S. Rossoff, *Handbook of Veterinary Drugs*, Springer-Verlag, New York, 1974, p. 375.
287. S. M. Finegold and I. Ziment, *Pediatr. Clin. N. Am.*, **15,** 95 (1968).
288. W. A. Goss, *Urol. Panam.*, **1,** 103 (1969).
289. W. A. Goss and T. M. Cook, "Nalidixic Acid—Mode of Action", in *Antibiotics*, Vol. 3, *Mechanism of Action of Antimicrobial and Antitumor Agents*, J. W. Corcoran and F. E. Hahn, Eds., Springer-Verlag, New York, 1975, p. 176.
290. B. B. Huff, Ed., *Physician's Desk Reference*, 30th ed., Medical Economics, Oradell, N.J., 1976, p. 1667.
291. A. Bauernfeind, *Antibiot. Chemother.* (Basel), **17,** 122 (1971).
292. W. A. Goss, W. H. Dietz, and T. M. Cook, *J. Bacteriol.*, **88,** 1112 (1964).
293. W. A. Goss, W. H. Dietz, and T. M. Cook, *J. Bacteriol.*, **89,** 1068 (1965).
294. G. J. Bourguignon, M. Levitt, and R. Sternglass, *Antimicrob. Agents Chemother.*, **4,** 479 (1973).
295. D. Kaminsky and R. I. Meltzer, *J. Med. Chem.*, **11,** 160 (1968).
296. F. J. Turner, S. M. Ringel, J. F. Martin, P. J. Storino, J. M. Daley, and B. S. Schwartz, *Antimicrob. Agents Chemother.*, **1967,** 475.

297. M. C. Crew, M. D. Melgar, L. J. Haynes, R. L. Gala, and F. J. DiCarlo, *Xenobiotica*, **1** (2), 193 (1971).
298. M. Fujihara, M. Otsuka, and Y. Sato, *Radioisotopes*, **24** (1), 12 (1975).
299. M. J. Kershaw and D. A. Leigh, *J. Antimicrob. Chemother.*, **1,** 311 (1975).
300. W. L. Staudenbauer, *Eur. J. Biochem.*, **62,** 491 (1976).
301. R. S. Pianotti, R. R. Mohan, and B. S. Schwartz, *J. Bacteriol.*, **95,** 1662 (1968).
302. M. Shimizu, Y. Sekine, H. Higuchi, H. Suzuki, S. Nakamura, and K. Nakamura, *Antimicrob. Agents Chemother.*, **1970,** 123.
303. S. Nakamura, M. Ishiyama, and M. Shimizu, *Progr. Chemother., Proc. 8th Int. Congr. Chemother.*, 1973, **1,** 432; *Chem. Abstr.*, **84,** 26413w (1976).
304. M. Shimizu, S. Nakamuru, and Y. Takase, *Antimicrob. Agents Chemother.*, **1970,** 117.
305. J. Matsumoto and S. Minami, *J. Med. Chem.*, **18,** 74 (1975).
306. M. Shimizu et al., *Antimicrob. Agents. Chemother.*, **1975,** 569.
307. C. F. Spenser, A. Engle, C. Yu, R. C. Finch, E. J. Watson, F. F. Ebetino, and C. A. Johnson, *J. Med. Chem.*, **9,** 934 (1966).
308. G. Y. Lesher, US Patents 3,313,817 (1967); 3,313,818 (1967); 3,324,135 (1967).
309. D. H. Holmes, P. W. Ensminger, and R. S. Gordee, *Antimicrob. Agents Chemother.*, **6,** 432 (1974).
310. H. Agui, T. Mitani, A. Izawa, T. Komatsu, and T. Nakagome, *J. Med. Chem.*, **20,** 791 (1977).
311. G. R. Clemo and H. McIlwain, *J. Chem. Soc.*, 479 (1938).
312. G. R. Clemo and A. F. Daglish, *J. Chem. Soc.*, 1481 (1950).
313. H. McIlwain, *Nature*, **148,** 628 (1941).
314. H. McIlwain, *J. Chem. Soc.*, 322 (1943).
315. C. N. Hand, *Nature*, **161,** 1010 (1948).
316. C. E. Coulthard, L. J. Hale, and M. R. Gurd, *Brit. J. Pharmacol.*, **10,** 394 (1954).
317. J. Francis, J. K. Landquist, A. A. Levi, J. A. Silk, and J. M. Thorp, *Biochem. J.*, **63,** 455 (1956).
318. T. D. Hennessey and J. R. Edwards, *Vet. Rec.*, **90,** 187 (1972).
319. M. L. Edwards, R. E. Bambury, and H. W. Ritter, *J. Med. Chem.*, **18,** 637 (1975).
320. G. W. Thrasher, J. E. Shively, C. E. Askelson, W. E. Babcock, and R. R. Chalquest, *J. Anim. Sci.*, **1969,** 208.
321. 1976 *Feed Additive Compendium*, Miller Publishing, Minneapolis, Minn., p. 176.
322. B. Roth, E. A. Falco, G. H. Hitchings, and S. Bushby, *J. Med. Pharm. Chem.*, **5,** 1103 (1962).
323. E. A. Falco, L. Goodwin, G. Hitchings, I. M. Rallo, and P. B. Russell, *Brit. J. Pharmacol.*, **6,** 185 (1951).
324. E. A. Falco, G. H. Hitchings, P. B. Russell, and H. Vander Werf. *Nature*, **164,** 107 (1949).
325. J. H. Darrell, L. P. Garrod, and P. M. Waterworth, *J. Clin. Pathol.*, **21,** 202 (1968).
326. J. R. May and J. Davies, *Brit. Med. J.*, **1972,** 376.
327. A. P. Ball and E. T. Wallace, *J. Int. Med. Res.*, **1974,** 18.
328. N. Datta and R. W. Hedges, *J. Gen. Microbiol.*, **72,** 349 (1972).
329. M. P. Fleming, N. Datta, and R. N. Grüneberg, *Brit. Med. J.*, **1972,** 726.
330. A. Lawrence, I. Phillips, and C. Nicol, *J. Infect. Dis.*, **128** (Nov. Suppl.), 673 (1973).
331. D. T. D. Hughes, *J. Infect. Dis.*, **128** (Nov. Suppl.), 701 (1973).
332. A. M. Geddes, R. Fothergill, J. A. D. Goodall, and P. R. Dorkin, *Brit. Med. J.*, **1971,** 451.
333. H. Nolte and H. Buttner, *Chemotherapy*, **18,** 274 (1973).
334. D. E. Schwartz and W. H. Ziegler, *Postgrad. Med. J.*, **45,** (Suppl.), 32 (1969).
335. V. Udall, *Postgrad. Med. J.*, **45** (Suppl.), 42 (1969).
336. V. Herbert, *J. Infect. Dis.*, **128** (Nov. Suppl.), 433 (1973).
337. W. Brumfitt and R. Pursell, *Brit. Med. J.*, **1972,** 673.
338. E. N. Whitman, *Postgrad. Med. J.*, **45** (Suppl.), 46 (1969).
339. J. J. Burchall and G. H. Hitchings, *Mol. Pharmacol.*, **1,** 126 (1965).
340. B. R. Baker and Beng-Thong Ho, *J. Pharm. Soc.*, **53,** 1137 (1964).
341. G. H. Hitchings and S. R. M. Bushby, *5th Int. Congr. Biochem.*, 1961, p. 165.
342. V. R. Potter, *Proc. Soc. Exp. Biol. Med.*, **76,** 41 (1951).
343. S. R. M. Bushby and G. H. Hitchings, *Brit. J. Pharmacol.*, **33,** 72 (1968).
344. W. L. Webb, in *Enzyme and Metabolic Inhibitors*, Vol. 1, Academic Press, New York, 1963, p. 498.
345. R. J. Rubin, A. Reynaud, and R. E. Handschumacher, *Cancer Res.*, 1002 (1964).

346. S. R. M. Bushby, *Postgrad. Med. J.*, **45** (Suppl.), 10 (1969).

347. M. Poe, *Science*, **194**, 533 (1976).

348. J. J. Burchall, in *Antibiotics*, Vol. 3, *Mechanism of Action of Antibiotics and Antitumor Agents*, J. W. Corcoran and F. E. Hahn, Eds., Springer-Verlag, New York, 1975, p. 304.

349. *J. Infect. Dis.*, **128**, Nov. Suppl. (1973).

350. W. Rehm, H. Thommen, and H. Weiser, *German Patent*. 1954232; through *Chem. Abstr.*, **73**, P 153390r (1970).

351. M. J. Katul and I. N. Frank, *J. Urol.*, **101**, 320 (1970).

352. W. Brumfitt, *Trans. Med. Soc. London*, **90**, 135 (1974).

353. F. M. Kahan and H. Kropp, *Abstr. 15th Intersci. Conf. Antimicrob. Agents Chemother.*, Washington, D.C., September 24–26, 1975, No. 100.

354. H. Kropp, F. M. Kahan, and H. B. Woodruff, in Ref. 353, No. 101.

355. J. Kollonitsch, L. Barash, N. P. Jensen, F. M. Kahan, S. Marburg, L. Perkins, S. M. Miller, and T. Y. Shen, in Ref. 353, No. 102.

356. F. M. Kahan, H. Kropp, H. R. Onishi, and D. P. Jacobus, in Ref. 353, No. 103.

357. J. Kollonitsch, F. M. Kahan, and H. Kropp, *Nature*, **243**, 346 (1973).

CHAPTER FIFTEEN

The β-Lactam Antibiotics

JOHN R. E. HOOVER

AND

GEORGE L. DUNN

Research and Development Division
Smith Kline and French Laboratories
Philadelphia, Pennsylvania 19101 USA

CONTENTS

1 INTRODUCTION, DEFINITION, SCOPE

The discovery of penicillin, the first antibiotic to find practical use in man, marked the beginning of an era that has since produced large numbers and types of such substances. In spite of the subsequent discovery and development of many new classes of antibiotics, two primal biosynthetic penicillins, benzylpenicillin and phenoxymethylpenicillin, are still considered to be drugs of choice for treating infections caused by gram-positive bacteria. And though these early biosynthetic penicillins have continued to find wide use in the clinic, many semisynthetic penicillins and cephalosporins with broader antibacterial activities and improved pharmacokinetic properties have been added to the group of antibiotics used in medical practice. Continued interest in this compound type has led to the more recent discovery of additional naturally occurring β-lactam-containing structures including the cephamycins, the nocardicins, clavulanic acid, and thienamycin. Of these, the cephamycins have also yielded a semisynthetic derivative that has been shown to be effective in controlling bacterial infections in man. Thus the β-lactam antibiotics have persisted as a dominant therapeutic class of drugs, and the size and scope of this group warrant a discussion of these antibiotics separately from the general review of the antibiotic field presented in Chapter 16.

Figure 15.1 illustrates the essential structural features of the naturally occurring forms of these antibiotics. The similarities in structure can be seen readily. All have a 4-membered lactam ring. With the exception of the nocardicins, the β-lactam ring is fused through the nitrogen and the adjacent tetrahedral carbon atoms to a second heterocyclic ring—a five-membered thiazolidine, pyrroline, or oxazolidine ring for the penicillins, thienamycin, and clavulanic acid, respectively, or a six-membered dihydrothiazine ring for the cephalosporins and cephamycins. A structural feature common to all is the carboxyl group on a carbon atom attached to the lactam nitrogen. Another feature shared by the penicillins, cephalosporins, cephamycins, and nocardicins is the acylated amino group on the carbon atom opposite the nitrogen of the β-lactam ring. The cephalosporins and the cephamycins have the same basic structure except that the cephamycins have a methoxy group instead of hydrogen on the amide-bearing carbon atom (C-7). The stereochemistry around the β-lactam ring of the penicillins and the cephalosporins is the same in both series; that is, the asymmetric centers at C-5 and C-6 in the penicillins correspond to those at C-6 and C-7 in the cephalosporins. This

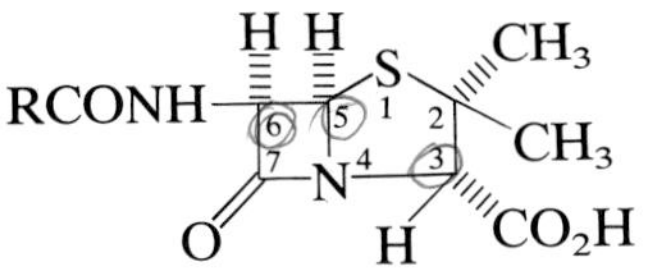

Pencillins

15.**1**

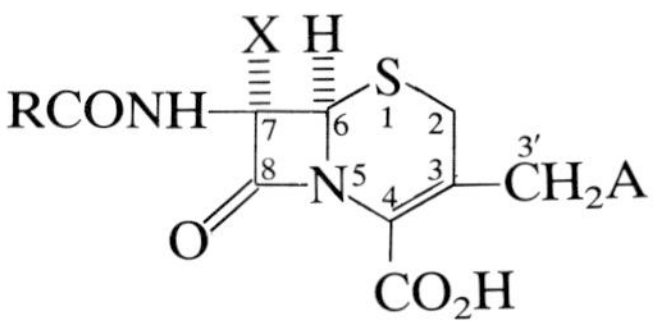

15.**2a** Cephalosporins (X = H)

15.**2b** Cephamycins ($X = OCH_3$)

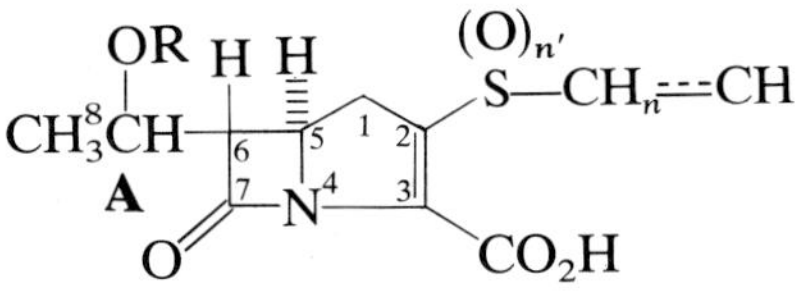

(Epi) Thienamycins

15.**3a** 6α-CH_3CHOH

15.**3b** 6β-CH_3CHOH

A = **R**, **S**; R = H, SO_3H; R^1 = H, $COCH_3$

$n = 1, 2; n' = 0, 1$

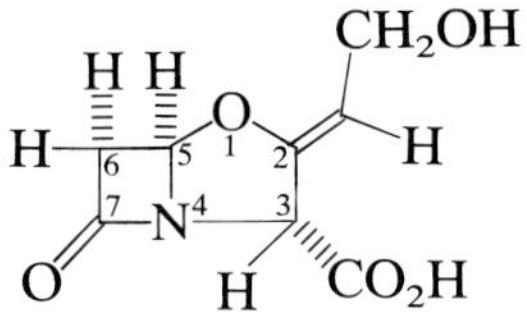

Clavulanic Acid

15.**4**

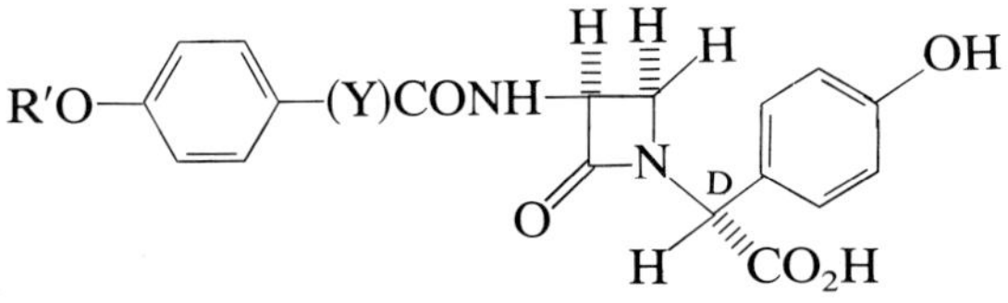

R′ = H, $HO_2CCH(NH_2)CH_2CH_2$-;

Y C=NOH (syn, anti), $CHNH_2$, C=O

Nocardicins A–G

15.**5**

Fig. 15.1 β-Lactam antibiotics.

correspondence, shown first by X-ray structure determinations (1, 2), has also been demonstrated by an elegant chemical conversion of the penicillin to the cephalosporin system (3). The amide-bearing carbon atom (C-6 of the penicillins and C-7 of the cephalosporins) has the L-configuration. The fused rings are, of course, not coplanar but are folded along the C-5 to N-4 axis of the penicillins and the C-6 to N-5 bond of the cephalosporins. The configuration of the fused rings is such that the hydrogen on the carbon atom at the ring junction is cis to the hydrogen on the amide-bearing carbon atom. In the penicillins the carbon atom carrying the carboxyl group (C-3) has the D-configuration, thus placing the carboxyl group on the opposite side of the ring system from the amide group at C-6. This asymmetric center does not exist for the cephalosporins (and cephamycins) because of the endocyclic double bond in the dihydrothiazine ring. The stereochemical placement of the ring substituents is designated by the α and β notations. Accordingly, the hydrogens on the β-lactam ring, the 7-methoxy group of the cephamycins, and the penicillin carboxyl are α-, and the (6- or 7-) acylamino groups are β-. The absolute stereochemistry of the penicillins is 3*S*:5*R*:6*R*: and for the cephalosporins it is 6*R*:7*R*. These similarities extend to the other naturally occurring β-lactam antibiotics. Thus the stereochemistry with respect to ring fusion and the attachment of the carboxyl group of clavulanic acid is the same as that of the penicillins (4), and although the nocardicins do not have the fused-ring arrangement, the acylamino- and carboxyl-carrying carbon atoms both have configurations congruent with the corresponding stereochemical centers of the other known structures in this group (5). The ring-juncture stereochemistry of thienamycin is the same as that of the other bicyclic systems, but the hydroxyethyl side chain is attached so that the lactam ring hydrogens are trans, in contrast to the cis relationship for these hydrogens on the penicillins and cephalosporins. Thienamycin analogs epimerized at the 6- and/or 8-positions have also been obtained from fermentation mixtures (6–8). This epimeric variation has not been encountered among the other natural β-lactam antibiotics.

In addition to the stereochemical and substituent correspondence already discussed, the penicillins, cephalosporins, and cephamycins have a further skeletal equivalence. Both ring systems are branched at the carbon atom beta to the carboxyl group. The structures are consistent with biogenesis from a common *N*-acyl-cysteinyl-valine percursor that cyclizes in different ways (9, 10), and labeling studies have demonstrated the incorporation of these amino acids into both structures. The biosynthesis of these antibiotics, about which a considerable amount is now known, has been extensively reviewed elsewhere (11, 12) and is not discussed here.

The nomenclature of the β-lactam antibiotics presents some thorny problems. For example, *Chemical Abstracts* indexes most penicillins as 4-thia-1-azabicyclo-[3.2.0]heptanes (15.**6**) and cephalosporins

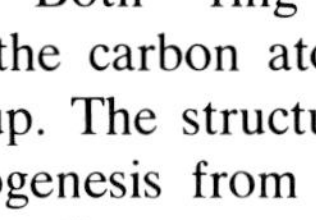

Penam

7-oxo-4-thia-1-azabicyclo[3.2.0]heptane

15.**6**

and cephamycins at 5-thia-1-azabicyclo-[4.2.0]oct-2-enes (15.**7**). Clavulanic acid is a 4-oxa-1-azabicyclo-[3.2.0]heptane. Using this system, penicillin G (15.**1,** R = $C_6H_5CH_2$) is 6-(2-phenylacetamido)-3,3-dimethyl-7-oxo-4-thia-1-azabicyclo[3.2.0]-heptane-2-carboxylic acid, and cephalosporin C (15.**2a,** R = $HO_2CCH(NH_2)(CH_2)_3$—, A = —$OCOCH_3$) is 3-(acetoxymethyl)-7-(D-5-amino-5-carboxyvaleramido)-8-oxo-5-thia-1-azabicyclo[4.2.0]oct-2-ene-2-carboxylic acid. Obviously the chemical substance names derived from this nomenclature system are too cumbersome for general use. One simplification designates the unsubstituted bicyclic ring systems of the penicillins, cephalosporins and thienamycins as penam (13), cepham (14), and 1-carbapenam, respectively (15.**6**–15.**8**). Thus

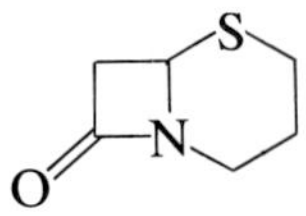

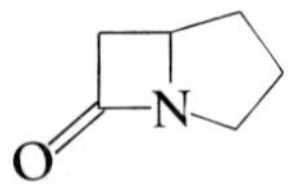

Cepham

8-oxo-5-thia-1-azabicyclo[4.2.0]octane

15.**7**

1-Carbapenam

15.**8**

the penicillins are generally 6-acylamino-2,2-dimethylpenam-3-carboxylic acids and the cephalosporins are 3-acetoxymethyl-7-acylamino-3-cephem-4-carboxylic acids. This nomenclature is widely used, especially in the chemically oriented literature dealing with the cephalosporins and cephamycins. A further simplification with narrower structural latitude is the use of the terms "penicillanic acid" and "cephalosporanic acid" to designate the penicillin and cephalosporin ring systems with the substituents indicated in structures 15.**9** and 15.**10**. Here the penicillins and

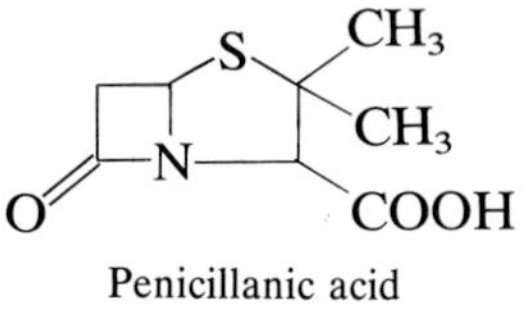

Penicillanic acid

15.**9**

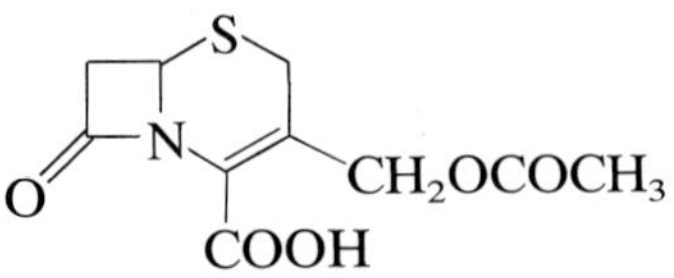

Cephalosporanic acid

15.**10**

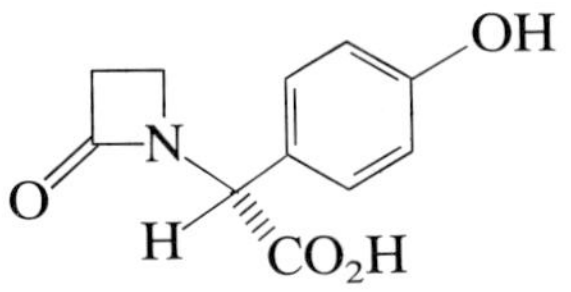

OH
N
O
H
CO_2H

Nocardicinic acid
15.**11**

cephalosporins are named as the appropriate acylaminopenicillanic and cephalosporanic acids. Using this system, thienamycins are named as 1-carbapenemic acids, and nocardicins as nocardicinic acids. Although convenient, this naming becomes restrictive for the cephalosporins (and cephamycins) in which the 3-acetoxymethyl grouping has been replaced by other substituents. For the penicillins, an old and straightforward naming system is widely used that relies on the fact that most of the variations of the penicillin structure are on the acyl group, the rest of the molecule remaining constant. In this case the carbonyl of the acyl group is included in the basic moiety name "penicillin" and penicillin G is named benzylpenicillin.

Since the cephamycins, the nocardicins, clavulanic acid, and thienamycin were discovered more recently than the penicillins and the cephalosporins, most of the present knowledge of the β-lactam antibiotics relates to the latter two antibiotic classes. The content of this chapter reflects this circumstance. For the most part, it deals with the information concerning the penicillins and cephalosporins; reference to the other members of the group are included only where appropriate information is available.

2 USE AND APPLICATION

The β-lactam antibiotics in use today are employed primarily for treating infectious diseases of bacterial origin in man and animals. To understand the use of such agents requires a knowledge of the infectious process and the application of various agents, whether synthetics, antibiotics, or biologicals, to the control of this process. Factors such as the metabolism of the antibiotic by the host, the metabolism and susceptibility of the invading organism, host defense mechanisms, drug distribution, binding, inactivation, and resistance, play a vital role in determining the effectiveness of the drug. Many of these concepts are discussed at length in Chapters 2–5 and 16. A few, including mechanism of action and enzymatic inactivation, are, of necessity, included in the discussions that follow. The reader is referred to the cited chapters for general background and for a review of the factors that result in the selection and use of β-lactams vis-à-vis other antibiotics.

In spite of the relative simplicity of their basic structures, a very large variety of β-lactam antibiotics, especially penicillins, cephalosporins, and cephamycins, exist today. Benzylpenicillin is the most commonly used member of this group. An idea of the antibacterial properties of this substance can be gained by examining the *in vitro* activities listed for it in Table 15.1. These values will also serve as a useful baseline in comparing the biological activities of the different penicillins, as well as the cephalosporins, cephamycins, and other β-lactam antibiotics. In general, benzylpenicillin is highly active against gram-positive bacilli and many, but not all, gram-positive and gram-negative cocci. One exception is the group of penicillinase-producing staphylococci, which are resistant because of their ability to destroy the antibiotic. Most gram-negative bacilli are resistant to benzylpenicillin at moderate levels although several, including *Escherichia coli, Proteus mirabilis,* and species of *Salmonella* and *Shigella*, are susceptible *in vitro* to high concentrations of the antibiotic (Table 15.1). Thus benzylpenicillin is used largely for the treatment of infections caused by gram-positive bacteria. Other penicillins, developed more recently, broaden this spectrum of activity to include gram-negative bacteria.

Table 15.1 Typical Minimum Inhibitory Concentrations (MIC) of Benzyl Penicillin and Cephalothin Against Representative Pathogenic Bacteria (15, 16)

	MIC, μg/ml	
Organism	Benzyl-penicillin	Cephalothin
Staphylococcus aureus (*S*)[a]	0.02–0.06	0.05–0.2
S. aureus (*R*)[b]	7.5–100	0.1–0.8
Streptococcus pyogenes	0.008–0.016	0.003–0.05
S. pneumoniae	0.006–0.015	0.02–0.15
S. faecalis	1.25–4	>100
Corynebacterium diphtheriae	0.036–3	0.16–0.63
Neisseria gonorrhoeae	0.03–0.1	0.25–0.5
Neisseria meningitidis	0.03	0.12–0.5
Hemophilus influenzae	0.5–3	2–8
Escherichia coli	16–>125	2–8
Salmonella typhi	2.5–16	0.5–2
Shigella sonnei	16	4–8
Proteus mirabilis	16–32	4
Proteus spp. (indole+)	16–>200	32–>200
Klebsiella pneumoniae	6.3	1–4
Serratia	>200	>200
Enterobacter spp.	>200	128–256
Pseudomonas aeruginosa	>200	>200

[a] *S* = nonpenicillinase producing.
[b] *R* = penicillinase producing.

The *in vitro* antibacterial activities of the most commonly used cephalosporin, cephalothin (15.**2a**; R = 2-thienymethyl, A = $OCOCH_3$), are included in Table 15.1. This provides a second baseline for comparing the antibacterial properties of the β-lactam antibiotics. Cephalothin is less active than benzylpenicillin against the cocci and gram-positive bacilli but, unlike benzylpenicillin, it is equally active against staphylococci that produce penicillinase and those that do not; and it is more active against certain of the gram-negative bacilli. There are some gram-negative bacteria against which neither benzylpenicillin nor cephalothin is active, for example, *Pseudomonas aeruginosa*. These properties of cephalothin are fairly typical of the cephalosporins and cephamycins. They generally have greater resistance to penicillinase than do the equivalent penicillin (although β-lactamases that inactivate cephalosporins have become an important factor in the design of new cephalosporins), and they inhibit certain gram-negative bacteria that are not susceptible to the penicillins at clinically significant levels. Since the remaining β-lactam antibiotics included in this chapter were discovered only recently, derivatives that may be useful clinically have not yet been described; but they are not without promise. The natural nocardicins have moderate antibacterial activities, primarily against gram-negative species, and are interesting because of their structural difference from the other members of this group. Clavulanic acid also appears to have only moderate antibacterial activity, but it is a powerful irreversible inhibitor of β-lactamases. Thus its principal use is likely to be to extend the antibacterial spectra of penicillins and cephalosporins to include bacteria that are resistant to the latter by virtue of β-lactamase production. Thienamycin, with a narrow range of stability, is reported to be highly active against a wide spectrum of microorganisms, including many not susceptible to the penicillins, cephalosporins, and cephamycins.

The penicillins are striking in their general lack of toxicity. An extreme example is carbenicillin, which is recommended in parenteral doses of up to 40 g/day for treating certain severe systemic infections. This lack of toxicity is impressive in normal individuals, but the wide use of these substances is accompanied by sufficient incidence of unpredictable adverse reactions to necessitate caution in their prescription. The most common adverse effect from the use of penicillins is an allergic reaction, which can range from a mild rash to fatal anaphylactic shock in rare cases. The cephalosporins are also considered to be particularly safe antibiotics, but they cannot be used with the level of inattention to potential toxicity applied to the penicillins. The cephalosporins have a lower incidence of allergic reactions than do the penicillins. Cross-allergenicity between the cephalosporins and penicillins has occurred, but its incidence is low, and cephalosporins have been used to treat patients with known allergy to penicillins. Because of the broad spectrum activity of these drugs, overgrowth by fungi or resistant bacteria can occur with prolonged use.

In general the β-lactam antibiotics are not active against other classes of organisms such as the amebae, fungi, plasmodia, viruses, or rickettsiae.

3 MECHANISM OF ACTION

Clinical control of the infectious process consists largely of an attempt to assist the host in establishing a tenable relationship with the parasite. In most cases this requires elimination of the parasite from the host, at least temporarily. The antibiotic is frequently a useful tool in accomplishing this end. Its utility hinges on some sort of toxicity differential between parasite and host. This, in turn, is dependent on exploitable differences in their metabolic patterns. In the case of the β-lactam antibiotics, the cell wall appears to be the target that permits the selective inhibition of the parasite in the presence of the host cells.

Bacteria have cell walls, but mammalian cells do not. A cell wall consists of a rigid structure that, among other things, protects the fragile cytoplasmic membrane from the high osmotic pressure within the cell. If faults are introduced into the cell wall, the cytoplasmic membrane may be damaged, and unless the cell is in a high osmotic environment, it will lyse. There is evidence that the β-lactam antibiotics generally exert their antibacterial activity by interfering with synthesis of the cell wall in susceptible organisms. Consequently, an understanding of the mode of action of these antibiotics requires some knowledge of the structure of the bacterial cell wall and how it is constructed.

A considerable amount is now known about the composition and organization of the bacterial cell wall, much of this as a result of studies on the mechanism of action of the penicillins. Not surprisingly, bacterial cell walls—for example, from different species—vary in the specific content and organization of their components, but their overall characteristics are sufficiently similar to allow a description of typical structures. The reader should bear in mind that the descriptions that follow are simplified and were selected to illustrate the process under discussion. A more complete account of the present knowledge regarding cell wall structures can be found in many reviews on the subject (17–20).

The cell wall is a complex structure made

up of a variety of polymeric materials including lipopolysaccharide (21), teichoic acid (22), and peptidoglycan (23, 24). Of these, the peptidoglycan is consistently present in the walls of bacterial cells; it is, in essence, a highly cross-linked giant molecule that surrounds the cell, providing rigidity and shape (25). The peptidoglycan is a branched polymer in which the backbone consists of alternating D-*N*-acetylglucosamine and *N*-acetylmuramic acid moieties linked β (1→4) in both cases (26, 27). Attached by way of the carboxyl of the muramic acid, which is the 3-D-lactyl ether of D-glucosamine, is a polypeptide chain of somewhat variable composition, depending on the bacterial species. In the case of *S. aureus* this peptide chain consists of L-alanine, D-glutamic acid, L-lysine, and D-alanine. In *E. coli* B it is L-alanine, D-glutamic acid, *meso*-diaminopimelic acid, and D-alanine. The amino acid sequences from the lactic acid moiety to the end of the chain are in the orders listed. The glutamic acid in *S. aureus* is linked by way of its γ-carboxyl group to the α-amino group of the lysine. Other variations of the chain occur among the different bacterial species. Finally, in *S. aureus* the peptidoglycan strands are cross-linked by bridges containing five glycine units. These bridges link the amino of the L-lysine of one peptide chain to the carboxyl of the terminal D-alanine of another. By contrast, in *E. coli* B peptidoglycan, the peptide chains are linked directly (without the pentaglycine bridges) by a bond from the terminal D-alanine of one chain to the *meso*-diaminopimelic acid of the second. The general features of this concept of the peptidoglycan for *S. aureus*, originally proposed by Wise and Park (28), are diagrammed in Fig. 15.2.

A rather complex series of reactions that occurs within the cell and at the cell membrane results in the formation of the cell wall structure (17, 29, 30). Key intermediates in the formation of the peptidoglycan are uridine nucleotides containing muramic acid and a variable polypeptide component. These nucleotides were first described by Park and Johnson (31), who observed their accumulation in cultures of *S. aureus* inhibited by penicillin. Later studies on their chemical nature (32) and their possible role in the metabolism of the cell led Park, Strominger, and Thompson (33, 34) to propose that these amino acid-containing nucleotides were cell wall precursors. Structure 15.**12** illustrates the nucleotide (33) having the most complete polypeptide chain.

The relationship of the composition of the acetylmuramyl pentapeptide of this nucleotide to a corresponding component of the peptidoglycan will be seen readily. It is important to the later discussion that the muramyl peptide portion of the nucleotide contains one D-alanine more than the corresponding component of the cell wall. A number of investigators have contributed to the present knowledge of the metabolic sequence leading to the UDP-*N*-acetylmuramyl pentapeptide and its incorporation into the peptidoglycan. These and many related studies have been reviewed recently by Blumberg and Strominger (17). In brief, UDP-*N*-acetylglucosamine is converted through an approximately five-step sequence to UDP-*N*-acetylmuramyl pentapeptide (15.**12**). The acetylmuramyl pentapeptide is transferred to membrane-bound phospholipid (C_{55}-isoprenyl alcohol) with retention of the high energy pyrophosphate linkage. While attached to this membrane component, an *N*-acetylglucosamine unit is added, then five glycine units are attached sequentially to the ε-amino grouping of the L-lysine in the pentapeptide chain. The disaccharide-pentapeptide-pentaglycine unit is finally transferred from the lipid carrier to an acceptor, presumably the growing oligomuropeptide chain. All that remains for formation of the peptidoglycan is the cross-linking of the glycine side chain to a

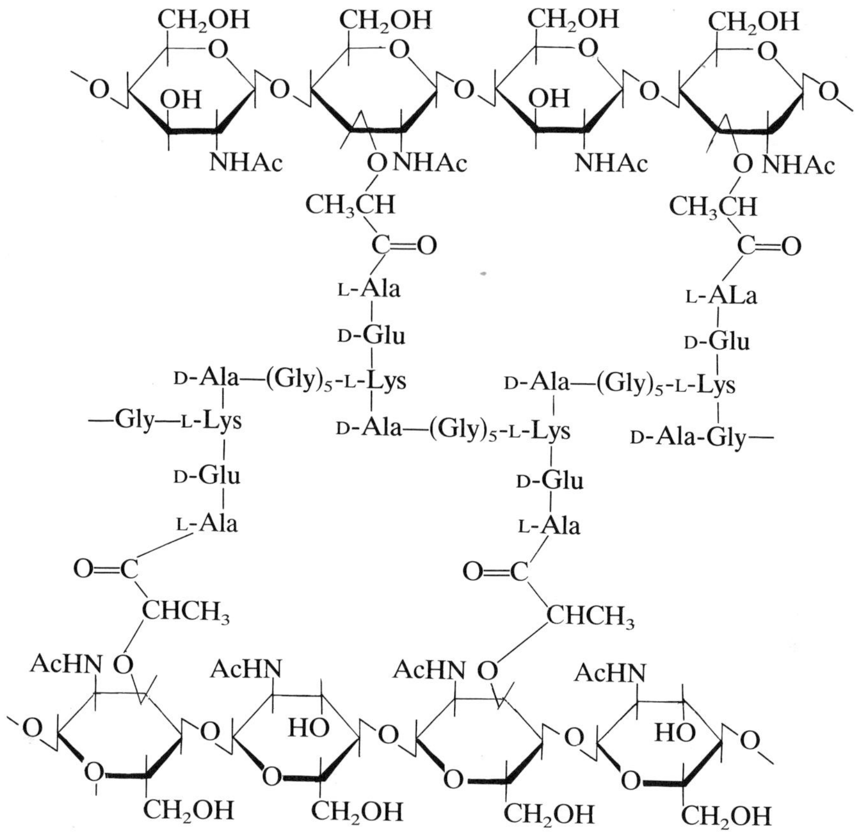

Fig. 15.2 Idealized structure of the cell wall peptidoglycan of *Staphylococcus aureus* as proposed by Wise and Park (28).

nearby pentapeptide, with the elimination of the terminal D-alanine unit from the latter (35, 36).

It is the last step in the synthetic sequence that has been most clearly shown to be sensitive to penicillins (37). The cross-linking reaction that attaches the pentaglycine bridge to the penultimate D-alanine of a neighboring pentapeptide chain is catalyzed by a membrane-bound D-alanine transpeptidase. The different transpeptidases studied have all been found to be penicillin sensitive. Those from *E. coli* and *S. aureus* are irreversibly inhibited (38, 40), but the transpeptidase from *Bacillus megaterium* is reported to be reversibly inhibited (41).

The cephalosporins (and presumably the cephamycins) appear to parallel the penicillins in this mechanism of action, although much less evidence has been obtained in support of this (42, 43).

This description of the mode of action of penicillins is an attractive model that has been widely accepted, but it understates the complexity of the relationships involved

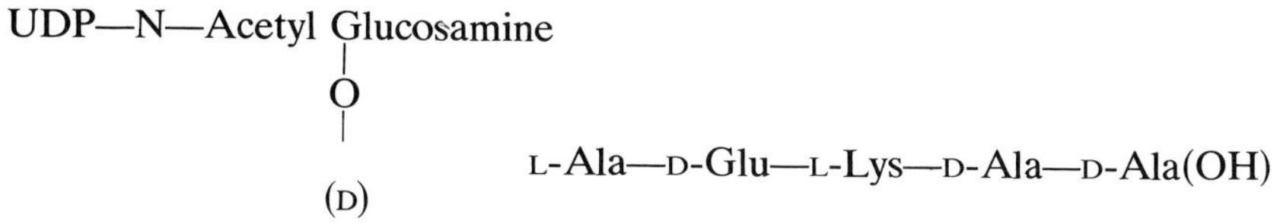

UDP—N—Acetyl Glucosamine
O
(D)
L-Ala—D-Glu—L-Lys—D-Ala—D-Ala(OH)

15.**12**

both in cell wall synthesis and in penicillin action. The regulation of cell wall synthesis is much more complex than the model indicates, involving control systems of unknown nature (therefore unknown susceptibility to the β-lactam antibiotics); these systems regulate, for example, the rate and extent of synthesis and the specific shape of the cell. The inhibition of the transpeptidase carries a degree of ambiguity *per se*, since the inhibition can be irreversible or reversible and it has been demonstrated that the inhibition of the cross-linking reaction is not necessarily lethal to the cell. In addition to the transpeptidases, investigators have identified other enzymes, both soluble and membrane bound, which act on the pentapeptide chain. They include D-alanine carboxypeptidases and endopeptidases (44–47). Both may have a role in controlling the transpeptidase cross-linking process by splitting the pentapeptide strand without forming a cross-link. These enzymes bind penicillins, but it has not been established whether this binding is involved in the killing of the cell by the antibiotic. Furthermore, on treatment with penicillins, cell membranes are found to bind the antibiotic at more sites than can be accounted for by the enzymes already mentioned, and at least part of the bound penicillin has no effect on cell growth (48). Likewise, differences have been observed in the changes that occur in cell morphology (formation of filaments or spheroplasts when susceptible bacteria are exposed to different β-lactam antibiotics or different concentrations of the same antibiotic). These studies imply involvement of different cell wall synthesis processes, or activation of feedback systems. For example, the morphology of *E. coli* cells inhibited by thienamycin is reported to be different from that of cells of the same species inhibited by cephalosporins (49), and the inhibition of gram-negative bacteria by the 6-amidino-penicillin, mecillinam (see Section 8.6), is believed to involve a mode of killing different from that of the 6-acylamino-penicillins (50). Thus it appears, that although the inhibition of D-alanine transpeptidase is a significant factor in the killing of bacteria by β-lactam antibiotics, other targets also exist that are not well characterized at this time.

The binding of the penicillins, whether to the transpeptidase or to other membrane binding sites, generally involves the formation of a covalent bond between the carbonyl group of the β-lactam ring and an unidentified group on the binding site. Products corresponding (chromatographically) to penicilloic acid (51, 52) and penicilloyl hydroxamate have been obtained when membrane-bound penicillin was released by treatment with alkali or hydroxylamine, respectively. The data from binding and subsequent release studies suggest that the penicillin is attached to the binding site as a thioester (52, 53). If this is the case, it is unclear whether the point of covalent attachment is directly to the acceptor site of the enzyme(s) (54) or to a nearby group, resulting in irreversible and inactivating changes in the conformation of the enzyme (55).

Several investigators have conjectured on the spatial requirements of the penicillins and cephalosporins that will rationalize a correspondence of their structures with cell wall components. Suggestions for structural analogy include the muramic acid moiety (56) and, assuming binding to transpeptidase as the principal mode of inhibition, the L-alanyl-γ-D-glutamyl (28) or the D-alanyl-D-alanine (35, 57) portions of the pentapeptide. The latter stress the cyclized dipeptide nature of these antibiotic structures. So far, knowledge of the mechanism of action of these antibiotics has contributed little to the design of more active analogs. The most active β-lactams, frequently with aromatic or heterocyclic rings, bear little resemblance to the cell wall components presumed to be involved in antibiotic action, and analogs designed to have closer structural analogy [e.g., 6-methylpenicillins (36)], in fact, exhibit lowered activity (58, 59).

In addition to providing the possibility of a favorable ratio of parasite-to-host toxicity through inhibition of biochemical systems present in the parasite but not in the host, this mechanism of action has another practical consequence. It is easily seen that the bacteria must be actively dividing, to permit these inhibitors of cell wall synthesis to effectively kill the cell. Thus resting cells, or cells concurrently inhibited by a second antibacterial agent (e.g., protein synthesis inhibitors) that arrests cell growth, are insensitive to the β-lactam antibiotics. This can account for "persistors" that survive the antibiotic treatment, although they remain sensitive to the drug. Likewise the simultaneous administration of penicillins and other antibiotics is usually contraindicated, although synergism between penicillins and aminoglycoside antibiotics has been described.

4 MECHANISMS OF BACTERIAL RESISTANCE: β-LACTAMASES

The susceptibility of bacteria to the β-lactam antibiotics may vary widely depending on the organism and the antibiotic structure. Bacterial resistance to the β-lactams can have various origins. In some cases the low sensitivity to the antibiotic is attributed to "intrinsic" resistance. Permeability barriers may prevent uptake of the antibiotic (60). The amount of antibiotic-sensitive, cell-wall synthesizing enzyme(s) produced by the organism may be large, or the enzyme may be produced in a modified, less sensitive form. Most of these intrinsic factors are still poorly understood, but they apparently account for the lack of susceptibility of many gram-negative bacteria that do not produce β-lactamases, for example, *S. typhi*, *H. influenzae*, and some strains of *P. mirabilis*. Probably the most important mechanism of resistance, about which there is now a considerable body of knowledge, is the conversion of these antibiotics to inactive substances by bacterially produced enzymes called β-lactamases. Some gram-positive organisms (penicillin-resistant *S. aureus*) appear to derive their resistance solely from the production of β-lactamases; for many gram-negative bacteria (*E. coli*, *P. aeruginosa*, *Shigella*, *Klebsiella*), resistance appears to depend on a combination of β-lactamase production and intrinsic resistance factors.

Almost as soon as the utility of the penicillins was discovered, an enzyme that could destroy these antibiotics was described (61). Since then many β-lactamases have been reported (62). These enzymes hydrolyze the β-lactam ring; individual enzymes may inactivate primarily penicillins, cephalosporins, or both. The penicillins are converted to inactive penicilloic acids (15.**13**); opening of the β-lactam ring of the cephalosporins is followed by more complex rearrangements. Production of the β-lactamase by the bacterium may be under chromosomal or R-plasmid (resistance factor) control. In some cases the β-lactamase is produced only in the presence of a β-lactam antibiotic (inducible); in others it is produced continuously (constitutive).

The β-lactamase may be excreted by the bacterium into the surrounding medium (extracellular). This is common with gram-positive bacteria. The enzyme acts on the antibiotic before it contacts the bacterial cell, thus helping to protect the entire bacterial population. With these organisms the level of sensitivity (MIC, *vide infra*) is influenced by the inoculum size. In gram-negative bacteria the β-lactamase is more commonly bound to the cell (intracellular). In this case the enzyme protects only the individual organism.

Later discussions reveal that the β-lactamases have played an important role in the development and use of the β-lactam antibiotics (penicillins, cephalosporins, and cephamycins). The transfer of resistance by way of β-lactamases between strains and even between species of bacteria has increased the problems of β-lactam antibiotic resistance so greatly that species previously easily controlled by these antibiotics have become significant medical problems (e.g., *Neisseria gonorrhae*, *H. influenzae*).

A second group of enzymes (acylases) are capable of hydrolyzing the acylamino side chains of the β-lactam antibiotics. These acylases are commonly obtained from gram-negative bacteria, but their role in bacterial resistance is less well established than that of the β-lactamases. These enzymes have found some commercial use for removing the acyl groups from natural penicillins. This use is discussed in a later section.

5 HISTORICAL BACKGROUND, STRUCTURE, AND SYNTHESIS

The discovery of an antibacterial substance from *Penicillia* by Sir Alexander Fleming in 1929 (63) and the subsequent recognition in 1940 by Florey, Chain, and Abraham, and their colleagues at Oxford University, of the potential utility of this substance for controlling infections in animals (64) and, shortly afterwards, in man (65) has been recounted many times (66). A detailed account by the principals in an autobigraphical review describes the early work on the penicillins (67).

The realization that penicillin was a useful drug occurred in the middle of World War II, and it triggered an immediate attempt to produce the antibiotic on large scale, both in the United States and in Britain. Many industrial concerns, universities, and hospitals in both countries, cooperated in this effort. Accompanying the attempted large-scale production of the antibiotic were widespread studies of its chemical properties and structure. Because of its strategic value, most of the results of this research were kept secret until the end of the war, when a complete chronological account of these efforts was included in the review already cited, and details of the chemical studies were also assembled and published (68).

Penicillin was first obtained as a product of the fungus *Penicillium notatum*. The early attempts to manufacture the drug utilized this organism on surface cultures that were not amenable to large-scale handling. The American workers, especially Coghill and his colleagues (69, 70) at the Northern Regional Research Laboratories in Illinois, quickly introduced modifications that made the commercial manufacture of penicillin a more feasible process. These improvements included the use of deep fermentations instead of surface cultures, the selection of high yielding strains of *P. chrysogenum* to replace the low yielding strain of *P. notatum*, and changes in the culture medium, notably the use of corn steep liquor to replace the less readily available yeast extract. As a result of these and subsequent technological advances, the yields in the fermentation mixture have gone from milligram to gram quantities per liter.

The chemotherapeutic properties of penicillin were demonstrated in 1940. In the years that followed, an intense effort was directed toward its purification and the elucidation of its basic structure. The correct structure, along with two isomeric ones, was suggested in 1943 by workers at Oxford and at Merck (71). However it proved unusually difficult to obtain unequivocal evidence regarding which of the proposed structures was correct, and it was 1945 before the combined results of chemical degradations and X-ray crystallography made it possible to be certain that the penicillins contained the β-lactam–thiazolidine ring system. A number of factors helped make this problem so formidable. Among them were the difficulty in

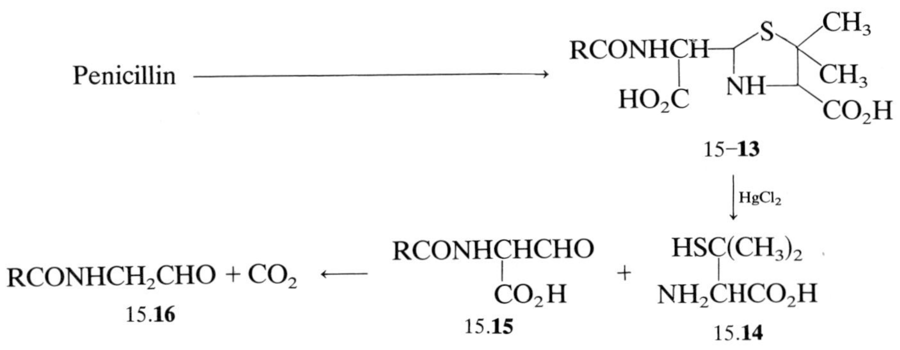

Penicillin ⟶ 15-**13** (RCONHCH(HO₂C)–thiazolidine with S, NH, CH_3, CH_3, CO_2H)

↓ $HgCl_2$

$RCONHCH_2CHO + CO_2$ ⟵ $RCONHCH(CO_2H)CHO$ + $HSC(CH_3)_2$–NH_2CHCO_2H

15.**16** 15.**15** 15.**14**

those days in obtaining pure samples because of the extreme lability of the molecule, and the unexpectedness of the β-lactam ring in a natural substance. The myriad reactions that led to the elucidation of the structures of the penicillins are detailed in the two volumes already cited. Only a few of the salient features are presented here.

Early work showed that a dibasic penicilloic acid (15.**13**) could be obtained by mild hydrolysis of the penicillins. Degradation of this with mercuric chloride gave the unnatural amino acid D-penicillamine (15.**14**) plus penaldic acid (15.**15**), which underwent decarboxylation to give as a net result of the reaction the corresponding penicilloaldehyde (15.**16**) and carbon dioxide. Construction of a possible structure from the ultimate fragments (less water) resulted in three likely possibilities: the correct β-lactam–thiazolidine system, an oxazolone structure (15.**17**), and a less likely tricyclic structure (15.**18**).

Although the properties of the penicillins did not support the presence of the basic center implied in the oxazoline structure, this was the one favored at first by most chemists as a more plausible ring system. Desulfurization studies carried out by the workers at Merck (72) supplied chemical evidence for the fused β-lactam ring. Dethiobenzylpenicillin (15.**19**) in which the β-lactam ring was preserved intact was shown to be a product from the treatment of benzylpenicillin with Rany nickel. Conclusive proof of the total penicillin structure was provided by X-ray crystallographic analysis of metal salts of the penicillins (1). These studies, of course, also furnished the relative stereochemical configuration of the asymmetric centers of the molecule.

As soon as reasonably pure samples of the penicillins were obtained, it became obvious that the penicillin initially crystallized by workers in the United States was different from the one being studied by the British investigators. There were differences in the ability to crystallize, in the chromatographic behavior, and in the properties of the respective benzylamine salts. Discrepancies in biological properties were

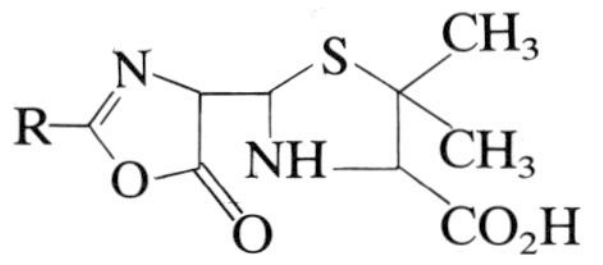

15.**17**

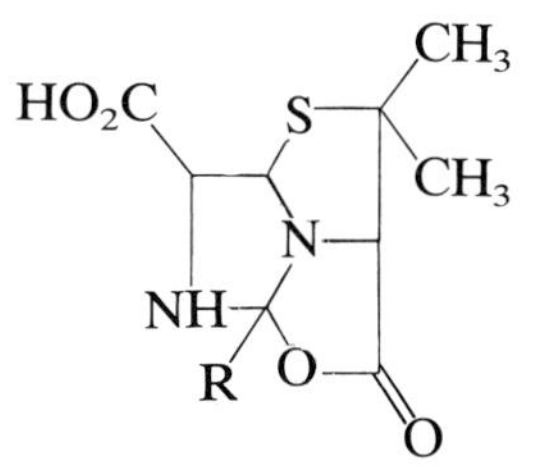

15.**18**

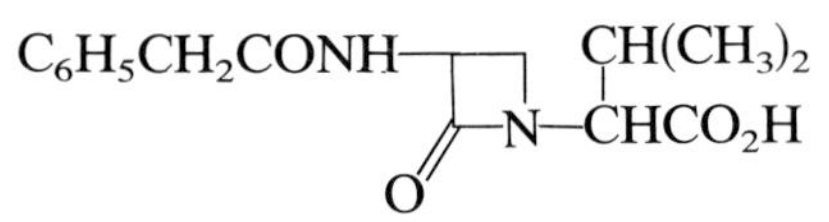

$C_6H_5CH_2CONH$–β-lactam–N–$CH(CH(CH_3)_2)CO_2H$

15.**19**

also observed. Strong hydrolysis of the penicillins, or their derived penillic acids, yielded phenylacetic acid in the case of the American preparations and 2-hexenoic acid from the British penicillin. It was found later that various penicillins differing only in the acyl side chain could be obtained from unaided fermentations depending on the strain of mold used and the composition of the fermentation mixture. Thus the substitution by the Americans of corn steep liquor for yeast extract had not only increased yields but had also resulted in a new penicillin, which eventually proved to be superior to the original. At least seven of the so-called natural penicillins have been described.

Even before the structures of the penicillins were known with certainty, attempts at synthesis were being made by fitting together the constituent parts of the molecule that had been characterized by the degradative studies. By and large, these attempts failed completely. In a few cases, antibiotic activities of reaction mixtures suggested that a trace of the penicillin might have been formed. Thus Folkers and his colleagues at Merck and Sir Robert Robinson and co-workers at Oxford attempted to synthesize penicillins based on the oxazolone structure (73); traces of penicillins (with the β-lactam ring) were formed, as shown by the antibacterial spectrum against various microorganisms, isotope dilution studies, and the fact that the activity could be destroyed by penicillinase. du Vigneaud and his colleagues (74), in an extension of this work, finally isolated in 0.008% yield the crystalline triethylamine salt of benzylpenicillin (75). Later efforts to synthesize the penicillins based on the correct β-lactam structure followed a more rational course (76, 77). Unfortunately, the yields did not exceed those obtained by du Vigneaud.

However with great tenacity Sheehan and his co-workers succeeded after 16 years in the preparation of totally synthetic penicillins, albeit still only in moderate to low overall yields. Sheehan's approach was the first to carry out the β-lactam ring closure on penicilloic acids in which alternative cyclization to an azlactone was minimized or impossible (13). This was accomplished by working with penicilloic acid derivatives in which the amino group was protected, for example, as the phthalimide (78), a benzyl or other alkyl- or arylsulfonamide (79), or an alkyl carbamate (80). The assembly of the appropriate penicilloic acid required, of course, consideration of the stereochemistry at three of the carbon atoms (78). The β-lactam ring closures were accomplished by the action of thionyl chloride on the penicilloic acid half-esters obtained by selective hydrolysis. The free penicillin was finally obtained by saponification of the resulting methyl ester or by hydrogenolysis of the benzyl ester. The general reaction sequence is outlined in Fig. 15.3. By using carbodiimides to accomplish the ring closure on penicilloic acid salts, rather than the esters, Sheehan and Hénery-Logan were able to synthesize phenoxymethylpenicillin in about 10% yield (cyclization step) and benzylpenicillin in 0.3% yield (81). This approach also allowed the total synthesis of 6-aminopenicillanic acid (82) by protecting the amino group with trityl during the ring closure, and an adaptation was used to convert benzylpenicillin to other analogs (83). In the latter case, the β-lactam ring was opened, the resulting penicilloic acid was modified, and subsequently the β-lactam ring was reclosed to give a new penicillin. Though of great academic interest, none of these reactions found commercial utility.

In 1959 Bachelor and his colleagues reported the isolation of the penicillin nucleus, 6-aminopenicillanic acid (6-APA; 15.**1**, RCO = H) from fermentations deficient in side chain precursors (84, 85). It was soon found that 6-APA could be produced more efficiently by removing the acyl

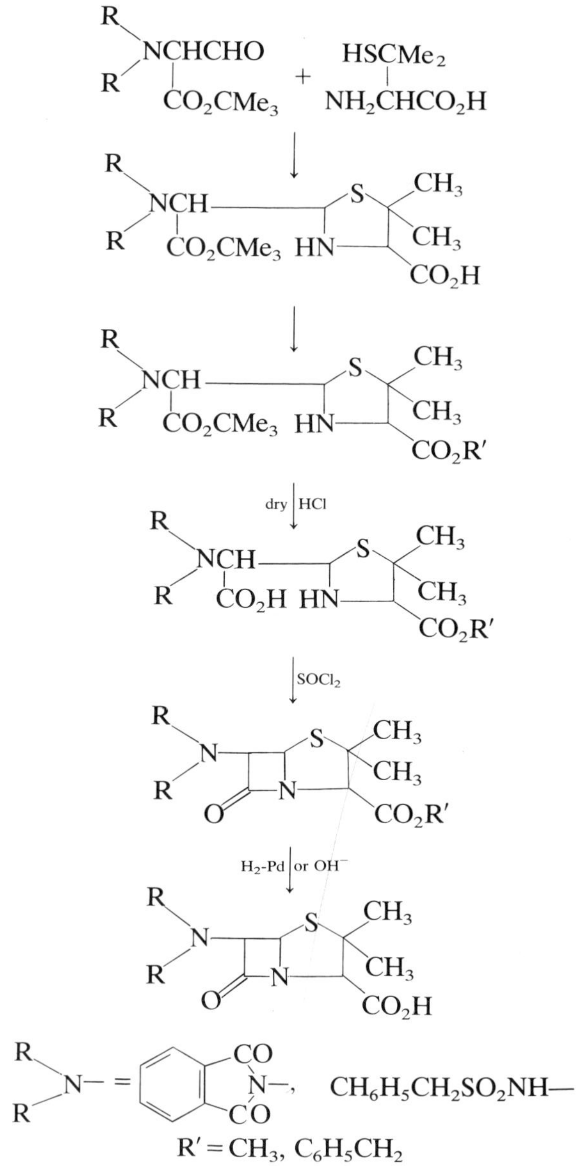

Fig. 15.3 Total synthesis of penicillin analogs (Sheehan).

group from various penicillins. The availability of 6-aminopenicillanic acid has resulted in the preparation and testing of literally thousands of penicillin analogs derived by acylation of the 6-amino group. The amino group has also been converted to a variety of other substituents.

The discovery and development of the cephalosporins began in 1948 with the finding by Brotzu that a *Cephalosporium* species produced antibiotic material that was active against certain gram-negative as well as gram-positive bacteria (86). This fungus was later found by the Oxford workers to produce at least six antibiotic substances. Five were steroidal (cephalosporin P_1–P_5) and active only against gram-positive bacteria (87–89). A study of the substances remaining after extraction of the cephalosporin P fraction from the antibiotic broth revealed the presence of a major hydrophilic component that was only one-hundredth as active against gram-positive organisms as penicillin G, but was 2–6 times as active against gram-negative organisms. This material was named cephalosporin N (90–92). It is probably the substance responsible for the broad spectrum activity of the antibiotic proparation originally described by Brotzu. Cephalosporin N was susceptible to degradation by penicillinase and was found to be D-4-amino-4-carboxybutyl penicillin, identical to Synnematin B, which had been described earlier (93, 94). It has been renamed penicillin N. In the process of studying the ion exchange chromatography of the products from the acid degradation of penicillin N, Abraham and Newton discovered a second hydrophilic antibiotic that had survived the degradation (95, 96). This material, which they named cephalosporin C, was apparently present only in minute amounts in the original fermentation mixture.

Chemical studies demonstrated a similarity between penicillin N and cephalosporin C (97). Thus cephalosporin C also contained a D-α-aminoadipic acid moiety, had an infrared absorption band at 5.62 μ indicative of the β-lactam ring, and yielded one mole of carbon dioxide on hydrolysis with hot acid. After Raney nickel desulfurization, hydrolysis yielded L-alanine, valine, and glycine. On the other hand, marked differences also existed. Hydrolysis of cephalosporin C did not produce penicillamine. The valine from desulfurization and hydrolysis was racemic. NMR studies indicated an absence of the geminal dimethyl group of the penicillins. Cephalosporin C displayed an ultraviolet absorption band at 260 nm, not shown by the penicillin nucleus. These, and other properties, led Abraham and Newton to suggest the correct structure for cephalosporin C (97). The structure was confirmed by X-ray crystallographic studies (2). This work has been reviewed in detail (10, 98).

The early work on cephalosporin C inadvertently produced derivatives resulting from the facile replacement of the acetoxy group on the C-3 methylene. These included the lactone (15.**20**) resulting from cyclization of the carboxyl with the adjacent hydroxymethyl that had been formed by hydrolytic removal of the acetoxy group. The lactone was named cephalosporin C_c. Pyridine used in ion exchange chromatography of cephalosporin C was found to displace the acetoxy group with quaternization of the nitrogen. This derivative (15.**21**) was given the cephalosporin C_A designation.

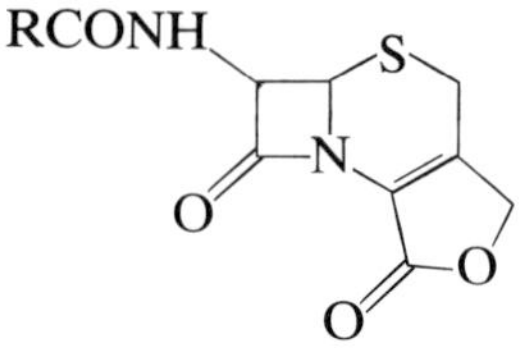

15.**20**

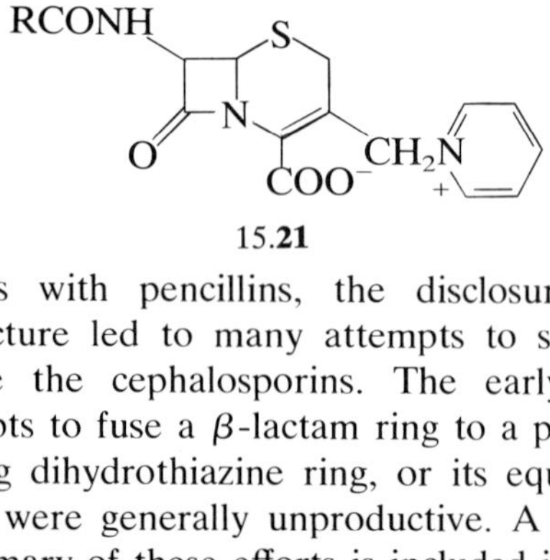

15.**21**

As with pencillins, the disclosure of structure led to many attempts to synthesize the cephalosporins. The early attempts to fuse a β-lactam ring to a preexisting dihydrothiazine ring, or its equivalent, were generally unproductive. A lucid summary of these efforts is included in the review on the cephalosporins already cited (98). Sheehan and Schneider, applying the general sequence used for the total synthesis of penicillin, succeeded in obtaining only traces of a cephalosporin analog (99). However using similar key intermediates (100), Heymès et al. successfully accomplished the total synthesis of analogs of cephalosporin C_c and a similar reaction sequence was described by Dolfini et al. (101).

Utilizing a completely different approach, Woodward and co-workers achieved an exquisite synthesis of cephalosporin C and the clinically useful analog, cephalothin (Fig. 15.4). In this sequence, the β-lactam ring, having substituents in the proper stereochemical configurations, was constructed first by a series of stereospecific reactions starting with the acetonide of L-cysteine. The dihydrothiazine ring was then added, with retention of the stereochemical configuration. Since both stereochemical centers of the cephalosporin nucleus are located on the β-lactam ring, this approach obviated the need for any resolution steps to obtain the natural isomer. The original article and the associated Nobel lecture (102, 103) provide an appreciation of the brilliant chemistry involved in this work.

More recently, cephalosporins and unnatural β-lactam-containing structures have been synthesized by other workers. Many of these substances were obtained by annelating various ring systems to the monocyclic β-lactam ring. The monocyclic β-lactams used for this were obtained by total synthesis or by opening the thiazolidine ring of penicillin sulfoxides as described later. In a few cases the β-lactam ring was generated from substituents attached to the preformed second ring. These syntheses are discussed in Section 12.

Initial attempts to improve cephalosporin C paralleled the earlier penicillin experiences. A substantial amount of work was

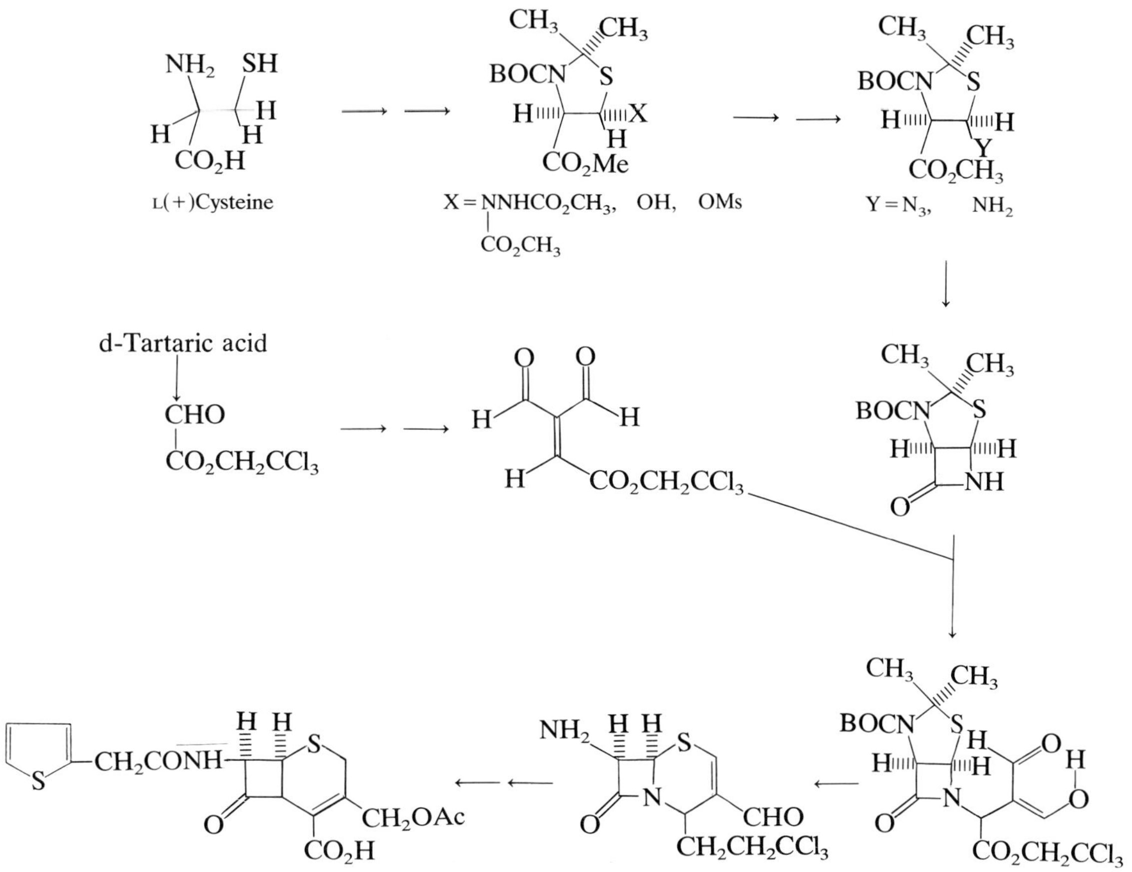

Fig. 15.4 Synthesis of cephalothin (Woodward).

directed toward replacing the 7-aminoadipic acid side chain, or modifying it appropriately. However cephalosporins modified at the 7-position were not obtained by adding side chain precursors to the fermentation, nor could 7-aminocephalosporanic acid (7-ACA) be produced by the biochemical methods used to obtain 6-APA. A practical chemical process to remove the aminoadipic acid side chain was reported by Morin and his coworkers in 1962 (14). Several related processes have since been developed (see Section 6).

7-Aminocephalosporanic acid, like 6-APA, has given rise to thousands of new semisynthetic cephalosporins. The cephalosporin structure offers more opportunities for chemical modification than the penicillins. In addition to the sulfur, double bond, carboxyl group, and unsubstituted positions, there are two side chains that especially lend themselves to chemical manipulation: the 7-acylamino and the 3-acetoxymethyl substituents. Most conceivable modifications have been tried through a huge investment in research on this chemical system by the academic and pharmaceutical communities.

The cephamycins were described almost simultaneously by workers at Lilly and at Merck in 1971 (104, 105). These antibiotics are produced by several *Streptomyces* species. Prior to this, β-lactam antibiotics had been obtained only from fungi. These antibiotics have the basic cephalosporin ring system with differences in the substituents at the 7α- and 3-positions. Again, the natural products from the fermentation have the D-α-aminoadipamido substituent at the 7-position. Very quickly the chemical experiences with the cephalosporins and penicillins were applied to the cephamycins to produce semisynthetic analogs (106, 107). These have been obtained by chemically introducing a methoxy grouping at the 7α-position of the cephalosporin ring system and by manipulating the 3- and 7-substituents of the natural cephamycins (108).

Thienamycin was first described by workers at Merck in 1976 (109). Like the cephalosporins and cephamycins, it was discovered as a fermentation product with broad antibacterial activity, in this case from *Streptomyces cattleya.* The nocardicins, described in 1975 by workers at Fujisawa, were discovered in a screen using a mutant of *E. coli* specifically supersensitive to β-lactams, and confirmed to be β-lactam-containing substances by inactivation with β-lactamases (5, 110, 111). Clavulanic acid, reported in 1976 by Beecham Laboratories, was discovered by still another approach, viz., through a program of screening for novel β-lactamase inhibitors. This material is only weakly active against bacteria and is produced along with penicillin N and two cephalosporins by *Streptomyces clavuligerus* (4, 112, 113). In addition to structures determination and initial biological studies, numerous descriptions of the isolation of naturally occurring analogs of thienamycin (epithienamycins, olivanic acids), and the synthesis of derivatives and analogs of both thienamycin and clavulanic acid have begun to appear.

6 BASIC STRUCTURAL VARIATIONS AND INTERCONVERSIONS

The β-lactam antibiotics now rank among the most extensively varied chemical systems in the field of medicinal chemistry. Limited structural variations, encountered in the earliest penicillin fermentations, were extended slightly by the addition of side chain precursors to the fermentation mixtures, and considerably by the chemical manipulation of 6-aminopenicillanic acid (6-APA) and 7-aminocephalosporanic acid (7-ACA). More recently, the use of penicillin sulfoxides and other penicillin and cephalosporin derivatives as versatile synthetic intermediates have led to still broader structural changes, and to entirely new fused ring systems. The subsequent discoveries of the cephamycins, nocardicins, clavulanic acid, and thienamycin have continued the impetus for a high chemical investment in structural modifications. Thus for more than 30 years the β-lactam antibiotics have been subjected to chemical modification. As a result, each position on the penicillin and cephalosporin rings has undergone alteration, with the exception of the 4(5)-bridgehead nitrogen atom. An impression of the extent of this work can be gained from Table 15.2, which is an incomplete listing of modifications that have been described in publications and patents. Most are single substituent changes; in some cases two or more substituents were changed simultaneously. Most of the modifications were accomplished without major disruption to the essential ring systems. Some involved rearrangement of or addition to the dihydrothiazine-ring double bond; and in an important group of reactions the ring fused to the β-lactam was opened and reclosed to a new one, for example, the rearrangement of penicillins to cephalosporins described below. Adequate treatment of this vast amount of chemical work is a formidable task even for monographs devoted solely to the subject (114). Access to detailed reviews of appropriate segments of this field can be obtained through the monograph and the review articles referenced in this chapter. Only the basic manipulations that have contributed to the development of derivatives with important biological properties, especially

Table 15.2 Chemical Modifications of Penicillins (P) and Cephalosporins (C)

P = [penam ring: S1, C2 bearing $CH_3\alpha$ and $CH_3\beta$, C3, N4, C5, C6, C7=O] C = [cephem ring: S1, C2, C3 bearing CH_2A (3′), C4, N5, C6, C7, C8=O]

Position	From	To
1	S	SO, SO_2, $\overset{+}{S}CH_3$
2-P	$(CH_3)_2$	H_2
2-C	H_2	=CHSAr; H, OAc; H, CH_3; CH_3, H; =CH_2; Br, CH_2Br; H, CH_2SR; CH_2SR, H; =CHSR; =O
2-α, β	H	OAc, Br, OCH_3
3-C	CH_2OAc	CHO, CO_2H, (=CH_2), OH, OR, Cl, F, NH_2, NHCOOR
3′	OAc	H, OH, OCOR, OR, SR, NC_5H_4X, S_2O_3Na, N_3, NH_2, CN, SO_nCH_3, S(C=NH)NR_2, S(C=S)NR_2, S(CS)OR, SCOR, SO_2Ar, Br, $OCONH_2$, OCONHR, *S*-heterocycle, NCS, Ar, heterocycle
3P, 4C	CO_2H	H, CO_2R, CO_2CH_2OCOR, $CONH_2$, CO_2OCOR, CONHCH(R)CO_2H, CO_2SiR_3, CON_3, CH_2OH, CH_2CO_2H, $COCHN_2$, $COCH_2Cl$, CN, tetrazole
5P, 6C	H	C_6H_5, OCH_3
6-β-P, 7-β-C	RCONH	H, NH_2, R^1CONH, R^2N—CH=N, ArC=N, R_2N, RNH, RSO_2NH, R_2PONH, RNHCONH, RNHCSNH, ROCONH, RCOO, $RCOCH_2$, RCON(NH_2)
6-α-P, 7-α-C	H	CH_3, OCH_3, RCONH, NH_2, Cl, OH, OCOR, CH_2OH, CH_2Cl, CH_2F, CH_2NH_2, CH_2CH_2CN, SCH_3, CH_2COOCH_3, CH_3Ar, CO_2H, CH_2COAr, CH(OH)$(CH_3)_2$, $NHCOOC_2H_5$
7-P, 8-C	=O	=S

those relating to the clinical use of these antibiotics, are discussed here.

6.1 6(7)-Acyl Group Variations

Of the many structural variations that have been performed, the most important in terms of numbers and useful biological properties have been those involving the 6- and 7-acylamino side chains of the penicillins, cephalosporins, and cephamycins. Nearly all the 6(7)-position manipulations that have produced analogs with significant antibacterial activities have entailed the introduction of a new acyl group at this position—*de novo*, by direct interchange, or by hydrolysis to the amine followed by reacylation.

6.1.1 FERMENTATION. The fermentations that produce the major β-lactam antibiotics fall into two general categories: the so-called penicillin type (*Penicillium* spp.) and the cephalosporin type (*Cephalosporium acremonium*, *Streptomyces* spp.) (115). The penicillin-type fermentation is characterized by the production of a range of penicillin antibiotics having various nonpolar side chains through the utilization of appropriate precursors. When side chain precursors are limited, these fermentations also accumulate 6-APA and isopenicillin N (having the L-aminoadipic acid side chain). The formation of benzylpenicillin in fermentations containing corn steep liquor is due to the presence in this material of phenylacetic acid precursors (70, 116). These findings led to the early production and, in some cases, the isolation of a number of modified penicillins by the addition of other appropriate side-chain precursors to the fermentation mixture (117–119). Although this approach generates new penicillins, it is severely limited in the type of side chain that can be introduced. Only derivatives with an unsubstituted methylene adjacent to the amide carbonyl, that is, monosubstituted acetamides, are obtained (120). It does allow limited introduction of side chains with ring substituents that can be converted to new chemical entities. For example, *p*-nitrobenzylpenicillin can be obtained by fermentation and hydrogenerated to *p*-aminobenzylpenicillin (penicillin T) (119). The more important penicillins that have been produced by precursor addition are included in Table 15.3, viz., analogs with side chains derived from phenylacetic acid (penicillin G), phenoxyacetic acid (penicillin V), and allylthioacetic acid (penicillin O).

The cephalosporin-type fermentations (*C. acremonium*, *Streptomyces* spp.) yield penicillin N (having the D-aminoadipic acid side chain) as the sole penicillin, but they give rise to a number of cephalosporins and cephamycins (Table 15.4). These fermentations display a greater versatility in the elaboration of other substituents on the fused rings, especially at the 3- and 7α-positions; since; however; they are insensitive to the addition of 7-acyl side chain precursors, the penicillin, cephalosporins, and cephamycins that are produced invariably have the D-aminoadipic acid group at the 7β-position (115). Thus in the early stages of the development of the cephalosporins, many attempts were made to produce modified analogs by direct fermentation, but they were uniformly unsuccessful. These failures, and the narrow limitations encountered in the variation of the penicillin structure through fermentation, resulted in the development of alternative methods for doing this that turned out to have significantly greater versatility.

Although it was surely present in earlier fermentations, the occurrence of 6-APA was first described in 1959 by Batchelor, Doyle, Nayler, and Rolinson (84), and it constituted a major breakthrough in penicillin structure modification. The discovery of this substance resulted from the observation that fermentation mixtures to which no side chain precursor was

Table 15.3 Biosynthetic Penicillins

Name	US Designation	British Designation	Side Chain
2-Pentenylpenicillin	F	I	$CH_3CH_2CH{=}CHCH_2$—
Pentylpenicillin	Dihydro F	Dihydro I	$CH_3(CH_2)_4$—
Heptylpenicillin	K	IV	$CH_3(CH_2)_6$—
Benzylpenicillin	G	II	$C_6H_5CH_2$—
p-Hydroxybenzylpenicillin	X	III	HO—$C_6H_4CH_2$—
D-4-Amino-4-carboxybutyl-penicillin	N[a]	—	D-HO_2C—$CH(NH_2)(CH_2)_3$—
L-4-Amino-4-carboxybutyl-penicillin	Iso-N	—	L-HO_2C—$CH(NH_2)(CH_2)_3$—
Phenoxymethylpenicillin	V	—	$C_6H_5OCH_2$—
Butylthiomethylpenicillin	—	BT	$C_4H_6SCH_2$—
Allylthiomethylpenicillin	O	AT	$CH_2{=}CHCH_2SCH_2$—
4-Carboxybutylpenicillin	—	—	$HOCO(CH_2)_4$—
p-Aminobenzylpenicillin	T	—	*p*-NH_2—$C_6H_4CH_2$—
p-Nitrobenzylpenicillin	—	—	*p*-NO_2—$C_6H_4CH_2$—

[a] Also known as Cephalosporin N and Synnematin B.

added (the biosynthesis of *p*-aminobenzylpenicillin was being studied) gave consistently higher results when assayed chemically than when assayed by biological methods. This suggested that there was a substance present in the fermentation that resembled penicillin chemically but was much less active biologically. it was suspected that this was 6-APA. Phenylacetylation followed by biological assay resulted in a dramatic increase in activity, supporting this supposition; this was verified by isolation and chemical studies (84, 85). Actually, 6-aminopenicillanic acid (then called "penicin") appears to have been produced earlier by Sakaguchi and Murao (131, 132), who had studied what appeared to be the deacylation and subsequent further decomposition of benzylpenicillin by penicillin acylases. Before the work by Batchelor and his colleagues, however, the significance of these studies had escaped general attention.

Before the consistent differences between the penicillin- and cephalosporin-type fermentations were fully recognized, many attempts were made to produce 7-ACA directly by fermentation. In view of the insensitivity of the cephalosporin-type fermentations to side chain precursors, it is not surprising that 7-ACA has not been obtained as a product of these fermentations.

6.1.2 ENZYMATIC CLEAVAGE. The direct fermentation of 6-APA in media deficient in side chain precursors is hampered by poor yields and difficult isolation procedures. It has been replaced by processes based on the chemical or enzymatic removal of the acyl group, usually from benzylpenicillin or phenoxymethylpenicillin. Penicillin acylases are produced by many living organisms including bacteria, fungi, and mammals (hog kidney acylase). They differ in the type of penicillin that can serve as substrate. Those derived from actinomycetes and filamentous fungi generally hydrolyze aliphatic and phenoxymethyl penicillins, but they split benzylpenicillin only slowly. Those of bacterial origin, for example, from the genera *Escherichia* and *Alcaligenes*, readily remove the phenylacetic acid side chain from benzylpenicillin, but they hydrolyze phenoxymethylpenicillin poorly. Some of these enzymes are bound to the cellular material, others are found mainly in the culture broths. Whole cell systems, as well as extracellular enzyme preparations in various stages of purification, have been used. The preparation and use of these penicillin acylases have been reviewed (133). Because of the structural similarities, one might expect the enzymatic methods that were used successfully to generate 6-APA to be applicable to the production of the analogous 7-ACA. However, as with the attempts to produce modified cephalosporins by direct fermentation, various attempts to find microorganisms, plant or animal tissues, or enzymes that could produce 7-ACA by cleavage of cephalosporin C (134–137) were unsuccessful. This failure to cleave off the cephalosporin C side chain by enzymes that readily remove the acyl groups from a variety of penicillins is notable. The complete lack of activity is attributable to the D-aminoadipic acid moiety rather than the cephalosporin nucleus, since synthetically introduced phenylacetyl and other nonpolar side chains are readily removed from the cephalosporin nucleus by penicillin acylases that are incapable of splitting cephalosporin C (138).

6.1.3 CHEMICAL CLEAVAGE. The inability to produce either modified cephalosporins or 7-ACA by biochemical techniques led to the production of 7-ACA from cephalosporin C by chemical means. Cephalosporin C, because of its moderate acid stability, can be hydrolyzed by dilute acid at room temperature (3 days) to 7-ACA in 0.6% yield (139). A slight improvement is realized if the side chain amino group is protected, for example, by attaching a 2,4-dinitrophenyl group (140) or by incorporating it into a hydantoin ring (141). Cleavage in 40–50% yields has been reported when diesters of cephalosporin C are allowed to stand in nonaqueous acetic acid or inert solvents for 4–20 days (142). The second ester group must then be cleaved to produce 7-ACA. None of these procedures represents a feasible method for producing 7-ACA in quantity.

The first practical chemical process for removing the side chain from cephalosporin C to give 7-ACA, developed by Morin et al. (14), is based on a peculiar property of the aminoadipamido group. Diazotization of the side chain amino group results in loss of nitrogen and intramolecular reaction of the derived carbonium ion with the amide carbonyl group (Fig. 15.5). This produces the cyclic iminolactone 15.**22.** In aqueous solution this imine hydrolyzes, and the resulting 7-ACA is destroyed by diazotization of the 7-amino group and loss of nitrogen. When formic acid is used as the solvent instead of water, and nitrosyl chloride is substituted for nitrous acid, hydrolysis of the imino ether can be delayed until the excess nitrosating agent is removed. This reduces the secondary diazotization of the 7-amino group, allowing yields of 7-ACA to be obtained. Addition of cosolvents such as acetonitrile or nitroparaffins to the reaction mixture results in higher yields (143).

This reaction provided the early means for the manufacture of semisynthetic cephalosporins. However a newer, extremely versatile chemical sequence is now also used that is not dependent on side chain cyclization and is capable of removing various acyl groups from both the penicillins and the cephalosporins (Fig. 15.5). In fact, it was originally developed for converting penicillins to 6-APA. The method, which allows the selective cleavage of the secondary amide linkage of the side chain without attack of the tertiary amide of the β-lactam ring, is based on the conversion of the side chain amide group to an

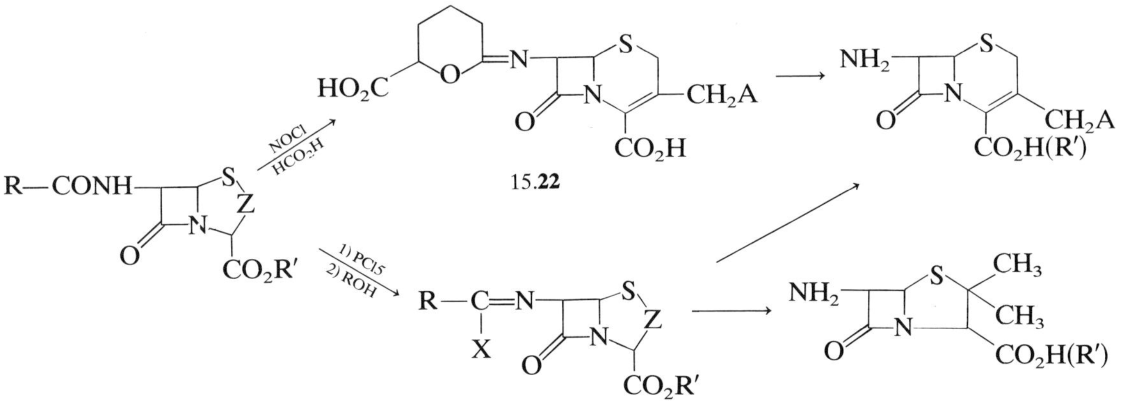

15.**23a,b**

Penicillins: R = $C_6H_5CH_2$, $C_6H_5OCH_2$; Z = —$C(CH_3)_2$
Cephalosporins: R = $R'O_2CCH(NH_2)(CH_2)_3$; Z = =$C(CH_2A)CH_2$—
R' = $Si(CH_3)_3$, $CH_2C_6H_4NO_2$, CH_2CCl_3; A = H, OAc, S-Het, etc.
X = Cl, OCH_3

Fig. 15.5 Chemical cleavage of 6(7)-acyl groups from penicillins and cephalosporins.

imino chloride (15.**23a,** X = Cl) using phosphorous pentachloride. This intermediate reacts readily with an alcohol to form the corresponding imino ether (15.**23b**, X = OR), which hydrolyzes on contact with water to the amine and the side chain acid ester (144). It is necessary to protect the carboxyl group before this reaction sequence is carried out. Benzyl esters were used initially, but it was found that silyl esters are the nearly ideal choice for this (145). They have sufficient chemical stability to allow the chemical manipulations described to be carried out in their presence, and they hydrolyze under conditions that are sufficiently mild to avoid opening of the β-lactam ring, in this case during the reaction workup that hydrolyzes the imino ether. Other agents have been used to convert the side chain carboxamide grouping to an imino ether (133).

When used to convert cephalosporin C to 7-ACA, this process is complicated by the presence of an amino and two carboxyl groups in the molecule. Fortunately, the use of silylation to protect the carboxyls allows the reaction with phosphorus pentachloride to be carried out without further protection of the amine. Indeed, the reported yields for removing the side chain using this sequence are significantly better than those reported for the nitrosyl chloride process. A considerable number of other groups for protecting the carboxyl and amino functions were investigated before and after the development of the silylation-based process (133).

Both the nitrosyl chloride and the phosphorous pentachloride procedures are applicable to the removal of the 7-acyl group on cephalosporins in which the acetoxy group of cephalosporin C has been displaced by one of a number of nucleophilic agents.

6.1.4 REACYLATION: SEMISYNTHETIC PENICILLINS AND CEPHALOSPORINS. The availability of 6-APA and 7-ACA removed the restrictions on the types of 6- or 7- side chain derivatives that can be obtained. Although the primary amino group can be reacted with many chemical reagents, the acylation of this group with carboxylic acids has been the most widely studied. The acylations can be accomplished using a variety of agents. In addition to acid chlorides and mixed anyhydrides, free carboxylic acids can be coupled using *N,N*-dicyclohexylcarbodiimide or a similar condensing agent. Activated esters with *N*-hydroxysuccinimide, *N*-hydroxyphthalimide and nitrophenols, cyclic anhydrides of amino acids, and other acylating agents commonly used in peptide synthesis can be employed as well. Direct coupling of acids to 6-APA has also been accomplished by enzymatic assistance achieved by reversing (through control of the pH) the penicillin acylase systems that split the penicillins (146, 147). Several less conventional methods for introducing desired acyl groups on the 6(7)-positions have also been described. These include direct acylation of benzylpenicillin iminochloride esters (15.**23a**, X = Cl) to give a diacyl derivative, followed by selective removal of the phenylacetyl group with thiophenolate (148). Alternatively, 6-APA esters have been converted to their 6-isocyanato analogs by treatment with phosgene and the isocyanate group is reacted with an appropriate organometallic compound (Grignard reagent) or side chain acid (—CO_2) to give the 6-acylamino derivative (149).

Many penicillins and cephalosporins of biological interest (e.g,, ampicillin, carbenicillin, cephalexin, cephamandole) have acylamino side chains with reactive substituents, notably amino, carboxyl, and hydroxyl groups. The acids used to prepare these antibiotics require the prior attachment of protective groupings capable of being removed without destruction of the β-lactam ring. Amino group snythons include benzyloxycarbonylamino (150), azide (151), *t*-butoxycarbonylamino (152, 153), Schiff bases from *o*-hydroxy aromatic aldehydes (2-hydroxy-1-naphthaldehyde) (154), and amine adducts with β-diketones, β-ketoamides and, especially, β-ketoesters (Dane salts) (155). The simple amine hydrochloride can be used when the side chain acid is activated as the acid chloride. Carboxyl protective groups include the benzyl, phenyl, 2,2,2-trichloroethyl, and simple aliphatic esters. Carbenicillin can be made using the mono or bis acid chloride of phenylmalonic acid; this is accompanied by some decarboxylation. The hydroxyl group has been protected as the formic acid (156) and dichloroacetic acid (157) esters and as the *O*-carboxyanhydride when the hydroxyl group is on the α-carbon atom. Acylations using acids with phenolic hydroxyls can be carried out without prior protection of the hydroxyl group. Many other protective groups are described in recent reviews on the penicillins and the cephalosporins (158, 114).

Some caution is required in the acylation 7-ACA, since under certain conditions (e.g., acid anhydrides and tertiary bases such as pyridine) double-bond isomerization to the Δ_2-isomer accompanies the acylation (159) (see below).

The 6- and 7-amino groups have also been converted to a wide variety of other acyl substituents, for example, ureas, thioureas, carbamates, acylureas, imides, sulfonamides, and phosphonyl and thionophosphonyl amides. The many other reactions used to convert the amino group to 6- and 7-substituents other than amides are discussed in a later section.

6.1.5 SEMISYNTHETIC CEPHAMYCINS. Acyl group variation on the cephamycins implies removal of the aminoadipic acid side chain and reacylation of the 7-amino function. However the presence of a geminal methoxy group raises the question of stability with respect to retention of these functional groups on the β-lactam ring. Surprisingly, 7α-methoxy-7β-amino analogs have sufficient stability to allow their isolation and acylation upon synthesis from 7-aminocephalosporanic acid derivatives under the conditions described in Section 6.4. However these structures are not stable enough to permit removal of the 7-acyl group from the natural analogs by the methods used for converting cephalosporin

C to 7-ACA. Thus when the imidoyl chloride from 7α-methoxy *N*-phthaloylcephalosporin C dibenzhydryl ester was treated with methanol and then water under conditions that produce 7-ACA in good yield, very little 7β-amino-7α-methoxy cephalosporanic acid benzhydryl ester was observed (160). If pyridine and phenoxyacetyl chloride were added before the water, 40% yield of the expected 7-phenoxyacetamido derivative was obtained, but the product was a mixture (1:2) of the 7α- and 7β-methoxy epimers. Semisynthetic cephamycins can be prepared without epimerization by reacting *N*-acyl (e.g., trichloroethoxycarbonyl or BOC) cephamycin diesters (e.g., benzhydryl) with acid chlorides in the presence of *N*-tri-methylsilytrifluroacetamide (in methylene chloride) to form 7-(*N*-protected aminoadipoyl-7-acyl imides. Removal (zinc and acetic acid or trifluoroacetic acid) of the *N*-acyl protecting group results in the loss of the aminoadipoyl group by way of cyclization to the lactam (benzhydryl 2-piperidone-6-carboxylate), and the semisynthetic cephamycin (ester) is obtained (161, 162).

6.2 3-Substituent Variations by Displacement of the Acetoxy Group

The scope of natural variation at the 3-position of the cephalosporin molecule, although broader than the single D-adipamido group at the 7-position, is still relatively narrow (Table 15.4). In spite of this, the second major locus of variation on the cephalosporins has been the side chain at the 3-position. Cephalosporin C has served as the primary source of cephalosporins with functionalization on the 3-substituent. Its natural 3-acetoxymethyl group is retained in a number of clinically important cephalosporins, but this substituent has also been converted to many other structures including several that are important clinically (methyl, carbamloxymethyl, alkoxymethyl, heterocyclicthiomethyl, pyridiniummethyl, alkoxy, and chloro) and many others that are of less

Table 15.4 Naturally Occurring Cephalosporins and Cephamycins

D-$HO_2CCH(NH_2)CH_2CH_2CH_2CONH$– [cephem nucleus: 7-X, 6-H, S, N, C=O, CO_2H, CH_2A]

Name	X	A	References
Cephalosporin C	H	$OCOCH_3$	10, 93
Deacetylcephalosporin C	H	OH	121, 122
Deacetoxycephalosporin C	H	H	123
—	H	$OCONH_2$	104
—	H	SCH_3	124
Cephamycin A	OCH_3	$OCOC(OCH_3){=}CHC_6H_4OSO_2OH(p)$	125–128
Cephamycin B	OCH_3	$OCOC(OCH_3){=}CHC_6H_4OH(p)$	125–128
Takeda C2801X	OCH_3	$OCOC(OCH_3){=}CHC_6H_3(OH)_2(m, p)$	129
Cephamycin C	OCH_3	$OCONH_2$	104, 125–128)
7α-Methoxycephalosporin C	OCH_3	$OCOCH_3$	104
—	OCH_3	H	130

biological interest. The easy displacement of the allylic acetoxy group from the natural acetoxymethyl side chain by nitrogen and sulfur nucleophiles (163) has provided access to many of these modified substituents. The early generation of the 3-pyridiniummethyl substituent (cephalosporin C_A, 15.**21**) through contact with warm pyridine acetate buffer used to elute cephalosporin C from ion exchange columns was mentioned earlier (164). This observation led to the important clinical cephalosporin analog cephaloridine and initiated other acetate displacement studies using many different nucleophiles.

The displacement of the 3′-acetoxy group tends to follow S_N1 kinetics. It does not occur with oxygen nucleophiles; it goes only very slowly with the corresponding cephalosporin sulfoxides, and not at all with the 4-carboxylic acid esters (and lactones). The 4-carboxylate group does not attack the 3-methylene during the displacement by nucleophiles to give the lactone. These characteristics, and the ease with which the displacement reactions occur, have been explained in terms of resonance stabilization through the dihydrothiazine ring and the carboxylate ion (15.**24**) (165, 166).

Nitrogen nucleophiles used to displace the 3′-acetoxy group include many substituted and unsubstituted pyridines, quinolines, pyrimidines, triazoles, pyrazoles, azide, and even aniline and methylaniline if the pH is controlled at 7.5 (164, 165, 167–172). Sulfur nucleophiles used in the displacement are legion, including alkyl thiols (*SR*), thiosulfate (S_2O_3Na), thio and dithio acids, carbamates and carbonates, thioureas, thioamides, and most important biologically, heterocyclic thiols (see Section 9).

In addition to simple displacement, certain bidentate nucleophiles react in a more complex manner. For example, with pyridine-2-thione, displacement of the acetoxy group by the sulfur atom is followed by an internal Michael addition of the pyridine nitrogen atom to the double bond with the formation of a spirocyclic derivative (165, 173).

In going from the fermentation-derived cephalosporin C to 3-substituted cephalosporins with significant antibacterial activities, it is sometimes necessary, of course, to replace the side chains at both the 7- and the 3′-positions. It is possible to carry out the reactions that achieve these conversions (acyl side chain removal, reacylation, displacement of the acetoxy group) in any of the several possible orders. For example, the acetate displacement reaction can be carried out on cephalosporin C, 7-aminocephalosporanic acid, or the appropriate 7-acylaminocephalosporanic acid.

6.3 3-Methyl Analogs: Conversion of Penicillins to Cephalosporins

Only a few cephalosporins are known to be efficiently absorbed when administered orally. The two clinical agents with the best absorption characteristics are derivatives of 7-amino-3′-deactoxycephalosporanic acid (7-ADCA), which has a methyl group at the 3-position. Deacetoxycephalosporin C has recently been identified as a constituent of product mixtures from cephalosporin-type fermentations (Table 15.4), but the

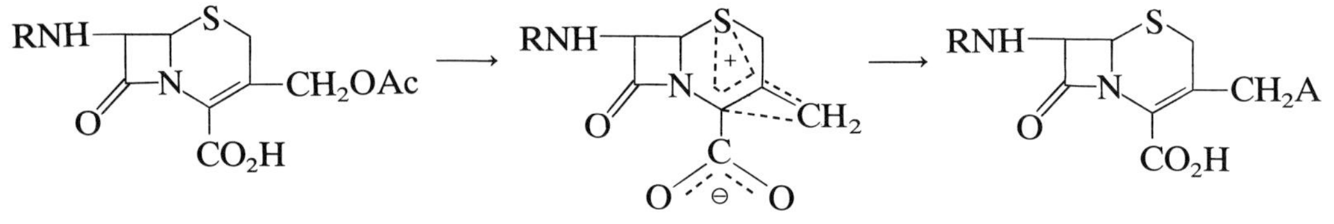

15.**24**

commercial 3-methyl analogs are not derived from this source. Deacetoxycephalosporins can be prepared by catalytic hydrogenolysis of the 3-acetoxymethyl cephalosporins (174, 3, 152). The reaction goes in moderate yield and requires relatively large amounts of noble metal catalyst (palladium). The hydrogenation conditions have been modified to achieve better yields (175), but these cephalosporins are more economically derived from penicillins by way of a ring expansion reaction. The latter reaction utilizes penicillin sulfoxides, which are readily obtained by oxidation of the penicillins or their carboxylic acid esters using reagents such as sodium metaperiodate, hydrogen peroxide, or organic peracids (176–179). The penicillins carrying an acylamino group on the 6-position normally give only the *S*-sulfoxide; the amide side chain directs the approach of the oxidant to the more hindered side of the ring sulfur atom. The less stable *R*-isomer can be obtained using analogs without hydrogen on the 6-position nitrogen atom as discussed later (180, 181). Not surprisingly, the sulfoxide configurations play a role in the course of these rearrangement reactions (181, 182).

The skeletal equivalence of the penicillins and cephalosporins was mentioned earlier. The conversion of the penicillanic acid to the cephalosporanic acid structure requires insertion of one of the *gem*-dimethyl groups on the penam ring into the thiazolidine ring to give the cepham ring system, generation of a double bond, and conversion of the second methyl group to a higher oxidation state by addition of an acetoxy group. In a reaction designed to introduce an acetoxy group (most likely at C-5), Morin and his colleagues treated penicillin V sulfoxide methyl ester (Fig. 15.6; 15.**25**, $R=C_6H_5OCH_2$, $R'=CH_3$) with acetic anhydride under the normal Pummerer conditions. No reaction occurred. However upon refluxing the sulfoxide with acetic anhydride, two new β-lactam-containing products were obtained in 60% yield, along with three minor products that no longer contained the β-lactam ring (3, 183). The products of interest (ratio 2:1) were the 2-β-acetoxymethylpenam (15.**26,** $R=C_6H_5OCH_2$, $R'=CH_3$) and the 3-β-acetoxycepham (15.**27,** $R=C_6H_5OCH_2$, $R'=CH_3$, $X=COCH_3$). When treated with triethylamine, the latter lost acetic acid and gave 7-phenoxyacetamino-deacetoxycephalosporanic acid methyl ester (15.**28**, $R=C_6H_5OCH_2$, $R'=CH_3$). When

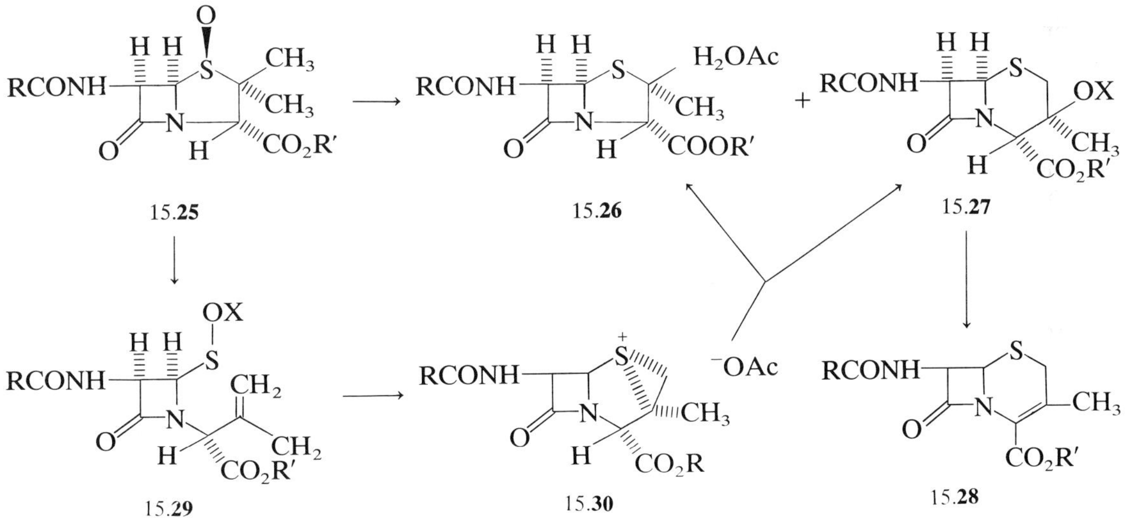

Fig. 15.6 Conversion of penicillin sulfoxides to deacetoxycephalosporins.

heated in toluene with a trace of *p*-toluensulfonic acid, the starting penicillin sulfoxide ester (15.**25**) gave this deacetoxycephalosporanic acid ester directly, in moderate yield. This reaction, carried out before the biological utility of the deactoxycephalosporins had been recognized, was of interest because it provided the first chemical correlation between the penicillin and cephalosporin structures. The identical cephalosporin (15.**28**) was obtained by hydrogenolysis of 7-phenoxyacetamidocephalosporanic acid methyl ester, establishing the correlation. Since this compound class has increased in commercial importance, the conversion described has been studied intensively and improved, so that it is now the primary industrial route to 7-ADCA and the deacetoxycephalosporins, cephalexin, and cephradine.

Although benzylpenicillin and phenoxymethylpenicillin are logical starting materials from an economic standpoint, the thiazolidine–dihydrothiazine ring expansion is quite general; thus these side chains can be replaced by other appropriate acylamino groups before conversion to the cephalosporins. Catalysts other than *p*-toluenesulfonic acid are also effective in accomplishing this rearrangement (184–186); the use of pyridine phosphate buffer in dioxane allows conversions on the order of 90% (185). In most cases (exception: sulfuric acid), decarboxylation occurs if the ring carboxyl group is not esterified. Easily removable groupings used for protecting the carboxyl include 2,2,2-trichloroethyl, *p*-nitrobenzyl, and trimethylsilyl. An interesting process uses excess silylating agent in the presence of organic amines to protect the carboxyl group and catalyze the ring expansion as well (186).

The mechanism of this ring expanison has been studied extensively (187–190); and it has been reviewed at length (191, 192). The original postulates of Morin (183) have been supported by subsequent studies of others. The reaction is believed to follow the sequence outlined in Fig. 15.6. Thermal opening of the penicillin sulfoxide ring is thought to occur through a reversible six-electron electrocyclic rearrangement, with the formation of a sulfenic acid by abstraction of an adjacent *cis*-methyl group hydrogen and formation of a double bond (15.**29**, X = H) (188, 190). Evidence of this equilibrium was provided by the formation of a deuterated β-methyl group when a penicillin sulfoxide ester was heated in the presence of D_2O (190). The initial step is accompanied or followed by formation of a reactive sulfenic acid derivative, e.g., by reaction with acetic anhydride in the sequence that was carried out originally (15.**29**, X = $COCH_3$). Evidence that this is a stepwise process with loss of the chirality of the sulfur atom has been presented by Cooper et al. (182). The mixed anhydride so formed converts the sulfur from a good nucleophile to an electrophile. This undergoes S_N^2 displacement by the olefinic double bond to form the episulfonium ion pair indicated in structure 15.**30**. It is the geometry of this episulfonium ion that controls the stereochemistry of the products (182). Opening of the episulfonium intermediate by the accompanying anion gives the functionalized penam (15.**26**) or cepham (15.**27**) by way of kinetic and thermodynamic control, respectively.

The sequential double application of these interconversions to produce 3-acetoxymethylcephalosporins fails in the more obvious approach, but a more complex successful route using these reactions has been described (189). A more promising method for converting penicillins to cephalosporins with functional groups on the 3-methylene, including acetoxy, involves rupture of the 1,2-carbon to sulfur bond of the penam ring system and trapping of the olefinic intermediate by incorporating the sulfur into a grouping that is more stable than the sulfenic acid mixed

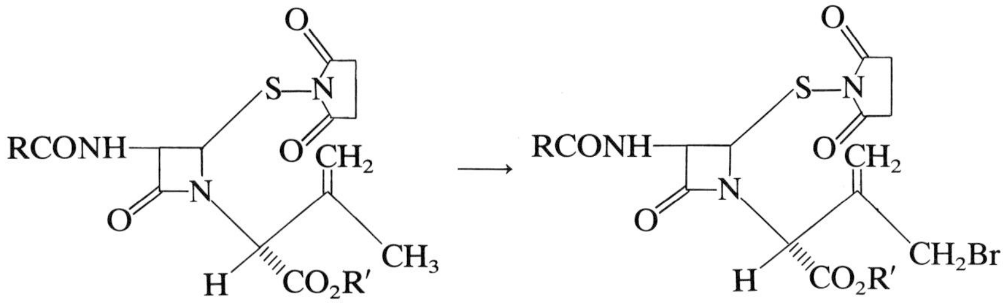

15.**31** → 15.**32**

anhydrides. Important intermediates of this type are the sulfenimides represented by 15.**31**. These substances undergo photolylic bromination of the methyl group, and the resulting bromomethyl derivatives (15.**32**) readily undergo allylic displacement by various nucleophiles. Removal of the imide moiety using an alkali metal or ammonium ion is reported to produce 3′-substituted cephalosporins in good yield (193).

The original demonstration of structural equivalence by chemical conversion of a penicillin to a cephalosporin (3), and the ring-opening reactions that resulted from this original discovery have led ultimately to the converse of the original sequence, viz., the conversion of a cephalosporin to a penicillin (194), though not a naturally occurring analog.

6.4 7α-Methoxylations: Cephamycins

Methods for replacing the α-aminoadipoyl side chain of the natural cephamycins with other acyl groups are discussed in Section 6.1. The limitations placed on these methods by the *gem*-aminomethoxy groups and the ready availability of the unmethoxylated cephalosporins have led to several methods for the stereospecific introduction of a methoxyl group into the 7α-position of cephalosporins. The first method reported involved the addition of bromine azide to benzyl-7-diazocephalosporanate to give the 7-azido-7-bromo adduct (15.**33** X, Y = N_3, Br) which, when reacted with silver fluoroborate in methanol, formed the 7β-azido-7α-methoxy cephalosporanate. Reduction of the azide, acylation, and removal of the benzyl group gave the desired 7α-methoxy cephalosporins (195). Several additional methods, developed subsequently, incorporate the addition of methanol from the less hindered α-face of a Schiff base anion at the 7-position. For example, the anion from 15.**34** (Z = C_6H_5CH) reacts with methyl methylthiosulfonate ($CH_3SSO_2CH_3$) to give the 7-methylthio derivative (15.**33**; X = SCH_3, Y = $C_6H_5CH{=}N$). Hydrolysis of the Schiff base and treatment of the amine with mercuric chloride in methanol gives the 7β-amino-7α-methoxy derivative (196). This anion can also be converted to the 7-bromo compound (NBS) that reacts with methanol in the presence of silver oxide to give the 7α-methoxy cephalosporin (197). Alternatively, the cephalosporin 7-acylamino side chain can be oxidized to an acylimine 15.**35** (Z = RCO) using *t*-butyl hypochlorite in methanol (containing lithium methoxide) with immediate capture of the solvent (198). In a parallel manner the Schiff base 15.**35**

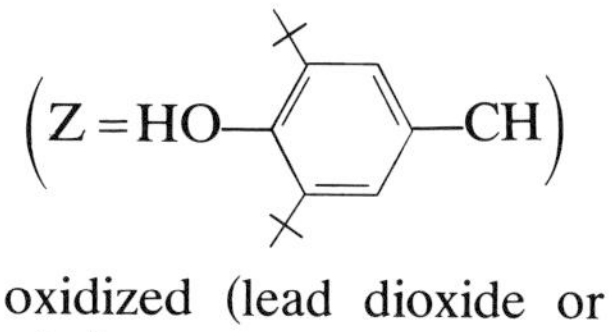

(Z = HO–[3,5-di-*t*-butylphenyl]–CH)

can be oxidized (lead dioxide or *t*-butyl hypochlorite) to the quinoidal compound 15.**35**

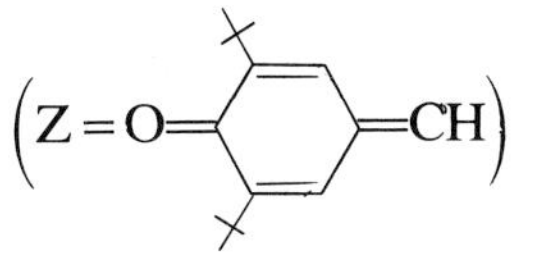

(Z = O=[quinonoid ring]=CH)

followed by addition of methanol (199).

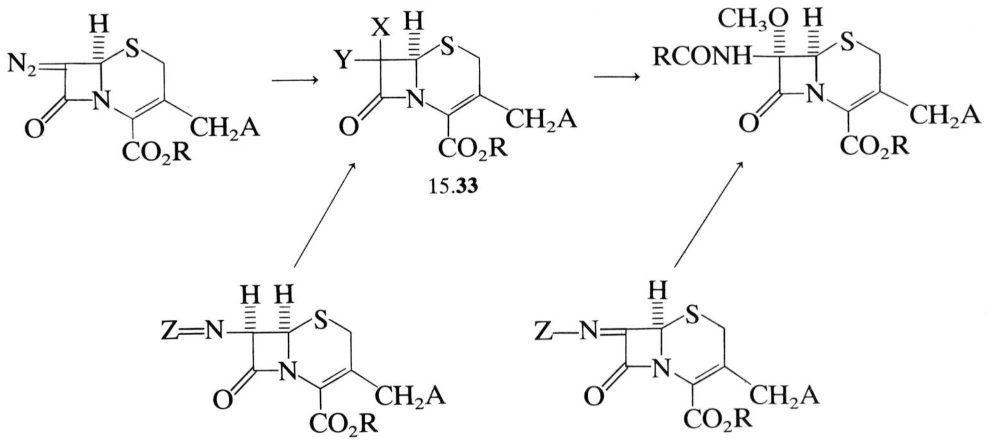

15.33

15.34

15.35

Two additional sequences proceed through imino structure 15.**35**. One starts with cephalosporins having an α-haloacetamido side chain at the 7-position, which after conversion to the imino chloride with PCl_5 (15.**34**); Z = RCHXCCl) undergoes a 1,4-elimination of hydrogen halide to give 15.**35** (Z = RCH═CCl). Addition of methanol to this imine gives a ketenime (15.**33**, Y = RCH═CHN, X = OCH_3)(200). A similar approach employs bromination of a 7-vinylidenamino cephalosporin with subsequent addition of methoxide (201).

7 STRUCTURE AND BIOLOGICAL PROPERTIES

Most of the chemical work on the β-lactam antibiotics has as the ultimate goal the discovery of agents that are suitable for clinical use. The first criterion for clinical effectiveness is the ability of the antibiotic to inhibit, and preferably kill, bacteria at acceptable concentrations of the drug (*in vitro* activity). But the behavior of the drug in the animal or human body is equally important. It must be nontoxic at the required dosage, and it must be capable of being transported from the site of administration to the site of infection, achieving a concentration greater than that required to inhibit the pathogenic organism. Thus an examination of structure-activity relationships requires the inclusion of pharmacokinetic characteristics as well as the *in vitro* activities of the antibiotics under study. Such studies may include laboratory-determined properties such as *in vitro* and *in vivo* antibacterial activities [minimum inhibitory concentrations (MIC), minimum bactericidal concentrations (MBC), maximum tolerated doses (MTD) and protective effectiveness (PD_{50}) in laboratory animals], serum levels (peak and duration, by parenteral and oral routes), tissue distribution, urinary excretion, metabolic products, serum and tissue binding, serum and tissue inactivation (e.g., MICs in the presence and absence of serum), and biliary excretion. The ability to resist inactivation by the target organism (effect of inoculum size, resistance to β-lactamases) is also important. Obviously, it is not possible to compare all such properties of all analogs. Thus the comparisons of structure-activity relationships that follow are, of necessity, not comprehensive but are organized around compounds and properties that are representative of general trends, or are of particular (clinical) interest. More complete data can be found in the original and review articles cited here.

Before considering the specific structure-activity relationships (SARs) and pharmacokinetic properties of the penicillins, cephalosporins, and the like, it may be instructive to examine the basic structural features that appear to be associated with the intrinsic antibacterial activities of these substances. Until recently, the SAR data suggested that the minimum requirements for significant antibacterial activity could be summarized by structure 15.**36**. These data

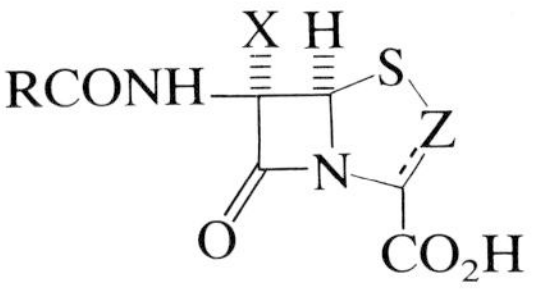

15.**36**

indicated the need for a fused ring to confer a degree of strain on the β-lactam. The requirement of the sulfur atom was assumed, but untested. The penicillins and cephalosporins (3-cephems) appear to be optimal in this respect, equipping the β-lactam ring with a high level of chemical reactivity, but retaining sufficient stability to survive the biological environment of the host. The isomeric 2-cephems were found to have a low level of antibacterial activity (159, 202). This property was attributed to a lower degree of strain on the β-lactam ring (203). Studies have been carried out that associate the level of antibacterial activity with β-lactam ring strain, reflected in the infrared absorption stretching frequency of the β-lactam carbonyl group (183).

The carboxyl group requirement is supported by the synthesis of many poorly active or inactive penicillin and cephalosporin derivatives with substituents other than this grouping at the 3(4)-positions. The single known exceptions are the penicillins and cephalosporins with a tetrazole ring at this position, described in Section 10.1. Similarly the acylamino group requirement is reinforced by many penicillin, cephalosporin, and cephamycin SAR studies. Exceptions to this requirement are penicillins in which the acylamino side chain is replaced by an amidine structure (15.**37**) (mecillinam). As mentioned else-

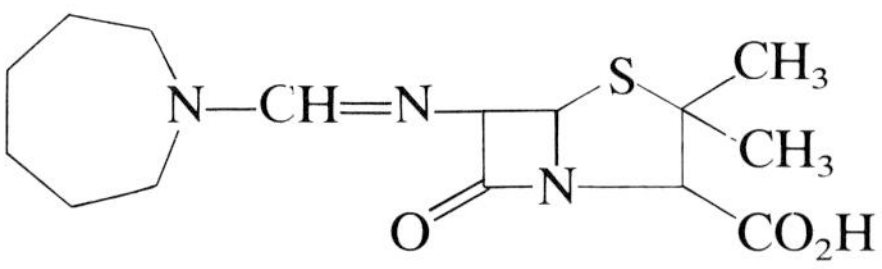

15.**37**

where, these derivatives interfere with cell wall synthesis, but they appear to have a mechanism of inhibition different from that of the 6-acylaminopenams. Some β-lactam-containing structures described recently further restrict 15.**36** as the synoptic structure associated with antibacterial activity. Semisynthetic and totally synthetic structures with new rings fused to the β-lactam, which display good antibacterial activities, indicate a lack of necessity for sulfur at the 1-position (15.**38**) (204), or carbon at the 2-position (15.**39**) (205). The

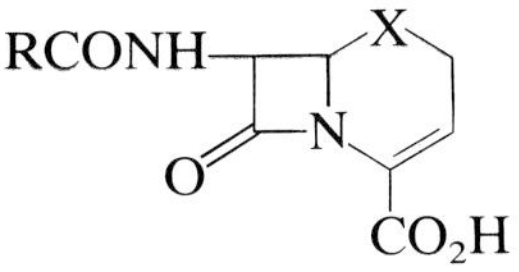

X = CH_2, O

15.**38**

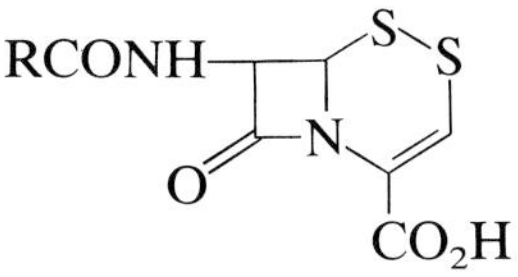

15.**39**

broad antibacterial activity of thienamycin violates the assumed requirement of the functionalized amino group in 15.**36**, but it supports the assumption that ring strain contributes to the level of biological activity observed. Conversely, the nocardicins would seem to negate the ring strain requirement for activity; but again, though the activity of the nocardicins appears to be directed at the cell wall, the activity observed differs in level and type from that exhibited by the bicyclic structures, and the specific location and mechanism of action are likely different.

8 THE PENICILLINS

Generally changes in the penicillin structure other than those involving the 6-acyl grouping have been unprofitable in terms of creating analogs with useful antibacterial activities. (Exceptions are the derivatives just discussed with a tetrazole ring in place of the carboxyl group and the 6-disubstituted amidino derivatives.) Indeed, the acyl groups that provide high levels of antibacterial activity fall within the relatively narrow structural limits of the carboxamides. Advantageous biological properties have not been observed with derivatives having other 6-acylamino structures such as sulfonamides (79), phosphonamides (206), imides (207), ureas (208, 209), and thioureas and urethanes (206). Most of the 6-acylamino groups of interest, though not all, are mono-or disubstituted acetic acid derivatives.

8.1 Biosynthetic Penicillins

Although 50 or so biosynthetic penicillins were obtained from unaided fermentations or through the addition of appropriate precursors, only three (penicillins G, V, and O) were ultimately produced commercially. Table 15.3 lists some of the more important of these early penicillins. Many of these penicillins (F, K, G, X) were similar in their *in vitro* antibacterial properties, but benzylpenicillin (G) was found to have superior activity *in vivo* and it was easier to manufacture on a large scale. Consequently, it attained a permanent place in clinical use, and it is still the one analog used most widely in the therapy of gram-positive infections. In general, it is an extremely nontoxic and safe chemotherapeutic agent. For example, the crystalline potassium or sodium salt can be given intramuscularly at levels of 1–7 g (2–12 million units; 1 mg of sodium benzylpenicillin = 1667 Oxford units) per day (meningococcal meningitis) or by continuous intravenous drip at levels of 3–12 g or more per day (enterococcal endocarditis). Because of rapid excretion through the kidney, and metabolic inactivation, the blood levels obtained by administering alkali metal salts of benzylpenicillin tend to fall off rapidly. After intramuscular injection, therapeutic serum levels usually last only about 3–6 hr. Salts with low aqueous solubilities allow intramuscular injection of large doses that persist for longer periods. The procaine salt of benzylpenicillin is the dosage form of this type most commonly used in clinical practice (210, 211). it is given intramuscularly at levels of 0.3–1.2 million units (0.2–0.8 g of penicillin) daily, and therapeutic levels persist for 8–12 hr. The benzathine (*N*, *N'*-dibenzylethylenediamine) salt is used in a similar manner (212). In an entirely different approach, higher and longer blood levels can be achieved by the concomitant administration of probenecid (4-carboxy-*N*, *N*-dipropylbenzenesulfonamide). This agent lowers the rate of excretion of the penicillin through the kidney.

In spite of its wide use, benzylpenicillin has a number of rather serious limitations. It has a narrow spectrum of activity (gram-positive bacteria) and it appears to be susceptible to all known β-lactamases. The allergic side effects (urticaria, anaphylaxis, etc.) associated with its use were mentioned earlier. Additionally, the geometry of the fused ring system suppresses the normal resonance of the β-lactam amide group. As a consequence, the β-lactam ring has a high chemical reactivity; on contact with alkali, penicilloic acids (15.**13**) are formed. Acid treatment results in rapid rearrangement to penillic acids (15.**41**, pH 2) and penicillenic acids (15.**42**, pH 4), with involvement of the side chain carbonyl (15.**40**) (203). Consequently, benzylpenicillin undergoes extensive degradation in the

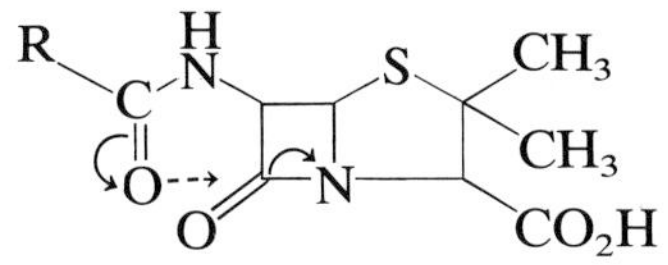

15.**40**

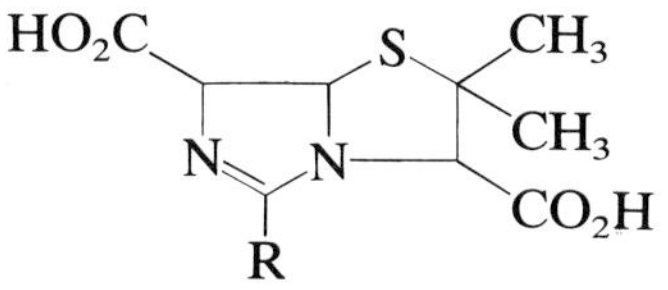

15.**41**

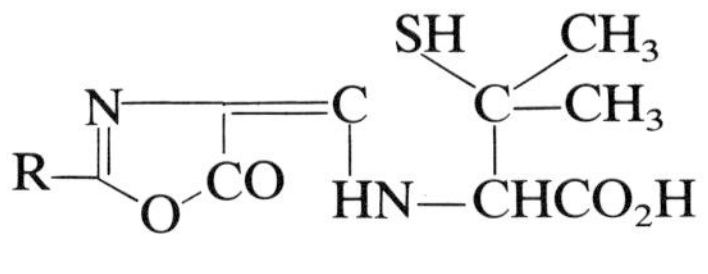

15.**42**

acidic milieu of the stomach. This results in erratic oral absorption and requires oral doses at least 5 times the recommended parenteral dose for therapeutic effectiveness (213).

Penicillins V and O were developed with the hope of overcoming some of these limitations. Penicillin O, originally considered to have a lower incidence of allergenic reactions associated with its use, is no longer manufactured. Phenoxymethylpenicillin (penicillin V) (119, 214) and other penicillins having a hetero atom on the α-carbon of the side chain, have better stability toward acids than has, for example, benzylpenicillin. The hetero atom apparently inhibits the participation of the side chain amide carbonyl in the electronic displacement that results in rearrangement to the penillic and penicillenic acids (215). The improved acid stability of phenoxymethylpenicillin results in a better resistance to inactivation by gastric fluids and, consequently, oral absorption is increased. The penicillinase susceptibility of this analog and its liability with respect to allergic side reactions are about equal to those of benzylpenicillin, and it is slightly less active *in vitro* than is benzylpenicillin. Nevertheless, because of its improved oral activity, it has enjoyed wide clinical use.

8.2 Semisynthetic Penicillins with Increased Acid Stability

The increased latitude in varying the acylamino side chain through the acylation of 6-APA resulted in more significant improvements in the biological properties of the derived penicillins, including greater penicillinase resistance and a broader spectrum of antibacterial activity. However the first semisynthetic penicillins to be prepared from 6-APA and studied in man were α-aryloxyalkylpenicillins (216). These are, obviously, analogs of phenoxymethylpenicillin, and they would be expected to share its advantages of increased acid stability and oral absorption. Three derivatives have been offered for clinical use: the next two higher homologs of penicillin V, phenethicillin and propicillin, and the α-phenyl analog, phenbenicillin (see Table 15.5). Claims for therapeutic superiority were based on *in vitro* activities very similar to those of phenoxymethylpenicillin, coupled with more efficient oral absorption resulting in blood levels that are higher and more prolonged than with the latter. For example, in one study 250 mg doses of the potassium salts of penicillin V, phenethicillin, and propicillin given in crossover studies to human volunteers resulted in 1 hr serum concentrations of 1.63, 5.26, and 6.22 μg/ml, respectively (217). These analogs were also shown to be slightly more resistant than penicillin V to low concentrations of penicillinase. With higher levels of the enzyme, these differences disappeared. Thus their advantage for treating mildly resistant staphylococcal infections is questionable. The more effective oral absorption is likewise offset to a large extent by

Table 15.5 Penicillins for Clinical Use

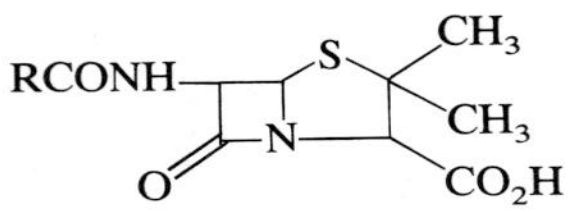

RCONH— (penam nucleus: S, N, O, CH_3, CH_3, CO_2H)

Generic Name	R	Generic Name	R
Narrow spectrum Benzylpenicillin	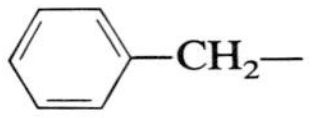 —CH_2—	Broad spectrum Ampicillin	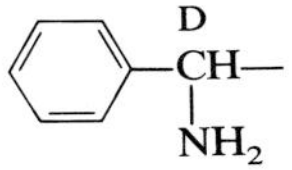 D —CH— NH_2
Phenoxymethylpenicillin	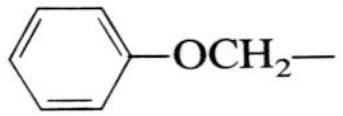 —OCH_2—	(Hetacillin, metampicillin) (Pivampicillin, talampicillin, bacampicillin)	(Side chain amine adducts) (Esters)
R′ Phenethicillin CH_3 Propicillin C_2H_5 Phenbenicillin C_6H_5	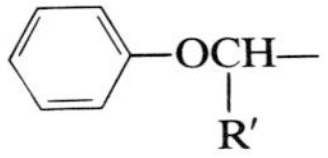 —OCH— R′	Amoxycillin	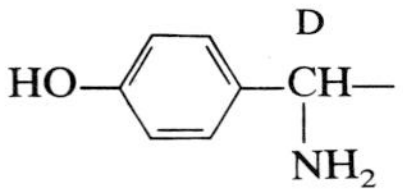 HO— D —CH— NH_2
β-Lactamase resistant Methicillin	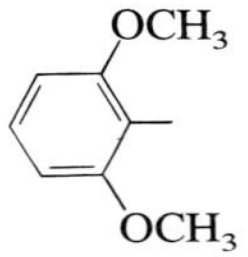 OCH_3 OCH_3	Epicillin	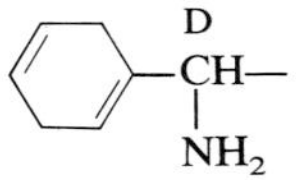 D —CH— NH_2
X Y Oxacillin H H Cloxacillin H Cl Dicloxacillin Cl Cl Flucloxacillin F Cl	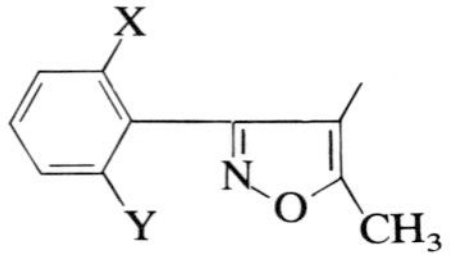 X Y N O CH_3	Broad spectrum—Narrow use Carbenicillin (and side chain esters)	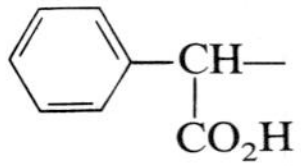 —CH— CO_2H
		Ticarcillin	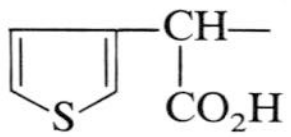 S —CH— CO_2H
Nafcillin	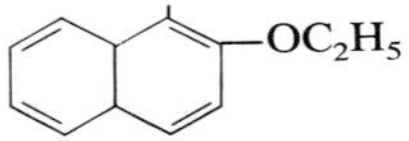 —OC_2H_5	Sulbenicillin	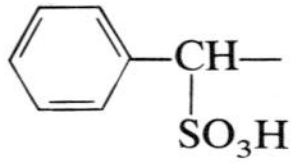 —CH— SO_3H
		Suncillin	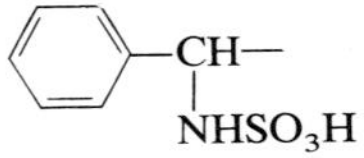 —CH— $NHSO_3H$

greater serum binding (218). The improvements in acid stability and oral absorption of the aryloxyalkylpenicillins are shared by the isomeric α-alkoxybenzylpenicillins. This is not particularly surprising, since they too have an oxygen atom on the α-carbon of the side chain. Thus 3,4-dichloro-α-methoxybenzylpenicillin has shown good therapeutic effectiveness and it has been used clinically in Europe (219, 220).

With the exception of phenoxymethylpenicillin, these compounds have an asymmetric carbon atom in the side chain. Although phenethicillin and propicillin having the side chains derived from the corresponding levorotatory phenoxyalkanoic acids have slightly better activities than do the opposite epimers, the commercially available products are epimeric mixtures.

The group of penicillins discussed in this section are by no means the only ones having greater stability to acids than benzylpenicillin. Good resistance to inactivation by acids is displayed by penicillins having various other substituents on the α-carbon of the side chain such as amino (ampicillin), chloro, benzyloxycarbonylamino (215), and guanidine (221). Likewise, penicillins with heterocyclic side chains such as isoxazolyl (oxacillin, cloxacillin) share this property. Many of these have other characteristics of greater importance, however, and they are discussed elsewhere in this chapter.

8.3 Semisynthetic Penicillins Resistant to Penicillinase

A more important development resulting from the availability of 6-APA has been the creation of semisynthetic penicillins that resist destruction by penicillinases. The widespread use of benzylpenicillin was accompanied by a steadily increasing incidence of infections by *Staphylococcus aureus*, which had become resistant to the penicillins through the ability to produce penicillianse. By 1960 this had become an alarming worldwide clinical problem, especially involving hospital patients where in some cases penicillin resistance was encountered in as high as 80% of the staphylococcal infections (222, 223). Many of these strains of *S. aureus* were both virulent and highly resistant to most or all of the other available antibiotics, making infection dangerous and treatment extremely difficult. Thus much of the early work on semisynthetic penicillins was directed toward the discovery of agents resistant to inactivation by penicillinase. In 1960 the penicillinase-resistant penicillin, methicillin, was introduced into clinical practice, followed by a number of analogs with increased intrinsic activity and good oral absorption properties. These penicillins have been supplemented by the cephalosporins, which are inherently resistant to penicillinase. Partly as a result of the availability of these agents, but probably for other reasons as well, the penicillin-resistant staphylococci have ceased to present the acute threat that they posed in 1960.

For the most part, resistance of penicillins to attack by penicillinase is associated with steric hindrance around the α-carbon atom of the acylamino group. Essentially all the penicillins reported to have significant levels of resistance carry acyl side chains in which the α-carbon atom is quaternary, either through multiple substitution or by incorporation into an aromatic or heterocyclic ring. The effect of simply increasing the level of substitution on methylpenicillin is illustrated in Table 15.6. Resistance to staphylococcal β-lactamase is only partial when one or two of the α-substituents are relatively small (e.g., trichloromethyl- and *t*-butylpenicillin), but it becomes essentially complete when all the substituents are bulky, as in triphenylmethylpenicillin. By contrast, diphenylmethylpenicillin and $\beta\beta\beta$-triphenylethylpenicillin are sensitive to penicillinase (224,

Table 15.6 Penicillins with Side Chains Derived from Multiply Substituted Acetic Acids: Effect of Substitution on Sensitivity to Penicillinase

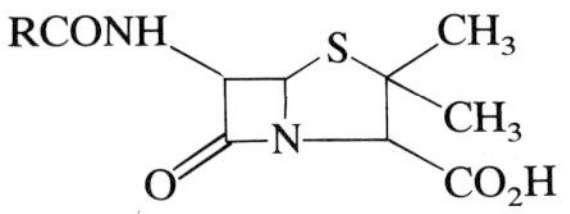

RCONH–(penam nucleus: S, CH_3, CH_3, CO_2H, N, O)

Resistant	Susceptible
$(C_6H_5)_3C$—	$C_6H_5OCH_2$—
$(C_6H_5)_2(Het)C$—[a]	$C_6H_5CH_2$—
$(C_6H_5)_2R'C$—	$(CH_3)_3C$—
$(C_6H_5)_2(RSO_2)C$—	Cl_3C—
$C_6H_5(R')_2C$—[b]	$(C_6H_5)_2CH$—
$(C_6H_5)_2(R'O)C$—[b]	$(C_6H_5)_3CCH_2$—
$(C_6H_5)_2(R'S)C$—[b]	

[a] Het = 2-thienyl, 2-furyl, 2-pyridyl, etc.

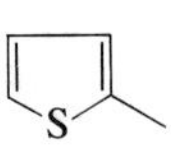

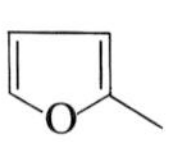

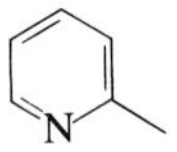

[b] $R' = CH_3$, C_2H_5, C_6H_{11}, $C_6H_5CH_2$, etc.

225). Usually the modifications of the penicillin side chain that favor resistance to penicillinase lower the intrinsic antibacterial activity of the molecule. This is the case here, where the increase in stability toward penicillinase achieved by adding large hydrophilic groups is accompanied by lower antibacterial activity and a narrower spectrum of activity. Still triphenylmethylpenicillin retains sufficient activity against the staphylococci to qualify it as a candidate for therapeutic use. However the *in vitro* activity it has is greatly diminished in the presence of serum, and it fails to protect laboratory animals against bacterial infection. Consequently neither it nor other analogs of this type have found commercial utility.

Penicillins in which the α-carbon atom of the side chain is incorporated into an aromatic or heterocyclic ring also have lower *in vitro* activities than their monosubstituted methylpenicillin analogs, and this side chain change does not, in itself, improve penicillinase resistance. Thus phenylpenicillin is significantly less active than the homologous benzylpenicillin, and its activity is confined to gram-positive bacteria that do not produce penicillinase. Substitution at the meta and para positions of the benzene ring does not greatly affect antibacterial activity or penicillinase susceptibility. However when steric hindrance is introduced by placing substituents on the ortho positions, there is again little change in the *in vitro* activity, but the resistance to penicillinase changes profoundly. It is this type of structure that has produced the clinically successful penicillinase-resistant penicillins, for example, methicillin 226–229), nafcillin (230–232), oxacillin (233–235), cloxacillin (236–238), dicloxacillin (239–241), and flucloxacillin (239, 242, 243) (see Table 15.5). In all these penicillins an aromatic ring is attached directly to the side chain amide carbonyl, and there is substitution at both positions ortho to the point of attachment. The ortho substituents can be alkyl, aryl, alkoxy, etc. (methicillin, the oxacillins), or a juncture with an annelated ring (nafcillin). The requirement of ortho substitution is readily seen in Table 15.7, which compares structures resistant to penicillinase with close analogs that are sensitive to the enzyme.

The size of the ring system plays an important role in determining the ability of the ortho substituent to confer penicillinase resistance on the structure. Phenylpenicillins, and equivalent heterocyclic analogs, have marked stability toward penicillinase when both ortho positions are occupied by any of a large variety of substituents (228, 244). In fact, with such ring systems (six- membered ring, or a fused ring system of equivalent or greater bulk) a single ortho-substituent of the proper type can be sufficient for good penicillinase resistance. The known examples of single ortho substituents capable of this include carboxyl (e.g., quinacillin, *vide infra*) and certain aromatic rings. Thus *o*-biphenylylpenicillin (diphenicillin, ancillin) (245) is stable toward penicillinase, but the analogous

Table 15.7 Aromatic and Heterocyclic Penicillins: Effect of Side Chain on Susceptibility to Penicillinase

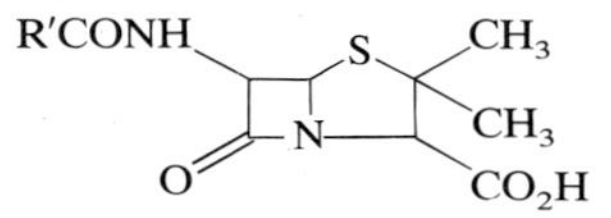

R′CONH, S, N, O, CH_3, CH_3, CO_2H

Resistant			Susceptible		
OCH_3, OCH_3 [a]	OR[b], OR, (X)	R, X		CH_3O, OCH_3	OCH_3, CH_2—, OCH_3
OC_2H_5 [c]	OR	OR, N, (R)		OCH_3	OCH_3
Y, Z, N, O, CH_3 [d]	H_3C, N, O	O, (R), R	N, O	N, O	H_3C, N, O, CH_3
[e]		N, N, CO_2H [f]			CH_2—

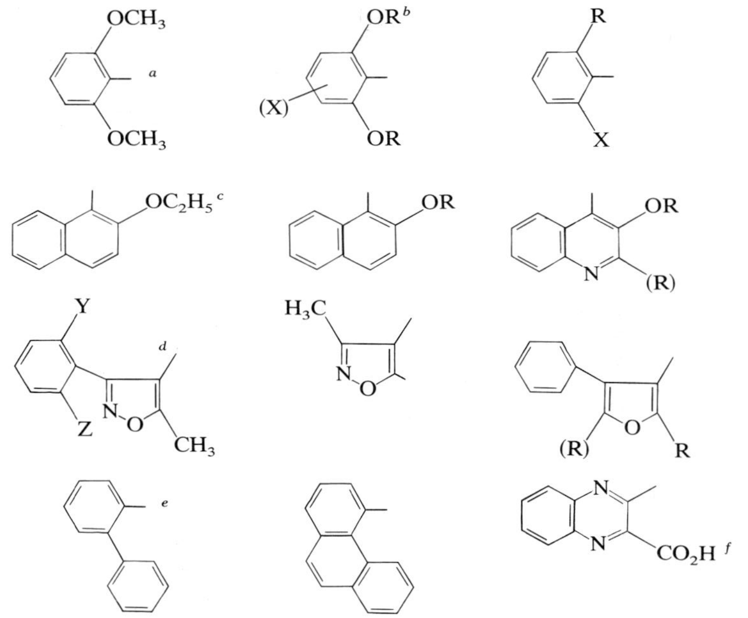

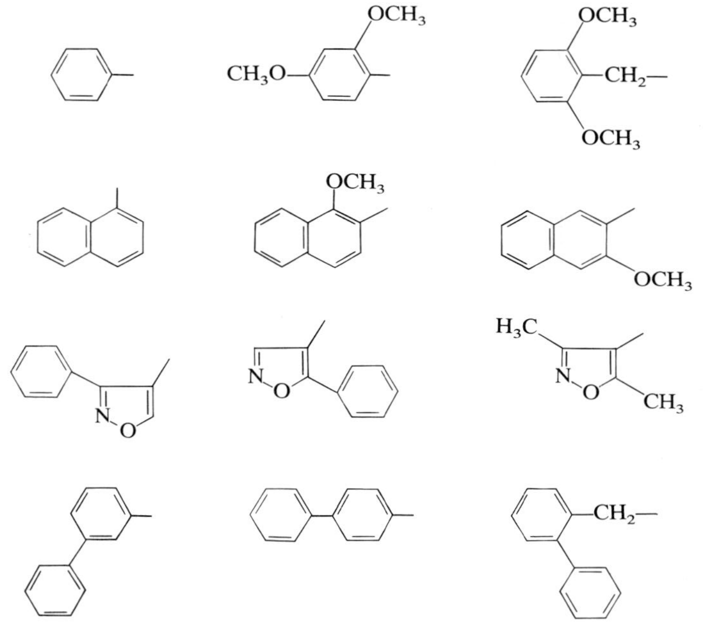

[a] Methicillin.
[b] R = alkyl; X = Br, Cl, NO_2, NH_2, etc.
[c] Nafcillin.
[d] The oxacillins.
[e] Diphenicillin.
[f] Quinacillin.

m-and *p*-biphenylylpenicillins, as well as *o*-biphenylylmethylpenicillin, are susceptible (Table 15.7) (246). Various aromatic and heterocyclic ring systems can substitute for either benzene ring in *o*-biphenylylpenicillin, provided they meet specific structural requirements (247, 248). An aromatic ring system is preferred, although analogs having a cyclohexyl ring in place of either benzene ring also possess moderate resistance to the enzyme.

Penicillins having a five-membered ring attached to the amide carboxyl group require bulkier substituents for significant penicillinase resistance. Thus neither a single ortho substituent of the type just described (e.g., phenyl) nor two *o*-methyl substituents confer penicillinase resistance on the isoxazolylpenicillin molecule. It is necessary that one of the substituents be more bulky than methyl. Very good resistance to penicillinase is realized when one of the two ortho substituents is phenyl and the other methyl (e.g., oxacillin)(233, 249). The phenyl group can be replaced by other aromatic rings (furyl, thienyl), but larger (naphthyl) or more polar (4-pyridyl) rings lower the *in vitro* activity. A methyl (or ethyl) substituent is fairly critical. If it is absent, the resistance to inactivation by penicillinase is lost, whereas its replacement by larger alkyl groups (isopropyl, *t*-butyl) or by phenyl results in retention of resistance to penicillinase but lower antibacterial activity (250).

Generally the *in vitro* activities of the 5-alkyl-3-aryl compounds are not significantly different from those of the 3-alkyl-5-aryl isomers. This rather definite substituent requirement for penicillinase resistance has been demonstrated for other penicillins having five-membered heterocyclic side chains such as 2,4-di- and 2,4,5-trisubstituted-3-furyl (252), 3,5-disubstituted-4-isothiazolyl (253, 254), 1,4-disubstituted-5-pyrazolyl (255), and 3-phenylsydnon-5-yl (256).

Methicillin (2,6-dimethoxyphenylpenicillin) was the first penicillinase-resistant penicillin to be used clinically. Its *in vitro* activity against typical penicillin-sensitive and penicillinase-producing strains of *S. aureus* is listed in Table 15.8, which compares the activity of benzylpenicillin with

Table 15.8 Typical *in Vitro* Activities of Benzylpenicillin and Penicillinase-Resistant Semisynthetic Penicillins Against Sensitive and Resistant (Penicillinase-Producing) *Staphylococcus aureus*

	MIC, μg/ml	
Penicillin	Sensitive	Resistant
Benzylpenicillin	0.005–0.05	5–>250
Triphenylmethyl-penicillin	0.3	0.3–0.6
Methicillin	0.5–2.5	1.25–3.7
Oxacillin group[a]	0.05–0.5	0.25–1.5
Nafcillin	0.2	0.6
Diphenicillin	0.2	0.5
Quinacillin	0.5	0.5

[a] Oxacillin, cloxacillin, dicloxacillin, flucloxacillin.

the penicillinase- resistant penicillins of importance to this discussion. Methicillin is less active than benzylpenicillin against susceptible staphylococci by a factor of 50–100 (MICs: 0.5–2.5 μg/ml vs. 0.005–0.05 μg/ml for benzylpenicillin). In addition, since methicillin is very rapidly inactivated by acids, it is poorly absorbed on oral administration. It must be administered by injection, in large doses, several times a day. As with the other penicillins of this group, it is virtually inactive against gram-negative bacteria, and it has relatively poor activity against some streptococci. On the other hand, it is markedly nontoxic, it is well absorbed after parenteral administration, and it is bactericidal at concentrations very near to its bacteriostatic level. Thus in spite of severe limitations it is still widely used as a life-saving drug.

The 2-alkoxy-1-naphthylpenicillins can be viewed as analogs of methicillin in which a fused ring contributes the steric effect supplied by one of the *o*-methoxy groups of methicillin. These penicillins and their corresponding quinoline analogs are stable to penicillinase, whereas the less hindered 1-naphthyl-, 3-methoxy-2-naphthyl-, and 4-quinolinylpenicillins are sensitive to the enzyme (230, 244) (Table 15.7). Nafcillin (2-ethoxy-1-naphthylpenicillin) is generally more effective than methicillin by a factor of 2–4 in the *in vitro* inhibition of *S. aureus.* Since it is more stable to acid than is methicillin, it is better absorbed when administered orally, but the absorption is irregular and incomplete (257). It is strongly bound by serum (50% serum reduces the *in vitro* antibacterial activity fourfold), and upon oral administration to mice it gives significantly lower blood levels than an equivalent dose of cloxacillin (*vide infra*). Yet the amount of nafcillin required to protect mice against staphylococcal infections is reported to be less than that required for cloxacillin (258). This unexpected behavior has been attributed to the recycling of nafcillin by biliary excretion to and resorption from the intestine, resulting in a persistence of the drug in the body for long periods (259).

From the large number of 3,5-disubstituted-4-isoxazolylpenicillins studied, four (oxacillin, cloxacillin, dicloxacillin, and flucloacillin) have been made available for clinical use. These penicillins are active *in vitro* at lower concentrations than methicillin (Table 15.8), and since they have good acid stability, they are readily absorbed from the gastrointestinal tract. Thus the recommended oral dose of, for example, oxacillin and cloxacillin, is half the intramuscular dose of methicillin (241, 260). These four penicillins illustrate the rather intricate interrelationships that are involved in the selection of β-lactam antibiotics for use in humans. All four analogs have essentially the same *in vitro* activities against the penicillin-senstive and penicillin-resistant staphylococci; the presence of one or two halogen atoms on the phenyl group has little effect on the intrinsic antibacterial activity. However these substituents on the phenyl group influence the efficiency of oral absorption. Thus the 1 hr serum level attained by a 500 mg oral dose of cloxacillin is approximately double that attained by the same dose of oxacillin (Table 15.9) (242). But a 250 mg dose of

Table 15.9 Mean Serum Concentrations of Isoxazolyl Penicillins 1 hr After Oral Administration to Fasting Volunteers[a]

Penicillin	Dose, mg	Total Level, μg/ml	Free Level, μg/ml
Oxacillin	500	4.9	0.34
Cloxacillin	500	9.2	0.55
Dicloxacillin	250	9.3	0.29
Flucloxacillin	250	8.8	0.46

[a] Adapted from Ref. 158.

either dicloxacillin or flucloxacillin provides essentially the same 1 hr serum concentration. However all these penicillins are extensively bound to serum proteins, and dicloxacillin is more highly bound than flucloxacillin. Consequently the lower dose of flucloxacillin, but not dicloxacillin, provides a 1 hr serum concentration of the "free' form of the drug roughly equivalent to that from the higher dose of cloxacillin (0.46 μ g/ml vs. 0.55 μ g/ml). In considering these nuances it should be borne in mind that human serum binding values for these four penicillins are 93.1, 94.0, 96.9, and 94.7%, respectively, as opposed to a value of 49% for methicillin.

The wide use of these semisynthetic penicillins has not resulted in the rapid emergence of *S. aureus* strains resistant to them, as feared originally. Methicillin-insensitive strains of *S. aureus* can be produced in the laboratory (usually with low virulence in man), and there have been scattered reports of relatively high incidences of natural methicillin-resistant staphylococcal infections, in individual hospitals in the United Kingdom and in the general population in parts of Europe (261). Studies on susceptibility indicate that in the United States the incidence went from about 0.4% in 1960 (262) to about 3% in 1971 (261). Although the methicillin-resistant strains produce large amounts of penicillinase, this does not appear to be the mechanism for their resistance, since they do not inactivate the penicillinase-resistant penicillins. The emergence of these strains is likely to be due to a process of selection of the few resistant organisms from a larger sensitive population rather than through induction of resistance in the latter.

8.4 Broad Spectrum Semisynthetic Penicillins

Except for a few species like *Neisseria, Hemophilus, Brucella,* and *Pasteurella,* the penicillins, at best, are intrinsically less active against gram-negative bacteria than they are against gram-positive organisms. The side chains on the penicillins described so far tend to accentuate this difference. Their hydrophobic character favors the activity against gram-positive organisms at the expense of activity against the gram-negative group. Introduction of hydrophobic substituents (e.g., chloro, alkyl, alkoxy) on these side chains generally depresses activity against gram-negative bacteria even further, but it has little effect on the activity against gram-positive organisms, or increases it slightly. Conversely, introduction of a hydrophilic group on the side chain can result in improvement of gram-negative activity. Thus penicillin N (Synnematin B) is 100 times less active than benzylpenicillin against gram-positive bacteria, but it is several times more active than penicillin G against coliform bacilli and certain other gram-negative organisms (263). *p*-Aminobenzylpenicillin (penicillin T) follows a similar pattern; it is only slightly less active than benzylpenicillin against the gram-positive organisms, and it is 2–4 times more active against some gram-negative bacteria (119). Acylation of the amino group of both penicillins N and T results in products having higher gram-positive and lower gram-negative activities (93, 119) (but compare the *n*-acylated ampicillins discussed below). The placement of the amino substituent is important since, unlike *p*-aminobenzylpenicillin, neither *o*- nor *m*-aminobenzylpenicillin has an antibacterial spectrum broader than that of benzylpenicillin (264).

The enhancement of gram-negative activity is most striking when the hydrophilic substituent is attached to the α-carbon of the side chain (Table 15.10). Although α-substituents on benzylpenicillin generally reduce activity against gram-negative bacteria, a few, notably amino, hydroxyl, carboxyl, sulfonyl, and sulfamyl, increase activity. This is the type of side chain that, so far, has been the source of the clinically important broad spectrum penicillins (Table 15.5). The penicillins of this type

Table 15.10 *In Vitro* Activities of α-Substituted Benzylpenicillins (158)

[Structure: C_6H_5–CH(X)CONH– penicillin nucleus with S, N, O, CH_3, CH_3, CO_2H]

X	MIC, μg/ml *S. aureus*	*E. coli*	*P. aeruginosa*
H	0.02	25	>500
Cl (D, L)	0.02	125	>500
CH_3 (D, L)	0.05	25	>500
OH (D)	0.05	5	>500
OH (L)	0.1	25	>500
NH_2 (D)	0.05	2.5	>500
NH_2 (L)	0.1	12.5	>500
CO_2H (D, L)	2.5	5	50
SO_3H (D, L)	2.5	2.5	50

that are currently available can be divided into two classes, exemplified by ampicillin and carbenicillin. Ampicillin (150, 265–269) is D-α-aminobenzylpenicillin (Table 15.5). It is the second most widely used penicillin in medical practice (270). Against gram-positive bacteria it has a level of activity approaching that of benzylpenicillin. It also shares with benzylpenicillin a high level of susceptibility to inactivation by penicillinases. it extends the antibacterial spectrum (Table 15.1) of benzylpenicillin—but only modestly—to include gram-negative bacteria that are not known to produce β-lactamases (e.g., *Salmonella typhi, Proteus mirabilis*), and a very limited group of β-lactamase producers (essentially *E. coli*).

Placement of the amino group on the α-carbon atom not only broadens the antibacterial spectrum but also increases the stability of the penicillin toward acids. Thus like phenoxymethylpenicillin, ampicillin is well absorbed on oral administration (peak serum levels at 2 hr are approximately 2.19 μg/ml; 250 mg dose in man) and significant serum concentrations are still present at 6 hr. Its sodium salt is used parenterally. Ampicillin is extremely nontoxic, but it is cross-allergenic with other penicillins. its good gram-positive activity and desirable pharmacokinetic properties contribute to its wide use in medical practice.

Carbenicillin (271–274) is α-carboxybenzylpenicillin. The side chain is racemic; when separated, the D- and L- isomers display only slight differences in biological activity, and they undergo rapid interconversion when in solution. This derivative of phenylmalonic acid has poor chemical stability, especially in the presence of acid, and it must be given by injection. At physiological pH where the side chain carboxyl group of carbenicillin is highly ionized, it is strongly hydrophilic as compared to the amino group of ampicillin. Thus it is not surprising that carbenicillin is much less active than ampicillin against gram-positive bacteria (the MIC against *S. aureus* Smith is 2.5 μg/ml vs. 0.02 μg/ml for benzylpenicillin and 0.05 μg/ml for ampicillin). In contrast to ampicillin, it is somewhat resistant to staphylococcal β-lactamase, as reflected in its MICs against benzylpenicillin-resistant strains of *S. aureus* (MICs: ampicillin/benzylpenicillin, > 500 μg/ml; carbenicillin, 50 μg/ml). The most important characteristic of carbenicillin is its broad activity against both gram-negative organisms that produce β-lactamases and those not known to elaborate these enzymes. Of the various gram-negative bacterial species, *Pseudomonas aeruginosa* is notable for its general lack of susceptibility to the β-lactam antibiotics. Carbenicillin is exceptional in exhibiting activity against this species (Table 15.10). It is also active against strains of indole-positive *Proteus, Serratia, Providentia, Citrobacter,* and several other newly emerging highly resistant pathogenic strains of enteric bacteria. Its activity against *P. aeruginosa* strains is modest by penicillin standards, with MICs that often range from 50 to 250 μg/ml. Thus the intravenous infusion of impressively high amounts of the drug is frequently required to achieve inhibitory concentrations in the body. Fortunately carbenicillin, like ampicillin, has an exceedingly low level of toxicity, which allows the administration of the large doses needed. Because of its effectiveness against *P. aeruginosa*, indole-positive *Proteus*; and the other resistant bacteria named above, carbenicillin and its close analogs with similar properties (Table 15.5), are indicated primarily for use in serious, often life-threatening, infections caused by this relatively narrow group of organisms.

In general these penicillins are relatively stable toward the β-lactamases produced by the gram-negative organisms that are sensitive to them, and their antibacterial activity is probably due in part to this greater resistance to enzyme inactivation; but the involvement of other factors such as cell wall permeability is also indicated by the sensitivity of the gram-negative organisms that are not known to produce β-lactamase but are resistant to benzylpenicillin. Likewise, the broader activity of these penicillins is not due solely to the hydrophilicity of the α-substituent. The stereochemistry of substituent attachment is important. The L-isomers of α-hydroxy and α-aminobenzylpenicillin are only about as active as benzylpenicillin against the gram-negative bacteria (275, 276) (Table 15.10). It is the D-isomers that show increased activity (e.g., MICs for the D- vs. the L-epimers of ampicillin: *E. coli*, 2.5 vs. 12.5 μg/ml; *Klebsiella pneumoniae*, 1.6 vs. 12.5 μg/ml; *Salmonella typhosa*, 1.6 vs. 12.5 μg/ml). This stereochemical specificity implies active participation of the side chain substituent at the receptor site level (but compare the activities of the D- and L-isomers of carbenicillin).

The success of ampicillin has led to many structural variations designed to improve its biological properties, and this has resulted in several analogs and derivatives of interest. These manipulations include side chain ring substitution (amoxycillin), replacement of the benzene ring by other cyclic systems (epicillin, BL-P875), homologation of the α-carbon (betacin), and conversion to *pro*-drug derivatives that release ampicillin on administration (hetacillin, metampicillin, pivampicillin, talampicillin).

For the broad spectrum penicillins substituted on the α-carbon of the side chain, the addition of a second substituent (viz., benzene- ring substitution) tends to reduce gram-negative activity. An important exception is the introduction of a hydroxyl group at the meta- or para-positions (an *o*-hydroxyl group reduces activity). Amoxycillin is the *p*-hydroxy derivative of ampicillin (276). It has essentially the same *in vitro* activity and serum levels as ampicillin when administered by injection, but it shows improved absorption on oral administration, giving higher serum levels and better urinary recovery than ampicillin (277). The benzene ring on the side- chain of these penicillins has been replaced by several other ring systems with retention of antibacterial activity. Epicillin is the 1,4-cyclohexadienyl analog of ampicillin (278–280). Its biological properties are virtually the same as those of ampicillin. A thiophene ring (either 2- or 3-thienyl) readily substitutes for the benzene ring in most cases. The 3-thienyl analog of ampicillin resembles the latter *in vitro* and gives higher oral blood levels in mice (281). Its behavior in man has not been reported. Other heterocyclic rings, for example, isothiazole (282), have also been reported to be capable of replacing the side- chain benzene ring. Insertion of a methylene group between the α-carbon of ampicillin and the benzene ring [6(D- or L-phenylalanylamino)penicillanic acid] lowers the gram-positive activity and results in gram-negative activities intermediate between those of benzylpenicillin and ampicillin. When the methylene group is inserted between the α-carbon atom and the amino group (D-α-phenyl-β-aminoethylpenicillin, betacin) the trend in gram-positive activity is the same, but the gram-negative activity is closer to that of ampicillin (283). However betacin is poorly absorbed when given orally (284).

Ampicillin has been converted to several derivatives which function as *pro*-drugs for the antibiotic. Two are adducts involving the side- chain amino group. Hetacillin [6-(2,2-dimethyl-5-oxo-4-phenyl-l-imidazolidinyl)penicillanic acid] is an acetone adduct (285). Although it has been reported to give higher and more prolonged blood levels than the parent antibiotic (286, 287), its pharmacokinetic properties are very close of those of ampicillin. Metampicillin is a similar adduct with formaldehyde (288, 289). Pivampicillin (290, 291), bacampicillin (292, 293) and talampicillin (294) represent attempts to improve oral absorption by esterification of the penicillin carboxyl group (15.**45**; see Section 10.1). These pivaloyloxymethyl, 1′-ethoxycarbonyloxyethyl, and phthalidyl esters of ampicillin give ampicillin serum concentrations (e.g., 6.7 μg/ml from talampicillin) in man 2–3 times greater than those obtained (e.g., 2.6 μg/ml) with an equivalent dose (250 mg) of ampicillin itself (290). Talampicillin is reported to release ampicillin at a faster rate than pivampicillin (294).

A considerable amount of structure-activity work has also been carried out on the carbenicillin structure. The most significant products from these studies involve benzene ring replacement by heterocycles (ticarcillin), replacement of the side chain carboxyl group by other acidic groupings (sulbenicillin, suncillin), and esterification of the side -chain carboxyl group (carbenicillin indanyl sodium, carfecillin). Ticarcillin is the 3-thienyl analog of carbenicillin. Its biological properties are essentially the same as carbenicillin's except that it is about twice as active as the latter against most strains of *P. aeruginosa in vitro*, and it is approximately twice as effective *in vivo* (295–297). Sulbenicillin (α-sulfobenzylpenicillin), with a more strongly acidic grouping on the side chain, might be expected to display biological properties somewhat different from those of carbenicillin. However the two penicillins have almost the same antibacterial activity and very similar pharmacokinetic properties (298–300). Sulbenicillin is more stable chemically and in contrast to carbenicillin, the D-isomer is reported to be more active than its epimer (298). Suncillin (α-sulfoaminobenzylpenicillin) also has an α-substituent containing a sulfonic acid group. It resembles sulbenicillin in its biological properties, being approximately equally active against *P. aeruginosa*, but it is less active against certain other gram-negative species (301–303). As expected, benzylpenicillins with other acidic α-substituents have been found to have similar properties. Perhaps of most interest is benzylpenicillin with an α-(5-tetrazolyl) group that resembles carbenicillin *in vitro* but is less active *in vivo* (Section 10.1). As with ampicillin, the carbenicillin side chain has been homologated, and hetero atoms have been inserted between the ring and the α-carbon. α-Carboxy-β-phenylethylpenicillin is essentially inactive against *P. aeruginosa*, and α-carboxyphenoxymethylpenicillin also has poor gram-negative activity. The chemical stability of carbenicillin can be improved by esterification of the side chain carboxyl group. The indanyl ester (carindacillin) is available for clinical use. This ester is absorbed orally (about 40%) and is rapidly hydrolyzed in serum to carbenicillin (serum peak, 6.7 μg/ml from dose equivalent to 500 mg of carbenicillin), but the relatively low serum levels of carbenicillin attained restrict its use (304–306). The phenyl ester (carfecillin) (307), selected from a study of 12 aromatic and aliphatic esters, behaves similarly to the indanyl ester; but it produces peak serum concentrations (7.0 μg/ml) at 1 hr post injection as opposed to a 2 hr peak for the indanyl ester.

One additional group of penicillins has been extensively investigated, largely because of the activity these analogs exhibit against *Pseudomonas* species. These are *N*-substituted derivatives of ampicillin. Ampicillin itself is inactive against *P. aeruginosa*. Simple *N*-acylation of the phenylglycine side chain tends to reduce its activity generally against the gram-negative bacteria (cf. penicillins N and T) (308), but much of this activity can be recovered when the complexity of the side chain is increased appropriately (309). However the original activity of ampicillin is usually not exceeded. Although broad gram-negative activity is lowered generally, acylation of ampicillin can result in derivatives that display significant activity against *P. aeruginosa*. Even relatively simple (pivaloyl, benzoyl) derivatives display slight, but measurable, activity (MIC: 250–800 μg/ml). Introduction of nitrogen into the acyl group (ureido, guanylureido, acylglycyl, etc.) and other similar manipulations can confer relatively good *in vitro* activity against *P. aeruginosa.* The effect of sulfonylation is similar. The α-sulfamic acid analog (—$NHSO_3H$, suncillin) was included with the benzylpenicillins having acidic α-substituents, but it is perhaps more logically an *N*-acylampicillin analog; the analogous benzylsulfonyl derivative displays slightly better *in vitro* activity than the sulfamic acid against, for example, *E. coli* and *P. aeruginosa* (MICs: *E. coli,* 25 vs. 125 μg/ml; *P. aeruginosa* 50 vs. 125 μg/ml, respectively). Unfortunately, the relatively good *in vitro* activities of these *N*-acylated ampicillins against *P. aeruginosa* is often lowered significantly in the presence of serum, and the effect of innoculum size on activity can be serious (310). Consequently, several of these penicillins have undergone clinical trials, but none have yet been cleared for marketing. Some of the *N*-acyl derivatives that have received attention because of their activity against *Pseudomonas* species are listed in Table 15.11.

8.5 Other 6-Acyl Group Modifications

The preceding discussion covers only a small (but biologically, the most important) part of the many variations of the 6-acylamino grouping that have been described. A few additional penicillins of interest are listed here without comment on their properties to provide literature access: α-hydrazinobenzyl (318), α-(arylideneiminoxy)benzyl (319), 3- and 4-pyridylmethyl (320, 321), isothiazolylmethyl (322), α-aminocycloalkyl (cyclacillin) (323, 324), α-azidobenzyl (325, 326), 3-amino-1-adamantylpenicillin (327), 6-phthalimidopenicillanic acid (328).

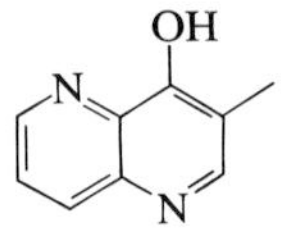

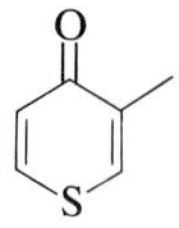

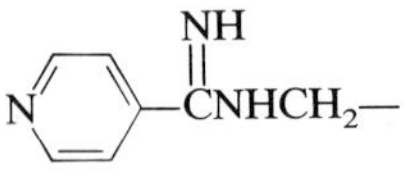

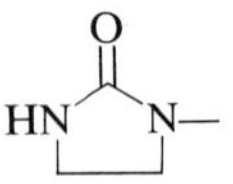

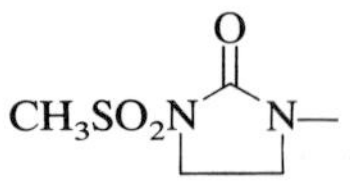

8.6 Mecillinam: 6β-Amidinopenicillanic Acids

Mecillinam—6β-[hexahydro-1H-azepin-1-yl)methyleneamino]penicillanic acid; FL 1060; 15.**37**—is not a 6-acylaminopenicillin analog, but it is more appropriately included here because of its biological properties and its structural similarity to the penicillins under consideration. This agent and close analogs display striking *in vitro* activity against a broad group of gram-negative bacteria, some of which are insensitive to ampicillin (329, 330). Its activity against gram-positive bacteria is much lower than that of ampicillin. The *in vitro*

Table 15.11 *N*-Acylated Ampicillins with Activity Against *Pseudomonas aeruginosa*

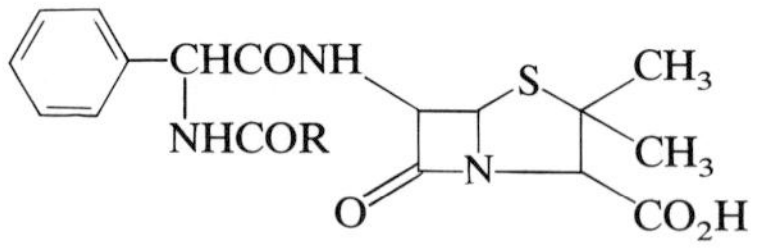

(Structure: phenyl–CHCONH–(penam with S, CH_3, CH_3, CO_2H, N, O), with NHCOR on the α-carbon)

R	Name	References
NH ‖ NH_2CNH—	BL-P1654	311
(OH, N, N ring structure)	Apalcillin	312
(O, S ring structure)[a]	Timoxicillin	313
(N ring)–C(=NH)$NHCH_2$—	Pirbenicillin	314
O, HN N— (ring)	Azlocillin	315
O, CH_3SO_2N N— (ring)	Mezlocillin	316
O O, Et—N N— (ring)	Piperacillin	317

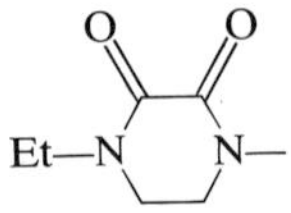

[a] This compound is the *p*-hydroxyphenyl analog.

gram-negative activity is affected by inoculum size, osmolality, and length of incubation (337). Although it inhibits bacterial cell wall synthesis, its mode of action differs from that of ampicillin (50). As a consequence, it has been found to be synergistic with several penicillins and cephalosporins when used in combination with them *in vitro* (332, 333) and *in vivo* (334) to inhibit various gram-negative bacteria. Synergy is also observed against *S. aureus*, but not other gram-positive organisms. It is not observed when this drug is used in combination with erythromycin or oxytetracycline. Synergy with gentamicin was very narrow (*E. coli*). The biological properties and clinical experiences with this drug have been summarized in a recent symposium (335).

9 THE CEPHALOSPORINS AND CEPHAMYCINS

Cephalosporin C is illustrative of the cephalosporins and cephamycins found in nature (Table 15.4). It has the α-aminoadipamido side chain at the 7-position and, so equipped, it leaves much to be desired as an antibiotic. Because of its polar nature it is difficult to isolate and purify. Its potency is low compared with other antibiotic agents; against penicillin-sensitive *S. aureus* it has less than 0.1% of the *in vitro* activity of benzylpenicillin. In addition, it is not absorbed orally. However it does have certain characteristics that appear to be inherent in the cephalosporin/cephamycin structure and offer the possibility of improving on the properties of the penicillins. It is extremely nontoxic, and it appears to have little cross-allergenicity with the penicillins (336). The β-lactam ring in cephalosporin C resists opening by both acid and penicillinase, and in this respect it is much more stable than when it is a part of the penicillin structure. The penicillinase resistance of cephalosporin C is of the order of that of oxacillin. Its potential for broad spectrum activity is somewhat ambiguous. The ratio of the gram-negative to gram-positive activity of cephalosporin C is much better than for benzylpenicillin. Because of its very low intrinsic activity, however cephalosporin C is actually less active than the latter against many gram-negative organisms. Thus the key to success in finding a real utility for the cephalosporins has rested in the ability to improve the intrinsic broad spectrum activity of this system without losing its favorable characteristics of low toxicity, low cross-allergenicity, and good stability toward acids and β-lactamases.

Although the structure-activity studies on the cephalosporins have largely paralleled the work on semisynthetic penicillins, the basic objectives have been somewhat different because of inherent differences in biological properties of the two antibiotic types. For example, the side chain modifications that increase penicillinase stability at the expense of intrinsic activity are unnecessary. Indeed, the primary objective of cephalosporin SAR studies has been the opposite: to increase the relatively low intrinsic activity of the natural cephalosporins as compared to the natural penicillins. As indicated earlier, the cephalosporins offer greater latitude for facile modification than do the penicillins; but similar to the latter, most modifications resulting in significantly improved biological properties fall within a relatively narrow range of structures. Again, studies involving 7-acyl group modifications have been the most profitable source of clinically useful antibiotics. Alteration of this side chain has played a significant role in influencing level and breadth of antibacterial activity. Changes in pharmacokinetic properties have been less substantial, with the narrow but very important exception of the orally absorbed 7-phenylglycyl type cephalosporins.

3-Position variations comprise the second most important type of alteration of the cephalosporin structure. Changes at this position have resulted occasionally in limited extension of the spectrum of activity [e.g. susceptibility of some *Enterobacter* to 3-(*N*-methyltetrazole)thiomethyl analogs], but they have been more useful in modifying the level of intrinsic activity [cf. 3-acetoxymethyl vs. 3-methyl cephalosporins and 3-(*N*-methyltetrazole)thiomethyl- vs. many other 3-heterocyclicthiomethyl cephalosporins) and the pharmacokinetic properties of the molecule.

Permissible variation at the third important locus of cephalosporin modification, the 7α-position, is extremely narrow, consisting essentially of hydrogen (cephalosporins) and methoxy (cephamycins). In essence, the 7-methoxy group influences the spectrum of antibacterial activity by increasing the resistance of the cephalosporin structure to attack by β-lactamases.

9.1 Modifications Involving the 7-Acylamino Side Chain

By analogy to penicillin N, which also has a D-α-aminoadipamido side chain and a low level of activity, it may be assumed that the low potency of cephalosporin C is attributable, at least in part, to this highly polar amino acid substituent. Since the removal or replacement of the aminoadipoyl moiety proved to be extremely difficult at first, attempts were made to improve the properties of cephalosporin C by direct chemical modification of the side chain. Simply acylation of the amino group generally results in an increase in gram-positive activity, but it is accompanied by a decrease in gram-negative potency (121, 337). The side chain amino and carboxyl groups have been simultaneously incorporated into heterocyclic rings, for example, hydantions, thiohydantions, and quinoxalines (338, 339). These derivatives are reported to have good activity against gram-positive bacteria coupled with a high level of penicillinase resistance. However none compares favorably with the clinically useful cephalosporins obtained by removing the aminoadipic acid structure and replacing it with a new acyl group. As with the penicillins, high antibacterial activity is observed essentially only when the new acyl groups are derived from carboxylic acids; 7-ureidocephalosporanic acid derivatives display fairly good broad spectrum activity (340), but cephalosporins with substituted urea and carbamate side chains at the 7-position have poor activity.

With respect to activity against gram-positive bacteria, a limited correlation between the penicillins and cephalosporins exists. Cephalosporins with carboxamido side chains that import high intrinsic activity to the penicillins tend to have relatively high potency against gram-positive organisms, although the correlation does not hold strictly between the two series. Table 15.12 lists several 7-acylaminocephalosporanic acids selected to illustrate this point. Like the penicillins, the highest antibacterial activities are observed when the side chain is derived from a monosubstituted acetic acid (e.g., compounds *3–8, 15–17)*. Multiple substitution on the α-carbon atom *(10–14)* or incorporation of this carbon into an aromatic ring (*9*) lowers the gram-positive activity. Within limits, substituents on the aromatic side chain ring (when present) that increase lipophilicity provide higher gram-positive activity and generally lower gram-negative activity (cf. *3, 7,* and *8)*. Other monosubstituted acetic acid side chains provide gram-positive activity equivalent to or, in many cases, better than that observed with the phenyl, phenoxy, and phenylthioacetyl analogs. These include side chains having a cyano *(17),* methylthio, trifluoromethylthio, or cyanomethylthio group, or various heterocyclic rings such as thianapthene *(6),* thiophene (*15*), tetrazole, sydnone, and pyridine (thio) (*16*). Many of these latter acyl groups also provide good levels of activity against gram-negative bacteria, resulting in analogs that are important clinically.

Table 15.12 Representative *In Vitro* Activities of Selected 7-Acylaminocephalosporanic Acids[a]

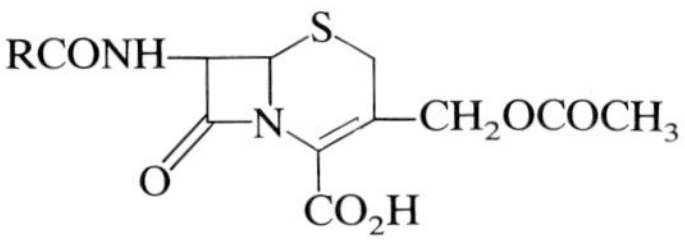

RCONH— S N —CH_2OCOCH_3 O CO_2H

Compound	R	MIC, μg/ml	
		S. aureus	*E. coli*
1	(Penicillin N)	180	160
2	$HO_2CCH(NH_2)(CH_2)_3$—	39	67
3	$C_6H_5CH_2$—	(0.5)[b]	27
4	$C_6H_5OCH_2$—	(0.2)[c]	140
5	$C_6H_5SCH_2$—	0.4	63
6	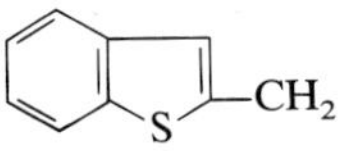 S —CH_2	0.1	62
7	*p*-$CH_3OC_6CH_2$	0.4	110
8	*p*-$ClC_6H_4CH_2$	<0.1	>200
9	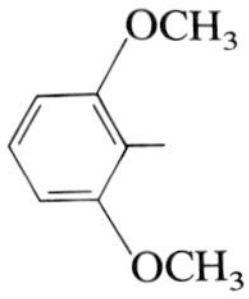 OCH_3 / OCH_3	18	>200
10	$C_6H_5CH(CH_3)$—	3.0	100
11	$C_6H_5CH(Cl)$—	2.5	25
12	$C_6H_5CH(CO_2H)$—	6.3	88
13	$C_6H_5CH(NH_2)$—	3.1	3.5
14	$C_6H_5CH(OH)$—	1.5	5.6
15	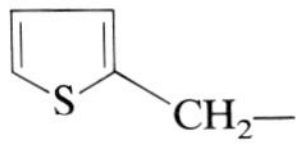 S CH_2—	0.5	6.4
16	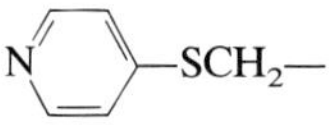 N —SCH_2—	0.4	17
17	$NCCH_2$—	0.6	12

[a] Data derived from Ref. 114, Ch. 12.

[b] Average value versus several strains of *S. aureus*; the reported value for the V32 strain of 6.0 μg/ml (114) does not correlate well with other reported data.

[c] Average value versus several strains of *S. aureus*.

It should be noted that although the gram-positive activities of these semi-synthetic cephalosporins are significantly improved over those of cephalosporin C, and the trends in activity roughly parallel those of the corresponding penicillins, these agents are consistently less active than the analogous penicillins against bacteria that are susceptible to the latter (gram-positive nonpenicillinase producers). This difference has been attributed to a greater affinity of the critical cell wall enzyme(s) for the penam than the cephem structure (39). Thus it has been suggested that differences in the efficiency of binding to the enzyme(s) (penam/cephem) are more likely determinants of intrinsic activity than differences in lactam ring reactivity (341). The possibility that greater penam reactivity accounts for the difference is not supported by studies based on rate of β-lactam ring hydrolysis, which indicate relatively equal reactivities for the β-lactam rings (pseudo-first-order rates of β-lactam hydrolysis, pH 10, 35°, log K/sec: benzylpenicillin, −4.3; phenylacetylaminocephalosporanic acid, −4.0) (342). But though "fit" appears to take precedence over reactivity in this case, the effects of ring strain and of 3-substituents on intrinsic activity, discussed below, suggest that the level of β-lactam ring reactivity is an important factor in the bioactivity of cephalosporins.

An examination of Table 15.12 reveals trends in the activity against gram-negative bacteria (*E. coli*) that again resemble some of the relationships between structure and activity seen with the penicillins, notably, the reduction of gram-negative activity when the lipophilicity of the side chain is increased and the enhancing effect of polar α-substituents (OH, NH_2). Even with the small number of analogs presented in the table, however, it can be seen that gram-negative activity is not a consistent characteristic of the cephalosporins, in spite of early expectations based on the properties of cephalosporin C. In fact, most cephalosporin analogs have relatively poor activity against gram-negative bacteria, and only a select few combine high intrinsic activity with a spectrum of susceptibility broad enough to make them candidates for clinical use. Table 15.13 lists some of the cephalosporin acyl groups associated with significant broad spectrum (especially gram-negative) activity. They include the side chains of the cephalosporanic acids that are sufficiently active *per se* to qualify for clinical use, as well as those of analogs, discussed next, on which the 3′-acetoxy group is replaced by other substituents. Most of these side chains are still mono- or disubstituted acetyl groups, but the phenyl-linked acetic acid moiety found on a large proportion of the penicillins (where gram-positive activity predominates) generally has additional α-carbon substitution (mandeloyl, phenylglycyl, etc.; side chains also found on broad spectrum penicillins). Its predominance has been replaced by acetyl groups linked to heterocyclic rings (thiophene, tetrazole, sydnone, etc.) or to small, frequently polar, groupings containing various hetero atoms (cyano, trifluoromethylthio, etc.). Notable departures from these general structures are the formyl group (of academic interest) and the α-oximino-containing side chains (cerfuroxime). The phenylmalonic acid and similar acyl groups of the carbenicillin type command less importance as cephalosporin side chains. Cephalosporin analogs with these side chains have broad spectrum activity, but the levels of intrinsic activity are low compared with the analogous penicillins, reflecting the inherent differences between the characteristics of penam and cepham systems.

It is not completely understood why the side chains in Table 15.13 confer broad spectrum activity on the cephalosporin structure while other similar acyl groups do not. The influence of the side chain on the permeability of the cephalosporin into the relatively complex gram-negative cell wall is likely to be important. Equally important may be a configuration that allows efficient binding to an appropriate enzyme involved in construction of the cell wall, while avoiding binding to a β-lactamase that may also be present and may have substrate configuration requirements closely resembling those of the cell wall synthesizing enzyme. A very recent study attempts to link the differences in bioactivity associated with different acyl groups to a relatively confined conformation of the side chain imposed by the steric properties of the latter and interactions with the rest of the

Table 15.13 Cephalosporin 7-Acyl Groups Associated with Broad Spectrum (Especially Gram-Negative) Activity

HCO	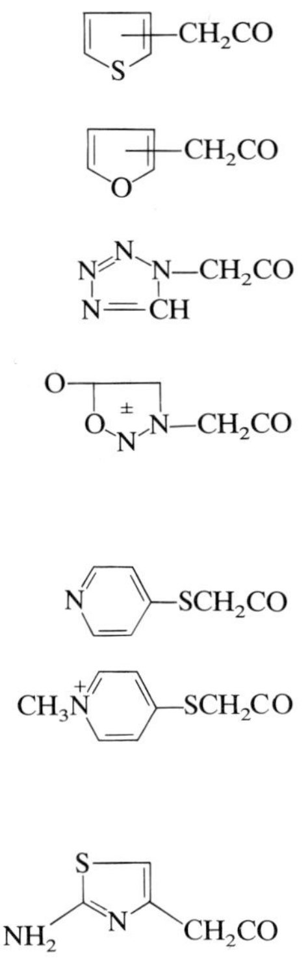 S —CH_2CO	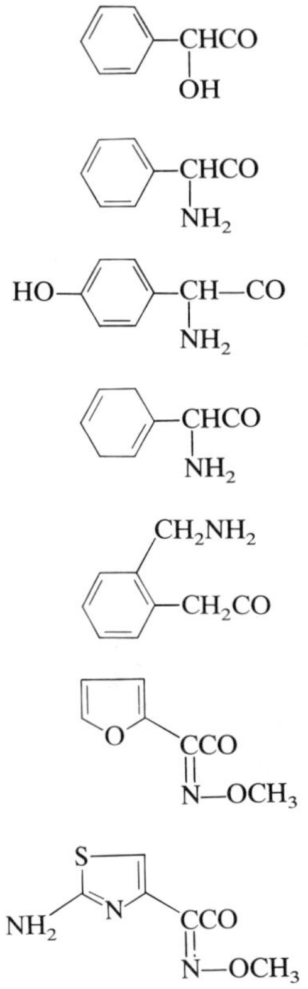 —CHCO, OH
$ClCH_2CO$	O —CH_2CO	—CHCO, NH_2
$Cl_2CHCHClCO$	N, N, N—CH_2CO, N═CH	HO— —CH—CO, NH_2
$NCCH_2CO$	O, O, ±, N, N—CH_2CO	—CHCO, NH_2
CH_3SCH_2CO		
$CH_3SO_2CH_2CO$	N —SCH_2CO	CH_2NH_2, —CH_2CO
$C_2H_5SOCH_2CO$	$CH_3\overset{+}{N}$ —SCH_2CO	O, CCO, N—OCH_3
CF_3SCH_2CO	S, NH_2, N, CH_2CO	S, NH_2, N, CCO, N—OCH_3
$NCCH_2SCH_2CO$		

molecule (343). In addition to this, the α-substituted mandeloyl and phenylglycyl side chains appear to have a separate role in assisting in the antibacterial action of the cephalosporin, since they are capable of conferring high activity on 3-methyl cephem derivatives where many other acyl groups provide only moderate or poor antibacterial activity.

9.2 Modifications Involving the 3-Substituent

The high reactivity of the β-lactam ring in the penicillins and cephalosporins has been associated with ring strain and with the lack of planarity of the amide nitrogen because of the constraints of the fused ring system (203). In the cephalosporins, the possibility for enamine resonance between the nitrogen atom's unshared electron pair and the olefinic π-orbital electrons provides an additional factor that contributes to the lability of the β-lactam amide group. The presence of enamine resonance is supported by the measurement of bond lengths using X-ray crystallography (344). Further support is provided by correlation of β-lactam absorption frequencies with various 3′-substituents ($OCOCH_3$ vs. H) (183). This resonance form is one of those advanced to account for the facile S_N1 displacement of the 3′-acetoxy group (structure 15.**24**). Thus although the study relating CNDO/2 calculations to the antibacterial activity of penicillins and cephalosporins, cited earlier (341), led to the conclusion that there is no evidence that the presence of acetate as a leaving group plays any role in the biological activity of cephalosporins, other studies using similar molecular orbital calculations (CNDO/2) (345), and correlation of substituent effects on the ease of base hydrolysis (346), imply the opposite. Whether the effects derive from the loss of the 3′-substituent, or only from its inductive effect on the β-lactam ring, the reactivity (rate of hydrolysis) of the β-lactam ring has been shown to correlate with the σ_I values of 3-methylene substituents (346, 347); and the rate of ring opening has been shown to be directly proportional to the intrinsic activity of cephalosporins against gram-negative bacteria (342).

The natural 3-acetoxymethyl grouping, which is retained on several cephalosporins in clinical use, is subject to metabolic alteration (hydrolysis) to give the corresponding 3′-alcohol with lowered antibacterial activity (348). This, in addition to the ability to influence intrinsic activity and pharmacokinetic properties, has encouraged broad variation of the 3′-substituent. Consequently many alterations have been carried out with extremely variable effects on biological activity. The number of examples becomes immense when modifications on both the 3- and 7-side chains are considered simultaneously. Therefore, a relatively small number of cephalosporins has again been selected for discussion (Table 15.14), primarily to illustrate trends or exemplify side chains of particular (clinical) interest. It should be kept in mind that although the examples in Table 15.14 have a thiopheneacetamide side chain, any 3-substituent change is likely to involve the preparation and testing of a large number of analogs having other 7-acyl groupings.

9.2.1 ESTERS. Deacetylcephalosporins (15.**2a** A = OH) are metabolic products of the 3-acetoxymethylcephalosporins and can be obtained for study by indirect methods (see Section 10.4). Their antibacterial activities (compound *1*, Table 15.14) are considerably lower than those of the parent acetoxymethyl analogs (e.g., *2*, cephalothin). The close homologous esters derived from the alcohol exhibit activities similar to those of the acetoxy derivatives, but activity decreases with chain length while binding increases. The benzoyl ester *(3)* displays improved gram-positive but lower gram-negative activity. The carbamyloxy substituent *(4)* occurs naturally (cephalosporins and cephamycins) and is part of the cefuroxime structure. It is resistant to metabolic attack, and cephalosporins with this substituent, or *N*-alkyl and acyl derivatives thereof, exhibit activities essentially equivalent to those of their 3-acetoxymethyl analogs (349).

9.2.2 NITROGEN NUCLEOPHILES. The early discovery that pyridine easily displaces the 3′-acetoxy group led to the marketing of cephaloridine (Table 15.14, compound *5*), the investigation of a large number of substituted 3-pyridiniummethyl cephalosporin analogs, and the introduction of other heterocyclic structures (pyrimidine, imidazole, etc.) on the 3′-position (see p. 108). Cephaloridine has activity against gram-negative bacteria resembling that of cephalothin *(2)* and excellent activity against gram-positive bacteria. The pyridiniummethyl group also provides several pharmacokinetic advantages (metabolic stability, water solubility, low serum binding, low pain on injection, good serum levels, etc.).

In most cases, substitution of the pyridine ring lowers activity against either gram-positive or gram-negative organisms, or both. Exceptions to this are the 3-bromo and several 4-substituted derivatives of cephaloridine. The 4-carboxamido derivative was found to be consistently the most active of this group, and it was assigned the

Table 15.14 Selected *in Vitro* Activities of Representative 3-Substituted-7-(2-Thiopheneacetamido)-3-Cephem-4-Carboxylic Acids (114)

(Structure: 2-thienyl–CH_2CONH– on 3-cephem nucleus with Z at C-3 and CO_2H at C-4)

Compound	Z	MIC, μg/ml S. aureus	MIC, μg/ml E. coli
1	CH_2OH	4.0	130
2	CH_2OCOCH_3	0.5	6.4
3	$CH_2OCOC_6H_5$	0.1	41
4	CH_2OCONH_2	0.5	15
5	$CH_2\overset{+}{N}$ (pyridinium)	0.4	3.3
6	CH_2N_3	(0.2)	—
7	$CH_2SCSOC_2H_5$	1.0	106
8	CH_2SCSN (piperazine) NCH_3	1.0	6
9	CH_2S–(5-methyl-1,3,4-thiadiazol-2-yl, N—N, S, CH_3)	0.3	5.7
10	CH_2S–(1-methyltetrazol-5-yl, N—N, N, N, CH_3)	0.3	1.0
11	CH_3	3.8	>50
12	CH_2OCH_3	0.5	39
13	CH_2SCH_3	3.1	>50

generic name cephalonium (169). Replacement of the pyridine moiety with other heterocyclic systems has not produced derivatives with a distinct advantage over cephaloridine.

Displacement of the acetoxy group by azide ion yields derivatives with relatively low gram-negative activity, but the gram-positive activity and serum binding are essentially unchanged (165). Several of these cephalosporin analogs have undergone extended evaluation, especially the 7-phenylglyoxylamide analog (350). The azide group has been reduced to a primary amine, which has been acylated by a variety of agents (351). None of these compounds show an overall activity superior to the acetoxymethyl analogs.

9.2.3 SULFUR NUCLEOPHILES. Early displacements of the 3′-acetoxy group with sulfur nucleophiles produced derivatives with undistinguished activities. For example, a large group of dithiocarbamate and xanthate derivatives [$Z = CH_2S(CS)NR_2$, $CH_2S(CS)OR$, e.g. compound 7] possess a fair degree of gram-positive activity; but they have generally poor gram-negative activity and suffer from serum inactivation (165, 167). The analog of cephalothin in which the dithiocarbamate group is derived from *N*-methylpiperidine (*8*) appears to be an exception. It has good gram-positive and gram-negative activity and little susceptibility to serum binding (167). A close analog with a different 7-acyl group and a quaternized methylpiperidine nitrogen has the generic name cephaclomezine (352). The derivatives obtained by displacement of the acetoxy group with aromatic and heterocyclic thioacids resemble their oxygen-containing analogs. The thiourea displacement products [$Z = CH_2S(CNH)NR_2$] have good gram-positive activity, with or without serum in the medium, but they are only moderately active against gram-negative bacteria (167). The Bunte salts ($Z = CH_2S_2O_3Na$) obtained by displacements with thiosulfate are poorly active and are bound by serum (353). Thioethers (especially 3-methylthiomethyl) have been prepared by 3′-acetoxy group displacements, and several derivatives with variation of the 7-acyl group have been evaluated (354). These cephalosporins and their oxygen analogs are discussed with the deacetoxymethyl cephalosporins.

By far the most important displacements by sulfur nucleophiles have been those using aromatic heterocyclic thiols. Many of these reactions generate thioethers with mediocre biological properties but, as with the 7-acyl group variations, a few result in enhancement of intrinsic activity, especially against gram-negative bacteria; and occasionally simultaneous improvement of such pharmacokinetic properties as the height and duration of serum levels is also observed. One cephalosporin of this type (cefazolin) is in wide clinical use, a second (cephamandole) was recently introduced into clinical practice, and several additional analogs (cefazaflur, cefatrizine, etc.) have undergone clinical evaluation. The relationships of the physiochemical properties of these 3-substituents to the biological activity and pharmacokinetic behavior of the cephalosporins have not yet been established quantitatively; however SAR studies with various acyl groups at the 7-position disclose interesting qualitative parallels in the trends of activity. These trends are illustrated in Table 15.15, which compares a selected group of 7-mandelamidocephalosporins. A similar SAR study of 3-heterocyclicthiomethyl-7-sydoneacetamido-3-cephem-4-carboxylic acids has been reported by the workers responsible for the discovery of cefazolin (355). The data in Table 15.15 were selected for use here because of the greater appropriateness of the mandelamido side chain. Among the 3-heterocyclicthiomethylcephalosporins with a five-membered heterocyclic ring, most are less active than the analog (*2*) with the 3-acetoxymethyl group, and, indeed, many are less active than the deacetoxymethyl derivative (*1*). The methyltetrazole (*3*), thiadiazole (*4*), and oxadiazole (*5*) derivatives have the best antibacterial activities *in vitro*, and they display the best PD_{50} values in infected mice. Similar trends are observed with 3-heterocyclicthiomethylcephalosporin analogs that have other 7-acyl groups in place of the D-mandeloyl moiety. In general, five-membered heterocycles appear to be more effective than those with a six-membered ring, although several recent studies report cephalosporins of the latter type with good broad spectrum activities. They include analogs with 2-pyridine-*N*-oxide, 3-(6-hydroxypyridazine, or 6-tetrazolo[4,5-6]pyridazine attached through a sulfur link to the 3′-position (356). The good activity of the cephalosporins carrying the bicyclic heteroaromatic substituent named is an exception to that observed with most analogs of this type.

Table 15.15 3-Heterocyclicthiomethyl Cephalosporins[a]

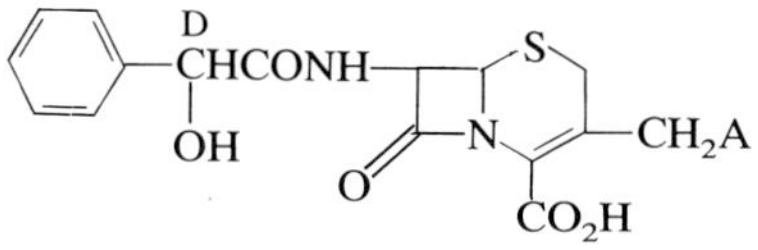

D, CHCONH, OH, S, N, CH_2A, O, CO_2H

Compound	A	In Vitro Activity: MIC, μg/ml		PD_{50} s.c. (*E. coli* in mouse), mg/kg
		S. aureus	*E. coli*	
1	H	6.3	12.5	25
2	$OCOCH_3$	1.6	1.6	6.2
3	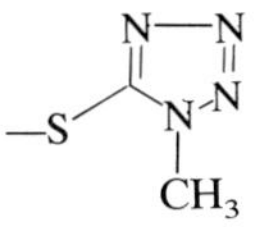 N—N, N, N, —S, CH_3	0.8	0.8	1.8
4	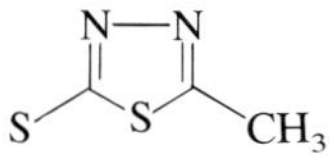 N—N, S, S, CH_3	0.4	1.6	3.6
5	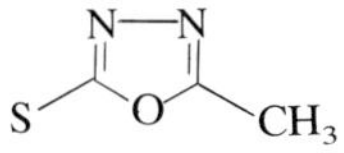 N—N, S, O, CH_3	0.8	3.1	5.5
6	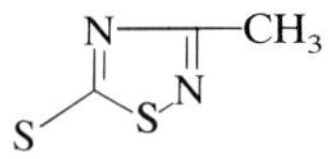 N, CH_3, N, S, S	6.3	6.3	50
7	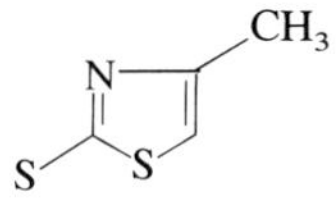 CH_3, N, S, S	3.1	6.3	152
8	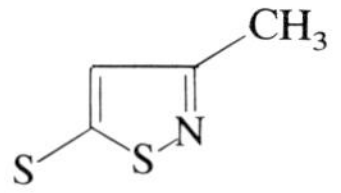 CH_3, N, S, S	3.1	50	50
9	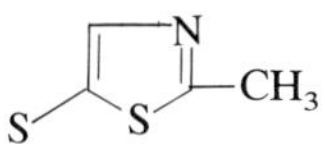 N, CH_3, S, S	6.3	100	—
10	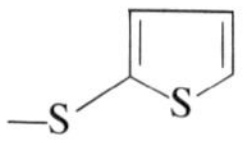 —S, S	6.3	200	—
11	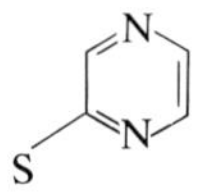 N, N, S	1.6	12.5	—

[a] Smith, Kline and French, unpublished data.

Although cefazolin (Table 15.16) is distinguished by the high serum levels it produces in laboratory animals and in man, improvement in pharmacokinetic properties does not necessarily parallel the enhancement of antibacterial activity. Except for cefatrizine, discussed below, these cephalosporins generally can be used only by injection, and the serum levels attained by this route are frequently low, especially with, for example, the methyltetrazole derivatives. On the other hand, the 3-tetrazolethiomethyl substituent can serve as a route to broad spectrum cephalosporins that produce high serum levels of long duration when injected into laboratory animals. This is accomplished by replacing the tetrazole *N*-methyl substituent with aliphatic groupings (C_1–C_4) carrying an acidic substituent (15.**43**, Z = e.g., CO_2H, SO_3H, $NHSO_3H$). In addition to exceptionally high serum levels these analogs are active

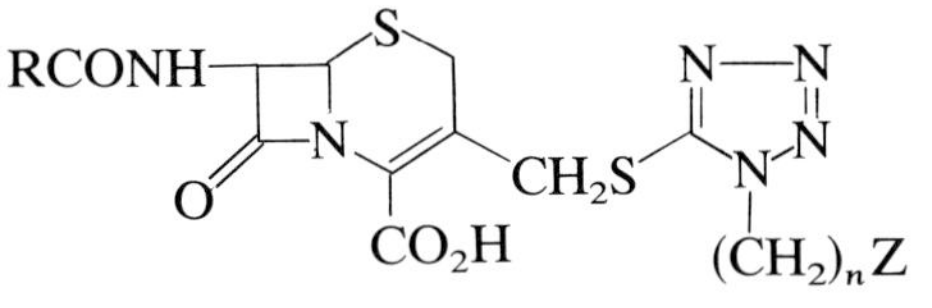

$n = 1$–4
Z = CO_2H, SO_3H, $NHSO_3H$, etc.
R = various

15.**43**

against several strains of gram-negative bacteria not generally susceptible to cephalothin, but they have poorer activity against the gram-positive bacteria. This enhancement of serum levels is observed with analogs having various acylamino groups on the 7-position. Two derivatives have been selected so far for extensive evaluation: ceforanide (15.**43,** R = *o*-NH_2-$CH_2C_6H_4CH_2$, $n = 1$, Z = CO_2H) (357, 358) and SK&F 75073 (15.**43**, R = $C_6H_5CH(OH)$, $n = 1$, Z = SO_3H) (359, 360).

A number of other variations of the 3-substituent that have resulted in significant changes in the biological properties of the cephalosporins have been achieved by chemical manipulations other than displacement of the 3′-acetoxy group. These include the 3-methylcephems (deacetoxycephalosporanic acids) and derivatives in which the complete acetoxymethyl group is replaced by, for example, hydrogen, alkoxy or halogen (fluorine, chlorine). These analogs are included in Section 9.4 on orally absorbed cephalosporins.

9.3 Injectable Clinical Cephalosporins

Tables 15.16 and 15.17 list the cephalosporins that are available for clinical use and those that have been subjected to extensive premarketing clinical evaluation. The spectra of antibacterial activities of the commercially available cephalosporins (Table 15.16) are almost identical, although there are quantitative differences in potency. All are characterized by high activity against a large number of gram-positive and gram-negative organisms, including penicillin-resistant staphylococci. Several of the cephalosporins in Table 15.17 extend the range of activity against the gram-negative bacteria beyond that obtained with the antibiotics listed in Table 15.16. The cephalosporins in both tables differ in pharmacokinetic properties that relate to parenteral and oral absorption, serum levels, biliary excretion, serum protein binding, and the like.

Cephalothin occupies a position among the cephalosporins similar to that of benzylpenicillin among the penicillins. Although marketed first and followed by analogs with improved properties, it continues to account for a significant part of cephalosporin use. It possesses broad spectrum activity with important exceptions in the gram-negative group (e.g., indole-positive *Proteus, Enterobacter, Serratia, Pseudomonas*) It has good resistance to staphylococcal penicillinase, which contributes to its broad use. Only about 2% of cephalothin is absorbed when it is given orally. Therefore it is administered intravenously or intramuscularly, where pain on injection is moderately high. Cephalothin is partially metabolized to the less active deacetylcephalothin. Cephapirin and cephacetrile are remarkably like cephalothin in their antimicrobial activities, pharmacokinetic behavior, and clinical indications. Cephaloridine displays better activity than cephalothin against the gram-positive cocci, it produces higher serum

Table 15.16 Clinically Important Cephalosporins

RCONH– (cephem nucleus: S, N, O=, CO_2H, CH_2A)

Generic Name	R	A	References
Injectables			
Cephalothin	2-thienyl–CH_2–	–$OCOCH_3$	361–363
Cephapirin	4-pyridyl–SCH_2–	–$OCOCH_3$	364–366
Cephacetrile	$N{\equiv}CCH_2$	–$OCOCH_3$	367–369
Cephaloridine	2-thienyl–CH_2–	–N^+ (pyridinium)	370–372
Cefazolin	tetrazol-1-yl–CH_2–	–S–(5-methyl-1,3,4-thiadiazol-2-yl), CH_3	373–377
Cephamandole (nafate)	phenyl–D-CH–OH(CHO)	–S–(1-methyltetrazol-5-yl), CH_3	156, 378, 379
Oral			
Cephaloglycin	phenyl–D-CH(–NH_2)–	–$OCOCH_3$	152, 380, 381
Cephalexin	phenyl–D-CH(–NH_2)–	–H	152, 382, 383
Cephradine	1,4-cyclohexadienyl–D-CH(–NH_2)–	–H	278, 279, 384

levels with equivalent doses, and it causes less pain on injection. These advantages are offset by a somewhat lower resistance to penicillinase and a renal toxicity liability that restricts its dosage to less than 4 g/day. Cefazolin is active against the gram-positive cocci at about the same level as cephalothin, but its activity against susceptible gram-negative pathogens is usually better. As with the other cephalosporins in this group, it is not appreciably absorbed when given orally. However, on intramuscular administration it gives serum levels that are 4 times the levels obtained with an equal dose of cephalothin. It has low renal toxicity in animals. Like cephaloridine, the 3-substituent is a type that resists metabolic removal.

Cefamandole has about the same activity as cefazolin against normally susceptible gram-negative bacteria such as *E. coli* and *K. pneumoniae*, but its activity extends to a

Table 15.17 Cephalosporins and Cephamycins with Clinical Evaluation

(General structure: RCONH–[X, H]–cephem nucleus with S, N, CO$_2$H and Z substituents)

Generic Name	R	X	Z	References
Injectable cephalosporins				
Cefazaflur	CF_3SCH_2—	H	$—CH_2S$–(1-methyltetrazol-5-yl)	385, 386
Cefuroxime	2-furyl–C(=$NOCH_3$)—	H	$—CH_2OCONH_2$	387–389
Cephanone	(sydnone)N—CH_2—	H	$—CH_2S$–(5-methyl-1,3,4-thiadiazol-2-yl) CH_3	355, 390
Cefotaxime	H_2N–(thiazol-4-yl)–C(=$NOCH_3$)—	H	$—CH_2OCOCH_3$	391
Oral cephalosporins				
Cefatrizine	HO–C_6H_4–CH(NH_2)—	H	$—CH_2S$–(1H-1,2,3-triazol-4-yl)	392–393
Cefachlor	C_6H_5–CH(NH_2)—	H	—Cl	394–396
Cefadroxil	HO–C_6H_4–CH(NH_2)—	H	$—CH_3$	397–399
Injectable cephamycin				
Cefoxitin	2-thienyl–CH_2—	OCH_3	$—CH_2OCONH_2$	161, 400–402

somewhat broader group of gram-negative organisms, including some strains of *Enterobacter* and indole-positive cocci is significantly lower than, for example, that of cephalothin, but is still sufficient for effective therapy. Peak serum levels (20 μg/ml; 1 g dose i.m.) are between those obtained with cephalothin (5–15 μg/ml) and cefazolin (40–50 μg/ml).

Four additional injectable cephalosporins that have undergone clinical evaluations are listed in Table 15.17. Cefuroxime extends the gram-negative spectrum less broadly than cefamandole but retains more gram-positive activity. Cefazaflur exhibits exceptionally high *in vitro* activities against gram-positive and gram-negative organisms and also extends the spectrum of activity against the latter, but less broadly than cephamandole. Cephanone displayed good *in vitro* activities and high serum levels on intramuscular injection, but it has been withdrawn from clinical trials. Cefotaxime is a very recent entry that shows great clinical promise. It displays impressively high *in vitro* activities against a very broad spectrum of bacteria. Its pharmacokinetic properties resemble those of cefamandole.

9.4. Oral Cephalosporins

Lack of oral activity, an almost universal characteristic of the cephalosporins, is shared by cephalosporin C and nearly all the semisynthetic cephalosporins. This is unexpected since these compounds have distinctly better acid stability than the penicillins, which are absorbed orally except when limited by instability to gastric acid. Obviously, this characteristic is associated with the cephalosporin nucleus, but the structural features of the β-lactam-dihydrothiazine ring system that account for the poor absorption from the gut are not known. And because of the generality of this characteristic among the cephalosporins, it is likewise unexpected that cephalexin and cephradine (Table 15.16) are absorbed orally with efficiencies (80% or better) greater than for the penicillins. These structurally related agents are very similar in their antimicrobial and pharmacokinetic properties (peak serum levels 20–30 μ g/ml with oral dose of 1 g) (403). They are generally less active *in vitro* than the clinically used injectable cephalosporins (Table 15.18), but they are less bound by serum proteins (5–20% vs 65% for cephalothin). Both are efficiently excreted through the kidney (80–100% recovery), giving high urine titers. They are indicated for treatment of mild to moderate infections, including infections of the urinary tract. Both can be adminstered orally; cephradine is also available in a dosage form suitable for injection. All the other cephalosporins that are now known to combine broad spectrum activity and oral absorption have similar 7-acyl groups of the D-phenylglycine type. As with the penicillins, the analogs with side chains having the L-configuration are less active (150, 152). Thus the 7-acyl group on cephaloglycin (Table 15.16) and cefachlor (Table 15.17) is D-phenylglycine; cefadroxil and cefatrizine (Table 15.17) carry the *p*-hydroxy-D-phenylglycine groups. The other acyl groups listed in Table 15.13, including the closely related D-mandelic acid moiety, do not provide derivatives capable of being absorbed orally.

Good oral absorption of cephalosporins

Table 15.18 Comparative Activities and Human Peak Serum Levels for Injectable and Oral Cephalosporins[a]

	MIC, μg/ml		Human Peak Serum Level, μg/ml[b]	
Cephalosporin	*S. aureus*	*E. coli*	i.m.	p.o.
Cephalothin	(0.5)	6.4	5–15	—
Cefazolin	0.6	1.0	40–50	0.7–0.9
Cephalexin/(cephradine)	4.8	9.7	(30–35)	20–30
Cephaloglycin	3.1	3.5	—	1.5

[a] Adapted from Refs. 114, (Ch. 12), 381, and 403.
[b] 1 g dose.

in humans has been ascribed to the presence in the structure of both the α-amino group on the 7-acyl substituent, and a small uncharged group at the 3-position (404). Indeed, the cephalosporins that exhibit the highest absorption efficiencies are derivatives of 7-ADCA, with a methyl group at the 3-position. Such derivatives, lacking a leaving group at the 3′-position, generally exhibit sharply reduced *in vitro* activities. Fortunately, the D-phenylglycinamide side chain not only provides for good oral absorption but, as mentioned earlier, 7-ADCA derivatives carrying this type of side chain exhibit activities against the gram-negative bacteria approaching those of cephalosporins with 3′-position functionalization. *In vitro* activity against gram-positive bacteria is lower, but usually within the clinically useful range. This capability of the 7-D-phenylglycine, and to a lesser extent the 7-D-mandeloyl group, extends to cephalosporins with other 3-substituents that would be expected to resemble the methyl group in their biological function. Thus although loss of the acetyl group from the 3-acetoxymethyl side chain in most cases results in a large drop in *in vitro* activity, the alcohol derived from cephaloglycin retains much of the activity of the parent (MICs: *S. aureus*, 3.1 vs. 2.8 μg/ml; *E. coli*, 3.5 vs. 12 μg/ml).

Nucleophilic 3′-substituents have been found to improve *in vitro* activity, but this advantage is counterbalanced by lower chemical stability, facilitated by a tendency for attack on the β-lactam carbonyl group by the α-amino group of the side chain. Thus cephaloglycin, which was developed before cephalexin, must be assayed *in vitro* by test methods designed to take into account its poor chemical stability; and it is poorly absorbed orally (10–25%). It affords serum levels (1.5 μg/ml peak, 1 g dose) significantly lower than those of cephalexin or cephradine, but urinary recoveries (6%) are measurable. Consequently, its use in the clinic is limited essentially to mild urinary tract infections. Other phenylglycl cephalosporins with substituents at the 3′-position that have been reported to produce serum levels on oral administration include analogs substituted with azide (405), methoxy (406), and methylthio (354) groups. In general, better *in vitro* activity is offset by lower absorption efficiency. A recent, thoroughly studied analog that violates the requirement, stated earlier, of a small nonpolar 3-substituent for efficient oral absorption is cefatrizine (Table 15.17). This analog, with *in vitro* activity against gram-negative bacteria significantly better than that of cephalexin (e.g., MICs using an *E. coli* sp., 1.5 vs. 6–12 μg/ml) affords serum levels in mice, both subcutaneously and orally, that are approximately double those obtained with cephalexin (20 mg/kg dose: i.m. peak serum levels, 54 vs. 28 μg/ml; p.o. peak serum levels, 44 vs. 18 μg/ml). These exceptionally high serum levels are dependent on the presence of both a 3-(1,2,3-triazole-4-thiomethyl) substituent and a *p*-hydroxyl group on the phenylglycine side chain at the 7-position (391). Peak serum concentrations in orally dosed mice for analogs without the *p*-hydroxyl group, or with a 2-methyl-1,3,4-thiadiazole or a 1-methyltetrazole ring in place of the 1,2,3-triazole moiety were 13, 24, and 7.6 μg/ml, respectively. Even though cefatrizine produces serum levels in man that are lower than predicted by the results in mice and other laboratory animals (407), its good *in vitro* activity and other promising biological properties have led to its extensive evaluation in the clinic (393).

Cefadroxil is a second orally absorbed cephalosporin with a *p*-hydroxyl group on the phenylglycine side chain. With *in vitro* activities essentially the same as those of cephalexin, it is reported to give peak serum concentrations in humans that are 75–80% of those of the latter. Because of a slower urinary excretion rate, however, the concentrations remain higher than those of cephalexin for a longer time (408).

Recently 7-phenylglycyl cephalosporin

analogs have been described on which the 3-acetoxymethyl substituent has been replaced *in toto* by hydroxyl, alkoxyl, and halo groups and by hydrogen (Section 10.4). Oral absorption of these derivatives has been reported, especially for the 3-methoxy (406) and 3-chloro analogs. The 3-deacetoxymethyl analog closely resembles cephalexin in its biological properties Cefachlor (Table 15.17) is reported to be more active microbiologically than cephalexin (395) and to produce peak serum levels in man that are 64% of those from an equivalent dose (250 mg) of cephalexin. Its clinical utility is currently being evaluated (396).

9.5 Cephamycins

A major limitation of the cephalosporins now in use is their sensitivity to inactivation by β-lactamases from many gram-negative bacteria, such as strains of *Enterobacter*, indole-positive *Proteus*, *Serratia*, *Providentia*, *Pseudomonas*, and many *Klebsiella* species. Cephamandole and cefuroxime are examples of cephalosporins that exhibit broader activity against gram-negative bacteria, including some of these β-lactamase-producing organisms. This broader activity is due, at least in part, to increased resistance to β-lactamases by virtue of the 7-acyl side chains of these cephalosporins. The cephamycins also resist many of the β-lactamases that can hydrolyze the commonly used cephalosporins. In this case resistance to these enzymes is due to the steric hindrance around the 7-position because of the 7α-methoxyl group. This broad resistance to enzyme attack is not always reflected in susceptibility of the β-lactamase-producing organism to the antibiotic. Nevertheless cephamycins, specifically cefoxitin, exhibit spectra of antibacterial activity that are broader than those of most cephalosporins.

Cephamycins A and B (Table 15.4) resemble cephalosporin C in that they have poor intrinsic activity against most bacteria, but cephamycin C, despite extremely poor activity against gram-positive bacteria, exhibits surprisingly good *in vitro* activity against many of the gram-negative species. Against various strains of susceptible *E. coli*, *K. pneumoniae*, *P. mirabilis* and the like, the MIC values of cephamycin C and cephalothin are within 1 or 2 twofold dilutions (128). Cephamycin C is extremely nontoxic, and it produces serum levels in mice (peak, 21 μg/ml with 20 mg/kg dose s.c.) of the order of those obtained with cephaloridine. Its *in vitro* effectiveness in mice is equal to that of cephalothin against gram-negative bacteria susceptible to the latter, and strikingly better against strains selected for their resistance to cephalothin through β-lactamase production. The *in vivo* protective activity against infections due to gram-positive bacteria is very low, as expected (130). Thus a major objective in modifying the cephamycin structure is to increase the antibacterial activity against gram-positive bacteria while retaining the gram-negative activity and the other desirable properties of cephamycin C.

Since structural modifications are more difficult than for the cephalosporins and penicillins, because of the 7α-methoxy and the 3-carbamyloxy substituents, published SAR studies on this antibiotic class remain relatively rare. Some 7- and 3-substituent modifications that have been reported are included in Table 15.19 (107, 162). The broader spectrum of antibacterial activity attainable with this structural type is reflected in the *in vitro* activity (MIC: 0.8–6.2) of a number of these derivatives against a β-lactamase-producing strain of *E. coli* resistant to cephalothin (MIC: 50 μg/ml). These data predict the creation of additional cephamycins with high levels of activity against the gram-positive and gram-negative bacteria.

Cefoxitin (Table 15.17) is the only semisynthetic cephamycin that has undergone extensive preclinical evaluation to date.

Table 15.19 Representative *in Vitro* Activities of Cephamycin Analogs (107, 162)

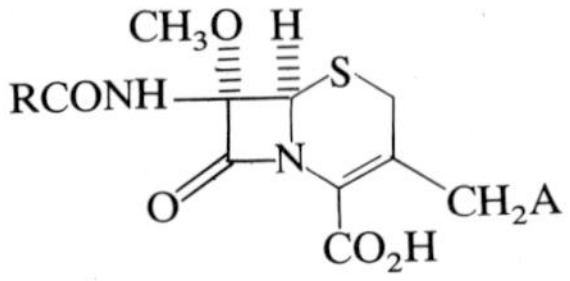

CH_3O H

RCONH — S — N — O — CH_2A

CO_2H

R	A	MIC, μg/ml		
		S. aureus	*E. coli*	*E. coli*[a]
Cephalothin		0.2	6.2	50
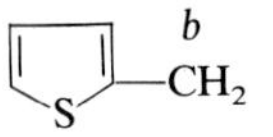 S —CH_2 [b]	$OCONH_2$	1.5	3.1	3.1
$HetSCH_2$[c]	$OCONH_2$	0.2–6.2	6.2–400	6.2–>400
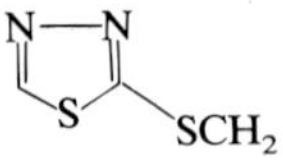 N—N, S, SCH_2	$OCONH_2$	1.5	3.1	3.1
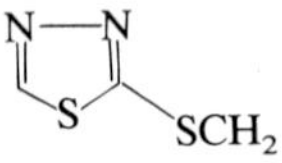 N—N, S, SCH_2	$OCOCH_3$	1.5	3.1	6.2
N—N, S, SCH_2	N_3	0.4	3.1	3.1
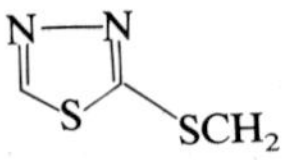 N—N, S, SCH_2	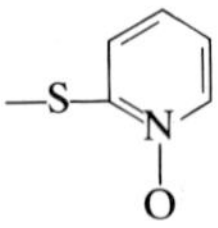 —S—, N, O	0.4	6.2	25
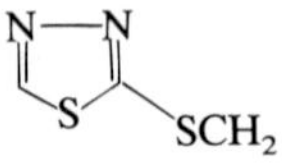 N—N, S, SCH_2	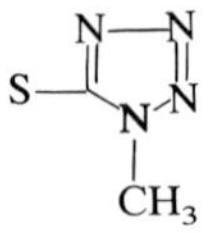 S—, N—N, N, N, CH_3	0.8	1.5	1.5
$NCCH_2SCH_2$	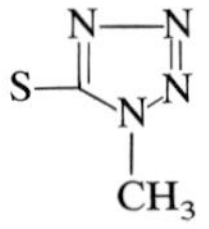 S—, N—N, N, N, CH_3	0.8	0.8	0.8

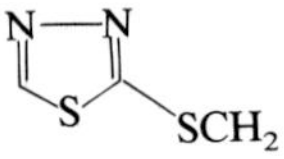

[a] β-lactamase producer.
[b] Cefoxitin.
[c] Other heterocyclicthioacetyl analogs similar to the following thiadizole derivative.

Reported *in vitro* activities compare favorably with those of the cephalosporins in clinical use (400). This activity extends to many resistant strains of *Enterobacter*, *Klebsiella*, *Proteus morganii*', and *Serratia*. Its activity against gram-positive bacteria more closely resembles that of cephalexin. Cefoxitin must be given intramuscularly (with much pain) or intravenously; it produces serum levels (peak, 20–25 μg/ml, 1 g dose i.m.) in the same range as cefamandole, intermediate between those of cephalothin and cefazolin (402). Its efficacy in man is now under investigation (402).

The high levels of antibacterial activity permitted by 7α-methoxy cephalosporins contrast sharply with the near inactivity of similar 6α-substituted penicillins (58). Again using base hydrolysis rates as an indicator, Indelicato and Wilham (409) have related the differences in bioactivity to changes in the reactivity of the β-lactam ring when such substituents are introduced. They propose that penicillins are sterically similar to isolated β-lactams that have one face hindered, and the cephalosporin structure resembles β-lactams with both faces unhindered. Thus 6α-substitution on penicillins results in a β-lactam hindered at both faces with lower overall reactivity, whereas after 7α-substitution on cephalosporins, the β-face of the lactam carbonyl is still unhindered, thus available for reaction. Indeed the polar effect of the methoxy substituent increases the β-lactam reactivity slightly. This would explain the differences in substituent effect and would favor the involvement of the β-face of cephalosporins in reactions with nucleophilic agents. It does not explain completely the lowered biological activities of cephalosporins substituted at the 7α-position by many substituents other than methoxyl.

10 OTHER MODIFICATIONS OF THE PENICILLINS, CEPHALOSPORINS, AND CEPHAMYCINS

The three preceding sections focused primarily on structural manipulations and biological properties that have led to clinically useful antibiotics or major trends in biological activity that were important in achieving this end. Many other structural changes have been carried out that have been less successful in this respect, and a few changes that have produced interesting biological results have entailed a body of work smaller than the material already discussed. This section summarizes some of the structural changes and resultant biological properties of the latter type.

10.1 Modification of the Carboxyl Group

A structural alteration that has led to derivatives with improved antibacterial properties is replacement of the carboxyl group by a 5-tetrazolyl moiety (15.**44**) (410, 411).

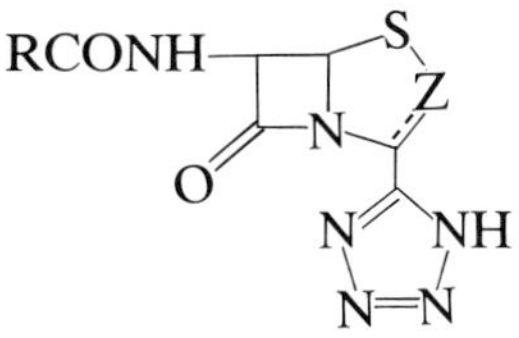

RCONH, S, Z, N, O, N, NH, N=N

15.**44**

These compounds, particularly in the penicillin series, are reported to have potent, broad spectrum antibacterial activity. Their synthesis is accomplished by conversion of a suitably protected penicillin or cephalosporin amide to the imino chloride, followed by reaction with azide ion to generate the tetrazole ring. When 6-tritylaminopenicillanic acid is used as starting material, the resulting 3-tetrazole derivative can be deblocked with hydrogen fluoride at low temperature to give the 6-amino derivative, used to prepare various 6-acyl analogs. The corresponding 7-amino-4-(5-tetrazolyl)-3-cephem can be made by a parallel route. This intermediate has also been derived from the 4-cyano derivative, which was derived in turn from the primary carboxamide. Detailed biological studies on many of these compounds have not yet appeared, but data on two penicillin analogs have been reported. The p-hydroxyphenylglycl analog is active against both gram-positive and gram-negative bacteria including *K. pneumoniae* and strains of *Enterobacter, Serratia, H. influenzae,* and *S. fecalis.* This compound is more resistant to β-lactamases than the corresponding penicillin, which may account, at least in part, for its improved activity. It displays excellent protective activity against experimental infections in mice, and it is well absorbed following oral or parenteral administration to mice and dogs, giving peak serum levels comparable to those of ampicillin. A second analog, the α-guanylureidophenylacetamido derivative, has even broader activity against gram-negative bacteria, including *Proteus* (indole positive) and *Pseudomonas* species. It is active only by the parenteral route, but it shows increased stability to β-lactamases. Clinical utility of these new agents has yet to be established.

Except for the tetrazole ring, chemical replacement of the carboxyl group of penicillins and cephalosporins has not produced derivatives with significant potential for clinical use. Thioacid analogs (COSH) of penicillins have about the same level of activity as the parent antibiotics against *S. aureus*; they have slightly increased resistance to β-lactamase, but they display reduced activity in the presence of serum (413). Esterification of the carboxyl group has resulted in a few derivatives that show improved oral absorption and distribution properties in man. Simple esters of penicillins lack significant *in vitro* antibacterial activity *per se*. The mouse has a specific serum esterase capable of hydrolyzing them to the free penicillin, but human tissues are incapable of doing this (414). However acyloxymethyl esters of penicillins (15.**45**)

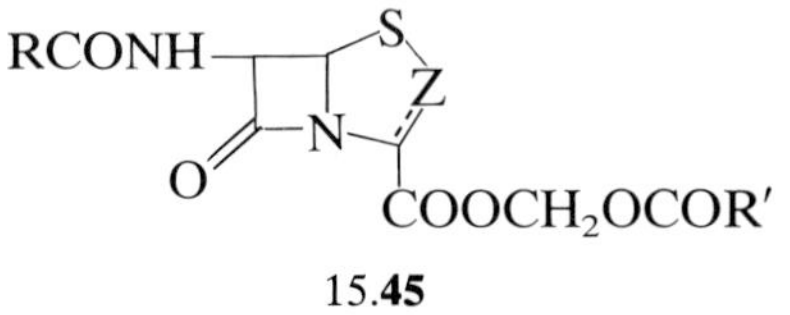

15.**45**

are susceptible to hydrolysis by human tissues (415). Presumably a nonspecific esterase cleaves the acyl group, and the resultant hydroxymethyl ester decomposes spontaneously to the penicillin and formaldehyde. On oral administration, the acetoxymethyl ester of penicillin G, penamecillin, gives penicillin G serum levels only slightly higher than those obtained from the free penicillin. In contrast, acyloxymethyl esters of ampicillin produce significantly improved serum levels of ampicillin. The utility of these and similar esters was described earlier in this chapter. Simple esters of cephalosporins likewise have poor activity *in vitro*, and though acyloxymethyl esters of cephalosporins are also easily hydrolyzed, none has achieved clinical significance (416).

The penicillin amides (417, 418) have modest intrinsic antibacterial activity, which is not the result of hydrolysis to the free acids. They also show some resistance to penicillinases, but they have not found any clinical application. Isomerization to biologically inactive Δ^2-cephalosporins frequently occurs when cephalosporins are converted to amides by reacting the activated carboxyl group (e.g., anhydride) with amines (202). However coupling of cephalothin with alanine using *N,N′*-dicyclohexylcarbodiimide gave the desired Δ^3-peptide. This product had a very low order of antibacterial activity. Although the mono- and disubstituted amides of penicillin are less active than their unsubstituted analogs, alkoxyamides (CONHOR) have good gram-positive activity and stability toward penicillinase (419). However they are bound by serum and are marginally active *in vivo* (420).

The carboxyl group of penicillins and cephalosporins can be converted to various substituents of lower oxidation state. Borohydride reduction of carboxyl-activated intermediates such as mixed anhydrides or acid chlorides gives the corresponding substituted methanols (421, 422). Penicillin 3-carboxaldehydes can be prepared by Raney nickel desulfurization of the thioacid (423). Cephalosporin 4-carboxaldehydes are synthesized by way of the diethylacetals by oxidation of the appropriate cephalosporin 4-methanol using DCC/DMSO (424). The homologous acetic acid analogs are obtained upon photolytic rearrangement of the intermediate diazoketones (425). Wittig reaction of the cephalosporin 4-carboxaldehydes with diphenyl methoxycarbonylmethylenetriphenylphosphorane, followed

followed by acid cleavage of the ester group, gives the vinylogous analog (424). None of these derivatives has useful antibacterial activity. The cephalosporin carboxyl group also has been replaed by a phosphonic acid moiety by a totally synthetic approach. The resulting compound is less active than the corresponding cephalosporin derivative (426).

Many penicillin and cephalosporin esters have been used as synthetic intermediates. Among the more important of these are esters that can be cleaved back to the free acids under mild conditions without disruption of the β-lactam ring. These include the benzyl (79, 177, 221), cyanomethyl (427), trimethylsilyl (428), and phenacyl (429) esters of penicillins, and the *t*-butyl (430), 2,2,2-trichloroethyl (102, 103), benzhydryl (431), *p*-methoxybenzyl (432), and *p*-nitrobenzyl (433) esters of cephalosporins. Many of the carboxyl-modified derivatives of the penicillins are discussed in a recent review article (158).

10.2 Modification and Replacement of the Amino Group

N-Alkylation of 6-APA has been accomplished by reductive condensation with aldehydes and ketones (434) and by treatment with diazoalkanes, which also esterify the carboxyl group (435). Monoalkylated, dialkylated, and quaternary derivatives of 6-APA have been prepared. The monoalkylated derivatives of benzyl- and phenoxymethylpenicillins show drastically reduced activities compared with penicillins G and V.

The 6(7)-amine has been replaced by a number of other functional groups. Modifications in which the 6(7)-acylamino group is replaced by an isosteric moiety illustrate the importance of the NH grouping for activity, since such analogs synthesized so far have greatly reduced activity (15.**46**).

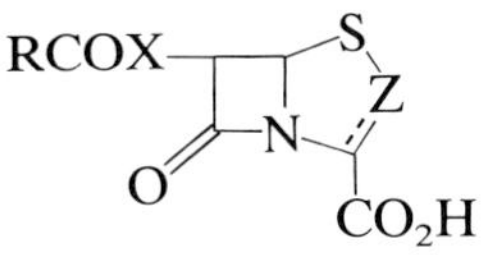

RCOX, S, Z, N, O, CO_2H

X=NHNH, CH_2, O

15.**46**

The NH group has been replaced by hydrazino and methylene groups, and by oxygen, all with the cis (natural) configuration on the β-lactam ring (436–438). The 6-hydrazino analog of penicillin G, prepared by reducing benzyl 6-diazopenicillinate with triphenylphosphine, followed by phenylacetylation, borohydride reduction, and dibenzylation, was only moderately active against a penicillinase-producing *S. aureus* strain. 7-Thienylacetylhydrazinocephalosporins have also been synthesized, but no biological results were reported (439). The 6(7)-hydroxypenicillins and cephalosporins and several of their acyl analogs were synthesized from diazo intermediates by mild acid hydrolysis to the 6(7)-α-hydroxy derivative, followed by oxidation to the 6(7)-ketone, borohydride reduction, and acylation. In both cases the α- and β-isomers were prepared. The α-isomers were inactive, the β-isomers displayed only moderate activity against a strain of *S. aureus.* An analog of penicillin V in which the amino group has been replaced by a methylene has been synthesized by reaction of the appropriate phosphorus ylid with a 6-ketopenicillin ester, followed by reduction and removal of the carboxyl protecting group. Only weak antibacterial activity was observed (437).

Treatment of 6-APA with nitrous acid in the presence of an appropriate anion produces 6-α-chloro, 6-α-bromo (440–442), and 6-α-iodopenicillin (443), along with 6,6-dibromo and diiodo derivatives. Reduction of 6-α-bromopenicillanic acid yields unsubstituted penicillanic acid. (444). As might be expected, all these derivatives are devoid of antibacterial activity. No deliberate effort to obtain the analogous cephalosporins has been reported, but 7-α-chlorocephalosporin was found as a by-product in the nitrosyl chloride deacylation of cephalosporin C (445). 7-Alkyl-7-deaminocephalosporins of undetermined stereochemistry have been prepared by reducing a 7-diazo intermediate with a trialkylborane (446). Most were inactive, but the adamantylmethylene derivative had low yet observable activity against gram-positive bacteria.

10.3 Other Modifications at the 6(7)-Position

A large variety of substituents have now been placed on the 6(7)α-position of penicillins and cephalosporins. With the exception of the 7α-methoxy group on the cephalosporin structure (see the cephamycin sections above), introduction of these substituents results in significantly lower antibacterial activity compared with the activity of the 6(7)α-unsubstituted counterpart. Several methods were used to accomplish this. Two of the more general methods were discussed earlier (pp. 111–112). One utilizes the reaction of 6(7)-anions, derived from 6(7)-imines (Schiff) bases) or isocyanides (447) and, for example, sodium hydride, with electrophillic agents (e.g., methyl iodide, benzyl chloroformate). In the second method these agents are added to 6(7)-aralkylimino or acylimino (448) penicillins and cephalosporins. An additional procedure employs direct carbamylation using *N*-chloro-*N*-sodioethane (449). Representative examples of substituents that have been attached to the penicillins and the cephalosporins include the following. *Penicillins:* D (450); Me (58, 451, 452); Et (451); CH_2Y, where Y = OH, NH_2, Cl, F (453, 454); CH_2OH, CH(OH)Me; CHO, COMe, CO_2Me, CO_2Na (454); CN (455); OH,OCHO (448); OR (96, 447, 455, 456); SMe (457); $NHCO_2Et$ (449). *Cephalosporins*: Me (58, 451, 452, 458); Et (451); CH_2OH (453); CN, $CH(CO_2Et)$; OCH_2CN, N_3 (459); CHO, COMe (452, 454); CO_2H (460); SMe (196, 459, 457); $NHCO_2Et$ (449); $PO(OMe)_2$ (461).

A number of penicillins and cephalosporins epimerized at the 6(7)-carbon have been described 15.**47**. For example,

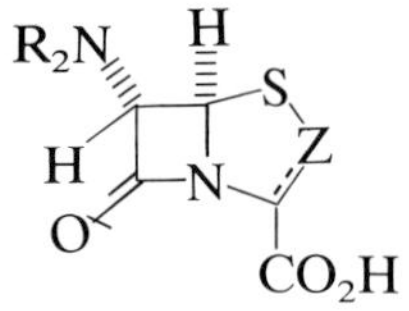

15.**47**

hetacillin is converted to its 6α-isomer, epihetacillin, in 85% yield on treatment with sodium hydroxide in aqueous solution; its methyl ester epimerizes similarly innonaqueous media (DMSO-trimethylamine) (462). The isomerization is accompanied by a loss of biological activity. Under the same conditions, benzylpenicillin and 6-APA do not epimerize (463). The epimeric 6-APA has been obtained by removal of the 7-acyl group of epihetacillin. Benzyl-6-epipenicillin derived from this is also biologically inactive. Conditions for epimerization of the 6-carbon of penicillins in an aqueous medium imply deprotonation and reprotonation; in nonaqueous media there is evidence for cleavage of the S-1 to C-5 bond by a β-elimination that generates a double bond in the β-lactam ring, followed by readdition of the resulting thiol to the double bond to give the epimeric product (463). Epimerization by way of the 6-anion is controlled by the electronegativity of the 6-substituent.

Penicillanic acids with primary amide (benzylpenicillin), amine, dimethylamine, and tritylamine substituents fail to epimerize with sodium hydroxide (464). Side chains reported to permit epimerization include, in addition to the hetacillin side chain, phthalimido (465), bromo (observed by way of deuterium exchange), and trimethylammonium (464). Epimerization of penicillin sulfoxide esters (with a secondary amide group such as phenoxyacetamido at the 6-position) has been accomplished under nonbasic conditions using *N,O*-bis-(trimethylsilyl)acetamide (466). This reaction is presumed to proceed through the silyl enol ether derived from the β-lactam carbonyl. Cephalosporins and their sulfoxides do not epimerize under these conditions. However a Morin ring expansion of the epimeric (6α) penicillin sulfoxide ester gave, on deblocking, the 7α-phenoxyacetamido-3-deacetoxycephalosporanic acid. Other cephalosporins epimerized at the 7-carbon have been prepared by total synthesis (100, 101). Additionally, cephalosporin sulfoxide esters (e.g., from cephalothin) give epimeric mixtures in the presence of trialkylamines in chloroform, whereas the unoxidized cephalosporins do not (467).

10.4 Other Modifications at the 3-Position of Cephalosporins

Although the versatility of the acetoxy group displacement provides access to many types of 3-substituents (see Section 6.2), limitations exist, and alternative methods for introducing new substituents on the 3-position have been developed. The 3-substituent types discussed here are divided into two classes, those attached to the 3-position by way of a methylene bridge (3′-substituted cephalosporins) and those attached directly to the ring.

10.4.1 SUBSTITUENTS ATTACHED THROUGH A 3-METHYLENE GROUP. The cephalosporins with variation of the 3′-acyloxy group, discussed elsewhere in this chapter, can be obtained by coupling aliphatic or aromatic carboxylic acids with 3-hydroxymethyl-3-cephems, or with 3-hydroxymethyl-2-cephems, followed by double bond isomerization (167, 168, 469). The intermediate Δ^3-alcohols cannot be prepared by direct chemical hydrolysis of the acetoxymethyl group; the β-lactam ring is opened with alkali and lactonization with the 4-carboxyl group occurs with acid. They are accessible by way of enzymatic deacetylation using esterases from orange peel (121) or from various microorganisms (470). The 3-hydroxymethyl-2-cephems are more stable than the Δ^3-isomers and are prepared from 3-acetoxymethyl-3-cephems by isomerization of the double bond, followed by mild alkaline (or enzymatic) hydrolysis (159, 431). The alcohol group reacts readily with isocyanates to give 3-carbamoyloxymethyl derivatives (471) and with diazoalkanes to produce cephalosporins having a 3-methoxymethyl substituent (472). The latter are more readily obtained from cephalosporins with a 3-halomethyl side chain. These versatile intermediates can be used to prepare 3′-substituted cephalosporins described in Section 6.2, as well as analogs such as 3-cyanomethylcephalosporins (473) that are not accessible by direct displacement of the 3′-acetoxy group. They are obtained in a number of ways, including (*a*) reaction of deacetylcephalosporanic acid esters (e.g., benzhydryl) with thionyl halides or their equivalent (472), (*b*) reaction of 3-methyl-2-cephems or 3-methyl-3-cephem sulfoxides with NBS using photochemical initiation (followed by double bond isomerization of the Δ-2 isomer) (406, 474), (*c*) direct displacement of the acetoxy or carbamoyloxy group from 2-cephems (the Δ-3 isomers do not react) with halogen in the presence of strong acids (HCl, HBr, HI) in nonpolar solvents (475, 476), (*d*) displacement of the 3′-acetoxy group using a boron trihalide (477), or (*e*) reaction of 3-exomethylene cephams (see below) with DBU-bromine or DBU iodine (478). In contrast to the acetoxy group, the 3′-halides undergo allylic displacements even when the 4-carboxyl group is esterified. The 3-halomethyl cephalosporins themselves are reported to have only weak antibacterial activity. Many other analogs obtained by way of 3′-halogen displacement—for example, 3-cyanomethyl (473) and 3-methoxymethylcephalosporins (406)—are less active *in vitro* than their 3-acetoxymethyl analogs, although in some cases substantial broad spectrum activity is retained.

Derived 3′-substituents can be reacted further. For instance, the 3′-azide has been reduced to the amine and cyclized by way of 1,3-dipolar additions to 1,2,3-triazoles and tetrazoles (479); the 3′-cyano group has been incorporated into a tetrazole ring as well, and in the presence of copper(II) salts the sulfide from displacement of the 3′-acetoxy group by 2-mercaptopyridine *N*-oxide undergoes facile displacement by methanol to give 3-methoxymethyl derivatives (480). Varied substituents can be introduced at the 3′-position by the addition of nucleophiles (e.g., azide, acetonitrile, phenol, ethylacetoacetate) to Δ^2-cephamycin carboxylic acid esters in the presence of Lewis acids (476), or by reacting "carbon nucleophiles" in trifluoroacetic acid with similar cephem esters (431). Subsequent double bond isomerization and ester hydrolysis give, for example, 3-arylmethyl and 3-heterocyclicmethyl cephalosporins. The 3-benzyl substituent has also been placed on the cephalosporin structure by synthesis from a penicillin-derived β-lactam intermediate (481). Some of these 3-arylmethyl and heterocyclicmethyl analogs are active against gram-positive bacteria, but most have poor activity against gram-negative species.

10.4.2 SUBSTITUENTS ATTACHED DIRECTLY TO THE RING. The 3-hydroxymethyl substituent (both Δ^2 and Δ^3-cephems) has been oxidized (CrO_3, DMSO-Ac_2O, DDQ) to the corresponding cephem-3-carboxaldehyde (15.**48,** Z = CHO) (482–484). These aldehydes serve as key intermediates for the synthesis of many 3-modified cephalosporins. Besides simple oximes (485, 486) and hydrazones (486), this group can be converted to 3-

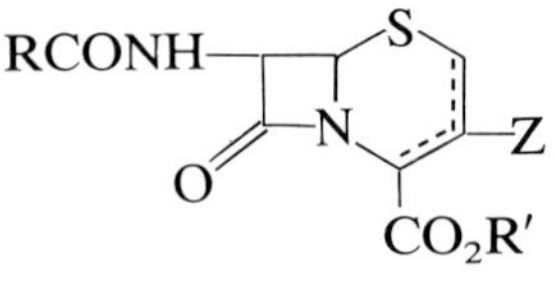

RCONH, S, N, O, Z, CO_2R'

15.**48**

diazomethyl (Z = CHN_2), oxonitrilomethyl (Z = $C{\equiv}\overset{+}{N}{-}\overset{-}{O}$), and N-methylnitrone (Z = $CH{=}\overset{+}{N}(CH_3)\overset{-}{O}$) groupings, which in turn undergo dipolar cyclo additions (with acetylenes, olefins, nitriles) to give cephalosporin analogs with a heterocyclic moiety attached directly to the 3-position (486, 487). Similar heterocyclic derivatives also are accessible by total synthesis (488). Although the gram-positive activity of these compounds is similar to that of cephalothin, activity against gram-negative organisms usually is greatly reduced. The 3-aldehyde reacts with Wittig-type ylids to give 3-vinyl cephalosporins (Z = CH═CHR), some of which have broad spectrum activity (489). Decarbonylation occurs to form the deacetoxymethyl-3-cephem (Z = H) when either 2- or 3-cephem-3-carboxaldehydes are treated with *tris*-triphenylphosphine rhodium chloride (484). These analogs can also be obtained from penicillins by a multistep synthesis (490). They retain significant antibacterial activity. Dehydration of the 3-aldehyde oxime produces the 3-cyano compound (485, 486).

Oxidation of the aldehyde leads to 3-cephem-3-carboxylic acids, esters, and amides (485, 491), which, in turn, can be converted to ketones, amines, and carbamates. None of these analogs has been reported to show enhanced antibacterial activity.

Synthesis of the versatile 3-*exo*-methylenecephams (15.**49**) provides access to

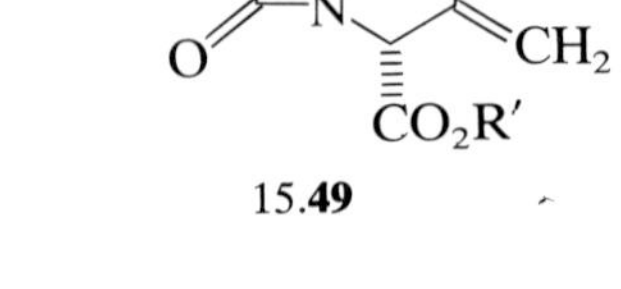

RCONH, S, N, O, CH_2, CO_2R'

15.**49**

many new analogs that would be difficult to prepare otherwise; indeed; some show improved antibacterial activity and may have clinical potential (e.g., cefachlor, Table 15.17). These intermediates are available by several methods: (*a*) reduction of 3-acetoxymethylcephalosporins by chromium(II) salts (492), (*b*) electrochemical reduction (493), and (*c*) desulfurization with Raney nickel of cephalosporins in which the acetoxy group has been displaced by a sulfur nucleophile such as 2-mercaptopyridine *N*-oxide (433). They also can be prepared directly from penicillin sulfoxides by ring expansion (494, 495). These exomethylene derivatives are devoid of antibacterial activity, even though the carboxyl-group configuration was shown to be the same as that in the penicillins (496–498). They can be isomerized to deacetoxycephalosporanic acids or ozonized to give 3-hydroxycephems (15.**48**, Z=OH) (394, 495, 499). The latter can also be obtained by ozonolysis of penicillin-ring-opened azetidinones followed by ring closure (495, 500). These hydroxy compounds have been converted to 3-methoxycepholosporins (15.**48**, Z=OCH_3) and 3-halocephalosporins (Z=Cl, Br), many of which show enhanced antibacterial activity (394, 499, 500). From the limited data available, the halo analogs appear to be consistently more active than the methoxy derivatives. The chemical reactivity of the β-lactam ring of 3-chloro-3-cephems is similar to that of the corresponding cephalosporanic acid and 12–15 times greater than deacetoxycephalosporanic acid (342). The increased β-lactam ring reactivity is reflected in higher antibacterial activities. Other groupings that have been derived from the 3-hydroxy substituent include fluorides (15.**48**, Z=F) (501), thioethers, sulfoxides, and sulfones (Z=SR, SOR, SO_2R), heterocyclicthioethers (Z=5-thio-1-methyltetrazole), amines (Z=NHR), and amides (Z=NHCOR) (502). Some of the analogs with these substituents are reported to have improved antibacterial activities.

10.5 Oxidation of the Sulfur Atom

A variety of agents (peracids, hydrogen peroxide, sodium metaperiodate, ozone, iodobenzene dichloride) will oxidize penicillin acids, esters, and amides to the corresponding sulfoxides (177, 179, 181, 189, 503). More vigorous conditions (potassium permanganate) are needed to produce the sulfones (177, 427). The role of the 7-acylamino side chain in determining the stereochemistry of the sulfoxide (*S*-isomer) 15.**25** obtained from the peracid or hydrogen peroxide oxidations was mentioned earlier (p. 109). Penicillins that have no amide N—H, for example, 6-phthalimido derivatives, do not hydrogen bond with the oxidant; hence steric effects predominate and the *R*-sulfoxide is formed as the major product (180, 181). The nature of the oxidizing agent also plays a role in determining the sulfoxide stereochemistry. Although peracid oxidation of penicillin G methyl ester gives exclusively the *S*-isomer, treatment with iodobenzene dichloride in aqueous pyridine yields a 1 : 1 mixture of sulfoxides. Oxidation of penicillin V with ozone in acetone-water likewise gives a 1 : 1 mixture of isomers, and 6-phthalimidopenicillanic acid yields only the *R*-sulfoxide (504). The *R*-sulfoxides also are accessible by acetone-sensitized photochemical inversion of *S*-sulfoxides (505); *R*-sulfoxides are thermally unstable and revert to the *S*-isomers in refluxing benzene (189, 503). The sulfoxides and sulfones of both benzyl- and phenoxymethylpenicillin show greatly reduced antibacterial activities (427), but the *R*-sulfoxide of penicillin V is reported to be 5 times more active than the *S*-isomer against gram-positive bacteria (506). Penicillin sulfoxides are of primary interest as intermediates in the conversion of penicillins to cephalosporins (see Section 6.3).

Cephalosporin sulfoxides can be obtained by the same methods described for penicillins. Peracid oxidation affords a mixture of *S*- and *R*-sulfoxides, the *S*-isomer predominating by a factor of 9:1 (507). In practice, oxidation of either the 2- or 3-cephem acids and esters produces the 3-cephem sulfoxide (508). The 2-cephem sulfoxides can be isolated from these oxidations, but they are unstable and rapidly isomerize to the 3-cephem sulfoxide when dissolved in hydroxylic solvents. Cephalosporin *R*-sulfoxides are obtained preferentially by oxidation of various cephalosporin intermediates with peracid (oxidation of a Schiff base), singlet oxygen or *N,N'*-dichlorourethane (509). Cephalosporin sulfones can be obtained by further oxidation of the sulfoxides with peracid (508). Cephalosporin sulfoxides cannot be reduced to the sulfides using common reducing agents (159), but if the sulfoxide is first activated by reacting it with an acid halide, presumably forming a sulfoxonium intermediate, it can be reduced by several types of reducing agents ($S_2O_4^{2-}$, I^-, Sn^{2+}, etc.) (508). Reagents such as phosphorus trichloride and phosphorus tribromide will effect this reduction without external activation, and phosphorus pentasulfide has been reported to reduce both penicillin and cephalosporin sulfoxides to the sulfides (510). The oxidation-reduction scheme has been used as a method of controlling the double bond position in cephalosporins. Cephalosporin *S*-sulfoxides show only weak antibacterial activity, but the *R*-sulfoxides of cephalothin and cephalexin show activity *in vitro* similar to that of the parent sulfides (509).

10.6 Other Modifications of the Penicillin and Cephalosporin Ring Systems

Whereas oxidation of the ring sulfur atom yields the sulfoxides and sulfones, other reactions (e.g., alkylation) involving the penicillin sulfur atom lead to cleavage of either the S-1 to C-2 or the S-1 to C-5 bond, depending on the reagent employed. For example, penicillin esters react with methyl iodide in the presence of base to give 2-methylthioazetidinones (15.**50**;

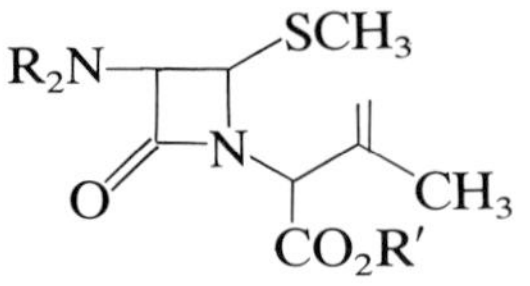

15.**50**

cleavage at S-1/C-2) (511). Treatment with chlorine or sulfuryl chloride affords 2-chloroazetidinones (15.**51**; cleavage at S-1/-C-5) (512). These azetidinones have been

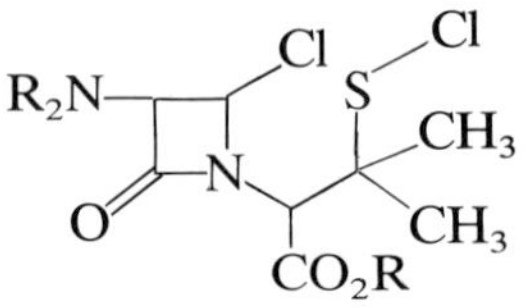

15.**51**

used as intermediates to synthesize novel fused-ring *β*-lactam systems. Cephalosporins behave differently. Alkylation of a cephalosporin ester with methylfluorosulfonate produces a stable 1-methylsulfonium salt, but the stereochemistry at C-6 is inverted (*β*-lactam hydrogens trans) (513). Scission of the S-1 to C-2 bond also occurs through base-catalyzed rearrangement of penicillin acid chlorides or mixed anhydrides to anhydropenicillins (15.**52**)

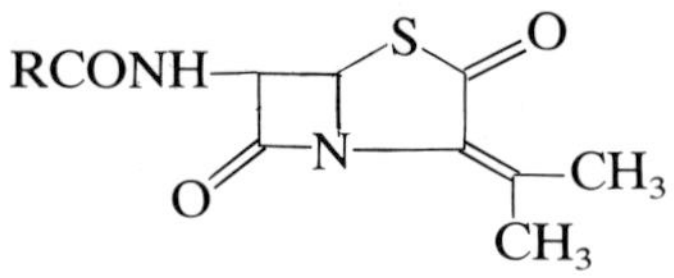

15.**52**

(514, 515). These compounds are biologically inactive, but the rearrangement is of interest as a possible route to the azetidinone intermediates used in the semisynthesis of new *β*-lactam-containing structures. The complete removal of sulfur from the penicillin thiazolidine ring (15.**19**) was accomplished very early in the studies on penicillins, using nickel desulfurization (72). Desthiobenzylpenicillin is biologically inactive.

The geminal methyl groups on C-2 of the penicillins make alterations at this position difficult. The 2-acyloxymethyl analogs (15.**26**), obtained as by-products from the ring expansion of penicillin sulfoxides to cephalosporins, were described earlier. The β-sulfoxides give 2β-acyloxymethyl derivatives; the α-sulfoxides lead to mixtures of 2α- and 2β-acyloxy analogs (189). Reoxidation of a 2-acyloxymethyl penicillin to its sulfoxide followed by a second treatment with anhydride can give 2,2-diacyloxymethyl derivatives (516). Similarly, 2-halomethyl derivatives are obtained by reacting the sulfoxides with an acyl halide in pyridine (517). Both 2-norphenoxymethylpenicillins (one methyl group replaced by hydrogen) and 2-bisnorphenoxymethylpenicillin (both methyls replaced by hydrogen) have been prepared by a total synthesis route similar to that used by Sheehan to synthesize penicillins (518). The nor analogs were only slightly less active than phenoxymethylpenicillin, but the bisnor compound was about 10 times less active than phenoxymethylpenicillin against a strain of *S. aureus.* A 2-bisnor-2-carbalkoxypenicillin, synthesized using a penicillin-derived monocyclic β-lactam intermediate, was inactive against gram-negative bacteria (519). Cephalosporin analogs, designated "cephalocillins," in which the C-2 hydrogens have been replaced by geminal methyl groups, were prepared by a semisynthetic approach (520). No biological results were reported for these compounds. However a 7-oximinoacyl derivative of 2α-methyl-3-cephem-4-carboxylic acid (FR 13374) has been reported to display biological properties superior to those of its 7-acylaminocephalosporanic acid analog (521). Unlike penicillins, the 2-position of the cephalosporins is much more amenable to substitution. 2-Alkoxy and 2-halo derivatives are obtained by treating cephalosporin esters with chlorine in the presence of an alcohol or with NBS (522, 523). The 2-methoxy derivatives can also be obtained using *N*-chloro-*N*-sodiourethane in methanol-acetonitrile (524). These substituents were shown to have the α-configuration exclusively. Substitution at C-4 with shift of the double bond to the 2-position is a frequent, and sometimes major, side reaction. However this circumstance is overcome when the 2-position is further activated by oxidation of the sulfide to the sulfoxide. Cephalosporin ester sulfoxides undergo the Pummerer reaction with acetic anhydride to give the 2α-acetoxy derivatives (525), which also can be obtained directly by treating the unoxidized dephalosporin with lead tetraacetate (507).

Under the conditions of the Mannich reaction (formaldehyde, secondary amine salts) cephalosporin sulfoxides give 2-exomethylene derivatives. The latter have been used as intermediates for synthesizing numerous 2-substituted analogs. Hydrogenation gives the epimeric 2-methyl analogs (526), which also can be prepared semisynthetically from penicillin (527) or by alkylation of 2-methylthiocephalosporins (528). Addition of thiols (but not amines or alcohols) to the 2-exomethylene cephalosporin sulfoxides yields 2-thiomethyl ethers, which on dehydration give 2-thiomethylene analogs (529). Reaction with sulfonium ylids gives 2-spirocyclopropyl derivatives (530), and reaction with diazo compounds gives pyrazolines (531). With bromine, vicinal dibromides are obtained. Michael reaction with nucleophiles such as malonate esters and nitromethane give products that have been used to synthesize C-2/C-3 tricyclic cephalosporins (532). Reduction of the sulfoxide affords the 2-exomethylene cephalosporins (526) also obtained by totally synthetic methods (533). All the cephalosporin analogs obtained by reduction of the sulfoxide and removal of the protecting groups showed reduced antibacterial activity.

Other reactions at the 2-position of cephalosporin sulfoxides include methylthiolation (528), Michael addition with acrylonitrile, formation of 2-carbonates with alkoxychloroformates, and interchange with tosyl azide to give 2-diazosulfoxides (534). Reaction with *t*-butyl hypochlorite in methanol gives 2,2-dichlorocephalosporin sulfoxides (530).

The lack of sufficient activation makes modification at the 5(6)-position difficult. Direct epimerization of the C-5(6)-hydrogen has not been reported, but the synthesis of 5-epipenicillins (15.**53**, Z = H) has been achieved by electrophillic cleavage of the S-1 to C-5 bond with chlorine, followed by recyclization of the 2-chloroazetidinone sulfenyl chloride (15.**51**) by treatment with stannous chloride (512, 535). 5-Epibenzylpenicillin is only 0.1% as active as benzylpenicillin. Analogous C-5 epimeric cephalosporins have not been made, but the promising biological characteristics of the 7-α-methoxy cephalosporins led to the preparation of 6α-methoxy cephalosporins (15.**53**, Z = OCH_3) by a totally synthetic route (536). Cycloaddition of azidoacetyl chloride with an appropriately substituted dihydrothiazine gave a 6α-methylthiocepham (Z = SCH_3). Conversion to the 6α-methoxy cepham by treatment with thallic nitrate in methanol followed by dehydration, reduction, acylation, and hydrogenolysis gave ($\pm$)-6α-methoxy cephalothin. This analog was very stable, but it had greatly reduced antibacterial activity.

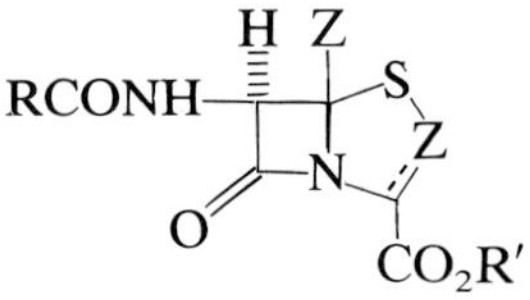

H Z
RCONH S
Z
N
O
CO_2R'

15.**53**

Replacement of the penicillin C-5 hydrogen with other functional groups has been accomplished only by total synthesis. A 5-phenylpenicillin methyl ester was inactive, but the configurations at both C-5 and C-6 were not determined (537). Against a strain of *S. aureus* 5α-phenylphenoxymethyl penicillin (15.**53**; R = $C_6H_5OCH_2$, Z = C_6H_5), synthesized later by an analogous route in which the key β-lactam-forming step involved cycloaddition of azidoacetyl chloride to an appropriately functionalized 2-thiazoline (538), had an MIC of 37 μg/ml compared to 0.025 μ g/ml for phenoxymethyl penicillin. Other 5(6)-substituted penams and cephams have been prepared (530), but none contain both the 3(4)-carboxyl group and the 6(7)-acylamino side chain required for antibiotic activity.

Replacement of the β-lactam carbonyl oxygen by sulfur has been accomplished in both the penicillin and cephalosporin series by treatment with boron sulfide (539). These analogs show greatly reduced antibacterial activity.

A ring modification of great promise is the recent replacement of the dihydrothiazine sulfur atom with oxygen (15.**2a,b**; S = O). 1-Oxacephalosporins have been prepared by total synthesis (204) and by semisynthesis from penicillins (540) via thiazolidine-ring-opened intermediates such as 15.**51**. The 1-oxacephalosporin analogs display activity trends congruent with SAR trends among the cephalosporins and cephamycins. However, their *in vitro* activities are consistently 4 to 10 times better (e.g., MIC values for cefamandole versus the 1-oxa-analog (μg/ml): *S. aureus*, 0.1 vs. 0.02; *E. coli* and *K. pneumoniae*, 0.4 vs. 0.05; *P. vulgaris* 0.8 vs. 0.1). In laboratory animals these analogs exhibit pharmacokinetic properties generally similar to those of the cephalosporins. The 1-oxacephalosporins contrast with 1-oxapenicillins and 1-carba-2-oxacephalosporins (541), which display intrinsic activities generally equal to or lower than the corresponding penicillins and cephalosporins.

11 NEWER β-LACTAM ANTIBIOTICS

The penicillins and cephalosporins have provided many clinically useful agents for treating bacterial infections, and new products with potentially greater usefulness continue to result from further investment in these chemical systems. But the maturity of this area of research and the growing versatility of β-lactam chemistry have led to increased emphasis on novel β-lactam-containing structures obtained by total and by semisynthesis. However recent discoveries of several new fermentation products promise to provide new impetus, and new directions, to research on β-lactam-containing systems obtained from natural sources.

11.1 Thienamycins

Thienamycin (15.**54**) (49, 109) shares two basic structural features with the penicillins

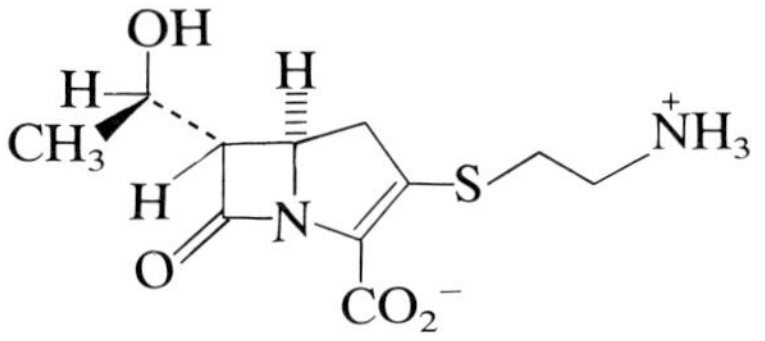

15.**54**

and cephalosporins—a bicyclic β-lactam-containing ring system and an appropriately attached carboxyl group. Otherwise it is a radical departure from the structures that have provided the useful β-lactam antibiotics over the past 35 years. The fused carbapenem ring containing a double bond implies a higher level of ring strain (and β-lactam ring reactivity) than would be considered acceptable for such a natural product. Perhaps more surprising is the absence of an acylamino side chain on the carbon adjacent to the β-lactam carbonyl. This carbon atom carries instead a 1-hydroxyethyl group, and the stereochemistry of attachment (α) is opposite to that of the penicillin and cephalosporin acylamino group (absolute stereochemistry: 5*R*:6*S*:8*S*). Several additional natural products containing the carbapenem ring system have also been described (6, 8, 542). They include stereoisomers of thienamycin epimerized at the 6-carbon (epithienamycin A and B, Beecham MM 13902 and MM 4550; 5- and 6-hydrogens cis as in the penicillins and cephalosporins) or the 8-carbon atom (epithienamycin C and D; 5- and 6-hydrogens trans as in thienamycin) and analogs (PS-5) without the hydroxyl function on the side chain (15.**55**; OX = H).

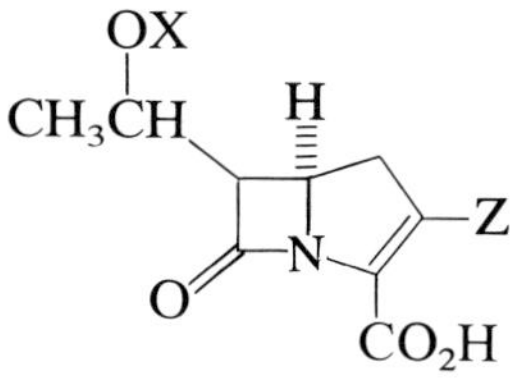

15.**55**

These fermentation products incorporate other structural variations (15.**55**: X = SO_3H; Z = $SCH_2CH_2NHCOCH_3$, $SCH{=}CHNHCOCH_3$, $S(O){=}CHNHCOCH_3$). The amino group of the aminoethylthio side chain generally carried an acetyl group. This side chain may be saturated (thienamycin, epithienamycin A and C), or it may contain a (trans) double bond (MM 13902, MM 4550, PS-5, epithienamycin B and D). All are sulfides except MM 4550, which is a sulfoxide. In MM 13902 and MM 4550 the hydroxyl group occurs as the sulfate ester.

Thienamycin is a potent antibacterial agent with an extraordinarily broad spectrum of activity against gram-positive and gram-negative bacteria; this includes *P. aeruginosa*, where it is more active than gentamicin, and anaerobes (especially *Bacteroides*), where its activity is somewhat greater than that of Clindamycin. An idea of this impressive activity is conveyed by

Table 15.20 Comparative *in Vitro* Activities of Thienamycin, Cephalothin, and Cefoxitin Against Selected Bacteria (109)

Bacteria	MIC, μg/ml		
	Thienamycin	Cephalothin	Cefoxitin
S. aureus (*S*)	0.02	0.09	3.1
S. aureus (*R*)[a]	0.01	1.0	0.6
E. coli (*S*)	0.8	6.3	1.6
E. coli (*R*)[b]	0.5	43	0.8
Proteus morganii	3.1	>400	12.5
Pseudomonas aeruginosa	3.0	—	—
Enterobacter cloacae (*S*)	0.5	1.8	0.8
E. cloacae (*R*)[b]	0.7	>120	70
Serratia sp.	3.1	>400	25

[a] Resistant to penicillins.
[b] Resistant to penicillins and cephalosporins.

Table 15.20, which compares *in vitro* activities of thienamycin with those of cephalothin and cefoxition against selected bacteria, including several chosen for their resistance to the penicillins and cephalosporins (109). Systemically thienamycin exhibits acceptable pharmacokinetic properties reflected in the *in vivo* protective effectiveness of this agent in laboratory animals, where it compares favorably with other antibiotics such as cephalothin, ampicillin, cefazolin, and gentamicin. [Typical s.c. PD_{50} values in mice for thienamycin vs. cephalothin: *S. aureus*, 0.26 vs. 2.1 mg/kg (×2); *E. coli* (*S*) 2.5 vs. 60 mg/kg (×2); *E. coli* (*R*), 9.9 vs.>500 mg/kg (×3). For thienamycin vs. gentamicin: *P. aeruginosa* (*S*), 2.4 vs. 9.4 mg/kg (×3); *P. aeruginosa* (*R*), 4.1 vs.>200 mg/kg (×3) (109).] Thienamycin is reported to have low toxicity comparable to the other β-lactam antibiotics. Serum levels in the monkey resemble those of the penicillins (5 mg/kg dose i.v.: peak serum concentrations, 25 μ g/ml; $t_{1/2}$, 11 min; urinary recovery, 57%).

In spite of its outstanding biological properties, thienamycin is not likely to be a clinically useful antibacterial agent *per se*, largely because of its poor stability in solution (109). In dilute solution (30 μg/ml) the stability profile of thienamycin resembles that of benzylpenicillin (maximum stability between pH 6 and 7; (0.3 *M* phosphate buffer), but the level of stability in terms of half-life is one-tenth of that of penicillin G. At higher concentrations, especially in unbuffered solution, thienamycin undergoes rapid self-inactivation, presumably forming an inactive dimer ($t_{1/2}$ at pH 7.0 and 25°C: 1 mg/ml, 100 hr; 57 mg/ml, 6 hr). The outlook for development of derivatives of this antibiotic with improved stability is very positive.

The epimeric analogs of thienamycin described here are also reported to exhibit potent antibacterial activities, but they display a wider variation in β-lactamase susceptibility than thienamycin (6). The latter is highly resistant to a wide spectrum of β-lactamases. This accounts at least in part for its broad antibacterial activity, which includes organisms such as *P. aeruginosa.* Thus the role of the hydroxyethyl group is not equatable to that of the acylamino side chain of the penicillins and cephalosporins.

Rather, it appears to contribute to the broad resistance of thienamycin to inactivation by β-lactamases (cf. the similar role of the 7α-methoxy group of the cephamycins). In support of this assumption, the thienamycin nucleus has 10–25% of the activity of thienamycin against non-β-lactamase producers, but it is inactive against organisms that produce this enzyme. On the other hand descysteaminyl thienamycin is resistant to β-lactamases with *in vitro* activities generally equal to or better than those of thienamycin (543). Several of the analogs described here are also powerful inhibitors of β-lactamases (542). This property and its potential utility for treating bacterial infections are discussed in the next section.

The derivatives of thienamycin and the other analogs in this group that have been described include, as expected, carboxylate esters and amides, esters and ethers of the side chain hydroyl and alkyl, and carboxamide and urethane derivatives of the side chain amino group. The cysteaminyl side chain has been reductively removed and the total synthesis of thienamycin, homothienamycin (poorly active), and the thienamycin nucleus have been described (543).

11.2 Clavulanic Acid

Clavulanic acid (15.**4**) is produced by *Streptomyces clavuligerus* along with penicillin N, 3-deacetoxycephalosporin C, the 3-carbamyloxymethyl analog of cephalosporin C, and its 7α-methoxy derivative (cephamycin C) (542). Like the other metabolic products from this fermentation, it contains a β-lactam ring and it exhibits measurable activity against gram-positive and gram-negative bacteria. However its *in vitro* activity is low, as might be expected on structural grounds (typical MIC values in μg/ml: *S. aureus*, 15; *K. pneumoniae*, 31; *E. coli*, 31, *P. aeruginosa*, 250) (544). It is a powerful irreversible inhibitor of β-lactamases produced by many gram-positive and gram-negative bacteria including those just named (plasmid mediated β-lactamase of *E. coli*) and *Proteus mirabilis*. It exhibits a lower level of inhibition of other β-lactamases such as those produced by *P. aeruginosa* and *Enterobacter*, and the chromosomally mediated enzyme of *E. coli*. Since many bacterial species are resistant to the β-lactam antibiotics because of their ability to produce β-lactamases, clavulanic acid and structures related to it may provide a means of removing this mechanism of resistance, thus extending the spectrum of antibacterial activity for these substances. This possibility is illustrated by the following MIC values, in micrograms per milliliter, obtained with ampicillin alone versus ampicillin in the presence of 5 μg/ml of clavulanic acid: *S. aureus*, 500/0.02; *K. Pneumoniae*, 250/0.1; *E. coli* (plasmid mediated resistance) > 2000/4; *E. coli* (chromosomally mediated resistance), 250/250; *P. aeruginosa* (carbenicillin in place of ampicillin) > 2000/500. Similar results are seen when cephaloridine is used as the antibiotic (544). However bacterial growth in the presence of subinhibitory mixtures of cephalosporins and clavulanic acid can result in regrowth of bacteria with marked resistance to the mixture (e.g., *K. pneumoniae*, MIC 8 → 1000 μg/ml) (545). This *in vitro* effect of clavulanic acid is reflected in a striking reduction of the dose of antibiotic required to protect mice infected with bacteria resistant to the latter when clavulanic acid is coadministered.

This phenomenon is not unique to clavulanic acid. The inhibition of these enzymes, for example, by β-lactamase-insensitive semisynthetic penicillins (methicillin, cloxacillin) and cephalosporins [7-2,6-dichlorobenzamide)cephalosporanic acid] had been examined earlier (546). A similar protective effect was observed both *in vitro* and *in vivo*, but the effect of

R—O—(C$_6$H$_4$)—(X)CONH—(β-lactam ring, N)—CH(COOH)—(C$_6$H$_4$)—OH

	X	R
A =	NOH ‖ —C—	$HO_2CCHCH_2CH_2$— (with NH_2 on CH)
B =	HON ‖ —C—	HO—$CCHCH_2CH_2$— (with NH_2 on CH)
C =	NH_2 | —CH—	$HO_2CCHCH_2CH_2$ (with NH_2 on CH)
D =	O ‖ —C—	$HO_2CCHCH_2CH_2$ (with NH_2 on CH)
E =	NOH ‖ —C—	H
F =	HON ‖ —C—	H
G =	—CH—	H

Fig. 15.7 Naturally occurring nocardicins (553).

clavulanic acid is more pronounced, probably because of the irreversibility of its binding to the enzyme. Penicillanic acid sulfone has now also been reported to irreversibly inhibit β-lactamases in a manner similar to clavulanic acid (547). A few other natural inhibitors of β-lactamases were reported (548) before clavulanic acid was discovered by a screening method designed to detect this type of activity (544), but they are less well characterized. Two additional inhibitors (MM 4550 and MM 13902) have been detected by this screen and characterized (8, 542)). Products of *Streptomyces olivaceus*, they are more active against bacteria (MICs 5–50 and $<5\ \mu$g—ml, respectively) than clavulanic acid. Since they have been found to be analogs of epithienamycin, they are described further under that heading.

In addition to the structure elucidation of clavulanic acid using, primarily, spectral and X-ray crystallographic data obtained from clavulanic acid esters (4), several chemically modified derivatives have been described, and the total synthesis of (2-methyl and 2,2-dimethyl) 7-oxo-4-oxa-1-azabicyclo[3.2.0]heptane analogs has been reported (549). Derivatives include the double-bond-isomerized isoclavulanic acid (113), deoxyclavulanic acid ($=CH-CH_3$); carboxylic acid, carbamate and sulfonate esters of the side chain hydroxyl; alkyl, acyloxyalkyl, and aralkyl esters, and the carboxamide (550). The side chain allylic alcohol has also been oxidized to the aldehyde (551), and the double bond has been hydrogenated (552) and epoxidized. Many of these derivatives in which the exocyclic double bond is retained function as β-lactamase inhibitors. The clinical usefulness of these derivatives, including clavulanic acid, and penicillanic acid sulfone remains to be demonstrated.

11.3 The Nocardicins

The structural variations among the naturally occurring nocardicins (A–G) are indicated in Fig. 15.7 (5, 553). The stereochemical correspondence of these structures with that of the penicillins was noted at the beginning of the chapter. The discussions of the relationships of β-lactam ring reactivity to the level of antibacterial activity of the penicillins and cephalosporins (e.g., p. 113), and the lack of bioactivity of desthiobenzylpenicillin (72), would not predict antibacterial activity as a property for this antibiotic group. Indeed, the spectrum of antibacterial activity exhibited by the nocardicins differs from that generally observed with the penicillins and cephalosporins; and although these antibiotics produce spheroplasts, indicating that their inhibitory effect derived from interference with cell wall synthesis (111), the specific mechanism of antibacterial action appears to differ from that of the penicillin as has been most extensively evaluated; some of its properties serve to illustrate the rather unusual antibacterial activities of this antibiotic class.

Nocardicin A is active *in vitro* against a fairly narrow group of gram-negative bacteria, essentially *P. aeruginosa*, *Proteus* species (except *P. morganii*) and *Neisseria* species. It does not exhibit significant activity *in vitro* against gram-positive bacteria (e.g., *S. aureus*) and most other gram-negative organisms (Table 15.21) (554). these *in vitro* activities are difficult to demonstrate, since the activity is influenced by inoculum size as well as by constituents in most assay media, including sodium chloride, some amino acids, sugars, and divalent cations (555). However in contrast to most other antibiotics, the *in vitro* activity of nocardicin A against, for example, *P. aeruginosa*, increases in the presence of serum; and though it has only weak activity against *E. coli* (Table 15.21), this activity is increased in the presence of polymorphonuclear leukocytes (554). Thus in spite of the very poor *in vitro* activities obtained in most assay media, nocardicin A, exhibits PD_{50} values in mice that are significantly better than those obtained with carbenicillin and cefazolin, not only against *P. aeruginosa* and species of *Proteus* but also against *E. coli* species that are insensitive to the antibiotic *in vitro* (556). Against *S. aureus*, the *in vitro* data are more predictive; nocardicin A does not protect mice against this gram-positive organism. Nocardicin A has a very low level of toxicity, similar to other β-lactam antibiotics, and it produces serum levels in laboratory animals 1.4–2.8 times higher than the levels achieved from an equivalent dose of carbenicillin. In these animals the serum half-life is about twice that of carbenicillin (557). The clinical utility of nocardicin A is yet to be determined.

In addition to structure determination

Table 15.21 Comparison of the *in Vitro* Activity of Nocardicin A with Carbenicillin

	MIC, μg/ml	
Organism	Nocardicin A	Carbenicillin
Staphylococcus aureus	800	0.78
Streptococcus pyogenes	200	0.2
Bacillus subtilis	50	0.2
Echerichia coli	100	12.5
Klebsiella pneumoniae	200	50
Serratia marcescens	800	12.5
Enterobacter aerogenes	200	6.2
Proteus mirabilis	1.56	0.78
P. vulgaris	1.56	0.39
Pseudomonas aeruginosa	12.5	50
Neisseria gonorrhoeae	1.56	—

(111), the oximino, amino, and carboxyl groups have been chemically modified directly, and 3-aminonocardicinic acid has been prepared by hydrolytic removal of the modified nocardicin acyl group as well as by total synthesis by several routes (553). As with the penicillins and cephalosporins, this intermediate is readily acylated to allow wide variation of the acyl side chain. Studies of the structure-activity relationships of nocardicin analogs have not yet been published.

REFERENCES

1. D. Crowfoot, C. W. Bunn, B. W. Rogers-Low, and A. Turner-Jones, in *The Chemistry of Penicillin*, H. T. Clarke, J. R. Johnson, and R. Robinson, Eds., Princeton University Press, Princeton, N.J., 1949, p. 310. The absolute stereochemistry of the penicillins could not be derived from this work.
2. D. C. Hodgkin and E. N. Maslen, *Biochem. J.*, **79,** 393 (1961).
3. R. B. Morin, B. G. Jackson, R. A. Mueller, E. R. Lavagnino, W. B. Scanlon, and S. L. Andrews, *J. Am. Chem. Soc.*, **85,** 1896 (1963).
4. T. T. Howarth, A. G. Brown, and T. J. King, *J. Chem. Soc., Chem. Commun.*, 266 (1976).
5. M. Hashimoto, T. Komori, and T. Kamiya, *J. Antibiot.* (Tokyo), **29,** 890 (1976).
6. E. O. Stapley. P. Cassidy, S. A. Currie, D. Daoust, R. Goegelman, S. Hernandez, M. Jackson, J. M. Mata, A. K. Miller, R. L. Monaghan, J. B. Tunae, S. B. Zimmerman, and D. Hendlin, Abstract No. 80, 17*th Interscience Conference on Antimicrobial Agents and Chemotherapy*, New York, 1977.
7. P. J. Cassidy, E. O. Stapley, R. Goegelman, T. W. Miller, B. Arison, G. Albers-Schönberg, S. B. Zimmerman, and J. Birnbaum, Abstract No. 81, 17*th Interscience Conference on Antimicrobial Agents and Chemotherapy*, New York, 1977.
8. A. G. Brown, D. F. Corbett, A. J. Eglington, and T. T. Howarth, *J. Chem. Soc., Chem. Commun.*, 523 (1977).
9. H. R. V. Arnstein and D. Morris, *Biochem. J.*, **76,** 357 (1960).
10. E. P. Abraham and G. G. F. Newton, *Adv. Chemother.*, **2,** 23 (1965).
11. A. L. Demain, *Lloydia*, **37,** 147 (1974); T. Kanzaki and Y. Fujisawa, *J. Takeda Res. Lab.*, **34,** 324–349 (1975).
12. P. A. Lempke and D. R. Brannon, in *Cephalosporins and Penicillins*, E. H. Flynn, Ed., Academic Press, New York, 1972, Ch. 9; D. J. Aberhart, *Tetrahedron*, **33,** 1545 (1977).
13. J. C. Sheehan, K. R. Hénery-Logan, and D. A. Johnson, *J. Am. Chem. Soc.*, **75,** 3292 (1953).
14. R. B. Morin, B. G. Jackson, E. H. Flynn, and R. W. Roeske, *J. Am. Chem. Soc.*, **84,** 3400 (1962).

15. K. Kucers and N. McK. Bennett, *The Use of Antibiotics*, 2nd ed., Heinemann, London, 1975, pp. 6, 128.
16. B. M. Barker and F. Prescott, *Antimicrobial Agents in Medicine*, Blackwell, London, 1973, pp. 213 ff.
17. P. M. Blumberg and J. L. Strominger, *Bacteriol. Rev.*, **38,** 291 (1974).
18. L. Glaser, *Ann. Rev. Biochem.*, **42,** 92 (1973).
19. D. J. Tipper, in *Subunits in Biological Systems*, G. D. Fasman and S. N. Timasheff, Eds., Dekker, New York, 1973, pp. 121, 331.
20. M. R. J. Salton, *The Bacterial Cell Wall*, Elsevier, New York, 1964.
21. H. Nikaido, *Advan. Enzymol.*, **31,** 77(1968).
22. J. Baddiley, in *Essays in Biochemistry*, Vol. 8, P. N. Campbell and F. Dickens, Eds., Academic Press, New York, 1972, p. 35.
23. K. H. Schleifer and O. Kandler, *Bacteriol. Rev.*, **36,** 407 (1972).
24. E. F. Gale, E. Cundliffe, P. E. Reynolds, M. H. Richmond, and M. J. Waring, in *The Molecular Basis of Antibiotic Action*, Wiley, New York, 1972, p. 49.
25. W. Weidel and H. Pelzer, *Advan. Enzymol.*, **26,** 193 (1964).
26. R. W. Jeanloz, N. Sharon, and H. M. Flowers, *Biochem. Biophys. Res. Commun.*, **13,** 20 (1963).
27. M. R. J. Salton and J. M. Ghuysen, *Biochim. Biophys. Acta*, **36,** 552 (1959).
28. E. M. Wise, Jr., and J. T. Park, *Proc. Nat. Acad. Sci., US*, **54,** 75 (1965).
29. J. L. Strominger, K. Izaki, M. Matsuhashi, and D. J. Tipper, *Fed. Proc.*, **26,** 9 (1967).
30. J. L. Strominger, *Johns Hopkins Med. J.* **133,** 63 (1973).
31. J. T. Park and M. J. Johnson, *J. Biol. Chem.*, **179,** 585 (1949).
32. J. T. Park, *J. Biol. Chem.*, **194,** 897 (1952).
33. J. T. Park and J. L. Strominger, *Science*, **125,** 99 (1957).
34. J. L. Strominger, J. T. Park, and R. E. Thompson, *J. Biol. Chem.*, **234,** 3263 (1959).
35. J. L. Strominger and D. J. Tipper, *Am. J. Med.*, **39,** 708 (1965).
36. D. J. Tipper and J. L. Strominger, *Proc. Nat. Acad. Sci., US*, **54,** 1133 (1965).
37. D. J. Tipper and J. L. Strominger, *J. Biol. Chem.*, **243,** 3169 (1968).
38. Y. Araki, R. Shirai, A. Shimada, N. Ishimoto, and E. Ito, *Biochem. Biophys. Res. Commun.*, **23,** 466 (1966).
39. K. Izaki, M. Matsuhashi, and J. L. Strominger, *J. Biol. Chem.*, **243,** 3180 (1968).
40. D. Mirelman and N. Sharon, *Biochem. Biophys. Res. Commun.*, **46,** 1909 (1972).
41. G. G. Wickus and J. L. Strominger, *J. Biol. Chem.*, **247,** 5297, 5307 (1972).
42. J. R. Edwards and J. T. Park, *J. Bacteriol.*, **99,** 459 (1969).
43. A. D. Russell and R. H. Fountain, *J. Bacteriol.*, **106,** 65 (1971).
44. Y. Araki, A. Shimada, and E. Ito, *Biochem. Biophys. Res. Commun.*, **23,** 518 (1966).
45. K. Izaki, M. Matsuhashi, and J. L. Strominger, *Proc. Nat. Acad. Sci., US*, **55,** 656 (1966).
46. H. Pelzer, *Z. Naturforsch.*, **18b,** 950 (1963).
47. R. Hartmann, J.-V. Höltje, and U. Schwarz, *Nature* (London), **235,** 426 (1972).
48. J. T. Park, J. R. Edwards, and E. M. Wise, *Ann N.Y. Acad. Sci.*, **235,** 300 (1974).
49. J. S. Kahan, F. M. Kahan, R. Goegelman, S. A. Currie, M. Jackson, E. O. Stapley, T. W. Miller, A. K. Miller, D. Hendlin, S. Mochales, S. Hernandez, and H. B. Woodruff, Abstract No. 227, *16th Interscience Conference on Antimicrobial Agents and Chemotherapy*, Chicago, 1976.
50. J. T. Park and L. Burmun, *Biochem. Biophys. Res. Commun.*, **51,** 863 (1973).
51. S. A. Schepartz and M. J. Johnson, *J. Bacteriol.*, **71,** 84 (1956).
52. P. J. Lawrence and J. L. Strominger, *J. Biol. Chem.*, **245,** 3653 (1970).
53. H. Suginaka, P. M. Blumberg, and J. L. Strominger, *J. Biol. Chem.*, **247,** 5279 (1972).
54. P. M. Blumberg, R. R. Yocum, E. Willoughby, and J. L. Strominger, *J. Biol. Chem.*, **249,** 6828 (1974).
55. H. J. Barnett, *Biochim. Biophys. Acta*, **304,** 332 (1973).
56. J. F. Collins and M. H. Richmond, *Nature* (London), **195,** 142 (1962).
57. J. T. Park, in *Biochemical Studies of Antimicrobial Drugs*, B. A. Newton and P. E. Reynolds, Eds., Cambridge University Press, Cambridge, 1966, p. 70.
58. E. H. W. Böhme, H. E. Applegate, B. Toeplitz, J. F. Dolfini, and J. Z. Gougoutas, *J. Am. Chem. Soc.*, **93,** 4324 (1971).
59. P. P. K. Ho, R. D. Towner, J. M. Indelicato, W. A. Spitzer, and G. A. Koppel, *J. Antibiot.* (Tokyo), **25,** 627 (1972).
60. J. T. Smith, J. M. Hamilton-Miller, and R. Knox, *J. Pharm. Pharmacol.*, **21,** 337 (1969).

61. E. P. Abraham and E. Chain, *Nature* (London), **146,** 837 (1940).

62. R. B. Sykes and M. Matthew, *J. Antimicrob. Chemother.*, **2,** 115 (1976).

63. A. Fleming, *Brit. J. Exp. Pathol.*, **10,** 226 (1929).

64. E. Chain, H. W. Florey, A. D. Gardner, N. G. Heatley, M. A. Jennings, J. Orr-Ewing, and A. G. Sanders, *Lancet*, **2,** 226 (1940).

65. E. P. Abraham, E. Chain, C. M. Fletcher, A. D. Gardner, N. G. Heatley, M. A. Jennings and H. W. Florey, *Lancet*, **2,** 177 (1941).

66. D. Wilson, *In Search of Penicillin*, Knopf, New York, 1976; Ronald Hare, *The Birth of Penicillin*, Allen & Unwin, London, 1970.

67. H. W. Florey, E. Chain, N. G. Heatley, M. A. Jennings, A. G. Sanders, E. P. Abraham, and M. E. Florey, *Antibiotics*, Vol. 2, Oxford University Press, London, 1949.

68. H. T. Clarke, J. R. Johnson, and R. Robinson, Eds., *The Chemistry of Penicillin*, Princeton University Press, Princeton, N.J., 1949.

69. A. J. Moyer and R. D. Coghill, *J. Bacteriol.*, **51,** 57, 79 (1946).

70. A. J. Moyer and R. D. Coghill, *J. Bacteriol.*, **53,** 329 (1947).

71. See Ref. 67, p. 667, and Ref. 68, p. 5.

72. E. Kaczka and K. Folkers, in Ref. 68, p. 243.

73. See Ref. 68, p. 8.

74. V. du Vigneaud, F. H. Carpenter, R. W. Holley, A. H. Livermore, and J. R. Rachele, *Science*, **104,** 431 (1946).

75. V. du Vigneaud, J. L. Wood, and M. E. Wright, in Ref. 68, p. 892.

76. A. H. Cook, *Q. Rev., Chem. Soc.*, **2,** 203 (1948).

77. O. Sus, *Justus Liebigs Ann. Chem.*, **571,** 201 (1951).

78. J. C. Sheehan and P. A. Cruickshank, *J. Am. Chem. Soc.*, **78,** 3677 (1956).

79. J. C. Sheehan and D. R. Hoff, *J. Am. Chem. Soc.*, **79,** 237 (1957).

80. W. A. Bolhofer, J. C. Sheehan, and E. L. A. Abrams, *J. Am. Chem. Soc.*, **82,** 3437 (1960).

81. J. C. Sheehan and K. R. Hénery-Logan, *J. Am. Chem. Soc.*, **79,** 1262 (1957); **81,** 3089 (1959).

82. J. C. Sheehan and K. R. Hénery-Logan, *J. Am. Chem. Soc.*, **81,** 5838 (1959).

83. J. C. Sheehan and J. P. Ferris, *J. Am. Chem. Soc.*, **81,** 2912 (1959).

84. F. R. Batchelor, F. P. Doyle, J. H. C. Nayler, and G. N. Rolinson, *Nature* (London), **183,** 257 (1959).

85. F. R. Batchelor, E. B. Chain, T. L. Hardy, K. R. L. Mansford, and G. N. Rolinson, *Proc. Roy. Soc.* (London), *Ser. B.*, **154,** 498 (1961).

86. G. Brotzu, *Ric. Nuovo Antibiot. Lav. Ist. Ig. Cagliari* (1948).

87. H. Crawford, N. G. Heatley, P. F. Boyd, C. W. Hale, B. K. Kelly, G. A. Smith, and N. Smith, *J. Gen. Microbiol.*, **6,** 47 (1952).

88. H. S. Burton and E. P. Abraham, *Biochem. J.*, **50,** 168 (1951).

89. H. S. Burton, E. P. Abraham, and H. M. E. Cardwell, *Biochem. J.*, **62,** 171 (1956).

90. E. P. Abraham, G. G. F. Newton, K. Crawford, H. S. Burton, and C. W. Hale, *Nature* (London), **171,** 343 (1953).

91. E. P. Abraham and G. G. F. Newton, *Biochem. J.*, **58,** 266 (1954).

92. E. P. Abraham, G. G. F. Newton, and C. W. Hale, *Biochem. J.*, **58,** 94 (1954).

93. G. G. F. Newton and E. P. Abraham, *Biochem. J.*, **58,** 103 (1954).

94. E. P. Abraham, G. G. F. Newton, J. R. Schenk, M. P. Hargie, B. H. Olson, D. M. Shuurmans, M. W. Fisher, and S. A. Fusari, *Nature* (London), **176,** 551 (1955).

95. G. G. F. Newton and E. P. Abraham, *Nature* (London), **175,** 548 (1955).

96. G. G. F. Newton and E. P. Abraham, *Biochem. J.*, **62,** 651 (1956).

97. E. P. Abraham and G. G. F. Newton, *Biochem. J.*, **79,** 377 (1961).

98. E. van Heyningen, *Advan. Drug Res.*, **4,** 1 (1967).

99. J. C. Sheehan and J. A. Schneider, *J. Org. Chem.*, **31,** 1635 (1966).

100. R. Heymès, G. Amiard, and G. Nominé, *Compt. Rend., Ser. C*, **263,** 170 (1966); G. Nominé, *Chim. Ther.*, **6,** 53 (1971).

101. J. E. Dolfini, J. Schwartz, and F. Weisenborn, *J. Org. Chem.*, **34,** 1582 (1969).

102. R. B. Woodward, K. Heusler, J. Gosteli, P. Naegeli, W. Oppolzer, R. Ramage, S. Ranganathan, and H. Vorbruggen, *J. Am. Chem. Soc.*, **88,** 852 (1966).

103. R. B. Woodward, *Science*, **153,** 487 (1964); K. Heusler, in *Topics in Pharmaceutical Sciences*, Vol. 1, D. Perlman, Ed., Wiley-Interscience, New York, 1968, p. 33.

104. R. Nagarajan, L. D. Boeck, M. Gorman, R. L. Hamill, C. E. Higgens, M. M. Hoehn, W. M. Stark, and J. G. Whitney, *J. Am. Chem. Soc.*, **93,** 2308 (1971).

105. E. O. Stapley, D. Hendlin, S. Hernandez, M. Jackson, J. H. Mater, A. K. Miller, H. B. Woodruff, T. W. Miller, G. Albers-Schonberg, B. H.

Arison, and J. L. Smith, Abstract No. 8, *11th Interscience Conference on Antimicrobial Agents and Chemotherapy*, Atlantic City, N.J., 1971.

106. H. R. Onishi, D. R. Daoust, S. B. Zimmerman, D. Hendlin, and E. O. Stapley, *Antimicrob. Agents Chemother.*, **5,** 38 (1974).

107. H. Nakao, H. Yanagisawa, B. Shimizu, M. Kaneko, M. Nagano, and S. Sugawara, *J. Antibiot.* (Tokyo), **29,** 554 (1976).

108. W. Brumfitt, J. Kosmidis, J. M. T. Hamilton-Miller, and J. N. G. Gilchrist, *Antimicrob. Agents Chemother.*, **6,** 290 (1974); Abstract No. 77, *16th Interscience Conference on Antimicrobial Agents and Chemotherapy*, Chicago, 1976.

109. See Ref. 49; and H. Kropp, J. S. Kahan, F. M. Kahan, J. Sundelof, G. Darland, and J. Birnbaum, Abstract No. 228, *16th Interscience Conference on Anitmicrobial Agents and Chemotherapy, Chicago*, 1976; G. Albers-Schonberg, B. H. Arison, E. Kaczka, F. M. Kahan, J. S. Kahan, B. Lago, W. M. Maiese, R. E. Rhodes and J. L. Smith, *ibid.*, Abstract No. 229; US Patent 3,950,357 (April 13, 1976), J. S. Kahan et al. (to Merck & Co., Inc.).

110. M. Hashimoto, T. Komori, and T. Kamiya, *J. Am. Chem. Soc.*, **98,** 3023 (1976).

111. H. Aoki, H. Sakai, M. Kohsaka, T. Konomi, J. Hosoda, Y. Kubochi, E. Iguchi, and H. Imanaka, *J. Antibiot.* (Tokyo), **29,** 492 (1976).

112. P. A. Hunter and C. Reading, Abstract No. 211, *16th Interscience Conference on Antimicrobial Agents and Chemotherapy*, Chicago, 1976.

113. A. G. Brown, T. T. Howarth, I. Stirling, and T. J. King, *Tetrahedron Lett.*, 4203 (1976).

114. E. H. Flynn, Ed., *Cephalosporins and Penicillins, Chemistry and Biology*, Academic Press, New York, 1972.

115. P. A. Fawcett and E. P. Abraham, *Biosynthesis*, **4,** 248 (1976).

116. T. H. Mead and M. W. Stack, *Biochem. J.*, **42** vxiii (1948).

117. Q. F. Soper, C. W. Whitehead, O. K. Behrens, J. J. Corse, and R. G. Jones, *J. Am. Chem. Soc.*, 70, 2849 (1948); see also previous papers in this series, cited therein.

118. J. A. Thorn and M. J. Johnson, *J. Am. Chem. Soc.*, **72,** 2052 (1950).

119. A. L. Tosoni, D. G. Glass, and L. Goldsmith, *Biochem. J.*, **69,** 476 (1958).

120. D. C. Mortimer and M. J. Johnson, *J. Am. Chem. Soc.*, **74,** 4098 (1952).

121. J. D. Jeffery, E. P. Abraham, and G. G. F. Newton, *Biochem. J.*, **81,** 591 (1961).

122. Y. Fujisawa, H. Shirafuji, M. Kida, K. Nara, M. Yoneda, and T. Kanzaki, *Nature* (London), *New Biol.*, **246,** 154 (1973).

123. C. E. Higgens, R. L. Hamill, T. H. Sands, M. M. Hoehn, N. E. Davis, R. Nagarajan, and L. D. Boeck, *J. Antibiot.* (Tokyo), **27,** 298 (1974).

124. T. Kanzaki, T. Fukita, H. Shirafuji, T. Fujisawa, and K. Kitano, *J. Antibiot.* (Tokyo), **27,** 361 (1974).

125. E. O. Stapley, M. Jackson, S. Hernandez, S. B. Zimmerman, S. A. Currie, S. Mochales, J. M. Mata, H. B. Woodruff, and D. Hendlin, *Antimicrob. Agents Chemother.*, **2,** 122 (1972).

126. T. W. Miller, R. T. Goegelman, R. G. Weston, I. Putter, and F. J. Wolf, *Antimicrob. Agents Chemother.*, **2,** 132 (1972).

127. A. K. Miller, E. Celozzi, E. A. Pelak, E. O. Stapley, and D. Hendlin, *Antimicrob. Agents Chemother.*, **2,** 281 (1972).

128. A. K. Miller, E. Celozzi, Y. Kong, B. A. Pelak, H. Kropp, E. O. Stapley, and D. Hendlin, *Antimicrob. Agents Chemother.*, **2,** 287 (1972).

129. H. Fukase, T. Hasegawa, K. Hatano, H. Iwasaki, and M. Yoneda, *J. Antibiot.* (Tokyo), **29,** 113 (1976).

130. Japanese Patent 74-102889 (September 28, 1974), H. Imanaka et al. (to Fujisawa Pharmaceutical Co., Ltd.).

131. K. Sakaguchi and S. Murao, *J. Agr. Chem. Soc., Japan* **23,** 411 (1950); *Chem. Abstr.*, **45,** 1197 (1951).

132. S. Murao, *J. Agr. Chem. Soc., Japan*, **29,** 400, 404 (1955); *Chem. Abstr.*, **51,** 8160 (1957).

133. F. M. Huber, R. R. Chauvette, and B. G. Jackson, in Ref. 114, p. 29.

134. E. P. Abraham and L. D. Sabath, *Enzymologia*, **29,** 221 (1965).

135. C. A. Claridge, J. R. Luttinger, and J. Lein, *Proc. Soc. Exp. Biol. Med.*, **113,** 1008 (1963).

136. A. L. Demain, R. B. Walton, J. F. Newkirk, and I. M. Miller, *Nature* (London), **199,** 909 (1963).

137. R. B. Walton, *Science*, **143,** 1438 (1964).

138. H. T. Huang, T. A. Seto, and G. M. Shull, *Appl. Microbiol.*, **11,** 1 (1963).

139. B. Loder, G. G. F. Newton, and E. P. Abraham, *Biochem. J.*, **79,** 408 (1961).

140. US Patent 3,207,755 (September 21, 1965), E. P. Abraham and G. G. F. Newton (to National Research Development Corp.).

141. US Patent 3,454,564 (July 8, 1969), E. Vischer et al. (to Ciba Corp.).

142. Belgian Patent 645,157 (September 14, 1964), (to CIBA, Ltd.).

143. US Patent 3,367,933 (February 6, 1968), S. Eardley et al. (to Glaxo Laboratories, Ltd.).

144. B. Fechtig, H. Peter, H. Bickel, and E. Vischer, *Helv. Chim. Acta*, **51,** 1108 (1968).

145. US Patents 3,499,909 (March 10, 1970), 3,575,970 (April 20, 1971), H. W. O. Weissenburger and M. G. van der Hoeven (to Kon. Ned. Gistern Spiritusfab.); Belgian Patent 719,712 (February 20, 1969), (to Glaxo Laboratories, Ltd.); Netherlands Patent 6,812,413 (March 3, 1969), (to CIBA, Ltd.); Ref. 26, p. 37.

146. G. N. Rolinson, F. R. Batchelor, D. Butterworth, J. Cameron-Wood, M. Cole, G. C. Eustace, M. V. Hart, M. Richards, and E. B. Chain, *Nature* (London), **187,** 236 (1960).

147. K. Kaufman, K. Bauer, and H. A. Offe, *Antimicrob. Agents Ann.*, 1 (1961).

148. I. Busko-Oszczapowicz, J. Kazimierczak, and J. Cieslak, *Rocz. Chem.*, **48,** 253 (1974).

149. G. A. Koppel, *Tetrahedron Lett.*, 2427 (1974); cf. Netherlands Patent 6808622 (December 23, 1969), (to Kon. Ned. Gistern Spiritusfab.).

150. F. P. Doyle, G. R. Fosker, J. H. C. Nayler, and H. Smith, *J. Chem. Soc.*, 1440 (1962).

151. B. Elkstrom, A. Gomez-Revilla, R. Mallberg, H. Thelin, and B. Sjoberg, *Acta Chem. Scand.*, **19,** 281 (1965).

152. J. L. Spencer, E. H. Flynn, R. W. Roeske, F. Y. Siu, and R. R. Chauvette, *J. Med. Chem.*, **9,** 746 (1966).

153. C. W. Ryan, R. L. Simon and E. M. van Heyningen, *J. Med. Chem.*, **12,** 310 (1969).

154. US Patent 3,230,214 (January 18, 1966), G. R. Fosker and J. H. C. Nayler (to Beecham Laboratories, Ltd.).

155. E. Dane and T. Dockner, *Chem. Ber.*, **98,** 789 (1965).

156. US Patent 3,641,021 (February 8, 1972), C. W. Ryan (to Eli Lilly & Co).

157. British Patent 962,024 (June 24, 1964), E. G. Brain and E. R. Stove (to Beecham Laboratories, Ltd.).

158. J. H. C. Nayler, in *Advances in Drug Research*, Vol. 7, N. J. Harper and A. B. Simmonds, Eds., Academic Press, New York, 1973, p. 1.

159. J. D. Cocker, S. Eardley, G. I. Gregory, M. E. Hall, and A. G. Long, *J. Chem. Soc. C.*, 1142 (1966).

160. W. H. W. Lunn, R. W. Burchfield, T. K. Elzey, and E. V. Mason, *Tetrahedron Lett.*, 1307 (1974).

161. S. Karaday, S. H. Pines, L. M. Weinstock, F. E. Roberts, G. S. Brenner, A. M. Hoinowski, T. Y. Cheng, and M. Sletzinger, *J. Am. Chem. Soc.*, **94,** 1410 (1972).

162. B. Shimizu, M. Kaneko, M. Kimura, and S. Sugawara, *Chem. Pharm. Bull.* (Tokyo), **24,** 2629 (1976).

163. C. F. Murphy and J. A. Webber, in Ref. 114, Chap. 4, cover the literature through 1971.

164. C. W. Hale, G. G. F. Newton, and E. P. Abraham, *Biochem. J.*, **79,** 403 (1961).

165. J. D. Cocker, B. R. Cowley, J. S. G. Cox, S. Eardley, G. I. Gregory, J. K. Lazenby, A. G. Long, J. C. P. Sly, and G. A. Somerfield, *J. Chem. Soc.*, 5015 (1965).

166. A. B. Taylor, *J. Chem. Soc.*, 7020 (1968).

167. E. van Heyningen, *J. Med. Chem.*, **8,** 22 (1965); E. van Heyningen and C. N. Brown, *ibid.*, **8,** 174 (1965).

168. R. A. Archer and B. S. Kitchell, *J. Org. Chem.*, **31,** 3409 (1966).

169. L. Spencer, F. Y. Siu, E. H. Flynn, B. G. Jackson, M. V. Sigal, H. M. Higgins, R. R. Chauvette, S. L. Andrews, and D. E. Bloch, *Antimicrob. Agents Chemother.*, 573 (1967).

170. L. B. Hogan, Jr., W. J. Hollaway, and R. A. Jakubowitch, *Antimicrob. Agents Chemother.*, 624 (1968).

171. J. Bradshaw, S. Eardley, and A. G. Long, *J. Chem. Soc. C*, 801 (1968).

172. US Patents 3,226,384 (December 28, 1965), E. P. Abraham et al., 3,228,934 (January 11, 1966), E. P. Abraham and G. G. F. Newton (to National Research Development Corp.); 3,278, 531 (October 11, 1966), J. S. G. Cox et al., British Patent 1,153,421 (May 29, 1969), B. Boothroyd et al., US Patent 3,821,206 (June 28, 1974), B. R. Cowley et al. (to Glaxo Laboratories, Ltd.); see Refs. 351, 370.

173. H. Fazakerley, D. A. Gilbert, G. I. Gregory, J. K. Lazenby, and A. G. Long, *J. Chem. Soc. C*, 1959 (1967).

174. R. J. Stedman, K. Swered, and J. R. E. Hoover, *J. Med. Chem.*, **7,** 117 (1964).

175. US Patents 3,773,761 (November 20, 1973), 3,856,704 (December 24, 1974), D. W. Blackburn et al. (to SmithKline Corp.).

176. P. Sykes and A. R. Todd, in Ref. 68, pp. 156, 946, 1008.

177. A. W. Chow, N. M. Hall, and J. R. E. Hoover, *J. Org. Chem.*, **27,** 1387 (1962).

178. E. Gaddal, P. Morch, and L. Tybring, *Tetrahedron Lett.*, 381 (1962).

179. J. M. Essery, K. Dadabo, W. J. Gottstein, A. Hallstrand, and L. C. Cheney, *J. Org. Chem.*, **30,** 4388 (1965).

180. R. D. G. Cooper, P. V. DeMarco, and D. O. Spry, *J. Am. Chem. Soc.*, **91,** 1528 (1969).

181. D. H. R. Barton, F. Comer, and P. G. Sammes, *J. Am. Chem. Soc.*, **91,** 1529 (1969).

182. R. D. G. Cooper, L. D. Hatfield, and D. O. Spry, *Acc. Chem. Res.*, **6,** 32 (1973).

183. R. B. Morin, B. G. Jackson, R. A. Mueller, E. R. Lavagnino, W. B. Scanlon, and S. L. Andrews, *J. Am. Chem. Soc.*, **91,** 1401 (1969).

184. D. H. R. Barton, M. Girijavallabban, and P. G. Sammes, *J. Chem. Soc., Perkin Trans.*, **1,** 929 (1972).

185. US Patents 3,725,397 (April 3, 1973), 3,852,295 (December 3, 1974), W. Graham and L. A. Wetherill (to Glaxo Laboratories, Ltd.).

186. Netherlands Patent 7211213 (August 17, 1972), (to Gist-Brocades N.V.).

187. D. H. R. Barton, D. C. T. Grieg, P. G. Sammes, M. V. Tayler, C. M. Cooper, G. Hewitt, and W. G. E. Underwood, *J. Chem. Soc., Chem. Commun.*, 1683 (1970).

188. R. D. G. Cooper and F. L. José, *J. Am. Chem. Soc.*, **92,** 2575 (1970).

189. D. O. Spry, *J. Am. Chem. Soc.*, **92,** 5006 (1970).

190. R. D. G. Cooper, *J. Am. Chem. Soc.*, **92,** 5010 (1970).

191. R. D. G. Cooper and D. O. Spry in Ref. 114, Ch. 5.

192. P. G. Sammes, *Chem. Rev.*, **76,** 113–155 (1976).

193. US Patents 3,962,277 (June 8, 1976), 3,966,738 (June 29, 1976), 4,007,202 (February 8, 1977), J. Verweij and H. S. Tan (to Gist-Brocades N.V.).

194. M. Yoshimoto, S. Ishihara, E. Nakayama, and N. Soma, *Tetrahedron Lett.*, 2923 (1972).

195. L. D. Cama, W. J. Leanza, T. R. Beattie, and B. G. Christensen, *J. Am. Chem. Soc.*, **94,** 1408 (1972).

196. T. Jen, J. Frazee, and J. R. E. Hoover, *J. Org. Chem.*, **38,** 2857 (1973).

197. L. D. Cama and B. G. Christensen, *Tetrahedron Lett.*, 3505 (1973).

198. G. A. Koppel and R. E. Koehler, *J. Am. Chem. Soc.*, **95,** 2403 (1973).

199. H. Yanagisawa, M. Fukushima, A. Ando, and H. Nakao, *Tetrahedron Lett.*, 2705 (1975); *J. Antibiot.* (Tokyo), **29,** 969 (1976).

200. Y. Sugimura, K. Iino, Y. Iwano, T. Saito, and T. Hiraoka, *Tetrahedron Lett.*, 1307 (1976).

201. T. Saito, Y. Sugimura, Y. Iwano, K. Iino, and T. Hiraoka, *J. Chem. Soc., Chem. Commun.*, 516 (1976).

202. R. R. Chauvette and E. H. Flynn, *J. Med. Chem.*, **9,** 741 (1966).

203. J. R. Johnson, R. B. Woodward, and R. Robinson, in Ref. 68, p. 440.

204. L. D. Cama and B. G. Christensen, *J. Am. Chem. Soc.*, **96,** 7582 (1974).

205. K. Heusler, in Ref. 114, p. 275.

206. B. K. Koe, T. A. Seto, A. R. English, and T. J. McBride, *J. Med. Chem.*, **6,** 653 (1963).

207. Y. G. Perron, W. F. Minor, L. B. Crast, A. Gourevitch, J. Lein, and L. C. Cheney, *J. Med. Pharm. Chem.*, **5,** 1016 (1962).

208. Y. G. Perron, W. F. Minor, L. B. Crast, and L. C. Cheney, *J. Org. Chem.*, **26,** 3365 (1961).

209. T. Naito, S. Nakagawa, J. Okumura, M. Konishi, and H. Kawaguchi, *J. Antibiot.* (Tokyo); *Ser. A*, **18,** 145 (1965).

210. C. J. Salivar, F. H. Hedger, and E. V. Brown, *J. Am. Chem. Soc.*, **70,** 1287 (1948).

211. N. P. Sullivan, A. T. Symmes, H. C. Miller, and H. W. Rhodehamel, Jr., *Science*, **107,** 169 (1948).

212. J. L. Szabo, C. D. Edwards, and W. F. Bruce, *Antibiot. Chemother.*, **1,** 499 (1951).

213. W. J. Martin, *Lancet*, **87,** 79 (1967).

214. W. W. Wright, A. Kirshbaum, B. Arret, L. E. Putnam, and H. Welch, *Antibiot. Med.*, **1,** 490 (1961).

215. F. P. Doyle, J. H. C. Nayler, H. Smith, and E. R. Stove, *Nature* (London), **191,** 1091 (1961).

216. Y. G. Perron, W. F. Minor, C. T. Holdrege, W. J. Gottstein, J. C. Godfrey, L. B. Crast, R. B. Babel, and L. C. Cheney, *J. Am. Chem. Soc.*, **82,** 3934 (1960).

217. G. M. Williamson, J. K. Morrison, and K. J. Stevens, *Lancet*, **1,** 847 (1961).

218. B. Lynn, *Antibiot. Chemother.*, **13,** 125 (1965).

219. H. Vanderhaeghe, P. Van Dijck, M. Claesen, and P. DeSomer, *Antimicrob. Agents Chemother.*, 581 (1962).

220. M. Claesen, P. J. Van Dijck, H. Vanderhaeghe, and P. DeSomer, *Antibiot. Chemother.*, **12,** 187, 192 (1962).

221. W. J. Leanza, B. G. Christensen, E. F. Rogers, and A. A. Patchett, *Nature* (London), **207,** 1395 (1965).

222. R. M. Thompson, J. W. Harding, and R. D. Simon, *Brit. Med. J.*, 708, ii (1960).

223. Y. M. Ridley, D. Barrie, K. Lynn and K. C. Stead, *Lancet*, **1,** 230 i (1970).

224. E. G. Brain, F. P. Doyle, K. Hardy, A. A. W. Long, M. D. Mehta, D. Miller, J. H. C. Nayler, M. J. Soulal, E. R. Stove, and G. R. Thomas, *J. Chem. Soc.*, 1445 (1962).

225. US Patent 3,245,983 (April 12, 1966), F. P. Doyle and J. H. C. Nayler (to Beecham Laboratories, Ltd.).

226. G. N. Rolinson, S. Stevens, F. R. Batchelor, J. C. Wood, and E. B. Chain, *Lancet*, **2,** 564 (1960).

227. P. Acred, D. M. Brown, D. H. Turner, and D. Wright, *Brit. J. Pharmacol.*, **17,** 70 (1961).

228. F. P. Doyle, K. Hardy, J. H. C. Nayler, M. J. Soulal, E. R. Stove, and H. R. J. Waddington, *J. Chem. Soc.*, 1453 (1962).

229. For initial references to the properties and clinical use of methicillin, see Editorial, *Brit. Med. J.*, **2,** 720 (1960).

230. S. B. Rosenman and G. H. Warren, *Antimicrob. Agents Chemother.*, 611 (1962) and two following papers.

231. J. A. Yurchenco, M. W. Hopper, and G. H. Warren, *Antibiot. Chemother.*, **12,** 535 (1962).

232. J. Smith and A. White, *Antimicrob. Agents Chemother.*, 354 (1963) and four following papers.

233. F. P. Doyle, A. A. W. Long, J. H. C. Nayler, and E. R. Stove, *Nature* (London), **192,** 1183 (1961).

234. A. Gourevitch, G. A. Hunt, T. A. Pursiano, C. C. Carmack, A. J. Moses, and J. Lein, *Antibiot. Chemother.*, **11,** 780 (1961).

235. J. O. Klein, L. D. Sabath, B. W. Steinhauer, and M. Finland, *New Engl. J. Med.*, **269,** 1215 (1963).

236. J. H. C. Nayler, A. A. W. Long, D. M. Brown, P. Acred, G. N. Rolinson, F. R. Batchelor, S. Stevens, and R. Sutherland, *Nature* (London), **195,** 1264 (1962).

237. G. T. Stewart, *Lancet*, 634 (1962-I).

238. P. A. Bunn and S. Milicich, *Antimicrob. Agents Chemother.*, 220 (1964).

239. US Patent 3,239,507 (March 8, 1966), J. H. C. Nayler (to Beecham Laboratories, Ltd.).

240. P. Naumann and B. Kempf, *Arzneim-Forsch.*, **15,** 139 (1964); C. Gloxhuber, H. A. Offe, E. Rauenbusch, W. Scholtan, and J. Schmid, *ibid.*, 322, and three following papers (331–348).

241. J. V. Bennett, C. F. Gravenkemper, J. L. Brodie, and W. M. M. Kirby, *Antimicrob. Agents Chemother.*, 257 (1965).

242. R. Sutherland, E. A. P. Croydon, and G. N. Rolinson, *Brit. Med. J.*, **4,** 455 (1970).

243. J. W. Harding and E. T. Knudsen, *Practitioner*, **205,** 801 (1970).

244. F. G. Brain, F. P. Doyle, M. D. Mehta, D. Miller, J. H. C. Nayler, and E. R. Stove, *J. chem. Soc.*, 491 (1963).

245. M. M. Dolan, A. Bondi, J. R. E. Hoover, R. Tumilowicz, R. C. Stewart, and R. J. Ferlauto, *Antimicrob. Agents Chemother.*, 648 (1962) and two following articles.

246. J. R. E. Hoover, A. W. Chow, R. J. Stedman, N. M. Hall, H. S. Greenberg, M. M. Dolan, and R. J. Ferlauto, *J. Med. Chem.*, **7,** 245 (1964).

247. R. J. Stedman, J. R. E. Hoover, A. W. Chow, M. M. Dolan, N. M. Hall, and R. J. Ferlauto, *J. Med. Chem*; **7,** 251 (1964).

248. A. W. Chow, N. M. Hall, J. R. E. Hoover, M. M. Dolan, and R. J. Ferlauto, *J. Med. Chem.*, **9,** 551 (1966).

249. F. P. Doyle, J. C. Hanson, A. A. W. Long, and J. H. C. Nayler, *J. Chem. Soc.*, 5845 (1963).

250. F. P. Doyle, J. C. Hanson, A. A. W. Long, J. H. C. Nayler, and E. R. Stove, *J. Chem. Soc.*, 5638 (1963).

251. J. H. C. Nayler, in Ref. 158, p. 65.

252. J. C. Hanson, J. H. C. Nayler, T. Taylor, and P. H. Gore, *J. Chem. Soc.*, 5984 (1965).

253. R. G. Micetich and R. Raap, *J. Med. Chem.*, **11,** 159 (1968).

254. M. S. Grant, D. L. Pain, and R. Slack, *J. Chem. Soc.*, 3842 (1965).

255. J. Koczka, O. Feher, and L. Vargha, in *Progress in Antimicrobial and Anticancer Chemotherapy*, Vol. 1, University of Tokyo Press, Tokyo, 1970, p. 44.

256. A. Pala, G. Coppi, A. Mantezani, and E. Crescenzi, *Chim. Ther.*, **4,** 26 (1969).

257. J. O. Klein and M. Finland, *Am. J. Med. Sci.*, **246,** 10 (1963).

258. M. W. Hopper, J. A. Yurchenco, S. B. Rosenman, A. L. Gillen, and G. H. Warren, *Antimicrob. Agents Chemother.*, 305 (1964).

259. S. S. Walkenstein, R. Wiser, E. LeBoutillier, C. Gudmundsen and H. Kimmel, *J. Pharm. Sci.*, **52,** 763 (1963).

260. P. Nauman, *Antimicrob. Agents Chemother.*, 937 (1966).

261. G. N. Rolinson and R. Sutherland, *Advan. Pharmacol. Chemother.*, **11,** 151 (1973), see p. 186.

262. M. P. Jevons, A. W. Coe, and M. T. Parker, *Lancet*, **1,** 904 (1963).

263. N. G. Heatley and H. W. Florey, *Brit. J. Pharmacol.*, **8,** 252 (1953).

264. K. E. Price, A. Gourevitch, and L. C. Cheney, *Antimicrob. Agents Chemother.*, 682 (1967).

265. G. N. Rolinson and S. Stevens, *Brit. Med. J.*, **2,** 191 (1961).

266. D. M. Brown and P. Acred, *Brit. Med. J.*, **2,** 197 (1961).

267. E. T. Knudsen, G. N. Rolinson, and S. Stevens, *Brit. Med. J.*; **2,** 198 (1961).

268. G. T. Stewart, H. M. T. Coles, H. H. Nixon, and R. J. Holt, *Brit. Med. J.*, **2,** 200 (1961); cf. Editorial, p. 223.

269. P. Bunn, J. O'Brien, D. Bentley, and H. Hayman, *Antimcrob. Agents Chemother.*, 323 (1963) and two following articles, pp. 339, 350.

270. Synthetic Organic Chemicals, US Production and Sales 1974, US International Trade Commission

Publication 776, Government Printing Office, Washington, D.C., 1976.

271. P. Acred, D. M. Brown, E. T. Knudsen, G. N. Rolinson, and R. Sutherland, *Nature* (London), **215,** 25 (1967).

272. E. T. Knudsen, G. N. Rolinson, and R. Sutherland, *Brit. Med. J.*, **3,** 75 (1967).

273. P. Nauman and B. Kempf, *Arzneim.-Forsch.*, **19** 1222 (1969).

274. W. M. M. Kirby, Chairman, Symposium on Carbenicillin, *J. Infect. Dis.*, **122,** Suppl. S1-116 (1970); 16 articles.

275. J. H. C. Nayler, in Ref. 158, p. 52.

276. US Patent 3,674,776 (July 4, 1972), A. A. W. Long and J. H. C. Nayler (to Beecham Laboratories, Ltd.).

277. H. Neu and E. B. Windshell, *Antimicrob. Agents Chemother.*, 407 (1971); and four following articles, pp. 411, 416, 423, 427.

278. J. E. Dolfini, H. E. Appelgate, G. Bach, H. Basch, J. Bernstein, J. Schwartz, and F. L. Weisenborn, *J. Med. Chem.*, **14,** 117 (1971).

279. H. Basch, R. Erickson, and H. Gadebusch, *Infect. Immunol.* **4,** 44 (1971); H. Gadebusch, G. Mirglia, F. Pansy, and K. Reny, *ibid.*, 50 (1971).

280. J. E. Beck, J. A. Hubsher, and D. L. Caloza, *Curr. Ther. Res.*, **13,** 530 (1971); P. D. Reyes-Javier, *ibid.*, **13,** 602 (1971); L. Landa, *ibid.*, **13,** 654 (1971).

281. K. E. Price, J. A. Bach, D. R. Chisholm, M. Misiek, and A. Gourevitch, *J. Antibiot.* (Tokyo), **22,** 1 (1969).

282. R. Raap, *J. Antibiot.* (Tokyo), **24,** 695 (1971).

283. E. Testa, G. Cignarella, G. Pifferi, S. Füresz, M. T. Timbal, P. Schiatti, and G. Maffi, *Farmaco, Ed. Sci.*, **19,** 895 (1964).

284. G. Acocella, G. C. Baroni, and F. B. Nicolés, *Curr. Ther. Res., Clin. Exp.*, **7,** 226 (1965).

285. G. A. Hardcastle, Jr., D. A. Johnson, C. A. Panetta, A. I. Scott, and S. A. Sutherland, *J. Org. Chem.*, **31,** 897 (1966).

286. P. A. Bunn, S. Milicich, and J. S. Lunn, *Antimicrob. Agents Chemother.*, 947 (1966).

287. S. B. Tuano, L. D. Johnson, J. L. Brodie, and W. M. M. Kirby, *New Engl. J. Med.*, **275,** 635 (1966).

288. B. Gradnik, A. Pedrazzoli, E. Ferrero, and V. Guzzon, *Farmaco, Ed. Sci.*, **26,** 520 (1971).

289. R. Sutherland, S. Elson, and E. A. P. Croydon, *Chemotherapy* (Basel), **17,** 145 (1972).

290. W. Von Daehne, E. Fredriksen, E. Gundersen, F. Lund, P. Morch, H. J. Petersen, K. Roholt, L. Tybring, and W. O. Godtfredsen, *J. Med. Chem.*, **13,** 607 (1970).

291. E. L. Foltz, J. W. West, I. H. Breslow, and H. Wallick, *Antimicrob. Agents Chemother.*, 442 (1971).

292. N. O. Bodin, B. Ekström, U. Forsgren, L. P. Jalar, L. Magni, C. H. Ramsay, and B. Sjöberg, *Antimicrob. Agents Chemother.*, **8,** 518 (1975).

293. H. O. Hallander, A. Flodström, and J. Sjövall, *Antimicrob. Agents Chemother.*, **11,** 185 (1977).

294. J. P. Clayton, M. Cole, S. W. Elson, and H. Ferres, *Antimicrob. Agents Chemother*, **5,** 670 (1974).

295. Netherlands Patent 68,05524 (April 18, 1967) (to Beecham Laboratories, Ltd.).

296. G. P. Bodey and B. Deerake, *Appl. Microbiol.*, **21,** 61 (1971); H. C. Neu and E. B. Winshell, *ibid.*, 66 (1971).

297. R. Sutherland, J. Burnett, and G. N. Rolinson, *Antimicrob. Agents Chemother.*, 390 (1971); P. Acred, P. A. Hunter, L. Mizen, and G. N. Rolinson, *ibid.*, 396 (1971).

298. S. Morimoto, H. Nomura, T. Ishiguro, T. Fugono, and K. Maeda, *J. Med. Chem.*, **15,** 1105 (1972); S. Morimoto, H. Nomura, T. Fugono, T. Azuma, I. Minami, M. Hon, and T. Masada, *ibid.*, **15,** 1108 (1972).

299. K. Tsuchiya, T. Oishi, C. Iwagishi, and T. Iwaki, *J. Antibiot.* (Tokyo), **24,** 607 (1971); T. Yamazaki and K. Tsuchiya, *ibid.*, **24**, 620 (1971); K. Tsuchiya, T. Yamazaki, A. Kuchimura, and T. Fugono, *ibid.*, **25,** 336 (1972).

300. M. Okoshi and Y. Naide, in *Advances in Antimcrobial Antineoplastic Chemotherapy*, Vol. I/2, Avicenum, 1972, p. 1005.

301. K. E. Price, D. R. Chisholm, F. Leitner, M. Misiek, and A. Gourevitch, *Appl. Microbiol.*, **17,** 881 (1969); G. P. Bodey and D. Stewart, *ibid.*, **18,** 76 (1969).

302. M. Barza, H. Berman, D. Michaeli, A. Molavi, and L. Weinstein, *Antimicrob. Agents Chemother.*, 341 (1971).

303. G. P. Bodey and V. Rodriguez, *Curr. Ther. Res.*, **12,** 363 (1970).

304. US Patents 3,557,090 (January 19, 1971), 3,574,189 (April 6, 1971), K. Butler (to Pfizer, Inc.).

305. A. R. English, J. A. Retsema, V. A. Ray, and J. E. Lynch, *Antimicrob. Agents Chemother.*, **1,** 185 (1972).

306. J. F. Wallace, E. Atlas, D. M. Bear, N. K. Brown, H. Clark, and M. Turck, *Antimicrob. Agents Chemother.*, 223 (1971); J. L. Bran, D. M. Karl and D. Kage, *Clin. Pharmacol. Ther.*, **12,** 525 (1971).

307. J. P. Clayton, M. Cole, S. W. Elson, K. D.

Hardy, L. W. Mizen, and R. Sutherland, *J. Med. Chem.*, **18,** 172 (1975).

308. F. Benigni, C. Botré, and I. R. Riceieu, *Farmaco, Ed. Sci.*, **20,** 885 (1965).

309. J. H. C. Nayler, in Ref. 158, p. 55.

310. S. Kurtz, K. Holme, and M. Turck, *Antimicrob. Agents Chemother.*, **7,** 215 (1975).

311. K. E. Price, F. Leitner, M. Misiek, R. Chisholm, and T. A. Pursiano, *Antimicrob. Agents Chemother.*, 17 (1971).

312. H. Noguchi, Y. Eda, H. Tobiki, T. Nakagome, and T. Komatsu, *Antimicrob. Agents Chemother.*, **9,** 262 (1976).

313. T. Kashiwagi, I. Isaka, N. Kawahara, K. Nakano, A. Koda, T. Ozasa, I. Souzu, Y. Murakami and M. Murakami, Abstract No. 222, 15*th Interscience Conference on Antimicrobial Agents and Chemotherapy*, Washington, D.C., 1975.

314. J. A. Retsema, A. R. English, and J. E. Lynch, *Antimicrob. Agents Chemother.*, **9,** 975 (1976).

315. D. Stewart and G. P. Bodey, *Antimicrob. Agents Chemother.*, **11,** 865 (1977).

316. G. P. Bodey and T. Pan, *Antimicrob. Agents Chemother.*, **11,** 74 (1977).

317. S. Mitsuhashi, I. Saikawa, and T. Yasuda, Abstract No. 349, 16*th Interscience Conference on Antimicrobial Agents and Chemotherapy, Chicago,* 1976.

318. G. LiBassi, R. Monguzzi, R. Broggi, G. Broccali, C. Carpi, and G. Pifferi, *J. Antibiot.* (Tokyo), **30,** 376 (1977).

319. P. Bamberg, B. Ekström, K. Undheim, and B. Sjöberg, *Acta Chem. Scand.*, **19,** 352 (1965).

320. R. J. Stedman, A. C. Swift, L. S. Miller, M. M. Dolan, and J. R. E. Hoover, *J. Med. Chem.*, **10,** 363 (1967).

321. P. Bamberg, B. Ekström, and B. Sjöberg, *Acta Chem. Scand.*, **21,** 2210 (1967).

322. R. Raap and R. G. Micetich, *J. Med. Chem.*, **11,** 70 (1968).

323. S. B. Rosenman, L. S. Weber, G. Owen, and G. H. Warren, *Antimicrob. Agents Chemother.*, 590 (1968).

324. H. E. Alburn, D. E. Clark, H. Fletcher, and N. H. Grant, *Antimicrob. Agents Chemother.*, 586 (1968).

325. B. Sjöberg, B. Ekström, and U. Fosgren, *Antimicrob. Agents Chemother.*, 560 (1968).

326. E. Hansson, L. Magni, and S. Wahlqvist, *Antimicrob. Agents Chemother.*, 569 (1968).

327. A. Reyn and M. W. Bentzon, *Brit. J. Vener. Dis.*, **44,** 140 (1968).

328. G. H. L. Nefkens, G.I. Tesser, and R. J. F. Nivard, *Rec. Trav. Chim. Pays-Bas*, **79,** 688 (1960); J. C. Sheehan and K. R. Hénery-Logan, *J. Am. Chem. Soc.*, **84,** 2983 (1962); Ref. 207.

329. F. Lund and L. Tybring, *Nature* (London), **236,** 135 (1972).

330. L. Tybring, *Antimicrob. Agents Chemother.*, **8,** 266 (1975).

331. D. Greenwood and F. O. Grady, *J. Clin. Pathol.*, **26,** 1 (1973).

332. L. Tybring and N. H. Melchior, *Antimcrob. Agents Chemother.*, **8,** 271 (1975).

333. V. Lorain and B. Atkinson, *Antimicrob. Agents Chemother.*, **11,** 541 (1977).

334. E. Grunsberg, R. Cleeland, G. Besked, and W. F. DeLorenzo, *Antimicrob. Agents Chemother.*, **9,** 589 (1976).

335. A. M. Geddes, R. Wise, et al., *J. Antimicrob. Chemother.*, **3** (Suppl. B), 1–160 (1977).

336. G. T. Stewart, *Lancet*, **1,** 509 (1962).

337. E. P. Abraham and G. G. F. Newton, *Biochem. J.*, **62,** 658 (1956).

338. US Patent 3,296,258 (January 3, 1967), E. Visher et al. (to Ciba Corp.).

339. US Patents 3,160,631 (December 8, 1964), L. H. Petersen and A. A. Patchett, 3,227,712 (January 4, 1966), A. A. Patchett and S. A. Harris (to Merck and Co., Inc.).

340. U.S. Patents 3,772,286 (November 13, 1973), 3,903,277 (September 2, 1975), J. R. E. Hoover (to SmithKline Corp.).

341. W. C. Topp and B. G. Christensen, *J. Med. Chem.*, **17,** 342 (1974).

342. J. M. Indelicato, A. Dinner, L. R. Peters, and W. L. Wilham, *J. Med. Chem.*, **20,** 961 (1977).

343. R. D. Cramer, III, unpublished data, SmithKline Corp.

344. R. M. Sweet and L. F. Dahl, *J. Am. Chem. Soc.*, **92,** 5489 (1970).

345. D. B. Boyd, R. B. Hermann, D. E. Presti, and M. M. Marsh, *J. Med. Chem.*, **18,** 408 (1975).

346. J. M. Indelicato, T. T. Norvilos, R. R. Pfeiffer, W. J. Wheeler, and W. L. Wilham, *J. Med. Chem.*, **17,** 523 (1974).

347. H. Bundgaard, *Arch. Pharm. Chem. Sci. Ed.*, **3,** 94 (1975).

348. R. R. Chauvette, E. H. Flynn, B. G. Jackson, E. R. Lavagnino, R. B. Morin, R. A. Mueller, R. P. Pioch, R. W. Roeske, C. W. Ryan, J. L. Spencer, and E. van Heyningen, *Antimicrob. Agents Chemother.*, 687 (1963).

349. M. Gorman and C. W. Ryan, in Ref. 114, p. 555.

350. US Patent 3,546,219 (December 8, 1970), A. G. Long et al. (to Glaxo Laboratories, Ltd.).

351. US Patent 3,274,186 (September 20, 1966), M.

D. Barker and G. A. Somerfield, (to Glaxo Laboratories, Ltd.).

352. M. Okui, K. Hattori, and M. Nishida, *J. Antibiot.* (Tokyo), **24,** 667 (1971).

353. A. L. Demain, J. F. Newkirk, G. E. Davies, and R. E. Harman, *Appl. Microbiol.*, **11,** 58 (1963).

354. C. F. Murphy, R. E. Koehler, and C. W. Ryan, Abstract No. 425, 14*th Interscience Conference on Antimicrobial Agents and Chemotherapy*, San Francisco, 1974; D. A. Preston and W. E. Wick, *ibid.*, Abstract No. 426; M. Gorman and C. W. Ryan, in Ref. 114, pp. 566, 568.

355. M. Kurita, T. Teraji, Y. Saito, H. Harada, K. Hattori, T. Kamiya, M. Nishida, and T. Takano in *Advances in Antimicrobial and Antineoplastic Chemotherapy*, Vol. I/2, Avicenum, 1972, p. 1055.

356. US Patent 3,878,204 (April 15, 1975), M. Ochiai (to Takeda Chemical Industries, Ltd.); C. H. O'Callaghan, R. B. Sykes, and S. E. Staniforth, *Antimicrob. Agents Chemother.*, **10,** 245 (1976); T. Naito, J. Okumura, K. Kasai, K. Masuko, H. Hoshi, H. Kamachi, and H. Kawaguchi, *J. Antibiot.* (Tokyo), **30,** 692 (1977); *ibid.*, **30,** 698 (1977); T. Naito, J. Okumura, H. Kamachi, H. Hoshi, and H. Kawaguchi, *ibid.*, **30,** 705 (1977).

357. W. J. Gottstein, M. A. Kaplan, J. A. Cooper, V. H. Silver, S. J. Nachfolger, and A. P. Granatek, *J. Antibiot.* (Tokyo), **29,** 1226 (1976).

358. F. Leitner, M. Misiek, T. A. Pursiano, R. E. Buck, D. R. Chisholm, R. G. DeRegis, Y. H. Tsai, and K. E. Price, *Antimicrob. Agents Chemother.*, **3,** 426 (1976); R. D. Meyer, *J. Antibiot.* (Tokyo), **30,** 326 (1977); see following articles in same journal, **30,** 576, 583 (1977).

359. D. A. Berges, G. L. Dunn, J. R. E. Hoover, S. J. Schmidt, G. W. Chan, J. J. Taggart, C. M. Kinzig, F. R. Pfeiffer, P. Actor, C. S. Sachs, J. V. Uri, and J. A. Weisbach, Abstract No. 87, 16*th Interscience Conference on Antimicrobial Agents and Chemotherapy*, Chicago, 1976.

360. P. Actor, J. V. Uri, I. Zajac, J. R. Guarini, C. S. Sachs, L. Phillips, D. A. Berges, G. L. Dunn, J. R. E. Hoover, and J. A. Weisbach, Abstract No. 86, 16*th Interscience Conference on Antimicrobial Agents and Chemotherapy*, Chicago, 1976.

361. R. R. Chauvette, E. H. Flynn, B. G. Jackson, E. R. Lavagnino, R. B. Morin, R. A. Mueller, R. P. Pioch, R. W. Roeske, C. W. Ryan, J. L. Spencer, and E. van Heyningen, *J. Am. Chem. Soc.*, **84,** 3401 (1962).

362. W. S. Boniece, W. E. Wick, D. H. Holmes, and C. E. Redman, *J. Bacteriol.*, **84,** 1292 (1962).

363. See series of introductory papers on cephalothin in *Antimicrob. Agents Chemother.*, 150, 695, 706, 716, 724, 787 (1963).

364. L. B. Crast, R. G. Graham, and L. C. Cheney, *J. Med. Chem.*, **16,** 1413 (1973).

365. D. R. Chisholm, F. Leitner, M. Misiek, G. E. Wright, and K. E. Price, *Antimicrob. Agents Chemother.*, 244 (1970); J. Axelrod, B. R. Meyers, and S. Z. Hirshman, *Appl. Microbiol.*, **22,** 904 (1971).

366. J. L. Bran, M. E. Levison, and D. Kage, *Antimicrob. Agents Chemother.*, **1,** 35 (1972); P. Weisner, R. MacGregor, D. Bear, S. Berman, K. Holmes and M. Turck, *ibid.*, **1,** 303 (1972).

367. US Patent 3,483,197 (December 9, 1969), H. Bickel et al. (to CIBA Corp.).

368. F. Knusel, E. A. Konopka, J. Gelzer, and A. Rosselet, *Antimcrob. Agents Chemother.*, 140 (1971); F. Kradolfer, W. Sackmann, O. Zak, H. Brunner, R. Hess, E. A. Konopka, and J. Gelzer, *ibid.*, 150; H. Neu and E. B. Winshell, *J. Antibiot.* (Tokyo), **25,** 400 (1972).

369. F. Kradolfer, T. Ahrens, J. Gelzer, W. Vischer, and W. Zimmerman, *Schweiz. Med. Wochenschr.*, **103,** 711 (1973); Symposium, *Arzneim.-Forsch*, **24,** 1446–1533 (1974), 22 articles.

370. British Patent 1,028,563 (May 4, 1966), V. Arkley et al. (to Glaxo Laboratories, Ltd.).

371. P. W. Muggleton, C. H. O'Callaghan, and W. K. Stevens, *Brit. Med. J.*, **2,** 1234 (1964); M. Barber and P. M. Waterworth, *ibid.*, 344 (1964); J. M. Murdock, C. F. Spiers, A. M. Geddes, and E. T. Wallace, *ibid.*, **2,** 1238 (1964); G. T. Stewart and R. J. Holt, *Lancet*, **2,** 1305 (1964).

372. For early American work on cephaloridine, see *Antimicrob. Agents Chemother.*, 724, 863, 879, 888, 901, 922, 933, (1966); 6, 88, 96, 101 (1967).

373. K. Kariyone, H. Harada, M. Kurita, and T. Takano, *J. Antibiot.* (Tokyo), **23,** 131 (1970).

374. M. Nishida, T. Matsubara, T. Murakawa, Y. Mine, and Y. Yokota, *J. Antibiot.* (Tokyo), **23,** 137 (1970); M. Nishida, T. Matsubara, T. Murakawa, Y. Mine, Y. Yokota, S. Goto, and S. Kuwahara, *ibid.*, **23,** 184 (1970); J. Kozatani, M. Okui, T. Matsubara, and M. Nishida, *ibid.*, **25,** 86 (1972).

375. M. G. Bergeron, J. L. Brusch, M. Barza, and L. Weinstein, *Antimicrob. Agents Chemother.*, **4,** 396 (1973).

376. K. Ries, M. E. Levison, and D. Kage, *Antimicrob. Agents Chemother.*, **3,** 168 (1973); K. Shibata and M. Fujii, *ibid.*, 467 (1971).

377. Symposium, *J. Infect. Dis.*, **128** (Suppl.), S307–S422 (1973), 22 articles; Y. Ueda, *Cefazolin*, Shinryo Sinsha, Osaka, 1977.

378. W. E. Wick and D. A. Preston, *Antimicrob. Agents Chemother.*, **1,** 221 (1972); for additional articles on cefamandole, see *ibid.*, **3,** 657 (1973); **8,** 679, 737 (1975); **9,** 690, 852, 994, 1019, 1066 (1976); **9,** 140 (1976); **9,** 65 (1976); **10,** 421, 457, 623, 733, 814 (1976); **12,** 67 (1977).

379. Abstracts Nos. 256–260. 16*th Interscience Conference on Antimicrobial Agents and Chemotherapy*, Chicago, 1976.

380. W. E. Wick and W. S. Boniece, *Appl. Microbiol.*, **13,** 248 (1965); J. Pitt, R. Siasco, K. Kaplan, and L. Weinstein, *Antimicrob. Agents Chemother.*, 630 (1968).

381. A. R. Ronald and M. Turck, *Antibiot. Agents Chemother.*, 82 (1967); J. M. Applestein, E. B. Crosby, W. D. Johnson, and D. Kaye, *Appl. Microbiol.*, **16,** 1006 (1968).

382. W. E. Wick, *Appl. Microbiol.*, **15,** 765 (1967); P. W. Muggleton, C. O'Callaghan, R. D. Foord, S. M. Kirby, and D. M. Ryan, *Antimicrob. Agents Chemother.*, 353 (1969); P. Braun, J. Tillotson, C. Wilcox, and M. Finland, *Appl. Microbiol.*, **16,** 1684 (1968).

383. R. S. Griffith and H. R. Black, *Clin. Med.*, **75,** 14 (1968); H. Clark and M. Turck, *Antimicrob. Agents Chemother.*, 296 (1969).

384. A. W. Bauer, W. M. Kirby, J. C. Sherris, and M. Turck, *Am. J. Clin. Pathol.*, **45,** 493 (1966).

385. R. M. DeMarinis, J. R. E. Hoover, G. L. Dunn, P. Actor, J. V. Uri, and J. A. Weisbach, *J. Antibiot.* (Tokyo), **28,** 463 (1975).

386. P. Actor, J. V. Uri, J. R. Guarini, I. Zajac, L. Phillips, C. S. Sachs, R. M. DeMarinis, J. R. E. Hoover, and J. A. Weisbach, *J. Antibiot.* (Tokyo), **28,** 471 (1975); P. Actor, D. H. Pitkin, G. Lucyszyn, and J. A. Weisbach, *Chemotherapy* (Basel), **5,** 253 (1976); C. Harvengt, H. Meunier and F. Lamy, *J. Clin. Pharmacol.*, **17,** 128 (1977).

387. US Patents 3,966,717 (June 29, 1976), 3,971,153 (August 10, 1976), M. C. Cook et al. (to Glaxo Laboratories, Ltd.).

388. C. H. O'Callaghan, R. B. Sykes, D. M. Ryan, R. D. Foord, and P. W. Muggleton, *J. Antibiot.* (Tokyo), **29,** 29 (1976); C. H. O'Callaghan, R. B. Sykes, A. Griffiths, and J. E. Thornton, *Antimicrob. Agents Chemother.*, **9,** 511 (1976); D. M. Ryan, C. H. O'Callaghan, and P. W. Muggleton, *ibid.*, **9,** 520 (1976).

389. R. D. Foord, *Antimicrob, Agents Chemother.*, **9,** 741 (1976); R. Norrby, R. D. Foord, and P. Hedlund, *J. Antimicrob. Chemother.*, **3,** 355 (1977); Abstracts Nos. 193, 344, *17th Interscience Conference on Antimicrobial Agents and Chemotherapy*, New York, 1977.

390. W. E. Wick and D. A. Preston, in Ref. 378; H. C. Neu and E. B. Winshell, *J. Antibiot.* (Tokyo), **26,** 153 (1973).

391. R. Heymès, A. Lutz, and E. Schrinner, *Infection*, **5,** 259 (1977); Abstracts Nos. 75–83, 133–135, 296–300, 18th Interscience Conference on Antimicrobial Agents and Chemotherapy, Atlanta, 1978.

392. G. L. Dunn, J. R. E. Hoover, D. A. Berges, J. J. Taggart, L. D. Davis, E. M. Dietz, D. R. Jakas, N. Yim, P. Actor, J. V. Uri, and J. A. Weisbach, *J. Antibiot.* (Tokyo), **29,** 65 (1976); P. Actor, J. V. Uri, L. Phillips, C. S. Sachs, J. R. Guarini, I. Zajac, D. A. Berges, G. L. Dunn, J. R. E. Hoover, and J. A. Weisbach, *J. Antibiot.* (Tokyo), **29,** 594 (1975); F. Leitner, R. E. Buck, M. Misiek, T. A. Pursiano, and K. E. Price, *Antimicrob. Agents Chemother.*, **7,** 298 (1975).

393. P. Actor, D. H. Pitkin, G. Lucyszyn, J. A. Weisbach, and J. Bran, *Antimicrob. Agents Chemother.*, **9,** 800 (1976); R. DelBusto, E. Haas, T. Madhavan, K. Burch, F. Cox, E. Fisher, E. Quinn, and D. Pohlod, *ibid.*, **9,** 397 (1976); Abstracts Nos. 185, 357, 359, 16*th Interscience Conference on Antimicrobial Agents and Chemotherapy*, Chicago, 1976.

394. R. R. Chauvette and P. A. Pennington, *J. Med. Chem.*, **18,** 403 (1975).

395. N. J. Bill and J. A. Washington, II, *Antimicrob. Agents Chemother.*, **11,** 470 (1977); H. R. Sullivan, S. L. Due, D. L. K. Kau, J. F. Quag, and W. M. Miller, *ibid.*, **10** 630 (1976); Abstracts Nos. 352–356, 16*th Interscience Conference on Antimicrobial Agents and Chemotherapy*, Chicago, 1976.

396. O. M. Korzeniowski, W. M. Scheld, and M. A. Sande, *Antimicrobial Agents Chemother.*, **12,** 157 (1977); Abstract Nos. 29, 228, 311, 343, 17*th Interscience Conference on Antimicrobial Agents and Chemotherapy*, New York, 1977.

397. US Patent 3,489,752 (January 13, 1970), L. B. Crast, Jr. (to Bristol Myers Co.).

398. R. E. Buck and K. E. Price, *Antimicrob. Agents Chemother.*, **11,** 324 (1977).

399. M. Pfeffer, A. Jackson, J. Ximenes, and J. P. DeMenzes, *Antimicrob. Agents Chemother.*, **11,** 331 (977); A. I. Hartstein, K. E. Patrick, S. R. Jones, M. J. Miller, and R. E. Bryant, *ibid.*, **12,** 93 (1977); Abstract, Nos. 361–365. 16*th Interscience Conference on Antimicrobial Agents and Chemotherapy*, Chigago, 1976.

400. H. Wallick and D. Hendlin, *Antimicrob. Agents Chemother.*, **5,** 25 (1974); A. K. Miller, E. Celozzi, Y. Kong, B. A. Pelak, D. Hendlin, and

E. O. Stapley, *ibid.*, **5,** 33 (1974); see also following articles same journal, **6,** 170, 320 (1974); **7,** 128 (1975); **8,** 224 (1975); **9,** 318, 506, 994, 1019 (1976); **11,** 26, 84, 679, 912, (1977); also, *J. Antibiot.* (Tokyo), **27,** 42 (1974); *ibid.*, **29,** 181 (1976); *Arzneim.-Forsch.* **27,** 89 (1977).

401. Reference 106; see also *Antimicrob. Agents Chemother.*, **6,** 170 (1974); **11,** 725 (1977).

402. Reference 108; see also *Antimicrob. Agents Chemother.*, **6,** 290, 338 (1974); A. M. Geddes, L. P. Schnurr, A. P. Ball, D. McGhie, G. R. Brookes, R. Wise, and J. Andrews, *Brit. Med. J.*, 1126 (1977); R. N. Heseltine, D. F. Busch, R. D. Meyer, and S. M. Finegold, *Antimicrob. Agents Chemother.*, **11,** 427 (1977).

403. M. Neuman, *Future Trends in Chemotherapy, Proc. Int. Symp. Drugs of Today*, **10,** Suppl., 11 (1974).

404. C. H. O'Callaghan, *J. Antimicrob. Chemother.*, **1,** 1 (1975).

405. D. Willner, C. T. Holdrege, S. R. Baker, and L. C. Cheney, *J. Antibiot.* (Tokyo), **25,** 64 (1972).

406. J. A. Webber, G. W. Huffman, R. E. Koehler, C. F. Murphy, C. W. Ryan, E. M. van Heyningen, and R. T. Vasileff, *J. Med. Chem.*, **14,** 113 (1971).

407. P. Actor et al., in Ref. 393.

408. M. Pfeffer et al., in Ref. 399.

409. J. M. Indelicato and W. L. Williams, *J. Med. Chem.*, **17,** 528 (1974).

410. US Patents 3,905,868 (September 16, 1975), J. J. Hamsher, 3,957,811 (May 18, 1976), S. Nakanishi (to Pfizer, Inc); 3,966,717 (June 29, 1976), M. C. Cook et al. (to Glaxo Laboratories, Ltd.); Belgian Patents 821,163 (April 17, 1975), 821,164 (April 17, 1975), 833,009 (March 3, 1976), (to Pfizer, Inc.).

411. A. R. English, J. A. Retsema, and J. E. Lynch, *Antimicrob. Agents Chemother.*, **10,** 132 (1976); Abstract No. 225, 16*th Interscience Conference on Antimicrobial Agents and Chemotherapy*, Chicago, 1976; G. P. Bodey, S. Weaver, and T. Pan, *J. Antibiot.* (Tokyo), **30,** 724 (1977).

412. W. J. Gottstein, R. B. Babel, L. B. Crast, J. M. Essery, R. R. Fraser, J. C. Godfrey, C. T. Holdredge, W. F. Minor, M. E. Neubert, C. A. Panetta, and L. C. Cheney, *J. Med. Chem.*, **8,** 794 (1965).

413. K. Meyer, G. L. Hobby, and E. Chaffee, *Science*, **97,** 205 (1943); J. Ungar, *Brit. J. Exp. Pathol.*, **28,** 88 (1947).

414. A. B. A. Jansen and T. J. Russell, *J. Chem. Soc.*, 2127 (1965); H. P. K. Agersborg, A. Batchelor, G. W. Cambridge, and A. W. Rule, *Brit. J. Pharmacol.*, **26,** 649 (1966).

415. W. V. Daehne, E. Frederiksen, E. Gundersen, F. Lund, P. Mørch, H. J. Petersen, K. Roholt, L. Tybring, and W. O. Godtfredsen, *J. Med. Chem.*, **13,** 607 (1970).

416. E. Binderup, W. O. Godfredsen, and K. Roholt, *J. Antibiot*, (Tokyo), **24,** 767 (1971).

417. R. P. Holysz and H. E. Stavely, *J. Am. Chem. Soc.*, **72,** 4760 (1950).

418. B. K. Koe, *Nature* (London), **195,** 1200 (1962).

419. E. Grunberg and G. Beskid, *Antimicrob. Agents Chemother.*, 619 (1967).

420. L. D. Broun, W. A. Zygmunt, and H. E. Stavely, *Appl. Microbiol.*, **17,** 339 (1969).

421. M. Claesen and H. Vanderhaeghe, *Bull. Soc. Chim. Belg.*, **73,** 647 (1964).

422. Y. G. Perron, L. B. Crast, J. M. Essery, R. R. Fraser, J. C. Godfrey, C. T. Holdredge, W. F. Minor, M. E. Neubert, R. A. Partyka, and L. C. Cheney, *J. Med. Chem.*, **7,** 483 (1964).

423. W. J. Gottstein, G. E. Bocian, L. B. Crast, K. Dadabo, J. M. Essery, J. C. Godfrey, and L. C. Cheney, *J. Org. Chem.*, **31,** 1922 (1966).

424. P. J. Beeby, *J. Med. Chem.*, **20,** 173 (1977).

425. T. Jen, B. Dienel, J. Frazee, and J. Weisbach, *J. Med. Chem.*, **15,** 1172 (1972).

426. B. G. Christensen and R. W. Ratcliffe, in *Annual Reports in Medicinal Chemistry*, Vol. 2, F. H. Clarke, Ed., Academic Press, New York, 1976, p. 271.

427. E. Guddal, P. Mørch, and L. Tybring, *Tetrahedron Lett.*, 381 (1962).

428. K. W. Glombitza, *Justus Liebigs Ann. Chem.*, **673,** 166 (1964).

429. J. C. Sheehan and G. D. Daves, *J. Org. Chem.*, **29,** 2006 (1964).

430. R. J. Stedman, *J. Med. Chem.*, **9,** 444 (1966).

431. H. Peter, H. Rodriguez, B. Muller, W. Sibral, and H. Bickel, *Helv. Chim. Acta*, **57,** 2024 (1974).

432. C. F. Murphy and R. E. Koehler, *J. Org. Chem.*, **35,** 2429 (1970).

433. R. R. Chauvette and P. A. Pennington, *J. Org. Chem.*, **38,** 2994 (1973).

434. T. Leigh, *J. Chem. Soc.*, 3616 (1965).

435. W. Dürckheimer and M. Schorr, *Justus Liebigs Ann. Chem.*, **702,** 163 (1967).

436. D. M. Brunwin and G. Lowe, *J. Chem. Soc., Chem. Commun.*, 192 (1972).

437. J. C. Sheehan and Y. S. Lo, *J. Org. Chem.*, **38,** 3227 (1973).

438. Y. S. Lo and J. C. Sheehan, *J. Am. Chem. Soc.*, **94,** 8253 (1972).

439. J. C. Sheehan, Y. S. Lo, and D. R. Ponzi, *J. Org. Chem.*, **42,** 1012 (1977).

440. G. Cignarella, G. Pifferi, and E. Testa, *J. Org. Chem.*, **27,** 2668 (1962).

441. D. Hauser and H. P. Sigg, *Helv. Chim. Acta*, **50,** 1327 (1967).

442. I. McMillan and R. J. Stoodley, *J. Chem. Soc. C*, 2533 (1968).

443. J. P. Clayton, *J. Chem. Soc., C*, 2123 (1969).

444. E. Evrard, M. Claesen, and H. Vanderhaeghe, *Nature* (London), **201,** 1124 (1964).

445. R. B. Morin, B. G. Jackson, E. H. Flynn, R. W. Roeske, and S. L. Andrews, *J. Am. Chem. Soc.*, **91,** 1396 (1969).

446. J. S. Wiering and H. Wynberg, *J. Org. Chem.*, **41,** 1574 (1976).

447. P. H. Bentley and J. P. Clayton, *J. Chem. Soc., Chem. Commun.*, 278 (1974).

448. R. A. Firestone and B. G. Christensen, *J. Org. Chem.*, **38,** 1436 (1973).

449. M. M. Campbell and G. Johnson, *J. Chem. Soc., Chem. Commun.*, 479 (1975).

450. R. A. Firestone and B. G. Christensen, *J. Chem. Soc., Chem. Commun.*, 288 (1976).

451. R. A. Firestone, N. Schelechow, D. B. R. Johnston, and B. G. Christensen, *Tetrahedron Lett.*, 375 (1972).

452. E. H. Bohme, H. E. Applegate, J. B. Ewing, P. T. Funke, M. S. Puar, and J. E. Dolfini, *J. Org. Chem.*, **38,** 230 (1973).

453. D. B. R. Johnston, S. M. Schmitt, R. A. Firestone, and B. G. Christensen, *Tetrahedron Lett.*, 4917 (1972).

454. G. H. Rasmusson, G. F. Reynolds and G. E. Arth, *Tetrahedron Lett.*, 145 (1975).

455. Y. S. Lo and J. C. Sheehan, *J. Org. Chem.*, **40,** 191 (1975).

456. W. A. Spitzer and T. Goodson, *Tetrahedron Lett.*, 273 (1973).

457. W. A. Slusarchyk, H. E. Applegate, P. Funke, W. Koster, M. S. Puar, M. Young, and J. E. Dolfini, *J. Org. Chem.*, **38,** 943 (1973).

458. H. Yanagisawa and H. Nakao, *Tetrahedron Lett.*, 1815 (1976).

459. H. Yanagisawa, M. Fukushima, A. Ando, and H. Nakao, *Tetrahedron Lett.*, 259 (1976).

460. W. A. Spitzer, T. Goodson, R. J. Smithey, and I. G. Wright, *J. Chem. Soc., Chem. Commun.*, 1138 (1972).

461. H. Yanagisawa and H. Nakao, *Tetrahedron Lett.*, 1811 (1976).

462. D. A. Johnson, D. Mania, C. A. Panetta, and H. H. Silvestri, *Tetrahedron Lett.*, 1903 (1968).

463. D. A. Johnson and D. Mania, *Tetrahedron Lett.*, 267 (1969).

464. J. P. Clayton, J. H. C. Nayler, R. Southgate, and E. R. Stove, *J. Chem. Soc., Chem. Commun.*, 130 (1969).

465. S. Wolfe and W. S. Lee, *J. Chem. Soc., Chem. Commun.*, 242 (1968).

466. G. E. Gutowski, *Tetrahedron Lett.*, 1779 (1970).

467. M. L. Sassiver and R. G. Shepherd, *Tetrahedron Lett.*, 3993 (1969).

468. S. Kukolja, *J. Med. Chem.*, **13,** 1114 (1970).

469. D. A. Berges, *J. Med. Chem.*, **18,** 1264 (1975).

470. B. J. Abbott and D. S. Fukuda, *Antimicrob. Agents Chemother.*, **8,** 282 (1975).

471. US Patents 3,355,452 (November 28, 1967) and 3,484,437 (December 16, 1969), J. Urech et al. (to CIBA Corp.).

472. US Patents 3,665,003 (May 23, 1972), J. Kennedy et al., 3,658, 799 (April 25, 1972), 3,948, 905 (April 6, 1976), S. Eardley et al. (to Glaxo Laboratories, Ltd.).

473. J. A. Webber and R. T. Vasileff, *J. Med. Chem.*, **14,** 1136 (1971).

474. C. F. Murphy and J. A. Webber, in Ref. 114, p. 156.

475. S. Karady, T. Y. Cheng, S. H. Pines, and M. Sletzinger, *Tetrahedron Lett.*, 2625 (1974).

476. S. Karady, T. Y. Cheng, S. H. Pines, and M. Sletzinger, *Tetrahedron Lett.*, 2629 (1974).

477. H. Yazawa, H. Nakamura, K. Tanaka, and K. Kariyone, *Tetrahedron Lett.*, 3991 (1974).

478. G. A. Koppel, M. D. Kinnick, and L. J. Nummy, *J. Am. Chem. Soc.*, **99,** 2822 (1977).

479. D. Willner, A. M. Jelenevsky, and L. C. Cheney, *J. Med. Chem.*, **15,** 948 (1972); US Patent 3,821,206 (June 8, 1974), B. R. Cowley et al. (to Glaxo Laboratories, Ltd.).

480. M. Ochiai, O. Aki, A. Morimoto, T. Okada, and T. Kaneko, *Tetrahedron Lett.*, 2345 (1972).

481. J. H. C. Nayler, M. J. Pearson, and R. Southgate, *J. Chem. Soc., Chem. Commun.*, 58 (1973).

482. J. W. Chamberlin and J. B. Campbell, *J. Med. Chem.*, **10,** 966 (1967).

483. US Patent 3,682,903 (August 8, 1972); H. Bickel et al. (to Ciba-Geigy Corp.).

484. H. Peter and H. Bickel, *Helv. Chim. Acta*, **57,** 2044 (1974).

485. H. Peter, B. Muller and H. Bickel, *Helv. Chim. Acta*, **58,** 2450 (1975).

486. J. L. Fahey, R. A. Firestone, and B. G. Christensen, *J. Med. Chem.*, **19,** 562 (1976).

487. D. O. Spry, *J. Org. Chem.*, **40,** 2411 (1975).

488. R. A. Firestone, N. S. Maciejewicz, and B. G. Christensen, *J. Org. Chem.*, **39,** 3384 (1974).

489. J. A. Webber, J. L. Ott and R. T. Vasileff, *J.*

Med. Chem., **18,** 986 (1975); US Patent 3,769,277 (October 30, 1973), A. G. Long and N. G. Wein (to Glaxo Laboratories, Ltd.).

490. R. Scartazzini and H. Bickel, *Helv. Chim. Acta,* **55,** 423 (1972).
491. D. O. Spry, *J. Chem. Soc., Chem. Commun.*, 1012 (1974).
492. M. Ochiai, O. Aki, A. Morimoto, T. Okada, and K. Morita, *Tetrahedron Lett.*, **31,** 115 (1975).
493. M. Ochiai, O. Aki, A. Morimoto, T. Okada, K. Shinozaki and Y. Asahi, *Tetrahedron Lett.*, 2341 (1972).
494. S. Kukolja, S. R. Lammert, M. R. B. Gleissner, and A. I. Ellis, *J. Am. Chem. Soc.*, **98,** 5040 (1976).
495. S. Kukolja, M. R. Gleissner, A. I. Ellis, D. E. Dorman, and J. W. Paschal, *J. Org. Chem.*, **41,** 2276 (1976).
496. D. O. Spry, *Tetrahedron Lett.*, 165 (1973).
497. M. Ochiai, O. Aki, S. Morimoto, and T. Okada, *Tetrahedron Lett.*, 3241 (1972).
498. M. Ochiai, E. Mizuta, O. Aki, A. Morimoto, and T. Okada, *Tetrahedron Lett.;* 3245 (1972).
499. R. Scartazzini and H. Bickel, *Helv. Chim. Acta,* **57,** 1919 (1974).
500. Y. Hamashima, T. Kubota, K. Ishikura, K. Minami, K. Tokura, and W. Nagato, *Heterocycles,* **5,** 419 (1976).
501. B. Muller, H. Peter, P. Schneider, and H. Bickel, *Helv. Chim.* Acta, **58,** 2469 (1975).
502. R. Scartazzini, P. Schneider, and H. Bickel, *Helv. Chim. Acta,* **58,** 2437 (1975).
503. D. H. R. Barton, F. Comer, D. G. T. Greig, P. G. Sammes, C. M. Cooper, G. Hewitt, and W. G. E. Underwood, *J. Chem. Soc. C,* 3540 (1971).
504. D. O. Spry, *J. Org. Chem.*, **37,** 793 (1972).
505. R. A. Archer and P. V. DeMarco, *J. Am. Chem. Soc.*, **91,** 1530 (1969).
506. M. Gorman and C. W. Ryan, in Ref. 114, Ch. 12, p. 540.
507. R. D. G. Cooper, P. V. DeMarco, C. F. Murphy, and L. A. Spangle, *J. Chem. Soc. C,* 340 (1970).
508. G. V. Kaiser, R. D. G. Cooper, R. E. Koehler, C. F. Murphy, J. A. Webber, I. G. Wright, and E. M. van Heyningen, *J. Org. Chem.*, **35,** 2430 (1970).
509. J. deKoning, A. F. Marx, M. M. Poot, P. M. Smid, and J. Verweij, presented at the symposium on "Recent Advances in the Chemistry of β-Lactam Antibiotics," sponsored by the Chemical Society (London) at Cambridge, England, June 1976.
510. R. G. Micetich, *Tetrahedron Lett.*, 971 (1976).
511. J. P. Clayton, J. H. C. Nayler, R. Southgate, and P. Tolliday, *J. Chem. Soc., Chem. Commun.*, 590 (1971).
512. S. Kukolja, *J. Am. Chem. Soc.*, **93,** 6267 (1971); **93,** 6269 (1971).
513. D. K. Herron, *Tetrahedron Lett.*, 2145 (1975).
514. S. Wolfe, J. C. Godfrey, C. T. Holdredge, and Y. G. Perron, *J. Am. Chem. Soc.*, **85,** 643 (1963).
515. S. Wolfe, *Can J. Chem.*, **46,** 459 (1968).
516. D. O. Spry, *J. Chem. Soc., Chem. Commun.*, 259 (1973).
517. H. Tanida, T. Tsuji, T. Tsushima, H. Ishitobi, T. Irie, T. Yano, H. Matsumura, and K. Tori, *Tetrahedron Lett.*, 3303 (1975).
518. P. J. Claes, J. Hoogruartens, G. Janssen, and H. Vanderhaeghe, *Eur. J. Med. Chem.*, **10,** 573 (1975); J. Hoogmartens, P. J. Claes and H. Vanderhaeghe, *J. Med. Chem.*, **17,** 389 (1974).
519. J. H. C. Nayler, presented at the symposium on "Recent Advances in the Chemistry of β-Lactam Antibiotics," sponsored by the Chemical Society (London) at Cambridge, England, June 1976.
520. R. Scartazzini, H. Peter, H. Bickel, K. Heusler, and R. B. Woodward, *Helv. Chim. Acta,* **55,** 408 (1972).
521. Y. Mine, T. Murakawa, T. Kamimura, T. Takaya, M. Nishida, and S. Kuwahara, Abstract No. 147, *17th Interscience Conference on Antimicrobial Agents and Chemotherapy,* New York, 1977; T. Murakawa, N. Okada, H. Sakamoto, Y. Mine, M. Nishida, S. Goto, and S. Kuwahara, *ibid.*, Abstract No. 148.
522. D. O. Spry, *Tetrahedron Lett.* 3717 (1972).
523. E. H. Bohme and J. E. Dolfini, *J. Chem. Soc., Chem. Commun.*, 941 (1972).
524. D. H. Brenner, M. M. Campbell, and G. Johnson, *Tetrahedron Lett.*, 2909 (1976).
525. R. D. G. Cooper, *MTP Int. Rev. Sci: Biochem., Ser.* 1, **6,** 247 (1973).
526. I. G. Wright, C. W. Ashbrook, T. Goodson, G. V. Kaiser, and E. M. van Heyningen, *J. Med. Chem.*, **14,** 420 (1971).
527. T. Kamiya, T. Teraji, M. Hashimoti, O. Nakaguchi, and T. Oku, *J. Am. Chem. Soc.*, **98,** 2342 (1976).
528. A. Yoshida, S. Oida, and E. Ohki, *Chem. Pharm. Bull. (Tokyo)*, **23,** 2507 (1975).
529. G. V. Kaiser, C. W. Ashbrook, T. Goodson, I. G. Wright, and E. M. van Heyningen, *J. Med. Chem.*, **14,** 426 (1971).
530. D. O. Spry, *Tetrahedron Lett.*, 2413 (1973).
531. J. Cs. Jaszberenyi and T. E. Gunda, in *Progress*

in Medicinal Chemistry, Vol. 12, G. P. Ellis and G. B. West, Eds., North-Holland, New York, 1975, p. 404.

532. D. O. Spry, *J. Chem. Soc., Chem. Commun.*, 671 (1973).

533. R. B. Woodward, K. Heusler, I. Ernest, K. Burri and R. J. Friary, F. Haviv, W. Oppolzer, R. Paioni, K. Syhora, R. Wenger, and J. K. Whitesell, *Nouv. J. Chim.*, **1,** 85 (1977).

534. D. H. Brenner and M. M. Campbell, *J. Chem. Soc., Chem. Commun.*, 538 (1976).

535. R. Busson and H. Vanderhaeghe, *J. Org. Chem.*, **41,** 2561 (1976).

536. F. Plavac, R. W. Ratcliffe, K. Hoogsteen, and B. G. Christensen, presented at the symposium on "Recent Advances in the Chemistry of β-Lactam Antibiotics," sponsored by the Chemical Society (London) at Cambridge, England, June 1976.

537. J. C. Sheehan, H. W. Hill, Jr., and E. L. Buhle, *J. Am. Chem. Soc.*, **73,** 4373 (1951); J. C. Sheehan and G. D. Laubach, *ibid.*, **73,** 4376 (1951).

538. H. Vanderhaeghe and J. Thomis, *J. Med. Chem.*, **18,** 486 (1975).

539. P. W. Wojtkowski, J. E. Dolfini, D. Kocy, and C. M. Cimarusti, *J. Am. Chem. Soc.*, **97,** 5628 (1975).

540. Y. Hamashima, M. Narisada, M. Yoshika, S. Uyeo, T. Tsuji, I. Kikkawa, and W. Nagata, Abstract No. 14, 176*th* National Meeting, American Chemical Society, Miami Beach, September 1978; T. Yoshida, M. Narisada, S. Matsuura, W. Nagata, and S. Kuwahara, Abstract No. 151, 18*th* Interscience Conference on Antimicrobial Agents, Atlanta, 1978; S. Matsuura, T. Yoshida, K. Sugeno, Y. Haradu, M. Harada, and S. Kuwahara, Abstract No. 152, *ibid.*

541. T. T. Conway, G. Lim, J. L. Douglas, M. Menard, T. W. Doyle, P. Rivest, D. Horning, L. R. Morris, and D. Cimon, *Can. J. Chem*, **56,** 1335 (1978), and preceding articles in this series.

542. A. G. Brown, D. Butterworth, M. Cole, G. Hanscomb, J. D. Hood, C. Reading, and G. N. Rolinson, *J. Antibiot.* (*Tokyo*), **29,** 668 (1976); K. Okamura, S. Hirata, Y. Okamura, Y. Fukagawa, Y. Shimauchi, K. Kouno, T. Ishikura, and J. Lein, *J. Antibiot.* (*Tokyo*), **31,** 480 (1978).

543. German Patents 2,652,674–2,652,677, 2,652,680 (June 2, 1977), (to Merck & Co., Inc.).

544. C. Reading and M. Cole, *Antimicrob. Agents Chemother.*, **11,** 852 (1977).

545. R. T. Jackson, L. F. Harris, and R. H. Alford, Abstract No. 63, *17th Interscience Conference on Antimicrobial Agents & Chemotherapy*, New York, 1977.

546. C. H. O'Callaghan, P. W. Muggleton, S. M. Kirby, and D. M. Ryan, *Antimicrob. Agents Chemother.*, 337 (1967); C. H. O'Callaghan and A. Morris, *ibid.*, **2,** 447 (1972).

547. A. R. English, J. A. Retsema, A. E. Girard, J. E. Lynch, and W. E. Barth, *Antimicrob. Agents Chemother.*, **14,** 414 (1978).

548. T. Hata, S. Omura, Y. Iwai, H. Ono, H. Takeshima, and H. Tamaguchi, *J. Antibiot.* (Tokyo), **25,** 473 (1972); H. Umezawa, S. Mitsuhashi, M. Hamada, S. Igobe, S. Takahashi, R. Utahara, Y. Osato, S. Yamazaki, H. Ogawura, and K. Maeda, *J. Antibiot.* (Tokyo), **26,** 51 (1973).

549. A. G. Brown, D. F. Corbett, and T. T. Haworth, *J. Chem. Soc., Chem. Commun.* 359 (1977).

550. German Patents. 2,616,087 (October 28, 1976), 2,517,316 (October 23, 1975), 2,629,926 (January 20, 1977), (to Beecham Group Ltd.)

551. Belgian Patent 846,678 (March 28, 1977), (to Beecham Group Ltd.)

552. German Patent 2,547,698 (April 29, 1976), (to Beecham Group Ltd.)

553. T. Kamiya, in Ref. 536.

554. M. Nishida, Y. Mine, S. Nonoyama, H. Kojo, S. Goto, and S. Kuwahara, *J. Antibiot.* (*Tokyo*), **30,** 917 (1977).

555. H. Kojo, Y. Mine, M. Nishida, and T. Yohota, *J. Antibiot.* (*Tokyo*), **30,** 926 (1977).

556. Y. Mine, S. Nonoyama, H. Kojo, S. Fukada, M. Nishida, S. Goto, and S. Kuwahara, *J. Antibiot.* (*Tokyo*), **30,** 932 (1977).

557. Y. Mine, S. Nonoyama, H. Kojo, S. Fukada, M. Nishida, S. Goto, and S. Kuwahara, *J. Antibiot.* (*Tokyo*), **30,** 939 (1977).

CHAPTER SIXTEEN

Nonlactam Antibiotics

U. HOLLSTEIN

Department of Chemistry
The University of New Mexico
Albuquerque, New Mexico 87131 USA

CONTENTS

1 INTRODUCTION

Nonlactam antibiotics are all antibiotics that do not contain the β-lactam ring found in penicillin, cephalosporin, and related compounds. Because of their special importance, the latter are discussed separately in

Chapter 15. Antibiotics are chemicals produced by microorganisms that inhibit the growth of other microorganisms. Synthetic compounds that possess such properties are not called antibiotics. Although true antibiotics have been used for more than 2000 years, their systematic study became possible only after Pasteur founded the science of bacteriology in the nineteenth century.

In 1877 Pasteur and Joubert observed that if "common bacteria" were introduced into a pure culture of anthrax bacilli, the latter died, and an otherwise deadly injection of anthrax bacilli into an animal was harmless if common bacteria were injected simultaneously. By 1890 impure pyocyanine, an antibacterial product from *Pseudomonas aeruginosa* was used in Germany in the treatment of diphtheria and other infectious diseases. However its clinical use was soon abandoned because of unsatisfactory results. The exciting story of the discovery in 1929 of penicillin, a β-lactam compound, by Alexander Fleming, its rediscovery in 1937 by H. W. Florey and E. B. Chain, and its first test in man in 1941 is referenced in Chapter 15, Section 5. One of the widest systematic searches for antimicrobial substances was undertaken by S. A. Waksman among the group of soil-inhabiting microbes known as actinomycetes or streptomycetes. In 1940 he reported the isolation of actinomycin, in 1942 streptothricin, and in 1943 streptomycin. Streptomycin turned out to be most useful in treating infectious diseases, especially tuberculosis. This discovery greatly stimulated a search among the actinomycetes for useful antibiotics, and this group of organisms is the source of most of the presently used antibiotics. Work on antibiotics now entered a new phase; the pharmaceutical industry used its large resources to screen many thousands of microorganisms for antibiotic production. Many hundreds of antibiotics were discovered, and more than 50 new antibiotics are reported every year.

Unfortunately because of the toxicity of most antibiotics, only a few of those mentioned in the literature can be used in medicine. Table 16.1 lists those presently manufactured on a commercial scale. Most are the products of microbial synthesis. Exceptions are semisynthetic compounds that are made by chemical manipulation of microbially produced antibiotics to derive compounds with additional useful properties (dihydrostreptomycin, dihydrodeoxystreptomycin, modified oxytetracyclines, and rifampicin).

Antibiotics possess a selective antibiotic spectrum: some affect primarily gram-positive bacteria, others act on gram-negative forms, and still others affect only certain fungi and yeasts. "Broad spectrum" antibiotics are those that inhibit gram-positive and gram-negative bacteria, and intracellular organisms as those of psittacosis, lymphogranuloma, or the rickettsiae.

Some microbial cultures yield more than one antibiotic, and some antibiotics are produced in families of closely related substances. In soils the proportion of antibiotic-producing organisms is quite high. When grown in laboratory media, nearly 50% of the streptomycetes and 40% of the fungi may be expected to produce some antibiotic activity. There is no convincing evidence of production of antibiotics by microorganisms growing in various types of soil. Addition of antibiotics to fresh soil samples almost invariably has resulted in the rapid disappearance of the antibiotic activity through microbial and chemical degradation.

Since antibiotic-producing microorganisms do not furnish antibiotics in their natural habitat, three widely used methods have been developed to detect their antibiotic activity. In the first, the soil is suspended in sterile water and portions of it are spread on the surface of nutrient agar plates. A large number of colonies are usually found a few days after incubation. Some of these microorganisms produce antibiotics and inhibit the growth of other organisms. This results in a cleared area around the antibiotic-producing organisms,

Table 16.1 Properties of Some Polypeptide Antibiotics

			Antibiotic Spectrum[a]					Chemical Status						
Name	Related to (or synonym)	Microbial Source	G+	G−	My	F	T	Purity[b]	Molecular Weight	Number of Amino Acid Residues	Structure Proposed	Chemical Synthesis	Number in Family	Reference
Actinomycins		*Streptomyces antibioticus, S. chrysomallus, S. galbus, S. kitasawaensis, S. latanus, S. michiganensis, S. murinus, S. parvullus, S. parvus*	×					1	1200	10	×	×	15	6
Aerosporin	Polymyxin A	*Bacillus polymyxa*		×				1	1225	10	×	×	7	7
Albomycin	Grisein, sideromycins	*S. subtropicalis*	×					1	1140	6	×		5	8
Amphomycin	Aspartocin, glumamycin	*S. canus*	×					1						9
Aspartocin	Amphomycin, glumamycin	*S. griseus* var. *spiralis, S. violaceus*	×					1						10
Bacillomycins	Fungistatin XG	*B. subtilis*				×		1					2	11
Bacitracins	Ayfivin	*B. licheniformis*	×					1	1410	11	×		5	12
Bottromycins		*S. bottropensis*	×	×				1	810	6	×		4	13
Capreomycins		*S. capreolus*	×	×	×			1	700	5			2	14
Circulins	Polymyxins	*B. circulans*		×				1	1240	10	×	×	2	15
Colistins	Polymyxin E	*B. colistinus*		×				1	1360	10	×	×	5	16
Destruxin B		*Oospora destructor*		(Insecticide)				1	584	5	×		1	17
Echinomycin	Levomycin, triostin, quinomycin	*S. echinatus*	×	×	×			1	1600	4	×		5	18
Edeine		*B. brevis*	×	×				1		5	×			19
Enniatins		*Fusarium orthoceras* var. *enniatinum, F. scirpi, F. lateritium*	×		×			1	640	6	×	×	5	20
Etamycin	Viridogrisein	*S. lavendulae*	×					1	800	8	×		1	21
Ferrimycins	Sideromycins	*S. griseoflavus, S. lavendulae, S. galilaeus*	×					1	600	6	×		4	22
Fungistatin	Antibiotic XG, bacillomycin	*B. subtilis*	×			×		3						23
Glumamycins	Amphomycin, aspartocin	*S. zaomyceticus*	×					1	1300	11	×			24
Gramicidin A		*B. brevis*	×					1	2000	15	×	×	6	25
Gramicidin J	Gramicidins	*B. brevis Nagano*	×					1	1140	10	×	×	1	26
Gramicidin S	Tyrocidine	*B. b. Gause-Brazhnikova*	×					1	1140	10	×	×	1	27
Ilamycins	Rufomycin	*S. islandicus*			×			1	960	6	×		2	28
Licheniformins		*B. licheniformis*			×			2	3800–4800				3	29
Malformin		*Aspergillus niger*	×	×	×	×		1	630	10	×	×	2	30
Micrococcin P	Micrococcin	*B. pumilis*	×					1						31
Mikamycin B's	Ostreogrycin B's, vernamycin B's	*S. mitakaensis*	×					1	900	7	×		4	32

Mycobacillin		*B. subtilis*				×		1	1525	13	×		1	33
Neocarzinostatin		*S. carzinostaticus*	×				×	2	9000					34
Nisins		*Streptococcus cremoris, S. lactis*	×					2	7000					35
Ostreogrycin B's	Mikamycin B's, staphylomycin S's, vernamycin B's	*Streptomyces ostreogriseus*	×					1	900	7	×		4	36
PA-114 B's	Mikamycin B's, PA-144 B's, E-129 B, ostreogrycin B's, Staphylomycin S's, vernamycin B's	*S. olivaceus*	×					2	700			4		37
Peptidolipine NA		*Nocardia asteroides*						1	919	7	×			38
Polymyxins	Aerosporins, Circulins, colistins	*B. polymyxa*		×				1	1150	10	×	×	8	39
Polypeptin	Polymyxin	*B. krzemieniewski*	×	×				1	1150	9			1	40
Pristinamycin 1's	Staphylomycin B's	*S. pristinae-spiralis*	×					1	900	7			4	41
Quinomycin	Echinomycin, triostin	*Streptomyces* species	×	×	×	×		1	850	8	×		5	42
Saramycetin		*S. saraceticus*				×		2	2000				1	43
Siomycin	Thiostrepton, Bryamycin	*S. sioyaensis*	×					1	1660				2	44
Staphylomycin S's	Vernamycin B's, mikamycin B's ostreogrycin B's PA-114 B's	*S. virginae*	×					1	900	7	×		4	45
						×		2	1850				2	46
Stendomycins		*Streptomyces* species	×					1					4	47
Streptogramins	Mikamycin B's, ostreogrycins, vernamycins	*S. graminofaciens*												48
Subtilins		*B. subtilis*	×					2	3600	26			2	48
Succinimycin	Sideromycins	*S. olivochromogenes*	×											49
Suzukacillin		*Trichoderma viride*	×					1	1600				1	50
Telomycin		*Streptomyces* species	×					1	1000	11	×		2	51
Thiostrepton	Bryamycin, siomycin	*S. azureus, S. hawaiiensis*	×					1	1650				2	52
Triostin	Echinomycin, quinomycin	*Staphylococcus aureus*	×	×	×		×	1	1630				5	53
Tyrocidines	Gramicidin S	*B. brevis*	×					1	1200	10	×	×	3	54
Tyrothricin	Gramicidin+, tyrocidine	*B. brevis*	×	×				(Mixture)						55
Valinomycin	Amidomycin	*S. fulvissimus*				×		1	1100	6	×	×	1	56
Vernamycin B's	Mikamycin B's, ostreogrycin B's, pristinamycin 1's, Staphylomycin S's	*S. loidensis*	×					1	900	7	×		4	57

[a] Antibiotic spectrum: G+ = activity mainly against gram-positive bacteria; G− = activity mainly against gram-negative bacteria; My = activity mainly against mycobacteria; F = activity mainly against fungi and yeasts; T = activity as an antitumor agent in laboratory studies.

[b] Purity: 1 = crystalline or greater than 95%; 2 = 50–95%; 3 = 25–50%.

and these colonies can be selected for further study. A second method involves the same general procedure, but confluent growth is prevented by using higher dilutions of the soils, resulting in fewer colonies per plate. After the colonies are formed, the plates are spread with a suspension of test bacteria (*Staphylococcus aureus* as gram-positive test bacteria, *Escherichia coli* as gram-negative test bacteria) or yeast (*Saccharomyces cerevisiae*). Areas of inhibition are noted, and colonies are selected for further examination. In the third method pure cultures of the microorganisms are streaked on agar plates. After a suitable interval of 4–10 days, the agar is crossed-streaked with a variety of test organisms. The extent of inhibition of growth of these organisms is studied, and if significant inhibition is noted, the antibiotic producer is selected for further study.

Since 4076 antibiotics were known at the end of 1972 (5a), there is a fair chance that a "new" antibiotic found as a metabolic product of a newly isolated microorganism may be related to a previously reported antibiotic. These relationships can be shown by a number of methods, including various types of chromatography, liquid-liquid countercurrent distribution, ionophoresis, and biological methods.

In the early years of the antibiotic era, many scientists hastily described their discoveries as "new". This led to much synonymy and consequent confusion. For instance, neomycin, a product from *Streptomyces fradiae* and other *Streptomyces* species is known as colimycin, dextromycin, flavomycin, fradiomycin, framycetin, mycifradin, and streptothricins B I and B II. Novobiocin has been called at one time or other albomycin, biotexin, cardelmycin, cathomycin, griseoflavin, inamycin, PA-93, streptonivicin, and vulcamycin.

Antibiotics have been named on a very subjective basis. The germs of the producing microorganism has been used: actinomycin from *Actinomyces antibioticus*, streptomycin from *Streptomyces griseus*, polymyxin from *Bacillus polymyxa*. Others have been named after the location of the soil sample: filipin after a streptomycete from a Philippine soil sample, foromacidin after a microorganism from the soil of the Roman Forum. A few enthusiasts have named their antibiotics after their laboratories: nystatin for New York State Board of Health Laboratories. Some antibiotics have been named after wives (perlinmycin), after secretaries (nancimycin), after a mother-in-law (seramycetin), after a patient Tracy (bacitracin). Among less serious examples are Etamycin (after culture number "8"), ayfivin (after culture "A-5"), rifamycin (after the movie *Rififi*) miamycin (after Miami Beach), and peliomycin and demetric acid (after a place and a god in Greek mythology). To avoid the confusion in naming antibiotics, the American Society for Microbiology appointed a committee to formulate a set of rules governing the naming of antibiotics. The rules include the following:

1. Cognizance should be given to the fact that antibiotics are often chemically related members of a family, and a name should be chosen which yields a root that can be modified so that the variants can be noted.
2. The name should be euphonious.
3. The chosen name should be based on the chemical structure, if a structure has been proposed.
4. If the structure is not known, the germs can be used as a root and the suffix "mycin" restricted to streptomycete products. Failing the use of the germs, the mode of action of the spectrum might be useful; geographic locations are not thought to be meaningful.

Antibiotics, their biosynthesis and their mechanism of action have been reviewed in recent years (1–5).

Recently Zähner (5b) concluded that the era of spectacular developments in the field of antibiotics appears to be over. Ever greater efforts are needed to find ever fewer new antibiotics. The view that well-considered hypotheses can lead as successfully as proven results to further research is supported by the establishment of the five theses. "Non-classical" screening methods and the search for secondary metabolites with unusual properties can provide a rich harvest. Zähner's theses are: (I) Only a small part of the conceivable fields for the introduction of antibiotics has so far been covered; (II) Only a small fraction of the natural antibiotics has so far been found; (III) The problems of antibiotic transport have been neglected far too long; (IV) Antibiotics are secondary metabolites whose importance to the producer cell should be sought at the levels of primary metabolism, regulation, transport, and differentiation or morphogenesis rather than in defense against competitors; and (V) Biological engineering processes also have their dangers.

2 PEPTIDE ANTIBIOTICS

During the past 40 years, since the discovery of tyrothricin, more than 200 peptide antibiotics have been described. The amino acid compositions of some 75 have been determined, and structures have been proposed for about 40 of the peptide antibiotics. However synthesis (and ultimate proof of structure) has been accomplished for only 10.

Among the reasons the study of the peptide antibiotics has gone so slowly are the following:

1. The compounds are highly toxic with low therapeutic indexes, discouraging further work.
2. They have relatively complicated structures, differing noticeably from the peptides isolated from animal and plant materials.
3. They are usually produced in small amounts in most fermentations, and usually a group of closely related substances are formed.

With the development of new separation and isolation techniques and advances in structure analysis and synthesis, a better approach to these interesting compounds has become available.

As a group, the peptide antibiotics have unique characteristics:

1. Most peptide antibiotic-furnishing microorganisms produce groups of chemically related substances rather than a single compound.
2. Many of the peptide antibiotics possess lipid moieties in addition to unnatural amino acids not found in peptides of animal and plant origin.
3. The same microbial peptides are produced by taxonomically different microorganisms.
4. The requirements for antimicrobial activity are extremely specific, and minor chemical modification often changes all biological properties.
5. Peptide antibiotics of rather varying structures may have the same mechanism of action in inhibiting the growth of microorganisms.

These generalizations are summarized in Tables 16.1 and 16.2. Most of the cultures producing such antibiotics as the actinomycins, the polymyxins, the vernamycins, the bottromycins, and the gramicidins synthesize a group of closely related compounds that vary only in one amino acid residue or even one methyl group. With very few exceptions, such as gramicidins A and D, the peptides are cyclic, and most are resistant to hydrolysis by animal and plant proteases. These features and their biosynthesis distinguish the peptide antibiotics from peptides found in plants and animals.

The antibiotic peptides contain a wide variety of unusual amino acids, some of

Table 16.2 Fatty Acids and Unusual Amino Acids Found in Peptide Antibiotics

Acid	Antibiotic
Fatty acids	
Aspartocin	13-Methyl-3-tetradecenoic; (+)-12-methyl-3-tetradecenoic acids
Destruxin B	D-α-Hydroxymethylvaleric acid
Enniatins	D-α-Hydroxyisovaleric acid
Glumamycin	3-Isotridecenoic acid
Polymyxins	6-Methyloctanoic; 6-methylheptanoic acids
Sporidesmolides	1-α-Hydroxyisovaleric acid
Amino acids	
Actinomycins	*N*-Methyl-L-valine; sarcosine; *N*-methyl-L-alanine; *N*-methyl-L-isoleucine
Aspartocin	D-α-Pipecolic; L-β-methylaspartic acids
Bottromycins	L-β-Dimethyl-α-aminobutyric; α-amino-β-phenylbutyric acids; β-methylphenylalanine; L-*cis*-3-methylproline
Capreomycins	β-Lysine
Cinnamycins	Lanthionine; β-methyllanthionine
Enniatins	*N*-Methyl-L-valine; *N*-methyl-L-isoleucine
Etamycin	L-α-*N*-Dimethylleucine; 3-hydroxypicolinic acid; phenylsarcosine
Ilamycins	*N*-Methyl-γ-formyl-L-norvaline; δ-dehydronorleucine; *N*-methyl-L-leucine; L-3-nitrotyrosine
Quinomycins	Quinoxalinecarboxylic acid: *N*-methyl-L-valine; *N*-methyl-L-isoleucine; *N*-dimethylcystine; L-*N*-methyl-β-dimethylisoleucine
Telomycin	L-β-Hydroxyleucine; L-*trans*-3-hydroxyproline; L-*cis*-3-hydroxyproline; L-tryptophan; β-methyltryptophan
Vernamycins	L-Phenylglycine; 3-hydroxypicolinic acid; 4-keto-L-pipecolic acid; *N*-methyl-L-phenylalanine; *N*-methyl-L-*p*-methylaminophenylalanine; *N*-methyl-L-*p*-dimethylaminophenylalanine

which are listed in Table 16.2. Certain of these have not been found elsewhere in natural products. The antibiotic peptides are also characterized by the presence of non-amino acid moieties: some of these are listed in Table 16.2. They also contain imino and *N*-methyl amino acids (Table 16.2). Possibly the formation of cyclic peptides is enhanced by the absence of amino hydrogen atoms, which could participate by way of hydrogen bonds in helix formation, or, owing to the occurrence of a ring, *N*-methyl groups may occur at sites that would be unavailable in helices. A connection between the frequent occurrence of imino acids and of rings must be suspected.

Many of the peptide antibiotics showed marked nephrotoxicity, and the generalization that "all peptide antibiotics are likely to be too toxic for systematic use" in clinical medicine was widely accepted. Thus many laboratories dropped peptide antibiotics from further study as soon as their peptide nature became apparent. Nevertheless, the following have been used in clinical medicine: bacitracins, cactinomycin (actinomycin C), capreomycin, cycloserine, dactinomycin (actinomycin D), gramicidins, mikamycins, polymyxins, pristinamycins, staphylomycins, tyrothricin, and viomycin.

Although there has been reluctance to study such compounds, the frequency of reports of new peptide antibiotics has grown in recent years. It is realized that antibiotics effective against *all* microorganisms are not likely to be found, and a reasonable effort should be concentrated on the more specialized antibiotics, including peptide types. There has been an improvement in separation techniques such as preparative thin layer chromatography, preparative ionophoresis, and new chromatographic supports, without which it would be impossible to collect sufficient amounts of pure materials for *in vivo* evaluations and determination of chemical structures.

Peptide antibiotics can be classified according to several principles. They can be divided into homeomeric (built up of only amino acids) and heteromeric peptides (containing amino acids *plus* other moieties). A further division leads to homodetic (amino acids in peptide linkages in the ring) and heterodetic peptides (rings containing other linkages). These classifications are illustrated in Fig. 16.1. Peptide antibiotics that contain hydroxy and amino acid residues joined by amide and ester bonds are called depsipeptides; these include actinomycin, angolide, emiatins, espirin, sporides, molides, and valinomycin.

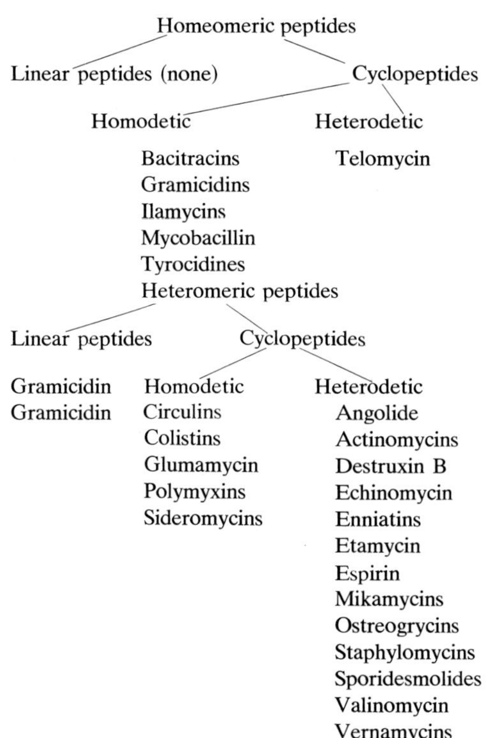

Fig. 16.1 Classification of peptide antibiotics.

2.1 The Actinomycin Group

The actinomycins are orange to red metabolites from various species of *Streptomyces*. Although these compounds are highly toxic, they have found usage in nontoxic dosages because of their antineoplastic effect. Actinomycins D (C_1) and C_3 are highly effective chemotherapeutic agents in the treatment of Wilms's tumor, trophoplastic tumors, and rhabdonyosarcoma (59). Current therapeutic efforts are largely directed at utilization of the drug in combination with other active agents against these tumor types.

The group name "actinomycin" was coined by Waksman, who discovered these antibiotics in cultures of *Actinomyces antibioticus* in 1940 (59). Early structure work by Todd and Johnson (60, 61) was soon followed by a major investigation by Brockmann starting in 1949 (62) and continuing to the present. In 1960 the constitution of the actinomycins had been well established, and a first total synthesis of an actinomycin had been achieved (63). The chemistry and mechanism of action of actinomycin has been reviewed recently (64).

Actinomycins are chromopeptides; that is, the molecule contains a chromophore moiety actinocin (3-amino-1,8-dimethyl-2-phenoxazone-4,5-dicarboxylic acid), carrying as amides two pentapeptides at its two carboxyl groups. The amino acids linked by amide bonds to the 4- and 5-carboxyls are always L-threonine, whose hydroxyl is always lactonized with the carboxyl of the fifth amino acid. The second amino acid can be D-valine or D-*allo*-isoleucine; the

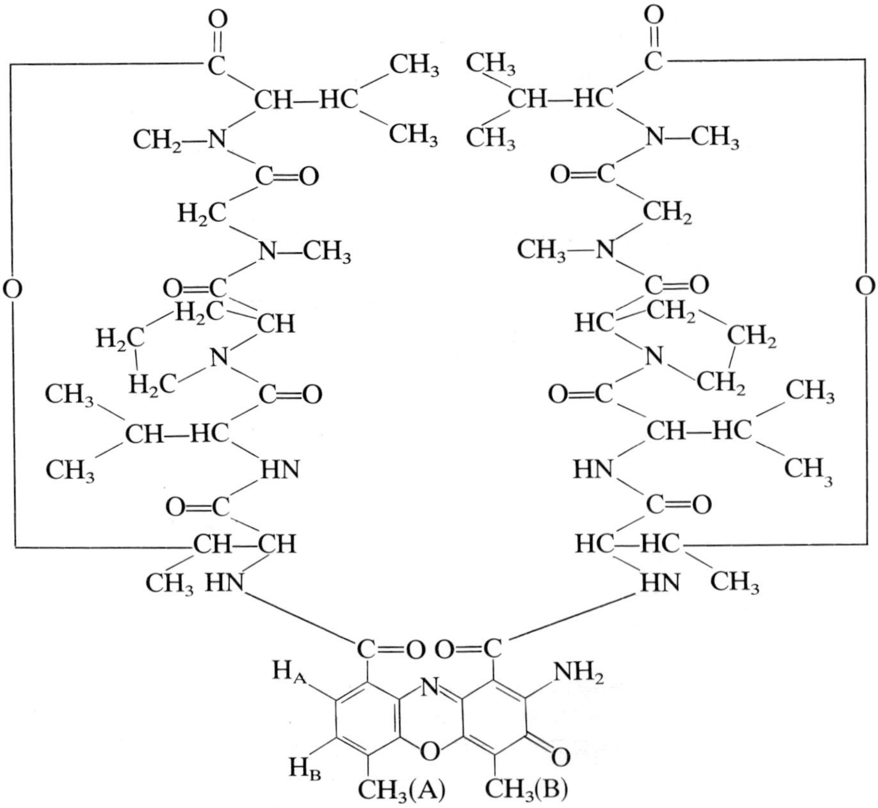

Fig. 16.2 Structure of actinomycin D: MeVal = *N*-MeVal = *N*-methylvaline, Sar = sarcosine: Pro = proline: Val = valine: Thr = threonine.

third can be L-proline, L-γ-hydroxyproline, L-γ-ketoproline, pipecolic acid, or sarcosine; the fourth is always sarcosine; and the fifth can be L-*N*-methylvaline or L-*N*-methylisoleucine. As an example, the structure of the presently most studied actinomycin D ("Dactinomycin", "Actinomycin C_1") is shown in Fig. 16.2. Table 16.3 lists the amino acid sequences in the α-chain, which is attached to the benzenoid portion, and the β-chain, which is attached to the quinoid portion of the phenoxazine. Controlled biosynthesis, a technique of predetermining the structure of a new antibiotic by furnishing specific chemical precursors to the antibiotic-producing microorganisms, has been applied successfully to the formation of modified forms of actinomycin. If an amino acid already present in actinomycin, or similar in structure, is supplied exogenously to the culture medium, it competes with the endogenously synthesized amino acid and is incorporated into the peptide chain, either with increased formation of a trace actinomycin component or with formation of a new actinomycin. Examples are two "new" actinomycins E_1 and E_2, which were formed in the presence of DL-Ile. In these compounds one or two molecules of MeIle replace one or two molecules MeVal. Other modifying amino acids are Sar, pipecolic acid, azetidine-2-carboxylic acid, and methyl- and halogenated prolines. For instance, *Streptomyces antibioticus* produces a mixture of actinomycins in the presence of

Table 16.3 Amino Acid Sequences in Different Antinomycins

Actinomycin	Chain	Amino Acid 1	2	3	4	5	Reference
C_1(IV, D, I_1, X_1)	α	Thr	Val	Pro	Sar	MeVal	
	β	Thr	Val	Pro	Sar	MeVal	
C_2(VI, I_2)	α	Thr	Val	Pro	Sar	MeVal	65
	β	Thr	*a*-ile	Pro	Sar	MeVal	
C_{2a}(i-C_2)	α	Thr	*a*-ile	Pro	Sar	MeVal	65
	β	Thr	Val	Pro	Sar	MeVal	
C_2(VII, I_3)	α	Thr	*a*-ile	Pro	Sar	MeVal	
	β	Thr	*a*-ile	Pro	Sar	MeVal	
II(F_8)	α	Thr	Val	Sar	Sar	MeVal	
	β	Thr	Val	Sar	Sar	MeVal	
E_1	α	Thr	*a*-ile	Pro	Sar	[MeVal	
	β	Thr	*a*-ile	Pro	Sar	Me-ile]	
E_2	α	Thr	*a*-ile	Pro	Sar	Me-ile	
	β	Thr	*a*-ile	Pro	Sar	Me-ile	
F_1	α	Thr	[Val	Sar	Sar	MeVal	
	β	Thr	*a*-ile]	Sar	Sar	MeVal	
F_2	α	Thr	[Val	[Pro	Sar	MeVal	
	β	Thr	*a*-ile]	Sar]	Sar	MeVal	
F_3	α	Thr	*a*-ile	Sar	Sar	MeVal	
	β	Thr	*a*-ile	Sar	Sar	MeVal	
F_4	α	Thr	*a*-ile	[Pro	Sar	MeVal	
	β	Thr	*a*-ile	Sar]	Sar	MeVal	
Pip/α	α	Thr	Val	[Pip	Sar	MeVal	
	β	Thr	Val	Oxopip]	Sar	MeVal	
Pip/β	α	Thr	Val	[Pro	Sar	MeVal	
	β	Thr	Val	Pip]	Sar	MeVal	
Pip 2	α	Thr	Val	[Pip	Sar	MeVal	
	β	Thr	Val	Pip]	Sar	MeVal	
$X_{o\alpha}$	α	Thr	Val	[Sar	Sar	MeVal	66
	β	Thr	Val	Hypro]	Sar	MeVal	
$X_{0\beta}$(I)	α	Thr	Val	[Pro	Sar	MeVal	66
	β	Thr	Val	Hypro]	Sar	MeVal	
$X_{0\gamma}$(III, F_9)	α	Thr	Val	[Sar	Sar	MeVal	66
	β	Thr	Val	Pro]	Sar	MeVal	
$X_{0\delta}$	α	Thr	Val	[Pro	Sar	MeVal	66
	β	Thr	Val	Hypro]	Sar	MeVal	
X_{1a}	α	Thr	Val	[Sar	Sar	MeVal	66
	β	Thr	Val	Oxopro]	Sar	MeVal	
X_2(V)	α	Thr	Val	[Pro	Sar	MeVal	
	β	Thr	Val	Oxopro]	Sar	MeVal	67, 68
Z_1	In unknown order: Thr, Val, MeAla, Sar, MeVal, 5-Me(?)4-Oxopro and an unidentified hydroxyamino acid						

pipecolic acid in which proline is replaced by the analog. The three new antibiotics are designated Pip 1α, Pip 1β, and Pip 2. Pip 1β and Pip 2 have molar ratios of pipecolic acid to proline of 1:1 and 2:0, respectively. Pip 1α contains one pipecolic acid and one 4-oxopipecolic acid (69–71).

Actinomycin binds strongly to DNA. This topic has been reviewed frequently in recent years (72–79) from a molecular point of view. Therefore the subject is dealt with only briefly here. Although cytostatic properties of actinomycin have been known since its discovery (80), the reasons for this, viz., the complexing of actinomycin with DNA (81) and the consequential inhibition of RNA synthesis (74, 75), did not become known until the early 1960s. The complex formation has been studied using spectrophotometric methods, buoyant density measurements, equilibrium dialysis, circular dichroism (CD) (91, 91a) and optical rotary dispersion (ORD) (82–84) melting temperature, and inhibition of DNA template controlled RNA synthesis. DNA-controlled DNA synthesis is also inhibited by much larger actinomycin concentrations, but the mechanism seems to be a different one. Whereas the former is a direct consequence of steric interference by the antibiotic, the latter seems to be a stabilization by DNA (85). Actinomycin also interferes with reactions in which DNA is modified, such as methylation (86).

Actinomycin complexes with DNA but not with RNA. The association constant is about $5 \times 10^6\, M^{-1}$. The DNA must be doubled stranded helical and must contain guanine residues (72). The maximum ratio of bound actinomycin per nucleotide pair runs from 0 at 0% dG content to about 0.16 at 50% dG in poly (dGC–dGC) with relative constant stoichiometry of binding in the middle range (~25% dG) of base composition, suggesting the involvement of more than one base pair, one of which is G-C, at the intercalation site (72). In DNA with adjacent dG's, less than half the sites are available for binding (86–88).

The conception of the actinomycin-DNA complex was further refined with the discovery that a 2-amino group on a purine was required for binding (84); 2,6-diaminopurine can replace the dG as binding factor. Two exceptions to the dG specificity are known. In one case the presence of dG is not required for binding. Single stranded poly-dI binds actinomycin, possibly because of a peculiar conformation of the polymer (89). In the other case the presence of dG is not sufficient for binding. Poly-d(A-T-C):poly-d(G-A-T) does not interact with actinomycin by spectrophotometric measurement, equilibrium dialysis, buoyant density, melting temperature, inhibition of RNA synthesis (89, 90), and circular dichroism (91). Again, this may be caused by a difference in conformation, or it may be because actinomycin requires a specific base sequence not present in this polytrimer. Actinomycin is bound more tightly to a polydeoxyribonucleotide that contains both purines and pyrimidines on both strands than to the isomer with all purines on one strand and all pyrimidines on one complementary strand (89).

Actinomycin interferes with the RNA chain elongation but not with the initiation or termination step. Kinetic studies have shown that specifically the CTP and GTP incorporation is slowed down (92). This result has a bearing on the alternative between an inside or outside model for binding (*vide infra*), since the data require the actinomycin not to be bound symmetrically with respect to a G-C pair and an adjacent pair.

During the last decade four models have been proposed for the complex between actinomycin and DNA (79, 93–96). In the first two, actinomycin is bound to the outside of the double-stranded DNA helix; the last two represent inside bound complexes whereby the chromophore intercalates between two successive base pairs. There are arguments pro and con on each type, but the most recent model (79, 96) has received a high level of confidence throughout the scientific community. It is based on the X-ray structure of a crystalline actinomycin-dG_2 complex (Fig. 16.3) and combines the guanine-2-amino group selectivity of the first two models with the intercalative feature of the third. The phenoxazinone chromophore intercalates between adjacent G-C pairs, where the guanine residues are on opposite strands. On each strand, intercalation takes place between a GpC (3′→5′) sequence. The 2-amino groups of guanine bind to $C{=}O_{Thr}$ of the peptide

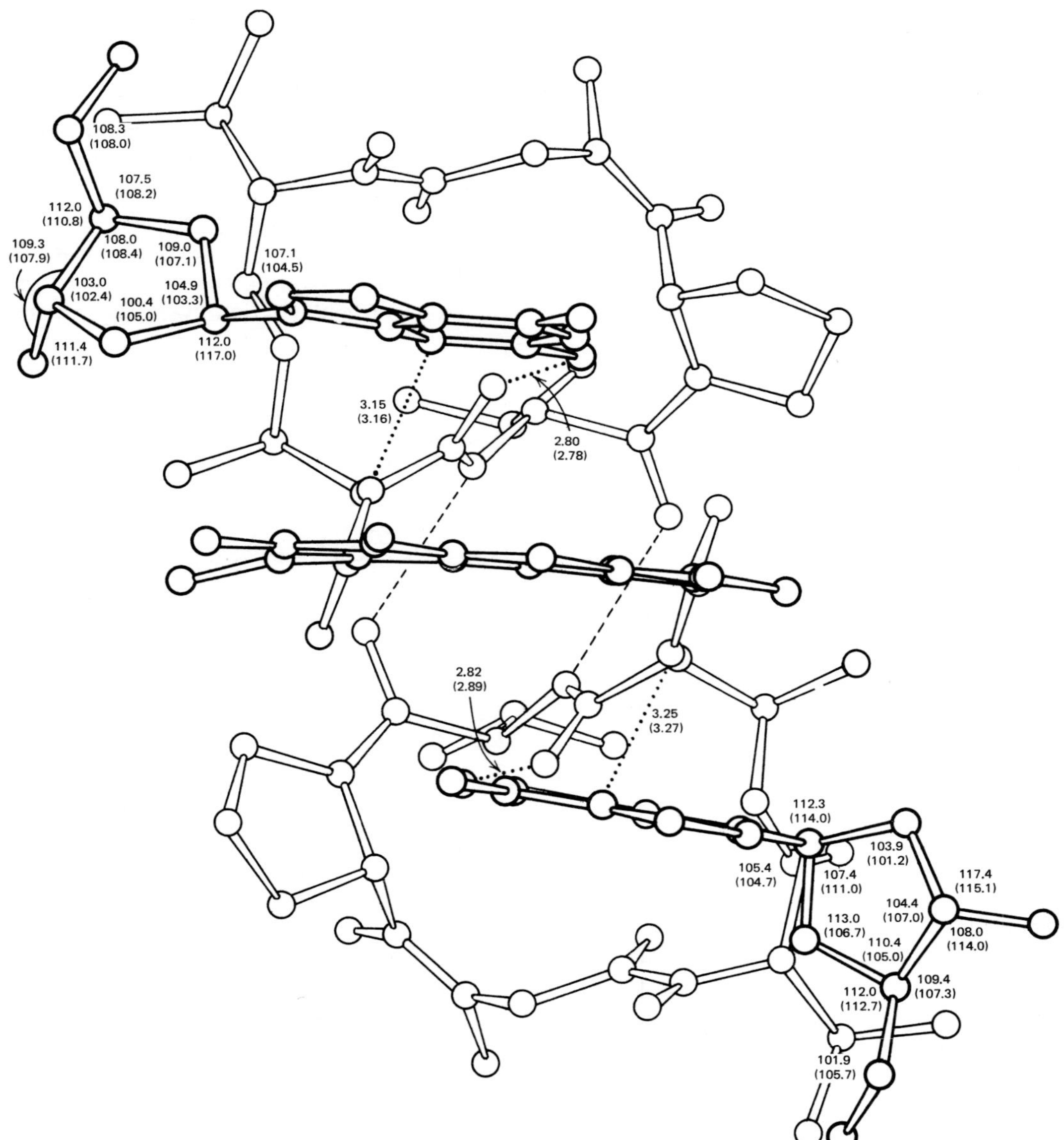

Fig. 16.3 Oakridge Thermal Ellipsoid Plot illustration of the actinomycin-2dG complex, viewed down its quasi-dyed axis. Dotted lines indicate hydrogen bonds connecting the pentapeptide chains with each other and with the deoxyguanosine molecules. Bond distances and angles obtained from the heavy atom analysis are shown in parentheses; those shown without parentheses have been obtained from the light-atom analysis (from Jain and Sobell (96) with permission).

rings that lie in the minor groove, trans with respect to the plane of the chromophore. The NH_{Val} is bound to the $C{=}O_{Val}$ of the other ring, and vice versa. Sobell's model has quasi-C_2-symmetry in the immediate vicinity of the actinomycin chromophore, as in the actinomycin-dG_2 complex. The model is supported by several studies using spectrophotometry of complexes of actinomycin with several deoxydinucleotides (e.g., pGpC) (97), by ^1H, ^{13}C, and ^{31}P NMR of the complexes of actinomycin with several deoxynucleotide 5′-monophosphates (98, 99) and with several deoxydinucleotides (100, 101), and by ^1H and ^{31}P NMR of the complex of actinomycin with the hexadeoxynucleotides D-ApTpGpCpApT and *d*-pGpCpGpCpGpC (102). The results seem to support an actinomycin-DNA model that was derived from the X-ray diffraction picture of the actinomycin-*d*G_2 complex. Although the supporting studies also allow for intercalation between other sequences GpN, the sequences CpN, specifically CpG, are not considered because of the restrictions imposed by the X-ray structure. A recent CD study, however, showed that CpG and GpC are both strong binding sequences (91, 91a). Data indicating that actinomycin binds most strongly to poly (*d*GC–*d*GC) (89) are often cited as evidence for the GpC intercalation model, but they are also consistent with the GpC and CpG intercalation.

Actinomycin is one of the most potent antitumor agents known. Unfortunately, it has found only limited use clinically because of its extreme toxicity. Numerous investigators have synthesized actinomycin analogs in the hope of enhancing the chemotherapeutic index. As the picture of the mechanism of action of actinomycin emerges, it becomes increasingly clear that the potency of actinomycin is due to its high specificity, which requires a precise and unique steric fit between the two molecules DNA and actinomycin. Any change in either molecule that will interfere with this sensitive geometry of the binding complex renders the system less active or inactive. It is remarkable that natural actinomycins seem already to provide an optimum combination between the antibiotic and the polydeoxyribonucleotide so that any attempt to enhance their activity has failed. Improvement of the chemotherapeutic index, however, is a different problem, which is related to a difference in cell membrane permeability of the healthy cell and the unwanted cell. Many possibilities remain open in this area. Fascinating suggestions have been made by Sobell (79), who ascertained on the basis of his model which groups could be altered without affecting the steric fit of the actinomycin-DNA complex.

Although the naturally occurring actinomycins differ only slightly in their activity, any changes in different portions of a synthetic actinomycin may affect its inhibitory activity to a greater or lesser extent (72, 95, 103). The presence of the unaltered $C_2{-}NH_2$ and $C_3{=}O$ groups and the intact pentapeptide lactones is essential. The activities of various actinomycins and actinomycin analogs are listed in Table 16.4.

2.2 Bacitracin

Bacitracin is an antibiotic produced by the Tracy I strain of *Bacillus subtilis*, isolated in 1943 from the damaged tissue and street dirt debrided from a compound fracture in a young girl named Tracy; hence the name bacitracin. The history, properties, and uses of bacitracin have been reviewed (119). The bacitracins are a group of polypeptide antibiotics; multiple components have been demonstrated in the commercial products. The major constituent is bacitracin A. Its probable structure is depicted in Fig. 16.4 (120). A unit of the antibiotic is equivalent to 26 μg of the USP Pharmacopoeia (USP) standard.

Table 16.4 Biological Activities of Natural Actinomycins and Synthetic Analogs

Compound	Activity, μg/ml[a]	Method of Expression	Reference
Actinomycin C_1	0.25	Concentration required to inhibit growth of *B. subtilis*	104
Actinomycin C_2	0.25		
Actinomycin C_3	0.25		
Actinomycin F_1	1.0		
Actinomycin $X_{0\beta}$	1.5		
Actinomycin $X_{0\delta}$	0.35		
N-Methylactinomycin C_2	1.0		
N-(β-Dimethylamino)actinomycin C_3	2.5		
Deaminoactinomycin C_3	10		
Chloroactinomycin C_3	10		
N-(*p*-Aminophenyl)actinomycin C_3	10		
N-Aminoactinomycin C_3	10		
Actinomycin C_1	70	100×MIC (*B. subtilis*) of actinomycin C_3: MIC of compound in first column	105
Actinomycin $X_{0\alpha}$	1.5		
Actinomycin $X_{0\beta}$	2.5		
Actinomycin $X_{0\gamma}$	30		
Actinomycin $X_{0\delta}$	40		
Actinomycin X_{1a}	70		
Actinomycin X_2	150		
Actinomycin C_1	$1:20\times10^6$	MIC (*B. subtilis*)	106
Actinomycin X_2	$1:30\times10^6$		
Actinomycin $X_{0\delta}$	$1:10\times10^6$		
Actinomycin $X_{0\beta}$	$1:0.5\times10^6$		
Actinomycin $X_{0\delta}$ acetate	$1:2.5\times10^6$		
Actinomycin $X_{0\beta}$ acetate	$1:1.5\times10^5$		
7-Bromoactinomycin C_3	$1:4\times10^6$		
7-Hydroxyactinomycin C_1, pH 6.0	$1:0.5\times10^6$		
7-Hydroxyactinomycin C_1, pH 7.1	$1:5\times10^3$		
7-Nitroactinomycin C_1	$1:10\times10^6$		
7-Aminoactinomycin C_2	$1:2\times10^5$		
7-Methoxyactinomycin C_1	$1:2\times10^6$		
Deaminoactinomycin C_2	$1:8\times10^3$		
3-Chloroactinomycin C_2	$1:2\times10^4$		
N-Methylactinomycin C_2	$1:2\times10^6$		
N-(β-Hydroxyethyl)actinomycin C_2	$1:6.4\times10^4$		
N-Dimethyleneactinomycin C_2	$1:4\times10^3$		
N-(β-Diethylaminoethyl)-actinomycin C_3	$1:20\times10^3$		
N-(*p*-Aminophenyl)actinomycin C_3	$1:3.2\times10^4$		
N-(β-Aminoethyl)actinomycin C_3	$1:6.4\times10^4$		
N-Trimethyleneactinomycin C_3	$1:6.4\times10^4$		
N-Isopropylactinomycin C_3	$1:5\times10^3$		
N-Cyclohexylactinomycin C_3	$1:5\times10^3$		
N-(α-Carbomethoxylethyl)-actinomycin C_3	$1:5\times10^3$		

Table 16.4 (*Continued*)

Compound	Activity, μg/ml[a]	Method of Expression	Reference
N-(β-Chloroethyl)actinomycin C_2	$1:6.4\times10^4$		
Actinocin	Inactive		
seco-Actinomycin C_3	Inactive		
Bis(*seco*-actinomycin C_3)	Inactive		
Actinomycinic (C_3) acid	Inactive		
Actinomycin C_1 with L-Ser instead of L-Thr	8X	MIC (*B. subtilis*) relative to actinomycin C_3	107
Actinomycin Z_1	50X	MIC (*B. subtilis*) relative to actinomycin C_3	67
Enantiomer of actinomycin C_1	Inactive	Activity against *B. subtilis*	108
7-Hydroxyactinomycin C_2	0.25%	Activity against *B. subtilis* relative to that of actinomycin C_3	109
7-Nitroactinomycin C_2	40%		
7-Aminoactinomycin C_2	1%		
7-Chloroactinomycin C_3	50%		
2-Deamino-2-chloro-7-bromoactinomycin C_3	Inactive		
7-Bromoactinomycin C_3	150%		
Actinocyl-gramicidin S	None	Complexing with DNA	110
Actinomycin C_3 with D-Leu instead of D-*a*-ile	25%	Activity against *B. subtilis* relative to that of actinomycin C_3	111
Actinomycin C_1 with L-Ser instead of L-Thr	20%		
Actinomycin C_1 or C_3 with D-Ala instead of D-val or D-*a*-ile	1%		
Actinomycin D	0.02	MIC against *B. subtilis*	70
Actinomycin pip 1α	0.25		
Actinomycin pip 1β	0.02		
Actinomycin pip 2	0.1		
Various actinomycins with α or β ring truncated or open	Inactive	Activity against *B. subtilis*	65
Various natural actinomycins	0.05–12	MIC against *B. subtilis*	112
4,6-Didemethylactinomycin C_1	0.01	Activity against *B. subtilis* relative to that of actinomycin C_1	113
4,6-Didemethyl-4,6-dimethoxyactinomycin C_1	0.01		
4,6-Didemethyl-4,6-diethyl-actinomycin C_1	0.5		
4,6-Didemethyl-4,6-di-*tert*-butylactinomycin C_1	0		
4,6-Didemethyl-4,6-dibromoactinomycin C_1	23%	Activity against *B. subtilis* relative to that of actinomycin C_1	114

Table 16.4 (*Continued*)

Compound	Activity, μg/ml[a]	Method of Expression	Reference
Actinomycin D-lactam	0.5	LD_{50} *Lactobacillus arabinosus*	115, 116
[$Gly^{4'}$, $Val^{5'}$]actinomycin D	0	Activity against *B. subtilis*	117
2-Deaminoactinomycin	50	Toxic dose level of actinomycin D against murine tumor systems	118
N^2-(γ-Hydroxypropyl) actinomycin	1	Antitumor activity of actinomycin D	

[a] Except where noted.

A variety of gram-positive cocci and bacilli, *Neisseria*, *Hemophilus influenzae*, and *Treponenon pallidum* are sensitive to 0.1 unit or less of bacitracin per milliliter. *Actinomyces* and *Furobacterium* are inhibited by concentrations of 0.5–5 units/ml. Enterobacteriaceae, *Pseudomonas*, *Candida*, *Torula*, and *Nocardia* are resistant to the drug. Current use is essentially restricted to topical application.

Its mechanism of action has been reviewed (121). The antibiotic provokes termination of the cell wall synthesis. It inhibits peptidoglycan synthetase in an *in vitro* system prepared from *E. coli* (122, 123). The inhibition of the hydrolysis of the pyrophosphate linkage of the P-P. lipid results in its accumulation, and since the transport P. lipid is no longer liberated, it cannot participate in a new cycle (124). In preparations obtained from *Bacillus licheniformis*, bacitracin inhibits the synthesis of TA only under conditions where the synthesis of peptidoglycan takes place (125). Bacitracin determines the characteristic functional alterations of the cell membrane. Like the surface active materials of the quaternary ammonium type, it provokes an increase of the entrance of colored tetracolium derivatives (126), and the exit of potassium (127) and material of the positive ninhydrin type (128). It is bacteriolytic for growing bacteria only. On the other hand, bacitracin inhibits the growth of intact bacteria as well as that of protoplasts (127). Under the action of bacitracin, L-forms of streptococci were obtained (129). Therefore the inhibition of the synthesis of the wall is only one consequence of a primary action at the membrane level (127). Yet

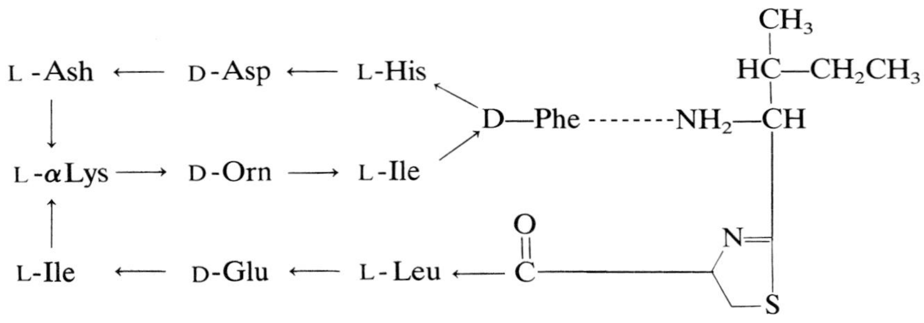

```
                                                              CH3
                                                              |
L-Ash  <--  D-Asp  <--  L-His                                HC—CH2CH3
  |                          \                                |
  v                           D—Phe --------NH2—CH
L-αLys -->  D-Orn  -->  L-Ile /                               |
  ^                                         O                 |
  |                                         ||            N=  |
L-Ile  <--  D-Glu  <--  L-Leu <-- C ————————————————— (       |
                                                          \__S
```

Fig. 16.4 Structure of bacitracin A.

the effect of bacitracin on the synthesis of the cell wall derives from a direct inhibitory action on the peptidoglycan synthetase. Among secondary actions, inhibition of protein synthesis (126, 130) and accumulation of nucleotides has been found. The antibiotic can act as chelating agent (131).

2.3 Tyrothricin

Tyrothricin is an antibiotic obtained from *Bacillus brevis*, a bacterium isolated from soil by Dubos, who discovered the microorganism and the bactericidal properties of its cultures. Tyrothricin contains two polypeptide components, *gramicidin* (about 20%) and *tyrocidin* (about 80%) (132). The antibacterial activity of tyrothricin is the resultant of the sum of the actions of gramicidin and tyrocidine; gramicidin is particularly active against gram-positive bacteria, whereas tyrocidine shares this activity and also inhibits some gram-negative bacilli. Gramicidin is considerably more active than tyrocidine against bacteria sensitive to both agents.

Tyrothricin is employed only locally in solution or as an ointment. The concentration of antibiotic is 0.5 mg/ml or 0.5 mg/g; higher concentrations may be irritating. Gramicidin is also a component of several antibiotic preparations for topical use.

Crude gramicidin contains at least four different antibiotics, called A, B, C, and D. Also, gramicidins J_1 and J_2 have been described as hexapeptides containing two ornithine residues per molecule (133). Table 16.5 gives the composition in amino acids of gramicidins A, B, C, and D. For a long time these peptides were thought to be cyclic because of the impossibility of rationalizing the C- and N-terminal amino acid. However it was shown that they are linear, where the terminal NH_2 group is amidified by formic acid (134). Deformylation of gramicidins furnishes the "*seco*-gramicidins". The structure of Valgramicidin A is HCO—L-Val—Gly—L-Ala—D-Leu—L-Ala—D-Val—L-Val—D-Val—L-Try—D-Leu—L-Try—D-Leu—L-Try—D-Leu—L-Try—$NHCH_2CH_2OH$, and that of gramicidin B is HCO—L-Val—Gly—L-Ala—D-Leu—L-Ala—D-Val—L-Val—D-Val—L-Try—D-Leu—L-Phe—D-Leu—L-Try—D-Leu—L-Try—NH—CH_2—CH_2OH. Both are pentapeptides containing one mole of ethanolamine (135). Gramicidin A is in reality a mixture of Val-gramicidin A and Ileu-gramicidin A, with the terminal *N*-formylated amino acid being either valine or isoleucine. The structures of gramicidins C and D have also been established (136).

Tyrocidin A is a decapeptide whose structure (Fig. 16.5) has been confirmed by synthesis (137). Tyrocidin B differs from tyrocidin A by simple replacement of a residue of L-phenylalanine by L-tryptophan. The structure of tyrocidin C is represented in Fig. 16.6. This cyclic peptide is opened by treatment with $LiAlH_4$, and the linear product thus formed is hydrolyzable by pepsin (138).

Table 16.5 Composition in Amino Acids of Gramicidins

	Number of Residues of						
Gramicidin	Gly	Ala	Val	Leu		Tyr	Ethanolamine
A	1	2	4	4		4	1
B	1	2	4	4	Phe 1	3	1
C	1	2	4	4	Tyr 1	6	1
D	1	2	3	4	Ileu 1	6	1

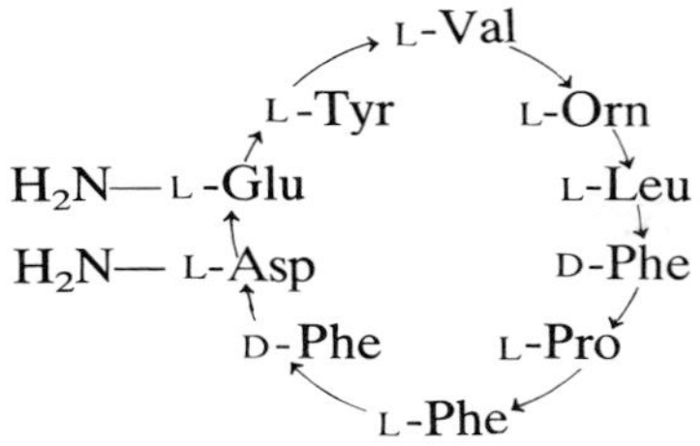

L-Val
L-Tyr L-Orn
H_2N—L-Glu L-Leu
H_2N—L-Asp D-Phe
D-Phe L-Pro
L-Phe

Fig. 16.5 Structure of tyrocidin A.

Tyrocidin and gramicidin have been reviewed (139).

An enzymatic system capable of synthesizing the tyrocidins has been obtained from *B. brevis*: to function, it needs the amino acids that enter into the composition of the tyrocidins, Mg^{2+}, and ATP. The synthesis of a peptide linkage consumes one mole of ATP (140). Under certain conditions such a noncellular extract can synthesize a single antibiotic, for example, tyrocidin D (141).

Numerous suggestions have been made with regard to the role these peptides could play in the physiology of the cell. In particular, it has been proposed that they could bind specifically to certain macromolecules, thus could intervene in the regulation of certain cellular activities (142).

Gramicidin A is a linear polypeptide composed of 15 amino acids alternating the L- and D-forms: HCO—L-Val—Gly—L-Ala—D-Leu—L-Ala—D-Val—L-Val—D-Val[L-Trp—D-Leu]$_3$—L-Trp—NH—CH_2-CH_2OH (143). The terminal NH_2 group is formylated; the terminal COOH group is amidified by ethanolamine. Gramicidin A

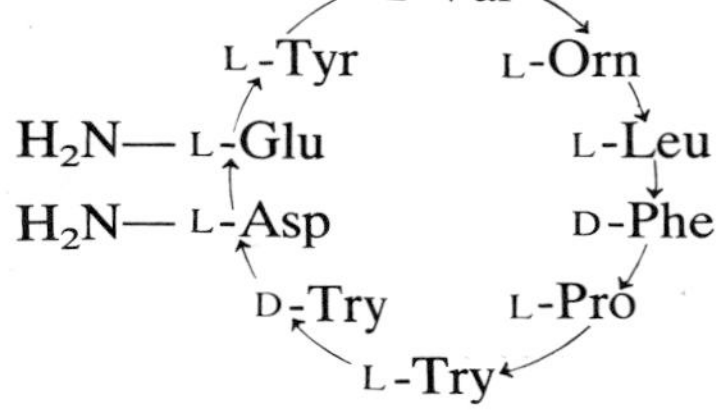

L-Val
L-Tyr L-Orn
H_2N—L-Glu L-Leu
H_2N—L-Asp D-Phe
D-Try L-Pro
L-Try

Fig. 16.6 Structure of tyrocidin C.

permits the establishment of an ion flux through a double layer membrane by the formation of conduction canals (144). For a double layer membrane of thickness of the order 40 Å, two antibiotic molecules are necessary to form a canal (145–147). The effect of gramicidin depends on the thickness of the double membrane. An interesting phenomenon is produced with the double layers composed of phosphatidylserine, for which the initial conduction rate is low. As a function of the number of created canals, the negative charges of the lipid are neutralized by the cations, which reduces the repulsion forces, decreases the thickness of the layer, and consequently tends to increase the conduction rate. A study of the structural conditions that permit the establishment of such a canal (148, 149) has provided a model in which gramicidin A should have a lipophilic conformation in a left-handed helix; two helices form a canal with the formyl groups head to head. In such a conformation, leading to a tetrahedral coordination of the ion, an easy displacement of the coordinations permits the movement of the ion along the canal.

2.4 Polymyxin and Colistin

The polymyxins, discovered in 1947, are a group of closely related substances (polymyxins A, B, C, D, E, M) elaborated by various strains of *Bacillus polymyxa*, an aerobic spore-forming rod found in soil. Polymyxin B is available for clinical use. The polymyxins, which are cationic detergents, are relatively simple basic peptides with molecular weight of about 1000. They readily form water-soluble salts with mineral acids.

Colistin is an antibiotic produced by *Bacillus* (*Aerobacillus*) *colistinus*, a microorganism isolated from a soil sample obtained from Fukushima Prefecture, Japan. Colistin is polymyxin E, identical to polymyxin B except for the substitution of a residue of D-leucine for that of D-phenylalanine. Solutions of colistin salts are relatively unstable above pH 6.

The *in vitro* and *in vivo* activity of polymyxin B and colistin is sharply restricted to gram-negative bacteria. *Enterobacter, Escherichia, Hemophilus, Klebsilla, Pasteurella, Salmonella, Shigella*, and *Vibrio* are sensitive to concentrations of 0.5–2.0 μg/ml. Many strains of *Pseudomonas aeruginosa* are inhibited *in vitro* by less than 8 μg/ml. *Brucella* is only moderately susceptible. Most strains of *Proteus* are unaffected by the drug. Some *Neisseria* are also resistant, and gram-positive bacteria are singularly unaffected. Orally administered polymyxin B markedly reduces but does not eliminate coliform microorganisms from the feces of man; the drug eradicates *P. aeruginosa* from the intestinal tract. Polymyxin B is rapidly bactericidal *in vitro*. Anionic substances, such as soap that bind to cationic surface-active agents impair the action of the drug. The development of bacterial resistance to polymyxin B is infrequent in most species. However insensitive strains are occasionally encountered among susceptible microorganisms. There is complete cross-resistance between polymyxin B and colistin.

The polymyxins constitute an extremely complex group of polypeptides; they are characterized by their cyclic structure, their basic properties, and the presence in their molecule of a branched fatty acid (6-methyl- or 7-methyloctanoic acid). Polymyxins B, D, and E are mixtures of two polymyxins that differ in the nature of the fatty acid: 6-methyl- or 7-methyloctanoic acid. The composition in amino acids is given in Table 16.6 and their structure is represented in Fig. 16.7 (150).

An excellent review gives all references

Table 16.6 Composition in Amino Acids of Polymyxins and Related Polypeptides (151)

	DAB[a]	L-Thr	Leu	Ileu	D-Phe	D-Ser	D-Val	Fatty Acid[b]
Polymyxin								
A	+	+	+(D)	—	—	—	—	Me-6
B_1	6	2	1(L)	—	1	—	—	Me-6
B_2	6	2	1(L)	—	1	—	—	Me-7
C	+	+	—	—	+	—	—	Me-6
D_1	5	3	1(D)	—	—	1	—	Me-6
D_2	5	3	1(D)	—	—	1	—	Me-7
M	6	3	1(D)	—	—	—	—	Me-6
Colistin								
A	6	2	1(L) 1(D)	—	—	—	—	Me-6
B	6	2	1(L) 1(D)	—	—	—	—	Me-7
Circulin								
A	6	2	1(D)	1	—	—	—	Me-6
B	6	2	1(D)	1	—	—	—	
Polypeptin	3	1	2(L)	1	1	—	1	?

[a] DAB = α, γ-diaminobutyric acid.
[b] Me-6 = 6-methyloctanoic acid; Me-7 = 7-methyloctanoic acid.

R
CH—NH
OC CO
H_2N— L-DAB CH—R′
H_2N— L-DAB NH
L-Thre L-DAB—NH_2
L-DAB NH_2 H CH_3
γ ↑ α
Z← L-Thre← L-DAB←CO—$(CH_2)_4$—CH—CH—CH_3
x y

Polymyxins			
B:	R = CH_3—$CH(CH_3)_2$	R′ = CH_2—C_6H_5	Z = L-DAB
D:	CHOH—CH_3	CH_2—$CH(CH_3)_2$	D-Ser
E:	CH_2—$CH(CH_3)_2$	CH_2—$CH(CH_3)_2$	L-DAB

In each case the methyl of the fatty acid can be in position *x* or *y*.

Colistin			
A:	CH_2—$CH(CH_3)_2$	$CH(CH_3)$—CH_2—CH_3	L-DAB

Fig. 16.7 Structures of polymyxins: in each polymyxin the methyl of the fatty acid can be in position *x* or *y*.

concerning the determination of the structure of polymyxins (and related polypeptides) and their syntheses (151). Among the most recent work is the structure determination of polymyxin D_1 (152). An NMR study of the conformation of these polymyxins in aqueous solution shows a pleated structure (153).

In the group of the polymyxins one can also include the circulin produced by *Bacillus circulans*. Chemically they are very similar, and they have the same antibiotic properties and the same relatively high toxicity.

The action of the polymyxins has been particularly studied by Newton (154). Polymyxins were treated with dansylchloride so that, on the average, only one dansyl group per molecule of polymyxin was introduced. In this manner, the dansylpolymyxin retains an antibiotic activity very similar to that of nontreated polymyxin. Dansyl-polymyxin is strongly fluorescent in the ultraviolet region. If the dansylpolymyxin is brought into contact with susceptible bacteria (*Bacillus megaterium*, *Sarcina lutea*, *Micrococcus lysodeikticus*), one can see in the fluorescence microscope that the antibiotic is fixed on the surface of the bacteria. When these are mechanically disintegrated, the antibiotic is found essentially in a fraction of small particles, sedimenting at only 100,000 g and very little above the cell wall. Polymyxin B interacts with both the polar and apolar regions of the phospholipids. The conformation of the antibiotic is not modified by this interaction (155). Polymyxins make the cell wall more vulnerable to attack by lysozyme (156). For further studies on the action of polymyxin B on bacterial membranes, see Ref. 157.

2.5 Antibiotic Polypeptides with a Lactone Ring

The polypeptide chain is cyclized by formation of an ester linkage between the carboxyl of the *C*-terminal amino acid and the

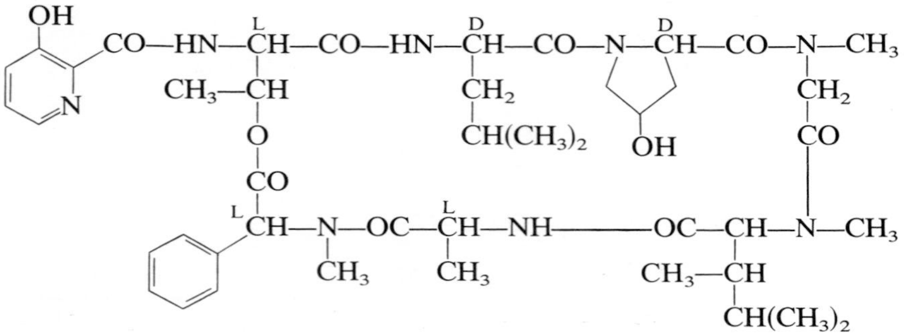

Fig. 16.8 Structure of etamycin.

hydroxyl of a hydroxylated amino acid present at the *N*-terminus. These antibiotics are all synthesized by *Streptomyces.*

2.5.1 ETAMYCIN OR VIRIDOGRISEIN. This antibiotic is produced particularly by *Streptomyces griseus.* It is very active *in vitro* against gram-positive bacteria and *Mycobacterium tuberculosis*, but it is relatively toxic (LD_{50}: 50 mg/kg, mouse, i.p.). Its structure was established in 1958 (Fig. 16.8) and confirmed by synthesis (158). The presence of *N*-methylated amino acids is characteristic for this group, as well as aromatic heterocyclic acids. For mode of action see Ref. 159.

2.5.2 STAPHYLOMYCIN S. This antibiotic is produced by *Streptomyces virginiae* in the form of a complex of several antibiotics. Staphylomycin S has synergistic action with staphylomycin M (identical to ostreogrycin A, *vide infra*) and is active against gram-positive bacteria. Its structure (Fig. 16.9, R = H) (160) has been confirmed by mass spectrometry (161).

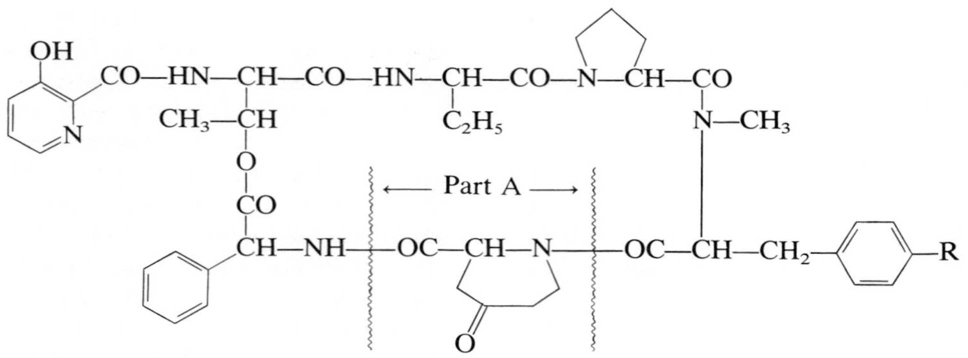

(254) R = H, staphylomycin S
R = —$N(CH_3)_2$, ostreogrycin B
R = —$N(CH_3)_2$, Part A = —OC—CH(CH_2—COOH)—NH— Doricin
R = H, Part A = —OC—CH—N— (pyrrolidine ring) Vernamycin B_α

Fig. 16.9 Structure of staphylomycin S and related substances.

Besides staphylomycin, also called virginiamycin S, three minor constituents have been isolated: virginiamycin S, ($C_{42}H_{47}N_7O_{10}$) and virginiamycins S_2 and S_3. Virginiamycin is identical with ostreogrycin B_1 or vernamycin B_γ or pristinamycin IC, virginiamycin differs only from ostreogrycin B_3 by the replacement of a dimethylaminophenyl group by a monomethylaminophenyl group (162). For mode of action, see Ref. 159.

2.5.3 OSTREOGYRYCIN. Ostreogrycin, produced by *Streptomyces ostreogriseus*, is also obtained in the form of a complex, from which ostreogrycins A_1, B_1, B_2, B_3, and G are isolated. Ostreogrycins A and G are chemically very close and show synergism in association with those of the B group. Ostreogrycin A is identical with staphylomycin M and is very close to virginiamycin M. Its structure appears in Fig. 16.10 (163, 164); Fig. 16.9 gives the structure of ostreogrycin B, which is chemically very close to staphylomycin S (164). Three other ostreogrycins are known: B_1, B_2, and B_3. They differ from ostreogrycin B by the replacement of the α-aminobutyric acid residue by alanine for ostreogrycin B_1, by replacement of the dimethylaminophenyl group by a monomethylaminophenyl group for ostreogrycin B_2, and by the presence of a hydroxyl on the piperidine, para to the carbon carrying the carboxyl, for ostreogrycin B_3 (165). For the mechanism of action, see Ref. 159.

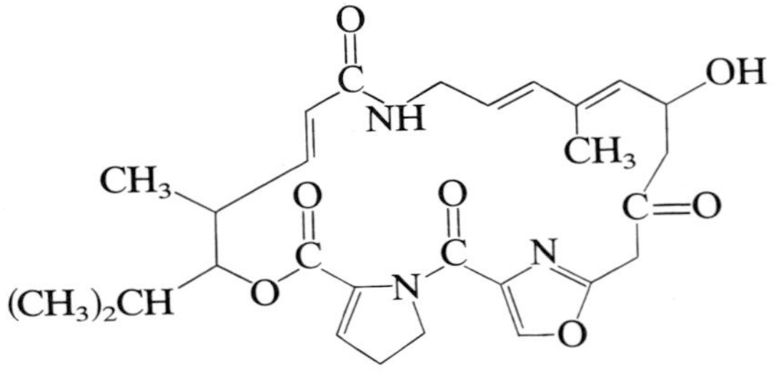

Fig. 16.10 Structure of ostreogrycin A.

2.5.4 DORICIN. Doricin has been isolated from *Streptomyces loidensis*, besides vernamycins. Its structure is represented in Fig. 16.9 with R = —$N(CH_3)_2$, and part A is replaced by an aspartic acid residue (166). For the mechanism of action see Ref. 159.

2.5.5 VERNAMYCIN. The antibiotic complex vernamycin is produced by *Streptomyces loidensis*. Vernamycin B has been isolated and subsequently separated into vernamycins B_α, B_β, B_γ, and B_δ. The structure of vernamycin B_α is represented in Fig. 16.9, where R = H and part A is replaced by a proline residue (167). Pristinamycin has been separated by thin layer chromatography into five fractions: I_A, I_B, I_C, II_A, and II_B. Pristinamycin I_A is identical to vernamycin B_α (and mikamycin B), and pristinamycin I_B is identical to vernamycin B_β (168). The mode of action has been described (159).

2.5.6 CYCLOHEPTAMYCIN. This antibiotic, $C_{48}H_{68}O_{12}N_2$, produced by *Streptomyces*, is active against gram-positive bacteria and mycobacteria. Its structure is represented in Fig. 16.11.

2.5.7 TELOMYCIN. This antibiotic is produced by *Streptomyces*. It is active against gram-positive bacteria (LD_{50}: 500 mg/kg, mouse, i.p.). The molecule contains several unusual amino acids not found in the proteins or the cell wall of the microorganism (169), and, in particular, a mixture of *cis*- and *trans*-3-hydroxyproline. Its structure appears in Fig. 16.12 (171); its NMR spectrum and conformation have been studied (170).

There exists a group of antibiotics that possess certain characteristics of the lactonic peptides (*N*-methylamino acids, aromatic acids) but whose macrocycle is of pure peptide nature. They are listed in Sections 2.5.8–2.5.10.

2.5.8 RUFOMYCIN A. This antibiotic, produced by *Streptomyces antratus*, is reduced

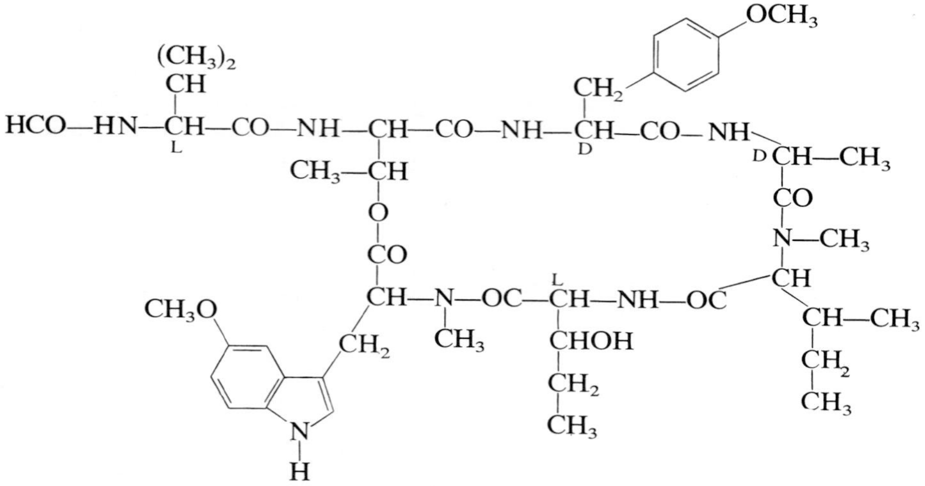

Fig. 16.11 Structure of cycloheptamycin.

by $NaBH_4$ into a more stable anhydro form. Its structure (Fig. 16.13), established in 1964 (172), shows a number of particularities, notably an *m*-nitrotyrosine residue and an *N*-methyl-δ-oxoleucine residue responsible for the presence of an aldehydic function ($NaBH_4$ reduction).

2.5.9 ILAMYCIN. Ilamycin has been isolated from *Streptomyces islandicus*. Its structure, close to that of rufomycin A, is shown in Fig. 16.13. It is active against mycobacteria. In the culture, it is accompanied by ilamycin B_2, which has no aldehyde function (173) but retains strong biological activity (174). Ilamycin B_1 differs from ilamycin B_2 by the tryptophan residue (part A, in Fig. 16.13), which carries on the indole nitrogen a dimethyl-vinylmethyl group (in place of the cyclized alcoholic chain). Its secondary structure has been studied by 300 MHz NMR (175).

2.5.10 STREPTOGRAMIME AND MIKAMYCIN. Both antibiotics show the synergism phenomenon. Mikamycin exhibits a complete cross-resistance with pristinamycin (176). Both antibiotics have been reviewed (177).

Formation of new ribosomes does not take place in *B. subtilis* in the presence of the lactone peptide antibiotics, but a ribosomal pattern similar to that of control cultures can be observed soon after removal of the inhibitors (178). An unusual 60 S peak has been described in sucrose density gradients of lysates from *B. subtilis* treated with streptogramin A antibiotics; this peak may be due to the formation of labile monosomes in the presence of the

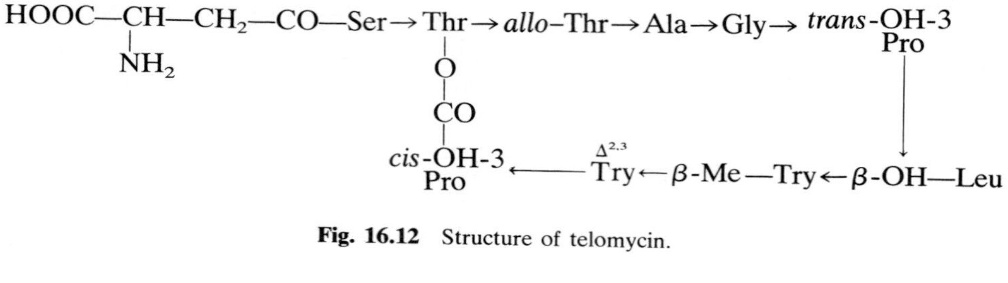

Fig. 16.12 Structure of telomycin.

HO, NO_2 (aromatic ring) —CH_2—CH—CO—NH—CH—CO—N(CH_3)—CH—CO—NH—CH—CH_2—$CH(CH_3)_2$

Part B

(CH—CH_3; CH(CH_3)—CH—CH_3, CHO; NH—CO; CO)

$(CH_3)_2CH$—CH_2—CH—N(CH_3)—OC—CH—NH—OC—CH—NH

(CH_2—indolyl; CH_2—CH=CH—CH_3)

Part A

Rufomycin A	part A	Without change	Part B, Without change
Ilamycin	part A:	OC—CH—NH— (CH_2; N; CH_3, CH_3; OH)	Part B, Without change
Ilamycin B_2			Part B, N-Methylleucine

Fig. 16.13 Structure of rufomycin and related antibiotics.

antibiotics that are transformed in the 60 S particles in the centrifugation procedure (179). The lactone peptide antibiotics are inhibitors of protein synthesis (180).

2.6 Gramicidin S

Gramicidin S was isolated in 1944 from a culture of *Bacillus brevis* obtained from the soil in the USSR (S corresponds to Soviet). This antibiotic is active against gram-positive cocci and some species of gram-negative bacteria. It is a cyclodecapeptide whose structure (Fig. 16.14) was established in 1945 (181). For the mode of action, see Ref. 139. Because of the relative simplicity of the structure, gramicidin S has been synthesized (182), and numerous analogs have been prepared with the goal of studying structure-activity relationships.

Gramicidin S is inactivated by acetylation, showing the importance of the basic free NH_2 groups. The open chain analog is weakly active (183). Replacement of L-Orn

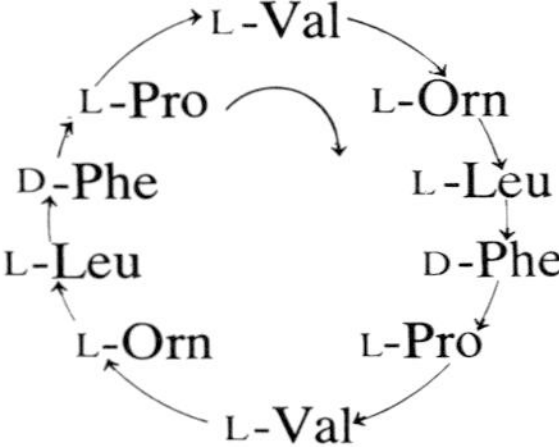

Fig. 16.14 Structure of gramicidin S.

```
L-Val ——→ L-Orn
  ↑          ↓
L-Pro      L-Leu
   ↖       ↙
     D-Phe
```

Fig. 16.15 Structure of cyclo-semi-gramicidin S.

by L-Lys does not change the activity. Replacement of L-Pro by glycine furnishes a more active antibiotic, called Gly^{5,10}-gramicidin S (184). Cyclo-semi-gramicidin S (Fig. 16.15) is devoid of activity at concentrations of 100 μg/ml (185). The negative result is probably explained by the fact that gramicidin S possesses a conformation (186) that is not found in the half-molecule; the importance of the conformation in the activity of these cyclic polypeptide antibiotics has been emphasized (187).

Replacement of the D-Phe by L-Phe furnishes an "all-L" gramicidin S that has no activity against *E. coli* and has little against gram-positive bacteria (188). Interesting studies concerning the stereoisomerism of these substances have been made (187). Based on the hypothesis that the antibiotic activity is due to a certain disposition in space of the polar groups with respect to each other, it has been observed that the retroenantiomer of Gly^{5,10}-gramicidin S (enantiomer of gramicidin S with the direction of peptide bonds reversed) possesses the same distribution of polar groups in space and the same activity as Gly^{5,10}-gramicidin S. Retrogramicidin S recently has been synthesized (189). These studies show the importance of the spatial disposition of the functional groups with respect to each other, so that the product conserves its spatial activity. They have contributed to further studies by X-ray diffraction or in solution by NMR spectroscopy (190).

Gramicidin S solubilizes lecithin dispersed in water (191) as well as dipalmitoyl lecithin (192). The particles obtained in the latter case seem to contain regions in which the lipid chains are in a double layer. This effect could serve as a model for that observed in bacterial membranes containing not lecithin but negatively charged phospholipids. The effect of this antibiotic on the permeability to ions in lipid double layers and the nature of its action have been studied (193, 194). The activity of gramicidin S depends, just as with the polymyxins, on the presence of free amino groups (195).

The conformations of *N*-methylleucine gramicidin-S and (di-*N*)-methylleucine gramicidin-S have been studied (196).

2.7 Albomycin

Albomycin belongs to a group of antibiotics called sideromycins, containing chelated iron. It was discovered by Gause (197) and its structure was investigated by Sormetal (198–200). It is active against gram-positive bacteria. Albomycin contains L-serine and N^{δ}-hydroxyl-L-ornithine. Moreover, a pyrimidine part and an atom of sulfur have been detected. The amino acid chain has been studied in desferrialbomycin through oxidation with performic acid; in this way the N^{γ}-hydroxyornithine residues are transformed into glutamic acid residues.

Albomycin has been separated into several similar antibiotics, differing in the nature of the pyrimidine part. Structures of albomycins δ_1, δ_2, and ε are represented in Fig. 16.16 (200). Between the pyrimidine part and the peptide (which chelates the ferric ion) is sulfur, in the form of a sulfuric acid residue. For a review, see Ref. 201.

Albomycin does not inhibit incorporation of amino acids into proteins in cell-free systems. It is suggested that albomycin interferes with the transport of metabolic precursors through bacterial membranes (202).

2.8 Bacteriocin

Bacteriocin is a high molecular weight, protein-like substance. It is capable of enzymatically hydrolyzing the constituents of

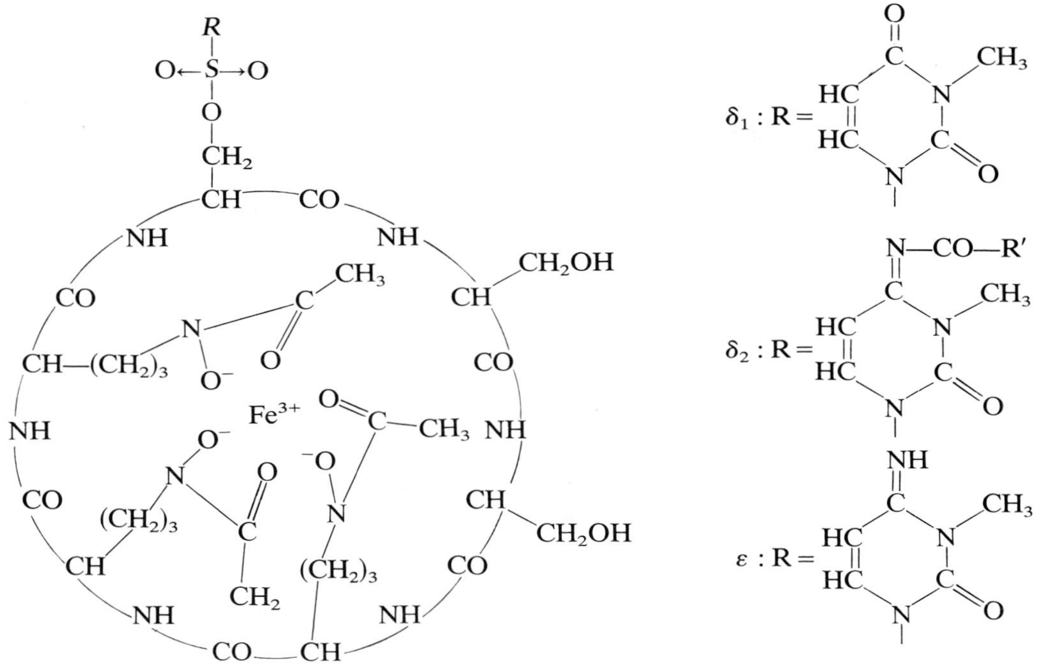

Fig. 16.16 Structure of albomycins.

the bacterial cell wall, and it inhibits the development of other bacteria of the *same species.* Chemically, these substances are still little known. A very well documented review was published in 1965 (203), and more recent works (204–208) exist.

2.9 Colicins 1972

Colicins are bactericidal proteins synthesized by certain strains of enteric bacteria and active against other strains of the same, or related, bacterial species. They fall into three groups, as defined by their predominant physiological effects: (1). inhibition of protein synthesis, (2). degradation of DNA, and (3). general blockage of energy-dependent cellular functions. Colicins of all three classes exert their effects by way of poorly understood processes involving the cell membrane (209–211).

2.10 Edeine

Bacillus brevis Vm4 produces a mixture of antibiotics from which have been isolated edeine A_1 and edeine B_1. The antibiotics (Fig. 16.17) have a basic character (more pronounced in edeine B_1) and furnish by hydrolysis unusual amino acids: β-tyrosine, isoserine, 2,6-diamino-7-hydroxyazelaic acid, as well as spermidine.

They have broad spectrum activity and inhibit gram-positive and gram-negative bacteria (212), mycoplasmas (213), fungi, and yeasts, as well as some mammalian neoplastic cells in tissue culture (214). The bacteriostatic concentrations of edeines are 4–8 μg/ml for *E. coli, Shigella typhimurium, Serrata marcescens, Sarcina lutea, Mycobacterium phlei, Bacillus subtilis,* and *Streptococcus hemolytus.* Higher concentrations are bactericidal.

Edeines have an effect on DNA synthesis and protein synthesis (215).

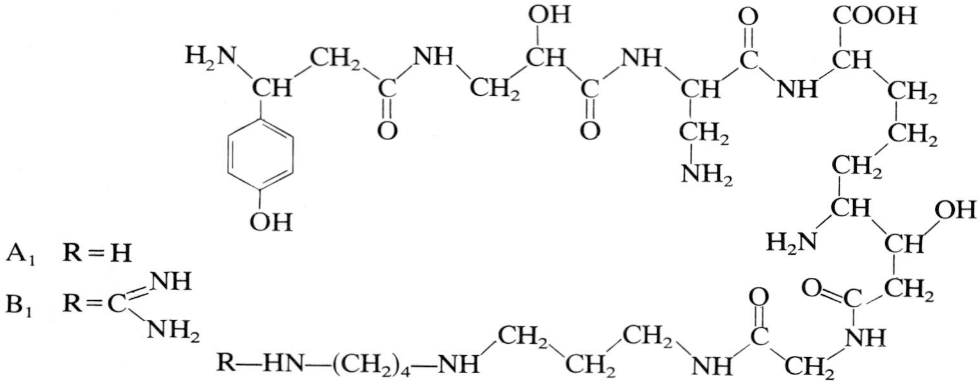

Fig. 16.17 Structure of edeines A_1 and B_1.

2.11 Phytoactin

Phytoactin is a noncyclic polypeptide that inhibits the growth of some fungi and bacteria. It neither affects the permeability of *Saccharomyces pastoriamus* to phosphorus-containing compounds nor its permeability to the uptake of inorganic phosphorus. Respiration is inhibited only to a small degree. With glucose ^{14}C as substrate, the synthesis of small molecules and polysaccharides is not inhibited. Protein synthesis is retarded somewhat, but the greatest effect is on the formation of RNA. Relatively long exposures of the yeast to phytoaction reduce RNA synthesis 80–90% (216).

2.12 Valinomycin

Valinomycin, produced by *Streptomyces fulvissimus* is active *in vitro* against the tuberculosis bacillus, and less active against other gram-positive bacteria. It is too toxic to be used practically. The molecule of valinomycin results from the coupling of 2 moles of L-valine, 2 moles of D-valine, 2 moles of L-lactic acid, and 2 moles of D-α-hydroxyisovaleric acid (Fig. 16.18) (217). Analogs of valinomycin have been synthesized (218). Its mode of action has been reviewed (219).

Valinomycin specifically chelates potassium ions, and the influence of this

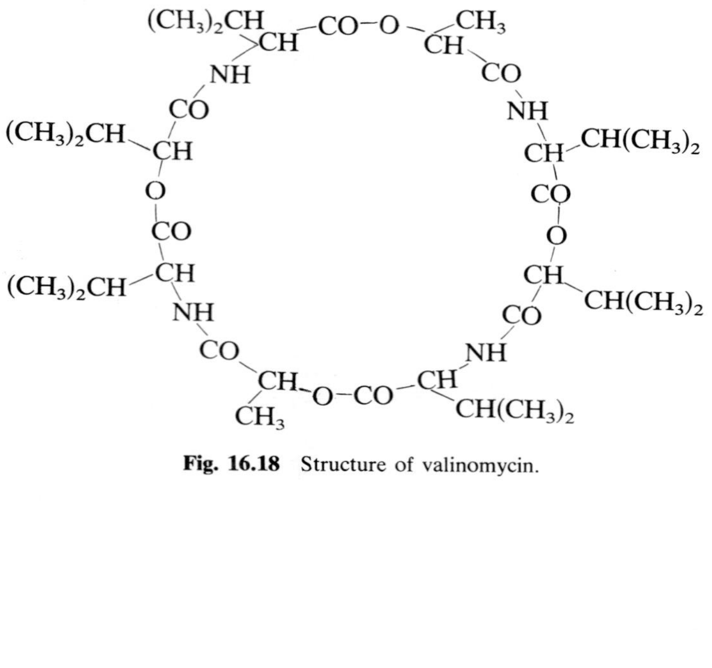

Fig. 16.18 Structure of valinomycin.

phenomenon on the conformation of the molecule has been studied (220). Valinomycin decouples oxidative phosphorylation and provokes the entrance of K^+. It modifies in a selective fashion the permeability of the membranes (221–232). Penetration of monovalent ions is correlated with the process of energy production. This problem has been studied with submitochondrial particles (226, 227, 233–239). A comparative study of the structure of valinomycin has permitted the elaboration of a model (240). Valinomycin does not possess an ionizable group and forms complexes with alkaline cations by oxygen bonds in a cavity of the molecule (226, 241–244). The specificity for the cation (K^+, Rb^+) is determined by the relative dimensions of the cavity and the hydrated or unhydrated ions (231, 245). Although the molecule itself is not charged, the complex acquires a net positive charge. It is probable that as in nonactin (which has effects similar to those of valinomycin), the hydrophobic part of the molecule is situated on the exterior of the spheroidal complex. Thus it is possible for it to penetrate the lipoprotein membrane.

The antibiotic therefore can be a cation transfer agent if the system is coupled to an energy source such that the ions are conducted against an electrochemical gradient. This system constitutes an "electrogene pump". The charged complex could be accompanied by an anion (e.g., a polycarboxylic acid from the Krebs cycle) for adequate concentrations of the antibiotic and, in that case, there should be stimulation of oxidative phosphorylation (246); for untimely penetration of K^+ there should thus be decoupling.

The conformation of valinomycin passes through an elongated form in the free state to an oblate spheroid form for the complex with K^+. This change of conformation corresponds to the rupture of two hydrogen bonds induced by the K^+ ion, and to a rearrangement allowing the establishment of six coordinated bonds. Figure 16.19 illustrates this behavior (247).

2.13 Viomycin

Viomycin is a strongly basic, complex antibiotic produced by an actinomycete. It is most active *in vitro* against *M. tuberculosis.* Almost all strains of this microorganism are inhibited by drug concentrations of 1–10 μg/ml. Viomycin is more tuberculostatic than aminosalicylic acid but less so than streptomycin; it is effective in the treatment of experimental tuberculosis produced by streptomycin-resistant microorganisms. Mycobacteria insensitive to kanamycin are also not susceptible to viomycin *in vitro.* On the other hand, viomycin-resistant strains may retain their sensitivity to kanamycin. The drug is not very active against the common gram-negative and gram-positive bacteria. Viomycin inhibits protein synthesis by *M. tuberculosis.*

By complete hydrolysis, viomycin liberates L-serine, L-2,3-diaminopropionic acid, L-β-serine, and a new substance, viomycidine, in molar ratio 2:1:1:1, as well as urea, carbon dioxide, and ammonia (248). Its structure (Fig. 16.20) has been established (249, 250). It is to be noted that its structure contains an α,β-unsaturated α-amino acid that also exists in capreomycin, ostreogrycin A, telomycin, stendomycin, nisine, and albonoursin.

2.14 Antimycins

Antimycins are produced by species of *Streptomyces* (*S. griseus, S. kitasawaensis, S. blastmyceticus*). The mixture of antibiotics can be fractionated into at least four constituents whose structures (Fig. 16.21) have been established (253, 254). Blastmycin and virosin are mixtures of antimycins. Antimycin A has been reviewed (255). Antimycins are active against yeasts and fungi

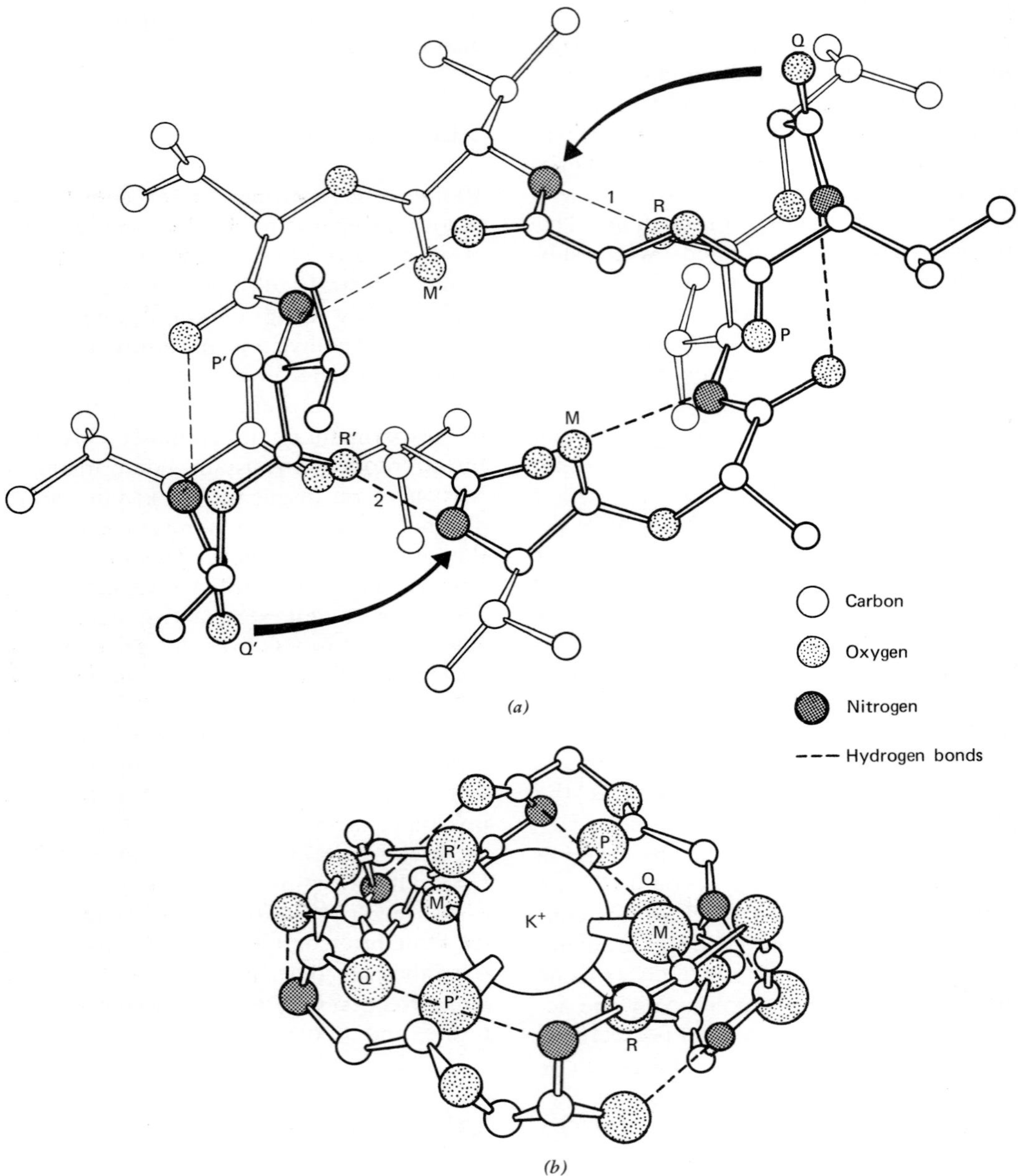

Fig. 16.19 Conformation of valinomycin alone (*a*) and of the K^+ complex (*b*). The carbonyl oxygens P,P′ and M,M′ are in the most exposed positions and can start the complexation with the potassium ion. The hydrogen bonds, marked 1 and 2, can be broken, allowing atoms R and R′ to furnish the rest of six coordinate bonds with the K^+ ion. The complexing of the molecule around the ion is produced by minor conformational changes that place atoms Q and Q′ such that, as indicated by the arrows, the hydrogen bonds of the complex are completely established. After Duax (247), with permission; copyright 1972 by the American Association for the Advancement of Science.

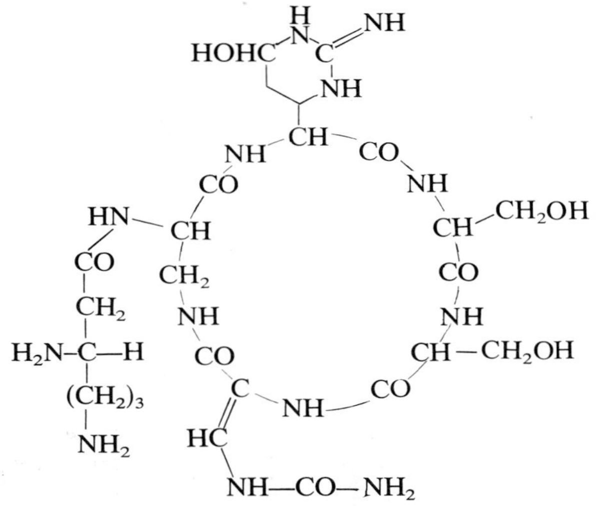

Fig. 16.20 Structure of viomycin.

and are rather toxic (LD_{100}: 30 mg/kg, rat, p.o.).

Antimycin blocks the transfer of electrons at the level of complex III between cytochromes *b* and c_1 (255–261). The manner of fixation and action at the level of the complex has been intensively studied (262–273). Antimycin also acts on photophosphorylation (274, 275).

2.15 Distamycin A and Netropsin

Distamycin A, produced by *Streptomyces distallicus*, possesses antitumor properties. Its structure is shown in Fig. 16.22 (276).

With the help of synthetic substances, structure-activity relations have been studied. Increase of the number of pyrrole units increases the antiviral activity. Substitution of the propionamidine group leads to more toxic derivatives. The product with five rings is 10 times as active as distamycin A. The formyl group is indispensable for activity. Replacement of the propionamidine group by an acetamidine residue is favorable. On the other hand, replacement of the propionamidine residue by butyramidine diminishes antiviral activity and increases toxicity (277, 278). The site of action of distamycin A has been studied (279).

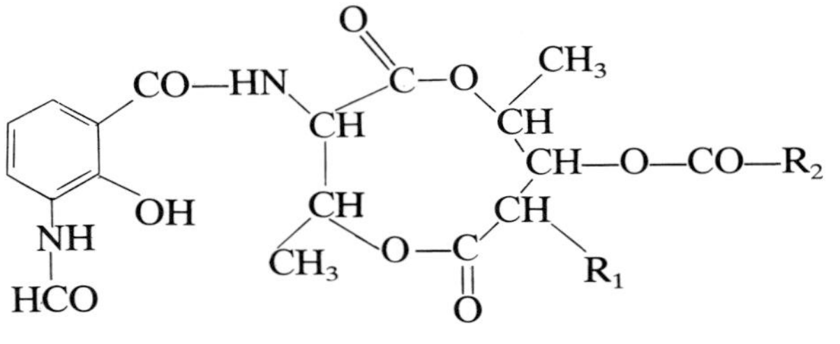

Antimycin A_1 $R_1 = n{-}C_6H_{13}$ $R_2 = CH_2{-}CH(CH_3)_2$
A_2 $n{-}C_4H_9$ $CH_2{-}CH(CH_3)_2$
Other antimycines $n{-}C_6H_{13}$ or $n{-}C_4H_9$ $CH_2{-}CH(CH_3)_2$ or $CH(CH_3){-}CH_2{-}CH_3$ or $CH(CH_3)_2$

Fig. 16.21 Structures of antimycins.

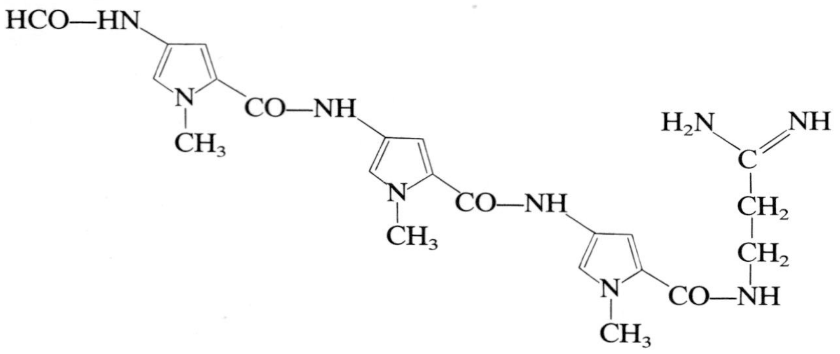

Fig. 16.22 Structure of distamycin A.

Netropsine, produced by *Streptomyces netropsis*, is active against bacteria and viruses. Its structure (Fig. 16.23) is similar to that of distamycin A (280).

Both distamycin and netropsin have been reviewed (281).

A total synthesis of distamycin A has been reported recently (281a).

2.16 Thiostrepton

The antibiotic thiostrepton, $C_{69}H_{84}N_{18}O_{18}S_5$, is produced by a streptomycete species and is active against gram-positive bacteria. This weakly basic polypeptide (Fig. 16.24) has been reviewed recently (282).

Thiostrepton inhibits the process of elongation with procaryotes by acting as an inhibitor of the EF_G and EF_{Tu} factors (283–287).

2.17 EM49

EM49 is a new family of similar peptide antibiotics, each an octapeptide acylated

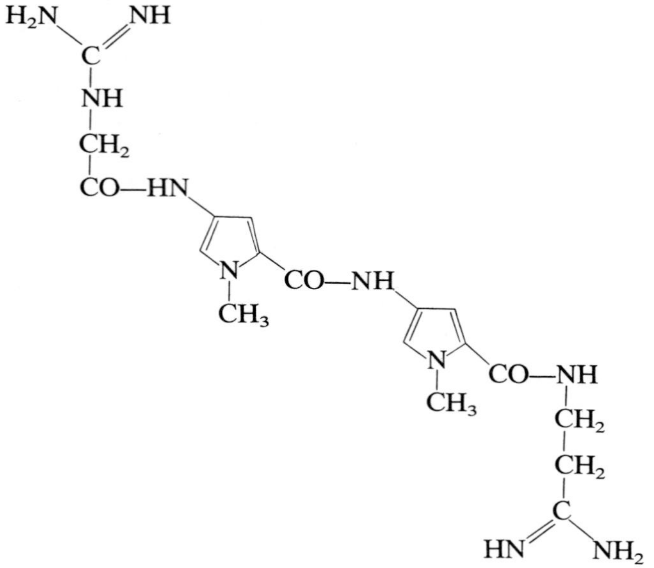

Fig. 16.23 Structure of netropsin.

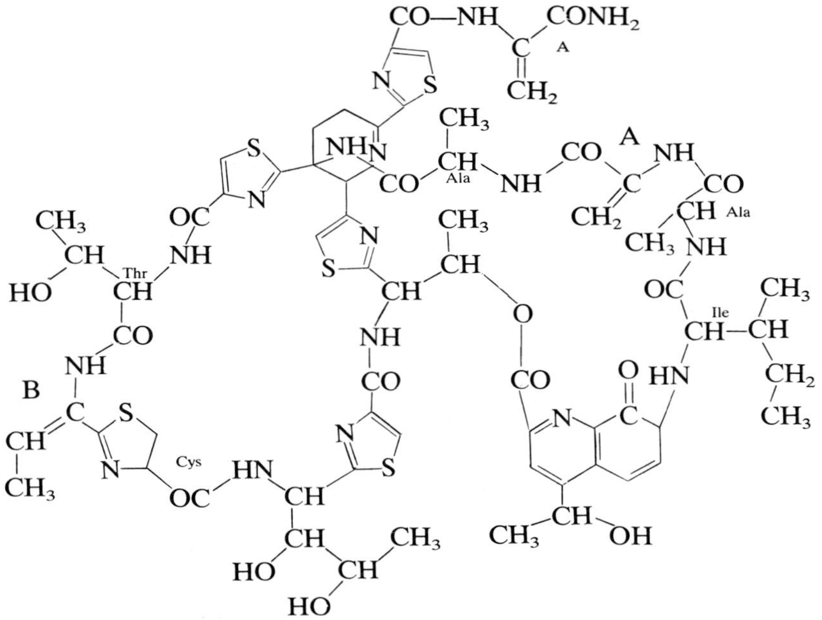

Fig. 16.24 Structure of thiostrepton.

with a β-hydroxy fatty acid. Its structure is given in Fig. 16.25 (288).

3 POLYENE ANTIFUNGAL ANTIBIOTICS

The polyene antifungal agents are a group of highly unsaturated antibiotics produced by various streptomycete strains. All are relatively insoluble in water, and many undergo light catalyzed autoxidation. They are pale yellow compounds having molecular weights on the order of 800. Table 16.7 lists the names, sources, and types of some of the polyenes.

This group is characterized by a lactonic

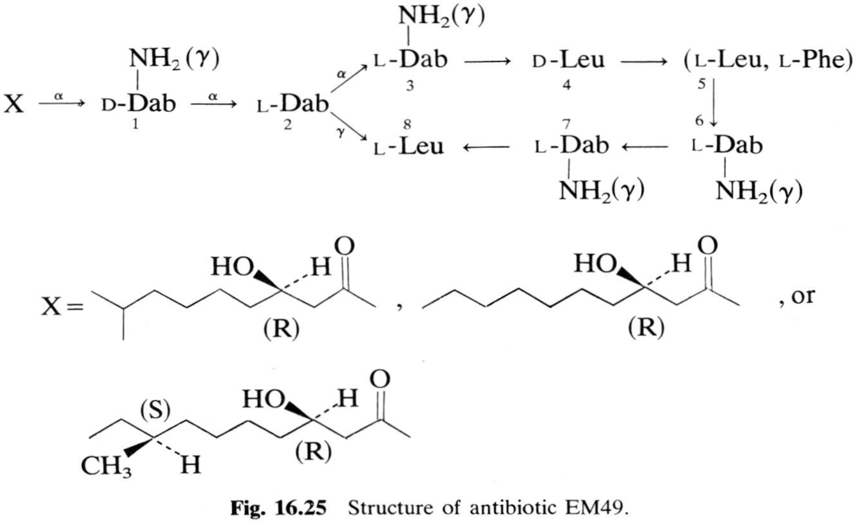

Fig. 16.25 Structure of antibiotic EM49.

Table 16.7 Characteristics of Some Polyene Antifungal Agents

Name (alternate)	Microbial Source	Other Antibiotics Found in Fermentation	Empirical Formula	Ionic Character	Mouse Toxicity: LD_{50}, mg/kg	Reference
Triene						
MM8	*Streptomyces* species		Not reported		Not reported	289
Tetraene						
Amphotericin A	*S. nodosus*	Amphotericin B	$C_{44}H_{75}NO_{17}$	Amphoteric	450 (i.p.)	290
Chromin	*S. antibioticus*			Acid	36	291
Endomycin A (helixin A)	*S. endus*, *S. antibioticus*	Helixin B, antibiotic 9-20F-1				292
Etruscomycin (lucensomycin, antibiotic Fl 1163)	*S. lucensis*		$C_{36}H_{57}NO_{17}$	Amphoteric	37 (i.p.)	293
Nystatin (fungicidin)	*S. noursei*, *S. albulus*, *Staphylococcus aureus*	Cycloheximide, E-73	$C_{46}H_{75}NO_{18-19}$	Amphoteric		294
PA-166	*Streptomyces* species		$C_{35}H_{53}NO_{14}$	Amphoteric	800 (s.c.)	295
Pimiricin (Tennecetin)	*S. natalensis*		$C_{33}H_{47}NO_{13}$	Amphoteric	650 (i.p.)	296
Protocidin	*Streptomyces* species		$C_{29}H_{45}NO_{13}$	Amphoteric	30 (i.v.)	297
Rimocidin	*S. rimosus*	5-Hydroxytetracycline	$C_{37}H_{59}NO_{13}$	Amphoteric	30 (i.v.)	298
Tetrin	*Streptomyces* species		$C_{31}H_{59}NO_{12}$			299
Pentaene						
Aliomycin	*S. acidomyceticus*	Acidomycin			45 (i.p.)	300
Capacidin	*S. noursei*		$C_{54}H_{65}N_2O_{18}$	Base	4 (i.p.)	301

Eurocidin	*S. eurocidicus* *S. albireticuli*	Azomycin, carbomycin, enteromycin, tertiomycin, actinomycin		Amphoteric	22 (i.p.)	302
Mycoticin A	*S. ruber*		$C_{36}H_{58}O_{10}$			303
Mycoticin B	*S. ruber*		$C_{37}H_{60}O_{10}$			304
PA-153	*Streptomyces* species		$C_{37}H_{61}NO_{14}$	Amphoteric		295
Methylpentaene						
Cabacidin	*S. gugeroti*		$C_{35}H_{60}O_{13}$	Nonionic		305
Filipin	*S. filipinensis*		$C_{37}H_{62}O_{12}$	Nonionic	17	306
Fungichromin	*S. cellulosae*	Fungichromatin	$C_{35}H_{58}O_{12} \cdot H_2O$	Nonionic	16 (i.p.)	307
Lagosin (pentamycin)	*S. pentaticus* *S. roseoluteus* *S. penticus*		$C_{35}H_{58}O_{12}$	Nonionic	33 (i.p.)	308
Hexaene						
Endomycin B (helixin B)	*S. endus*, *S. hygroscopicus*	Helixin A		Amphoteric		309
Heptaene						
Amphotericin B	*S. nodosus*	Amphotericin A	$C_{46}H_{73-75}NO_{18-20}$	Amphoteric	280 (i.p.)	310
Ascosin	*S. canescus*			Amphoteric	22 (i.p.)	311
Candicidin B	*S. griseus*			Amphoteric	79 (i.p.)	312
Gerobriecin	*S. jujuy*		$C_{35}H_{55}NO_{13}$			313
Hamycin	*S. pimprina*	Hamycin X		Amphoteric		314
PA-150	*Streptomyces* species		$C_{54}H_{82}N_2O_{18}$	Amphoteric	2.2 (s.c.)	295
Perimycin (fungimycin, aminomycin, NC-1968)	*S. coelicolor* var. *aminophilus*					315
Trichomycin A (hamycin?)	*S. hachijoensis*		$C_{61}H_{86}N_2O_{21} \cdot H_2O$	Amphoteric	2 (i.p.)	316

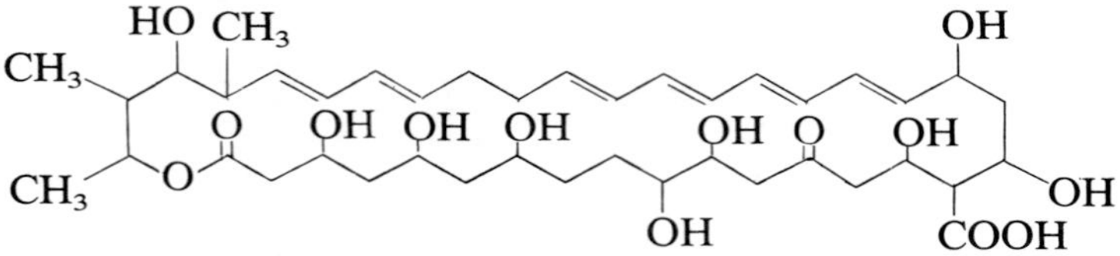

Fig. 16.26 Structure of nystatinolide (nystatin A_1).

macrocycle, almost without methyl substituents and possessing at least four conjugated double bonds. The entire group has been reviewed (317).

Polyenes function by modification of membrane permeability to ions. Their action is reversed by sterols. They appear to become attached to the sterol constituents of the fungal cell wall, which explains their lack of activity toward bacteria that do not have sterols. Filipin lyses *Mycoplasma laidlawii* only if this organism is grown in the presence of cholesterol (318). Certain species of *Pythium*—namely, those not containing sterols in their membrane—are insensitive to filipin (319). The antibiotics lyse erythrocytes (320, 321). The addition of cholesterol can prevent hemolysis. This interaction with sterols has been confirmed by studies with sterols, free or bound to the membrane (322–328). For example, the interaction of nystatin with sterols induces a modification of the membrane permeability to ions. The hypothesis has been advanced that aggregates of the antibiotic form pores of about 8 Å diameter (322, 329).

3.1 Nystatin

The antibiotic nystatin, produced by *Streptomyces noursei*, is one of the oldest known in this the polyene antifungal group. Nystatin has fungicidal activity *in vivo*, but, like most of the polyenes, it is rather toxic (LD_{50}: 20–26 mg/kg, mouse, i.p.). By acid hydrolysis it liberates mycosamine, which is glycosidically linked to the 19-hydroxyl of the aglycone nystatinolide (Fig. 16.21) (330).

The ketone at C-13 forms a hemiacetal with the 17-hydroxyl (331, 332). Nystatin has been separated into two conjugated tetraenes, nystatin A_1 (Fig. 16.26) and nystatin A_2 (333).

Ribonucleic acid synthesis is dependent on exogenous triphosphates in nystatin-treated cells of *Kluyveromyces lactis* (334).

3.2 Pimaricin

Pimaricin, $C_{33}H_{47}NO_{13}$ is produced by *Streptomyces natalensis.* Acid hydrolysis liberates mycosamide. Its structure (Fig. 16.27*a*) has been elucidated by a series of studies (335–338).

3.3 Lucensomycin

The antibiotic lucensomycin, also called etruscomycin, is produced by *Streptomyces lucensis.* Its structure appears in Fig. 16.27*b*.

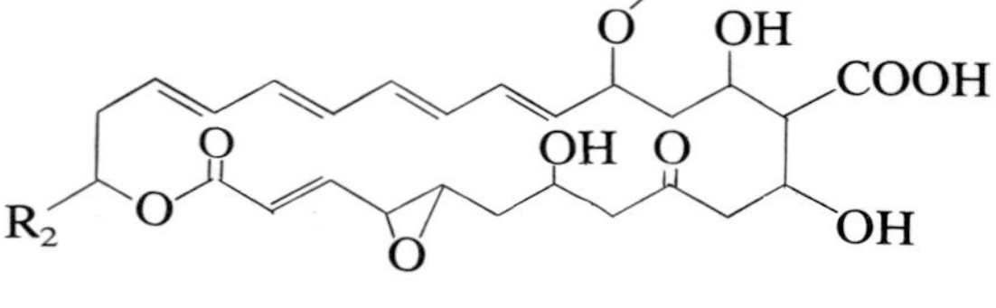

Fig. 16.27 Structure of pimaricin, *a*: R_1 = D-mycosamine, $R_2 = CH_3$; lucensomycin, *b*: R_1 = D-mycosamine, $R_2 = nC_4H_9$.

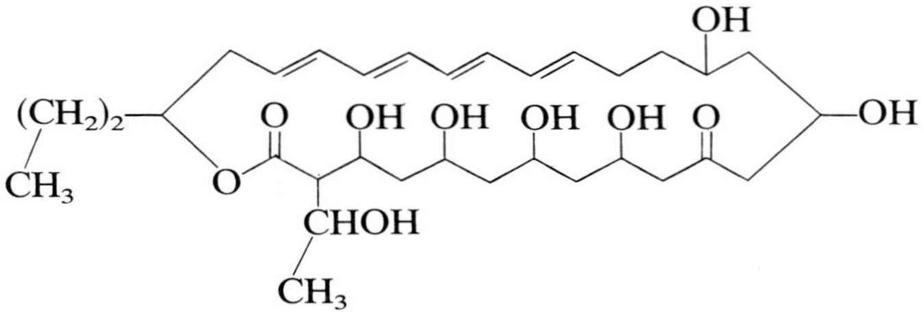

Fig. 16.28 Structure of rimocidinolide.

3.4 Rimocidin

Rimocidin, produced by *Streptomyces rimosus*, contains D-mycosamine, which is glycosidically linked to an aglycon with 32 carbons (Fig. 16.28).

3.5 Amphotericin B

The antibiotic amphotericin B is the glycoside of D-mycosamine with a macrolide containing seven conjugated double bonds. Its structure was established by X-ray analysis (Fig. 16.29), (339). The methyl ester hydrochloride of amphotericin B is significantly less toxic than the parent compound (340).

The alteration of tyrosine aminotransferase activity in hepatoma cells in tissue culture by amphotericin B (341), the characterization of the binding of amphotericin B to *Saccharomyces cerevisiae*, and the relationship to the antifungal effects (342) have been investigated.

3.6 Primycin

An actinomycete isolated from the intestine of an insect produces this antibiotic, which is active against gram-positive bacteria and mycobacteria. It is an α-D-arabinofuranoside of a macrolide that lacks conjugated double bonds. It also possesses a guanidinium group (Fig. 16.30) (343).

3.7 Levorins A and B

Streptomyces levoris furnishes two pentaene antibiotics containing mycosamine (344). Their structures are unknown.

3.8 Candidin

Streptomyces viridoflavus produces three heptaene antibiotics. The principal constituent, candidin, is built up from a molecule mycosamine linked glycosidically to an aglycon containing seven conjugated

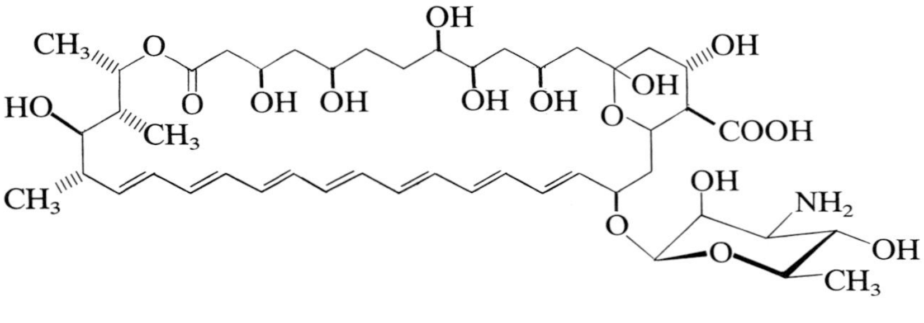

Fig. 16.29 Structure of amphotericin B.

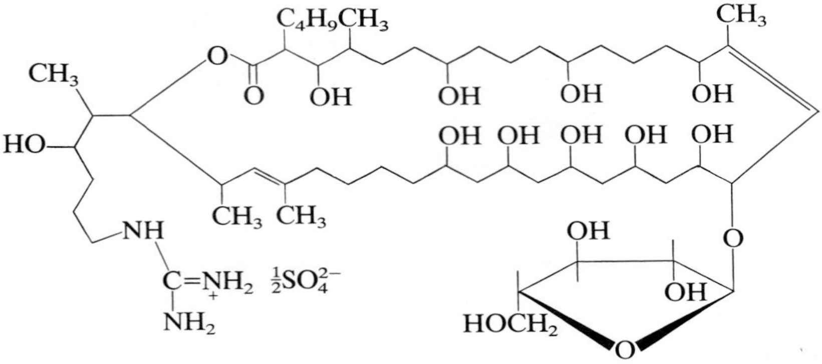

Fig. 16.30 Structure of primycin.

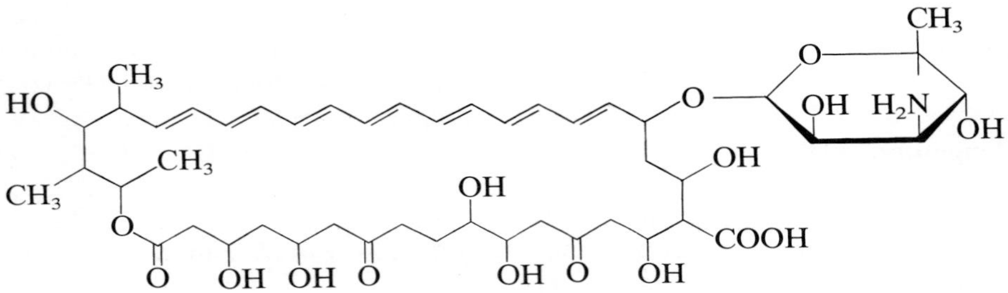

Fig. 16.31 Structure of candidin.

double bonds and two keto functions (Fig. 16.31) (345).

3.9 Lagosin

Lagosin is produced by *Streptomyces*. It contains five conjugated double bonds, and its structure is depicted in Fig. 16.32*a* (346). It contains numerous hydroxyl functions attached to the odd numbered carbons. Pentamycin as well as fungichromin have been identified with Lagosin (347, 348).

3.10 Filipin

This antibiotic, produced by *Streptomyces*, is a 14-desoxylagosin (Fig. 16.32*b*) (349,

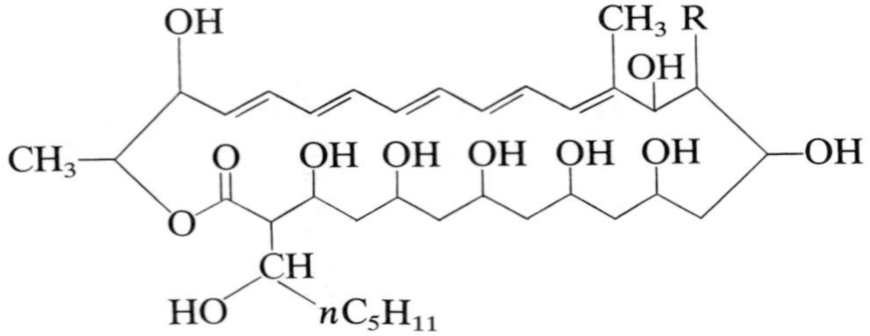

Fig. 16.32 Structures of lagosine (R = OH) and filipin (R = H).

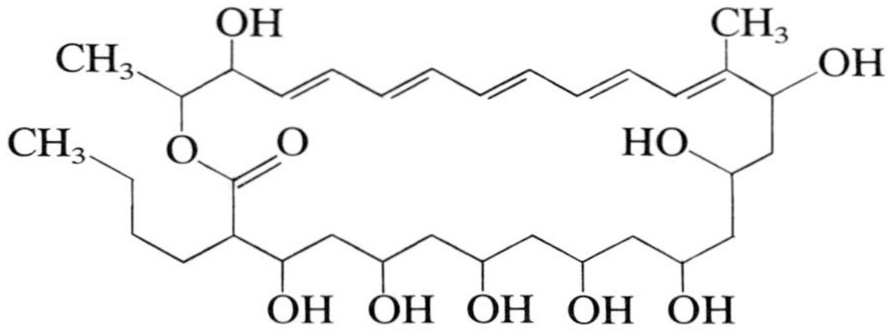

Fig. 16.33 Structure of chainin.

350). The crude preparation of the antibiotic contains at least eight pentaenes of the filipin type (351).

3.11 Chainin

A pentaene antibiotic, lacking the glycidic bond, has been isolated from a species of *Chainia* (Fig. 16.33) (352).

3.12 Mycoticin

Mycoticin is a product of *Streptomyces*. In effect, it is a mixture of two homologs (Fig. 16.34) (353).

3.13 Flavofungin

This antibiotic is produced by *Streptomyces flavofungini*. It contains a mixture of two substances, 1a and 1b. Flavofungin 1b has one CH_2 group more than flavofungin 1a. Their planar structures are identical with those of the mycoticins a and b (354), and there must be a stereoisomeric relationship.

4 MACROLIDE ANTIBIOTICS

The macrolide antibiotics are characterized by a macrocyclic lactone, various ketonic and hydroxyl functions, and a glycosidically bound deoxy sugar. The macrolides are of great interest because of their antibacterial activity, primarily against gram-positive bacteria and *Mycoplasma* species. Table 16.8 gives the names and some properties of a number of the better characterized macrolides. Mass spectral comparison of microgram quantities of the pure macrolides is often the most definitive method of identification (385). The first distinguishing chemical feature of these macrolides was the presence of unusual 6-deoxy sugars. Several of these have been isolated from various members of the group, and with the exception of oleandrose, which had been noted previously in plants, none had been found in other natural products. Table 16.9 lists the structures of these sugars and their sources. The extensive chemical investigation of these sugars has been the subject of several reviews (386–388). The macrolide antibiotics and their

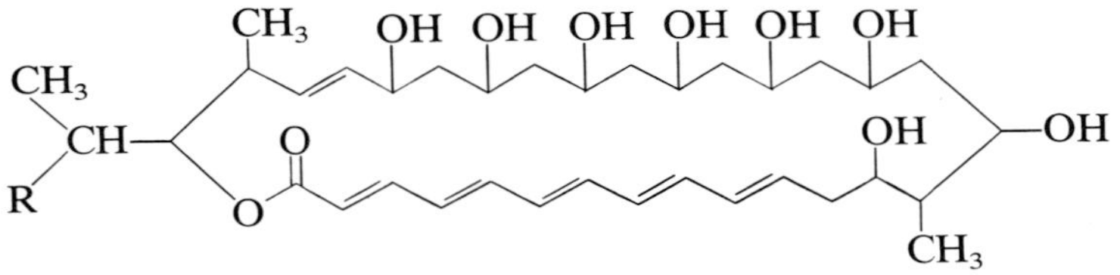

Fig. 16.34 Structure of mycoticin: *a*, $R=CH_3$; *b*, $R=C_2H_5$.

Table 16.8 Properties of Some Macrolide Antibacterial Antibiotics

Name	Organism Producing Antibiotic	Number of Atoms in Macrolide Ring	Empirical Formula	Reference
Acumycin	*Streptomyces giseoflavus*		$C_{38}H_{61}NO_{12}$	355
Aldgamycin C	*S. lavendulae*		$C_{36}H_{60}O_{14}$	356
Amaromycin	*S. flavochromogenes*		$C_{25}H_{36}NO_{18}$	357
Angolamycin	*S. eurythermus*		$C_{50-1}H_{89-2}NO_{18}$	358
Bandamycin A	*S. goshikiensis*		Not reported	359
Bandamycin B	*S. goshikiensis*		Not reported	359
Carbomycin A	*S. halstedii*	16	$C_{42}H_{67}NO_{16}$	360
Carbomycin B	*S. halstedii*	16	$C_{42}H_{67}NO_{15}$	361
Chalcomycin	*S. bikiniensis*	16	$C_{35}H_{56}O_{14}$	362
Cirramycin A	*S. cirratus*		$C_{27}H_{45}NO_{8}$	363
Cirramycin B	*S. cirratus*		$C_{36}H_{59}NO_{12}$	364
Erythromycin A	*S. erythreus*	14	$C_{37}H_{67}NO_{13}$	365
Erythromycin B	*S. erythreus*	14	$C_{37}H_{67}NO_{12}$	366
Erythromycin C	*S. erythreus*	14	$C_{36}H_{65}NO_{13}$	367
Lankamycin	*S. violaceoniger*	14	$C_{42}H_{72}O_{16}$	368
Leucomycin A_1	*S. kitasatoensis*		$C_{46}H_{81}NO_{17}$	369
Leucomycin B_1	*S. kitasatoensis*		$C_{35}H_{59}NO_{13}$	370
Methymycin	*Streptomyces* M-2140	12	$C_{25}H_{43}NO_{7}$	371
Narbomycin	*S. narbonensis*	14	$C_{28}H_{47}NO_{7}$	372
Neomethymycin	*Streptomyces* M-2140	12	$C_{25}H_{43}NO_{7}$	373
Neutramycin	*S. rimosus*		$C_{34}H_{54}O_{14}$	374
Niddamycin	*S. djakartensis*	16	$C_{40}H_{65}NO_{14}$	375
Pikromycin (proactinomycin A)	*S. felleus*	12	$C_{25}H_{43}NO_{7}$	376
Proactinomycin	*Nocardia gardneri*	12	$C_{24}H_{41}NO_{6}$	377
Relomycin	*S. hygroscopicus*	14	$C_{45}H_{79}NO_{17}$	378
Shincomycin A	*S. flavochromogenes*		$C_{52}H_{89}NO_{19}$	379
Spiramycin A	*S. ambofaciens*	17	$C_{43}H_{74}N_2O_{14}$	380
Spiramycin B	*S. ambofaciens*	17	$C_{45}H_{76}N_2O_{15}$	381
Spiramycin C	*S. ambofaciens*	17	$C_{46}H_{78}N_2O_{15}$	382
Tertiomycin A	*S. albireticuli*		$C_{42}H_{69}NO_{16}$	383
Tertiomycin B	*S. albireticuli*		$C_{43}H_{77}NO_{17}$	384
Tylosin	*S. fradiae*		$C_{45}H_{77}NO_{17}$	385

mechanism of action have also been reviewed (389, 390).

Recent progress in macrolide synthesis by Masamune has been published (390a).

4.1 Methymycin

Methymycin is produced by an unidentified *streptomycete*. It possesses a basic character

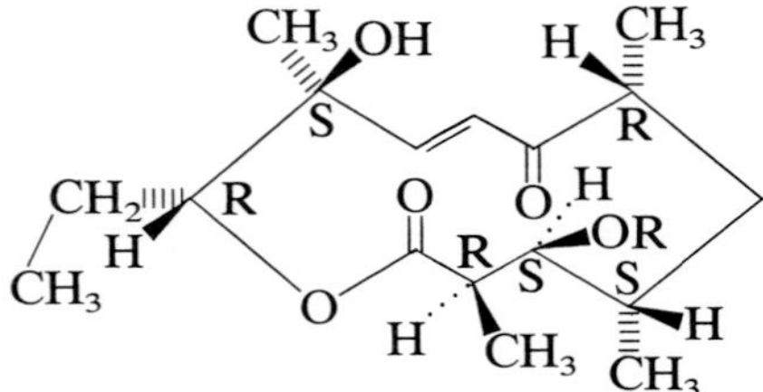

Fig. 16.35 Structure of methinolide (R = H) and methymycin [R = β-desosaminyl].

Table 16.9 Some Sugars Found in the Macrolide Antibiotics

Sugar	Antibiotic Origin	Empirical Formula	Structural Formula
L-Cladinose	Erythromycin	$C_8H_{16}O_4$	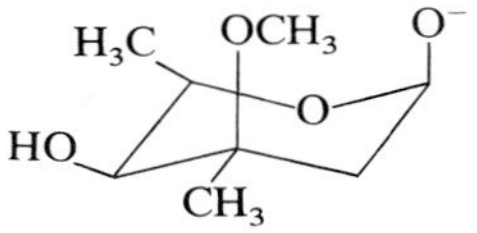 H₃C, OCH₃, O⁻, O, HO, CH₃
L-Arcanose	Lankamycin	$C_8H_{16}O_4$	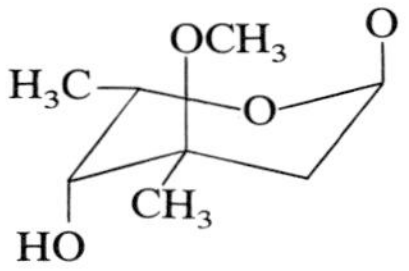 OCH₃, O, H₃C, O, CH₃, HO
L-Mycarose	Carbomycin, tylosin, spiramycin, leucomycin, erythromycin C, angolamycin	$C_7H_{14}O_4$	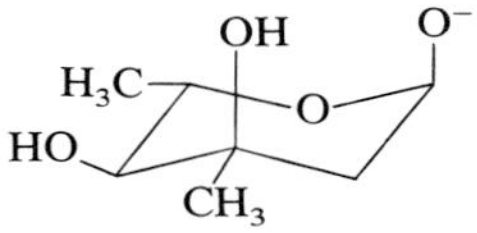 OH, O⁻, H₃C, O, HO, CH₃
L-Oleandrose	Oleandomycin	$C_7H_{14}O_4$	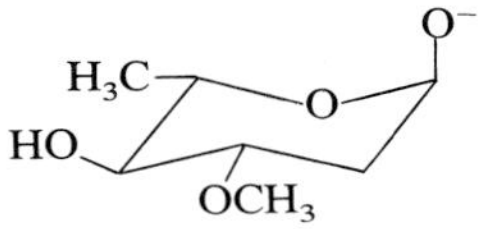 O⁻, H₃C, O, HO, OCH₃
D-Chalcose (lankavose)	Chalcomycin, lankamycin	$C_7H_{14}O_4$	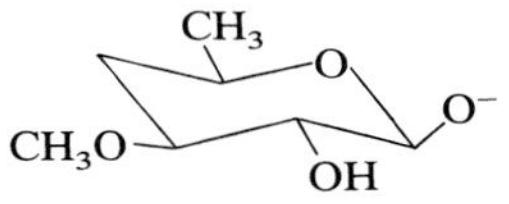 CH₃, O, O⁻, CH₃O, OH
D-Mycinose	Chalcomycin, tylosin	$C_8H_{16}O_5$	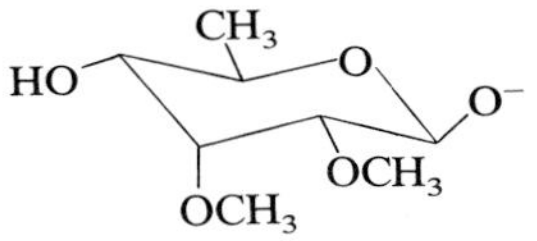 CH₃, HO, O, O⁻, OCH₃, OCH₃
D-Desosamine	Erythromycins A, B, C; methymycin, narbomycin, neomethymycin, oleandomycin, pikromycin	$C_8H_{17}NO_3$	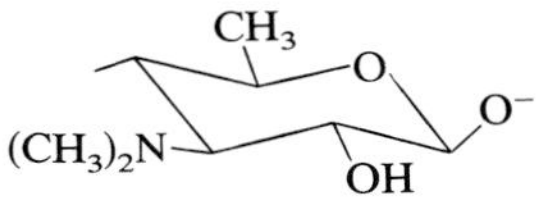 CH₃, O, O⁻, (CH₃)₂N, OH
D-Mycaminose	Carbomycin, leucomycin, spiramycin, tylosin	$C_8H_{17}NO_4$	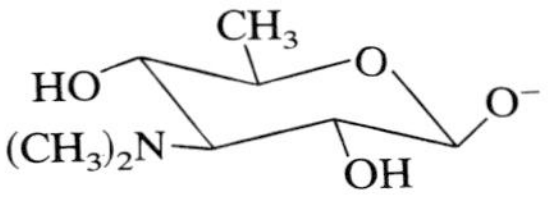 CH₃, O, HO, O⁻, (CH₃)₂N, OH
D-Forosamine	Spiramycin	$C_8H_{17}NO_2$	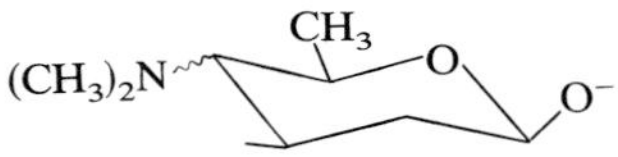 CH₃, O, (CH₃)₂N, O⁻

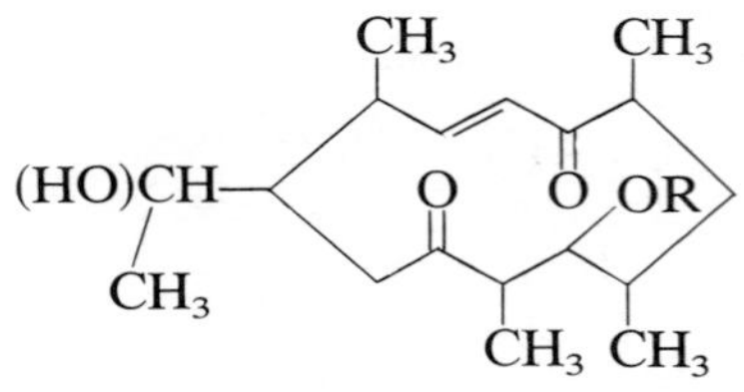

Fig. 16.36 Structure of neomethymycin.

and gives mono salts. Heating briefly in 5*N* hydrochloric acid cleaves off a sugar, identified as desosamine and the aglycone methinolide. The structures are represented in Fig. 16.35 (391–393).

Methymycin is accompanied in the culture filtrate by an isomer, neomethymycin (Fig. 16.36) (391) and a third isomer, 10-desoxymethymycin (394).

4.2 Picromycin

Picromycin (or albomycetin or amaromycin) presents the same antibiotic properties as methymycin, but is relatively toxic. By acid hydrolysis picromycin yields desosamine and the aglycone kromycin. Studies (395, 396) have shown that its structure (Fig. 16.37) is similar to that of narbomycin: it is a glycoside of hydroxynarbocine (397).

Picromycin has been synthesized from narbonolide (398).

4.3 Lancamycin

Lancamycin is produced by *Streptomyces violaceoniger*. It lacks nitrogen and is not

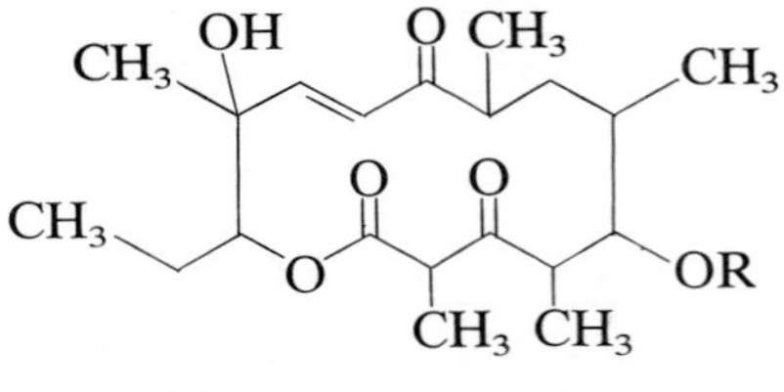

Fig. 16.37 Structure of picromycin (R = desosaminyl).

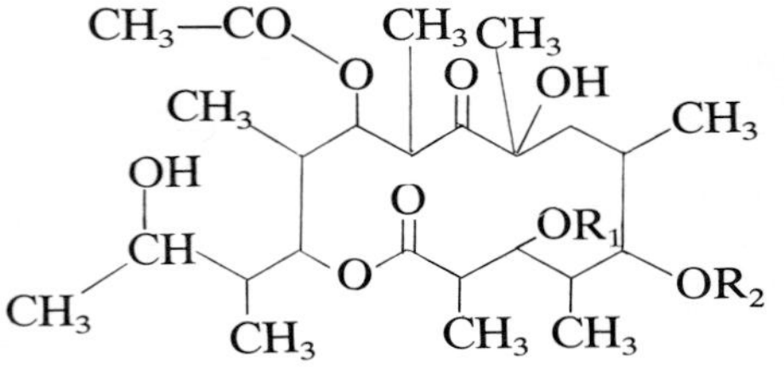

Fig. 16.38 Structure of lancamycin: R_1 = 4-acetylarcanose; R_2 = lancavose.

basic, as the macrolides usually are. Upon acid hydrolysis it liberates two sugars: lancavose (identical with chalcose) and 4-acetylarcanose. Its structure is represented in Fig. 16.38 (399).

A new macrolide antibiotic, 3″-de-*O*-methyl-2″, 3″-anhydro-lancamycin, has been isolated from *S. Violaceoniger* (400).

4.4 Oleandomycin

Oleandomycin has been isolated from *Streptomyces antibioticus*; it is basic because of its amino sugar and shows synergistic action with tetracycline (LD_{50}: 550 mg/kg mouse, i.v.). Acid hydrolysis yields two sugars: oleandrose (α-glycosidically bound) and D-desosamine (β-glycosidically bound). Its structure and its stereochemistry have been established (Fig. 16.39) (401–403). Oleandomycin is used against infections by organisms that are resistant to other antibiotics, in particular, infections of the biliary and urinary tracts.

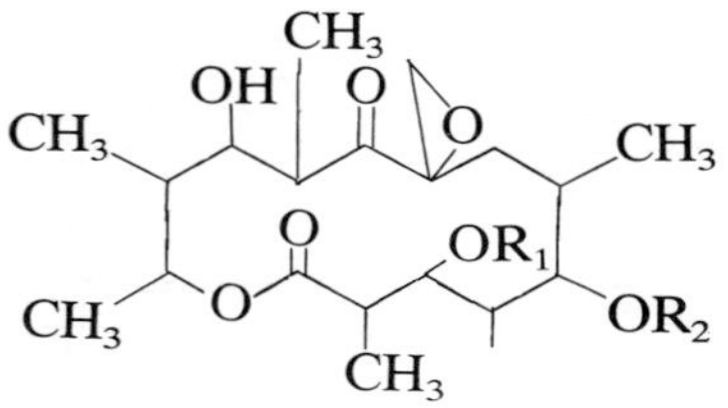

Fig. 16.39 Structure of oleandomycin: $R_1 = \alpha$-L-oleandrose; $R_2 = \beta$-D-desosamine.

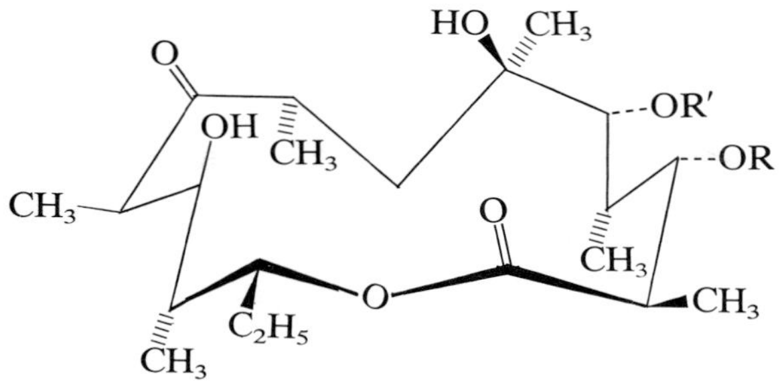

Fig. 16.40 Structure of erythromycin A_1 : R = cladinose, R′ = desosamine.

4.5 Erythromycin

From the filtrate of a *Streptomyces erythreus* culture, an antibiotic fraction is isolated that can be separated into erythromycins A, B, and C. Erythromycin A is a much used antibiotic, especially against gram-positive bacteria, such as staphylococci resistant to penicillin. Its toxicity is relatively low (LD_{50}: 1800 mg/kg, mouse, s.c.). By careful acid hydrolysis it liberates the sugar eladinose; more drastic hydrolysis yields the basic sugar desosamine. The stereochemistry (404) and the nature of the glycosidic bonds (405) have been established. The stereo structure of erythromycin A is represented in Fig. 16.40 (406), Erythromycin B contains one oxygen less than erythromycin A (Fig. 16.41). Erythromycin C differs from erythromycin A by replacement of cladinose by nonmethoxylated mycarose.

The erythromycins and their mechanism of action have been recently reviewed (407, 408). Erythromycin, as well as other macrolide antibiotics, inhibits protein synthesis by binding to 50 S ribosomal subunits of sensitive microorganisms. Erythromycin can interfere with the binding of chloramphenicol, which also acts at this site. The association between erythromycin and the ribosomes is reversible but takes place only when the 50 S subunit is free from tRNA molecules bearing nascent peptide chains. The production of small peptides goes on normally in the presence of the antibiotic, but that of highly polymerized homopeptides is suppressed. Gram-positive bacteria accumulate about 100 times more erythromycin than do gram-negative organisms (409–413). The effect of leukomycins and analogs on binding [^{14}C]-erythromycin to *E. coli* ribosomes has been studied (414). Oxime derivatives of erythromycin inhibit Rous Sarcoma virus reverse transcriptase activity and focus formation (415).

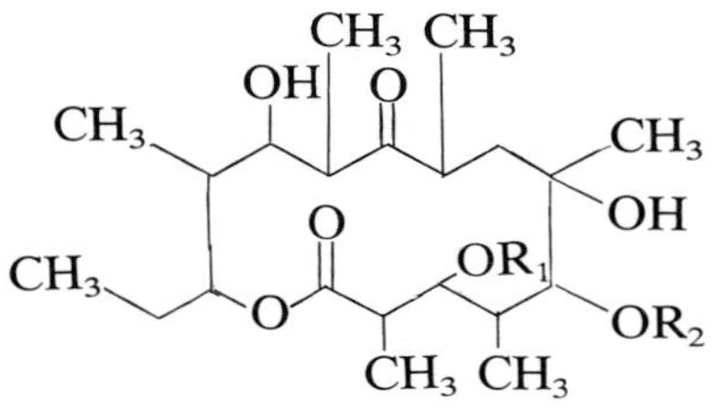

Fig. 16.41 Structure of erythromycin B : R_1 = cladinose, R_2 = desosamine.

The conformation and conformational flexibility of erythronolide, the 14-membered aglycon ring of the erythromycins, have been investigated (416, 417).

Erythromycin antibiotics have been chemically modified, and structure-activity relationships have been studied (418).

4.6 Carbomycin

This antibiotic is isolated from *Streptomyces halstedii* and is better known under the

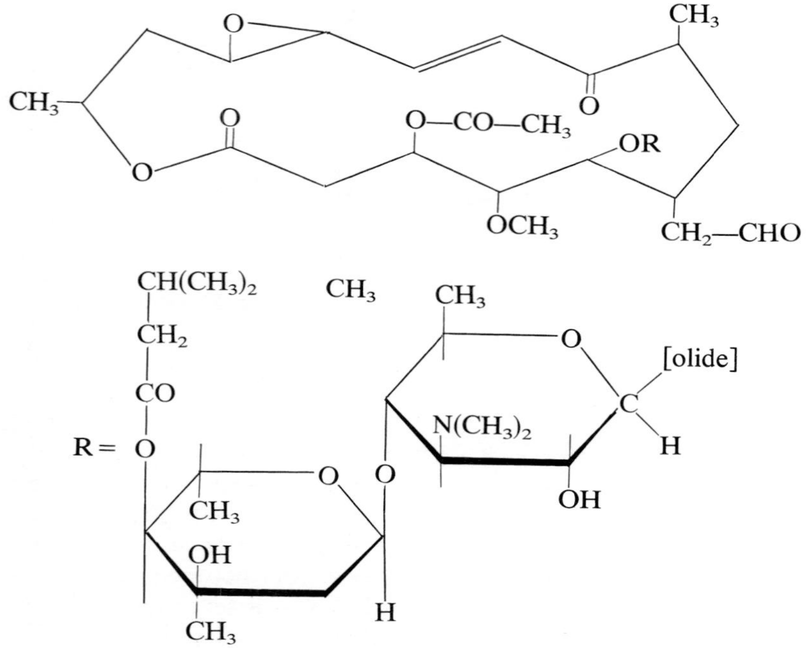

Fig. 16.42 Structure of carbomycin.

commercial name Magnamycin. It is active against gram-positive bacteria, gram-negative cocci, amebas, and some rickettsiae (LD_{50}: 550 mg/kg, mouse, i.v.; 3500 mg/kg, mouse, p.o.). Carbomycin possesses 2 molecules of sugar in the form of a disaccharide (Fig. 16.42) (419–421). Treatment of carbomycin with potassium iodide in acetic acid transforms the epoxide into a double bond, leading to a compound identical with natural carbomycin B (422).

4.7 Spiramycins

These antibiotics are isolated simultaneously under the name of foromacidins. They are produced by *Streptomyces* and are separated into three very similar compounds, spiramycins A, B, and C (423, 424). Hydrolysis yields three sugars: mycarose, mycaminose, and forosamine (isomycamine) (425). The structures appear in Fig. 16.43 (426–428).

4.8 Chalcomycin

Chalcomycin is produced by an unidentified *Streptomyces* and contains the sugars mycinose and chalcose (or lankavose) (Fig. 16.44) (429). Chalcomycin has been reviewed (430).

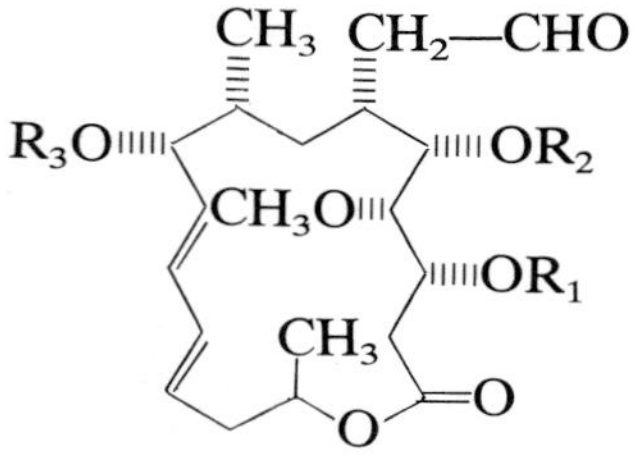

Fig. 16.43 Structure of spiramycins. Spiramycin S, A: R_1=H; B: R_1=CO—CH_3; C: R_1=CO—CH_2—CH_3; R_2 = mycaroside of mycaminose; R_3 = forosamine.

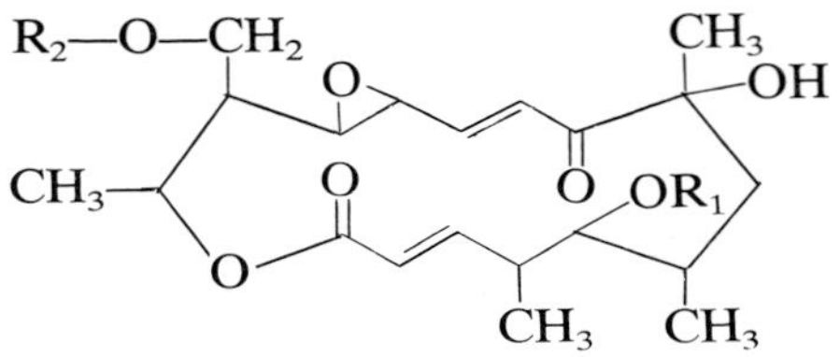

Fig. 16.44 Structure of chalcomycin: R_1 = chalcose, R_2 = mycinose.

4.9 Borrelidin

Borrelidin, represented in Fig. 16.45, has been isolated from *Streptomyces rochei.* It

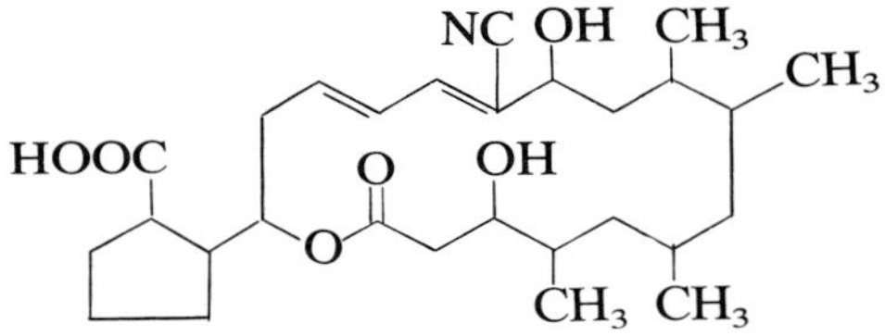

Fig. 16.45 Structure of borrelidin.

has a strong *in vitro* activity against *Coryne bacterium* species and certain viruses and has been reviewed (432).

4.10 Tylosin

Tylosin is produced by *Streptomyces fradiae.* It has three typical macrolide sugars: mycarose, mycaminose, and mycinose. Figure 16.46 shows its structure (433).

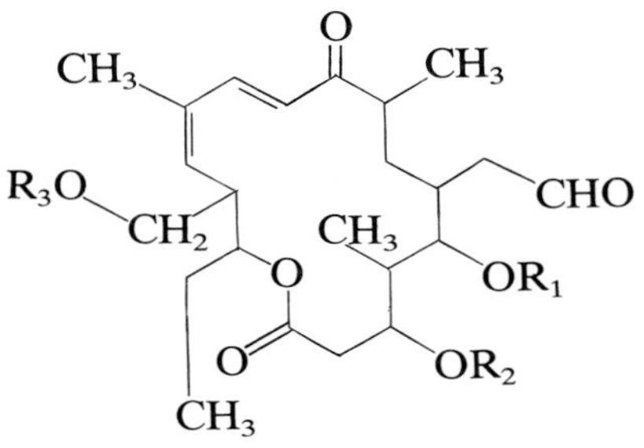

Fig. 16.46 Structure of tylosin: R_1, R_2 = H, or mycarosyl-mycaminosyl; R_3 = mycinosyl.

4.11 Angolamycin

Produced by an actinomycete, angolamycin is an antibiotic active against gram-positive bacteria. It contains the sugars L-mycarose, D-mycinose, and angolosamine (434).

4.12 Nonactin

This compound (Fig. 16.47), produced by streptomycetes, possesses a large antibiotic spectrum and recently has been synthesized (435). The mechanism of action has been reviewed (436). Nonactin can transport K^+ ions across a membrane. Its antibiotic activity is probably due to its interference with ion transport phenomena.

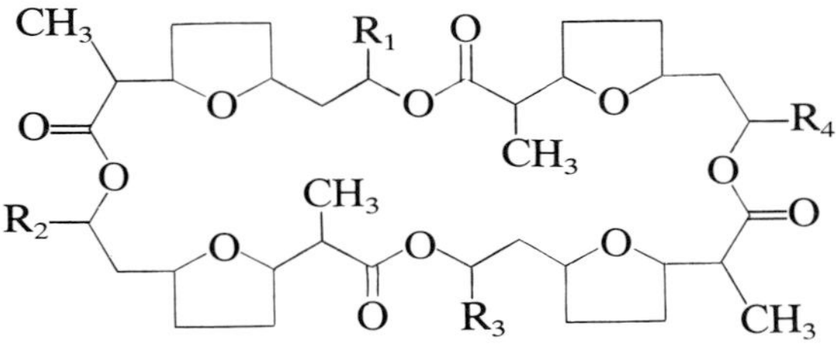

Fig. 16.47 Structure of nonactin: $R_1 = R_2 = R_3 = R_4 = CH_3$.

4.13 Oligomycins

Oligomycins, produced by *Streptomyces diastatochromogenes,* are essentially antifungal. They are rather toxic (LD_{50}: 1.5 mg/kg, mouse, i.v.). Oligomycins have been separated into three components (437). Oligomycin A contains five methyl groups. Oligomycin B (Fig. 16.48) shows the absence of a sugar. Its structure has been established by X-ray diffraction (438). Oligomycin C has six methyl groups.

The mechanism of action of the oligomycins has been reviewed (439). They inhibit oxidative phosphorylation. Presumably this inhibition is caused by blocking at the level of the reaction:

$$X{\sim}I + Pi \rightleftarrows X{\sim}P + I$$

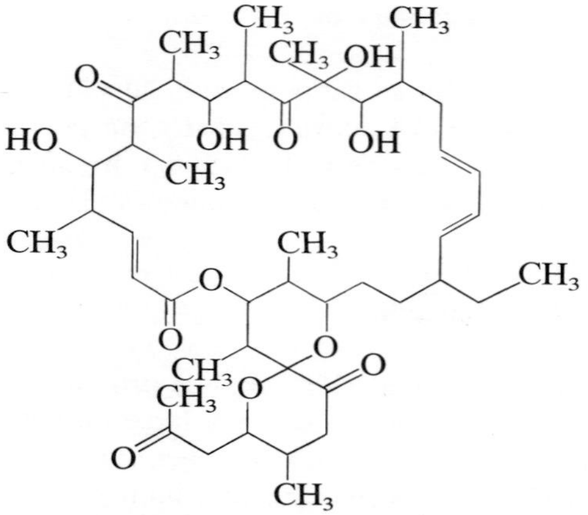

Fig. 16.48 Structure of oligomycin B.

without provoking decoupling. The ATPase activity in relation to the coupling process in the entire mitochondria is inhibited by oligomycin. The coupling factor F_1 presents an ATPase activity that is insensitive to oligomycin. From F_1 one can obtain a reconstitution of a system in which the sensitivity of the ATPase activity to oligomucin is restored by the F_C factor (440–442), which corresponds to the partially purified OSCP factor (443, 444). This factor could be the target of the antibiotic.

Oligomycin interacts with the pathway of mitochondrial energy transfer (445).

4.14 Maridomycin

A new macrolide antibiotic, maridomycin, which is mainly active against gram-positive bacteria, was isolated from a culture filtrate of *Streptomyces hygroscopicus* (446—448).

4.15 XK-41 Complex

The antibiotic XK-41 complex, isolated from a *Micromonospora* species, consists of five major components, A, B, C_1, C_2, and 4″-propionylmegalomicin A, depicted in Fig. 16.49 (449).

5 AMINOGLYCOSIDE ANTIBIOTICS

The streptomycins, neomycins, paromomycins, gentamicins, and kanamycins, which comprise the aminoglycoside group of clinically important antibiotics, have many

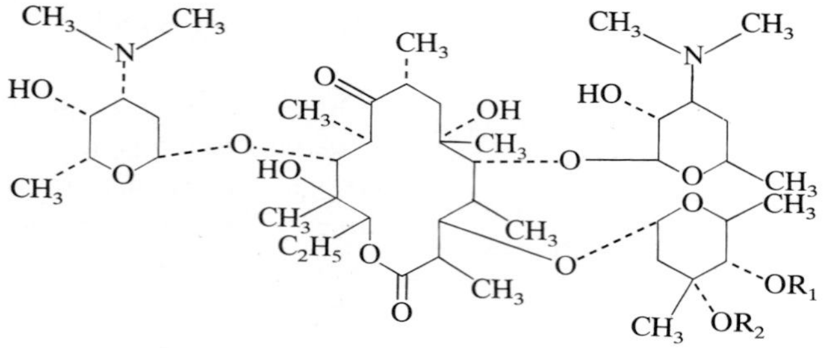

Component	Empirical Formula	R_1	R_2	Designation
XK-41-A	$C_{49}H_{86}N_2O_{17}$	CH_3CH_2CO—	CH_3CO-	Megalomicin C_2
XK-41-A_2	$C_{48}H_{84}N_2O_{17}$	CH_3CO—	CH_3CO—	Megalomicin C_1
XK-41-B_1	$C_{46}H_{82}N_2O_{16}$	CH_3CO—	H—	Megalomicin B
XK-41-B_2	$C_{47}H_{84}N_2O_{16}$	CH_3CH_2CO—	H—	—
XK-41-C	$C_{44}H_{80}N_2O_{15}$	H—	H—	Megalomicin A

Fig. 16.49 Structures of the components of the XK–41 complex.

chemical and antimicrobial features in common: they are all mixtures of closely related, water-soluble, basic carbohydrates that form crystalline salts. The streptomycins contain streptidine, which is a diguanidyl derivative of a 1,3-diaminohexose (streptamine), and each of the other members of the group listed in Table 16.10 contains a 2-deoxystreptamine or related unit. All these antibiotics show antimicrobial activity, and paromomycin also inhibits *Entameba histolytica.* None of the aminoglycoside antibiotics is absorbed from the alimentary tract, and neomycin has been used widely in the treatment of intestinal infections and chemosterilization of the bowel prior to surgery of that organ. Aminoglycosides and their mode of action have been reviewed recently (469).

The structure-activity relationships among the aminoglycosides, especially the role of hydroxyl and amino groups, have been studied (470).

5.1 Streptomycin

Streptomycin, the first antibiotic discovered in this group and the most important from the point of view of practical applications was isolated from *Streptomyces griseus* (471). Streptomycin is active against gram-positive and gram-negative bacteria as well as mycobacteria and spirochetes. Since *S. griseus* is sensitive to streptomycin, the producing cultures must be resistant (472).

Streptomycin (Fig. 16.50) contains three basic groups and forms a trihydrochloride. The drug has three components: streptidine, streptose, and *N*-methyl-L-glucosamine. The nature of the glycosidic linkages has been elucidated (473). Streptomycin has been synthesized (474).

Certain strains of *Streptomyces* (in particular *S. humidus*) produce a streptomycin in which the free aldehyde group of the streptose residue has been reduced to a primary alcohol. This transformation can also be carried out by catalytic hydrogenation. The antibiotic activity of dihydrostreptomycin is comparable to that of streptomycin, with the advantage that it is stable in alkaline media. Streptomycin, dihydrostreptomycin, and their mechanisms of action have been recently reviewed (475). Dihydrostreptomycin has an effect on the ribosome function (476, 477).

Streptomycin and other aminoglycosides act directly on the ribosome, where they inhibit protein biosynthesis and decrease the fidelity of translation of the genetic code. The major result of streptomycin action appears to be the prevention of amino acid polymerization after formation of the initiation complex (478). The site of action of streptomycin is the 30 S ribosomal subunit, and mutations in the gene coding for a specific protein of this subunit (P10) control the binding of the antibiotic to the ribosome and the sensitivity of the microorganism to the drug (479). Although isolated P10 does not itself bind to streptomycin, this protein appears to form a crucial portion of the binding site or to control access of the drug to such a site.

The binding of streptomycin to sensitive ribosomes also causes misreading of the genetic code, perhaps by causing distortion of critical components of the protein synthetic apparatus. Thus specific aminoacyl tRNA may fail to recognize its proper codon on mRNA, with the result that incorrect amino acids are inserted into the peptide chain (480). Although misreading was originally thought to account for the *lethal* action of aminoglycosides on bacteria, this does not appear to be the case; the bactericidal property of the aminoglycosides is still unexplained.

Misreading of the genetic code may, however, account for the phenomenon of bacterial *dependence* on streptomycin, a condition that may be acquired as a single-step mutational event. If there is a mutation at some other site in the bacterial genome that would effectively prevent

Table 16.10 Relationships Among the Aminoglycoside Antibacterial Antibiotics

Name	Synonyms or Closely Related Compounds	Source	Chemical Features		Reference
			Base	Amino Sugar	
Aminosidin	Catenulin, hydroxymycin, paromomycin	*Streptomyces chrestomyceticus*	Deoxystreptamine	Unidentified	450
Bluensomycin	U-12898	*S. bluensis* var. *bluensis*	Bluensidin	L-*N*-Methylglucosamine	451
Gentamicin A		*Micromonospora purpurea*	Deoxystreptamine	2-Amino-2-deoxy-glucose, 3-*N*-methyl-3-deoxyglucose	452
Gentamicin C_1		*M. purpurea*	Deoxystreptamine	Garosamine	453
Gentamicin C_2		*M. purpurea*	Deoxystreptamine	Unknown	454
Glebomycin		*S. hygroscopicus* forma *glebosus f. nov.*	(Unknown; gives Sakaguchi test)		455
Hygromycin	Homomycin 17-3-18B	*S. hygroscopicus*	Neoinosamine-2	Unknown	456
Hygromycin B		*S. hygroscopicus*	Neoinosamine-2	Unknown	457
Kanamycin A		*S. kanamyceticus*	Deoxystreptamine	3-Aminoglucose, 6-aminoglucose	458
Kanamycin B		*S. kanamyceticus*	Deoxystreptamine	3-Aminoglucose, plus unknown amino sugar	459
Kanamycin C		*S. kanamyceticus*	Deoxystreptamine	3-Aminoglucose, D-glucosamine	460

Neomycin B	Streptothricin B I	*S. fradiae*	Deoxystreptamine	2,6-Diaminoglucose, neosamine B	461
Neomycin C	Streptothricin B II	*S. fradiae*	Deoxystreptamine	2,6-Diaminoglucose, neosamine C	462
Paromomycin I	Zygomycin A_1, monomycin	*S. rimosus forma paromomycinus S. pulveraceus*	Deoxystreptamine	D-Glucosamine, neosamine B	463
Paromomycin II	Zygomycin A_2	*S. rimosus* forma *paromomycinus, S. pulveraceus*	Deoxystreptamine	D-Glucosamine, neosamine C	464
Streptomycins					
Streptomycin	Streptomycin A	*S. griseus, S. mashuensis*	Streptidine	L-*N*-Methylglucosamine	465
Mannosidostreptomycin	Streptomycin B	*S. griseus, S. bikiniensis*	Streptidine	L-*N*-Methylglucosamine	466
Hydroxystreptomycin	Reticulin	*S. griseocarneus, S. reticuli*	Streptidine	L-*N*-Methylglucosamine	467
Dihydrostreptomycin		*S. humidus*, also produced by chemical reduction of streptomycin	Streptidine	L-*N*-Methylglucosamine	468

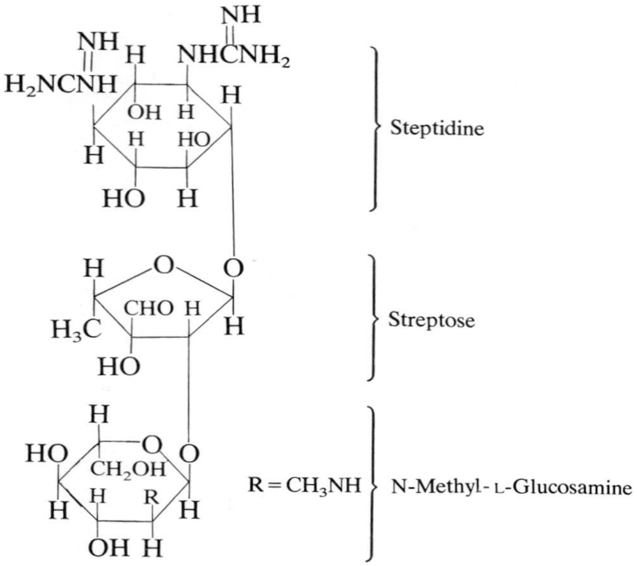

Fig. 16.50 Structure of streptomycin.

growth (e.g., an amino acid substitution in a protein essential for normal metabolism), streptomycin-induced misreading of the mutation could result in an acceptable correction of the defect (phenotypic suppression). Bacteria could then resume growth only in the presence of the aminoglycoside. The prolonged use of streptomycin may lead to a permanent damage of the eighth cranial nerve. Damage to the auditory branch is associated with permanent impairment of hearing and vestibular damage, with equilibrium problems. Because of these limitations, streptomycin is often regarded only as an adjunct to the nonchemotherapeutic forms of treatment of tuberculosis. Dihydrostreptomycin affects the auditory branch of the eighth nerve, whereas streptomycin appears to be more toxic for the vestibular branch.

5.2 Kanamycin

This antibiotic, produced by *Streptomyces kanamyceticus*, was discovered by Umezawa in 1957. Less than a year after its isolation, kanamycin was sold industrially.

Kanamycin is tetrabasic and very stable in the pH range 2.0–11.0. It has a large antibiotic spectrum, similar to that of streptomycin. The structure of kanamycin A (Fig. 16.51) was established independently by an American-Canadian group (481) and a Japanese group (482); it has been confirmed by synthesis (483). Kanamycin A is accompanied in the culture filtrate by kanamycin B and kanamycin C (Fig. 16.51). Structure-activity relations in 1-*N*-acylkanamycin have been studied (484). The synthesis and activity of 4′-deoxykanamycin A has been investigated (485). Kanamycin has a broad range of activity against gram-positive and gram-negative microorganisms. Sensitive bacteria include *E. coli*, *Entrobacter* (*Aerobacter*) *aerogenes*, *K. pneumoniae*, *Proteus* species, *Citrobacter* (*Paracolobactum*), *Salmonella*, *Shigella*, *Vibrio*, *Neisseria*, *Crucella*, *M. tuberculosis*, atypical mycobacteria, and *Staphylococcus aureus*. Most strains of

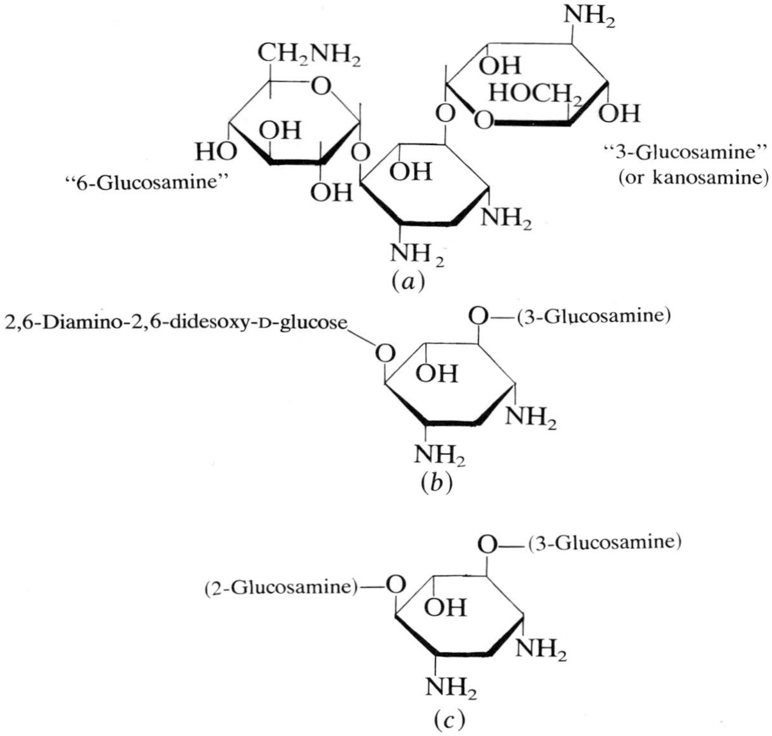

Fig. 16.51 Structures of kanamycins. (*a*) Kanamycin A. (*b*) Kanamycin B. (*c*) Kanamycin C.

staphylococci are inhibited by 1 μg/ml or less; some are suppressed only by concentrations of 2-5 μg/ml. Tubercle bacilli are suppressed by 2.5–10 μg/ml. Pneumococci, *Alcaligenes*, and *Streptomyces pyogenes* are generally insensitive. Resistant microorganisms include *Pseudomonas*, other streptococci, *Bacteroides*, clostridia and other anaerobes, yeast, and fungi (486).

Kanamycin has an effect on protein synthesis (487).

5.3 Paromomycin

This aminoglycoside antibiotic, isolated from cultures of *Streptomyces rimosus*, is amebicidal both *in vitro* and *in vivo*. It acts directly on amebas but is also antibacterial to normal and pathogenic microorganisms in the gastrointestinal tract. The structure of paromomycin I is represented in Fig. 16.52 (488). Paromomycin II differs from its I isomer by replacement in the paromobiosamine fragment of diaminodidesoxy-L-idose by 2,6-diamino-2,6-didesoxyglucose, which corresponds to the change of a single asymmetric center in the entire molecule (489).

5.4 Neomycin

In 1949 Waksman and Lechevalier isolated a soil organism, *Streptomyces fradiae*, which produced a new antibiotic that in crude form contained an antifungal compound (fradicin) and a group of antibacterial substances that were labeled "neomycin". Purified in the same year, neomycin was

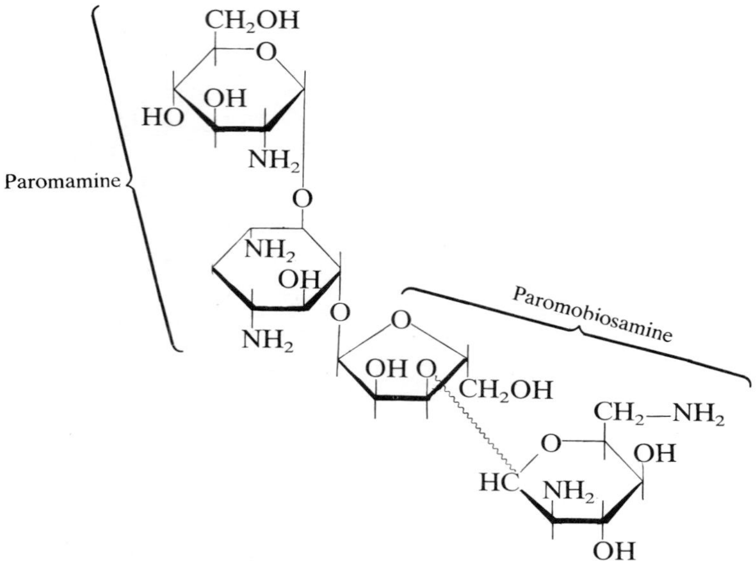

Fig. 16.52 Structure of paromomycin I.

found to be a complex of three components, neomycins A, B, and C, having different antimicrobial activities. Commercial preparations consist almost entirely of neomycin B. Neomycin is a polybasic substance that readily forms salts with a variety of acids. Neomycin A is neamine (deoxystreptamine linked to 2,6-diamino-2,6-dideoxy-D-glucose) (Fig. 16.53) (490). Neomycins B and C are isomeric; each contains neamine and neobiosamine (D-ribose linked to a diaminohexose). Their structures appear in Fig. 16.54 (490).

Neomycin is a broad spectrum antibiotic. Its antimicrobial activity is presumably exerted by a mechanism analogous to that discussed for streptomycin. Susceptible

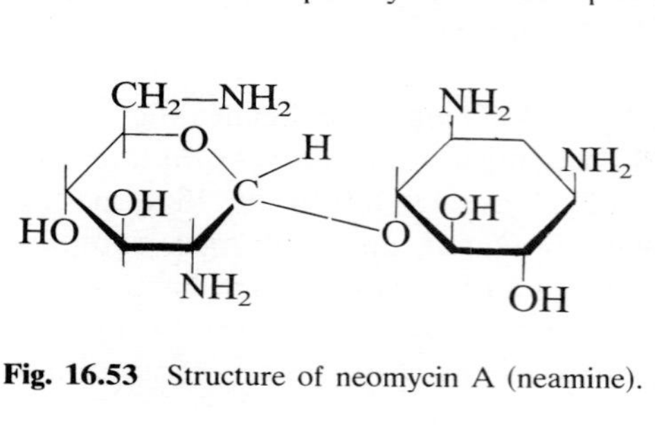

Fig. 16.53 Structure of neomycin A (neamine).

microorganisms are usually inhibited by concentrations of 5–10 μg/ml or less. Gram-negative species that are highly sensitive are *E. coli*, *Enterobacter* (*Aerobacter*) *aerogenes*, *K. pneumonia*, *Pasteurella*, *Proteus vulgaris*, *Salmonella*, *Shigella*, *H. influenza*, *N. meningitidis*, *Viprie cholerae*, and *Bordetella pertussis*. Gram-positive microorganisms that are inhibited include *Bacillus anthracis Corynebacterium diphtheriae*, *Staphylococcus aureus*, *Streptococcus fecalis*, *Listeria monocytogenes*, and *M. tuberculosis*, *Borrelia* and *Leptospira interrogans* (*icterohemorrhagiae*) are also suppressed. The sensitivity of *P. aeruginosa* to neomycin is variable but not very high. Group A *Streptomyces pyogenes*, the *viridans* group of *streptococci*, fungi, and viruses are resistant (491, 492). Neomycin is active against tubercle bacilli, regardless of their susceptibility to streptomycin. Neomycin-resistant microorganisms are less susceptible to streptomycin; cross-resistance is induced to a greater degree by neomycin than by streptomycin. Analytical studies on neomycin have been reviewed.

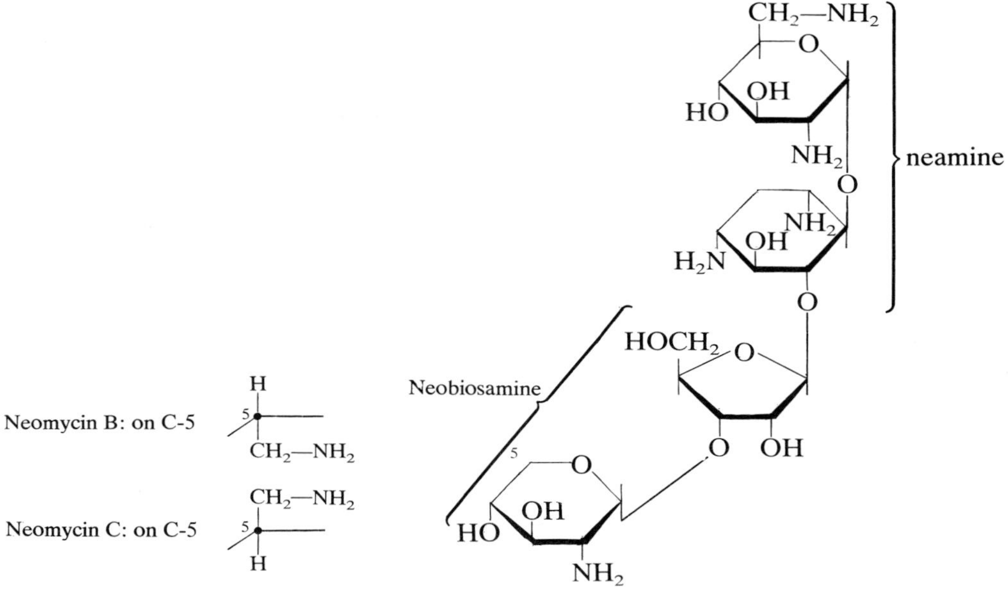

Fig. 16.54 Structures of neomycins B and C.

5.5 Gentamicin

Gentamicin is a broad spectrum antibiotic derived from the actinomycete *Micromonospora purpurea.* The drug was first studied and described by Weinstein in 1963 (494) and isolated, purified, and characterized by Rosselot the following year (495). It is currently of great value in the therapy of severe infections due to gram-negative bacteria, and it is the most important of the aminoglycosides.

Crude gentamicin has been separated into several components. Gentamicin A results from an α-glycosidically bound D-glucosamine and a β-glycosidically bound *N*-methyl-3-amino-3-desoxy-D-xylopyranose (gentosamine) to hydroxyls 4 and 6, respectively, of desoxystreptamine (496, 497). Gentamicins C are glycosides of parosamine and particularly diamino sugars (purpurosamines) with 2-desoxystreptamine (498) (Fig. 16.55). Separation and structure determination of gentamicins A_1, A_2, A_3, and A_4 has been carried out (499).

The three components of gentamicin

Gentamycin

	R_1	R_2
C_1	CH_3	CH_3
C_{1a}	H	H
C_3	CH_3	H

Fig. 16.55 Structure of gentamicins C.

have nearly identical antimicrobial activity *in vitro*. It is generally agreed that about 95% of *P. aeruginosa* are inhibited by 10 μg/ml or less of the drug. *E. coli, Klebsiella,* and *Enterobacter* (*Aerobacter*) are also highly sensitive. Almost all penicillin-sensitive and some methicillin-resistant strains of *S. aureus* are suppressed by a concentration of 5 μg/ml or less. Group A streptococci, *S.* (*D*) *pneumoniae, Pasturella multocida, H. influenzae, Acinetobacter* (*Mina-Herellea* group), and *Bacteroides* are reasonably sensitive to gentamicin. *Serratia* species (nonpigmented) are inhibited by concentrations of 1.5 μg/ml or less. Most strains of indole-negative *Proteus* are highly sensitive; the susceptibility of the indole-producing strains is variable. *Mycobacterium tuberculosis* and *Mycoplasma pneumoniae* are highly sensitive. *Citrobacter* (*Paracolobactrum*), *Proteus inconstans, Salmonella, Shigella, Listeria, Brucella,* and some types of streptococci are variably susceptible. *Neisseria gonorrheae, N. meningitidis, Pseudomonas pseudomallei, Clostridium,* and *Corynebacterium* are relatively resistant. The drug is bactericidal in concentrations 2–3 times those required to produce bacteriostasis (500–503). Gentamicin is more active in alkaline media. The concentration of divalent cations in the medium alters the results of sensitivity tests of *P. aeruginosa* to the drug (504). Although heparin decreases the antimicrobial activity of gentamicin, the concentration of heparin in the blood of patients given this agent for anticoagulation is too low to produce this effect (505). The antibacterial activity of gentamicin appears to be additive with ampicillin or kanamycin against *Proteus,* and with colistin against *Pseudomonas.* A supra-additive effect is produced by a combination of gentamicin with cephalothin or penicillin against enterococci, and with carbenicillin against gram-negative bacilli. However this varies with the bacterial species and even with individual strains (506–509). The combination of carbenicillin and gentamicin is highly effective for experimental *Pseudomonas* infection in rats. Concurrent use of chloramphenicol or a tetracycline with gentamicin may lead to a reduction in antimicrobial efficacy (510, 511).

Gentamicin and its mode of action, which is quantitatively similar to that of the other aminoglycoside antibiotics, have been recently reviewed (475).

6 TETRACYCLINES

The development of the tetracycline antibiotics was the result of a systematic screening, for antibiotic-producing microorganisms, of soil specimens collected from many parts of the world. The first of these compounds, chlortetracycline, was introduced in 1948. Two years later oxytetracycline became available. Elucidation of the chemical structure of these agents confirmed their similarity and furnished the basis for the production of a third member of this group, tetracycline, in 1952. In 1957 a new family of tetracyclines was developed, characterized chemically by the absence of the ring-attached methyl group present in the others. One of these, demethylchlortetracycline, subsequently given the official name demeclocycline, became available for general use in 1959. The next compound to appear was rolitetracycline, a soluble derivative of tetracycline. Other congeners, certain of which have useful properties, have continued to be developed: methacycline, a derivative of oxytetracycline, was introduced in 1961; doxycycline became available in 1966, and minocycline in 1972.

Soon after their initial development, the tetracyclines were found to be highly effective against rickettsiae, a number of gram-positive and gram-negative bacteria, and the agents responsible for lymphogranuloma venereum, inclusion conjunctivitis, and psittacosis; hence they became

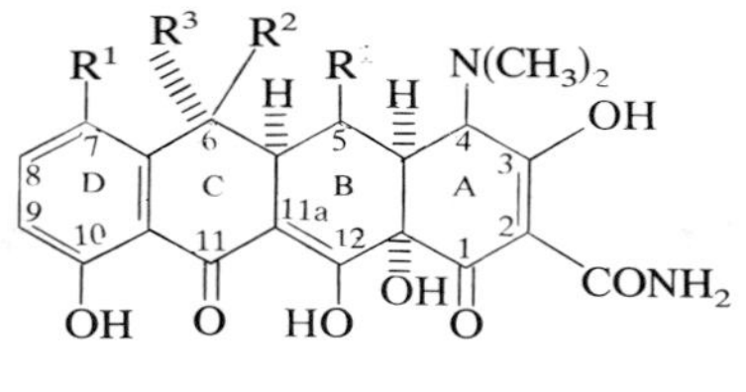

Name	R^1	R^2	R^3	R^4	Other games
Tetracycline	H	OH	CH_3	H	Achromycin
7-Chlortetracycline	H	OH	CH_3	Cl	Aureomycin
5-Oxytetracycline	OH	OH	CH_3	H	Terramycin
6-Demethyl-7-chloro tetracycline	H	OH	H	Cl	Declomycin, demeclocycline
6-Demethyl-6-deoxy 5-hydroxy-6-methylene tetracycline	OH		$=CH_2$	H	Methacycline
6-Deoxy-5-oxytetra cycline	OH	H	CH_3	H	Doxycycline
Rolitetracycline	H	OH	CH_3	H	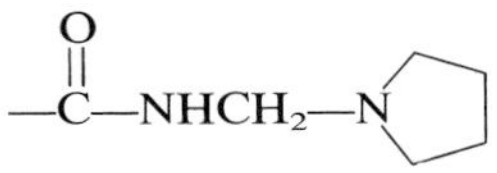 —C(=O)—$NHCH_2$—N(pyrrolidine) at position 2
Minocycline	H	H	H	$N(CH_3)_2$	

Fig. 16.56 Structures of tetracyclines.

known as "broad spectrum" antibiotics. With establishment of their *in vitro* antimicrobial activity, effectiveness in experimental infections, pharmacological properties, the tetracyclines rapidly gained wide use in therapy (512–514).

Chlortetracycline and oxytetracycline are elaborated by *Streptomyces aureofaciens* and *S. rimosus*, respectively. Tetracycline is produced semisynthetically from chlortetracycline; it had also been obtained from a species of *Streptomyces*. Demeclocycline is the product of a mutant of the strain *S. aureofaciens* from which chlortetracycline was first obtained. Rolitetracycline, methacycline, doxocycline, and minocycline are all semisynthetic derivatives.

The tetracyclines are closely congeneric derivatives of the tetracyclic naphthacene carboxamide. Their structural formulas appear in Fig. 16.56.

Streptomyces flavovirens produces an antibiotic pillaromycin A that consists of an aglycone related to the tetracyclines with an unusual sugar (Fig. 16.57) (515).

The tetracyclines have been reviewed several times in recent years (516–520). An excellent review on structure-activity relations has been published (521).

Recent investigations into the mode of action of the tetracyclines (522, 523) lend support to previous observations (524–526) that they inhibit the protein synthesis of

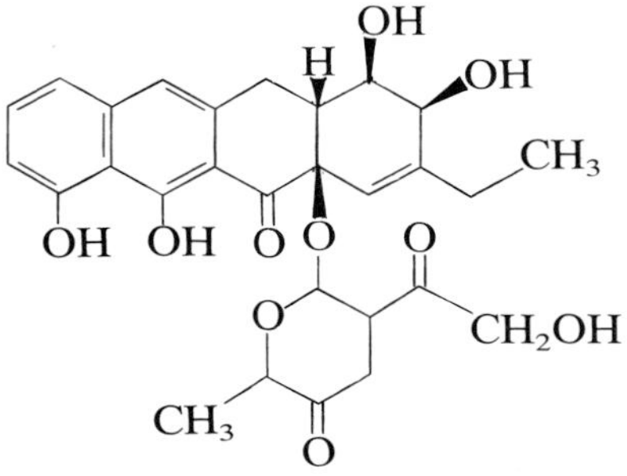

Fig. 16.57 Structure of pillaromycin A.

sensitive bacteria. This inhibition is reported to interfere with a variety of biochemical systems: cell wall synthesis (527), biosynthesis of bacterial respiratory systems (516), and similar systems (528).

Current views on the mechanisms of protein synthesis propose that these biochemical reactions occur on the ribosomes. Addition of a tetracycline molecule to the protein synthesizing system on the ribosomes prevents the approach of the aminoacyl-tRNA to the ribosome site, with a resultant break in the normal protein synthesis of a pathogenic organism (529, 530). Although there is good evidence (531) that this interference with protein synthesis is the primary mechanism of tetracycline antibacterial action, other unrelated reactions are affected by the presence of a tetracycline molecule. The process (532) by which peptides are released from the transferring RNA when synthesis is completed appears to be inhibited by the tetracyclines and tetracyclines block the exchange reaction between ribosomal subunits (533).

7 STEROIDAL ANTIBIOTICS

Three steroids show an antibiotic activity mainly against gram-positive bacteria: *Staphylococcus aureus*, *Corynebacterium diphtheriae*, and *Clostridium tetani.*

Helvolic acid (Fig. 16.58) is produced by

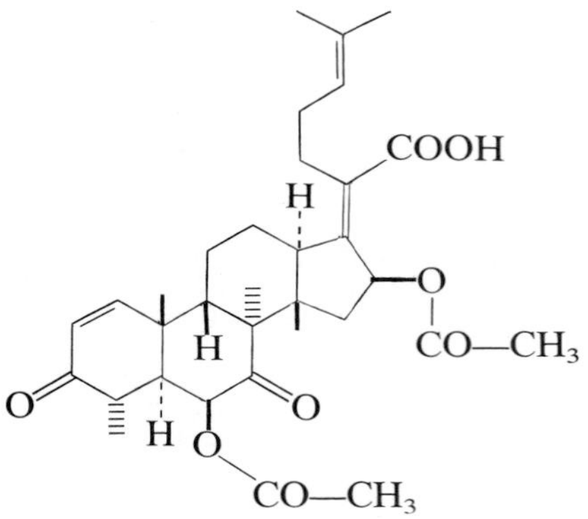

Fig. 16.58 Structure of helvolic acid.

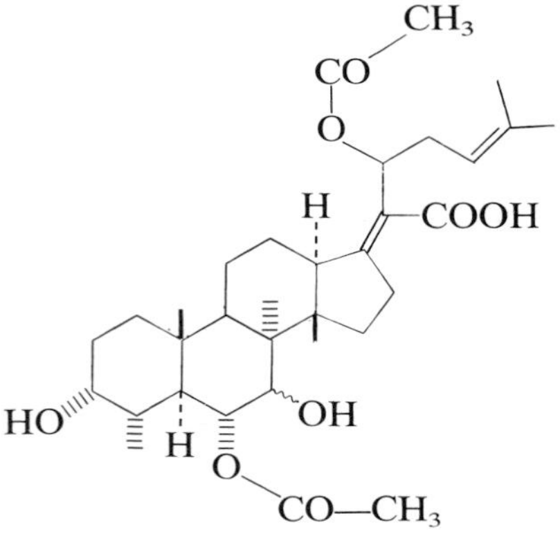

Fig. 16.59 Structure of cephalosporin P_1.

Aspergillus fumigatus (534, 535). Cephalosporin P_1 (Fig. 16.59) is produced by *Cephalosporium synnematum* (536–538).

Fusidic acid (Fig. 16.60), produced by *Fusidium coccineum*, shows a cross-resistance with cephalosporin P_1 (539).

One of the remarkable features of these molecules is the unusual trans-syn-trans-anti-trans stereochemistry, which differs fundamentally from that of steroids, which usually have the trans-anti-trans-anti-trans arrangement. Consequently, ring B of the antibiotics is forced into the boat conformation.

Cephalosporin P_1 is about twice as active as helvolic acid, and fusidic acid is 10 times as active as cephalosporin P_1. These antibiotics are active against gram-positive bacteria in concentration of 0.02–0.2 μg/ml

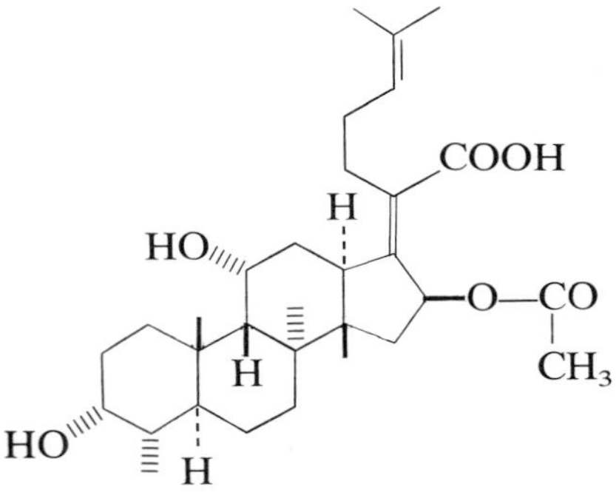

Fig. 16.60 Structure of fusidic acid.

and against *M. tuberculosis* at a concentration of 1 μg/ml. They have relatively low toxicity (fusidic acid, LD_{50}: 200 mg/kg, mouse, i.v.). The antibiotics are inactivated by the bacterial enzyme *P*-cephalosporinase (536). Fusidic acid, the only steroidal antibiotic used therapeutically, is utilized in its sodium salt form (fucidin).

Fusidic acid reversibly inhibits the process of translocation at the level of systems containing procaryote ribosomes as well as eucaryote ribosomes (540–557). *In vitro* as well as with protoplasts, this antibiotic acts by inhibiting the dissociation of the ternary complex formed on the subunit 50 S:50 S-EF_G-GDP. After formation of the 50 S-EF_G-GTP complex, it allows for a hydrolysis cycle, thus a translocation. Consequently, after the formation of the initiation complex, the fixation of the first aminoacyl-tRNA is not inhibited; in the course of the elongation of the polypeptide chain, the peptidyl-tRNAs are blocked at the P position, and the binding of the aminoacyl-tRNA is thus prevented by the 50 S-EF_G-DGP complex. The utilization of this antibiotic has led to an extension of the study of numerous problems concerning the elongation process. Fusidic acid binds to the 50 S ribosome subunit and to the γ-core, which does not contain any more peptidyl transferase (557).

8 ANSAMYCINS

Ansamycins are compounds containing an aromatic ring system spanned (*ansa* = handle) by a long macrocyclic bridge. They were discovered in 1957 (558), and their structure was elucidated in 1963 (559). The rifamycins might easily have escaped detection altogether, since rifamycin B, the compound produced by *Streptomyces mediterranei* sp. n., has no antibacterial activity. However it is readily oxidized to the active compound rifamycin S, which inhibits the growth of gram-positive bacteria at concentrations as low as 0.00025 μg/ml. Rifamycins and other ansamycins have been reviewed recently (560). Recent data indicate that some of the analogs of rifampin and the streptovaricins can significantly suppress cell-mediated immunity and suggest that other ansamycins may have significant immunosuppressant activity (561).

8.1 Rifamycin

The antibiotic rifamycin is produced by *Streptomyces mediterranei.* The crude product shows a strong activity against gram-positive bacteria and mycobacteria. Since it has relatively low toxicity, it offers good protection for infected animals (562, 563). Paper chromatography shows that this antibiotic is a mixture of five closely related substances, rifamycins A, B, C, D, and E. If the streptomyces are cultured in a medium to which 0.2% barbital (sodium diethyl barbiturate) has been added, 95% of the antibiotic product consists of rifamycin B, which is easily isolated because of its strongly acidic properties. Rifamycin B in aqueous solution is quickly transformed in a more active product: rifamycin O. After 72 hr the aqueous solution contains a still more active product: rifamycin S, which, however, is more toxic than the starting material (LD_{50}: 120 mg/kg, mouse, i.v.). Reduction of rifamycin S leads to rifamycin SV. The structural relationships are shown in Fig. 16.61.

Rifamycin Y is a by-product of the preparation of rifamycin B in the presence of barbital. The structure of rifamycin YO (Fig. 16.62), which derives from rifamycin Y in the same way as rifamycin O derives from rifamycin B, has been established (564). Rifampicin (Fig. 16.61) is a semi-synthetic derivative of rifamycin, prepared from rifamycin SV (565).

Rifampicin inhibits DNA-dependent RNA polymerase of mycobacteria and

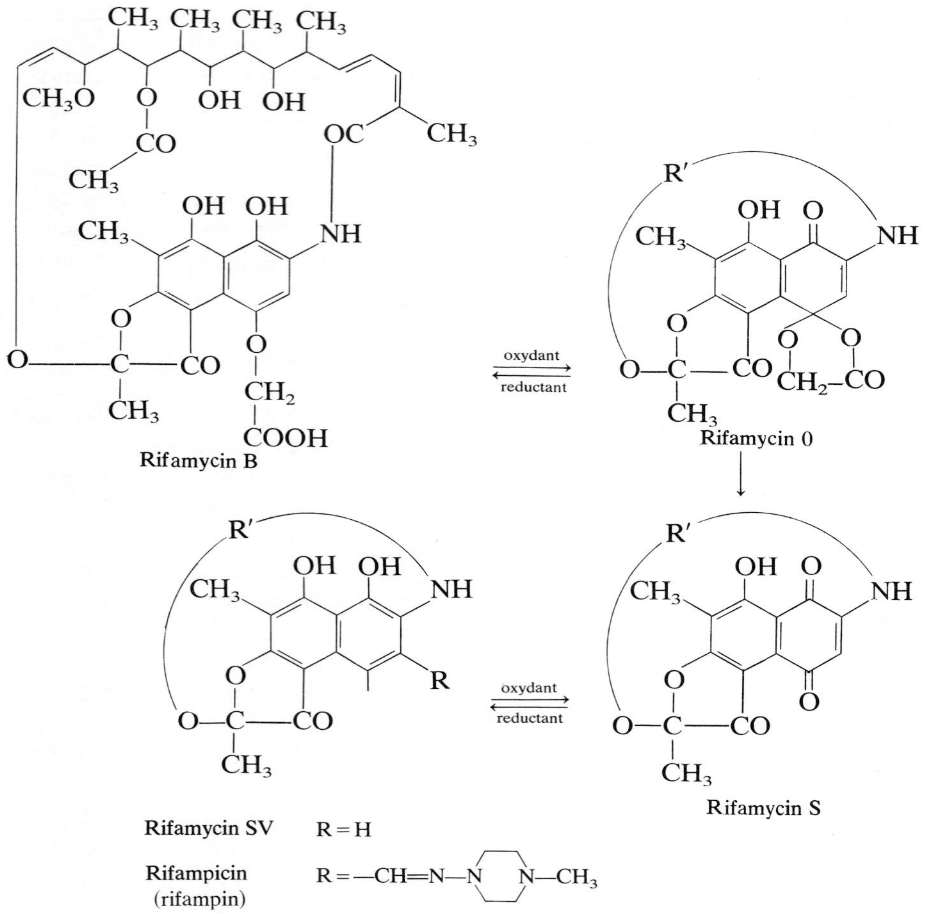

Rifamycin B

Rifamycin 0

Rifamycin S

Rifamycin SV R = H

Rifampicin (rifampin) R = —CH=N—N N—CH_3

Fig. 16.61 Structures of rifamycins.

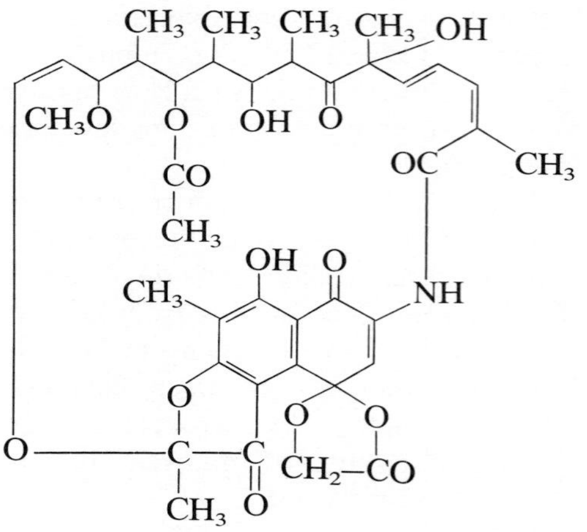

Fig. 16.62 Structure of rifamycin YO.

other microorganisms, leading to suppression of initiation of chain formation (but not chain elongation) in RNA synthesis. More specifically, the β-subunit of this complex enzyme is the site of action of the drug. RNA polymerase from mammalian cells does not bind rifampin, and RNA synthesis is correspondingly unaffected (566, 567).

Dissociation kinetics of complexes between rifamycin and DNA-dependent RNA polymerase from *E. coli* have been studied (568). The synthesis of several new rifamycin derivatives has been accomplished. The overall conformation of the ansa bridge is affected by C-3 substitution.

The conformational changes probably affect the enzyme-inhibitory activity of these derivatives (569).

The inhibition of ribonucleic acid synthesis in *Saccharomyces cerevisiae* by amphotericin B and rifampin was studied (570, 571). The kinetics of the rifampin-RNA polymerase complex has been investigated (572). Rifampicin has an effect on *in vitro* RNA synthesis of *Streptomyces mediterranei* (573).

8.2 Streptovaricins

Streptomyces spectabilis produces a mixture of orange antibiotics, active *in vivo* against *M. tuberculosis*. Yet the clinical use of these antibiotics has provided disappointing results. By partition chromatography or countercurrent distribution, six antibiotics, streptovaricin A, B, C, D, E, and G, have been isolated (574). The structures in Fig. 16.63 (575) have been proposed. The relative biological activities of individual streptovaricins have been measured (576). The effect of the intrinsic helicity of the ansa rings on the biological activities of the streptovaricins has been examined (577).

8.3 Geldamycin

This antibiotic, produced by *Streptomyces hygroscopicus* var. *geldanus* possesses activity especially against protozoa. Geldamycin has a benzoquinone (instead of a naphthoquinone system). Its structure is represented in Fig. 16.64 (578). The synthesis and bioactivities of geldamycin derivatives have been reported (579).

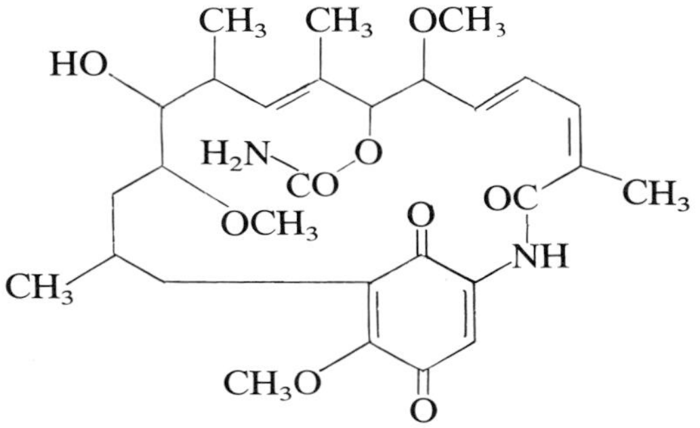

Fig. 16.64 Structure of geldamycin.

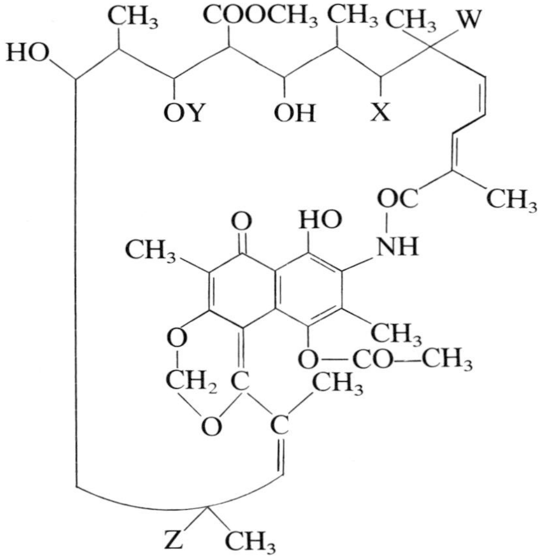

	W	X	Y	Z
A....	OH	H, OH	CH_3—CO	OH
B....	H	H, OH	CH_3—CO	OH
C....	H	H, OH	H	OH
D....	H	H, OH	H	H
E....	H	=O	H	OH
G....	OH	H, OH	H	OH

Fig. 16.63 Structures of streptovaricins.

9 GLUTARIMIDS

Several strains of *Streptomyces* produce antifungal antibiotics that are 3-substituted glutarimids. A review on the glutarimid antibiotics has been published (580).

9.1 Cycloheximide or Actidione

This antibiotic, produced by *Streptomyces griseus*, is active against fungi, protozoa and algae, but its elevated toxicity limits its application in agriculture. On the other hand, cycloheximide is the most potent substance known in eradicating rats: rats would rather die of thirst than drink water containing 4–5 ppm cycloheximide (581). Its structure (582) and stereochemistry (583) are represented in Fig. 16.65. The synthesis of cycloheximide and of some stereoisomers has been carried out (584).

The site of action of this antibiotic has not been precisely determined. It inhibits the process of translocation of ribosomes along the mRNA chain—thus its reading and association of ribosome units on new mRNA chains to form polysomes.

Cycloheximide has no effect on the activation of amino acids, nor on the formation of aminoacyl-tRNA in *Saccharomyces pastorianus* (585, 586) and in an acellular system of rat liver (587). Cycloheximide does not provoke the detachment of polypeptide chains during the synthesis, nor the destruction of the existing polysomes, *in vivo* as well as *in vitro*, but it inhibits the reformation, or the initiation, of polysomes from mRNA and of ribosomes (588–593). Cycloheximide inhibits the translocation reaction in eucaryote systems and probably the initiation. Puromycin reacts with the peptidyl-tRNA at the P position to form a peptidyl-puromycin. On polysomes freshly prepared from rat liver, 20% of the total peptidyl-tRNA are at the P position and can give rise to the "puromycin reaction". The fraction placed in the A position must be translocated to become reactive with puromycin. Under the experimental conditions used, cycloheximide prevents this fraction from becoming so active; it inhibits the translocation (594). The translocation is dependent on the TF_2 enzyme, which requires mercapto groups. The inhibition by cycloheximide is prevented by high concentrations of reduced glutathion (GSH) (594, 595). This explains the contradictory results obtained in studies in the presence of GSH at low (590) and at high concentrations (589).

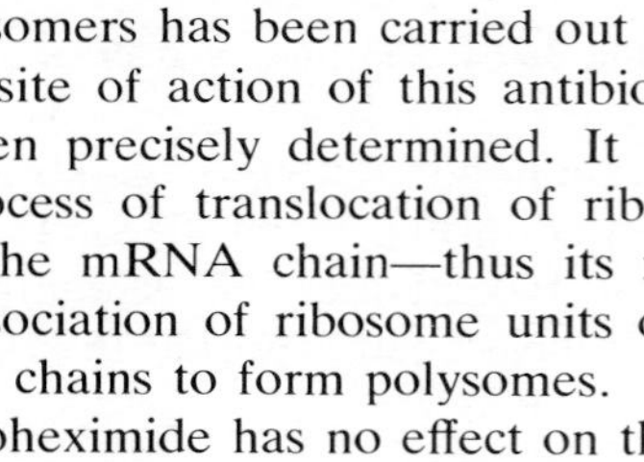

In intact rabbit reticulocytes as well as in an acellular system derived therefrom, cycloheximide affects both initiation and elongation, the latter being more sensitive (592, 596).

Although the antibiotic inhibits the translocation, it has no effect on the ribosome dependent GTPase activity of TF_2. It acts directly on the ribosomes at the level, or in the vicinity of the P site (597). This leads to the inhibition of the entrance of tRNA into this site at the moment of initiation or translocation (596). In effect, cycloheximide inhibits the nonenzymatic fixation (at high Mg^{2+} concentration) of nonacylated $tRNA^{Phe}$, which takes place at the P position, as well as its enzymatic detachment, dependent on T II and the presence of Phe-$tRNA^{Phe}$. The resistance of certain mutants of *S. cerevisiae* to the antibiotic is connected with the 60 S ribosome subunits (598).

Comparison of cycloheximide and other antibiotics of this family, as well as synthetic derivatives, shows that the imide, the

Fig. 16.65 Structure of cycloheximide.

hydroxyl, and the keto carbonyl group are indispensable for antibiotic activity (599). Cycloheximide also causes a decrease in the rate of protein degradation in cultured fetal mouse hearts (600).

9.2 Naramycin B

Naramycin B (Fig. 16.66) is a stereoisomer of cycloheximide. *Streptomyces griseus* produces also inactone (Fig. 16.67) (601), whose hydrogenation leads to a mixture of cycloheximide and naramycin B.

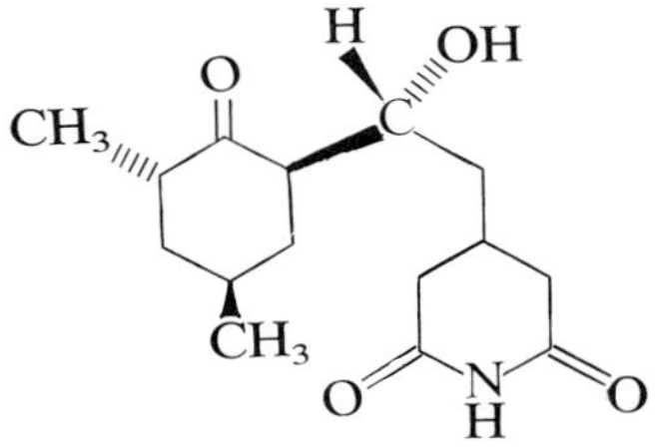

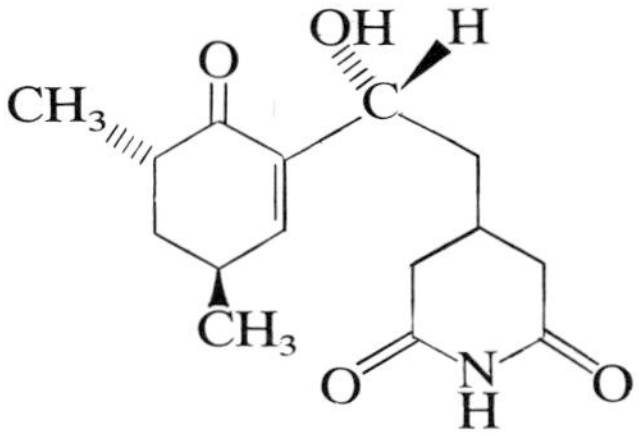

Fig. 16.66 Structure of naramycin B.

Fig. 16.67 Structure of inactone.

9.3 Antitumor E-73

This substance (Fig. 16.68), produced by *Streptomyces albulus*, possesses antitumor activity but is too toxic to be used practically (602).

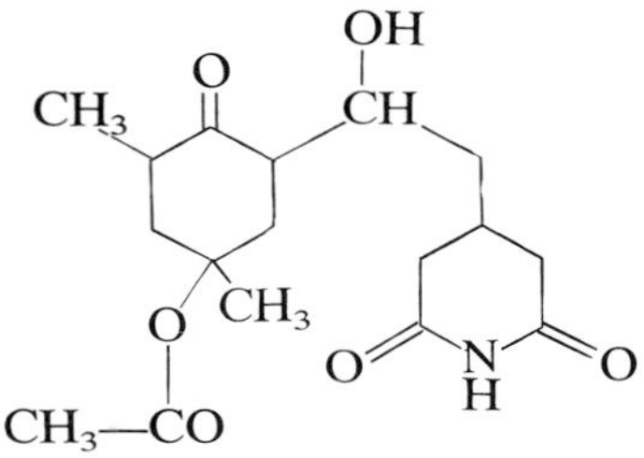

Fig. 16.68 Structure of antitumor E-73.

9.4 Streptovitacins

Streptomyces griseus also produces a family of hydroxylated substances, the streptovitacins, possessing antitumor activity (Fig. 16.69). Their stereochemistry is the same as that of cycloheximide (604).

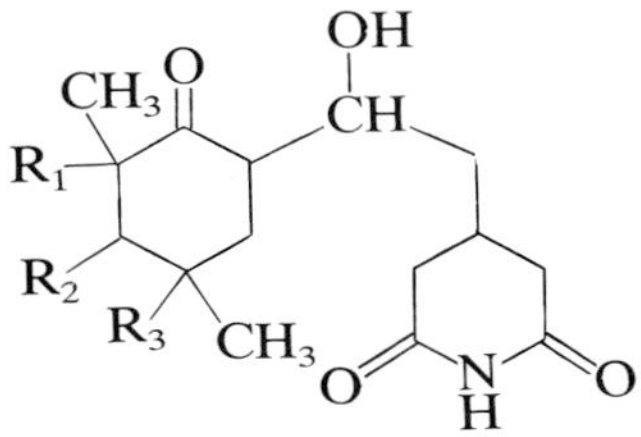

Fig. 16.69 Structure of streptovitacin A ($R_1 = R_2 =$ H, $R_3 =$ OH); B ($R_1 = R_3 =$ H, $R_2 =$ OH); C ($R_2 = R_3 =$ H, $R_1 =$ OH); and D, structure not established (603).

10 NUCLEOSIDE ANTIBIOTICS

Certain antibiotics present a large analogy in structure with the purine or pyrimidine bases, or with their nucleosides. These substances have been reviewed (605).

10.1 Puromycin

Puromycin is produced by *Streptomyces alboniger.* It is a dibasic product. Its structure (Fig. 16.70) (606) has been verified by synthesis (607). Numerous analogs of puromycin have been synthesized to facilitate study of structure-activity relations (608). Puromycin is active against gram-positive bacteria and trypanosomes. It also possesses antitumor activity. Lethal doses in the mouse are as follows: LD_{50}, 350 mg/kg i.v., 525 mg/kg, i.p.; 675 mg/kg, p.o.

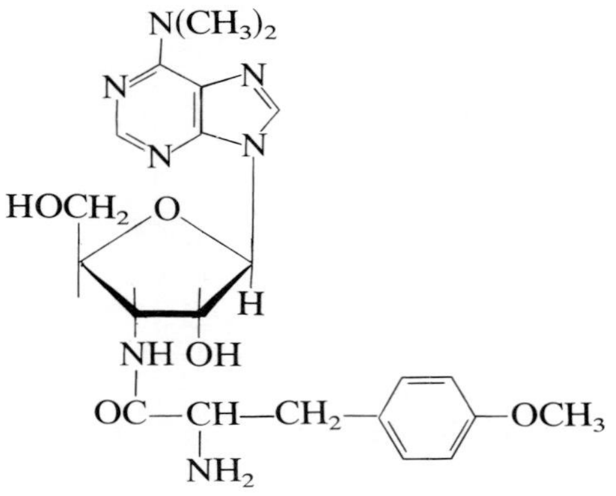

Fig. 16.70 Structure of puromycin.

Puromycin inhibits protein synthesis. It acts by accepting the peptidyl group carried by tRNA placed at the P site. The peptidyl-puromycin thus formed detaches itself from the ribosome.

There is a structural similarity between puromycin and the terminal aminoacyl-adenosine group of the tRNA, which carries an amino acid or a polypeptide chain (609). On the ribosomes are attached 2 molecules of tRNA; one carries the polypeptide chain of the protein to be synthesized, the other the amino acid that follows in the sequence. The new peptide bond is made between the acyl group of the polypeptide chain and the amino group of the new amino acid to be incorporated. It is transferred from the polypeptide chain of amino acids to the aminoacyl-tRNA, which then carries a chain of $n+1$ amino acids. After translocation, the process repeats for the amino acid $n+2$ of the sequence. It may be considered that by an analogous mechanism, puromycin behaves as the aminoacyl-tRNA that carries the amino acid $n+1$, and while it substitutes on it, it binds to the polypeptide chain and detaches the latter from the ribosome, thus interrupting the protein synthesis. The length of the detached polypeptide is a function of the moment at which puromycin has been added. This precise conception is based on a number of the following experimental data.

Puromycin acts hardly at all during the early stages of the establishment of the peptide bond. It does not inhibit the activation of the amino acids (609), nor the attachment of the aminoacyl-tRNA and of nRNA to the ribosomes (610). *In vitro* and *in vivo* puromycin causes the liberation of polypeptides of different length, and *in vitro* it inhibits the formation of long peptides. It leads to an accumulation of unused aminoacyl-tRNA (611–614). One molecule of puromycin is attached to the carboxyl terminal of each detached chain by an ester linkage (611, 615, 616). The ester linkage of the polypeptide with puromycin is made by transfer from that which it has with its tRNA under the influence of peptidyl transferase. Puromycin can act by direct interaction with the terminal part of peptidyl-tRNA in the P position rather than by displacement of the aminoacyl-tRNA in the A position. *This reaction has great experimental importance in that it permits the characterization of the positioning and the adjustment at the P position* of a peptidyl-tRNA, of F-meth-$tRNA_f^M$ or of the analog of the Ac-phe-$tRNA^{Phe}$ initiation (617).

It has been shown (618–623) that under certain conditions the polypeptide of a peptidyl-oligonucleotide obtained from a peptidyl-tRNA can transfer the polypeptide to puromycin in the presence of ribosomes; similarly, the 50 S ribosome subunit catalyzes the formation of *N*-formylmethionylpuromycin, for example, from *N*-formylmethionylhexanucleotide CAACCA-f-meth, the terminal fragment of *N*-formylmethionyl-tRNA. This transfer reaction to puromycin can operate from acetylphenylalanyl-$tRNA^{Phe}$ or terminal fragments carrying Ac-Phe. The "fragment reaction" catalyzed by the isolated, large 50 S subunit is dependent on the presence of methanol or ethanol in the reaction medium. The "fragment reaction" takes also place with the β-core of the 50 S subunits, but not with the γ-core (624). This kind of result with a fragment of tRNA carrying its amino acid whose α-NH_2 is formylated or acetylated has the advantage of simplifying the system of the study of the function of the peptidyl-transferase by reducing the interactions of the 50 S tRNA subunit. Puromycin is a precise tool in the study of the process of the formation of the peptide linkage in bacteria and eucaryotes.

By utilizing synthetic analogs of puromycin (612, 625, 626), the structural elements required for antibiotic activity have been determined. Both the aminonucleoside and the aminoacyl residue must be present. Neither the 2′- nor the 5′-isomer is active. The amino acid residue must be in the L-configuration. Puromycin analogs differing in the aminoacyl residue (glycyl, leucyl, tryptophanyl) show weak or no activity. Only the tyrosyl or phenylalanyl residue possess considerable activity.

Puromycin analogs have an effect on peptidylpuromycin synthesis on polyribosomes (627).

10.2 Tubercidin

This antibiotic, produced by *Streptomyces tubercidicus* also possesses antitumor properties. Its structure (Fig. 16.71) (628) has been confirmed by synthesis (629). Very similar to tubercidin are the antibiotics toyocamycin (Fig. 16.71) and sangivamycin (Fig. 16.71) (630).

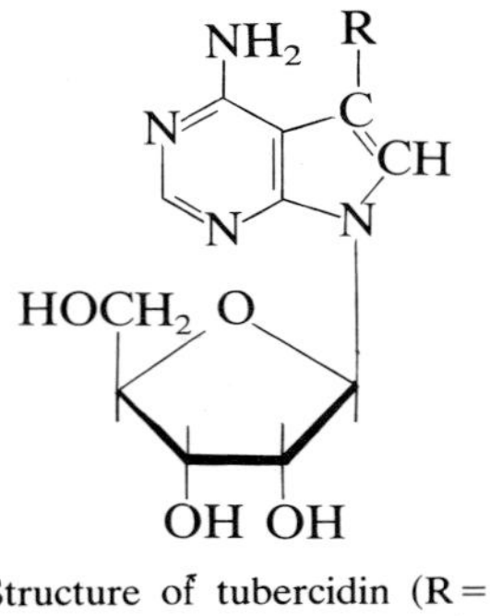

Fig. 16.71 Structure of tubercidin (R = H), toyocamycin (R = CN), and sangivamycin (R = $CONH_2$).

In animal cells the RNA of the 45 S precursor of the ribosome RNA, synthesized in the presence of low concentrations of toyocamycin, is specifically inhibited. Toyocamycin is probably phosphorylated and incorporated in the 28 S and 18 S RNA. On the other hand, mRNA synthesized under the same conditions is normally recovered at the polyribosome level (631, 632).

10.3 Angustmycin and Psicofuranine

This antibiotic, also called decoyinin, is produced as a mixture by *Streptomyces hygroscopius* var. *angustmycetius.* Its structure appears in Fig. 16.72 (633–635).

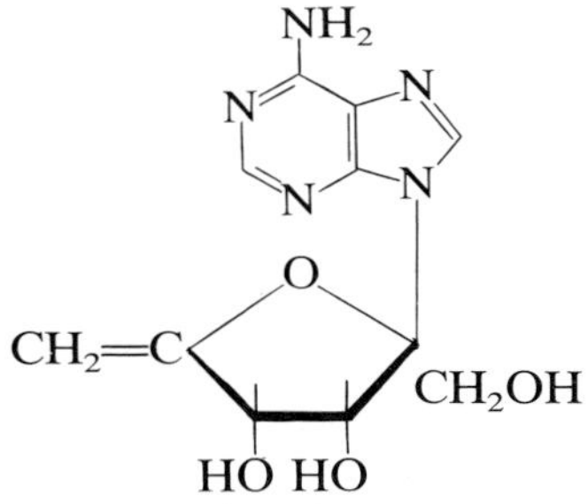

Fig. 16.72 Structure of angustmycin.

Angustmycin C or psicofurarine (636) is depicted in Fig. 16.73 (637). It possesses a relatively weak antibiotic activity *in vitro*; *in vivo* it is active against *Streptococcus hemolyticus.* Moreover, it possesses antitumor activity (LD_{50} : 10,000 mg/kg,

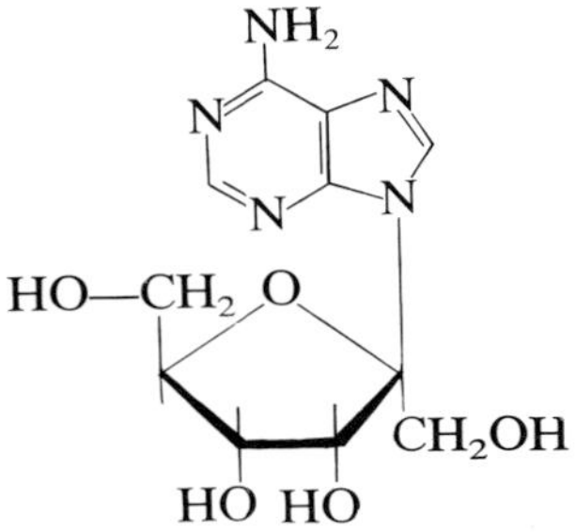

Fig. 16.73 Structure of angustmycin C.

mouse, p.o.). Streptomyces transform angustmycin C into angustmycin A: in the microorganism these two antibiotics are thus in equilibrium (638).

Angustmycin C inhibits xanthosine-5′-phosphate aminase, thus the transformation of xanthosine-5′-phosphate into guanosine-5′-phosphate. The inhibition is not competitive. The point of impact of the antibiotic has been determined (639–641). Angustmycin attaches itself to the enzyme at a site away from the enzymatic site (642–646). This fixation is dependent on the substrate xanthosine-5′-phosphate and pyrophosphate, one of the reaction products.

10.4 Cordycepin

Cordycepin is produced by *Cordyceps militaris* and *Aspergillus nidulans* (647). It is active *in vitro* against *Bacillus subtilis* (648). It is a 3′-deoxyadenosine (Fig. 16.74) (649–651).

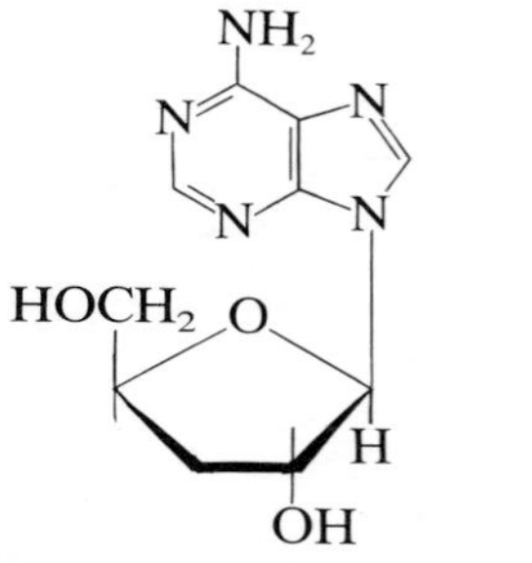

NH_2 N N N N $HOCH_2$ O H OH

Fig. 16.74 Structure of cordycepin.

Cordycepin is phosphorylated in the cell to cordycepin triphosphate and causes the inhibition of RNA synthesis (652). During growth of the RNA chain, cordycepin monophosphate is incorporated in the chain and arrests the growth because of its lack of the 3′-OH group (653, 654) (Fig. 16.75).

10.5 Blasticidin S

Blasticidin S has been isolated from the filtrate of a *Streptomyces griseochromogenes* culture. It is active against a variety of bacterial species and against the fungus *Piricularia oryzae.* Its structure (655) and stereochemistry (656) have been established (Fig. 16.76). The mechanism of action of blasticidin S has been reviewed (657).

The nucleoside moeity of blasticidin H, pentopyranamine D, has been synthesized (658).

10.6 Gougerotin

This antibiotic is also called asteromycin. Its structure appears in Fig. 16.77.

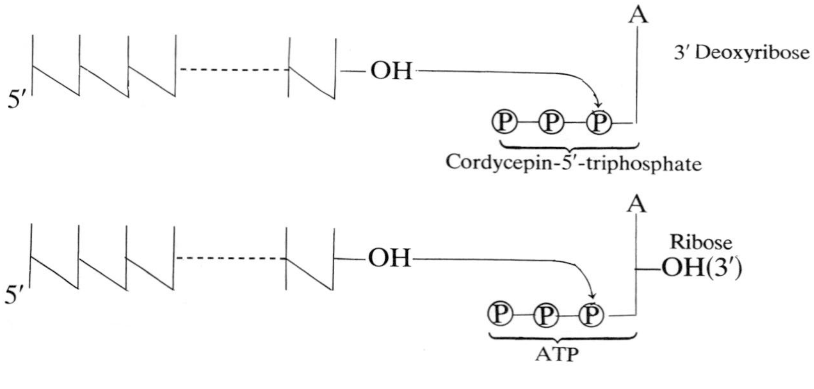

5′ OH A 3′ Deoxyribose Ⓟ–Ⓟ–Ⓟ Cordycepin-5′-triphosphate

5′ OH A Ribose OH(3′) Ⓟ–Ⓟ–Ⓟ ATP

Fig. 16.75 Mechanism of action of cordycepin.

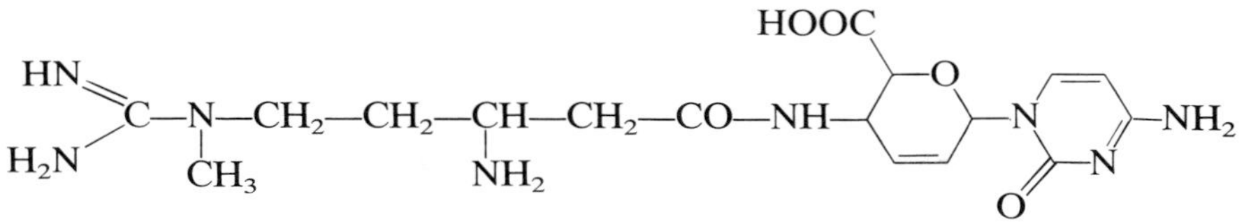

Fig. 16.76 Structure of blasticidin S.

Gougerotin possesses a large antibiotic spectrum, but its activity is weak and it is somewhat toxic. Its mechanism of action has been reviewed (659).

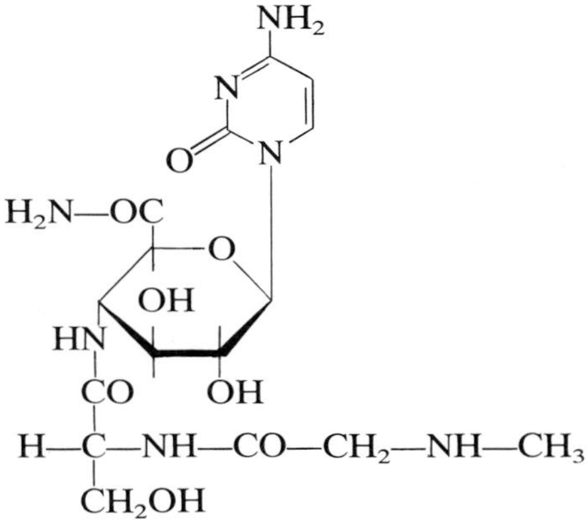

Fig. 16.77 Structure of gougerotin.

10.7 Polyoxins

The polyoxins constitute a group of antibiotics used as agricultural fungicides in Japan. They are produced by *Streptomyces cacaoi* var. *asoensis.* These antibiotics are virtually inactive against yeast and bacteria. Polyoxins C and I are presented in Fig. 16.78; other forms appear in Fig. 16.79 (660).

10.8 3′-Amino-3′-deoxyguanosine

The antibiotic 3′-amino-3′-deoxyguanosine has been recently reviewed (660). Its structure is shown in Fig. 16.80.

10.9 Nucleocidin

The partial structure of nucleocidin is shown in Fig. 16.80*a*. This antibiotic has been reviewed (661).

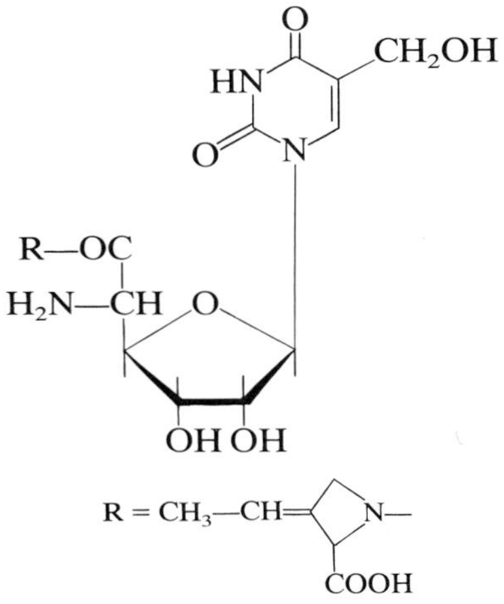

Fig. 16.78 Structures of polyoxins C (R = —OH) and I.

10.10 Amicetin

Amicetin is produced by several *Streptomyces* species (*S. vinaceus-diappus, S. fasciculatus, S. plicatus*). *In vitro,* it is active against gram-positive bacteria; *in vivo* it is inactive against tuberculosis. Its structure appears in Fig. 16.81 (662, 663).

10.11 Sparsomycin

Sparsomycin is produced by *Streptomyces sparsogenes.* Its structure (Fig. 16.81*a*) is

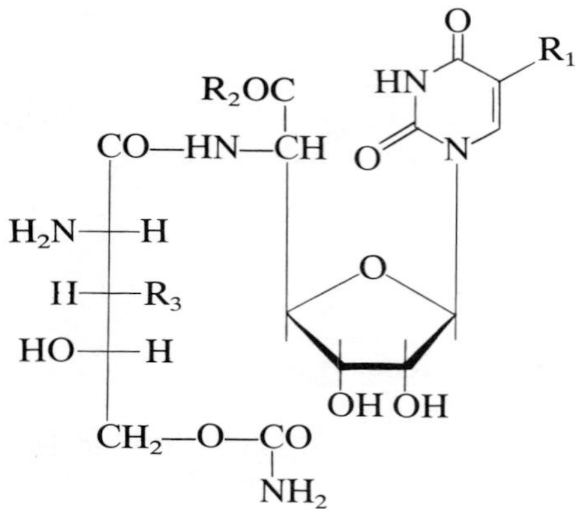

R_1	R_2	R_3	Polyoxin
$—CH_2OH$	X[a]	—OH	A
$—CH_2OH$	—OH	—OH	B
—COOH	—OH	—OH	D
—COOH	—OH	—H	E
—COOH	X[a]	—OH	F

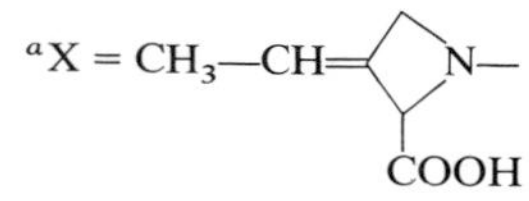

[a]X = $CH_3—CH=$(azetidine ring with COOH)N—

Fig. 16.79 Structures of polyoxins A, B, D, E, and F.

unusual in that it contains a dithioacetal, in which one sulfur is in the form of a sulfoxide (664). It is active against gram-positive and gram-negative bacteria and possesses *in vivo* antitumor activity (665). It inhibits the formation of the peptide linkage at the level of the 70 S ribosome systems (procaryotes) (666–670).

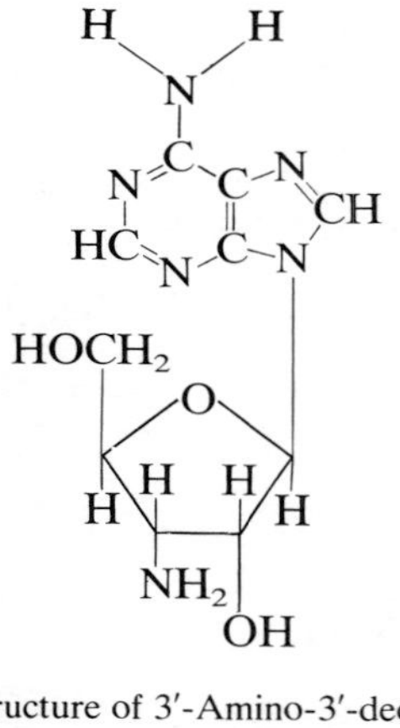

Fig. 16.80 Structure of 3′-Amino-3′-deoxyguanosine.

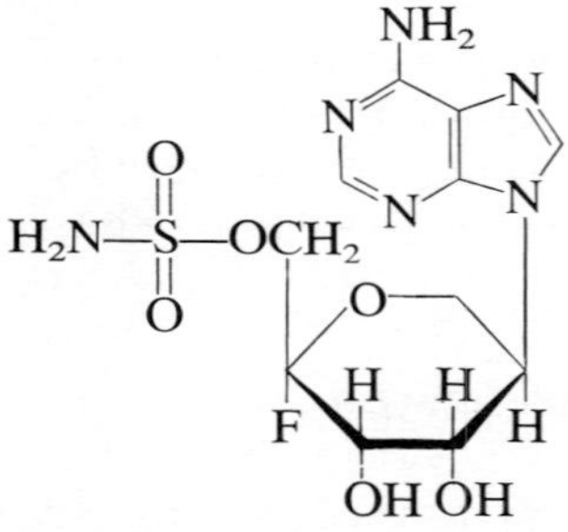

Fig. 16.80*a* Partial structure of nucleocidin.

11 ANTHRACYCLINE ANTIBIOTICS

This group of antibiotics, mostly tetracyclic, are derived from anthraquinone, and generally are produced by *Streptomyces.* A general review has been published (671). The anthraquinones bind to DNA by intercalation, but synthetic planar naphthacenequinones stack externally on DNA (672).

11.1 Daunomycin

This antibiotic, also called daunorubicin or rubidomycin, is produced by *Streptomyces peucitius.* It has antitumor activity (acute leukemia, children's neuroblastoma) and the structure is shown in Fig. 16.82. Daunomycin and adriamycin (see Section 11.2) have been reviewed (673).

Although the mechanism of action is not yet fully established, studies of daunomycin involving X-ray diffraction and DNA model building suggests that the anthracycline antibiotics bind tightly with DNA. It has been proposed that intercalation occurs

Fig. 16.81 Structure of amicetin.

Fig. 16.81*a* Structure of sparsomycin.

between adjacent base pairs on a DNA strand. The amino sugar daunosamine plays an essential role in this binding. The DNA helix is untwisted to permit intercalation, producing a longer, thinner molecule and causing inhibition of the template activity of DNA (674). The binding of daunomycin to DNA has been investigated calorimetrically and spectroscopically (675). The effects of the stereochemical configuration on the interaction of some daunomycin derivatives with DNA have been studied (676).

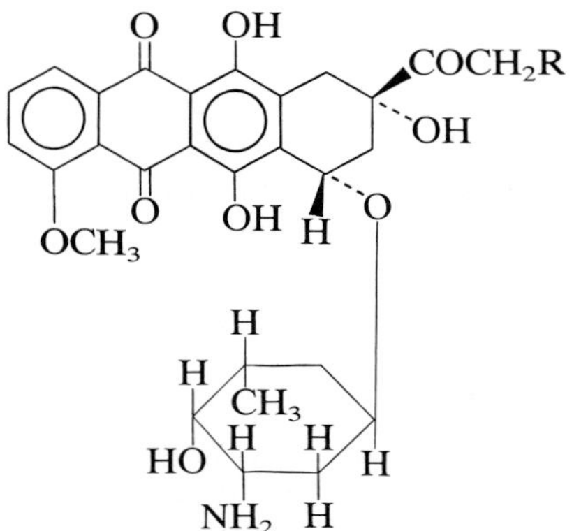

Fig. 16.82 Structure of daunomycin (R = H) and adriamycin (R = OH)

11.2 Adriamycin

This antibiotic, sometimes called doxorubicin, is also produced by *S. peucetius* and is very similar in structure to daunomycin (Fig. 16.82). It was developed in Italy (677) and has an impressive record of activity against a wide spectrum of tumors, despite a relatively brief period of clinical testing (679, 680). Adriamycin has been reviewed (673, 678).

Adriamycin has recently been approved by the US Food and Drug Administration as a prescription drug for use in cancer therapy. It displays a more favorable therapeutic index than daunomycin in different experimental tumors (681, 682) and has been shown to be effective in the clinical treatment of leukemia and solid tumors (683, 684).

The drug is thought to achieve its anticancer effect at the cellular level by blocking the synthesis of RNA copies of DNA. This blockage is due to the binding of the drug to DNA. Various physicochemical studies of the adriamycin-DNA complex, such as sedimentation, viscosity, spectrophotometry, unwinding of the open chain and closed, circular, supercoiled DNA helix, reduced availability of the phenolic hydroxyls to OH^- ions, loss of characteristic polarographic behavior of the quinone, and X-ray diffraction, have indicated a plausible model for the complex. The planar moiety of the molecule is intercalated between two successive base pairs on the DNA helix, an interaction that is sustained by weak hydrophobic stabilization. In addition, electrostatic interaction exists between the protonated amino group of the sugar residue and the ionized DNA phosphate group; hydrogen bonding is involved also (685). It is still undecided if a true DNA base specificity exists for bound adriamycin. Binding sites on DNA for the structurally related daunomycin and actinomycin (whose selectivity for deoxyguanosine residues is well established) are different (686). Daunomycin displays little base specificity as determined by the decrease in buoyant density of different native DNAs in a CsCl gradient or by the degree of inhibition of DNA-directed RNA polymerase reaction, using different DNA primers. CD spectra have shown that complex formation is little dependent on the GC content. On the other hand, a specific interaction with adenine-thymine base pairs is indicated by the selective inhibition of exogenous templates in the tumor viruses DNA polymerase reaction (685). It has been shown that daunomycin and adriamycin facilitate actinomycin D binding to poly d(A−T) (685a).

At present there is no satisfactory explanation for the surprisingly and markedly different clinical antitumor activities of daunomycin and adriamycin. It is possible, however, that differences in their metabolic degradation may be responsible. Both antibiotics are subject to rapid and extensive metabolism. In a single passage through the liver, about 60% of adriamycin is extracted, metabolized, and excreted in the bile; at least six metabolites have been identified, the principal being adriamycinol. This product results from the reduction of the keto group on C-13 by an enzyme found in leukocytes and erythrocytes, and presumably in malignant tissues. An analogous daunomycin analog, daunomycinol, has been demonstrated, and it displays antitumor activity. Responsiveness to daunomycin of patients with acute myelocytic leukemia has been correlated with the presence of the enzyme, referred to as daunorubicin reductase. In addition to the reduction products, several aglycone metabolites of these antibiotics have been identified.

Resistance is observed to the anthracyclenes. As yet, however, there is no clear biochemical explanation of the resistance mechanism. Complete cross-resistance has been reported between daunomycin and adriamycin in leukemia L 1210 sublines. Interestingly, cross-resistance has also been described between daunomycin, antinomycin, and the vinca alkaloids, which raises the possibility that alteration of cellular permeability may be involved.

The synthesis and antitumor properties of new glycosides of daunomycinone and adriamycinone have been described (687, 688).

Since adriamycin is only available in short supply and shows dose related cardio toxicity, intense attempts have been made in recent years by various groups to synthesize adriamycin and analogs. The main

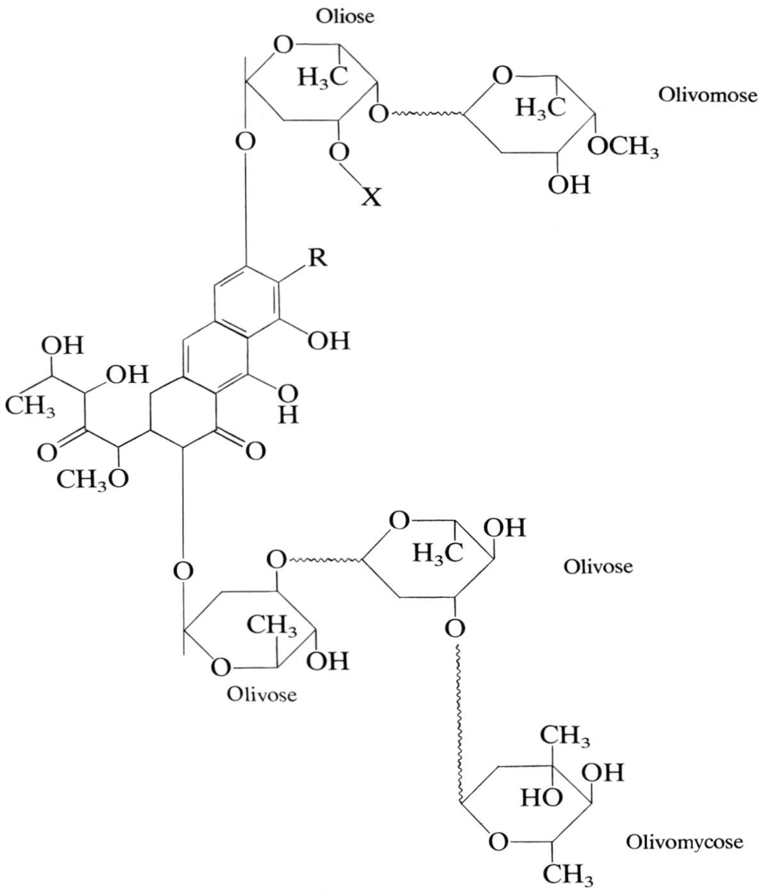

Fig. 16.83 Structures of olivomycins (R = H) and chromomycins ($R = CH_3$).

synthetic problem is one of regiospecificity in the construction of the aglycone ring system (688a).

11.3 Olivomycin, Chromomycin, and Mithramycin

Olivomycin, chromomycin, and mithramycin form a group of antibiotics of similar structure, possessing anti-tumor activity. A review has been published in 1965 (689). They are built up from a tricyclic aglycone (which is not an anthraquinone) bound to several molecules of unusual sugars. The olivomycins have been isolated from *Streptomyces olivoreticuli* (690), and the chromomycins from *S. griseus* (691). Their structures are shown in Fig. 16.83, and their various substituents are listed in Table 16.11. The stereochemistry of chromomycinone (Fig. 16.84) has been elucidated (692, 693).

Mithramycin, or aureolic acid, is built up from an aglycone, chromomycinone, bound on one side to a disaccharide of D-olivopyranose, and on the other side to a trisaccharide formed by D-mycarose, D-oliose, and D-olivose (693).

These antibiotics inhibit the biosynthesis

Table 16.11 Substituents in Olivomycins and Chromomycins

Compound	X	Y
Olivomycin		
A	CH_3CO—	4-α-Isobutyryl-olivomycosyl
B	CH_3CO	4-α-Acetyl-olivomycosyl-
C	H	4-α-Isobutyryl-divomycosyl
D	CH_3CO	H-
Chromomycin		
A_2	CH_3CO	4-α-Isobutyryl-olivomycosyl-
A_3	CH_3CO	4-α-Acetyl-olivomycosyl-
A_4	CH_3CO	H-
Desacetyl-A_3	CH_3CO-	α-Olivomycosyl-

of DNA and DNA-dependent RNA in bacteria as well as in animal cells. Their mechanism of action (694) and the physicochemical properties of their complexes with DNA are similar (695–697). In particular, the conditions for the complex formation with chromomycin A_3 are the following: (1) the DNA should not be denaturated, (2) divalent ions (Mg^{2+}, Mn^{2+}, Co^{2+}, Zn^{2+}) should be present in stochiometric amount with regard to the antibiotic, and (3) guanine should be present in the DNA molecule. The quantity of the bound pigment is related to the percentage of guanine in the DNA. The 2-amino group in the guanine is required for binding (698).

The divalent ions play an interesting role in the formation of the complexes. They intervene in the spectral change of the antibiotic. Moreover, these pigments are strong chelating agents (e.g., olivomycin). In spite of the existence of common sites of DNA binding for chromomycin A_3 and mithramycin, it seems that certain sequences of the nucleic acid bind specifically each of these antibiotics (695–697).

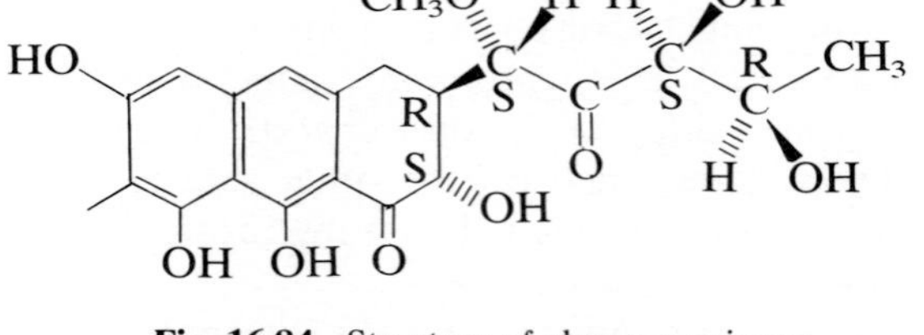

Fig. 16.84 Structure of chromomycinone.

Chromomycin A_3, because it has the shortest polysaccharide chains, has the largest affinity for DNA and is the most active in this series (697). Chromomycin and mithramycin do not intercalate in the complex formation (699).

11.4 Nogalamycin

Nogalamycin, produced by *Streptomyces nogalater* var. *nogalater*, is an antitumor antibiotic. Its structure is shown in Fig. 16.85 (699a).

Nogalamycin interacts with DNA, presumably by intercalation (700, 701). The earlier proposed intercalation model (702) has been modified (703).

11.5 Leukaeomycin

A *Streptomyces* strain belonging to *S. griseus* produces the antitumor antibiotic leukaeomycin. Four components were isolated: leukaeomycin B_1 (= rubomycin B), B_2 (daunosaminyldaunomycin), C (= daunomycin), and D (dihydrodaunomycin) (704).

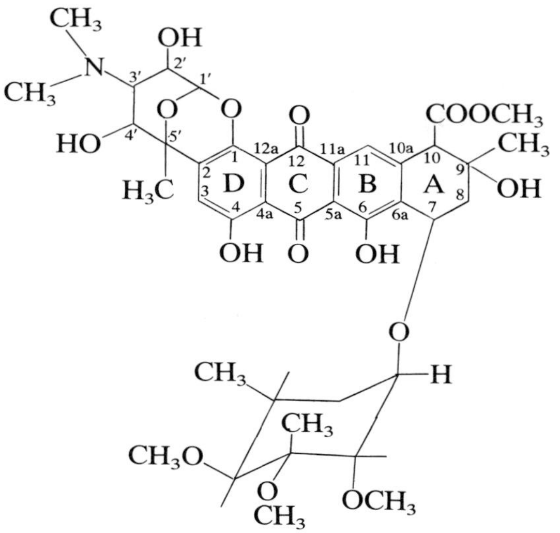

Fig. 16.85 Structure of nogalamycin.

11.6 Steffimycin

Steffimycin (U-20661) was discovered in 1967 (705) from cultures of *Streptomyces steffisburgensis.* A second member of this family, steffimycin B, came from a new species of streptomyces designated *S. elgreteus,* which also produces steffimycin (706). Their structures appear in Fig. 16.86.

Steffimycin B is active in inhibiting the growth of L-1210 mouse leukemia cells *in vitro.* It binds to double-stranded DNA, as evidenced by difference spectroscopy and an increase of the thermal stability of DNA in the presence of the antibiotic. It impairs the replicative and transcriptive template functions of DNA. The marginal decrease of template activity of poly (dG) · poly (dC) in the presence of **steffimycin** B for RNA polymerase and full template activity for DNA polymerase I suggests that **steffimycin** B interacts predominantly with adenine and thymine or base pairs thereof in the double-stranded DNA helix. Poly [d(A-T)] primed reactions with both enzymes are strongly impaired in the presence of **steffimycin** B (707, 708).

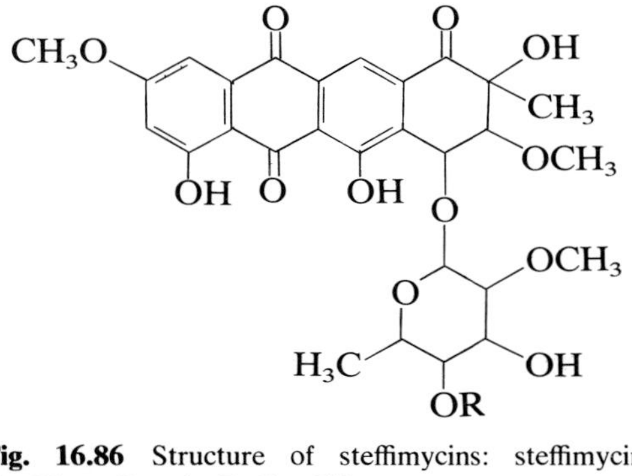

Fig. 16.86 Structure of steffimycins: steffimycin, R = H; steffimycin B, $R = CH_3$.

11.7 Carminomycin I

Carminomycin I (Fig. 16.87) was isolated from *Actinomadura carminata.* Carminomycin I was found to be more effective than the related antibiotics daunomycin and adriamycin in inhibiting DNA synthesis and growth of murine lymphoid leukemia L 1210. It gave evidence of less severe cardiotoxicity and seems to be better absorbed from the gastrointestinal tract than daunomycin. In view of its promising antineoplastic activity, this anthracycline is now the subject of clinical trials in the Soviet Union (709).

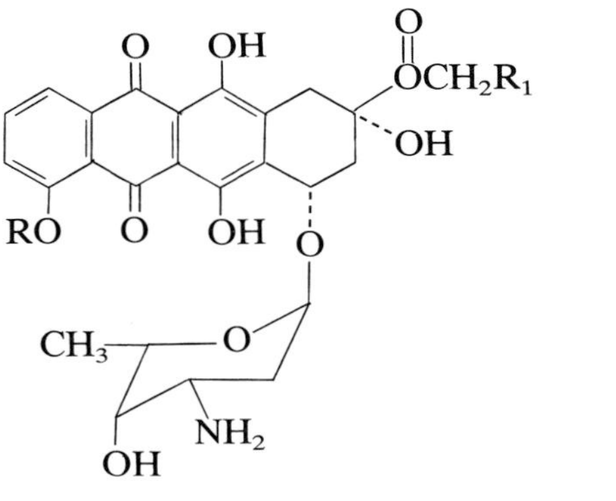

Fig. 16.87 Structure of carminomycin I: $R = R_1 = H$.

12 PHENAZINES

A number of phenazine derivatives, produced by a variety of bacteria, possess antibiotic properties, especially against gram-positive bacteria. Their structures are tabulated in Table 16.12 and their origins in Table 16.13. Iodinin is active against gram-positive bacteria, mycobacteria, and fungi. In the 1,6-dihydroxyphenazine series, the activity falls off with decreasing *N*-oxide groups. Lomofungin is active against gram-positive or gram-negative bacteria and fungi.

Table 16.12 Structures of Naturally Occurring Phenazines

	R_1	R_2	R_3	R_4	R_5	R_6	R_7	R_8	R_9
Pyocyanine	H	—	O^-	H	H	H	N^+-Me	H	H
1-Phenazinol	H	—	OH	H	H	H	—	H	H
Iodinin	H	N→O	OH	H	H	H	N→O	OH	H
Oxychlororaphin	$CONH_2$	—	H	H	H	H	—	H	H
Phenazine-1-carboxylic acid	COOH	—	H	H	H	H	—	H	H
Pigment A		N^+-Me		NH_3^+				(—COO^-, —Cl^-)	
Aeruginosin B	COOH	—	H	H	NH_2	H	N^+-CH_3	H	SO_3
Griseolutin A	COOH	—	OCH_3	H	H	CH_2—O—CO—CH_2OH	—	H	H
Griseolutin B	COOH	—	OCH_3	H	H	CH_2—O—COH—CH_2OH	—	H	H
1,6-Dihydroxyphenazine	OH	—	H	H	H	OH	—	H	H
Chlororaphin	Molecular compound of 3x oxychlororaphin + 1x dihydrochlororaphin								
Tubermycin A	COOH		(—C_6H_8)						
2-Phenazinol	H	—	H	OH	H	H	—	H	H
1,6-Phenazinediol-5-oxide	H	—	OH	H	H	H	N→O	OH	H
1-Phenazinol-10-oxide	H	—	OH	H	H	H	N→O	H	H
6-Methoxy-1-phenazinol	H	—	OH	H	H	H	—	OMe	H
1,6-Dimethoxyphenazine	H		OMe	H	H	H	—	OMe	H
Myxin	H	N→O	OH	H	H	H	N→O	OMe	H
2-Hydroxy-1-carboxyphenazine	H	—	COOH	OH	H	H	—	H	H
3-Hydroxyphenazine-1-carboxylic acid	COOH	—	H	H	H	H	—	H	OH

Table 16.12 (*Continued*)

	R_1	R_2	R_3	R_4	R_5	R_6	R_7	R_8	R_9
Phenazine-1,6-dicarboxylic acid	COOH	—	H	H	H	COOH	—	H	H
9-Hydroxyphenazine-1-carboxylic acid	COOH	—	OH	H	H	H	—	H	H
2,9-Dihydroxyphenazine-	OH	—	H	OH	H	H	—	H	H
2,9-Dihydroxyphenazine-1-carboxylic acid	OH	—	COOH	OH	H	H	—	H	H
4,7-Dihydroxyphenazine-5-oxide	H	—	H	H	H	OH	N→O	H	OH
2-Amino-9-hydroxyphenazine	OH	—	H	NH_2	H	H	—	H	H
Lomofungin	OH	—	$COOCH_3$	H	H	OH	—	CHO	OH

Table 16.13 Origins of Phenazines

		Producing Organism							
Metabolite	References	*Sporangium* species	*Nocardiaceae* strain	*Brevibacterium iodinum*	*Waksmania aerata*	*Chromobacterium iodinum*	*S. mitakiensis*	*S. thioluteus*	*S. griseoluteus*
Pyocyanine	710–716								
1-Phenazinol	716–718							×	
Iodinin	719–721			×	×	×		×	
Oxychlororaphin	722								
Phenazine-1-carboxylic acid	718, 721, 723–725		×				×	×	
Pigment A	726								
Aeruginosin B	726–728								
Griseolutin A	729–732								×
Griseolutin B	732, 733								×
1,6-Dihydroxyphenazine	718, 720, 721, 734		×	×	×			×	
Chlororaphin	722, 735								
Tubermycin A	723						×		
2-Hydroxyphenazine	736								
1,6-Phenazinediol-5-oxide	721		×	×				×	
1-Phenazinol-10-oxide	721		×						
6-Methoxy-1-phenazinol	718							×	
1,6-Dimethoxyphenazine	718							×	
Myxin	737, 738	×							
2-Hydroxy-1-carboxyphenazine	739								
3-Hydroxyphenazine-1-carboxylic acid	740								
Phenazine-1,6-dicarboxylic acid	741								
9-Hydroxyphenazine-1-carboxylic acid	741								

Table 16.13 (*Continued*)

Metabolite	References	Producing Organism: *Streptomyces chromofuscus*	*P. iodinum*	*P. chlororaphis*	*P. aureofaciens*	*Pseudomonas aeruginosa*	*Aspergillus sclerotiorum*	Unidentified bacterium	*Streptomyces lomondensis*
2,9-Dihydroxyphenazine	741								
2,9-Dihydroxyphenazine-1-carboxylic acid	741								
4,7-Dihydroxyphenazine-5-oxide	741								
2-Amino-9-hydroxyphenazine	741								
1-Carbomethoxy-6-formyl-4,7,9-trihydroxyphenazine (lomofungin)	742								
Pyocyanine	710–716					×			
1-Phenazinol	716–718					×			
Iodinin	719–721		×						
Oxychlororaphin	722			×		×			
Phenazine-1-carboxylic acid	718, 721, 723–725			×	×				
Pigment A	726					×			
Aeruginosin B	726–728					×			
Griseolutin A	729–732								
Griseolutin B	732, 733								
1,6-Dihydroxyphenazine	718, 720, 721, 734								
Chlororaphin	722, 735			×		×			
Tubermycin A	723								
2-Hydroxyphenazine	736				×				
1,6-Phenazinediol-5-oxide	721								
1-Phenazinol-10-oxide	721								
6-Methoxy-1-phenazinol	718								
1,6-Dimethoxyphenazine	718								
Myxin	737, 738								
2-Hydroxy-1-carboxyphenazine	739				×				
3-Hydroxyphenazine-1-carboxylic acid	740						×		
Phenazine-,16-dicarboxylic acid	741							×	
9-Hydroxyphenazine-1-carboxylic acid	741							×	
2,9-Dihydroxyphenazine	741							×	
2,9-Dihydroxyphenazine-1-carboxylic acid	741							×	
4,7-Dihydroxyphenazine-5-oxide	741							×	
2-Amino-9-hydroxyphenazine	741							×	
1-Carbomethoxy-6-formyl-4,7,9-trihydroxyphenazine (lomofungin)	742								×

Phenazines interact with DNA, presumably by intercalation, inhibiting RNA synthesis (743–746).

13 QUINOXALINE ANTIBIOTICS

These antibiotics are characterized by two quinoxalines connected by a (quasi)-symmetrical octapeptide dilactone ring, bridged in the center. Because of the unique biochemical consequences (*vide infra*) of the two planar chromophores, they are not classified under the polypeptide antibiotics. Quinoxaline antibiotics have been reviewed (747).

13.1 Echinomycin

Echinomycin is produced by *Streptomyces echinatus.* Its recently revised structure appears in Fig. 16.88 (748). From a culture of *Str. aureus* there have also been isolated quinomycin A (=echinomycin), B_0, C, B, and E. These compounds differ in one or two amino acids. The molecule of echinomycin shows a twofold axis of rotational symmetry for the cyclic octapeptide dilactone and its attached quinoxaline-2-carboxylic acid chromophores, whereas the sulfur-containing bridge introduces an element of asymmetry. In respect of this pseudosymmetrical appearance, as well as the sequence of amino acid residues in the two halves, there are obvious parallels with the structure of actinomycin (Section 2.1).

Echinomycin has long been known to bind to DNA, but the nature of its interaction remains obscure. It is an extremely potent inhibitor of RNA synthesis, some 4–5 times more potent than actinomycin D *in vivo*, and there is every indication that its antitumor activity results from its binding to DNA (747). Echinomycin is a bifunctional intercalating antibiotic. That both planar chromophores are capable of intercalation, possibly in a symmetry-related fashion, has been shown by studies with supercoiled circular PM2 DNA. The helix unwinding angle of the complex of this DNA with echinomycin is almost twice that with ethidium, an established monofunctional intercalating drug. The two intercalation sites are presumably distinct, because

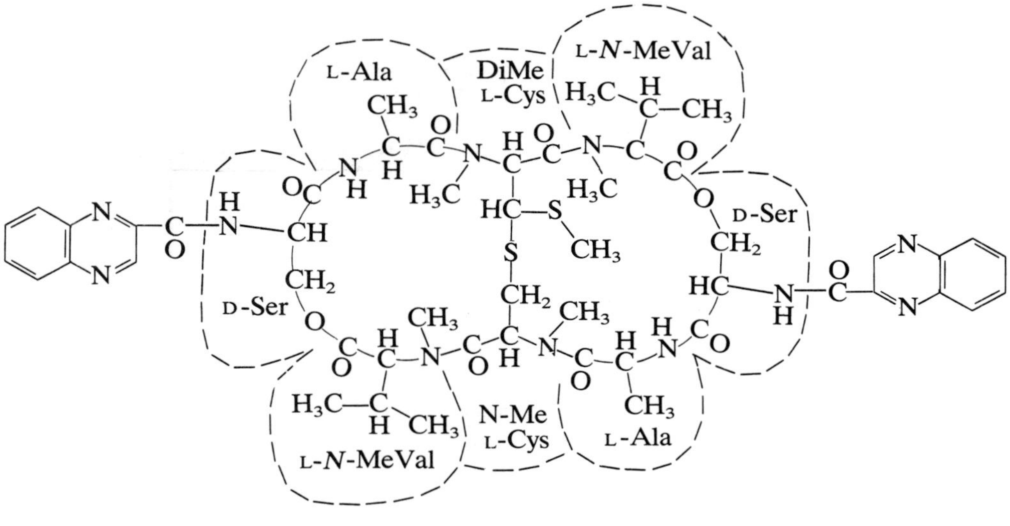

Fig. 16.88 Structure of echinomycin.

it is inconceivable that both chromophores could be accommodated in the space between two adjacent base pairs. In the extreme case where one chromophore demanded one specific site and the other chromophore the same specific site in antiparallel fashion, the binding specificity of this drug would be phenomenal. Such seems not to be the case. Some studies have indicated a weak specificity for G-C pairs, whereas other studies showed binding to poly (dG) · poly (dC), poly d(G-C), and poly d(A-T), albeit with widely different binding constants. By contrast, poly (dA) · poly (dT), poly (dI) · poly (dC), poly d(I-C), and poly (rA) · poly (rU) showed barely detectable binding. Since coliphage T2 DNA, whose major groove is largely filled with glucosyl substituents, binds echinomycin well, it is likely that the nonintercalating peptide moiety lies in the minor groove. In that case the 2-amino group of guanine could have an important influence on the binding of echinomycin (749–751). Recent CD studies have confirmed the binding pattern to DNAs containing dA, dT, dC, and dG (751a).

13.2 Triostins

Chemically similar to the quinomycins, the triostins are also found in the cultures of *Str. aureus.* Triostin A (Fig. 16.89), B_0, B, and C have been separated. They differ in one or two amino acids.

Triostin A binds to DNA, in a fashion similar to that of echinomycin. (751b). However, unlike echinomycin, the largest binding constant for triostin A is for poly d(A−T).

Synthetic des-N-tetra methyl-triostin A also has been shown to be a bifunctional intercalator (751c).

14 IONOPHORES

A number of antibiotics are characterized by a polyether structure. They cause leakage of ions through the cell membrane. Thus they behave similarly to the crown ethers.

Of the 30 structurally defined carboxylic acid ionophores A23187 and recently reported X-14547A contain nitrogen (751d).

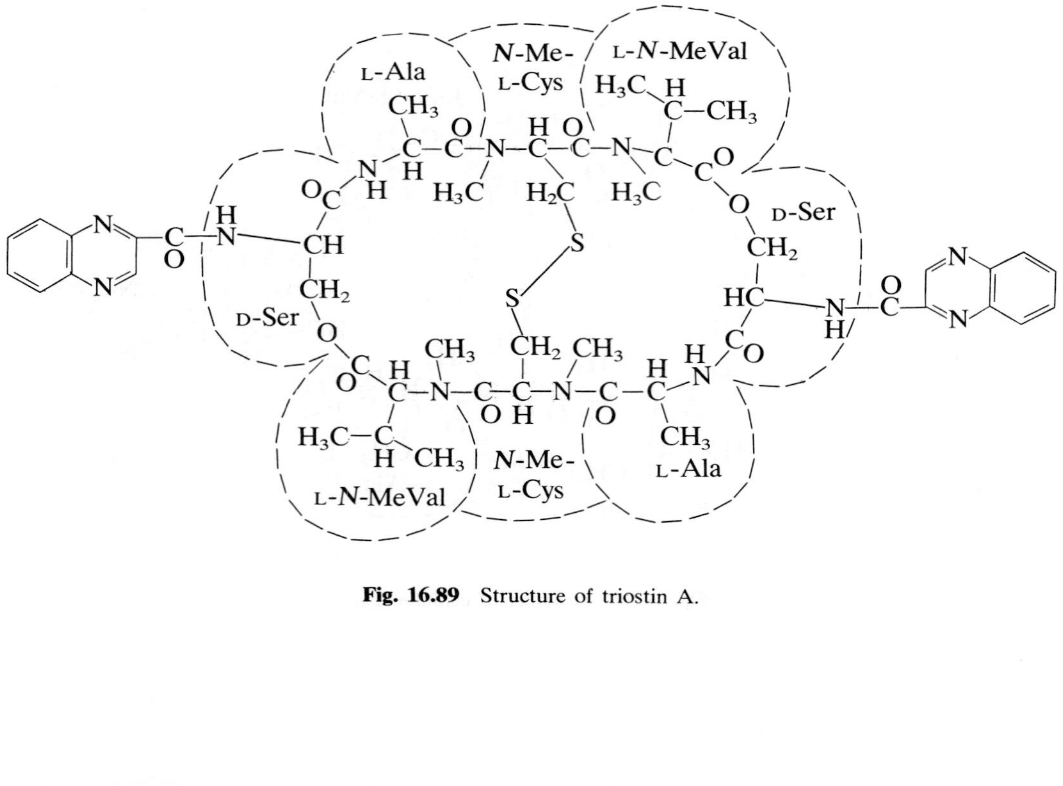

Fig. 16.89 Structure of triostin A.

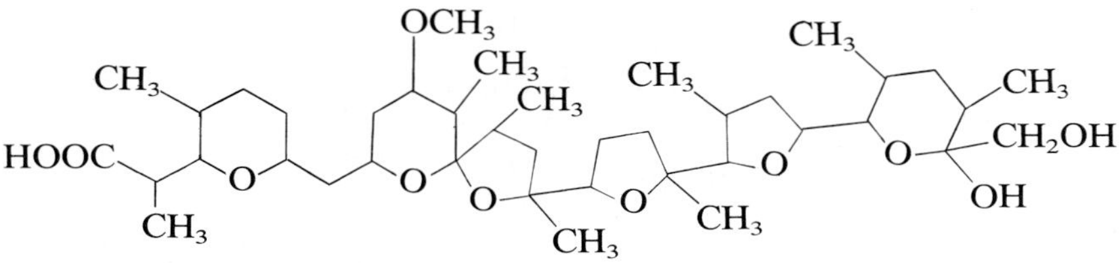

Fig. 16.90 Structure of polyetherin.

14.1 Polyetherin A

Polyetherin A is produced by *Streptomyces hygroscopicus* and possesses the structure shown in Fig. 16.90 (752). This antibiotic is identical with nigericin (753), produced by a *Streptomyces* strain from the soil of the Niger (754).

The mechamism of action of nigericin is similar to that of valinomycin (see Section 2.12).

14.2 Monensin

Monensin, initially called monensic acid, is produced by *Streptomyces cinnamonensis.* It is particularly active against coccidiae. The structure of monensin (Fig. 16.91) has been confirmed by an X-ray diffraction study of its silver salt, which shows a chelate-type structure with the molecule curved around the silver atom (755). Monensin inhibits the growth of gram-positive bacteria. It induces the uptake of K^+ and the ejection of H^+ in mitochondria and uncouples oxidative phosphorylation (756).

14.3 Antibiotic X-537 A

This antibiotic, also called habalocide, is produced by a *Streptomyces* strain. It is active against chicken coccidiae. Its structure (Fig. 16.92) contains a benzene ring (757).

15 NONCLASSIFIABLE ANTIBIOTICS

The many antibiotics whose unrelated structures stand alone and do not fall in the categories of Sections 2–14 are discussed presently.

15.1 Actinomycetin

Actinomycetin is a high molecular weight protein that enzymatically hydrolyzes the constituents of bacterial cell walls. It is produced by *Streptomyces albus* (758).

15.2 Actithiazic Acid

Streptomyces virginiae and *S. lavendulae* produce actithiazic acid, which is active *in*

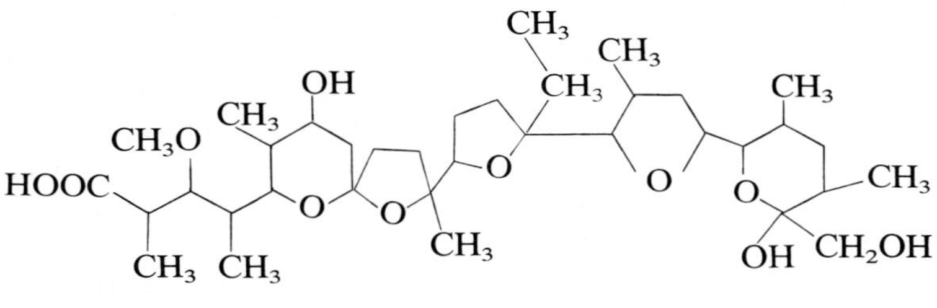

Fig. 16.91 Structure of monensin.

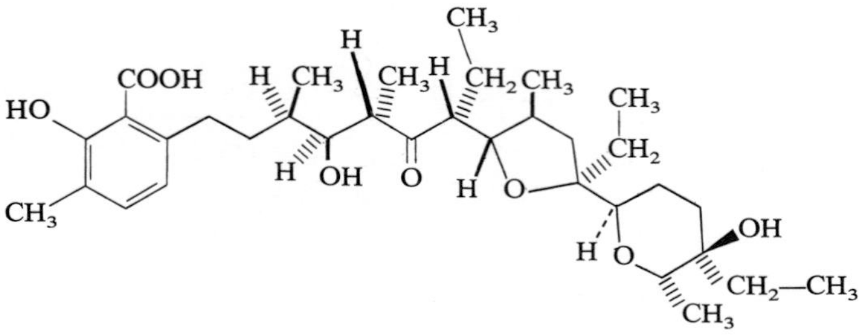

Fig. 16.92 Structure of antibiotic X-537A.

vitro, but not *in vivo*, against mycobacteria. The structure of this antibiotic (Fig. 16.93) contains sulfur (759). Its mechanism of action has been reviewed (760).

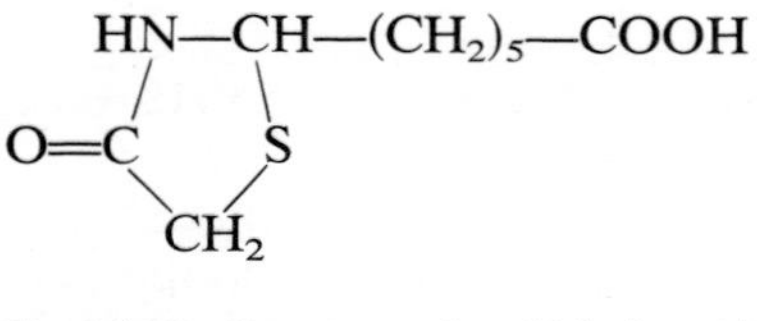

Fig. 16.93 Structure of actithiazic acid.

15.3 Althiomycin

Althiomycin was isolated from *Streptomyces*. It inhibits the growth of gram-positive and gram-negative bacteria. The structure of its acetyl derivative (Fig. 16.94) shows the presence of sulfur. Its mechanism of action has been reviewed (761).

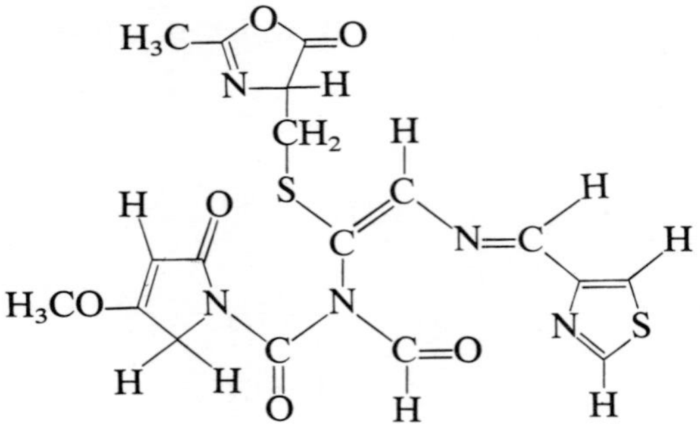

Fig. 16.94 Structure of acetylalthiomycin.

15.4 Anthramycin

Produced by *Streptomyces refluineus*, anthramycin is of interest because of its antitumor properties. Its structure (Fig. 16.95) (762) has been confirmed by synthesis (763). The anthramycin molecule reacts specifically with DNA to form a nearly irreversible complex. It is suggested that this binding is covalent. The molecular mechanism of this binding, however, is still conjectural (764).

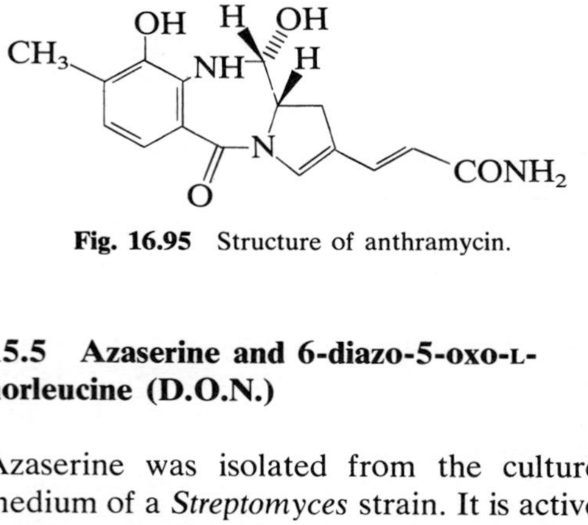

Fig. 16.95 Structure of anthramycin.

15.5 Azaserine and 6-diazo-5-oxo-L-norleucine (D.O.N.)

Azaserine was isolated from the culture medium of a *Streptomyces* strain. It is active against gram-positive bacteria, mycobacteria, some rickettsiae, and amebas. Of particular interest, however, is its antitumor activity (LD_{50}: 60–120 mg/kg, mouse, i.v.). Its structure (Fig. 16.96), which is that of a diazoacetate of L-serine, has been confirmed by synthesis (765).

6-Diaza-5-oxo-L-norleucine, also called D.O.N., is produced by an unidentified

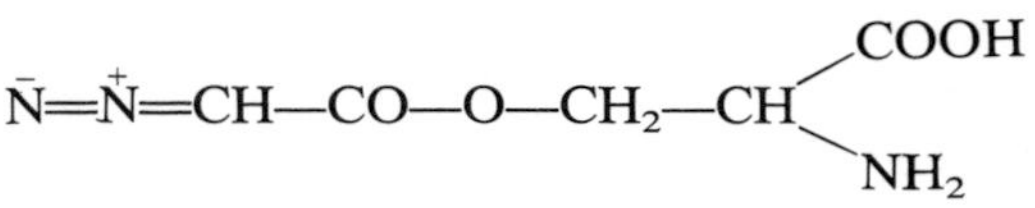

$$\bar{N}{=}\overset{+}{N}{=}CH{-}CO{-}O{-}CH_2{-}CH(COOH)(NH_2)$$

Fig. 16.96 Structure of azaserine.

Streptomyces strain. It is especially active against gram-positive bacteria (in particular, the diphtheria bacillus) and some gram-negative bacteria. Like azaserine, it possesses antitumor properties. Its structure (Fig. 16.97) (766, 767) is very similar to that of azaserine. Since azaserine and D.O.N. act by inhibiting the utilization of glutamine,

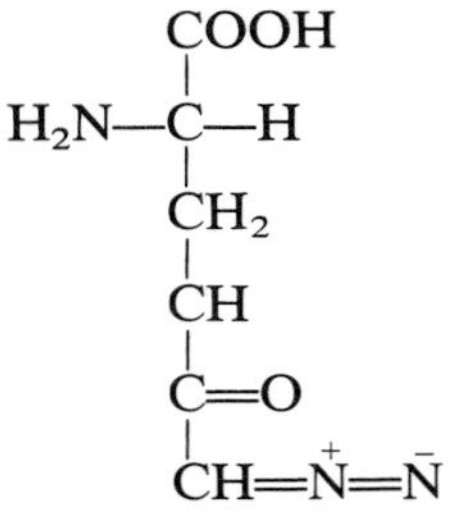

$$HOOC{-}CH(NH_2){-}CH_2{-}CH_2{-}C({=}O){-}CH{=}\overset{+}{N}{=}\bar{N}$$

Fig. 16.97 Structure of D.O.N.

the length of the chain is important: diazo-5-oxo-4-norvaline has no antibiotic activity. Both antibiotics have been reviewed (768).

By alkylation of an SH group, azaserine blocks the enzyme that catalyzes the conversion of formylglycineamide ribotide and the corresponding amidine in the biosynthesis of inosinic acid, which is the precursor of guanylic and adenylic acids. This reaction (Fig. 16.98) requires glutamine as the donor of the amide group. The elucidation of the mechanism of action of azaserine is largely due to Buchanan (769–772). Simultaneously with the inhibition of the synthesis of purines, there is an accumulation of formylglycinamide ribotide (I). The transformation of (I) into (II) requires the presence of glutamine. Azaserine behaves like a competitive inhibitor of glutamine with regard to the enzyme that affects this reaction. Azaserine binds specifically and irreversibly to the thiol of a single cysteine at the enzymatic site (770). The mode of action of azaserine is the same with bacteria and with animal cells. Azaserine can act on other enzymes (773, 774). D.O.N. also inhibits other enzymes, such as the transaminase that transforms fructose-6-phosphate to glucosamine-6-phosphate (775). The competition with glutamine is not the only action of azaserine. It also possesses mutagenic activity (776–778).

15.6 Bleomycins

The bleomycins, produced by *Streptomyces verticillatus*, contain copper. Hydrolysis furnishes several basic glycopeptides that

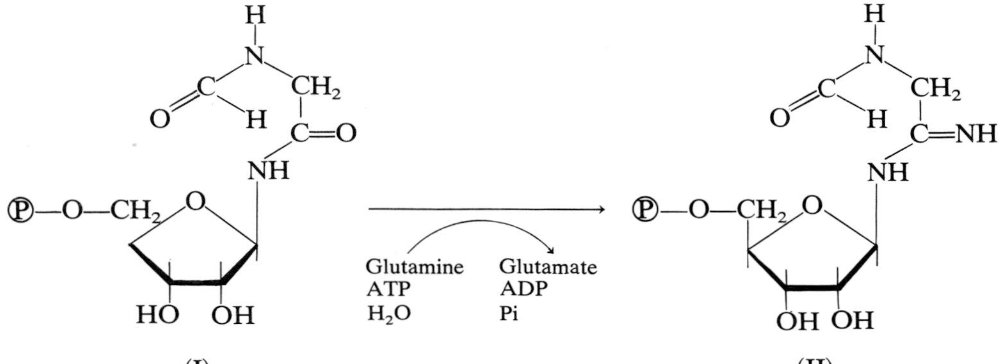

(I) ⟶ (II)

Glutamine, ATP, H_2O → Glutamate, ADP, Pi

Fig. 16.98 Biosynthesis of inosinic acid.

differ from one another in their terminal amine moieties. Present information indicates that a common chemical structure occurs where modifications of the radical R yield different bleomycins (779, 780). Very recently this structure has been revised (Fig. 16.99) (780a, 780b).

The bleomycins include a potentially important new group of clinically active antitumor agents. A complex mixture has recently been approved by the US Food and Drug Administration as a prescription drug for use in cancer chemotherapy. It is to be expected that highly purified and chemically modified bleomycins will become available that perhaps will differ from present preparations in their antineoplastic spectra and toxic manifestations. Reviews of the bleomycins have been published recently (781–784).

Bleomycins have attracted great interest because of their activity in a variety of human tumors, including squamous carcinomas of skin, head, neck, and lungs, in addition to lymphomas and testicular tumors. In comparison with many other antineoplastic agents, the bleomycins in current use have minimal myelosuppressive and immunosuppressive activities. They do, however, cause unusual cutaneous and pulmonary toxicity. Since the toxic manifestations of the bleomycins do not overlap significantly with those of most other drugs, and since their apparent mechanism of action is also unique (*vide infra*), it seems likely that the bleomycins will find an important place in combination chemotherapy.

It has been possible to prepare bleomycinic acid, where the radical R is a hydroxyl group. Nine naturally occurring bleomycins have been isolated in pure

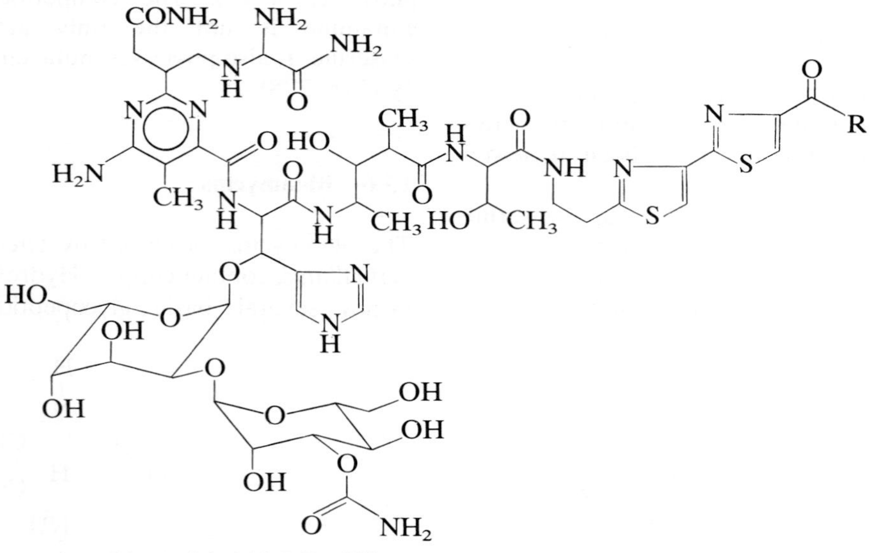

Bleomycinic acid R = OH

Bleomycin A_2 R = $NHCH_2CH_2CH_2{-}\overset{+}{S}(CH_3)_2$

Bleomycin B_2 R = $NHCH_2CH_2CH_2CH_2NHC(=NH)NH_2$

Fig. 16.99 Structures of bleomycins.

form, and chemical addition of various amines to bleomycinic acid has made possible the synthesis of at least 100 artificial bleomycins. The composition of the bleomycins can also be modified by the addition of specific amines to the fermentation mixtures. Of the natural components, bleomycin A_2 is the principal component of the bleomycin mixture presently used. It appears that large numbers of natural and semisynthetic bleomycins will become available for experimental and perhaps clinical study.

Although the bleomycins have been shown to have a number of interesting biochemical properties, it seems most likely that their cytotoxic action is related to their ability to cause chain scission and fragmentation of DNA molecules. Marked chromosomal abnormalities have also been described that probably are due to the damage to DNA.

Bleomycin B_2 in very low concentrations can bind to DNA and cause nicking. It has been proposed that a chemical reaction occurs between a reactive group on the bleomycin and the DNA, causing the nick (782). Furthermore, an ATP-dependent DNA ligase isolated from a rat hepatoma is markedly inhibited by low concentrations of bleomycin. Since DNA ligases play an important role in DNA replication, recombination, and repair, it appears that in the presence of a bleomycin, the repair of chain scission caused by the reaction of the drug or perhaps by an endonuclease cannot be performed, leading to progressive fragmentation of the DNA chain.

Of considerable interest is the apparent mechanism of the selective action of the bleomycins against squamous cell carcinomas and their toxicity to lung and skin. Evidence indicates that enzymes in most tissues, with the exception of lung and skin, can rapidly inactivate the bleomycins. Furthermore, it has been shown that sarcomas inactivate bleomycin more readily than do carcinomas. The mechanism of the enzymatic inactivation is not yet established, although it appears to involve a deamination or a peptidase reaction.

Studies with synchronized cells have indicated that the bleomycins block the cell cycle, causing accumulation of cells, some severely injured, at G_2. Other studies have shown that cells in mitosis are most sensitive to these antibiotics (781–783). A stimulatory effect of bleomycin on the synthesis of acidic glycosaminoglycans in cultured fibroplasts derived from rat carrageenin granuloma has been noted (785).

Interactions of DNA with bleomycin by UV and CD measurements have been reported (786).

The effect of chelating agents and metal ions on the degradation of DNA by bleomycin has been studied (786a).

Bleomycin and Fe(II) together act to cause the highly efficient degradation of adenovirus-2 DNA to acid soluble products when the drug and the metal ion are present in a one- to twofold excess of DNA (786b).

Tallysomycin, a new antitumor antibiotic complex, related to bleomycin, has recently been discovered (786c).

15.7 Boromycin

Streptomyces antibioticus contains in its mycelium a colorless substance, boromycin, which possesses inhibitory activity against the growth of gram-positive bacteria. Its structure (Fig. 16.100) contains boron. The structural complex is largely spherical, with a lipophilic surface and a cavity in which the valine side chain is placed (787). Its mechanism of action has been reviewed (788).

15.8 Bruneomycin

Bruneomycin is produced by *Streptomyces albus* var. *bruneomycini* and is structurally related to streptonigrin (789).

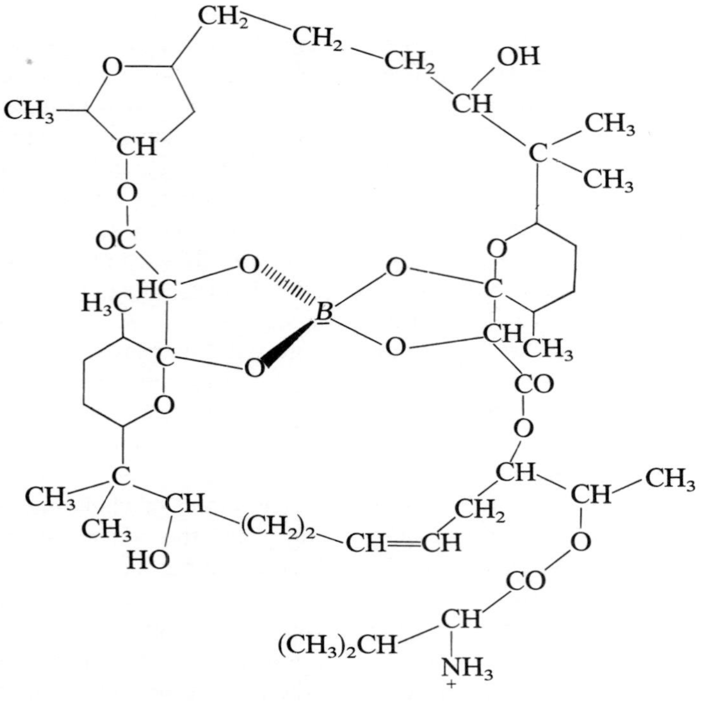

Fig. 16.100 Structures of boromycin.

15.9 Carzinophilin

Carzinophilin, an antitumor compound used clinically in Japan, is produced by *Streptomyces sahachiroi* (790). The antibiotic, $C_{50}H_{58}N_5O_{18}$, inhibits gram-positive and acid-fast bacteria *in vitro.* A clinical study showed improvement in patients suffering from mesenchymal tumors, sarcoma, malignant lymphogranulomatosis, and cancer of the skin, when the drug was given by intravenous injection (791). The toxicity in mice is 0.15 mg/kg, i.v.

15.10 Cellocidin

Cellocidin ($H_2NCOC{\equiv}CCONH_2$), an antibiotic from *Streptomyces chibaensis* (792) with antibacterial activity, is produced in tonnage amounts by chemical synthesis (793) in Japan for use against the rice plant bacterial plant pathogens. Antitumor activity has been noted *in vitro*, but no successes have been observed in testing *in vivo* against Ehrlich ascites carcinoma.

15.11 Chloramphenicol

Chloramphenicol (Fig. 16.101) is an antibiotic produced by *Streptomyces venezuelae*, an organism first isolated in 1947 from a soil sample collected in Venezuela.

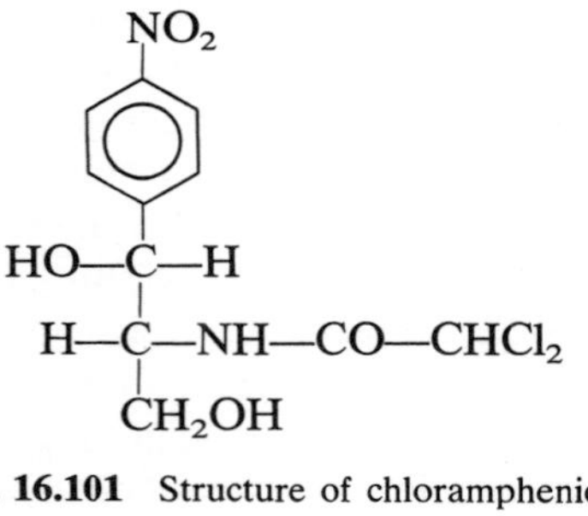

Fig. 16.101 Structure of chloramphenicol.

Filtrates of liquid cultures of the organisms were found to possess marked effectiveness against several gram-negative bacteria and also to exhibit antirickettsial activity. A crystalline antibiotic substance was then isolated and named "chloromycetin" because it contained chlorine and was obtained from an actinomycete. When the structural formula of the crystalline material was determined, the antibiotic was prepared synthetically. By 1948 chloramphenicol was being produced in amounts sufficient for general clinical use and was found to be of value in the therapy of a variety of infections. By 1950, however, it became evident that the drug could cause serious and fatal blood dyscrasias.

Chloramphenicol possesses a fairly wide spectrum of antimicrobial activity. It is primarily bacteriostatic, although it may be bactericidal to certain species under some conditions. Among the bacteria inhibited by relatively low concentrations of the antibiotic *in vitro* are *Enterobacter* (*Aerobacter*) *aerogenes*, *E. coli*, *K. pneumoniae*, *Bordetella pertussis*, *H. influenza*, *Pasteurella*, *Pseudomonas mallei*, *P. pseudomallei*, *Bacteroides*, *Salmonella typhi* and other species, *Proteus* (certain strains), *Neisseria*, *Shigella*, *Brucella*, and *Vibrio cholerae*. Some streptococci and staphylococci are suppressed by higher concentrations. *Actinomyces*, *Bacillus anthracis*, *Corynebacterium diphtheriae*, *Clostridium*, *Listeria*, *Bartonella*, and *Leptospira* are sensitive to moderate concentrations.

In general, the results of chloramphenicol therapy of bacterial infections in experimental animals parallel the *in vitro* results. Chloramphenicol exerts marked prophylactic and therapeutic effects in experimental infections produced by all rickettsiae. The drug, as a rule, merely suppresses rickettsial growth, thus permits the development of immunity that is responsible for recovery. Chloramphenicol is also effective against chlamydia and mycoplasma.

Some species of bacteria, but not rickettsiae, may be made resistant to chloramphenicol *in vitro* by serial culture in increasing concentrations of the drug. Bacterial resistance to chloramphenicol *in vivo* is a problem of increasing clinical importance, for both gram-positive and gram-negative microorganisms. Insensitivity to the drug of *E. coli*, *Salmonella*, and other gram-negative bacteria is due to the presence of a specific resistance (R) factor acquired by conjugation. The resistance of such strains to chloramphenicol appears to be attributable to the presence of a specific acetyltransferase, which inactivates the drug by using acetyl coenzyme A as the donor of the acetyl group (794). The enzyme is constitutive in *E. coli*. Resistance of staphylococci to this antibiotic has also increased in incidence; it varies from one hospital to another and is as high as 50% or more in some. Shaw and Brodsky demonstrated that resistant *Staphylococcus aureus* contains an inducible form of chloramphenicol acetyltransferase (795).

Chloramphenicol and its mechanism of action have been reviewed recently (796). Chloramphenicol inhibits protein synthesis in bacteria and in cell-free systems. It acts primarily on the 50S ribosomal subunit and shares this site of action with macrolide antibiotics and lincomycin. The activity of peptidyl transferase, which catalyzes peptide bond formation, is suppressed, although ribosomes may still bind to and move along strands of mRNA. Ribosomal translocation thus appears to be uncoupled from peptide bond synthesis (797–800).

The effects on mammalian cells, including some of the hematological abnormalities observed in clinical practice, are also thought to be related primarily to inhibition of protein synthesis. However Godchaux and Herbert (801) have suggested that the mechanism of action of chloramphenicol on reticulocytes is different from that on bacterial cells. The main effect on reticulocytes is inhibition of the conversion of polysomes to single ribosomes and a decrease in the content of ATP. The synthesis of both RNA and protein is inhibited. It is also clear that chloramphenicol can inhibit mitochondrial protein synthesis in higher cells (802); it is hypothesized that mitochondrial ribosomes resemble bacterial ribosomes (both are 70S) more than they do the 80S cytoplasmic ribosomes of mammalian cells.

Chloramphenicol acetyltransferases specified by fi^- (F-fertility-noninhibiting) R factors were compared with those specified by the fi^+ R factors R1, 222, and R6-S (803). The mechanism of chloramphenicol resistance in staphylococci has been described in terms of characterization and hybridization of variants of chloramphenicol acetyltransferase (804). *E. coli* membrane proteins are stable during chloramphenicol treatment (805). The following structure-activity relationships have been recognized.

1. Replacement of the nitro group with a number of other substituents including CN, $CONH_2$, SO_2NHR, NH_2, OH, $N(CH_3)_2$, NHR, $NHCH_2R$, Br, Cl, I, F, SO_2R, C_6H_5, C_6H_4R, and various heterocyclic groups, resulted in some reduction or complete loss of antibacterial activity. This confirms the hypothesis that electronegativity, molecular volume, and perhaps the ability to participate in *p*-quinoid-type systems are important factors in determining activity. The methylthiol and methylsulfonyl compounds were among the most promising analogs of the group, but interest waned with the demonstration of undesirable toxic properties. Shifting the nitro group from the *p*-position also reduces the antibacterial activity.
2. The phenyl group has been replaced with other aromatic or alicyclic groups such as naphthyl, nitronaphthyl, pyridyl, quinolyl, thienyl, furyl, nitrofuryl, nitrothienyl, and cyclohexyl. Only the nitrothienyl compound had antibacterial activity, and it was less potent than chloramphenicol (805a–805e).
3. Only the D-*threo* compound of the four stereoisomers is antibacterially active (805f–h). The primary alcohol group also seems to be needed, since its deletion or replacement with alkyl decreases potency. Extending the propanediol side chain by branched alkyl groups is similarly detrimental to the activity of the compounds.
4. Replacement of the dichloroacetyl group with such acyls as dibromoacetyl resulted in some loss of potency, but major activities were still retained (805i). Even the acetamide (nonhalogen) compound has marked antibiotic properties.

15.12 Cycloserine

Cycloserine is produced by a whole series of *Streptomyces* species (in particular, *S. lavendulae, S. orchidaceus, S. garyphalus, S. roseochromogenes*). It is very active *in vitro* against mycobacteria, but much less active *in vivo*, particularly in animals whose serum contains D-alanine, e.g., mice, guinea pigs (806) (LD_{50}: 1800 mg/kg, mouse, i.v., and 5300 mg/kg, mouse, p.o.). Its structure (Fig. 16.102) contains an asymmetric carbon. The natural compound corresponds to D-serine (807, 808). Cycloserine can be synthesized (809). L-Cycloserine possesses antibiotic activity, acting by a different mechanism, and the racemic form possesses superior antibiotic activity (synergism).

The mechanism of action of cycloserine has been reviewed (810). The antibiotic acts on the synthesis of the bacterial cell

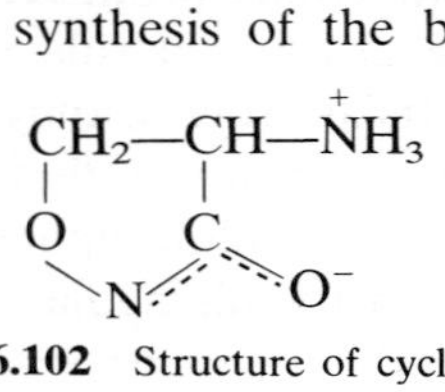

$$\begin{array}{l} CH_2—CH—\overset{+}{N}H_3 \\ \;|\qquad\;\; | \\ O \qquad C \\ \;\diagdown N \overset{\cdot\cdot\cdot}{\diagup}\;\overset{\cdot\cdot\cdot}{\diagdown} O^- \end{array}$$

Fig. 16.102 Structure of cycloserine.

wall. It is a competitive inhibitor of L-alanine racemase and of D-Ala-D-Ala synthetase. The L-alanine racemase inhibition has been shown in *S. aureus* and *S. fecalis* (811–814). On the other hand, L-cycloserine is not an inhibitor. Since the racemase can have as substrate D- or L-alanine, this inactivity of L-cycloserine implies that the difference in conformation between the L- and D-forms of the antibiotic is not of the same order as that between D- and L-alanine. D-Cycloserine, which does inhibit, is noteworthy in having an affinity for the enzyme ($K_i = 5.10^{-5}$), 100 times larger than its affinity for the natural substrate ($K_m = 5.10^{-3}$). Comparison of the conformations of D- and L-alanine and D- and L-cycloserine can explain these facts.

Strominger's hypothesis implies the existence of a single site on the alanine racemase to which L- and D-alanine bind in the same conformation. If L-cycloserine does not inhibit the enzyme of *Staphylococcus aureus* and *Streptococcus fecalis*, it inhibits that of *E. coli* and *B. subtilis*. Lambert and Neuhaus (815), following a study of the racemase of *E. coli*, suggested that the hypothesis of Strominger is not general, and it is possible in this case that there are two distinct sites for the binding of L- and D-alanine. Johnson et al. had already proposed a model for the racemase of *Lactobacillus fermenti* (816) and had sketched two forms of the enzyme: one that binds D-alanine, and the other for L-alanine.

D-Cycloserine does not inhibit the enzyme that activates for the incorporation of teichoic acids (817). Alanine-racemase is an enzyme that requires pyridoxal phosphate as coenzyme. Cycloserine can form a Schiff's base (818, 819) with this coenzyme. It is possible that the antibiotic gives rise to inhibition by acting on pyridoxal phosphate (645).

D-Ala-D-Ala synthetase is competitively inhibited by cycloserine with *Staphylococcus aureus* (918) and with *Streptococcus fecalis* (820). Here, again, the affinity of the inhibitor for the enzyme ($K_i \sim 2.10^{-5}$) is 100 times larger than that of the substrate D-Ala (3.10^{-3}). Strominger's hypothesis, based on conformational considerations, is applicable. The work by Neuhaus and Lynch (820) is, in this respect, affirmative. This double inhibition results in the accumulation of a nucleotide: the uridine diphosphate of (*N*-acetyl-muramyl)-L-Ala-D-Glu-L-Lys, which lacks the D-Ala-D-Ala terminal.

15.13 Flavensomycin

Flavensomycin has been isolated from *Streptomyces griseus* (821). It is active against fungi and gram-positive bacteria (LD_{50}: 1 mg/kg, mouse, i.p.). Its partial structure appears in Fig. 16.103. Its mechanism of action has been reviewed (822).

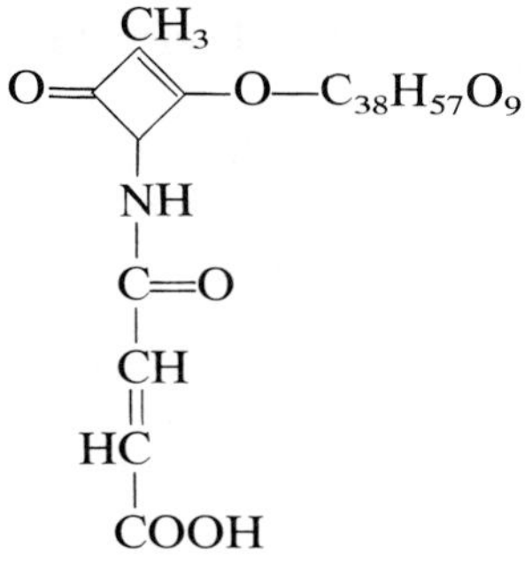

CH_3

O= [cyclobutene ring] —O—$C_{38}H_{57}O_9$

NH—C(=O)—CH=CH—COOH

$C_{38}H_{57}O_9$: ca. 10 (C—CH_3); ca. 1 (C—$CH(CH_3)_2$); ca. 3 (OCH_3); ca. 6 (active H); 4 (reducible double bonds)

Fig. 16.103 Partial structure of flavensomycin.

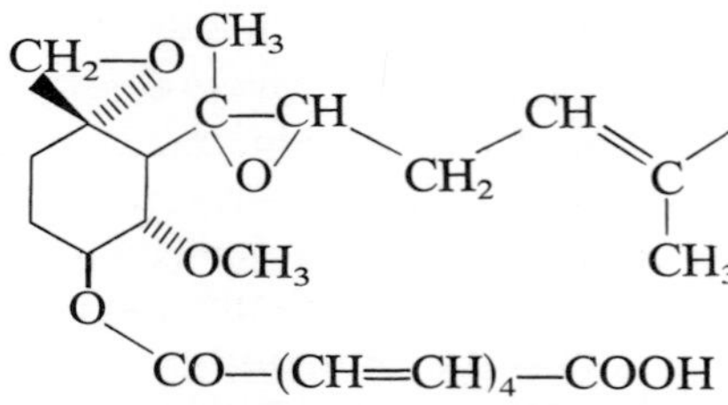

Fig. 16.104 Structure of fumagillin.

15.14 Fumagillin

Fumagillin (Fig. 16.104) (823) is produced by *Aspergillus fumigatus.* It is active against protozoa (in particular *Entameba histolytica* and *Trichomonas vaginalis*). In man it is used against intestinal amebiasis and has low toxicity (LD_{50}: 800 mg/kg, mouse, s.c.).

15.15 Griseofulvin

Griseofulvin was first isolated from *Penicillium griseofulvum dierckx* by Oxford and co-workers in 1939. Because it was ineffective against bacteria, no further attention was paid to it for some time. In 1946 Brian and associates found a substance in *P. janczewski* that produced shrinking and stunting of fungal hyphae; they named this the curling factor; it was later found to be griseofulvin. During the next 10 years the antibiotic was widely employed in the treatment of a variety of fungal diseases in plants and ringworm of cattle. In the course of a search for potential therapeutic compounds for the management of fungal infections of the feet of Scottish miners, Gentles (824) observed that griseofulvin cured experimentally produced mycotic disease of guinea pigs. Soon, thereafter, the drug was widely subjected to clinical trial and became available for general use. Figure 16.105 gives the structure of griseofulvin.

Griseofulvin inhibits the growth *in vitro* of various species of dermatophytes *Microsporum, Epidermophyton,* and *Trichophyton.* It has no effect on bacteria or on other

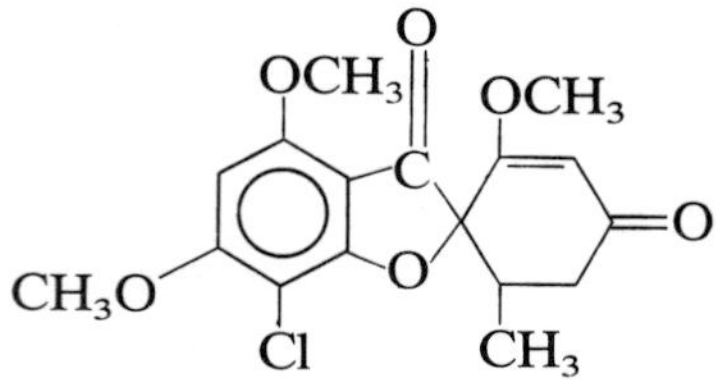

Fig. 16.105 Structure of griseofulvin.

fungi, yeasts, *Actinomycins,* or *Nocardia.* Griseofulvin is fungistatic and not fungicidal. Young, actively metabolizing cells are killed by the drug, but the older more dormant elements are less intensely affected.

Trichophyton, Epidermophyton, and *Microsporum* can be made resistant to griseofulvin *in vitro.* Animals infected with resistant strains develop infections similar to those produced by sensitive strains. With a few exceptions, isolates from humans receiving the antibiotic appear to retain their sensitivity to the drug when examined *in vitro.* The mycelia of *Microsporum* and *Trichophyton* destroy griseofulvin; the relationship of this phenomenon to fungal resistance to griseofulvin is presently not established.

Actively growing cultures of *Microsporum gypseum* take up very large quantities of griseofulvin, and the drug is bound to cellular lipids. The details of the fungistatic actions of the antibiotic are unfortunately unclear (825, 826). For a recent review, see Ref. 827.

15.16 Hadacidin

Hadacidin has been isolated from cultures of a number of species of *Penicillium* (in particular *P. frequentans* and *P. aurantioviolaceum*). It possesses antitumor properties. Its structure (Fig. 16.106) is that of

$$HOOC\text{—}CH_2\text{—}N(OH)\text{—}CHO$$

Fig. 16.106 Structure of hadacidin.

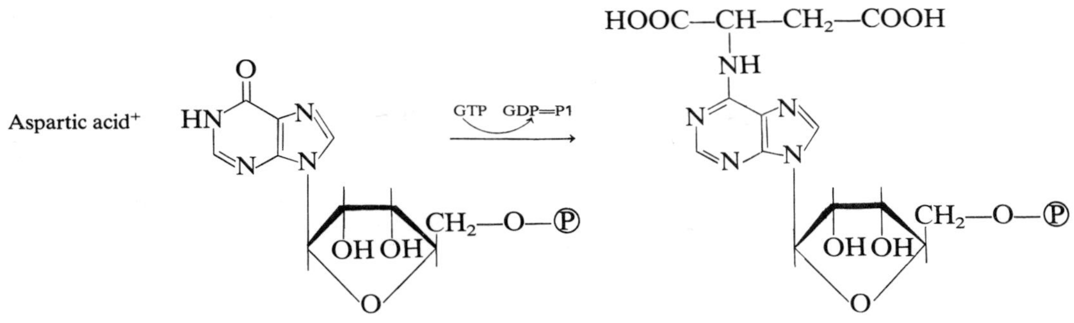

Aspartic acid$^+$ [Inosinic acid] $\xrightarrow{\text{GTP} \quad \text{GDP=P1}}$ [Adenyl-succinic acid]

Inosinic acid

Adenyl-succinic acid

Fig. 16.107 Synthesis of adenylic acid from inosinic acid.

an *N*-formylhydroxyaminoacetic acid. It acts as an analog of aspartic acid and blocks the synthesis of adenylic acid from inosinic acid (Fig. 16.107). This mechanism of action has essentially been elucidated by Shigeura and Gordon (828, 829).

15.17 Kanchanomycin

Kanchanomycin is an antibiotic of unknown structure, produced by a *Streptomyces* species. It is bactericidal and tumoricidal for neoplastic cells in culture at extremely low concentrations (830, 831). Kanchanomycin is of particular interest because it appears to inhibit *in vitro* RNA and DNA synthesis in two distinctive ways (832).

15.18 Lincomycin

Lincomycin is an antibiotic elaborated by an actinomycete, *Streptomyces lincolnensis*, so named because it was isolated from soil collected near Lincoln, Nebraska. The drug was first reported in the literature in 1962. Lincomycin is a derivative of the amino acid *trans*-L-4-*n*-propylhygrinic acid, attached to a sulfur-containing derivative of an octose. The structural formula of lincomycin is depicted in Fig. 16.108.

Concentrations of lincomycin less than 0.5 μg/ml inhibit the multiplication *in vitro* of *Streptomyces* (D.) *pneumoniae*, group A *S. pyogenes*, the *viridans* group of streptococci, and *Bacillus anthracis*. However some strains of pneumococci and group A streptococci are resistant. The drug is without effect on enterococci. *Corynebacterium diphtheriae*, *Clostridium tetani*, and *C. perfringens* are suppressed by concentrations lower than 2 μg/ml. Susceptibility of *Staphylococcus aureus* to the drug is variable; most strains are sensitive to about 2 μg/ml, but about 15% of strains grow in a concentration of 5 μg/ml. A number of strains of staphylococci that are resistant to

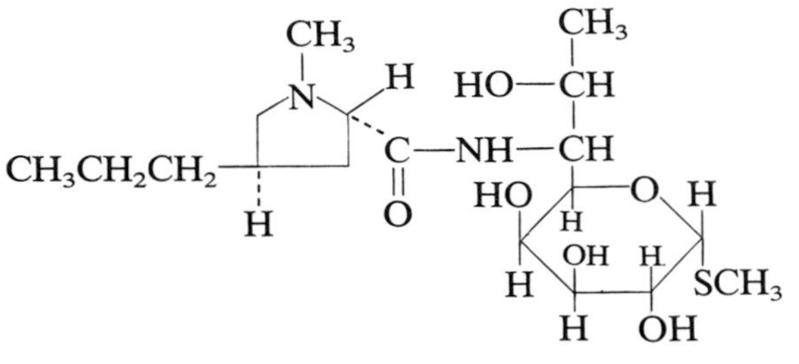

Fig. 16.108 Structure of lincomycin.

methicillin or erythromycin are also resistant to lincomycin. The antibiotic is active against some but not all types of Bacteroides; in one study, only 7% of strains of *Bacillus fragilis* were found to be susceptible to the drug (833). Lincomycin is bacteriostatic for *Actinomyces* in a concentration of 0.125–0.25 μg/ml. Mycoplasma are inhibited, but not nearly as effectively as by erythromycin. T strains of *M. hominis* are not susceptible. Lincomycin is not inhibitory for most strains of *Neisseria gonorrheae*, *H. influenzae*, and enterococci. Most gram-negative bacilli and all viruses and fungi are resistant (834, 835).

Lincomycin binds exclusively to the 50S subunit of bacterial ribosomes and suppresses protein synthesis. Although lincomycin, erythromycin, and chloramphenicol are not structurally related, they all act at this site, and the binding of one of these antibiotics to the ribosome may inhibit the reaction of the other. There are no clinical indications for the concurrent use of these antibiotics (836, 837).

Chlorination of lincomycin at the 7-carbon results in clindamycin. Both compounds bind to plasma protein (838). Both lincomycin and clindamycin have an effect on peptide chain initiation (839).

In various studies lincomycin has been chemically modified (840). Among the compounds that have been made are 2,7-dialkylcarbonate esters (841), (7*S*)-7-alkoxy-7-deoxy–analogs (842), 7-*O*-methyl and 6-de-(1-hydroxyethyl) analogs (843), and *N*-dimethyllincomycin (844).

15.19 Micrococcin

This antibiotic, produced by a species of *Micrococcus*, yields upon hydrolysis thiazole derivatives (Fig. 16.108*a*), among others. A recent review presents its chemistry and mode of action (845).

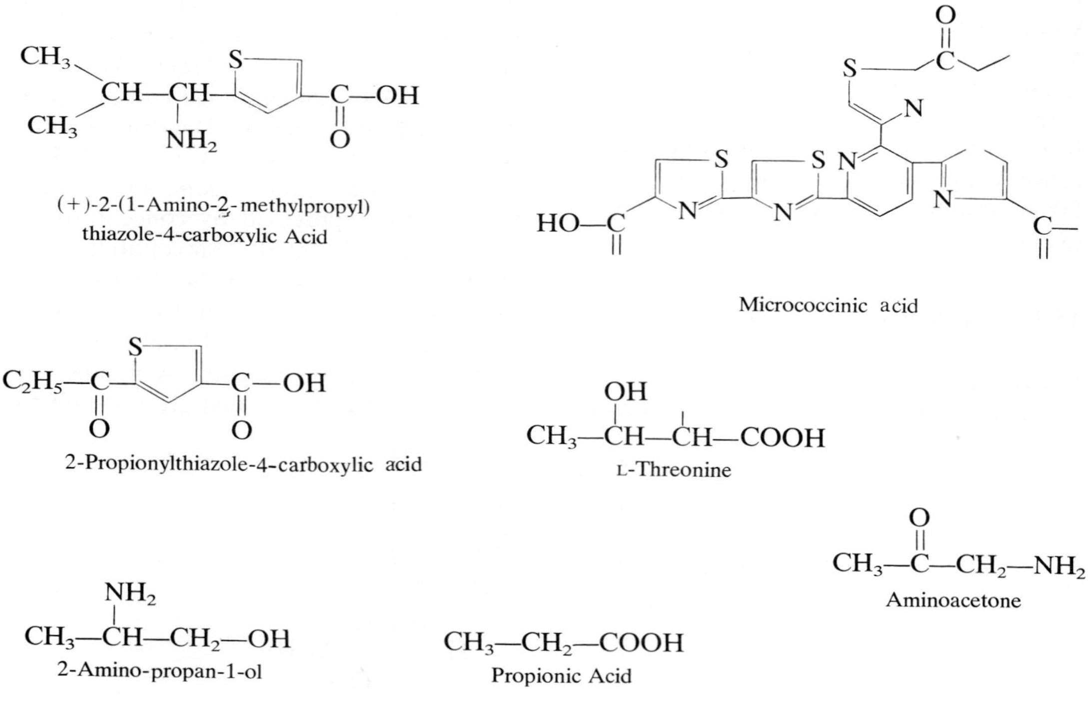

(+)-2-(1-Amino-2-methylpropyl) thiazole-4-carboxylic Acid

Micrococcinic acid

2-Propionylthiazole-4-carboxylic acid

$CH_3—CH(OH)—CH(NH_2)—COOH$

L-Threonine

$CH_3—CO—CH_2—NH_2$

Aminoacetone

$CH_3—CH(NH_2)—CH_2—OH$

2-Amino-propan-1-ol

$CH_3—CH_2—COOH$

Propionic Acid

Fig. 16.108*a* Hydrolytic fragments from micrococcin.

15.20 Mitomycins and Porfiromycin

Streptomyces caespitosus produces a mixture of antibiotics called mitomycins. From the mixture have been isolated mitomycins A, B, C, R, and Y (846). In addition to a powerful antibacterial activity, common to these substances, mitomycin C possesses antitumor activity. The compounds are rather toxic: LD_{50} with mice, i.v., is 2 mg/kg for mitomycin A, 10 mg/kg for mitomycin B, and 5 mg/kg for mitomycin C. Besides mitomycins A, B, and C, *S. verticillatus* produces porfiromycin, which is closely related structurally (Fig. 16.109). The structure of mitomycin A has been confirmed by X-ray diffraction of its *N*-brosyl derivative (847). Elimination in mitomycin A of the C_{10}-methoxyl with double bond formation between C-9 and C-10 furnishes a derivative that retains powerful antibiotic activity (848).

Mitomycins and porfiromycins (849) are antibiotics that can affect the development of bacteria as a function of the concentration of the antibiotic and the bacterial species, as well as normal and neoplastic cells of mammals.

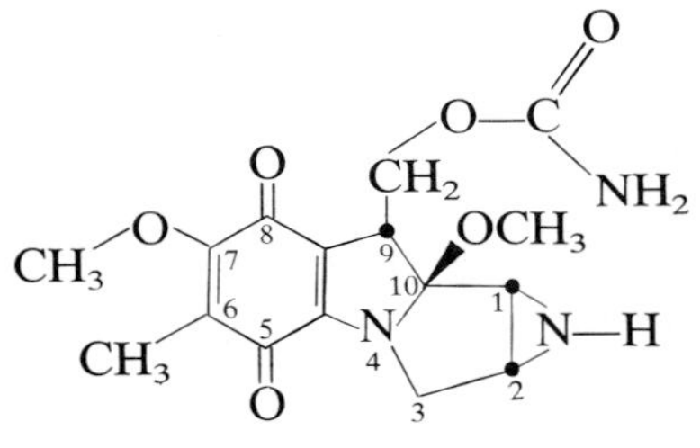

(*a*)

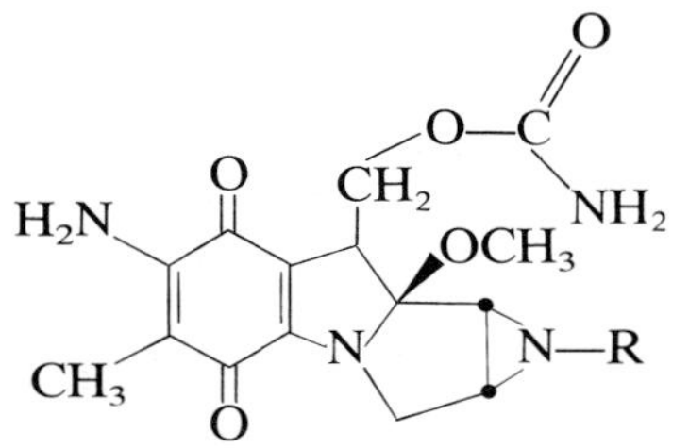

(*b*)

Fig. 16.109 Structures of mitomycins and porfiromycin. (*a*) Mitomycin A. (*b*) Porfiromycin ($R = CH_3$) and mitomycin C ($R = H$).

Under reduced activated form the mitomycins are activated and bind to nucleic acids by alkylation. The presence of at least two binding functions allows the antibiotic molecule to establish bridges, particularly between the two complementary strands of the double helix DNA. They do not bind to nucleic acids *in vitro* unless they undergo activation because of reduction. This reduction can be effected chemically by borohydride, hydrosulfite, or by hydrogen over palladium, and enzymatically by an extract of *B. subtilis* (the reaction is said to be catalyzed by a reductase quinone in presence of NADPH) (850, 851). The reduction product is very labile, and the alkylation reaction must take place in a few seconds following reduction. Numerous chemical studies have led to the determination of the sites of the reduced molecule that are capable of reacting with the nucleic acids. The activation steps are pictured in Fig. 16.110.

Mitomycin can alkylate nucleic acids either by one of its alkylating functions or by two such functions, thus creating a bridge between the two strands of the double DNA helix (850, 851). By isolating mitomycin linked to two guanines, it has been shown that mitomycin can link to two guanines in the RNA chain (852). The number of mitomycin molecules that establish a bridge represents only a small fraction of those that bind to the nucleic acid. Using ^{14}C-marked mitomycin, the extent of fixation of the antibiotic on purified DNA has been studied (853, 854). Under the experimental conditions, one molecule of mitomycin is bound per 2500 pairs of nucleotides, and one molecule in 5 or 10 forms a bridge between the two chains. It seems that the number of bridges *in vivo* is higher, nevertheless it is rather low. One cannot speak of base specificity, although the number of bridges rises with the G-C content of the DNA. It is possible that the

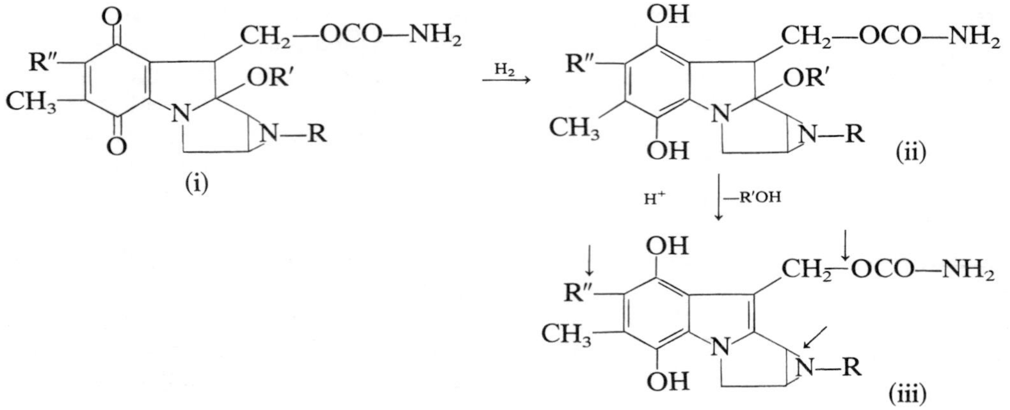

Fig. 16.110 Activation steps of mitomycins; in formula III the arrows indicate the possible reactive sites (851).

reaction simply is faster with guanine (852). The oxygen at position 6 in guanine could be involved in this reaction, but N_7 is probably not involved (855).

One of the most interesting physicochemical effects brought to light is the behavior of the DNA molecules during thermal denaturation (850–854). DNA can be "melted"; that is. the two strands come apart. Under slow cooling, the two strands link up again, to a large degree by virtue of hydrogen bonds, but reassociation is not possible under very fast cooling, and the two strands remain separated in this condition. It has been shown that in the presence of mitomycin, thermal denaturation leads to fusion of DNA, but the two strands remain bound together by the mitomycin bridges, and these bridges allow renaturation during a very rapid cooling process.

It can easily be seen that the bridging of the two complementary DNA chains constitutes an obstacle to replication as well as to the proper functioning of the DNA-dependent RNA polymerase. Thus there is an inhibition of RNA synthesis (856, 857). Still, it is not certain that the action of mitomycin is exclusively due to the alkylation reaction. Nonalkylating substances with a quinone ring inhibit the synthesis of nucleic acids (858). Moreover, a repair process at the level of the bridges intervenes, since mitomycin can inhibit replication only in a transitory fashion (858). It is remarkable that treatment with mitomycin provokes a rise in nuclease activity toward DNA in connection with the repair process. This is also true for RNA (859).

Recently the reaction of mitomycin C with DNA has been examined by ethidium fluorescence assay (860). The proportional decrease in fluorescence with pH strongly suggests that the alkylation is due to the aziridine moiety of the antibiotic.

There is a reversible conversion of mitomycin C into sodium 7-aminomitosane-9a-sulfonate (861).

15.21 Nalidixic Acid

Nalidixic acid is a synthetic product. It is particularly active against gram-negative bacteria *in vitro* and *in vivo* (LD_{50}: 3300 mg/kg, mouse, p.o.; 176 mg/kg, mouse, i.v.). Its structure shows a naphthyridine skeleton (Fig. 16.111).

Nalidixic acid selectively blocks DNA replication in susceptible bacteria in a manner as yet undefined (862). Recent work on its mechanism of action has been reported (863–865).

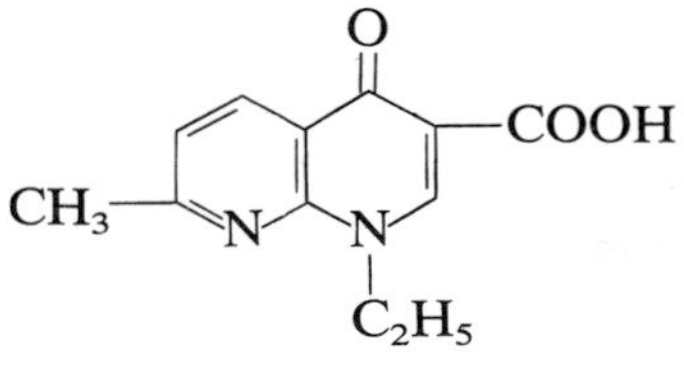

Fig. 16.111 Structure of nalidixic acid.

There is a bactericidal effect of combinations of nalidixic acid and various antibiotics on Enterobacteriaceae (866).

15.22 Novobiocin

This antibiotic is produced by several species of *Streptomyces*, in particular *S. spheroides* and *S. niveus*. It is also known under the names cathomycin, streptonivicin, and cardelmycin. Novobiocin (Fig. 16.112) is active against gram-negative bacteria, but especially against gram-positive bacteria, in particular staphylococci; it is active *in vitro* at a concentration 0.07–0.15 μg/ml in the case of staphylococci, but only at 1–15 μg/ml in the case of streptococci (LD_{50}: 470 mg/kg, mouse, i.v.; 262 mg/kg, mouse, i.p.; 962 mg/kg, mouse, p.o.). Guinea pigs are more sensitive (LD_{50}: 11.5 mg/kg, i.v.). With dilute base, novobiocin is isomerized to isonovobiocin through migration of the carbamyl group; isonovobiocin has no antibiotic activity. Several novobiocin syntheses have been accomplished (867).

The mode of action of novobiocin has been reviewed (868). Novobiocin and its combination with tetracycline, chloramphenicol, erythromycin, and lincomycin has an effect on the microbial generation of *E. coli* (869).

15.23 Pactamycin

Pactamycin (Fig. 16.113) is produced by *Streptomyces pactum*. Besides its activity against gram-positive and gram-negative bacteria, it possesses *in vivo* activity against numerous types of tumors (LD_{50}: 15.6 mg/kg, mouse, i.v.). Pactamycin and sparsomycin exert a synergistic effect on mycoplasma-induced lethal toxicity of mice (870).

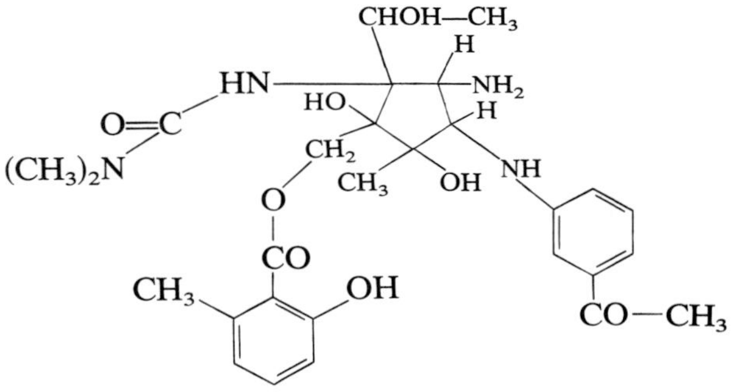

Fig. 16.113 Structure of pactamycin.

Pactamycin has been shown to act primarily by inhibiting protein synthesis in intact cells and in extracts of microorganisms and animals. The ribosomes have been implicated as the site of action of the antibiotic. Pactamycin selectively blocks polypeptide chain initiation (872).

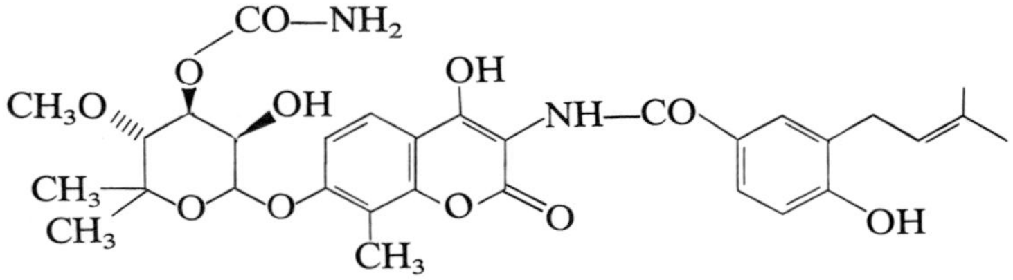

Fig. 16.112 Structure of novobiocin.

15.24 Patulin

Produced by *Penicillium patulum*, by *Aspergillus clavatus*, and by other species of these microorgansims, patulin is active *in vitro* against various gram-positive and gram-negative bacteria. *In vivo* it exhibits little activity and is too toxic to be used. Since it has been isolated from various microorganisms, it also carries the names clavicin, clavatin, claviformin, penicidin, expansin, and mycoin. Its structure is depicted in Fig. 16.114 (873).

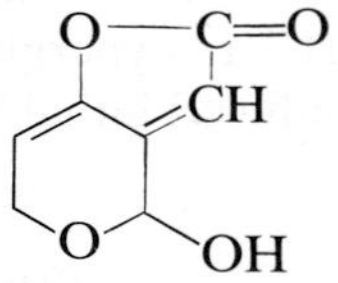

Fig. 16.114 Structure of patulin.

Patulin inhibits the cells and/or nuclear division, but the observations regarding the precise nature of its action are quite conflicting (874).

15.25 Pluramycin

Pluramycin A, obtained from the culture broth of *Streptomyces pluricolorescens*, is a basic antibiotic. Its molecular formula is $C_{20}H_{25}NO_5$. Another antibiotic, designated pluramycin B, was isolated from the same culture filtrate in a crude form. Both pluramycins A and B inhibit growth of bacteria and tumor cells. The LD_{50} of pluramycin A ascorbate to mice are 1.0 mg/kg, i.v., and 6.6 mg/kg, i.p. (875).

15.26 Protoanemonin

Protoanemonin is an antibiotic substance produced mainly by species of Ranunculaceae. Its structure (Fig. 16.115) is that of α-hydroxyvinylacrylic acid. Protoanemonin inhibits growth of gram-positive and

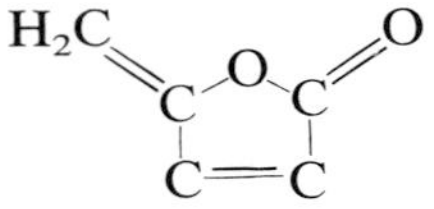

Fig. 16.115 Structure of protoanemonin.

gram-negative bacteria, and of fungi, but the degree of inhibition varies widely.

There have been no systematic studies on the mode of action of protoanemonin. There is some evidence that protoanemonin inhibits growth by reaction with sulfhydryl enzymes (876).

15.27 Pyrrolnitrin

Pseudomonas pyrrocinia produces this antibiotic, which has antifungal character (LD_{50}: 500 mg/kg, mouse, i.p.). The structure in Fig. 16.116 has been proposed for pyrrolnitrin (877).

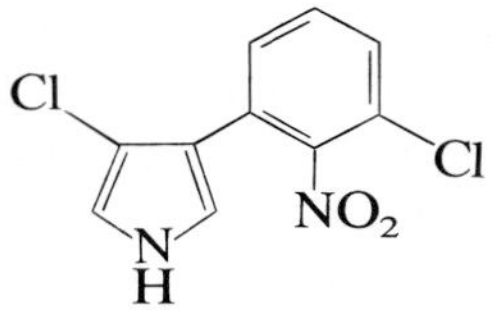

Fig. 16.116 Structure of pyrrolnitrin.

15.28 Sarkomycin

Sarkomycin is produced by *Streptomyces erythrochromogenes*. It is active against bacteria, yeasts, and fungi. Moreover, sarkomycin possesses antitumor activity (LD_{50}: 800–1600 mg/kg, mouse, i.v.; 4800–6800 mg/kg, mouse, p.o.). Its structure is represented in Fig. 16.117 (878). Because

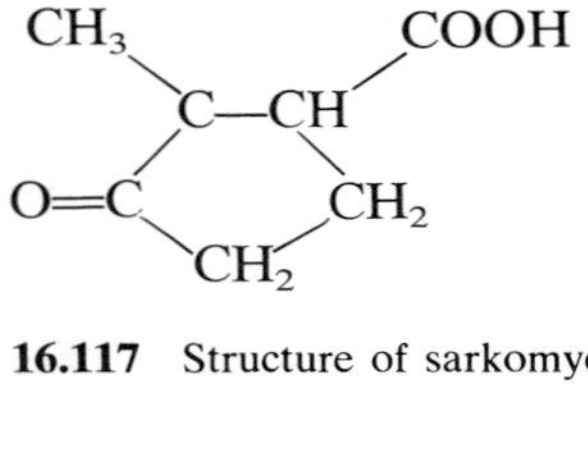

Fig. 16.117 Structure of sarkomycin.

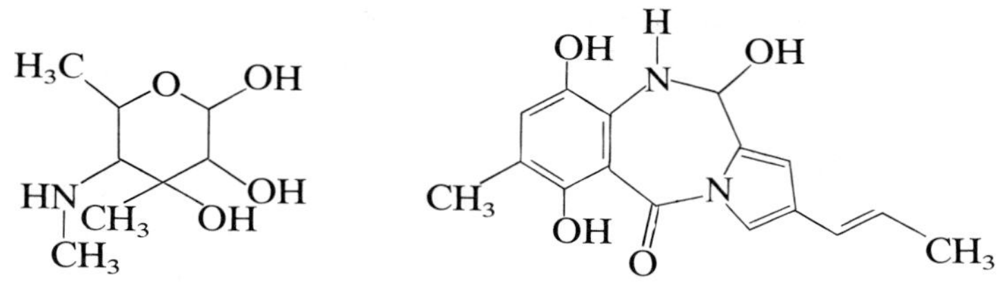

Fig. 16.118 Structures of (*a*) amino sugar and (*b*) aglycone of sibiromycin.

of its antitumor properties and its relatively simple structure, numerous derivatives have been synthesized (879). Catalytic hydrogenation of sarkomycin yields *trans*-2-methyl-3-cyclopentanone carboxylic acid, which has no antibacterial activity but retains antitumor activity (880, 881).

This antibiotic inhibits the synthesis of DNA in cells of Ehrlich ascites carcinoma (882). Cysteine, glutathion, and mercaptoethanol are antagonists (883, 884).

15.29 Sibiromycin

The antitumor antibiotic sibromycin is a glycoside of a new amino sugar sibirosamine. The aglycone is a derivative of 1,4-benzdiasepine (Fig. 16.118) (885–887). It is produced by an actinomycete *Streptosporangium sibiricum* and was first detected by its capacity to inhibit the multiplication of suspended ascites tumor cells. Sibiromycin inhibits growth of *Bacillus*

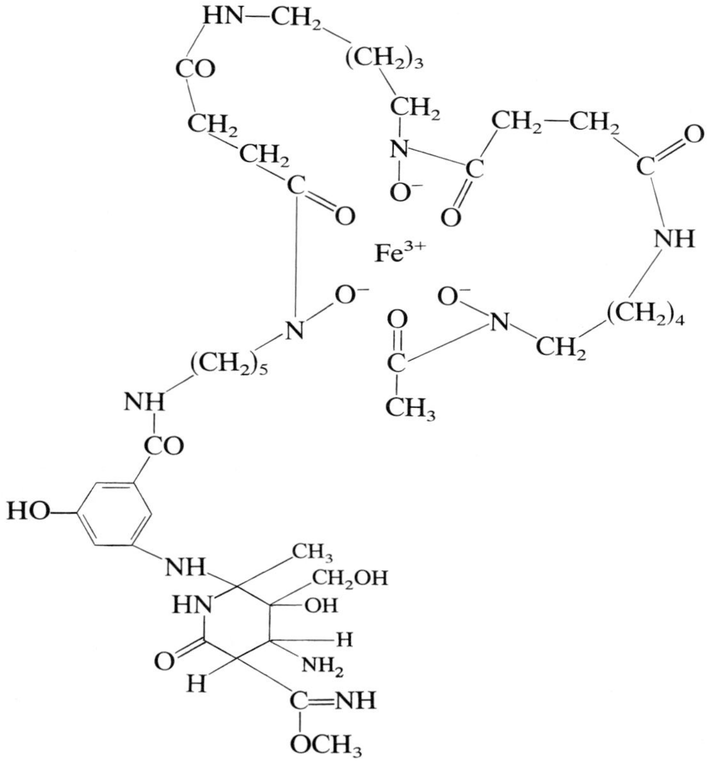

Fig. 16.119 Structure of ferrimycin A_1 (891, 892).

mycoides and *B. subtilis* (0.3 μg/ml), *Staphylococcus aureus* (1 μg/ml), and *E. coli* (20 μg/ml). When sibiromycin was administered to mice intravenously, intraperitoneally, subcutaneously, and orally, the LD_{50} were found to be 58, 32, 84, and 459 μg/ml, respectively. Sibiromycin interacts specifically with DNA (888).

15.30 Sideromycins

The sideromycins whose first representative was discovered by Waksman in 1947 in a culture of *Streptomyces griseus* (889) and described under the name of griseine, are essentially active against gram-positive bacteria; in some cases they are also active against gram-negative bacteria. In animals, for example, ferrimycin A (Fig. 16.119) is 10–50 times more active than penicillin (890). Sideromycins are well tolerated by animals. Their two principal inconveniences are the difficulty of isolation from culture media, and the fast establishment of a resistance by bacteria (891).

The mode of action of sideromycins has been reviewed recently (893).

15.31 Tenuazonic Acid

This antibiotic is produced by *Alternaria tenuis*. It is believed to be the first substituted tetramic acid isolated from natural sources (Fig. 16.120) (894). The structure has been verified by synthesis (895). Tenuazonic acid inhibits the growth of human adenocarcinoma growing in the embryonated egg. The compound is inactive against several species of bacteria and yeast.

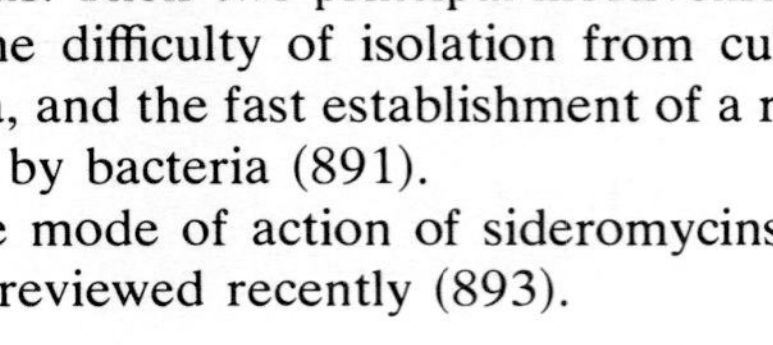

Fig. 16.120 Structure of tenuazonic acid.

The principal site of action in mammalian cells appears to be related to the suppression of protein synthesis; more precisely, the inhibition of release of nascent proteins from the microsomes into the cell's sap. Tenuazonic acid appears to have no direct effect on nucleic acid synthesis (896). Tenuazonic acid analogs have been made by microbial production (897).

15.32 Trichothecin

This antifungal antibiotic was isolated from culture filtrates of *Trichothecium roseum*. A structure (Fig. 16.121) has been proposed (898). Trichothecin is of no therapeutic value in animals because of its extreme toxicity. Very little is known about its mode of action (899).

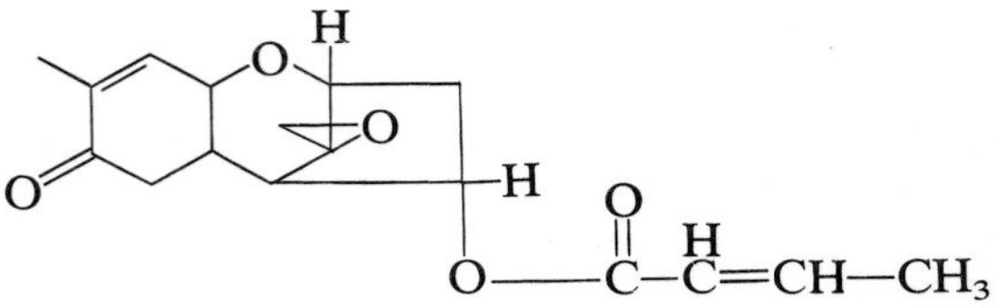

Fig. 16.121 Structure of trichothecin.

15.33 Usnic Acid

Usnic (or usninic) acid is an antibiotic produced by many species of lichens (*Cladonia cristatella*). Its structure is given in Fig. 16.122. It is active against gram-positive

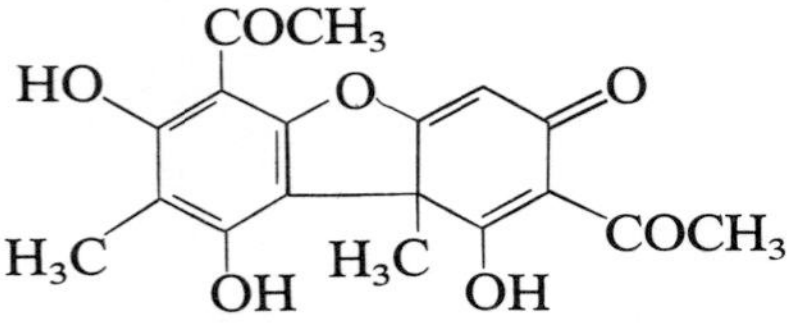

Fig. 16.122 Structure of usnic acid.

bacteria such as *B. subtilis*, *Sarcina lutea*, staphylococci, *Corynebacterium diphtheriae*, *Hemophilus pertussis*, and *M. tuberculosis* at about 1 ppm. Most gram-negative bacteria, filamentous fungi, and yeasts are not inhibited (LD_{50}: 25 mg/kg, mouse, i.v.).

Though very little work has been done to elucidate the mechanism of action of usnic acid, it appears to be at some site in the terminal electron transport system. Since usnic acid inhibits respiration and uncouples oxidative phosphorylation, inhibition may be associated with the energy-transforming system in the terminal respiratory pathway (900).

15.34 Vancomycin

Vancomycin is an antibiotic produced by *Streptomyces orientalis*, an actinomycete isolated from soil samples obtained in Indonesia and India. Vancomycin is a complex amphoteric glycopeptide chemically related to ristocetin, a defunct antibiotic, the ristomycins, and the actinoidins. A tentative structure has been proposed for ristomycin A (Fig. 16.123) (901, 902), but the structures of the other antibiotics have not been determined.

The primary activity of vancomycin is against gram-positive bacteria. Many strains of streptococci and staphylococci are sensitive *in vitro* to concentrations of 0.5–5 μg/ml. Some strains of *Staphylococcus aureus* have been found to be resistant to clinically achievable concentrations of the antibiotic. Combinations of this drug with streptomycin or gentamicin act synergistically against many but not all strains of enterococci (903, 904). The drug is rapidly bactericidal. Cross-resistance with other antimicrobial agents has not been demonstrated.

The mechanism of action of vancomycin has been reviewed (905). It has been shown that this antibiotic is a transfer inhibitor for the disaccharide-pentapeptide from the lipid intermediate to the acceptor in a system functioning *in vitro* and isolated from

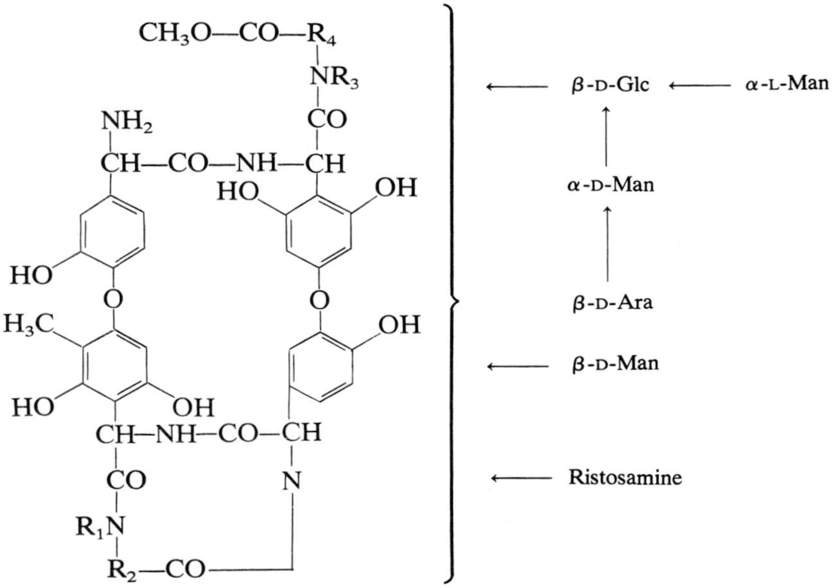

Fig. 16.123 Structure of the aglycone of ristomycin A. A similar type of structure might be found in vancomycin, the ristocetins, and the actinoidins.

$$CH_3(CH_2)_3CHOHCH{=}\underset{\displaystyle CH_3}{\underset{|}{C}}CH{=}CHCH{=}CHCON\langle\text{(cyclic, }O{=})\rangle$$

Fig. 16.124 Structure of variotin.

E. coli. Although this substance acts under certain conditions on the protoplasts (906, 907), it is probable that the primary effect is at the level of the cell wall synthesis (905, 908, 909). It had already been shown that the inhibition by ristocetins of growth of *Staphylococcus aureus* is due to the inhibition of cell wall synthesis. Strominger and co-workers (910, 911) have characterized this action as an inhibition of the transfer reaction of the disaccharide-pentapeptide from the lipid intermediate to the acceptor.

Vancomycin and ristocetin bind to the cell wall and can also form a complex with (UDP)*N*-acetylmuramyl-pentapeptide (909, 912–919). The inhibitory effect of vancomycin in an acellular system of *B. megaterium* is reversed by the presence of an analog of the polypeptide chain that is not bound to the mucopeptide: the diacetyl-L-diaminobutyryl-D-alanyl-D-alanine. The two antibiotics have a greater affinity for the cell wall than for the precursor of the peptidoglycan. Their absorption on the membrane is probably responsible for their effect (912). Vancomycin inhibits peptidoglycan synthesis in *Gaffkya homari* (920).

There is synergism of vancomycin-gentamicin and vancomycin-streptomycin against enterococci (921).

15.35 Variotin

Variotin is an antifungal substance produced by strains of *Paecilomyces varioti* Bainier var. *antibioticus* (922). Its structure (Fig. 16.124) has been determined (923). Variotin inhibits the growth of mycosis-causing fungi. It has essentially no activity against *Geotrichum, Nocardia, Aspergillus,* or *Candida,* but it is used clinically in Japan and in Europe for the treatment of infections caused by *Trichophyton, Microsporum,* and *Epidermophyton.*

REFERENCES

1. *Antibiotics,* Vol. 1, *Mechanism of Action,* D. Gottlieb and P. D. Shaw, Eds., Springer-Verlag, New York, 1967.
2. *Antibiotics,* Vol. 2, *Biosynthesis,* D. Gottlieb and P. D. Shaw, Eds., Springer-Verlag, New York, 1967.
3. *Antibiotics,* Vol. 3, *Mechanism of Action of Antimicrobial and Antitumor Agents,* J. W. Corcoran and F. E. Hahn, Eds., Springer-Verlag, New York, 1975.
4. E. F. Gale, E. Cundliffe, P. E. Reynolds, M. H. Richmond, and M. J. Waring, *The Molecular Basis of Antibiotic Action,* Wiley, New York, 1972.
5. J. Asselineau and J. P. Zalta, *Les Antibiotiques, Structure et Exemples de Mode d'Action,* Hermann, Paris, 1973.

5a. J. Berdy, *Adv. Appl. Microbiol;* **18,** 309 (1974).

5b. H. Zähner, *Angew. Chem. Int. Ed. Engl.,* **16,** 687 (1977).

6. A. W. Johnson, in *The Actinomycins,* S. A. Waksman, Ed., Wiley-Interscience, New York, 1968, p. 33.
7. G. Brownlee, *Ann. N.Y. Acad. Sci.,* **51,** 875 (1949).
8. J. Turkova, O. Mikes, and F. Sorm, *Collect. Czech. Chem. Commun.,* **29,** 280 (1964).
9. B. Heinemann, M. A. Kaplan, R. D. Muir, and I. R. Hooper, *Antibiot. Chemother.,* **3,** 1239 (1953).
10. W. K. Hausmann, A. H. Struck, J. H. Martin, R. H. Barrit, and N. Bohonos, *Antimicrob. Agents Chemother.,* 352 (1964).
11. R. A. Turner, *Arch. Biochem. Biophys.,* **60,** 364 (1956).
12. I. M. Lockhart and E. P. Abraham, *Biochem. J.,* **58,** 633 (1954).

13. J. M. Waisvisz, M. G. van der Hoeven, J. van Peppen, and W. C. M. Zwennis, *J. Am. Chem. Soc.*, **79,** 4520 (1957).
14. E. B. Herr. *Antimicrob. Agents Chemother.*, 201 (1963).
15. D. H. Peterson and L. M. Reineke, *J. Biol. Chem.*, **181,** 95 (1949).
16. S. Wilkinson and L. A. Lowe, *J. Chem. Soc.*, 4107 (1964).
17. S. Kuyama and S. Tamura, *Agr. Biol. Chem.*, **29,** 168 (1965).
18. R. Corbaz, L. Ettlinger, E. Gaumann, W. Keller-Schierlein, F. Kradolfer, L. Neipp, V. Prelog, P. Reusser, and H. Zahner, *Helv. Chim. Acta*, **40,** 199 (1957).
19. G. Roncari, Z. Kurylo-Borowska, and L. C. Graig, *Biochemistry*, **5,** 2153 (1966).
20. P. A. Plattner, K. Vogler, R. O. Studer, P. Quitt, and W. Keller-Schierlein, *Helv. Chim. Acta*, **46,** 927 (1963).
21. J. C. Sheehan, H. G. Zachau, and W. B. Lawson, *J. Am. Chem. Soc.*, **80,** 3349 (1958).
22. H. Bickel, E. Gaumann, G. Nussberger, P. Reusser, E. Vischer, W. Voser, A. Wettstein, and H. Zahner, *Helv. Chim. Acta*, **43,** 2105 (1960).
23. G. L. Hobby, P. P. Regna, N. Dougherty, and W. E. Steig, *J. Clin. Invest.*, **28,** 927 (1948).
24. M. Fujino, M. Inoue, J. Ueyangi, and A. Miyake, *Bull. Chem. Soc. Japan*, **38,** 515 (1965).
25. B. Witkop, S. I. Ishii, R. Sarges, F. Sakiyama, L. K. Ramachandran, and E. Gross, *Angew. Chem.*, **76,** 793 (1964).
26. S. Otani and Y. Saito, *Proc. Jap. Acad.*, **30,** 191 (1954).
27. R. Consken, A. H. Gordon, A. J. P. Martin, and R. L. M. Synge, *Biochem. J.*, **41,** 596 (1947).
28. T. Takita, K. Ohi, Y. Okami, K. Maeda, and H. Umezawa, *J. Antibiot.* (Tokyo), *Ser. A*, **15,** 46 (1962).
29. R. K. Callow and T. S. Work, *Biochem. J.*, **51,** 558 (1952).
30. S. Marumo and R. W. Curtis, *Phytochemistry*, **1,** 245 (1961).
31. P. Brooks, A. T. Fuller, and J. Walker, *J. Chem. Soc.*, 689 (1957).
32. K. Watanabe, H. Yonehara, H. Umezawa, and Y. Sumiki, *J. Antibiot.* (Tokyo), *Ser. A*, **13,** 293 (1960).
33. S. K. Majumdar and S. K. Bose, *Biochem. J.*, **74,** 596 (1960).
34. K. Kumagai, Y. Ono, T. Nishikawa, and N. Ishida, *J. Antibiot.* (Tokyo), *Ser. A*, **19,** 69 (1966).
35. N. J. Berridge, G. G. F. Newton, and E. P. Abraham, *Biochem. J.*, **52,** 529 (1952).
36. F. W. Eastwood, B. K. Snell, and A. Todd., *J. Chem. Soc.*, 2286 (1960).
37. W. D. Celmer and B. A. Sobin, *Antibiot. Ann. 1955–1956*, 437 (1956).
38. M. Guinand and G. Michel, *Biochim. Biophys. Acta*, **125,** 75 (1966).
39. K. Vogler and R. O. Studer, *Experientia*, **22,** 345 (1966).
40. W. K. Hausmann and L. C. Craig, *J. Biol. Chem.*, **198,** 405 (1952).
41. J. Preud'homme, A. Belloc, Y. Charpentier, and P. Tarridec, *Compt. Rend.*, **260,** 1309 (1965).
42. K. Katagiri and K. Sugiura, *Antimicrob. Agents Chemother.*, 162 (1962).
43. J. Berger, L. H. Sternback, M. Muller, E. R. LaSala, E. Grunberg, and M. W. Goldberg, *Antimicrob. Agents Chemother.*, 436 (1962).
44. H. Nishimura, S. Okatmoto, M. Mayama, H. Ohtsuka, K. Nakajima, K. Twara, M. Shimohira, and N. Shimaoka, *J. Antibiot.* (Tokyo), *Ser. A.*, **14,** 255 (1961).
45. H. Vanderhaeghe and G. Parmentier, *J. Am. Chem. Soc.*, **82,** 4414 (1960).
46. M. Bokanszky, I. Muramatsu, A. Bodanszky, M. Lukin, and M. R. Doubler, *J. Antibiot.* (Tokyo), *Ser. A*, **21,** 77 (1968).
47. J. Charney, W. P. Fisher, C. Curran, R. A. Machlowitz, and A. A. Tytell, *Antibiot. Chemother.*, **3,** 1283 (1953).
48. A. Stracher and L. C. Craig, *J. Am. Chem. Soc.*, **81,** 696 (1959).
49. T. H. Haskell, R. H. Bunge, J. C. French, and Q. R. Bartz, *J. Antibiot.* (Tokyo), *Ser. A*, **16,** 67 (1963).
50. T. Ooka, Y. Shimojima, T. Akomoto, I. Takeda, S. Senoh, and J. Abe, *Agr. Biol. Chem.*, **30,** 700 (1966).
51. J. Sheehan, D. Mania, S. Nakamura, J. A. Stock, and K. Maeda, *J. Am. Chem. Soc.*, **90,** 462 (1968).
52. M. Bodanszky, J. Fried, J. T. Sheehan, N. J. Williams, J. Alicino, A. I. Cohen, B. T. Keeler, and C. A. Birkhimer, *J. Am. Chem. Soc.*, **86,** 2478 (1964).
53. H. Otsuka and J. Shoji, *J. Antibiot.* (Tokyo), *Ser. A*, **19,** 128 (1966).
54. T. P. King and L. C. Craig, *J. Am. Chem. Soc.*, **77,** 6627 (1955).
55. R. J. Dubos and R. D. Hotchkiss, *J. Exp. Med.*, **73,** 629 (1941).

56. M. M. Shemyakin, N. A. Aldanova, E. I. Vinogradova, and M. Yu Feigina, *Tetrahedron Lett.*, 1921 (1963).
57. M. Bodanszky and M. A. Ondetti, *Antimicrob. Agents Chemother.*, 360 (1964).
58. J. Meienhofer, *J. Am. Chem. Soc.*, **92,** 3771 (1970).
59. S. A. Waksman and H. B. Woodruff, *Proc. Soc. Exp. Biol. Med.*, **45,** 609 (1940).
60. C. E. Dagliesh and A. R. Todd, *Nature* (London), **164,** 830 (1949).
61. C. E. Dagliesh, A. W. Jonson, A. R. Todd, and L. C. Vining, *J. Chem. Soc.* 2946 (1950).
62. H. Brockmann and N. Grubhofer, *Naturwissenschaften*, **36,** 376 (1949).
63. H. Brockmann, W. Sunderkotter, K. W. Ohly, and E. Boldt, *Naturwissenschaften*, **47,** 230 (1960).
64. U. Hollstein, *Chem. Rev.*, **74,** 625 (1974).
65. H. Lackner, *Chem. Ber.*, **103,** 2476 (1970).
66. H. Brockmann and J. H. Manegold, *Chem. Ber.*, **95,** 1081 (1962).
67. H. Brockmann and J. H. Manegold, *Hoppe-Seyler's Z. Physiol. Chem.*, **343,** 86 (1966).
68. H. Brockmann and E. A. Stahler, *Naturwissenschaften*, **52,** 391 (1965).
69. J. V. Formica, *Diss. Abstr.*, **B28** (8), 3398 (1967).
70. J. V. Formica, A. J. Shatkin, and E. Katz, *J. Bacteriol.*, **95,** 2139 (1968).
71. J. V. Formica and E. Katz, *J. Biol. Chem.*, **248,** 2066 ((1973).
72. E. Reich and I. H. Goldberg, *Progr. Nucleic Acid Res.*, **3,** 183 (1964).
73. E. Reich, *Symp. Soc. Study Dev. Growth*, **23,** 73 (1964).
74. E. Reich, A. Cerami and D. C. Ward, in Ref. 1, p. 714.
75. G. Hartmann, W. Behr, K. A. Beissner, K. Honikel, and A. Sippel, *Angew. Chem., Int. Ed. Engl.*, **7,** 693 (1968).
76. I. H. Goldberg and P. A. Friedman, *Ann. Rev. Biochem.*, **40,** 772 (1971).
77. I. H. Goldberg and P. A. Friedman, *Pure Appl. Chem.*, **28,** 499 (1971).
78. E. F. Gale, E. Cundliffe, P. E. Reynolds, M. H. Richmond, and M. J. Waring, *The Molecular Basis of Antibiotic Action*, Wiley, New York, 1972, p. 220.
79. H. Sobell, *Progr. Nucleic Acid Res. Mol. Biol.*, **13,** 153 (1973).
80. H. J. Robinson and S. A. Waksman, *J. Pharm. Exp. Ther.*, **74,** 25 (1942).
81. W. Kersten, H. Kersten, and H. M. Rauen, *Nature* (London), **187,** 60 (1960).
82. M. F. Perutz, *Nature* (London), **201,** 814 (1964).
83. R. B. Homer, *Arch. Biochem. Biophys.* **129,** 405 (1969).
84. A. Cerami, E. Reich, D. C. Ward, and I. H. Goldberg, *Proc. Nat. Acad. Sci. US*, **57,** 1030 (1967).
85. E. Reich, *Science*, **143,** 684 (1964).
86. R. W. Hyman and N. Davidson, *Biochem. Biophys. Res. Commun.*, **26,** 116 (1967).
87. N. R. Ringertz and L. Bolund, *Biochim. Biophys. Acta*, **174,** 147 (1969).
88. R. W. Hyman and N. Davidson, *Biochim. Biophys. Acta*, **228,** 38 (1971).
89. R. D. Wells and J. E. Larson, *J. Mol. Biol.*, **49,** 319 (1970).
90. R. D. Wells, *Science*, **165,** 76 (1969).
91. F. S. Allen, R. P. Moen, and U. Hollstein, *J. Am. Chem. Soc.*, **98,** 864 (1976).
91a. F. S. Allen, M. B. Jones, and U. Hollstein, *Biophys, J.*, **20,** 69 (1977).
92. R. W. Hyman and N. Davidson, *J. Mol. Biol.*, **50,** 421 (1970).
93. L. Hamilton, W. Fuller, and E. Reich, *Nature* (London), **198,** 538 (1963).
94. G. V. Gurskii, *Mol. Biol.*, **3,** 749 (1969); *Mol. Biol.* (USSR), **3,** 292 (1970).
95. W. Müller and D. M. Crothers, *J. Mol. Biol.*, **35,** 251 (1968).
96. H. M. Sobell and S. C. Jain, *J. Mol. Biol.*, **68,** 1, 21 (1972).
97. T. R. Krugh, *Proc. Nat. Acad. Sci., USA*, **69,** 1911 (1972).
98. T. R. Krugh and J. W. Neely, *Biochemistry*, **12,** 1775 (1973).
99. D. J. Patel, *Biochemistry*, **13,** 1476 (1974).
100. T. R. Krugh and J. W. Neely, *Biochemistry*, **12,** 4418 (1973).
101. D. J. Patel, *Biochemistry*, **13,** 2388 (1974).
102. D. J. Patel, *Biochemistry*, **13,** 2396 (1974).
103. H. Brockmann, *Fortschr. Chem. Org. Naturst.*, **18,** 1 (1960).
104. E. Reich, I. H. Goldberg, and M. Rabinowitz, *Nature* (London), **196,** 743 (1962).
105. H. Brockmann and J. H. Manegold, *Chem. Ber.*, **95,** 1081 (1962).
106. W. Müller, *Naturwissenschaften*, **49,** 156 (1962).
107. H. Brockmann and H. Lackner, *Tetrahedron Lett.*, 3523 (1974).
108. H. Brockmann and W. Schramm, *Tetrahedron Lett.*, 2331 (1966).

109. H. Brockmann, W. Müller, and H. Peterssen-Borstel, *Tetrahedron Lett.*, 3531 (1966).

110. A. B. Mauger and R. Wade, *J. Chem. Soc. C*, 1406 (1966).

111. H. Brockmann and H. Lackner, *Chem. Ber.*, **101,** 1312 (1968).

112. E. Katz, in Ref. 2, p. 276.

113. H. Brockmann and F. Seela, *Chem. Ber.*, **104,** 2751 (1971).

114. F. Seela, *J. Med. Chem.*, **15,** 684 (1972).

115. E. Atherton and J. Meienhofer, *J. Am. Chem. Soc.*, **94,** 4759 (1972).

116. E. Atherton, R. P. Patel, Y. Sano, and J. Meienhofer, *J. Med. Chem.*, **16,** 355 (1973).

117. C. W. Mosher and L. Goodman, *J. Org. Chem.*, **37,** 2928 (1972).

118. S. Moore, M. Kondo, M. Copeland, and J. Meienhofer, *J. Med. Chem.*, **18,** 1098 (1975).

119. E. Jawetz, *Pediatr. Clin. N. Am.*, **8,** 1057 (1961).

120. R. E. Galardy, M. P. Printz, and L. C. Craig, *Biochemistry*, **10,** 2429 (1971).

121. D. R. Storm, *Ann. N.Y. Acad. Sci.*, **235,** 387 (1974).

122. J. L. Strominger, K. Izaki, M. Matsuhashi, and D. J. Tipper, *Fed. Proc.*, **26,** 9 (1967).

123. K. Izaki, M. Matsuhashi, and J. L. Strominger, *Proc. Nat. Acad. Sci., US*, **55,** 656 (1966).

124. G. Siewert and J. L. Strominger, *Proc. Nat. Acad. Sci. US*, **57,** 767 (1967).

125. R. G. Anderson, H. Hussey, and J. Baddiley, *Biochem. J.*, **127,** 11 (1972).

126. J. L. Smith and E. D. Weinberg, *J. Gen. Microbiol.*, **28,** 559 (1962).

127. R. Hancock and P. C. Fitz-James, *J. Bacteriol.*, **87,** 1044 (1964).

128. V. Helms and E. D. Weinberg, in *Antimicrobial Agents and Chemotherapy, 1962*, American Society for Microbiology, Ann Arbor, Mich., 1963, p. 241.

129. J. Rotta, W. W. Karakawa, and R. M. Krause, *J. Bacteriol.*, **89,** 1581 (1965).

130. E. J. Gale and J. P. Folkers, *Biochem. J.*, **53,** 493 (1953).

131. E. D. Weinberg, in *Antimicrobial Agents and Chemotherapy, 1967*, American Society for Microbiology, Ann Arbor, Mich., 1965, p. 120.

132. R. J. Dubos and R. D. Hotchkiss, *J. Exp. Med.*, **73,** 629 (1941).

133. T. Kato and N. Izumiya, *J. Biochem.* (Japan), **59,** 629 (1966).

134. R. Sarges and B. Witkop, *J. Am. Chem. Soc.*, **86,** 1861 (1964).

135. A. W. Chow, N. M. Hall, and J. R. E. Hoover, *J. Org. Chem.*, **27,** 1381 (1962).

136. R. Sarges and B. Witkop, *Biochemistry*, **4,** 2491 (1965).

137. M. Ohno and N. Izumiya, *J. Am. Chem. Soc.*, **88,** 376 (1966).

138. M. A. Ruttenberg, T. P. King, and L. C. Craig, *Biochemistry*, **4,** 11 (1965).

139. F. E. Hunter, Jr., and L. S. Schwartz, in Ref. 1, pp. 636, 642.

140. K. Fujikawa, T. Suzuki, and K. Kurahashi, *Biochim. Biophys. Acta*, **161,** 232 (1968).

141. R. K. Rao, N. V. Bhagavan, K. R. Rao, and J. B. Hall, *Biochemistry*, **7,** 3072 (1968).

142. E. D. Weinberg, *Antibiotics*, **2,** 240 (1967).

143. R. Sarges and B. Witkop, *J. Am. Chem. Soc.*, **86,** 1861, 1862 (1964).

144. S. Hladky and D. A. Haydon, *Nature*, **225,** 451 (1970).

145. M. C. Goodall, *Biochim. Biophys. Acta*, **219,** 470 (1970).

146. M. C. Goodall, *Biochim. Biophys. Acta*, **219,** 28 (1970).

147. D. C. Tosteron, T. E. Andreoli, M. Tiefferberg, and P. Cook, *J. Gen. Physiol.*, **51,** 3735 (1968).

148. D. W. Urry, *Proc. Nat. Acad. Sci. US*, **68,** 672 (1971).

149. D. W. Urry, M. C. Goodall, J. D. Glikson, and D. F. Mayers, *Proc. Nat. Acad. Sci., US*, **68,** 1907 (1971).

150. L. C. Vining and D. W. S. Westlake, *Can. J. Microbiol.*, **10,** 705 (1964); R. MacGrath, L. C. Vining, F. Sala, and D. W. S. Westlake, *Can. J. Biochem.*, **46,** 587 (1968).

151. K. Vogler and R. O. Struder, *Experientia*, **22,** 345 (1966); H. Paulus, *Antibiotics*, **2,** 254 (1967).

152. K. Hayashi, Y. Sukita, K. Isukamoto, and T. Suzuki, *Experientia*, **22,** 355 (1966).

153. T. M. Chapman and R. M. Golden, *Biochem. Biophys. Res. Commun.*, **46,** 2040 (1972).

154. B. A. Newton, *Bacteriol. Rev.*, **20,** 14 (1956); M. R. W. Brown and W. M. Watkins, *Nature* (London), **227,** 1360 (1970).

155. W. Pache, D. Chapman, and R. Hillaby, *Biochim. Biophys. Acta*, **255,** 358 (1972).

156. G. H. Warren, J. Gray, and J. A. Yurchenko, *J. Bacteriol.*, **74,** 788 (1957).

157. P. R. G. Schindler and M. Teuber, *Antimicrob. Agents Chemother.*, **8,** 95 (1975); A. Galizzi, G. Cacco, A. G. Siccardi, and G. Mazza, *ibid.*, **8,** 366 (1975); M. Teuber and J. Bader, *ibid.*, **9,** 26 (1976).

158. J. C. Sheehan and S. L. Ledis, *J. Am. Chem. Soc.*, **95,** 875 (1973).

159. D. Vasquez, in Ref. 1, p. 387; in Ref. 3, p. 521.

160. H. Vanderhaeghe and G. Parmentier, *Bull. Soc. Chim. Belg.*, **68,** 716 (1959).

161. A. A. Kiryushkin, V. M. Burikov, and B. V. Rosinov, *Tetrahedron Lett.*, 2675 (1967); F. Compernolle, H. Vanderhaeghe, and G. Janssen, *Org. Mass Spectrom.*, **6,** 151 (1972).

162. H. Vanderhaeghe, G. Janssen, and F. Compernolle, *Tetrahedron Lett.*, 2687 (1971).

163. G. R. Delpierre, F. W. Eastwood, C. E. Gream, D. G. I. Kingston, P. Sarin, Lord Todd, and D. H. Williams, *Tetrahedron Lett.*, 369 (1966); *J. Chem. Soc.*, 1653 (1966).

164. F. W. Eastwood, B. K. Snell, and A. Todd, *J. Chem. Soc.*, 2286 (1960).

165. B. R. Cox, F. W. Eastwood, B. K. Snell, and A. Todd, *Chem. Commun.*, 1623 (1970).

166. M. Bodanszky and J. C. Sheehan, *Antimicrob. Agents Chemother.*, 38 (1963).

167. M. A. Ondetti and P. L. Thomas, *J. Am. Chem. Soc.*, **87,** 4373 (1965); R. Charles-Sigler and E. Gil-Av, *Tetrahedron Lett.*, 4231 (1966).

168. J. Preud'homme, P. Terridec, and A. Belloc, *Bull. Soc. Chim. Fr.*, 585 (1968).

169. F. Irreverre, *Biochim. Biophys. Acta*, **117,** 485 (1966).

170. N. G. Kumar and D. W. Urry, *Biochemistry*, **12,** 3811, 4392 (1973).

171. R. J. Holt and G. T. Stewart, *Biochim. Biophys. Acta*, **100,** 235 (1965).

172. H. Iwasaki and B. Witkop, *J. Am. Chem. Soc.*, **86,** 4698 (1964).

173. A. W. Chow, N. M. Hall, and J. R. E. Hoover, *J. Org. Chem.*, **27,** 1381 (1962).

174. T. Takita, H. Naganawa, K. Maeda, and H. Umezawa, *J. Antibiot.* (Tokyo), *Ser. A*, **17,** 129 (1964).

175. L. W. Cary, T. Takita, and M. Ohnishi, *FEBS Lett.*, **17,** 145 (1971); *Tetrahedron Lett.*, 3189 (1970); 2221 (1971).

176. K. Okamoto, Y. Kakita, S. Tateishi, and S. Nakasawa, *Nippon Kagaku Ryogakukai Zasshi*, **15,** 21 (1967); *Chem. Abstr.*, **66,** 73.515u (1967).

177. N. Tanaka, in Ref. 3, p. 487; D. Vasquez, in Ref. 3, p. 521.

178. C. Cocito, *Biochimie*, **55,** 153 (1973).

179. C. Cocito, *Biochimie*, **55,** 309 (1973).

180. D. Vasquez, "The Streptogramin Family of Antibiotics", in Ref. 3, p. 521.

181. A. H. Gordon, A. J. P. Martin, and R. L. M. Synge, *Biochem. J.*, **41,** 596 (1947).

182. R. Schwyzer and P. Sieber, *Helv. Chim. Acta*, **40,** 624 (1957); H. Klostermeyer, *Chem. Ber.*, **101,** 2823 (1968); G. Losse and K. Neubert, *Tetrahedron Lett.*, 1267 (1970).

183. B. F. Erlanger and L. Goode, *Science*, **131,** 669 (1960).

184. H. Aoyagi, T. Kato, M. Ohno, M. Kondo, and N. Izumiya, *J. Am. Chem. Soc.*, **86,** 5701 (1964).

185. M. Waki and N. Izumiya, *J. Am. Chem. Soc.*, **89,** 1278 (1967).

186. A. M. Liquori, P. de Santis, A. L. Kovacs, and L. Mazarella, *Nature* (London), **211,** 1039 (1966); A. M. Liquori, and F. Conti, *Nature* (London), **217,** 635 (1968); see also D. Balasubramanian, *J. Am. Chem. Soc.*, **89,** 5445 (1967); F. Quadrifoglio and D. W. Urry, *Biochem. Biophys. Research Commun.*, **29,** 785 (1967); R. Schwyzer and U. Ludescher, *Biochemistry*, **7,** 2519 (1968); S. Laiken, M. Printz, and L. C. Craig, *J. Biol. Chem.*, **244,** 4454 (1969).

187. M. M. Shemyakin, Y. A. Ovchimikov, V. T. Ivanov, and I. D. Ryabova, *Experientia*, **23,** 326 (1967); M. M. Shemyakin, Y. A. Ovshimikov, and V. T. Ivanov, *Angew. Chemie Inter. Ed. Engl.*, **8,** 492 (1969).

188. M. Rothe and F. Eisenbeis, *Angew. Chem. Int. Ed. Engl.*, **7,** 883 (1968).

189. M. Waki and N. Izumiya, *Tetrahedron Lett.*, 3083 (1968).

190. M. Ohnishi and D. W. Urry, *Biochem. Biophys. Res. Commun.*, **36,** 185 (1969); R. Schwyzer and U. Ludescher, *Helv. Chim. Acta*, **52,** 2033 (1969); G. Camiletti, P. de Santis, and R. Rizzo, *Chem. Commun.*, 1073 (1970); Y. A. Ovchimikov, V. T. Ivanov, V. F. Bystrov, A. I. Miroshnikov, E. N. Shepel, N. D. Abdullaev, E. S. Efremov, and L. B. Senyavina, *Biochem. Biophys. Research Commun.*, **39,** 217 (1970).

191. E. G. Finer, A. Hanser, and D. Chapman, *Chem. Phys. Lipids*, **3,** 386 (1969).

192. W. Pache, D. Chapman, and R. Hillaby, *Biochim. Biophys. Acta*, **255,** 358 (1972).

193. M. C. Goodall, *Biochim. Biophys. Acta*, **219,** 470 (1970).

194. M. C. Goodall, *Biochim. Biophys. Acta*, **219,** 28 (1970).

195. F. M. Harold, *Advan. Microbiol. Physiol.*, **4,** 45 (1970).

196. D. J. Patel and A. E. Tonelli, *Biopolymers*, **15,** 1623 (1976).

197. G. F. Gause, *Brit. J. Med.*, 1177 (1955).

198. J. Turková, O. Mikeš, and F. Šorm, *Experientia*, **19,** 633 (1963).

199. O. Mikeš, J. Turková, and F. Šorm, *Coll. Czech. Chem. Commun.*, **28,** 1747 (1963).

200. O. Mikeš, J. Turková, and F. Šorm, *Coll. Czech. Chem. Commun.*, **30,** 118 (1965).

201. H. Maehr, *Pure Appl. Chem.*, **28,** 603 (1971).

202. J. Voříšek and D. Grunberger, paper presented at the Ninth International Congress on Microbiology, Moscow, July 1966.

203. P. Reeves, *Bacteriol. Rev.* **29,** 24, (1965).

204. J. Foulds, *J. Bacteriol.*, **110,** 1001 (1972).

205. J. Konisky, *J. Biol. Chem.*, **247,** 3750 (1972).

206. I. B. Holland, in Ref. 1, p. 684.

207. W. G. Iverson and N. F. Millis, *Can. J. Microbiol.*, **22,** 1040 (1976).

208. J. Kramer and H. Brandis, *Antimicrob. Agents Chemother.*, **7,** 117 (1975).

209. L. W. Wendt, in Ref. 3, p. 588.

210. L. W. Wendt, in Ref. 3, p. 588.

211. T. Beppu, H. Yamamoto, and K. Arima, *Antimicrob. Agents Chemother.*, **8,** 617 (1975).

212. Z. Kurylo-Borowska, *Bull. State Inst. Mar. Trop. Med., Gdansk, Poland*, **10,** 83 (1959).

213. J. Borysiewicz, *Appl. Microbiol.*, **14,** 1049 (1966).

214. Z. Kurylo-Borowska, *Biochim. Biophys. Acta*, **61,** 897 (1962).

215. Z. Kurylo-Borowska, in Ref. 3, p. 129.

216. J. P. Lynch and H. D. Sisler, *Phytopathology*, **57,** 367 (1967).

217. H. Brockmann and G. Schmidt-Kastner, *Chem. Ber.*, **88,** 57 (1955).

218. M. M. Shemyakin, E. I. Vinogradova, M. Y. Feigina, N. A. Aldanova, Y. B. Shvetsov, and L. A. Fonina, *Zh. Obsch. Khim.*, **36,** 1391 (1966).

219. F. E. Hunter, Jr., and L. S. Schwartz, in Ref. 1, p. 631.

220. M. Ohnishi and D. W. Urry, *Biochem. Biophys. Research Commun.* **36,** 185 (1969); M. Pinkerton, L. K. Steinrauf, and P. Dankins, *ibid.*, **35,** 512 (1969); V. T. Ivanov, I. A. Laine, N. D. Abdulaev, L. B. Senyavina, E. M. Popov, Y. A. Ovchimikov, and M. M. Shemyakin, *ibid.*, **34,** 803 (1969).

221. *Membranes, Models, and the Formation of Biological Membranes*, L. Bolis and B. A. Pethica, Eds., North-Holland, Amsterdam, 1968.

222. B. C. Pressman, *Proc. Nat. Acad. Sci., US*, **53,** 1076 (1965).

223. E. J. Harris and K. van Dam. *Biochem. J.* **106,** 759 (1968).

224. E. J. Harris, R. Cockrell, and B. C. Pressman, *Biochem. J.*, **99,** 200 (1966).

225. E. J. Harris, M. P. Hoffer, and B. C. Pressman, *Biochemistry*, **6,** 1348 (1967).

226. R. S. Cockrell, E. J. Harris, and B. C. Pressman, *Nature*, **215,** 1487 (1967).

227. R. S. Cockrell, E. J. Harris, and B. C. Pressman, *Biochemistry*, **5,** 2326 (1966).

228. W. McMurray and R. W. Begg, *Arch. Biochem. Biophys.*, **84,** 546 (1959).

229. C. Moore and B. P. Pressman, *Biochem. Biophys. Res. Commun.*, **15,** 562 (1964).

230. A. A. Lev, V. A. Cottlib, and E. P. Buzuhsky, *J. Evolution Biochem. Physiol.*, **2** 109 (1966).

231. P. Mueller and D. D. Rudin, *Biochem. Biophys. Res. Commun.*, **26,** 398 (1968).

232. J. B. Chappel and K. Haarhoff, in *Biochemistry of Mitochondria*, E. Slater, Ed., Academic Press, New York, 1966, p. 75.

233. S. Papa, J. M. Tager, F. Guerrieri, and E. Quliarello, *Biochim. Biophys. Acta*, **172,** 184 (1969).

234. S. Papa, F. Guerrieri, L. Rossi-Bernardi, and J. M. Tager, *Biochim. Biophys. Acta*, **197,** 100 (1970).

235. R. S. Cockrell and E. Racker, *Biochem. Biophys. Res. Commun.*, **35,** 414 (1969).

236. M. Montal, B. Chance, and C. P. Lee, *J. Membrane Biol.*, **2,** 201 (1970).

237. L. L. Grimus, *Biochim. Biophys. Acta*, **216,** 1 (1970).

238. L. E. Bakeeva, L. L. Grimus, A. A. Jasaitis, V. V. Kuliene, D. O. Levitsky, E. A. Liberman, I. I. Severina, and U. P. Skulachev, *Biochim. Biophys. Acta*, **216,** 13 (1970).

239. B. C. Pressman, E. J. Harris, W. S. Jagger, and J. M. Johnson, *Proc. Nat. Acad. Sci. US*, **58,** 1949 (1967).

240. B. C. Pressman, in *Mitochondria Structure and Function*, L. Eruster and Z. Drahota, Eds., Academic Press and Publishing House of the Czechoslovak Academy of Sciences, London and Prague, 1968.

241. L. A. R. Pioda, H. A. Wacrer, R. E. Dohner, and W. Simon, *Helv. Chim. Acta*, **50,** 1373 (1967).

242. B. T. Kilbourn, J. D. Dunitz, L. A. R. Pioda, and W. Simon, *J. Mol. Biol.*, **30,** 559 (1967).

243. M. M. Shemyakin, Y. A. Ovshimikov, V. K. Ivanov, A. M. Antanov, I. I. Shkrob, A. V.

Hikhaleva, and G. G. Malenkov, *Biochem. Biophys. Res. Commun.*, **29,** 834 (1967).

244. V. T. Ivanov, I. A. Laine, N. D. Abdulaev, L. B. Senyavina, E. M. Dolov, Y. A. Ovchimikov, and M. M. Shemyakin, *Biochem. Biophys. Res. Commun.*, **34,** 803 (1969).

245. B. C. Pressman and E. J. Harris, *Abstracts of the Seventh International Congress of Biochemistry, Tokyo, 1967*, Vol. 5, p. 900.

246. E. J. Harris, K. Vendam, and B. C. Pressman, *Nature*, **213,** 1126 (1967).

247. W. L. Duax, H. Hauptman, C. M. Weeks, and D. A. Norton, *Science*, **176,** 911 (1972); see also G. D. Smith and W. L. Duax, *Proceedings of the Ninth Jerusalem Conference*, 1977.

248. J. R. Dyer, H. B. Hayes, E. G. Miller, and R. F. Nassar, *J. Am. Chem. Soc.*, **86,** 5353 (1964).

249. B. W. Bycroft, D. Cameron, L. R. Croft, A. Hassanali-Walji, A. W. Johnson, and T. Webb, *Tetrahedron Lett.*, 5901 (1968); 2539 (1969).

250. B. W. Bycroft, D. Cameron, L. R. Croft, A. Hassanali-Walji, A. W. Johnson, and T. Webb, *Experientia*, **27,** 501 (1971); *J. Chem. Soc. Perkin Trans. I*, 827 (1972); B. W. Bycroft, *Chem. Commun.*, 660 (1972).

251. P. G. Caltrider, in Ref. 1, p. 677.

252. Y. F. Liou and N. Tanaka, *Biochem. Biophys. Res. Commun.*, **71,** 477 (1976).

253. F. M. Strong, J. P. Dickie, M. E. Loomans, E. E. van Tamelen, and R. S. Dewey, *J. Am. Chem. Soc.*, **82,** 513 (1960).

254. A. J. Birch, D. W. Cameron, R. W. Rickards, and Y. Hirada, *Proc. Chem. Soc.*, 22 (1960).

255. J. S. Rieske, in Ref. 1, p. 542.

256. D. E. Green, B. Mackler, R. Repaske, and H. R. Mahler, *Biochim. Biophys. Acta*, **15,** 435 (1964).

257. H. W. Clark, H. A. Newfeld, C. Widher, and E. Stotz, *J. Biol. Chem.*, **210,** 851 (1954).

258. B. Chance and G. R. Williams, *Advances in Enzymology*, Wiley-Interscience, New York, Vol. 17, 1956, p. 65.

259. D. Keilin and E. F. Hartree, *Nature*, **176,** 200 (1955).

260. R. W. Estabrook, *Biochim. Biophys. Acta*, **60,** 236 (1962).

261. R. W. Estabrook, *Fed. Proc.*, **14,** 45 (1955).

262. J. S. Rieske and W. S. Zangg, *Biochem. Biophys. Res. Commun.*, **8,** 421 (1962).

263. B. Chance and G. R. Williams, *J. Biol. Chem.*, **217,** 429 (1955).

264. B. Chance, *J. biol. Chem.*, **233,** 1223 (1958).

265. J. S. Rieske, H. Baum, C. D. Stoner, and S. Lipton, *J. Biol. Chem.*, **242,** 4854 (1967).

266. J. S. Rieske, S. Lipton, H. Baum, and I. Silman, *J. Biol. Chem.*, **242,** 4888 (1967).

267. H. Baum, J. S. Rieske, H. I. Silman, and S. H. Lipton, *Proc. Nat. Acad. Sci. US*, **57,** 798 (1967).

268. M. Reporter, *Biochemistry*, **5,** 2416 (1966).

269. R. W. Estabrook, *J. Biol. Chem.*, **227,** 1093 (1967).

270. A. M. Pumphrey, *J. Biol. Chem.*, **237,** 2384 (1962).

271. H. Baum and J. S. Rieske, *Biochem. Biophys., Res. Commun.*, **24,** 1 (1966).

272. Z. Kaniuga, J. Bryla, and E. C. Slater, in *Inhibitors: Tools in Cell Research*, Ph. Bücher and H. Sies, Eds., Springer-Verlag, Berlin, 1969, p. 296.

273. J. Bryla, Z. Kaniuga, and E. C. Slater, *Biochim. Biophys. Acta*, **189,** 317, 327 (1969).

274. H. Baltscheffsky, *Acta Chem. Scand.*, **14,** 264 (1960).

275. M. Nishimura, *Biochim. Biophys. Acta*, **66,** 17 (1963).

276. F. Arcamone, S. Penco, P. Orezzi, V. Nicoleilla, and A. M. Pirelli, *Nature* (London), **203,** 1064 (1964).

277. P. Chandra, A. Götz, A. Wacker, M. A. Verini, A. M. Casazza, A. Fioretti, F. Arcamone, and M. Ghione, *FEBS Lett.*, **16,** 249 (1971).

278. P. Chandra, A. Götz, A. Wacker, M. A. Verini, A. M. Casazza, A. Fioretti, F. Arcamone, and M. Ghione, *FEBS Lett.*, **9,** 327 (1972); *Z. Physiol. Chem.*, **353,** 393 (1972).

279. A. G. Siccardi, E. Lanza, E. Nielson, A. Galizzi, and G. Mazza, *Antimicrob. Agents Chemother.*, **8,** 370 (1975).

280. S. Nakamura, H. Youchara, and H. Umezawa, *J. Antibiotics* (Tokyo), *Ser. A*, **17,** 220 (1964); M. Julia and N. Preau-Joseph, *Bull. Soc. Chim. Fr.*, 4348 (1967).

281. F. E. Hahn, in Ref. 3, p. 79.

281a. M. Bialer, B. Yagen, and M. Mechonlam, *Tetrahedron*, **37,** 2399 (1978).

282. S. Pestka and J. W. Bodley, in Ref. 3, p. 551.

283. J. H. Highland, L. Lin, and J. W. Bodley, *Biochemistry*, **10,** 4404 (1971).

284. J. Modelell, B. Cabrer, A. Pameggiani, and D. Vasquez, *Proc. Nat. Acad. Sci. US*, **68,** 1796 (1971).

285. D. Richter, L. Lin, and J. Bodley, *Arch. Biochem. Biophys.*, **147,** 186 (1971).

286. M. Springer, J. Dondon, M. Graffe, and M. Grunberg-Manago, *Biochimie*, **53,** 1047 (1971).

287. M. Grunberg-Manago, J. Dondon, and M. Graffe, *FEBS Lett.*, **22,** 217 (1972).

288. W. L. Parker and M. L. Rathnum, *J. Antibiotics* (Tokyo), **28,** 379 (1975).

289. J. J. Armstrong, J. F. Grove, W. B. Turner, and G. Ward, *Nature* (London), **206,** 399 (1965).

290. J. Vandeputte, J. L. Wachtel, and E. T. Stiller, *Antibiot. Ann., 1955–1956,* 587 (1956).

291. S. Wakaki, K. Hamada, S. Akanabe, and T. Asahina, *J. Antibiot.* (Tokyo), *Ser. A,* **6,** 145 (1953).

292. L. C. Vining and W. A. Taber, *Can. J. Chem.*, **35,** 1461 (1957).

293. F. Arcamone and M. Perego, *Ann. Chim.*, **49,** 345 (1959).

294. J. D. Dutcher, G. Boyack, and S. Fox. *Antibiot, Ann. 1953–1954,* 191 (1954).

295. B. K. Koe, F. W. Tanner, K. V. Rao, B. A. Sobin, and W. D. Celmer, *Antibiot. Ann. 1957–1958,* 897 (1958).

296. A. P. Struyk, I. Hoette, G. Drost, J. M. Waisvisz, T. van Eek, and J. C. Hoogerheide, *Antibiot. Ann. 1957–1958,* 878 (1958).

297. J. M. J. Sakamoto, *J. Antibiot.* (Tokyo), *Ser. A,* **10,** 128 (1957).

298. J. W. Davisson, F. W. Tanner, A. C. Finlay, and I. A. Solomons, *Antibiot. Chemother.*, **1,** 289 (1951).

299. K. L. Rinehart, V. F. German, W. P. Tucker, and D. Gottlieb, *Justus Liebigs Ann. Chem.*, **668,** 77 (1963).

300. M. Igarashi, K. Ogata, and A. Miyake, *J. Antibiot.* (Tokyo), *Ser. B,* **9,** 101 (1956).

301. R. Brown and E. L. Hazen, *Antibiot. Chemother.*, **10,** 702 (1960).

302. T. Osato, M. Ueda, S. Fukuyama, K. Yagishita, Y. Okami, and H. Umezawa, *J. Antibiot., Ser. A* (Tokyo), **8,** 105 (1955).

303. R. C. Burke, J. H. Swartz, S. S. Chapman, and W. Huang, *J. Invest. Dermatol.*, **23,** 163 (1954).

304. H. H. Wasserman, J. E. VanVerth, D. J. McCaustland, I. J. Borowitz, and B. Kamber, *J. Am. Chem. Soc.*, **89,** 1535 (1967).

305. K. Ogata, S. Igarashi, and Y. Nakao, Japanese Patent 9245 (1958).

306. G. B. Whitfield, T. D. Brock, A. Ammann, D. Gottlieb, and H. E. Carter, *J. Am. Chem. Soc,*, **77,** 4799 (1955).

307. A. C. Cope, R. K. Bly, E. P. Burrows, O. J. Ceder, E. Ciganek, B. T. Gillis, R. F. Porter, and H. E. Johnson, *J. Am. Chem. Soc.*, **84,** 2170 (1962).

308. C. J. Bissell, D. L. Fletcher, A. M. Mortimer, W. K. Anslow, A. H. Campbell, and W. H. C. Shaw, British Patent 884,711 (1961).

309. C. Leben, C. J. Stessel, and G. W. Keitt, *Mycologia*, **44,** 159 (1952).

310. R. Donovick, B. A. Steinberg, J. D. Dutcher, and J. Vandeputte, *G. Microbiol.*, **2,** 147 (1956).

311. R. J. Hickey, C. J. Corum, P. H. Hidy, I. R. Cohen, U. F. B. Nager, and E. Kropp, *Antibiot. Chemother.*, **2,** 472 (1952).

312. L. C. Vining, W. A. Taber, and F. J. Gregory, *Antibiot. Ann. 1954–1955,* 980 (1955).

313. M. S. Cataldi, V. Lopez, J. Pahn, and O. L. Galmarini, US Patent 3,159,541 (1964).

314. M. J. Thirumalacher, S. K. Menon, and V. V. Bhatt, *Hind. Antibiot. Bull.*, **3,** 136 (1961).

315. E. Borowski, C. P. Schaffner, and H. Lechevalier, *Antimicrob. Agents Ann.*, 532 (1960).

316. S. Hosoya, N. Komatsu, M. Soeda, T. Yanaguchi, and Y. Sonoda, *J. Antibiot.* (Tokyo), *Ser. A,* **5,** 564 (1952).

317. W. Oroshnik and A. D. Mebane, *Progr. Chem. Org. Nat. Prod.*, **21,** 17 (1963); D. Perlman, *Prog. Ind. Microbiol.*, **6,** 1 (1967); S. C. Kinsky, in Ref. 1, pp. 122, 749.

318. M. M. Weber and S. C. Kirisky, *J. Bacteriol.*, **89,** 306 (1965).

319. E. Schlosser and D. Gottlieb, *J. Bacteriol.*, **91,** 1080 (1966).

320. E. Schlosser and D. Gottlieb, *Z. Naturforsch.*, **21b**, 74 (1966).

321. S. C. Kinsky, R. A. Demel, and L. L. M. Van Deenen, *Biochim. Biophys. Acta,* **135,** 835 (1967).

322. R. A. Denel, L. L. M. Van Deenen, and S. C. Kirisky, *J. Biol. Chem.*, **240,** 2749 (1965).

323. S. C. Kirisky, S. A. Lux, and L. L. M. Van Deenen, *Fed. Proc.*, **25,** 1503 (1966).

324. S. C. Kinsky, *Ann. Rev. Pharmacol.*, **10,** 119 (1970).

325. A. W. Norman, R. A. Demel, and L. L. M. Van Deenen, *Fed. Proc.*, **30,** 1282 (1971).

326. A. W. Norman, R. A. Demel, B. de Kruyff, and L. L. M. Van Deenen, *J. Biol. Chem.*, **247,** 1918 (1972).

327. F. Schroeder, J. F. Holland, and L. L. Bieber, *J. Antibiot.* (Tokyo), **24,** 846 (1971).

328. F. Schroeder, J. F. Holland, and L. L. Bieber, *Biochemistry,* **11,** 3105 (1972).

329. S. Hladky and D. A. Haydon, *Nature,* **225,** 451 (1970).

330. D. R. Walter, J. D. Dutcher, and O. Wintersteiner, *J. Am. Chem. Soc.*, **79,** 5076 (1957); D.

S. Manwaring, R. W. Rickards, and B. T. Golding, *Tetrahedron Lett.*, 5319 (1969).

331. C. N. Chong and R. W. Rickards, *Tetrahedron Lett.*, 5145 (1970).

332. C. N. Chong and R. W. Rickards, *Tetrahedron Lett.*, 5053 (1972).

333. E. Borowski, J. Zielinski, L. Falkowski, T. Ziminski, J. Golik, P. Kolodziejczyk, E. Jereczek, M. Gdulewicz, Y. Shenin, and T. Kotienko, *Tetrahedron Lett.*, 685 (1971).

334. G. Badaracco and G. Cassani, *Antimicrob. Agents Chemother.*, **9,** 748 (1976).

335. J. B. Patrick, R. P. Williams, and J. S. Webb, *J. Am. Chem. Soc.*, **80,** 6689 (1958).

336. O. Ceder, J. M. Waisvisz, M. G. Van der Hoeve, and R. Ryhage, *Acta Chem. Scand.*, **18,** 126 (1964).

337. O. Ceder and B. Hansson, *Tetrahedron*, **23,** 3753 (1967).

338. B. T. Golding, R. W. Rickards, W. E. Meyer, J. B. Patrick, and M. Barber, *Tetrahedron Lett.*, 3551 (1966).

339. W. Mechlinski and C. P. Schaffner, *Tetrahedron Lett.*, 3873 (1970).

340. G. R. Keim Jr., J. W. Pontsiaka, J. Kirpan, and C. H. Keysser, *Science*, **179,** 584 (1973).

341. S. T. Donta, *Antimicrob. Agents Chemother.*, **5,** 240 (1974).

342. J. Kotler-Brajtburg, G. Medoff, D. Schlessinger, and G. S. Kobayashi, *Antimicrob. Agents Chemother.*, **6,** 770 (1974).

343. J. Aberhart, R. C. Jain, T. Fehr, P. de Mayo, and I. Szilagyi, *J. Chem. Soc. Perkin Trans. I*, 816 836 (1974).

344. E. Borowski, M. Malishkyna, S. Soloviev, and T. Ziminsky, *Chemotherapia*, **10,** 176 (1965); *Chem. Abstr.*, **64,** 13,349 (1966).

345. E. Borowski, L. Falkowski, J. Golik, J. Zielinski, T. Ziminski, W. Mechlinski, E. Jereczek, P. Kolodziejczyk, H. Adlercreutz, D. P. Schaffner, and S. Neelakantan, *Tetrahedron Lett.*, 1987 (1971).

346. M. C. Whiting, *Chem. Ind.* (London), 416 (1961).

347. C. J. Bessel, D. L. Fletcher, A. M. Mortimer, W. K. Anslow, H. C. Campbell, and W. H. C. Shaw, British Patent 884,711 (1962); *Chem. Abstr.*, **56,** 10,713 (1962).

348. A. C. Cope, R. K. Bly, E. P. Burrows, and O. J. Ceder, *J. Am. Chem. Soc.*, **84,** 2170 (1962).

349. R. L. Wagner, F. A. Hochstein, K. Murai, N. Messina, and P. P. Regna, *J. Am. Chem. Soc.*, **75,** 4684 (1953).

350. R. B. Woodward, *Angew. Chem.*, **69,** 50 (1957).

351. M. E. Bergy and T. E. Eble, *Biochemistry*, **7,** 653 (1968).

352. R. C. Pandey, N. Narasimhachari, K. L. Rinehart, and D. S. Millington, *J. Am. Chem. Soc.*, **94,** 4306 (1972).

353. H. H. Wasserman, J. E. Van Verth, D. J. Caustland, I. J. Borowitz, and B. Kamber, *J. Am. Chem. Soc.*, **89,** 1535 (1967).

354. R. Bognăr, S. Makleit, K. Zsupán, B. O. Brown, W. J. S. Lockley, T. B. Toube, and B. C. L. Weedon, *J. Chem. Soc. Perkin Trans. I*, 1848 (1972).

355. H. Bickel, E. Gaumann, R. Hutter, W. Sackmann, E. Vischer, W. Voser, A. Wettstein, and H. Zahner, *Helv. Chim. Acta*, **45,** 1396 (1962).

356. M. P. Kinstmann, L. A. Mitscher, and N. Bohonos, *Tetrahedron Lett.*, 839 (1966).

357. T. Hata, Y. Sano, H. Tatsuta, H. Sugawara, A. Matsumae, and K. Kanamori, *J. Antibiot.* (Tokyo), *Ser. A*, **8,** 9 (1955).

358. R. Cobaz, L. Ettlinger, E. Gaumann, W. Keller-Schierlein, L. Neipp, V. Prelog, P. Reusser, and H. Zahner, *Helv. Chim. Acta*, **38,** 1202 (1955).

359. S. Kondo, J. J. Sakamoto, and H. Yumoto, *J. Antibiot.* (Tokyo), *Ser. A*, **14,** 365 (1961).

360. R. L. Wagner, F. A. Hochstein, K. Murai, N. Messina, and P. P. Regna, *J. Am. Chem. Soc.*, **75,** 4684 (1953).

361. F. A. Hochstein and K. Murai, *J. Am. Chem. Soc.*, **76,** 5080 (1954).

362. R. P. Frohardt, R. Pittilo, and J. Ehrlich, US Patent 3,065,137 (1962).

363. H. Kawaguchi, H. Koshiyama, and M. Okanishi, US Patent 3,159,540 (1964).

364. H. Koshiyama, M. Okanishi, T. Ohmori, T. Miyaki, H. Tsukiura, M. Matsuzake, and H. Kawaguchi, *J. Antibiot.* (Tokyo), *Ser. A*, **16,** 59 (1963).

365. E. H. Flynn, M. V. Sigal, P. F. Wiley, and K. Gerzon, *J. Am. Chem. Soc.*, **76,** 3121 (1954).

366. P. F. Wiley, M. V. Sigal, O. Weaver, R. Monahan, and K. Gerzon, *J. Am. Chem. Soc.*, **79,** 6079 (1957).

367. P. F. Wiley, R. Gale, C. W. Pettinga, and K. Gerzon, *J. Am. Chem. Soc.*, **79,** 6070 (1957).

368. W. Keller-Schierlein and G. Roncari, *Helv. Chim. Acta*, **47,** 78 (1964).

369. T. Watanabe, *Bull. Chem. Soc. Japan*, **33,** 523 (1960).

370. J. Abe, Y. Iida, M. Fukumura, T. Takeda, K. Satake, and T. Watanabe, *J. Antibiot.* (Tokyo), *Ser. A*, **16,** 214 (1963).

371. C. Djerassi and J. A. Zderic, *J. Am. Chem. Soc.*, **78,** 6390 (1956).

372. R. Corbaz, L. Ettlinger, E. Gaumann, W. Keller-Schierlein, F. Kradolfer, E. Kyburz, L. Neipp, V. Prelog, R. Reusser, and H. Zahner, *Helv. Chim. Acta*, **38,** 935 (1955).

373. C. Djerassi, O. Halpern, D. I. Wilkinson, and E. J. Eisenbraun, *Tetrahedron*, **4,** 369 (1958).

374. M. P. Kunstmann and L. A. Mitscher, *Experientia*, **21,** 372 (1965).

375. G. Huber, K. H. Wallhaeuser, L. Fries, A. Steigler, and H. L. Weidenmueller, *Arzneim.-Forsch.*, **12,** 1191 (1962).

376. H. Brockmann and R. Oster, *Chem. Ber.*, **90,** 605 (1957).

377. H. W. Florey, M. A. Jennings, and A. G. Sanders, *Brit. J. Exp. Pathol.*, **26,** 337 (1945).

378. H. A. Whaley, E. L. Patterson, A. C. Dornbush, E. J. Backus, and N. Bohonos, *Antimicrob. Agents Chemother.*, **1963,** 45 (1964).

379. N. Nishimura, K. Kumagai, and N. Ishida, *J. Antibiot.* (Tokyo), *Ser. A*, **18,** 251 (1965).

380. S. Pinnert-Sindico, L. Ninet, J. Preud'homme, and C. Cosar, *Antibiot. Ann. 1954–1955*, 724 (1955).

381. R. Paul and S. Tchelitcheff, *Bull. Soc. Chim. Fr.*, 443 (1957).

382. M. E. Kuehne and B. W. Benson, *J. Am. Chem. Soc.*, **87,** 4660 (1965).

383. T. Osato, M. Ueda, S. Fukuyama, K. Yagishita, Y. Okami, and H. Umezawa, *J. Antibiot.* (Tokyo), *Ser. A*, **8,** 105 (1955).

384. A. Miyake, H. Iwasaki, and T. Takewaka, *J. Antibiot.* (Tokyo), *Ser. A*, **12,** 59 (1959).

385. R. B. Morin and M. Gorman, *Tetrahedron Lett.*, 2339 (1964).

386. R. B. Morin and M. Gorman, *Encyclopedia of Chemical Technology*, Vol. 12, 2nd ed., Interscience Publishers, 1967, p. 638.

387. W. D. Celmer, in *Biogenesis of Antibiotic Substances*, Z. Vanek and Z. Hostalek, Eds., Czechoslovak Academy of Sciences, Prague, 1965, p. 99.

388. W. Keller-Schierlein, *Fortschr. Chem. Org. Naturst.*, **30,** 313 (1973).

389. D. Vazquez, in Ref. 3, p. 459.

390. J. C. H. Mao and E. E. Robishaw, *Biochemistry*, **10,** 2054 (1971).

390a. S. Masamune, Award Address, ACS Award Symposium, March 14, 1978, Anaheim, California. *Aldrichimica Acta*, **11,** 23 (1978).

391. C. Djerassi, O. Halpern, D. I. Wilkinson, and E. J. Eisenbraun, *Tetrahedron*, **4,** 369 (1958).

392. D. G. Manwaring, R. W. Rickards, and R. M. Smith, *Tetrahedron Lett.*, 1029 (1970).

393. S. Masamune, C. U. Kim, K. E. Wilson, G. O. Spessard, P. E. Georghion, and G. S. Bates, *J. Am. Chem. Soc.*, **97,** 3512 (1975).

394. A. Kinumaki and M. Suzuki, *Chem. Commun.*, 744 (1972).

395. H. Muxfeldt, S. Schrader, P. Hansen, and H. Brockmann, *J. Am. Chem. Soc.*, **90,** 4748 (1968).

396. R. W. Rickardts, R. M. Smith, and J. Majer, *Chem. Commun.*, 1049 (1968).

397. R. E. Hughes, H. Muxfeldt, C. Tsai, and J. Stezowski, *J. Am. Chem. Soc.*, **92,** 5267 (1970).

398. I. Maezawa, T. Hori, A. Kinumaki, and M. Suzuki, *J. Antibiot.* (Tokyo), **26,** 771 (1973).

399. R. S. Egan and J. R. Martin, *J. Am. Chem. Soc.*, **92,** 4129 (1970).

400. J. R. Martin, R. S. Egan, A. W. Goldstein, S. L. Muller, W. Keller-Schierlein, L. A. Mitscher, and R. L. Foltz, *Helv. Chim. Acta*, **59,** 1886 (1976).

401. F. A. Hochstein, H. Els, W. D. Celmer, B. L. Shapiro, and R. B. Woodward, *J. Am. Chem. Soc.*, **82,** 3225 (1960).

402. W. D. Celmer and D. C. Hobbs, *Carbohydr. Res.*, **1,** 137 (1965).

403. W. D. Celmer, *J. Am. Chem. Soc.*, **87,** 1797 (1965).

404. W. D. Celmer, *J. Am. Chem. Soc.*, **87,** 1801 (1965).

405. D. R. Harris, S. G. McGeachin, and H. H. Mills, *Tetrahedron Lett.*, 679 (1965).

406. T. J. Perun and R. S. Egan, *Tetrahedron Lett.*, 387 (1969).

407. N. L. Oleinick, in Ref. 3, p. 396.

408. *Drug Action and Drug Resistance in Bacteria*, S. Misuhashi, Ed.; University of Tokyo Press, Tokyo, 1971, pp. 123, 153.

409. J. C. H. Mao and R. G. Wiegand, *Biochim. Biophys. Acta*, **157,** 404 (1968).

410. K. Tanaka, H. Teraoka, M. Tamaki, E. Otaka, and S. Osawa, *Science*, **162,** 576 (1968).

411. B. Weisblum and J. Davis, *Bacteriol, Rev.*, **32,** 493 (1968).

412. J. C. H. Mao and M. Putterman, *J. Mol. Biol.*, **44,** 347 (1969).

413. Z. Vogel, T. Vogel, and D. Elson, *FEBS Lett.*, **15,** 249 (1971).

414. S. Pestka, A. Nakagawa, and W. Omura, *Antimicrob. Agents Chemother.*, **6,** 606 (1974).

415. P. P. Hung, *J. Gen. Virol.*, **26,** 135 (1975).

416. R. S. Egan, T. J. Perun, J. R. Martin, and L. A. Mitscher, *Tetrahedron*, **29,** 2425 (1973).

417. R. S. Egan, J. R. Martin, T. J. Perun, and L. A. Mitscher, *J. Am. Chem. Soc.*, **97,** 4578 (1975).

418. Y. C. Martin, P. H. Jones, T. J. Perun, W. E. Grundy, S. Bell, R. R. Brower, and N. L. Shipkowitz, *J. Med. Chem.*, **15,** 635 (1972).

419. R. L. Wagner, F. A. Hochstein, K. Murai, N. Messina, and P. P. Regna, *J. Am. Chem. Soc.*, **75,** 4684 (1953).

420. R. B. Woodward, *Angew. Chem.*, **69,** 50 (1957).

421. R. B. Woodward, L. S. Weiler, and P. C. Dutta, *J. Am. Chem. Soc.*, **87,** 4662 (1965).

422. F. A. Hochstein and K. Murai, *J. Am. Chem. Soc.*, **76,** 5080 (1954).

423. R. Paul and S. Tchelitcheff, *Bull. Soc. Chim. Fr.*, **443,** 734, 1059 (1957); 150 (1960).

424. R. Corbaz, L. Ettlinger, E. Gaumann, W. Keller-Schierlein, F. Kradolfer, E. Kyburz, L. Neipp, V. Prelog, A. Wettstein, and H. Zahner, *Helv. Chim. Acta*, **39,** 304 (1956).

425. C. L. Stevens, G. E. Gutowsky, K. G. Taylor, and C. P. Bryant, *Tetrahedron Lett.*, 5717 (1966).

426. M. E. Kuehne and B. W. Benson, *J. Am. Chem. Soc.*, **87,** 4660 (1965).

427. S. Omura, A. Kakagawa, M. Otani, T. Hata, H. Ogura, and K. Furuhata, *J. Am. Chem. Soc.*, **91,** 3401 (1969).

428. L. A. Freiberg, R. S. Egan, and W. H. Washburn, *J. Org. Chem.*, **39,** 2474 (1974).

429. P. W. K. Woo, H. W. Dion, and Q. R. Bartz, *J. Am. Chem. Soc.*, **84,** 1512 (1962).

430. D. C. Jordan, in Ref. 1, p. 446.

431. W. Keller-Schierlein, *Experientia*, **22,** 355 (1966).

432. K. Poralla, in Ref. 3, p. 365.

433. R. B. Morin and M. Gaman, *Tetrahedron Lett.*, 2339 (1964); 4737 (1970).

434. M. Brufani and W. Keller-Schierlein, *Helv. Chim. Acta*, **49,** 1962 (1966).

435. U. Schmidt, J. Gombos, E. Haslinger, and H. Zak, *Chem. Ber.*, **109,** 2628 (1976).

436. P. D. Shaw, in Ref. 1, pp. 649, 759.

437. S. Masamune, J. M. Sehgal, E. E. van Tamelen, F. M. Strong, and W. H. Peterson, *J. Am. Chem. Soc.*, **80,** 6092 (1958).

438. M. von Glehn, R. Norrestam, P. Kierkegaard, L. Maron, and L. Ernster, *FEBS Lett.*, **20,** 267 (1972).

439. P. D. Shaw, in Ref. 1, p. 585.

440. Symposium on Energy Coupling in Electron Transport, *Fed. Proc.*, **26,** no. 5 (1967).

441. B. Bulos and E. Racker, *J. Biol. Chem.*, **243,** 3891 (1968).

442. B. Bulos and E. Racker, *J. Biol. Chem.*, **243,** 3901 (1968).

443. A. Tzagloff, D. H. MacLennan, and K. H. Bryington, *Biochemistry*, **7,** 1596 (1968).

444. D. H. MacLennan and A. Tzagloff, *Biochemistry*, **7,** 1603 (1968).

445. C. K. Ramakrishna Kurup and D. R. Sanadi, *Arch. Biochem. Biophys.*, **176,** 218 (1976).

446. S. Harada, M. Muroi, M. Kondo, T. Tsuchiya, T. Matsuzawa, T. Fugono, T. Kishi, and J. Ueyanagi, *Antimicrob. Agents Chemother.*, **4,** 140 (1973).

447. M. Kondo, K. Ishifuji, K. Tsuchiya, S. Goto, and S. Kuwahara, *Antimicrob. Agents Chemother.*, **4,** 156 (1973).

448. M. Kondo, T. Oishi, K. Tsuchiya, S. Goto, and S. Kuwahara, *Antimicrob. Agents Chemother.*, **4,** 149 (1973).

449. R. S. Egan, S. L. Mueller, L. A. Mitscher, I. Kawamoto, R. Okachi, H. Kato, S. Yamamoto, S. Takasawa, and T. Nara, *J. Antibiot.* (Tokyo), **27,** 544 (1974).

450. F. Arcamone, C. Bertazzoli, M. Ghione, and T. Scott, *G. Microbiol.*, **7,** 251 (1959).

451. B. Bannister and A. D. Argoudelis, *J. Am. Chem. Soc.*, **85,** 234 (1963).

452. H. Maehr and C. P. Schaffner, *J. Am. Chem. Soc.*, **89,** 6787 (1967).

453. M. J. Weinstein, G. M. Luedemann, E. M. Oden, and G. H. Wagman, *Antimicrob. Agents Chemother.*, **1963,** 1 (1964).

454. H. Maehr and C. P. Schaffner, *J. Chromatogr.*, **30,** 572 (1967).

455. M. Okanishi, H. Koshiyama, T. Ohmori, M. Matsuzaki, S. Ohashi, and H. Kawaguchi, *J. Antibiot.* (Tokyo), *Ser. A*, **15,** 7 (1962).

456. R. L. Mann and D. O. Woolf, *J. Am. Chem. Soc.*, **79,** 120 (1957).

457. R. L. Mann and W. W. Bromer, *J. Am. Chem. Soc.*, **80,** 2714 (1958).

458. H. Umezawa, M. Ueda, K. Maeda, K. Yagishita, S. Kondo, Y. Okami, R. Utahara, Y. Osato, K. Nitta, and T. Takeuchi, *J. Antibiot.* (Tokyo), *Ser. A*, **10,** 181 (1957).

459. H. Ogawa, T. Ito, S. Inoue, and S. Kondo, *J. Antibiot.* (Tokyo), *Ser. A*, **11,** 72 (1958).

460. H. Ogawa, T. Ito, S. Inoue, and S. Kondo, *J. Antibiot.* (Tokyo), *Ser. A*, **11,** 166 (1958).

461. J. D. Dutcher, N. Hosansky, M. N. Donin, and O. Wintersteiner, *J. Am. Chem. Soc.*, **73,** 1384 (1951).

462. K. L. Rinehart, Jr., M. Hichens, A. D. Argoudelis, W. S. Chilton, H. E. Carter, M. P. Georgiadis, C. P. Schaffner, and R. T. Schillings, *J. Am. Chem. Soc.*, **84,** 3218 (1962).

463. T. H. Haskell, J. C. French, and Q. R. Bartz, *J. Am. Chem. Soc.*, **81,** 3482 (1959).

464. S. Horii, H. Hitomi, and A. Miyake, *J. Antibiot.* (Tokyo), *Ser. A,* **16,** 144 (1963).

465. R. U. Lemieux and M. L. Wolfrom, *Advan. Carbohydr. Chem.* **3,** 337 (1948).

466. J. Fried and H. Stavely, *J. Am. Chem. Soc.*, **74,** 5461 (1952).

467. F. H. Stodola, O. L. Shotwell, A. M. Borud, R. G. Benedict, and A. C. Riley, *J. Am. Chem. Soc.*, **73,** 2290 (1951).

468. F. Kavanagh, E. Grinnan, E. Allanson, and D. Tunin, *Appl. Microbiol.*, **8,** 160 (1960).

469. N. Tanaka, in Ref. 3, p. 340.

470. R. Benveniste and J. Davies, *Antimicrob. Agents Chemother.*, **4,** 402 (1973).

471. A. Schatz, E. Bugie, and S. A. Waksman, *Proc. Soc. Exp. Biol. Med.*, **55,** 66 (1944).

472. J. B. Walker, *Lloydia*, **34,** 363 (1971).

473. I. J. McGilveray and K. L. Rinehart, *J. Am. Chem. Soc.*, **87,** 4003 (1965).

474. S. Mezawa, Y. Takahashi, T. Usui, and T. Tsuchiya, *J. Antibiot.* (Tokyo), **27,** 997 (1974).

475. D. Schlessinger and G. Medoff, in Ref. 3, p. 535.

476. M. Kogut and E. Prizant, *Antimicrob. Agents Chemother.*, **7,** 341 (1975).

477. D. Lando, M. A. Cousin, T. Ojasoo, and J. P. Raynaud, *Eur. J. Biochem.*, **66,** 597 (1976).

478. B. Weisblum and J. Davies, *Bacteriol. Rev.*, **32,** 493 (1968).

479. M. Nomura, S. Miaushima, M. Ozaki, P. Traub, and C. W. Lowry, *Cold Spring Harb. Symp. Quant. Biol.*, **34,** 49 (1969).

480. J. Davies and B. D. Davis, *J. Biol. Chem.*, **243,** 3312 (1968).

481. M. J. Cross, O. B. Fardig, D. L. Johnson, H. Schmitz, D. F. Whitehead, I. R. Hooper, and R. U. Lemieux, *J. Am. Chem. Soc.*, **80,** 2342, 4115, 4741 (1958).

482. H. Ogawa, T. Ito, S. Inoue, and S. Kando, *J. Antibiot.* (Tokyo), *Ser. A*, **11,** 70, 72, 166 (1958).

483. A. Hasegawa, N. Kurihara, D. Nishimura, and M. Nakajima, *Agr. Biol. Chem.*, **32,** 1130 (1968).

484. H. Yamashita, T. Yamasaki, K. Fujisawa, and H. Kawaguchi, *J. Antibiot.*, (Tokyo), **27,** 851 (1974).

485. T. Naito, S. Nakagawa, Y. Abe, K. Fujisawa, and H. Kawaguchi, *J. Antibiot.* (Tokyo), **27,** 838 (1974).

486. Conference on Kanamycin (various authors). Appraised after eight years of clinical application. *Ann. N.Y. Acad. Sci.*, **132,** 773 (1966).

487. M. Suzuki, *J. Antibiot.* (Tokyo), **23,** 99 (1970).

488. T. H. Haskell and S. Hanessian, *J. Org. Chem.*, **28,** 2598 (1963).

489. K. L. Rinehart, M. Hichens, A. D. Argoudelis, W. S. Chilton, H. E. Carter, M. Georgiadis, C. P. Schaffner, and R. T. Schillings, *J. Am. Chem. Soc.*, **84,** 3218 (1962).

490. K. L. Rinehart, *The Neomycins and Related Antibiotics*, Wiley, New York, 1964.

491. S. A. Waksman and H. A. Lechevalier, *Science*, **109,** 305 (1949).

492. S. A. Waksman, E. Katz, and H. Lechevalier, *J. Lab. Clin. Med.*, **36,** 93 (1950).

493. W. T. Sokilski, *Anal. Microbiol.*, **2,** 2825 (1972).

494. M. J. Weinstein, G. M. Luedeman, E. M. Oden, G. H. Wagman, J. P. Rosselot, J. A. Marquez, C. T. Conglio, W. Chasney, H. L. Herzog, and J. Black, *J. Med. Chem.*, **6,** 463 (1963).

495. J. P. Rosselot, J. Marquez, E. Meseck, A. Murawski, A. Hamdan, C. Joyner, R. Schmidt, D. Migliore, and H. L. Herzog, in *Antimicrobial Agents and Chemotherapy, 1963.* J. C. Sylvester, Ed., American Society for Microbiology, Ann Arbor, Mich., 1964, p. 14.

496. H. Maehr and C. P. Schaffner, *J. Am. Chem. Soc.*, **89,** 6787 (1967).

497. H. Maehr and C. P. Schaffner, *J. Am. Chem. Soc.*, **92,** 1697 (1970).

498. D. J. Cooper, P. J. L. Daniels, M. D. Yudis, H. M. Marigliano, R. D. Guthrie, and S. T. K. Bukhari, *J. Chem. Soc. C*, 2876, 3126 (1971).

499. T. L. Nagabhushan, W. N. Turner, P. J. L. Daniels, and J. B. Morton, *J. Org. Chem.*, **40,** 2830, 2835 (1975).

500. J. O. Klein, T. C. Eickhoff, and M. Finland, *Am. J. Med. Sci.*, **248,** 528 (1964).

501. M. J. Weinstein, G. M. Luedeman, E. M. Oden, and G. H. Wagman, in *Antimicrobial Agents and Chemotherapy, 1963,* J. C. Sylvester, Ed., American Society for Microbiology, Ann Arbor, Mich., 1964, p. 1.

502. M. Finland, *Med. Times, N.Y.*, **97,** 161 (1969).

503. International Symposium on Gentamicin (various authors), *J. Infect. Dis.*, **119,** 341 (1969).

504. V. M. Zimelis and G. G. Jackson, *J. Infect. Dis.*, **127,** 663 (1973).

505. C. Regamey, D. Schaberg, and W. M. M. Kirby, *Antimicrob. Agents Chemother.*, **1,** 329 (1972).

506. N. Rosdahl and V. F. Thompson, *Acta Pathol. Microbiol. Scand.*, **B, 79,** 333 (1971).

507. Second International Symposium on Gentamicin (various authors), *J. Infect. Dis.*, **124,** Suppl. Sl (1971).

508. C. Watanakunakorn, *J. Infect. Dis.*, **124,** 581 (1971).

509. C. Regamey, R. C. Gordon, and W. M. M. Kirby, *Clin. Pharmacol. Ther.*, **14,** 396 (1973).

510. C. Cox, *Med. Clin. N. Am.*, **54,** 1305, (1970).

511. M. A. Sande and J. W. Overton, *J. Infect. Dis.*, **128,** 247 (1973).

512. H. F. Dowling, *Tetracycline*, Medical Encylopedia, Inc., New York, 1955.

513. M. H. Lepper, *Aureomycin (Chlortetracycline)*, Medical Encyclopedia, Inc., New York, 1956 (769 references).

514. M. M. Musselman, *Terramycin (oxytetracycline)*, Medical Encyclopedia, Inc., New York, 1956 (664 references).

515. J. O. Pezzanite, J. Clardy, P.-Y. Lau, G. Wood, D. L. Walker, and B. Fraser-Reid, *J. Am. Chem. Soc.*, **97,** 6250 (1975).

516. A. I. Laskin, in Ref. 1, pp. 331, 752.

517. T. Money and A. I. Scott, *Progr. Org. Chem.*, **7,** 1 (1968).

518. H. Muxfeldt and R. Bangert, *Fortschr. Chem. Org. Naturst.*, **21,** 80 (1963).

519. D. L. Clive, *Quart. Rev.* (London), **22,** 435 (1968).

520. J. J. Hlavka and J. H. Boothe, *Progr. Drug Res.*, **17,** 210 (1973).

521. R. K. Blackwood and A. R. English, *Advan. Appl. Microbiol.*, **13,** 237 (1970).

522. G. Suarez and D. Nathans, *Biochem. Biophys. Res. Commun.*, **18,** 743 (1965).

523. A. Cammarata, S. J. Yan, J. H. Collett, and A. N. Martin, *Mol. Pharmacol.*, **6,** 61 (1970).

524. R. Rendi and S. Ochoa, *J. Biol. Chem.*, **237,** 3711 (1962); *Science*, **133,** 1367 (1961).

525. T. J. Franklin, *Biochem. J.*, **87,** 449 (1963); **84,** 110P (1962).

526. T. Akiba and T. Yokota, *Igaku To Seibutsugaku*, **64,** 34, 39 (1962).

527. J. Park, *Biochem. J.*, **70,** 2P (1958).

528. J. Snell and L. Cheng, *Dev. Ind. Microbiol.*, **2,** 107 (1961).

529. G. Suarez and D. Nathans, *Biochem. Biophys. Res. Commun.*, **18,** 793 (1965).

530. R. Connamacher and H. Mandel, *Biochim. Biophys. Acta*, **166,** 475 (1968).

531. A. Larkin and J. Laro, *Antibiot. Chemother.*, **17,** 1 (1971).

532. Z. Vogel, *Biochemistry*, **8,** 5161 (1969).

533. R. Kaempfer, *Proc. Nat. Acad. Sci., US*, **61,** 106 (1968).

534. N. L. Allinger and J. L. Coke, *J. Org. Chem.*, **26,** 4522 (1961).

535. S. Okuda, S. Iwasaki, M. I. Sair, Y. Machida, A. Inoue, K. Tsuda, and Y. Nakayama, *Tetrahedron Lett.*, 2295 (1967); W. von Daehne, H. Lorch, and W. O. Godtfredsen, *Tetrahedron Lett.*, 4843 (1968); S. Iwasaki, M. I. Sair, H. Igasashi, and S. Okuda, *Chem. Commun.*, 1119 (1970).

536. E. P. Abraham, *Biochemistry of Some Peptide and Steroid Antibiotics*, Wiley, New York, 1957.

537. B. M. Baird, T. G. Holsall, E. R. H. Jones, and G. Lowe, *Chem. Ind.* (London), 257 (1961); *Proc. Chem. Soc.* 16 (1963).

538. T. S. Chou, E. J. Eisenbraun, and R. T. Rapala, *Tetrahedron Lett.*, 409 (1967).

539. N. Tanaka, in Ref. 3, p. 436.

540. N. Tanaka, T. Kinoshita, and H. Mazukawa, *Biochem. Biophys. Res. Commun.*, **30,** 278 (1968).

541. C. L. Harvey, S. G. Knight, and C. J. Sih, *Biochemistry*, **5,** 3320 (1966).

542. A. L. Haenni and J. Lucas-Lenard, *Proc. Nat. Acad. Sci., US*, **61,** 1363 (1968).

543. S. Petska, *Proc. Nat. Acad. Sci., US*, **61,** 726 (1968).

544. M. Malkin and F. Lipman, *Science*, **164,** 71 (1969).

545. D. Richter, L. Lin, and J. Bodley, *Arch. Biochem. Biophys.*, **147,** 186 (1971).

546. D. Richter and F. Lipmann, *Biochemistry*, **9,** 5065 (1970).

547. U. Albrecht, K. Prenzel, and D. Richter, *Biochemistry*, **9,** 316 (1970).

548. J. W. Bodley, F. J. Zieve, L. Lin, and S. T. Zieve, *Biochem. Biophys. Res. Commun.*, **37,** 437 (1969).

549. J. W. Bodley and L. Lin, *Nature*, **227,** 60 (1970).

550. J. W. Bodley, F. J. Zieve, and L. Lin, *J. Biol. Chem.*, **245,** 5662 (1970).

551. J. W. Bodley, L. Lin, M. Salas, and M. Tao, *FEBS Lett.*, **11,** 153 (1970).

552. N. Brot, C. Spears, and H. Weissnach, *Arch. Biochem. Biophys.*, **43,** 286 (1971).

553. J. Mondollel, D. Vasquez, and R. E. Monro, *Nature New Biol.*, **230,** 109 (1971).

554. J. Mondolell, B. Cabrer, A. Pameggiani, and D.

Vasquez, *Proc. Nat. Acad. Sci., US*, **68,** 1796 (1971).

555. E. Cundliff, *Biochem. Biophys. Res. Commun.*, **44,** 912 (1971); **46,** 1794 (1972).
556. B. S. Baliga, S. A. Cohen, and H. N. Nunro, *FEBS Lett.*, **8,** 249 (1970).
557. M. Springer, J. Dondon, M. Graffe, and M. Grunberg-Manago, *Biochimie*, **53,** 1047 (1971).
558. P. Sensi, A. M. Greco, and R. Ballotta, *Antibiot. Ann.* 262 (1959–1960).
559. V. Prelog, *Pure Appl. Chem.*, **7,** 551 (1963).
560. W. Wehrli and M. Staehelin, in Ref. 3, p. 252.
561. J. E. Kasik, M. Mowick, and J. S. Thompson, *Antimicrob. Agents Chemother.*, **9,** 470 (1976).
562. P. Sensi, in *Research Progress in Organic Biological and Medicinal Chemistry*, U. Gallo and L. Santamaria, Eds., North-Holland, Amsterdam, 1964, p. 337; P. Sensi and J. E. Thiemann, *Progr. Ind. Microbiol.*, **6,** 21 (1967).
563. S. Riva and L. G. Silvestri, *Ann. Rev. Microbiol.*, **26,** 199 (1972).
564. S. Harada, E. Higashide, T. Fugono, and T. Kishi, *Tetrahedron Lett.*, 2239 (1969); M. Uramoto, N. Otake, Y. Ogawa, and H. Yonehara, *Tetrahedron Lett.*, 2249 (1969).
565. W. Lester, *Ann. Rev. Microbiol.*, **26,** 85 (1972).
566. W. Zillig, K. Zechel, D. Rabussay, M. Schachner, U. S. Sehti, P. Palm, A. Heil, and W. Seifert, *Cold Spring Harb. Symp. Quant. Biol.*, **35,** 47 (1970).
567. K. Konno, K. Oizumo, and S. Oka, *Ann. Rev. Respir. Dis.*, **107,** 1006 (1973).
568. W. Stender and K. H. Scheit, *Eur. J. Biochem.*, **65,** 333 (1976).
569. M. F. Dampier, C. W. Chen, and H. W. Whitlock, Jr., *J. Am. Chem. Soc.*, **98,** 7064 (1976).
570. E. Battaner and B. Vijaya Kumar, *Antimicrob. Agents Chemother.*, **5,** 371 (1974).
571. P. V. Venkov, G. I. Milche, and A. A. Hadjiolov, *Antimicrob. Agents Chemother.*, **8,** 627 (1975).
572. J. C. Handschin and W. Wehrli, *Eur. J. Biochem.*, **66,** 309 (1976).
573. S. Watanabe and K. Tanaka, *Biochem. Biophys. Res. Commun.*, **72,** 522 (1976).
574. K. L. Rinehart, P. K. Martin, and C. E. Coverdale, *J. Am. Chem. Soc.*, **88,** 3149 (1966).
575. K. L. Rinehart, H. H. Mathur, K. Sasaki, P. K. Martin, and C. E. Coverdale, *J. Am. Chem. Soc.*, **90,** 6241 (1968); K. L. Rinehart, M. L. Maheshwari, F. J. Antosz, H. H. Mathur, K. Sasaki, and R. J. Schacht, *ibid.*, **93,** 6273 (1971).
576. K. L. Rinehart, Jr., F. J. Antosz, K. Sasaki, P. K. Martin, M. L. Maheshwari, F. Reusser, L. H. Li, D. Moran, and P. F. Wiley, *Biochemistry*, **13,** 861 (1974).
577. K. L. Rinehart, Jr., W. M. Knoll, K. Kakinuma, F. J. Antosz, I. C. Paul, A. H. J. Wang, F. Reusser, L. H. Li, and W. C. Krueger, *J. Am. Chem. Soc.*, **97,** 196 (1975).
578. K. Sasaki, K. L. Rinehart, G. Slomp, M. F. Grostic, and E. C. Olson, *J. Am. Chem. Soc.*, **92,** 7591 (1970).
579. M. W. McMillan, K. L. Rinehart, Jr., F. Reusser, and L. H. Li, *Abstr. Pap. Meet. Am. Chem. Soc.*, 166, 70 (1973).
580. F. Johnson, *Progr. Chem. Org. Nat. Prod.*, **29,** 140 (1971).
581. J. F. Welch, *J. Agr. Food Chem.*, **2,** 142 (1954).
582. J. H. Ford and B. E. Leach, *J. Am. Chem. Soc.*, **69,** 474 (1947).
583. F. Johnson, N. A. Starkovsky, and W. D. Gurowitz, *J. Am. Chem. Soc.*, **87,** 3492 (1965).
584. F. Johnson, N. A. Starkowsky, A. C. Paton, and A. A. Carlson, *J. Am. Chem. Soc.*, **88,** 149 (1966); *J. Org. Chem.*, **31,** 1327 (1966).
585. M. R. Siegel and H. D. Sisler, *Nature*, **200,** 675 (1963).
586. M. R. Siegel and H. D. Sisler, *Biochim. Biophys. Acta*, **87,** 70, 83 (1964).
587. M. L. Ennis and M. Lubin, *Science*, **146,** 1474 (1964).
588. F. O. Wettstein, H. Noll, and S. Penman, *Biochim. Biophys. Acta*, **87,** 525 (1964).
589. A. R. Williamson and R. Schweet, *J. Mol. Biol.*, **11,** 358 (1965).
590. B. Colombo, L. Felicetti, and C. Baglioni, *Biochem. Biophys. Res. Commun.*, **18,** 389 (1965); *Biochim. Biophys. Acta*, **119,** 120 (1966).
591. A. C. Trakatellis, M. Montjar, and A. E. Axelrod, *Biochemistry*, **4,** 2065, (1965).
592. S. Y. Lin, R. D. Mosteller, and B. Hardesty, *J. Mol. Biol.*, **21,** 51 (1966).
593. W. Godchaux, S. D. Adamson, and E. Herbert, *J. Mol. Biol.*, **27,** 57 (1967).
594. B. S. Baliga, S. A. Cohen, and H. N. Nunro, *FEBS Lett.*, **8,** 249 (1970).
595. H. Munro, B. S. Baliga, and A. W. Pronczuk, *Nature*, **219,** 944 (1968).
596. T. G. Obrig, W. J. Culp, W. L. McKeehan, and B. Hardesty, *J. Biol. Chem.*, **244,** 4480 (1969).
597. W. McKeehan and B. Hardesty, *Biochem. Biophys. Res. Commun.*, **36,** 625, (1969).

598. S. S. Rao and A. P. Grollman, *Biochem. Biophys. Res. Commun.*, **29,** 696 (1967).
599. M. Suzuki, *Yakugaku Zasshi,* **80,** 1217 (1960).
600. K. Wildenthal and E. E. Griffin, *Biochim. Biophys. Acta,* **444,** 519 (1976).
601. R. Paul and S. Tschelitcheff, *Bull. Soc. Chim. Fr.*, 1316 (1955).
602. K. V. Rao, *J. Am. Chem. Soc.*, **82,** 1129 (1960).
603. R. R. Herr, *J. Am. Chem. Soc.*, **81,** 2595 (1959).
604. F. Johnson, L. G. Duquette, and H. E. Hennis, *J. Org. Chem.*, **33,** 904 (1968).
605. R. J. Suhadolnik, *Nucleoside Antibiotics,* Wiley, New York, 1970.
606. C. W. Waller, P. W. Fryth, B. L. Hutchins, and J. H. Williams, *J. Am. Chem. Soc.*, **75,** 2025 (1953).
607. B. R. Baker, R. E. Schaub, J. P. Joseph, and J. H. Williams, *J. Am. Chem. Soc.*, **77,** 12 (1955).
608. A. O. Hawtrey, S. I. Biedron, and S. H. Eggers, *Tetrahedron Lett.*, 1693 (1967); F. W. Lichtenthaler and H. P. Albrecht, *Angew. Chem. Int. Ed.*, **7,** 457 (1968).
609. N. B. Yarmolinski and G. L. de la Haba, *Proc. Nat. Acad. Sci., US,* **45,** 1721 (1959).
610. G. J. Spyrides, *Proc. Nat. Acad. Sci., US,* **51,** 1220 (1964).
611. D. Allen and P. C. Zamechik, *Biochim. Biophys. Acta,* **55,** 865 (1962).
612. D. Nathans and A. Neidle, *Nature,* **197,** 1076 (1962).
613. D. Nathans, J. E. Allende, T. W. Conway, G. Y. Spyrides, F. Lipmann, in *Symposium on Information Macromolecules,* H. J. Vogel, U. Brisson, and J. O. Lapman, Eds., New York, Academic Press, 1963.
614. W. Gilbert, *J. Mol. Biol.*, **6,** 389 (1963).
615. D. Nathans, *Proc. Nat. Acad. Sci., US,* **51,** 585 (1964).
616. J. D. Smith, R. R. Trout, G. M. Blackburn, and R. E. Monro, *J. Mol. Biol.*, **13,** 617 (1965).
617. M. Springer, J. Dondon, M. Graffe, and M. Grunberg-Manago, *Biochimie,* **53,** 1047 (1971).
618. R. E. Munro, *J. Mol. Biol.*, **26,** 147 (1967).
619. R. E. Munro and K. A. Marker, *J. Mol. Biol.*, **25,** 347 (1967).
620. R. E. Monro, J. Cerna, and K. A. Marker, *Proc. Nat. Acad. Sci., US,* **61,** 1048 (1968).
621. R. E. Monro and D. Vasquez, *J. Mol. Biol.*, **28,** 161 (1967).
622. R. E. Monro and K. A. Marker, *J. Mol. Biol.*, **25,** 347 (1967).
623. R. E. Monro, in *Methods in Enzymology,* K. Moldave and L. Grossman, Eds., Vol. 20, *Nucleic Acids and Protein Synthesis,* Part C, Academic Press, p. 472, 1971.
624. D. Vasquez, T. Saebelin, H. L. Cema, E. Battaner, R. Fernandez-Nuñoz, and R. E. Monro, in *Macromolecular Biosynthesis and Function,* S. Ochoa, C. F. Heredia, C. Ascensio, and D. Nachmanson, Eds, FEBS, New York, Academic Press, 1970, p. 109.
625. B. L. Hutchins, "Puromycin", in *Chemistry and Biology of Purines,* G. E. W. Wolstenholme, and C. H. O'Connor, Eds, Boston; Little, Brown, 1957.
626. N. Dickie, C. S. Alexander, and H. T. Nagasawa, *Biochim. Biophys. Acta,* **95,** 156 (1965).
627. S. Pestka, R. Vince, S. Daluge, and R. Harris, *Antimicrob. Agents Chemother.*, **4,** 37 (1973).
628. S. Suzuki and S. Marumo, *J. Antibiot.* (Tokyo), *Ser. A.*, **14,** 34 (1961).
629. Y. Mizuno, M. Ikehara, and K. Watanabe, *Chem. Pharm. Bull.* (Tokyo), **11,** 1091 (1963).
630. H. Seto, N. Otaka, and H. Yonehara, *Agr. Biol. Chem.*, **32,** 1292, 1299 (1968).
631. A. Tavitian, C. S. Uretsky, and G. Acs. *Biochim. Biophys. Acta,* **157,** 33 (1968); **179,** 50 (1969).
632. L. V. Crawford and M. J. Waring, *J. Mol. Biol.*, **25,** 23 (1967).
633. H. Y. Yüntsen, *J. Antibiot.* (Tokyo), *Ser. A,* **11,** 79 (1958).
634. H. Hoeksema, G. Slomp, and E. E. van Tamelen, *Tetrahedron Lett.*, 1787 (1964); J. R. McCarthy, R. K. Robins, and M. J. Robins, *J. Am. Chem. Soc.*, **90,** 4993 (1968).
635. A. J. Guarino, in Ref. 1, p. 464.
636. L. J. Hanka, in Ref. 1, p. 457.
637. W. Schroeder, *J. Am. Chem. Soc.*, **81,** 1767 (1959).
638. B. M. Chassy, T. Sugimoro, and R. J. Suhadolnik, *Biochim. Biophys. Acta,* **130,** 12 (1966).
639. L. Slechta, *Biochem. Pharmacol.*, **5,** 96 (1960).
640. L. Slechta, *Biochem. Biophys. Res. Commun.*, **3,** 596 (1960).
641. L. J. Hanka, *J. Bacteriol.*, **80,** 30 (1960).
642. H. S. Moyed, *Cold Spring Harb. Sympos. Quant. Biol.*, **26,** 323 (1961).
643. T. T. Fukuyama and H. S. Moyed, *Biochemistry,* **3,** 1488 (1964).
644. S. Udaka and H. S. Moyed, *J. Biol. Chem.*, **238,** 2797 (1963).
645. H. Kuramitsu and H. S. Moyed, *Biochim. Biophys. Acta,* **85,** 504 (1964).
646. H. Kuramitsu and H. S. Moyed, *J. Biol. Chem.*, **241,** 1596 (1966).

647. C. A. Dekker, *J. Am. Chem. Soc.*, **87,** 4027 (1965).

648. H. R. Bentley, K. G. Cunningham, and F. S. Spring, *J. Chem. Soc.*, 2299, 2301 (1951).

649. E. A. Kaczka, N. R. Tremer, B. Arison, R. W. Walker, and K. Folkers, *Biochem. Biophys. Research Commun.*, **14,** 456 (1964).

650. S. Hanessian, D. C. de Jongh, and J. A. McCloskey, *Biochim. Biophys. Acta*, **117,** 480 (1966).

651. A. J. Guarino, in Ref. 1, p. 468, 756.

652. S. Frederiksen and H. Klenow, *Biochem. Biophys. Res. Commun.*, **17,** 165 (1964).

653. H. Klenow and S. Frederiksen, *Biochim. Biophys. Acta*, **87,** 495 (1964).

654. H. Shigeura and G. Boxer, *Biochem. Biophys. Res. Commun.*, **17,** 165 (1964).

655. N. Otake, S. Takeuchi, T. Endo, and H. Yonehara, *Tetrahedron Lett.*, 1405, 1411 (1965).

656. J. J. Fox and K. A. Watanabe, *Tetrahedron Lett.*, 897 (1966).

657. T. Misato, in Ref. 1, p. 434.

658. K. A. Watanabe, T. M. K. Chiu, U. Reichman, C. K. Chu, and J. J. Fox, *Tetrahedron*, **32,** 1493 (1976).

659. M. Yukoda, in Ref. 3, p. 448.

660. H. T. Shigeura, in Ref. 3, p. 12.

661. J. R. Florini, in Ref. 1, p. 427.

662. C. L. Stevens, K. Nagarajan, and T. H. Haskell, *J. Org. Chem.*, **27,** 2991 (1962).

663. D. Gottlieb, in Ref. 1, p. 762.

664. P. F. Wiley and F. A. MacKellar, *J. Am. Chem. Soc.*, **92,** 417 (1970).

665. L. Slechta, in Ref. 1, p. 410, 756.

666. J. Jayaraman and I. H. Goldberg, *Biochemistry*, **7,** 418 (1968).

667. I. H. Goldberg and K. Mitsugi, *Biochemistry*, **6,** 383 (1967).

668. B. L. Colombo, L. Felicetti, and C. Baglioni, *Biochim. Biophys. Acta*, **119,** 109 (1966).

669. A. C. Trakatellis, *Proc. Nat. Acad. Sci., US*, **59,** 854 (1968).

670. B. S. Baliga, S. A. Cohen, and H. N. Nunro, *FEBS Letters*, **8,** 249 (1970).

671. H. Brockmann, *Fortschr. Chem. Org. Naturst.* **21,** 121 (1963).

672. J. C. Double and J. R. Brown, *J. Pharm. Pharmacol.*, **28,** 166 (1976).

673. A. DiMarco, F. Arcamone, and F. Zunino, in Ref. 3, p. 101.

674. W. J. Pigram, W. Fuller, and L. D. Hamilton, *Nature New Biol.*, **235,** 17 (1972).

675. F. Quadrifoglio and V. Crescenzi, *Biophys. Chem.* **2,** 64 (1974).

676. F. Zumino, R. Gambetta, A. DiMarco, G. Luoni, and A. Zacarra, *Biochem. Biophys. Res. Commun.*, **69,** 744 (1976).

677. F. Arcamone, G. Cassinelli, G. Fantini, A. Grein, P. Orezzi, C. Poli, and C. Spalla, *Biotechnol. Bioeng.*, **11,** 1101 (1969).

678. *International Symposium on Adriamycin*, S. K. Karter, A. DiMarco, M. Ghione, I. H. Krakoff, and G. Mathé, Eds., Springer-Verlag, Berlin, 1972.

679. B. A. Chabner, C. E. Myers, C. N. Coleman, and D. G. Johns, *New Engl. J. Med.*, **292,** 1107, 1159 (1975).

680. A. DiMarco, in *Antineoplastic and Immunosuppressive Agents*, Part 2, A. C. Sartorelli and D. G. Johns, Eds., Springer-Verlag, Berlin, 1975, p. 593.

681. A. DiMarco, M. Gaetani, and B. Scarpinato, *Cancer Chemother. Rep.*, **53,** 33 (1969).

682. J. S. Sandberg, F. L. Howesden, A. DiMarco, and A. Golding, *Cancer Chemother. Rep.*, **54,** 1 (1970).

683. G. Bonadonna, S. Monfardini, M. DeLena, F. Fossati-Bellani, and C. Beretta, *Cancer Res.*, **30,** 2572 (1970).

684. E. Middleman, J. Luce, and E. Frei, *Cancer*, **28,** 844 (1971).

685. A. DiMarco and F. Arcamone, *Arzneim.-Forsch.*, **25,** 368 (1975).

685a. T. R. Krugh and M. A. Young, *Nature*, **269,** 627 (1977).

686. A. Rusconi, *Biochim. Biophys. Acta*, **123,** 627 (1966).

687. F. Arcamone, S. Penso, A. Vigevani, S. Redaelli, and G. Franchi, *J. Med. Chem.*, **18,** 703 (1975).

688. F. Arcamone, A. Bargiotti, G. Cassinelli, S. Redaelli, S. Hanessian, A. DiMarco, A. M. Casazza, T. Dasdia, A. Necco, P. Reggiani, and R. Supino, *J. Med. Chem.*, **19,** 733 (1976).

688a. F. S. Swenton and P. W. Raynolds, *J. Am. Chem. Soc.*, **100,** 6188 (1978) and references therein.

689. G. F. Gause, *Advan. Chemother.*, **2,** 179 (1965).

690. Y. A. Berlin, O. A. Chupronova, B. A. Klyashchitskii, M. N. Kolosov, G. Y. Peck, L. A. Piotrovich, M. M. Shemyakin, and I. V. Vasina, *Tetrahedron Lett.*, 1425 (1966).

691. M. Miyamoto, Y. Kawematsu, K. Kawaghima, M. Shinohara, and K. Nakanishi, *Tetrahedron Lett.*, 545 (1966); *Tetrahedron*, **23,** 421 (1967).

692. M. Miyamoto, K. Morita, Y. Kawamatsu, K. Kawashima, and K. Nakanashi, *Tetrahedron*

Lett., 411 (1967); N. Narada, K. Nakanashi, and S. Tatsuoka, *J. Am. Chem. Soc.*, **91,** 5896 (1969).

693. G. P. Bakhaeva, Y. A. Berlin, E. F. Boldyreva, O. A. Chuprunova, M. N. Kolosov, V. S. Soifer, T. E. Vasiljeva, and I. V. Yartseva, *Tetrahedron Lett.*, 3595 (1968); Y. A. Berlin, M. N. Kolosov, and L. A. Piotrovich, *ibid.*, 1329 (1970).
694. D. Ward, E. Reich, and I. H. Goldberg, *Science*, **149,** 1259 (1965).
695. W. Kersten, H. Kersten, and W. Szybalski, *Biochemistry*, **5,** 236 (1965).
696. M. Kamiyama, *Biochem., Japan*, **63,** 566 (1968).
697. W. Berk, K. Honikel, and G. Hartman, *Eur. J. Biochem.*, **9,** 82 (1969).
698. A. Cerami, E. Reich, D. G. Ward, and I. H. Goldberg, *Proc. Nat. Acad. Sci., US*, **57,** 1036 (1967).
699. M. Waring, *J. Mol. Biol.*, **54,** 247 (1970). (a) P. F. Wiley, R. B. Kelly, E. L. Caron, V. H. Wiley, J. H. Johnson, F. A. MacKeller, and S. A. Mizsak, *J. Am. Chem. Soc.*, **99,** 542 (1977).
700. B. K. Bhuyan and C. G. Smith, *Proc. Nat. Acad. Sci., US*, **54,** 566 (1965).
701. R. T. Neogy, K. Chowdhury, and G. G. Thakurta, *Biochim. Biophys. Acta*, **299,** 241 (1973).
702. E. Kersten, H. Kersten, and W. Szybalski, *Biochemistry*, **5,** 236 (1966).
703. G. C. Das, S. Dasgupta, and N. N. Das Gupta, *Biochim. Biophys. Acta*, **353,** 274 (1974).
704. D. Strauss and W. Fleck, *Z. Allg. Mikrobiol.*, **15,** 615 (1975).
705. M. E. Bergy and F. Reusser, *Experientia*, **23,** 254 (1967).
706. T. F. Brodasky and F. Reusser, *J. Antibiot.* (Tokyo), **27,** 809 (1974).
707. R. C. Kelly, I. Schletter, J. M. Koert, F. A. Mackellar, and P. F. Wiley, *J. Org. Chem.*, **42,** 3591 (1977).
708. F. Reusser, *Biochim. Biophys. Acta*, **383,** 266 (1975).
709. G. R. Pettit, J. J. Einck, C. L. Herald, R. H. Ode, R. B. Von Drelle, P. Brown, M. G. Brazhnikova, and G. F. Gause, *J. Am. Chem. Soc.*, **97,** 7387 (1975).
710. H. Hilleman, *Ber.*, **71B,** 46 (1938).
711. G. Farber, *Sh. Cescoslov. Akad. Zemed.*, **23,** 355 (1951); *Chem. Abstr.* **45,** 9605 (1951).
712. W. S. Moos and J. W. Rowen, *Arch. Biochem. Biophys.*, **43,** 88 (1953).
713. M. V. Burton, J. J. R. Campbell, and B. A. Eagles, *Can. J. Res.*, **26C,** 15 (1948).
714. A. C. Blackwood and A. C. Neish, *Can. J. Microbiol.*, **3,** 165 (1957).
715. N. Grossowicz, P. Hayat, and Y. S. Halpern, *J. Gen. Microbiol.*, **16,** 576 (1957).
716. L. H. Frank and R. D. DeMoss, *J. Bacteriol.*, **77,** 776 (1959).
717. G. M. Badger, R. S. Pearce, and R. Pettit, *J. Chem. Soc.*, **3204** (1951).
718. N. N. Gerber, *J. Org. Chem.* **32,** 4055 (1967).
719. G. R. Clemo and A. F. Daglisch, *J. Chem. Soc.*, 1481 (1950).
720. T. Irie, E. Kurosawa, and I. Nagaoka, *Bull. Chem. Soc. Japan*, **33,** 1057 (1960).
721. N. N. Gerber, *Biochemistry*, **5,** 3824 (1966).
722. F. Kogl and J. J. Postowski, *Ann.*, **480,** 280 (1930).
723. K. Isono, K. Anzai, and S. Suzuki, *J. Antibiot.* (Tokyo), *Ser. A*, **11,** 264 (1959).
724. A. J. Kluyver, *J. Bacteriol.*, **72,** 406 (1956).
725. W. C. Haynes, *J. Bacteriol.*, **72,** 412 (1956).
726. G. Holliman, *Chem. Ind.* (London), 1668 (1957).
727. R. B. Herbert and F. G. Holliman, *Tetrahedron*, **21,** 663 (1965).
728. R. B. Herbert and F. G. Holliman, *Proc. Chem. Soc.*, **19,** (1964).
729. S. Nakamura, K. Maeda, T. Osato, and H. Umezawa, *J. Antibiot.* (Tokyo), *Ser. A*, **10,** 265 (1957).
730. H. Umezawa, *J. Antibiot.* (Tokyo), **4,** 34 (1951).
731. T. Osato, K. Maeda, and H. Umezawa, *J. Antibiot.* (Tokyo), *Ser. A*, **7,** 15 (1954).
732. S. Nakamura, *Chem. Pharm. Bull.* (Japan), **6,** 539, 543, 547 (1958).
733. K. Yakishita, *J. Antibiot.* (Tokyo), *Ser. A*, **13,** 83 (1960).
734. H. Akabori and M. Nakamura, *J. Antibiot.* (Tokyo), *Ser. A*, **12,** 17 (1959).
735. C. Dufraisse, A. Etienne, and E. Toromanoff, *Compt. Rend.*, **235,** 920 (1952).
736. M. E. Levitch and P. Reitz, *Biochemistry*, **5,** 689 (1966).
737. M. Weigele and W. Leimgruber, *Tetrahedron*, 715 (1967).
738. H. P. Sigg and A. Roth, *Helv. Chim. Acta*, **50,** 716 (1967).
739. E. S. Olson and J. H. Richards, *J. Org. Chem.*, **32,** 2887 (1967).
740. J. C. Hill and J. T. Johnson, *Mycologia*, **61,** 452 (1969).
741. N. N. Gerber, *J. Heterocycl. Chem.*, **6,** 297 (1969).

742. C. D. Tipton and K. L. Rinehart, Jr., *J. Am. Chem. Soc.*, **92,** 1425 (1970).

743. U. Hollstein and R. J. Van Gemert, *Biochemistry*, **10,** 497 (1971).

744. U. Hollstein and P. L. Butler, *Biochemistry*, **11,** 1345 (1972).

745. S. C. Kuo, F. R. Cano, and J. O. Lampen, *Antimicrob. Agents Chemother.*, **3,** 716 (1973).

746. F. R. Cano, S. C. Kuo, and J. O. Lampen, *Antimicrob. Agents Chemother.*, **3,** 723 (1973).

747. K. Katagiri, T. Yoshida, and K. Sato, in Ref. 3, p. 234.

748. A. Dell, D. H. Williams, H. R. Morris, G. A. Smith, J. Feeney, and G. C. K. Roberts, *J. Am. Chem. Soc.*, **97,** 2497 (1975).

749. M. J. Waring and L. P. G. Wakelin, *Nature*, 252, 653 (1974).

750. L. P. G. Wakelin and M. J. Waring, *Biochem. J.*, **157,** 721 (1976).

751. M. J. Waring, L. P. G. Wakelin, and J. S. Lee, *Biochim. Biophys. Acta*, **407,** 200 (1975).

751a. H. B. Jones, F. S. Allen, and U. Hollstein, unpublished results.

751b. J. S. Lee and M. J. Waring, *Biochem. J.*, **173,** 115 (1978).

751c. *Ibid.*, 129 (1978).

751d. J. W. Westley, R. H. Evans, Jr., C.-M. Liu, T. Hermann, and J. F. Blount, *J. Am. Chem. Soc.*, **100,** 6784 (1978) and references therein.

752. T. Kubota, S. Matsutani, M. Shiro, and H. Koyama, *Chem. Commun.*, 1541 (1968).

753. P. D. Shaw, in Ref. 1, p. 613.

754. L. K. Steinrauf, M. Pinkerton, and J. W. Chamberlin, *Biochem. Biophys. Research Commun.*, **33,** 29 (1968); T. Kubota and S. Matsutani, *J. Chem. Soc. C*, 695 (1970).

755. A. Agtarap, J. W. Chamberlin, M. Pinkerton, and L. Steinrauf, *J. Am. Chem. Soc.*, **89,** 5737 (1968).

756. E. F. Gale, E. Cundliffe, P. E. Reynolds, M. H. Richmond, and M. J. Waring, *The Molecular Basis of Antibiotic Action*, Wiley, New York, 1972, p. 151.

757. J. W. Westley, R. H. Evans, T. Williams, and A. Stempel, *Chem. Commun.*, 71 (1970); C. A. Maier and I. C. Paul, *ibid.*, 181 (1971); E. C. Bissel and I. C. Paul, *ibid.*, 967 (1972).

758. P. G. Caltrider, in Ref. 1, p. 681.

759. W. D. Celmer and I. A. Solomons, *J. Am. Chem. Soc.*, **74,** 2946 (1952); **75,** 105 (1953).

760. P. G. Caltrider, in Ref. 1, p. 666.

761. S. Pestka, in Ref. 3, p. 323.

762. W. Leimgruber, A. D. Batcho, and F. Schenker, *J. Am. Chem. Soc.*, **87,** 5793 (1965).

763. W. Leimgruber, A. D. Batcho, and R. C. Czajkowski, *J. Am. Chem. Soc.*, **90,** 5641 (1968).

764. K. W. Kohn, in Ref. 3, p. 3.

765. J. A. Moore, J. R. Dioe, E. D. Nicolaides, R. D. Westland, and E. L. Wittle, *J. Am. Chem. Soc.*, **76,** 2884, 2887 (1954).

766. H. A. Dewald and A. M. Moore, *J. Am. Chem. Soc.*, **80,** 3941 (1958).

767. S. E. de Voe and N. Bohonos, *Antibiotics Ann.*, 730 (1956–1957).

768. R. F. Pittillo and D. E. Hunt, in Ref. 1, p. 481.

769. J. M. Buchanan, in *The Chemistry and Biology of Purines*, G. E. W. Wolstenholme and C. M. O'Connor, Eds., Churchill, London, 1957, p. 233.

770. T. C. French, E. G. David, and J. M. Buchanan, *J. Biol. Chem.*, **238,** 2171, 2178, 2186 (1963).

771. S. C. Hartman, B. Levenberg, and J. M. Buchanan, *J. Am. Chem. Soc.*, **77,** 501 (1955).

772. S. C. Hartman, B. Levenberg, and J. M. Buchanan, *J. Biol. Chem.*, **221,** 1057 (1956).

773. K. P. Chakraborty and R. B. Hurlbert, *Biochim. Biophys. Acta*, **47,** 607 (1961).

774. S. C. Hartman, *J. Biol. Chem.*, **238,** 3036 (1963).

775. S. Harbon, G. Herman, and H. Clauser, *Biochemistry*, **5,** 3309 (1966).

776. R. K. Barclay, E. Garfinkel, and M. A. Phillips, *Cancer Res.*, **22,** 809 (1962).

777. A. Weissbach and A. Lisio, *Biochemistry*, **4,** 196 (1965).

778. M. N. Lipsett and A. Weissbach, *Biochemistry*, **4,** 206 (1965).

779. H. Umezawa, Y. Suhara, T. Takita, and K. Maeda, *J. Antibiot.* (Tokyo), *Ser. A*, **17,** 194 (1964).

780. G. Koyama, H. Nakamura, Y. Muraoka, T. Takita, K. Maeda, and H. Umezawa, *Tetrahedron Lett.*, 4635 (1968).

780a. T. Takita, Y. Muraoka, T. Nakatani, A. Fujii, Y. Umezawa, H. Naganawa, and H. Umezawa, *J. Antibiotics* (Japan), **31,** 801 (1978).

780b. N. J. Oppenheimer in *Bleomycin: Chemical Biochemical and Biological Aspects,* S. M. Hecht, Ed., Springer Verlag, New York, N.Y. (in press) 1979.

781. H. Umezawa, *Biomedicine*, **18,** 459 (1973).

782. H. Umezawa, "Principles of Antitumor Antibiotic Therapy", in *Cancer Medicine*, J. F. Holland and E. Frei III, Eds., Lea & Febiger, Philadelphia, 1973, p. 817.

783. H. Umezawa, in Ref. 3, p. 21.

784. B. A. Chabner, C. E. Myers, C. N. Coleman, and

D. G. Johns, *New Engl. J. Med.*, **292,** 1107, 1159 (1975).

785. K. Otsuka, S. I. Murota, and Y. Mori, *Biochim. Biophys. Acta*, **444,** 359 (1976).

786. W. C. Krueger, L. M. Pschigoda, and F. Reusser, *J. Antibiot.* (Tokyo), **26,** 424 (1973).

786a. E. A. Sausville, J. Peisach, and S. B. Horwitz, *Biochemistry*, **17,** 2740 (1978).

786b. E. A. Sausville, R. W. Stein, J. Peisach, and S. B. Horwitz, *Biochemistry*, **17,** 2746 (1978).

786c. H. Imanishi, M. Ohbayashi, Y. Nishiama, and H. Kawaguchi, *J. Antibiotics*, **31,** 667 (1978).

787. J. D. Dunitz, D. M. Hawley, D. Mikloš, D. N. J. White, Y. Berlin, R. Marušić, and V. Prelog, *Helv. Chim. Acta*, **54,** 1709 (1971).

788. W. Pache, in Ref. 3, p. 585.

789. G. F. Gause, *Chem. Ind.* (London), 1506 (1966).

790. T. Hata, J. Koga, Y. Sano, K. Kanamori, A. Matsumae, R. Sugawara, T. Hoshi, and T. Shima, *J. Antibiot.* (Tokyo), *Ser. A.*, **7,** 107 (1954).

791. N. Shimada, M. Uekusa, T. Denda, Y. Ishii, T. Lizuka, Y. Sato, T. Hatori, M. Fukui, and M. Sudo, *J. Antibiot.* (Tokyo), *Ser. A*, **8,** 67 (1955).

792. S. Suzuki, G. Nakamura, K. Okuma, and Y. Tomiyama, *J. Antibiot.* (Tokyo), *Ser. A*, **11,** 81 (1958).

793. S. Suzuki and K. Okuma, *J. Antibiot.* (Tokyo), *Ser. A*, **11,** 84 (1958).

794. W. V. Shaw, *Ann. N.Y. Acad. Sci.*, **182,** 234 (1971).

795. W. V. Shaw and R. F. Brodsky, *J. Bacteriol.*, **95**; 28 (1968).

796. S. Pestka, in Ref. 3, p. 370.

797. A. S. Weisberger, *Ann. Rev. Med.*, **18,** 483 (1967).

798. B. Weisblum and J. Davies, *Bacteriol. Rev.*, **32,** 493 (1968).

799. C. Gurgo, D. Aprion, and D. Schlessinger, *J. Mol. Biol.*, **45,** 205 (1969).

800. S. Pestka, *Ann. Rev. Microbiol.*, **25,** 487 (1971).

801. W. Godchaux III and E. Herbert, *J. Mol. Biol.*, **21,** 537 (1966).

802. L. W. Wheeldon and A. L. Lehninger, *Biochemistry*, **5,** 3533 (1966).

803. T. J. Foster and W. V. Shaw, *Antimicrob. Agents Chemother.*, **3,** 99 (1973).

804. L. S. Sands and W. V. Shaw, *Antimicrob. Agents Chemother.*, **3,** 299 (1973).

805. A. N. Baccus and G. T. Javor, *Antimicrob. Agents Chemother.*, **8,** 387 (1975). (a) G. Carrara and G. Weitnauer, *Gazz. Chim. Ital.*, **81,** 142 (1951). (b) I. Hagedorn and H. Tönjes, *Pharmazie*, **11,** 409 (1956). (c) K. Hayes and G. Gever, *J. Org. Chem.*, **16,** 269 (1951). (d) M. C. Rebstock, H. M. Crooks, Jr., J. Controulis, and Q. R. Bartz, *J. Am. Chem. Soc.*, **71,** 2458 (1949). (e) S. Van der Meer, H. Kofman, and H. Veldstra, *Rec. Trav. Chim. Pays-Bas*, **72,** 236 (1953). (f) M. C. Rebstock, *J. Am. Chem. Soc.*, **73,** 3671 (1951). (g) M. C. Rebstock, G. W. Moersch, A. C. Moore, and J. M. Vandenbelt, *J. Am. Chem. Soc.*, **73,** 3666 (1951). (h) M. C. Rebstock and A. C. Moore, *J. Am. Chem. Soc.*, **75,** 1685 (1953). (i) M. C. Rebstock, *J. Am. Chem. Soc.*, **72,** 4800 (1950).

806. P. D. Hoeprich, *J. Biol. Chem.*, **240,** 1654 (1965).

807. P. H. Hidy, E. B. Hodge, V. V. Young, R. L. Harned, G. A. Brewer, W. F. Philipps, W. F. Runge, H. E. Stavely, A. Pohland, H. Boaz, and H. R. Sullivan, *J. Am. Chem. Soc.*, **77,** 2345 (1955).

808. H. Hoeksema, *J. Am. Chem. Soc.*, **90,** 755 (1968).

809. C. H. Stammer, A. N. Wilson, F. W. Holly, and K. Folkers, *J. Am. Chem. Soc.*, **77,** 2346 (1955).

810. F. C. Neuhaus, in Ref. 1, p. 40.

811. J. L. Strominger, R. H. Threnn, and S. S. Scott, *J. Am. Chem. Soc.*, **81,** 3803 (1959).

812. J. L. Strominger, E. Ito, and R. H. Threnn, *J. Am. Chem. Soc.*, **82,** 998 (1960).

813. J. L. Strominger, K. Izaki, M. Matsuhashi, and D. J. Tipper, *Fed. Proc.*, **26,** 9 (1967).

814. W. A. Wood and I. C. Gunsalus, *J. Biol. Chem.*, **190,** 403 (1951).

815. M. P. Lambert and F. C. Neuhaus, *J. Bacteriol.*, **110,** 978 (1972).

816. M. M. Johnston and W. F. Diven, *J. Biol. Chem.*, **244,** 5414 (1969).

817. F. C. Neuhaus and J. L. Lynch, *Biochem. Biophys. Res. Commun.*, **8,** 377 (1962).

818. E. Ito, T. Aoki, M. Yamamoto, M. Yuasa, H. Mizobata, and K. Tone, *Med. J. Osaka Univ.*, **9,** 23 (1958).

819. U. Roze and J. L. Strominger, *Fed. Proc. Abstr.*, **22,** 423 (1963).

820. F. C. Neuhaus and J. L. Lynch, *Biochemistry*, **3,** 471 (1964).

821. C. I. Chacko and D. Gottlieb, *Phytopathology*, **55,** 587 (1965).

822. D. Gottlieb, in Ref. 1, p. 617.

823. D. S. Tarbell, R. M. Carman, D. D. Chapman, K. R. Huffman, and N. J. McCorkindale, *J. Am.*

Chem. Soc., **82,** 1005 (1960); N. J. McCorkindale and J. G. Sime, *Proc. Chem. Soc.*, 331 (1961).

824. J. C. Gentles, *Nature* (London), **182,** 476 (1958).
825. M. A. El-Nakeeb and J. O. Lampen, *J. Bacteriol.*, **89,** 564 (1965).
826. F. M. Huber and D. Gottlieb, *Can. J. Microbiol.*, **14,** 111 (1968).
827. F. M. Huber, in Ref. 3, p. 606.
828. H. T. Shigeura and C. N. Gordon, *J. Biol. Chem.* **237,** 1932, 1937 (1962).
829. H. T. Shigeura, in Ref. 1, p. 451.
830. W. C. Liu, W. P. Cullen, and K. V. Rao, *Antimicrob. Agents Chemother.*, 767 (1962).
831. J. R. Bateman, A. A. Marsh, and J. L. Steinfeld, *Cancer Chemother. Rep.* No. 44, 25 (1965).
832. I. H. Goldberg, in Ref. 3, p. 166.
833. V. L. Sutter, Y. Y. Kwok, and S. M. Finegold, *Antimicrob. Agents Chemother.*, **3,** 188 (1973).
834. B. R. Meyers, K. Kaplan, and L. Weinstein, *Appl. Microbiol.*, **17,** 653 (1969).
835. J. M. S. Dixon and A. E. Lipinski, *Antimicrob. Agents Chemother.*, **1,** 333 (1972).
836. F. N. Chang and B. Weisblum, in Ref. 1, p. 440.
837. R. Fernandez-Nuñoz, R. E. Munro, R. Torres-Pinedo, and D. Vasquez, *Eur. J. Biochem.*, **23,** 185 (1971).
838. W. T. Sokilski, *Infection and Antimicrobial Agents*, Vol. 3, Proceedings of the First Intersectional Congress of IAMS, 1975, pp. 547–556.
839. F. Reusser, *Antimicrob. Agents Chemother.*, **7,** 32 (1975).
840. C. Lewis, *Fed. Proc.*, **33,** 2303 (1974).
841. A. A. Sinkula and C. Lewis, *J. Pharm. Sci.*, **62,** 1757 (1973).
842. B. Bannister, *J. Chem. Soc. Perkin Trans. I*, 360 (1974).
843. B. Bannister, *J. Chem. Soc. Perkin Trans. I*, 1676 (1973).
844. A. D. Argoudelis, L. E. Johnson, and T. R. Pyke, *J. Antibiot.* (Tokyo), **26,** 429 (1973).
845. S. Pestka, in Ref. 3, p. 480.
846. T. Hata, Y. Sano, R. Sugawara, A. Matsumae, K. Kamamori, T. Shima, and T. Hoshi, *J. Antibiot.* (Tokyo), *Ser. A*, **9,** 141 (1956).
847. A. Tulinksy and J. H. van den Hende, *J. Am. Chem. Soc.*, **89,** 2905 (1967).
848. J. B. Patrick, R. P. Williams, W. E. Meyer, W. Fulmor, D. B. Cosulich, R. W. Broschard, and J. S. Webb, *J. Am. Chem. Soc.*, **86,** 1889 (1964).
849. W. Szybalski and V. N. Iyer, in Ref. 1, p. 211; M. J. Waring, "Cross-Linking and Intercalation in Nucleic Acids", *16th Symposium of the Society for General Microbiology*, 1966, p. 235.
850. V. N. Iyer and W. Szybalski, *Proc. Nat. Acad. Sci., US*, **50,** 355 (1963).
851. V. N. Iyer and W. Szybalski, *Science*, **145,** 55 (1964).
852. M. N. Lipsett and A. Weissback, *Biochemistry*, **4,** 206 (1965).
853. W. Szybalski and V. N. Iyer, *Fed. Proc.*, **23,** 946 (1964).
854. V. N. Iyer and W. Szybalski, *Microbiol. Genet. Bull.*, No. 21, 16 (1964).
855. M. Tomaz, *Biochim. Biophys. Acta*, **213,** 288 (1970).
856. H. Kersten, W. Kersten, G. Leopold, and B. Schniders, *Biochim. Biophys. Acta*, **80,** 521 (1964).
857. J. Smith-Kieland, *Biochim. Biophys. Acta*, **119,** 486 (1966).
858. H. Kersten and W. Kersten, *Inhibitors: Tools in Cell Research*, Th. Bucher and H. Sies, Eds., Springer-Verlag, Berlin, 1969, p. 16.
859. H. Suzuki and W. W. Kilgoore, *Science*, **146,** 1585 (1964).
860. J. W. Lown, A. Begleiter, D. Johnson, and A. R. Morgan, *Can. J. Biochem.*, **54,** 110 (1976).
861. U. Hornemann, Y. K. Ho, J. K. Mackey, Jr., and S. C. Srivastava, *J. Am. Chem. Soc.*, **98,** 7069 (1976).
862. W. A. Goss and T. M. Cook, in Ref. 3, p. 174.
863. C. A. Michels, J. Balmire, B. Goldfinger, and J. Marmur, *Antimicrob. Agents Chemother.*, **3,** 562 (1973).
864. G. J. Bourguignon, M. Levitt, and R. Sternglanz, *Antimicrob. Agents Chemother.*, **4,** 479 (1973).
865. J. F. de Castro, J. F. O. Carvalho, N. Moussatche, and F. T. de Castro, *Antimicrob. Agents Chemother.*, **7,** 487, (1975).
866. J. Michel, R. Luboshitzky, and T. Sacks, *Antimicrob. Agents Chemother.*, **4,** 201 (1973).
867. B. P. Vaterlaus, K. Doebel, J. Kiss, A. I. Rachlin, and H. Spiegelberg, *Experientia*, **19,** 383 (1963).
868. T. D. Brock, in Ref. 1, pp. 651, 760.
869. E. A. Garrett and C. M. Loon, *Antimicrob. Agents Chemother.*, **4,** 626 (1973).
870. M. G. Gabridge, *Antimicrob. Agents Chemother.*, **5,** 453 (1974).
871. P. F. Wiley, H. K. Jahnke, F. MacKellar, R. B. Kelly, and A. D. Argoudelis, *J. Org. Chem.*, **35,** 1420 (1970).
872. I. H. Goldberg, in Ref. 3, p. 498.
873. R. B. Woodward and G. Singh, *J. Am. Chem. Soc.*, **72,** 1428 (1950).

874. J. Singh, in Ref. 1, p. 621.
875. N. Tanaka, in Ref. 1, p. 166.
876. P. G. Caltrider, in Ref. 1, p. 671.
877. K. Arima, H. Imanaka, M. Kousaka, A. Fukuta, and G. Tamura, *Tetrahedron Lett.*, 737 (1966).
878. O. Yonemitsu, Y. Sato, S. Nishioka, and Y. Ban, *Chem. Ind.* (London), 490 (1963).
879. A. Caputo, B. Giovanella, and R. Giuliani, *Nature* (London), **190,** 819 (1961).
880. W. B. Wheatley, C. T. Holdredge, and L. Walsh, *J. Org. Chem.*, **21,** 485 (1956).
881. R. K. Hill, P. J. Foley, and L. A. Gardella, *J. Org. Chem.*, **32,** 2330 (1967).
882. S. C. Sung, in Ref. 1, pp. 5, 751.
883. S. C. Sung and J. H. Quastel, *Cancer Res.*, **23,** 1549 (1963).
884. H. H. Keir and J. B. Shepherd, *Biochem. J.*, **95,** 483 (1965).
885. M. G. Brazhnikova, I. N. Kovsharova, N. V. Konstantinova, A. S. Mesentsev, V. V. Proshlyakova, and I. V. Tolstykh, *Antibiotiki*, **15,** 297 (1970).
886. A. S. Mesentsev, V. V. Kulyaeva, L. M. Rubasheva, M. G. Brazhnikova, O. S. Anisinova, T. V. Veasova, and Y. N. Sheinker, *Khim. Prir. Soedin.*, **5,** 650 (1971).
887. A. S. Mesentsev, L. M. Rubasheva, V. V. Kulyaeva, M. G. Brazhnikova, O. S. Anisimova, T. V. Vlasova, and Y. N. Sheinker, *Khim. Prir. Soedin.*, **7,** 234 (1973).
888. G. F. Gause, in Ref. 3, p. 269.
889. F. A. Kuehl, M. N. Bishop, L. Chaiet, and K. Folkers, *J. Am. Chem. Soc.*, **73,** 1770 (1951).
890. H. Bickel, E. Gaumann, W. Keller-Schierlein, V. Prelog, E. Vischer, A. Wettstein, and H. Zahner, *Experientia*, **16,** 129 (1960).
891. W. Keller-Schierlein, V. Prelog, and H. Zahner, *Fortschr. Chem. Org. Naturst.*, **22,** 279 (1964).
892. H. Bickel, P. Mertens, V. Prelog, J. Seibl, and A. Walser, *Tetrahedron*, Suppl. 8, Part I, 171 (1966).
893. F. Knusel and W. Zimmermann, in Ref. 3, p. 653.
894. C. E. Stickings, *Biochem. J.*, **72,** 332 (1959).
895. S. A. Harris, L. V. Fischer, and K. Folkers, *J. Med. Chem.*, **8,** 478 (1965).
896. H. T. Shigeura, in Ref. 1, p. 360.
897. S. Gatenbeck and J. Sierankiewicz, *Antimicrob. Agents Chemother.*, **3,** 308, (1973).
898. J. Gutzwiller, R. Mauli, H. P. Sigg, and C. Tam, *Helv. Chim. Acta*, **47,** 2234 (1964).
899. P. G. Caltrider, in Ref. 1, p. 674.
900. P. D. Shaw, in Ref. 1, p. 611.
901. N. N. Lomakina, R. Bognar, M. G. Brazhnikova, F. Sztaricskai, and L. I. Muravyeva, *Abstracts, 7th International Symposium on the Chemistry of Natural Products*, Riga, 1970, p. 625.
902. N. N. Lomakina, I. Muravieva, and M. S. Yurina, *Antibiotiki*, **15,** 21 (1970).
903. C. Watanakunakorn and C. Bakie, *Antimicrob. Agents Chemother.*, **4,** 120 (1973).
904. G. O. Westenfelder, R. Y. Paterson, B. E. Reisberg, and G. M. Carlson, *J. Am. Med. Assoc.*, **223,** 37 (1973).
905. D. C. Jordan and P. E. Reynolds, in Ref. 3, p. 704.
906. M. D. Yudkin, *Biochem. J.*, **89,** 290 (1963).
907. D. C. Jordan and H. D. C. Mallory, *Antimicrob. Agents Chemother.*, **1961,** 218 (1962).
908. P. E. Reynolds, *Biochim. Biophys. Acta*, **237,** 239, 255 (1971).
909. H. R. Perkins, *Biochem. J.*, **111,** 195 (1969).
910. J. L. Strominger, K. Izaki, M. Matsuhashi, and D. J. Tipper, *Fed. Proc.*, **26,** 9 (1967).
911. K. Izaki, M. Matsuhashi, and J. L. Strominger, *Proc. Nat. Acad. Sci. US*, **55,** 656 (1966).
912. G. K. Best, M. K. Grastie, and R. D. McConnel, *J. Bacteriol.*, **102,** 476 (1970).
913. G. Wickus, and J. S. Strominger, *Fed. Proc.*, **30,** abstr. 1174 (1971).
914. B. Oppenheim, Y. Burstein, and A. Patchornik, *Israel J. Biochem.*, **10,** 43 (1972).
915. H. J. Rogers, *Bacteriol. Rev.*, **74,** 194 (1970).
916. H. Sandermann, *FEBS Lett.*, **21,** 254 (1972).
917. V. Braun and H. Wolff, *Eur. J. Biochem.*, **14,** 387 (1970).
918. R. G. Anderson, H. Hussey, and J. Baddiley, *Biochem. J.*, **127,** 11 (1972).
919. M. Nieto and H. R. Perkins, *Biochem. J.*, **124,** 845 (1971).
920. W. P. Hammes and F. C. Neuhaus, *Antimicrob. Agents Chemother.*, **6,** 722 (1974).
921. C. Watanakunakorn and C. Bakie, *Antimicrob. Agents Chemother.*, **4,** 120 (1973).
922. H. Yonehara, S. Takeuchi, H. Umezawa, and Y. Sumiki, *J. Antibiot.* (Tokyo), *Ser. A*, **12,** 109 (1959).
923. S. Takeuchi and H. Yonehara, *J. Antibiot.* (Tokyo), *Ser. A*, **14,** 44 (1961).

CHAPTER SEVENTEEN

Antimycobacterial Agents

PIERO SENSI

Research Laboratories,
Gruppo Lepetit S.p.A.
Milan, Italy

and

GIULIANA GIALDRONI–GRASSI

Department of Chemotherapy,
University of Pavia,
Pavia, Italy

CONTENTS

1 INTRODUCTION

Some species of mycobacteria are pathogenic for several animal species and are responsible for two important human chronic diseases, tuberculosis and leprosy, as well as for other less widespread but severe infections generally called mycobacterioses. *Mycobacterium leprae*, identified by Hansen in 1871, and *M. tuberculosis* (Koch, 1882) were among the first bacteria recognized as causative agents of human diseases. Yet despite the early discovery of the etiological agents of the infections, only in the past three decades have drugs highly effective in the treatment of mycobacterial diseases been discovered.

The introduction of chemotherapy for mycobacterial infections brought about a dramatic decrease in the mortality and morbidity of the illnesses. These successes notwithstanding, mycobacterial infections still require particular attention as a worldwide, challenging health problem. One important area of research in fighting these diseases is to determine the best way to utilize the available drugs. Clinical evaluation of the various chemotherapeutic regimens is a complex problem.

Although some general guidelines for the therapy are accepted everywhere, great effort must be made to adapt these guidelines to the socioeconomical situations and to pathological variants existing in the various countries. It is still necessary to search for new antimycobacterial agents for many reasons, e.g., the acquisition by the infecting organisms of resistance to the present drugs, drug side effects, and the unsatisfactory status of present treatments of leprosy and atypical mycobacterioses.

Research programs involving blind screening for new antimycobacterial drugs and for improving the evaluation criteria are under way in many laboratories. In addition, knowledge of specific constituents of the mycobacterial cell and of their biochemical roles has advanced considerably in the recent years and may permit a more rational approach to the design of new drugs acting on specific targets. Also, knowledge of the mechanism of action of the available drugs and of the biochemical mechanisms of resistance to them may be used as a basis for designing new and better weapons to fight the mycobacterial diseases.

2 THE MYCOBACTERIA

Mycobacteria are transition forms between bacteria and fungi. The genus *Mycobacterium* belongs to the order Actinomycetales, family Mycobacteriaceae, characterized by nonmotile, nonsporulating rods that resist decolorization with acidified organic solvents (1). For this reason they are also called "acid fast" bacteria. Some mycobacterial species are pathogenic for man. Among these *M. tuberculosis hominis*, *M. t. bovis*, and *M. leprae* are the most important. A recently identified variety, *M. africanum*, endowed with characteristics intermediate between those of *M. tuberculosis hominis* and *M. bovis*, is also pathogenic for man (2).

Other so-called atypical mycobacterial species have been classified by Runyon into four groups, according to their growth rates and pigment production (3). The characteristics of the groups and the species that can be pathogenic for man (given in parentheses) are the following. Group 1 includes the so-called photochromogenic mycobacteria that show a yellow pigmentation after exposure to light (*M. kansasii*, *M. marinum*, *M. ulcerans*). Group 2 includes the so-called scotochromogenic mycobacteria that show a yellow pigmentation even when kept in darkness (*M. scrofulaceum*, *M. aquae*). Group 3 includes nonchromogenic mycobacteria (*M. intracellulare*, *M. avium*, *M. xenopi*). Group 4 includes fast-growing mycobacteria (*M. fortuitum*, *M. abscessus*).

M. tuberculosis hominis is a nonmotile bacillus 1–2 μ long and 0.3–0.6 μ wide. It can be demonstrated in pathologic specimens by means of specific staining procedures, the most widely used being the Ziehl–Neelsen method. It is acid-fast and acid-alcohol-fast. *In vitro* culture of tubercle bacilli is slow and sometimes difficult. The nutritional requirements are not particularly complex, but the content of the medium greatly influences the composition of the mycobacterial cell. The most common media used for the isolation of *M. tuberculosis* from pathological specimens and for its maintenance are solid media, with egg yolk as a base (Petragnani, Lowenstein–Jensen, IUTM media). In these media the culture begins to appear 12–15 days after inoculation, but full growth is obtained after 30–40 days. When inoculation is made with pathological material from patients, observation must be prolonged. The most widely used maintenance liquid media are synthetic media containing albumin (Dubos, Youmans, 7 HT media). They usually allow rapid growth (8–10 days), and addition of Tween 80 makes it is possible to obtain uniformly dispersed growth (4, 5).

In vivo pathogenic activity of tubercle bacilli is demonstrated in guinea pigs. Infection in the rabbit, which is susceptible to *M. bovis* infection but scarcely or not at all to *M. hominis*, is employed to differentiate the two infections.

M. leprae, or the Hansen bacillus, is resistant to acid and to alcohol and requires the Ziehl–Neelsen method of staining to be recognized. It is found in lepromatous lesions, where it is arranged mostly in clumps. It is 1–8 μ long, nonmotile, and nonsporeforming. The most important drawback for the accumulation of knowledge about the biology, the susceptibility to antibiotics, and the epidemiology of the disease is the impossibility of cultivating this mycobacterium *in vitro*. Tests in animals have been improved in the recent years, but they are complex and can be performed only in the specialized laboratories.

The biochemical constitution of mycobacteria is very complex, and an enormous amount of work has been done in this field. Novel chemical structures have been discovered, but the relationships between these and the pathogenic and biological activities of mycobacteria have not yet been satisfactorily elucidated (6–12). Information about metabolism of mycobacteria is extremely voluminous, but the overall picture of the mycobacterial metabolism is far from complete (10, 12).

Metabolism of carbohydrates and lipids, electron transport, and oxidative phosphorylation have been extensively studied; research into nucleic acids and protein synthesis is at a less advanced stage. To go deeply into these subjects is beyond the scope of this book. However it is appropriate to indicate here some metabolic aspects and functional structures specific to mycobacteria that might be potential targets for antimycobacterial drugs.

Some interesting differences exist in the metabolic properties of tubercle bacilli grown *in vivo* and *in vitro*, which must be considered when the practical value of antimycobacterial agents designed and tested in laboratory must be assessed in practice. Populations of *M. tuberculosis* H37 Rv grown in the lungs of mice and populations grown *in vitro* show two different phenotypes, Phe I and Phe II, with marked differences in the metabolism of certain energy sources, in the production of detectable sulfolipids, or in immunogenicity (Phe II is a better immunogen than Phe I) (13–15). Since the shift from Phe I to Phe II is readily reversible, it can be deduced that the genome of H37 Rv remains the same (16). Phe I is unable to bind neutral red (17, 18) and is resistant to 4% sodium hydroxide at 37° for 4 hr (19–21), suggesting that a modification in its surface has occurred, probably because of the presence of a coating layer, rendering the surface components of Phe II that react with neutral red unavailable (18, 22).

Further differences have been observed between virulent and avirulent strains of mycobacteria. The differences in oxidative metabolism are quantitative and cannot account for the capacity of virulent mycobacteria to grow in host tissue, where the oxygen tension is low. By contrast, there are

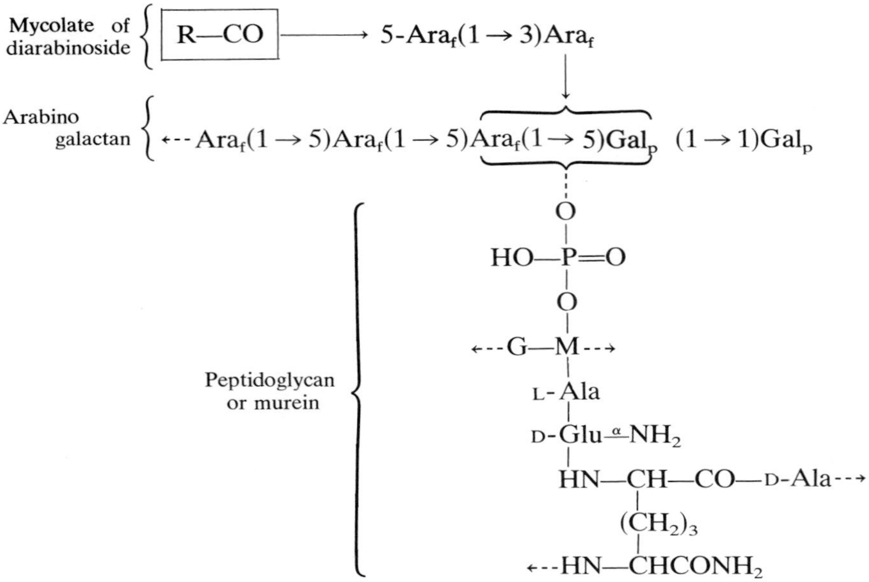

Mycolate of diarabinoside { R—CO ⟶ 5-$Ara_f(1 \rightarrow 3)Ara_f$

Arabino galactan { ←-- $Ara_f(1 \rightarrow 5)Ara_f(1 \rightarrow 5)Ara_f(1 \rightarrow 5)Gal_p$ $(1 \rightarrow 1)Gal_p$

Peptidoglycan or murein { O—HO—P=O—O—←--G—M--→ / L-Ala / D-Glu—α—NH_2 / HN—CH—CO—D-Ala--→ / $(CH_2)_3$ / ←--HN—$CHCONH_2$

17.**1**

some qualitative differences in amino acid metabolism. The virulent strains (H37 Rv) possess one type of asparaginase, and the avirulent one (H37 Ra) possesses two asparaginases. The avirulent strain has an aspartotransferase that transfers the aspartyl moiety of asparagine to hydroxylamine, whereas the avirulent strain does not (23–25).

A great deal of research effort has been focused on the constituents of the mycobacterial cell wall, since they are responsible for many of the pathogenic effects of tubercle bacilli. The two major components of the mycobacterial cell wall are a peptidoglycan (mucopeptide or murein) and a glycolipid in a tentative structure, outlined in 17.**1** (26–28). The murein consists of a repeating disaccharide unit, in which *N*-acetyl-D-glucosamine (G) is linked in a 1–4 linkage to *N*-acetyl-D-muramic acid (M) attached to L-alanine-D-glutamic acid-NH_2-*meso*-diaminopimelic acid-NH_2-D-alanine. This unit is linked to a glycolipid that contains mycolic acids esterified to an arabinogalactan. The nature of the linkage of the glycolipid to the peptidoglycan has not been clearly elucidated, although some data suggest that it might be a phosphodiester linkage (7).

Mycolic acids are α-branched, β-hydroxylated long-chain fatty acids (29), of which three principal groups are known: the corynomycolic acids, ranging from C_{28} to C_{36}, the nocardic acids, ranging from C_{40} to C_{60}, and the mycobacterial mycolic acids, ranging from C_{60} to C_{90} (29, 30).

Mycolic acids can also be detected in the skin lesions of patients suffering from lepromatous leprosy, indicating that the agent of leprosy is a mycobacterium containing it (31).

The chemical structures of methoxylated mycolic acid and β-mycolic acid extracted from *M. tuberculosis* var. *hominis* are shown in 17.**2** and 17.**3** (32).

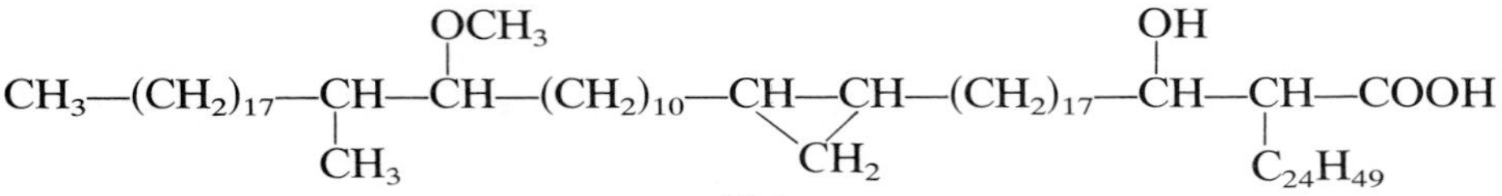

$$CH_3—(CH_2)_{17}—CH(CH_3)—CH(OCH_3)—(CH_2)_{10}—CH—CH(CH_2)—(CH_2)_{17}—CH(OH)—CH(C_{24}H_{49})—COOH$$

17.**2**

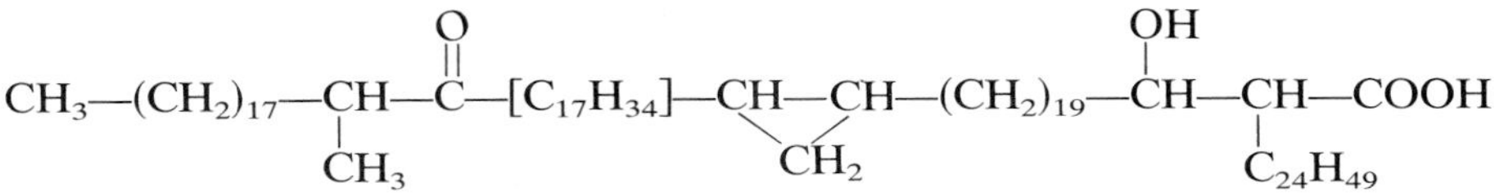

$$CH_3-(CH_2)_{17}-\underset{\underset{CH_3}{|}}{CH}-\overset{\overset{O}{\|}}{C}-[C_{17}H_{34}]-\underbrace{CH-CH}_{CH_2}-(CH_2)_{19}-\overset{\overset{OH}{|}}{CH}-\underset{\underset{C_{24}H_{49}}{|}}{CH}-COOH$$

17.3

The mycolic acids are linked through their carboxy groups to the end terminal 5-OH groups of the D-arabinofuranose (Ara_f) molecules, branches of the arabinogalactan of the cell wall (33–35). Mycolic acids are known to be acid fast, since they bind fuchsin and the binding is acid fast. Thus it seems that acid fastness of mycobacteria depends on two mechanisms: the capacity of the mycobacterial cell to take fuchsin into its interior, and the capacity of mycolic acids to form a complex with the dye (12, 36, 37).

In addition to the lipid murein part of the rigid structure, there is a series of soluble lipid compounds that seem to be located in or on the outer part of the cell wall: waxes D, cord factor, mycosides, sulfolipids, phospholopids (7–9).

The so-called waxes D are ether-soluble, acetone-insoluble, chloroform-extractable peptidoglycolipid components of the mycobacterial cell, probably an autolysis product of the cell wall (38). Since from a chemical point of view they are esters of mycolic acids with arabinogalactan linked to a mucopeptide containing *N*-acetylglucosamine, *N*-glycolylmuramic acid, L- and D-alanine, *meso*-diaminopimelic acid, and D-glutamic acid, it has been suggested that they are materials synthesized in excess of those needed for insertion into the cell wall (9, 12, 39). The constitution of wax D differs in the different varieties and strains of mycobacteria.

Cord factor is a toxic glycolipid (6,6′-dimycolate of trehalose, 17.**4**), to which has been attributed (40, 41) the responsibility for the phenomenon of cording—that is, the capacity of *M. tuberculosis* to grow in serpentine cords, a capacity that is correlated with its capacity to kill guinea pigs (42, 43). The detergent properties of cord factor and its location on the outer cell wall have led to the suggestion that it may play a role in facilitating the penetration of certain molecules necessary for growth of mycobacteria (12).

Mycosides are glycolipids and peptidoglycolipids type-specific of mycobacteria (44)

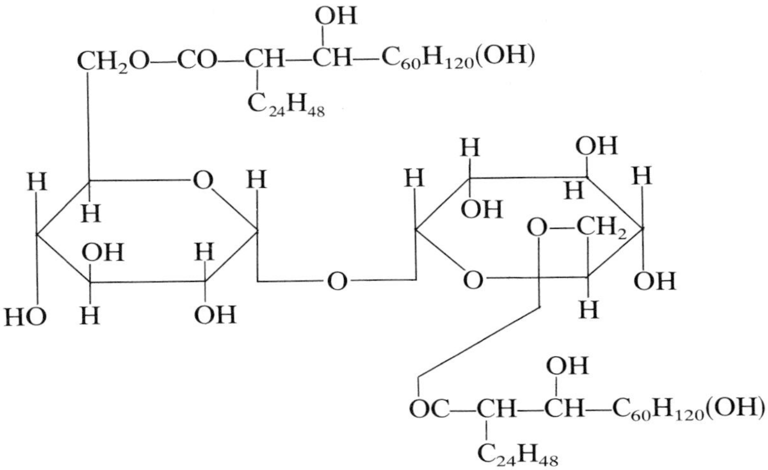

$CH_2O-CO-CH(C_{24}H_{48})-CH(OH)-C_{60}H_{120}(OH)$

H, O, H, H, OH, H, HO, H, OH — O — H, H, OH, H, OH, H, $O-CH_2$, H, O, OH, H

$OC-CH(C_{24}H_{48})-CH(OH)-C_{60}H_{120}(OH)$

17.4

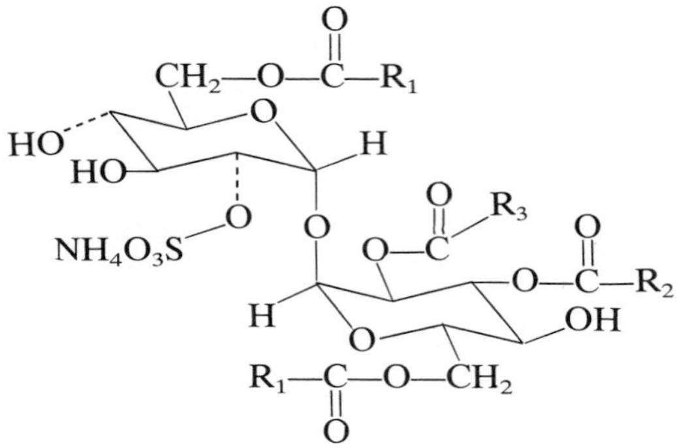

$$R_1 = C_{15}H_{31}\text{—}\underset{|}{\overset{OH}{CH}}\text{—}\left[\overset{CH_3}{\underset{}{CH}}\text{—}CH_2\right]_7\text{—}\overset{CH_3}{CH}\text{—}$$

$$R_2 = C_{15}H_{31}\text{—}CH_2\text{—}\left[\text{—}\overset{CH_3}{CH}\text{—}CH_2\right]_6\text{—}\overset{CH_3}{CH}\text{—}$$

$$R_3 = C_{15}H_{31}\text{—}$$

17.**5**

that often have in common terminal saccharide moieties containing rhamnoses *O*-methylated in various positions (45). They can be distinguished according to two main categories (30): those in category 1 are phenolic glycolipids with branched-chain fatty acids, those in category 2 are peptidoglycolipids consisting of a sugar moiety, a short peptide, and a fatty acid. The biological activity of mycosides is still obscure. They probably have a role in cellular permeability (46). Glycolipids or peptidoglycolipids are responsible for the ropelike appearance that is evident in one of the outer layers of mycobacteria when they are visualized by the technique of negative staining (12).

The sulfolipids (which are 2,3,6,6′-tetraesters of trehalose, 17.**5**), (9, 17), to which are attributed the cytochemical neutral- red fixing activity of viable, cord-forming tubercle bacilli, seem to play a role in conferring virulence to tubercle bacilli and influencing their pathogenicity (47), acting synergistically with the cord factor (48).

The phospholipids (cardiolipin, phosphatidylethanolamine-glycosyl diglyceride, and phosphatidylinositol -mono- and oligomannosides) were considered to be antigenic substances elaborated by *M. tuberculosis*, but the most purified preparations have been shown to behave only as haptens (9, 29, 49).

Even though from the enormous amount of work that has been summarized here, some suggestions have been made about the biological activities of the lipids of the tubercle bacillus, a clear structure-function relationship has not yet been delineated. Nor has it been determined which structural features can produce favorable or detrimental effects.

Other interesting substances isolated from mycobacteria are the mycobactins, which are a group of bacterial growth factors that occur only in the genus *Mycobacterium* (6). The isolation of the mycobactins was followed by the identification of growth factors in other microorganisms, the lsideramines, which differ from mycobactins but share with them some common properties, the most relevant being strong chelating capacity for ferric iron.

At least nine mycobactin groups have been isolated from different mycobacteria. They have the same basic constitution, with some variations in details of structure. Mycobactin P (17.**6**), isolated in 1946, was the first example of a natural product with an exceptional iron-chelating activity, and its structure was the first to be determined. Mycobactin S (17.**7**) is the most active of these factors, showing growth stimulation at concentrations as low as 0.3 ng/ml. Mycobactin M (17.**8**) is a representative of the structure of M-type factors.

The most biochemically unusual product in the structure of mycobactins is N^6-hydroxylysine, which is present in the

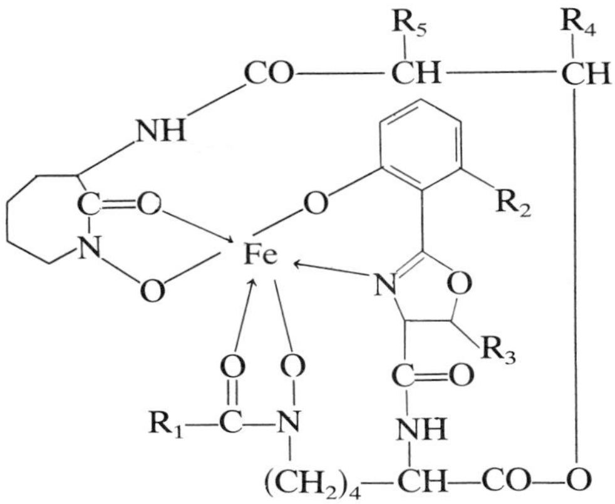

$R_1 = C_{17}H_{34}$, $R_2 = CH_3$, $R_3 = H$, $R_4 = C_2H_5$, $R_5 = CH_3$ **17.6**

$R_1 = C_{17}H_{34}$, $R_2 = H$, $R_3 = H$, $R_4 = CH_3$, $R_5 = H$ **17.7**

$R_1 = CH_3$, $R_2 = H$, $R_3 = CH_3$, $R_4 = C_{17}H_{34}$, $R_5 = CH_3$ **17.8**

molecule in both acyclic and cyclic forms. All the known mycobactins contain either a salicylic acid or a 6-methylsalicylic acid moiety. The oxazoline rings derive from 3-hydroxy amino acids, either serine or threonine. The biochemical function of mycobactins seems to be related to the metabolism of iron.

Mycobacteria responds to iron deficiency by producing salicylic or 6-methylsalicylic acid, together with mycobactins that have a very great affinity for ferric iron. It has been suggested that in the mycobacteria, salicylic or methylsalicylic acid mobilizes the iron in the environment and that mycobactins are concerned with the active transport of iron into the cell.

3 NATURE OF THE DISEASES AND EPIDEMIOLOGY

Tuberculosis is sometimes an acute but more frequently a chronic communicable disease that derives its character from several properties of the tubercle bacillus, which in contrast with many common bacterial pathogens, multiplies very slowly, does not produce exotoxins and does not stimulate an early reaction from the host. The tubercle bacillus is also an intracellular parasite, living and multiplying inside macrophages. The virulent bacilli in the small tubercles and in the macrophages represent a reservoir for invasion into other parts of the organ or in other organs, with damaging effects that may have fatal consequences.

The invasion of the body by the infective agent, generally through inhalation, does not produce any immediate short-term effect, and the tubercle bacillus can remain dormant in the lungs of the host for a long period. In fact, the first contact of the human organism with tubercle bacilli, which usually takes place in infancy or adolescence, normally does not produce any clinical manifestation. The anatomic lesion induced by proliferation of mycobacteria and the reactive regional adenitis are called "primary complex". At that moment the subject shows a positive tuberculin test (a cutaneous reaction obtained by injection or percutaneous application of culture filtrates of mycobacteria or of their purified protein content), which indicates a state of hypersensitivity to the tubercle bacillus, not necessarily a state of immunity. Usually the primary complex remains clinically silent, but it can also progress and evolve to a state of disease. Chronic pulmonary tuberculosis in adults may be due to reactivation of the primary infection or to exogenous reinfection.

A typical characteristic of tuberculosis is the formation in the infected tissue of nodular formations called tubercles, which can have different sizes and different modes of diffusion, giving rise to various clinical forms called miliary, infiltrate, lobar tuberculosis, and so on. The disease progresses by means of ulceration, caseation and cavitation, with bronchogenic spread of infectious material. Healing may occur at any stage of the disease by processes of resolution, fibrosis, and calcification.

Control of the disease has been achieved in part through mass vaccination with BCG (the bacillus of Calmette and Guérin, an attenuated strain of *M. tuberculosis bovis*), but above all through correct application of active chemotherapeutic agents. Chemotherapeutic treatment now available enables one to stop the propagation of the disease in a high percentage of cases, by killing the pathogenic bacilli, thus permitting the organism to repair or to confine the pathological alterations. Another important consequence of chemotherapeutic treatment is the prevention of dissemination of virulent bacilli to other persons.

In spite of the efficacious drugs now available for the treatment of tuberculosis, this illness is present all over the world. In the developing countries it still represents a dramatic social problem. In countries with high standards of living, mortality has dropped to very low values, but morbidity shows a less impressive decrease (50).

Data from the World Health Organization indicate that each year there are more than 480,000 new cases of tuberculosis in Europe and about 3.2 million in the whole world. The number of persons with contagious tuberculosis in the world is of the order of 15–20 million, and the number of deaths per year due to this illness is of the order of 600,000. These figures are certainly underestimates, because they are based on cases with microbiological or histological documentation (51).

Atypical mycobacterioses are less frequent than tuberculosis, but there are geographic areas where their incidence is rather high. For example, *M. kansasii* is prevalent in central United States, and *M. ulcerans* in Australia and Africa. The more affected organs are lungs and neck lymph nodes, but urogenital, skin, bone joint, and disseminated miliary infections have also been reported. The severity of these illnesses is aggravated by the poor efficacy of drugs developed for the treatment of tuberculosis. More extensive studies of potential new drugs are certainly necessary in this field.

Leprosy is a chronic disease caused by *M. leprae*, a mycobacterium that multiplies even more slowly than the tubercle bacilli. Common belief to the contrary, the organism has low pathogenicity and infectiveness. It can live dormant for years in the invaded organism and does not show recognizable signs during the first stages of its propagation.

There are various clinical types of leprosy. In the most severe lepromatous disease the bacilli massively infiltrate the skin, which becomes thickened, glossy, and corrugated. Then other tissues are invaded, mainly peripheral nerves and bones, as a consequence, atrophy of skin and muscle, ulcerations, and amputation of small bones occur. The microorganism is detectable in smears from skin and mucosa.

The tuberculoid leprosy is characterized by the presence of skin macules with clear centers, insensitive to pain stimuli. *M. leprae* is generally detectable only during reactive phases. The final stages are similar to the lepromatous leprosy. There are also borderline forms that present characteristics common to lepromatous and tuberculoid leprosy.

Leprosy was an epidemic disease in Europe in medieval times but now is confined to some tropical areas, especially India, the Philippines, South America, and tropical Africa. Social and economic poverty is the main reason for the prevalence of this disease, which has the greatest distribution in underdeveloped countries. A total of 10–20 million persons in the world appear to be affected by leprosy. Chemotherapy offers a great possibility for eradication of the disease, but unfortunately only 20% of the affected people are able to receive the proper treatment (52, 53).

4 LABORATORY MODELS FOR SCREENING AND EVALUATING ANTIMYCOBACTERIAL AGENTS

In the search for new antimycobacterial agents, demonstration of *in vitro* activity against the virulent strain of *M. tuberculosis* H_{37} Rv in one of the simplest preliminary tests. Although much more predictive than other *in vitro* models using avirulent or fast-growing mycobacteria (*M. smegmatis*, *M. phlei*), the *in vitro* test with *M. tuberculosis* gives a large number of false positive and, unfortunately, also some false negative results. Despite these limitations, the *in vitro* test, with various modifications of the inoculum size, the culture media, and the observation time, is still used in many laboratories for the blind primary screening of a large number of compounds. It is also used in antibiotic screening, where thousands of fermentation broths must be tested, and a primary screen using *in vivo* models is a practical impossibility.

The *in vitro* test gives only an indication of activity; quantitative evaluation of the potential usefulness of the new products must be obtained through *in vivo* tests. These are performed, generally speaking, by inoculating virulent mycobacteria strains into laboratory animals, administering the product to a group of them, and comparing the course of infection in treated and untreated animals. There are a variety of procedures for performing these tests, differing with respect to animal species (mouse, guinea pig, rabbit, etc.), mycobacterial strain and size of inoculum, route of product administration, and evaluation of the results. The most current procedure uses mice infected with the human virulent mycobacterial strain, evaluating the results in terms of ED_{50}, survival time, the pathology of the lung, or bacterial count. The products active in the mice are then evaluated in other *in vivo* tests using more sophisticated techniques.

The best species for extrapolation of the results to humans is the rhesus monkey, *Macaca mulata* (54, 55). Experimental tuberculosis in this species closely parallels the human disease and, in spite of the difficulties in terms of time, space, and cost of the test, it is advisable to perform it, especially when doubtful results have been obtained from other species. In any case, extrapolation to the human disease of the results obtained in animals requires comparison of the kinetics and metabolism of the product in the different animal species and in humans. Differences in activity are sometimes clearly related to differences in the metabolic behaviors.

In the case of leprosy, up to 16 years ago, no screening or evaluation models were available using the pathogenic agent *M. leprae*, which could not be cultivated *in vitro* or transmitted to animals. Therefore the experimental infection of rodents with *M. lepraemurium* was used for evaluating the effect of potential drugs, although this model shows a low predictivity for activity in humans. For example, dapsone is inactive and isoniazid very active in this test, whereas the opposite is true for human leprosy. Only in 1960 was local infection in the mouse footpad with *M. leprae* set up (56). This model has been successfully used, with various procedural modifications, for screening and evaluation of drugs (57, 58). Thymectomy and body irradiation of mice inoculated with *M. leprae* provokes dissemination of bacilli (59), and this may be a model for a generalized infection. Another model of experimental leprosy was set up using the armadillo, which develops a severe disseminated lepromatoid disease several months after inoculation with a suspension of human leprosy bacilli (60, 61).

These recent animal models represent a great improvement for the evaluation of antileprotic agents, but they are too time-consuming for the screening of a large number of compounds. The search for short-term models is necessary, and there are indications that it may be feasible to use some *in vitro* tests on both *M. leprae* (62) and *M. lepraemurium* (63), but more extensive confirmation is needed. It has been also proposed to test compounds against *Mycobacterium species 607* (64), because a correlation has been observed between minimum inhibitory concentration for this species *in vitro* and the mouse footpad test with *M. leprae* (65).

Activity of products against atypical mycobacteria is generally tested *ad hoc*, *in vitro*, or *in vivo*, and the compounds selected for this purpose are those showing antitubercular action. There is no indication of extensive research aimed at finding specific chemotherapeutic agents for the treatment of atypical mycobacterioses, given their present relatively low incidence and the variety of the pathogenic agents. On the other hand, the severity of these infections and the apparent increase in their frequency should stimulate more research activity in this area.

The inclusion of a number of atypical mycobacteria in the large antibacterial screening programs of new compounds could provide leads for finding new, more active chemotherapic agents for the diseases caused by these microorganisms. On the other hand, there is certainly need for more knowledge on the biochemistry and physiology of the atypical mycobacteria and on their pathogenic behavior in laboratory animals.

5 SEARCH FOR AND DISCOVERY OF ANTIMYCOBACTERIAL DRUGS

Using the laboratory models available for testing and evaluating products, the medicinal chemist has fundamentally two possible approaches in the search for antimycobacterial drugs. The first approach is the blind screening of a large number of compounds, which permits the detection of a certain number of structures endowed with antimycobacterial activity. Chemical modification of these "lead" structures, accompanied by careful studies of structure-activity relationships, can yield the optimal derivative for therapeutic use. The second approach, more challenging from the scientific point of view, is based on designing drugs to act selectively on biochemical targets specific for the particular microorganism.

The antimycobacterial drugs presently in therapeutic use (Table 17.1) have been obtained mainly by the first approach. Dapsone (4,4′-diaminodiphenylsulfone) (66, 67), a breakthrough in the chemotherapy of mycobacterial infections and still the drug of choice for the treatment of leprosy, was synthesized as an analog of the antibacterial sulfonamides. Thiacetazone (68), thiambutosine (69), and thiocarlide (70) are chemical modifications of the thiosemicarbazone structure, which had proved to have antituberculous activity. Isoniazid (71) is the result of intensive research built around the finding of weak antituberculous activity of nicotinamide (72), and pyrazinamide (73) also originated from nicotinamide through chemical modification of the heterocyclic nucleus. Analogously, the observation of tuberculostatic activity of thioisonicotinamide (74) gave rise to ethionamide (75).

The observation that salicylic acid increases the oxygen consumption of tubercle bacilli and the hypothesis that related substances might have a reverse effect (76) yielded *p*-aminosalicylic (PAS) acid (77),

Table 17.1 Antimycobacterial Drugs in Therapeutic Use

Drug	Year of Discovery	Main Indication(s)
Dapsone	1939	Leprosy
Streptomycin	1944	Tuberculosis
p-Aminasalicylic acid	1946	Tuberculosis
Thioacetazone	1946	Tuberculosis, leprosy
Viomycin	1951	Tuberculosis
Pyrazinamide	1952	Tuberculosis
Isoniazid	1952	Tuberculosis
Thiambutosine	1953	Leprosy
Cycloserine	1955	Tuberculosis
Ethionamide	1957	Tuberculosis, leprosy
Kanamycin	1957	Tuberculosis
Clofazimine	1957	Leprosy
Capreomycin	1960	Tuberculosis
Ethambutol	1961	Tuberculosis
Rifampicin	1965	Tuberculosis, leprosy

which does not, in fact, affect the respiration of the mycobacterium. Ethambutol (78) was discovered as result of chemical modifications of the *N,N'*-dialkylethylenediamine structures, which had shown antituberculous activity (79).

Streptomycin (80), cycloserine (81), viomycin (82), and kanamycin (83) were discovered in the course of screening for new antibiotics, and it is certainly not unimportant that they show activity also against other microorganisms commonly used in the primary tests of fermentation broths. Chemical modification of their structures did not yield superior derivatives.

Rifampicin (84) is a semisynthetic antibiotic derived from the natural fermentation product rifamycin B, which, having very limited antibacterial activity, was submitted to extensive studies of chemical modification to improve its properties (85, 86).

Clofazimine (87), now extensively used in the therapy of leprosy, was selected among several diaminophenazines known to be antituberculous agents *in vitro*, as are many other basic dyes (88).

Although screening for antimycobacterial agents will continue to be a possible way to discover useful new drugs, the increasing knowledge of the biochemistry of the mycobacteria makes possible a more rational approach to the problem. In particular, the studies of the biosynthesis of the unique constituents of the mycobacterial cell will indicate the targets for inhibitors of the biosynthetic pathways present specifically in the microorganisms of the mycobacterium species.

Selective inhibitors could open new horizons in the therapy of mycobacterial infections because they will be ineffective on the eukaryotic cells of the host, therefore potentially will have little toxicity. Furthermore, since they will be ineffective also on the other microorganisms, they will not alter the normal microbial flora. From the available information on the biochemistry of mycobacteria, which has been previously summarized, some potential targets for specific antituberculous agents can be listed. For example, the mycolic acids seem to be fatty acids present only in mycobacteria, suggesting that the mycolate synthetase might be a target for specific tuberculostatics. In fact, among the various mechanisms of action proposed for isoniazid, the inhibition of mycolic acid synthesis is a very recent one and is gaining more favor. This inhibition has been observed in *M. tuberculosis BCG* (89) and *M. tuberculosis* H37 Rv (90, 91), not in isoniazid-resistant strains.

Another specific constituent of pathogenic mycobacteria is the cord factor, and more extensive studies on its biosynthesis might indicate the possibility of inhibiting its formation.

Inhibitors of either the formation or the function of mycobactins are also of potential practical interest in view of the stimulating role played by these factors in the growth of mycobacteria. The discovery of the competitive inhibition of mycobactin P by chromic mycobactin P in the growth of *M. paratuberculosis* is an interesting approach. Unfortunately chromic mycobactin P does not antagonize the growth of other mycobacteria, probably because these microorganisms overcome the inhibitory effect by making greater quantities of mycobactins or different ones (92).

Attempts have also been made to find antagonist analogs, but the complexity of the molecule makes the task very difficult. The closest structural analog so far synthesized, similar to mycobactin T but lacking the iron chelating groups, has no antimycobacterial activity (93). On the other hand, recent findings offer a plausible explanation of why PAS is much more effective as a bacteriostatic against mycobacteria than against other bacteria, namely, that it acts through a specific inhibition of mycobactin synthesis, probably by a mechanism of noncompetitive inhibition (94–96).

Another specific target for antimycobacterial drugs is the DNA-dependent RNA polymerase (DDRP), the enzyme that synthesizes RNA by using DNA as template. Rifamycins are potent and specific inhibitors of bacterial DDRP without having an effect on the mammalian DDRP (97, 98), and the same mechanism is the basis of their action against mycobacteria (99–104).

Also, the folate biosynthesis in mycobacterial organisms could be a target for potential new drugs. In the search for potential antileprotic agents, several compounds of the diphenylsulfone class have been examined for their ability to suppress growth of *Mycobacterium species 607*, presumably by way of inhibition of the synthesis of the dihydrofolate, and some 2,4-diamino-6-substituted pteridines have been studied as potential inhibitors of the reduction of dihydrofolate to tetrahydrofolate in the same organism (105).

For the drugs in therapeutic use, preliminary or definitive indications of their mechanisms of action have been reached a posteriori. The active substances, besides being important as chemotherapeutic agents, often constitute tools for a better understanding of the biochemistry of mycobacteria, consequently for defining specific targets for the design of new drugs.

Although some important clues have appeared in the fields of specific biochemical pathways inside the mycobacteria and of the mechanism of action of mycobacterial drugs, little progress has been made till now in overcoming the problem of drug resistance in mycobacteria. From the "fluctuation test" it appears that *M. tuberculosis* mutates spontaneously and at random to resistance to isoniazid, streptomycin, ethambutol, and rifampicin (106), and that is in a genotype form. Apparently, factors other than random mutation may be involved in resistance; these factors lack genetic control and are probably involved in cytoplasm or enzyme mechanisms.

A better knowledge of the mechanism of mycobacterial resistance to a drug could indicate the direction in which to search for new products specifically overcoming this mechanism. In the case of aminoglycoside antibiotics, the mechanism of resistance in Enterobacteriaceae and some *Pseudomonas* strains has been extensively studied, and the inactivating enzymes have been identified. Chemical modifications at the site of attack of inactivating enzymes gave new products that were active against resistant strains (107). However little information has been collected about the genetic control of resistance to aminoglycoside antibiotics in *M. smegmatis* (108–110).

Unfortunately, present knowledge of the genetic mechanisms and genotypical systems governing resistance in mycobacteria is limited because of the difficulty of using mycobacteria in classical genetic techniques. Therefore, at present, the delay or prevention of the evolution toward resistance of mycobacterial flora, and the formation of atypical strains, is accomplished only through combination therapy, based on the complementary action of the constituents. It is well known that in this case the probability of a concomitant mutation toward resistant strains is much lower than the probability of mutation to resistance to a single drug.

6 AVAILABLE ANTIMYCOBACTERIAL DRUGS AND RELATED PRODUCTS

Among the several thousand compounds screened for antimycobacterial activity, only few have had therapeutic indices sufficient to warrant introducing them into clinical use. These drugs are described in some detail, together with general information about the chemical analogs, mechanisms of action, pharmacokinetics and metabolism, clinical use, and untoward effects. The information, in very summary form, is intended to cover the aspects that are useful for understanding the role of each product in current therapy, the limitations of use, and the need for improvement or for further studies.

The drugs have been subdivided arbitrarily into synthetic products and antibiotics, and within these two categories they are listed in a quasi-chronological order, with products having structural similarities grouped with the representative first introduced into therapy.

6.1 Synthetic Products

6.1.1 SULFONES. The sulfones were synthesized on analogy of sulfonamides, which had no antimycobacterial activity. The first sulfones prepared, 4,4′-diaminodiphenylsulfone (dapsone) (17.**9**) and its glucose bisulfite derivative, glucosulfone sodium (17.**10**), were found to be active in suppressing experimental tuberculous infections (66, 67).

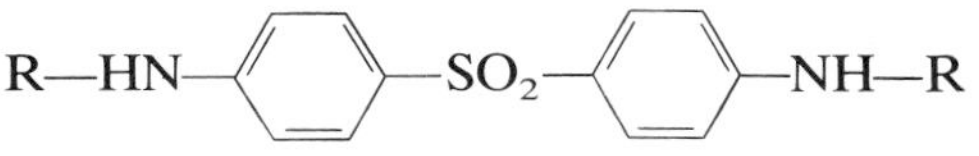

R—HN—⟨C₆H₄⟩—SO_2—⟨C₆H₄⟩—NH—R

R = H

17.**9**

R = CH(CHOH)$_4$CH$_2$OH
  |
  SO_3Na

17.**10**

Their usefulness in the chemotherapy of human tuberculosis was very limited, but the discovery of some effect of 17.**10** in leprosy experimentally induced in rats (111) opened the way to their successful introduction into the treatment of human leprosy. Since it was considered that 17.**10** is active after metabolic conversion to dapsone, intensive studies have been carried out, varying the structure of the latter to find optimal activity and to improve its low solubility. Various substitutions on the phenyl rings have yielded products less active than dapsone. The only product of this type that has some clinical use is acetosulfone sodium, which contains one $SO_2N(Na)COCH_3$ substituent in the ortho position to the sulfone group. Its antibacterial effect seems to be due to the unchanged drug. Substitutions in both the amino groups gave rise to products that are in general active only if they are converted metabolically to the parent dapsone.

Substitution on the amino groups to improve solubility yielded products such as the above-mentioned glucosulfone, the methanesulfonic acid derivative (sulfoxone

$R = CH_2SO_2Na$

17.**11**

sodium, aldesulfone), 17.**11**, and the cinnamaldehyde–sodium bisulfite addition product (sulfetrone sodium, solasulfone), 17.**12**, which have limited use in leprosy

$$R = \underset{\displaystyle SO_3Na}{\underset{|}{CH}}—CH_2—\underset{\displaystyle SO_3Na}{\underset{|}{CH}}—C_6H_5$$

17.**12**

treatment. They act through their metabolic conversion to dapsone in the body. Several methanesulfonic acid derivatives of 4,4′-diaminodiphenylsulfone have been tested for their ability to be metabolized to dapsone (112).

The 4,4′-dacetyldiaminodiphenylsulfone, acedapsone, 17.**13**, has low activity *in vitro*,

$R = COCH_3$

17.**13**

but it is used as an injectable depot sulfone, which releases dapsone at a steady rate over several weeks. The advantage of this type of depot usage is evident, especially in prophylaxis of people exposed to risk (113).

Although a large number of sulfones have been synthesized and tested as potential antileprotic agents, dapsone remains the drug most useful clinically. Dapsone is a bacteriostatic agent for *M. leprae* at concentration estimated to be of the order of 0.01–0.02 μg/ml (114), when the microorganism has been isolated from untreated patients. *M. leprae* becomes resistant to dapsone and its congeners. Dapsone is usually administered orally at a daily dose of 100 mg. It is nearly completely absorbed from the gastrointestinal tract, well distributed into all tissues, and excreted in high percentage in the urine as the mono-*N*-sulfamate and other unidentified metabolities (114). It is monoacetylated in man. The characteristics of dapsone acetylation parallel those of isoniazid and sulfametazine, thereby establishing genetic polymorphism for the acetylation of dapsone in man (115). Two metabolic factors, greater acetylation and greater clearance of dapsone from the circulation may contribute to emergence of dapsone-resistant *M. leprae* (116).

Acedapsone is administered intramuscularly in oily suspension at a dose of 225 mg every 7 weeks. From the site of injection, the product is slowly released, and the plasma contains mainly dapsone and its monoacetyl derivative, the ratio of these two products depending on whether the patient is a slow or rapid acetylator, as in the case of dapsone.

Several severe untoward effects are caused by dapsone and its analogs. Besides frequent gastrointestinal and central nervous system disturbances, the most common is hemolysis. There are indications that individuals with a glucose-6-phosphate dehydrogenase deficiency are more susceptible to hemolysis during sulfone therapy, although this statement is controversial (117). It is assumed that dapsone interferes with incorporation of *p*-aminobenzoic acid into dehydrofolate, in analogy with the action of sulfonamides in other bacterial systems. This mechanism of action of dapsone has been proved for *E. coli* (118), and the finding of cross-resistance to sulfones and sulfonamides in *Mycobacterium species 607* indirectly confirms their similarity of action (64). Unfortunately, the inability to cultivate *M. leprae in vitro* makes it very difficult to ultimately verify that dapsone acts through the proposed mechanism on this organism.

6.1.2 *p*-AMINOSALICYLIC ACID AND ANALOGS. The observation that benzoates and salicylates have a stimulatory effect on the respiration of mycobacteria (76) suggested that analogs of benzoic acid might interfere with the oxidative metabolism of the bacilli. When various compounds structurally related to benzoic acid were tested. it was found that some of them had limited antituberculous activity; *p*-aminosalicylic acid (17.**14**) was the most active (77).

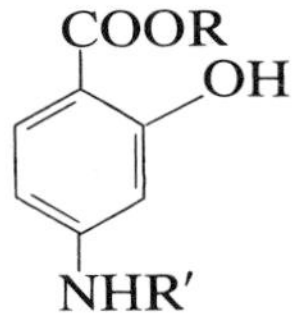

COOR, OH, NHR′ (benzene ring structure)

R	R′	
H	H	17.**14**
C_6H_5	H	17.**15**
H	COC_6H_5	17.**16**
H	$COCH_3$	17 **17**
H	$COCH_2NH_2$	17.**18**

The discovery of PAS cannot be quoted as an example of biochemically oriented chemotherapeutic research because in fact its mechanism of action is not by way of the respiration of mycobacteria.

The *in vitro* and *in vivo* antimycobacterial activity of a simple molecule such as PAS stimulated the synthesis, and testing of many derivatives. This extensive research failed to give rise to better drugs but did provide knowledge of the structural requirements for activity in the series. Modification of the position of the hydroxy and amino groups with respect to the carboxy group resulted in a sharp decrease in activity. The amino group confers a distinct pharmacodynamic property to the molecule, eliminating the antipyretic and analgesic activities of salicylic acid and giving the specific tuberculostatic activity. Further nuclear substitution and replacement of the amino, hydroxy, or carboxy groups with other groups yielded inactive or poorly active products. Also, functional derivatives on the amino, hydroxy, and carboxy groups of PAS are generally inactive, unless they are converted *in vivo* into the active molecule. Among the latter, the phenylester (17.**15**) and benzamidosalicylic acid (17.**16**) must be mentioned.

PAS has bacteriostatic activity *in vitro* on *M. tuberculosis* at a concentration of the order of 1 μg/ml. It is active only against growing tubercle bacilli, being inactive against intracellular organisms. Other microorganisms are not affected by the compound. Also, most of the atypical mycobacteria are insensitive to the drug. Although active against *M. leprae* in the mouse footpad test (119), it is not used in the current treatment of leprosy.

PAS is readily absorbed by the gastrointestinal tract and well distributed throughout the body. It is quickly eliminated through the urine in form of inactive metabolites, the *N*-acetyl (17.**17**) and *N*-glycyl (17.**18**) derivatives. For this reason it is administered orally in a daily dose of 8–12 g. The side effects of PAS in the gastrointestinal tract and the poor acceptance by the patients are due to the high dosage. The search for derivatives with more adequate pharmacokinetic properties has given products such as 17.**15** and 17.**16** (the second used as calcium salt), which seem to release PAS slowly, giving more prolonged blood levels. However their use in the therapy is very limited.

The initial use of PAS alone in the treatment of tuberculosis was followed by the emergence of mutants resistant to it. It is now used in combination with other and more potent antituberculous agents to increase their efficacy and prevent or delay development of bacterial resistance to them. In the case of the combination of PAS with isoniazid, the higher plasma concentration of the latter is due to competition in the acetylation reaction.

The mechanism of action of PAS is not clear. It was demonstrated earlier that *p*-aminobenzoic acid antagonizes the antibacterial activity of PAS *in vitro* and *in vivo*. This property can perhaps be explained by the finding that PAS is taken up into cells by an active process, possibly by the route used for assimilation of *p*-aminobenzoic acid. The formation of mycobactin, an ionophore for iron transport, is strongly inhibited by PAS, and the bacteriostatic activity of PAS might be due to the inhibition of the metabolic pathway for iron uptake (94–96).

6.1.3 THIOACETAZONE, THIOCARLIDE, THIAMBUTOSINE. The synthesis of a series of thiosemicarbazones as intermediates in the preparation of analogs of sulfathiadiazole (68, 120), which has weak antituberculous activity (121), led to the discovery of the thiosemicarbazone of *p*-acetamidobenzaldehyde (thioacetazone, amithiozone), 17.**19,** the most active substance *in vitro* and *in vivo* of the series (122–124).

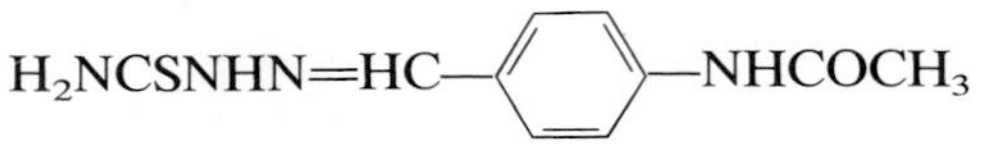

$H_2NCSNHN{=}HC{-}C_6H_4{-}NHCOCH_3$

17.**19**

In the search for better products, many modifications of the thioacetazone molecule have been made. The studies clearly indicate that the activity resides in the thiosemicarbazone structure of the aromatic aldehydes. In fact, several products with modified aromatic moieties, including some heteroxyclic nuclei, have been found to be active. Some of them have been tested clinically with positive results, but thioacetazone is the only thiosemicarbazone still in clinical use. Its good activity *in vitro* and *in vivo*, and the lack of cross-resistance to isoniazid and streptomycin, indicate the use of thioacetazone as a drug to combine with these drugs to delay bacterial resistance. Despite relatively low toxicity in laboratory animals, thioacetazone has limitations in clinical use because of serious side effects, such as gastrointestinal disorders, liver damage, and anemia, when administered to humans at the initially proposed daily dose of 300 mg. A review of the side effects and efficacy of thioacetazone in relation to the dosage indicates that the drug has an activity comparable to that of PAS and an acceptable toxicity when administered at lower dosage (125).

A dose of 300 mg of isoniazid plus 150 mg of thioacetazone is a cheap and acceptable combination for long-term therapeutic treatment after the initial treatment with three drugs. This schedule is used in developing countries (126), although there are considerable differences in side effects among patients from different geographic areas (127). The reported effectiveness in leprosy (128) notwithstanding, thioacetazone is of limited usefulness in the treatment of this disease because of its side effects and the emergence of resistance of *M. leprae* to the drug.

The mechanism of action of thioacetazone is not known. Its tuberculostatic activity is not counteracted by *p*-aminobenzoic acid (129) and there is a partial cross-resistance to antituberculous thioureas. Treatment with thioacetazone may produce thioacetazone-resistant strains, some of which are also resistant to ethionamide (130).

Several thioureas that are structurally related to thiosemicarbazones, have been found to be active *in vitro* and *in vivo* against *M. tuberculosis*, the most active being the 1,3-diphenylthioureas with *p*-alkoxy groups in one or both the aromatic nuclei. Of these, thiocarlide (17.**20**) and thiambutosine (17.**21**) have been introduced into clinical use.

Thiocarlide shows some efficacy against experimental tuberculosis in mice (131) and is active against tubercle bacilli resistant to PAS, streptomycin, and isoniazid (132,

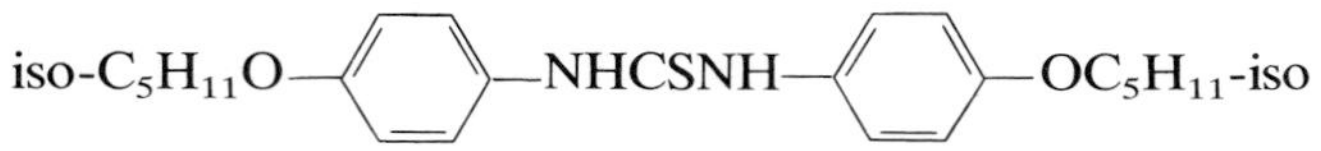

$\text{iso-}C_5H_{11}O{-}C_6H_4{-}NHCSNH{-}C_6H_4{-}OC_5H_{11}\text{-iso}$

17.**20**

$n\text{-}C_4H_9\text{-}O{-}C_6H_4{-}NHCSNH{-}C_6H_4{-}N(CH_3)_2$

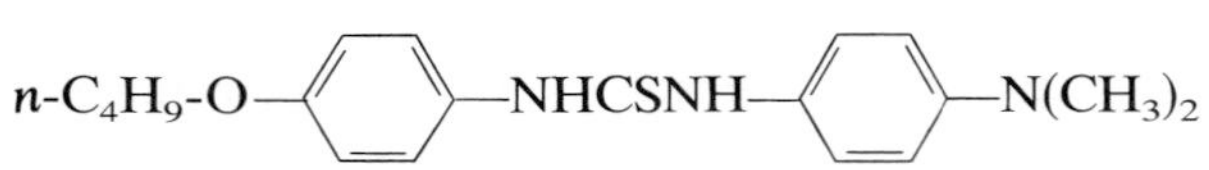

17.**21**

133); but several clinical trials have indicated little or no usefulness in the treatment of human tuberculosis, even in combination with other drugs (134). Its use is now very limited. From a theoretic point of view, however, it is interesting that thiocarlide acts through inhibition of mycolic acid synthesis, as part of a more general inhibition of the free lipids of *M. tuberculosis* (135).

Thiambutosine has given disappointing results in clinical use for tuberculosis, but it was found to be active in the treatment of leprosy (136), though inferior to dapsone (137). It is used for patients who do not tolerate the latter (138).

6.1.4 ISONIAZID, ETHIONAMIDE, PYRAZINAMIDE. After the early report that nicotinamide possesses tuberculostatic activity (72, 139), several compounds related to it were examined. Attention was aimed at the isonicotinic acid derivatives and, in view of the already established antitubercular activity of thiosemicarbazones, the thiosemicarbazone of isonicotinaldehyde was prepared. When the isonicotinyl hydrazide (isoniazid, 17.**22**), prepared as an intermediate in the synthesis of the aldehyde was tested, it proved to be a very potent antitubercular agent *in vitro* and *in vivo* (71, 140, 141).

The outstanding antituberculous activity of isoniazid in experimental infections, confirmed by the clinical trials, stimulated the study of chemical modifications of this simple molecule.

At least 100 analogs were prepared, but any structural change caused a reduction in or loss of activity. Among the modified forms that retained appreciable activity, the N^2-alkyl derivatives should be mentioned. In particular the N^2-isopropyl derivative (iproniazide, 17.**23**), was found to be very active *in vivo*. Extensive clinical trials proved the therapeutic effectiveness of iproniazid and revealed its psychomotor stimulant effect, caused by the inhibition of monoamine oxidase (142). Use of iproniazid in the treatment of tuberculosis or of psychotic and neurotic depression was discontinued because of the hepatic toxicity of the drug. Although acetyl isoniazid (17.**24**) is inactive, its hydrazones constitute a group of isoniazid congeners that have activity of the same order as the parent compound. The activity of these compounds generally is related to the rate of their hydrolysis to the parent compound. Some hydrazones have been introduced into therapeutic use, such as the 3,4-dimethoxybenzylidene (verazide, 17.**25**) and the 3-methoxy-4-hydroxy-benzylidene (phthivazid, 17.**26**) derivatives, but their

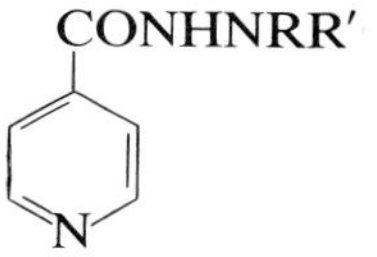

CONHNRR′ (4-pyridyl)

R	R′	
H	H	17.**22**
H	$CH(CH_3)_2$	17.**23**
H	$COCH_3$	17.**24**
	= CH—(3-OCH_3, 4-OCH_3-phenyl)	17.**25**
	= CH—(3-OCH_3, 4-OH-phenyl)	17.**26**

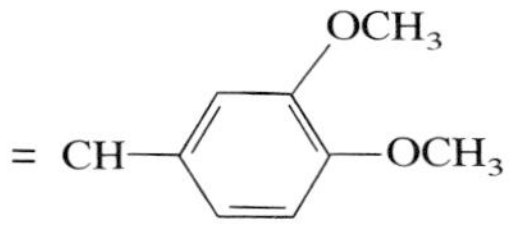

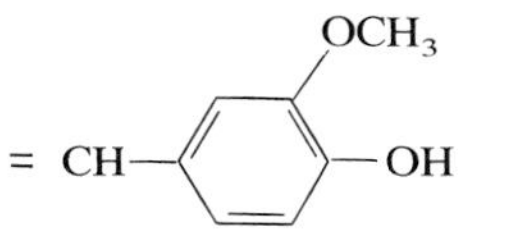

utility is questionable, and products of this kind now have very limited or no application. The injectable streptomycylidene isoniazid is an example of an incorrect medicinal chemical approach, because the compound in fact acts as a combination of the two components, which in addition are not in the right ratio for proper therapeutic use.

Isoniazid has bacteriostatic and bactericidal activity *in vitro* against *M. tuberculosis* and also against strains resistant to other antimycobacterial drugs. The minimal inhibitory concentration for the human strain is of the order of 0.05 μg/ml. It acts on growing cells and not on resting cells and is effective also against intracellular bacilli. Its effect on the atypical mycobacteria is marginal or nonexistent.

Isoniazid is very active in the various models of experimental tuberculosis in animals. It shows limited activity against *M. leprae* in the mouse footpad test (143), but it is essentially inactive in human leprosy (144). The drug is readily absorbed from the gastrointestinal tract and diffuses very well into all organs, in various degrees. It is commonly used in adult patients at doses of the order of 5–8 mg/kg, but this dosage can be increased in children or in very severe cases.

Isoniazid is one of the most effective antituberculous drugs but, when it is administered alone, a quick emergence of resistant strains follows. Therefore isoniazid is administered with other antituberculous drugs, which delay the emergence of resistant tubercle bacilli. The drug has relatively low toxicity. Peripheral neuritis and stimulation of the central nervous system are common side effects. Isoniazid seems to compete with pyridoxal phosphate, and the concurrent administration of the latter has been suggested to prevent isoniazid toxicity (145, 146).

Isoniazid is excreted mainly in the urine, where it is found in part in unchanged form, together with various inactive metabolites: *N*-acetyl isoniazid, monoacetyl hydrazine, diacetyl hydrazine, isoniazid hydrazones with pyruvic and α-ketoglutaric acid, isonicotinic acid, and isonicotinylglycine. The primary metabolic route that determines the rate at which isoniazid is eliminated from the body is acetylation to acetyl isoniazid. There are large differences among individuals in the rate at which isoniazid is acetylated. The acetylation rate of isoniazid appears to be under genetic control (147, 148), and individuals can be slow or rapid acetylators of the drug. The serum half-lives of isoniazid in a large number of subjects show a bimodal distribution, the isoniazid half-lives of rapid metabolizers ranging from about 45 to 110 min and those of slow metabolizers from 2 to 4.5 hr (149). The rate of acetylation appears to be conditioned by race. The proportion of slow acetylators varies from 10% among Japanese and Eskimos to 60% among Negroes and Caucasians. The isoniazid acetylator status of tuberculosis patients treated with isoniazid-containing regimens seems to be relevant only for once-weekly treatments with the drug (150).

Several hypothesis have been put forward concerning the mechanism of action of isoniazid. The most convincing ones take into account that the activity of this drug is specific against mycobacteria at very low concentrations. Recent investigations in this direction have indicated that the action of isoniazid is on the biosynthethic pathway to the mycolic acids (89, 91, 151, 152). In particular, it seems that isoniazid blocks the synthesis of fatty acids longer than C_{26} in chain length (153). Scanning electron microscopy shows impressive changes in mycobacterial cells exposed to concentrations of isoniazid that inhibit mycolic acid synthesis. There is complete loss of some areas of outer membrane, as well as development of thin spots in the cell wall associated with bulging (154). A further proof of the interaction of isoniazid with mycolic acid seems to be the loss of acid fastness of cells susceptible to isoniazid (155).

Another hypothesis suggests that isonicotinic acid is responsible for the inhibitory effect of isoniazid on mycobacteria (156–158). Isoniazid is said to penetrate the cell, where it is oxidized enzymatically to isonicotinic acid, which at the intracellular pH is nearly completely ionized and cannot return across the membrane; consequently it accumulates inside the cell. Isonicotinic acid is then quaternized and competes with nicotinic acid through the formation of an analog of nicotinamide–adenine dinucleotide, which does not have the activity of the natural coenzyme. Alteration of the metabolic functions of the cell follows, particularly with respect to lipid metabolism. A study of quantitative structure-activity correlations among a series of 2-substituted isonicotinic acid hydrazides gave evidence that the reactivity of the pyridine nitrogen atom, measured through the reaction rates for quaternization, is essential for the biological activity of compounds of this kind and seems to support the hypothesis that isonicotinic acid derivatives are incorporated into a nicotinamide–adenine dinucleotide analog (158).

These data could be perhaps reconciled with the previous hypotheses, including that of the formation of yellow pigments (159), and with the findings of other authors indicating a decrease in nicotinamide–adenine dinucleotide synthesis following treatment with isoniazid. However it is not explained why the inhibition of the synthesis of nicotinamide–adenine dinucleotide by isoniazid is of the same order in sensitive and resistant strains (160). Further studies are necessary for clarification of the primary site of action of isoniazid in *M. tuberculosis.*

As mentioned earlier, the discovery of isoniazid was the consequence of research based on the weak antitubercular activity of nicotinamide. This lead was pursued in various directions, and among the earliest modifications, thioisonicotinamide (17.**27**) (74, 161, 162) appeared to have the intriguing property of an *in vivo* efficacy superior to that expected from the *in vitro* activity.

The hypothesis that some metabolic product of the drug was responsible for the activity *in vivo* stimulated the synthesis, as well as the testing of a series of potential thioisonicotinamide metabolites and various other derivatives. Among the latter, an increased activity was observed for the 2-alkyl derivatives (75). 2-Ethyl thioisonicotinamide (ethionamide, 17.**28**) and the 2-*n*-propyl analog (prothionamide, 17.**29**) were selected for clinical use. Of these two drugs, ethionamide has been more extensively studied, and prothionamide seems to possess biological properties very similar to it.

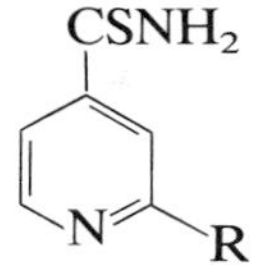

$CSNH_2$

R = H	17.**27**
R = C_2H_5	17.**28**
R = n-C_3H_7	17.**29**

At concentrations of the order of 0.6–2.5 μg/ml, ethionamide is active *in vitro* against *M. tuberculosis* strains, either sensitive or resistant to isoniazid, streptomycin, and *p*-aminosalicylic acid. Administered orally, it is very effective in the treatment of experimental tuberculosis in animals. It shows also activity against atypical mycobacteria, especially those belonging to the photochromogenic group.

Although activity against *M. leprae* in animal infections has been reported, ethionamide is rarely used in the therapeutic treatment of leprosy. In the case of tuberculosis, the drug is given orally at doses varying from 125 mg to a maximum of 1 g daily. It is rapidly absorbed and widely distributed in the body. It provokes various side effects at the gastric level and has some hepatic toxicity. Bacterial resistance develops quickly when ethionamide is given alone; therefore it is used in combination with other antimycobacterial drugs.

Ethionamide has a short-half life and is rapidly excreted in the urine, but only a minor percentage is in the form of unaltered product. A series of metabolites has been found in the urine: the active sulfoxide, the 2-ethyl isonicotinic acid and amide, and the corresponding dihydropyridine derivatives (163). The antibacterial action of ethionamide seems to be due to an inhibitory effect on the mycolic acid synthesis, with a concomitant effect on the non-mycolic acid bound lipids (135). This pattern is like that shown by isoniazid. In studies of chemical modifications of the nicotinamide structure, other heterocyclic nuclei have been investigated, and the 2-carboxamidopyrazine (pyrazinamide, 17.**30**) was synthesized (73, 164, 165).

Pyrazinamide is active *in vitro* mainly at slightly acidic pH and is active also against intacellular bacilli.

The activity of the drug in experimental infections is evident in the first period of treatment, when the microorganisms are sensitive to the drug. In the long-term treatments, resistance develops.

Pyrazinamide is absorbed well from the gastrointestinal tract and is excreted with the urine, mainly in the form of inactive metabolites, pyrazinoic acid, and 5-hydroxypyrazinoic acid (166). The oral daily dosage is 20–35 mg/kg.

The present use of pyrazinamide is limited because of its various severe side effects, the most relevant and frequent one being hepatic toxicity.

Compounds with other substitutions on the pyrazine nucleus or other carboxamido heterocycles were found to be inactive or less active than pyrazinamide. The only analog, developed because of its potential superiority over pyrazinamide, was morphazinamide (*N*-morpholinomethylamide of pyrazinoic acid, 17.**31**) (167). Interest in

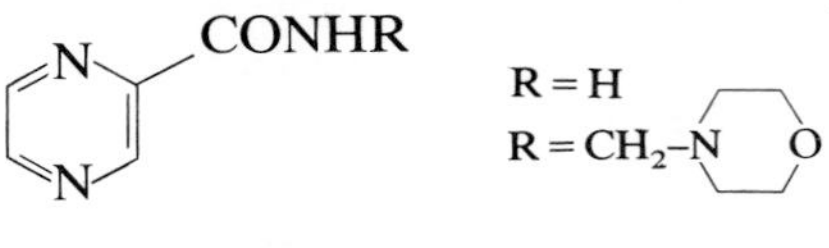

CONHR

R = H 17.**30**

R = CH_2–N O 17.**31**

this drug ceased when it was ascertained that the activity and toxicity parallel those of pyrazinamide, to which morphazinamide is converted *in vivo* (1968).

6.1.5 CLOFAZIMINE. Clofazimine belongs to a very peculiar class of phenazines, the so-called riminophenazines. Studies on these compounds derived from the original observation that treating a solution of 2-aminodiphenylamine with ferric chloride produced a red crystalline precipitate that completely inhibited the growth of tubercle bacilli H37 Rv strain *in vitro*, and was not inactivated by human serum (169–171). The *in vivo* activity was moderate and the toxicity very low. Such a compound, named B-283 (17.**32**), was the leading structure for a series of riminophenazines, which are alkyl or aryl imino derivatives.

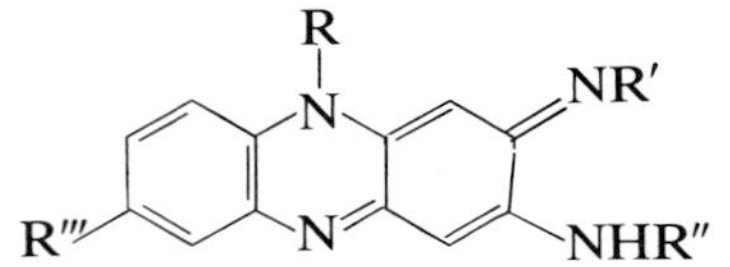

R	R′	R″	R‴	
	H		H	17.**32**
p-ClC_6H_4	$CH(CH_3)_2$	*p*-ClC_6H_4	H	17.**33**
C_6H_5	cyclohexyl (CH ring: CH_2—CH_2, CH_2, CH_2—CH_2)	C_6H_5	Cl	17.**34**

Among the first compounds synthesized on the track of B-283, the compound B-663, later on named clofazimine (17.**33**), was the most active (172, 173). Its *in vitro* inhibitory activity against *M. tuberculosis* is at concentrations of 0.1–0.5 μg/ml. Strains resistant to isoniazid, and/or streptomycin, PAS, and thioacetazone, are susceptible to the drug. Also atypical mycobacteria belonging to Runyon groups I, II, III, and IV are susceptible to this compound. B-663 has not only a bacteriostatic but also a bactericidal action (but the latter is rather slow), and only on multiplying mycobacteria. In the treatment of murine tuberculosis, clofazimine was found to be more active than isoniazid on a weight-for-weight basis, but much more active on molar basis (174). This high activity of clofazimine in tuberculosis infections was confirmed in other experiments with mice, hamsters, and rats. Much higher doses of clofazimine were necessary to achieve a therapeutic effect of the drug with guinea pigs and monkeys. Limited trials in chronic human pulmonary tuberculosis indicated that clofazimine had no significant effect on the disease at doses up to 10 mg/kg.

In experimental infections with atypical mycobacteria, clofazimine was found to be much more active against *M. kansasii* than was isoniazid (174). Other studies have shown that clofazimine is also active in experimental infections with *M. johnei* (175), *M. ulcerans* (176), *M. lepraemurium* (177, 178) and *M. leprae* (179–186). In particular, *M. leprae* seems to be about 10 times more susceptible to clofazimine than *M. tuberculosis* (143). The marked activity against leprosy was confirmed in clinical trials (179, 180–185). Generally speaking, the activity of clofazimine is similar to that of dapsone.

Dapsone-resistant mutants are susceptible to clofazimine. During treatment of lepromatous leprosy with clofazimine, the characteristic inflammatory reaction "erythema nodosum leprosum" (ENL) seldom develops; if clofazimine is combined with dapsone, the latter agent no longer causes ENL. This makes the concurrent use of corticosteroids unnecessary. It was suggested that clofazimine would have a corticosteroidlike antiinflammatory action (186). In a dye-hyaluronidase spreading test, clofazimine had a hyaluronidase-inhibitory effect, after single oral application of 100–200 mg in humans (187). In agreement with these results, it was found that clofazimine [50–100 mg/(kg)(day)] inhibited rat adjuvant arthritis and the inflammatory paw swelling following an adjuvant injection (188). It did not inhibit the primary antibody response to sheep erythrocites or the tuberculin skin response. Thus clofazimine seems to have antiinflammatory but not immunosuppressive activity.

In laboratory animals, clofazimine has a very low acute and subacute toxicity (189). In the clinical use, all patients develop ruddiness of the skin followed by hyperpigmentation (186).

Clofazimine has a peculiar pharmacokinetic pattern, characterized by slow absorption, low blood concentration, high macrophage concentration, and extremely slow excretion. All riminophenazines are very soluble in fats and in micronized form are well absorbed by the intestine. Derivatives with hydrophylic groups are either less active or inactive. Riminophenazines, once absorbed by the intestine, are carried in the blood flow by lipoprotein and inglobed by macrophages. After continued oral administration, the macrophages appear as red-orange phagosomes. Therefore the compounds have a diffusion that is mainly intracellular. They are stored in the body for a long time, and this confers on them some prophylactic action (174).

To obtain compounds with better pharmacodynamic properties, which would be cheaper and possibly more useful than clofazimine in the therapy of tuberculosis, a number of new riminophenazines were designed. The compound B-1912 (17.**34**) was selected, showing a higher serum level and lower level in the tissues (except than in lipids) than clofazimine. In *M. leprae* infections experimentally induced in mice, it was shown that clofazimine and B-1912 have the same activity (190). The compound is still under investigation.

The mechanism of action of riminophenazines has not been clearly elucidated because of the low solubility of these compounds in aqueous media. The activity seems to allow correlation with the *p*-quinoid system: in fact, when this is removed by reductive acylation, activity disappears. The mycobacteria, under anaerobic conditions, reduce the quinoid system. It has been shown that 20% of the respiratory hydrogen can be transferred from a respiratory enzyme to clofazimine (171).

6.1.6 ETHAMBUTOL. Extensive studies of the chemical and biological properties of compounds related to alkylenediamine were carried out after the discovery during screening of the antimycobacterial activity of *N,N'*diisopropylethylendiamine (17.**35**) (78, 191). This compound was found to be active both *in vitro* and *in vivo*, with a therapeutic index of the same order as that of streptomycin.

Chemical modifications from this lead, attempted with the aim of obtaining the product with the highest therapeutic index,

$$RNHCH_2CH_2NHR$$

$R = CH(CH_3)_2$	17.**35**
$R = CH(C_2H_5)CH_2OH$	17.**36**
$R = CH(C_2H_5)CHO$	17.**37**
$R = CH(C_2H_5)COOH$	17.**38**

gave indications of the structural requirements for antimycobacterial activity. Most relevant are the following: the presence of the two basic amine centers, the distance between the two carbons, and the presence of a simple, small, branched alkyl group on each nitrogen.

A correlation between metal chelation of compounds of this structure and antimycobacterial activity suggested the utility of synthesizing products with hydroxy substitution on the *N*-alkyl groups as more effective metal chelators and possibly more active antimycobacterial agents. The most active of these derivatives was the *dextro* isomer of *N,N'*bis(1-hydroxy-2-butyl) ethylenediamine (ethambutol, 17.**36**). The *meso* isomer is less active, the *levo* almost inactive. Also, hydroxy substitution on other alkyl groups (isopropyl, *t*-butyl) or in other positions of the butyl group gave inactive products. These data appear in contrast with the working hypothesis of a correlation between metal chelation and antimycobacterial activity. Various other modifications of the structure of ethambutol gave inactive products, with few exceptions. The OCH_3, OC_2H_5, and $HNCH_3$ derivatives have the same activity *in vivo* as the parent compound because dealkylation occurs in the body. In addition, the monohydroxy unsymmetrical analog has activity equal to ethambutol, but it is more toxic.

Ethambutol inhibits *in vitro* the growth of most of the human strains of *M. tuberculosis* at concentrations of the order of 1 μg/ml. Strains resistant to other antimycobacterial agents are just as sensitive to ethambutol. Among the other mycobacteria, the bovine and photochromogenic bacilli are sensitive to ethambutol, and the scotochromogenic and nonchromogenic mycobacteria are variably sensitive to it (192).

Ethambutol is not active in the experimental mouse infection with *M. leprae* (143). and is not used in the treatment of human leprosy. The efficacy of ethambutol against *M. tuberculosis in vivo* was proved in various experimental models in animals and confirmed in the clinical trials in human tuberculosis.

In current therapeutic use, the drug is administered at daily doses of 15–25 mg/kg, in combination with other antituberculous agents, to prevent emergence of resistant strains (193, 194). The drug is well absorbed from the gastrointestinal tract. About half the ingested dose is excreted as active drug in the urine, where there are also minor quantities of two inactive metabolites, the dialdehyde (17.**34**) and the dicarboxylic acid (17.**38**) derivatives (195, 196). Ethambutol is rather well tolerated and produces few side effects. The effect of decreasing the visual acuity is controversial and probably correlated with dosage and duration of the therapeutic use.

The primary mechanism of action of ethambutol on mycobacteria is not understood. The growth inhibition by ethambutol is largely independent of concentration, being more related to the time of exposure. It seems that most of the ethambutol taken up by mycobacteria has no direct role in growth inhibition, and there is no information on the subcellular components responsible for critical ethambutol binding (197,

198). Treatment of mycobacteria with ethambutol results in inhibition of protein and DNA synthesis, and it was proposed that ethambutol interferes with the role of polyamines and divalent cations in ribonucleic acid metabolism (199–201). Other authors have found an inhibitory effect of ethambutol on phosphorylation of specific compounds of intermediary metabolism, under conditions of endogenous respiration (202). Further studies are necessary to clarify the primary action of the drug.

6.2 Antibiotics

6.2.1 STREPTOMYCIN, KANAMYCIN, AND OTHER AMINOGLYCOSIDE ANTIBIOTICS. Streptomycin was discovered in 1944 as a fermentation product of *Streptomyces griseus* (80). It belongs to the family of so-called aminoglycoside antibiotics, which includes kanamycin, gentamicin, neomycin, amikacin, nebramycin, paromomycin, kasugamycin, and spectinomycin. The chemical structure of streptomycin is *N*-methyl-L-glucosaminidostreptosidostreptidine. It is made up of three components: streptidine, streptose, and *N*-methyl-L-glucosamine (17.**39**). The intact molecule is necessary for antibacterial action.

R^1	R^2	R^3	
—CHO	H	H	17.**39**
—CHO	H	CH_2OH, O, OH OH, HO, O (mannosyl ring)	17.**40**
—CHO	—OH	H	17.**41**
CH_2OH	H	H	17.**42**

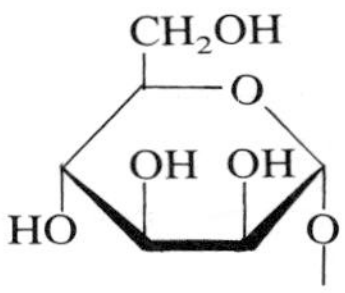

Mannosidostreptomycin (17.**40**), is another antibiotic, produced together with streptomycin by *S. griseus*, which has not found clinical application because it is less active than streptomycin itself. Hydroxystreptomycin (17.**41**), produced by *S. griseocarneus*, has biological properties similar to those of streptomycin, with no advantages over it. In the attempt to improve activity and/or decrease toxicity of streptomycin, some chemical modification have been performed (e.g., on aldehyde or guanidino functions), which yielded generally less active products. One chemical derivative of streptomycin, dihydrostreptomycin (17.**42**), obtained by catalytic hydrogenation of the carbonyl group of streptose, has almost the same antibacterial activity as the parent compound, and investigators hoped that it would differ from the parent in having lower toxicity. Later clinical experience did not confirm this evaluation (203).

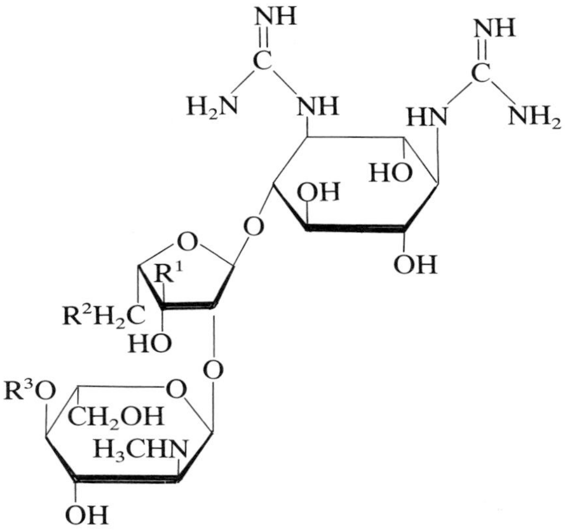

Streptomycin is both bacteriostatic and bactericidal for the tubercle bacillus *in vitro*, according to the concentration of antibiotic. Concentrations of streptomycin of the order of 1 μg/ml inhibit the growth of *M. tuberculosis* H 37 Rv. Atypical mycobacteria are not susceptible to streptomycin. The antibacterial activity of streptomycin is not restricted to *M. tuberculosis* but includes a variety of gram-positive and gram-negative bacteria, as well.

The most important clinical use of

streptomycin is in the therapy of tuberculosis, and it was the first really effective drug for this disease. The investigation of the mechanism of action of streptomycin has involved a number of very elegant studies of microbiological chemistry and molecular biology that have led to a succession of hypotheses and to a continuous increase in knowledge not only of the mode of action of the antibiotic, but also of the biology of the bacteria.

After the first hypotheses, which attributed the activity of streptomycin to some effects on terminal respiration (204) or on the bacterial membrane (205) or to an interaction with DNA (206), it was finally ascertained that the drug is a specific inhibitor of protein biosynthesis in intact bacteria (207, 208).

The ribosome, and particularly its 30S subunit, is the site of action of the antibiotic (209, 210) and, after careful disassemblage of 30S ribosomes, a protein designated as P10 was determined to be the genetic locus responsible for the phenotypic expression of sensitivity and resistance to and dependence on streptomycin (211). The antibiotic induces a misreading of the genetic code, as demonstrated through studies of the erroneous incorporation of amino acids in cell-free ribosome systems (212). It was deduced that the misreading *in vivo* was the cause of the bactericidal effect of streptomycin, since it resulted in "flooding the cell" with erroneous, hence nonfunctional, proteins. However it was subsequently demonstrated that this could not be the case because in the intact bacteria the antibiotic inhibits the synthesis of proteins (213).

The ultimate mode by which streptomycin exerts its bactericidal activity has not been elucidated. Two hypotheses have been put forward: one suggesting that streptomycin specifically inhibits initiation of protein synthesis (214) (this is supported by the involvement of protein P10, the site of action of streptomycin, in the initiation reaction), the other suggesting that it inhibits peptide chain elongation, that is, the synthesis of peptide bonds at any time during the growth of the peptide chain (215, 216).

As noted before, sensitivity and resistance to and dependence on streptomycin all seem to be expressed in the ribosome and apparently are multiple alleles of a single genetic locus. Streptomycin-resistant mutant cells arise spontaneously in a bacterial culture, with a frequency that is relatively low (217).

In the phenomenon of streptomycin dependence, bacteria require streptomycin to grow; these bacteria also arise by spontaneous mutations (218), and the mechanism of their behavior is also related to the reading of codons. This can be done correctly only in the presence of streptomycin, which overcomes an undiscriminating restriction (caused by mutation) leading to a mutant in which the ribosomal screen does not allow normal translation for growth (213–219).

In addition, resistance to streptomycin can be transferred by means of R-factors or plasmids, namely, by extrachromosomal DNA carrying multiple antibiotic resistance (220). The mode of transmission of resistance is particularly frequent among enterobacteria. The mechanism by which this type of resistance is expressed toward aminoglycosides is an enzymatic inactivation.

So far nine main aminoglycoside-inactivating enzymes are known: four phosphotransferases, three acetyltransferases, and two adenyltransferases. Since they act by inactivating some chemical group that is common to different aminoglycosides, bacterial strains that produce only one of them can be resistant to all aminoglycosides possessing the same chemical group (cross-resistance). Streptomycin can be inactivated by streptomycin-adenyltransferase and streptomycin-phosphotransferase, which usually do not affect other aminoglycosides except spectinomycin (221).

In mycobacteria, the incorporation of ^{14}C-phenylalanine into proteins directed by RNA from *M. smegmatis* and the incorporation of various ^{14}C-amino acids into proteins from *M. tuberculosis* H 37 Rv have been studied in the presence of streptomycin. The results confirmed that both sensitivity and resistance to streptomycin are ribosomal (109). What role the extrachromosomal resistance in mycobacteria plays has not been assessed, despite indications that such a role does exist (108).

From a pharmacological point of view, streptomycin behaves like the other members of the group. It is not absorbed from the gastrointestinal tract, and therefore it must be administered parenterally. Serum peak levels are reached in 1–2 hr, and the values are 9–15 μg/ml after administration of 0.5 g and 15–27 μg/ml after administration of 1 g. Its half-life is 2–3 hr. The serum protein binding of streptomycin is 25–35%, that of dihydrostreptomycin 15% (222).

Streptomycin diffuses slowly into the pleura, better into the peritoneal, pericardial, and synovial fluids. It does not penetrate into spinal fluid, unless the meninges are inflamed. Urinary elimination is rapid, and 70% of the drug is excreted in unmodified form in the first 24 hr.

The most important toxic effects of streptomycin involve the peripheral and central nervous systems. The eighth pair of cranial nerves is the most frequently injured by prolonged administration of streptomycin, especially in its vestibular portion, causing equilibrium disturbances to appear. Treatment with 2–3 g a day for 2–4 months produces this type of side effect in about 75% of patients, but the incidence is much less when administration is 1 g a day. Dihydrostreptomycin was thought to be less toxic than streptomycin, but clinical use showed that it causes severe damage to the cochlear portion of the eighth cranial nerve, often inducing irreversible impairment of auditory function. For this reason dihydrostreptomycin has been discarded. Other side effects are a hypersensitivity reaction and renal damage.

Since the introduction of other broad spectrum antibiotics, the use of streptomycin in the treatment of other infections is limited to diseases in which other alternatives are lacking and the sensitivity of the infective organism indicates the choice and eventually the use of this drug in combination with other antibiotics. Thus the therapeutic use of streptomycin is mainly restricted to tuberculosis, in combination with other antituberculous drugs, according to the schedules commonly accepted for treatment of this disease.

Another aminoglycoside antibiotic used in the therapy of tuberculosis was isolated as a fermentation product of *Streptomyces kanamyceticus* in 1957 and named kanamycin. It consist of three components; kanamycins A, B, and C. Kanamycin A (17.**43**) is the largest part of the mixture (98%). The molecule contains deoxystreptamine, instead of the streptidine present in the streptomycin molecule, and two amino sugars: kanosamine and 6-glucosamine. It is water soluble and stable at both acid and basic pH as well as at high temperature.

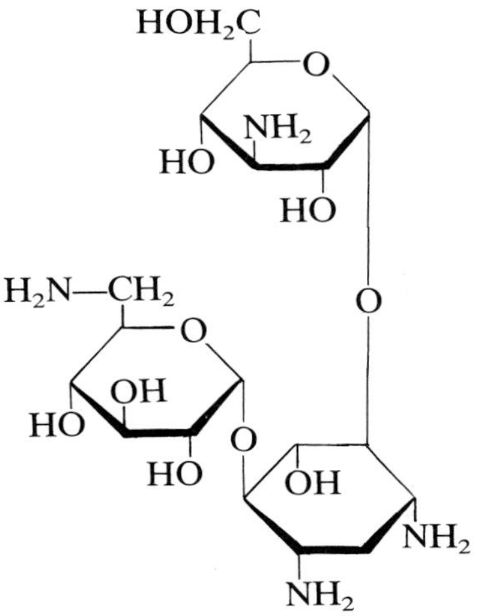

17.**43**

It has a quite broad spectrum of activity, including gram-positive cocci and gram-negative bacteria and, in addition, *M.*

tuberculosis and some atypical mycobacteria. Its activity against *M. tuberculosis* is weaker than that of streptomycin (223). The bactericidal concentrations are close to the bacteriostatic ones, but they are very hard to achieve *in vivo* (224).

The mechanism of action of kanamycin is similar to that of streptomycin, since it produces a misreading on the genetic code, interacting with 30 S ribosomal subunit in more than one site (whereas streptomycin is bound only to one site), and inhibits protein synthesis (225–227). All aminoglycoside antibiotics that cause miscoding contain a 2-deoxystreptamine or streptidine residue (streptomycin, kanamycin, neomycin, paromomycin, gentamicin, and hygromycin B); kasugamycin and spectinomycin, which lack this residue, do not induce miscoding (228). Kanamycin, like streptomycin and other aminoglycosides, blocks both initiation and elongation of peptide chains (229). The mechanism of action of kanamycin was confirmed in mycobacteria. *In vitro* studies on cell-free preparations of *M. bovis* have shown that kanamycin inhibits polypeptide synthesis, followed by breakdown of polysomes and detachment of mRNA (230). A kanamycin-induced increase in ^{14}C-isoleucine incorporation by poly-U-directed ribosomes indicated a misreading of the genetic code, but this did not seem to be directly related to the bactericidal action of the antibiotic. Resistance to kanamycin can be acquired *in vitro* in a stepwise fashion by subculturing bacteria in increasing concentration of antibiotic.

In addition to the chromosomal resistance, a resistance to kanamycin can be acquired by conjugation, thrôugh the transfer of extrachromosomal DNA, the so-called R-factors or plasmids, coding aminoglycoside-inactivating enzymes (phosphotransferases, acetyltransferases, and nucleotidyltransferases). Kanamycin A can be inactivated by neomycin–kanamycin phosphotransferases I and II, kanamycin acetyltransferase, and gentamicin adenyltransferases. Cross-resistance will appear to any other aminoglycoside antibiotic that may be inactivated by the same enzyme (221). Cross-resistance is total with neomycin and paromomycin. With streptomycin, a "one-way resistance" is observed, namely, strains resistant to kanamycin and neomycin are usually resistant to streptomycin, whereas streptomycin-resistant strains are usually susceptible to kanamycin and gentamicin. It has been suggested that this is due to different sites of action of the antibiotics on the ribosomes (231). Thus in therapy it is advisable to administer streptomycin before kanamycin.

From a pharmacokinetic point of view, kanamycin behaves very similarly to the other aminoglycosides: it is not absorbed when given by the oral route, but it is rapidly absorbed after intramuscular administration, reaching high peak serum level 2–3 hr after administration (232). There is almost no serum protein binding (222). Diffusion into cerebrospinal fluid is poor (236) when meninges are normal but increases when they are inflamed. Kanamycin diffuses quite well into pleural, peritoneal, synovial, and ascitic fluids (233, 234), but poorly into bile, feces, amniotic fluid, and so on. It is excreted by the kidney, mainly by glomerular filtration (50–80%), and for the most part in unmodified form. Kanamycin is used in therapy of infections caused by penicillin-resistant *Staphylococcus aureus* (now less frequently used because of the availability of penicillinase-resistant penicillins and other antistaphylococcal antibiotics) or to gram-negative bacilli, such as *E. coli*, *Klebsiella*, *Enterobacter*, and *Proteus*. It has no activity against *Pseudomonas*. It has been used in the therapy of tuberculosis, in combinations with other antituberculous drugs. The common dose is 15 mg/(kg)(day), but a total dose of 1.5 g must not be exceeded.

Drawbacks to the use of kanamycin are its ototoxicity and nephrotoxicity (234).

Cochlear and vestibular functions are damaged in about 5% of patients, but the percentage increases proportionally to the total dose administered. Thus in prolonged treatments, as in the case of tuberculosis, patients must be closely followed. Nephrotoxicity can be prevented if dosage to patients with decreased renal function is reduced according to the decrease in creatinine clearance or the increase in creatininemia (232). Kanamycin can produce phenomena of neurotoxicity, with curarelike effects due to neuromuscular blockade.

6.2.2 VIOMYCIN AND CAPREOMYCIN. Viomycin a basic peptide antibiotic (17.**44**) was discovered independently by two groups of investigators (82, 235) from an actinomycete named *Streptomyces puniceus* by one group and *S. floridae* by the other. Viomycin is relatively more active against the mycobacteria than against other species. It inhibits protein synthesis (236) but has no or very little miscoding activity (226). Viomycin reduced the amounts of dihydrostreptomycin bound to ribosomes of *M. smegmatis*, although they have different modes of action, perhaps because of a significant interaction between the binding sites of viomycin and streptomycin on ribosomes (237). Viomycin-resistant mutants isolated from *M. smegmatis* have altered ribosomes (238): one of these mutants had altered 50S subunits: others had altered 30S subunits. The genetic locus for viomycin-capreomycin resistance (*vic* locus) in *M. smegmatis* consisted of two groups, *vic*-A and *vic-B*. It is likely that alterations in the 30S subunit conferred by *vic*-B and alterations in the 50S subunit conferred by *vic*-A interact in response to viomycin (110). There is a one-way cross-resistance with kanamycin: viomycin-resistant strains may retain their susceptibility to kanamycin, but kanamycin-resistant strains are also resistant to viomycin. It is interesting to note that in *M. smegmatis*, the genetic locus for neomycin-kanamycin resistance (*nek* locus) is not linked to *str*-locus (for streptomycin resistance) as in *E. coli* but is linked to *vic*-locus (110).

On the whole, although viomycin is a peptide antibiotic, it behaves very like the aminoglycosides from an antibacterial and also a pharmacological point of view. The absorption and excretion of viomycin are similar to those of streptomycin. The usual daily dose is 1 g, i.m. Side effects produced by viomycin are severe and frequent: vestibular and auditory impairment, renal damage, and disturbance in the electrolyte balance have a very high incidence during viomycin therapy. For these reasons the drug is very seldom used.

Capreomycin is a polypeptide complex

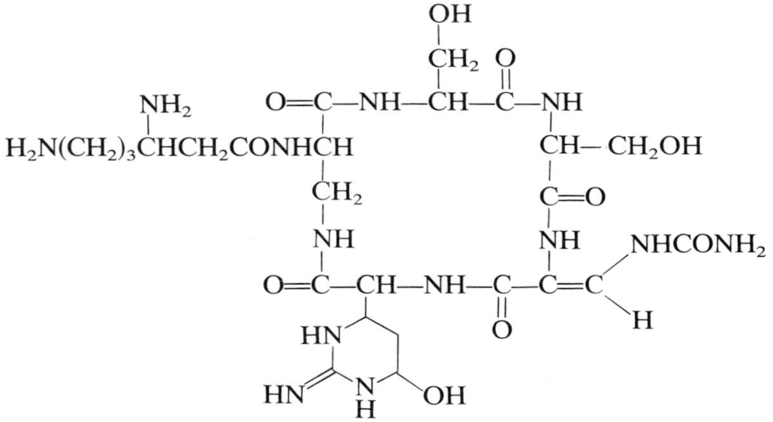

```
                                  OH
                                  |
                                  CH2  O
                                  |    ||
          NH2         O=C—NH—CH—C—NH
          |             |                 |
H2N(CH2)3CHCH2CONHCH                 CH—CH2OH
                        |                 |
                        CH2               C=O
                        |                 |
                        NH                NH     NHCONH2
                        |                 |     /
                  O=C—CH—NH—C—C=C
                          /        ||       \
                     HN            O         H
                     |
              HN=C   N      OH
                     H
```

17.**44**

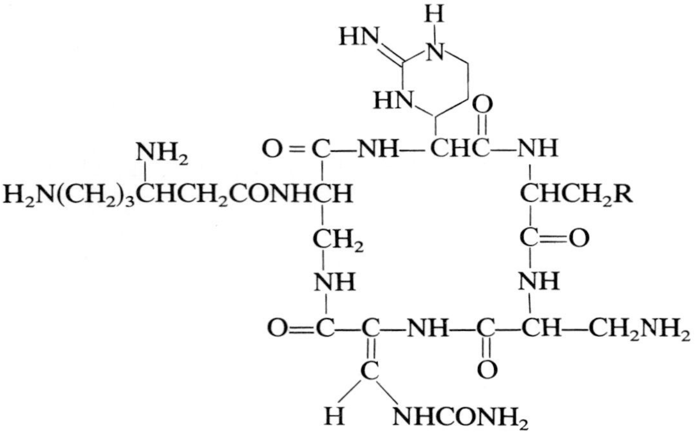

R = H
R = OH } 17.**45**

17.**46**

isolated from *Streptomycin capreolus* (239). The structure of some components of the complex (17.**45**), indicates the similarity with viomycin. It is active only against *M. tuberculosis* and some atypical mycobacteria, particularly *M. kansasii.* In its antibacterial and pharmacological activities it is very similar to the aminoglycosides.

Cross-resistance to kanamycin, neomycin, and viomycin has been described, and the phenomenon of partial "one-way resistance" to kanamycin has been demonstrated. Capreomycin-resistant strains are not always fully resistant to kanamycin, but kanamycin-resistant strains are always resistant to capreomycin.

The most common side effects are some damage to the auditory and renal functions and, sometimes, the appearance of anorexia with vomiting. The common daily dosage is 1 g, i.m. Its use is restricted to retreatment of chronic cases with resistant mycobacterial flora.

6.2.3 CYCLOSERINE. D-Cycloserine was isolated independently by several groups of workers from cultures of *Streptomyces garyphalus, S. orchidaceus,* and *S. lavendulae* (81, 240, 241). On the basis of degradation studies and physicochemical properties, the structure of D-4-amino-3-isoxazolidone (17.**46**) was assigned to this antibiotic (242, 243).

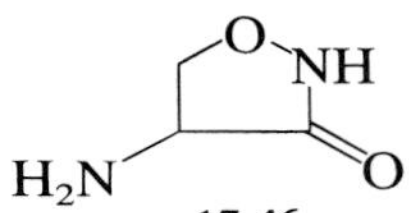

The structure was confirmed by synthesis (244), and various methods of preparation have been reported subsequently, which have also been used to prepare L-cycloserine from L-serine. Cycloserine inhibits *M. tuberculosis* at concentrations of 5–20 μg/ml. Strains resistant to other antimycobacterial drugs have the same sensitivity to cycloserine. The antibiotic is also active *in vitro* against a variety of gram-positive and gram-negative microorganisms, but only in culture media free of D-alanine, which antagonizes the antibacterial activity of cycloserine (245, 246). *In vivo,* cycloserine was ineffective against experimental tuberculosis in mice and was marginally effective in guinea pigs, but some activity was found against the disease induced in the monkey. The drug is more effective in man than in animals. The explanation of the different responses resides in the different pharmacokinetic properties of cycloserine in the various animal species. When given orally to man, cycloserine is well and quickly absorbed from the gastrointestinal tract and is well distributed in the body fluids and tissues. The usual dose for adults is 250 mg twice a day orally, always in combination with other effective tuberculostatic agents. About half the ingested dose is excreted unchanged in the urine in 24 hr. A part of the antibiotic is metabolized into products not yet identified.

Cycloserine produces in the central nervous system severe side effects that can also generate psychotic states with suicidal tendencies and epileptic convulsions. Therefore its use is limited only to cases in which other drugs cannot be used.

The mechanism of action of cycloserine on mycobacteria has not been studied, but it has been proved in other bacterial species that this antibiotic interferes with the synthesis of the cell wall. In fact, cycloserine induces the formation of protoplasts in *E. coli.* Microorganisms treated with cycloserine accumulate a muramic-uridine-nucleotide-peptide, which differs from that produced by penicillin in the absence of the terminal D-alanine dipeptide. The inhibition of alanine racemase, which converts L-alanine into D-alanine, is probably the primary action of cycloserine (247–249). It is rather surprising that synthetic L-cycloserine has antibacterial activity also, but presumably it acts through a different mechanism of action that has not been clarified.

Some chemical variations of the structure of cycloserine failed to yield products with improved antimycobacterial activity.

6.2.4 RIFAMPICIN.* The rifamycin antibiotics were discovered as metabolites of a microorganism originally considered to belong to the genus *Streptomyces* and subsequently reclassified as a *Nocardia* (*N. mediterranea*) (250–252). The crude material extracted from the fermentation broths contained several rifamycins (rifamycin-complex) (86). Only rifamycin B was isolated as a pure crystalline substance, and it is essentially the only component found when sodium diethylbarbiturate is added to the fermentation media (253).

Rifamycin B (17.**47**) has the unusual property that in oxygenated aqueous solutions, it tends to change spontaneously into other products with greater antibacterial activity (rifamycin O, 17.**48**; rifamycin S, 17.**49**). Rifamycin SV (17.**50**), was obtained from rifamycin S (85, 86, 254) by mild reduction. The structures of rifamycin

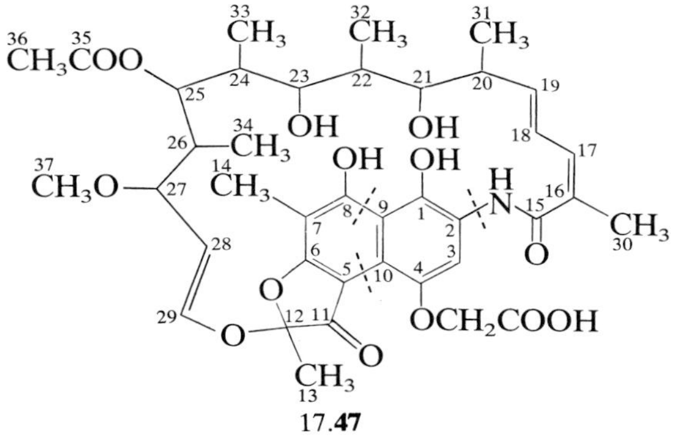

17.**47**

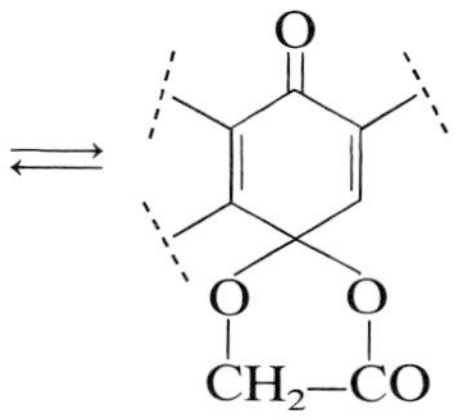

17.**48**

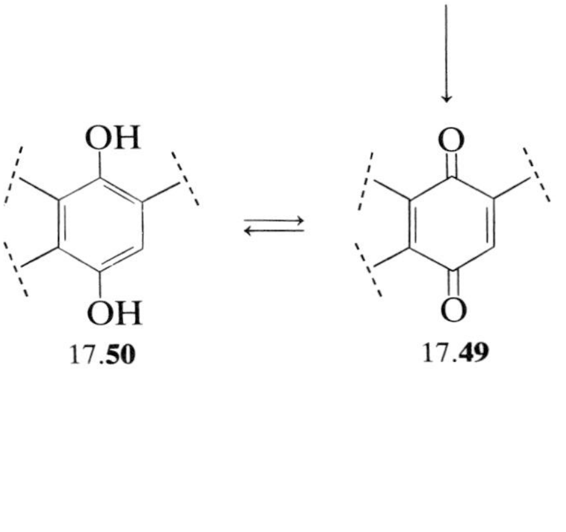

17.**50**

17.**49**

* The United States adopted name is rifampin.

B and of the related compounds involved in the "activation" process have been elucidated by chemical and X-ray crystallographic methods (255–257).

The rifamycins are the first natural substances to have been assigned an *ansa* structure consisting of an aromatic moiety spanned by an aliphatic bridge. At present several natural substances with ansa structures are known, and for those that are metabolites of Actinomycetales, the general name of "ansamycins" has been proposed (258). Streptovaricins (259, 260), tolypomycins (261, 262), and halomycins (263) are other ansamycins, structurally and biogenetically related to rifamycins, which also have in common activity against mycobacteria, gram-positive and, to a lesser extent, gram-negative bacteria.

Among the first rifamycins, the sodium salt of rifamycin SV was considered for clinical use because of its high antibacterial activity *in vitro*, low toxicity, and good local tolerance when dissolved in polyvinylpyrrolidone solutions (264–267). Rifamycin SV is partially and very irregularly absorbed from the gastrointestinal tract. When administered parenterally, the drug is rapidly eliminated through the bile (266). Thus in spite of the high *in vitro* activity against *M. tuberculosis* (of the order of 0.1 μg/ml) (267), the doses of rifamycin SV required to control experimental tuberculosis in the animal are very high (265). Also in human tuberculosis, rifamycin SV gives modest results (268–270). Only topical treatment of pleuropulmonary and extrapulmonary tuberculosis gave good results in the majority of cases (271).

Several authors (272–278) obtained encouraging results in short-term treatments of leprosy: the results obtained with 1–6 months of treatment were comparable to those obtained with 9 months of treatment with other antileprosy drugs, including sulfones (273). Improvements from the clinical and bacteriological standpoints were observed in patients treated for 8 months with rifamycin SV, 0.5–1 g daily (277), but some patients developed erythema nodosum leprosum. These preliminary results notwithstanding, rifamycin SV is not in current therapeutic use for leprosy, mainly because the need for frequent intramuscular injections makes the treatment unacceptable.

Several hundred derivatives of rifamycin B have been prepared with the aim of obtaining a compound that would have the following advantages over rifamycin SV: oral absorption and more prolonged therapeutic levels in the host, higher activity in the treatment of mycobacterial infections, and higher activity in infections caused by gram-negative bacteria (84).

Chemical modifications have been made on the glycolic chain of rifamycin B, on the aliphatic ansa, and on the chromophoric nucleus. A great deal of information about the structure-activity relationships has been obtained (84, 279, 280). All rifamycins possessing a free carboxy group are partially or totally inactive because they do not enter into bacterial cell. The minimal requirements for activity appear to be the presence of two free hydroxyls in positions 21 and 23 on the ansa chain and of two polar groups (either free hydroxyl or carbonyl) at positions 1 and 8 of the naphthoquinone nucleus, together with a conformation of the ansa chain that results in certain specific geometrical relationships among these four functional groups.

This conclusion is based on the following data. (*a*) Substitution or elimination of the 21- or 23-hydroxyls gives inactive products. (*b*) Modifications of the ansa chain that alter its conformation (e.g., 16–17 and 18–19 mono- and diepoxy derivatives) give inactive or less active products. Also, the stepwise hydrogenation of the ansa chain double bonds results in a gradual decrease in activity as a consequence of the increase in flexibility of the ansa diverging from the most active conformation. (*c*) The oxygenated function at carbons 1 and 8 must be either free hydroxyl or carbonyl for maintaining the biological activity. (*d*) All modifications at the 3(4)-positions that do not interfere with the previous requirements do not affect the activity of the products (84, 279, 280).

The nature of the substituents at the 3(4)-positions influences the physicochemical properties of the derivatives, especially lipophilicity. The various derivatives show a minor degree of variation in antibacterial activity against intact cells, because the transport through bacterial wall and membrane is the major factor affected by these substituents (281). Other biological characteristics influenced by the various modifications of the 3(4)-positions are absorption from the gastrointestinal tract and the kinetics of elimination.

Among the earlier derivatives of the glycolic side chain, the diethylamide of rifamycin B, rifamide (17.**51**), had a better therapeutic index than rifamycin SV (282). It was introduced into clinical use in some countries, but it still suffers from most of the limitations of use of rifamycin SV (283).

When the 3-formylrifamycin SV (17.**52**) was prepared by oxidation of *N*-dialkylaminomethyl rifamycin SV (284), it was found that many of its *N,N*-disubstituted hydrazones had very high activity, both *in vitro* and *in vivo*, against *M. tuberculosis* and gram-positive bacteria, and moderate activity against gram-negative bacteria. For some of these derivatives the *in vivo* activity in animal infections was of the same order whether the products were administered orally or parenterally, indicating good absorption from the gastrointestinal tract (84).

The hydrazone of 3-formylrifamycin SV with *N*-amino-*N*′-methylpiperazine (rifampicin, 17.**53**) (84, 285) was the most active *in vivo* and was selected for clinical use. Rifampicin is active *in vitro* against *M. tuberculosis* at concentrations below 1 μg/ml in semisynthetic media. It is active against other gram-positive bacteria at lower concentrations and against gram-negative bacteria at concentrations of 1–20 μg/ml. Rifampicin is active at the same concentrations against strains resistant to other antibiotics and antimycobacterials. The bactericidal activity of rifampicin is demonstrated at concentrations close to the static ones. It is possible to isolate strains resistant to rifampicin from mycobacterial cultures exposed to the antibiotic, but the frequency of resistant mutants to rifampicin in sensitive populations of *M. tuberculosis* is lower than to other antimycobacterial drugs (286). Rifampicin is also active against many atypical mycobacteria, although at concentrations generally higher than those effective against *M. tuberculosis*.

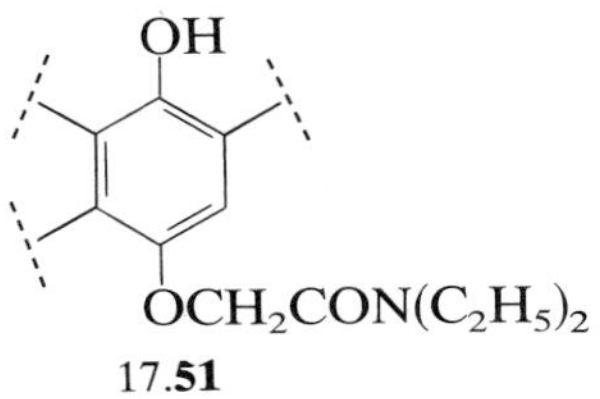

OH

$OCH_2CON(C_2H_5)_2$

17.**51**

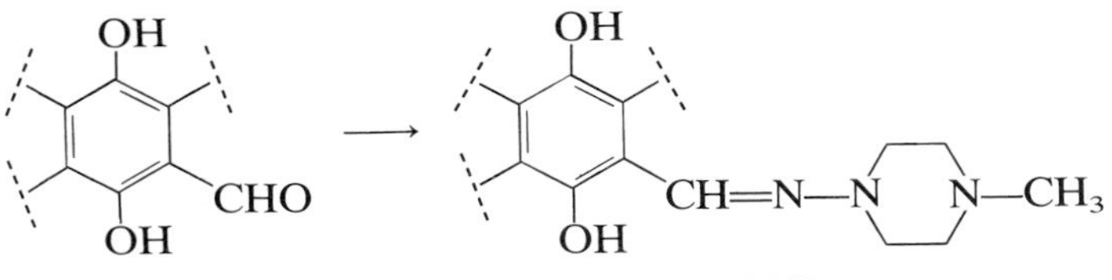

OH CHO OH → OH $CH{=}N{-}N\quad N{-}CH_3$ OH

17.**52** 17.**53**

Among the atypical mycobacteria tested, *M. kansasii* and *M. marinum* are the most sensitive (287).

There is no evidence of cross-resistance among rifampicin and other antibiotics or antituberculous drugs (288). Transfer of resistance to rifampicin could not be obtained.

Preliminary laboratory studies on the *in vivo* antituberculous activity (289) showed that the efficacy of rifampicin in experimental infections in mice was comparable to that of isoniazid and markedly superior to that of streptomycin, kanamycin, and ethionamide. In guinea pigs it was comparable to streptomycin. Rifampicin is also remarkably active in experimental infections due to gram-positive and gram-negative bacteria (289).

The excellent antituberculous activity of rifampicin *in vivo* was confirmed by other experiments in many laboratories using various animal models (mice, guinea pigs, rabbits) and various schedules of treatment and criteria of evaluation (290–300). The overall results indicate that rifampicin has a high bactericidal effect and a therapeutic efficacy of the order of that of isoniazid and superior to all the other antituberculous drugs. The combination of rifampicin plus isoniazid has been shown to produce a more rapid, complete, and durable sterilization of infected animals than other combinations (293). Rifampicin has a very low toxicity according to acute, subacute, and chronic toxicity studies in several animals species (84, 301). Results of animal and human studies showed no toxic effect on ear (302) and eye. After oral administration, rifampicin has excellent absorption in animals and man (303). In humans, after administration of 150 and 300 mg, serum levels reach maximum values around the second hour and persist, as appreciable values beyond the eighth and twelfth hour, respectively. When the dose is increased, serum levels are very high and long lasting. Generally the serum levels found at the beginning of treatment are higher than the levels that gradually set in as treatment continues. This phenomenon occurs during the first few weeks of treatment (304, 305). The half-life of rifampicin is of the order of 3 hr and increases in patients with biliary obstruction or liver diseases (306–308). Rifampicin shows a very good distribution in the tissues and crosses the blood-brain barrier. It reaches good antibacterial levels in cavern exudate and in pleural fluid.

Rifampicin is eliminated through both the bile and the urine. It appears rapidly in the bile, where it reaches very high concentrations that last even when the antibiotic is not measurable in the serum. After reaching the threshold of hepatic eliminatory capacity, biliary levels do not increase with an increased dosage, but serum and urinary levels do.

In man, rifampicin is mainly metabolized to 25-*O*-desacetylrifampicin (309), which is only slightly less active than the parent drug against *M. tuberculosis*, but considerably less active against some other bacteria. Both rifampicin and desacetylrifampicin are excreted in high concentrations in the bile. Rifampicin is reasorbed from the gut, forming an enterohepatic cycle, but the desacetyl derivative is poorly absorbed, thus is excreted with the feces. Rifampicin has a stimulating effect on microsomal drug metabolizing enzymes (310).

Many clinical trials have confirmed the efficacy of rifampicin in a variety of bacterial infections (311). In particular, rifampicin is now largely used for the treatment of human tuberculosis both for newly diagnosed patients and for patients whose primary chemotherapy has failed. In the normal treatment rifampicin is administered orally at dose of 600 mg daily in combination with other antituberculous drugs, mainly isoniazid. Adverse reactions to daily rifampicin are uncommon and usually trivial. The most frequent ill effects are cutaneous reactions and gastrointestinal disturbances. Rifampicin can also disturb liver function, but the risk of its causing serious or permanent liver damage is small, particularly among patients with no previous history of liver disease.

In the case of intermittent therapy, when the drug is given three times, twice, or once a week, a high incidence of severe untoward effects (such as the "flulike" syndrom and cytotoxic reactions) may result. These adverse reactions seem to be associated with rifampicin dependent antibodies, suggesting their immunological basis. However with proper adjustment of the size of each single dose, of the interval between doses, and of the length of treatment, it has been possible to develop intermittent regimens with rifampicin that are highly effective and acceptably safe (312).

Rifampicin in very active against *M. leprae*, suppressing the multiplication and the viability of the bacilli infecting laboratory animals (313–317). In human leprosy (313–319), the treatment with rifampicin alone or in combination with other antileprosy drugs gave very favorable results in almost all the patients. In particular, the variations of the morphological index and, when carried out, the mouse footpad inoculation, showed the rapid and constant bactericidal action of rifampicin. The same effect was observed in many patients who had become resistant to other antileprosy drugs.

Rifampicin, like the other rifamycins, acts on the bacteria by inhibiting specifically the activity of the enzyme DNA-directed RNA-polymerase (DDRP). The mammalian DDRP is resistant even to very high concentrations of rifamycins (97, 98). In bacteria the rifamycins inhibit the initiation of RNA synthesis, forming a rather stable equimolecular complex with bacterial DDRP, but they have no effect on chain elongation. Bacterial mutants resistant to rifamycins possess an altered RNA polymerase that is not inhibited by rifamycins. Most of the studies on the mechanism of action of rifamycins have been performed using *E. coli* (320–323). The inhibitory effect of rifampicin on DDRP as the cause of its bactericidal activity has been verified on several mycobacterial species, e.g., *M. smegmatis*, *M. bovis BCG*, *M. tuberculosis* (99–102). Also in the case of *M. tuberculosis*, rifampicin inhibits the initiation of the RNA chain, but not its elongation.

Electron microscopy studies (103, 104) have shown that treatment of cells of *M. tuberculosis* with rifampicin causes a loss of the compact structure of the cytoplasm. Ribosomes become irregular, and the normal structure of mesosomes disappears. However nucleus, cytoplasmic membrane, and cell wall seem to be normal. The changes are apparently due to the blocking effect of rifampicin on RNA polymerase, which in turn leads to disturbances in protein synthesis. The rate of incorporation of ^{14}C-rifampicin is similar in both resistant and susceptible strains of *M. phlei*.

The mechanism of resistance probably involves a change in the structure of RNA polymerase, rather than differences in cell permeability. However both a strain of *M. intracellulare* and a strain of *M. smegmatis*, ATCC 607, which were resistant to rifampicin, demonstrated a permeability barrier, and the RNA polymerase was found to be susceptible to rifampicin. Probably different causes of resistance in mycobacteria must be considered (324).

7 PRESENT STATUS OF THE CHEMOTHERAPY OF TUBERCULOSIS AND LEPROSY

Chemotherapy has been the most potent and useful tool for modifying the evolution and prognosis of tuberculosis, having reached the goal of eradicating tuberculosis from some countries. To be efficacious, however, certain rules must be followed in its application, because of the biology of the tubercle bacillus and the chronicity of the disease. It must be emphasized that the success of chemotherapy is strictly related to the appropriate use of combinations of drugs. It is a fundamental rule to use at least two or, better, three drugs, to avoid the emergence of bacterial resistance, which is the principal cause of therapeutic failure. In fact, mutants resistant to one or possibly to more drugs are present in the bacterial population and will prevail when sensitive organisms have been killed by the active drug (325). Since chemotherapy is prescribed after diagnosis of the disease without knowing the susceptibility of the mycobacteria, it is considered safer to administer three drugs, to avoid the risk of possible ineffectiveness of more than one drug. Later, in a maintenance regimen, a double-drug regimen may be indicated.

During the last 15 years different combinations and different regimens have been tried, with effective treatments of 90–100% of the cases. The choice of combinations and regimens has been based on the properties of the different drugs, particularly on their bactericidal activity, intracellular penetrability, resistance patterns of mycobacteria, *in vivo* activities, pharmacological and pharmacokinetic behavior, and toxicity (326).

The triple-drug combination most commonly used in the past for initial treatment has been streptomycin (1 g/day, i.m.) isoniazid (300–800 mg, p.o.), and *p*-aminosalicylic acid (12–15 p.o. or by i.v. infusion) for 30–90 days.

The maintenance regimen that usually followed the first phase was planned according to the results of the antibiogram and consisted of two or three drugs, for example, streptomycin and isoniazid, then isoniazid and ethambutol for 18–24 months or more, shifting to other possible associations every 3–6 months to avoid the prevalence of surviving resistant mutants (327, 328).

A new direction to antituberculous therapy was given in 1967 by the introduction into therapy of rifampicin. This drug has a very high bactericidal activity against mycobacteria, which, in addition, shows a low rate of development of resistance to it. Since then, the drugs of first choice for the initial treatment have been isoniazid, rifampicin, streptomycin, and ethambutol. Drugs of second choice are pyrazinamide, ethionamide (and its congener prothionamide), kanamycin, cycloserin, viomycin, and capreomycin (329–331). The less effective drugs, *p*-aminosalicylic acid and thioacetazone, are less frequently used, with the exception of thioacetazone (332–335), which because of its cheapness is still widely employed in some parts of the developing world.

Because of the high therapeutic activity of the combination of the first-choice drugs and particularly of the isoniazid-rifampicin-ethambutol combination, some trials have been performed in which the drugs were administered intermittently, that is, 2–3 times a week, at the usual daily dosage used in the traditional regimens. Better results are obtained when the intermittent administration is preceded by 1–3 months of continuous administration (336–344). The aim of this regimen is to reduce the dosage of the drugs, to avoid or decrease toxic side effects. Even though the therapeutic results are satisfactory, various aspects of this therapeutic modality remain to be assessed to reduce the high incidence of severe phenomena of hypersensitivity to rifampicin (312, 345–349).

Recently attempts have been made all over the world to shorten the period of therapy (350–352). The most successful regimens for short-course treatment of tuberculosis include rifampicin and isoniazid. In fact, the treatments based on the isoniazid-streptomycin combination with the addition of a third drug (*p*-aminosalicylic acid, ethambutol, or thioacetazone) must be continued for at least 18 months to minimize or avoid relapses after discontinuation, while the treatments based on the isoniazid-rifampicin combination with the addition of a third drug for the first 2–3 months achieve the same or better results in 6–9 months.

It has been suggested that certain drug combinations are so highly effective in short-course therapy because of the presence of at least two bactericidal drugs (352). It has also been postulated that the possibility of obtaining good results in short treatment is linked to bactericidal activity against both dividing and resting bacilli (353). On this regard, the combination of rifampicin with pyrazinamide is taken in serious consideration. In fact, since rifampicin kills bacilli *in vitro* after very short exposure, it might be capable of killing persisting bacilli that start to multiply (354, 355). On the other hand, pyrazinamide, since it penetrates cells and is active in the acid intracellular environment, is in a position to kill intracellular resting bacilli (356). In conclusion, both for doctrinal implications and from the clinical results, the short-course treatment of tuberculosis is a very promising new approach, which may well be a new important turning point in the struggle against this disease.

In the treatment of leprosy, sulfones—particularly dapsone—continue to be the drugs of choice, even though their efficacy cannot be considered to be satisfactory. In fact, it usually takes more than 5 years of continuous therapy to render lepromatous patients bacilli negative. On the other hand, these drugs prevent the evolution of the indeterminate form of leprosy to the lepromatous type (357–362).

Other drugs endowed with activity against *M. leprae*, and usually employed when resistance to dapsone appears, are clofazimine, thiambutosine, long-acting sulfonamides, thioacetazone, ethionamide, and rifampicin. Their activities and their roles in routine therapy have not yet been assessed.

So far, the treatment of choice in routine treatment of leprosy is the oral administration of dapsone at a dosage of 6–10 mg/kg, from the beginning of therapy, with a weekly maximum dosage that must not exceed 600 mg. Some investigators and the US Public Health Service suggest that therapy be started with a gradually increasing dosage (358). The total weekly dose can be divided so that it is given once per day for 6 days of the week; or twice a week or even once a week.

Because of the social and environmental conditions in which leprosy develops, the conduct of therapy must be adapted to the actual possibilities with respect to the sanitary facilities of the region in which the patients live. It is essential to convince patients that continuity of therapy is of vital importance.

Intramuscular treatment can be given with acedapsone, a depot form of dapsone, which can be administered every 15 days. It is recommended that all outpatients on oral dapsone should also receive acedapsone every 10–12 weeks (225 mg in adults), after sulfone allergy has been excluded (359, 362–364).

Dapsone resistance has been reported, but it seems to occur in a limited number of cases, and the existence of this condition is based on clinical observation. Because of the difficulties in testing the sensitivity of *M. leprae* to chemotherapeutic agents, this assumption cannot be exhaustively documented. There are remarkable differences in the rates of development of resistance depending on the countries in which the investigations are carried out.

Dapsone-resistant leprosy can be treated with thiambutosine orally (from 0.5 g at the beginning to 1.5 g daily) or intramuscularly (maximum dosage, 1 g once a week). At present the most common trend is to administer the drugs in combination, particularly, rifampicin-clofazimine and/or thioacetazone, rifampicin-ethionamide and/or thioacetazone, clofazimine-ethionamide-thioacetazone, and so on. It is at present suggested that these combinations also be used in untreated cases to prevent resistance. Whether these regimens can achieve better results must be assessed through extensive trials. On the basis of the results so far obtained in the therapy of tuberculosis with drug combinations, it seems reasonable to expect that in leprosy also they will achieve more radical and rapid negativation than does monochemotherapy.

Reactions during chemotherapy are of two main types, namely, erythema nodosum leprosum, and reversal reactions; and they are usually controlled with prednisolone. In the most severe cases of ENL, thalidomide can be efficacious, but its administration must be restricted to the cases not responding to other drugs and must be strictly supervised because of its well-known teratogenic activity (357).

REFERENCES

1. G. S. Wilson and A. A. Miles, *Topley and Wilson's Principles of Bacteriology and Immunity,* Arnold., London, 1975.
2. M. Castets, N. Rist, and H. Boisvert, *Bull. Soc. Med. Afr. Noire Lang. Fr.,* **16,** 221 (1969).
3. E. H. Runyon, *Advn. Tuberc. Res.,* **14,** 235 (1965).
4. R. Buttiaux, H. Beerens, and A. Tacquet, *Manuel de Techniques Bactériologiques,* 4th ed., Flammarion Medécine Sciences, Paris, 1974.
5. G. Canetti and J. Grosset, *Techniques et Indications des Examens Bactériologiques en Tuberculose,* Editions de la Tourelle, St. Mandé, 1968.
6. G. A. Snow, *Bacteriol. Rev.,* **34,** 99 (1970).
7. E. Lederer, *Pure Appl. Chem.,* **25,** 135 (1971).
8. E. Lederer, A. Adam, R. Ciorbarn, J. F. Petit, and J. Wietzerbin, *Mol. Cell. Biochem.,* **7,** 87 (1975).
9. M. B. Goren, *Bacteriol. Rev.,* **36,** 33 (1972).
10. T. Ramakrishnan, M. Suryanarayana Murthy, and K. P. Gopinathan, *Bacteriol. Rev.,* **36,** 65 (1972).
11. L. P. Macham and C. Ratledge, *J. Gen. Microbiol.,* **89,** 379 (1975).
12. L. Barksdale and K. S. Kim, *Bacteriol. Rev.,* **41,** 217 (1977).
13. W. Segal and U. Block, *J. Bacteriol.,* **72,** 132 (1956).
14. W. Segal and U. Block, *Am. Rev. Tuberc. Pulm. Dis.,* **75,** 495 (1957).
15. W. Segal and W. T. Miller, *Proc. Soc. Exp. Biol. Med.,* **118,** 613 (1965).
16. W. Segal, *Proc. Soc. Exp. Biol. Med.,* **118,** 214 (1965).
17. G. Middlebrook, C. M. Coleman, and W. B. Schaefer, *Proc. Nat. Acad. Sci.,* US, **45,** 1801 (1959).
18. W. Segal, *Am. Rev. Respir. Dis.,* **91,** 285 (1965).
19. K. Kanai, *Japan J. Med. Sci. Biol.,* **20,** 401 (1967).
20. K. Kanai, *Japan J. Med. Sci. Biol.,* **20,** 73 (1967).
21. K. Kanai, *Japan J. Med. Sci. Biol.,* **20,** 91 (1967).
22. E. Kondo, K. Kanai, K. Nishimura, and T. Tsumita, *Japan J. Med. Sci. Biol.,* **23,** 315 (1970).
23. K. Kanai, E. Wiegeshaus, and D. W. Smith, *Japan J. Med. Sci. Biol.,* **23,** 327 (1970).
24. H. N. Jayaram, T. Ramakrishnan, and C. S. Vaidyanathan, *Arch. Biochem. Biophys.,* **126,** 165 (1968).
25. H. N. Jayaram, T. Ramakrishnan, and C. S. Vaidyanathan, *Indian J. Biochem.,* **6,** 106 (1969).
26. S. Kotani, T. Kitaura, T. Hirano, and A. Tanaka, *Biken's J.* **2,** 129 (1959).
27. K. Takaya, K. Hisatsune, and J. Inoue, *J. Bacteriol.,* **59,** 388 (1966).
28. F. Kanetsuna, *Biochim. Biophys. Acta,* **158,** 130 (1968).
29. J. Asselineau, *The Bacterial Lipids,* Hermann, Paris, and Holden Day, San Francisco, 1966, p. 176.
30. E. Lederer, *Chem. Phys. Lipids,* **1,** 294 (1967).
31. A. H. Etémadi and J. Convit, *Infect. Immun.* **10,** 236 (1974).
32. A. H. Etémadi, *Exp. Ann. Biochem. Med.,* **28,** 77 (1967).
33. J. Azuma and Y. Yamamura, *J. Biochem.,* **52,** 200 (1962).
34. J. Azuma and Y. Yamamura, *J. Biochem.,* **53,** 275 (1963).
35. N. P. V. Acharya, M. Senn, and E. Lederer, *C. R. Acad. Sci., Paris, Ser. C,* **264,** 2173 (1967).
36. J. W. Berg, *Proc. Soc. Exp. Biol. Med.,* **84,** 196 (1953).
37. J. W. Berg, *Yale J. Biol. Med.,* **26,** 215 (1953).
38. J. Markovits, E. Vilkas, and E. Lederer, *Eur. J. Biochem.,* **18,** 287 (1971).
39. F. Kanetsuma, *Biochim. Biophys. Acta,* **98,** 476 (1965).
40. H. Bloch, *J. Exp. Med.,* **91,** 197 (1950).

41. H. Noll, H. Bloch, J. Asselineau, and E. Lederer, *Biochim. Biophys. Acta*, **20,** 299 (1956).
42. E. Dàrzins and G. Fahar, *Dis. Chest*, **30,** 642 (1956).
43. G. Middlebrook, R. J. Dubos, and C. Pierce, *J. Exp. Med.*, **88,** 521 (1948).
44. D. W. Smith, H. M. Randall, A. P. McLennan, and E. Lederer, *Nature*, **186,** 887 (1960).
45. A. P. McLennan, D. W. Smith, and H. M. Randall, *Biochem. J.*, **80,** 309 (1961).
46. G. Lanéelle and J. Asselineau, *Eur. J. Biochem.*, **5,** 487 (1968).
47. P. R. S. Gangadharam, M. L. Cohn, and G. Middlebrook, *Tubercle*, **44,** 452 (1963).
48. M. Kato and M. B. Goren, *Japan J. Med. Sci. Biol.*, **27,** 120 (1974).
49. P. Pigretti, E. Vilkas, E. Lederer, and H. Bloch, *Bull. Soc. Chim. Biol.*, **47,** 2039 (1965).
50. A. M. Lowell, in *Tuberculosis*, American Public Health Association, Ed., Harvard University Press, Cambridge, Mass., 1969.
51. P. T. Chapman, in *Communicable and Infectious Diseases*, 7th ed., F. H. Top and P. F. Wehrle, Eds., Mosby., St Louis, 1972, p. 694.
52. L. M. Bechelli and V. Martinez Dominguez, *Bull. W. H. O.*, **34,** 811 (1966).
53. L. M. Bechelli and V. Martinez Dominguez, *Bull. W. H. O.*, **46,** 523 (1972).
54. L. H. Schmidt, *Am. Rev. Tuberc.*, **74,** 138 (1956).
55. L. H. Schmidt, *Ann. N. Y. Acad. Sci.*, **135,** 747 (1966).
56. C. C. Shepard, *J. Exp. Med.*, **112,** 445 (1960).
57. C. C. Shepard and Y. T. Chang, *Proc. Soc. Exp. Biol. Med.*, **109,** 636 (1962).
58. R. J. W. Rees, *J. Exp. Pathol.*, **45** (1960).
59. R. J. W. Rees, J. M. H. Pearson, and M. F. R. Waters, *Brit. Med. J.*, **1,** 89 (1970).
60. W. F. Kirchheimer and E. E. Storrs, *Int. J. Lepr.*, **39,** 693 (1971).
61. E. E. Storrs, G. P. Walsh, H. P. Burchfield, and C. H. Binford, *Science*, **183,** 851 (1974).
62. T. Murohashi and K. Yoshida, *Acta Leprol.*, **54,** 31 (1974).
63. E. E. Camargo, S. M. Larson, B. S. Teper, and H. N. Wagner, *Int. J. Lepr.*, **43,** 234 (1975).
64. W. T. Colwell, G. Chan, V. H. Brown, J. I. De Graw, J. H. Peters, and N. E. Morrison, *J. Med. Chem.*, **17,** 142 (1974).
65. N. E. Morrison, *Int. J. Lepr.*, **39,** 34 (1971).
66. N. Rist, *C. R. Soc. Biol.*, **130,** 972 (1939).
67. W. H. Feldman, H. C. Hinshaw, and H. E. Moses, *Proc. Staff Meet. Mayo Clin.*, **15,** 695 (1940).
68. R. Behnisch, F. Mietzsch, and H. Schmidt, *Am. Rev. Tuberc.*, **61,** 1 (1950).
69. C. F. Huebner, J. L. Marsh, R. H. Mizzoni, R. P. Mull, D. C. Schroeder, H. A. Traxell, and C. R. Scholtz, *J. Am. Chem. Soc.*, **75,** 2274 (1953).
70. N. P. Buu-Hoi and N. D. Xuong, *Compt. Rend.*, **237,** 498 (1953).
71. H. H. Fox, *Science*, **116,** 129 (1952).
72. V. Chorine, *Compt. Rend.*, **220,** 150 (1945).
73. S. Kushner, H. Dalalian, J. L. Sanjurio, F. L. Bach, Jr., S. R. Safir, V. K. Smith, Jr., and J. H. Williams, *J. Am. Chem. Soc.*, **74,** 3617 (1952).
74. T. S. Gardner, E. Wenis, and J. Lee, *J. Org. Chem.*, **19,** 753 (1954).
75. F. Grumbach, N. Rist, D. Libermann, M. Moyeaux, S. Cals, and S. Clavel, *Compt. Rend.*, **242,** 2187 (1956).
76. F. Bernheim, *J. Bacteriol.*, **41,** 385 (1941).
77. J. Lehmann, *Lancet*, **1,** 15 (1946).
78. J. P. Thomas, C. O. Baughn, R. G. Wilkinson, and R. G. Shepherd, *Am. Rev. Respir. Dis.*, **83,** 891 (1961).
79. R. G. Wilkinson, R. G. Shepherd, J. P. Thomas, and C. Baughn, *J. Am. Chem. Soc.*, **83,** 2212 (1961).
80. A. Schatz, E. Bugie, and S. A. Waksman, *Proc. Soc. Exp. Biol. Med.*, **55,** 66 (1944).
81. R. L. Harned, P. H. Hidy, and E. K. La Baw, *Antibiot. Chemother.*, **5,** 204 (1955).
82. A. C. Finlay, G. L. Hobby, F. Hochstein, T. M. Lees, T. F. Lenert, J. A. Menas, S. Y. P'An, P. P. Regna, Y. B. Routien, B. A. Sabin, K. B. Tat, and Y. H. Kane, *Am. Rev. Respir. Dis.*, **63,** 1 (1951).
83. H. Umezawa, M. Ueda, K. Maeda, K. Yagishita, S. Korido, Y. Okami, R. Utahara, Y. Osato, K. Nitta, and T. Tacheuchi, *J. Antibiot. (Tokyo), Ser A*, **10,** 181 (1957).
84. P. Sensi, N. Maggi, S. Furesz, and G. Maffii, *Antimicrob. Agents Chemother.*, **1966,** 699.
85. P. Sensi, M. T. Timbal, and G. Maffii, *Experientia*, **16,** 412 (1960).
86. P. Sensi, A. M. Greco, and R. Ballotta, *Antibiot. Ann.*, 262 (1959–1960).
87. V. C. Barry, J. G. Belton, M. L. Conalty, J. M. Denneny, D. W. Edward, J. F. O'Sullivan, D. Twomey, and F. Winder, *Nature*, **179,** 1013 (1957).
88. P. D'Arcy Hart, *Brit. Med. J.*, **2,** 849 (1946).
89. F. G. Winder and P. B. Collins, *J. Gen. Microbiol.*, **63,** 41 (1970).

90. L. Wang and K. Takayama, *Antimicrob. Agents Chemother.*, **2,** 438 (1972).
91. K. Takayama, E. Lee Armstrong, and H. L. David, *Am. Rev. Respir. Dis.*, **110,** 43 (1974).
92. G. A. Snow, *Biochem. J.*, **115,** 199 (1969).
93. J. G. D. Carpenter and J. W. Moore, *J. Chem. Soc.*, 1610 (1969).
94. C. Ratledge and B. J. Marshall, *Biochim. Biophys. Acta*, **279,** 58 (1972).
95. C. Ratledge and K. A. Brown, *Am. Rev. Respir. Dis.*, **106,** 774 (1972).
96. K. A. Brown and C. Ratledge, *Biochim. Biophys. Acta*, **385,** 207 (1975).
97. G. Hartmann, K. O. Honikel, F. Knussel, and J. Nuesch, *Biochim. Biophys. Acta*, **145,** 843 (1967).
98. H. Umezawa, S. Mizuno, H. Yamazaki, and K. Nitta, *J. Antibiot. (Tokyo)*, **21,** 234 (1968).
99. R. J. White, G. C. Lancini, and L. Silvestri, *J. Bacteriol.*, **108,** 737 (1971).
100. P. Mison and L. Trnka, *Collect. Czech. Chem. Commun.*, **37,** 1049 (1972); *Chem. Abstr.*, **76,** 150433 (1972).
101. K. Konno, K. Oizumi, and S. Oka, *Am. Rev. Respir. Dis.*, **107,** 1006 (1973).
102. K. Konno, Y. Oizumi, I. Hayashi, S. Oka, and O. Sutemi, *Kekkakui*, **47,** 255 (1972); through *Chem. Abstr.*, **78,** 326 (1973).
103. K. Konno, K. Oizumi, F. Arji, J. Yamaguchi, and S. Oka, *Am. Rev. Respir. Dis.*, **107,** 1002 (1973).
104. R. Radanov, N. Spasova, and E. Kalfin, *Pneumol. Ftiziatr.*, **13,** 18 (1976); through *Chem. Abstr.*, **85,** 137907 (1977).
105. J. I. De Graw, V. H. Browa, W. T. Colwell, and N. E. Morrison, *J. Med. Chem.*, **17,** 144 (1974).
106. H. L. David, *Appl. Microbiol.*, **20,** 810 (1970).
107. K. E. Price, D. R. Chrisholm, M. Misiek, F. Leitner, and Y. H. Tsai, *J. Antibiot. (Tokyo)*, **25,** 709 (1972).
108. M. Alberghina, G. Nicoletti, and A. Torrisi, *Chemotherapy*, **19,** 148 (1973).
109. M. S. Shaila, K. P. Gopinathan, and T. Ramakrishnan, *Antimicrob. Agents Chemother.*, **4,** 205 (1973).
110. T. Yamada, K. Masuda, Y. Mizuguchi, and K. Suga, *Antimicrob. Agents Chemother.*, **9,** 817 (1976).
111. E. V. Cowdry and C. Ruangsiri, *Arch. Pathol.*, **32,** 632 (1941).
112. Y. Kurono, K. Ikeda, and K. Uekama, *Chem. Pharm. Bull. (Tokyo)*, **22,** 1261 (1974).
113. Editorial, *Lancet*, **2,** (7723), 534 (1971).
114. C. C. Shepard, *Ann. Rev. Pharmacol.*, **9,** 37 (1969).
115. R. Gelber, J. H. Peters, G. R. Gordon, A. J. Glazko, and L. Levy, *Clin. Pharmacol. Ther.*, **12** (2), 225 (1971).
116. J. H. Peters, *Am. J. Trop. Med. Hyg.*, **23,** 222 (1974).
117. J. H. S. Pettit and J. Chin, Editorial, *Lancet*, **2,** (7628), 1014 (1969).
118. J. L. McCullough and T. H. Moren, *Antimicrob. Agents Chemother.*, **3,** 665 (1973).
119. R. J. Rees, *Trans. Roy. Soc. Trop. Med. Hyg.*, **61,** 581 (1967).
120. R. Behnisch, F. Mietzsch, and H. Schmidt, *Angew. Chem.*, **60,** 113 (1948).
121. G. Domagk, R. Behnisch, F. Mietzsch, and H. Schmidt, *Naturwissenschaften*, **33,** 315 (1946).
122. G. Domagk, *Am. Rev. Tuberc.*, **61,** 8 (1950).
123. R. Donovik and J. Bernstein, *Am. Rev. Tuberc.*, **60,** 539 (1949).
124. D. M. Spain, W. G. Childress, and J. S. Fischer, *Am. Rev. Tuberc.*, **62,** 144 (1950).
125. H. Blaha, *Med. Welt*, **25,** 915 (1974).
126. W. H. O., *Tech. Rep.*, **552,** (1974).
127. *Bull. W. H. O.*, **47,** 211 (1972).
128. J. Lowe, *Lancet*, **2,** 1065 (1954).
129. G. Domagk, *Schweiz. Z. Pathol. Bakteriol.*, **12,** 575 (1949).
130. *Brit. Med. J.*, **1,** (5948), 33 (1975).
131. E. Freerksen and M. Rosenfeld, *Beitr. Klin. Tuberk.*, **127,** 386 (1963), through *Chem. Abstr.*, **60,** 4659c (1964).
132. L. Trnka, R. Urbancik, and H. Polenska, *Rozh. Tuberk.*, **23,** 147 (1963), through *Chem. Abstr.*, **59,** 8016 (1963).
133. S. Oka, K. Konno, M. Kudo, K. Oizumi, and S. Yamaguchi, *Japan J. Chest Dis.*, **23,** 326 (1964).
134. Editorial, *Tubercle*, **46,** 298 (1965).
135. G. Winder, P. B. Collins, and D. Whelan, *J. Gen. Microbiol.*, **66,** 379 (1971).
136. T. F. Davy, *Lepr. Rev.*, **29,** 25 (1958).
137. J. Stecca and P. Homen de Mello, *Int. J. Lepr.*, **31,** 548 (1963).
138. *W. H. O., Tech. Rep*, **459** (1970).
139. D. McKenzie, L. Malone, S. Kushner, J. J. Oleson, and Y. Subbarow, *J. Lab. Clin. Med.*, **33,** 1249 (1948).
140. J. Bernstein, W. A. Lott, B. A. Steinberg, and H. L. Yale, *Am. Rev. Tuberc.*, **65,** 357 (1952).
141. H. A. Offe, W. Siekfen, and G. Domagk, *Z. Naturforsch.*, **7b,** 446, 462 (1952).

142. E. A. Zeller, J. Barsky, J. R. Fouts, W. F. Kirchheimer, and L. S. Van Orden, *Experientia*, **8,** 349 (1952).

143. C. C. Shepard and Y. T. Chang, *Int. J. Lepr.*, **32,** 260 (1964).

144. J. A. Doull, J. N. Rodriguez, A. R. Davison, J. G. Tolentino, and J. V. Fernandez, *Int. J. Lepr.*, **25,** 173 (1957).

145. R. R. Ross, *J. Am. Med. Assoc.*, **168,** 273 (1958).

146. J. M. Robson and F. M. Sullivan, *Pharmacol. Rev.*, **15,** 169 (1963).

147. W. Mandel, D. A. Heaton, W. F. Russel, and G. Middlebrook, *J. Clin. Invest.*, **38,** 1356 (1959).

148. S. Sunahara, M. Urano, and M. Ogawa, *Science*, **134,** 1530 (1961).

149. H. Tiitinen, *Scand. J. Respir. Dis.*, **50,** 110 (1969).

150. G. A. Ellard, *Clin. Pharmacol. Ther.*, **19,** 610 (1976).

151. F. G. Winder and P. B. Collins, *Am. Rev. Respir. Dis.*, **100,** 101 (1969).

152. K. Takayama, *Ann. N.Y. Acad. Sci.*, **235,** 426 (1974).

153. K. Takayama and H. K. Schones, *Fed. Proc.*, **33,** 1425 (1974).

154. K. Takayama, L. Wang, and R. S. Merkal, *Antimicrob. Agents Chemother.*, **4,** 62 (1973).

155. D. Kock-Weser, R. H. Ebert, W. R. Barclay, and V. S. Lee, *J. Lab. Clin. Med.*, **42,** 828 (1953).

156. J. K. Seydel, E. Wempe, and H. J. Nestler, *Arzeneim.-Forsch.*, **18,** 362 (1968).

157. H. J. Nestler, *Arzneim.-Forsch.*, **16,** 1442 (1966).

158. J. K. Seydel, K. J. Schaper, E. Wempe, and H. P. Cordes, *J. Med. Chem.*, **19,** 483 (1976).

159. J. Youatt and S. Tham, *Am. Rev. Respir. Dis.*, **100,** 25, 31 (1969).

160. K. S. Sriprakash and T. Ramakrishnan, *Indian J. Biochem.*, **6,** 49 (1969).

161. R. I. Meltzer, A. D. Lewis, and J. A. King, *J. Am. Chem. Soc.*, **77,** 4062 (1955).

162. N. Rist, F. Grumbach, and D. Libermann, *Am. Rev. Tuberc.*, **79,** 1 (1959).

163. A. Bieder, P. Brunel, and L. Mazeau, *Ann. Pharm. Fr.*, **24,** 493 (1966).

164. L. Malone, A. Schurr, H. Lindh, D. McKenzie, J. S. Kiser, and J. H. Williams, *Am. Rev. Tuberc.*, **65,** 511 (1952).

165. E. F. Rogers, W. J. Leanza, H. J. Becker, A. R. Matzuk, E. C. O'Neill, A. J. Basso, G. A. Stein, M. Solotorovsky, F. G. Gregory, and K. Pfister, *Science*, **116,** 253 (1952).

166. I. M. Weiner and J. P. Tinker, *J. Pharmacol. Exp. Ther.*, **180,** 411 (1972).

167. E. Felder, D. Pitré, and U. Tiepolo, *Minerva Med.*, **53,** 1699 (1962).

168. L. Trnka, J. Kuska, and A. Havel, *Chemotherapia*, **9,** 158 (1965).

169. V. C. Barry, J. G. Belton, J. F. O'Sullivan, and D. Twomey, *J. Chem. Soc.*, 896 (1956).

170. V. C. Barry, M. L. Conalty, and E. E. Graffney, *J. Pharm. Pharmacol.*, **8,** 1089, (1956).

171. V. C. Barry, J. G. Belton, M. L. Conalty, and D. Twomey, *Nature (London)*, **162,** 622 (1948).

172. V. C. Barry, *Sci. Proc. Roy. Dubl. Soc. Ser. A*, **3,** 153 (1969).

173. W. A. Vischer, *Arzneim.-Forsch.*, **18,** 1529 (1968).

174. W. A. Vischer, *Arzneim.-Forsch.*, **20,** 714 (1970).

175. N. J. L. Gilmour, *Brit. Vet. J.*, **122,** 517 (1966).

176. H. F. Lunn and R. J. W. Rees, *Lancet*, **1,** 247 (1964).

177. Y. T. Chang, *Antimicrob. Agents Chemother.*, 294 (1962).

178. Y. T. Chang, *Int. J. Lepr.*, **34,** 1 (1966).

179. Y. T. Chang, *Int. J. Lepr.*, **35,** 78 (1967).

180. R. Y. W. Rees, *Int. J. Lepr.*, **33,** 646 (1965).

181. J. M. Gangas, *Lepr. Rev.*, **38,** 225 (1967).

182. J. H. S. Pettit and R. J. W. Rees, *Int. J. Lepr.*, **34,** 391 (1966).

183. J. H. S. Pettit, R. J. W. Rees, and D. S. Ridley, *Int. J. Lepr.*, **35,** 25 (1967).

184. A. G. Warren, *Lepr. Rev.*, **39,** 61 (1968).

185. F. M. Imkamp, *Lepr. Rev.*, **39,** 119 (1968).

186. S. G. Browne, *Advan. Pharmacol. Chemother.*, **7,** 211 (1969).

187. H. Mathies and U. Ress, *Arzneim.-Forsch.*, **20,** 1838 (1970).

188. H. L. F. Currey and P. Fowler, *Brit. J. Pharmacol.*, **45,** 676 (1972).

189. E. G. Steuger, L. Aeppli, E. Peheim, and P. E. Thomann, *Arzneim.-Forsch.*, **20,** 794 (1970).

190. C. C. Shepard, L. L. Walker, R. M. van Landingham, and M. A. Redus, *Proc. Soc. Exp. Biol. Med.*, **137,** 728 (1971).

191. E. G. Wilkinson, M. B. Cantrall, and R. G. Sheperd, *J. Med. Chem.*, **5,** 835 (1962).

192. A. G. Karlson, *Am. Rev. Respir. Dis.*, **84,** 905 (1961).

193. R. F. Corpe and F. A. Blalcock, *Dis. Chest*, **48,** 305 (1965).

194. I. D. Bobrowitz and K. S. Go Kulanathan, *Dis. Chest*, **48,** 239 (1965).

195. V. A. Place and J. P. Thomas, *Am. Rev. Respir. Dis.*, **87,** 901 (1963).
196. E. A. Peets, W. M. Sweeney, V. A. Place, and D. A. Buyske, *Am. Rev. Respir. Dis.*, **91,** 51 (1965).
197. W. H. Beggs and F. A. Andrews, *Am. Rev. Respir. Dis.*, **108,** 691 (1973).
198. W. H. Beggs and F. A. Andrews, *Antimicrob. Agents Chemother.*, **5,** 234 (1974).
199. M. Forbes, N. A. Kuck, and E. A. Peets, *J. Bacteriol.*, **84,** 1099 (1962).
200. M. Forbes, N. A. Kuck, and E. A. Peets, *J. Bacteriol.*, **89,** 1299 (1965).
201. M. Forbes, N. A. Kuck, and E. A. Peets, *Ann. N.Y. Acad. Sci.*, **135,** 726 (1966).
202. H. Reutgen and H. Iwainsky, *Z. Naturforsch.*, **27b,** 1405 (1972).
203. H. Shubin, *Antibiot. Ann.*, 437 (1954–1955).
204. W. B. Geiger, *Arch. Biochem.*, **15,** 227 (1947).
205. D. Anand, B. D. Davies, and A. K. Armitage, *Nature*, **185,** 23 (1960).
206. S. S. Cohen, *J. Biol. Chem.*, **166,** 393 (1946).
207. F. E. Hahn and J. Ciak, *Bacteriol. Proc.*, **1959,** 131.
208. C. R. Krishna Murthi, *Biochem. J.*, **76,** 362 (1960).
209. C. R. Spotts and R. Y. Stamier, *Nature*, **192,** 633 (1961).
210. E. C. Cox, J. R. White, and J. G. Flakes, *Proc. Nat. Acad. Sci., US*, **51,** 703 (1964).
211. M. Ozaki, S. Mizushima, and M. Nomura, *Nature*, **222,** 333 (1969).
212. J. Davies, D. S. Jones, and H. G. Khorana, *J. Mol. Biol.*, **18,** 48 (1966).
213. D. Elseviers and L. Gorini, in *Drug Action and Drug Resistance in Bacteria*, Vol. 2, *Aminoglycoside Antibiotics*, S. Mitsuhashi, Ed., University Park Press, Baltimore, 1975, p. 147.
214. L. Luzzato, D. Apirion, and D. Schlessinger, *Proc. Nat. Acad. Sci., US*, **60,** 873 (1968).
215. J. Modollel and B. D. Davis, *Proc. Nat. Acad. Sci., US*, **61,** 1270 (1968).
216. J. Modollel and B. D. Davis, *Nature*, **224,** 345 (1969).
217. H. B. Newcombe and M. H. Nyholm, *Genetics*, **35,** 603 (1950).
218. H. B. Newcombe and R. Haxizko, *J. Bacteriol.*, **57,** 565 (1949).
219. J. G. Flakes, E. C. Cox, M. L. Witting, and J. R. White, *Biochem. Biophys. Res. Commun.*, **7,** 390 (1962).
220. H. Unezawa, M. Okamishi, S. Kondo, K. Hamona, R. Utahara, and K. Maeda, *Science*, **157,** 1559 (1967).
221. R. Benveniste and J. Davies, *Ann. Rev. Biochem.*, **42,** 471 (1973).
222. R. C. Gordon, C. Regamey, and W. M. M. Kirby, *Antimicrob. Agents Chemother.*, **2,** 214 (1972).
223. Conference on Kanamycin, *Ann. N.Y. Acad. Sci.*, **132,** 773 (1966).
224. E. M. Yow and H. Abu-Nassar, *Antibiot. Chemother.*, **11,** 148 (1963).
225. D. Apirion and D. Schlessinger, *J. Bacteriol.*, **96,** 768 (1968).
226. J. Davies, L. Gorini, and D. B. Davis, *Mol. Pharmacol.*, **1,** 93 (1965).
227. H. Masukawa, N. Tanaka, and H. Umezawa, *J. Antibiot. (Tokyo)*, **21,** 517 (1968).
228. J. Davies, P. Anderson, and B. D. Davis, *Science*, **149,** 1096 (1965).
229. N. Tanaka, Y. Yoshida, K. Sashikata, H. Yamaguchi, and H. Umezawa, *J. Antibiot. (Tokyo)*, **19,** 65 (1966).
230. K. Konno, K. Oizumi, N. Kumano, and S. Oka, *Am. Rev. Respir. Dis.*, **108,** 101 (1973).
231. D. H. Starkey and E. Gregory, *Can. Med. Assoc. J.*, **105,** 587 (1971).
232. J. T. Doluisio, L. W. Dittert, and J. C. La Piana, *J. Pharmacokinet. Biopharmaceut.*, **1,** 253 (1973).
233. L. L. McDonald and J. W. St. Geme, *Antimicrob. Agents Chemother.*, **2,** 41 (1972).
234. E. Kuntz, *Klin. Wochenschr.*, **40,** 1107 (1962).
235. Q. R. Bartz, J. Ehrlich, J. D. Mold, M. A. Penner, and R. M. Smith, *Am. Rev. Tuberc. Pulm. Dis.*, **63,** 4–6 (1951).
236. N. Tanaka and S. Igusa, *J. Antibiot. (Tokyo)*, **21,** 239 (1968).
237. K. Masuda and T. Yamada, *Biochim. Biophys. Acta*, **435,** 333 (1976).
238. T. Yamada, K. Masuda, K. Shoj, and M. Hari, *J. Bacteriol.*, **112,** 1 (1972).
239. E. B. Herr, Jr., and M. O. Redstone, *Ann. N.Y. Acad. Sci.*, **135,** 940 (1966).
240. D. A. Harris, R. Ruger, M. A. Reagan, F. J. Wolf, R. L. Peck, H. Wallick, and H. B. Woodruff, *Antibiot. Chemother.*, **5,** 183 (1955).
241. G. Shull and J. Sardinas, *Antibiot. Chemother.*, **5,** 398 (1955).
242. F. A. Kuehl, F. J. Wolf, N. R. Trenner, R. L. Peck, R. H. Buhs, I. Putter, R. Ormond, J. E. Lyons, L. Chaiet, E. Howe, B. D. Hunnewell, G. Downing, E. Newstead, and K. Folkers, *J. Am. Chem. Soc.*, **77,** 2344 (1955).

243. P. H. Hidy, E. B. Hodge, V. V. Young, R. L. Harned, G. A. Brewer, W. F. Phillips, W. F. Runge, H. E. Stavely, A. Pohland, H. Boaz, and H. R. Sullivan, *J. Am. Chem. Soc.*, **77,** 2345 (1955).
244. C. H. Stammer, A. N. Wilson, C. F. Spencer, F. W. Bachelor, F. W. Holly, and K. Folkers, *J. Am. Chem. Soc.*, **79,** 3236 (1957).
245. P. D. Hoeprich, *Arch. Intern. Med.*, **112,** 405 (1963).
246. P. D. Hoeprich, *J. Lab. Clin. Med.*, **62,** 657 (1963).
247. J. L. Strominger, E. Ito, and R. H. Threnn, *J. Am. Chem. Soc.*, **82,** 998 (1960).
248. J. L. Strominger, R. H. Threnn and S. S. Scott, *J. Am. Chem. Soc.*, **81,** 3083 (1959).
249. F. C. Neuhaus and J. L. Lynch, *Biochemistry*, **3,** 471 (1964).
250. P. Sensi, P. Margalith, and M. T. Timbal, *Farmaco, Ed. Sci.*, **14,** 146 (1959).
251. P. Margalith and G. Beretta, *Mycopathol. Mycol. Appl.*, **8,** 321 (1960).
252. J. E. Thiemann, G. Zucco, and G. Pelizza, *Arch. Microbiol.*, **67,** 147 (1969).
253. P. Margalith and H. Pagani, *Appl. Microbiol.*, **9,** 325 (1961).
254. P. Sensi, R. Ballotta, A. M. Greco, and G. G. Gallo, *Farmaco, Ed. Sci.*, **16,** 165 (1961).
255. W. Oppolzer, V. Prelog, and P. Sensi, *Experientia*, **20,** 336 (1964).
256. M. Brufani, W. Fedeli, G. Giacomello, and A. Vaciago, *Experientia*, **23,** 508 (1967).
257. J. Leitich, W. Oppolzer, and V. Prelog, *Experientia*, **20,** 343 (1964).
258. W. Oppolzer and V. Prelog, *Helv. Chim. Acta*, **56,** 2287 (1973).
259. P. Siminoff, R. M. Smith, W. T. Sokolski, and G. M. Savage, *Am. Rev. Respir. Dis.*, **75,** 579 (1957).
260. K. L. Rinehart, M. L. Maheshwari, K. Sasaki, A. J. Schacht, H. H. Mathur, and F. J. Antosz, *J. Am. Chem. Soc.*, **93,** 6273 (1971).
261. T. Kishi, M. Asai, M. Muroi, S. Harada, E. Mizuta, S. Teroo, T. Miki, and K. Mizuno, *Tetrahedron Lett.*, **1969,** 91.
262. T. Kishi, S. Harada, M. Asai, M. Muroi, and K. Mizuno, *Tetrahedron Lett.*, **1969,** 97.
263. A. K. Ganguly, S. Szmulervicz, O. Z. Sarre, D. Greeves, J. Morton, and J. Glotten, *J. Chem. Soc. Commun.*, **1974,** 395.
264. G. Maffii, P. Schiatti, G. Bianchi, and M. G. Serralunga, *Farmaco, Ed. Sci.*, **16,** 235 (1961).
265. M. T. Timbal and A. Brega, *Farmaco, Ed. Sci.*, **16,** 191 (1961).
266. G. Maffii, G. Bianchi, P. Schiatti, and G. G. Gallo, *Farmaco, Ed. Sci.*, **16,** 246 (1961).
267. M. T. Timbal, R. Pallanza, and G. Carniti, *Farmaco, Ed. Sci.*, **16,** 181 (1961).
268. B. Rescigno, *Arch. Tisiol.*, **18,** 238 (1963).
269. V. Monaldi, *Chemotherapia* (Basel), **7,** 569 (1963).
270. A. Tacquet, *Chemotherapia* (Basel), **7,** 492 (1963).
271. N. Bergamini and G. Fowst, *Arzneim.-Forsch.*, **796,** 953 (1965).
272. L. De Souza Lima and D. V. A. Opromolla, *Chemotherapia* (Basel), **7,** 668 (1963).
273. D. V. A. Opromolla and L. De Souza Lima, *Dia Méd.*, **37,** 700 (1965).
274. F. P. Merklen and F. Cottenot, *Bull. Soc. Fr. Dermatol.*, **70,** 528 (1963).
275. D. V. A. Opromolla, L. De Souza Lima, and G. Caprara, *Lepr. Rev.*, **36,** 123 (1965).
276. M. Silva and J. B. Risi, *Rev. Bras. Med.*, **20,** 194 (1963).
277. G. Farris and A. Baccaredda-Boy, *Int. J. Lepr.*, **31,** 560 (1963).
278. F. P. Merklen and F. Cottenot, *Presse Med.*, **72,** 48 (1964).
279. P. Sensi, *Pure Appl. Chem.*, **35,** 383 (1973).
280. G. Lancini and W. Zanichelli, in *Structure-Activity Relationship Among the Semisynthetic Antibiotics*, D. Perlman, Ed., Academic Press, New York, 1977, p. 531.
281. G. Pelizza, G. C. Lancini, G. C. Allievi, and G. G. Gallo, *Farmaco, Ed. Sci.*, **28,** 298 (1973).
282. P. Sensi, N. Magzi, R. Ballotta, S. Furesz, R. Pallanza, and V. Arioli, *J. Med. Chem.*, **7,** 596 (1964).
283. G. Maffii and P. Schiatti, *Toxicol. Appl. Pharmacol.*, **8,** 138 (1966).
284. N. Maggi, R. Pallanza, and P. Sensi, *Antimicrob. Agents Chemother.*, **1965,** 765.
285. N. Maggi, C. R. Pasqualucci, R. Ballotta, and P. Sensi, *Chemotherapia*, **11,** 285 (1966).
286. L. Verbist and A. Gyselen, *Am. Rev. Respir. Dis.*, **98,** 923 (1968).
287. J. K. McClatchy, R. F. Wagonner, and W. Lester, *Am. Rev. Respir. Dis.*, **100,** 234 (1969).
288. P. W. Steinbrück, *Acta Tuberc. Pneumol. Belg.*, **60,** 413 (1969).
289. R. Pallanza, V. Arioli, S. Furesz, and G. Bolzoni, *Arzneim.-Forsch.*, **17,** 529 (1967).

290. F. Grumbach and N. Rist, *Rev. Tuberc.* (Paris), **31,** 749 (1967).
291. L. Verbist, *Acta Tuberc. Pneumol. Belg.*, **60,** 390 (1969).
292. F. Grumbach, G. Canetti, and M. Le Lirzin, *Tubercle* (London), **50,** 280 (1969).
293. F. Grumbach, G. Canetti, and M. Le Lirzin, *Rev. Tuberc. Pneumol.* (Paris), **34,** 312 (1970).
294. F. Kradolfer and R. Schnell, *Chemotherapy* (Basel), **15,** 242 (1970).
295. F. Kradolfer, *Am. Rev. Respir. Dis.*, **98,** 104 (1968).
296. F. Kradolfer, *Antibiot. Chemother.* (Basel), **16,** 352 (1970).
297. V. Nitti, E. Catena, A. Ninni, and A. Di Filippo, *Arch. Tisiol.*, **21,** 867 (1966).
298. V. Nitti, E. Catena, A. Ninni, and A. Di Filippo, *Chemotherapia*, **12,** 369 (1967).
299. V. Nitti, *Antibiot. Chemother.* (Basel), **16,** 444 (1970).
300. M. Lucchesi and P. Mancini, *Antibiot Chemother.* (Basel), **16,** 431 (1970).
301. S. Furesz, *Antibiot. Chemother.* (Basel), **16,** 316 (1970).
302. P. Kluyskens, *Acta Tuberc. Pneumol. Belg.*, **60,** 323 (1969).
303. S. Furesz, R. Scotti, R. Pallanza, and E. Mapelli, *Arzneim.-Forsch.*, **17,** 726 (1967).
304. G. Curci, A. Ninni, and F. Iodice, *Acta Tuberc. Pneumol. Belg.*, **60,** 276 (1969).
305. G. Acocella, V. Pagani, M. Marchetti, G. B. Baroni, and F. B. Nicolis, *Chemotherapy* (Basel), **16,** 356 (1971).
306. M. G. Meyer-Brunot, K. Schmid, and H. Keberle, paper presented at Fifth International Congress of Chemotherapy, Vienna, 1967.
307. G. Acocella, L. Bonollo, M. Garimoldi, M. Mainardi, L. T. Tenconi, and F. B. Nicolis, *Gut*, **13,** 47 (1972).
308. L. Dettli and F. Spina, *Farmaco, Ed. Sci.*, **23,** 795 (1968).
309. N. Maggi, S. Furesz, R. Pallanza, and G. Pelizza, *Arzneim.-Forsch.*, **19,** 651 (1969).
310. W. Zilly, D. D. Breimer, and E. Richter, *Clin. Pharmacokinet.*, **2,** 61 (1977).
311. G. Binda, E. Domenichini, A. Gottardi, B. Orlandi, E. Ortelli, B. Pacini, and G. Fowst, *Arzneim.-Forsch.*, **21,** 796 (1971).
312. D. J. Girling, *J. Antimicrob. Chemother.*, **3,** 115 (1977).
313. R. J. Rees, J. M. H. Pearson, and M. F. R. Waters, *Brit. Med. J.*, **1,** 89 (1970).
314. G. R. F. Hilson, D. K. Banerjee, and J. B. Holmes, *Int. J. Lepr.*, **39,** 349 (1971).
315. C. C. Shepard, L. L. Walker, R. M. Van Landingham, and M. A. Redus, *Am. J. Trop. Med. Hyg.*, **20,** 616 (1971).
316. S. R. Pattyn, *Int. J. Lepr.*, **41,** 489 (1973).
317. S. R. Pattyn and E. J. Saerens, *Ann. Soc. Belg. Med. Trop.*, **54,** 35 (1974).
318. D. L. Leiker, *Int. J. Lepr.*, **39,** 462 (1971).
319. R. J. W. Rees, M. F. R. Waters, H. S. Helmy, and J. M. H. Pearson, *Int. J. Lepr.*, **41,** 682 (1973).
320. S. Riva and L. G. Silvestri, *Ann. Rev. Microbiol.*, **26,** 199 (1972).
321. W. Wehrli and M. Staehelin, in *Antibiotics, Vol. 3, Mechanism of Action of Antimicrobial and Antitumor Agent.* J. W. Corcoran and H. Hahn, Eds., Springer-Verlag, Berlin, 1975, pp. 252–268.
322. U. J. Lill and G. R. Hartmann, *Eur. J. Biochem.*, **38,** 336 (1973).
323. W. Stender, A. A. Stutz, and K. H. Scheit, *Eur. J. Biochem.*, **56,** 129 (1975).
324. J. Hui, N. Gordon, and R. Kajioka, *Antimicrob. Agents Chemother.*, **11,** 773 (1977).
325. V. C. Barry, Ed., *Chemotherapy of Tuberculosis*, Butterworths, London, 1964.
326. Commission du Traitement de l'Union Internationale contre la Tuberculose, *Rev. Fr. Mal. Respir.*, **4,** 157 (1976).
327. International Union against Tuberculosis, *Bull. Union Against Tuberc.*, **34,** 79 (1966).
328. Medical Research Council, Tuberculosis Chemotherapy Trials Committee, *Tubercle*, **43,** 201 (1962).
329. W. Fox, *Am. Rev. Respir. Dis.*, **97,** 767 (1968).
330. W. Fox, *Bull. Union Int. Contre Tuberc.*, **47,** 51 (1972).
331. R. S. Mitchell, *New Eng. J. Med.*, **276,** 842, 905 (1967).
332. East African/British Medical Research Council, *Tubercle*, **47,** 1 (1966).
333. East African/British Medical Research Council, *Tubercle*, **51,** 353 (1970).
334. Singapore Tuberculosis Services/Brompton Hospital/British Medical Research Council, *Tubercle*, **52,** 88 (1971).
335. Singapore Tuberculosis Services/Brompton Hospital/British Medical Research Council, *Tubercle*, **55,** 251 (1974).
336. G. Decroix, B. Kreis, C. Sors, J. Birenbaum, M. Le Lirzin, and G. Canetti, *Rev. Tuberc. Pneumol.*, **33,** 751 (1969).

337. G. Decroix, B. Kreis, C. Sors, J. Birenbaum, M. Le Lirzin, and G. Canetti, *Rev. Tuberc. Pneumol.*, **35,** 39 (1971).

338. J. M. Dickinson and D. Mitchinson, *Tubercle*, **51,** 82 (1970).

339. W. Fox, *Postgrad. Med. J.*, **47,** 729 (1971).

340. H. Eule, E. Wernes, K. Winsel, and H. Jwainzy, *Tubercle*, **55,** 81 (1974).

341. A Cooperative Tuberculosis Chemotherapy Study in Poland, *Tubercle*, **57,** 1 (1976).

342. L. Verbist, S. Mbete, H. Van Landuyt, T. Darras, and A. Gyselen, *Chest*, **61,** 555 (1972).

343. Tuberculosis Chemotherapy Center, Madras, *Tubercle*, **54,** 23 (1973).

344. Tuberculosis Chemotherapy Center, Madras, *Brit. Med. J.*, **1,** 7 (1973).

345. G. Poole, P. Stradling, and S. Worlledge, *Brit. Med. J.*, **3,** 343 (1971).

346. N. Riske and K. Mattson, *Scand. J. Respir. Dis.*, **53,** 87 (1972).

347. M. Zierski, *Scand. J. Respir. Dis.*, **84** Suppl., 166 (1973).

348. Hong Kong Tuberculosis Treatment Services/British Medical Research Council, *Tubercle*, **55,** 193 (1974).

349. Hong Kong Tuberculosis Treatment Services/British Medical Research Council, *Tubercle*, **57,** 81 (1975).

350. G. Brouet, *Bull. Union Int. Contre Tuberc.*, **49,** 1 (1974).

351. British Thoracic and Tuberculosis Association, *Lancet*, **2,** 1102 (1976).

352. W. Fox and D. A. Mitchinson, *Am. Rev. Respir. Dis.*, **111,** 325 (1975).

353. W. Fox, *Proc. Roy. Soc. Med.*, **70,** 4 (1977).

354. J. M. Dickinson, P. S. Jackett, and D. A. Mitchinson, *Am. Rev. Respir. Dis.*, **105,** 519 (1972).

355. D. A. Mitchinson, *Bull. Int. Union Contre Tuberc.*, **43,** 322 (1970).

356. J. M. Dickinson and D. A. Mitchinson, *Tubercle*, **51,** 82 (1970).

357. OMS, *Sér. Rapp. Techn.*, **607** (1977).

358. C. S. Shepard, *Ann. Rev. Pharmacol.*, **9,** 37 (1969).

359. R. G. Cochrane and T. I. Davey, *Leprosy in Theory and Practice*, Williams and Wilkins, Baltimore, 1964.

360. S. G. Browne, *Int. J. Lep.*, **39,** 406 (1971).

361. D. L. Leiker, *Int. J. Lep.*, **39,** 462 (1971).

362. W. H. Jopling and R. M. Harman, in *Textbook of Dermatology*, A. Rook, D. S. Wilkinson, and F. Y. G. Ebling, Eds., Blackwell, Oxford/Edinburgh, 1972, p. 680.

363. J. A. Doull, *J. Am. Med. Assoc.*, **173,** 363 (1970).

364. A. Luger, *Wien. Klin. Wochenschr.*, **87,** 161 (1971).

365. C. C. Shepard, *Int. J. Lepr.*, **39,** 340 (1971).

366. M. F. R. Waters and H. S. Helmy, *Lepr. Rev.*, **46,** 299 (1974).

367. J. M. H. Pearson, R. J. W. Rees, and M. F. R. Waters, *Lancet*, **2,** 69 (1975).

368. T. W. Meade, J. M. H. Pearson, R. J. W. Rees, and W. R. S. North, *Int. J. Lepr.*, **41,** 684 (1973).

369. J. H. Peters, C. C. Shepard, G. R. Gordon, V. A. Rojas, and C. Elizondo, *Int. J. Lepr.*, **44,** 143 (1976).

370. J. M. H. Pearson, W. F. Ross, and R. J. W. Rees, *Int. J. Lepr.*, **44,** 140 (1976).

CHAPTER EIGHTEEN

Antimalarials

THOMAS R. SWEENEY

and

RICHARD E. STRUBE

Division of Experimental Therapeutics,
Walter Reed Army Institute of Research,
Washington, D.C. 20012 USA

CONTENTS

1 INTRODUCTION

Malaria is the only disease that over the years has evoked the concerted attention of governments. Progress in combating the disease that has been made as the result of this attention can be attributed largely to the exigencies of war or conquest. Thus the Spanish, in about 1640, took cinchona bark to Europe; the Dutch government, near the turn of the century, supported the cultivation of cinchona trees in Java; the German government recognized the importance of a synthetic drug development program to eliminate dependence on imported cinchona products during World War I; the Allied powers inaugurated a vigorous antimalarial synthesis program after the Japanese conquered Java in World War II; and finally, the United States sponsored an extensive antimalarial research program as the result of troubles with drug-resistant malaria during the conflict in Southeast Asia. Indeed the US Army bore the brunt of the fight against drug-resistant malaria and continued its efforts long after the cessation of hostilities.

1.1 The Global Problem

Despite the outstanding progress of the World Health Organization program to eradicate malaria, initiated in 1955, the situation has deteriorated in the last several years, and although there have been tremendous net gains, malariologists no longer predict the eradication of the disease in the foreseeable future. The social, economic, financial, administrative, and personnel requirements for successful eradication programs are beyond the capabilities of some countries, and little additional progress can be expected in the immediate future. Factors that have contributed to the dampening of the optimism of the late 1950s include the migration of nomadic peoples and workers, the transportation by high speed jet aircraft of infected persons and mosquitoes, urbanization, with the concomitant concentration of people and changes in the breeding and feeding patterns of the vector,* the decreased availability of DDT (18.**1**), the development of resistance to insecticides by the vector, and particularly forboding, the inexorable spread of drug-resistant strains of the malaria parasite. Fortunately, the parasite is quite host specific. Some primates apparently can harbor the parasites that cause human malaria, but the prospect of zoonosis is vanishingly small. The series of reports from the World Health Organization (1a, b) discuss the many facets of the global problem of malaria.

1.2 The Disease

Today malaria is primarily a disease of warm climates, although around the turn of

* The terminology of malaria is defined in the Appendix.

this century it was also common in temperate zones. Nevertheless, malaria is still the most prevalent of infectious diseases, and more than one billion people live in malarious regions. Until the nineteenth century the disease was attributed to the effect of unwholesome emanations from swamps and stagnant waters and was called marsh fever, paludism, and malaria (*mal aria*, Ital.). In 1880 the French Army physician Laveran noticed pigmented bodies in the red blood cells of malarial patients and he identified *plasmodia* as the causative agent of the disease. Later Ross, a British Army surgeon in India, demonstrated that the *Anopheles* mosquito is the transmitter of the disease, and these investigations won for him the Nobel prize in 1902 (2). It is now known that malaria is a disease resulting from infection by protozoa of the genus *Plasmodium*. In nature, man contracts malaria by the bite of a mosquito carrying the infective forms of the malaria parasite (sporozoites). In turn, the mosquito is infected by the sexual form of the parasite (gametocyte) when it takes a blood meal from an infected human. Four species of human malaria parasites are known: *Plasmodium falciparum*, *P. vivax*, *P. malariae*, and *P. ovale*. The first two species, *P. falciparum* and *P. vivax*, account for more than 95% of prevalent cases of malaria, the latter being the most widely distributed. The disease caused by *P. falciparum* is often called malignant tertian malaria, tropical malaria or pernicious malaria, and if not promptly treated is usually fatal to nonimmune persons. Corpuscles infected with this parasite tend to clump together and adhere to the linings of blood capil-

Table 18.1 Common Malarial Plasmodia of Mammals and Birds

	Host	
Plasmodium Species	Natural	Experimental
Human malarias		
P. falciparum	Man	Chimpanzee (splenectomized) Owl monkey (aotus)
P. vivax	Man	Chimpanzee (splenectomized) Owl monkey (aotus)
P. malariae	Man	Chimpanzee (splenectomized)
P. ovale	Man	Chimpanzee (splenectomized)
Monkey malarias		
P. knowlesi	Kra-monkey	Various monkeys
P. cynomolgi	Kra-monkey	Various monkeys
Rodent malarias		
P. berghei	Tree rat	Mouse, rat
P. vinckei	Tree rat	Mouse, rat
P. chabaudi[a]	Tree rat	Mouse, rat
Bird malarias		
P. relictum	Sparrow	Canary, pigeon, siskin
P. praecox[b]	Sparrow	Canary, pigeon, siskin
P. cathermerium	Sparrow	Canary, pigeon, duck
P. gallinaceum	Domestic fowl	Chick
P. lophurae	Pheasant (Borneo)	Canary, chick, duck
P. fallax	Owl	Turkey

[a] Should be considered a subspecies of *P. vinckei* (3).

[b] Probably a subspecies of *P. relictum* (4a).

laries, which may cause blockage. When this happens in the brain, the condition is known as cerebral malaria. Vivax malaria, also called benign tertian malaria, or simple tertian malaria, evokes milder clinical attacks than does falciparum malaria and has a low mortality rate even in untreated adults; however the symptoms may then recur (relapse) sporadically for some time within at least 2 years after the original infection (see Section 2.2). Malaria caused by *P. malariae*, known as quartan malaria, is a mold form of the disease with an uneven global distribution, readily susceptible to chemotherapy if treated early but noted for its chronicity. *P. ovale* is also a mild infection, geographically rather restricted and susceptible to chemotherapy.

In addition to the four species of plasmodia infecting humans, there are plasmodia that infect apes, monkeys, rodents, birds, lizards, and frogs. Table 18.1 lists the plasmodia of man and those used most often in malaria research. A tremendous amount of work has been done on the bird malarias, because until the discovery of rodent malarias, *i.e.*, prior to 1948, birds were the most convenient model for screening potential antimalarial compounds.

2 BIOLOGICAL PRINCIPLES

2.1 The Vector of Human Malaria: *Anopheles*

Approximately 3000 species of mosquitoes are known, and some 400 of them belong to the genus *Anopheles*. About 100 *Anopheles* species can carry the malaria parasites of primates, including man; however not all are equally implicated as vectors because much depends on the feeding habits of the species and their association with man. A case in point is the situation in Africa, where there are some 100 species of *Anopheles* but only 15–20 species are believed to be important vectors of human malaria, with members of the *A. gambiae* complex (six species) apparently the most important. The life cycle of human malaria parasites is confined to man and the female anopheline mosquito. The reason for such specificity is not yet clearly understood, but it is particularly intriguing in view of other relationships that have been established between other genera of mosquitoes and vertebrates.

Both the male and female mosquito feed on suitable flowers and fruits as a source of carbohydrate to replenish their energy. For the development of eggs in the female mosquito, however, components are needed that are obtained from the blood of vertebrates. Only the female mosquito is equipped with piercing mouthparts and, consequently, it is the female that transmits the disease. After being fertilized, the female mosquito deposits a batch of eggs on the surface of water, and a few days later larvae appear. The larvae pass through four developmental stages before metamorphosing to the pupal stage, from which the adult mosquitoes emerge.

2.2 The Life Cycle of Human Plasmodia

After Ross demonstrated (6a), around 1900, that the *Anopheles* mosquito is the vector in malaria, almost 50 years passed before the complete life cycle of the malaria parasite was elucidated (5). To have a better understanding of the action of antimalarial drugs, a brief discussion of the life cycle of the malaria parasites is essential.

Malaria parasites are intracellular protozoans whose life cycle involves an asexual development in a vertebrate host and a sexual development in the body of a mosquito (Fig. 18.1). When an infected mosquito bites for the purpose of taking a blood meal, it injects sporozoites, the infective stage of the parasite, into the blood stream of the vertebrate. After a period of

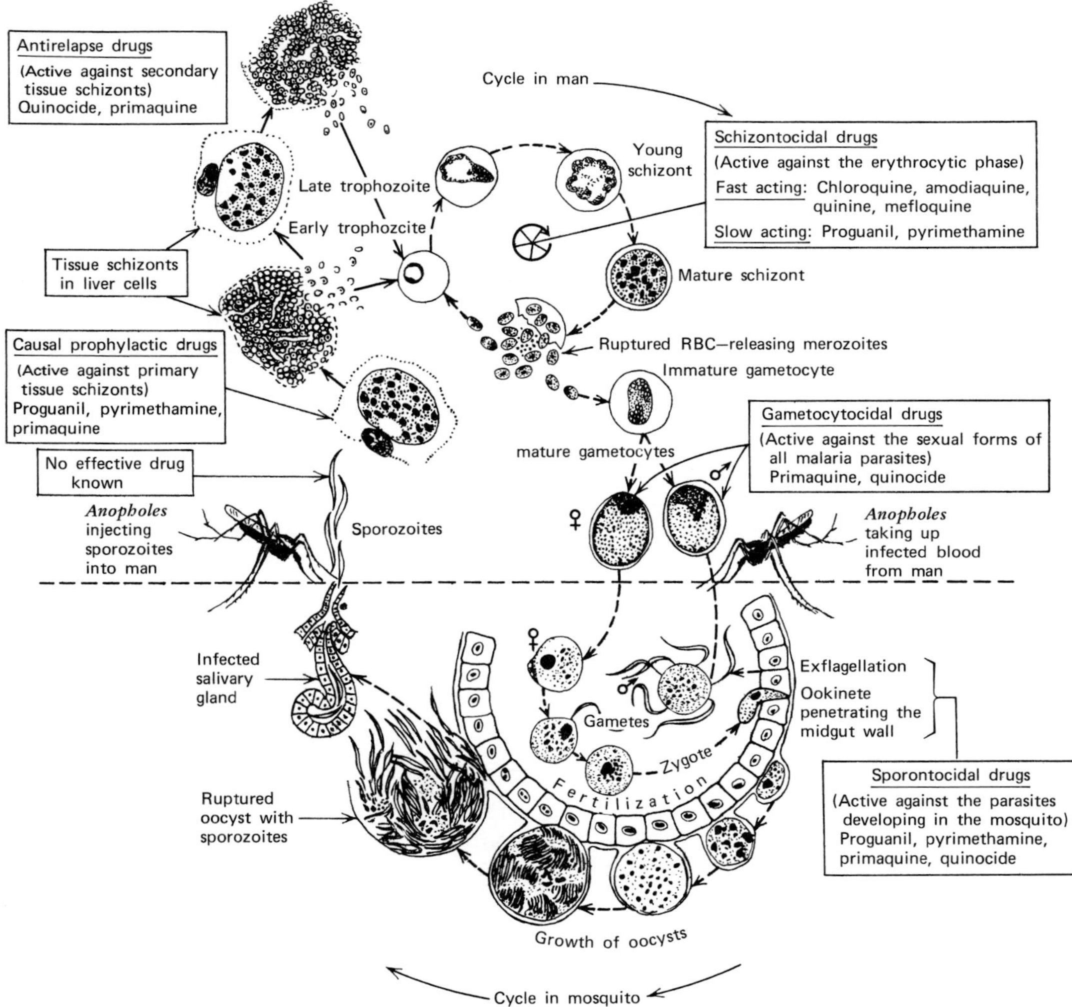

Fig. 18.1 Life cycle of the malaria parasite and classification of antimalarial drugs. After L. J. Bruce-Chwatt, *Bull. W. H. O.*, **27,** 288 (1962). For a recent interpretation of tissue schizonts, see F. E. G. Cox, *Nature*, **266,** 408 (1977).

less than an hour, the sporozoites are sequestered in the parenchymal cells of the liver, where they undergo asexual division to form merozoites. In a matter of days the parasitized hepatocytes rupture, releasing the merozoites into the bloodstream, where most of them soon invade erythrocytes. Until very recently, it was generally accepted that some of the released parasites invade fresh liver cells to begin another asexual division. These developing stages (exoerythrocytic or ee forms) in the liver are designated, respectively, as primary if derived directly from sporozoites and secondary if developed from the primary forms. No overt symptoms of the disease have become evident at this time.

However there is now a growing belief that continuous exoerythrocytic cycles do not occur in any species of human malaria and that relapses can be attributed to differences in the time taken for different sporozoites to develop (7). Within the red cells the parasite grows and divides; the enlarged erythrocyte eventually ruptures and releases the parasites, whereupon they invade fresh red cells to begin the cycle again. It is the periodic rupture of the parasitized red cells with the sudden release of parasites, parasite waste products, and cellular debris that gives rise in the host to the episodes of chills and fever so characteristic of malaria. Although the timing of the erythrocytic cycle, hence the bouts of chills and fever, is often erratic with new infections, it tends to become synchronized and, because of this periodicity, the type of malaria was originally identified as "tertian" for a 3-day cycle and "quartan" for a 4-day cycle. For reasons not understood, some of the intraerythrocytic merozites develop into sexual forms, both male and female, called gametocytes. These forms do not develop further in man but are the infective stage for the mosquito. When they are imbibed with the blood meal by an anopheline mosquito, the female gametocyte is fertilized by the male through a process of exflagellation in the stomach of the mosquito. The resulting zygote develops in the stomach wall to an oocyst that within 20 days, depending on temperature and species, ruptures to release sporozoites. These forms migrate to the salivary gland of the mosquito where they are ready to begin the cycle again.

Various species of the malaria parasite can have specific characteristics that differ from the general cycle shown in Fig. 18.1, and, as will become apparent, these differences can have important chemotherapeutic consequences. *P. falciparum*, for example, has no extended development in liver cells and following rupture of the parasitized liver cells this organism invades erythrocytes exclusively. Thus theoretically, elimination of the erythrocytic form of *P. falciparum* would effect a radical cure. There are, however, persisting erythrocytic forms of the parasite that if not destroyed, can develop and bring about recrudescences that except for mechanism, can be considered to be relapses. *P. vivax* and *P. ovale* are true relapsing malarias, i.e., they have a prolonged or secondary tissue phase in their development, and eradication of the erythrocytic forms of the parasite will not effect a radical cure. The fourth type of human malaria, *P. malariae*, is noted for persistent relapses and was originally thought to be a true relapsing malaria. However it now appears that it is a nonrelapsing malaria with extremely long-lasting erythrocytic forms.

The development of malaria parasites in other vertebrates, such as birds and rodents, is similar but not identical to that of man (6b).

2.3 Resistance Phenomena Associated with Malaria

2.3.1 RESISTANCE TO PLASMODIAL DRUGS. Resistance to antimalarial drugs is defined as the "ability of a parasite strain to survive and/or to multiply despite the administration and absorption of a drug given in doses equal to, or higher than, those usually recommended, but within the limits of tolerance of the subject" (1c). This definition applies for all species and all development stages of malaria parasites, although in practice is most commonly applied to the blood schizonts. From patients, strains of plasmodia have been isolated that are less sensitive to a particular drug than is usually the case. The difference in responsiveness was recognized at the beginning of this century with quinine (18.**27**), the only valuable antimalarial drug then available. In some cases of falciparum malaria considerably higher doses of quinine had to be administered to cure patients. Another case in point is that of the West African strains of *P. falciparum*, which are relatively insensitive to chlorproguanil (18.**96**). This type

Table 18.2 Degree of Resistance to Quinine, Chloroquine, and Proguanil of Asian Strains of *P. falciparum*

P. falciparum Strain	Quinine	Chloroquine	Proguanil	Reference
Vietnam (Smith)	R III	R III	R III	8
Vietnam (Marks)	R I	R III	R III	9
Malaya II	S	R III	R II	10
Malaya (Camp.)	R I	R I	R I	11
Philippines (Per.)	R I	R I	S	12
Cambodia II	S	R I	R I	10

of natural resistance should not be confused with resistance developed by exposure to drugs. The sensitivity of strains to a particular drug may differ considerably, therefore a grading system is used (1c); a strain can be sensitive (S), slightly resistant (R I), moderately resistant (R II) or highly resistant R III). Table 18.2 shows the profile of response to various drugs by several strains of *P. falciparum* isolated from patients. Besides the difference in drug sensitivity, strains may differ in other respects, such as the immune response induced in the host or the degree of pathogenicity. With regard to the pathogenicity of a strain, it should be stressed that a higher resistance of a strain to a drug is not necessarily linked with a higher virulence.

Drug resistance in malaria became a problem after the introduction of pyrimethamine (18.**25**) and other antifolic drugs (see Section 6). Soon after the introduction of proguanil (18.**22**), resistance to it was observed in both falciparum and vivax malaria, but the occurrence of resistance to these drugs was not considered to be a serious problem because the resistant parasites were still responsive to other drugs, such as chloroquine (18.**16**), quinacrine (18.**14**), and quinine (18.**27**). However the situation became alarming after 1960 when many cases of chloroquine-resistant *P. falciparum* infections were reported from South America and the Far East. Chloroquine resistance in nature has been encountered only with *P. falciparum* strains, whereas resistance to antifolate drugs has been established for all human plasmodia studied (4b). Cross-resistance among antimalarial drugs occurs and, as one might expect, compounds with similar modes of action—consequently, more or less similar chemical structures—are, as a rule, cross-resistant (see Sections 5 and 6). Thus in human malaria, the main types of drug resistance are against (*a*) antifolate drugs, (*b*) chloroquine, quinacrine, and structurally related drugs, or (*c*) both these types. Although resistance to quinine has not yet become a serious problem, a decrease in sensitivity to this drug has been reported (4c, 13).

The natural development of resistant strains of human plasmodia to the 8-aminoquinoline type of drugs, such as primaquine (18.**17**), is not as clear-cut as it is for the antifolate drugs and the 4-aminoquinolines. The introduction of a primaquine-resistant strain of *P. vivax* in man has been reported (14), but its resistance was demonstrated only for the asexual blood forms, not for the tissue forms of the parasite where the principal action of primaquine occurs (see Section 7.1.2). Although not demonstrated directly, it may well be that a resistance to primaquine in the tissue forms of *P. vivax* can be developed, since Bishop (304c) demonstrated the transmission of primaquin-resistant *P. gallinaceum* through mosquitos and

Beaudin (15) established that the tissue stages of bird malaria parasites, *P. fallax* (turkey) and *P. gallinaceum* (*chicken*), *could be made resistant to primaquine.*

Resistance to the antifolate drugs, viz., the sulfonamides, sulfones, and dihydrofolate reductase (DHFR) inhibitors (see Section 6), is relatively easy to induce, and resistance to the latter class has been correlated geographically with their use. However the trend today is to administer the DHFR-inhibiting drugs in combination with a sulfonamide because of the greater effectiveness of the combination, especially against drug-resistant strains of the parasite, and a decreased tendency to induce resistance.

The occurrence of resistance may be restricted to certain geographical areas. For example, chloroquine-resistant strains of *P. falciparum* are present in the Far East and South America but, with the possible exception of Ethiopia (16a, 17), not in Africa. One may speculate that the geographical segregation of malaria parasites will diminish with the spreading of the vector by the present fast and voluminous world air travel. In the laboratory, techniques have been developed for producing drug-resistant strains which are being used widely to study the mechanism of drug resistance and for testing chemicals in anticipation of the discovery of drugs active against such strains (see Section 3).

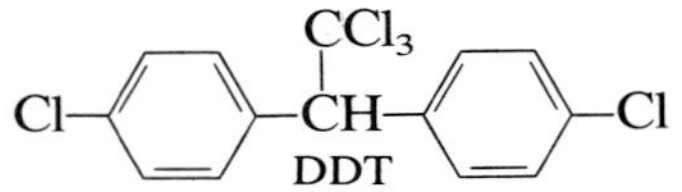

2.3.2 RESISTANCE OF THE VECTOR TO INSECTICIDES. The situation of mosquito resistance to insecticides, particularly, DDT (18.**1**), dieldrin (18.**2**), chlordane (18.**3**), and γ-HCH (18.**4**), is complicated because a distinction exists between physiological and behavioristic resistance. In the latter case mosquitoes have developed the ability to escape from areas sprayed with insecticides without detectable change in their physiological susceptibility. Nevertheless, resistance to insecticides has been defined as "the development of an ability in a strain of insects to tolerate doses of toxicants which are lethal to the majority of individuals in a normal population of the same species." For mosquitoes, the ability to tolerate at least a four fold increase in the lethal dose of the insecticide is necessary to indicate resistance, whereas for the mosquito larvae at least a ten fold increase is necessary (18a). The occurrence of insecticide-resistant mosquitoes is worldwide, and Table 18.3 shows a number of regions where malaria vectors, resistant to DDT and dieldrin have been detected. Up to 1975, *Anopheles* species reported to be resistant numbered 42 (1d). Resistance to one of the chlorinated hydrocarbon insecticides—for instance, DDT—does not imply resistance to all other insecticides of this type. Two different groups of chlorinated hydrocarbon insecticides exist, namely, (1) DDT and its analogs, and (2) cyclodiene derivatives (dieldrin, chlordane), and γ-HCH. Mosquitoes resistant to DDT are still sensitive to dieldrin and γ-HCH, and conversely, resistance to dieldrin does not affect susceptibility to DDT significantly. However cross-resistance to insecticides within a group does exist.

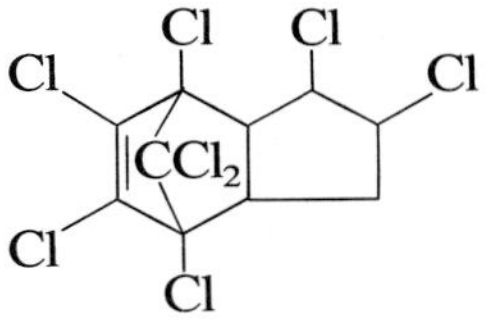

DDT
18.**1**

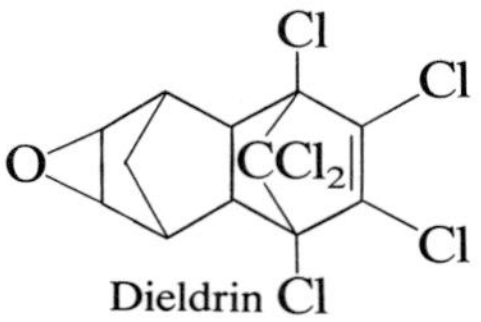

Dieldrin
18.**2**

18.**3**

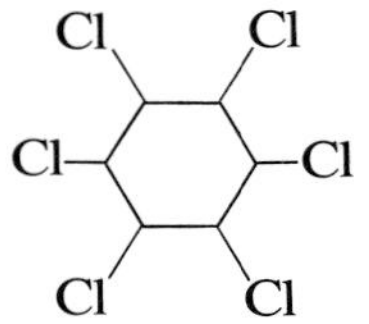

γ-HCH
18.**4**

Table 18.3 Regions and Year of First Reported Resistance to DDT and to Dieldrin in Anopheles Species[a]

Main Regions	Year		*Anopheles* Species
	DDT	Dieldrin	
Greece, Turkey	1950	1952	*sacharovi*
Egypt	1959	1959	*pharoensis*
West Africa	1967	1955	*gambiae*
India, Afghanistan	1960	1958	*culicifacies*
India, Persian Gulf	1955	1959	*stephensi*
Indonesia (Java)	1962	1960	*aconitus*
Venezuela, Colombia	1961	1959	*albitarsis*
Central America	1958	1958	*albimanus*
Mexico	1959	1953	*quadrimaculatus*
Mexico	1967	1958	*pseudopunctipennis*

[a] Compiled from Ref. 18.

Studies performed on flies (19, 20) indicated that in DDT-resistant flies, the enzymatic conversion of DDT to inactive DDE (18.**5**) increased. According to Perry

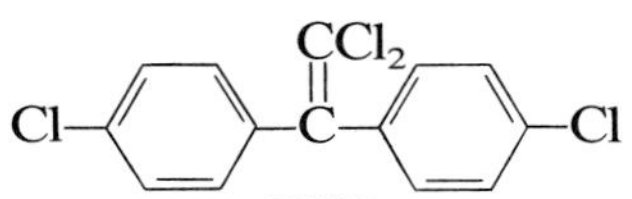

$$Cl-C_6H_4-C(=CCl_2)-C_6H_4-Cl$$

DDE

18.**5**

(21) and Gartrell and Ludvik (22), the detoxification of DDT by conversion to DDE is also more pronounced in DDT-resistant mosquitoes. However other mechanisms (23, 24) may also be involved.

Insecticides other than the chlorinated hydrocarbons are also in use, namely, the organophosphorus compounds such as malathion (18.**6**) and fenitrothion (18.**7**),

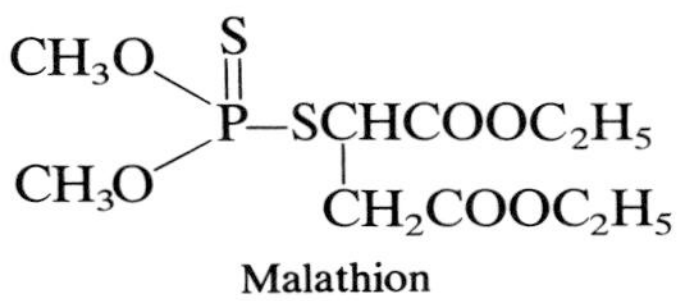

$$(CH_3O)_2P(=S)-SCH(COOC_2H_5)CH_2COOC_2H_5$$

Malathion

18.**6**

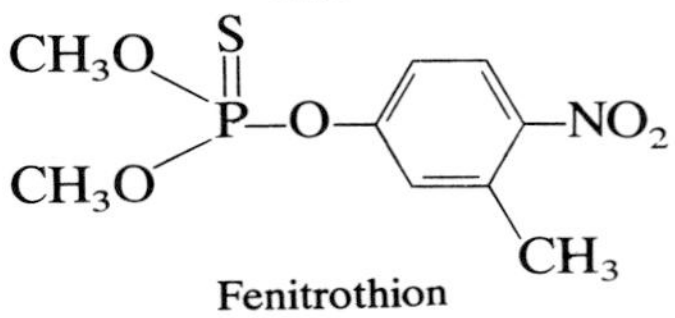

$$(CH_3O)_2P(=S)-O-C_6H_3(CH_3)-NO_2$$

Fenitrothion

18.**7**

$$C_6H_4(OCONHCH_3)(OCH(CH_3)_2)$$

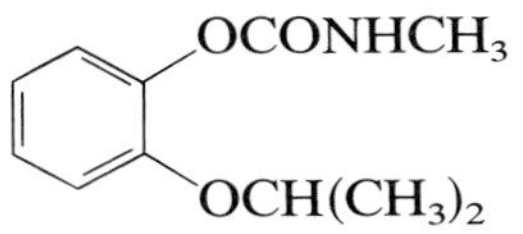

Propoxur

18.**8**

and the carbamates such as propoxur (18.**8**) (1e). The latter insecticide has been used in Central America where *A. albimanus* was resistant to the chlorinated hydrocarbon insecticides. Resistance to propoxur developed fast, probably because of the abundant applications of carbamates in agriculture where mosquito control is a greater problem than in nonagricultural areas.

The modes of action of the phosphorus and carbamate insecticides are similar and are based on the inhibition of acetylcholinesterase. As would be expected, there is cross-resistance to these two groups of insecticides. In the resistant strain of mosquito, a mutant acetylcholinesterase is present that is inhibited more slowly by the insecticide than is the enzyme from the susceptible strain. [For further reading about the mode of action of insecticides, see Albert (25a).] It seems that the successive application of agents from each of the three groups of insecticides, viz., the DDT-type, the cyclodiene-type including γ-HCH, and the acetylcholinesterase-type, for a number of mosquito generations, will prevent the development of resistance in mosquitoes. It should be mentioned that a change to another type of insecticide may gradually reverse resistance (18b).

2.4 The Immunology of Malaria

The use of antimalarial drugs, which is discussed in this chapter, is but one part of the total effort against malaria. On another front much progress has been made in the understanding of the immunology of malaria. The mechanisms of resistance to malaria and how the parasite manages to circumvent the immune systems of the host are important questions. Great benefits would derive from the development of a vaccine against malaria and from an understanding of the role of immunological effects in the pathogenesis of such pernicious phenomena associated with malaria as anemia, renal failure, and cerebral complications. A short but comprehensive report on the status of developments in malaria immunology is available (1f).

3 EVALUATION OF COMPOUNDS FOR ANTIMALARIAL ACTIVITY

The complicated life cycle of the malaria parasite (Fig. 18.1) suggests several phases during which the parasite might be vulnerable to drug action. Thus a prophylactic agent that would attack the parasite during its short transit in the blood, before it is sequestered in the liver, would be desirable. This type of drug is not known. Other possibilities are agents that would attack the tissue stage or the erythrocytic stage. It would also be desirable to have agents that would act on the sexual forms, the gametocytes, to interrupt the transmission of the disease. There are drugs that are effective against one or more of these stages, but no drug is known that is usefully effective against all stages. In the testing of compounds, different procedures are required depending on the phase of the life cycle of the parasite it is desired to interrupt, the type of malaria being investigated (i.e., relapsing or nonrelapsing), and the host that is used (mouse, chick, monkey, etc.).

The testing of compounds against experimentally established infections is made the more difficult because the various species of plasmodia are highly selective with respect to their host and cross-infection is possible only between closely related hosts. The natural transmission of monkey malaria to man has been recorded, but it is extremely rare. A milestone in malaria research was reached recently when human malaria was experimentally so well established in owl monkeys that the testing in this model of all candidate compounds for clinical study in the present US Army antimalarial program became possible (*vide infra*).

In the past, all experimental chemotherapy had to be conducted with nonhuman malarias in birds or animals. Peters (26) has viewed the primary screening of compounds for antimalarial activity as divided into three periods: 1926–1935, when canaries were used in various modifications of a test described by Roehl (27); 1935–1948, when based on the work of Brumpt (28) with *P. gallinaceum* in chicks, the use of fowls became popular; and the present period, beginning in 1948, in which the use of *P. berghei* in albino mice has become widely accepted, the latter model being based on the work of Vincke and Lips (29) and Vincke (30). Birds were used exclusively for the primary screens in the large antimalarial effort of World War II, although the shortcomings of such screens were recognized (31a). For advanced testing, the monkey is used as the host in such models as *P. cynomolgi* or *P. knowlesi* in the rhesus and *P. falciparum* in the owl monkey. The *P. cynomolgi*-rhesus model parallels to a great extent a *P. vivax* infection in man and hence can be used to study the causal prophylactic and antirelapse properties of a compound. This relationship was early recognized by Schmidt (32) who, with his associates, developed the model for the evaluation of blood schizontocidal activity as well as causal prophylactic and curative activity (462). This model proved to be very valuable in advancing the chemo-therapy of malaria. The *P. knowlesi*-rhesus model has properties similar to a *P. falciparum* infection in man (4f). It has been used to some extent for the evaluation of compounds and has also proved to be very useful in basic parasitological studies. The monkey as a host, however, presents problems because of the difficulties and expense connected with procurement, handling, husbandry and colony maintenance, and the relatively large quantity of drug required; for a primary screen, therefore, the use of monkeys is not feasible. For economy, convenience, and general reliability in the screening of large numbers of compounds, *P. berghei* in the laboratory mouse is, today, the model of choice. Despite some shortcomings and some still unanswered questions, the benefits derived from the use of this model have established its preeminence.

The actual mechanics of testing vary widely. If it is desired to test a drug for activity against sporozoites or against primary tissue forms or against secondary tissue forms, i.e., for curative activity against relapsing malarias, it is necessary either to inoculate the host with sporozoites obtained from infected mosquitoes or to allow infected mosquitoes to feed on the host. If it is desired to investigate suppressive curative activity only, i.e., activity against the erythrocytic forms of the parasite without involvement of tissue forms, inoculation with parasitized blood usually suffices. Compounds can be administered orally, intraperitioneally, subcutaneously, or intravenously, in single or multiple doses. Each route has its advantages and disadvantages, and each has its advocates. Various end points have been used for assessing the effectiveness of drugs. The end points are, of course, relative to the end points for the controls. When testing for prophylactic or curative activity of compounds against relapsing malarias using sporozoite-induced infections (i.e., for tissue schizontocidal activity), delay in patency, failure to develop an infection for a given time, often confirmed by subinoculation of blood from the host animal into clean animals, and microscopic examination of liver slices for the presence of parasites have all been used as criteria of effectiveness. With blood-induced infections, various end points can be used. For routine screening a fixed range of doses can be used, and one can simply quote the dose, expressed as milligrams per kilogram of body weight (mg/kg) required to bring about a particular effect—for example, the minimum curative dose or the minimum dose that will extend the mean survival time of the treated animals for a given period beyond that of the controls (i.e., a minimum effective dose). Alternatively, the end point can be expressed as the percentage of the blood cells parasitized at various times after compound administration or as the drug dose required to suppress the parasitemia to a given level (e.g., an SD_{50}). Activity is sometimes quoted in terms of the activity of a standard drug, i.e., the ratio of the dose of the standard to the dose of the experimental drug to bring about a certain effect. Quinine (18.**27**) was used as the standard in the World War II antimalarial program, which use led to the well-known "Quinine Equivalent." For compounds of special interest, which have gone beyond routine testing, the well-known therapeutic index can be obtained. It is often of interest to know whether a strain of parasite resistant to a given drug is also resistant to a new compound, particularly if the new compound is of the same chemical class. A certain degree of such cross-resistance in structurally similar compounds is usually the rule. For example, a sulfone-resistant strain of *Plasmodium* will show some resistance to other sulfones; a chloroquine-resistant strain will show some resistance to other 4-aminoquinolines. Strains of *P. berghei* resistant to all the standard antimalarial drugs have been developed and maintained by Thompson et al. (32a). It must be kept in mind, however, that these drug-resistant strains are maintained under drug pressure and, in this sense, are not normal parasites. If the drug resistance becomes unrealistically high, a cross-resistance to a new drug may be misleading (33). An excellent discussion of the evaluation of antimalarials is given by Davey (34), and more recent work by Thompson and Werbel (35a) and Peters (26) is valuable. Test systems used in the World War II program are described in the compendium edited by Wiselogle (31b).

Test systems are still being refined and developed (37, 38). The primary test system in the present US Army Antimalarial Drug Development Program for the routine screening of large numbers of compounds utilizes *P. berghei* in mice and is described by Osdene et al. (39).

Although the well-established antimalarial drugs in use today have evolved from drug evaluation using avian, monkey, and rodent malarias, the shortcomings of such test systems, with respect to their worth in predicting activity in man, have long been appreciated. The ultimate test of a potential antimalarial lies in seeing how effective it is in humans. However such testing in humans is becoming increasingly more complicated and expensive because of new regulations and social attitudes toward the use of volunteers. In addition, the geographic spread of multi-drug-resistant strains of parasites has emphasized the need to develop drugs that will be effective against such strains. This has complicated testing because of the inherent danger of introducing such strains into nonimmune subjects. Clearly an animal system that could accommodate human malarias and could predict with some degree of assurance the behavior of a drug against the parasite in the human host is urgently needed.

A step in this direction was made when it was shown that a *P. falciparum* infection could be established in splenectomized chimpanzees (40–44). However the cost and difficulties involved in working with chimpanzees militated against the use of these animals in any drug development program. The white-banded gibbon was also successfully infected (45). Shortly thereafter Young et al. (46) demonstrated that a *P. vivax* infection could be established in the owl monkey (*Aotus trivirgatus*), and Geiman and Meagher (47) showed that a *P. falciparum* infection could also be established. This pioneering work culminated in a lengthy period of research and development by Schmidt (48), who delveloped and standardized conditions whereby human malarias, both drug-sensitive and drug-resistant strains, could be used in the owl monkey to test new antimalarials reliably and continuously. Tests using the owl monkey became a key part of the army's antimalarial drug development program. This achievement represents a milestone in the evaluation of antimalarial drugs.

In attempts to circumvent the expense and time required for *in vivo* testing of potential drugs, a variety of *in vitro* systems have been investigated. Such systems may employ parasitized erythrocytes or erythrocyte-free parasites. The effect of drugs on measurable parameters such as glucose utilization (49), parasite maturation (50), incorporation of methionine into protein (51), incorporation of adenosine into nucleic acids (51, 52), and lactic acid production (49, 53) have all been used. An automated system for measuring the ability of compounds to inhibit glucose consumption and lactic acid production was reported (49). An *in vitro* test that proved to be very useful in the army's antimalarial program was that of Rieckmann et al. (50), who measured the effect of drugs on the maturation of *P. falciparum*, both chloroquine-sensitive and chloroquine-resistant strains, in defibrinated parasitized blood.

In vitro screening of antimalarials has certain advantages, including cost, rapidity, and a requirement for a very small amount of compound. However such screening also has drawbacks: standardization of conditions can be difficult, a gross indication of toxicity is not obtained, and the compound may be missed if its activity is dependent on the formation of a metabolite.

4 THE MAIN ANTIMALARIAL DRUGS: HISTORICAL DEVELOPMENT

The oldest remedy for malaria, known at least since 200 BC, is the drug *Ch'ang Shan* which was prepared from powdered roots of *Dichroa febrifuga* Lour and later (54) from hydrangea leaves. The most active component, febrifugine (18.**9**) (55), was

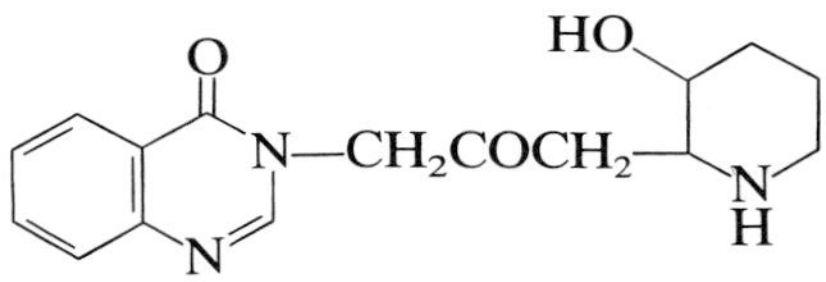

Febrifugine
18.**9**

isolated by Jang and co-workers in 1958 (56, 57); its constitution was established by degradation (55, 58–63) and by synthesis in 1952 (64). Febrifugine is highly active in experimental malaria, but unfortunately it is also highly toxic (65, 66). Baker (67–73) and others (74, 76, 77, 110c) synthesized many congeners but none of these compounds was superior to febrifugine (35b). Clinical investigations of febrifugine against falciparum and vivax infections had limited success (78–80).

A better remedy was prepared from the bark of the wild cinchona trees of Peru. After preparations from the bark had been used in Europe as a specific malaria remedy for more than 200 years, the cultivation of the trees was accomplished successfully in Java around 1880, making this Indonesian island the main producer of the bark. The chief antimalarial compounds present in the bark are quinine and quinidine (Fig. 18.4), and cinchonidine (18.**10**) and cinchonine (18.**11**). Quinine (18.**27**), the most valuable

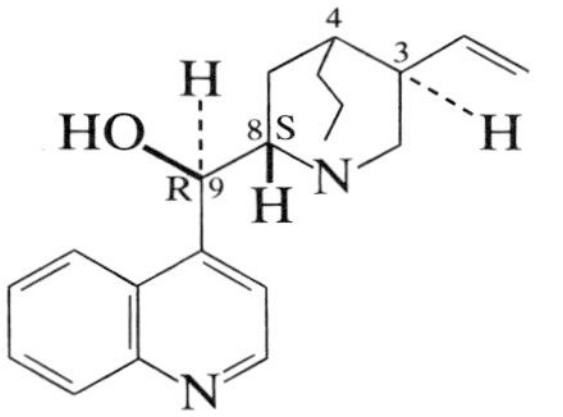

Cinchonidine
18.**10**

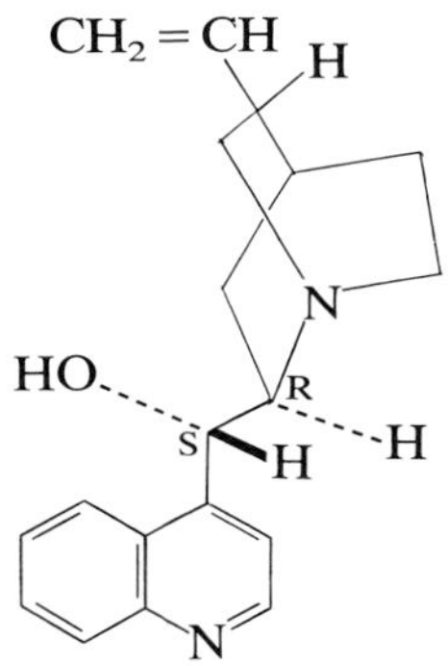

Cinchonine
18.**11**

component, was isolated in 1820, and its structure was elucidated about 100 years later (81). It took almost another half-century before a total synthesis of quinine was accomplished (82), but this synthesis and others (82a) are too complex and expensive to provide a practical source of the drug. Until 1932 quinine and related alkaloids were the sole antimalarial drugs active against the intraerythrocytic form of the parasite (see Section 5.2).

The first synthetic compound investigated for its potential antimalarial property was the dye methylene blue (18.**12a**). This compound was selected at the time dyes were being investigated for their ability to

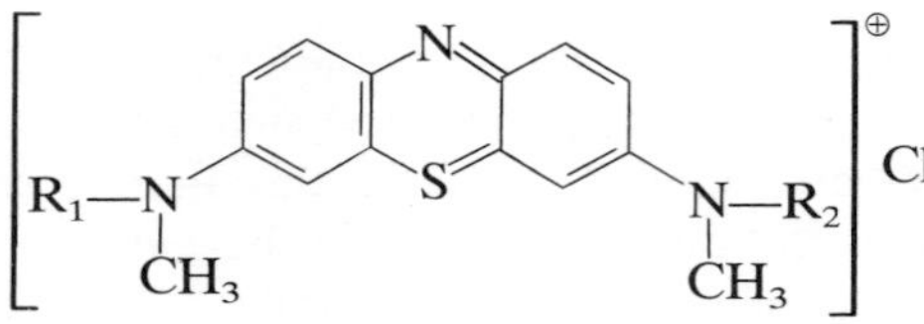

$$\left[R_1-N(CH_3)-\text{phenothiazinium}-N(CH_3)-R_2 \right]^{\oplus} Cl^{\ominus}$$

a, $R_1 = R_2 = CH_3$ (methylene blue)
b, $R_1 = CH_3$, $R_2 = CH_2CHN(C_2H_5)_2$

18.**12a**,
18.**12b**,

stain microorganisms as a means of identification. Methylene blue was one of the basic dyes that was strongly bound by plasmodia; it proved to be active *in vitro* and showed relatively low toxicity. Since a method had not yet been developed for testing chemicals for their antimalarial activity *in vivo*, methylene blue could be tried only on patients suffering from malaria. In 1891 Guttmann and Ehrlich (83) evaluated this compound in man and observed some beneficial effect. Twenty years later, Kopanaris (84) demonstrated the activity of quinine against bird malaria, and Marks (85) showed that methylene blue was also active. Consequently, chemists began to design potential antimalarial agents based on modifications of quinine and methylene blue (see Section 7.1). These investigations led to the syntheses of compounds having the 6-methoxyquinoline moiety of quinine as well as the diethylaminoalkylamino type of side chain, which had been shown to enhance the activity of methylene blue such as present in 18.**12b**. The culmination of such research by Schulemann, Schönhöfer, and Roehl was the drug pamaquine (plasmoquine) (18.**13**), which was introduced in

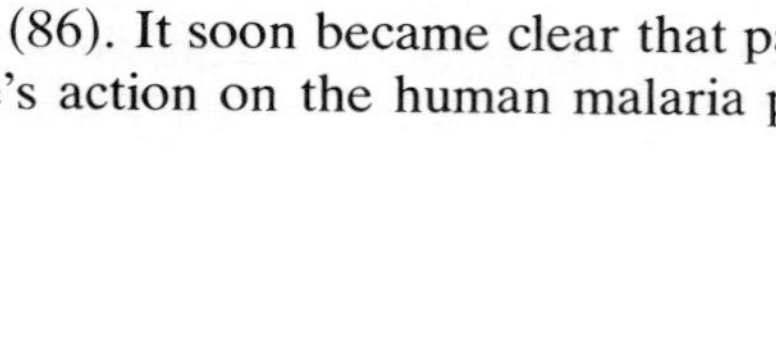

CH_3O — quinoline (positions 1–8) — $HNCH(CH_2)_3N(C_2H_5)_2$ with CH_3

Pamaquine

18.**13**

1926 (86). It soon became clear that pamaquine's action on the human malaria parasite differed from that of quinine; in addition, pamaquine proved to be quite toxic. Hence the search for drugs with quininelike action (blood schizonticidal drugs, see Section 2.2) was continued. An outstanding group of compounds with this action was found in the 9-dialkylaminoalkylamino acridines (87) from which emerged the drug quinacrine (Atebrin) (18.**14**) in 1932 (88).

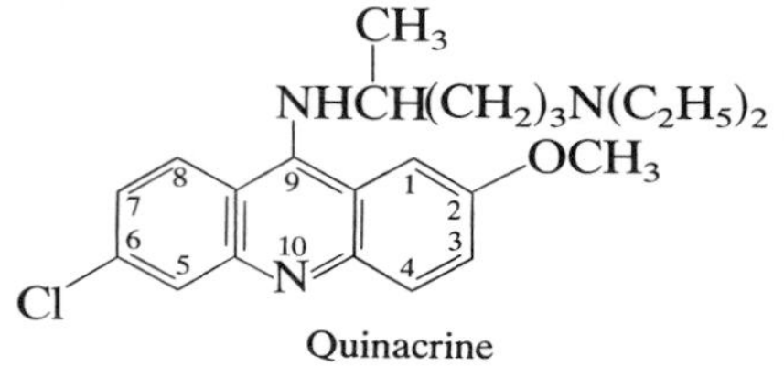

$NHCH(CH_3)(CH_2)_3N(C_2H_5)_2$ at position 9, OCH_3, Cl — acridine (positions 1–10)

Quinacrine

18.**14**

Structurally this drug encompasses the 6-methoxy-4-quinolyl moiety of quinine and the basic side chain of pamaquine; it is appreciably more effective and less toxic than quinine.

Another class of compounds structurally related to quinacrine is the 4-aminoquinolines (see Section 5.2), which were first investigated in Germany, and later in the Soviet Union and the United States. The Germans used sontoquine (18.**15**) as their drug of choice in the North

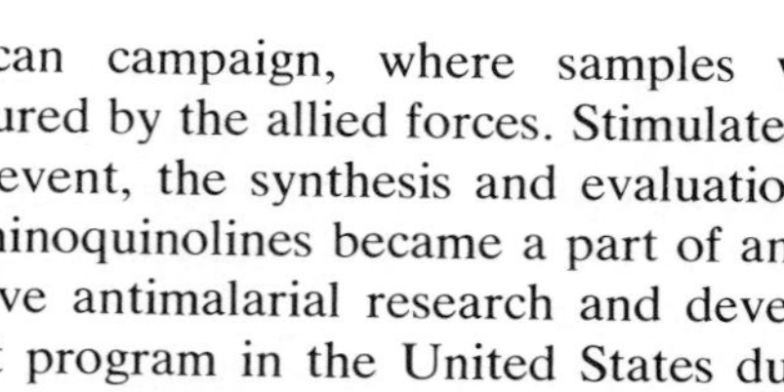

$HNCH(CH_3)(CH_2)_3N(C_2H_5)_2$, CH_3, Cl — quinoline

Sontoquine

18.**15**

African campaign, where samples were captured by the allied forces. Stimulated by this event, the synthesis and evaluation of 4-aminoquinolines became a part of an extensive antimalarial research and development program in the United States during the years 1941–1945. Through this program several drugs were developed, most notably chloroquine (18.**16**) (89) and

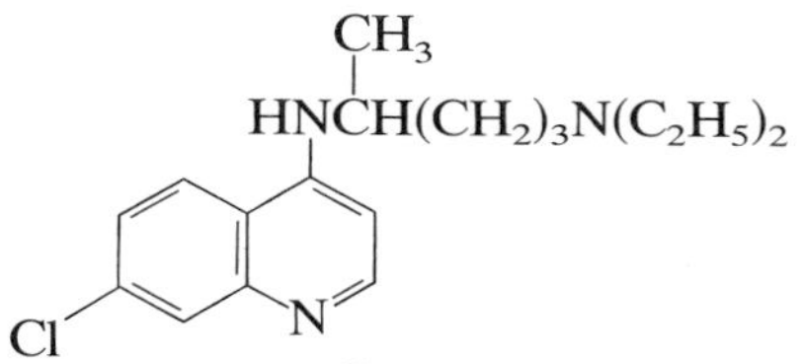

Chloroquine
18.**16**

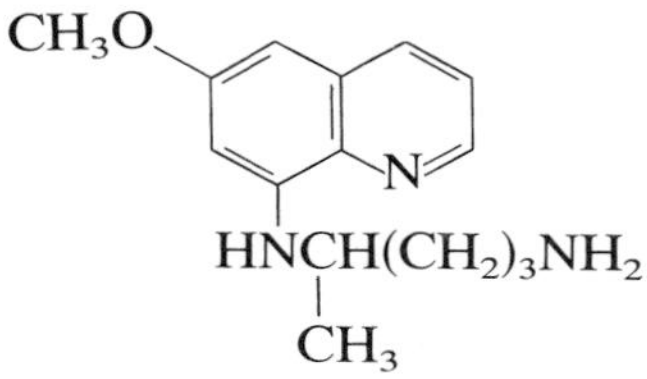

Primaquine
18.**17**

primaquine (18.**17**) (90). Chloroquine was first investigated in Germany in the late 1930s, but because of its toxicity (unpublished studies) it was not considered to be an outstanding drug. Intensive pharmacological and clinical studies carried out in the United States showed that chloroquine was extremely valuable, and it now is the most widely used of antimalarial drugs (see Section 5.2.2). The other drug, primaquine, is structurally closely related to pamaquine (18.**13**) and is presently the drug of choice against relapsing vivax malaria (see Section 7.1.3).

Shortly afterward it was shown that Prontosil (18.**18**) was converted in animals to sulfanilamide (18.**19**) and that the entire structure was not necessary for antibacterial action. The antimalarial activity of Prontosil was demonstrated against *P. falciparum* and *P. knowlesi* (91) and against *P. vivax* (92, 93). One of its metabolites, sulfanilamide, was itself shown to have appreciable antimalarial activity (94), a finding that ushered in a succession of studies on the synthesis and testing of sulfonamides that despite the shortcomings of these drugs when used alone, has now been phased into the present era of sulfonamide–dihydrofolate reductase inhibitor combinations (see Section 6.1.2).

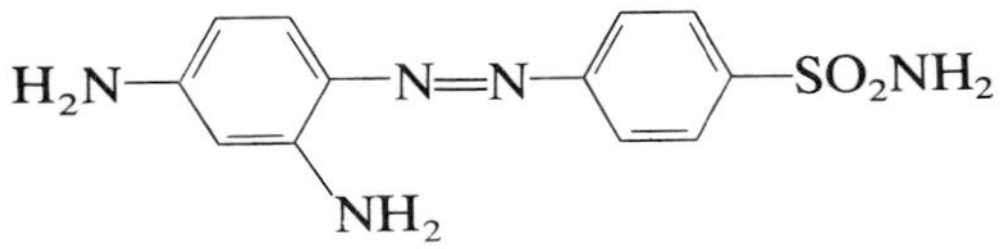

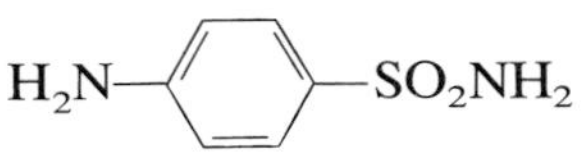

Prontosil
18.**18**

Sulfanilamide
18.**19**

The recognition of the antileprotic diaminodiphenylsulfone (DDS, dapsone) (18.**20a**) as an antimalarial drug dates from the work of Coggeshall et al. (95) who, looking for a compound better than but related to sulfanilamide, tested a derivative of DDS, sodium glucosulfone (18.**21**), in man.

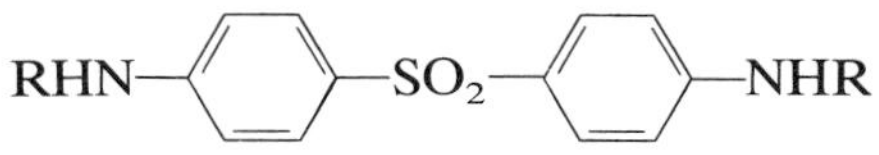

18.**20**

	R	
18.**20a**	H	DDS
18.**20b**	HCO	DFDDS
18.**20c**	CH_3CO	DADDS

Sodium glucosulfone
18.**21**

Concurrent with the American research on antimalarials that was carried out during World War II, British workers at Imperial Chemical Industries, Ltd., discovered a new type of antimalarial drug. Their work was based on an attempt to combine what were believed to be important features of sulfanilamidopyrimidines, which were

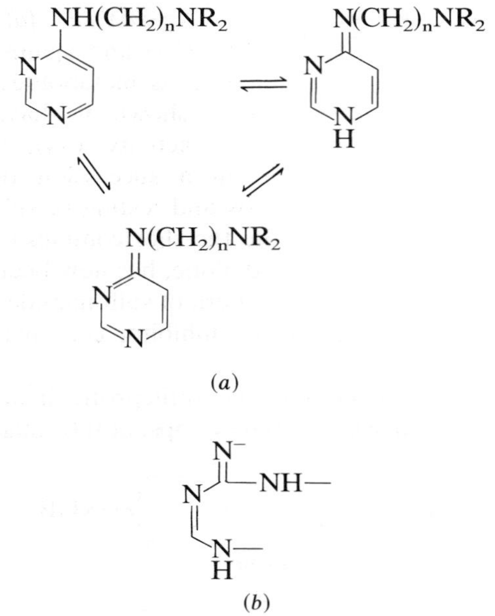

(*a*)

(*b*)

Fig. 18.2 (a) Tautomeric system of 4-aminopyrimidines. (b) Prototropic pyrimidine system.

known to have antimalarial activity, and quinacrine. The pyrimidine ring was chosen from the sulfonamides as the site for attachment of the basic alkylaminoalkyl side chain. This system would also have the advantage of being capable of a tautomerism, which was considered at the time to have an important association with antimalarial activity (96) (Fig. 18.2*a*). This approach was productive in that a variety of active structures were uncovered. In an attempt (97) to simplify the molecule, it was reasoned that the entire pyrimidine may not be necessary as long as the prototropic system is present (Fig. 18.2*b*). Further structural modifications around the biguanide moiety eventually led to the antimalarial drug chlorguanide (proguanil, 18.**22**) (98a).

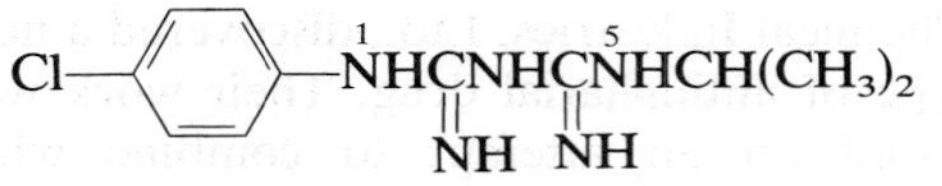

Chlorguanide (Proguanil)
18.**22**

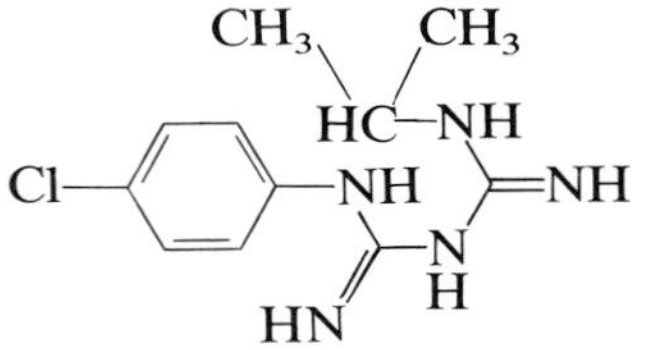

Chlorguanide (Proguanil)
18.**22a**

While the work on chlorguanide was proceeding in England, a group in the United States at the Wellcome Research Laboratories was studying the effect of 2,4-diaminopyrimidines and condensed pyrimidine systems on the growth of *Lactobacillus casei.* These substances were found to be growth inhibitory, especially those heavily weighted in the 5-position. When these analogs showed no untoward toxicity, it was realized that chemotherapeutic agents might emerge from the group of compounds. The formal structural analogy of certain of the inhibitors, e.g., 2,4-diamino-5-(*p*-chlorophenoxyl)pyrimidine (18.**23**) and chlorguanide, drawn as 18.**22a**,

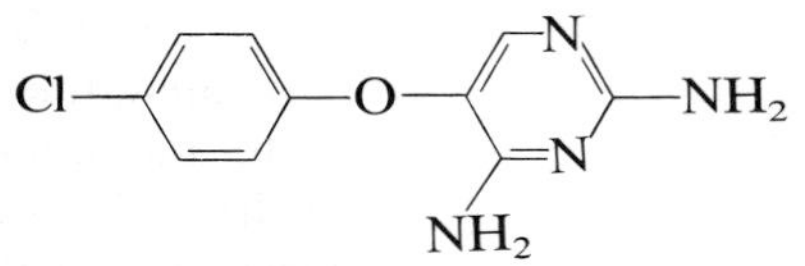

2,4-Diamino-5-(*p*-chlorophenoxyl)pyrimidine
18.**23**

prompted the testing of the pyrimidines for antimalarial activity (99). Interestingly, the analogy is much closer than had at first been believed in view of the fact that the active form of chlorguanide (18.**22a**) is the cyclic triazine, cycloguanil (18.**24**). The encouraging activity prompted (99, 100) the

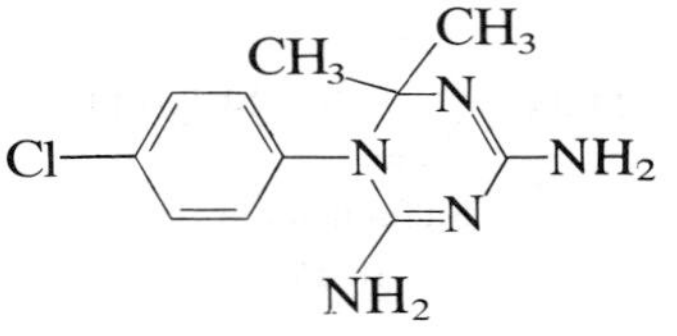

Cycloguanil
18-**24**

synthesis of a large number of analogs, and the evolutionary path led, with increasing antimalarial activity, through a series of 2,4-diaminopyrimidines containing a substituted 5-benzyl group to a series in which the bridge between the rings was eliminated, the 5-phenyl series. The greater activity imparted to the various series by the presence of a 6-alkyl substituent on the pyrimidine ring was early established. The final choice of the compound pyrimethamine (18.**25**) for advanced studies

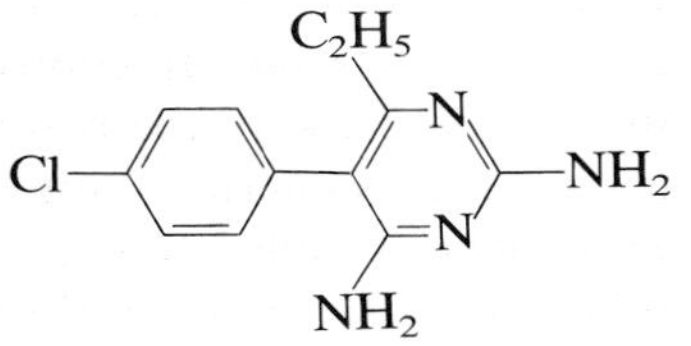

Pyrimethamine
18.**25**

was based on its consistency of activity against several experimental malarias, not solely on its absolute level of activity (101).

As a consequence of the appearence of chloroquine-resistant strains of *P. falciparum* in Southeast Asia and the military involvement of the United States in this area, the US Army Medical Research and Development Command began in 1963 a vigorous program of research and development on new antimalarial drugs. Because quinine was still beneficial in the treatment of chloroquine-resistant falciparum malaria, although the presence of less sensitive strains of *P. falciparum* to quinine was known (13), a major effort was undertaken to develop a superior quinine type (amino alcohol) of drug (see Section 5.1). This work culminated in the development of mefloquine (Fig. 18.5).

5 FAST-ACTING BLOOD SCHIZONTOCIDAL DRUGS

5.1 Amino Alcohols

The best known amino alcohol type of drug is quinine (18.**27**), which is the chief alkaloid of the bark of *Cinchona ledgeriana*. Since its synthesis is too complex and expensive for practical use, the bark of the cinchona tree is still the main source of the drug. Numerous attempts to modify the structure of quinine to obtain better antimalarial drugs of the amino alcohol type had not been successful until mid-1960, when the US Army Medical Research and Development Command sponsored an extensive research and development program that led to the discovery of a number of amino alcohols that were highly active against chloroquine-resistant strains of *P. falciparum*.

5.1.1 STRUCTURE-ACTIVITY RELATIONSHIPS. The general structure of antimalarial agents belonging to this type appears in Fig. 18.3.

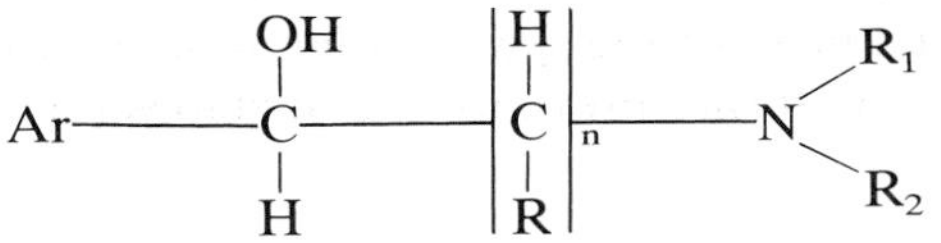

Fig. 18.3 General structure of the amino methanols listed in Tables 18.4 and 18.5: Ar is a substituted aromatic nucleus; 4-quinolyl, 1-naphthyl, 9-phenanthryl, 9-anthryl, 12-chrysenyl, 2-phenyl-4-pyridyl; *n* is 1 or 2, R and R_1 are hydrogen or alkyl; R_2 is alkyl; R, R_1, and R_2 can form a substituted quinuclidine nucleus; R and R_2 can form a piperidyl nucleus.

The structure of quinine, with its four asymmetric enters at C_3, C_4, C_8, and C_9, has been examined thoroughly to establish the parts of the molecule responsible for the antimalarial activity. Particularly from the work of Ainley and King (102) and Buttle et al. (103), it became clear that the asymmetry at positions 3 and 4 is not essential for antimalarial activity.* For instance, both racemates of compound 18.**26**, which lack these two asymmetric centers,

* The degree of activity depends on the test system used. In this discussion of the effect of asymmetry on the antimalarial activity, a compound is considered to be active if activity has been reported in any test system, and inactive if no activity could be established.

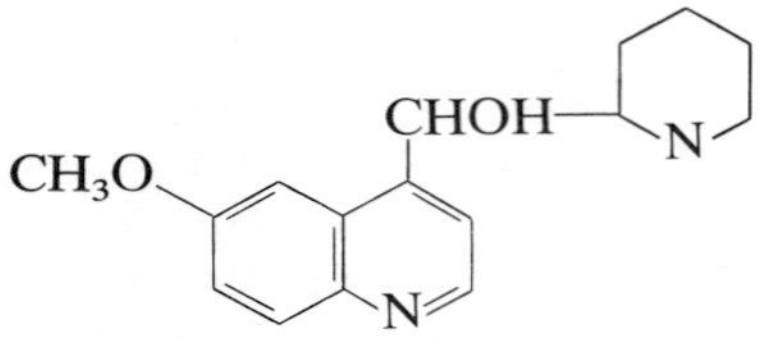

18.**26**

were found to be slightly active (102, 104). However the configurations at position 8 and 9 affect the juxtaposition of the hydroxy group and the nonaromatic nitrogen atom, a relationship that seems to be associated with antimalarial activity. Because of the presence of these two asymmetric centers, two erythro forms, quinine (18.**27**) and quinidine (18.**28**), and two threo forms, 9-epiquinine (18.**29**) and 9-epiquinidine (18.**30**) exist. Figure 18.4 shows the stereochemical relationships of these compounds (105, 106). It is likely that the bulkiness of the quinuclidine moiety in the threo forms prevents the juxtaposition of the hydroxy group and the nitrogen atom of the quinuclidine nucleus that is necessary for activity. Support for this view is obtained when the rigid quinuclidine nucleus is replaced with the more flexible piperidyl group, since both the erythro and threo forms of 18.**26** were found to be slightly active (102). Although these two racemates have not been resolved into their optically active components, the two racemates with an identical side chain (Fig. 18.5) have been resolved (107). In this case, all four forms were found to be equally active (Table 18.4: 18.**31**–18.**34**). In contrast, it is significant that only one of the two possible racemates of the isomeric 3′-piperidyl-4-quinolinemethanol (Table 18.4: 18.**35**) was found to be active. Here again, the inactivity of one of the racemates can be associated with the unfavorable orientation of the hydroxy group and the piperidyl nitrogen atom. Cheng (109), using Dreiding

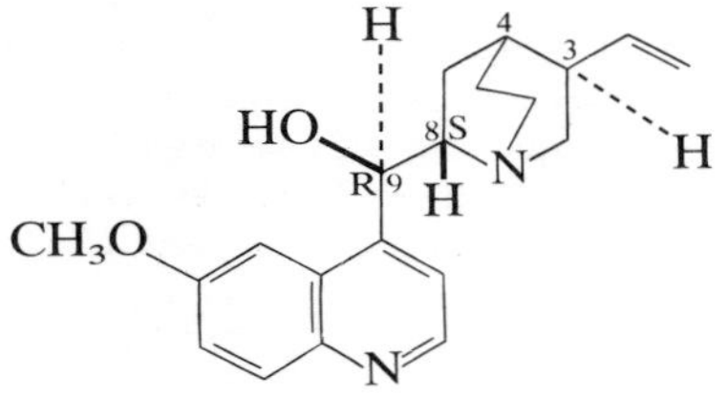

Quinine
18.**27**

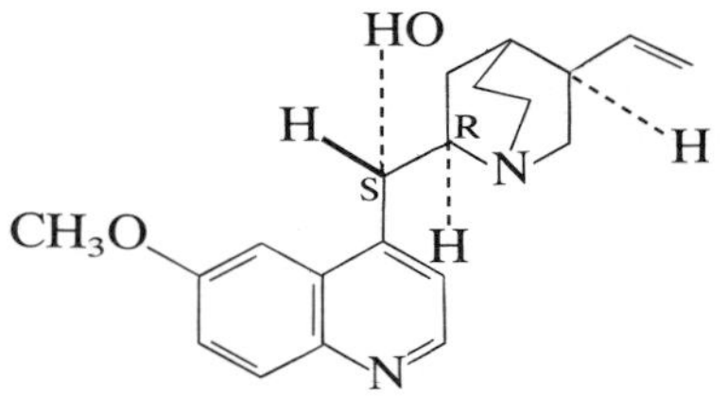

Quinidine
18.**28**

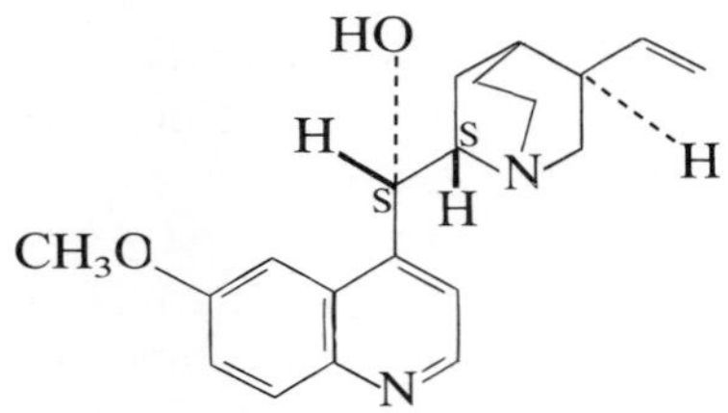

9-Epiquinine
18.**29**

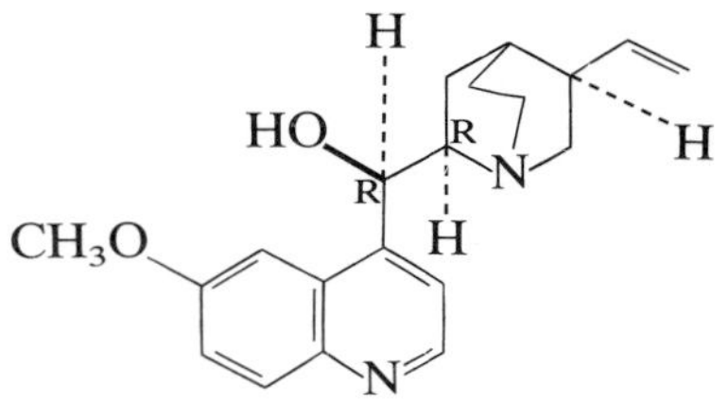

9-Epiquinidine
18.**30**

Fig. 18.4 Configuration at C_8 and C_9 of quinine-type of alkaloid. These isomers have identical configuration at the asymmetric centers C_3 and C_4 (81); consequently they are not enantiomers. The erythro forms, quinine and quinidine are active; the threo forms, 9-epiquinine and 9-epiquinidine are inactive (for activity, see Table 18.4).

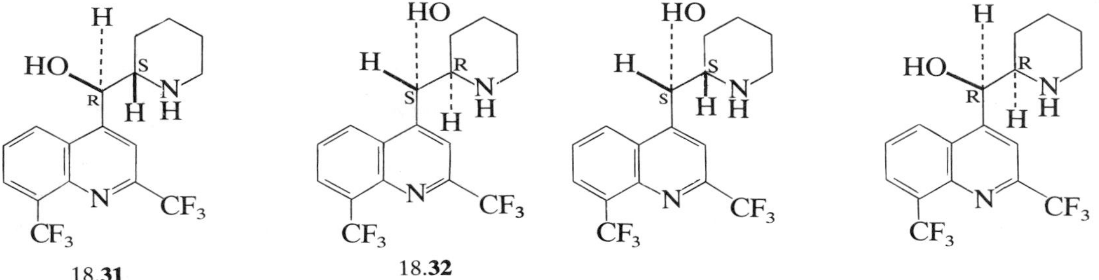

Fig. 18.5 Configuration at the two asymmetric centers of mefloquine-type compounds. Mefloquine consists of equal parts of 18.**31** and 18.**32**. Enantiomers are the erythro forms 18.**31** and 18.**32**, and the threo forms 18.**33** and 18.**34**. The four isomers are active (for activity, see Table 18.4).

Table 18.4 4-Quinolinemethanols

CHOHR (at C-4 of the quinoline ring; positions 2, 6, 8 marked)

R:

A	B	C	D	E
—(quinuclidinyl)—$CH{=}CH_2$	2-piperidyl	4-methyl-2-piperidyl	—(quinuclidinyl)—C_2H_5	$CH_2N(C_4H_9)_2$

Compound Number	Structure	Q^a *P. lophurae*, Duck	MED^b *P. berghei*, Mouse	References
18.**31**–18.**34**	2,8-diCF_3; **B**		10	107, 108
18.**35**	2,8-diCF_3; **C**;			
	Racemate a		*ca.* 40,	110a
	Racemate b		inactive	110a
18.**27**	6-OCH_3; **A** (quinine)	1.0	<1280>640	31c, 4d
			200^c	112
18.**10**	Desmethoxyquinine or cinchonidine	1.5		31d
18.**36**	6-OCH_3; **D** (dihydroquinine)	1.0	100^c	31c, 112
18.**26**	6-OCH_3; **B** (both racemates)	0.3		31e
18.**37**	6-Cl; **D**		100^c	112
18.**38**	6-Cl; **B**	0.3		31f
18.**39**	6,8-diCl; **B**	1.5		31g
18.**40**	6,8-diCl; 2-phenyl; **B**	2.0	<20	31h
18.**41**	6,8-diCl; 2-(3′, 4′-Cl_2-phenyl); **E**	20	5	31i, 113
18.**28**	6-OCH_3; **A** (quinidine)	1.0		31c
18.**29**	6-OCH_3; **A** (9-epiquinine)	Inactive		31c
18.**30**	6-OCH_3; **A** (9-epiquinidine)	Inactive		31c

[a] Q = quinine equivalent = minimum effective dose of quinine/minimum effective dose of agent.
[b] MED = minimum effective dose = the dose (mg/kg) needed to double the mean survival time (days) of treated mice relative to the controls (39, 4d).
[c] MED = the lowest dose (mg/kg) preventing detectable parasitemia on day 5 after inoculation (112).

molecular models, studied the respective orientations and demonstrated that for antimalarial activity, the distance between the oxygen and the nonaromatic nitrogen should be about 3 Å. He postulated (110a) that a compound will be inactive if this distance is greater in the compound's favored conformation. His postulate was found to be in agreement with the energy conformational studies of Loew and Sahakian (111) on the phenanthrene amino alcohols 18.**42** and 18.**43** (Table 18.5), which also have the 2′- and 3′-piperidyl side chain, respectively. Apparently, in all active amino alcohol-type antimalarials the orientation of the hydroxy hydrogen and the amine nitrogen should be such that hydrogen bonding is possible.

Table 18.5 Prominent 9-Phenanthryl, 9-Anthryl, 1-Naphthyl, 12-Chrysenyl, and 4-Pyridyl Amino Alcohols

Compound Number	Structure	MED[a] *P. berghei*, Mouse	References
	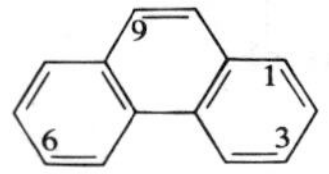 (phenanthrene ring, positions 1, 3, 6, 9)		
18.**42**	3,6-diCF$_3$-9-CHOH(2′-Piperidyl)		
	Racemate a	10	107, 123
	Racemate b	10	107
18.**43**	3,6-diCF$_3$-9-CHOH(3′-Piperidyl)		
	Racemate a	ca. 40	110b, 111
	Racemate b	Inactive	110b, 111
18.**44**	6-Br-9-CHOHCH$_2$N(C$_7$H$_{15}$)$_2$	40	122, 123
18.**45**	1,3-diCl-6-CF$_3$-9-CHOHCH$_2$CH$_2$N(C$_4$H$_9$)$_2$	5	124
18.**46**	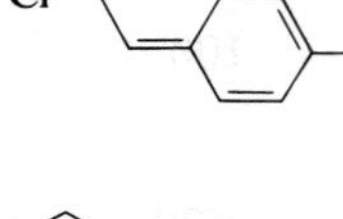 (10-Cl-anthracene) 9-CHOHCH$_2$N(C$_4$H$_9$)$_2$	20	125
18.**47**	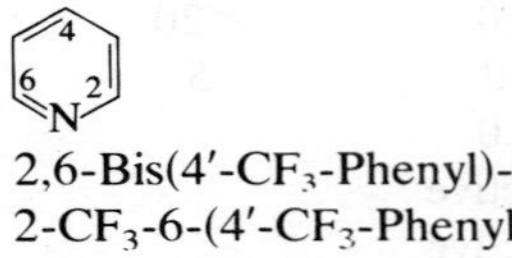 (naphthalene with 3,4-diCl-phenyl) 1-CHOHCH$_2$N(C$_4$H$_9$)$_2$	<10	126
18.**48**	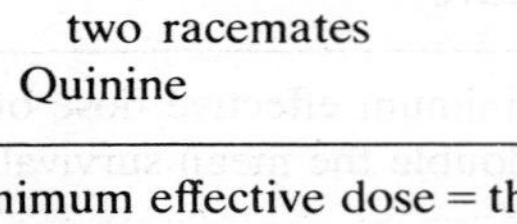 (Cl- and CF$_3$-chrysene) 12-CHOHCH$_2$N(C$_4$H$_9$)$_2$	20	113
	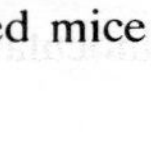 (pyridine ring, positions 2, 4, 6)		
18.**49**	2,6-Bis(4′-CF$_3$-Phenyl)-4-CHOHCH$_2$CH$_2$N(C$_4$H$_9$)$_2$	20	124
18.**50**	2-CF$_3$-6-(4′-CF$_3$-Phenyl)-4-CHOH(2′-piperidyl), two racemates	5–20	127
18.**27**	Quinine	<1280>640	4d

[a] MED = minimum effective dose = the dose (mg/kg) needed to double the mean survival time (days) of the treated mice relative to the controls (39, 4d).

The presence of the methoxy group in quinine is not essential for activity because the alkaloid cinchonidine, a desmethoxy quinine, is also active (Table 18.4; 18.**10**). Replacement of the methoxy group by a chloro atom in the quinine-related compounds 18.**36** and 18.**26** gives 18.**37** and 18.**38**, respectively, which are both active (Table 18.4). Activity is usually enhanced by the introduction of a halogen at position 8, viz., compounds 18.**38** and 18.**39** (Table 18.4). A further increase in activity resulted from the introduction of a phenyl group at position 2 as seen in 18.**40** (Table 18.4). In general, blocking of position 2 of the quinoline ring with a phenyl group, but not with an aliphatic hydrocarbon group, led to highly active compounds, such as 18.**40** and 18.**41** (Table 18.4). The rationale for the blocking of position 2 was based on an attempt to increase activity by preventing biological oxidation at this position, since it was known that 2-hydroxyquinine, a metabolite of quinine (114), is less active than quinine (115). Unfortunately, all highly active 2-phenyl-4-quinolylamino alcohols were also highly phototoxic in mice (116). A few selected compounds of this type were also tested in swine for phototoxicity, and interestingly, 18.**41** (117) proved to be relatively low in phototoxicity (118). In man, its phototoxicity was considerably less (119, 120) than that of 18.**40** (121), which had been evaluated in the clinic earlier. More recently, it was discovered that high activity without phototoxicity could be attained by blocking position 2 with a trifluoromethyl group, a finding that eventually led to the development of mefloquine (Fig. 18.5), in the course of a search for compounds active against infections with chloroquine-resistant strains of *P. falciparum* (113).

In the extensive antimalarial screening program in the United States during World War II, it was found that in addition to the quinoline amino alcohols, certain amino alcohols having a phenanthrene or naphthalene nucleus were slightly active against *P. gallinaceum* in chicks. This discovery stimulated the subsequent synthesis and investigation of a great number of amino alcohols with aromatic ring systems other than quinoline. The structures and activity in mice of a number of the more interesting compounds of these types are listed in Table 18.5. These compounds were selected from a large number of agents investigated in the US Army Antimalarial Program. In contrast to the 2-phenyl-4-quinolylamino alcohols, these compounds have little or no phototoxicity (113).

An interesting attempt to arrive at potential antimalarial agents of the amino alcohol type was undertaken by Henry (128), who assumed that these agents intercalate between the base pairs of the DNA double helix of the parasite (see Section 5.3.1.2 and Fig. 18.12). In such intercalation the DNA becomes extended, and Henry suggested that the more fully the volume between the DNA base pairs was occupied, the more active the compound would be when compounds with similar amino alcohol side chains were compared. The relationship of the intercalative positions of the diverse aromatic nuclei shown in Table 18.4 and 18.5 is illustrated schematically in Fig. 18.6. Such a scheme was considered in designing structures of potentially active agents (113). It should be emphasized that

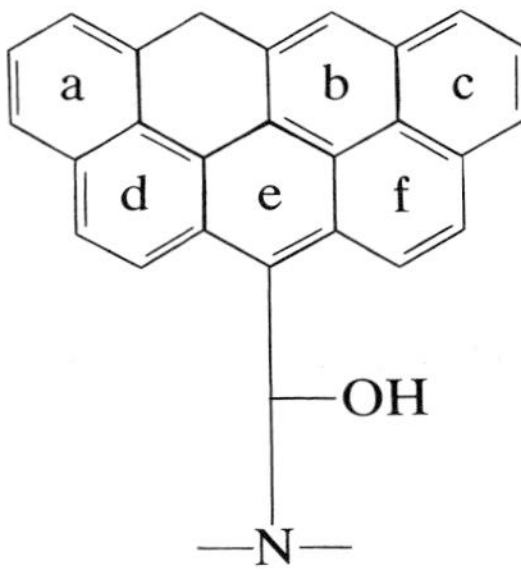

Fig. 18.6 Phenylnaphthyl amino alcohols or phenylquinolyl amino alcohols: d, e, c; 9-phenanthryl amino alcohols: d, e, b; 2,6-diphenyl-4-pyridyl amino alcohols: a, e, c; anthryl amino alcohols: d, e, f; chrysenyl amino alcohols: d, e, b, c.

this model was used as a working hypothesis, and it may well be that intercalation in DNA is not the primary antimalarial mechanism. Indeed, the highly active quinolylamino alcohol, mefloquine (Fig. 18.5), was reported not to bind to DNA (129, 223, 224) (see Section 5.3.1.2).

In addition to the two efforts already mentioned to achieve outstanding antimalarials of the amino alcohol type, mathematical approaches were explored (130, 131); unfortunately, the calculations did not result in the discovery of a better drug.

5.1.2 DRUGS. For centuries quinine and quinine-containing products have been used as antimalarials, and until the early 1930s quinine was the sole drug available for the treatment of malaria. At present quinine is rarely used alone except in regions of the world where the synthetic antimalarials are unavailable or too expensive. A less expensive but equally effective form of quinine is the product Totaquine, which contains approximately 10% quinine and 75% of other cinchona alkaloids. The therapeutic properties of quinine have been described extensively (132–134); and thus only a brief description of the use of quinine as an antimalarial drug is presented below.

Quinine is a fast-acting blood schizontocidal drug, and in its action resembles other fast-acting blood schizontocides such as quinacrine 18.**14**), chloroquine (18.**16**), and amodiaquine (18.**51**); however it is less effective and more toxic than the others. It produces a radical cure of falciparum malaria, but it does not prevent relapses in vivax malaria because it does not have tissue schizontocidal activity. Quinine has gametocytocidal activity against *P. vivax* and *P. malariae* but not *P. falciparum*. Resistance of *P. falciparum* to quinine is not as prevalent as that to the abovementioned synthetic, fast-acting blood schizontocides, although it has been observed (1g). Particularly good results against recrudescences from drug-resistant strains of *P. falciparum* were obtained by Hall (135a) using infused quinine; such an administration was more effective than oral administration because higher plasma levels of drug were obtained. Combinations of quinine with other antimalarial drugs have also been studied (1h), but none of these combinations is commercially available. Quinine combinations with pyrimethamine (18.**25**) were markedly effective against chloroquine-resistant strains of *P. falciparum*. Hall warned against the use of combinations containing quinine and chloroquine (18.**16**) because of the observed antagonistic effect (135b).

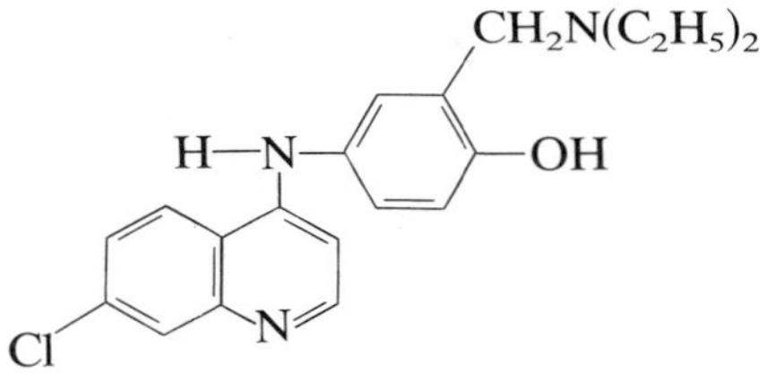

$CH_2N(C_2H_5)_2$ H—N OH Cl N

18.**51**

No other amino alcohol has been used routinely as an antimalarial drug, but several have been investigated in man (31j, 136). The most interesting new compound is mefloquine (Fig. 18.5), which may reach drug status. This investigational drug may well become the drug of choice for the treatment of drug-resistant infections of *P. falciparum* (136).

5.2 9-Aminoacridines and 4-Aminoquinolines

The first synthetic antimalarial drug with blood schizontocidal activity was discovered in Germany in 1932 (88, 137) and was marketed under the name of Atebrin (18.**14**). The adopted international nonproprietary name is mepacrine, and in the United States Pharmacopeia it is listed as quinacrine.

Table 18.6 Activity Against Avian Malarias of Prominent 9-(4-Diethylamino-1-methylbutyl-amino)acridines

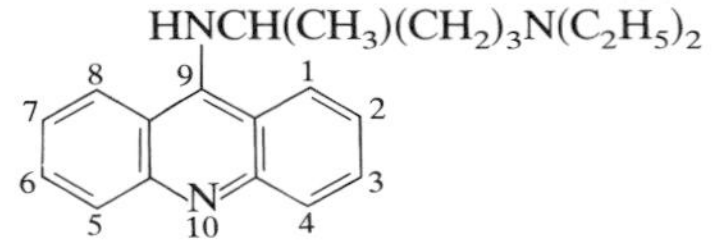

$HNCH(CH_3)(CH_2)_3N(C_2H_5)_2$

Compound Number	Structure	TI[a]	Q[b]	Reference
18.**14**	2-OCH_3; 6-Cl (quinacrine)	16.9[c]	—	138a
		30	—	87
		—	6	31k
18.**52**	2-OC_6H_{13}; 6-Cl	15	—	87
18.**53**	2-SCH_3; 6-Cl	15	—	87
18.**54**	2-CH_3; 6-Cl	15	—	87
18.**55**	2-OCH_3; 6-CN	—	3	31k

[a] TI = therapeutic index against *P. relictum* in canaries.
[b] Q = quinine equivalent against *P. lophurae* in ducks.
[c] *P. gallinaceum* in chicks.

As a consequence of the Japanese occupation of Java during World War II, the Allies were deprived of their main source of quinine and were forced to find a substitute. They developed their own process for the manufacture of quinacrine (18.**14**), and this drug was extensively used during the war. Nevertheless, a search for a superior antimalarial continued in Germany, and from a great number of 4-aminoquinolines investigated, both before and during World War II, sontoquine (18.**15**) was selected for field studies in North Africa. Samples of sontoquine were obtained in Tunis by the Allied forces, and this drug and quinacrine stimulated the synthesis and evaluation of numerous congeners in the United States. Numerous 9-aminoacridines (approximately 300) and 4-aminoquinolines (approximately 250) were investigated (31k, 138a), and a literature study made at the time revealed that at least a similar number of these types had been evaluated in Germany and in the Soviet Union.

5.2.1 STRUCTURE-ACTIVITY RELATIONSHIPS. Tables 18.6 and 18.7 give the structures and activities against avian malarial infections of a number of prominent 9-aminoacridines. Besides quinacrine other acridine antimalarials were evaluated clinically, such as the compounds 18.**56** (25b); 18.**57**,

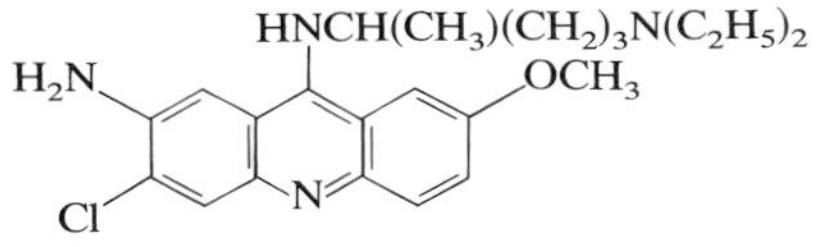

$HNCH(CH_3)(CH_2)_3N(C_2H_5)_2$ H_2N OCH_3 N Cl

18.**56**

and 18.**58** (139), 18.**61** (311), 18.**62** (140) (Table 18.7); 18.**63** (141); 18.**64** (142); and

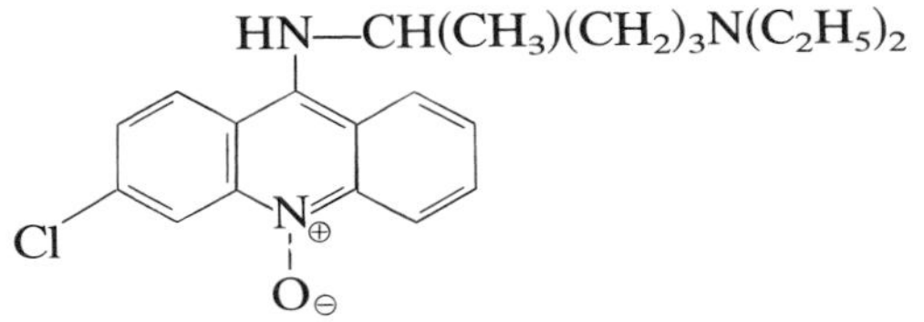

$HN—CH(CH_3)(CH_2)_3N(C_2H_5)_2$ Cl $N^{\oplus}$ $O^{\ominus}$

Desmethoxyquinacrine-*N*-oxide

18.**63**

$HN—CH(CH_3)(CH_2)_3N(C_2H_5)_2$ N OCH_3 N Cl

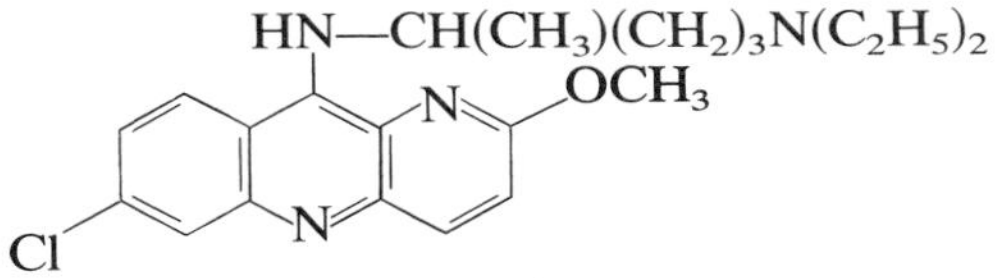

Azacrine

18.**64**

18.**71** (31m) (Table 18.8a) but none has superseded quinacrine. Desmethoxyquinacrine-*N*-oxide (18.**63**) behaved like quinacrine, but it lacked the skin-coloring property of quinacrine (143). Azacrine (18.**64**) was found to be as active as quinacrine, but it was inferior to the 4-aminoquinolines, chloroquine (18.**16**) and amodiaquine (18.**51**) (142).

The 4-aminoquinoline-type antimalarial drugs are structurally related to the 9-aminoacridines, which may be considered to be condensates of two 4-aminoquinolines; for instance, quinacrine consists of a 7-chloro-4-aminoquinoline (chloroquine) condensed with a 6-methoxy-4-aminoquinoline. Of these two compounds, chloroquine is by far the more potent agent

Table 18.7 Activities Against Avian Malarias of Prominent 2-Methoxy-6-chloro-9-aminoacridines

(Structure: 2-methoxy-6-chloro-9-(HNR)-acridine; substituents HNR, OCH_3, Cl, N)

Compound Number	Structure R	TI[a] P. relictum, Canary (87)	TI[a] P. gallinaceum, Chick (138a)	TI[a] P. praecox, Siskin (144, 139)	Q[b] P. lophurea, Duck (31k)
18.**14**	$CH(CH_3)(CH_2)_3N(C_2H_5)_2$ (quinacrine)	30	16.9	15	6
18.**57**	$(CH_2)_3N(C_2H_5)_2$ (acrichin N5)	15	—	15	3
18.**58**	$(CH_2)_4N(C_2H_5)_2$ (acrichin N8)	8	—	20	3
18.**59**	$CH(CH_3)(CH_2)_2N(C_2H_5)_2$	30	—	6.6	1.5
18.**60**	$CH(CH_3)(CH_2)_3N(CH_3)(C_2H_5)$		7.3	—	4
18.**61**	phenyl ring with $CH_2N(C_2H_5)_2$ and —OH	—	12.3	—	4
18.**62**	cyclohexyl ring with —$N(C_2H_5)_2$	30 (Ref. 140)	—	—	3

[a] TI = therapeutic index.
[b] Q = quinine equivalent = minimum effective dose of quinine/minimum effective dose of agent.

(18.**65** and 18.**16**, Table 18.8a). The congeneric 6-chloroacridine (18.**71**) is less active than chloroquine, but is is the most active monochloroacridine (Table 18.8a). The quinoline ring system seems to be inherently more active than the acridine for a given side chain; for instance, the introduction of the side chains listed in Table 18.7 into the 4-amino group of 7-chloro-4-aminoquinoline led to compounds that were more potent against duck malaria than were the corresponding acridines (Table 18.8b). The structural relationship between the 4-aminoquinolines and 9-aminoacridines is also apparent in the possible tautomerism (Fig. 18.7). Schönhöfer (96) had postulated that the formation of such quinone-type structures was a prerequisite for high antimalarial activity.

The majority of the 9-aminoacridines and 4-aminoquinolines synthesized had a dialkylaminoalkylamino side chain, and the most active compounds were those having 2–5 carbon atoms between the nitrogen atoms. A particularly favorable therapeutic index was obtained with the 4-diethylamino-1-methylbutylamino side chain, which is present in quinacrine, chloroquine, and sontoquine. Because of the asymmetric carbon in the side chain, these drugs are racemic mixtures. The racemates of quinacrine (149) and chloroquine (150) have been resolved, and no difference in antimalarial activity has been found between the enantiomers of the respective drugs (151, 31o). However in the case of quinacrine the dextrorotatory isomer was found to be less toxic in man and bird than the levorotatory

Table 18.8 Activity of 4-Aminoquinolines and 9-Aminoacridines Against *P. lophurea* in Duck (31)

(a)

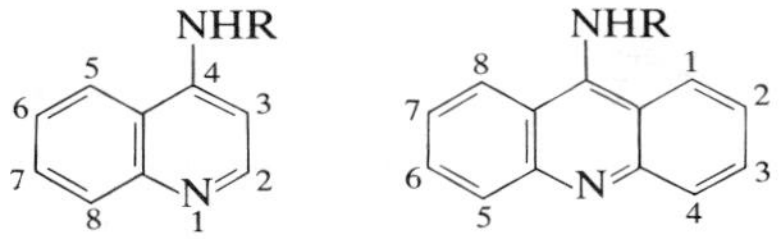

A, B; $R = CH(CH_3)(CH_2)_3N(C_2H_5)_2$

Compound Number	Structure	Q^a
18.**65**	**A**, 6-OCH_3	2
18.**66**	**B**, 7-OCH_3	2
18.**67**	**A**, 5-Cl	0.6
18.**68**	**B**, 8-Cl	—[b]
18.**69**	**A**, 6-Cl	2
18.**70**	**B**, 7-Cl	0.6
18.**16**	**A**, 7-Cl	15
18.**71**	**B**, 6-Cl	3
18.**72**	**A**, 8-Cl	<0.4
18.**73**	**B**, 5-Cl	0.8

(b)

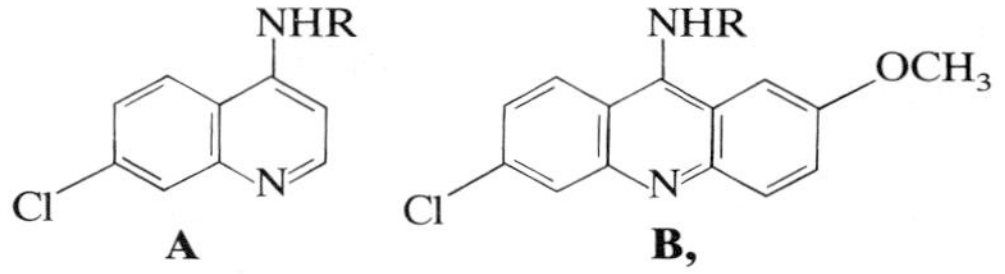

A; **B**, (OCH_3)

Compound Number	Structure	Q^a
18.**16**	**A**, $CH(CH_3)(CH_2)_3N(C_2H_5)_2$	15
18.**14**	**B**, $CH(CH_3)(CH_2)_3N(C_2H_5)_2$	6
18.**74**	**A**, $(CH_2)_3N(C_2H_5)_2$	6
18.**57**	**B**, $(CH_2)_3N(C_2H_5)_2$	3
18.**75**	**A**, $(CH_2)_4N(C_2H_5)_2$	15
18.**58**	**B**, $(CH_2)_4N(C_2H_5)_2$	3
18.**51**	**A**, 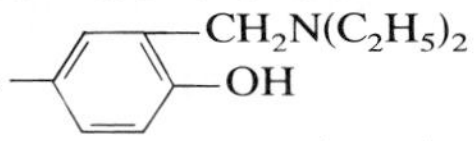 phenyl-3-$CH_2N(C_2H_5)_2$-4-OH	15
18.**61**	**B**, 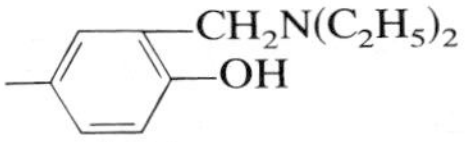 phenyl-3-$CH_2N(C_2H_5)_2$-4-OH	4
18.**52**	**A**, 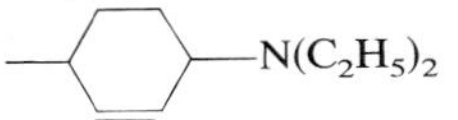 cyclohexyl-$N(C_2H_5)_2$	15
18.**62**	**B**, 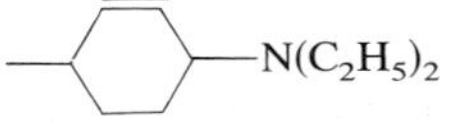 cyclohexyl-$N(C_2H_5)_2$	3

[a] Q = Quinine equivalent = minimum effective dose of quinine/minimum effective dose of agent.
[b] Not reported.

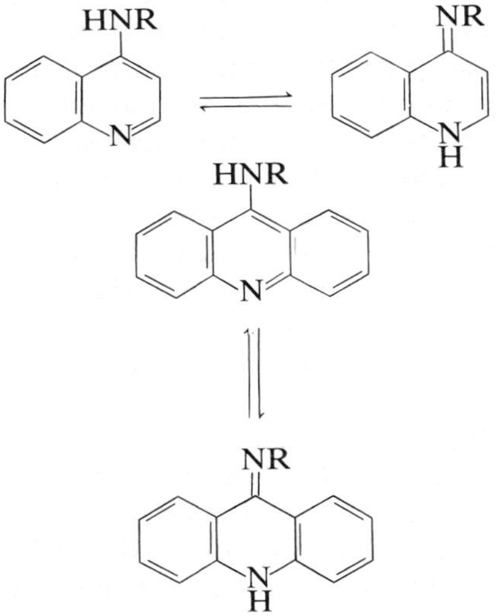

Fig. 18.7 Tautomerism of 4-aminoquinolines and 9-aminoacridines.

form (151), whereas no difference in toxicity was observed for the chloroquine isomers (310). The introduction of an unsaturated bond in the 4-diethylamino-1-methylbutylamino side chain (18.**79**) was

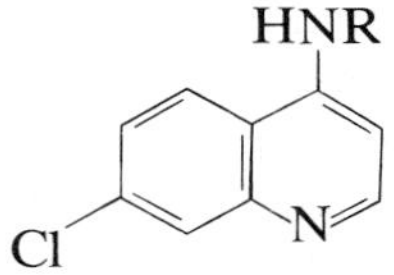

	R
18.**79a**	$CH(CH_3)C{\equiv}CCH_2N(C_2H_5)_2$
18.**79b**	$CH(CH_3)CH{=}CHCH_2N(C_2H_5)_2$

18.**79**

not detrimental to the antimalarial activity against *P. berghei* in mice (152). Quite a different type of side chain was introduced by Burckhalter in 18.**51**, 18.**61**, and 18.**77**.

His rationale for incorporating the α-dialkylamino-*o*-cresol moiety in these compounds was based on his discovery of a new class of antimalarial agents (153) represented by 18.**80** and 18.**81**. It is

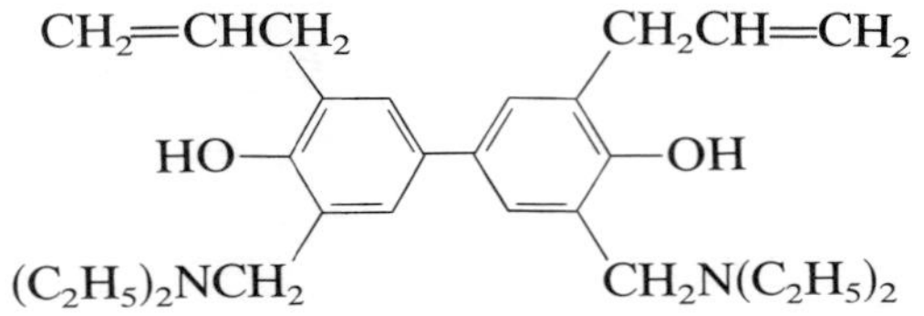

$$\text{18.80: } 4,4'\text{-biphenyl with } CH_2{=}CHCH_2\text{, HO, }(C_2H_5)_2NCH_2 \text{ on one ring and } CH_2CH{=}CH_2\text{, OH, } CH_2N(C_2H_5)_2 \text{ on the other}$$

18.**80**

$$\text{18.81: biphenyl with } C(CH_3)_3\text{, OH, } CH_2N(C_2H_5)_2$$

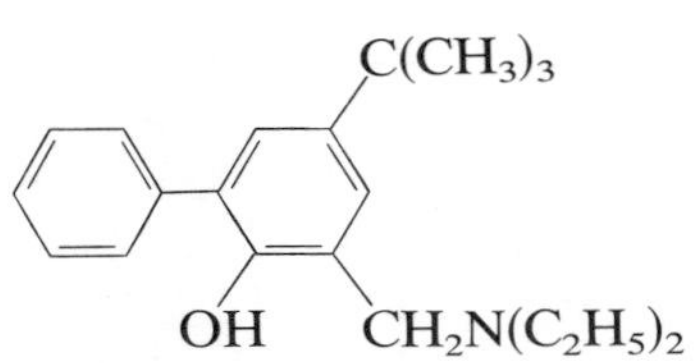

18.**81**

noteworthy that in 18.**51**, 18.**61**, and 18.**77** the number of carbon atoms between the nitrogen atoms is still the preferred number, 4.

An interesting structural similarity seen from the Dreiding molecular models of 4-aminoquinolines, 9-aminoacridines and febrifugine (18.**9**) was reported by Cheng (154). When the quinazoline ring of febrifugine was superimposed on the quinoline ring of chloroquine (18.**16**), with ring nitrogens of position 1 adjacent to each other, the side chains could be superimposed nicely, with the aliphatic nitrogens of the side chains falling side by side. Such a similarity of the structures may imply that the antimalarial mode of action of febrifugine is similar to that of chloroquine.

Bass et al. (155) carried out regression analyses on a great number of 4-aminoquinolines to study structure-activity relationships. Their findings were, by and large, in agreement with the model proposed previously by Hahn (156; see Section 5.3.1.2).

The 4-aminoquinolines and 9-aminoacridines, as well as the amino alcohols (see Section 5.1), are all fast-acting blood schizontocides and their mode of action is discussed in Section 5.3).

5.2.2 DRUGS. Chloroquine (18.**16**), the present drug of choice (132), was first made and studied in Germany in 1934 but apparently was rejected in favor of sontoquine (18.**15**) (148). It is active against the erythrocyte forms of human malarial parasites, and therefore effects a radical cure of susceptible falciparum malaria. However it suppresses only relapsing malarias, such as vivax, because it lacks tissue schizontocidal activity. Since chloroquine is fast acting, it is used for acute attacks of malaria. It is also used in combination with the tissue schizontocide primaquine (18.**17**), when relapsing malarias may be involved. Moreover, this combination is effective against gametocytes of all species because chloroquine is gametocytocidal for parasites other than *P. falciparum*, whereas primaquine is active against the gametocytes of both *P. vivax* and *P. falciparum*. The combination is also recommended for malaria prophylaxis except when chloroquine-resistant strains of *P. falciparum* may be present. Chloroquine alone is not recommended as a causal prophylactic drug because it is inactive against preerythrocytic forms of malaria parasites. However, as mentioned, it is an effective suppressive drug against susceptible strains and will prevent clincial symptoms as long as it is taken.

Other well-known drugs with action similar to chloroquine are the 9-aminoacridines, quinacrine (132) and its 7-amino (derivative (18.**56**) (25b), as well as the 4-aminoquinolines, hydroxychloroquine (18.**76**), amodiaquine (18.**51**), and amopyroquine (18.**77**) (Table 18.9). Of these drugs, quinacrine is less effective than chloroquine and definitely more toxic. Moreover, it has the disadvantage of imparting a yellow color to the skin. The other 4-aminoquinoline drugs are at least as

Table 18.9 Prominent 7-Chloro-4-aminoquinoline Drugs

(Structure: 7-chloroquinoline with HNR at position 4; position 3 marked)

Compound Number	Name	R	References
18.**15**	Sontoquine	$CH(CH_3)(CH_2)_3N(C_2H_5)_2$, 3-$CH_3$	31n
18.**16**	Chloroquine	$CH(CH_3)(CH_2)_3N(C_2H_5)_2$	31o
18.**76**	Hydroxychloroquine	$CH(CH_3)(CH_2)_3N(C_2H_5)(CH_2CH_2OH)$	145a, 146
18.**51**	Amodiaquine	4-hydroxyphenyl with $CH_2N(C_2H_5)_2$ at 3-position; —OH	31p, 145b, 147
18.**77**	Amopyroquine	4-hydroxyphenyl with CH_2N(pyrrolidinyl) at 3-position; —OH	145c, d
18.**78**	12,278 RP	$CH(CH_3)CH_2$—N(piperazine)N—CH_2—$(CH_3)HC$ (bisquinoline)	35c

good as chloroquine, but the earlier introduction and extensive experience with chloroquine made the latter the drug of choice. Amodiaquine (18.**51**) has been reported (157) to be somewhat effective against chloroquine-resistant strains of *P. falciparum*, but at doses presently prescribed the cure rate is not sufficiently high for it to be recommended for use against such strains. Activity against resistant strains of *P. falciparum* was achieved by using a combination of chloroquine, primaquine, and dapsone (18.**20a**) (1i); such a combination and others are under investigation but are not commercially available as drugs.

5.3 Mode of Action

5.3.1 CLUMPING AND ACCUMULATION PHENOMENA. Interest in studying the mode of action of antimalarial drugs was revived after 1960 as a result of the discovery of chloroquine-resistant strains of *P. falciparum* (4e). To gain an insight into the mode of action of drugs, such as chloroquine, amodiaquine, quinacrine, and quinine, *in vivo* as well as *in vitro*, studies have been conducted with various malarial parasites, viz., *P. falciparum* (infects man), *P. knowlesi* (infects monkeys), *P. berghei* (infects rodents), and *P. gallinaceum* (infects birds). The rodent parasite has been used extensively because it can be handled conveniently in the laboratory. Although this parasite has some characteristics that are similar to those of primate plasmodia, due caution should be used in drawing conclusions about the mode of action of a drug against human malaria based on experimental results gathered from studies performed on nonhuman models (158).

The pigmented bodies discovered in 1880 by Lavernan in the red blood cells of patients were identified by him as plasmodia. It is now known that the pigment in the plasmodia is a breakdown product of hemoglobin from the red blood cells. The intraerythrocytic parasite ingests hemoglobin and converts it to amino acids (159) and a pigment (160). This pigment consists of a porphyrin moiety attached to peptides (161, 162) and is located in discrete areas of the parasite called food, or digestive, vacuoles (163), which seem to be analogous to mammalian secondary lysosomes (164, 165). In these vacuoles hemoglobin and pigmented components are present in variable ratios. However the exact composition of the final colored degradation product, called hemozoin, has not yet been established (166).

Chloroquine brought about a fusion of the food vacuoles of parasites in infected mouse erythrocytes, both *in vitro* (167, 168) and *in vivo* (169, 170), within 60 min, to form the so-called autophagic vacuoles. It is within the latter that degradation of ribosomal RNA takes place (171) and aggregation of hemozoin occurs. This chloroquine-induced aggregation, or clumping, is the first morphological effect detectable by electron microscopy (170). *In vivo* clumping occurred within 30 min after the treatment of infected mice (*P. berghei*) with a therapeutically effective dose of chloroquine, whereas *in vitro* the onset was observed within 10 min (173). The concentration of chloroquine that produced 50% clumping *in vitro* was about 4.5×10^{-8} *M*. Energy is required for clumping (174, 175), and for this process to occur the parasite, or host cell–parasite complex, must be able to synthesize RNA and proteins (173, 175). The basicity of the drug seemed to play a part because clumping also occurred to some extent by increasing the pH of the medium in which the parasitized erythrocytes were suspended (176). This effect may be an indication that clumping is not directly related to the antimalarial action of chloroquine. In addition, other 4-aminoquinolines also induced clumping of pigment, whereas quinine and other arylamino alcohols were competitive clumping inhibitors (177, 178). These clumping phenomena indicated that a relationship exists between the 4-aminoquinolines and amino alcohols in that both these drug types may bind to the same receptor.

Chloroquine-induced clumping may be a process that interferes with hemoglobin degradation in the parasite, though no proof of this has been presented. Nevertheless, Howells et al. (179) postulated that interference with the formation of hemoglobin breakdown products by chloroquine may deprive the parasite of essential amino acids despite the possibility that the parasite can obtain adequate amounts of amino acids from the blood and by *de novo* biosynthesis (see Section 10.2). Several investigators (170, 180) have associated the amount of pigment present in the parasite with its sensitivity to chloroquine, but this relationship was later disputed (181) (see Section 5.3.2).

Another property of the fast-acting blood schizontocidal drugs is their high accumulation in parasitized erythrocytes. This phenomenon has been observed in *P. berghei* (182), *P. knowlesi* (183a), *P. falciparum* (184), and *P. gallinaceum* (185). Fitch (184, 186) studied the *in vitro* uptake of various concentrations of ^{14}C-chloroquine by erthyrocytes infected with *P. berghei* or *P. falciparum.* He identified three drug binding sites (receptors) having different drug affinities; one was located in the erythrocyte itself, and two were in the parasite (187). In the case of *P. berghei* and chloroquine, the high affinity receptor reached 50% saturation at an external chloroquine concentration of about 10^{-8} *M* at pH 7.2 and 22° or an estimated apparent intrinsic association constant (*K*) of 10^{8} M^{-1}. For the two other receptors he found *K* values of about 10^{5} and 10^{3} M^{-1}; the latter was presumably associated with the erythrocyte, probably on the erythrocyte membrane (188), since its presence was demonstrated in unparasitized cells.

Whether the two parasite-associated binding sites are present on protein, nucleic acid, or some other macromolecule, is unknown, but according to Kramer and Matusik (187), the high affinity receptor seemed to be associated with parasite membrane, whereas the low affinity receptor ($K = 10^5\ M^{-1}$) was located in the parasite cytoplasm. It seems that the high affinity receptor is a part of the food vacuole of the parasite (189–191), and the high affinity site and the clumping site are probably identical (173). The chloroquine concentration affecting the low affinity receptor is in the inhibiting range of nucleic acid syntheses (192), and since nucleic acid synthesis is essential for clumping, this concentration will also inhibit the clumping induced by lower concentrations of chloroquine. It may well be that the low affinity binding site in the cytoplasm of the parasite is associated with the inhibition of nucleic acid synthesis by chloroquine (173).

Fitch and co-workers (189, 193) also investigated the *in vitro* accumulation of ^{14}C-chloroquine in mouse erythrocytes infected with *P. berghei* when the media were varied with respect to pH, temperature, added substrates (e.g., glucose), and such glycolysis inhibitors as iodoacetate and sodium fluoride. Just as clumping was affected by the pH of the medium, so was the accumulation of the drug, higher accumulation occurring at higher pH levels. Low temperature (2°), low pH, or the presence of inhibitors of glycolysis, decreased chloroquine accumulation, whereas the presence of substrates such as glucose increased the accumulation without appreciably affecting the affinity. Glucose had a similar effect on the accumulation of chloroquine in monkey erythrocytes infected with a chloroquine-sensitive strain of *P. falciparum* (for a discussion of resistant strains, see Section 5.3.2). Since the concentration of ATP is very low in infected mouse erythrocytes compared with noninfected cells, but increases considerably when glucose is added to the medium, it may well be that glucose serves as a source of energy (ATP) necessary for the processes leading to increased chloroquine uptake (194).

Besides studying the accumulation of chloroquine in parasitized erythrocytes of the mouse, Fitch demonstrated that a number of other 4-aminoquinolines and arylamino alcohols interact reversibly with the same binding sites, indicating that these compounds may have similar modes of action. This finding is in agreement with the conclusion drawn from clumping experiments (177, 178).

The aforementioned investigations were concerned with the immediate effect of chloroquine, quinine, and their congeners on the parasite. The effect of the 4-aminoquinoline type of compounds was morphologically manifested by pigment clumping, whereas quinine and other amino alcohols did not show this effect and actually inhibited, competitively, chloroquine-induced clumping. The immediate morphological effect of quinine seemed to be on the membrane surrounding the food vacuole of the parasite (190). After a longer time interval it is clear, as the next section discusses, that 4-aminoquinolines and amino alcohols profoundly affect the biosynthesis and degradation of the nucleic acids of the parasite.

5.3.2 EFFECT OF DRUGS ON THE BIOSYNTHESIS AND DEGRADATION OF NUCLEIC ACIDS. Following Clark's (195a) significant observation that quinine ($10^{-5}\ M$) inhibited completely, *in vitro*, the incorporation of ^{32}P-labeled phosphate into DNA, Schellenberg and Coatney (196) administered ^{32}P phosphate and antimalarial drugs to chicks infected with *P. gallinaceum*, and after 24 hr they determined the radioactivity of the DNA of the parasite. The results showed that chloroquine and quinine inhibited markedly the biosynthesis of DNA.

Warhurst and Williamson (171) studied

in vivo the effect of chloroquine on plasmodial RNA. Rhesus monkeys infected with *P. knowlesi* were injected intraperitoneally with chloroquine, and 60, 75, and 90 min thereafter the composition of the RNA of the host-cell-free parasite was determined electrophoretically. The results revealed that in the presence of chloroquine and after the formation of the autophagic vacuole, a progressive degradation of ribosomal RNA occurred, and it was suggested that digestion of ribosomes may take place in the autophagic vacuole. From *in vitro* studies with *Bacillus megaterium*, Ciak and Hahn (197) had obtained similar findings earlier. In the absence of chloroquine, they did not observe a release of radioactivity to the surrounding medium of cells containing radiolabeled RNA, whereas in the presence of chloroquine such a release occurred, indicating a degradation of RNA. Moreover, chromatographic studies of the RNA of *B. megaterium* showed clearly that in the presence of chloroquine, a degradation of RNA had taken place and that the ribosome content of the cells had decreased progressively during the chloroquine treatment.

In vitro studies with cultures of *P. berghei* (192, 198a) and *P. knowlesi* (199–201) showed that radiolabeled nucleic acids were biosynthesized when cultures of parasites were treated with radiolabeled precursors of nucleic acids, such as adenosine or orotic acid. Van Dyke and co-workers observed that quinacrine (18.**14**), chloroquine (18.**16**), amodiaquine (18.**51**), and quinine (18.**27**) inhibited the incorporation of ^{3}H-labeled adenosine into nucleic acids of *P. berghei* developing in erythrocytes (192) or in erythrocyte-free (198a) cultures. The inhibiting effect of quinacrine occurred at significantly lower concentrations than was the case for the other drugs. Gutteridge et al. (201) also studied the effect of chloroquine on the incorporation of labeled adenosine by *P. knowlesi.* During the first hours therapeutically active concentrations of chloroquine ($\geq 10^{-6}$ *M*) had a negligible effect on the synthesis of DNA and RNA, but after 16 hr more than an 80% inhibition of DNA and RNA synthesis was noted in the presence of 10^{-6} *M* chloroquine. Also, after 16 hr this concentration markedly inhibited the synthesis of proteins and lactate. Polet and Barr (199) demonstrated the inhibiting effect of chloroquine and dihydroquinine (18.**36**) on nucleic acid biosynthesis of *P. knowlesi*, using labeled orotic acid as the nucleic acid precursor (for nucleic acid biochemistry of plasmodia see Section 10.1).

5.3.3 DRUG INTERACTION WITH ISOLATED NUCLEIC ACIDS. Since Parker's (202, 203) discovery of a stronger interaction between chloroquine and beef spleen DNA than between chloroquine and RNA, the interaction of chloroquine and structurally related compounds with DNA has been studied extensively by various physiochemical methods (204, 215). Based on spectrophotometric investigations, Cohen and Yielding (206) concluded that the binding of chloroquine and its congeners with DNA occurred at two places, a weakly reacting site devoid of purine residues, and a strongly reacting site associated with the purines of DNA. The same authors (207) demonstrated also that these compounds inhibited DNA and RNA polymerases; the inhibition appeared to be related to the interaction of the compounds (4-aminoquinolines) with the DNA used as a primer in DNA polymerase reactions. O'Brien et al. (208) confirmed these studies for chloroquine and, in addition, observed a similar behavior for quinacrine and quinine. These three drugs inhibited the DNA-primed DNA polymerase reaction to a greater extent than the DNA-primed RNA polymerase reaction.

With regard to the binding of blood schizontocidal drugs to DNA, the work of Hahn and co-workers is particularly noteworthy. From viscosity measurements, sedimentation experiments, and alterations in dichroism, they concluded that a chloroquine-DNA complex was formed by intercalation, a process in which the aromatic moiety of the drug inserts itself between the base pairs of the double-stranded DNA, with a corresponding extension, and unwinding, of the DNA backbone. In addition, they demonstrated that for 4-aminoquinoline-type compounds, a relationship exists between antimalarial activity, the length of the carbon chain between the nitrogens of the side chain, and the change in "melting temperature" (ΔT_m) of DNA and the DNA-compound complex. It was postulated that the basic side chain of chloroquine falls outside the contour of the DNA base pairs and binds ionically with the phosphate of the complementary strands of DNA across the minor groove of the double helix (Fig. 18.12) (209–211) and, based on spectrophotometric studies (208), the electrostatic attraction between the 7-chloro atom of chloroquine and the 2-amino group of DNA-guanine was though to be of special importance in the binding process (212). Thus chloroquine complex formation with synthetic double helical polymers of the DNA type, such as deoxyguanylic acid and deoxycytidylic acid (dGdC), was found to occur, whereas no complex was formed with a copolymer of deoxyinosinic acid and deoxycytidylic acid (dIdC); guanine (G) contains an NH_2 group in position 2 of the purine ring, whereas inosine (I) lacks this group. This interaction between the 7-chloro atom of chloroquine and the NH_2 group of guanine in DNA was consistent with the Hückel molecular orbital calculation of Singer and Purcell (213), who concluded that the 2-amino group of guanine was a major contributor to the electron-donor property of guanine. Orbital calculations by Pullman and Pullman (214) showed that the guanine-cytosine (GC) base pair is a better electron donor and acceptor than the adenine-thymine (AT) pair.

Márquez et al. (215) investigated the interaction of DNA with a few bis(7-chloro-4-quinolyl) analogs and, based on changes in melting temperature, inhibition of the RNA polymerase, and spectrophotometric studies, concluded that only one of the quinoline rings was involved in the intercalative process. Moreover, they demonstrated that coplanarity between the quinoline rings was not a prerequisite for binding to DNA, whereas such coplanarity seemed to be important in the amodiaquine-type of compounds (216). With amodiaquine (18.**51**) itself, both the quinoline ring and the aromatic ring of the side chain were thought to be intercalated, in contrast to chloroquine, in which the side chain falls outside the DNA contour.

Evidence of an intercalation of the acridine nucleus of quinacrine (18.**14**) was reported first by Lerman (217) and later was investigated by others (208, 218). From a study of the absorption spectra there seemed to be no specific site on the DNA bases that contributed to the intercalative binding of quinacrine, as was found to be the case for chloroquine (208) and quinine (219). However because of the proximity of the basic moieties of DNA and an intercalated compound, it should be expected that strong interaction exists between the π-orbitals of the intercalated compound and the bases of DNA. According to Hückel molecular orbital calculations (213), quinacrine should be both a better electron donor and electron acceptor than chloroquine; consequently the former should be bound more firmly than the latter in the intercalating process by π-complex formation.

The binding of quinine to DNA was found to be basically similar to that of chloroquine; the quinoline ring of quinine was intercalated between the base pairs of the double-stranded DNA, and the side chain was thought to fall outside the contour of the DNA base pairs. The hydroxyl group of quinine participated through hydrogen bonding, whereas the basic part of the side chain, the quinuclidine moiety, was electrostatically attracted to the phosphate groups. The presence of these bonds was verified through spectrophotometric studies (219, 220).

The interaction of amino alcohols other than quinine with DNA has also been investigated; compounds 18.**40**, Table 18.4 (221) and 18.**42**, Table 18.5 (178), as well as a number of naphthothiophenethanolamines (222), formed complexes with DNA. Mefloquine (Fig. 18.5), however, did not bind calf thymus DNA (223) and *E. coli* DNA (224); it was assumed that the bulky trifluoromethyl groups of mefloquine prevented intercalation, and the authors supported their assumption with model building studies. These observations suggest that the intercalating process may not necessarily be prerequisite for activity of the fast-acting blood schizontocidal drugs. One may question the significance of these mefloquine investigations because plasmodial DNA was not used. However the binding of chloroquine to plasmodial DNA (*P. knowlesi*) was investigated by Gutteridge et al. (201), who found that the binding affinity is of the same order as that for mammalian DNA. Further studies are necessary to explain the exceptional behavior of mefloquine.

5.3.4 DRUG EFFECTS ON PROTEIN SYNTHESIS. The interaction of antimalarial drugs with DNA will result in an inhibition of DNA replication, with consequent inhibition of RNA transcription and protein synthesis. A study of the *in vitro* inhibitory effect of chloroquine on the synthesis of DNA, RNA, and protein in *P. knowlesi* (183b, 201), showed that after 16 hr at a high chloroquine concentration (10^{-6} *M*), the production of all three was markedly reduced; but at a lower concentration (10^{-7} *M*) the synthesis of DNA and RNA was more inhibited than was protein synthesis. The production of the nucleic acids was established by measuring the incorporation of radiolabeled adenosine and orotic acid (18.**122**, in Fig. 18.13), whereas protein synthesis was determined by measuring the incorporation of radiolabeled 1-isoleucine (see Sections 9.1 and 9.2).

Other investigators showed that there were other ways by which chloroquine could inhibit protein synthesis. The *in vivo* studies of Warhurst and Williamson (171) on the effect of chloroquine on the ribosomal RNA of *P. knowlesi* have already been mentioned. Furthermore by studying the transport of a number of radiolabeled amino acids into normal and duck erythrocytes infected by *P. lophurae*, as well as into the free parasites, Sherman and Tanigoshi (225) found that the fast-acting blood schizontocidal drugs chloroquine and quinine inhibited the uptake of certain amino acids into all these cells. Surprisingly, quinacrine was ineffective.

5.3.5 OTHER CONSIDERATIONS. In addition to the aforementioned phenomena associated with chloroquine, viz., clumping of hemazoin, accumulation in infected red cells, and inhibition of nucleic acid and protein synthesis, other biochemical effects of this drug have been reported; none of them, however, is believed to be the major mode of action of the drug as an antimalarial agent. For instance, chloroquine inhibited the incorporation of ^{14}C-labeled acetate into the lipids of *P. fallax* (226) and the production of free fatty acids in intraerythrocytic *P. berghei* (227). The latter effect may be the result of the inhibition of the lipolytic activity of phospholipase A, an enzyme apparently essential for the hydrolysis of host lipids, which could be a source of the free fatty acids for the plasmodium (227).

Markus and Ball (228) also suggested that the fast-acting blood schizontocidal drugs quinine, chloroquine, and quinacrine owe their antimalarial effectiveness, in part, to their ability to reduce the availability of free fatty acids to the parasite because the drugs were found to be antilipolytic. However Hellerman et al. (229) showed that the common denominator for antilipolytic activity was the presence of a quinoline or acridine nucleus, regardless of antimalarial activity.

More recently Laser et al. (230) have shown that depending on the ratio of fatty acid to protein (hemoglobin), a variety of antimalarials may either inhibit or stimulate hemolysis, and they have proposed a new mode of antimalarial action for quinine and other blood schizontocidal drugs. As discussed later (Section 9.3), there is a rise in the free fatty acid content of both the erythrocytes and the plasma of an infected host. Under normal physiological conditions these fatty acids are bound to protein—in particular, to serum albumin—and in this state they are unable to exert their potent lytic activity, which thus allows the full development of the erythrocytic stage of the parasite. In the presence of quinine or a blood schizontocidal drug, a drug–fatty acid complex is formed that is hemolytic, although less so than the free fatty acids. Thus the action of the drug, by complexing with the fatty acids, is to relieve the inhibition of the lytic action of the fatty acids that is caused by their binding with protein. Lysis of the immaturely parasitized cell would follow, with fatal interruption of the life cycle. A number of standard antimaliarials of different types were tested for this ability to stimulate hemolysis *in vitro* in the erythrocyte–fatty acid system; *cis*-vaccenic acid was used as the lytic agent. However factors other than the rate of hemolysis are obviously involved with antimalarial activity, since 4,7-dichloroquinoline, which has no antimalarial activity, was the most effective of the compounds tested.

The effect of the fast-acting blood schizontocidal drugs on isolated enzyme systems has also been studied, particularly the enzymes involved in the carbohydrate metabolism of the parasite (see Section 9.4). The contribution of these effects to antimalarial activity is still questionable.

5.3.6 RESISTANCE TO 4-AMINOQUINOLINES. The discovery of chloroquine-resistant strains of *P. falciparum* in South America came quite as a surprise because numerous attempts to develop chloroquine-resistant strains of *P. gallinaceum* in the laboratory had failed or had produced only a low order of resistance (231). However after the introduction of the rodent malaria parasites *P. berghei* and *P. vinckei* as experimental models, it was observed that a high order of resistance to this drug can be developed relatively easily in these plasmodia compared to *P. gallinaceum* (232, 233). In these chloroquine-resistant plasmodia, pigment formation was absent or highly reduced (233, 234); therefore the absence of pigment was associated with chloroquine resistance. Although this was the case for induced chloroquine resistance in plasmodia, pigment was found to be present in the naturally chloroquine-resistant strains of *P. falciparum, e.g.*, the Malayan Camp strain (235) and in *P. berghei yoeli* (236).

At one time chloroquine resistance was attributed to the formation of a complex between chloroquine and ferrihemic acid (hematin) because *in vitro* studies had shown that such a complex was less active than chloroquine itself (180, 237). Ferrihemic acid was assumed to be a hemoglobin breakdown product of the parasite, but it has not been found in malaria parasites (166). However if a complex were to be formed *in vivo* between chloroquine and a malaria pigment (not the chloroquine-hematin complex), the production of an excess amount of this pigment by the parasite might be assumed to render it more resistant to the drug. This chloroquine-deactivation postulate was challenged by Macomber et al. (170, 182) after they found that erythrocytes infected with a resistant strain of *P. berghei* accumulated considerably less chloroquine than a chloroquine-susceptible strain. They suggested that chloroquine resistance was the result of an impairment of the drug accumulation mechanism. Fitch concluded from his *in vitro* studies on chloroquine-sensitive (CS) and chloroquine-resistant (CR) strains of *P. berghei* (186) and *P. falciparum* (184) that the lower accumulation of chloroquine by the resistant strain could be attributed to a deficiency of high affinity drug receptor sites (see Section 5.3.1) and tentatively named this deficiency as the cause of resistance to chloroquine. Fitch (193, 238) also studied the uptake of amodiaquine (18.**51**) on CS and CR strains of these plasmodia and found that for *P. falciparum* ^{14}C-amodiaquine was accumulated to a greater extent than ^{14}C-chloroquine, although the apparent association constant for the binding of both drugs was approximately $10^7\,M^{-1}$. Furthermore ^{14}C-chloroquine was taken up to a lesser extent by the CR strain than by the CS strain, whereas with ^{14}C-amodiaquine there was no apparent difference. These differences in accumulation of chloroquine and amodiaquine may account for the superiority of the latter drug in the treatment of simian and human infections with CR strains of *P. falciparum* (238). It may well be that further modification of the diethylamino-*o*-cresol moiety of amodiaquine will augment this favorable accumulation (193) and will lead to compounds with a higher chemotherapeutic index. Fitch et al (189, 193, 194, 239) also found that the addition of glucose to the medium stimulated the accumulation of ^{14}C-chloroquine and ^{14}C-amodiaquine by the high affinity uptake process in CS strains of these plasmodia, although the effect was less pronounced with ^{14}C-amodiaquine. In contrast, glucose stimulated the accumulation of ^{14}C-amodiaquine, but not ^{14}C-chloroquine in CR strains of *P. falciparum.*

Howells et al. (179) postulated that the acquisition of chloroquine resistance by *P. berghei* was associated with the presence of a Krebs citric acid cycle in the CR, but not in the CS strain. This postulate was based on histochemical identification of succinate dehydrogenase within CR parasites and the knowledge that a Krebs cycle exists in the sporogonic stages of the parasite (240). However Howells later discarded this postulate because additional investigations did not substantiate the presence in the Krebs cycle of succinate and isocitrate dehydrogenases, the involved enzymes (241a, 242).

Another explanation of chloroquine resistance was offered by Rollo (243), who proposed it to be the consequence of an unknown metabolic change in the resistant parasites that may raise the intracellular pH. As a result, there would be a lower accumulation of the drug in the parasite and more would remain in the relatively higher acid environment of the cell. Rollo's hypothesis was challenged by Williams and Fanimo (244), who used ^{14}C-5,5-dimethoxyazolidine-2,4-dione for determining the internal pH of cells (245). Their results show that the internal pH of CR strains of *P. berghei* is slightly lower than that of CS strains, therefore Rollo's hypothesis is not supported by the evidence.

6 ANTIFOLATES

Folic acid (FA) (Fig. 18.8, 18.**82**) or its derivatives is present in all living things, and has a wide variety of biochemical functions. Both mammals and plasmodia require FA in its tetrahydro cofactor form (FAH_4) (18.**83**) for essential metabolic processes. Mammals can utilize FA, which is normally obtained in sufficient quantities in the diet, as a precursor for the biosynthesis of FAH_4. FA is reduced enzymatically to 7,8-dihydrofolic acid (FAH_2) (18.**84**), then further to 5,6,7,8-tetrahydrofolic acid (FAH_4). These reductions are accomplished

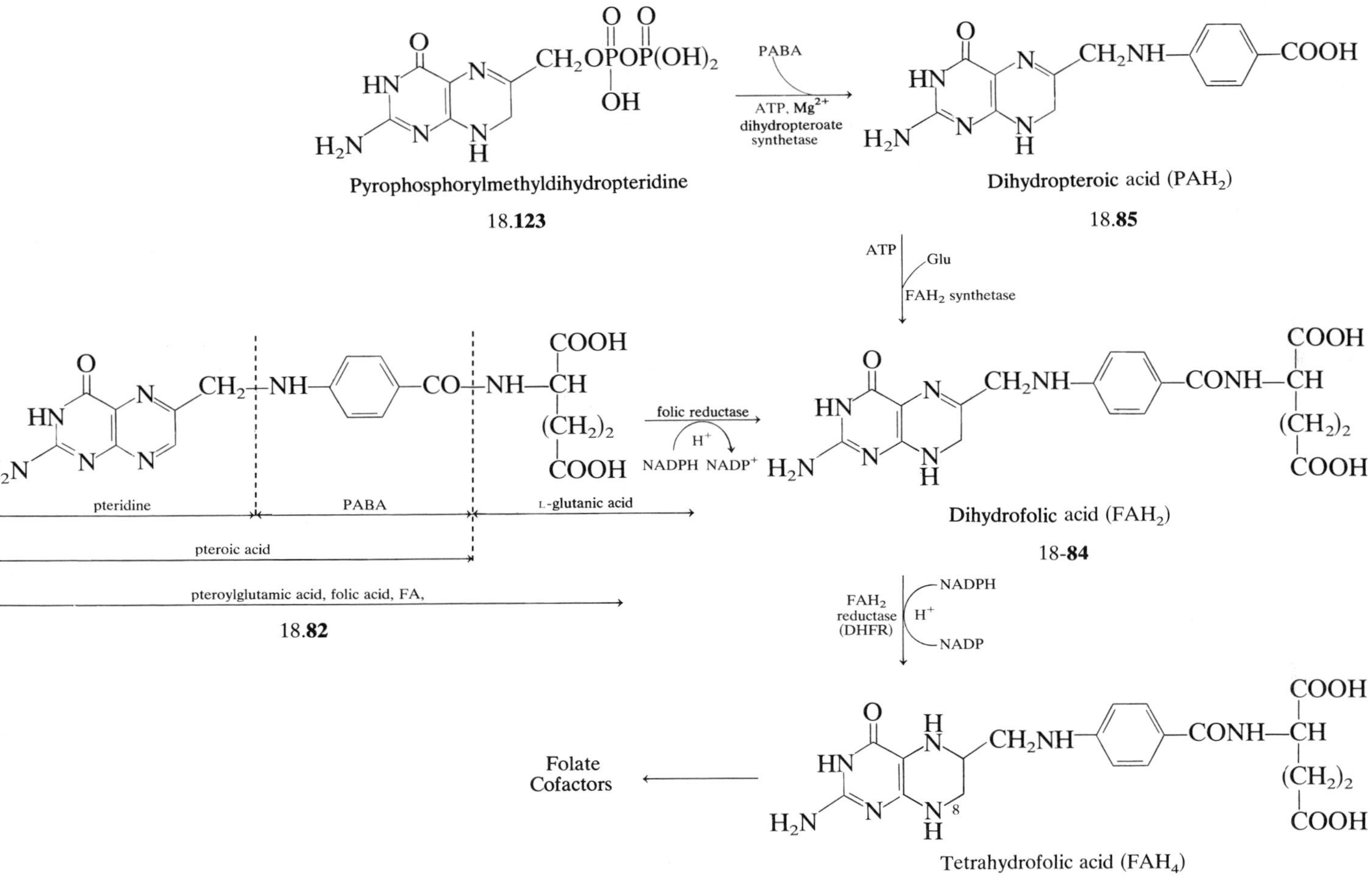

Fig. 18.8 Biosynthesis of tetrahydrofolic acid.

by a single enzyme, which is referred to as folate reductase if the substrate is FA or as dihydrofolate reductase if the substrate is FAH_2.

Since plasmodia cannot utilize FA efficiently enough to provide required FAH_2, they must synthesize FAH_2 *de novo.* It is this difference that chemotherapy seeks to exploit. Drugs that interrupt the biosynthesis of FAH_4 are known collectively as antifolates, although they may interrupt the biosynthetic sequence at different places. The sulfonamides and sulfones interrupt the biosynthesis of the intermediate dihydropteroic acid (PAH_2) (18.**85**), whereas the biguanide, triazine, and pyrimidine class of antifolates interrupt the enzymatic reduction of FA or FAH_2 (Fig. 18.8) (see Sections 6.1 and 6.2). The antifolates, as blood schizontocides, are much slower acting than the amino alcohols, 9-aminoacridines, and 4-aminoquinolines.

6.1 Sulfonamides and Sulfones

Sulfonamides and sulfones may be considered together because of their mode of action, narrow spectrum of activity, ease of induction of resistance, and slow clincial response. The prototype compounds of these classes are sulfanilamide (18.**19**) and 4,4′-diaminodiphenyl sulfone (DDS, dapsone, 18.**20a**).

6.1.1 STRUCTURE-ACTIVITY RELATIONSHIPS. The testing of the antimalarial activity of sulfonamides has disclosed a tremendous variation in the susceptibility of various species of plasmodia to this class of compounds. In general the sulfonamides (Table 18.10) are much less effective against avian malarias than against mammalian. *P. knowlesi* in the monkey and *P. berghei* in the mouse are very susceptible. In his survey of antimalarials, Coatney (138b) analyzed the structure-activity relationships among a large number of sulfonamides tested orally in chicks against blood-induced *P. gallinaceum.* Sulfanilamide (18.**19**), which was used as the standard for comparison, had definite antimalarial action but a low therapeutic index. The introduction of substituents on the sulfonamide nitrogen, e.g., alkyl, acyl, and aryl, generally reduced both toxicity and activity. Sulfonamides possessing a heterocyclic substituent were exceptions to this generalization. In the latter class toxicity was usually appreciably reduced, whereas both therapeutic and prophylactic antimalarial activity was sometimes increased markedly. For example, the therapeutic index of sulfadiazine (18.**86**) was 12 times greater than the standard. The introduction of halogen on the heterocyclic moiety further increased activity, so that a higher therapeutic index was maintained despite increased toxicity. The pyrazinyl and quinoxalyl substituents were very effective; sulfapyrazine (18.**87**) had the highest therapeutic index among the compounds tested. Relatively ineffective were carbazolyl, quinolyl, isoquinolyl, and thiazolyl; the polycyclic aromatic hydrocarbons, naphthyl, anthryl, and phenanthryl, were essentially inactive. Substitution on the aromatic amino group or on both nitrogens usually decreased activity.

The presence of a free aromatic amino group was apparently important to activity. Replacement of this group by nitro, hydroxyl, or methyl, or insulating it from the ring by one or two methylene groups, decreased or abolished activity. Movement of the aromatic amino group to the meta position decreased or abolished activity. Metachloridine (18.**88**), a metanilamide

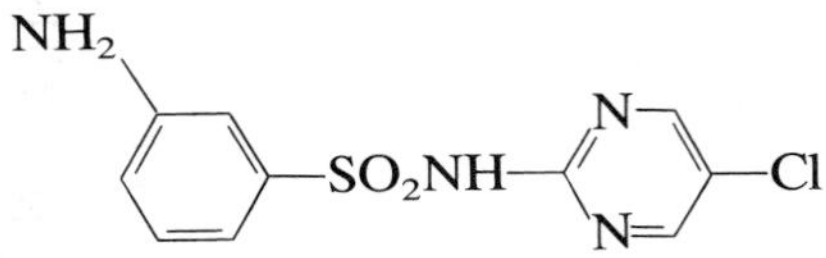

NH_2 —SO$_2$NH— N N —Cl

Metachloridine

18.**88**

(246), is an exception, and in contrast to the *p*-aminobenzensulfonamides, it is more

Table 18.10 Sulfonamides Used in Malaria

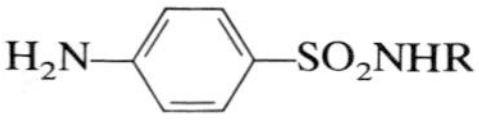

$H_2N-C_6H_4-SO_2NHR$

Compound Number	Name	R
18.**86**	Sulfadiazine	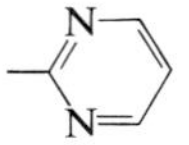 N, N
18.**87**	Sulfapyrazine	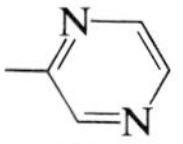 N, N
18.**89**	Sulfamethoxypyridazine	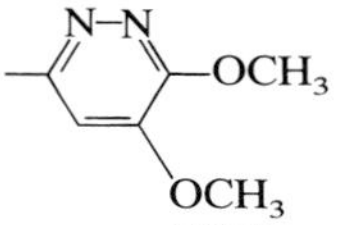 N–N, OCH_3
18.**90**	Sulfadimethoxine	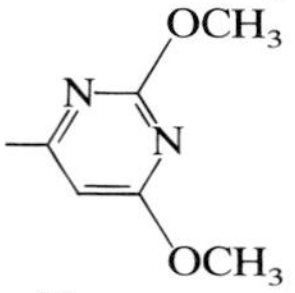 OCH_3, OCH_3, N, N, OCH_3
18.**91**	Sulfadoxine	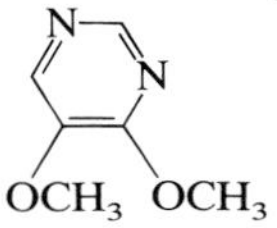 N, N, OCH_3, OCH_3
18.**92**	Sulfalene	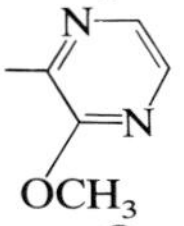 N, N, OCH_3
18.**94**	Sulfisoxazole	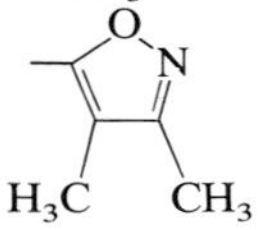 O, N, H_3C, CH_3
18.**97**	Sulfamethoxazole	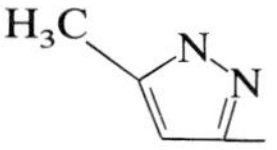 H_3C, N, N

effective against avian than against mammalian malarias.

A number of investigations of structure–antimalarial activity relationships in DDS-related compounds have been made (247–254). It appears that in general, diphenyl sulfones having an aromatic amine on each ring, at least one of which is free or potentially free, metabolically, will show antimalarial activity. DADDS (18.**20**c), however, does not protect rats from challenge by *P. berghei*, although the compound is very active in mice. The difference in activity is attributed to the inefficiency of the deacetylation process in rats, which prevents the reaching of an effective blood level of the drug (255). Some modifications, though conforming to the generalization, are inactive, e.g., the introduction of nitro groups in the 3,3′-positions of DDS (18.**20**a) abolishes activity (247a), as do certain modifications of one of the amino groups (247b).

6.1.2 DRUGS. The sulfonamides and sulfones have been reported to interfere with the maturation of the preerythrocytic and erythrocytic stages of both rodent (256a) and avian malarias (257); in addition, they effectively interfere with the development of sporozoites in the mosquito (36). However they are not effective against the preerythrocytic forms of human malarias, hence are not causal prophylactics against relapsing malarias.

To date, four longer acting sulfonamides have been tested alone against human malaria: sulfamethoxypyridazine (18.**89**), sulfadimethoxine (18.**90**), sulfadoxine (18.**91**), and sulfalene (18.**92**). The latter two are superior to the others, but use has been limited, and results have not been encouraging compared with the sulfonamide–dihydrofolate reductase (DHFR) inhibitor combinations.

The activity of the sulfonamides and sulfones is markedly potentiated by DHFR inhibitors, and the trend today is definitely toward the use of combinations of a sulfonamide or a sulfone with a DHFR inhibitor. Such combinations have been highly successful against *P. falciparum* malaria, even against chloroquine-resistant and pyrimethamine-resistant strains. To ensure that the blood residence time of the sulfonamide is in phase with the relatively long-lasting pyrimethamine (18.**25**), medium or long-acting sulfonamides are preferred when combinations with pyrimethamine are used. Combinations that have given positive clinical results are sulfadoxine (18.**91**) with pyrimethamine (marketed as Fansidar) (258–268), sulfalene (18.**92**) with pyrimethamine (269, 270), sulfalene (18.**92**) with trimethoprim (18.**93**) (271, 272), and dapsone (18.**20a**) with pyrimethamine (260, 273). Despite such encouraging results, failures have been reported with the combinations sulfalene-trimethoprim (18.**92**, 18.**93**) (274, 275)

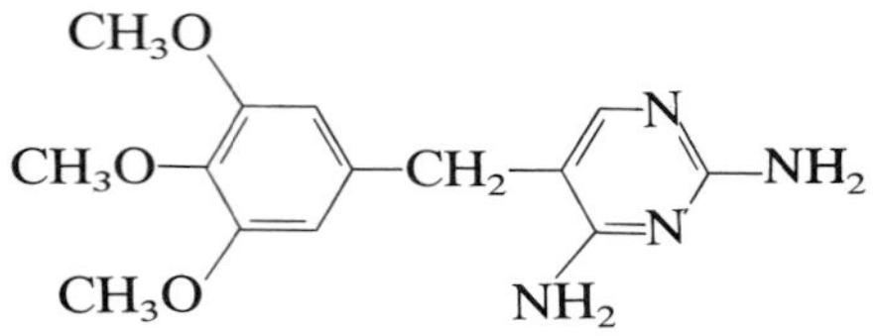

CH_3O / CH_3O— / CH_3O (3,4,5-trimethoxyphenyl)—CH_2—(pyrimidine, N, N)—NH_2, NH_2

Trimethoprim
18.**93**

and sulfalene-pyrimethamine (18.**92**, 18.**25**) (75). For an excellent review, see Richards (276). There has been a strong warning (1j) that sulfones and sulfonamides, either alone or in potentiating combinations with DHFR inhibitors, should not be used prophylactically in areas with chloroquine-sensitive strains of *P. falciparum*, not only because of the reliability of the 4-aminoquinolines and the risk of inducing resistance in the malaria parasite, but also because of the danger of inducing resistance in pathogenic bacteria.

Numerous two- and three-drug combinations of quinine, chloroquine, or amodiaquine with sulfonamides, sulfones, or DHFR inhibitors have been tried and, in general, have been very effective. Thus the combination of pyrimethamine with quinine proved to be more effective than quinine alone against chloroquine-resistant *P. falciparum* (277, 278) and became the standard therapy in Vietnam, where it was used in several thousand cases (279). Other combinations included quinine pyrimethamine, and sulfadiazine (278); quinine, pyrimethamine, and dapsone (277, 280); chloroquine, primaquine, and dapsone (281–283); chloroquine, DFDDS (18.**20b**), and primaquine (284, 285); chloroquine, pyrimethamine, and sulfisoxazole (18.**94**) (286); and chloroquine, pyrimethamine, and sulfalene (18.**92**) (269). A 4-aminoquinoline has been included in these combinations to bring about a more rapid response of the infection to the drugs; the effects appear to be additive, and no claims for potentiation in humans have been made.

The drug DDS (18.**20a**) (284) has been tried rather extensively in the field, with generally positive results; for a review, see Powell (287). It is more effective against *P. falciparum* than against *P. vivax*. There is the risk of its inducing hemolysis in G6PD-deficient individuals (see also Section 7.1.3). Two derivatives of DDS have been used as drugs in man, viz., the diformyl derivative (18.**20b**) (284) and the diacetyl derivative (acedapsone, DADDS, 18.**20c**) (284, 288). The SD_{50} of DFDDS (18.**20b**) in mice infected with *P. berghei* was shown by Aviado (289a) to be only half that of DDS, but the LD_{50} was 1.8 times higher, giving DFDDS a considerably higher therapeutic index. Against multiresistant strains of *P. falciparum*, DFDDS had an antimalarial action similar to that of DDS, but more prolonged; when used alone as a curative drug, it was only partially successful and action was slow (284). Prophylactically it was also partially successful. Antimalarial action is much improved when it is used in combination with sulfalene, chloroquine, or pyrimethamine (262, 284, 288, 290, 291). The diacetyl derivative DADDS (18.**20c**) has remarkable repository antimalarial activity (292–295). In a study of the potential repository activity of a large series of sulfanilylanilides, DADDS showed the longest duration of action. Mice were protected for 6–14 weeks against challenges with *P. berghei*, and monkeys for 2–8 months against challenges with *P. cynomolgi*. The repository combination of DADDS with cycloguanil (18.**24**) pamoate is superior and has received considerable attention.

6.1.3 MODE OF ACTION. Pteroylglutamic acid, commonly known as folic acid (18.**82**, Fig. 18.8), is a vitamin whose structure may be viewed as having three constituent parts, viz., a 2-amino-4-hydroxypteridine nucleus and a glutamic acid moiety linked through *p*-aminobenzoic acid (PABA). In nature it exists as a family of compounds, with the glutamic acid moiety linked to other glutamic moieties, in various numbers, through peptide bonds (conjugates). Mammals require FA as an essential growth factor, and it is ordinarily obtained in ample quantities from the diet. This acid serves as a precursor to the coenzyme 5,6,7,8-tetrahydrofolic acid, FAH_4 (18.**83**). The reduction of FA to FAH_4 is effected in a stepwise process through 7,8-dihydrofolic acid (18.**84**) by a single reductase called folate reductase or dihydrofolate reductase, depending on the substrate involved. The tetrahydrofolate, through several derivatives, is then involved in a number of enzymatic reactions effecting one-carbon transformations in purines, pyrimidines, and several amino acids, hence ultimately in the biosynthesis of nucleic acids and proteins.

From a consideration of a body of experimental evidence, much of it derived from bacterial studies (296), it can be reasonably concluded that the malaria parasite must synthesize folate-derivative cofactors *de novo* because it is unable to utilize, efficiently, preformed FA as a precursor for the biosynthesis of the cofactor FAH_4. Thus, dietary studies (297) showed that *P. berghei* did not thrive in mice that were fed a PABA-deficient diet but did well when the diet was supplemented with PABA. Furthermore, PABA was completely effective in promoting the development of *P. berghei* in mice that were fed a FA-deficient diet, but FA only partially substituted for PABA on a diet deficient in the latter compound. The action of sulfonamides in inhibiting malarial infections of mice infected with *P. berghei* (298) and in chicks infected with *P. gallinaceum* was found to be more easily reversed by PABA than by FA.

These reversal data indicate that the weak activity of FA may be due to its being a source of PABA after metabolic degradation. Such an indirect action is supported by *in vitro* studies (299) in which the stimulation of growth of *P. hexamerium* by FA was evident only after a 24 hr lag period.

Ferone and Hitchings (300) demonstrated unequivocally in *in vitro* experiments with both infected erythrocytes and free parasites that *P. berghei* was incapable of converting more than trace amounts of FA to the FA cofactor, folinic acid (5-formyl FAH_4). The possibility of cell membranes complicating the interpretation was eliminated by showing that disrupted cell preparations were equally ineffective. Dihydrofolic acid (18.**84**), on the other hand, was converted to folinic acid in good yield by both infected red cells and free parasites.

Following the isolation of the enzyme dihydropteroate synthetase from *P. chabaudi* by Walter and Königk (301) and the demonstration that both sulfanilamide (18.**19**) and sulfaguanidine (18.**95**) were

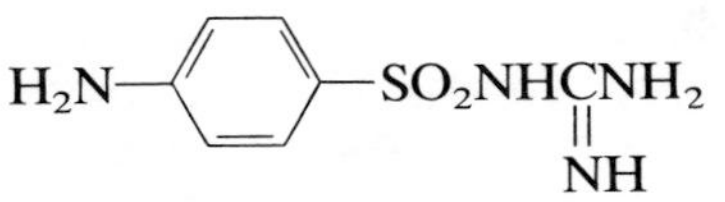

$$H_2N-C_6H_4-SO_2NHC(=NH)NH_2$$

Sulfaguanidine
18.**95**

effective inhibitors of this enzyme, it was shown by Ferone (302) that cell-free extracts of *P. berghei* are capable of synthesizing dihydropteroic acid (18.**85**) and dihydrofolic acid (18.**84**) from 2-amino-4-(hydroxy-6-hydroxymethyl-7,8-dihydropteridine and PABA or *p*-aminobenzoylglutamate, respectively. Hydroxymethyldihydropteridine is initially converted to the pyrophosphorylmethyldihydropteridine (18.**123**), which in turn is condensed with PABA by dihydropteroate synthetase (Fig. 18.8). This synthesis was shown to be inhibited by several sulfonamides as well as by DDS (18.**20a**), which was competitive with PABA.

More recently, dihydropteroate synthetase has been isolated from *P. berghei* by McCullough and Maren (303) and some of its properties described. Both sulfanilamide and sulfaguanidine inhibited the enzyme, and it was suggested that both are competitive inhibitors.

The antimalarial activity of DDS (18.**20a**) against *P. berghei* can be completely antagonized by PABA (255, 304a). In the same way, a number of studies on various malaria parasites have shown that PABA can antagonize the action of sulfonamides (305–310). The compound metachloridine (18.**88**) is of interest in that it was 6 times as effective as sulfadiazine (18.**86**) and 16 times as effective as quinine when tested against *P. gallinaceum* in chicks (246); but unlike the 4-aminosulfonamides, this activity was only reduced, rather than abolished, by PABA. In addition, metachloridine was active against several sulfadiazine-resistant strains of plasmodia (311) but ineffective against species of sulfonamide-sensitive bacteria. As with sulfonamides in general, metachloridine was not effective in preventing infections or in curing two strains of vivax malaria (257). Its mode of action is not well understood.

The accumulated evidence, nevertheless, indicates that the biochemical action of the sulfonamides can be attributed to interference with the biosynthetic reaction of 2-amino-4-hydroxy-6-hydroxymethyl-7, 8-dihydropteridine pyrophosphate (18.**123**) with PABA to yield dihydropteroic acid (18.**85**, ig. 18.8). Because the host cannot synthesize FAH_2 *de novo* and must utilize preformed FA, interruption of the biosynthesis of FAH_2 is lethal only to the plasmodia (Fig. 18.9). In contrast to the classical competitive inhibitor mechanism, there is evidence that the sulfonamides can complete with PABA as substrates and can participate in the biosynthetic reaction in place of PABA to yield fraudulent dihydropteroic acid derivatives (312–314), which may inhibit conversion of dihydropteroate

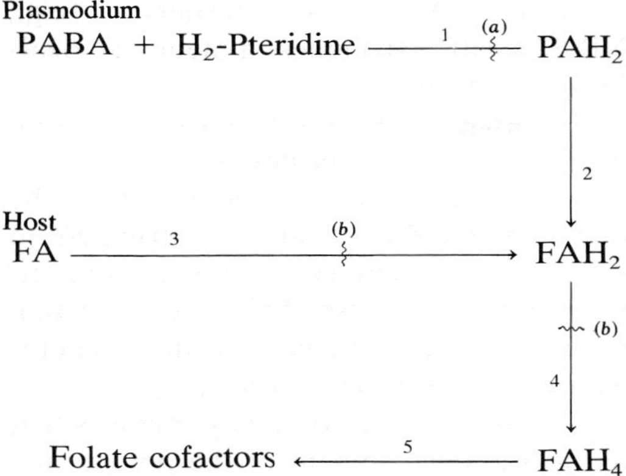

Fig. 18.9 Schematic representation of folate biosynthetic pathways: 1, dihydropteroate synthetase; 2, FAH_2 synthetase; 3, folate reductase; 4, dihydrofolate reductase; 5, one-carbon transfer reactions. (a) Site of action of sulfonamides and sulfones. (b) Site of action of FA and FAH_2 reductase inhibitors (e.g., pyrimethamine).

to FAH_2 or metabolic reactions involving FAH_2 (315). Such a reaction appears to play a very minor role compared to the inhibition of the synthetase.

In addition to the antimalarial action of DDS wherein it interferes with the utilization of PABA in the biosynthesis of FAH_2, it has been suggested (316) that DDS may also inhibit the biosynthesis indirectly through the inhibition of parasite glycolysis. Such inhibition is effected by interfering with the transport of glucose across the erythrocyte membrane, thus restricting the availability of glucose to the parasite. Several pieces of *in vitro* evidence obtained from *P. berghei*-infected rat erythrocytes support this mechanism: increasing the medium glucose concentration reverses the inhibition; DDS has no effect on the glucose metabolism of the erythrocyte-freed parasite; DDS inhibits the glucose uptake of unparasitized red cells. In further support of this mechanism it was found (317) that DDS was less effective in depressing a malaria infection in hyperglycemic mice than in normoglycemic mice. Furthermore, parasitized blood cells from *P. berghei*-infected normoglycemic rats that had been treated with DDS appeared to consume less glucose than identically parasitized cells from untreated rats.

6.1.4 RESISTANCE TO SULFONAMIDES AND SULFONES. The mechanisms by which malaria parasites evade the antimalarial action of sulfonamides and sulfones have not received the experimental attention that has been given to the mechanisms of resistance to FAH_2 reductase inhibitors. Trager has suggested (318) that the sulfonamide-resistant parasites may be able to function at much lower levels of folates than the normal strains. Since the incorporation of PABA occurs before the reduction of FAH_2 in the metabolic chain, a smaller PABA requirement would be reflected in a smaller FAH_4 requirement and strains resistant to sulfonamides would be expected to be resistant to FAH_2 reductase inhibitors; but as Trager points out, the converse would not be required. In general this pattern of cross-resistance seems to be borne out, although caution in generalization is necessary, given the complicated patterns of cross-resistance reported in the various strains of both single- and multiple-resistant parasites.

It has also been suggested that resistance to sulfonamides may arise from an ability of the parasite to obtain its FAH_2 by way of the reaction of *p*-aminobenzoyl glutamic acid (PABG) with 2-amino-4-hydroxy-6-hydroxymethyl-7,8-dihydropteridine pyrophosphate (18.**123**, Fig. 18.8). This mechanism seems to be unlikely, since both PABG and PABA serve as substrates for the enzyme dihydropteroate synthetase obtained from *P. gallianceum*, *P. lophurae*, and *P. knowlesi* (319).

Although resistance to sulfonamide–dihydrofolate reductase combinations has been reported (75, 274, 320), it does not seem to be prevalent at present.

6.2 Biguanides, Dihydrotriazines, and 2,4-Diaminopyrimidines

6.2.1 STRUCTURE-ACTIVITY RELATIONSHIPS. The course of events that led to proguanil (18.**22**, chlorguanide) has been outlined in the historical discussion (Section 4). A great many modifications of the proguanil structure were subsequently synthesized (321–324), but no real improvement in activity was obtained. The presence of an *N*-1 aryl group was important, but the introduction of a second one decreased activity. Alkyl substituents on *N*-1, *N*-2, or *N*-4 led to decreased activity. Although the replacement of the isopropyl group on *N*-5 by a normal group gave compounds of essentially equal activity, the introduction of shorter or longer groups resulted in decreased activity.

It was shown very early that proguanil had essentially no activity against *P. gallinaceum in vitro* (325) but that an active metabolite was present in the sera of monkeys treated with the drug (326, 327). Subsequently, a metabolite, identified as 4,6-diamino-1-(*p*-chlorophenyl)-1,2-dihydro-2,2-dimethyl-*s*-triazine (18.**24**, cycloguanil), was isolated from the urine of proguanil-treated rabbits and humans and was shown to be highly active against *P. gallinaceum in vivo* and *in vitro* (328, 329). Based on such evidence, it now seems to be generally accepted that the activity of proguanil can be attributed to the cyclic metabolite, cycloguanil, although Smith and co-workers (330) concluded from a study of the metabolism of both proguanil and cycloguanil in monkeys and man that the activity of proguanil against primate malarias must be attributed in part to the parent drug. The structural relationship of cycloguanil to proguanil can be seen when the structure of the latter is drawn in the curved form (18.**22a**). If activity is to be attributed entirely to the dihydrotriazine metabolite, it is difficult to understand the activity of proguanil analogs in which the terminal *N*-5 is tertiary [e.g., $NR_1R_2{=}N(CH_3)_2$] unless a metabolic dealkylation occurs.

Accumulated evidence, much of it from bacterial studies, indicates that the activity of biguanides and triazines, like the diaminopyrimidines, can be attributed to their ability to antagonize the enzyme dihydrofolate reductase. This mode of action is discussed in connection with pyrimethamine (18.**25**) in Section 6.2.3.

The investigations of the pyrimidines that led to the development of the potent, and now well-established antimalarial pyrimethamine (98b) have been outlined in the historical discussion of Section 4. As mentioned, three series of 5-substituted 2,4-diaminopyrimidines were studied, and despite some deviations, structure-activity relationship among these series (i.e., the phenoxy, benzyl, and phenyl series) were quite parallel. The best activity was obtained when the amino groups were unsubstituted and there was no spacer between the rings. The presence of electron-attracting groups such as chloro and nitro on the phenyl ring enhanced activity, especially when they were in the para position (331–334), and an alkyl group in the 6 position had a marked effect on activity.

6.2.2 DRUGS. Proguanil (18.**22**) (326) is effective against the asexual blood forms of all human malarial parasites, and because of the absence of secondary, or persisting, exoerythrocytic forms of the parasite in *P. falciparum* malaria, it is radically curative against this infection. The drug is effective against the primary tissue form of *P. falciparum* but not of *P. vivax*; it is not gametocytocidal but does interfere with the development of the parasite within the mosquito and, therefore, with the transmission of the disease. It is slow acting, hence is not recommended for acute attacks of malaria. Daily administration is recommended because the drug is promptly eliminated from the body. The only other biguanide that has been used as a drug is chlorproguanil (18.**96**). It is eliminated

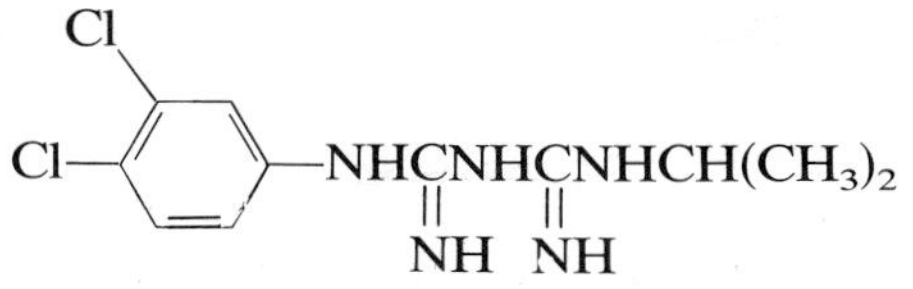

$$\text{3,4-}Cl_2C_6H_3\text{—NHC(=NH)NHC(=NH)NHCH(CH}_3)_2$$

Chlorproguanil

18.**96**

more slowly than proguanil but appears to have no outstanding advantage; proguanil has enjoyed much wider use.

The activity of the proguanil metabolite cycloguanil (18.**24**) stimulated the synthesis and testing of many dihydrotriazines (335, 336) and, in general, they showed greater activity than the corresponding biguanides against avian malarias (304b, 328, 337–339) but not against simian infections (339–342) or human malaria (330). The relatively lower effectiveness of cycloguanil in man has been attributed to its rapid elimination (330, 343). Because of the ease of elimination and its lower effectiveness compared to proguanil, none of the water-soluble salts of cycloguanil has developed into a useful drug. However a long-acting, injectable, repository form of cycloguanil, the pamoic acid salt (cycloguanil embonate), has been developed (344, 364) and gave protection for several months to monkeys that were challenged with blood-induced (344) and sporozoite-induced (346) *P. cynomolgi* infections. Furthermore, a single intramuscular injection of the salt is capable of providing protection to humans for many months against proguanil-susceptible strains of all four types of malaria. Numerous reports are available (342–357).

Although the effectiveness of cycloguanil embonate when used in man is well established, the drug is not without untoward side effects, notably pain and tenderness at the site of injection. The severity of such side effects can be markedly reduced by employing a careful injection technique, as pointed out by Clyde (358) in his review and compilation of statistics on tolerance and side effects of the drug. Nevertheless, "difficulties in injecting the drug, painful reactions at the injection site, the inherent risk of bacterial infection, and the lack of protection against parasite strains resistant to proguanil and pyrimethamine have led to discontinuation of this formulation" (1k).

A combination of cycloguanil embonate with the long-acting repository drug acedapsone (18.**20c**) is also used. The combination usually gives better results than either drug alone. It is effective against pyrimethamine- and proguanil-refractory *P. falciparum* but less so against *P. vivax* strains that are similarly resistant (358). The tolerance for the combination, in humans, which was reviewed by Clyde (358), is similar to that for cycloguanil embonate alone, and the problems associated with field use are essentially those mentioned previously for cycloguanil embonate alone.

On a dose-for-dose basis, pyrimethamine is the most potent suppressive antimalarial in clinical use today. It is an effective radical curative drug against susceptible *P. falciparum*. Unlike proguanil, it has a long biological half-life, and a 25 mg dose once a week is considered to be an effective suppressive prophylactic. The drug also has an effect on the gametocytes of susceptible strains of *P. falciparum*, making them noninfective to mosquitoes, hence interrupting the life cycle of the parasite. Unfortunately, pyrimethamine is slow acting and must be used along with a fast-acting blood schizonticide against fulminating infections. It has also been recognized that resistant strains can emerge rather promptly when suboptimal doses of the drug are administered. Resistance to the DHFR inhibitors is known for the three most prevalent human malarial parasites and has been found in Southeast Asia, East and West Africa, the Middle East, and South America. Cross-resistance among the DHFR inhibitors is the rule (359–362). The trend today is to use pyrimethamine in combination with a sulfa drug, and some very effective combinations have been reported (Section 6.1.2.

In some later work on the 2,4-diamino-5-benzylpyrimidine type of antifolate, there was obtained 2,4-diamino-5-(3,4,5-trimethoxybenzyl)pyrimidine (18.**93**, trimethoprim) (363, 364a). The compound was originally synthesized as an antibacterial and is used principally in this way; it is marketed in a combination with sulfamethoxazole (18.**97**, Table 18.10), in the ratio of 1 to 5, under the proprietary name of Septra®. Surprisingly, trimethoprim is essentially inactive when tested against *P. berghei* in the mouse (365); however it has undergone considerable testing in both monkeys and man. It was first tested in man by Martin and Arnold (365), who found it effective against both a completely drug-susceptible and a chloroquine- and pyrimethamine-resistant strain of *P. falciparum.* Even better results were obtained by these workers when trimethoprim was used in combination with sulfalene (271). Subsequent work in the rhesus monkey (366) demonstrated a considerable cross-resistance between trimethoprim and phrimethamine. Disparate reports on the effectiveness of the trimethoprim-sulfalene combination against both susceptible and drug-resistant strains of *P. falciparum* (275, 316, 367–370) leave the future of the drug rather clouded. Nevertheless, along with the more widely prescribed pyrimethamine, it is the only other pyrimidine antimalarial in clinical use today.

6.2.3 MODE OF ACTION. A considerable body of experimental evidence indicates that the biguanides, the dihydrotriazines, and the 2,4-diaminopyrimidines have similar antifolate action. The biguanides are believed to exert their antimalarial effect mainly through the action of a dihydrotriazine metabolite, a DHFR inhibitor. The one-carbon transfer reactions involving purines, pyrimidines, and some amino acids require folic acid (18.**82**) in its reduced (tetrahydro) form (step 5 in Fig. 18.9), a requirement common to animals, bacteria, and protozoa. The reductase inhibitors, therefore, exert their effect on plasmodia by blocking the conversion of FAH_2 to FAH_4 (step 4, Fig. 18.9). Since this reaction, unlike the *de novo* biosynthesis of FAH_2, is essential to both host and parasite, the role of chemotherapy in this area has been concentrated on the discovery of selective inhibitors. The reductase inhibitors that are important from the standpoint of antimalarial use are the "small molecule" antifolates (296), e.g., pyrimethamine, as opposed to those that are closely related structurally to the substrate, e.g., methotrexate (18.**98**). In the "small molecule" antifolates the substituted pyrimidine moiety has been retained, but the remainder of the FA molecule has been greatly simplified. Although the inhibitors closely related to FA in structure are highly active, the close structural relationship imparts a universality in their binding; therefore they show little discrimination in their binding to reductases from different sources (319, 371, 372). Differences in their antifolate activity may be due mainly to differ-

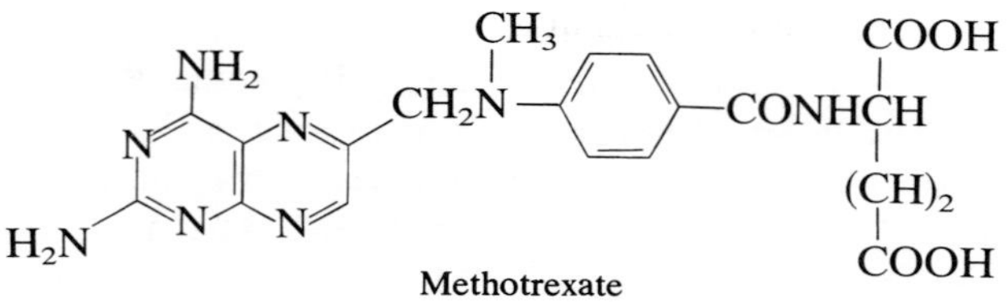

Methotrexate
18.**98**

ences in the mechanism of cellular transport rather than marked differences in binding (296). Nevertheless, the successful use of methotrexate (18.**98**) against *P. vivax* has been reported; clearance of parasitemia was achieved, but not radical cure (373), indicating that the drug does not have tissue schizontocidal activity.

In the same way that the role of PABA and the sulfonamides implied the synthesis of folate cofactors *de novo* (Section 6.1), so does the demonstration that *P. berghei* can carry out the conversion of FAH_2 to N^5-formyl-FAH_4 (folinic acid) (300) suggest the presence of a reductase. However the isolation of dihydrofolate reductase from *P. berghei* was not reported until 1969, when Ferone, Burchall, and Hitchings isolated it and studied its characteristics (319). The enzyme possessed properties distinctly different from those of FAH_2 reductases derived from other sources, including a molecular weight of about 190,000 and a distinct profile of sensitivity to several FAH_2 reductase inhibitors.

The selective binding of the drug to the parasite FAH_2 reductase can be appreciated from the data in Table 18.11. For example, the enzyme from the mouse erythrocytes requires a concentration of pyrimethamine, the most potent of the antimalarials listed, that is 2000 times greater than that needed for the enzyme from the parasite for a 50% inhibition. Also apparent from the table is the positive correlation between the *in vivo* antimalarial activity of the compounds and the 50% inhibitory values for the parasite enzyme. Similar data have been reported for a series of dihydrotriazines (319). The good correlation of the concentration of drugs required to inhibit the isolated enzymes with the chemotherapeutic activity, plus the much greater binding of the drugs to the parasite FAH_2 reductase as compared to the host FAH_2 reductase, suggests that the basis of the antimalarial chemotherapeutic activity is the selective inhibition of parasite FAH_2 reductase.

Further support for this conclusion has been forthcoming from the work of Gutteridge and Trigg (375), who isolated a FAH_2 reductase from the primate malarial parasite *P. knowlesi* and showed that the properties of the enzyme are remarkably similar to those of the *P. berghei* FAH_2 reductase. The 50% inhibitory concentrations for several antifolates were shown to parallel those for the *P. berghei* FAH_2 reductase. Finally Platzer (376) has reported that FAH_2 reductase from the avian malaria parasite *P. lophurae* had a much higher sensitivity to pyrimethamine than did the FAH_2 reductase from the host (duck) erythrocytes.

As discussed earlier, the malaria parasite cannot utilize exogenous FA as a precursor to the coenzyme FAH_4 but must obtain the

Table 18.11 Comparison of the Effects of Three Antifolate-type Antimalarials *in Vivo* and on Host and Parasite Reductase (319, 374)

Compound Number	Name	Concentration ($\times 10^{-9}$ *M*) for 50% Inhibition: *P. berghei*	Concentration ($\times 10^{-9}$ *M*) for 50% Inhibition: Mouse Erythrocytes	ED_{50}[a], mg/kg
18.**25**	Pyrimethamine	0.5	1000	0.15
18.**24**	Cycloguanil	3.6	1600	0.85
18.**93**	Trimethoprim	70.0	10^6	75.0

[a] The ED_{50} is the dose of drug that reduced the parasitemia of treated animals to 50% that of the controls.

latter by way of the biosynthesis of FAH_2 as shown in Fig. 18.8. The mammalian host, on the other hand, utilizies exogenous FA; and this distinction forms the basis of the chemotherapeutic action of the sulfonamides. Both the host and the parasite, however, depend on their respective FAH_2 reductases for the conversion of FAH_2 to FAH_4 (Fig. 18.9), and the chemotherapeutic action of the reductase inhibitors depends on the selectively greater inhibition of the parasite reductase, a selection that can be made most effectively by the small molecule antifolates. A number of derivatives of FAH_4 (folate cofactors) then participate in a host of enzymatic reactions involving one-carbon transfers in the biosynthesis of purines, the interconversions among several amino acids, and the biogenesis of the methyl group of thymine.

The question is, how does the blocking of the conversion of FAH_2 to FAH_4 bring about the death of the parasite? Certainly the parasite requires purines and pyrimidines as building blocks for the replication of DNA and the synthesis of RNA. However numerous studies (192, 198b, 377a,–c; 378a, 379–381, 483) indicate that it is the present view that the parasite cannot synthesize purines *de novo* but must obtain them by a salvage pathway, either from the host erythrocyte or from degradation of the host nucleic acids. Thus, for the parasite, the process of obtaining purines would be exempt from an FAH_4 requirement. Pyrimidine nucleosides, unlike the purine nucleosides, are not taken up from an exogenous source by free parasites (379), although they do enter the parasitized erythrocyte (382), and it appears that the parasite must synthesize the needed pyrimidines *de novo* (377a, 378a, 379, 382, 383). There has been an indication, however, that the parasite can utilize exogenous cytidine and that thymidine can be incorporated into the late stage of parasite growth (see Section 10.1).

FAH_4 is not involved in the *de novo* synthesis of the pyrimidine ring but is involved through one of its cofactors, N^5,N^{10}-methylenetetrahydrofolate, in a one-carbon transfer reaction that effects the methylation of deoxyuridylate (deoxyuridine-5′-phosphate, dUMP) to form deoxythymidylate (deoxythymidine-5′-phosphate, dTMP). The transfer is catalyzed by thymidylate synthetase (Fig. 18.10). FAH_4 is oxidized in the process to FAH_2, and the latter must be reduced by FAH_2 reductase before it can again participate in the biosynthesis of dTMP. Thus the interruption of this cycle accounts very well for the potent activity of the FAH_2 reductase type of antimalarials.

Until recently, evidence for amino acid transformations involving FAH_4 cofactors has been lacking for the malaria parasite, although the parasite can utilize exogenous amino acids (375, 384–387, 388a, 389–392) obtained from the host cell. The *in*

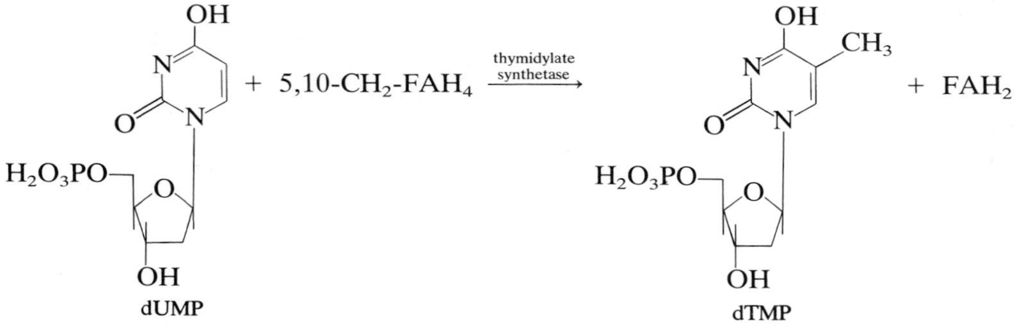

Fig. 18.10 Biosynthesis of deoxythymidylate.

vitro finding (385) that in the absence of methionine in the growth medium, the growth of *P. knowlesi* was still 52% of the control, indicated that the parasite must have obtained the amino acid sufficient for this growth either from hydrolysis of erythrocyte protein or biosynthetically. That the biosynthesis of methionine, involving a one-carbon transfer, can indeed be accomplished by *P. knowlesi,* was subsequently shown by Smith et al. (393). When monkey erythrocytes infected by *P. knowlesi* were cultured *in vitro* with L-[3-^{14}C]-serine, radioactivity was detected in approximately equivalent amounts in methionine and thymidylic acid in acid hydrolysates of washed erythrocytes, which indicated that the biosynthetic pathway serine, 5,10-methylenetetrahydrofolate, 5-methyltetrahydrofolate, methionine, is operative in *P. knowlesi.*

It thus appears that in the parasite, the step in the synthetic pathway to nucleic acid that is most vulnerable to the FAH_2 reductase inhibitors is the synthesis of deoxythymidylate (Fig. 18.10). Therefore the antiparasitic action of the FAH_2 reductase inhibitors would be the result of the FAH_4 pool not being replenished by the reduction of FAH_2 to FAH_4. Deprived of the cofactor, the synthesis of deoxythymidylate through the action of thymidylate synthetase would cease, as would, ultimately, the synthesis of DNA. However given the lack of correspondence between the periodicity of DNA synthesis and pyrimethamine activity, and the inability to demonstrate an effect of the drug on DNA production in radiotracer experiments, Coombs (394) has questioned whether the mode of action of pyrimethamine does involve inhibition of DNA synthesis.

6.2.4 DRUG RESISTANCE. The propensity of the dihydrofolate-type antimalarials to induce drug resistance and cross-resistance is well known (11). In an investigation of this phenomenon, Ferone (374) obtained an FAH_2 reductase from a pyrimethamine-resistant strain of *P. berghei* that was developed by constant exposure to partially inhibitory doses of the drug over a period of 50 weeks. A number of differences were noted between the enzymes from the resistant strain and the susceptible strain. The specific activity of the reductase from the resistant strain was eleven fold higher than that from the susceptible strain. The turnover numbers for the two enzymes, however, were almost identical, which indicated that the greater specific activity of the resistant strain enzyme must be attributed to an increased number of catalytic sites, not to an increase in activity per site. Other differences found between the two enzymes were a 12.4 higher K_m value for the resistant strain, a distinctly different pattern of chloride effects, higher K_i values for pyrimethamine and other antifolates for the resistant strain and, finally, a competitive inhibition of the FAH_2 reductase from the susceptible strain and a noncompetive inhibition from the resistant strain. From these studies, Ferone proposed that the resistance is due mainly to the combined effects of an increase in enzyme content and a decrease in inhibitor binding and suggested that the differences observed in the two enzymes is of genetic origin.

Similar changes were noted in the reductase from pyrimethamine-resistant *P. vinckei* (395).

In consideration of sulfonamide resistance in the malaria parasite and cross-resistance to FAH_2 reductase inhibitors, Trager (318) has hypothesized that the phenomenon may be based on the ability of the resistant parasites to function on a much lower level of folates than is required by the normal strains (see Section 6.1.4).

An interesting phenomenon was observed by Yoeli et al. (396), who reported the transference of resistance to pyrimethamine between two species of rodent malaria, *in vivo*. This has been investigated by Ferone et al. (395), who inoculated mice concurrently with both pyrimethamine-resistant *P. vinckei* and pyrimethamine-sensitive *P. berghei* and allowed the mixed infection to develop. When the mixed infection was passed from the mice to hamsters, a pyrimethamine-resistant strain of *P. berghei* was isolated from the hamsters. The development of the infection in the hamster was, in effect, a "biological filtration" because *P. vinckei* is incapable of growth in the hamster. The properties of the FAH_2 reductase from the sensitive strain of *P. berghei* were markedly different from those of the resistant strain of *P. berghei* isolated from the hamster. It was concluded from the experiments that, as with bacteria, the transfer of genetic material among plasmodia is possible. However in view of a lack of confirmatory evidence (397–401), this genetic transfer or "synpholia" is still controversial, and additional research is needed.

7 TISSUE SCHIZONTOCIDAL DRUGS

7.1 8-Aminoquinolines

The shortage of quinine in Germany during World War I provided the impetus for the Germans to search for a synthetic substitute. In spite of much excellent synthetic work performed in the quinine area, a quininelike antimalarial drug could not be developed (402), and other leads were pursued. Besides quinine, two other compounds were known to have limited antimalarial activity, namely, arsphenamine (Salvarsan) (18.**99**) and methylene blue

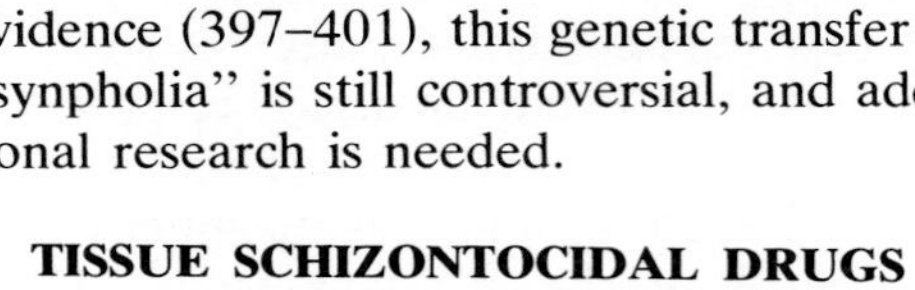

HO—C_6H_3(—NH_2)—As=As—C_6H_3(—NH_2)—OH

Arsphenamine (Salvarsan)

18.**99**

(18.**12a**) (403). Modification of methylene blue produced a slight improvement in activity with the analog (18.**12b**). This modification was followed by the introduction of the diethylaminoethyl moiety of 18.**12b** into aminoquinolines. Compounds of this type may be considered to incorporate moieties of the active compound 18.**12b** and quinine. The first one synthesized was 18.**100**, which Roehl found to be active in

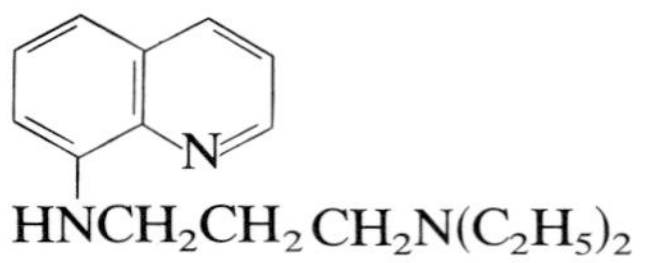

$HNCH_2CH_2CH_2N(C_2H_5)_2$

18.**100**

canaries infected with *P. relictum* (404). This new lead prompted an extensive synthetic research program in which 8-aminoquinolines were made with a great number of different alkylamino side chains and substituents in the quinoline nucleus (402). Unfortunately, most of the original German research was never published and undoubtedly much of this work has been repeated by later investigators.

In 1925 the drug plasmochin, later also called pamaquine (18.**13**) (Table 18.12) was introduced as the first synthetic antimalarial drug. It very soon became clear that the action of pamaquine on malarial parasites is different from that of quinine, particularly in reducing the relapses associated with vivax malaria. At the beginning of World War II, pamaquine was the only antirelapse drug known; it was used in combination with quinine or quinacrine, the two blood schizontocides known at that time (88). Because of its toxicity, however, pamaquine fell into disrepute. Its use in the US Army was discontinued (405), and other superior 8-aminoquinolines were developed in the United States and in the Soviet Union, such as those listed in Table 18.12; primaquine (18.**17**) is now the antirelapse drug of choice. An isomer of primaquine is used in Russia under the name quinocide (18.**101**, Table 18.12).

7.1.1 STRUCTURE-ACTIVITY RELATIONSHIPS. It is difficult to give a clear picture of the

Table 18.12 8-Aminoquinolines Active Against *P. vivax* in Man

(Structure: 6-methoxy-8-(HNR)-quinoline; CH_3O at position 6, HNR at position 8)

Compound Number	R	Generic Name	References[a]
18.**13**	$CH(CH_3)(CH_2)_3N(C_2H_5)_2$	Pamaquine	90, 403
18.**17**	$CH(CH_3)(CH_2)_3NH_2$	Primaquine	90
18.**102**	$CH(CH_3)(CH_2)_3NHCH(CH_3)_2$	Isopentaquine	90
18.**103**	$(CH_2)_3N((C_2H_5)_2$	Plasmocide, rhodoquine	147b
18.**104**	$(CH_2)_5NHCH(CH_3)_2$	Pentaquine	406, 407
18.**101**	$(CH_2)_3CH(CH_3)NH_2$	Quinocide	147b

[a] See also: G. Covell, G. R. Coatney, J. W. Field, and J. Singh, *Chemotherapy of Malaria*; World Health Organization, Geneva, 1955, selected bibliography p. 107.

structure-activity relationships of the 8-aminoquinolines for several reasons. First, results reported by various investigators were often obtained by different test methods: for example, Fourneau et al. (408) used sparrows infected with *Haemoproteus*; Bovet et al. (409) used canaries infected with *P. relictum*; Magidson et al. (410) used siskins infected with *P. praecox*; and Coatney et al. (138c) used chickens infected with *P. gallinaceum*. Moreover, the results were expressed in different ways; thus Coatney et al. (138c) determined the minimum effective doses and toxicities, whereas Wiselogle (31q) reported quinine equivalents. This situation did not improve even after the introduction of rodent malaria test systems because the 8-aminoquinolines such as pamaquine (18.**13**) and primaquine (18.**17**), which were highly active in bird malarias, were considerably less effective against the rodent malarial parasities (289b), and, again, activities were expressed by other indices (4d). Second, there are indications, discussed later, that the 8-aminoquinolines are not active as such, but rather are converted to the active compounds by the host. And, finally, the 8-aminoquinolines affect, albeit to different degrees, several stages of the life cycle of the malarial parasite, which makes the structure-activity relationship more confusing. Despite these difficulties, a number of statements regarding structure-activity relationships can be abstracted from the literature (31, 138d, 402, 408, 410–412). The reader should, however, keep in mind that these statements refer to avian malarias and that structure-activity relationships with mammalian models may not be identical.

1. Compounds with a high chemotherapeutic index had a methoxy group at position 6 of the quinoline nucleus. This group, however, was not indispensable to antimalarial activity, and it may be substituted by H, OH, or low OR groups. The 2-, 4-, or 6-methoxy analogs of 8-diethylaminopropylaminoquinoline were all active; the 6-methoxy was the most active but had the lowest therapeutic index. The introduction of a second methoxy group at positions 2 or 5 in 6-methoxy-8-diethylaminopropylaminoquinoline increased the therapeutic index (138d).
2. Optional activity was obtained with 2–6

methylene groups between the two nitrogens of the side chain. Homologs with an even number of methylene groups were found to be less active than those with an odd number. The introduction of additional hetero atoms in the basic side chain did not result in promising compounds.

3. For activity, the terminal aliphatic amino group may be primary, secondary, or tertiary, but the aromatic amine must be secondary.
4. Although only a relatively small number of 6-methoxy-8-aminoquinolines with additional substituents in the quinoline nucleus have been studied, it seems that certain additional substituents at the 4- and 5-positions may be beneficial, as suggested by the compounds shown in Table 18.13, and number of 5-phenoxy derivatives of primaquine recently tested against *P. berghei* in mice (413). Despite the relatively high toxicity of primaquine in chicks, it proved to be superior to other compounds in Table 18.13 that were tested clinically (90, 405–407).

It should be emphasized that these structure-activity relationships of the 8-aminoquinolines may predominantly be associated with blood schizontocidal action, whereas the main value of this class of compounds rests on tissue schizontocidal activity.

7.1.2 MODE OF ACTION. The investigations of Greenberg et al. (414) gave strong evidence that the 8-aminoquinoline antimalarial drugs are not active *per se*, but rather, it

Table 18.13 Activity of 8-Aminoquinolines Against *P. gallinaceum* in Chicks

(CH_3O, 5, 4 — quinoline ring, N, HNR)

Compound Number[a]	Survey Number[b]	Structure: R	Structure: 4	Structure: 5	MTD[c], mg/g	METD[d], mg/g	TI[e]
18.**105**	15333[f]	$(CH_2)_5NHCH(CH_3)_2$		$O-C_6H_4-OCH_3$	0.023	0.00013	177.0
18.**106**	15332[f]	$(CH_2)_5NHCH(CH_3)_2$		$O-CH_3$	0.011	0.00013	84.6
18.**107**	14011	$(CH_2)_6N(C_2H_5)_2$	CH_3		0.049	0.00083	59.0
18.**104**	13276	$(CH_2)_5NHCH(CH_3)_2$			0.0057	0.0001	57.0
18.**108**	15302[f]	$(CH_2)_5NHCH(CH_3)_2$	CH_3		0.014	0.00025	56.0
18.**109**	13129	$(CH_2)_4$–(piperidin-2-yl, HN)			0.012	0.00024	50.0
18.**17**	13272	$CH(CH_3)(CH_2)_3NH_2$			0.006	0.0002	30.0

[a] Compounds in this table have a therapeutic index (TI) of at least 50% over that of primaquine (18.**17**) and were selected from Coatney et al. (138d).

[b] The survey numbers are those used for these compounds in the compilations of Wiselogle (31) and Coatney et al. (138d).

[c] MTD = maximum tolerated dose.

[d] METD = minimum effective therapeutic dose.

[e] TI = MTD/METD.

[f] Not listed in Wiselogle (31).

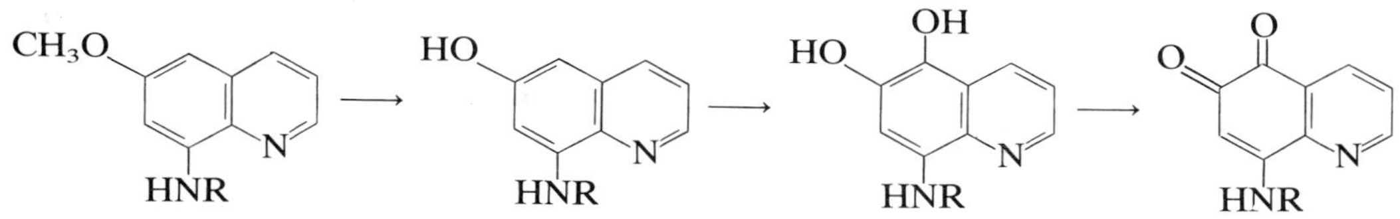

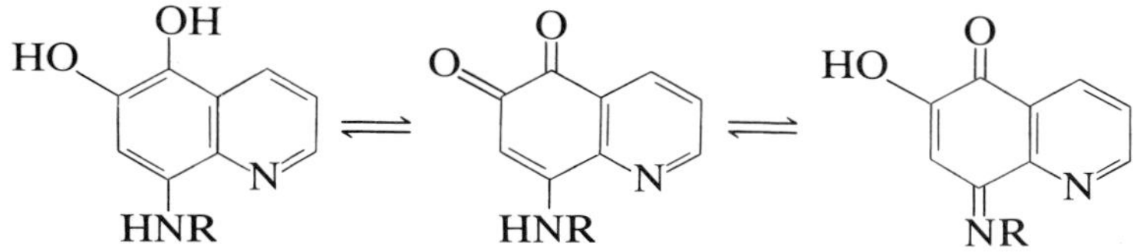

Fig. 18.11 Metabolism of 8-aminoquinolines: R represents the basic side chain present in the more common 8-aminoquinoline drugs.

is their metabolites that are the active compounds. They demonstrated that *in vitro*, pentaquine (18.**104**) and primaquine (18.**17**) were inactive against *P. gallinaceum*, whereas metabolites of these drugs were active. The 6-hydroxy and 5,6-dihydroxy derivatives are the likely metabolites. Smith (415) studied the metabolism of radiolabeled pentaquine in the rhesus monkey, and based on his findings and on the earlier results of Josephson et al. (416) with pamaquine (18.**13**), concluded that these drugs were metabolized to a 5,6-quinolinequinone by the route depicted in Fig. 18.11*a*. Data for a number of related compounds that were investigated for both *in vitro* and *in vivo* activity against *P. gallinaceum* appear in Table 18.14. Although the *in vivo* formation of the quinone has been questioned (35d), it is conceivable that an equilibrium is established (Fig. 18.11*b*) that would be capable of disrupting biological oxidation-reduction systems. This effect may be basically responsible for the antimalarial action of the 8-aminoquinoline drugs and (*vide infra*) for their undesirable hemolytic properties (417).

Morphological studies of Aikawa and Beaudoin (418) and Howells et al. (419) showed that the earliest changes observed in avian and rodent parasites after exposure to certain 8-aminoquinolines occurred in the mitochondria of the exoerythrocytic forms and in the mitochondrialike organelles of the erythrocytic forms. These *in vitro* studies indicated that the 8-aminoquinoline drugs [e.g., primaquine (18.**17**)] are themselves active antimalarial agents (420), although the possibility of the formation of active metabolities in the tissue culture cannot be precluded (421). Studies with primaquine showed that this drug did not affect the mitochondria of the host cells nor those of the sporogonic stages (*P. berghei*) in the mosquito (420). Aikawa and Beaudoin (418) postulated that these compounds disrupt the oxidative processes of the parasite mitochondria, leading to death. They hypothesized that the susceptibility of the exoerythrocytic forms is due to the supposedly greater sensitivity of their mitochondria to oxidative damage as opposed to the mitochondrialike organelles of the erythrocytic forms. A similar action on the exoerythrocytic states of *P. vivax* could account for the radical curative effect of the 8-aminoquinolines.

No convincing report has appeared showing the development of primaquine-resistant strains in nature, but such strains have been developed experimentally in

Table 18.14 Comparison of *in Vitro* and *in Vivo* Activity of 8-Aminoquinolines Against *P. gallinaceum* in Chick Erythrocytes

(8-aminoquinoline structure: positions 5 and 6 marked; 8-substituent HNR)

Compound Number	Structure: R	5	6	Activity of *P. gallinaceum*: *In Vitro*	*In Vivo*	References
18.**110**	$(CH_2)_3N(C_2H_5)_2$		OH	+	+	414
18.**111**	$(CH_2)_3N(C_2H_5)_2$		$OCOCH_3$	+	+	414
18.**104**	$(CH_2)_5NHCH(CH_3)_2$		OCH_3	−	+	414
18.**112**	$(CH_2)_5NHCH(CH_3)_2$		OH	+	+	414
18.**113**	$(CH_2)_5NHCH(CH_3)_2$	OH[a]	OH	+	+	414
18.**114**	$(CH_2)_5NHCH(CH_3)_2$	OH[a]	OCH_3	+	—[b]	414
18.**106**	$(CH_2)_5NHCH(CH_3)_2$	OCH_3	OCH_3	—[b]	+	138d
18.**115**	$CH(CH_3)(CH_2)_3N(C_2H_5)_2$	=O (quinone)	=O	+	—[b]	53e, 416

[a] 5-OH Compounds are very unstable, and the possibility that degradation products are responsible for the activity should be kept in mind.
[b] Not reported.

both man and animals (14). Thus a strain of *P. vivax* has been reported to show a significant increase in trophozoite-resistance to primaquine in humans (15).

For additional reading on the mode of action of these drugs, see Refs. 35d, 256b, 421, and 422.

7.1.3 DRUGS. During World War II and shortly thereafter a great number of 8-aminoquinolines were evaluated in man; the best known compounds are shown in Table 18.12. Primaquine (18.**17**) is the present drug of choice in the United States and Western Europe. Quinocide (18.**101**), an isomer of primaquine, has been used in the Soviet Union and Eastern Europe, but it has a lower therapeutic index than primaquine (35e).

Primaquine is active against secondary tissue schizonts (secondary or late developing exoerythrocytic forms), therefore it is used in achieving a radical cure of relapsing malaria such as *P. vivax*. It is also active as a causal prophylactic against the primary exoerythrocytic forms of all human malarial parasites. At tolerated doses, primaquine is relatively ineffective against the blood schizonts of human malarias, and, consequently, it is not satisfactory for treatment of acute attacks of malaria. However it is used in combination with fast-acting blood schizontocides such as quinine (18.**17**), chloroquine (18.**16**), or amodiaquine (18.**51**), but not in combination with quinacrine (18.**14**) because the latter drug apparently potentiates the hemolytic properties of primaquine (35f). The combination of primaquine (45 mg base) and chloroquine (300 mg base) given weekly is widely used for protection against vivax malaria (423), but it is not satisfactory in preventing infections with chloroquine-resistant *P. falciparum*. Although at tolerated doses, primaquine does not possess appreciable blood schizontocidal activity, it is highly active against the gametocytes of all species of human malaria parasites, particularly against those of *P. falciparum*, including the chloroquine-resistant strains (424).

The toxicity of primaquine and other 8-aminoquinoline antimalarial drugs can involve the gastrointestinal tract, the central nervous system, and the erythrocytes. In the case of primaquin administered in therapeutic doses, the first two types of toxicity can be very annoying but they are reversed upon termination of therapy. Especially noteworthy is the specific life-threatening effect on the red blood cells. The life span of human erythrocytes is approximately 120 days; after this time they are removed from the circulation. The formation of new red cells in the bone marrow maintains the number of these cells at a required level. However untoward events, such as the presence of certain drugs or chemicals in the bloodstream, can shorten the life span of erythrocytes. If the loss of erythrocytes is not compensated for by production in the bone marrow, anemia develops. The destruction of the red cells by certain drugs, including the 8-aminoquinolines, occurs with the liberation of hemoglobin, and this process (hemolysis) takes place particularly easily in patients with a genetic deficiency of the enzyme glucose-6-phosphate dehydrogenase (G6PD) (425). The deficiency itself is usually without demonstrable adverse effect, although there are indications of a decreased life expectancy (426). This abnormality is rare among Caucasians and occurs predominantly in persons who live in areas, or whose ancestors had lived in areas, with endemic aalaria (e.g., American Negroes). It is estimated that more than 100 million people in the world have this abnormality (427). The enzyme G6PD plays a crucial role in the oxidation-reduction processes of the erythrocytes, and if the amount of this enzyme is insufficient, the red cell is prone to undergo biochemical change leading to hemolysis. The oxidative metabolites of 8-aminoquinolines (Fig. 18.11*b*) seem to impair this oxidation-reduction system, particularly in G6PD-deficient persons (428).

Persons whose erythrocytes are deficient in G6PD are relatively more resistant to infections with *P. falciparum* (429). Studies of Theakston et al. (430) indicated that *P. falciparum* requires this enzyme and obtains it from the host erythrocytes, thus suggesting that relatively low amounts of G6PD in the erythrocytes retard the normal growth of the parasites. However other studies by Powell (431) and Segal (432) and co-workers showed that G6PD-deficient persons are not, *per se*, more than normally resistant to falciparum malaria.

For additional reading on the subject of G6PD, see Refs. 417, 433, and 434.

Because of the presence of an asymmetric carbon atom in primaquine, this drug consists of equal parts of D- and L-isomers (435). Studies of Schmidt et al. (436) show that the activities of these isomers against *P. cynomolgi* in rhesus monkeys is essentially identical but the D-form is 3–5 times less toxic than the L-form. This property would be of particular value if this result was also found in man.

8 MISCELLANEOUS COMPOUNDS

An appreciable number of compounds with diverse structures have been reported to have antimalarial properties in one or more animal models and have been subjected to various degrees of investigation. Thompson and Werbel (35g) have reviewed such structures. Because of the limitations of this chapter, we discuss only some of the better known ones that have been studied in man. Some of these have been selected from a listing by the World Health Organization (1m); compounds that have been discussed elsewhere in the text are not mentioned.

8.1 Antibiotics

An excellent account of the use of antibiotics in the treatment of malaria up to 1952 was given by Coatney and Greenberg (437). Of the 31 antibiotics tested in lower animals, 8 exhibited some antimalarial action. Penicillin, streptomycin, dehydrostreptomycin, and bacitracin were all inactive against blood-induced avian infection. Although there was some variation in effectiveness relative to quinine (18.**27**), chloramphenicol, chlortetracycline, and terramycin were all active therapeutically and prophylactically against *P. cathemerium*, *P. gallinaceum*, and *P. berghei*; chlortetracycline was the most active of the three against all three parasites. The same three antibiotics were also the only ones of those tested that were active in man. From a review of 90 infected patients treated with antibiotics, however, these authors concluded that the antibiotics then available were of no practical value against acute attacks of malaria, since they were slow acting, not truly curative, and not causally prophylactic, hence offered no advantage over the drugs in use.

This view has prevailed until recent years when the emergence of drug-resistant strains of *P. falciparum* prompted a reappraisal of antibiotics. Most of the investigations have been carried out on tetracycline and its derivatives, doxycycline and minocycline. Rieckmann et al. (438), using volunteers infected with a chloroquine-susceptible, a moderately chloroquine-resistant, or a highly chloroquine-resistant strain of *P. falciparum* found that tetracycline appeared to be about equally effective against the erythrocytic forms of the three strains and cured most cases if administered daily over at least a 5 day period. However the drug had no effect on the course of the disease for the first 2 or 3 days; hence it was concluded that it should not be used alone for treatment of an acute attack. Clyde et al. (439), obtained similar results with both tetracycline and doxycycline. These workers also tested the antibiotics against vivax malaria and found that although infections were slowly cleared, they invariably recurred. In addition, the compounds were shown to have no prophylactic effect against vivax malaria and no sporontocidal effect upon *P. falciparum*, i.e., they did not affect the development of gametocytes in the mosquito. Willerson et al. (440), who tested minocycline against multi-drug-resistant falciparum malaria, found this drug to have similar characteristics. In addition to effecting radical cures, it protected volunteers after challenge with infected mosquitoes. Like the other tetracyclines, it is slow acting and without gametocytocidal or sporontocidal effect. In studies (441, 442) of acutely ill patients infected with *P. falciparum*, in an area where chloroquine-resistant falciparum malaria was endemic, excellent results were obtained with sequential quinine-tetracycline and quinine-minocycline treatment. When the quinine treatment was followed by a conventional chloroquine treatment instead of tetracycline, results (6) were not nearly so good (41.6% cures vs. 96.6% cures). Excellent results were obtained by Rieckmann et al. (443) with combinations of tetracycline with amodiaquine or quinine.

The mode of action of these antibiotics against plasmodia is known. The clumping of pigment in growing intraerythrocytic trophozoites of *P. berghei* that occurs after chloroquine treatment (see Section 5.3.1) requires protein synthesis, RNA synthesis, and energy (444–446). However neither tetracycline (446) nor minocycline (447) inhibited such clumping *in vitro* at a concentration of 10^{-4} *M*, and it was concluded that the drugs did not gain access to the growing trophozoites, or that they did not affect cytoplasmic ribosomal protein synthesis in the parasite. Erythromycin, on the other hand, did inhibit chloroquine-induced pigment clumping at 10^{-4} *M* (445), which seems to indicate a direct action on the malaria parasite. The antimalarial action of the antibiotics *in vivo* is complicated somewhat by their action on the intestinal flora of the mice, thus affecting the nutritional state of the host and parasite.

Lincomycin (18.**116a**) is a water-soluble

	R_1	R_2	R_3	R_4
18.**116a**	OH	H	CH_3	nC_3H_7
18.**116b**	H	Cl	CH_3	nC_3H_7
18.**116c**	H	Cl	H	nC_5H_{11}

antibiotic that is very effective against gram-positive organisms (448, 449). Displacement of the 4-hydroxyl group of lincomycin by chlorine (18.**116b**, clindamycin) (452) or the introduction of chlorine in this position in semisynthetic derivatives (451) results in 7-deoxy-7(*S*)-chloro lincomycin analogs that have improved antibacterial activity, are more rapidly absorbed, and give higher blood levels and better tissue penetration compared to the nonchlorinated analog (450). In addition, the introduction of the chlorine conferred an activity against the rodent malaria parasite *P. berghei*, which was not present in the parent lincomycin (18.**116a**) (450, 453); additional modification of the structure by elimination of the *N*-1′-methyl and substitution of an *n*-pentyl group for the *n*-propyl at C-4′ (18.**116c**) resulted in a further marked increase in antiplasmodial activity. It is especially noteworthy that the chloro derivative of lincomycin (18.**116b**) was also active against chloroquine- and DDS-resistant strains of *P. berghei* (453).

The antimalarial activity of the chloro analogs of lincomycin were studied using *P. cynomolgi* in rhesus monkeys by Powers (454) and by Schmidt et al. (455), The latter investigators found that both clindamycin (18.**116b**) and 18.**116c** exhibited significant blood schizontocidal activity but were slow to clear parasitemia. Both compounds effected marked delays in patency against a challenge with sporozoites, and 18.**116c** was capable of providing complete protection to some of the challenged monkeys. However neither compound was regularly effective in curing sporozoite-induced infection, but both were as effective against a sporozoite challenge with a pyrimethamine-proguanil-resistant strain as against a susceptible strain. On the basis of his studies, Schmidt et al. (455) concluded that 18.**116c** is a more effective agent than clindamycin (18.**116b**).

More recently Powers and Jacobs (456) studied the activity of clindamycin and 18.**116c** against a blood-induced human malaria using as a model the chloroquine-resistant Oak Knoll strain of *P. falciparum* in the owl monkey. Although changes in parasite morphology were seen within 24 hr after administration of the first dose of drug and trophozoites were cleared from the peripheral blood by the end of a 7 day treatment, an actual decrease in parasitemia was not apparent until after 48 hr, an indication that the drugs were slow in acting. Curative activity was dose related, but not the speed of clearance of parasites. Gametocytes persisted after clearance of the asexual forms of the parasite but the infectivity of these gametocytes was not determined.

The good results obtained when the slow acting antibiotics tetracycline or minocycline were used in conjunction with quinine (141) prompted the evaluation of the slow-acting clindamycin (18.**116b**) in combination with quinine against three multi-drug-resistant strains of *P. falciparum* in man (457). Although quinine alone was not curative against these strains, the combination was; and it appears that clindamycin may have a shorter course of therapy than is required by tetracycline.

The accelerated response of *P. falciparum* to clindamycin in man brought about by the combination with quinine was also noted by Clyde et al. (458), although the proportion of cures was not clearly affected. When a combination of chloroquine and the antibiotic was tested against the relapsing malaria *P. vivax*, relapses occurred in all cases, indicating that the antibiotic was not active against the secondary tissue form of the parasite. Mild to severe gastric intolerance was noted with the use of clindamycin (457, 458), and Clyde et al. (458) have suggested that despite its effectiveness, the antibiotic is unlikely to be recommended for treatment of falciparum malaria because of other serious side effects.

The mode of action of the chlorolincomycin derivatives against plasmodia has not been established. However lincomycin (18.**116a**) does inhibit bacterial protein synthesis without interfering with DNA and RNA synthesis (459) and the site of action has been shown to be at the 50S ribosomal level (460). Lewis (453) has suggested that since the overall protein-synthesizing mechanisms of various organisms have been found to be similar, the inhibitory mechanism for bacteria is similar to that for plasmodia, and the action against the latter organisms is due to the inhibition of protein syntheses at the ribosomal level.

8.2 RC-12

The compound RC-12 (18.**117b**) resulted from the discovery almost a half-century ago that certain pyrocatechol amine derivatives had antimalarial activity (364b).

Early structure-activity studies (461) resulted in an analog of RC-12 (18.**117a**, dimeplasmin) that was more active than pamaquine against trophozoite-induced infections in birds, but subsequent trials in

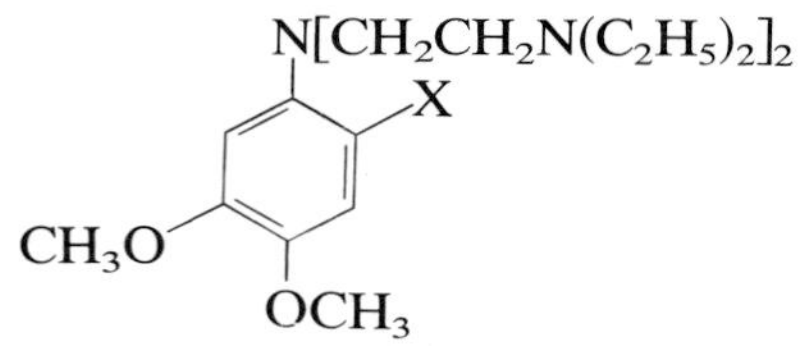

$N[CH_2CH_2N(C_2H_5)_2]_2$

X

CH_3O

OCH_3

	X
18.**177a**	H
18.**177b**	Br(RC-12)

18.**117**

humans were disappointing and interest in the pyrocatechols waned. Then in 1965 it was reported (16b) that the compound RC-12 had an effect against the exoerythrocytic forms of *P. cathemerium* in the canary. Shortly thereafter Schmidt et al. (462) concluded on the basis of studies in the monkey that the compound had little promise as a suppressive but significant promise as a prophylactic or radical curative agent especially, e.g., in cases where there is chloroquine resistance, need for a faster curative agent, or fear of enhanced susceptibility to the hematotoxicity of primaquine. Subsequent studies by Sodeman et al. (463), showed that single weekly doses of 25 mg/kg body weight of RC-12 usually prevented the development and/or maturation of exoerythrocytic stages of *P. cynomolgi* in rhesus monkeys. However, this treatment was not uniformly successful, leaving the usefulness of the compound open to some doubt. In a recent study with human volunteers, Clyde et al. (464), working with the Chesson strain of *P. vivax*, showed that the naphthalene disulfonate salt of RC-12 failed to protect volunteers when they were exposed to infected mosquitoes. Thus with this failure in a clinical trial, the erratic course of RC-12 may have to come to an end.

8.3 α,α,α,α′,α′,α′-Hexachloroxylene Derivatives

The compound 1,4-bis(trichloromethyl)-benzene (18.**118**, Hetol® was reported by

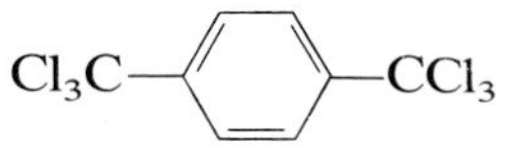

Cl_3C–C_6H_4–CCl_3

Hetol®
18.**118**

Elslager et al. (345) to be about twice as potent as quinine against *P. berghei* when administered continuously in the diet. A number of related compounds were also synthesized and tested, but none proved to be as active as 18.**118** (345). Hetol® was well tolerated when tested in volunteers. However against a chloroquine-resistant strain of *P. falciparum* it produced only a temporary suppression of the parasitemia in one of two subjects who received 4 g daily for 3 days; similarly, a single dose of 4 g produced only temporary suppression of parasitemia in a volunteer infected with drug-sensitive *P. falciparum* (465). The drug brought about the clearance of a blood-induced *P. vivax* infection but was not curative at a dose of 4.5 g daily for 4 days (465). Because of the slow action of the drug, the large dose required, and the failure to cure infections, development of the compound has been discontinued.

8.4 Menoctone

The naphthoquinone hydrolapachol (18.**119a**) and two related quinones, originally prepared by Hooker, were found to

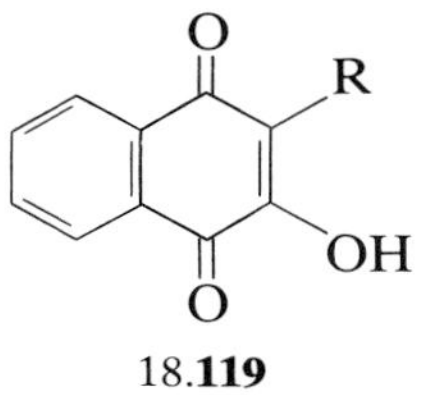

18.**119**

	R
18.**119a**	$-CH_2CH_2CH(CH_3)_2$
18.**119b**	$-CH_2CH_2CH_2C_6H_{11}$
18.**119c**	$-CH_2(CH_2)_7C(OH)(nC_5H_{11})_2$
18.**119d**	$-CH_2(CH_2)_7C_6H_{11}$

have antimalarial activity after they had been made part of the Harvard University collection. This discovery resulted in a tremendous research effort during World War II for improved compounds of this type (see references in Ref. 35h); a great many analogs with antimalarial activity were obtained. Two of these early compounds, which were active against *P. lophurae*, were tested in man; only one, 18.**119b**, showed even weak activity against *P. vivax* and *P. falciparum* (466). In contrast to their metabolism in ducks and chickens, 18.**119a** and 18.**119b** are rapidly degraded in man. Introduction of a hydroxyl group into the side chain increased the metabolic stability of 18.**119b** but reduced antimalarial activity. However this loss in activity could be compensated for by increasing the length of the chain, thus restoring the proper hydrophilic-lipophilic balance. Compound 18.**119c** represents such a balance; it had high potency against *P. lophurae* in ducks and was reported to be both suppressive and curative in man when administered intravenously (466). Because of the development of other potent antimalarials during the war, and because quinones had to be administered parenterally, interest in them waned. It was not until 1964, when chloroquine-resistant malaria became a serious problem, that interest was renewed. By this time the mouse had superseded the bird as the model of choice for testing antimalarial activity, and the former appears to be superior to the latter as a model for the testing of quinones.

Using blood-induced *P. berghei* infections in mice, Berberian and Slighter (467) tested quinone homologs with side chains longer than those that had been studied earlier by Fieser. The compounds were administered intragastrically, twice daily for 4 consecutive days, beginning immediately after infection. Several series of side chains were studied, viz., *n*-alkyl, isoalkyl, phenylalkyl, adamantylalkyl, and cyclohexylalkyl. In four of the five series, peak activity occurred when the methylene group in the chain between the quinone and the terminal methyl or alicyclic moiety numbered 8 or 9. It is interesting that the compounds selected for clinical trials in Fieser's studies based on activity against avian parasites showed little or no activity in this study. In general, the activity against the intraerythrocytic form of the parasite was minimal, and only 3 compounds out of the 32 tested produced cures. One of the better 3-substituted alkyl-2-hydroxy-1,4-naphthoquinones that was studied, 18.**119d** (menoctone), was selected for testing against sporozoite-induced *P. berghei* in mice to see whether it had prophylactic activity (468). The test indicated that on a weight basis, menoctone was superior to primaquine (18.**17**) as a causal prophylactic, and was considerably less toxic, as well. An interesting potentiation of the blood schizontocidal action of menoctone against *P. berghei* in mice was noted by Peters (26b) when this drug was administered along with cycloguanil (18.**24**).

The blood schizontocidal and causal prophylactic activity of menoctone against *P. berghei* in mice was not carried over to humans. A daily oral dose of 500 mg for 3 days exerted only slight blood schizontocidal activity in patients infected with the Malaya (Camp) strain of *P. falciparum*, and no definite gametocytocidal or sporontocidal effects. The drug also failed to show any causal prophylactic activity against a drug-sensitive or drug-resistant *P. falciparum* (465, 1n). It has been suggested that poor absorption from the gastrointestinal tract, which is characteristic of compounds of this type, may account for the apparent inactivity of menoctone in humans (1n). However it should also be noted that naphthoquinones are strongly bound to plasma proteins; the order, as judged by dialysis experiments was human > monkey > duck (469), and quinones so complexed are less active against parasitized red cells than are free quinones.

The mode of antimalarial action of the 2-hydroxy-3-alkyl-1,4-naphthoquinones is not known. However, these quinones are potent inhibitors of the respiration of parasitized red blood cells. Wendel (470) found that a large percentage of the quinones he tested depressed the oxygen uptake *in vitro* of cells parasitized with *P. knowlesi* or *P. lophurae* and that the relative antirespiratory activity roughly paralleled the antimalarial activity as judged by suppression of *P. lophurae* infections in ducks. In another series of quinones, Fieser and Heymann (471) did not find an exact parallelism between *in vitro* and *in vivo* activity, but high *in vivo* activity was always reflected in high *in vitro* activity. However no parallelism was found between *in vivo* antimalarial activity and antirespiratory activity against the succinate oxidase system (472).

Parasitized red cells are characterized by an abnormal content of coenzyme Q (CoQ, ubiquinone, 18.**120**). Thus in addition to

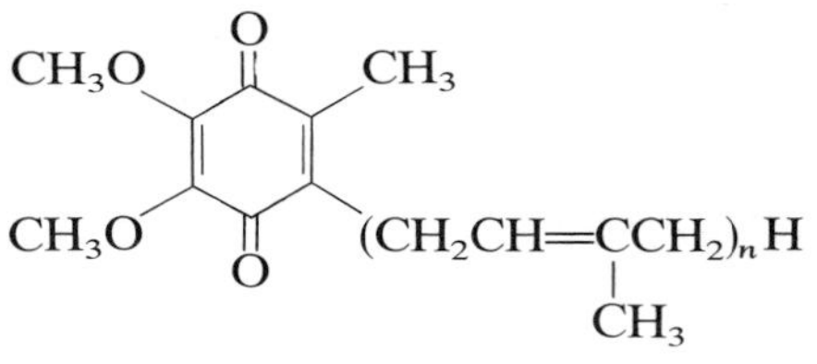

Ubiquinone
18.**120**

CoQ_{10} (18.**120**, $n = 10$) found in normal duck blood, *P. lophurae*-parasitized blood contained CoQ_8 (18.**120**, $n = 8$) and CoQ_9 (18.**120**, $n = 9$) (473, 474). Similarly, whereas CoQ_8, CoQ_9, and CoQ_{10} are normally present in the blood of both the normal rhesus monkey and the mouse, the concentration of CoQ_8 was greater in monkey blood parasitized with *P. knowlesi* or *P. cynomolgi* and mouse blood parasitized with *P. berghei* (475). No evidence for the presence of K vitamins was obtained in the blood of ducks, mice, or monkeys, normal or parasitized. It has also been shown that menoctone (18.**119d**) inhibits, *in vitro*, the mitochondrial oxidation of DPNH and succinate by coenzyme Q, and it has been suggested from the evidence above that menoctone may exert at least part of its antimalarial activity through the inhibition of electron transport involving CoQ (18.**120**), thus interfering with the biosynthesis or function of CoQ in the metabolism of the parasite. The active metabolites of the 8-aminoquinolines, the 5,6-quinolinequinones, would also have the ability to participate in biological redox system (see Section 7.1.2).

8.5 Clociguanil (WR-38,839) and WR-99210

Clociguanil (18.**121a**) (476) is a DHFR inhibitor that is closely related to cycloguanil

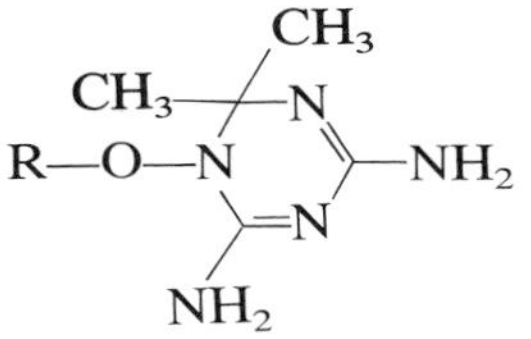

CH_3 CH_3 N R—O—N NH_2 N NH_2

18.**121**

	R
18.**121a**	$—CH_2$—(3,4-dichlorophenyl) (Cl, Cl)
18.**121b**	$—(CH_2)_3—O—$(2,4,5-trichlorophenyl) (Cl, Cl)

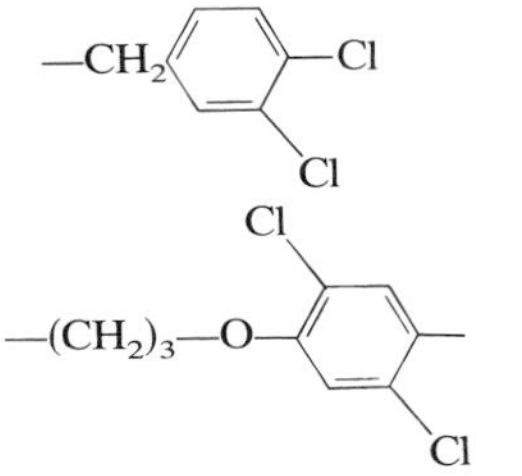

(18.**24**). Originally synthesized for antimicrobial studies (477). it was subsequently found to be highly active against both pyrimethamine-sensitive and -resistant strains of *P. berghei* in the mouse and active against chloroquine-sensitive and -resistant or pyrimethamine-sensitive and -resistant *P. falciparum* in the owl monkey (1o). In man a combination with sulfadiazine (18.**86**) was more effective than clociguanil alone against drug-resistant malaria and, particularly significant, the combination protected all patients against infection when they were exposed to mosquitoes heavily infected with drug-resistant malaria, whereas the drugs given alone at similar or higher doses failed to prevent infection. Thus there seems to be a synergistic effect against the preerythrocytic tissue forms of the parasite (478). A related drug (18.**121b**, WR-99210) has been approved for human trials (465).

9 BIOCHEMISTRY OF PLASMODIA

Table 18.1 indicates that malarial parasites are rather natural-host specific; therefore it is not surprising to see differences in the biochemistry of the various plasmodia. This is, for instance, most pronounced when comparing the biochemistry of the bird malarial parasite *P. lophurae* with the rodent malarial parasite *P. berghei.* The first, when developing in the nucleated avian erythrocytes, may utilize the Krebs cycle (479), whereas the latter, when present in the nonnucleated mammalian erythrocytes, does not possess such a cycle (240). The avian parasite *P. cathemerium* probably does not possess the enzyme adenosine deaminase, but *P. berghei* and *P. vinckei* have a high content of this enzyme (377a). One would also expect differences in the biochemistry of plasmodia developing in the mosquito host and in the vertebrate host. As mentioned, intraerythrocytic *P. berghei* does not utilize the Krebs cycle, but when in the mosquito, it probably does utilize this cycle because the oocysts of the parasite contain the Krebs cycle enzymes succinate dehydrogenase and isocitrate dehydrogenases (241b).

Most of the biochemical studies of malarial parasites have been performed on the intraerythrocytic stage, and this stage is discussed mainly.

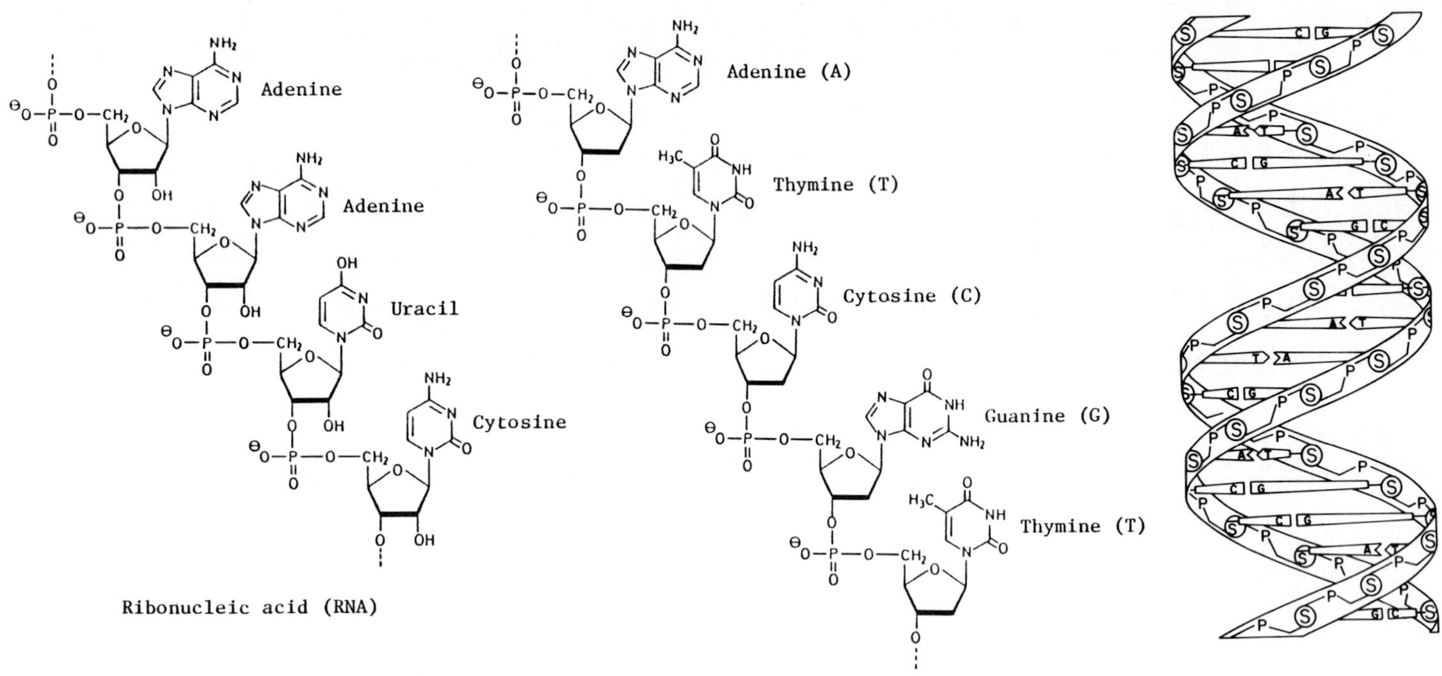

Fig. 18.12 Structures of RNA, DNA, and the stereo representation of the DNA double helix: nucleosides (base and sugar): RNA: adenosine, uridine, and cytid DNA: deoxyadenosine, Thymidine, and deoxycytidine.

9.1 Nucleic Acids

For the formation of plasmodial nucleic acids DNA and RNA, the malarial parasite needs to have available the constituents, viz., purines (adenine and guanine), pyrimidines (cytosine, thymine, and uracil), ribose sugars, and phosphate (Fig. 18.12). Of these compounds, the parasite is unable to synthesize purines, *de novo* [*P. berghei* (480); *P. lophurae* (378a)] and the ribose sugars [*P. gallinaceum*, *P. berghei*, *P. knowlesi*, *P. falciparum* (485)] and obtains these compounds, together with the phosphate [*P. gallinaceum* (195*a*, b, *P. lophurae* (378b), *P. berghei* (196, 481)] from the hosts, whereas the pyrimidines are synthesized within the parasities. Walsh and Sherman (378a) demonstrated that pyrimidine syntheses, as determined by the incorporation of $^{14}C\text{-}NaHCO_3$ into the pyrimidines cytosine, uracil, and thymine, was slight in normal duck erythrocytes, whereas both *P. lophurae*-infected erythrocytes and the free parasites had high rates of incorporation of labeled carbon in these pyrimidines. Several investigators found that radiolabeled, naturally occurring pyrimidines do not enter the free parasites [*P. berghei* (379, 482)] or the intraerythrocytic parasites [*P. berghei* (377a, 379, 382), *P. vinckei* (377a), *P. knowlesi* (199, 483, 484)]; the pyrimidines and nucleosides investigated were thymine (199, 379, 382, 483), thymidine (377a, 483), uracil (199, 483), uridine (199, 377a, 379, 483), cytidine (379, 382, 483), and 2′-deoxycytidine (483). However studies with *P. knowlesi* showed that the pyrimidine derivative orotic acid (18.**122**, Fig. 18.13) could be taken up (199, 483, 484) and that this plasmodium could utilize thymidine and uridine to some degree (484). Because of the capability of malarial parasites to synthesize pyrimidines *de novo*, the required enzymes for these conversions should be present, and a number of these enzymes have been isolated from plasmodia—for instance, aspartate transcarbamylase [*P. berghei* (379)], orotidine-5′-monophosphate pyrophosphorylase, and thymidylate synthetase [*P. lophurae* (378a)] (Figs. 18.10 and 18.13).

The malarial parasite procures needed purines from the host erythrocytes. The latter are also incapable of *de novo* purine biosynthesis and obtain them from the liver, a purine-synthesizing tissue (486).

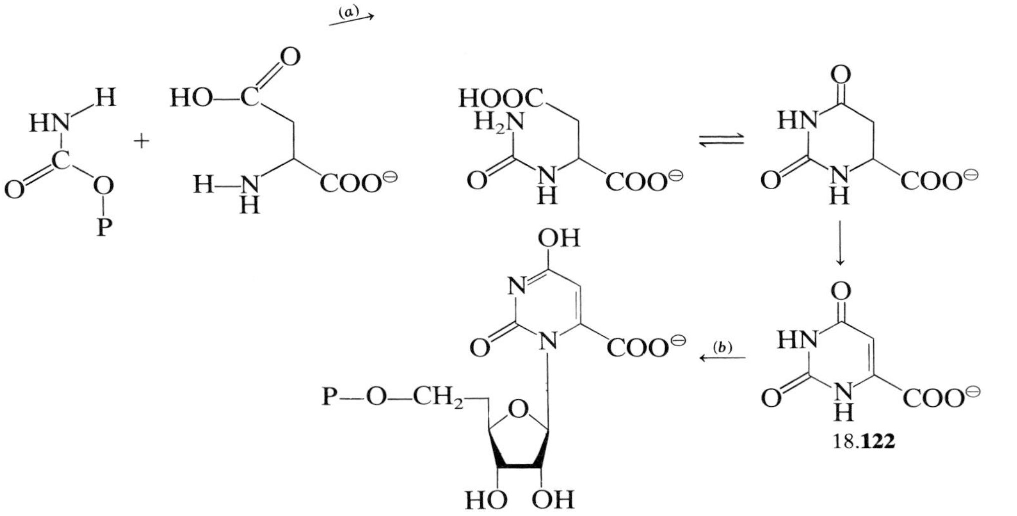

Fig. 18.13 Pyridine biosynthesis. (*a*) Aspartate transcarbamylase (ACTase), (*b*) Orotidine-5′-monophosphate pyrophosphorylase (OMPase).

Numerous studies have been conducted on the uptake and utilization by various malarial parasites of naturally occurring purines. The research utilized radiolabeled adenine (199, 379, 482, 483, 487, 488), adenosine (377a, b; 379, 380, 382, 482, 483, 487), deoxyadenosine (379, 483, 487), guanine (483, 488), guanosine (379, 382, 483, 488), inosine (482, 488), hypoxanthine (377a, b; 482, 483, 488), xanthine and xanthosine (488), and a number of nucleotides (487, 488). The earliest *in vitro* studies on the utilization of radiolabeled adenosine and hypoxanthine for the biosynthesis of nucleic acids by *P. berghei* and *P. vinckei* were done by Büngener and Nielsen (377b), who concluded that the purine requirements of the parasite could be satisfied by the transformation of adenosine by adenosine kinase to adenosine monophosphate (AMP) and by the conversion of hypoxanthine to inosine monophosphate (IMP) by hypoxanthine phosphoribosyltransferase. The former conversion occurs in both normal and parasitized cells, wheras the latter occurs only in parasitized cells (Fig. 18.14).

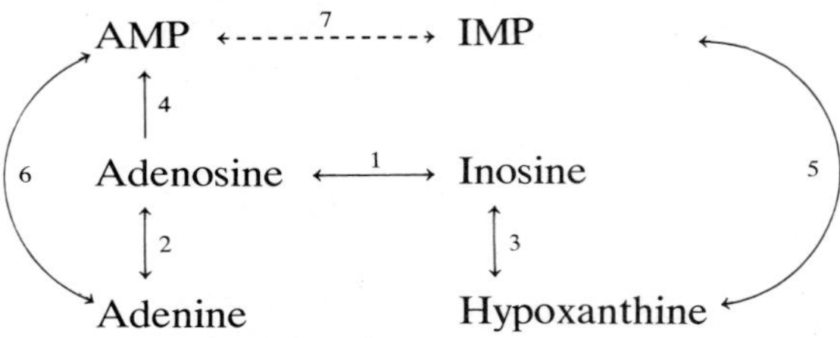

Fig. 18.14 Purine interconversion: 1, adenosine deaminase; 2, 3, purine nucleoside phosphorylase; 4, adenosine kinase; 5, hypoxanthine/guanine phosphoribosyltransferase (HGPRTase); 6, adenine phosphoribosyltransferase (APRTase), For step 7, see Ref. 507.

Tracy and Sherman's studies (488) with *P. lophurae* showed that compared to other purines, adenosine, inosine, and hypoxanthine were best taken up and incorporated into nucleic acid, and they expressed the possibility that adenosine may be deaminated to inosine shortly before or during uptake by the parasites. Xanthine and xanthosine were poorly taken up and not incorporated in nucleic acid. The nucleotides IMP, AMP, and ATP were only slightly incorporated into nucleic acids; This was attributed to poor uptake by normal red cells, parasitized red cells, and free parasites. The conversion of adenosine to inosine was earlier postulated by Van Dyke and Szustkiewicz (489); later Van Dyke and co-workers (380, 482) concluded that adenosine is metabolized by *P. berghei* to inosine and finally to hypoxanthine, a process that occurs external to or on the membrane of, the parasite. Inside the parasite, hypoxanthine is converted to IMP and further, successively, to AMP, ADP, and ATP. Carter et al. (490) demonstrated that erythrocyte-free *P. berghei* phosphorylated adenosine to ATP and subsequently incorporated it into nucleic acids, but these processes occurred only when glucose was present in the medium.

The enzymes involved in the biochemical conversions of purines have been extensively studied in animal tissue (491), but so far only a few of these enzymes have been isolated from plasmodia. The conversion of adenosine to inosine requires the enzyme adenosine deaminase, which Büngener (492) found to be present in *P. berghei, P. vinckei, and P. cynomolgi.* He also established the presence of purine nucleoside phosphorylase in the rodent parasite. The presence of these two enzymes led Büngener to postulate that the parasites might convert adenosine to hypoxanthine and IMP, which, as mentioned before, was substantiated by Van Dyke (482). Other enzymes, viz., adenosine kinase (493), hypoxanthine–guanine phosphoribosyltransferase (HGPRTase), and adenine phosphoribosyltransferase (APRTase) (301b) were concentrated from *P. chabaudi.* Figure 18.17 summarizes the metabolic relationship of these enzymes.

Several investigators studied the effect of chemicals on the incorporation of radiolabeled orotic acid (18.**122**, Fig. 18.13) and adenosine into nucleic acid. Inhibition of such incorporation was interpreted as an inhibition of the growth of the parasite. Van Dyke et al. (52) developed an *in vitro* antimalarial drug screening system based on the ability of chemical agents to inhibit the incorporation of adenosine-8-^{3}H into nucleic acids of the malarial parasite *P. berghei* (see Section 3). McCormack et al. (51) studied the inhibitory effect of a number of purine nucleosides, purine bases, and orotic acid analogs on the incorporation of adenosine-8-^{14}C and orotic acid-6-^{14}C into nucleic acids of *P. knowlesi.* They observed high inhibitory effects with many of the compounds, particularly 3′-deoxyadenosine, adenine xyloside, puromycin, tubercidin, 1,3-dimethyl-2-oxy-6-thio-8-(3′-hydroxy-n- propyl)purine, and 5-fluoroortic acid. Other *in vitro* experiments involved the study of the effect on nucleic acid production of chloroquine (18.**16**) 167, 183b, 192, 198a, 200, 201), amodiaquine (18.**51**) (198a), quinacrine (18.**14**) 192, 198a), dihydroquinine (18.**36**) (183b), quinine (18.**27**) (192, 198a), and chloroguanide (18.**22**) (198a), using red cells infected by *P. berghei* or *P. knowlesi.* All these drugs inhibited nuclei acid synthesis, but to different degrees (see also Section 5.3.1). For the effect of amino acid antagonists on nuclei acid production, see Section 9.2.

In constrast to the extensive literature on the pyrimidine and purine requirements of intraerythrocytic malarial parasites, few publications are concerned with these requirements for the parasite developing in the mosquito. Several investigators found that the oocyst stages (Fig. 18.1) of the malarial parasites *P. berghei* (494, 495) and *P. cynomolgi* (496) were incapable of incorporating tritium-labeled thymidine into nucleic acids, but that tritium-labeled adenosine was incorporated. It seems, therefore, that the invertebrate sporogonic stage and the vertebrate intraerythrocytic stage of malarial parasites rely on the *de novo* synthesis of pyrimidines and exogenous sources for purines. As mentioned before, orotic acid (18.**122**) can be taken up by the intraerythrocytic parasites (199, 483, 484), but this does not seem to be the case for the sporogonic stages (495) in the mosquito vector.

9.2 Amino Acids and Proteins

The amino acids required for the biosynthesis of proteins are obtained from host protein (hemoglobin), from extracellular sources (i.e., plasma), and from *de novo* biosynthetic processes. Most of these amino acids are derived by the proteolytic digestion [*P. berghei, P. knowlesi* (497)] of red cell hemoglobin [*P. lophurae* (388a), *P. gallinaceum* (498), *P. berghei* (159), *P. knowlesi* (499)]. Polet and Conrad (500) found that 1-isoleucine, an amino acid not present as a building block in human and monkey hemoglobin, is essential for the growth of erythrocytic forms of *P. knowlesi,* and they showed that optimum *in vitro* growth necessitated an exoerythrocytic source of 1-isoleucine, 1-methionine, 1-cystine, 1-tyrosine, 1-arginine, 1-glutamine 1-histidine, and 1-lysine, because thes amino acids were not adequately present in the host hemoglobin. The growth, as measured by the amount of radiolabeled orotic acid (18.**122**) incorporated into plasmodial DNA, was particularly inhibited by the absence of the first three amino acids; this observation supported earlier work on the essentiality of methionine for growth (392). Studies on the nutritional requirements for *in vitro* cultivation of *P. knowlesi* (501, 502) and *P. falciparum* (502) showed that isoleucine and methionine had be present for intracellular *in vitro* development of the parasites. These two amino acids were avidly accumulated by intraerythrocytic *P. knowlesi* and markedly incorporated into the parasite's proteins (199, 385, 500b,

503). Studies of Sherman et al. (504) revealed that there exists a striking difference in the uptake of radiolabeled amino acids by erythrocyte-free *P. lophurae*, infected erythrocytes, and normal duck erythrocytes; thus isoleucine and methionine enter the normal erythrocyte by a carrier-mediated process and the infected erythrocyte by diffusion. It seems that the transport carriers of the erythrocyte are affected in some unknown way by the intra-erythrocytic parasite.

The third source of amino acids for the parasite is *de novo* biosynthesis. *In vitro* experiments with intraerythrocytic and erythrocyte-free *P. lophurae* (505) revealed that the carbon of ^{14}C-bicarbonate was incorporated into glutamic acid, aspartic acid, and alanine. Radiolabeled keto acids were also formed, suggesting the occurrence of transamination. Polet et al. (506) investigated the *in vitro* biosynthesis of amino acids from uniformly ^{14}C-labeled glucose, -pyruvate, and -acetate by intraerythrocytic *P. knowlesi*, and found radioactivity in glutamic acid, aspartic acid, and alanine when labeled glucose or pyruvate were present. With labeled acetate they identified labeled glutamic acid and aspartic acid but not labeled alanine. No radioactivity was detectable in any of the other 13 amino acids examined.

Based on the knowledge that 1-isoleucine and 1-methionine are essential amino acids for plasmodial growth (*P. knowlesi*), that these amino acids are not amply available to the parasite, and that they are avidly incorporated into plasmodial proteins, it was anticipated that antagonists of these amino acids may have antimalarial activity. McKee and Geiman (392) found that *in vitro* growth of *P. knowlesi* was markedly inhibited by methoxine and ethionine and that this effect was annulled by adding extra methionine. Polet and Conrad (385, 500b) studied three antagonists of 1-isoleucine: 1-*O*-methylthreonine (L-OMT), alloisoleucine, and *N*-acetylisoleucine. L-OMT strongly inhibited the incorporation of labeled 1-isoleucine and 1-methionine into plasmodial proteins, as well as the incorporation of labeled orotic acid into plasmodial DNA; 1-isoleucine was the only amino acid capable of reversing this inhibition. Alloisoleucine had a marked inhibitory effect on the incorporation of 1-isoleucine in proteins, but it had only a slight effect on the incorporation of orotic acid in DNA; *N*-acetylisoleucine as ineffective.

The inhibitory effect on the incorporation of ^{14}C-isoleucine into plasmodial proteins was investigated by Schnell and Siddiqui (390) for puromycin, cycloheximide, and chloramphenicol—antibiotics known to inhibit protein synthesis in other biological systems. They found that puromycin had a strong inhibitory effect on ^{14}C-isoleucine incorporation into proteins of *P. knowlesi* and *P. falciparum*, whereas chloramphenicol did not inhibit protein synthesis. Cycloheximide, tested with *P. falciparum* only, was found to have a strong inhibitory effect.

For the effect on protein synthesis of antimalarial drugs such as chloroquine (18.**16**), dihydroquinine (18.**36**), and quinacrine (18.**14**), see Section 5.3.1.

9.3 Lipids

Compared to some other areas of malaria parasite metabolism, the study of lipid metabolism has been neglected. It is not surprising therefore that no antimalarial drugs have been forthcoming that are based on the antagonism of the lipid metabolic system.

During the growth of the intraerythrocytic parasite both *in vitro* and *in vivo*, there is a severalfold increase in the lipid content of the infected cell compared to the normal cell (508–512). This lipid is probably associated with the parasite membrane; in the development of the malaria parasite from the ring trophozoite to the segmented schizont there is a ten- to fifteenfold increase in the membrane surface area (513), hence a large requirement for lipids. The neutral lipids of the parasite consist of cholesterol, cholesterol esters, diglycerides, triglycerides, and fatty acids; the phospholipids present are phosphatidylcholine, phospatidylinositol, phosphatidylethanolamine, phosphatidylaerine, phosphatidylglycerol, and phosphatidic acid.

Avian malaria parasites, unlike mammalian, incorporate a large amount of ^{14}C into their free fatty acids (FFA) (226, 514, 515) when infected red cells are incubated with ^{14}C-acetate. This would imply *de novo* fatty acid synthesis, but it must be remembered that nucleated fowl erythrocytes have the ability to biosynthesize fatty acids *de novo*; thus the acetate incorporation may be partly a reflection of biosynthesis by the host cell or the result of chain elongation of the fatty acids (516). The avian parasite *P. fallax* in turkey erythrocytes took up ^{14}C-fatty acids during incubation, indicating the need for preformed FFA (226).

There is considerable evidence that mammalian parasites do not synthesize their fatty acids *de novo*. Thus Cenedella (511) showed that intraerythrocytic *P. berghei* incorporated ^{14}C from labeled glucose mainly into the glyceryl portion of the phospholipids rather than the fatty acid moiety, based on the assumption that glucose is the main carbon source for fatty acid synthesis, he concluded that the parasite obtains the bulk of its fatty acids for phospholipid synthesis from its environment. Rock (516a) also found that ^{14}C from labeled glucose and glycerol was incorporated into the phospholipids of intraerythrocytic or free *P. knowlesi in vitro*, principally into the glyceryl moiety. Acetate-^{14}C incorporation, in contrast, occurred primarily in the acyl portion of the phospholipids, rather than in the glyceryl moiety, and was not incorporated in detectable amounts into the neutral lipids. The lack of incorporation of ^{14}C from acetate into the neutral lipids again suggests that the parasite may obtain its fatty acids preformed from the host membranes or plasma; the incorporation of acetate into the acyl portion of the phospholipids may be explained on the basis of chain elongation, a process consistent with the increase in the levels of acetate incorporation with the addition of ATP, COA, or NADH. Other lines of evidence also indicate that the parasite depends on the host for its fatty acids. For example, intraerythrocytic *P. knowlesi* rapidly incorporated 10–15 times as much ^{14}C-labeled palmitic, oleic, and stearic acids as did the host erythrocyte, and 80% of the activity appeared in the phospholipids of the parasite; the remaining 20% appeared in the neutral lipid diglycerides, triglycerides, and unesterified fatty acids (516b). This apparent dependence of the parasite on preformed fatty acids was also indicated by studies of the *in vitro* growth requirements of *P. knowlesi* for fatty acids (517, 518). Finally, Cenedella (227) has shown that the FFA produced in large quanity by *P. berghei*-parasitized rat erythrocytes during incubation has the same relative composition as the FFA in unparasitized and parasitized cells. This indicated that the increase in fatty acids was the result of hydrolysis of the host cell lipids rather than *de novo* synthesis. Such a process not only could supply the parasite with the fatty acids required for phospholipid synthesis, it also could explain the increased fragility of parasitized cells.

In addition to the preformed fatty acids the parasite obtains from the host cell for its phospholipid synthesis, Rock (516a) has shown that ^{14}C-labeled glycerol, glucose, ethanolamine, and choline are rapidly incorporated by *P. knowlesi* from incubation media; neither normal nor infected host cells incorporated these precursors. Between 80 and 95% of the ^{14}C incorporated appears in three major lipid classes, viz.

phosphatidylcholine, phosphatidylinositol, and phosphatidylethanolamine, whereas the remainder is found in the di- and triglycerides. These results suggest that the parasite obtains these precursors from the host erythrocyte or from the surrounding plasma. It has also been shown by Rock et al. (519) that 80–100 times as much ^{33}P-orthophosphate is incorporated into the membrane phospholipids of *P. knowlesi* during *in vitro* incubation as is incorporated into the membranes of the host red cell, and most of the ^{33}P that is taken up by the parasite appears in the same three major phospholipid classes. The host cell, in contrast, incorporates it only into phosphatidic acid; Rock (519) has suggested that the presence of microsomal enzymes with phosphate cytidyl transferase activity could explain this difference. From a study of the effects of various substrates and inhibitors on ^{33}P incorporation into the parasite membrane phospholipids, it appears that anaerobic glycolysis is predominant in the *in vitro* metabolism of this parasite and that the incorporation of ^{33}P may be through incorporation into host erythrocyte or parasite ATP and substrate phosphorylation.

The sterol components of the neutral lipids of the parasite are mainly free cholesterol and cholesterol esters (508, 516a, 520). From the work of Trigg (521) it appears that the parasite must obtain its sterols directly from the host. He studied the uptake by *P. knowlesi*, of two known sterol precursors, acetate and mevalonate, as well as the uptake of cholesterol, and found that only cholesterol was incorporated into the sterol fraction of the parasite. There still seems to be some question, however, since Gutierrez (226) earlier had shown that ^{14}C-acetate as incorporated into the cholesterol fraction of the avian parasite *P. fallax*.

There is a growing body of evidence, therefore, that the intrusion of the malaria parasite brings about profound changes in the lipid metabolism of the red cells of the host. To date, unfortunately, we have no antimalarial drugs based on the antagonism of the pathological metabolic changes induced by the parasite. Assuming that the parasite must obtain most of its required free fatty acids from the plasma, Cenedella (522) reasoned that if the plasma level of the free fatty acids could be reduced sufficiently, the phospholipid, hence the membrane synthesis of the parasite, might be impaired, with lethal results. When this hypothesis was tested on male rats infected with *P. berghei*, using ethyl(*p*-chlorophenoxy)isobutyrate, a well-tolerated drug known to reduce lipid and fatty acid levels in plasma, only equivocal results were obtained.

9.4 Carbohydrates

The glucose metabolism of malaria parasites has been only partly elucidated. The importance of the Embden-Meyerhof pathway has been established for some time; but there is much equivocal experimental evidence, and it is still questionable whether the parasite has a functioning pentose phosphate pathway. The requirement for pentoses for nucleic acid syntheses seems to indicate that the pentose phosphate pathway, as possibly the sole source of these sugars, plays an essential role. At this time, from studies in several species of parasites, both avian and mammalian, the acculated evidence indicates that the parasite is dependent on the pentose phosphate pathway of the host erythrocyte (485).

The metabolic pathway beyond glycolysis is still largely unknown, particularly in the mammalian parasites. It does seem clear, however, that there are some fundamental differences between the processes occurring in the avian and in the mammalian parasites. The former species appear to have an active Krebs cycle, whereas it appears that the latter species do not have a functional cycle. It has been demonstrated that carbon dioxide fixation can occur in the mammalian parasite, and it has been suggested (532) that if carbon dioxide fixation occurs at a significant level, the part of the Krebs cycle sequence from malate to α-ketoglutarate through citrate must function. The metabolism of the malaria parasite has been reviewed by Fletcher and Maegraith (523).

Selected established antimalarial drugs have been shown to inhibit certain enzymes involved in plasmodial carbohydrate metabolism under experimental conditions. Fraser and Kermack (524) studied the inhibition of hexokinase from *P. berghei* by a number of antimalarials. With the exception of proguanil (18.**22**), all active antimalarials, including chloroquine (18.**16**), mepacrine (quinacrine, 18.**14**), azacrine (18.**64**), quinine (18.**27**), and a number of diaminodihydrotriazines, inhibited the enzymes. The exceptional behavior of proguanil may be attributed to the necessity of metabolic conversion to the dihydrotriazine (18,**24**) for antimalarial action, since the latter compound was active. Unfortunately solubility problems precluded the testing of pyrimethamine (18.**25**). Some compounds that are devoid of antimalarial activity also showed appreciable enzyme inhibitory activity. Other studies had also shown the inhibitory effect of quinacrine on hexokinase of avian parasites (525, 526). Quinacrine had also been shown to inhibit avian plasmodium 6-phosphofructokinase and triose phosphate dehydrogenase (526) as well as lactic dehydrogenase (525). Working with *P. berghei*, freed from host reticulocytes, Bowman et al. (527) concluded that the enzyme most sensitive to quinacrine is 6-phosphofructokinase with hexokinase inhibited to a lesser extent. Ali et al. (528) using *P. knowlesi*-infected rhesus monkeys and infected erythrocytes, reported that chloroquine (18.**16**) inhibited the utilization of glucose, as well as oxygen uptake and lactate production. Plasmodial fixation of carbon dioxide with phosphoenolpyruvate to form oxaloacetate can be inhibited by chloroquine and quinine (529). Subsequently, Siu (530) has demonstrated the presence of phosphoenolpyruvic carboxylase and carboxykinase activity in cell-free preparations from *P. berghei*-infected mouse erythrocytes. Both these enzymes are involved in carbon dioxide fixation, and their activity can be inhibited by chloroquine and quinine.

The significance of such findings with respect to the antimalarial action of the drugs is, of course, unknown. Because of species specificity, both qualitative and quantitative, any progress in understanding the biochemistry of the malaria parasites on the basis of host interaction will be slow, and the application of such knowledge to drug design seems to be some distance away.

APPENDIX

TERMINOLOGY OF MALARIA*

CURE, CLINICAL. Relief of symptoms of a malaria attack (e.g., by chemotherapeutic action against asexual erythrocytic parasites) without complete elimination of the infection.

CURE, RADICAL. Complete elimination of the malaria parasite from the body so that relapses cannot occur.

CURE, SUPPRESSIVE. Complete elimination of the parasite from the body by means of continuous suppressive treatment.

ERYTHROCYTIC. Developing within red blood cells; applied to stages of the malaria parasite.

* Terms have been selected and simplified from the World Health Organization monograph "Terminology of Malaria and of Malaria Eradication," Geneva, 1963.

EXFLAGELLATION. Extrusion and liberation of microgametes (flagella) by male gametocytes (see Fig. 18.1).

EXOERYTHROCYTIC. Developing in tissues outside the red blood cells.

GAMETE. Mature sexual form, male or female. In malaria parasites the female gametes (macrogametes) and male gametes (microgametes) normally develop in the mosquito (see Fig. 18.1).

GAMETOCYTE. Parent cell of a gamete. In malaria parasites the female gametocytes macrogametocytes) and male gametocytes (microgametocytes) develop in the red blood cell. Very young gametocytes usually cannot be distinguished from trophozoites (see Fig. 18.1).

GAMETOCYTOCIDE. Drug that destroys the sexual forms of malaria parasites.

MALARIA, BENIGN TERTIAN. Synonym for vivax malaria.

MALARIA, CEREBRAL. Form of pernicious malaria associated with cerebral symptoms and due to infection with *Plasmodium falciparum.*

MALARIA, FALCIPARUM. Malaria infection caused by *Plasmodium falciparum*; also called tropical malaria; subtertian malaria.

MALARIA, INDUCED. Malaria infection properly attributable to the effect of a blood transfusion or other form of parenteral inoculation, but not to normal transmission by the mosquito.

MALARIA, QUARTAN. Synonym for infections with *P. malariae.* Recurring every third day (every 72 hr). Recurrence on two successive days, with one-day free intervals, is known as double-quartan periodicity.

MALARIA, SUBTERTIAN. Synonym of falciparum malaria.

MALARIA, TERTIAN. Synonym of vivax malaria.

MALARIA, TROPICAL. Synonym of falciparum malaria.

MALARIA, VIVAX. Malaria infection caused by *Plasmodium vivax*; also called (benign) tertian malaria.

MEROZOITE. Product of segmentation of a tissue schizont, or of an erythrocytic schizont before entering a new host cell. Merozoites are found either separated from or contained in the original schizont (see Fig. 18.1).

OOCYST. Fertilized female cell (zygote), developing in malaria parasites from the ookinete (see Fig. 18.1).

OOKINETE. Motile vermicule stage of the malaria parasite, following fertilization the macrogamete and preceding oocyst formation (see Fig. 18.1).

PREERTYTHROCYTIC. Existing before the infection of erythrocytes.

PROPHYLAXIS. Any method or protection from or prevention of disease; when applied to chemotherapy it is commonly designated "drug prophylaxis" or "chemoprophylaxis."

PROPHYLAXIS, CAUSAL. Complete prevention of erythrocytic infection by the administration of drugs that destroy either the sporozoites or the primary tissue forms of the malaria parasite.

RECRUDESCENCE. Renewed manifestation (of clinical symptoms and/or parasitemia) of malarial infection, separated from previous manifestations of the same infection by an interval greater than those due to the normal periodicity of the paroxysms brought about by surviving erythrocytic forms of the parasite.

RELAPSE. Renewed manifestation (of clinical symptoms and/or parasitemia) of malarial infection, separated from previous manifestations of the same infection by an interval greater than those due to the normal periodicity of the paroxysms brought about by release of secondary or slow developing tissue forms of the parasite from the liver.

SCHIZONT. Intracellular asexual form of the malaria parasite, developing either in tissue or in blood cells (see Fig. 18.1).

SCHIZONTOCIDE. Drug that destroys the asexual forms of malaria parasites. Schizontocides are distinguished as blood schizontocides and tissue schizontocides. When 'schizontocide" is used alone, it usually refers to a blood schizontocide (i.e., one that acts on the erythrocytic asexual parasites). Tissue schizontocides are drugs that destroy the exoerythrocytic stages of the parasite. If they act on the primary exoerythrocytic forms, they are referred to as primary tissue schizontocides ("causal prophylatic drugs"); if on the secondary forms, as secondary tissue schizontocides.

SPOROGONY. In the mosquito, the process of development that follows sexual union of gametes and ends with the formation of sporozoites.

SPORONTOCIDE. Drug that when given to the malaria-infected vertebrate host, prevents or interrupts the development of the parasite in mosquitoes feeding on that host.

SPOROZOITE. Final stage of sporogony of *Plasmodium* in the mosquito; the infective form of the malaria parasite occurring either in a mature oocyst before its rupture or in the salivary glands of the mosquito (see Fig. 18.1).

SUPPRESSION. See under Treatment, suppressive.

TERTIAN. Recurring every other day (every 48 hr).

TISSUE STAGES. Schizogonic stages of malaria parasites occurring in cells other than erythrocytes in the vertebrate host.

TREATMENT, SUPPRESSIVE. Treatment aimed at preventing or eliminating clinical symptoms and/or parasitemia by early destruction of erythrocytic parasites. It does not necessarily prevent or eliminate the infection.

TROPHOZOITE. Strictly, any asexual and growing parasite with undivided nucleus. In malaria terminology, generally used to indicate intracellular erythrocytic forms in their early stages of development. Trophozoites may be in either a ring stage or an early ameboid or solid stage, but they always have the nucleus still undivided (see Fig. 18.1).

VECTOR. In malaria, any species of mosquito in which the plasmodium completes its sexual cycle in nature, thus is able to transmit the disease.

ZYGOTE. Product of the union of the male and female gametes (see Fig. 18.1).

REFERENCES

1. *World Health Organization Technical Report Series.* (a) No. 443 (1967). (b) No. 537 (1974), (c) No. 529, p. 30 (1973), (d) No. 585, p. 11, Table 1 (1976), (e) No. 513, pp. 17–19 (1973), (f) No. 579 (1975), (g) No. 529, p. 14 (1973), (h) No. 529, pp. 19–22 (1973), (i) No. 529, p. 23 (1973), (j) No. 529, p. 24 (1973), (k) No. 529, p. 17 (1973), (1) No. 529, p. 48 (1973), (m) No. 529, pp. 83, 85 (1973), (n) No. 529, p. 70 (1973), o) No. 529, p. 67 (1973).
2. L. J. Bruce-Chwatt, *Brit. Med. J.*, No. 3, 464 (1972).
3. J. Bafort, *Nature* (London), **217,** 1264 (1968).
4. W. Peters, *Chemotherapy and Drug Resistance in Malaria*, Academic Press, New York, 1970. (a) p. 64, (b) Ch. 12, (c) pp. 426–439, (d) p. 94, (e) pp. 540–601, (f) p. 110.
5. P. C. C. Garnham, *Malaria Parasites and Other Haemosporida*, Blackwell, Oxford, 1966.
6. P. F. Russell, L. S. West, R. D. Manwell, and G. McDonald, *Practical Malariology*, Oxford University Press, New York, London, 1963: (a) p. 11, (b) pp. 35–40.
7. F. E. G. Cox, *Nature* (London), **266,** 408 (1977).
8. D. F. Clyde, R. M. Miller, H. L. DuPont, and R. B. Hornick, *J. Am. Med. Assoc.*, **213,** 2041 (1970).

9. K. H. Rieckmann, *J. Am. Med. Assoc.*, **217,** 573 (1971).
10. P. G. Contacos, J. S. Lunn, and G. R. Coatney, *Trans. Roy. Soc. Trop. Med. Hyg.*, **57,** 417 (1963).
11. R. L. DeGowin, and R. D. Powell, *Am. J. Trop. Med. Hyg.*, **14,** 519 (1965).
12. D. F. Clyde, V. C. McCarthy, G. T. Shute, and R. P. Sangalang, *J. Trop. Med. Hyg.*, **74,** 101 (1971).
13. J. V. McNamara, K. H. Rieckmann, H. Fischer, T. A. Stockert, P. E. Carson, and R. D. Powell, *Ann. Trop. Med. Parasitol.*, **61,** 386 (1967).
14. J. Arnold, A. S. Alving, and C. B. Clayman, *Trans. Roy. Soc. Trop. Med. Hyg.*, **55,** 345 (1961).
15. R. L. Beaudoin, C. P. A. Strome, T. A. Tubergen, and F. Mitchell, *Exp. Parasitol.*, **28,** 280 (1970).
16. L. J. Bruce-Chwatt, *Trans. Roy. Soc. Trop. Med. Hyg.* (a) **64,** 776 (1970), (b) **59,** 104 (1965).
17. D. T. Dennis, E. B. Doberstyn, A. Sissay, and G. K. Tesfai, *Trans. Roy. Soc. Trop. Med. Hyg.*, **68,** 241 (1974).
18. A. W. A. Brown and R. Pal, *Insecticide Resistance in Anthropods*, World Health Organ., Geneva, 1971, (a) pp. 23, 24, (b) p. 167.
19. J. Sternburg, C. Kearns, and H. Moorefield, *J. Agr. Food Chem.*, **2,** 1125 (1954).
20. F. Winteringham and J. Barnes, *Physiol. Rev.*, **35,** 701 (1955).
21. A. A. Perry, *Bull. W. H. O.*, **22,** 743–756 (1960).
22. F. E. Gartrell and G. F. Ludvik, *Am. J. Trop. Med. Hyg.*, **3,** 817 (1954).
23. N. Frontali and S. Carta, *Riv. Parasitol.*, **20,** 107 (1959).
24. A. Lipke and J. Chalkley, *Bull. W. H. O.*, **30,** 57 (1964).
25. A. Albert, (a) *Selective Toxicity*, 5th ed., Chapman and Hall., London, 1973 (b) *The Acridines*, 2nd ed., St. Martin's Press, New York, 1966, p. 428.
26. W. Peters, *Trans. Roy. Soc. Trop. Med. Hyg.* (a) **61,** 400 (1967), (b) **64,** 462 (1970).
27. W. Roehl, *Arch. Schiffs-U. Tropenhyg.*, **30,** 311 (1926).
28. E. Brumpt, *C. R. Hebd. Séances Acad. Sci. Paris*, **200,** 783 (1935).
29. I. H. Vincke and M. Lips, *Ann. Soc. Belg. Med. Trop.*, **30,** 79 (1948).
30. I. H. Vincke, *Indian J. Malariol.*, **8,** 257 (1954).
31. F. Y. Wiselogle, Ed., *A Survey of Antimalarial Drugs*, 1941–1945, Edwards, Ann Arbor, Mich., 1946. (a) Vol. 1, Ch. 2, (b) Vol. 1, Ch. 6, (c) Vol. 2, p. 1097, (d) Vol. 2, p. 1064, (e)Vol. 2, p. 1093, (f) Vol. 2, p. 1073, (g) Vol. 2, p. 1081, (h) Vol. 2, p. 1082, (i) Vol. 2, p. 1088, (j) Vol. 1, pp. 309–362, (k) Vol. 2, pp. 1323–1382; Vol. 1, pp. 153–163, (l) Vol. 1, p. 373, (m) Vol. 1, p. 371, (n) Vol. 1, p. 380, (o) Vol. 1, p. 388, (p) Vol. 1, p. 398, (q) Vol. 1, p. 62.
32. L. H. Schmidt and C. S. Genther, *J. Pharmacol. Exptl. Therap.*, **107,** 61 (1953).
32a. P. E. Thompson, B. Olszewski, A. Bayles, and J. A. Waitz, *Am. J. Trop. Med. Hyg.*, **16,** 133 (1967).
33. P. E. Thompson and A. L. Ager, *Ninth International Congress on Tropical Medicine and Malaria*, Athens, October 14–21, 1973.
34. D. G. Davey, in *Experimental Chemotherapy*, R. J. Schnitzer and F. Hawking, Eds., Academic Press, New York, 1963, p. 487.
35. P. E. Thompson and L. M. Werbel, *Antimalarial Agents*, Academic Press, New York, 1972. (a) p. 46, (b) p. 317, (c) p. 157, (d) p. 112, (e) p. 107, (f) p. 143, (g) p. 339, (h) p. 320.
36. L. A. Terzian, N. Stahler, and A. T. Dawkins, Jr., *Exp. Parasitol.*, **23,** 56 (1968).
37. K. G. Gregory and W. Peters, *Ann. Trop. Med. Parasitol.*, **64,** 15 (1970).
38. H. Most and W. A. Montuori, *Am. J. Trop. Med. Hyg.*, **24,** 179 (1975).
39. T. S. Osdene, P. B. Russell, and L. Rane, *J. Med. Chem.*, **10,** 431 (1967).
40. R. S. Bray, *Am. J. Trop. Med. Hyg.*, **7,** 20 (1958).
41. R. S. Bray, *Ergeb. Mikrobiol. Immun. Exp. Ther.*, **36,** 169 (1963).
42. J. Rhodhain and J. Judin, *Ann. Soc. Belg. Med. Trop.*, **44,** 531 (1964).
43. E. H. Sadun, R. L. Hickman, B. T. Wellde, A. P. Moon, and I. O. K. Udeozo, *Mil. Med.* **131** (Suppl.), 1250 (1966).
44. R. L. Hickman, W. S. Gochenour, J. D. Marshall, and N. B. Guillored, *Mil. Med.*, **131** (Suppl.), 935 (1966).
45. R. A. Ward, J. H. Morris, D. J. Gould, A. T. C. Bourke, and F. C. Cadigan, *Science*, **150,** 1604 (1965).
46. M. D. Young, J. A. Porter, and C. M. Johnson, *Science*, 153, 1006 (1966).
47. Q. M. Geiman and M. J. Meagher, *Nature* (London), **215,** 437 (1967).
48. L. H. Schmidt, *Trans. Roy. Soc. Trop. Med. Hyg.*, **67,** 446 (1973).

49. R. J. Cenedella, L. H. Saxe, and K. van Dyke, *Chemotherapy*, **15,** 158 (1970).

50. K. H. Rieckmann, J. V. McNamara, H. Frischer, T. A. Stockert, P. E. Carson, and R. D. Powell, *Am. J. Trop. Med. Hyg.*, **17,** 661 (1968).

51. G. J. McCormick, C. J. Canfield, and G. P. Willet, *Antimicrob. Agents Chemother.*, **6,** 16 (1974).

52. K. van Dyke, C. Szustkiewicz, R. Cenedella, amd L. H. Saxe, *Chemotherapy*, **15,** 177 (1970).

53. C. J. Canfield, L. B. Altstatt, and V. B. Elliot, *Am. J. Trop. Med. Hyg.*, **19,** 905 (1970).

54. F. Ablondi, S. Gordon, J. Martin, II, and J. H. Williams, *J. Org. Chem.*, **17,** 14 (1952).

55. J. B. Koepfli, J. F. Mead, and J. A. Brockman, Jr., *J. Am. Chem. Soc.*, **69,** 1837 (1947); **71,** 1048 (1949).

56. C. S. Jang, F. Y. Fu, C. Y. Wang, K. C. Huang, *G. Lu, and T. C. Chou, Science*, **103,** 59 (1946).

57. C. S. Jang, F. Y. Fu, K. C. Huang, and C. Y. Wang, *Nature* (London), **161,** 400 (1948).

58. T. Q. Chou, F. Y. Fu, and Y. S. Kao, *J. Am. Chem. Soc.*, **70,** 1765 (1948).

59. J. B. Koepfli, J. A. Brockman, Jr., and J. Moffat, *J. Am. Chem. Soc.*, **72,** 3323 (1950).

60. B. L. Hutchings, S. Gordon, F. Ablondi, C. F. Wolf, and J. H. Williams, *J. Org. Chem.*, **17,** 19 (1952).

61. R. K. Hill and A. G. Edwards, *Chem. Ind.* (London), 858 (1962).

62. D. F. Barringer, Jr., G. Berkelhammer, S. D. Carter, L. Goldman, and A. E. Lanziloth, *J. Org. Chem.*, **38,** 1933 (1973).

63. D. F. Barringer, Jr., G. Berkelhammer, and R. S. Wayne, *Org. Chem.*, **38,** 1937 (1973).

64. B. R. Baker, R. E. Schaub, F. J. McEvoy, and J. H. Williams, *J. Org. Chem.*, **17,** 132 (1952).

65. J. F. B. Edeson and T. Wilson, *Trans. Roy. Soc. Trop. Med. Hyg.*, **49,** 543 (1955).

66. F. G. Henderson, C. L. Rose, P. N. Harris, and K. K. Chen, *J. Pharmacol. Exp. Ther.*, **95,** 191 (1949).

67. B. R. Baker, J. P. Joseph, R. E. Schaub, F. J. McEvoy, and J. H. Williams, *J. Org. Chem.*, **17,** 157 (1952); **18,** 138 (1953).

68. B. R. Baker, M. V. Querry, A. F. Kadish, and J. H. Williams, *J. Org. Chem.*, **17,** 35 (1952); **17,** 52 (1952).

69. B. R. Baker, M. V. Querry, R. E. Schaub, and J. H. Williams, *J. Org. Chem.*, **17,** 58 (1952).

70. B. R. Baker, M. V. Querry, R. Pollikoff, R. E. Schaub, and J. H. Williams, *J. Org. Chem.*, **17,** 68 (1952).

71. B. R. Baker, R. E. Schaub, M. V. Querry, and J. H. Williams, *J. Org. Chem.*, **17,** 77 (1952); **17,** 97 (1952).

72. B. R. Baker, R. E. Schaub, and J. H. Williams, *J. Org. Chem.*, **17,** 109 (1952); **17,** 116 (1952).

73. B. R. Baker, R. E. Schaub, J. P. Joseph, F. J. McEvoy, and J. H. Williams, *J. Org. Chem.*, **17,** 141 (1952); **17,** 149 (1952); **17,** 164 (1952); **18,** 133 (1953).

74. M. Fishman and P. A. Cruickshank, *J. Med. Chem.*, **13,** 155 (1970); *J. Heterocycl. Chem.*, **5,** 467 (1968).

75. G. M. Trenholme, R. L. Williams, H. Frischer, P. E. Carson, and K. H. Rieckmann, *Ann. Intern. Med.*, **82,** 219 (1975).

76. Y. K. Lu and O. Y. Magidson, *Zh. Obshch. Khim.*, **29,** 3299 (1959).

77. O. Y. Magidson and Y. K. Lu, *Zh. Obshch. Khim.*, **29,** 2943 (1959).

78. R. N. Chaudhuri, B. N. Dutta, and N. K. Chakravarty, *Indian Med. Gazz*, **89,** 660 (1954).

79. G. R. Coatney, W. C. Cooper, W. B. Culwell, W. C. White, and C. A. Imboden, Jr., *J. Nat. Malar Soc.*, **9,** 183 (1950).

80. V. A. Trevino, L. Amanda Reyes, and M. F. Mendoza, *Rev. Inst. Solubr. Enfer. Trop.* (Mex.), **13,** 253 (1953).

81. R. B. Turner and R. B. Woodward, in *The Alkaloids*, Vol. 3, Academic Press, New York, 1953, p. 25.

82. R. B. Woodward and W. von E. Doering, *J. Am. Chem. Soc.*, **66,** 849 (1944); **67,** 860 (1945).

82a. See publication of M. R. Uskokovic et al., *Helv. Chim. Acta*, **56,** 1485–1503 (1973); *J. Am. Chem. Soc.*, **100,** 576–592 (1978).

83. P. Guttmann and P. Ehrlich, *Berl. Klin. Wochenschr.*, **28,** 953 (1891).

84. P. Kopanaris, *Arch. Schiffs. Trop-Hyg.*, **15,** 586 (1911).

85. W. Kikuth and W. Menk, *Chemotherapie der wichtigsten Tropenkrankheiten. Die Chemotherapie der Malaria*, S. Hirzel, Leipzig, 1943, p. 45.

86. P. Mühlens, *Naturwissenchaften*, **14,** 1162 (1926).

87. H. Mauss, in *Medizin und Chemie*, Vol. 4, Verlag Chemie, Berlin, 1942, pp. 60–72.

88. H. Mauss and F. Mietzsch, *Klin. Wochenschr.*, **12,** 1276 (1933).

89. R. F. Loeb, W. M. Clark, G. R. Coatney, L. T. Coggeshall, F. R. Dieuaide, A. R. Dochez, A. G. Hakansson, E. K. Marshall, C. S. Marvel, O. R. McCoy, J. J. Sapero, W. H. Sebrell, J. A. Shannon, and G. A. Carden, *J. Am. Med. Assoc.*, **130,** 1069 (1946).

90. W. C. Cooper, A. V. Myatt, T. Hernandez, G. M. Jeffery, and G. R. Coatney, *Am. J. Trop. Med. Hyg.*, **2,** 949 (1953).

91. R. H. Hill and H. M. Goodwin, Jr., *South. Med. J.*, **30,** 1170 (1937).

92. A. Diaz de Leon, *Bol. Of. Sanit. Pan Am.*, **16,** 1039 (1937).

93. A. Diaz de Leon, *Medicina* (Mexico City), **18,** 89 (1938).

94. L. T. Coggeshall, *Proc. Soc. Exp. Biol. Med.*, **38,** 768 (1938).

95. L. T. Coggeshall, J. Mair, and C. A. Best, *J. Am. Med., Assoc.*, **117,** 1077 (1941).

96. F. Schönhöfer, *Hoppe-Seyler's Z. Physiol. Chem.*, **274,** 1 (1942).

97. F. H. S. Curd, D. G. Davey, and F. L. Rose, *Ann. Trop. Med. Parasitol.*, **39,** 208 (1945).

98. F. H. S. Curd and F. L. Rose, *J. Chem. Soc.* (a) 729 (1946), (b) 574, 586 (1948).

99. L. G. Goodwin, *Nature* (London), **164,** 1133 (1949).

100. E. A. Falco, G. H. Hitchings, P. B. Russell, and H. Vanderwerff, *Nature* (London), **164,** 107 (1949).

101. G. H. Hitchings, *Trans Roy. Soc. Trop. Med. Hyg.*, **46,** 467 (1962).

102. A. D. Ainley and H. King, *Proc. Roy. Soc., Ser. B*, **125,** 60 (1938).

103. G. A. H. Buttle, T. A. Henry, and J. W. Trevan, *Biochem. J.*, **28,** 426 (1934).

104. H. King and T. S. Works, *J. Chem. Soc.*, 1307 (1940).

105. G. G. Lyle and L. K. Keefer, *Tetrahedron*, **23,** 3253 (1967).

106. J. Gutzwiller and M. R. Uskoković, *Helv. Chim. Acta*, **56,** 1494 (1973).

107. F. I. Carroll and J. T. Blackwell, *J. Med. Chem.*, **17,** 210 (1974).

108. C. J. Ohnmackt, A. R. Patel, and R. E. Lutz, *J. Med. Chem.*, **14,** 926 (1971).

109. C. C. Cheng, *J. Pharm. Sci.*, **60,** 1596 (1971).

110. Ping-lu Chien and C. C. Cheng, *J. Med. Chem.* (a) **19,** 170 (1976), (b) **16,** 1093 (1973), (c) **13,** 867 (1970).

111. G. H. Loew and R. Sahakina, *J. Med. Chem.*, **20,** 103 (1977).

112. A. Brossi, M. Uskoković, J. Gutzwiller, A. U. Krettli, and Z. Brener, *Experientia*, **27,** 1100 (1971).

113. R. E. Strube, *J. Trop. Med. Hyg.*, **78,** 171 (1975).

114. J. Mead and J. B. Koepfli, *J. Biol. Chem.*, **145,** 507 (1944).

115. F. E. Kelsey, F. K. Oldham, W. Cantrell, and E. M. K. Geiling, *Nature* (London), **157,** 440 (1946).

116. W. E. Rothe and D. P. Jacobus, *J. Med. Chem.*, **11,** 366 (1968).

117. R. E. Lutz, P. S. Bailey, M. T. Clark, J. F. Codington, A. J. Deinet, J. A. Freek, G. H. Harnest, N. H. Leake, T. A. Martin, R. J. Rowlett, J. M. Salsbury, N. H. Shearer, J. D. Smith, and J. W. Wilson, *J. Am. Chem. Soc.*, **68,** 1813 (1946).

118. W. W. Bay, C. A. Gleiser, A. Chester, R. G. Feldman, K. R. Pierce, and K. M. Charlton, *US C. F. S. T. I.*, AD 1969 No. 701055; *Chem. Abstr.*, **73,** 75504 (1970).

119. D. C. Martin, J. D. Arnold, D. F. Clyde, M. A. Ibrahim, P. E. Carson, K. H. Rieckmann, and D. Willerson, Jr., *Antimicrobiol. Agents Chemother.*, **3,** 214 (1973).

120. C. J. Canfield, A. P. Hall, B. S. MacDonald, D. A. Newman, and J. A. Shaw, *Antimicrob. Agents Chemother.*, **3,** 224 (1973).

121. T. N. Pullman, L. Eichelberger, A. S. Alving, R. Jones, B. Craig, and C. M. Whorton, *J. Clin. Invest.* **27,** Suppl., 12 (1948).

122. E. L. May and E. Mosettig, *J. Org. Chem.*, **11,** 627 (1946).

123. E. A. Nodiff, K. Tanabe, C. Syefried, S. Matsuura, Y. Kondo, E. H. Chenand, and M. P. Tyagi, *J. Med. Chem.*, **14,** 921 (1971).

124. W. T. Colwell, V. Brown, P. Christie, J. Lange, C. Reece, K. Yamamoto, and D. W. Henry, *J. Med. Chem.*, **15,** 771 (1972).

125. J. T. Traxler, E. P. Lira, and C. W. Huffman, *J. Med. Chem.*, **15,** 861 (1972).

126. J. S. Gillespie, S. P. Acharya, D. A. Shamblee, and R. E. Davis, *J. Med. Chem.*, **18,** 1223 (1975).

127. M. P. LaMontagne, A. Markovac, and P. Blumbergs, *J. Med. Chem.*, **17,** 519 (1974).

128. D. W. Henry, *Abstracts*, 13th National Medical Chemistry Symposium, American Chemical Society, Washington, D.C., 1972, pp. 41–50.

129. M. W. Davidson, B. G. Griggs, D. W. Boykin, and W. D. Wilson, *Nature* (London), **254,** 632 (1975).

130. P. N. Craig, *J. Med. Chem.* (a) **15,** 144 (1972), (b) **16,** 661 (1973).

131. W. P. Purcell and K. Sundaram, *J. Med. Chem.*, **12,** 18 (1969).

132. I. M. Rollo, in *The Pharmacological Basis of Therapeutics* 5th Ed., L. S. Goodman and A. Gilman, Eds., Macmillan, New York. 1975, Ch. 52.

133. L. H. Schmidt, in *The Alkaloids*, Vol. 5, R. H. F. Manske, Ed., Academic Press, New York, 1953, Ch. 41.

134. G. M. Findlay, *Recent Advances in Chemotherapy*, Vol. 2, 3rd ed., Blakiston, Philadelphia, 1951.

135. A. P. Hall, (a) *Am. J. Trop. Med. Hyg.*, **21,** 851 (1972). (b) *Trans Roy. Soc. Trop. Med. Hyg.*, **67,** 425 (1973).

136. R. S. Rozman and C. J. Canfield, *Advances in Pharmacology and Chemotherapy*, Academic Press, New York, 1978.

137. W. Kikuth, *Deut. Med. Wochenschr.*, **58,** 530 (1932).

138. G. R. Coatney, W. C. Copper, M. B. Eddy, and J. Greenberg, Public Health Monograph No. 9, Government Printing Office, Washington, D.C., 1953. (a) Chs. 4, 6. (b) Ch. 10. (c) Ch. 1. (d) Ch. 5, (e) Chs. 2, 3.

139. I. L. Krichevshii, O. Y. Magidson, E. P. Halperin, and A. M. Grigorovskii, *Ber. Ges. Physiol. Exp. Pharmakol.*, **83,** 220 (1934); *Chem. Abstr.*, **31,** 3208 (1937).

140. L. M. Asano, Y. Kameda, O. Tamemasa, N. Ishii, and T. Chida, *Jap. J. Exp. Med.*, **20,** 779 (1950); *Chem. Abstr.*, **46,** 6650f (1952).

141. E. T. Reid, R. J. Fraser, and F. B. Wilford, *Cent. Afr. J. Med.*, **9,** 478 (1963).

142. J. F. B. Edeson, *Ann. Trop. Med. Parasitol.*, **48,** 160 (1954).

143. P. E. Thompson, J. E. Meisenhelder, H. H. Najarian, and A. Bayles, *Am. J. Trop. Med. Hyg.*, **10,** 335 (1961).

144. O. Y. Magidson and A. M. Grigorovskii, *Chem. Ber.*, **69B,** 396 (1936).

145. M. T. Hoekenga, *Am. J. Trop. Med. Hyg.* (a) **4,** 221 (1955). (b) **3,** 833 (1954). (c) **6,** 986 (1957). (d) **11,** 1 (1962).

146. M. Nieto-Caicedo, *Am. J. Trop. Med. Hyg.*, **5,** 681 (1956).

147. J. Hill, in *Experimental Chemotherapy*, Vol. 1, R. E. Schnitzer and F. Hawking, Eds., Academic Press, New York, 1963. (a) pp. 532–541. (b) pp. 524–532.

148. G. R. Coatney, *Am. J. Trop. Med. Hyg.*, **12,** 121 (1963).

149. B. R. Brown and D. L. Hammick, *J. Chem. Soc.*, 99 (1948).

150. B. Kiegel and L. T. Sherwood, Jr., *J. Am. Chem. Soc.*, **71,** 1129 (1949).

151. G. F. Gause, *Nature* (London), **156,** 784 (1945).

152. T. Singh, R. G. Stein, and J. H. Biel, *J. Med. Chem.*, **12,** 368 (1969).

153. J. H. Burckhalter, F. H. Tendick, E. M. Jones, W. F. Holcomb, and A. L. Rawlins, *J. Am. Chem. Soc.*, **68,** 1894 (1946).

154. C. Cheng, *J. Theor. Biol.*, **59,** 497 (1976).

155. G. E. Bass, D. R. Hudson, J. E. Parker, and W. P. Purcell, *J. Med. Chem.*, **14,** 275 (1971).

156. F. E. Hahn, R. L. O'Brien, J. Ciak, J. L. Allison, and J. G. Olenick, *Mil. Med.*, **131,** Suppl., 1071 (1966).

157. A. P. Hall, H. E. Segal, E. J. Pearlman, P. Phintuyothin, and S. Kosakal, *Am. J. Trop. Med. Hyg.*, **24,** 575 (1975).

158. C. D. Fitch, *Proc. Helminthol. Soc. Wash.*, **39,** (special issue), 265 (1972).

159. R. J. Cenedella, H. Rosen, C. R. Angel, and L. H. Saxe, *Am. J. Trop. Med. Hyg.*, **17,** 800 (1968).

160. I. W. Sherman, J. B. Mudd, and W. Trager, *Nature* (London), **208,** 691 (1965).

161. T. Deegan and B. G. Maegraith, *Ann. Trop. Med. Parasitol.*, **50,** 194 (1956).

162. G. A. Moore and B. Boothroyd, *Ann. Trop. Med. Parasitol.*, **68,** 489 (1974).

163. M. Aikawa, *Exp. Parasitol.*, **30,** 284 (1971).

164. C. de Duve and R. Wattiaux, in *Ann. Rev. Physio.*, **28,** 435 (1966).

165. M. Aikawa and P. E. Thompson, *J. Parasitol.*, **57,** 603 (1971).

166. A. F. W. Morselt, A. Glastra, and J. James, *Exp. Parasitol.*, **33,** 17 (1973).

167. C. A. Homewood, D. C. Warhurst, and V. C. Baggaley, *Trans. Roy. Soc. Trop. Med. Hyg.*, **65,** 10(1971).

168. D. C. Warhurst and S. C. Thomas, *Biochem. Pharmacol.*, **24,** 2047 (1975).

169. D. C. Warhurst and D. J. Hockley, *Nature* (London), **214,** 935 (1967).

170. P. B. Macomber, H. Sprinz, and A. J. Tousimis, *Nature* (London), **214,** 937 (1967).

171. D. C. Warhurst and J. Williamson, *Chem.-Biol. Interactions*, **2,** 89 (1970).

172. D. C. Warhurst and B. L. Robinson, *Life Sci.*, **10,** 755 (1971).

173. D. C. Warhurst, C. A. Homewood, and V. C. Baggaley, *Ann. Trop. Med. Parasitol.*, **68,** 265 (1974).

174. C. A. Homewood, D. C. Warhurst, W. Peters, and V. C. Baggaley. *Proc. Helminthol. Soc. Wash.*, **39** (special issue), 382 (1972).

175. C. A. Homewood and E. M. Atkinson, *Trans. Roy. Soc. Trop. Med. Hyg.*, **67,** 26 (1973).

176. C. A. Homewood, D. C. Warhurst, W. Peters, and V. C. Baggaley, *Nature* (London) **235,** 50 (1972).
177. D. C. Warhurst, C. A. Homewood, W. Peters, and V. C. Baggaley, *Proc. Helminthol. Soc. Wash.*, **39** (special issue), 259 (1972).
178. M. Porter and W. Peters, *Ann. Trop. Med. Parasitol.*, **70,** 259 (1976).
179. R. E. Howells, W. Peters, C. A. Homewood, and D. C. Warhurst, *Nature* (London) **228,** 625 (1970).
180. S. N. Cohen, K. O. Phifer, and K. L. Yielding, *Nature* (London), **202,** 805 (1964).
181. R. Ladda and H. Sprinz, *Proc. Roy. Soc. Exp. Biol. Med.*, **130,** 524 (1969).
182. P. B. Macomber, R. L. O'Brien, and F. E. Hahn, *Science*, **152,** 1374 (1966).
183. H. Polet and C. F. Barr, *J. Pharmacol. Exp. Ther.* (a) **168,** 187 (1969).(b) **164,** 380 (1968).
184. C. D. Fitch, *Science*, **169,** 289 (1970).
185. J. Ceithaml and E. A. Evans, *Arch. Biochem. Biophys.*, **10,** 397 (1946).
186. C. D. Fitch, *Proc. Nat. Acad. Sci., US*, **64,** 1181 (1969).
187. P. A. Kramer and J. F. Natusik, *Biochem. Pharmacol.*, **20,** 1619 (1971).
188. A. D. Inglot and E. Wolna, *Biochem. Pharmacol.*, **17,** 269 (1968).
189. C. D. Fitch, N. G. Yunis, R. Chevli, and Y. Gonzalez, *J. Clin. Invest.*, **54,** 24 (1974).
190. E. E. Davies, D. C. Warhurst, and W. Peters, *Ann. Trop. Med. Parasitol.*, **69,** 147 (1975).
191. M. Aikawa, *Am. J. Pathol.*, **67,** 277 (1972).
192. K. van Dyke, C. Szustkiewicz, C. H. Lantz, and L. H. Saxe, *Biochem. Pharmacol.*, **18,** 1417 (1969).
193. C. D. Fitch, Y. Gonzalez and R. Chevli, *J. Pharmacol. Exp. Ther.*, **195,** 397 (1975).
194. C. D. Fitch, R. Chevli, and Y. Gonzalez, *J. Pharmacol. Exp. Ther.*, **195,** 389 (1975).
195. D. E. Clarke, *J. Exp. Med.* (a) **96,** 451 (1952). (b) **96,** 439 (1952).
196. K. A. Schellenberg and G. R. Coatney, *Biochem. Pharmacol.*, **6,** 143 (1961).
197. J. Ciak and F. E. Hahn, *Science*, **151,** 347 (1966).
198. C. H. Lantz and K. van Dyke, *Biochem. Pharmacol.* (a) **20,** 1157 (1971). (b) **21,** 891 (1972).
199. H. Polet and C. F. Barr, *Am. J. Trop. Med. Hyg.*, **17,** 672 (1968).
200. D. C. Warhurst, *Trans. Roy. Soc. Trop. Med. Hyg.*, **63,** 4 (1969).
201. W. E. Gutteridge, P. I. Trigg, and P. M. Bayley, *Parasitology*, **64,** 37 (1972).
202. F. S. Parker and J. L. Irvin, *J. Biol. Chem.*, **199,** 897 (1952).
203. J. L. Irvin, E. M. Irvin, and F. S. Parker, *Science*, **110,** 426 (1949).
204. N. B. Kurnick and I. E. Radcliffe, *J. Lab. Clin. Med.*, **60,** 669 (1962).
205. D. Stollar and L. Levine, *Arch. Biochem. Biophys.*, **101,** 335 (1963).
206. S. N. Cohen and K. L. Yielding, *J. Biol. Chem.*, **240,** 3123 (1965).
207. S. N. Cohen and K. L. Yielding, *Proc. Nat. Acad. Sci. US*, **54,** 521 (1965).
208. R. L. O'Brien, J. G. Olenick, and F. E. Hahn, *Proc. Nat. Acad. Sci. US*, **55,** 1511 (1966).
209. J. L. Allison, R. L. O'Brien, and F. E. Hahn, *Science*, **149,** 1111 (1965).
210. J. L. Allison, R. L. O'Brien, and F. E. Hahn, *Antimicrob. Agents Chemother.*, 310 (1966).
211. R. L. O'Brien, J. L. Allison, and F. E. Hahn, *Biochim. Biophys. Acta*, **129,** 622 (1966).
212. R. L. O'Brien and F. E. Hahn, *Antimicrob. Agents Chemother.*, 315 (1966).
213. J. A. Singer and W. P. Purcell, *J. Med. Chem.*, **10,** 754 (1967).
214. B. Pullman and A. Pullman, *Quantum Biochemistry*, Wiley-Interscience, New York, 1963, pp 218, 219.
215. V. E. Marquez, J. W. Cranston, R. W. Ruddon, and J. H. Burckhalter, *J. Med. Chem.*, **17,** 856 (1974).
216. V. E. Marquez, J. W. Cranston, R. W. Ruddon, L. B. Kier, and J. H. Burckhalter, *J. Med. Chem.*, **15,** 36 (1972).
217. L. S. Lerman, *Proc. Nat. Acad. Sci. US*, **49,** 94 (1963).
218. A. K. Krey and F. E. Hahn, *Mol. Pharmacol.*, **10,** 686 (1974).
219. R. D. Estensen, A. K. Krey, and F. E. Hahn, *Mol. Pharmacol.*, **5,** 532 (1969).
220. F. E. Hahn, *Progr. Antimicrob. Anticancer Chemother.*, **10,** 636 (1974).
221. *F. E. Hahn and C. L. Fean, Antimicrob. Agents Chemother.*, **1969,** 63 (1970).
222. J. W. Panter, D. W. Boykin, and W. D. Wilson, *J. Med. Chem.*, **16,** 1366 (1973).
223. M. W. Davidson, B. G. Griggs, D. W. Boykin, and W. D. Wilson, *J. Med. Chem.*, **20,** 1117 (1977).
224. W. Peters, R. E. Howells, J. Portus, B. L. Robinson, S. Thomas, and D. C. Warhurst, *Ann. Trop. Med. Parasitol.*, **71,** 407 (1977).
225. I. W. Sherman and L. Tanigoshi, *Proc. Helminthol. Soc. Wash.*, **39** (special issue), 250 (1972).

226. J. Gutierrez, *Am. J. Trop. Med. Hyg.*, **15,** 818 (1966).
227. R. J. Cenedella, J. J. Jarrell, and L. H. Saxe, *Exp. Parasitol.*, **24,** 130 (1969).
228. H. B. Markus and E. G. Ball, *Biochim. Biophys. Acta*, **187,** 486 (1969).
229. L. Hellerman, M. R. Bovarnick, and C. C. Porter, *Fed. Proc.* **5,** 400 (1946).
230. H. Laser, P. Kemp, N. Miller, D. Lander, and R. Klein, *Parasitology*, **71,** 167 (1975).
231. A. P. Ray and G. K. Sharma, *Nature* (London), **178,** 1291 (1956).
232. S. P. Ramakrishnan, S. Prakash, and D. S. Choudhury, *Nature* (London), **179,** 975 (1957).
233. K. G. Powers, P. L. Jacobs, W. C. Good, and L. C. Koontz, *Exp. Parasitol.*, **26,** 193 (1969).
234. W. Peters, K. A. Fletcher, and W. Stäubli, *Ann. Trop. Med. Parasitol.*, **59,** 126 (1965).
235. J. V. McNamara, K. H. Rieckmann, and R. D. Powell, *Ann. Trop. Med. Parasitol.*, **61,** 125 (1967).
236. D. Warhurst and R. Killick-Kendrick, *Nature* (London), **213,** 1048 (1967).
237. F. W. Schueler and W. F. Cantrell, *J. Pharmacol. Exp. Ther.*, **143,** 278 (1964).
238. C. D. Fitch, *Antimicrob. Agents Chemother.*, **3,** 545 (1973).
239. C. D. Fitch, R. Chevli, and Y. Gonzalez, *Antimicrob. Agents Chemother.*, **6,** 757 (1974).
240. R. E. Howells, *Ann. Trop. Med. Parasitol.*, **64,** 181 (1970).
241. R. E. Howells and L. Maxwell, *Ann. Trop. Med. Parasitol.* (a) **67,** 285 (1973). (b) **67,** 279 (1973).
242. E. E. Davies, *Ann. Trop. Med. Parasitol.*, **68,** 283 (1974).
243. I. M. Rollo, *Fed. Proc.*, **27,** 537 (1968).
244. S. G. Williams and O. Fanimo, *Ann. Trop. Med. Parasitol.*, **69,** 301 (1975).
245. W. J. Waddell and R. G. Bates, *Physiol. Rev.*, **49,** 285 (1969).
246. J. P. English, J. H. Clark, R. G. Shepherd, H. W. Marson, J. Krapcho, and R. O. Roblin, Jr., *J. Am. Chem. Soc.* **68,** 1039 (1946).
247. H. Bader, J. F. Hoops, J. H. Biel, H. H. Koelling, R. G. Stein, and T. Singh, *J. Med. Chem.*, **12** (a) 709, (b) 1108 (1969).
248. I. C. Popoff and G. H. Singhal, *J. Med. Chem.*, **11,** 631 (1968).
249. G. H. Singhal, P. M. Thomas, and I. C. Popoff, *J. Heterocycl. Chem.*, **5,** 411 (1968).
250. I. C. Popoff, G. P. Singhal, and A. R. Engle, *J. Med. Chem.*, **14,** 550 (1971).
251. I. C. Popoff, A. R. Engle, R. L. Whitaker, and G. H. Singhal, *J. Med. Chem.*, **14,** 1166 (1971).
252. B. Serafin and T. Urbanski, *J. Med. Chem.*, **12,** 336 (1969).
253. E. F. Elslager, A. A. Phillips, and D. F. Worth, *J. Med. Chem.*, **12,** 363 (1969).
254. E. F. Elslager and A. A. Phillips, *J. Med. Chem.*, **12,** 519 (1969).
255. B. P. Vogh and L. N. Gleason, *J. Pharmacol. Exp. Ther.*, **177,** 301 (1071).
256. W. Peters, in *Advances in Parasitology*, Vol. 12, B. Dawes, Ed. Academic Press, New York, 1974. (a) p. 85. (b) pp. 78–81.
257. G. R. Coatney and W. C. Cooper, *J. Parasitol.*, **34,** 275 (1948).
258. A. B. G. Laing, *Med. J. Malay*, **23,** 5 (1968).
259. Chun-Chantholl, *Bull. Soc. Pathol. Exot.*, **61,** 858 (1968).
260. A. B. G. Laing, *Bull. W. H. O.*, **43,** 513 (1970).
261. H. E. Segal, P. Chinvanthananond, B. Laixuthal, E. J. Pearlman, A. P. Hall, P. Phintuyothin, A. Na-Nakorn, and B. F. Castaneda, *Trans. Roy. Soc. Trop. Med. Hyg.*, **69,** 139 (1975).
262. E. B. Doberstyn, A. P. Hall, K. Vetvutanapibul, and P. Sonkom, *Am. J. Trop. Med. Hyg.*, **25,** 14, (1976).
263. B. Simpson, W. S. Jamieson, and A. H. Dimind, *Trans. Roy. Soc. Trop. Med. Hyg.*, **66,** 222 (1972).
264. A. Depinay, L. Holzer, and H. Felix, *Bull. Soc. Pathol. Exot.*, **65,** 409 (1972).
265. T. Muto, I. Ebisawa, and G. Mitsui, *Jap. J. Exp. Med.*, **41,** 459 (1971).
266. A. Z. Shafei, *J. Trop. Med. Hyg.*, **78,** 190 (1975).
267. P. J. Bartelloni, T. W. Sheehy, and W. D. Tigertt, *J. Am. Med. Assoc.*, **199,** 173 (1967).
268. T. P. H. McKelvey et al., *Trans. Roy. Soc. Trop. Med. Hyg.*, **65,** 286 (1971).
269. J. Storey, A. Rossi-Espagnet, S. P. H. Mandel, T. Matsushima, P. Lietaert, D. Thomas, S. Brøgger, C. Duby, and G. Gramiccia, *Bull. W. H. O.*, **49,** 275 (1973).
270. G. Catarinella and L. Donno, *J. Trop. Med. Hyg.*, **74,** 243 (1971).
271. D. C. Martin and J. D. Arnold, *J. Am. Med. Assoc.*, **203,** 476 (1968).
272. W. Chin, D. M. Bear, E. J. Colwell, and S. Kosakal, *Am. J. Trop. Med. Hyg.*, **22,** 308 (1973).
273. A. O. Lucas, R. G. Hendrickse, O. A. Okubadejo, W. H. G. Richards, R. A. Neal, and B. A. K. Kofie, *Trans. Roy. Soc. Trop. Med. Hyg.*, **63,** 216 (1969).
274. D. F. Clyde, *J. Am. Med. Assoc.*, **209,** 563 (1969).

275. C. J. Canfield, E. G. Whiting, W. H. Hall, and B. S. MacDonald, *Am. J. Trop. Med. Hyg.*, **20,** 524 (1971).
276. W. H. G. Richards, *Advan. Pharmacol. Chemother.*, **8,** 121 (1970).
277. R. E. Blount, *Arch. Intern. Med.*, **119,** 557 (1967).
278. T. W. Sheehy and R. C. Reba, *Ann. Intern. Med.*, **66,** 616 (1967).
279. T. W. Sheehy, R. C. Reba, and G. R. Parks, *South. Med. J.*, **62,** 152 (1969).
280. O. J. Martelo, M. Smoller, and T. A. Saladin, *Arch. Intern. Med.*, **123,** 383 (1969).
281. R. B. Eppes, J. V. McNamara, R. L. DeGowin, P. E. Carson, and R. D. Powell, *Mil. Med.*, **132,** 163 (1967).
282. R. J. T. Joy, J. E. McCarty, and W. D. Tigertt, *Mil. Med.*, **134,** 493 (1969).
283. R. J. T. Joy, W. R. Gardner, and W. D. Tigertt, *Mil. Med.*, **134,** 497 (1969).
284. D. F. Clyde, C. C. Rebert, V. C. McCarthy, A. T. Dawkins, and S. A. Cucinell, *Mil. Med.*, **135,** 527 (1970).
285. D. Willerson, Jr., K. H. Rieckmann, L. Kass, P. E. Carson, H. Frischer, and J. E. Bowman, *Am. J. Trop. Med. Hyg.*, **21,** 138 (1972).
286. S. J. Berman, *J. Am. Med. Assoc.*, **207,** 128 (1969).
287. R. D. Powell, R. L. DeGowin, R. B. Eppes, J. V. McNamara, and P. E. Carson, *Int. J. Lepr.* **35,** 590 (1967).
288. D. F. Clyde, C. C. Rebert, V. C. McCarthy, and R. M. Miller, *Mil. Med.*, **136,** 836 (1971).
289. D. M. Aviado, *Exp. Parasitol.*, (a) **20,** 88 (1967). (b) **25,** 399 (1969).
290. D. F. Clyde, C. C. Rebert, V. C. McCarthy, and R. M. Miller, *Mil. Med.*, **138,** 418 (1973).
291. E. J. Pearlman, W. Thiemanum, and B. F. Castaneda, *Am. J. Trop. Med. Hyg.*, **24,** 901 (1975).
292. E. F. Elslager and D. F. Worth, *Nature* (London), **206,** 630 (1965).
293. E. F. Elslager, Z. B. Gavrilis, A. A. Phillips, and D. F. Worth, *J. Med. Chem.*, **12,** 357 (1969).
294. P. E. Thompson, B. Olszewski, and J. A. Waitz, *Am. J. Trop. Med. Hyg.*, **14,** 343 (1965).
295. P. E. Thompson, *Int. J. Lepr.* **35,** 605 (1967).
296. G. H. Hitchings and J. J. Burchall, *Advan. Enzymol.*, **27,** 417 (1965).
297. R. L. Jacobs, *Exp. Parasitol.*, **15,** 213 (1964).
298. J. P. Thurston, *Parasitology*, **44,** 99 (1954).
299. S. Glenn and R. D. Manwell, *Exp. Parasitol.*, **5,** 22 (1956).
300. R. Ferone and G. H. Hitchings, *J. Protozool.*, **13,** 504 (1966).
301. R. D. Walter and E. Königk, *Z. Tropenmed. Parasitol.* (a) **22,** 256 (1971). (b) **25,** 227 (1974).
302. R. Ferone, *J. Protozool.*, **20,** 459 (1973).
303. J. L. McCullough and T. H. Maren, *Mol. Pharmacol.*, **10,** 140 (1974).
304. A. Bishop, *Parasitology*, (a) **55,** 407 (1965). (b) **34,** 1 (1942), (c) **57,** 755 (1967).
305. E. K. Marshall, Jr., J. T. Litchfield, Jr., and H. J. White, *J. Pharmacol. Exp. Ther.*, **75,** 89 (1942).
306. J. Maier and E. Riley, *Proc. Soc. Exp. Biol. Med.*, **50,** 152 (1942).
307. A. O. Seeler, O. Graessle, and E. D. Dusenbery, *J. Bacteriol.*, **45,** 205 (1943).
308. A. P. Richardson, R. I. Hewitt, L. D. Seager, M. M. Brooke, F. Martin, and H. Maddux, *J. Pharmacol. Exp. Ther.*, **87,** 203 (1946).
309. J. P. Thurston, *Lancet*, **2,** 438 (1950).
310. J. P. Thurston, *Brit. J. Pharmacol.*, **5,** 409 (1950).
311. W. Peters, *Trop. Dis. Bull.*, **64,** 1145–1175, see p. 1165 (1967).
312. G. M. Brown, *J. Biol. Chem.*, **237,** 536 (1962).
313. G. M. Brown, *Int. J. Lepr.* **35,** 580 (1967).
314. L. Bock, G. H. Miller, K. J. Schaper, and J. K. Seydel, *J. Med. Chem.*, **17,** 23 (1974).
315. R. M. Hutchinson, *Biochem. J.*, **99,** 23P (1966).
316. R. J. Cenedella and J. J. Jarrell, *Am. J. Trop. Med. Hyg.*, **19,** 592 (1970).
317. R. J. Cenedella and L. H. Saxe, *Am. J. Trop. Med. Hyg.*, **20,** 530 (1971).
318. W. Trager, *Trans. Roy. Soc. Trop. Med. Hyg.*, **66,** 800 (1972).
319. R. Ferone, J. J. Burchall, and G. H. Hitchings, *Mol. Pharmacol.*, **5,** 49 (1969).
320. W.-P. Fung, *Aust. N. Z. J. Med.*, 3, 262 (1971).
321. F. H. S. Curd, J. A. Hendry, T. S. Kenny, A. G. Murray, and F. L. Rose, *J. Chem. Soc.*, 1630 (1948).
322. A. F. Crowther, F. H. S. Curd, D. N. Richardson, and F. L. Rose, *J. Chem. Soc.*, 1636 (1948).
323. S. Birtwell, F. H. S. Curd, J. A. Hendry, and F. L. Rose, *J. Chem. Soc.*, 1646 (1948).
324. A. D. Ainley, F. H. S. Curd, and F. L. Rose, *J. Chem. Soc.*, 98 (1949).
325. I. M. Tomkin, *Brit. J. Pharmacol.*, **1,** 163 (1946).
326. F. Hawking and W. L. M. Perry, *Brit. J. Pharmacol.*, **3,** 320 (1948).
326a. N. H. Fairley, *Trans. Roy. Soc. Trop. Med. Hyg.*, **40,** 105 (1946).

327. H. C. Carrington, A. F. Crowther, D. G. Davey, A. A. Levi and F. L. Rose, *Nature* (London), **168,** 1080 (1951).

328. A. F. Crowther and A. A. Levi, *Brit. J. Pharmacol.*, **8,** 93 (1953).

329. E. S. Josephson, D. J. Taylor, J. Greenbert, and G. R. Coatney, *J. Infect. Dis.*, **93,** 257 (1953).

330. C. C. Smith, J. Ihrig, and R. Menne, *Am. J. Trop. Med. Hyg.*, **10,** 694 (1961).

331. E. A. Falco, L. G. Goodwin, G. H. Hitchings, I. M. Rollo, and P. B. Russell, *Brit. J. Pharmacol.*, **6,** 85 (1951).

332. E. A. Falco, P. B. Russell, and G. H. Hitchings, *J. Am. Chem. Soc.*, **73,** 3753 (1951).

333. E. A. Falco, S. DuBreuil, and G. H. Hitchings, *J. Am. Chem. Soc.*, **73,** 3758 (1951).

334. P. B. Russell and G. H. Hitchings, *J. Am. Chem. Soc.*, **73,** 3763 (1951).

335. E. J. Modest, *J. Org. Chem.*, **21,** 1 (1956).

336. E. J. Modest and P. Levine, *J. Org. Chem.*, **21,** 14 (1956).

337. C. P. Nair and A. P. Ray, *Indian J. Malariol.*, **10,** 11 (1956).

338. J. Singh, P. C. Basu, and A. P. Ray, *Indian J. Malariol.*, **6,** 145 (1952).

339. J. Singh, H. L. Bami, G. R. Chandrasekhar, and A. P. Ray, *Indian J. Malariol.*, **8,** 1 (1954).

340. J. Singh, A. P. Ray, and G. R. Chandrasekhar, *Indian J. Malariol.*, **7,** 117 (1953).

341. A. P. Ray, C. P. Nair, M. K. Menon, and B. G. Misra, *Indian J. Malariol.*, **8,** 209 (1954).

342. L. H. Schmidt, T. L. Loo, R. Radkin, and H. B. Hughes, *Proc. Soc. Exp. Biol. Med.*, **80,** 367 (1953).

343. G. I. Robertson, *Trans. Roy. Soc. Trop. Med. Hyg.*, **51,** 488 (1957).

344. P. E. Thomspon, B. J. Olszewski, E. F. Elslager, and D. F. Worth, *Am. J. Trop. Med. Hyg.*, **12,** 481 (1963).

345. E. F. Elslager, M. P. Hutt, and L. M. Werbel, *J. Med. Chem.*, **13,** 542 (1970).

346. L. H. Schmidt, R. N. Rossan, and K. F. Fisher, *Am. J. Trop. Med. Hyg.*, **12,** 494 (1963).

347. G. R. Coatney, P. G. Contacos, and J. S. Lunn, *Am. J. Trop. Med. Hyg.*, **13,** 386 (1964).

348. R. D. Powell, R. L. DeGowin, and R. B. Eppes, *Am. J. Trop. Med. Hyg.*, **14,** 913 (1965).

349. I. A. McGregor, K. Williams, G. H. Walker, and A. K. Rahman, *Brit. Med. J.*, **1,** 695 (1966).

350. P. G. Contacos, G. R. Coatney, J. S. Lunn, and J. W. Kelpatrick, *Am. J. Trop. Med. Hyg.*, **13,** 386 (1964).

351. J. S. Lunn, W. Chin, P. G. Contacos, and G. R. Coatney, *Am. J. Trop. Med. Hyg.*, **13,** 783 (1964).

352. G. R. Coatney, P. G. Contacos, J. S. Lunn, J. W. Kelpatrick, and H. A. Elder, *Am. J. Trop. Med. Hyg.*, **12,** 504 (1963).

353. K. H. Rieckmann, *Am. J. Trop. Med. Hyg.*, **15,** 833 (1966).

354. R. H. Black, B. B. Dew, W. B. Hennessy, B. McMillan, and D. C. Torpy, *Med. J. Aust.*, **2,** 588 (1966).

355. W. Chin, J. S. Lunn, J. Buxbaum, and P. G. Contacos, *Am. J. Trop. Med. Hyg.*, **14,** 922 (1965).

356. P. G. Contacos, G. R. Coatney, J. S. Lunn, and W. Chin, *Am. J. Trop. Med. Hyg.* (a) **14,** 925 (1965), (b) **15,** 281 (1966).

357. A. B. G. Laing, G. Pringle, and F. E. T. Lane, *Am. Soc. Trop. Med. Hyg.*, **15,** 838 (1966).

358. D. F. Clyde, *J. Trop. Med. Hyg.*, **72,** 81 (1969).

359. G. I. Robertson, D. G. Dawey, and N. H. Fairley, *Brit. Med. J.*, **2,** 1255 (1952).

360. T. Hermandez, A. J. Myatt, G. R. Coatney, and G. M. Jeffery, *Am. J. Trop. Med. Hyg.*, **2,** 797 (1953).

361. S. A. Jones, *Brit. Med. J.*, **1,** 977 (1953).

362. S. A. Jones, *Trans. Roy. Soc. Trop. Med. Hyg.*, **52,** 547 (1958).

363. B. Roth, E. A. Falco, G. H. Hitchings, and S. R. M. Bushby, *J. Med. Chem.*, **5,** 1103 (1962).

364. U.S. Patent 3,074,947 (1963).

365. D. C. Martin and J. D. Arnold, *J. Clin. Pharmacol.*, **7,** 336 (1967).

366. L. H. Schmidt, J. Harrison, R. Ellison, and P. Worchester, *Proc. Exp. Biol. Med.*, **131,** 294 (1969).

367. D. C. Martin and J. D. Arnold, *J. Clin. Pharmacol. J. New Drugs*, **9,** 155 (1969).

368. W. E. Rothe, D. P. Jacobus, and W. G. Walter, *Am. J. Trop. Med. Hyg.*, **18,** 491 (1969).

369. L. Donno, V. Sanguineti, M. L. Ricciardi, and M. Soldat, *Am. J. Trop. Med. Hyg.*, **18,** 182 (1969).

370. M. Rey, C. Lapix, I. D. Mar, R. Michel, and R. Rombourg, *Bull. Soc. Med. Afr. Noire Lang. Fr.* **16,** 9 (1969).

371. G. H. Hitchings and J. J. Burchall, *Fed. Proc.* **25,** 881 (1966).

372. R. Heischkeil, *Z. Tropenmed. Parasitol.*, **24.** 505 (1973).

373. T. W. Sheehy and H. Dempsey, *J. Am. Med. Assoc.*, **214**, 109 (1970).

374. R. Ferone, *J. Biol. Chem.*, **245,** 850 (1970).

375. W. E. Gutteridge and P. I. Trigg, *Parasitology*, **62,** 431 (1971).
376. E. G. Platzer, *J. Parasitol.*, **56,** No. 4, Sect. 11, Part 1, 267 (1970).
377. W. Büngener and E. Nielsen, *Z. Tropenmed. Parasitol.* (a) **18,** 456 (1967); (b) **19,** 185 (1968), (c) **20,** 67 (1969).
378. C. J. Walsh and I. W. Sherman, *J. Protozool.* (a) **15,** 763 (1968), (b) **15,** 503 (1968).
379. K. van Dyke, G. C. Tremblay, C. H. Lantz, and C. Szustkiewicz, *Am. J. Trop. Med. Hyg.*, **19,** 202 (1970).
380. M. S. P. Manandhar and K. van Dyke, *Exp. Parasitol.*, **37,** 138 (1975).
381. W. Büngener, *Ninth International Congress on Tropical Medicine and Malaria*, Athens, October 14–21, 1973.
382. K. D. Neame, P. A. Brownbill, and C. A. Homewood, *Parasitology*, **69,** 329 (1974).
383. R. S. Krooth, K. D. Wure, and R. Ma, *Science*, **164,** 1073 (1968).
384. G. A. Butcher and S. Cohen, *Parasitology*, **62,** 309 (1971).
385. H. Polet and M. E. Conrad, *Mil. Med.*, **134,** 939 (1969).
386. I. W. Sherman, J. A. Ruble, and L. Tanigoshi, *Mil. Med.*, **134,** 954 (1969).
387. I. W. Sherman, L. Tanigoshi, and B. J. Mudd, *Int. J. Biochem.*, **2,** 27 (1971).
388. I. W. Sherman and L. Tanigoshi, *Int. J. Biochem.* (a) **2,** 41 (1971) (b) **1,** 635 (1970).
389. W. Trager, *J. Protozool.*, **18,** 392 (1971).
390. J. V. Schnell and W. A. Siddiqui, *Proc. Helminthol. Soc. Wash.* **39** (*special issue*), 201 (1972).
391. R. W. McKee, L. M. Gieman, and T. S. Cobbey, *Fed. Proc.*, **6,** 276 (1947).
392. R. W. McKee and L. M. Geiman, *Fed. Proc.* **7,** 172 (1948).
393. C. C. Smith, G. J. McCormick, and C. J. Canfield, *Exp. Parasitol.*, **40,** 432 (1976).
394. G. H. Coombs, Technical Report ERO-5-74, 248, May 1974.
395. R. Ferone, M. O'Shea, and M. Yoeli, *Science*, **167,** 1263 (1970).
396. M. Yoeli, R. S. Upmanis, and H. Most. *Parasitology*, **59,** 429 (1969).
397. S. M. Diggins, and K. G. Gregory, *Trans. Roy. Soc. Trop. Med. Hyg.*, **64,** 468, (1970).
398. S. M. Diggins, W. E. Gutteridge, and P. I. Trigg, *Nature* (London), **228**, 579 (1970).
399. D. Walliker, R. Carter, and S. Morgan, *Parasitology*, **66,** 309 (1971).
400. D. Walliker, R. Carter, and S. Morgan, *Nature* (London), **232,** 561 (1971).
401. C. Schoenfeld, H. Most, and N. Entner, *Exp. Parasitol.*, **36,** 265 (1974).
402. W. Schulemann, *Proc. Roy. Soc. Med.*, **25,** 897 (1932).
403. W. Schulemann, F. Schönhöfer, and A. Wingler, *Klin. Wochenschr.*, **11,** 381 (1932).
404. W. Roehl, *Naturwissenschaften*, **14,** 1156 (1926).
405. A. S. Alving, T. N. Pullman, B. Craige, Jr., R. Jones, Jr., C. M. Whorton, and L. Eichelberger, *J. Clin. Invest.*, **27,** 34 (1948).
406. B. Craige, Jr., L. Eichelberger, R. Jones, Jr., A. S. Alving, T. N. Pullman, and C. M. Whorton, *J. Clin. Invest.*, **27,** 17 (1948).
407. A. S. Alving, B. Craige, Jr., R. Jones, Jr., C. M. Whorton, T. N. Pullman, and L. Eichelberger, *J. Clin. Invest.*, **27,** 25 (1948).
408. E. Fourneau, J. Tréfouel, D. Bovet, and G. Benoit, *Ann. Inst. Pasteur*, **46,** 514 (1931); **50** 731 (1933).
409. D. Bovet, G. Benoit, and R. Altman, *Bull. Soc. Pathol. Exot.*, **27,** 236 (1934).
410. O. Y. Magidson and I. T. Strukov, *Arch. Pharm.* (Weinheim), **271,** 359 (1933); *Chem. Abstr.* **27,** 5112 (1933), 569 (1933); **28,** 1770 (1934).
411. O. Y. Magidson, O. I. Madaeva, and M. V. Rubzov, *Arch Pharm.* (Weinheim), **273,** 320 (1935); *Chem. Abstr.*, **29,** 7013 (1935).
412. O. Y. Magidson and M. D. Boboshev, *J. Gen. Chem.* (*USSR*), **8,** 899 (1938); *Chem Abstr.*, **33,** 1327 (1939).
413. E. H. Chen, A. J. Saggiomo, K. Tanabe, B. L. Verma, and E. A. Nodiff, *J. Med. Chem.*, **20,** 1107 (1977).
414. J. Greenberg, D. J. Taylor, and E. S. Josephson, *J. Infect. Dis.*, **88,** 163 (1951).
415. C. C. Smith, *J. Pharmacol. Exp. Ther.*, **116,** 67 (1956).
416. E. S. Josephson, D. J. Taylor, J. Greenberg, and A. P. Ray, *Proc. Soc. Exp. Biol. Med.*, **76,** 700 (1951).
417. A. R. Tarlov, G. J. Brewer, P. E. Carson, and A. S. Alving, *Arch. Intern. Med.*, **109,** 209 (1962).
418. M. Aikawa and R. L. Beaudoin, *Mil. Med.*, **134,** 986 (1969).
419. R. E. Howells, W. Peters, and J. Fullard, *Ann. Trop. Med. Parasitol.*, **64,** 203 (1970).
420. E. E. Davies, R. E. Howells, and W. Peters, *Ann. Trop. Med. Parasitol.*, **65,** 461 (1971).
421. D. C. Warhurst, in *Chemotherapeutic Agents in Study of Parasites*, Vol. 11, A. E. R. Taylor and R. Muller, Eds., Blackwell, Oxford, 1973, p. 6.

422. K. A. Conklin and S. C. Chou, *Proc. Helminthol. Soc. Wash.* **39** (special issue), 261 (1972).

423. P. G. Contacos, W. E. Collins, W. Chin, M. H. Jeter, and P. E. Briesch, *Am. J. Trop. Med. Hyg.*, **23,** 310 (1974).

424. K. H. Rieckmann, J. V. McNamara, L. Kass, and R. D. Powell, *Mil. Med.*, **134,** 802 (1969).

425. P. E. Carson, C. L. Flanagan, C. E. Ickes, and A. S. Alving, *Science*, **124,** 484 (1956).

426. N. L. Petrakis, S. L. Wiesenfeld, B. J. Sams, M. F. Collen, J. L. Cutler, and A. B. Siegelaub, *New Engl. J. Med.*, **282,** 767 (1970).

427. P. A. Marks and J. Banks, *Ann. N.Y. Acad. Sci.*, **123,** 198 (1965),

428. G. Cohen and P. Hochstein, *Biochemistry*, **3,** 895 (1964).

429. A. G. Motulsky, *Am. J. Trop. Med. Hyg.*, **13,** 147 (1964).

430. R. D. G. Theakston, K. A. Fletcher, and G. A. Moore, *Ann. Trop. Med. Parasitol.*, **70,** 125 (1976).

431. R. D. Powell and G. J. Brewer, *Am. J. Trop. Med. Hyg.*, **14,** 358 (1965).

432. H. E. Segal, W. W. Noll, and W. Thiemanun, *Proc. Helminthol. Soc. Wash.*, **39** (special issue), 79 (1972).

433. E. Beutler, *Pharmacol. Rev.*, **21,** 73 (1969).

434. H. N. Kirkman, in *Advances in Human Genetics*, Vol. 2, Plenum Press, New York, 1971, Ch. 1.

435. F. I. Carroll, B. Berrang, and C. P. Linn, *Chem. Ind.* (NY), **7,** 477 (1975).

436. L. H. Schmidt, S. Alexander, L. Allen, and J. Rasco, *Antimicrob. Agents Chemother.*, **12,** 51 (1977).

437. G. R. Coatney and J. Greenberg, *Ann. N.Y. Acad. Sci.*, **55,** 1075 (1952).

438. K. H. Rieckmann, R. D. Powell, J. V. McNamara, D. Willerson, Jr., L. Kass, H. Frischer, and P. E. Carson, *Am. J. Trop. Med. Hyg.*, **20,** 811 (1971).

439. D. F. Clyde, R. M. Miller, H. L. DuPont, and R. B. Hornick, *J. Trop. Med. Hyg.*, **74,** 238 (1971).

440. D. Willerson, Jr., K. H. Rieckmann, P. E. Carson, and H. Frischer, *Am. J. Trop. Med. Hyg.*, **21,** 857 (1972).

441. E. J. Colwell, R. L. Hickman, R. Intraprasert, and C. Tirabutana, *Am. J. Trop. Med. Hyg.*, **21,** 144 (1972).

442. E. J. Colwell, R. L. Hickman, and S. Kosakal, *J. Am. Med. Assoc.*, **220,** 684 (1972).

443. K. H. Rieckmann, W. D. Willerson, Jr., P. E. Carson, and H. Frischer, *Proc. Helminthol. Soc. Wash.*, **39** (Special issue), 339 (1972).

444. D. C. Warhurst, B. L. Robinson, R. E. Howells, and W. Peters, *Life Sci.*, **10,** 761 (1971).

445. D. C. Warhurst and V. C. Baggaley, *Trans. Roy. Soc. Trop. Med. Hyg.*, **66,** 5 (1972).

446. D. C. Warhurst, *Symp. Brit. Soc. Parasitol.*, **11,** 1 (1973).

447. J. B. Kaddu, D. C. Warhurst, and W. Peters, *Ann. Trop. Med. Parasitol.*, **68,** 41 (1974).

448. D. J. Mason, A. Dietz, and C. BeBoer, *Antimicrob. Agents Chemother.*, 554 (1963).

449. C. Lewis, H. W. Clapp, and J. E. Grady, *Antimicrob. Agents Chemother.*, 570 (1963).

450. C. Lewis, *J. Parasitol.*, **54,** 169 (1968).

451. B. J. Magerlein, R. D. Birkenmeyer, and F. Kagan, *J. Med. Chem.*, **10,** 355 (1967).

452. B. J. Magerlein, R. D. Birkenmeyer, and F. Kagan, *Antimicrob. Agents Chemother.*, 726 (1967).

453. C. Lewis, *Antimicrob. Agents Chemother.*, 537 (1967).

454. K. G. Powers, *Am. J. Trop. Med. Hyg.*, **18,** 485 (1969).

455. L. H. Schmidt, J. Harrison, R. Ellison, and P. Worcester, *Am. J. Trop. Med., Hyg.*, **19,** 1 (1970).

456. K. G. Powers and R. L. Jacobs, *Antimicrob. Agents Chemother.*, **1,** 49 (1972).

457. L. H. Miller, R. H. Glew, D. J. Wyler, W. A. Howard, W. E. Collins, P. G. Contacos, and F. A. Neva, *Am. J. Trop. Med. Hyg.*, **23,** 565 (1974).

458. D. F. Clyde, R. H. Gilman, and V. C. McCarthy, *Am. J. Trop. Med. Hyg.*, **24,** 369 (1975).

459. J. J. Josten and P. McAllen, *Biochem. Biophys. Res. Commun.*, **14,** 241 (1964).

460. F. N. C. Chang, C. J. Sih, and B. Weisblum, *Proc. Nat. Acad. Sci., US*, **55,** 431 (1966).

461. F. Schönhöfer, Office of Technical Services Report, RB-85033, 1948; *FIAT, Rev. Ger. Sci.*, 1939–1946.

462. L. H. Schmidt, R. N. Rossan, R. Fradkin, J. Woods, W. Schulemann, and L. Kratz, World Health Organization Publication WHO/Mal/532.65, Geneva; and *Bull. W. H. O.*, **34,** 783 (1966).

463. T. M. Sodeman, P. G. Contacos, W. E. Collins, C. S. Smith, and J. R. Jumper, *Bull. W. H. O.*, **47,** 425 (1972).

464. D. F. Clyde, V. C. McCarthy, and R. M. Miller, *Trans. Roy. Soc. Trop. Med. Hyg.*, **68,** 167 (1974).

465. C. J. Canfield and R. S. Rozman, *Bull. W. H. O.* **50,** 203 (1974).

466. L. F. Fieser, J. P. Schirmer, S. Archer, R. R. Lorenz, and P. I. Pfaffenbach, *J. Med. Chem.*, **10,** 513 (1967).

467. D. A. Berberian and R. G. Slighter, *J. Parasitol.*, **54,** 999 (1968).

468. D. A. Berberian, R. G. Slighter, and H. W. Freele, *J. Parasitol.*, **54,** 1181 (1968).

469. H. Heymann and L. F. Fieser, *J. Pharmacol.*, **94,** 97 (1948).

470. W. B. Wendel, *Fed. Proc.*, **5,** 406 (1946).

471. L. F. Fieser and H. Heymann, *J. Biol. Chem.*, **176,** 1363 (1948).

472. H. Heymann and L. F. Fieser, *J. Biol. Chem.*, **176,** 1359 (1948).

473. P. J. Rietz, F. S. Skelton, and K. Folkers, paper presented at *153rd National Meeting of the American Chemical Society, Miami Beach,* April 1967.

474. P. J. Rietz, F. S. Skelton, and K. Folkers, *Int. J. Vitam. Res.*, **37,** 405 (1967).

475. F. S. Skelton, P. J. Rietz, and K. Folkers, *J. Med. Chem.*, **13,** 602 (1970).

476. South African Patent 68/7,449, Vitamins, Ltd. (1969).

477. P. Mamalis, L. Jeffries, S. Price, M. J. Rix, and D. J. Outred, *J. Med. Chem.*, **8,** 684 (1965).

478. K. H. Rieckmann, D. Willerson, Jr., and P. E. Carson, *Trans. Roy. Soc. Trop. Med. Hyg.*, **65,** 533 (1971).

479. I. W. Sherman, J. A. Ruble, and I. P. Ting, *Exp. Parasitol.*, **25,** 181 (1969).

480. K. van Dyke, G. C. Tremblay, C. Szustkiewicz, and L. H. Saxe, *J. Protozool.*, **15,** 23 (1968).

481. P. R. Whitfield, *Aust. J. Sci.*, **6,** 591 (1953).

482. K. van Dyke, *Z. Tropenmed. Parasitol.*, **26,** 232 (1975).

483. W. E. Gutteridge and P. I. Trigg, *J. Protozool.*, **17,** 89 (1970).

484. K. A. Conklin, S. C. Chou, W. A. Siddiqui, and J. V. Schnell, *J. Protozool.*, **20,** 683 (1973).

485. R. D. G. Theakston and K. A. Fletcher, *Life Sci.*, **10,** 701 (1971).

486. J. B. Pritchard, F. Chavez-Peon, and R. D. Berlin, *Am. J. Physiol.*, **219,** 1263 (1970).

487. C. H. Lantz, K. van Dyke, and G. Carter, *Exp. Parasitol.*, **29,** 402 (1971).

488. S. M. Tracy and I. W. Sherman, *J. Protozool.*, **19,** 541 (1972).

489. K. van Dyke and C. Szustkiewicz, *Mil. Med.*, **134,** 1000 (1969).

490. G. Carter, K. van Dyke, and H. F. Mengoli, *Proc. Helminthol. Soc. Wash.*, **39** (special issue), 241 (1972).

491. A. W. Murray, D. C. Elliott, and M. R. Atkinson, *Progr. Nucleic Acid Res. Mol. Biol.*, **10,** 87 (1970).

492. W. Büngener, *Z. Tropenmed. Parasitol.*, **18,** 48 (1967).

493. G. Schmidt, R. D. Walter, amd E. Königk, *Z. Tropenmed. Parasitol.*, **25,** 301 (1974).

494. E. E. Davies and R. E. Howells, *Trans. Roy. Soc. Trop. Med. Hyg.*, **67,** 20 (1973).

495. R. L. Jacobs, L. H. Miller, and L. C. Koontz, *J. Parasitol.*, **60,** 340 (1974).

496. M. S. Omar, R. W. Gwadz, and L. H. Miller, *Z. Tropenmed. Parasitol.*, **26,** 303 (1975).

497. L. Cook, P. T. Grant, and W. O. Kermack, *Exp. Parasitol.*, **11,** 372 (1961).

498. J. W. Moulder and E. A. Evans, *J. Biol. Chem.*, **164,** 145 (1946).

499. J. D. Fulton and P. T. Grant, *Biochem. J.*, **63,** 274 (1956).

500. H. Polet and M. E. Conrad, *Proc. Soc. Exp. Biol. Med.* (a) **127,** 251 (1968), (b) **130**, 581 (1969).

501. W. A. Siddiqui, J. V. Schnell, and G. M. Geiman, *Mil. Med.*, **134,** Suppl. 929 (1969).

502. W. A. Siddiqui and J. V Schnell, *Proc. Helminthol. Soc. Wash.* **39** (special issue), 204 (1972).

503. G. J. McCormick, *Exp. Parasitol.*, **27,** 143 (1970).

504. I. W. Sherman, R. A. Virkar, and J. A. Ruble, *Comp. Biochem. Physiol.*, **23,** 43 (1967).

505. I. W. Sherman and I. P. Ting, *Nature* (London), **212,** 1387 (1966).

506. H. Polet, N. D. Brown, and C. R. Angel, *Proc. Roy. Soc. Exp. Biol. Med.*, **131,** 1215 (1969).

507. I. Lukow, G. Schmidt, R. D. Walter, and E. Königk, *Z. Tropenmed. Parasitol.*, **24,** 500 (1973).

508. D. B. Morrison and H. A. Jesskey, *Fed. Proc.*, **6,** 279 (1947).

509. C. W. Lawrence and R. J. Cenedella, *Exp. Parasitol.*, **26,** 181 (1969).

510. E. G. Ball, R. W. McKee, C. B. Aenfinsen, W. O. Cruz, and Q. M. Geiman, *J. Biol. Chem.*, **175,** 547 (1948).

511. R. J. Cenedella, *Am. J. Trop. Med. Hyg.*, **17,** 680 (1968).

512. K. N. Rao, D. Subrahmanyam, and S. Prakash, *Exp. Parasitol.*, **27,** 22 (1970).

513. R. C. Rock and J. Standefer, *J. Parasitol.*, **56,** 287 (1970).

514. W. G. Brundage, C. M. Hyland, and G. T. Dimopoullos, *Am. J. Trop, Med. Hyg.*, **18,** 657 (1969).

515. C. L. S. Hardy, L. T. Hart, G. T. Dimopoullos, and E. N. Lambremont, *Exp. Parasitol.*, **37,** 193 (1975).

516. R. C. Rock, *Comp. biochem. Physiol.* (a) **40B,** 557 (b) 893 (1971).

517. W. A. Siddiqui, J. V. Schnell, and Q. M. Geiman,, *Science*, **156,** 1623 (1967).

518. P. I. Trigg, *Parasitology*, **59,** 915 (1969).

519. R. C. Rock, J. Standefer, and W. Little, *Comp. Biochem. Physiol.*, **40B,** 543 (1971).

520. W. R. Wallace, J. F. Finerty, and G. T. Dimopoullos, *Am. J. Trop. Med. Hyg.*, **14,** 715 (1965).

521. P. I. Trigg, *Ann. Trop. Med. Parasitol.*, **62,** 481 (1968).

522. R. J. Cenedella, J. J. Jarrell, and L. H. Saxe, *Mil. Med.*, **134** (special issue), No. 10, 1045 (1969).

523. A. Fletcher and B. Maegraith, *Advan. Parasitol.*, **10,** 31 (1972).

524. D. M. Fraser and W. O. Kermack, *Brit. J. Pharmacol.*, **12,** 16 (1957).

525. J. F. Speck and E. A. Evans, *J. Biol. Chem.*, **159,** 71 (1945).

526. P. B. Marshall, *Brit. J. Pharmacol.*, **3,** 1 (1948).

527. I. B. R. Bowman, P. T. Grant, W. O. Kermack, and D. Ogston, *Biochem. J.*, **78,** 472 (1961).

528. S. N. Ali, K. A. Fletcher, and B. G. Maegraith, *Trans. Roy. Soc. Trop. Med. Hyg.*, **63,** 4 (1969).

529. P. M. L. Siu, *Fed. Proc.*, **25,** 756 (1966).

530. P. M. L. Siu, *Comp. Biochem. Physiol.*, **23,** 785 (1967).

CHAPTER NINETEEN

Antiamebic Agents

WILLIAM J. ROSS

Lilly Research Centre, Limited
Erl Wood Manor
Windlesham
Surrey, GU20 6PH,
England

CONTENTS

1 INTRODUCTION

Amebiasis, in the widest sense of the word, implies infection of a host by any parasitic ameba; however the term is generally restricted to the harboring in man of *Entameba histolytica*, with or without clinical manifestations. Seven species of ameba are natural parasites of man: *E. histolytica*, *E. hartmanni*, *E. coli*, *E. gingivales*, *Endolimax nana*, *Iodameba buetschlii*, and *Dientameba fragilis*. *E. gingivalis* is an inhabitant of the mouth, whereas the others inhabit the colon. Only *E. histolytica* is recognized as being pathogenic to man and, in many individuals, it too may live as a harmless commensal. *Dientameba fragilis* is regarded as nonpathogenic, but there is some evidence that it may cause diarrhea (1). *E. histolytica* is a microscopic, one-celled animal of the phylum Protozoa, class Rhizopoda, family Amebidae, which has five successive stages in its life cycle, namely, the trophozoite, precyst, cyst, metacyst, and metacystic trophozoite, all of which occur in the human intestine. The parasite enters a new host by the oral route at the cyst stage, and contaminated drinking water, food, direct fecal contact, person-to-person contact, flies, and cockroaches have been implicated in the transmission of the cysts (2).

The prevalence of amebiasis, which occurs throughout the world, varies greatly from country to country but is generally associated with poor economic and sanitary conditions. However there is some confusion about the exact clinical classification of amebiasis because *E. histolytica* may be present in a host without overt signs of disease. The following classification is used by an expert committee of the World Health Organization (2).

1. *Asymptomatic.*
2. *Symptomatic.*
   a. Intestinal amebiasis: (i) dysentery, (ii) nondysenteric colitis, (iii) ameboma, and (iv) amebic appendicitis.
   b. Extraintestinal amebiasis: (i) hepatic acute nonsuppurative, and (ii) liver abscess.
3. *Cutaneous.* Involvement of other organs (e.g., lung, brain, and spleen) without obvious liver involvement.

Hepatic amebiasis is the commonest form of extraintestinal amebic disease. The epidemiology and clinical manifestations of the disease have been reviewed (3), and a regime for the comparative evaluation of amebicidal drugs in the clinic has been described (4).

2 CHEMOTHERAPY OF AMEBIASIS

The search for antiamebic agents may be pursued using either *in vitro* or *in vivo* techniques. The *in vitro* techniques, which entail growing *E. histolytica* on complex culture media and determining the minimum inhibitory concentration (MIC) for the test compounds, have been described in detail by Woolf (1). *In vitro* testing is generally a prelude to *in vivo* testing in laboratory animals. Weanling rats infected with *E. histolytica* are used for the assessment of drug activity against intestinal amebiasis, whereas infected hamsters are normally used to study hepatic amebiasis (1, 4).

In assessing the merits of potential drugs for treating amebiasis, it should be borne in mind that the ideal amebicide should be active within the bowel lumen, in the bowel wall, and systemically, particularly in the liver.

2.1 The Ipecac Alkaloids

The merits of powdered ipecacuanha root as a medicinal agent have been known to the natives of Brazil since ancient times, and its use spread to Europe after the Spanish and Portuguese conquest of South America. The alkaloid emetine, isolated from the powdered root of *Cephaelis ipecacuanha* or *C. acuminata*, was first described by Pelletier in 1817. However the *in vitro* amebicidal properties of emetine were first recognized about 60 years ago (6) and subsequently used in the clinic on patients suffering from acute amebic dysentery or hepatitis (7). The gross structure of emetine was finally elucidated in 1949 (8, 9) and the structure 19.**1** is now accepted as the configuration of the natural alkaloid

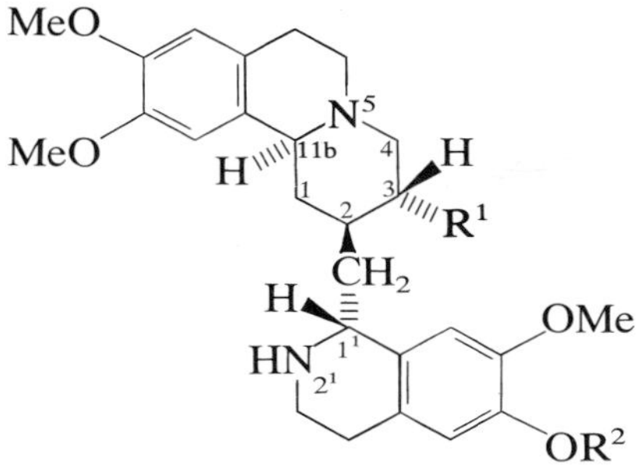

19.**1** $R^1 = C_2H_5$; $R^2 = CH_3$
19.**2** $R^1 = H$; $R^2 = CH_3$
19.**3** $R^1 = CH_3$; $R^2 = CH_3$
19.**4** $R^1 = C_2H_5$; $R^2 = H$

(−)emetine (10–13). A stereochemically favorable synthesis of (−)emetine has been achieved (14) and is now used on a commercial scale.

Since emetine has four asymmetric centers at positions 2, 3, 11b, and 1′, a number of stereoisomers are possible. However the antiamebic activity of (−)emetine is highly stereospecific because all the stereoisomers of emetine tested for amebicidal activity *in vitro* or *in vivo* are less active than the natural alkaloid (15–18). Quaternization of the 5- and 2′-nitrogens of (−)emetine results in a weakly amebicidal compound, but quaternization of N-5 only, improves activity relative to (−)emetine (19).

Great importance has been attached to the ethyl group at C-3, and it has been reported that (±)-3-desethylemetine (19.**2**) (bisnoremetine) has almost no activity *in vivo* (20). However the configuration of this compound was not clearly defined, and subsequent work demonstrated that both (±)bisnoremetine (19.**2**) and (±)noremetine (19.**3**) possess modest antiamebic activity *in vivo* (21). Thus the nature of the C-3 substituent does not appear to be as critical as originally supposed, and this is supported by the fact that (±)2,3-nordehydrometine (19.**10**) is an active amebicide *in vivo* (22). However introduction of various oxygen-bearing substituents at positions 2 and 3 leads to a marked decrease in activity (23). A range of $N^{2'}$-substituted derivatives of emetine have been synthesized, varying from (−)$N^{2'}$-methylemetine, which possesses little activity *in vitro* (24) or *in vivo* (25), to (−)$N^{2'}$-butylemetine and (−)$N^{2'}$-(3-hydroxybutyl)emetine, which exhibit one-half and equivalent activity, respectively, compared to the natural alkaloid (16, 23). None of these compounds appears to have been introduced clinically.

Cleavage of the tetrahydroisoquinoline ring in (−)-emetine leads to (−)-1′,8a'-secoemetine (19.**5**), which possesses modest antiamebic activity *in vivo*, but a series of analogs (19.**6**–19.**8**) was inactive (21).

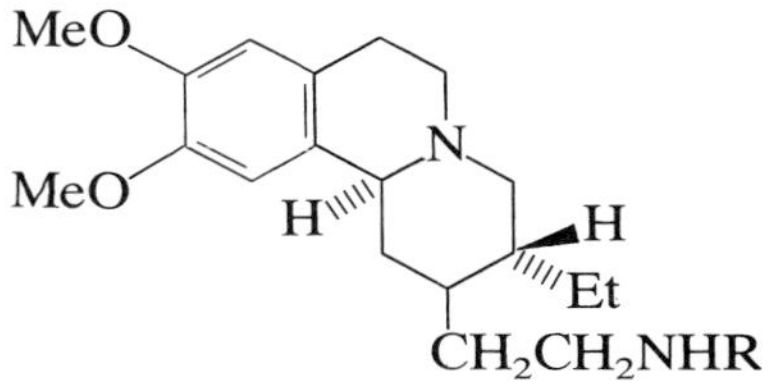

19.**5** R = —CH_2CH_2—(3,4-dimethoxyphenyl)

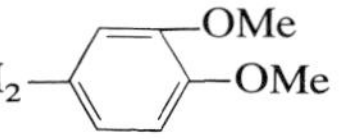

19.**6** R = —CH_3
19.**7** R = —$CH_2CH_2CH_3$
19.**8** R = —CH_2—Ph

An interesting compound, $N^{2'}$-acetyl-N-methyl-11^b-N^5-*secoemetine* (19.**9**) possesses *in vitro* activity (26, 27) but does not appear to have been tested *in vivo*.

Despite the vast number of emetine derivatives that have been synthesized, only one compound, (±)2,3-dehydroemetine (19.**11**), has proved worthy of detailed clinical evaluation. The synthesis,

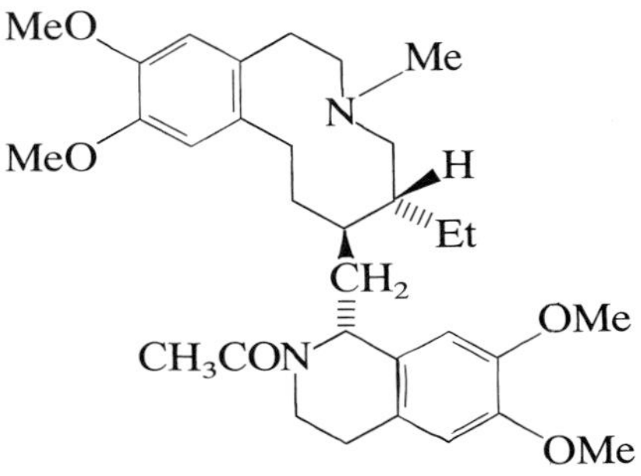

19.**9**

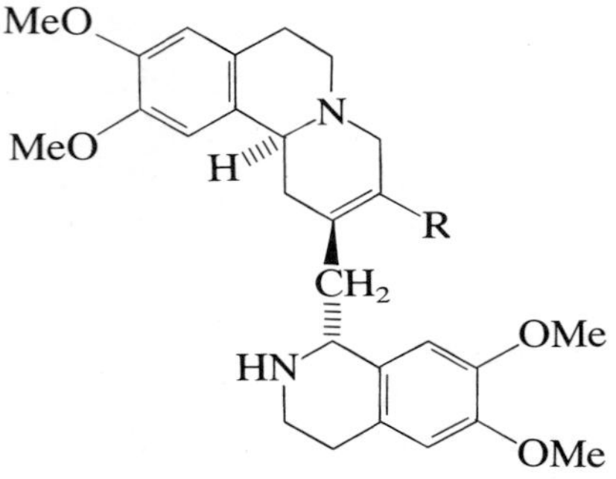

(Structures represent one of two enantiomers)

19.**10** R = —CH_3
19.**11** R = —C_2H_5

stereochemistry (23, 28–32), and antiamebic properties (23, 24, 28, 33) of dehydroemetine and related compounds are the subject of many papers. Detailed clinical studies (34, 35) have shown that (±)-dehydroemetine possesses antiamebic activity equal to natural (−)emetine and also appears to be better tolerated and more rapidly excreted than the natural alkaloid (36).

In laboratory experiments in which the antiamebic properties of natural(−)-emetine and (±)-2,3-dehydroemetine and (−)-2,3-dehydroemetine were compared, all three compounds had similar activity *in vitro* against *E. histolytica* and possessed comparable activity against experimental amebic liver abscess in hamsters. However comparisons of activity against rat cecal infections with *E. histolytica* showed that (−)-2,3-dehydroemetine and (−)emetine had similar activity but were twice as active as the racemate. Short-term chronic toxicity studies indicated the racemate to have only half the toxicity of (−)-2,3-dehydroemetine; consequently the activity and toxicity of the racemate are attributed to the (−)enantiomer (37).

The pharmacology and clinical use of emetine and (±)-dehydroemetine have been reviewed (38). To improve the activity of emetine in acute intestinal amebiasis, a complex with bismuth iodide (EBI) has been used clinically but has found favor only with British clinicians (38).

The modes of action of (−)-emetine and (±)-2,3-dehydroemetine and related compounds have been studied in some detail, and it appears that all the active compounds inhibit protein synthesis in certain mammalian and other cells (24, 39, 40).

Certain other compounds related to (−)-emetine possess amebicidal activity. Variations in the substituents in the aromatic portion of the isoquinoline moiety can be tolerated without loss of activity. Cephaeline (19.**4**), a minor ipecac alkaloid, has antiamebic activity, as have the carboline alkaloids tubulosine (19.**12**) (41) and deoxytubolosine (19.**13**) (42). However it

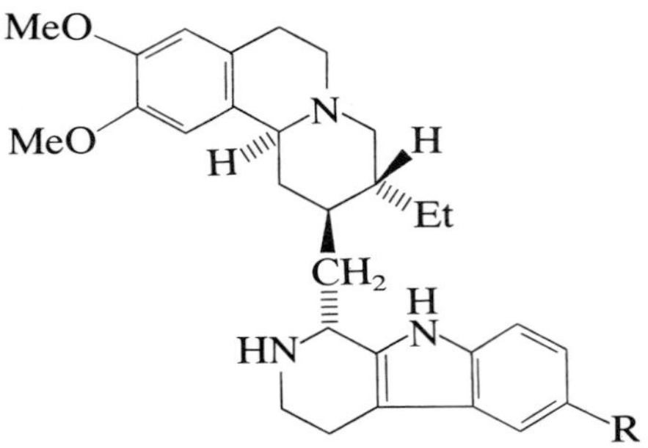

19.**12** R = OH
19.**13** R = H

should be emphasized that these compounds all have the same absolute configuration as natural emetine.

The discovery of antiamebic activity in tubulosine (19.**12**) confirmed the predictions of Grollman (41). He observed that (−)emetine and certain other ipecac alkaloids show configurational similarities to (−)-cycloheximide (19.**14**) and the glutarimide antibiotics and display similar effects on protein synthesis. This led to the proposal that structure 19.**15** contains the topochemical requirements for amebicidal activity and for the inhibition of protein synthesis (41).

Although the structure of emetine was not known with certainty until 1949, attempts were made to prepare simple

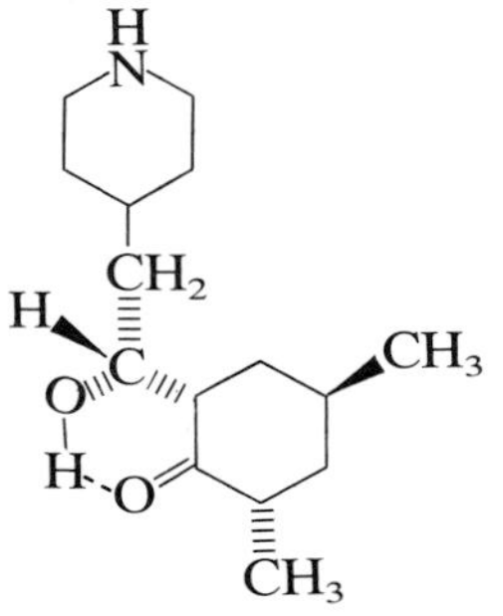

19.**14**

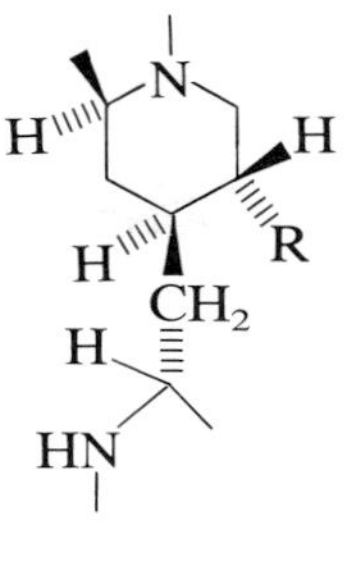

19.**15**

amines that would mimic the antiamebic properties of the alkaloid. Vast numbers of these compounds were prepared, but although some showed useful amebicidal activity *in vitro*, none proved to be clinically worthwhile.

Typical examples are 1,10-bis(dialkylamino)decane (19.**16**) (42) and *N,N'*-bis-(2-ethylbutyl)-3,10-dimethylaminododecane (19.**17**) (43).

$$(C_5H_{11})_2N(CH_2)_{10}N(C_5H_{11})_2$$

19.**16**

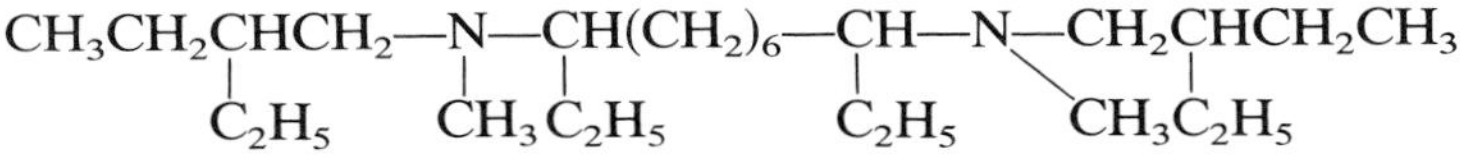

19.**17**

However in view of the apparent strict stereochemical requirements for amebicidal activity in the emetine series, it is hardly surprising that this approach did not yield useful products (1, 43–46).

2.2 *Holarrhena* Alkaloids

Extracts of plants of the *Holarrhena* species have played an important part in Ayurvedic medicine on the Indian subcontinent for more than 1500 years. In particular, the extracts of *H. antidysenterica* bark, known variously as kurchi, conessi, or telicherry bark, have been employed in the treatment of amebic dysentery. A number of alkaloids have been isolated from kurchi, but the major alkaloid is conessine (19.**18**) (47–50),

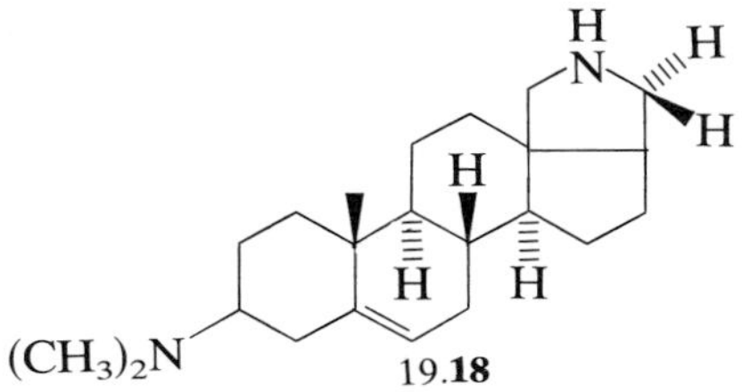

19.**18**

which has been used in the treatment of both intestinal and extraintestinal amebiasis in man (51–53).

Conessine has been used little outside the old French colonial territories and India, partly because of its known neurological toxicity (54, 55). Conessine has low *in vitro* activity against *E. histolytica* but is active against amebiasis in rats (1). By analogy with EBI, a preparation called "kurchibismuth iodide" has been used successfully (56) but did not overcome the toxicity problems.

Various derivatives of conessine have been synthesized, but they were inferior as amebicides (57, 58).

2.3 Amaroids

The amaroids are phenanthropyran-2-one derivatives allied to the triterpenoids. They occur as glycosides in various simaroubaceous plants. Extracts of the bark, fruit, or seeds of the simarouba have been used in the treatment of dysenteric conditions in the Americas, Europe, Africa, and Asia for many years.

The most interesting amebicidal compound isolated from the simarouba is glaucarubin (19.**19**), which possesses potent activity against *E. histolytica in vitro* and in rats, guinea pigs, and dogs (59–61).

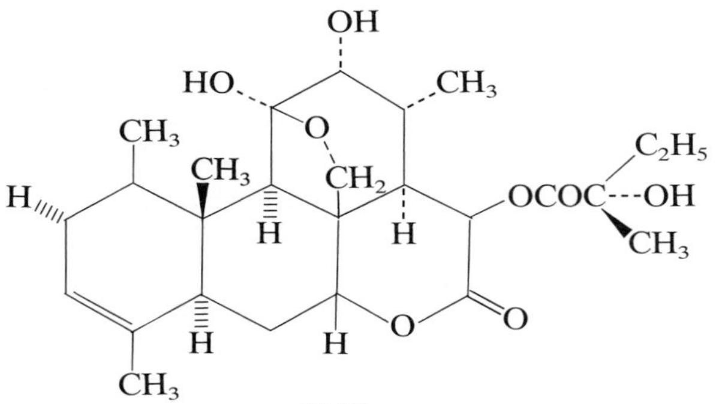

19.**19**

The structure of glaucarubin has been defined as 19.**19** by X-ray analysis (63). Numerous clinical trials have been conducted with glaucarubin, and it appears to be useful in the treatment of both chronic and acute intestinal amebiasis (64–66). However glaucarubin does not appear to have become established in clinical practice. A related compound, quassin (19.**20**) (67), which is present in the heartwood of *Quassia amara*, possesses significant amebicidal activity *in vitro* and in man (68, 69), but this property has not been pursued further.

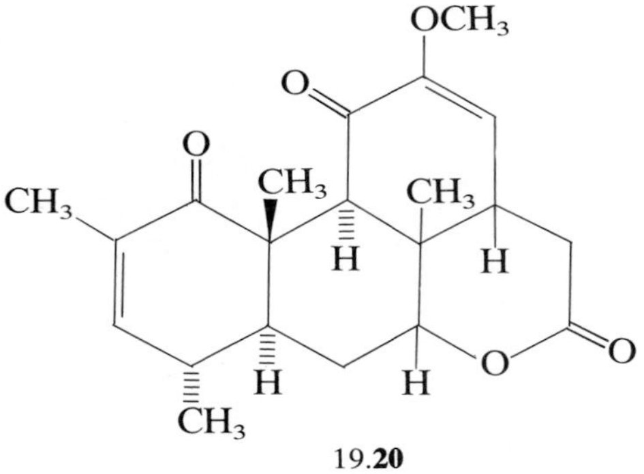

19.**20**

A variety of active principles have been isolated from the seed of *Brucea javanica* and *Brucea sumatrana*, and extracts are known under various names such as Ko-sam, Ya-Tan-Tzu, and Koo-Sheng-Tse. Amebicidal activity has been claimed for these decoctions (70). A compound, thought to have structure 19.**21**, has been isolated from *B. sumatrana* (71); but it is not clear whether the amebicidal properties of Ko-sam are due to such compounds.

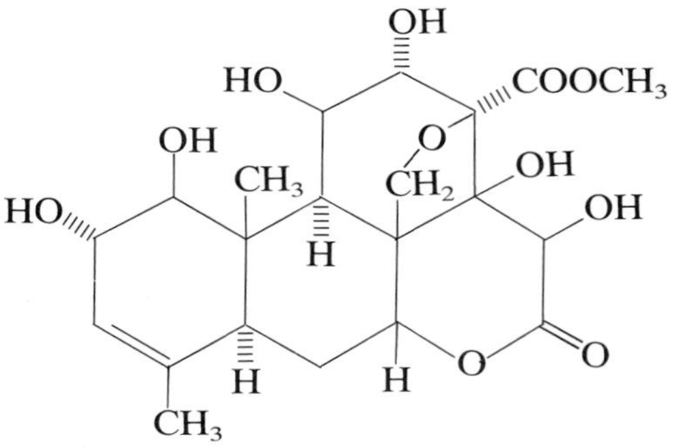

19.**21**

2.4 Miscellaneous Natural Products

The alkaloid berberine (19.**22**), which occurs in the plant *Berberis aristata* Linn (72), has antiamebic activity *in vitro* and in experimental amebiasis. The sulfate is active *in vitro* only at high concentrations (1000 μg/ml) but is effective in preventing

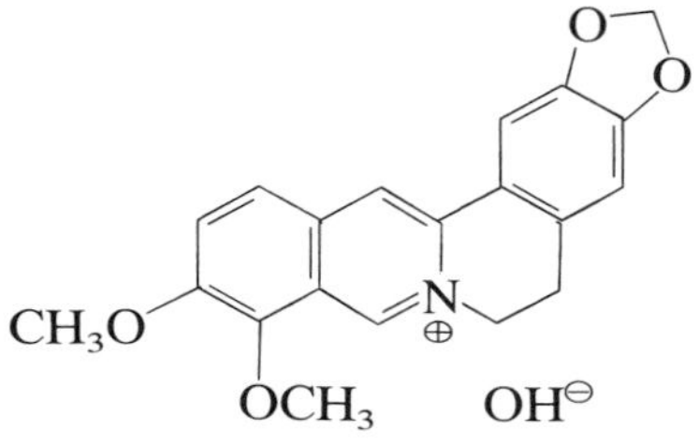

19.**22**

the development of experimental hepatic amebiasis in hamsters and intestinal amebiasis in rats (72). The clinical studies said to be underway (72) have not been reported.

Powdered leaf of henna, *Lawsonia alba* (73), and extracts of *Euphorbia hirta* (74) are claimed to be effective against intestinal amebiasis in man (73, 74). Similarly, extracts of *Chrysanthellum procumbens* (75) and *Anenome chinensis* (76) exhibit amebicidal activity.

2.5 Antibiotics

In the therapy of amebiasis, antibiotics have been used as supportive therapy for the control of the bacteria associated with the ameba. Although some antibiotics have a direct amebicidal action, the majority of those that act on *E. histolytica* do so indirectly by modifying the bacterial flora of the bowel. After the value of penicillin and the sulfonamides in amebic dysentery had been demonstrated (77), many combinations of antibiotics were tried. However it was soon shown that the tetracyclines were the antibiotics of choice, and these appeared to affect *E. histolytica* indirectly by acting on the bacterial flora of the bowel (78–80). The amebicidal properties of a large number of antibiotics have been listed (1, 81), and since their action is thought to be indirect, these are not discussed further.

However some antibiotics appear to have a direct effect on *E. histolytica*; these include fumagillin, a metabolite of *Aspergillus fumigatus* (19.**23**), which is very active

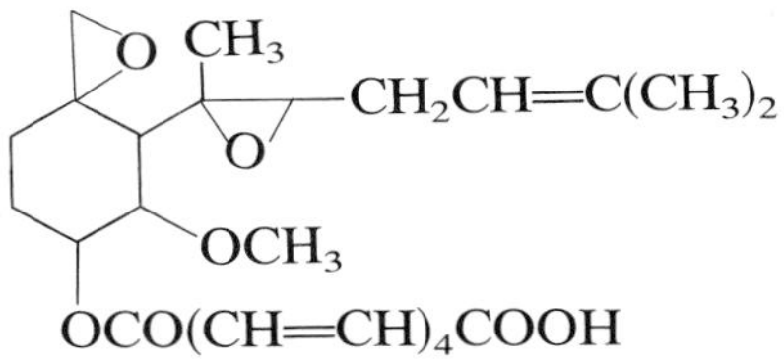

O CH_3 $CH_2CH{=}C(CH_3)_2$ O OCH_3 $OCO(CH{=}CH)_4COOH$

19.**23**

against *E. histolytica in vitro* (82). It is active against experimental amebiasis in rats and rabbits (82) and monkeys (83). However the compound that has recently been synthesized (84) appears to be too toxic for general use in man (1).

Paromomycin (19.**24**), a metabolite of *Streptomyces rimosus* (85), appears to have a direct effect on *E. histolytica in vitro* (86) and to be more active than emetine *in vitro* (87, 88). Paromomycin is active against experimental intestinal amebiasis in rats (89) and is effective against experimental amebic abscess in hamsters when dosed parentally (86, 87) but not orally. Paromomycin has been used successfully in the clinic for acute and chronic intestinal amebiasis (88–92).

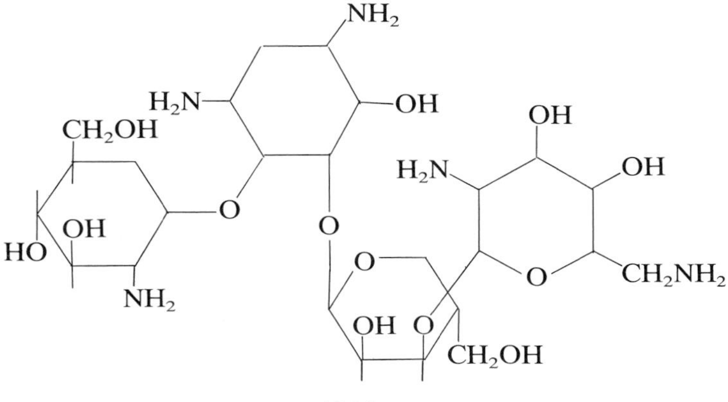

NH_2 H_2N OH CH_2OH OH H_2N OH O O OH HO O O CH_2NH_2 NH_2 OH O CH_2OH

19.**24**

Anisomycin (19.**25**), a metabolite of various *Streptomyces* species, which, like (−)-cycloheximide (19.**14**) and (−)emetine (19.**1**), appears to inhibit protein synthesis in various cell systems (93), possesses significant activity against *E. histolytica in vitro* and *in vivo* (94–96). Numerous derivatives and analogs of anisomycin have been prepared, but none has proved to be useful as an amebicide (97–99).

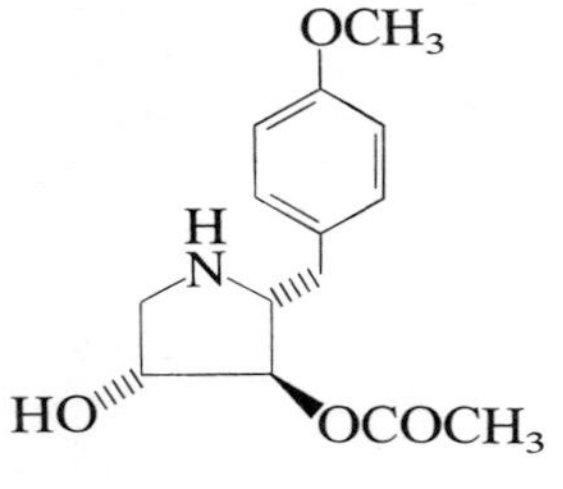

19.**25**

Dactylarin (19.**26**), a metabolite of *Dactylaria lutea*, has *in vitro* activity against *Entameba invadens* (100) and, in view of its structural relationship to the antifungal griseofulvin, may warrant more detailed investigation.

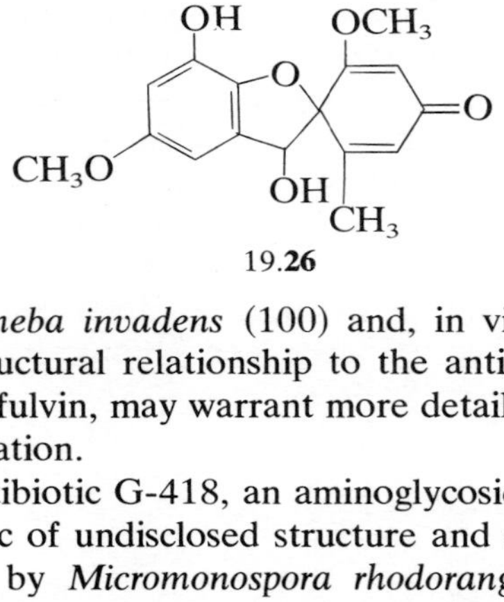

19.**26**

Antibiotic G-418, an aminoglycoside antibiotic of undisclosed structure and elaborated by *Micromonospora rhodorangea*, is claimed to be more active against cecal amebiasis in rats than paromomycin (19.**24**) or metronidazole (19.**65**) (101). Various viomycin derivatives are claimed to be amebicidal (102), as is the cytotoxic antibiotic anthramycin methyl ether (19.**27**) (103, 104).

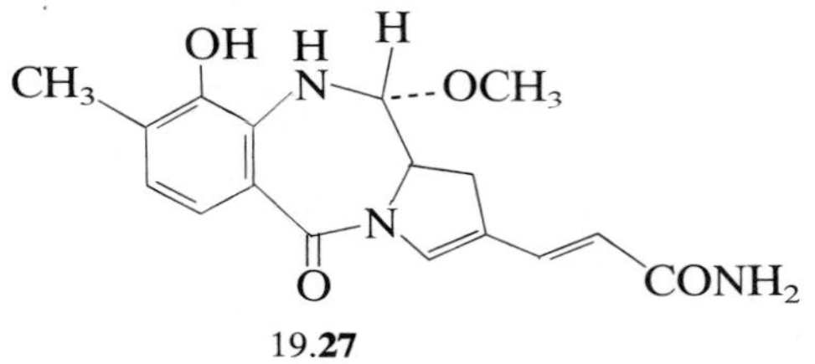

19.**27**

2.6 Quinoline Derivatives

2.6.1 HYDROXYQUINOLINES. Quinoline derivatives have been used for many years as antiamebic agents and, indeed, iodinated hydroxyquinolines were among the first synthetic agents to be used in the treatment of the disease. Three iodinated 8-quinolinols have been used for many years in the treatment of intestinal amebiasis, these being sodium 7-iodo-8-quinolinol-5-sulfonate (chiniofon, 19.**28**), 5-chloro-7-iodo-8-quinolinol (iodochlorohydroxquin, clioquinol, Vioform, 19.**29**), and 5,7-diiodo-8-quinolinol (Embequin, diiodohydroxyquinoline, 19.**30**). The compounds are ineffective against extraintestinal amebiasis.

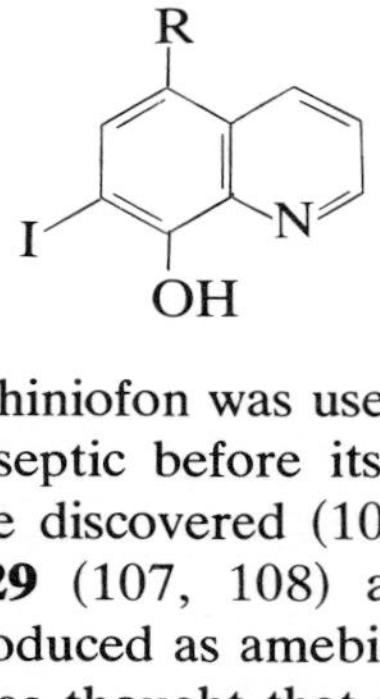

19.**28** R=SO_3Na
19.**29** R=Cl
19.**30** R=I

Chiniofon was used for many years as an antiseptic before its amebicidal properties were discovered (105, 106). Subsequently, 19.**29** (107, 108) and 19.**30** (109) were introduced as amebicidal agents. Originally it was thought that the amebicidal properties of iodinated hydroxyquinolines were due to the release of elemental iodine in the host. However this suggestion was discredited when it was found that large doses of elemental iodine or sodium iodide failed to cure intestinal amebiasis in dogs, whereas iodinated 8-hydroxyquinolines were curative (109). Additionally many noniodinated 8-hydroxyquinolines were found to be active against *E. histolytica in vitro* and in experimental amebiasis in rats and dogs (110, 111).

Of particular significance are 5,7-dichloro-2-methyl-8-quinolinol (chloroquinaldol, 19.**31**) (112, 113) and 5,7-dibromo-8-quinolinol (broxiquinolina, 19.**32**) (114, which are effective in man.

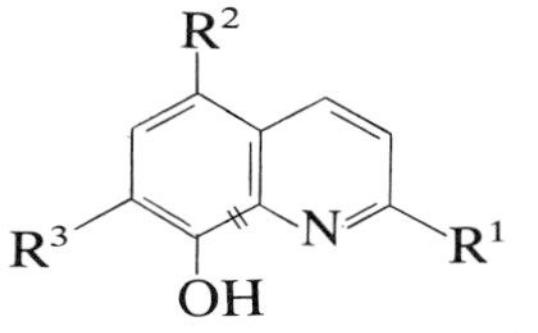

19.**31** $R^1 = CH_3$; $R^2 = R^3 = Cl$
19.**32** $R^1 = H$; $R^2 = R^3 = Br$

Application of the Mannich reaction to 8-hydroxyquinoline led to a series of compounds possessing high *in vitro* activity against *E. histolytica.* The most important compound, 19.**33**, proved to have activity

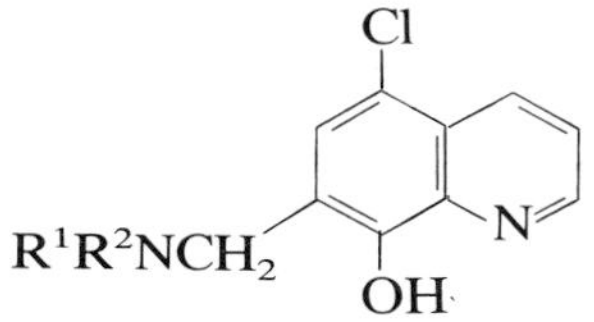

19.**33** $R^1 = R^2 = C_2H_5$
19.**34** $R^1 = H$; $R^2 = (C_2H_5)_2N(CH_2)_3$

in hepatic amebiasis in hamsters and was effective against intestinal amebiasis in man (109, 115).

As a consequence of this observation, a wide range of Mannich bases derived from 8-hydroxyquinolines were prepared (116–118) and investigated as amebicides. The most important series of compounds to emerge consisted of those having general structure 19.**35**, with the best activity being

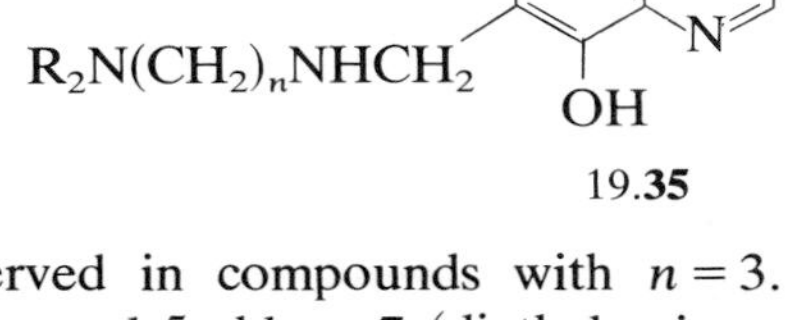

19.**35**

observed in compounds with $n = 3$. One compound, 5-chloro-7-(diethylaminopropylamino)methyl-8-hydroxyquinoline (19.**34**, clamoxyquin), as the hydrochloride salt, is active against hepatic amebiasis in hamsters and intestinal amebiasis in rats and dogs (118, 119).

Clamoxyquin (19.**34**) as the hydrochloride or pamoate salt has proved to be effective and was well tolerated in clinical trials against various forms of human intestinal amebiasis (120–123). The mode of action of the 8-hydroxyquinolines, especially chiniofonm (19.**28**), has been investigated (124), and the antiamebic effects appear to be exerted by chelation of ferrous iron necessary for amebal growth. Latour and Reeves (124) demonstrated that the growth of *E. histolytica* in a medium containing the amino acids L-cysteine, L-glutamic acid, and L-arginine depended directly on the concentration of added iron. However, the ferric iron chelators Chel DP and Versene Fe-3 Specific, had little effect on amebal growth, whereas the ferrous iron chelators, *o*-phenanthroline and chiniofon (19.**28**) markedly inhibited amebal growth. This observation was interpreted as indicating that the antiamebal properties of the 8-hydroxyquinolines was the result of their ferrous iron binding properties. The chelation theory is supported by the observation that various iodinated 5- and 8-hydroxyisoquinolines (125) and Mannich bases of 4-, 5-, 6-, and 7-hydroxyquinolines possess little antiamebic activity (126).

2.6.2 AMINOQUINOLINES AND RELATED COMPOUNDS. A number of antimalarial compounds of the aminoquinoline class possess significant activity against hepatic amebiasis in hamsters and in man. The most important compounds are chloroquine (19.**36**), and amodiaquine (19.**37**), hydroxychloroquine (19.**38**), sontoquine (19.**39**), and quinacrine (19.**40**) (5, 127, 128). However only chloroquine has found acceptance in the treatment of amebiasis. It is active against hepatic amebiasis in hamsters (5, 127) but has little or no activity when tested against intestinal infections in animals. Chloroquine is used for the treatment of extraintestinal amebiasis in man (2) but has poor activity against the intestinal form of the disease, presumably because it is so readily absorbed and does not reach the lower bowel in effective concentrations. To overcome this problem, chloroquine may be dosed in combination with a lumenal or contact amebicide such as chiniofon (129) or glycobiarsol (19.**86**) (130).

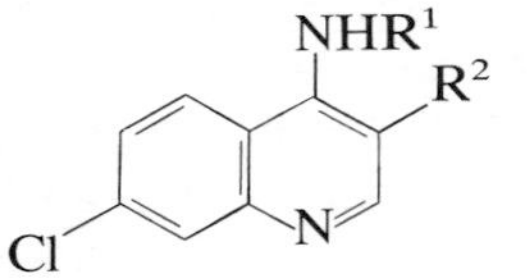

19.**36** $R^1 = -CH(CH_3)(CH_2)_3N(C_2H_5)_2$; $R^2=H$

19.**37** $R^1 =$ 4-hydroxy-3-($CH_2N(C_2H_5)_2$)phenyl; $R^2=H$

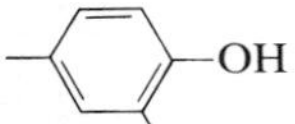

19.**39** $R^1 = -CH(CH_3)(CH_2)_3N(CH_2CH_2OH)(C_2H_5)$; $R^2=H$

19.**38** $R^1 = -CH(CH_3)(CH_2)_3N(C_2H_5)_2$; $R^2=Me$

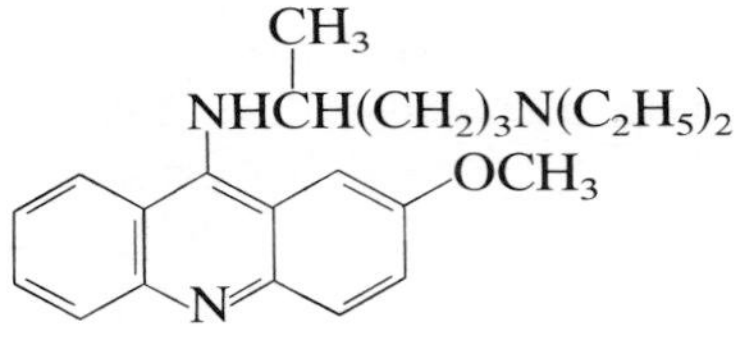

19.**40**

Despite the investigation of several hundred other new aminoquinoline and aminoacridine derivatives as amebicides, none has emerged to displace chloroquine in this class of compound (131–141).

Quinacrine possesses excellent antimalarial activity (see Chapter 18) and, as a consequence of its discovery, large numbers of related compounds have been prepared. In particular, a series of benz(c)acridines were prepared (142–144) which were devoid of antimalarial properties but, surprisingly, were active against experimental amebiasis. One compound in particular was selected for more detailed studies, and this compound, 7-{3-(octylamino)propyl}aminobenzacridine (19.**41**), proved to be efficacious against hepatic amebiasis in hamsters

$NH(CH_2)_3NH(CH_2)_7CH_3$

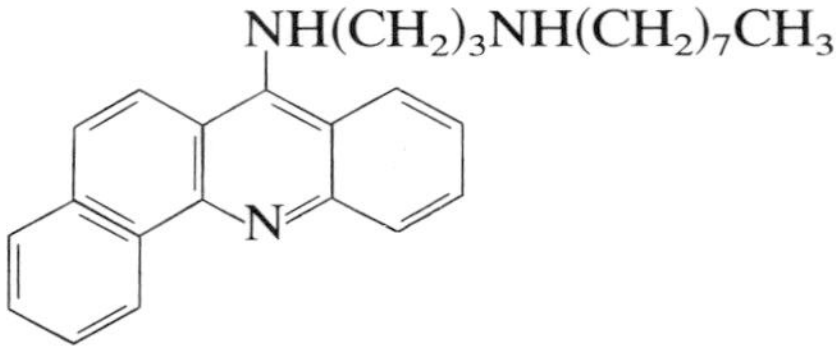

19.**41**

and intestinal amebiasis in rats and dogs (145). Clinical studies indicated that 19.**41** was effective in man against both amebic liver abscess and intestinal amebiasis (146, 147). However the compound has not come into general use.

A wide range of basically substituted heterocycles directly or indirectly related to the quinolines and acridines has been investigated for amebicidal activity, particularly by Elslager and his colleagues (see Ref. 148 for leading references), but none has been sufficiently interesting to warrant investigation in man.

2.7 *Ortho*-Aminomethylphenols

The interest engendered by the discovery of potent antimalarial activity in Mannich bases of the amodiaquin (19.**37**) type prompted the investigation of simple phenolic Mannich bases as antiparasitics. Few of these compounds possessed significant antimalarial activity. However one compound, 6,6′-diallyl-α,α′-bis(diethylamino)-4,4′-bi-*o*-cresol (bialamicol, biallylamicol, Camoform, 19.**42**) (149) exhibited moderate amebicidal activity *in vitro* and was effective against hepatic amebiasis in hamsters and intestinal amebiasis in rats and dogs (150).

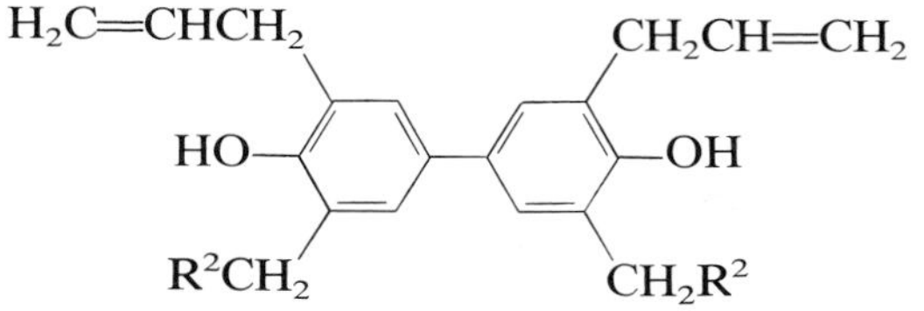

19.42 $R^2 = N(C_2H_5)_2$

19.43 $R^2 = $ —N (pyrrolidinyl)

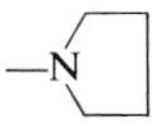

Subsequent clinical trials confirmed the amebicidal activity of 19.**42** against intestinal and hepatic amebiasis in man (151–153). Variation of the aminoalkyl side chain of 19.**42** led to a number of analogs possessing amebidical activity *in vitro*, but the best compound (19.**43**), when tested against intestinal amebiasis in rats, did not compare favorably with biallylamicol (137, 155).

2.8 Quinones and Hydroquinones

The discovery of the phenanthroline-quinone group of amebicides resulted from investigations related to the 8-quinolinols (see Section 2.6). The most interesting compounds are 4,7-phenanthroline-quinone (Entobex, phanquone, 19.**44**) and its monosemicarbazone (19.**45**) (155).

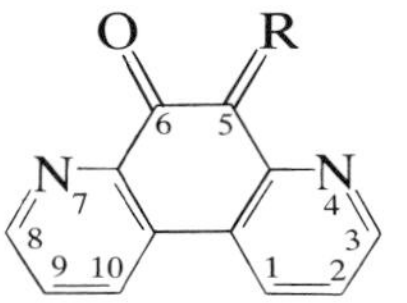

19.**44** R = O
19.**45** R = $NNHCONH_2$
19.**46** R = NOH

Entobex (19.**44**) is active against *E. histolytica in vitro* and against intestinal amebiasis in the rat, as was the semicarbazone (19.**45**). Activity was retained when the 1-position of 19.**44** was substituted by a methyl group, but the 3-methyl derivative was less active (156). The monooxime (19.**46**) has moderate activity in the rat, whereas the hydroquinone derived from 19.**44** was amebicidal *in vitro* but poorly active *in vivo* (157).

Entobex and its monosemicarbazone have been the subject of many clinical trials against intestinal amebiasis and, on balance, it appears that Entobex itself is more active than the semicarbazone and may also produce fewer side effects (1, 38, 157–162). A number of clinicans have reported that a combination of Entobex and iodochlorhydroxyquinoline (19.**29**, Vioform) is even more effective (162–164).

Investigations into compounds related to Entobex found that 1,10-, 1,7-, and 4,7-phenanthrolines were essentially devoid of antiamebic properties; of the monosubstituted compounds, only 5-hydroxy-4,7-phenanthroline (19.**47**) displayed significant

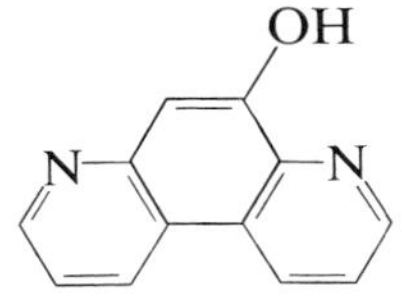

19.**47**

activity (165). This compound is directly related to the 8-hydroxy quinolines (see Section 2.6.1).

2.9 Haloacetamides

The development of the haloacetamides as amebicides resulted from the observation that certain phenylthiazolidine 1,1-dioxides possessed significant amebicidal activity against *E. criceti* infections in hamsters (166, 167). Of the numerous compounds tested, 2-(3,4-dichlorophenyl)-4-thiazolidinone-1,1-dioxide (19.**48**) was the most active, and this led to the preparation of a

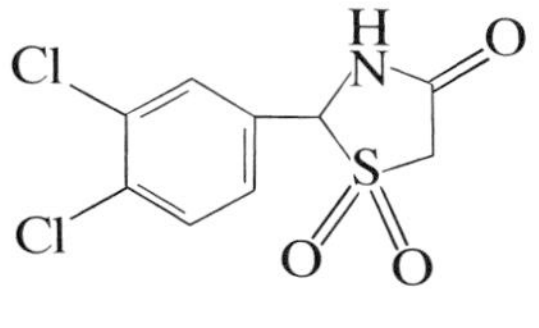

19.**48**

variety of compounds theoretically derived from that structure (168–173).

Removal of the —SO_2— moiety resulted in a series of active benzyl acetamides of general structure 19.**49** (168). It was found

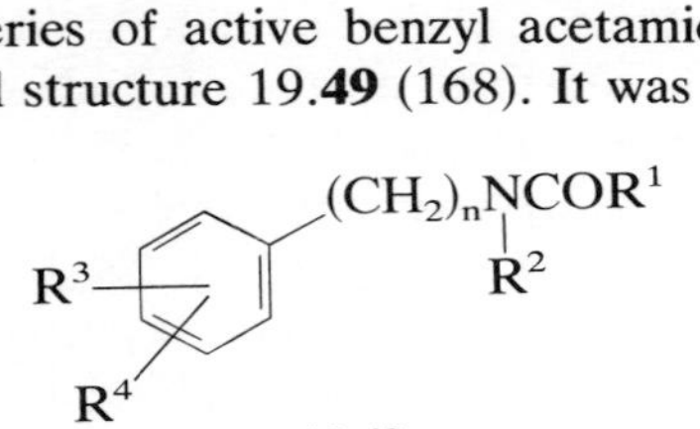

$$\text{R}^3,\text{R}^4\text{-C}_6\text{H}_3\text{-(CH}_2)_n\text{N(R}^2)\text{COR}^1$$

19.**49**

that in general, compounds with $n = 1$ and R^1 = dihalomethyl were more active than those with R^1 = trihalomethyl or halomethyl (168).

Various substitution patterns are allowable for R^3, R^4, but in the series where R^1 is dichloromethyl and R^2 alkyl, hydroxyalkyl, acyloxyalkyl, cyanoalkyl, carbamoylalkyl, or alkoxyalkyl, optimum activity was observed with R^3, R^4 = 2,4-dichloro, 4-butoxy or 4-isopropyl. The most important compound to emerge was 2,2-dichloro-*N*-(2,4-dichlorobenzyl)-*N*-(2-hydroxyethyl)-acetamide (19.**50**, chlorbetamide, Pontalin, Mantomide). This compound has good *in vitro* activity against *E. histolytica* and *in vivo* activity against *E. criceti* infections in hamsters (166) and *E. histolytica* infections in rats (174, 175) but is ineffective against hepatic amebiasis in hamsters (176). Clinical results with chlorbetamide have been equivocal, some clinicians achieving success against chronic amebiasis (177, 178) but others obtaining less favorable results (179). Replacement of the 2,4-dichloro functions of chlorbetamide (19.**50**) by a

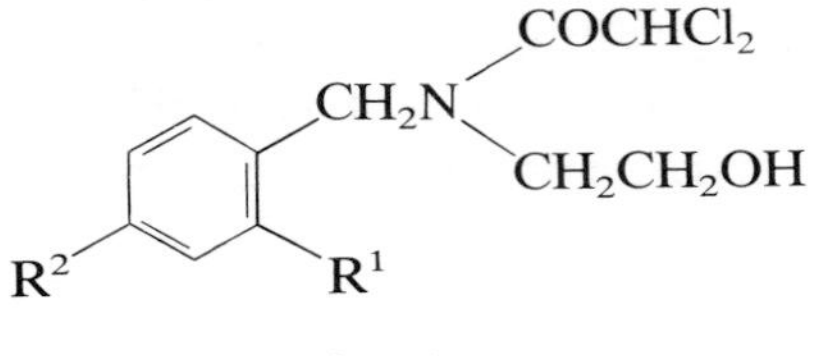

$$\text{R}^2,\text{R}^1\text{-C}_6\text{H}_3\text{-CH}_2\text{N(COCHCl}_2)\text{CH}_2\text{CH}_2\text{OH}$$

19.**50** $R^1 = R^2 = Cl$
19.**51** $R^1 = H$; $R^2 = CH_3SO_2$

4-methylsulfonyl group led to compound 19.**51**, which was 4 times as active as chlorbetamide agains *E. histolytica* infections in rats (180, 181). As with the chlorbetamide series, the dichloroacetamide derivatives were superior to the monochloroacetamides or simple acetamides. Compound 19.**51** was tried in man with disappointing results (181).

In another variation of the theme, the aromatic ring of chlorbetamide was replaced by a wide range of heterocyclic nuclei (176). The most promising compound, 2,2-dichloro-*N*-(2-hydroxyethyl)-*N*-(4-pyridylmethyl)acetamide (19.**52**) was active

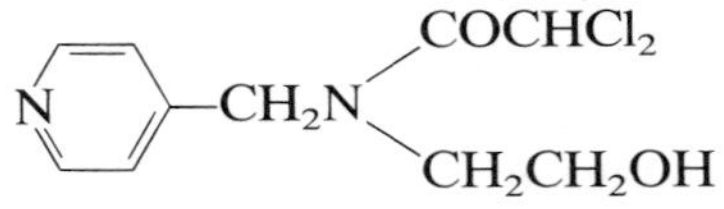

$$\text{NC}_5\text{H}_4\text{-CH}_2\text{N(COCHCl}_2)\text{CH}_2\text{CH}_2\text{OH}$$

19.**52**

against intestinal amebiasis in rats but was ineffective against hepatic amebiasis in hamsters (176).

The observations that the optical isomers of the antibiotic *threo*-chloramphenicol (19.**53**, chloromycetin) were equiactive

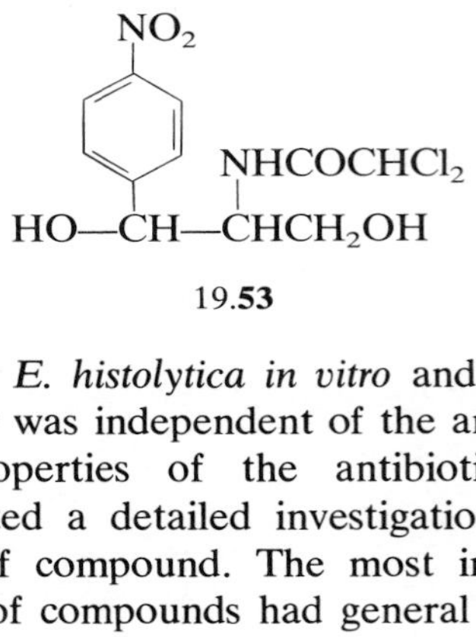

$$\text{O}_2\text{N-C}_6\text{H}_4\text{-CH(OH)-CH(NHCOCHCl}_2)\text{CH}_2\text{OH}$$

19.**53**

against *E. histolytica in vitro* and that this activity was independent of the antibacterial properties of the antibiotic (182), prompted a detailed investigation of this class of compound. The most interesting series of compounds had general structure 19.**54**.

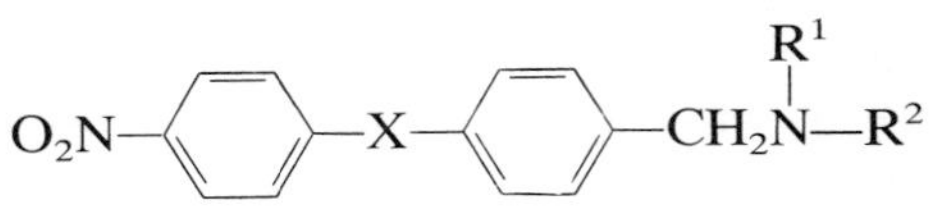

$$\text{O}_2\text{N-C}_6\text{H}_4\text{-X-C}_6\text{H}_4\text{-CH}_2\text{N(R}^1)\text{-R}^2$$

19.**54**

In this class, the most promising compounds had $X = O$ and $R^1 = CH_2CH_2OH$ or a simple variant thereof and $R^2 = COCHCl_2$. The compound with the best amebicidal activity *in vitro* and *in vivo* was 2,2-dichloro-*N*-(2-hydroxyethyl)-*N*-{(4-nitrophenoxy)-benzyl}-acetamide (19.**55**,

$O_2N-C_6H_4-O-C_6H_4-CH_2N(COCHCl_2)-CH_2CH_2OH$

19.**55**

chlorphenoxamide, clefamide, Mebinol) 183). The sulfide-linked analog of chlorphenoxamide (19.**54**, X = S; $R^1 = CH_2CH_2$-OH, $R^2 = COCHCl_2$) had *in vitro* activity similar to that of 19.**55** but was less effective in rats.

Numerous reports have confirmed the clinical efficacy of chlorphenoxamide in the treatment of intestinal amebiasis in man, and it has been proposed for use as a chemoprophylactic in endemic areas (38, 184, 185). A wide range of compounds related to chlorphenoxamide have been synthesized and tested for amebicidal activity (186–189), and the propiophenone (19.**56**) is reported to be active in the clinic against intestinal amebiasis (190, 191).

$Cl-C_6H_4-COCH(NHCOCHCl_2)CH_2Cl$

19.**56**

As a consequence of the discovery of chlorphenoxamide, a wide range of *N,N'*-disubstituted-*N,N'*-bis(2,2-dichloroacetyl)-diamines were prepared (192–194); these compounds exhibited good antiamebic properties but also possessed antispermatogenic characteristics (195, 196). It was possible to separate these properties, and the best antiamebic compound in this series proved to be 19.**57**.

$(C_2H_5)(Cl_2CHCO)N(CH_2)_{10}-N(C_2H_5)(COCHCl_2)$

19.**57**

$(CH_3CH_2OCH_2CH_2)(Cl_2CHCO)NCH_2-C_6H_4-CH_2N(CH_2CH_2OCH_2CH_3)(COCHCl_2)$

19.**58**

The replacement of the polymethylene chain by an aromatic ring led to much more important amebicidal compounds, namely, those derived from 4-aminomethylbenzylamine. The best compound proved to be *N-N'*-(4-phenylenedimethylene)bis{2, 2-dichloro-*N*-(2-ethoxyethyl)acetamide} 19.**58**, teclozan, Falmonox) (192). This compound is active against *E. histolytica in vitro* and against *E. criceti* infections in hamsters (193, 194). Detailed studies in humans have established the utility of teclozan in the treatment of acute and chronic intestinal amebiasis (197–199), and its effectiveness as a prophylactic has been reported (200).

In another series of compounds of general structure 19.**49**, where $n = 0$, it was found that compounds with R^1 = dichloromethyl, R^2 = alkyl and R^3, R^4 selected from halogen, hydroxyl, alkoxy, nitro, etc., possessed excellent *in vitro* activity against *E. histolytica* (200) but were less active against intestinal amebiasis in the rat (38). The compound most effective in rats was 2,2-dichloro-4-hydroxy-*N*-methylacetanilide (19.**59**, diloxamide, Entamide) (202–204).

$RO-C_6H_4-N(CH_3)COCHCl_2$

19.**59** R = H

19.**60** R = 2-furyl-CO—

However diloxanide was ineffective against hepatic amebiasis in hamsters (205).

Clinical trials demonstrated that although diloxanide was effective against chronic intestinal amebiasis, its activity in acute amebic dysentery and systemic amebiasis was less than desirable (38). A study was undertaken to determine whether more or less soluble derivatives of diloxanide were superior as amebicides (206). The soluble piperazinium sulfate ester was less active *in vivo* in rats than diloxanide itself, but the benzoate ester was equiactive with diloxanide in this test. More insoluble esters of diloxanide were prepared, and it was found that the 2-furoate ester (19.**60**, diloxanide furoate) was about 10 times as active as diloxanide *in vitro* and 2–4 times as active in intestinal amebiasis of the rat. Clinical trials demonstrated that diloxanide furoate was superior to diloxanide, the benzoate ester, and the piperazinium sulfate in acute amebiasis (38, 207–210). The metabolism of diloxanide and its furoate have been studied in man, and both are excreted as diloxanide glucuronide in the urine (38).

2.10 Nitroheterocyclic Compounds

2.10.1 NITROTHIAZOLES. The discovery of the antibacterial properties of the nitrofurans (211) stimulated interest in nitroheterocycles in general as chemotherapeutic agents, and soon various compounds were discovered that possessed antiparasitic activity (see Chapter 20 for details). The discovery of the potent *in vitro* and systemic trichomonicidal properties of 2-amino-5-nitrothiazole (19.**61** entramin, Enheptin) (212) resulted in the synthesis of

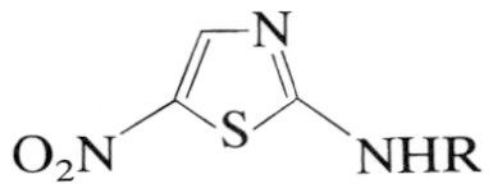

O_2N (thiazole, S, N) NHR

19.**61** R=H
19.**62** R=$COCH_3$

various simple derivatives. The most interesting compound proved to be 2-acetamido-5-nitrothiazole (19.**62**, aminitrozole, Tritheone). In addition to trichomonicidal properties, this compound was effective against intestinal amebiasis in rats and dogs (212). In a separate investigation, the clinically effective schistosomicide 1-(5-nitro-2-thiazolyl)-2-imidazolidinone (19.**63**, niridazole, Ambilhar) (213) was shown

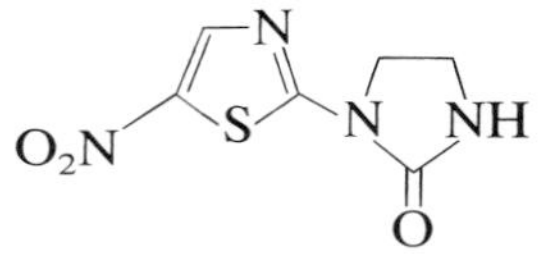

O_2N (thiazole, S, N) N NH, O

19.**63**

to be a potent systematically active amebicide (214). Niridazole is active against *E. histolytica in vitro* and is effective against intestinal amebiasis in rats and guinea pigs and hepatic amebiasis in hamsters (215).

Subsequent clinical trials have confirmed the efficacy of niridazole in the treatment of amebic dysentery and amebic liver abscess in humans (215, 217), but it must be used with care because of its side effects, which include psychoses and epileptiform fits (218). However niridazole was the first individual compound to approach the requirments of the ideal amebicide as defined in Section 1. Many other 2-amino-5-nitrothiazoles have been prepared, principally to investigate their antischistosomal properties, but they have also been examined as amebicides (219, 220).

Compound 19.**64** possesses activity similar to that of niridazole against hepatic

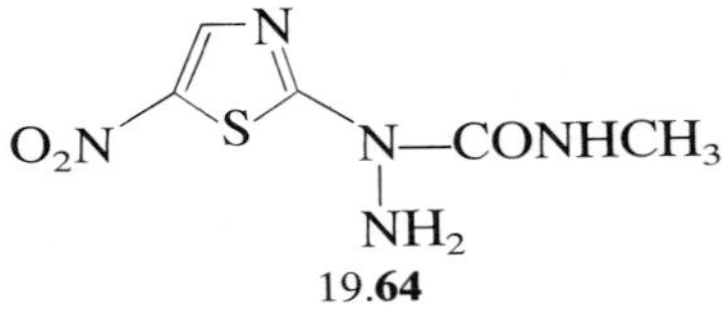

O_2N (thiazole, S, N) N—$CONHCH_3$, NH_2

19.**64**

amebiasis in hamsters and intestinal amebiasis in rats, but although relatively nontoxic to mice, its toxicity in rats precluded further development as an amebicide (221).

2.10.2 NITROIMIDAZOLES. The discovery of the antibacterial and antitrichomonal properties of the antibiotic azomycin (222) led to the investigation of nitroimidazoles as antiparasitic agents (see Chapter 20 for details). The discovery of the antitrichomonal properties of metronidazole (19.**65**,

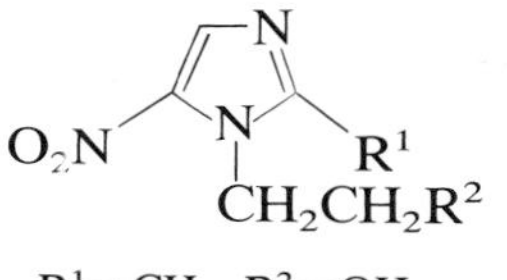

19.**65** $R^1 = CH_3$, $R^2 = OH$
19.**66** $R^1 = CH_3$, $R^2 = SO_2CH_2CH_3$
19.**67** $R^1 = H$, $R^2 =$ —N(morpholino)O
19.**68** $R^1 = CH_3$, R^2 — (pyridyl)N

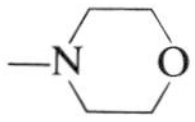

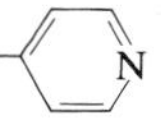

Flagyl) (223, 224) revolutionized the treatment of that disease. Although the amebicidal properties of metronidazole were described in the original paper (223), it was not tried in the clinic until some years later. In laboratory tests, metronidazole is effective against intestinal amebiasis in rats and hepatic amebiasis in hamsters and is active against *E. histolytica in vitro* (223, 224). The initial clinical trials of metronidazole indicated that it was capable of curing invasive amebic dysentery and amebic liver abscess (225) at nontoxic doses. Subsequent clinical trials have established metronidazole (Flagyl, Rhône-Poulenc) as the drug of choice in the treatment of all forms of amebiasis (4, 226–229).

Variation of the structure of metronidazole, principally to improve trichomonacidal activity and metabolic stability, led to the discovery of tinidazole (19.**66**, Fasigyn, Tricolam, Simplotan), nimorazole (19.**67**, nitrimidazine), and panidazole (19.**68**). Tinidazole (19.**66**) is active against *E. histolytica in vitro*, cecal amebiasis in rats, and hepatic amebiasis in hamsters (230, 231). Clinical trials have established the value of tinidazole in the treatment of intestinal and hepatic amebiasis in humans (232). Similarly, nimorazole (19.**67**) has been shown to possess antiamebic activity *in vitro* (233) and is claimed to be active against intestinal and hepatic amebiasis in humans (234). The metabolism of 19.**65**, 19.**66**, and 19.**67** is discussed in Chapter 20. Panidazole (19.**68**) has activity comparable to that of metronidazole against hepatic amebiasis in hamsters (235). In another variation on the structure of metronidazole, it was found that 19.**69** possessed the same

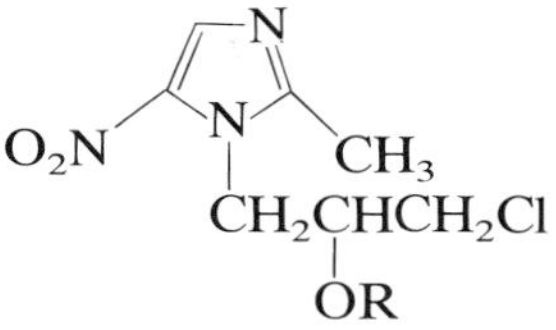

19.**69** R = H
19.**70** $R = CH_3$

spectrum of activity as metronidazole against experimental amebiasis in rats and hamsters (236–238). This compound is currently under clinical trial (239).

The corresponding methyl ether (19.**70**) also possesses antiamebic properties (240). In a paper (241) describing the most interesting nitroimidazoles prepared by the Merck organization, compounds 19.**71** (flunidazole), 19.**72** ("MF" nitroimidazole), 19.**73** ("MCA" nitroimidazole), and 19.**74**

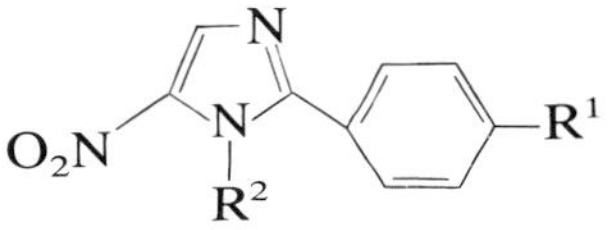

19.**71** $R^1 = F$, $R^2 = CH_2CH_2OH$
19.**72** $R^1 = F$, $R^2 = CH_3$
19.**73** $R^1 = CONH_2$, $R^2 = CH_3$

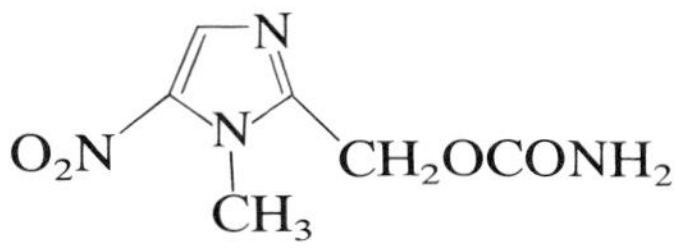

19.**74**

(ronidazole, Ridzole) were shown to be exceedingly potent amebicides *in vitro* and systemically. Although 19.**73** appears to be the most active of these compounds against experimental amebiasis in rats, 19.**71** (flunidazole, MK 910) was chosen for clinical evaluation. The clinical results with this compound were equivocal. Some clinicians (242–244) found it effective against intestinal and hepatic amebiasis in humans, whereas others (245) found it effective against amebic liver abscess but less so against the intestinal form of the disease.

In comparative tests against experimental intestinal amebiasis in rats and hepatic amebiasis in hamsters, the nitroimidazole 19.**75** was shown to be superior to most of

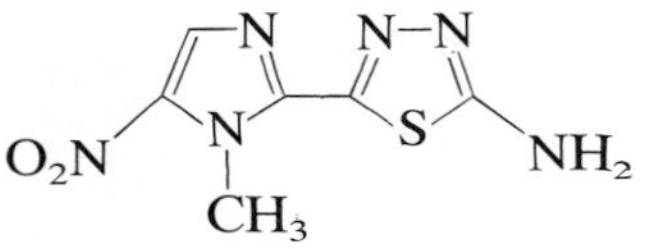

19.**75**

the standard amebicides except emetine (246). In another series of compounds it was found that the styryl imidazole derivatives 19.**76** and 19.**77** were particularly active against intestinal and hepatic amebiasis (247, 248).

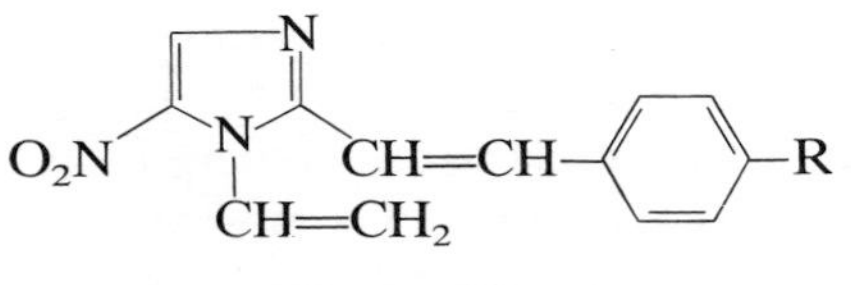

19.**76** R = CH_3
19.**77** R = CH_2OH

However neither compound has been subjected to clinical evaluation.

In two large series of nitrated bisimidazoles, it was found that 19.**78** possessed the best activity against intestinal amebiasis in rats, although a considerable number of the compounds were active against *E. histolytica in vitro* (249, 250).

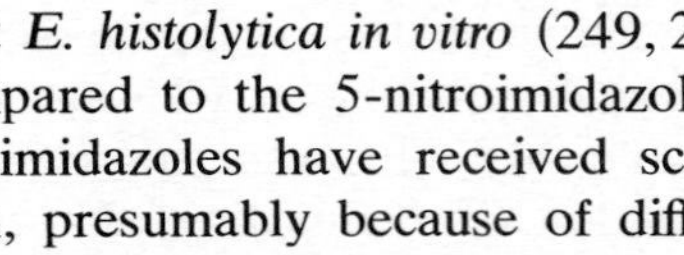

19.**78**

Compared to the 5-nitroimidazoles, the 2-nitroimidazoles have received scant attention, presumably because of difficulties in synthesis. Nevertheless, such compounds may possess useful antiprotozoal activity as shown by 19.**79** [1-(2-nitro-1-imidazolyl)-3-methoxy-2-propanol] whose activity against intestinal amebiasis in rats is similar to that of metronidazole (251, 252).

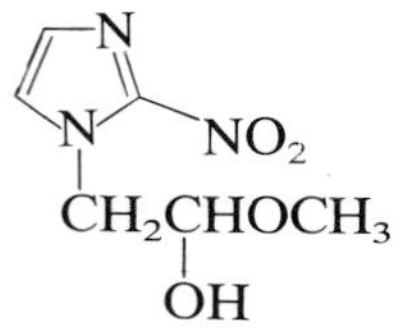

19.**79**

2.10.3 MISCELLANEOUS NITROHETEROCYCLES. Despite their wide spectrum of biological activity, the nitrofurans have claimed little attention as amebicides. Two such compounds have exhibited interesting amebicidal properties. The complex compound L(+)-*threo*-2(5-nitro-2-furyl)-5-(4-nitrophenyl)-2-oxazoline-4-methanol (19.**80**) shows good activity against intestinal amebiasis in rats and dogs (253), and 4-hydroxybenzoic acid (5-nitrofurfurylidene) hydrazide (Ercefuryl, 19.**81**) is active against amebic dysentery in man (254).

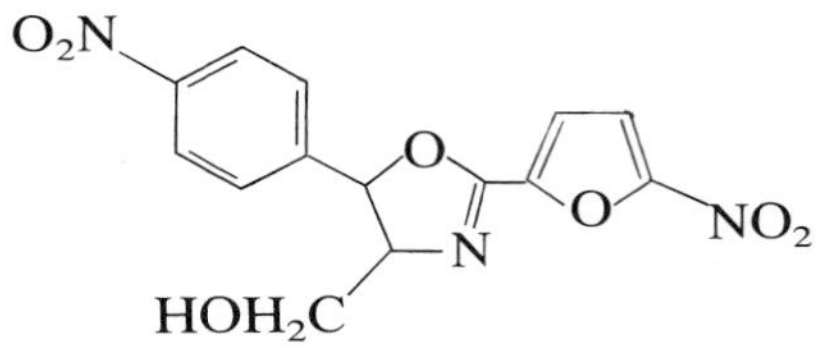

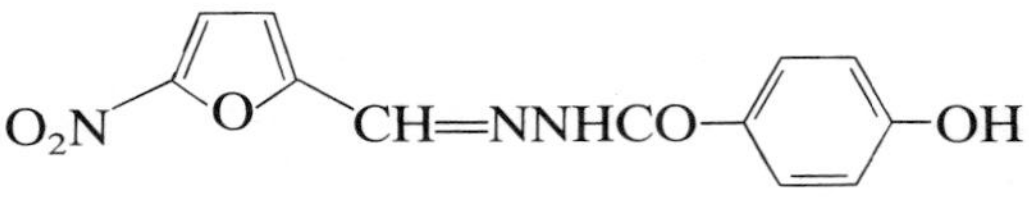

19.**80**

19.**81**

Many other nitroheterocycles have been investigated for antiamebic properties, including nitropyrroles (255) and nitropyridines (256, 257). The most interesting compound appears to be the nitropyridine 19.**82**, which was the most active of a large series, but limited clinical

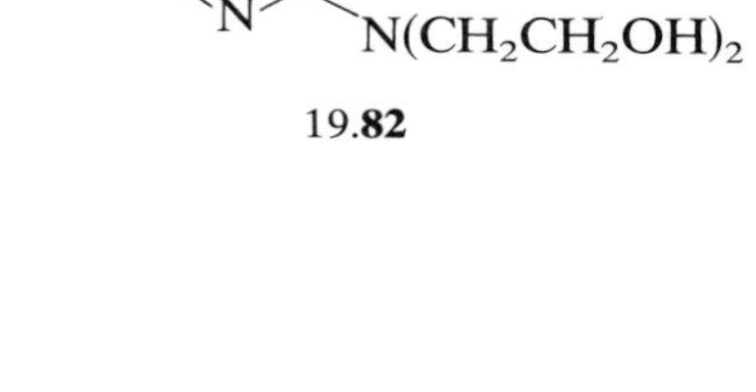

19.**82**

trials were disappointing (257). Also, the nitropyrrole 19.**83** has good activity against

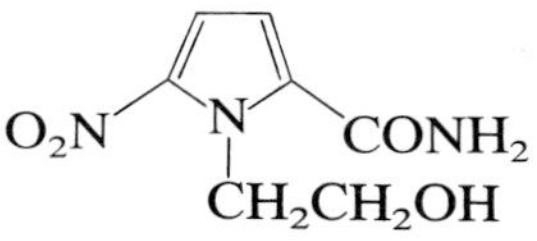

$$O_2N\text{-pyrrole}(N\text{-}CH_2CH_2OH)\text{-}CONH_2$$

19.**83**

intestinal amebiasis in rats and hepatic amebiasis in hamsters (255).

2.11 Organometallic Compounds

2.11.1 ARSENIC DERIVATIVES. Historically, organoarsenic compounds have played a significant role in the therapy of parasitic diseases, particularly trypanosomiasis (see Chapter 20 for details) and, to a lesser extent, amebiasis. Arsenical drugs have been used successfully in the treatment of intestinal amebiasis for many years but, to all intents and purposes, have been displaced by more modern and less toxic drugs.

The first arsenical to be used in treating amebiasis was 3-acetamido-4-hydroxyphenylarsonic acid (19.**84** acetarsone,

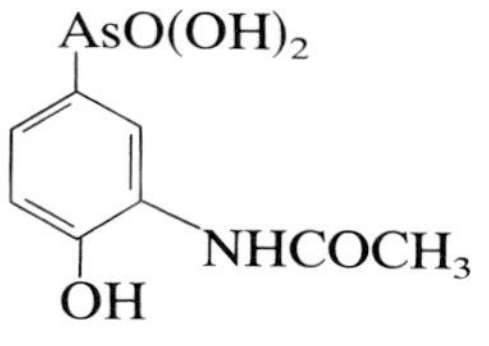

$$AsO(OH)_2\text{-}C_6H_3(NHCOCH_3)(OH)$$

19.**84**

Acetarsol, Stovarsol). This compound has poor *in vitro* activity against *E. histolytica* (258) but is effective against intestinal amebiasis in rats (259). However acetarsol is rather toxic and has fallen into disuse in the treatment of human amebiasis (1). Of more significance in the therapy of amebiasis is 4-ureidophenyl arsonic acid acid (19.**85**, carbarsone), which is still

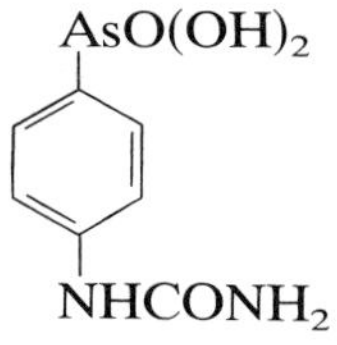

$$AsO(OH)_2\text{-}C_6H_4\text{-}NHCONH_2$$

19.**85**

available and used clinically (260). Carbarsone has poor *in vitro* activity against *E. histolytica* but is effective in large doses against intestinal amebiasis in rats (261). Clinical results with carbarsone have been variable, and the cure rate in intestinal amebiasis has not been impressive (1).

Bismuthoxy - 4 - *N* - glycolylarsanilate (19.**86**, glycobiarsol, Milibis, Wia) is active

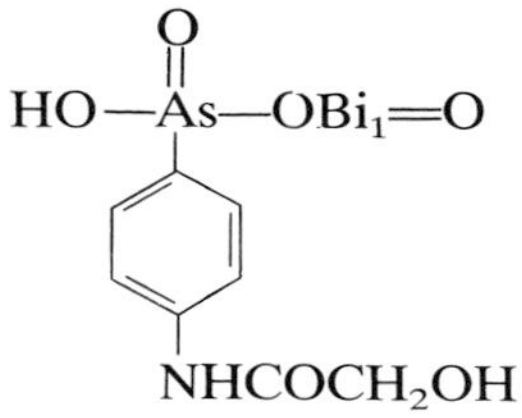

$$HO\text{—}As(=O)(\text{—}OBi_1{=}O)\text{-}C_6H_4\text{-}NHCOCH_2OH$$

19.**86**

against *E. histolytica in vitro* (262) and is effective against natural *E. criceti* infections in hamsters (262). Clinical trials showed glycobiarsol to be highly effective in subacute amebiasis in man (263).

In another variation of the carbarsone molecule, the dimeric structure, bis(4-arsonophenylamino)-1,2-ethane (19.**87**, diphetarsene, Bémarsal) was found to be clinically effective against intestinal infections (264).

The combination of a sulfonamide and a pentavalent arsenic moiety in one compound produced the interesting compound sulfarside (19.**88**), which is effective against

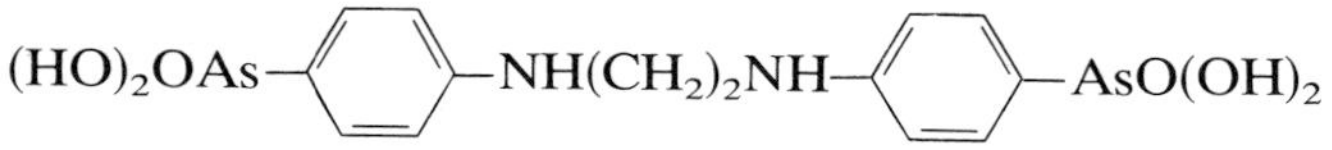

$$(HO)_2OAs\text{-}C_6H_4\text{-}NH(CH_2)_2NH\text{-}C_6H_4\text{-}AsO(OH)_2$$

19.**87**

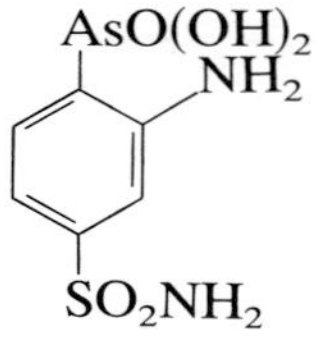

19.**88**

experimental amebiasis in rats (265) and intestinal amebiasis in man (266).

Trivalent arsenic compounds are more toxic than the corresponding pentavalent compounds but generally are more active against parasites. Various trivalent arsenicals, such as carbarsone oxide (19.**89**) and the thioarsenites 19.**90** and 19.**91**, have

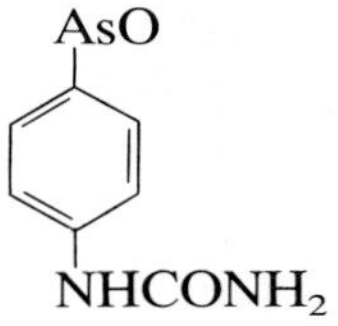

19.**89** 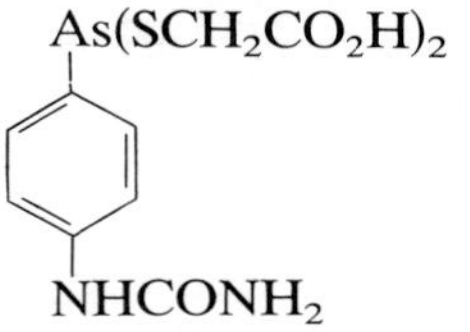 19.**90**

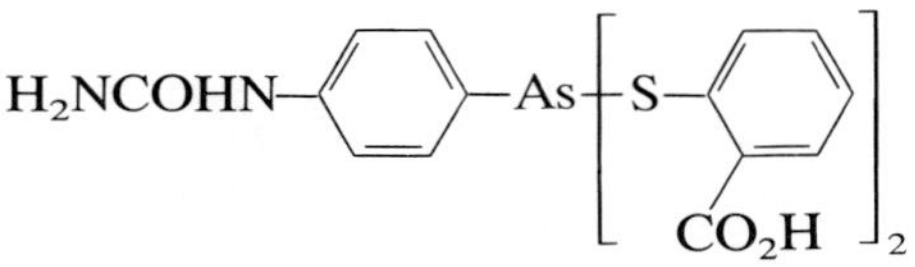

19.**91**

been investigated as amebicides but have never enjoyed widespread use.

Probably the most interesting of these compounds is arsthinol (19.**92**, balarsen),

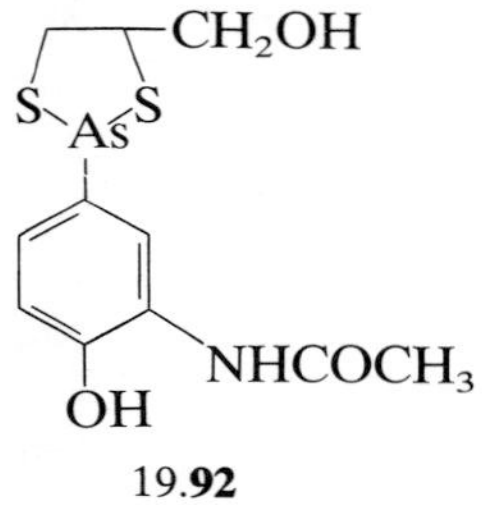

19.**92**

which proved to be effective against intestinal amebiasis in man (267, 268).

Many other arsenical compounds possess antiamebic activity but are not in clinical use (1).

2.11.2 ANTIMONY DERIVATIVES. Although useful in other protozoal infections, the antimonials have played little part in the chemotherapy of amebiasis. However one compound, 2-carboxymethylmercaptobenzene stibonic acid (19.**93**), is active against

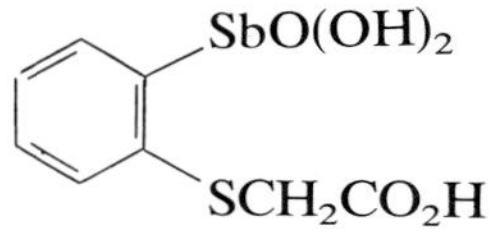

19.**93**

E. histolytica in vitro and against intestinal amebiasis in rats (269). Clinical efficacy was demonstrated against intestinal amebiasis, but untoward side effects were observed (270).

REFERENCES

1. G. Woolfe, in *Experimental Chemotherapy*, Vol. 1, R. J. Schnitzer and F. Hawking, Eds., Academic Press, New York, 1963, pp. 355–443.
2. Anonymous, *Amoebiasis, World Health Organization Technical Report Series* No. 421 (1969).
3. R. Eldson-Dew, in *Advances in Parasitology*, Vol. 6, B. Dawes, Ed., Academic Press, New York, 1968, pp. 1–62.
4. B. K. Vakil and N. J. Dalal, in Vol. 18, *Progress in Drug Research*, E. Jucker, Ed., Birkhäuser-Verlag, Basel, 1974, pp. 353–364.
5. J. W. Reinertson and P. E. Thompson, *Proc. Soc. Exp. Biol. Med.*, **76,** 518–521 (1951).
6. E. B. Vedder, *J. Trop. Med.*, **15,** 313 (1912).
7. L. Rogers, *Brit. Med. J.*, **1,** 1424 (1912).
8. M. Pailer and K. Porschinski, *Monatsh. Chem.*, **80,** 94 (1949).
9. A. R. Battersby and H. T. Openshaw, *J. Chem. Soc.*, 3207–3216 (1949).
10. A. R. Battersby, R. Binks, and G. C. Davidson, *J. Chem. Soc.*, 2704–2711 (1959).
11. A. R. Battersby and S. Garratt, *J. Chem. Soc.*, 3512–3521 (1959).
12. A. Brossi, A. Cohen, J. M. Osbond, P. Plattner, O. Schnider, and J. C. Wickens, *J. Chem. Soc.*, 3630–3632 (1959).
13. A. Brossi, Z. Brener, J. Pellegrino, H. Stohler, and J. R. Frey, *Experientia*, **16,** 62 (1960).
14. H. T. Openshaw and N. Whittaker, *J. Chem. Soc.*, 1461–1471 (1963).
15. M. Barash, J. M. Osbond, and J. C. Wickens, *J. Chem. Soc.*, 3530–3543 (1959).

16. D. E. Clark, R. F. K. Meredith, A. C. Ritchie, and T. Walker, *J. Chem. Soc.*, 2490–2499 (1962).

17. A. Brossi, Z. Brener, J. Pellegrino, H. Stohler, and J. R. Frey, *Experientia*, **16,** 62 (1960).

18. See Ref. 13.

19. W. Balamuth and A. Lasslo, *Proc. Soc. Exp. Biol. Med.*, **80,** 705 (1952).

20. M. Barash and J. M. Osbond, *J. Chem. Soc.*, 2157–2168 (1959).

21. H. T. Openshaw, N. C. Robson, and N. Whittaker, *J. Chem. Soc. C*, 101–105 (1969).

22. A. Brossi, *Pure Appl. Chem.*, **19,** 77–88 (1969).

23. A. C. Ritchie, D. R. Preston, T. Walker, and K. D. E. Whiting, *J. Chem. Soc.*, 3385–3393 (1962).

24. A. P. Grollman, *Proc. Nat. Acad. Sci., US*, **56,** 1867 (1966).

25. T. A. Henry, *The Plant Alkaloids*, 4th ed., Blakiston, Philadelphia, 1949.

26. D. Herbst, R. Rees, G. A. Hughes, and H. Smith, *J. Med. Chem.*, **9,** 864–868 (1966).

27. J. P. Yardley, R. Rees, and H. Smith, *J. Med. Chem.*, **10,** 1088–1091 (1967).

28. A. Brossi, M. Baumann, and O. Schnider, *Helv. Chim. Acta*, **42,** 1515–1522 (1959).

29. A. Brossi, M. Baumann, L. H. Chopard-dit-Jean, J. Würsch, F. Schneider, and O. Schnider, *Helv. Chim. Acta*, **42,** 772–788 (1959).

30. A. Brossi and F. Burkhardt, *Experientia*, **18,** 211–212 (1962).

31. A. Brossi, M. Baumann, F. Burkhardt, R. Richle, and J. R. Frey, *Helv. Chim. Acta*, **45,** 2219–2226 (1962).

32. D. E. Clark, P. G. Holton, R. F. K. Meredith, A. C. Ritchie, T. Walker, and K. D. E. Whiting, *J. Chem. Soc.*, 2479–2490 (1962).

33. H. H. Salem, Z. G. Hayatee, A. M. Awaness, and G. Al-Allaf, *Trans. Roy. Soc. Trop. Med. Hyg.*, **62,** 406–412 (1968).

34. J. Herrero, A. Brossi, M. Faust, and J. R. Frey, *Ann. Biochem. Exp. Med.*, **20** (Suppl.), 475–480 (1960).

35. F. Blanc, Y. Nosny, M. Armengaud, M. Sankale, M. Martin, and G. Charmot, *Presse Med.*, **69,** 1548–1550 (1961).

36. D. E. Schwartz and J. Herrero, *Am. J. Trop. Med. Hyg.*, **14,** 78–83 (1965).

37. R. Johnson and R. A. Neal, *Ann. Trop. Med. Parasitol.*, **62,** 455–461 (1968).

38. G. Woolf, in *Progress in Drug Research*, Vol. 8, E. Jucker, Ed., Birkhäuser-Verlag, Basel, 1965, pp. 13–52.

39. A. P. Grollman, *J. Biol. Chem.*, **243,** 4089–4094 (1968).

40. N. Entner and A. P. Grollman, *J. Protozool.*, **20,** 160–163 (1973).

41. A. P. Grollman, *Science*, **157,** 84–85 (1967).

42. D. M. Hall, S. Mahboob, and E. E. Turner, *J. Chem. Soc.*, 1956–1957 (1952).

43. W. A. Beppler and L. B. Schweiger, *Antibiotics Chemother.*, **7,** 513–520 (1957).

44. H. H. Anderson and E. Hansen, *Pharmacol. Rev.*, **2,** 399–439 (1950).

45. J. H. Chapman, P. G. Holton, A. C. Ritchie, T. Walker, G. B. Webb, and K. D. E. Whiting, *J. Chem. Soc.*, 2471–2479 (1962).

46. J. A. Goodson, L. G. Goodwin, J. H. Gorvin, M. D. Goss, K. S. Kirby, J. A. Lock, R. A. Neal, T. M. Sharp, and W. Solomon, *Brit. J. Pharmacol.*, **3,** 49–62 (1948), and references cited therein.

47. B. Bailey, R. D. Haworth, and J. McKenna, *J. Chem. Soc.*, 967–976 (1954).

48. R. D. Haworth, J. McKenna, R. G. Powell, and G. H. Whitfield, *J. Chem. Soc.*, 1115–1129 (1953).

49. R. D. Haworth, J. McKenna, and G. H. Whitfield, *J. Chem. Soc.*, 1110–1115 (1953).

50. R. D. Haworth, J. McKenna, and G. H. Whitfield, *J. Chem. Soc.*, 1102–1110 (1953).

51. M. Alain, E. Massal, R. Tonzin, and L. Porte, *Med. Trop.*, **9,** 5 (1949).

52. C. Durieux, J. Trenous, F. Tanguy, C. Robin, and A. Raoult, *Med. Trop.*, **8,** 7–21 (1948).

53. J. Soulage, *Med. Trop.*, **9,** 39 (1949).

54. R. Crosnier, *Bull. Soc. Pathol. Exot.*, **45,** 86 (1952).

55. O. Stephenson, *Brit. J. Pharmacol.*, **3,** 237–242 (1948).

56. J. Druey, *Ann. Biochem. Exp. Med.*, **20** (Suppl.), 423 (1960).

57. D. P. Dodgson and R. D. Haworth, *J. Chem. Soc.*, 67–71 (1952).

58. J. McConnel, V. Petrow, and B. Sturgeon, *J. Chem. Soc.*, 3332–3334 (1953).

59. D. J. Taylor and J. Greenberg, *Am. J. Hyg.*, **56,** 58–60 (1952).

60. A. C. Cuckler, S. Kuna, C. W. Mushett, R. H. Silber, R. B. Stebbins, H. C. Stoerk, R. N. Arison, F. Cuchie, and C. M. Malanga, *Arch. Int. Pharmacodyn.*, **114,** 307–321 (1958).

61. A. C. Cuckler and C. C. Smith, *Fed. Proc.*, **8,** 284 (1949).

62. B. P. Phillips, *Am. J. Trop. Med.*, **31,** 561–565 (1951).

63. G. Kartha and D. J. Haas, *J. Am. Chem. Soc.*, **86,** 3630–3634 (1964).
64. F. van Assendelft, J. W. Miller, D. T. Mintz, J. A. Schlack, P. Ottolenghi, and H. Most, *Am. J. Trop. Med. Hyg.*, **5,** 501–503 (1956).
65. A. Woodruff, S. Bell, and D. Schofield, *Trans. Roy. Soc. Trop. Med. Hyg.*, **50,** 114 (1956).
66. E. C. del Pozo and M. Alcaraz, *Am. J. Med.*, **20,** 412–414 (1956).
67. Z. Valenta, A. H. Gray, D. E. Orr, S. F. Papadopoulos, and C. Podesva, *Tetrahedron*, **18,** 1433 (1962).
68. N. Amin, M. Mahfouz, and M. A. F. Sheif, *Quart. J. Pharm. Pharmacol.*, **18,** 116–121 (1945).
69. T. Geissmann, *Ann. Rev. Pharmacol.*, **4,** 305–316 (1964).
70. W. C. Kuzell, W. B. Layton, W. D. Frick, and W. C. Cutting, *Am. J. Trop. Med.*, **21,** 731–738 (1941).
71. W. Stocklin and T. A. Geissman, *Tetrahedron Lett.*, 6007–6010 (1968).
72. T. V. Subbiah and A. H. Amin, *Nature* (London), **215,** 527–528 (1967).
73. M. E. Hanke and S. M. Talant, *Trans. Roy. Soc. Trop. Med. Hyg.*, **55,** 56 (1961).
74. M. Martin, J. Ridet, A. Chartol, J. Biot, L. Porte, and A. Bezon, *Med. Trop.*, **24,** 250 (1964). See *Trop. Dis. Bull.*, **61,** 1215 (1964).
75. P. Couderc, *Belgian Patent* No. 605, 440 (1961).
76. M. S. Kiang, T. L. Chiang, T. C. Fang, and F. H. Yu, *Chem. Abstr.*, **53,** 11646 (1949).
77. W. H. Hargreaves, *Lancet*, **2,** 68 (1945).
78. V. McVay, R. L. Laird, and D. H. Sprunt, *Science*, **109,** 590–592 (1949).
79. T. G. Armstrong, A. J. Wilmot, and R. Elsdon-Dew, *Lancet*, **2,** 10 (1950).
80. H. Most and F. Van Assendelft, *Ann. N.Y. Acad. Sci.*, **53,** 427 (1950).
81. E. F. Elslager, in *Medicinal Chemistry*, Part I; 3rd ed., A. Burger, Ed., Wiley, New York, 1970, pp. 535–540.
82. M. C. McCowen, M. E. Callender, T. Rennell, and J. F. Lawliss, *J. Science*, **113,** 202–203 (1951).
83. H. H. Anderson, A. K. Hrenoff, J. Van D. Anderson, M. Nakamura, and A. N. Contopoulous, *Am. J. Trop. Med. Hyg.*, **1,** 552–558 (1952).
84. E. J. Corey and B. Snider, *J. Am. Chem. Soc.*, **94,** 2549–2550 (1972).
85. R. T. Shillings and C. P. Schaffner, *Antimicrob. Agents Chemother.*, 274–285 (1961).
86. G. L. Coffey, L. E. Anderson, M.-W. Fisher, M. M. Galbraith, A. B. Hillegas, D. L. Krohberger, P. E. Thompson, K. S. Weston, and J. Ehrlich, *Antibiot. Chemother.*, **9,** 730–738 (1959).
87. P. E. Thompson, A. Bayles, S. F. Herbst, B. Olszewski, and J. E. Meisenhelder, *Antibiot. and Chemother.*, **9,** 618–626 (1959).
88. K. O. Courtney, P. E. Thompson, R. Hodgkinson, and J. R. Fitzsimmons, *Ann. Biochem. Exp. Med.*, **20,** 449 (1960).
89. K. O. Courtney, P. E. Thompson, R. Hodgkinson, and J. R. Fitzsimmons, *Antibiot. Ann.*, 304 (1959–1960).
90. E. D. Wagner and H. S. Burnett, *Trans. Roy. Soc. Trop. Med. Hyg.*, **55,** 428 (1961).
91. S. Bell and A. W. Woodruff, *Am. J. Trop. Med. Hyg.*, **9,** 155–157 (1960).
92. C. H. Carter, A. Bayles, and P. E. Thompson, *J. Trop. Med. Hyg.*, **11,** 448 (1962).
93. A. P. Grollman, *J. Biol. Chem.*, **242,** 3226–3233 (1967).
94. J. E. Lynch, A. R. English, H. Bauck, and H. Deligianis, *Antibiot. Chemother.*, **4,** 844 (1954).
95. J. E. Lynch, E. C. Holley, and J. E. Margison, *Antibiot. Chemother.*, **5,** 508 (1955).
96. B. A. Sobin and F. W. Tanner, *J. Am. Chem. Soc.*, **76,** 4053 (1954).
97. J. J. Beereboom, K. Butler, F. C. Pennington, and I. A. Solomons, *J. Org. Chem.*, **30,** 2334–2342 (1965).
98. J. P. Schaefer and P. J. Wheatley, *J. Org. Chem.*, **33,** 166–169 (1968).
99. M. Nabil Aboul-Enein, M. Khalifa, and S. M. El-Difrawy, *Pharm. Acta Helv.*, **48,** 405–411 (1973).
100. M. Kettner, *J. Antibiot.* (Tokyo), **26,** 692–969 (1973).
101. D. Loebenkerg, M. Counelis, and J. A. Waitz, *Antimicrob. Agents Chemother.*, **7,** 811–815 (1975).
102. T. Miura, *J. Antibiot.* (Tokyo), **26,** 528–530 (1973).
102. W. Leimgruber, A. D. Batcho, and F. Schenker, *J. Am. Chem. Soc.*, 87, 5793–5795 (1965).
104. E. Grunberg, H. N. Prince, E. Titsworth, G. Beskid, and M. D. Tendler, *Chemotherapia*, **11,** 249–260 (1966).
105. A. Küster, *Klin. Wochenschr.*, **41,** 1125 (1904).
106. P. Mühlens and W. Menk, *Münch. Med. Wochenschr.*, **68,** 802 (1921).
107. H. H. Anderson, N. A. David, and D. A. Koch, *Proc. Soc. Exp. Biol. Med.*, **28,** 484 (1931).
108. H. H. Anderson and D. A. Koch, *Proc. Soc. Exp. Biol. Med.*, **28,** 838 (1931).

109. A. C. Tenney, *Ill. Med. J.*, **70,** 145 (1936).

110. P. E. Thompson, J. W. Reinertson, A. Bayles, D. A. McCarthy, and E. F. Elslager, *Am. J. Trop. Med. Hyg.*, **4,** 224–228 (1955).

111. See Ref. 44.

112. G. M. Findlay, *Recent Advances in Chemotherapy*, 3rd ed., Vol. 1, Churchill, London, 1950, pp. 191–233.

113. H. Wenger, *Indian J. Med. Sci.*, **6,** 246–249 (1952).

114. M. Payet, P. Pene, Rouget-Campana, and C. Barthe, *Bull. Med. A.O.F.*, **10,** 165 (1953).

115. J. H. Burckhalter and W. H. Edgerton, *J. Am. Chem. Soc.*, **73,** 4837–4839 (1951).

116. A. F. Helin and C. A. Van der Werf, *J. Org. Chem.*, **17,** 229–232 (1952).

117. W. H. Edgerton and J. H. Burckhalter, *J. Am. Chem. Soc.*, **74,** 5209–5210 (1952).

118. J. H. Burckhalter, W. S. Bringar, and P. E. Thompson, *J. Org. Chem.*, **26,** 4070–4078 (1961).

119. P. E. Thompson, A. Bayles, P. McCloy, and J. E. Meisenhelder, *J. Parasitol.*, **51,** 817 (1965).

120. R. Hugenot, E. Granotier, and J. P. Farges, *Thérapie*, **20,** 329 (1965).

121. L. S. Grant, E. A. Belle, and C. Ramprashad, *W. Indian Med. J.*, **17,** 31 (1968).

122. R. Cavier and F. Gandon, *Thérapie*, **18,** 1153 (1963).

123. F. Fernandez, *Semana Med. Mex.*, **49,** 328 (1966).

124. N. G. Latour and R. E. Reeves, *Exp. Parasitol.*, **17,** 203 (1965).

125. F. Schenker, R. A. Schmidt, W. Leimgruber, and A. Brossi, *J. Med. Chem.*, **9,** 46–48 (1966).

126. J. S. Tandon, R. N. Iyer, and R. Gopalachari, *Ann. Biochem. Exp. Med.* (Calcutta) (Suppl.), **20,** 505 (1960).

127. P. E. Thompson and J. W. Reinertson, *Am. J. Trop. Med.*, **31,** 707–717 (1951).

128. G. A. H. Williams, *Brit. J. Pharmacol.*, **14,** 488–492 (1959).

129. L. Pfannemueller, *Lancet*, **1,** 934 (1956) and references cited therein.

130. D. A. Berberian, E. W. Dennis, R. Korns, and D. Angelo, *J. Am. Med. Assoc.*, **148,** 700 (1952).

131. E. W. Dennis, D. A. Berberian, and S. S. Hansen, *Am. J. Trop. Med.*, **29,** 683 (1949).

132. E. A. Steck and L. T. Fletcher, *J. Org. Chem.*, **24,** 701 (1959).

133. M. V. Rubtsov, G. N. Pershin, N. A. Yanbaktin, L. A. Pelenitsina, T. J. Gurevich, N. A. Novitskaya, S. N. Milovanova, and S. A. Vickkavova, *J. Med. Pharm. Chem.*, **2,** 113 (1960).

134. E. F. Elslager and F. M. Tendick, *J. Med. Pharm. Chem.*, **5,** 1149 (1962).

135. E. F. Elslager, R. E. Bowman, F. H. Tendick, D. J. Tivey, and D. F. Worth, *J. Med. Pharm. Chem.*, **5,** 1159 (1962).

136. E. F. Elslager, F. W. Short, and F. H. Tendick, *J. Heterocycl. Chem.*, **5,** 599 (1968).

137. E. F. Elslager and F. H. Tendick, *J. Med. Pharm. Chem.*, **5,** 646 (1962).

138. E. F. Elslager, *J. Org. Chem.*, **27,** 4346 (1962).

139. E. F. Elslager, E. H. Gold, F. H. Tendick, L. M. Werbel, and D. F. Worth, *J. Heterocycl. Chem.*, **1,** 6 (1964).

140. N. B. Ackerman, D. K. Haldorsen, F. H. Tendick, and E. F. Elslager, *J. Med. Chem.*, **11,** 315 (1968).

141. E. F. Elslager and D. F. Worth, *J. Med. Chem.*, **12,** 955 (1969).

142. E. F. Elslager, A. Moore, F. W. Short, M. J. Sullivan, and F. H. Tendick, *J. Am. Chem. Soc.*, **79,** 4699 (1957).

143. F. W. Short, E. F. Elslager, A. M. Moore, M. J. Sullivan, and F. H. Tendick, *J. Am. Chem. Soc.*, **80,** 223 (1958).

144. E. F. Elslager, F. W. Short, M. J. Sullivan, and F. H. Tendick, *J. Am. Chem. Soc.*, **80,** 451–455 (1958).

145. P. E. Thompson, D. A. McCarthy, J. W. Reinertson, A. Bayles, and H. Najarian, *Antibiot. Chemother.*, **8,** 37 (1958).

146. R. A. Radke, *Gastroenterology*, **36,** 509 (1959).

147. A. J. Wilmot, S. J. Powell, I. MacLeod, and R. Elsdon-Dew, *Ann. Trop. Med. Parasitol.*, **56,** 303 (1962).

148. See Ref. 141.

149. J. H. Burckhalter, F. H. Tendick, E. M. Jones, W. F. Holcomb, and A. L. Rawlins, *J. Am. Chem. Soc.*, **68,** 1894 (1946).

150. P. E. Thompson, J. W. Reinertson, D. A. McCarthy, A. Bayles, and A. R. Cook, *Antibiotic. Chemother.*, **5,** 433 (1955).

151. D. M. Forsyth, *Trans. Roy. Soc. Trop. Med. Hyg.*, **56,** 400 (1962).

152. H. Barrios, *Gastroenterology*, **27,** 81 (1954).

153. R. V. Taylor, *Am. J. Gastroenterology*, **26,** 713 (1956) and references cited therein.

154. E. L. Elslager and F. H. Tendick, *J. Med. Pharm. Chem.*, **5,** 646 (1962).

155. J. H. Burckhalter, R. I. Leib, Y. S. Chough, and R. F. Tietz, *J. Med. Chem.*, **6,** 89 (1963).

156. P. Schmidt and J. Druey, *Helv. Chim. Acta*, **40,** 350 (1957).
157. F. Kradolfer and L. Neipp, *Antibiot. Chemother.*, **8,** 297 (1958).
158. P. Sen and N. Sanyal, *Bull. Calcutta School Trop. Med.*, **4,** 81 (1956).
159. S. Sen, A. Mukherjee, N. Sanyal, G. N. Sen, and H. N. Ray, *Bull. Calcutta School Trop. Med.*, **3,** 75 (1955).
160. N. Das, *J. Indian Med. Assoc.*, **31,** 355 (1958).
161. P. K. Chatterjee, S. Mucherjee, S. Ghose, K. P. Dalta, and S. Sircar, *J. Indian Med. Assoc.*, **30,** 251 (1958).
162. P. K. Chatterjee, *Ann. Biochem. Exp. Med.* (Calcutta) (Suppl.), **20,** 471 (1960).
163. P. K. Ghosh and S. Gupta, *Ann. Biochem. Exp. Med.* (Calcutta) (Suppl.), **20,** 461 (1960).
164. J. G. Parekh and B. D. Patel, *Ann. Biochem. Exp. Med.* (Calcutta) (Suppl.), **20,** 465 (1960).
165. J. Druey, *Ann. Biochem. Exp. Med.* (Calcutta) (Suppl.), **20,** 423 (1960).
166. E. W. Dennis and D. A. Berberian, *Antibiot. Chemother.*, **4,** 554 (1954).
167. A. R. Surrey and R. A. Cutler, *J. Am. Chem. Soc.*, **76,** 578 (1954).
168. A. R. Surrey, *J. Am. Chem. Soc.*, **76,** 2214–2216 (1954).
169. A. R. Surrey and M. K. Rukwid, *J. Am. Chem. Soc.*, **77,** 3798–3801 (1955).
170. A. R. Surrey, G. Y. Lesher, and S. O. Winthrop, *J. Am. Chem. Soc.*, **77,** 5406–5408 (1955).
171. A. R. Surrey and G. Y. Lesher, *J. Am. Chem. Soc.*, **78,** 2573–2576 (1956).
172. A. R. Surrey, A. J. Olivet, S. O. Winthrop, and G. Y. Lesher, *J. Am. Chem. Soc.*, **78,** 3834–3836 (1956).
173. A. R. Surrey, S. O. Winthrop, M. K. Rukwid, and B. F. Tullar, *J. Am. Chem. Soc.*, **77,** 633–641 (1955).
174. V. D. Nosina, V. F. Gladkikh, and O. I. Kellina, *Med. Parazitol. Parazitar. Bolezn.* **25,** 252 (1956), *Chem. Abstr.*, **51,** 5297b (1957).
175. G. Woolfe, *Trans. Roy. Soc. Trop. Med. Hyg.*, **51,** 320 (1957).
176. E. F. Elslager, E. L. Benton, F. W. Short, and F. H. Tendick, *J. Am. Chem. Soc.*, **78,** 3453 (1956).
177. E. H. Loughlin and W. G. Mullin, *Antibiot. Chemother.*, **4,** 570 (1954).
178 G. McHardy, G. E. Welch, D. C. Browne, J. E. Blum, and R. J. McHardy, *Antibiot. Ann.* (1954–1955), 863 (1955).
179. R. D. Ganatra, N. A. Paralker, and R. A. Lewis, *Antibiot. Med. Clin. Ther.*, **3,** 253 (1956).
180. D. A. A. Kidd and D. E. Wright, *J. Chem. Soc.*, 1420 (1962).
181. D. A. A. Kidd and G. H. Smith, *Brit. J. Pharmacol.*, **18,** 128 (1962).
182. I. de Carneri, *Farmaco* (Pavia), **11,** 926 (1956).
183. W. Logeman, L. Almirante, and I. de Carneri, *Farmaco* (Pavia), *Ed. Sci.*, **13,** 139 (1957).
184. I. de Carneri, G. Coppi, L. Almirante, and W. Logemann, *Trans. Roy. Soc. Trop. Med. Hyg.*, **53,** 120 (1959).
185. I. de Carneri, *Bull. W.H.O.*, **23,** 103 (1960).
186. I. de Carneri, *Z. Tropenmed. Parasitol.*, **9,** 32 (1958).
187. W. Logemann, L. Almirante, and I. de Carneri, *Farmaco* (Pavia) *Ed. Sci.*, **13,** 139 (1958).
188. W. Logemann, F. Lauria, G. Tosolini, and I. de Carneri, *Farmaco* (Pavia) *Ed. Sci.*, **13,** 129 (1958).
189. W. Logemann, L. Almirante, S. Galimberte, and I. de Carneri, *Brit. J. Pharmacol.*, **17,** 286 (1961).
190. J. R. Shah, B. M. Amin, and E. Bonvini, *Indian J. Med. Sci.*, **12,** 655 (1958).
191. S. P. Mehta, F. T. Padoria, U. S. Shah, and M. M. Rathi, *J. Indian Med. Assoc.*, **32,** 197 (1959).
192. A. R. Surrey and J. R. Mayer, *J. Med. Pharm. Chem.*, **3,** 409, 419 (1961).
193. D. A. Berberian, R. G. Slighter, and A. R. Surrey, *Antibiot. Chemother.*, **11,** 245 (1961).
194. D. A. Berberian, R. G. Slighter, and E. W. Dennis, *Am. J. Trop. Med. Hyg.*, **10,** 503 (1961).
195. F. Coulston, A. L. Beyler, and H. P. Drobeck, *Toxicol. Appl. Pharmacol.*, **3,** 1 (1961).
196. A. L. Beyler, G. O. Potts, F. Coulston, and A. R. Surrey, *Endocrinology*, **69,** 819 (1961).
197. A. Moura Simas and H. L. Ferreira, *Hosp. Rio de Janeiro*, **62,** 1343 (1962).
198. R. Reis Goncalves and O. Miller, *Hosp. Rio de Janeiro*, **63,** 1305 (1963).
199. J. O. Machada, S. Silva, and F. J. R. Gomes, *Hosp. Rio de Janeiro*, **72,** 53 (1967).
200. R. D. Botero and H. Zuluaga, *Abstracts, Eighth International Congress on Tropical Medicine and Malaria*, Teheran 1968, p. 1176.
201. N. W. Bristow, P. Oxley, G. A. M. Williams, and G. Woolfe, *Trans. Roy. Soc. Trop. Med. Hyg.*, **50,** 182 (1956).
202. N. W. Bristow, P. Oxley, G. A. H. Williams, and G. Woolfe, *Trans. Roy. Soc. Trop. Med. Hyg.*, **50,** 182 (1956).
204. G. Woolfe, R. P. Everest, G. A. H. Williams, and E. C. Wilmshurst, *Trans. Roy. Soc. Trop. Med. Hyg.*, **61,** 427 (1967).

205. See Ref. 128.
206. P. T. Main, N. W. Bristow, P. Oxley, T. I. Watkins, G. A. H. Williams, E. C. Wilmshurst, and G. Woolfe, *Ann. Biochem. Exp. Med.*, **20,** 441 (1960).
207. A. W. Woodruff and S. Bell, *Trans. Roy. Soc. Trop. Med. Hyg.*, **54,** 389 (1960).
208. P. D. Marsden, *Trans. Roy. Soc. Trop. Med. Hyg.*, **54,** 396 (1960).
209. L. B. Nevill, *Trans. Roy. Soc. Trop. Med. Hyg.*, **56,** 81 (1962).
210. S. Bell, *Trans. Roy. Soc. Trop. Med. Hyg.*, **61,** 506 (1967).
211. M. C. Dodd and W. Stillman, *H. Pharmacol. Exp. Ther.*, **82,** 11 (1944).
212. A. C. Cuckler, A. B. Kupferberg, and N. Millman, *Antibiot. Chemother.*, **5,** 540–550 (1955).
213. C. R. Lambert, M. Wilhelm, H. Striebel, F. Kradolfer, and P. Schmidt, *Experientia*, **20,** 452 (1964).
214. F. Kradolfer and R. Jarumilinta, *Ann. Trop. Med. Parasitol.*, **59,** 210–302 (1965).
215. S. J. Powell, I. McLeod, A. J. Wilmot, and R. Elsdon-Dew, *Acta Trop. Suppl. 9,* 95–101, (1966).
216. R. Hugonot and S. Delons, *Acta Trop. Suppl. 9,* 110–119 (1966).
217. R. Jarumilinta, *Acta Trop. Suppl. 9,* 102–109 (1966).
218. See Ref. 2.
219. M. Avramoff, S. Adler, and A. Foner, *J. Med. Chem.*, **10,** 1138–1143 (1967).
220. L. M. Werbel, E. F. Elslager, A. A. Phillips, D. F. Worth, P. J. Islip, and M. C. Neville, *J. Med. Chem.*, **12,** 521–524 (1969).
221. S. S. Berg and M. P. Toft, *Eur. J. Med. Chem.*, **10,** 268–272 (1975).
222. C. Cosar and L. Julon, *Ann. Inst. Pasteur*, **96,** 238 (1959).
223. C. Cosar, P. Ganter, and L. Julon, *Presse Med.*, **69,** 1069 (1961).
224. C. Cosar, C. Cusan, R. Horclois, R. M. Jacob, J. Robert, S. Tchelitcheff, and R. Vaupré, *Arzneim.-Forsch.*, **16,** 23–29 (1966).
225. S. J. Powell, I. McLeod, A. J. Wilmot, and R. Elsdon-Dew, *Lancet*, **2,** 1329 (1966).
226. S. J. Powell, in *Current Therapy*, H. F. Conn. Ed., Saunders, Philadelphia, 1969, pp. 3–6.
227. S. J. Powell, *Bull. N.Y. Acad. Med.*, **47,** 469–477 (1971).
228. R. B. Khambatta, *Ann. Trop. Med. Parasitol.*, **62,** 139 (1968).
229. S. J. Powell, A. J. Wilmot, and R. Elsdon-Dew, *Ann. Trop. Med. Parasitol.*, **61,** 511 (1967).
230. H. L. Howes, J. E. Lynch, and J. L. Kilvin, *Antimicrob. Agents Chemother.*, 261 (1970).
231. M. W. Miller, H. L. Howes, Jr., R. V. Kasubick, and A. R. English, *J. Med. Chem.*, **13,** 849–852 (1970).
232. P. R. Sawyer, R. N. Brogden, R. M. Pinder, T. M. Speight, and G. S. Avery, *Drugs*, **11,** 423–440 (1976).
233. P. N. Giraldi, V. Mariotti, G. Nannini, G. P. Tosolini, E. Dradi, W. Logemann, I. de Carneri, and G. Monti, *Arzneim.-Forsch.*, **20,** 52–55 (1970).
234. P. N. Giraldi, G. P. Tosolini, E. Dradi, G. Nannini, R. Longo, G. Meinardi, G. Monti, and I. de Carneri, *Biochem. Pharmacol.*, **20,** 339–349 (1971).
235. S. Pickholz, M. Shapero, D. M. Ryan, H. S. Jefferies, and B. T. Warren, *Experientia*, **26,** 1025 (1970).
236. E. Grunberg, R. Cleeland, H. N. Prince, and E. Titsworth, *Proc. Soc. Exp. Biol. Med.*, **133,** 490–492 (1970).
237. A. Brossi, *Pure Appl. Chem.*, **19,** 70–78 (1969).
238. M. Hoffer and E. Grunberg, *J. Med. Chem.*, **17,** 1019–1020 (1974).
239. S. J. Powell, *Advan. Pharmacol. Chemother.*, **10,** 91–103 (1972).
240. E. Grunberg, G. Beskid, R. Cleeland, W. F. De Lorenzo, E. Titsworth, H. J. Scholer, R. Richle, and Z. Brener, *Antimicrob. Agents Chemother.*, 513–519 (1968).
241. A. C. Cuckler, C. M. Malanga, and J. Conroy, *Am. J. Trop. Med. Hyg.*, **19,** 916–925 (1970).
242. M. V. Chari and B. N. Gadiyar, *Am. J. Trop. Med. Hyg.*, **19,** 926–928 (1970).
243. S. K. Batra, N. K. Ajmani, D. R. Rellan, and H. K. Chuttani, *J. Trop. Med. Hyg.*, **75,** 16–18 (1972).
244. N. K. Ajmani, S. K. Batra, and H. K. Chuttani, *J. Trop. Med. Hyg.*, **75,** 40–41 (1972).
245. S. J. Powell and R. Elsdon-Dew, *Am. J. Trop. Med. Hyg.*, **20,** 839–841 (1971).
246. S. Carbajal, S. Pidacks, H. Steinmann, H. Maxon, and A. Wazniak, *Antimicrob. Agents Chemother.*, 541–544 (1969).
247. W. J. Ross, W. B. Jamieson, and M. C. McCowen, *J. Med. Chem.*,**15,** 1035 (1972).
248. W. J. Ross, W. B. Jamieson, and M. C. McCowen, *J. Med. Chem.*, **16,** 347–352 (1973).
249. P. Melloni, E. Dradi, and W. Logemann, *J. Med. Chem.*, **15,** 926–930 (1972).

250. P. Melloni, R. Metelli, D. Fusar Bassini, C. Confalonieri, W. Logemann, I. de Carneri, and F. Trane, *Arzneim.-Forsch.*, **25,** 9–14 (1975).

251. E. G. Grunberg, R. Beskid, R. Cleeland, W. F. De Lorenzo, E. Titsworth, H. J. Scholer, R. Richle, and Z. Brener, *Antimicrob. Agents Chemother.*, 513–519 (1968).

252. H. N. Prince, E. Grunberg, E. Titsworth, and W. F. De Lorenzo, *Appl. Microbiol.*, **18,** 728–730 (1969).

253. E. F. Elslager, in *Medicinal Chemistry*, 3rd ed., A. Burger, Ed., Wiley, New York, 1970, Ch. 19, p. 543.

254. A. Portal and M. Castellan, *Presse Med.*, **72,** 2457 (1964).

255. F. Benazet, C. Cosar, P. Ganter, L. Julon, P. Populaire, and L. Guillaume, *Compt. Rend., Ser. D*, **263,** 609 (1966).

256. A. R. Brown, F. C. Copp, and A. R. Elphick, *J. Chem. Soc.*, 1544–1548 (1957).

257. R. A. Neal and P. Vincent, *Brit. J. Pharmacol.*, **10,** 434 (1955).

258. L. G. Goodwin, C. A. Hoare, and T. M. Sharp, *Brit. J. Pharmacol.*, **3,** 44–48 (1948).

259. W. R. Jones, *Brit. J. Pharmacol.*, **2,** 217–220 (1947).

260. *Physician's Desk Reference*, 30th ed., B. R. Huff, Ed., Medical Economics., Oradell, N.J., 1976.

261. W. R. Jones, *Ann. Trop. Med. Parasitol.*, **40,** 130–140 (1946).

262. E. W. Dennis, D. A. Berberian, and S. S. Hansen, *Am. J. Trop. Med.*, **29,** 683–689 (1949).

263. D. A. Berberian, *J. Clin. Invest.*, **27,** 525 (1948).

264. J. Schneider and R. Dupoux, *Bull. Soc. Pathol. Exot.*, **46,** 550–561 (1953).

265. J. Schneider and R. Montezin, *Compt. Rendu.*, **323,** 2370 (1951).

266. J. Schneider and R. Dupoux, *Bull. Soc. Pathol. Exot.*, **44,** 741 (1951).

267. J. S. Levy and R. W. Talley, *Gastroenterology*, **22,** 588–595 (1952).

268. E. H. Loughlin, A. A. Joseph and W. G. Mullin, *Antibiot. Chemother.*, **4,** 570–573 (1954).

269. R. J. Schmitzer, D. R. Kelly, G. Soo-Hoo, E. Grunberg, and C. Unger, *Arch. Int. Pharmacodyn. Ther.*, **85,** 100–111 (1951).

270. D. T. Mintz, J. W. Miller, P. Ottolenghi, J. Schorck, F. Van Assendelft, and H. Most, *Am. J. Trop. Med. Hyg.*, **5,** 497–500 (1956).

CHAPTER TWENTY

Chemotherapy of Trypanosomiasis and Other Protozoan Diseases

WILLIAM J. ROSS

Lilly Research Centre, Limited
Erl Wood Manor
Windlesham
Surrey, GU20 6PH, England

CONTENTS

1 INTRODUCTION

The infectious protozoan diseases affecting man and his domestic animals described in this chapter are not regarded in the same emotive light as the scourge of malaria (Chapter 18), nor are they as widespread or numerous as bacterial or viral diseases. Nevertheless, they cause untold misery, death, and economic loss in many parts of the world. Although these diseases are more prevalent in the subtropical and tropical areas of the globe, the increase in international air travel exposes large numbers of people, sometimes unwittingly, to contact with protozoal diseases.

The protozoa, which comprise the first phylum of the animal kingdom, are divided into four classes: Sarcodina, Mastigophora, Sporozoa, and Ciliophora. Members of each class are responsible for protozoan diseases in man and animals. They infect mainly the intestinal tract, the vagina, the urethra, the blood, and the blood-forming organs, although other organs may also be parasitized. The most important serious protozoan diseases of man are malaria, (Chapter 18), amebiasis (Chapter 19), trypanosomiasis, and leishmaniasis. Indeed, so serious is the incidence of the latter two diseases that they are currently the subject of a World Health Organization "Special Programme for Research and Training in Tropical Diseases" (1).

Hemoflagellates of the genus *Trypanosoma* cause African sleeping sickness in man (*T. gambiense* and *T. rhodesiense*) and nagana (*T. congolense* and *T. brucei*) in domestic animals in tropical Africa. The vector for these diseases is the tsetse fly, and control of the disease is often accompanied by attempted elimination of this vector. Other species of trypanosomes cause various protozoan diseases such as mal de caderas (*T. equinum*), dourine (*T. equiperdum*), and surra (*T. evansi*) in other parts of the world. Chagas' disease of man, found in Central and South America, is caused by *T. cruzi*, which is transmitted by the bite of triatomid bugs.

Hemoflagellate parasites of the genus *Leishmania* cause the disfiguring diseases of oriental sore or cutaneous leishmaniasis and espundia or mucocutaneous leishmaniasis. The vectors for these diseases are sandflies, which transmit the parasites from gerbils and dogs to man.

Domestic fowl suffer from coccidiosis, a disease of vast economic importance caused by various species of *Eimeria*. Turkeys are susceptible to the intestinal flagellate *Histomonas meleagridis*, which causes a form of enterohepatitis known as "turkey blackhead". *Eimeria zürnii* causes "red dysentery", a disease that is frequently fatal to calves. *Balantidium coli*, an intestinal ciliate parasite of man, is transmitted from pigs, which harbor the parasite in their intestines.

Trichomoniasis is caused by *Trichomonas vaginalis* and is the most common parasitic disease of women in the temperate zone. *Trichomonas foetus* causes a venereal disease of cattle that results in sterility and abortion in cows. Tick-borne diseases caused by protozoa are of significant economic importance. Texas fever, a disease of cattle, is caused by *Babesia bigemina*, and *B. ovis* causes hemoglobinuric fever in European cattle. Malignant jaundice in dogs is caused by *B. canis*. Occasionally, humans may suffer from babesiasis. East coast fever, an acute disease of ruminants on the eastern coast of Africa, is caused by *Theileria parva* Anaplasmosis is a disease of cattle and other ruminants, the most important parasite being *Anaplasma marginale.*

Toxoplasmosa gondii, a protozoan of undetermined classification, affects many orders of mammals. The definitive host has recently been identified as the domestic cat, and transmission of the parasite to the human fetus has serious consequences.

The chemotherapy of the following diseases is discussed in some detail: trypanosomiasis, coccidiosis, trichomoniasis, leishmaniasis, histomoniasis, babesiasis, anaplasmosis, toxoplasmosis, balantidiasis, giardiasis, and theileriasis.

2 TRYPANOSOMIASIS

Trypanosomiasis is a group of closely related diseases of man and animals caused by infection with the species of the genus *Trypanosoma.* Two general forms of the disease are recognized, African trypanosomiasis occurring mainly but not exclusively in tropical Africa, and American trypanosomiasis or Chagas' disease, which occurs mainly in Central and South America. African trypanosomiasis, particularly the animal forms of the disease, has had great economic, social, and political impact in the past. Indeed this group of diseases have, to a large extent, determined which areas of Central Africa can be inhabited by man and his domestic animals, resulting in overpopulation and land exhaustion in noninfected areas. In addition, by limiting the production of beef cattle, the trypanosomiases have played an important role in the chronic protein deficiency frequently seen in the tropical African population. It is estimated that in nearly 4 million square miles south of the Sahara, the disease affects millions of people directly or indirectly, either through poor health or through loss of meat, milk, manure, and animal labor (2).

Trypanosomes occur in various vertebrates including mammals, birds, fish, amphibians, and reptiles. Vectors of the disease are various bloodsucking invertebrates, especially insects that transmit the infection to new vertebrate hosts. The principal vectors of pathogenic trypanosomes in Africa are various species of the genus *Glossina* (tsetse flies), although other bloodsucking flies may also be implicated.

The diseases of man caused by trypanosomes are West African or Gambian sleeping sickness, East African or Rhodesian sleeping sickness, and American trypanosomiasis or Chagas' disease of South and Central America. Gambian sleeping sickness is caused by *Trypanosoma gambiense,* Rhodesian sleeping sickness by *T. rhodesiense,* and Chagas' disease by *T. cruzi. T. gambiense* and *T. rhodesiense* appear to be morphologically indistinguishable (3), but nevertheless the resultant diseases have striking differences. In general, human trypanosomiasis, attributed to infection with *T. gambiense,* is of the more chronic type, whereas that due to *T. rhodesiense* is more acute. Man is the only important reservoir of infection of *T. gambiense,* and the disease is transmitted by the bite of an infected tsetse fly, *Glossina palpalis* or wet fly (4). *Glossina morsitans, G. pallidipes,* and *G. swynnertoni* are the vectors for Rhodesian sleeping sickness, and apart from man, the important reservoirs of the disease are the game animals eland, bushbuck, impala, and common duiker (4). The clinical manifestations and diagnosis of Gambian and Rhodesian sleeping sickness are described in detail by Apted (5).

T. brucei, a trypanosome morphologically indistinguishable from *T. gambiense* and *T. rhodesiense,* is transmitted to horses, mules, cattle, sheep, goats, pigs, dogs, and cats by *G. morsitans,* giving rise to the disease known as nagana (from a corruption of the

Zulu words meaning weakness). The disease is characterized by fever, anemia, edema, cachexia, and, frequently, paralysis and partial blindness in the affected animal; it occurs throughout tropical Africa.

T. congolense, a trypanosome with a geographical distribution similar to that of *T. brucei*, is responsible for the most important form of African trypanosomiasis in domestic animals. The manifestations of the disease are similar to those characteristic of nagana, with which it is frequently confused. *T. vivax* is widely distributed throughout the tsetse fly areas of Africa and also occurs in the West Indies and in Central and South America, where it is transmitted by tabanid flies. This trypanosome is pathogenic to cattle, sheep, goats, horses, and camels, and the disease is known as souma or nagana in Africa or secadera in South America.

T. evansi is the causative organism of surra disease, which occurs throughout the Middle East, Soviet Middle Asia, Iran, India, South east Asia, and parts of China. *T. evansi* is pathogenic to all domestic animals, but man is not susceptible to it. The most severe forms of the disease, which is transmitted by bloodsucking horseflies (tabanids), occur in horses, camels, and dogs. Although cattle and pigs are susceptible to *T. evansi*, the disease is mild and generally symptomless. Two trypanosomes, *T. hippicum* and *T. venezuelense*, which are morphologically indistinguishable from *T. evansi*, give rise to serious diseases in horses and dogs in Central America and Venezuela. *T. hippicum* is the causative agent of murrina or derrengadera, which affects horses and mules; *T. venezuelense* causes a disease resembling surra in horses and dogs. The former organism is transmitted by bloodsucking flies, and the latter by a rather more exotic vector, the vampire bat. Yet another disease of horses of South America, mal de caderas, is caused by *T. equinum*, an organism transmitted by the bite of stable flies (*Stamoxys*). Cattle, sheep, and goats are also susceptible but have the disease in a mild form.

Dourine, a venereal disease of horses and donkeys, is caused by *T. equiperdum* and is transmitted by direct contact during sexual congress. Formerly, the disease was found throughout the world, but control measures and the decline in the equine population has reduced the incidence. In Africa, the disease is prevalent mainly in countries bordering the Mediterranean Sea.

T. suis, a little known trypanosome, causes a disease of domestic pigs in Tanzania. The organism is highly pathogenic to young pigs but causes only a mild chronic disease in adults. The disease is cyclically transmitted by the bite of the tsetse fly *G. brevipalpis*. A rather more important trypanosome is *T. simiae*, which is a specific parasite of pigs and highly pathogenic to the domestic pig, in which it causes an acute and fatal disease of about 4 days' duration. The disease is common throughout most of tropical Africa and is transmitted by diverse species of *Glossina*.

South American trypanosomiasis or Chagas' disease is caused by *T. cruzi* and afflicts about 7 million people (6). Although the disease was first described in 1909, it was not recognized as a serious infectious disease until the 1930s, and by then improved diagnostic techniques were available (7). The disease occurs mainly in rural areas and is associated with poor sanitary conditions. The vectors for *T. cruzi* are reduviid bugs (*Triatoma* or *Panstrongylus*), which bite the host, then deposit infected semiliquid feces on the site. This causes local irritation, and infection occurs when the wound is rubbed. In most cases the site of entry is the ocular conjunctiva, and the resultant edema and conjunctivitus give rise to the classical Romaña sign of Chagas' disease (7). In the life cycle of *T. cruzi* in man, there are two forms that are readily distinguishable; (1) the trypanosome or blood form, and (2) the leishmanial (amastigote) or intracellular form. The principal organ involved in acute Chagas' disease is the heart, although other tissues may also be parasitized. The condition is acute mainly in children, but it becomes chronic, and the infected person may die of cardiac disease some 10–20 years later (7). The pathology has been reviewed in detail (7), and comparisons with African trypanosomiasis have been discussed (6).

In addition to the pathogenic trypanosomes, there are various nonpathogenic species such as *T. lewisi*, which has a cosmopolitan distribution in wild rats, and *T. rangeli*, which is distributed throughout Central and South America, the hosts being man, dogs, cats, and monkeys.

2.1 Chemotherapy of Trypanosomiasis

The majority of pathogenic trypanosomes can be adapted to infect small laboratory animals such as mice, rats, guinea pigs, and rabbits; consequently, the screening of compounds for activity is conducted in these species. Preliminary work is usually carried out in mice, the infection being induced by the intraperitoneal injection of blood containing the trypanosomes. However the important trypanosomes *T. vivax* and *T. simiae* are not readily amenable to such adaption, although under specialized conditions infections in rats and rabbits have been achieved (8, 9). The natural strains of the trypanosomes are not usually fatal to mice or rats but, with repeated syringe passage, the virulence of the trypanosomes increases greatly, eventually resulting in adapted or "laboratory" strains, which kill the animal in 3–5 days. These "laboratory" strains can then be used for the evaluation of compounds under standardized conditions. The tests are of fairly long duration, 30 days in the case of the *T. rhodesiense*, *T. gambiense*, and *T. congolense* group, and 60 days in the case of *T. cruzi*. Detailed test procedures have been described (10, 11). As indicated, the "laboratory" strains of trypanosomes are highly pathogenic to laboratory animals; but because they have been syringe passaged many times in rats or mice, they differ considerably from the "wild" strains of trypanosome encountered in the field. Consequently it is imperative to study the effect of "active" compounds on recently isolated strains before progression to the clinic or field. Various specialized tests have also been devised for investigating the prophylactic activity of drugs (especially important in animal trypanosomiasis), penetration of the compound across the blood–brain barrier and into the cerebrospinal fluid (important for late-stage human trypanosomiasis), and development of drug resistance (10). *In vitro* techniques are also available for drug evaluation; however such approaches are useful only for the determination of direct trypanocidal activity and are not necessarily indicative of *in vivo* activity, since the procedure does not detect compounds that require chemical modification in the animal or have a delayed action (*vide infra*).

The early history of trypanocidal drugs is synonymous with the name of Paul Ehrlich. While studying the staining of tissues with dyes, Ehrlich observed the preferential staining of the malaria parasite with methylene blue. This observation led Ehrlich and his associates (12, 13) to study a wide range of synthetic dyes and related compounds as trypanocidal agents, laying the foundations for the discovery and introduction of suramin (20.**6**) as a clinically effective drug for African sleeping sickness. Ehrlich, with his work on the effect of arsenic compounds (14) on trypanosomes, and Thomas (15) with his discovery of the trypanocidal activity and low toxicity of Atoxyl (*p*-aminobenzenearsonic acid), stimulated a line of research that led to tryparsamide (20.**8**) and other organoarsenicals that with suramin, have been the mainstay of effective drug control of sleeping sickness during the last 50 or 60 years.

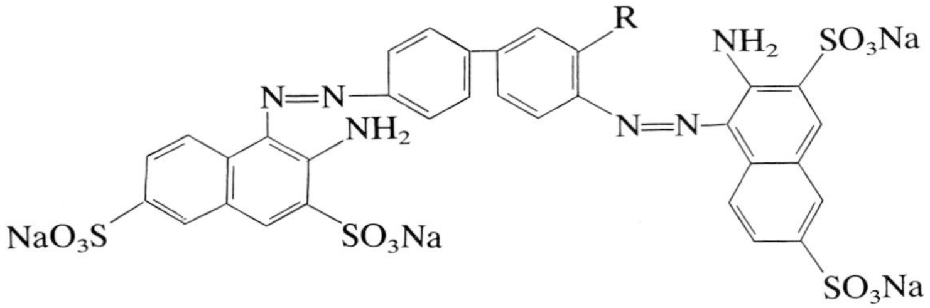

20.1 R = H
20.2 R = SO_3Na

In view of the many types of compound tested against the important strains of trypanosomes, the discussion of the chemotherapy of trypanosomiasis is based on general chemical families reported to have laboratory or clinical activity.

2.1.1 AZO DYES AND SURAMIN. Ehrlich's observation of the staining of the malaria parasite in histological sections by methylene blue led him to investigate the effects of dyes on other parasites, particularly trypanosomes. He and his associates began by studying the recently introduced cotton-substantive dyes derived from Congo red. After examining more than 100 dyes in mice infected with *T. equinum*, the causative organism of mal de caderas, weak activity was found in the dye benzopurpurin, later known as nagana red (20.**1**). Modification of the structure led to trypan red (20.**2**), which proved to be both curative and prophylactic (13) in mice infected with *T. equinum* but not against other trypanosomal infections (16).

Subsequently other workers discovered trypan blue (17) (20.**3**) and afridol violet (18) (20.**4**), which possessed superior antitrypanosomal properties in infected laboratory animals, but neither compound was introduced clinically.

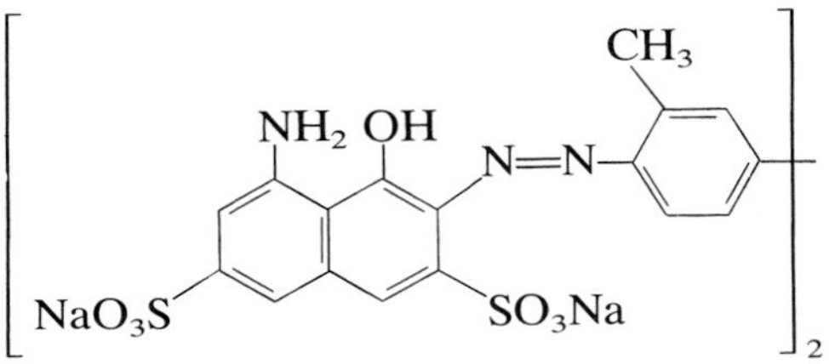

20.**3**

As a result of extensive investigations in this area, it was apparent that activity resided only in compounds that carried sulfonic acid substituents in the 3,6-position of the naphthylamine residues, but probably of equal interest was the presence of a diphenyl urea function instead of diphenyl as the central nucleus in afridol blue.

Highly colored dyes as therapeutic agents for man or domestic animals have obvious disadvantages, which the chemists at the German firm of Bayer sought to overcome. The rationale for their work was that if the trypanocidal action of the dyes was due to binding on tissues of parasites, compounds with similar affinities but lacking the chromophoric azo linkages could be expected to possess similar biological activity. One of the first active compounds found was a colorless analog (20.**5**) of trypan red, which nevertheless possessed the urea linkages found in afridol violet.

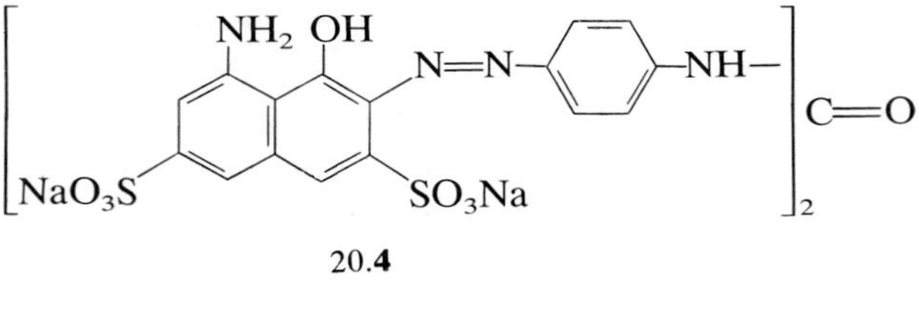

20.**4**

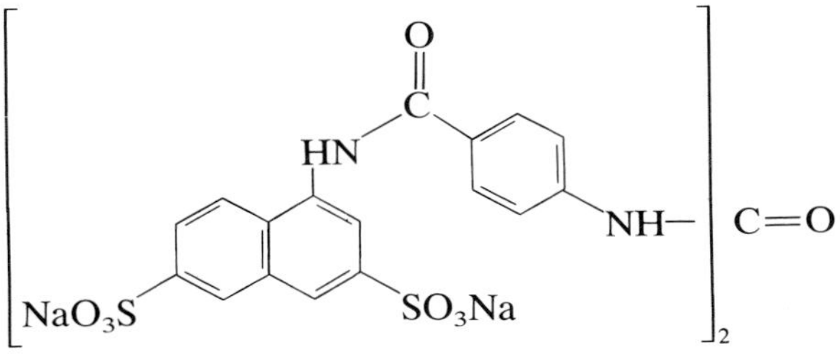

20.5

Subsequent work showed that the introduction of a further sulfonic acid group into the naphthylamine ring and the use of *m*-aminobenzoyl instead of *p*-aminobenzoyl residues as linking groups improved trypanocidal activity. This research culminated in the introduction of suramin (20.**6**) (19) as an effective agent for the treatment of early cases of human African trypanosomiasis.

In addition to its use in acute cases of sleeping sickness, suramin exerts a prolonged prophylactic action against various trypanosome infections (20). Suramin is very active against *T. brucei*, *T. gambiense*, *T. rhodesiense*, *T. equiperdum*, and *T. equinum* (21) but is relatively ineffective against *T. vivax* and *T. congolense* and is not active against *T. cruzi*. Despite the superficial complexity of suramin, minor changes in the structure results in loss of trypanocidal activity. Removal of the two methyl groups all but abolishes activity, and this property suggests a crucial role for these groups as with the antischistosomal compound lucanthone (22), where a methyl group must be oxidized to give the active species, hycanthone (see Chapter 21). However the mode of action of suramin is unknown. The structural requirements for persistence are much less specific than those for trypanocidal activity and can probably be met by any symmetrical, high molecular weight, polysulfonated compound. Attempts to obtain active analogs by replacing the naphthalene trisulfonic acid portion of the molecule with heterocyclic nuclei have been unsuccessful (23).

Following a fortuitous observation by Lourie (24), various suramin complexes with basic trypanocidal drugs [e.g., quinapyramine (20.**33**) and pentamidine (20.**21**)] have been investigated as depot preparations, particularly for the prevention of *T. vivax* and *T. congolense* infections in cattle (25).

Unfortunately, an unacceptable incidence of severe local reactions in patients after intramuscular injection precluded wide spread usage of these complexes in human practice.

2.1.2 ARSENICALS AND ANTIMONIALS. The use of inorganic arsenicals and antimonials in medicine has a long history, starting with

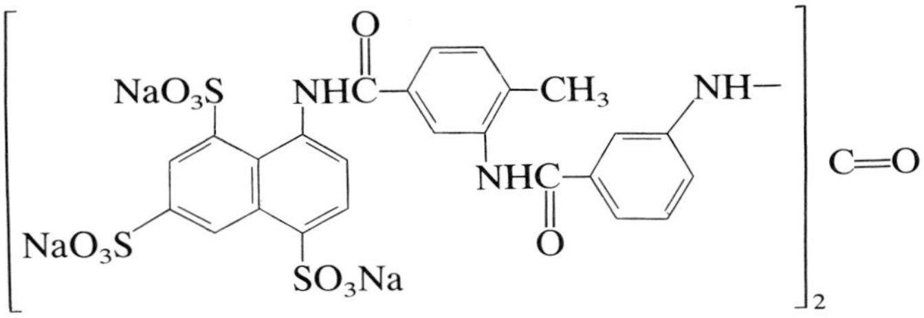

20.6

Hippocrates some 2500 years ago and continuing to the present day. Fowler's solution (of potassium arsenite) and orpiment (arsenic trisulfide) were used in conjunction with the benzidine dyes in the early days of the chemotherapy of trypanosomiasis. Tartar emetic (potassium antimony tartrate) was shown to be trypanocidal in 1908 (26), and for the following 40 years was the only readily available treatment for animal trypanosomiasis in various parts of Africa. However, the main use for antimonials has been in the treatment of leishmaniasis (see Section 5).

The seminal observation that led to the development of organoarsenic compounds as trypanocidal agents was that of Wolferstan Thomas who, in 1905, introduced Atoxyl (20.**7**) (15) as an effective trypanocidal agent for use in man. Initially there was some doubt about the structure of Atoxyl, but the structure was shown by Ehrlich to be 20.**7**, and subsequently Ehrlich was able, by varying the structure, to produce less toxic and more active compounds. Atoxyl soon fell into disfavor because it was rapidly shown to have disturbing toxic effects in man, particularly on the optic nerve.

However, from this work only one compound emerged, tryparsamide (20.**8**) (27),

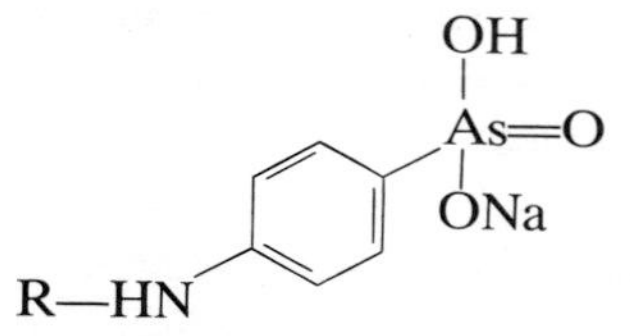

20.**7** R = H

20.**8** R = CH_2CONH_2

which has survived in clinical use to the present day. Since its introduction in 1919, this drug has been the mainstay in the treatment of Gambian sleeping sickness. A related compound orsanine (20.**9**, sodium 2-hydroxy-4-acetamidophenylarsonate) has also been used clinically (28) but failed to establish itself in practice.

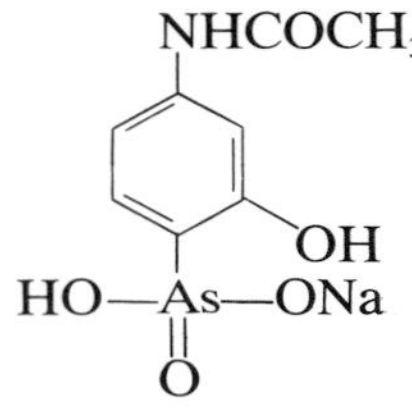

20.**9**

Tryparsamide and orsanine have only moderate trypanocidal activity, but they can penetrate the central nervous system, and this is of particular importance in late stage trypanosomiasis. As with Atoxyl, the major side effect in man is optic atrophy and blindness. Resistance to tryparsamide and related compounds is frequently seen in strains of trypanosomes (30, 31).

Early in his studies, Ehrlich had shown that pentavalent arsenic compounds were inactive *in vitro* and that their *in vivo* activity was probably due to reduction to the trivalent form, which was the true active agent (31). This was confirmed by a detailed study demonstrating that whereas compounds containing pentavalent arsenic had only slight trypanocidal activity, those containing trivalent arsenic (—AsO, —As=As—) were more active (32). The arsenoxide 3(4-arsenophenyl)butyric acid (20.**10**, Butarsen) was found to have excellent trypanocidal properties but proved

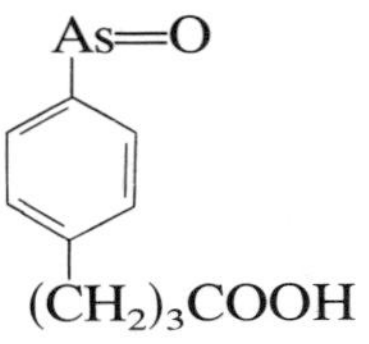

20.**10**

effective only in the early stages of sleeping sickness and did not come into general use (33, 34). However arsenoxides are much more toxic than arsonates, and many attempts have been made to prepare less toxic trivalent derivatives. Two such compounds, (20.**11**) and (20.**12**) derived from tryparsamide (20.**8**) and stovarsol (20.**116**), respectively, were tested against sleeping

$$\text{NHCH}_2\text{CONH}_2\text{-C}_6\text{H}_4\text{-As}(\text{S-CH}_2\text{-CH(CH}_2\text{OH)-S})$$

20.**11**

$$\text{HO-C}_6\text{H}_3(\text{NHCOCH}_3)\text{-As}(\text{S-CH}_2\text{-CH(CH}_2\text{OH)-S})$$

20.**12**

sickness in man but appear to offer no advantages over tryparsamide (34).

The search for less toxic forms of Atoxyl-derived compounds continued, and a major advance in therapy followed with Friedheim's introduction of the Melarsen series of compounds for the treatment of human trypanosomiasis (35). Melarsen, sodium *N*-(4,6-diamino-*s*-triazin-2-yl)-arsanilate (20.**13**) possesses activity against tryparsamide-resistant *T. gambiense* infections and particularly against late stage *T. rhodesiense* infections and, despite toxic side effects, still remains clinically useful. Melarsen may be reduced to the arsenoxide which, on condensation with BAL, gives the important compound Mel B (melarsoprol) (20.**14**). A further development in this area was the preparation of Mel W (20.**15**), a less toxic and more water-soluble derivative (37).

Many trials with these compounds have established their usefulness in human sleeping sickness, especially in the treatment of late stage disease (37–39). The spectrum of activity of the trypanocidal arsenicals is similar to that of suramin (see Section 2.1) but with the advantages that they penetrate the central nervous system. Resistance may develop to the Melarsen series, and such strains are also resistant to tryparsamide. The mode of action of the arsenical trypanocides has been investigated by numerous authors (see Ref. 34 for relevant references) but is not known with any great precision. The cytotoxicity of the arsenicals is thought to be due to inactivation of sulfhydryl groups on enzymes in the parasite by trivalent arsenic, but specificity of action appears to be controlled by the structure of the nonmetallic part of the drug molecule. (40, 41). A reanalysis of the data using Hansch analysis or related techniques might well be profitable in the design of more effective drugs. Whereas antimonials have an important role to play in other parasitic diseases, they have achieved only limited use in the therapy of human trypanosomiasis. The stibonic acid analog of Melarsen (isolated as a polymer known as MSb) has excellent prophylactic activity, either orally or parenterally, in experimental trypanosome infections (41, 42); it has proved clinically effective (44) against *T.*

$$(\text{H}_2\text{N})_2\text{C}_3\text{N}_3\text{-NH-C}_6\text{H}_4\text{-R}$$

20.**13** $R = As(=O)(ONa)_2$

20.**14** $R = As(S-CH_2-CH(CH_2OH)-S)$

20.**15** $R = As(S-CH(COOK)-CH(COOK)-S)$

gambiense infections. The trivalent analog of MSb has also been prepared and, on reaction with BAL, gives the antimony equivalent of Mel B (20.**14**), with which it has comparable activity (44). However the antimonials have not become established in practice.

2.1.3 DIAMIDINES. The multiplication of trypanosomes *in vivo* requires considerable glucose and is reduced by injection of insulin into the host animal (45). This led to the testing of the synthetic hypoglycemic 1,10-bis(guanidino)decane (20.**16**, Synthalin) against experimental *T. brucei* infections; results were favorable (46). Further investigation demonstrated that Synthalin was highly trypanocidal *in vitro* by direct action in the presence of glucose (47), indicating that the activity was not due to its hypoglycemic properties.

$$HN{=}C(NH_2)NH(CH_2)_{10}NHC(NH_2){=}NH$$

20.**16**

Synthesis of compounds of general structure 20.**17** (48), 20.**18** (49), and 20.**19** (48) led to compounds possessing high *in vitro* activity but with limited activity against *T. rhodesiense* infections in mice.

$$R(CH_2)_nR$$

20.**17** R = $-C(NH_2){=}NH$

20.**18** R = $-NHC({=}S)-NH_2$

20.**19** R = $-NHC(NH_2){=}NH$

Maximum activity in the bisguanidines and bisamidines was observed with $n = 10$–14, and in the bisisothioureas at $n = 6$.

The preparation of aromatic diamidines led to a major advance in the development of therapeutically useful compounds. The starting point was 20.**20** (50, 51), which was active against *T. equiperdum* and *T. rhodesiense* infections in mice. Development of the series led to the discovery of pentamidine (20.**21**), which is still in widespread clinical use. It has served for mass prophylaxis in the control of Gambian sleeping sickness (52) and has been employed in conjunction with tryparsamide for the treatment of early cases of the disease (36). However pentamidine is only used against *T. rhodesiense* infections to a very limited extent.

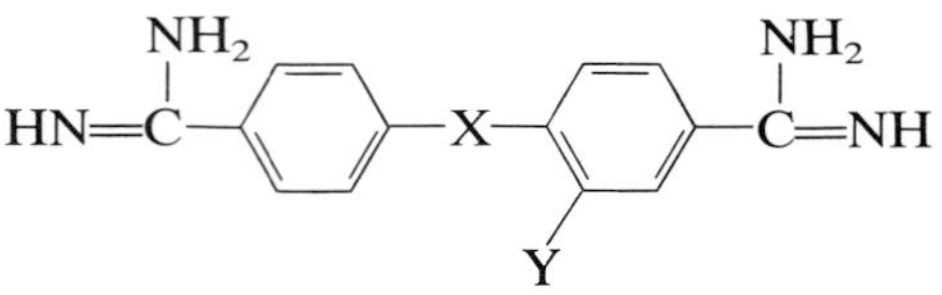

$$HN{=}C(NH_2)-C_6H_4-X-C_6H_3(Y)-C(NH_2){=}NH$$

	X	Y
20.**20**	X = $-CH_2-$	Y = H
20.**21**	X = $-O(CH_2)_5O-$	Y = H
20.**22**	X = $-O(CH_2)_3O-$	Y = H
20.**23**	X = $-CH{=}CH-$	Y = H
20.**24**	X = $-C(CH_3){=}C(CH_3)-$	Y = H
20.**25**	X = $-O-$	Y = H
20.**26**	X = $-N{=}NNH-$	Y = H
20.**27**	X = $-CH{=}CH-$	Y = OH

Related compounds that have been studied clinically but not introduced commercially include propamidine (20.**22**) (50), stilbamidine (20.**23**) (53), dimethylstilbamidine (20.**24**) (53), and phenamidine (20.**25**) (50). The use of stilbamidine was fraught with toxicity problems due mainly to the photochemical dimerization of the compound to a cyclobutane derivative (54). This disadvantage was overcome in 20.**24** (54), which was more active than stilbamidine but was very difficult to synthesize economically, and by the preparation of 2-hydroxystilbamidine (20.**27**) (54). Nevertheless neither compound has become established in practice. The chemical, pharmacological, and clinical aspects of this general class of compound have been reviewed extensively (10, 34, 56, 57).

Investigation of more complex linking groups between the amidine functions led to the discovery of the interesting compound 20.**28** (58) which possesses activity against *T. congolense*.

The obvious familial relationship of

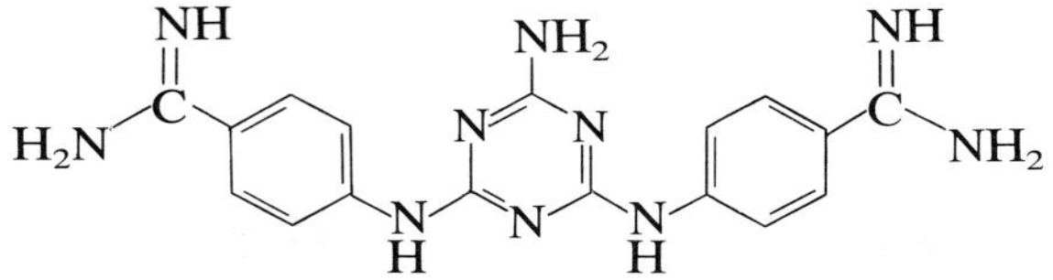

20.**28**

20.**26** to the latter compound can be readily discerned but, in fact, the discovery of 4,4′-diazoaminodibenzamidine diaceturate (20.**26**, diminazene, Berenil) (59, 60) resulted from a dissection into chemically and therapeutically equivalent portions (58, 59) of the bisaminoquinoline group of compounds (see Section 2.4).

Diminazene is widely used against cattle trypanosomiasis, particularly *T. congolense* and *T. vivax* infections (61) but is inactive against *T. simiae* infections in pigs (2). It may have some value in the treatment of early cases of human *T. gambiense* and *T. rhodesiense* sleeping sickness (2). The main reason for the success of diminazene is due to its high activity against cattle infections resistant to other drugs, and despite widespread use, little drug resistance has developed (2). The lack of prophylactic activity in diminazene is undoubtedly due to the rapidity with which it is degraded and excreted.

Diamidines of general structure (20.**29**) have pronounced activity against trypanosomes of the *brucei-evansi* group (62, 63) and *T. congolense* (64) *in vivo*. The most important compound is 20.**30** which, as its dilactate, appears to be active against late stage Rhodesian sleeping sickness (65).

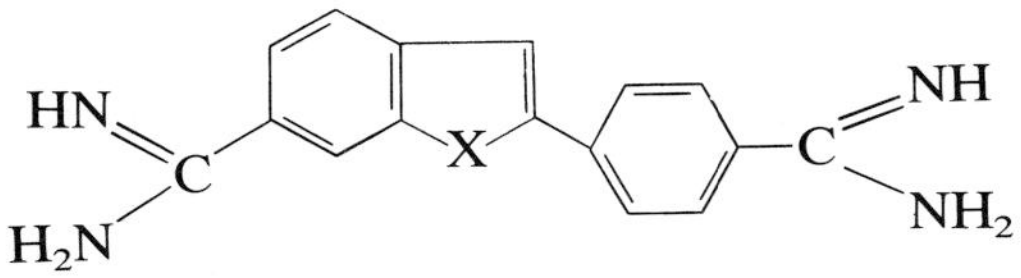

20.**29** X = O, S or NH
20.**30** X = S

2.1.4 QUINOLINE AND RELATED COMPOUNDS. During the course of his investigations into the properties of dyes, Erhlich discovered the trypanocidal activity of acriflavine (a mixture of 3,6-diaminoacridine and its N^{10}-methochloride) (66). A great number of derivatives of acriflavine were prepared, including the 6-nitro and 9-dialkyl amino derivatives, which had enhanced activity (67). Acriflavine is active against *T. rhodesiense* in mice (68) but has never been used in practice. Consideration of the structure led to the preparation of styryl and anilquinolinium salts, a number of which showed prophylactic activity against *T. brucei* infections in mice but were inactive against *T. congolense* and *T. vivax* (69). However none was introduced into practice because many of them produce local systemic toxic reactions.

The investigation of the derivatives of aminoquinolines led to the discovery of surfen (20.**31**) and surfen C (20.**32**) (70).

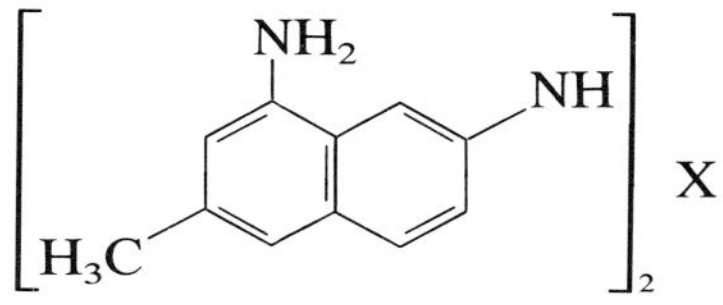

20.**31** X = —C=O

20.**32** X = (triazine, NH$_2$)

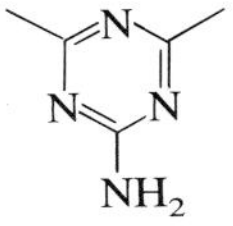

The latter compound was the first nonmetallic compound to show marked activity against *T. congolense* infections in field practice but did not achieve widespread use because of the introduction of more effective trypanocides. Variations of the structure of surfen C and the aminoacridines led to a weakly active trypanocidal compound that gave quinapyramine (20.**33**) upon quaternization (71, 72).

This compound, as its chloride, is active

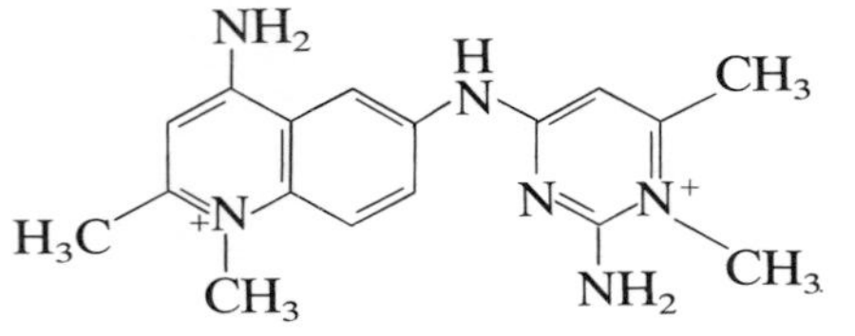

20.**33**

against mouse infections of *T. congolense*, *T. equiperdum*, *T. evansi*, *T. rhodesiense*, *T. gambiense*, and *T. brucei* (73, 74). In field practice, quinapyramine, as its sulfate, chloride, or mixture of both, has established itself as a standard drug for the treatment and prophylaxis of trypanosomiasis in domestic animals. The chloride is curative for *T. congolense* and *T. vivax* infections in cattle, *T. evansi* infections in camels, and *T. evansi* and *T. equiperdum* in equines (2). The chloride is prophylactic in pigs against *T. simiae*, as is a mixture of the chloride and the sulfate in cattle against *T. congolense* and *T. vivax* (2).

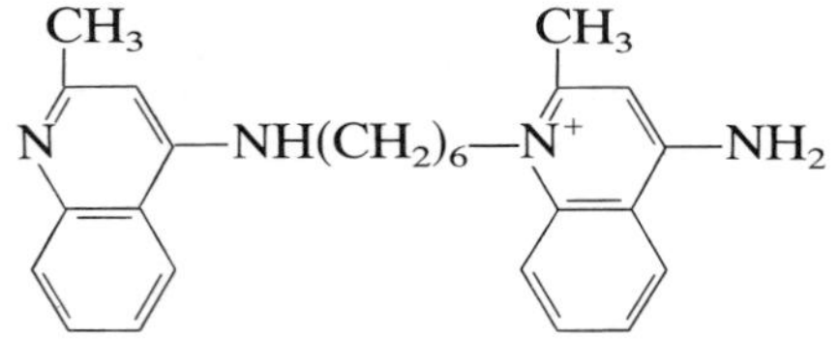

20.**34**

A related compound, cinnoline "528", N',N^3-bis(4-amino-6-cinnolyl) guanidine dimethiodide, which was prepared in an attempt to simplify the phenanthridinium quaternary salts (see Section 2.5) was shown to possess trypanocidal activity similar to that of quinapyramine, but it was unsatisfactory in field trials (75, 76). The quinaldinium compound tozocide (20.**34**) was shown to be trypanocidal (77), but despite variation of the structure, no compound superior to quinapyramine was obtained (8, 79).

A series of malonamides derived from 4,6-diaminoquinoline have been studied in experimental *T. cruzi* infections (70, 81), and 20.**35** has undergone clinical evaluation, though results were unsatisfactory (82).

2.1.5 PHENANTHRIDINIUM DERIVATIVES. The phenanthridine nucleus (20.**36**) (Table 20.1) is isomeric with acridine and contains both quinoline and isoquinoline rings, which, as discussed in Section 2.1.4, are associated with trypanocidal activity. Detailed investigation of this class of compound uncovered interesting trypanocidal activity (83) and, as with the acridines, quaternization resulted in increased trypanocidal activity, particularly against *vivax-congolense* infections in mice (84). The first compounds introduced for field use were phenidium chloride and dimidium bromide (Table 20.1), which were shown to have marked activity against *T. congolense* and *T. vivax* infections in African cattle (84). Unfortunately, treatment with dimidium was often followed by delayed toxic reactions some 2–3 months after administration, particularly when it had been necessary to use higher doses to overcome drug-resistant trypanosomes (85). The high trypanocidal activity of phenylphenanthridinium salts substituted by amino groups in the 2- and 7- positions (numbering in 20.**36** as used by the original workers) was confirmed by extensive studies by various workers (86–88). The study of the trypanocidal properties of a homologous series of quaternary N^{10}-alkyl derivatives led to the discovery of ethidium (homidium). This compound was markedly

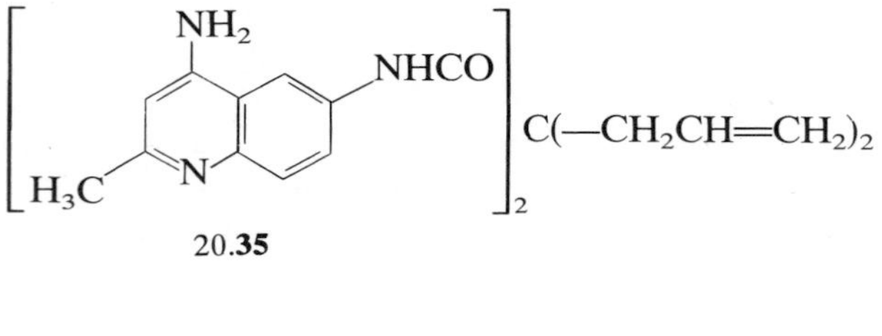

20.**35**

Table 20.1 Phenanthridinium Trypanocides

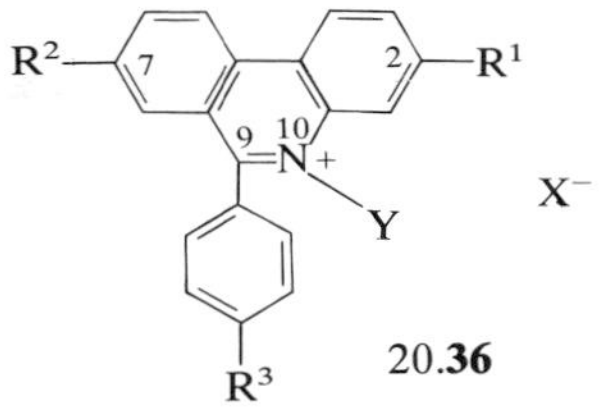

20.**36**

Name	R^1	R^2	R^3	Y	X
Phenidium	H	NH_2	NH_3	CH_3	Cl—
Dimidium	NH_2	NH_2	H	CH_3	Br—
Ethidium	NH_2	NH_2	H	C_2H_5	Br—
Prothidium	NH_2	—[a]	NH_2	CH_3	Br—
Metamidium[b]	NH_2	NH_2	H	C_2H_5	Cl—
Isometamidium	NH_2	—[c]	H	C_2H_5	Cl—

[a] 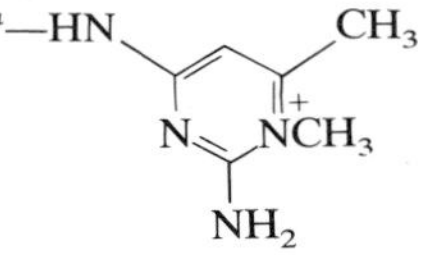 —HN, CH_3, NCH_3, N, NH_2 (pyrimidinium)

[b] 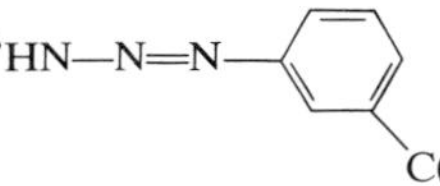 HN—N=N— (phenyl) C(=NH)NH_2 is at position 1, 3, 6 or 8

[c] As for note *b*; but at position 7.

more active against *T. congolense* and *T. gambiense* infections in mice than was the parent dimidium (89, 90). Subsequent field trials in cattle infected by *T. congolense* confirmed the superiority of ethidium over dimidium and also attested to the lack of toxic side effects of the latter. No satisfactory explanation is available for the fundamental change in activity and toxicity found in going from a quaternary *N*-methyl group to an *N*-ethyl function. Similar enhancement of activity by changing the nature of the quaternary group in other phenanthridinium compounds was observed (91), but none was sufficiently active to displace ethidium.

Introduction of the pyrimidyl moiety of quinapyramine (20.**33**) into a phenanthridinium nucleus related to phenidium resulted in prothidium, a compound with remarkable prophylactic and curative properties against *T. congolense* (92, 93). Depending on the degree of challenge, a single intramuscular injection of this compound protects animals for up to 4 months (6).

The introduction of the *m*-amidinophenyldiazoamino moiety of diminazene (20.**26**) into the phenanthridine nucleus gave metamidium and isometamidium (93) (Table 20.1). Both compounds are very active against *T. congolense* and *T. vivax* infections in cattle and have the added advantage of activity against quinapyramine-, homidium-, and prothidium-resistant trypanosomes (2). More details of these important drugs may be found in various reviews (10, 34, 94).

2.1.6 NITROHETEROCYCLIC COMPOUNDS. Soon after the discovery of the antibacterial activity of the nitrofurans (95) these compounds were tested against trypanosomal infections in laboratory animals. Nitrofurazone (20.**37**, 5-nitro-2-furaldehyde semicarbazone) was found to be curative for experimental *T. equiperdum* infections in mice (96, 97). Subsequent studies demonstrated the activity of nitrofurazone against experimental infections of *T. gambiense* infections in mice (98) and *T. gambiense* and *T. rhodesiense* in guinea pigs (99). Clinical trials in man established nitrofurazone as a useful drug for the treatment of relapsed cases of African sleeping sickness resistant to suramin, pentamidine, and melarsprol (100, 101). Nitrofurazone was suppressive but not curative for *T. cruzi* infections in mice (102).

An analog of nitrofurazone, furadroxyl (20.**38**), was shown to be active against *T. equiperdum*, *T. gambiense*, and *T. rhodesiense* infections in rats and mice but was inactive against *T. cruzi* (103). The carbazate 20.**38** is active against *T. congolense*, *T. gambiense*, *T. rhodesiense*, and *T. cruzi* infections in mice (104). Furaltadone (20.**39**) has been used successfully in the clinic (105). Undoubtedly the most important nitrofuran in the context of trypanosomiasis therapy is nifurtimox (20.**41**), the first compound to exhibit proved utility in the therapy of acute and chronic Chagas' disease. An extensive series of papers describes the synthesis of nifurtimox and various analogs (106–110) and the pharmacological and clinical properties of the compound. It is active against various strains of *T. cruzi* in laboratory animals and seems to be the long-awaited breakthrough in the treatment of the disease (111, 112).

Members of a series of nitrofurans of which 20.**42** is the best example are active against *T. cruzi* infections in mice (113). Nitrofurylthiazoles, represented by 20.**43**, have shown excellent activity against several different strains of *T. cruzi* in mice, including tissue forms of *T. cruzi* (Peru) (114). The metabolism of the compound has been studied (115) and as expected, the nitrofuran ring was degraded to a 3-cyanopropionyl group. Surprisingly, however, the morpholine ring was oxidized to a compound isolated as the lactone 20.**43** (R = O).

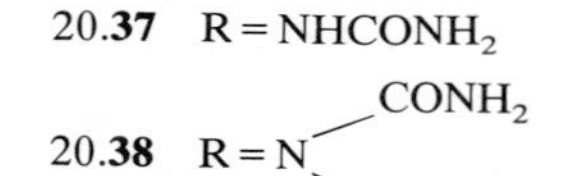

O_2N–(furan)–CH=NR

20.**37** R = $NHCONH_2$

20.**38** R = $N(CONH_2)(CH_2CH_2OH)$

20.**39** R = $NHCOOCH_2CH_2OH$

20.**40** R = —N(oxazolidinone)–CH_2N(morpholine)

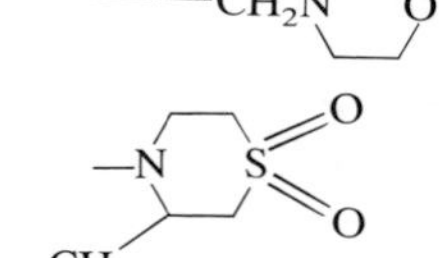

20.**41** R = —N(thiomorpholine S,S-dioxide), —CH_3

20.**42** R = NH–(methylpyrazolopyrimidine), CH_3

O_2N–(X-ring)–(thiophene)–CH=N–N(morpholine, =R)

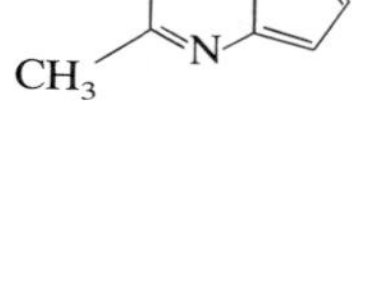

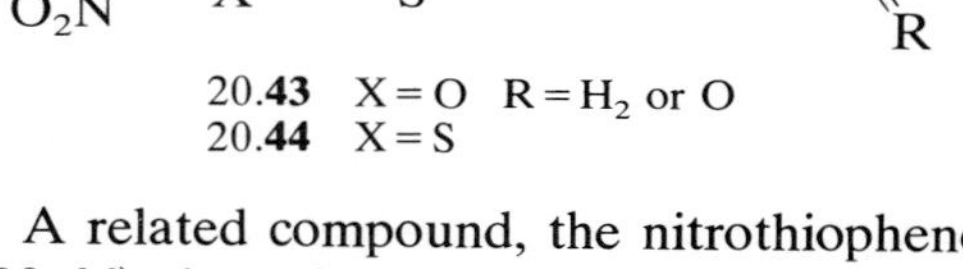

20.**43** X = O R = H_2 or O
20.**44** X = S

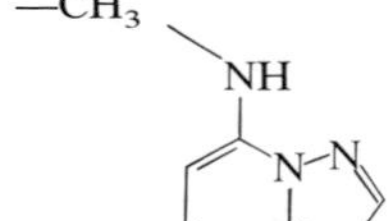

A related compound, the nitrothiophene (20.**44**), is active against *T. cruzi* and *T. rhodesiense* infections in mice (116). The antischistosomal compound 20.**45** (SQ 18,506) possesses activity against *T. rhodesiense* infections in mice (117) and is active against *T. cruzi* infections in mice and in human heart cells (118). The activity

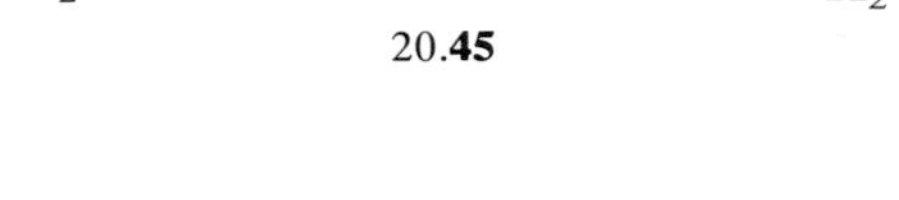

O_2N–(furan)–CH$\overset{t}{=}$CH–(oxadiazole N–O, N)–NH_2

20.**45**

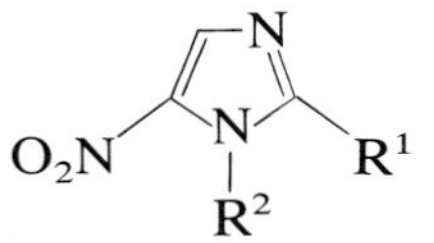

20.46 R^1 = —C$_6$H$_4$—F; R^2 = —CH_2CH_2OH

20.47 R^1 = —C$_6$H$_4$—F; R^2=CH_3

20.48 R^1 = —C$_6$H$_4$—$CONH_2$; R^2=CH_3

20.49 R^1 = —CH_2OCONH_2; R^2 = CH_3

20.50 R^1 = —CH=CH—C$_6$H$_4$—COOH; R^2 = —CH=CH_2

20.51 R^1 = CH=CH—C$_6$H$_4$—CH=NNHCOCH$_2$N(CH$_3$)$_2$; R^2 = —CH=CH_2

20.52 R^1 = —CH=CH—C$_6$H$_4$—C(=NH)NH$_2$; R^2 = —CH=CH_2

20.53 R^1 = 2-amino-1,3,4-thiadiazol-5-yl (N—N, S, NH_2); R^2 = —CH_3

20.54 R^1 = thiazolyl—CH=NN(thiomorpholine S,S-dioxide); R^2 = —CH_3

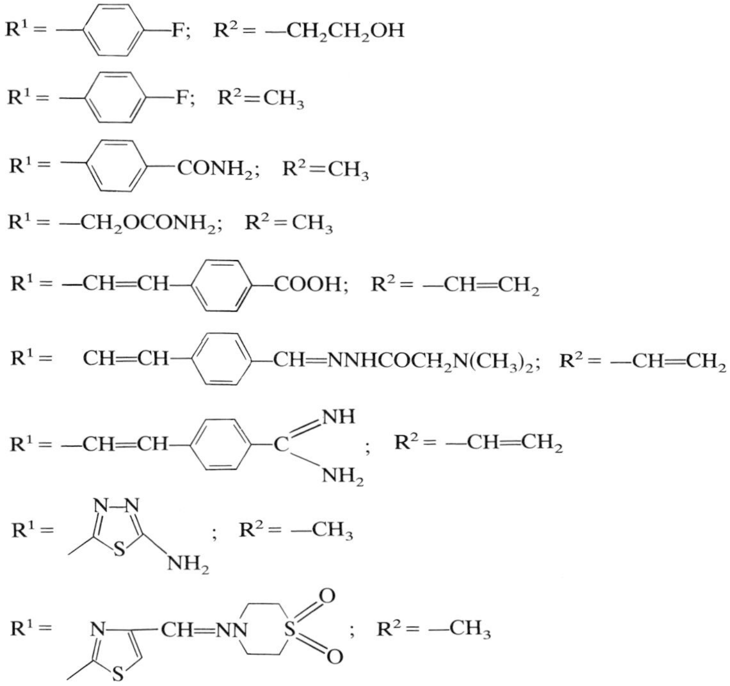

compares favorably with that of nifurtimox, and the compound is undergoing clinical trials (118).

Although nitroimidazoles have more importance in other protozoal diseases (e.g, amebiasis and trichomoniasis), some exhibit significant antitrypanosomal activity. The nitroimidazoles 20.**46** (flunidazole), 20.**47** ("MF" nitroimidazole), 20.**48** ("MCA" nitroimidazole), and 20.**49** (ronidazole) all cure *T. brucei* infections in mice (119). In another series of nitroimidazoles it was found that 20.**50** possessed the best antitrypanosomal activity against *T. rhodesiense*, *T. gambiense*, *T. congolense*, and *T. cruzi* infections in mice (120, 121).

Compound 20.**50** was also curative for *T. vivax* in calves upon multiple intravenous dosing (121). Studies of the metabolism of 20.**50** disclosed that it is excreted as the glycine and glucuronide derivatives of the 4-carboxylic acid function (122). The mode of action of 20.**50** against trypanosomes appears to be inactivation of glycolytic enzymes within the parasites (123). Replacement of the carboxyl function of 20.**50** by a hydrazone moiety (20.**51**) or amidine function 20.**52** (121) gave compounds whose activity was similar to that of suramin and pentamidine against *T. rhodesiense* infections in mice.

The nitroimidazole 20.**53** displays activity against *T. equiperdum* and *T. cruzi* infections in mice (124). The nitroimidazolylthiazole 20.**54**, a compound related to the nitrofuran 20.**43**, and utilizing the nifurtimox side chain, has excellent activity against three recently isolated strains of *T.*

cruzi in mice (114). In laboratory tests, the compound had comparable activity to that of nifurtimox (114).

2.1.7 ANTIBIOTICS AND MISCELLANEOUS COMPOUNDS. The major groups of antibiotics have all been tested against trypanosomes *in vitro* and *in vivo* but with few exceptions are inactive. Puromycin (125, 126) (20.**55**) has a wide spectrum of antitrypanosomal activity and has been extensively studied in laboratory animals. It is active against murine infections of *T. equiperdum, T. equinum, T. evansi, T. gambiense,* and *T. rhodesiense* but not against *T. congolense* (125, 127, 128). Puromycin has been the subject of limited clinical trials against Gambian sleeping sickness, but the results were not promising (129). The mode of action of puromycin is thought to involve interference with tRNA in the parasite, and this hypothesis receives some support from the observation that the trypanocidal activity is selectively antagonized by adenine *in vivo* and *in vitro* (130, 131).

Removal of the *O*-methyltyrosyl residue of puromycin gives the 9-(3-amino-3-deoxy-β-D-ribosyl) derivative of 6-dimethylaminopurine (132), known as "aminonucleoside".

Aminonucleoside is severalfold more active than puromycin against *T. equiperdum*

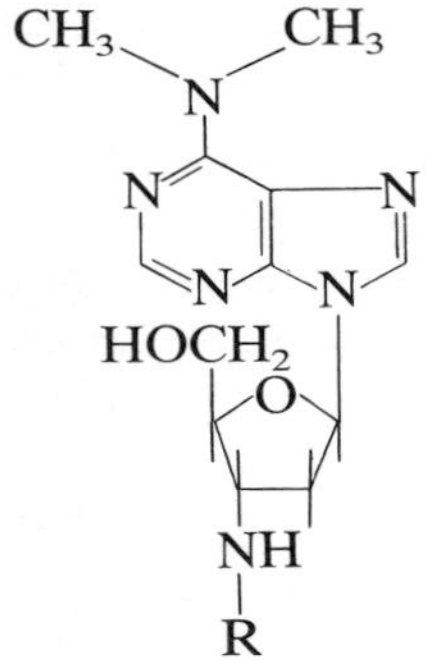

CH_3 CH_3 N N N N N $HOCH_2$ O NH R

20.**55** R = $COCHCH_2$–C_6H_4–OCH_3 (NH_2)

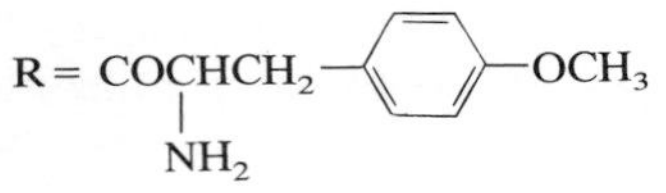

20.**56** R = H

infections in mice. Structural modification led to aminonucleoside analogs substituted in the 6- position by diethylamino- and dipropylamino groups that were 16–32 more active against *T. equiperdum* infections in mice (132).

Nucleocidin (20.**57**) (133) is more active against *T. congolense* than against *T. gambiense* in rats and mice (134) and, in addition, is active against *T. equiperdum* (135) and *T. equinum* infections in mice (134). Field trials against *T. vivax* and *T. congolense* infections in cattle and *T. simiae* infections in pigs showed some therapeutic but noncurative activity (136, 137).

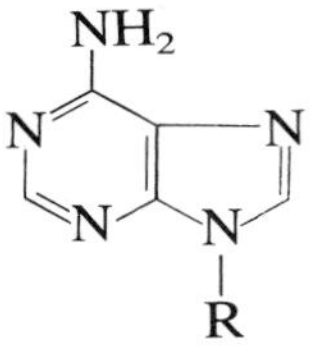

NH_2 N N N N R

20.**57** R = $CH_2SO_2NH_2$ O F HO OH

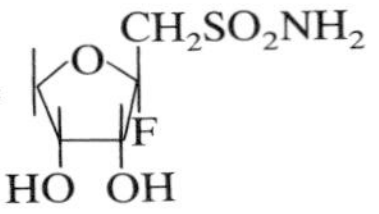

20.**58** R = CH_2OH O OH

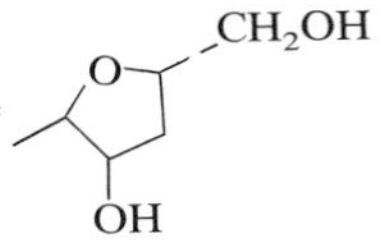

A related compound, cordycepin 20.**58** (138), has high specific activity against *T. congolense* infections in mice (139).

The well-known polyene antibiotic, amphotericin B (20.**59**), which has been in use for many years as a systemic antifungal agent (140), possesses significant activity against *T. cruzi* infections in mice (141). The mode of action of the compound is thought to involve the rupture of cytoplasmic membranes of trypanosomal cells (141).

An interesting biochemical approach to the chemotherapy of trypanosomiasis involves the blocking of the carbohydrate metabolism of the trypanosomes (142). Simultaneous administration of salicylhydroxamic acid and glycerol to rats and

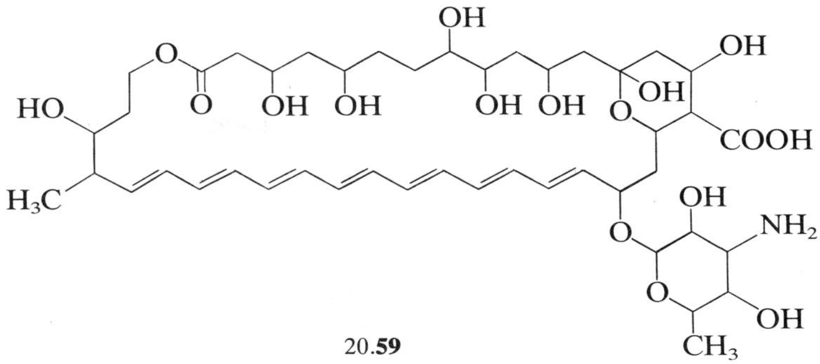

20.**59**

mice infected with *T. brucei* or *T. rhodesiense* results in the blocking of the aerobic and anaerobic glucose catabolism of the parasite, which is rapidly destroyed. However relapses occurred in the animals after some days. Nevertheless, this approach, based on interference with the peculiar carbohydrate catabolic pathway of trypanosomes, promises a more rational approach to the chemotherapy of the disease than hitherto has been available.

3 COCCIDIOSIS

The coccidia are microscopic protozoan parasites, belonging to the genera *Eimeria* and *Isospora*. These parasites infect vertebrates and invertebrates, sometimes causing serious or fatal diseases, particularly in domestic animals. From a commercial point of view, *Eimeria* infections are the more important. Poultry, cattle, and sheep can be seriously affected by *Eimeria* species. Since coccidiosis of chickens is virtually universal, the coccidia pose a serious economic threat to the world's poultry farmers (143, 144).

Chickens may be infected by any one of nine species of *Eimeria*, either alone or in combination, the most important being *E. brunetti, E. necatrix, E. acervulina, E. maxima, E. mivati,* and *E. tenella* (145, 146). The various species of *Eimeria* invade different regions of the digestive tract. This has some therapeutic importance, since some drugs are more active against cecal coccidiosis than against infections in other regions of the digestive tract. *E. acervulina* is found in the upper part of the small intestine; *E. necatrix* and *E. maxima* usually occur in the middle section of the intestine. *E. tenella* and *E. brunetti* occupy the lowest part of the digestive tract, the ceca, but the latter parasite also infects the rectum and cloaca (147). *E. tenella* is generally used for chemotherapeutic screening purposes (148).

Young turkeys are susceptible to seven species of *Eimeria*, but *E. gallopavonis, E. meleagrimitis,* and *E. adenoeides* are the most important (149). Whereas turkey poults readily contract the disease, older turkeys rarely become infected, possibly indicating an increase in resistance with age (150) or, alternatively, acquired immunity due to subclinical infections. Young calves may be infected with *E. bovis* or *E. zürnii*, the latter frequently causing fatalities (151). Lambs are often infected by *E. parva, E. pallida,* and other *Eimeria* species (152).

3.1 Chemotherapy of Coccidiosis

3.1.1 SULFONAMIDES AND OTHER *p*-AMINOBENZOIC ACID ANTAGONISTS. The introduction of the sulfonamides in 1940 for the control of coccidiosis in poultry (153, 154) transformed the control of the disease from empirical therapy to preventive medicine. Some sulfa drugs are still widely used today, but usually as a component in a

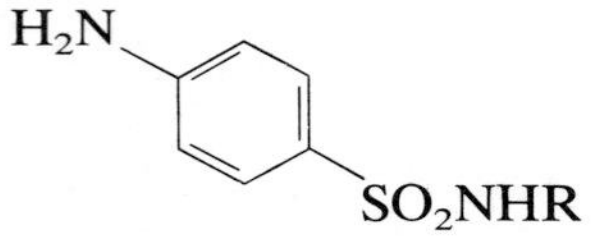

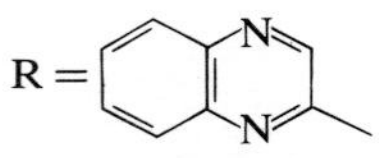

H_2N — SO_2NHR

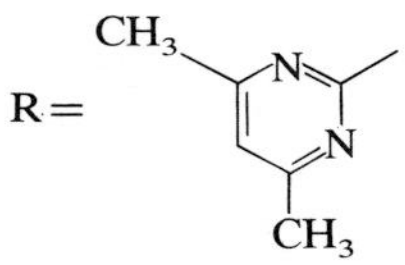

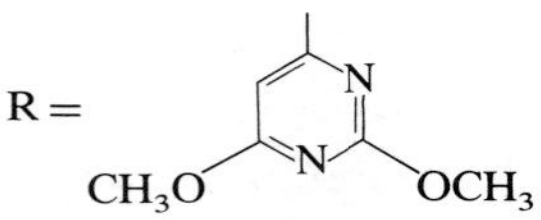

R = 20.60

R = 20.61

R = 20.62

R = 20.63

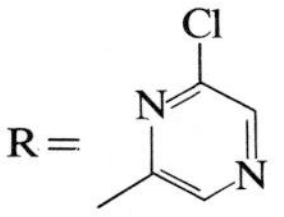

mixture of anticoccidial agents. Until recently, the most commonly used were sulfaquinoxaline (20.**60**) and sulfamethazine (20.**61**). The latter compound controls coccidiosis in sheep (151), whereas sulfaquinoxaline controls the disease in chicken and turkey poults when administered in the diet (150). Despite the introduction of new classes of anticoccidials, the sulfa drugs still play a part in the control of the disease. The emphasis has now shifted toward the use of the long-acting sulfa drugs exemplified by sulfadimethoxine (20.**62**) (155) and sulfachlorpyrazine (20.**63**) (156).

The anticoccidial activity of sulfa drugs is antagonized by *p*-aminobenzoic acid (PAB) (157), indicating that these compounds interfere with the PAB–folic acid metabolic pathway in the parasite. As a consequence, it would be expected (151) that other antifolate compounds would possess anticoccidial activity. Indeed this has proved to be the case, and it has been shown that compounds derived from the 2,4-diaminopyrimidine and the 2,2-dialkyl-1-aryl-4,6-diamino-1,2-dihydro-*s*-triazine class of antifolates have anticoccidial activity. In the former group, the most important compounds are 5(4-chlorophenyl)-2,4-diamino-6-ethylpyrimidine (20.**64**, pyrimethamine) (145), 5(3,4-dimethoxybenzyl)-2,4-diaminopyrimidine (20.**65**, diaverdine) (145), and 5(3,4-dimethoxy-2-methyl-benzyl-2,4-diaminopyrimidine (20.**66**, ormetoprim) (145).

In the dihydrotriazine series 1-(4-chlorophenyl)-4,6-diamino, 2,2-dimethyl 1,2-*s*-triazine (20.**67**), a metabolite of chloroguanide and its congener (20.**68**) are the most active (151).

Since the diaminopyrimidines and the sulfonamides interfere with the PAB–folic acid metabolic sequence at different stages, the former potentiate the activity of the sulfa drugs. As a result, much lower doses of each compound are needed to achieve control of the disease. Typical combinations that have been used are pyrimethamine (20.**64**) or diaverdine (20.**65**) plus sulfaquinoxaline (20.**60**) and ormetoprim (20.**66**), plus sulfadimethoxine (20.**62**)

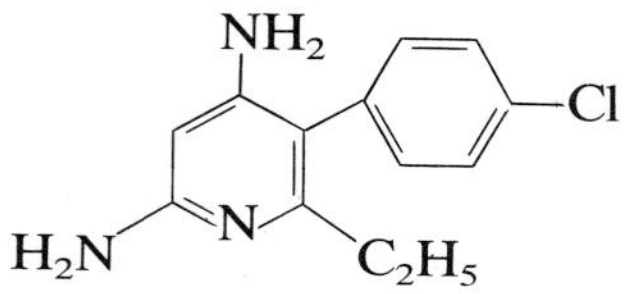

20.64

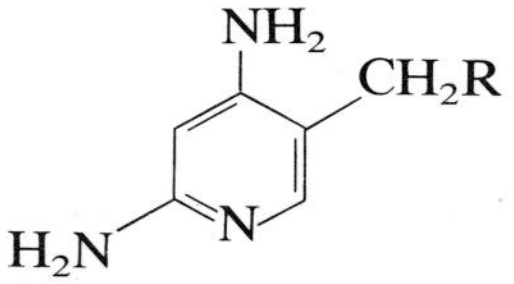

20.65 R =

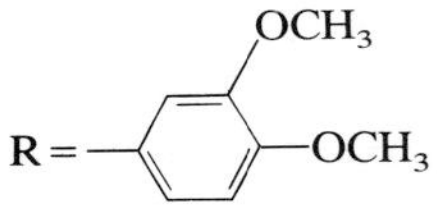

20.66 R =

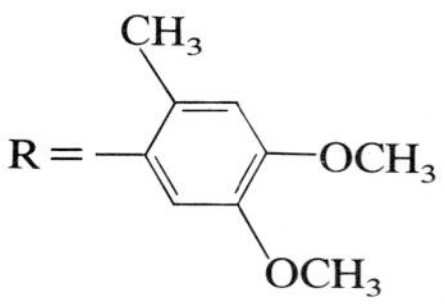

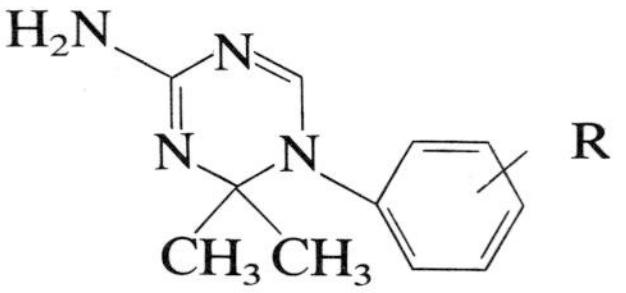

20.67 R=4—Cl

20.68 R=3,4-diCl

(158). The role of sulfonamides and potentiated mixtures with other antifolates has been comprehensively reviewed (145).

Compounds other than antifolates may also enhance the activity of sulfonamides, since a mixture of sulfamethazine (20.**61**) and 1,1′-dimethyl-4,4′-bipyridylium dichloride is much more active than the sulfonamide alone (159). The bipyridylium compound is inactive at nontoxic doses. In addition to the classical antifolates, a number of substituted *p*-aminobenzoic acids have been investigated for anticoccidial activity. The most active compound appears to be ethyl 2-ethoxy-4-acetamidobenzoate (20.**69**, ethopabate) (159, 160).

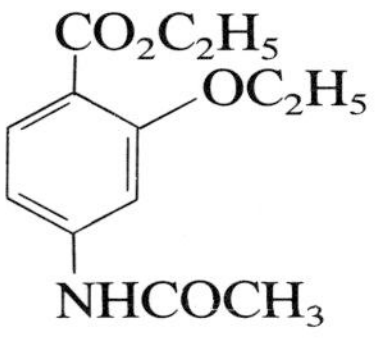

$CO_2C_2H_5$, OC_2H_5, $NHCOCH_3$

20·**69**

3.1.2 THIAMINE ANTAGONISTS AND RELATED COMPOUNDS. During work on thiamine antagonists (161, 162) it was found that amprolium (20.**70**) and many related compounds possessed anticoccidial properties. The exact mode of action of amprolium is uncertain, but it is believed that compared to the host, it preferentially reduces the uptake of thiamine (20.**72**) by the parasite (161). As a result of the success of amprolium, other thiamine analogs have been investigated, including the ethyl congener (20.**71**) of amprolium (163), 5-chloroethylthiamine (20.**73**, beclotiamine) dimethalium (20.**74**), and methylsulfinylethylthiamine (20.**75**), all of which display anticoccidial properties (164).

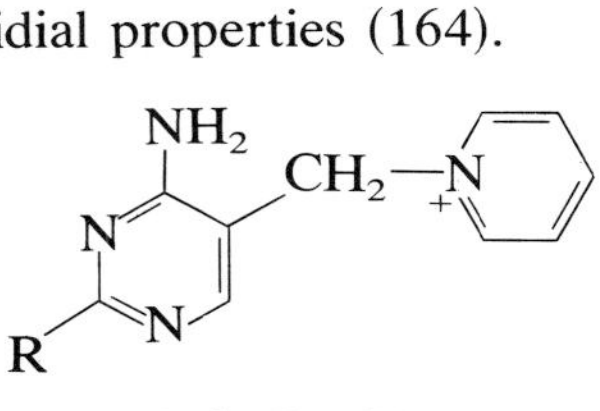

NH_2, CH_2—$\overset{+}{N}$, N, N, R

20.**70** $R = C_3H_7$
20.**71** $R = C_2H_5$

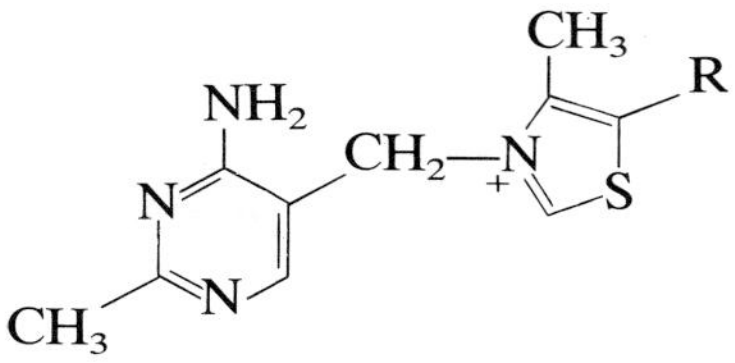

CH_3, R, NH_2, CH_2—$\overset{+}{N}$, S, N, N, CH_3

20.**72** $R = CH_2CH_2OH$
20.**73** $R = CH_2CH_2Cl$
20.**74** $R = CH_3$
20.**75** $R = CH_2CH_2SOCH_3$

Whereas large doses of amprolium cause polyneuritis in chickens, beclotiamine does not have this effect (165), and 20.**75** displays weak thiamine-like activity (166). A detailed study of amprolium analogs (167) demonstrated that the 4-aminopyrimidine moiety is essential for good anticoccidial activity, but a wide range of heterocyclic nuclei can substitute for the pyridinium group. Thiamine analogs in which the thiazole ring has been opened to give structures 20.**76** (167) and 20.**77** (168) are claimed to be anticoccidials.

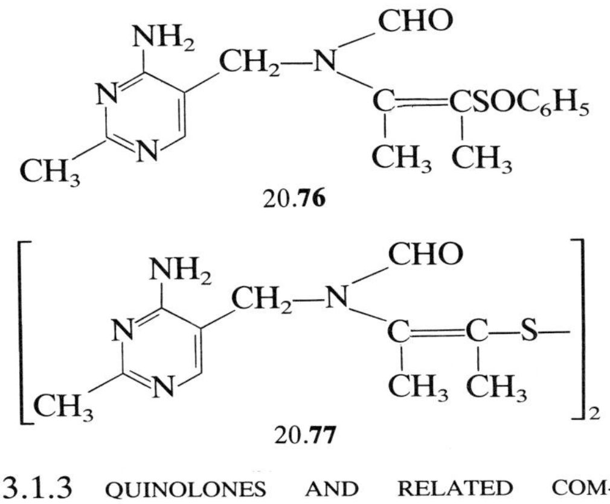

NH_2, CH_2—N, CHO, N, N, CH_3, C═$CSOC_6H_5$, CH_3 CH_3

20.**76**

[NH_2, CH_2—N, CHO, N, N, CH_3, C═C—S—, CH_3 CH_3 $]_2$

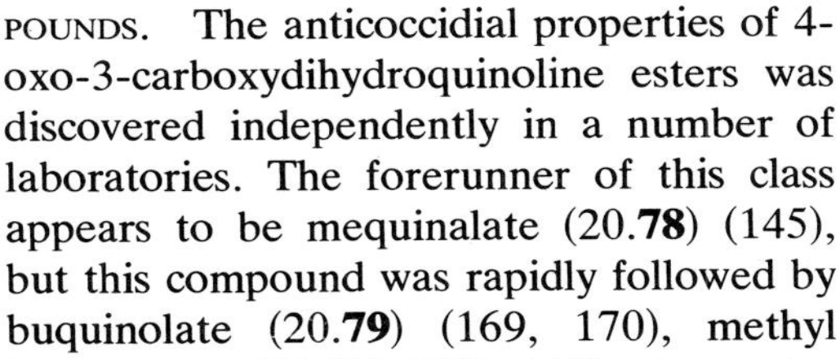

20.**77**

3.1.3 QUINOLONES AND RELATED COMPOUNDS. The anticoccidial properties of 4-oxo-3-carboxydihydroquinoline esters was discovered independently in a number of laboratories. The forerunner of this class appears to be mequinalate (20.**78**) (145), but this compound was rapidly followed by buquinolate (20.**79**) (169, 170), methyl benzoquate (20.**80**) (171, 172), decoquinate (20.**81**) (173), cyproquinate (20.**82**) (174), and amquinolate (20.**83**) (175), representing the best of very large series of

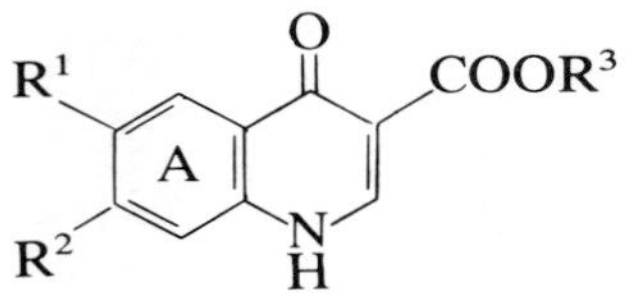

20.**78** $R^1 = R^2 = (CH_3)_2CHO$; $R^3 = CH_3$
20.**79** $R^1 = R^2 = (CH_3)_2CHCH_2O$; $R^3 = C_2H_5$
20.**80** $R^1 = C_4H_9$; $R^2 = C_6H_5CH_2O$; $R^3 = CH_3$
20.**81** $R^1 = C_{10}H_{21}O$; $R^2 = C_2H_5O$; $R^3 = C_2H_5$
20.**82** $R^1 = R^2 = c\text{-}C_3H_5CH_2O$; $R^3 = C_2H_5$
20.**83** $R^1 = C_3H_7$; $R^2 = (C_2H_5)_2N$; $R^3 = CH_3$

compounds. Structure-activity relationships have been discussed in detail (176–178). A wide range of substituents can be tolerated in the A-ring without loss of activity. Interestingly, the free acids are inactive. The mode of action of this class of compound is unknown, but at least with decoquinate there is a suggestion that the drug interferes with the synthesis of the nucleic acid in the protozoan cell (179). Despite their low toxicity and high activity, the quinolones suffer a grave disadvantage in that *Eimeria* species rapidly develop resistance to them (180).

Although 3,5-dichloro-2,6-dimethyl-4-pyridone (20.**84**, metichlorpindol, clopidol)

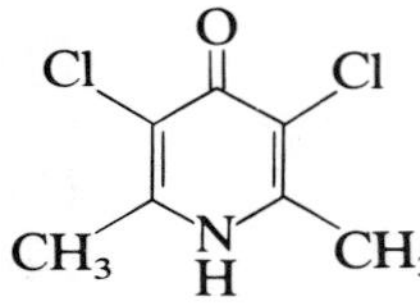

20.**84**

(181, 182) bears a superficial relationship to the quinolones (183), its mode of action as an anticoccidial must differ from that of the quinolones, since it has been shown that strains of *E. acervulina* that resist quinolones are not resistant to clopidol (181).

Synergism between the two classes of compounds has been observed (182).

Another group of compounds related to the quinolones are derivatives of the antimalarial drug febrifugine (20.**85**). The best compounds appear to be 20.**86** and 20.**87** (183).

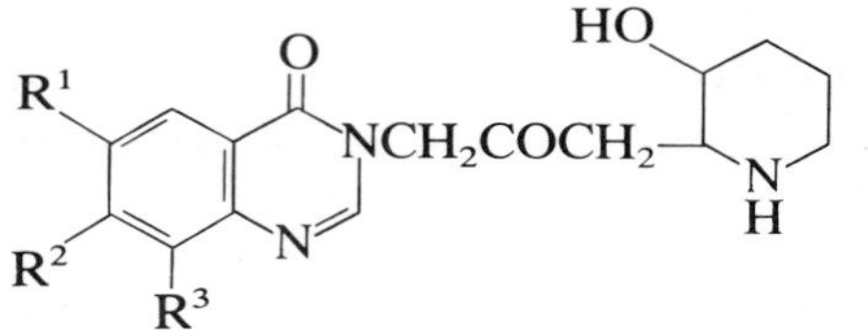

20.**85** $R^1 = R^2 = R^3 = H$
20.**86** $R^1 = R^3 = Cl$; $R^2 = H$
20.**87** $R^1 = Cl$; $R^2 = Br$; $R^3 = H$

3.1.4 NITROBENZAMIDES. A wide range of nitrobenzamides have been shown to have useful anticoccidial activity. The most important compounds are 3,5-dinitro-2-methylbenzamide (20.**88**, zoalene) (184), 3,5-dinitrobenzamide (20.**89**, nitromide) (185), and 4-nitro-2-chlorobenzamide (20.**90**, alkomide) (186). Although it is

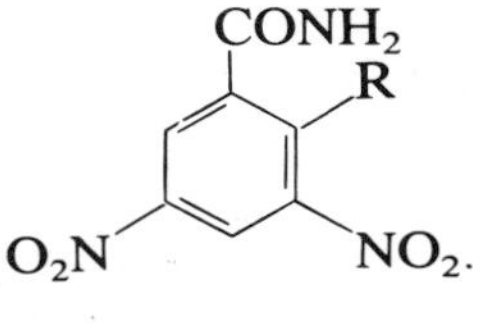

20.**88** R = Me
20.**89** R = H

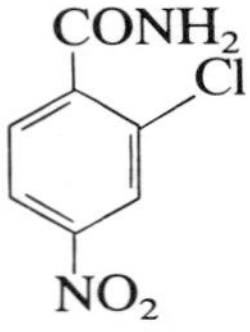

20.**90**

known that the nitro group is essential for significant anticoccidial activity (187), there is no direct evidence that the compounds act as antifolates as do the related aminobenzoic acids (*vide supra*). Detailed studies of the requirements for activity in this class of compound have been undertaken (187–190).

3.1.5 GUANIDINES. Robenidine, 1,3-bis(4-chlorobenzylideneamino)guanidine hydrochloride, 20.**91**, one of the most recently

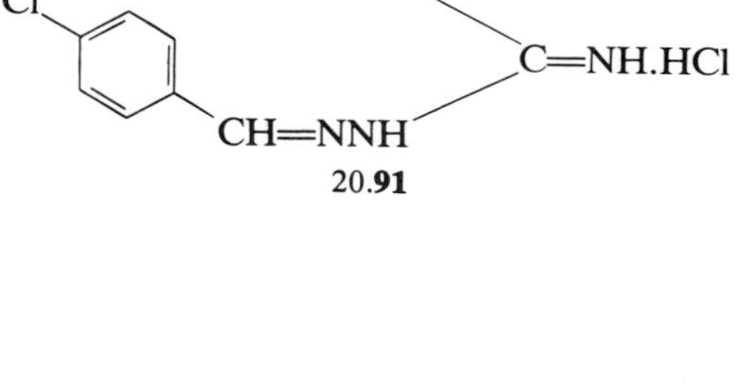

20.**91**

introduced compounds, shows efficacy against all pathogenic *Eimeria* species in chickens (191, 192). The compound is metabolized to 4-chlorobenzoic acid and is excreted mainly as 4-chlorohippuric acid (193). The mode of action of robenidine has been investigated, and it appears to affect all stages of the life cycle of the parasite (194).

3.1.6 IONOPHORIC ANTIBIOTICS. Monensin (20.**92**), a product of the fermentation of *Streptomyces cinnamonensis* (195), belongs to a group of polyether antibiotics first isolated some 25 years ago (196, 197). In common with a number of other fermentation products, these compounds, which are termed ionophores, render cations lipid soluble, enabling them to pass across cell membranes. Two modes of transport for the cations are apparent: the antibiotic either forms channels in the membrane or acts as a mobile carrier. The polyether antibiotics belong to the latter group and possess the remarkable ability to render mitochondrial membranes permeable to certain cations by passive diffusion down the concentration gradient (198–200). The determination of the structure of monensin (201) and the demonstration of its anticoccidial activity (202) and that of three other ionophoric antibiotics, X206, dianemycin, and nigericin (203), stimulated interest in this general class of compound. However only monensin has been marketed, although detailed studies on the anticoccidial properties of lasalocid (20.**93**) (69) a metabolite of *Streptomyces lasaliensis*, and salinomycin (20.**94**) (205) have been carried out.

Of these three compounds, the anticoccidial properties of monensin are best documented, particularly with regard to coccidiosis in poultry (206–208).

Monensin possesses excellent activity against *E. bovis* infections in cattle (209) and natural infections of *E. parva*, *E. pallida*, *E. ovina*, *E. ninakohyakimovae*, and *E. ahsata* in lambs (210).

Other ionophoric antibiotics claimed to

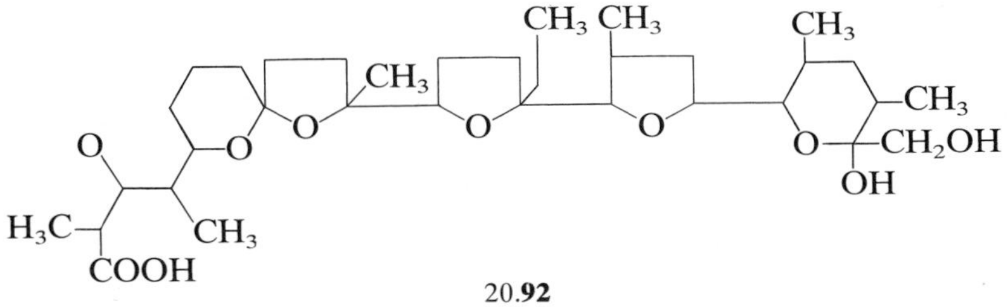

20.**92**

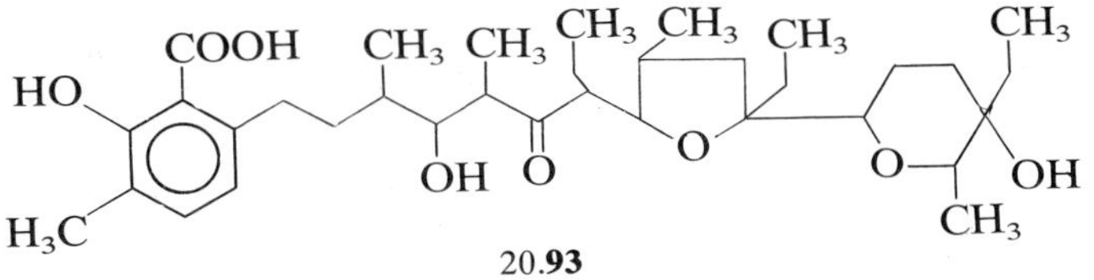

20.**93**

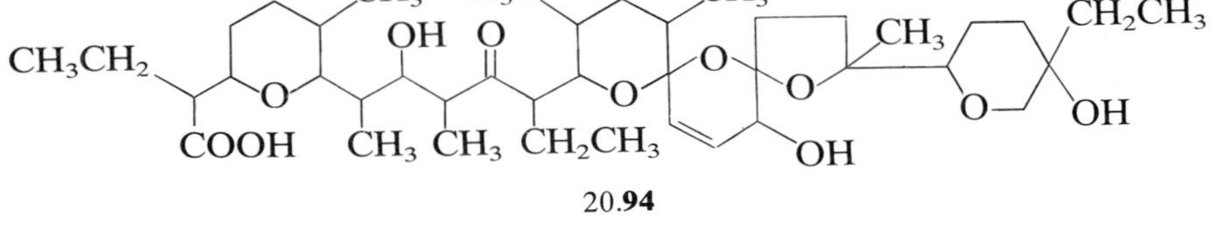

20.**94**

have anticoccidial properties include dianemycin (211), nigericin (212), lysocellin (213, 214), and laidlomycin (215).

The polyether antibiotics are poorly absorbed from the intestinal tract of the chicken and are selectively toxic to *Eimeria* species.

Although the mode of action of monensin on *Eimeria* species is not known in detail, possibly its effect is through the disruption of the normal metabolism of the parasite by altering the permeability of membranes to sodium, potassium, hydrogen, and other ions (200).

3.1.7 MISCELLANEOUS COMPOUNDS. In addition to the compounds already described in Section 3, diverse types of organic derivatives have useful anticoccidial properties. In particular, 3-nitro-4-hydroxyphenylarsonic acid (216, 217) and related compounds (218) possess commercially useful anticoccidial activity. The antibacterial nitrofurans, 5-nitro-2-furaldehyde semicarbazone (20.**37**, nitrofurazone) and *N*-(5-nitro-2-furfurylidene)-3-amino-2-oxazolidinone (furazolidine) are used in combination with other drugs as therapeutic anticoccidials (219, 220).

Nicarbazin is obtained by cocrystallizing from methanol a 1:1 mixture of 4,4′-dinitrocarbanilide and 4,6-dimethyl-2-pyrimidinol (221). Whereas the carbanilide has anticoccidial properties, the pyrimidinol is inactive (222); however the molecular complex is 10 times as active as the carbanilide alone. Mechanical mixing of the components does not enhance activity.

Various bisthiosemicarbazones (223), in particular bitipazone (20.**95**), are claimed to have useful anticoccidial properties. A

CH_3 C=NNHCSNHCH$_2$CH$_2$N (piperidine)
C=NNHCSNHCH$_2$CH$_2$N (piperidine) CH_3

20.**95**

number of hydroxyquinones, as exemplified by (20.**96**), originally prepared as antimalarials, are active against *E. brunetti* and *E. tenella* infections in chicks (224).

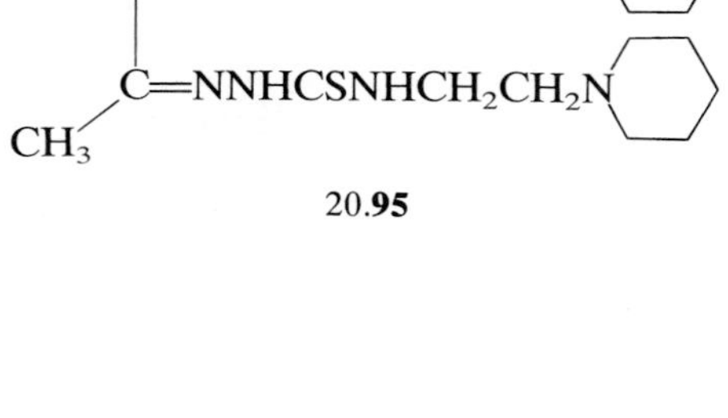

O, O, $(CH_2)_3$, OCH, C_3H_7, C_3H_7

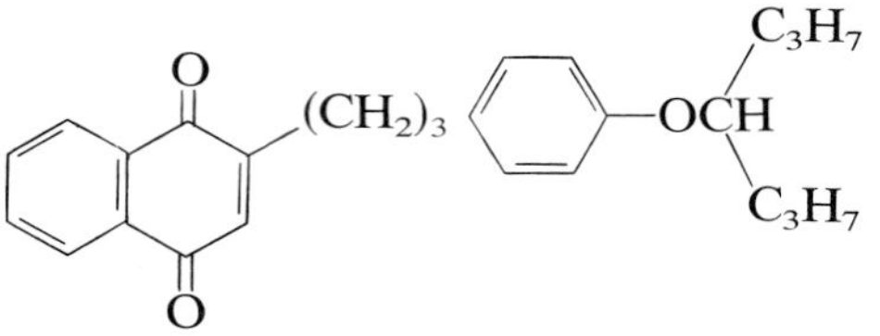

20.**96**

3,3′-Dinitrodiphenyl disulfide (nitrophenide) (225), *p*-dimethylaminobenzonitrile (226), and 5-dimethylamino-5,6-dihydro-6-methoxy-2-methyl-2-(4′-biphenylyl)2*H*-pyran-3(4*H*)-one (20.**97**) (227) and related compounds are active against *E. tenella* infections in chicks.

O, $N(CH_3)_2$, OCH_3, O, CH_3

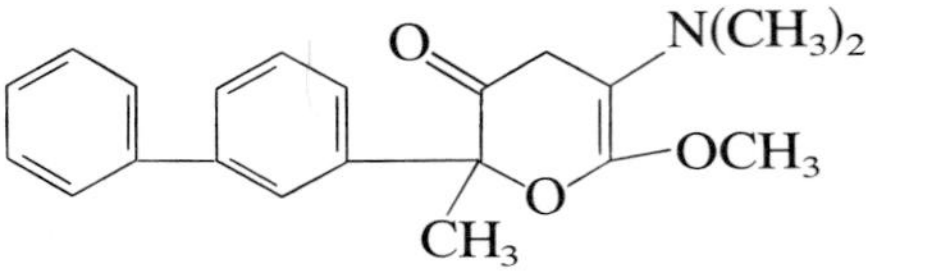

20.**97**

4 TRICHOMONIASIS

Trichomonads are parasitic flagellates, widely distributed in the animal kingdom. They are found most commonly on the mucosal surfaces of the intestinal or genitourinary tract, giving rise to the disease trichomoniasis. Only *Trichomonas vaginalis*, *T. foetus*, and *T. gallinae* are considered to be pathogenic. *T. hominis* and *T. tenax* are harmless commensals of the intestine and mouth of man, respectively. *T. vaginalis* is a parasite of the human genitourinary tract but generally causes overt trichomaniasis only in the female. *T. foetus* is a parasite of the genitourinary tract of cattle and is a common cause of abortion. *T. gallinae* is a parasite of the intestinal tract of domestic fiowl. All three species have been adapted to mice for chemotherapeutic screening purposes, but generally *T. vaginalis* and *T. foetus* are used (229). In addition, *in vitro* systems utilizing these organisms have been developed and are widely used for screening purposes (228, 229).

4.1 Chemotherapy of Trichomoniasis

4.1.1 NITROTHIAZOLES. Until the advent of systemically active trichomonacides, the chemotherapy of trichomoniasis presented a difficult problem. Although a number of compounds were known to act as topical trichomonacides, relapses were common, despite prolonged treatment (230). The first group of compounds to display systemic activity against *Trichomonas* infections in mice were derivatives of 2-amino-5-nitrothiazole (20.**98**, entramin). A detailed investigation of this group of compounds (231, 232) demonstrated that although the parent compound 20.**98** and numerous acylated derivatives were active, the acetamido compound (20.**99**, acinitrazole) possessed the best *in vitro* and *in vivo* activity against *T. vaginalis* and *T. foetus.* However clinical trials with acinitrazole were disappointing (233, 234).

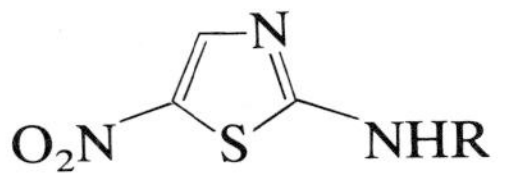

20.**98** R = H
20.**99** $R = COCH_3$
20.**100** $R = CONHC_2H_5$

Nevertheless, the demonstration of *in vivo* activity in this class of nitroheterocycle stimulated investigations in the general area and a group of 5-nitrothiazoles of general structure 20.**101**, which possess interesting *in vitro* and *in vivo* trichomonacidal activity, have been described (235).

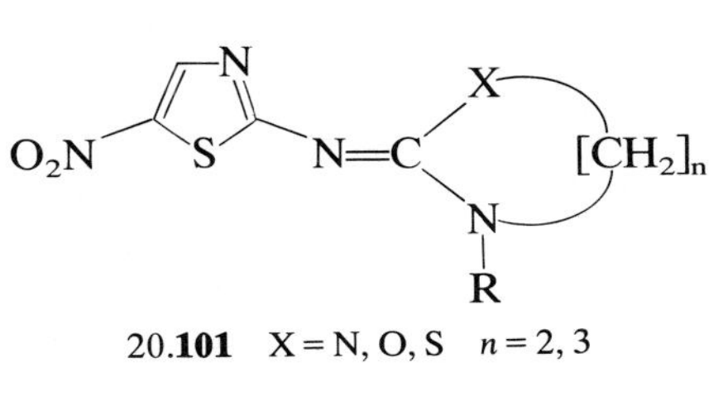

20.**101** X = N, O, S $n = 2, 3$

An analysis of the *in vitro* activity of the compounds against *T. foetus* indicated that the order was S, O, N, but *in vivo* experiments with the same organism in mice revealed good activity in all three series. The mode of action of these nitrothiazoles appears to be through interference with nitroreductase enzymes in the parasite. The metabolism of the compounds has also been investigated and partly explains the variation between *in vitro* and *in vivo* activities in the three series (235). Many other nitrothiazoles have been investigated for antitrichomonal activity, the most notable being the antischistosomal and antiamebic agent, niridazole (20.**102**, Ambilhar) and related ureas (236). Other nitroheterocyclic compounds have been examined for antitrichomonal activity and two, 2-amino-5-nitropyridine and 2-amino-5-nitro-pyrimidine, possess activity similar to that of acinitrazole (237). Replacement of the amino group by a hydroxyl function in these compounds enhances activity in the pyridine case, but the pyrimidine and thiazole analogs are inactive (237).

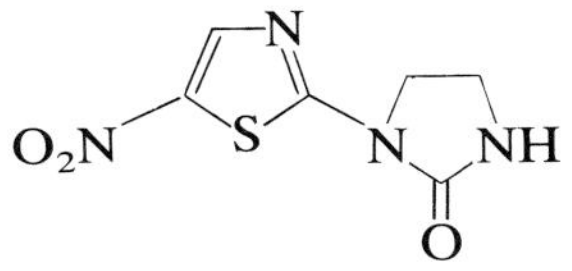

20.**102**

4.1.2 NITROIMIDAZOLES. Whereas the nitrothiazoles failed to live up to their early promise as trichomonacides, the observation of antiparasitic activity with certain nitroimidazoles has resulted in a plethora of compounds possessing interesting biological properties. The seminal observation was the discovery of antitrichomonal activity in the antibiotic azomycin (20.**103**) (238, 239).

Although 2-nitroimidazole derivatives

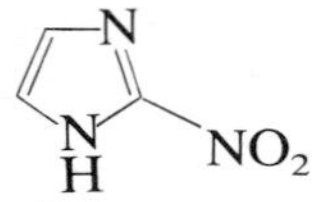

20.**103**

can be prepared, they are relatively inaccessible compared to the corresponding 4(5)-nitroimidazoles, and detailed investigation of the latter compounds by two separate groups of workers led to the discovery of compounds possessing potent systemic antitrichomonal activity. Workers at Rhône-Poulenc discovered metronidazole (20.**104**) (240), which is now the drug of choice for the treatment of human trichomoniasis (241–243).

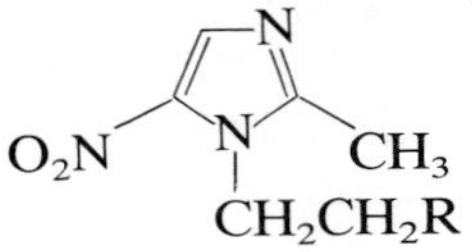

20.**104** R = OH
20.**105** R = SO_2CH_3
20.**106** R = $NHC(=S)OCH_3$
20.**107** R = $OC(=S)NHCH_3$

Structure activity studies by this group led to the conclusion that, in general, 1-substituted 5-nitroimidazoles possessed antitrichomonal activity superior to that of the 4-nitro analogs (244). Concurrently, a group at Merck were investigating imidazoles as antiparasitic agents, having observed that imidazole 4,5-dicarboxamide (glycarbylamide) possessed interesting anticoccidal activity (245). Modification of this structure led to 1-methyl-4-nitroimidazole-5-carboxamide, which displayed moderate activity against *T. foetus* in mice (246). Further investigations resulted in the discovery of a wide range of very active 2-substituted 1-methyl-5-nitroimidazoles, particularly 1-(2-hydroxyethyl)-2-(*p*-fluorophenyl)-5-nitroimidazole (20.**46**, flunidazole) (247), 1-methyl-2-(*p*-fluorophenyl)-5-nitroimidazole (20.**47**, MK 910) (248), the 2-carbamoyloxymethyl (20.**49**, ronidazole), and 2-morpholinomethyl derivatives (249). Perschin (250) compared 20 of the 5-nitroimidazoles in terms of their antitrichomonal activity.

Investigation of the metabolism of metronidazole in humans and laboratory animals has shown that the compound gives three major metabolites, 1-(2-hydroxyethyl)-2-hydroxymethyl-5-nitroimidazole, 1-(2-hydroxyethyl)-2-carboxy-5-nitroimidazole, and 1-(carboxymethyl)-2-methyl-5-nitroimidazole, all of which are inactive against *T. vaginalis* (251, 253). However no evidence has been presented to indicate that substantial reduction of the nitro group occurs, as with the nitrothiazoles. This vulnerability of metronidazole to oxidative metabolism has prompted the investigation of related compounds that possess greater metabolic stability. Replacement of the vulnerable 1-(2-hydroxyethyl) group by a cyanoethyl function led to a series of 1-(2-cyanoethyl)-2-alkyl-5-nitroimidazoles possessing significantly greater activity against *T. foetus* infections in mice than does metronidazole (254). A smooth bell-shaped curve is obtained when log K (partition coefficient in n-octanol–aqueous buffer) is plotted against $1/CD_{50}$ for this series of compounds. Other series of compounds show similar relationships, with certain variations in the shape of the curve due to variation of parameters other than partition coefficient. From these observations, it appears that the simplest structural requirement for biological activity is the 1-alkyl-5-nitroimidazole unit and that the nitro group should not be sterically crowded (254). Development of this theme resulted in the discovery of tinidazole (20.**105**) (255) and nitrimidazine (20.**108**, nimorazole) (256) and their introduction as effective therapy for human trichomoniasis (257, 258). Both compounds are significantly less readily metabolized in animals than is metronidazole (259, 260). In humans, tinidazole appears to be excreted unchanged (261), but nitrimidazine is metabolized to 20.**109** and 20.**110** (260).

Investigation of the requirements for antitrichomonal activity in the sulfone

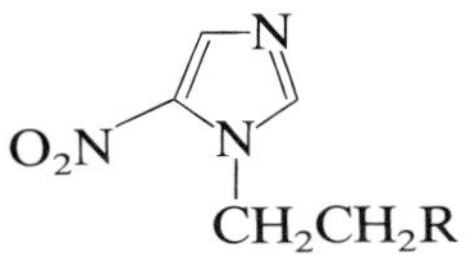

20.**108** R = morpholino; 20.**109** R = 3-oxomorpholino; 20.**110** R = morpholino N-oxide
O_2N ... CH_2CH_2R

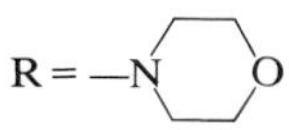

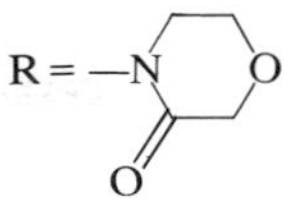

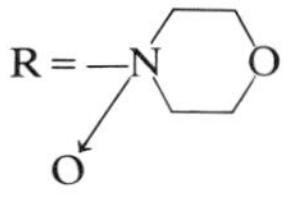

series of compounds related to tinidazole demonstrated that within narrow structural limits, the activity was directly proportional to the octanol-water partition coefficient (262). The biological properties of tinidazole have been reviewed in detail (263). Yet another series of compounds derived from metronidazole is exemplified by 20.**106** and 20.**107**, both of which have excellent activity against *T. vaginalis* infections in mice (264).

A wide range of 1-substituted 5-nitroimidazoles of general structure 20.**111** have

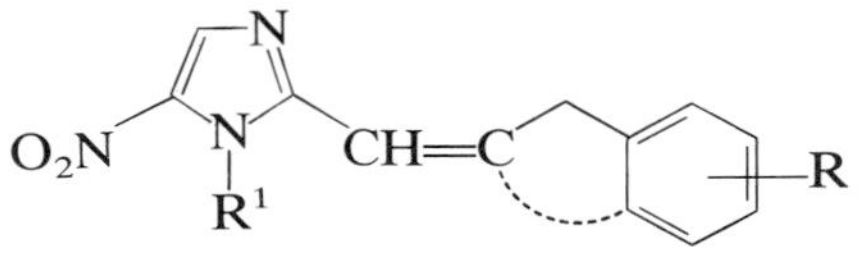

20.**111**

been investigated, and many possess activity similar to that of metronidazole (265).

The nitroimidazole analog of furaltadone (20.**112**) shows useful antitrichomonal activity (266). The enantiomers of this compound were prepared but were equipotent

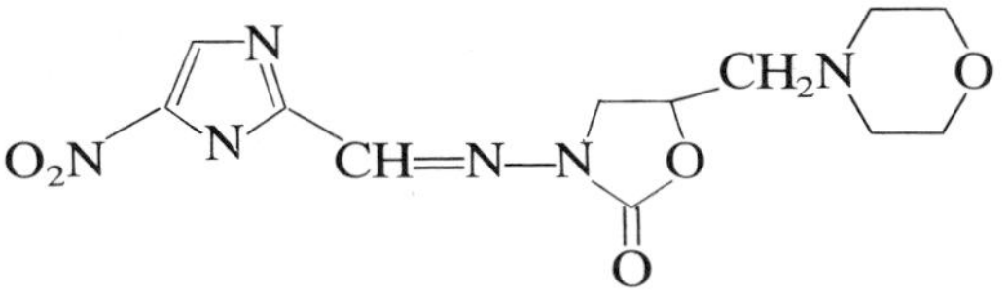

20.**112**

as trichomonacides (267). In general, it can be stated that 1-substituted 5-nitroimidazoles possess intrinsic antitrichomonal activity, and by variation of the substituents, it is possible to obtain compounds having useful systemic activity in animals or in man. Despite the detailed investigation of numerous nitroimidazoles, metronidazole remains the drug of choice for the treatment of human trichomoniasis.

4.1.3 MISCELLANEOUS COMPOUNDS. Although the hunt for effective antitrichomonals has centered on the nitroimidazoles during the last 15 years, many other nitroheterocyclic compounds have been found to possess significant activity in experimentally induced trichomoniasis infections. These include a wide range of nitrofurans (268–270), nitrothiophenes (270), nitropyrazoles (272), and nitropyrroles (273, 274). In the last group, 1-(2-hydroxyethyl)-5-nitropyrrole-2-carboxamide appears to be equipotent with metronidazole in *T. vaginalis* infections that were induced experimentally.

Other structures claimed to possess antitrichomonal properties are listed by Steck (57).

5 LEISHMANIASIS

The leishmaniases are a complex of diseases caused by the leishmania, which are intracellular parasites belonging, in common with the trypanosomes, to the highly infectious family of hemoflagellates. The parasites are transmitted by the bite of sandflies (*Phlebotomus* spp.) or possibly by direct contact. Natural hosts for the leishmania are man, dogs, and gerbils. Leishmaniasis afflicts millions of people throughout Asia, the Middle East, Africa, southern Europe, and Latin America and remains one of the world's major communicable diseases (1). Two forms of the disease are recognized; (1) visceral leishmaniasis, caused by members of the *Leishmania donovani* complex, principally found in the Old World and known as kala-azar (black fever) (275), and (2) mucocutaneous leishmaniasis, caused by the *L. tropica*, *L. mexicana*, and *L. braziliensis* complexes. The *L. tropica* complex gives rise to a disease known as oriental sore which may be "dry" or "moist" and is found in Asia. The New World leishmania complexes, *L. mexicana* and *L. braziliensis*, lead to diseases known variously as "chiclero's ear" or "ulcer", Bay sore, espundia, and uta (276). The chemotherapy of the diseases has been reviewed in depth (57, 277, 278).

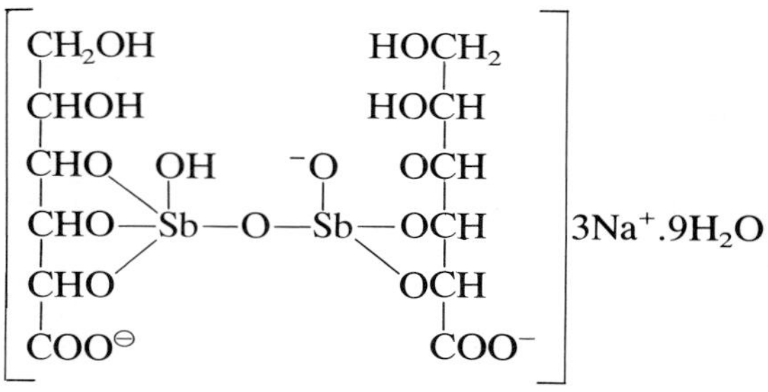

5.1 Antimonials

The introduction of tartar emetic in 1912 for the treatment of mucocutaneous leishmaniasis (279) heralded a new era in the treatment of the disease. This compound, which had already been successfully used in trypanosomiasis (280), and many other trivalent antimony compounds including sodium antimonyl tartrate, sodium antimony bis(pyrocatechol-3,5-disulfonate) (stibophen), and lithium antimony thiomalate (anthiomaline), were investigated for clinical efficacy in leishmaniasis. Although these compounds are somewhat less toxic than tartar emetic, they are still too toxic, as well as insufficiently potent, to be satisfactory (277).

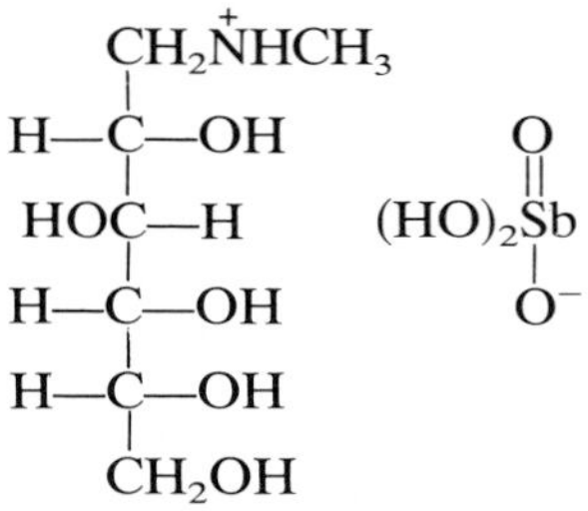

Until about 1924 tests for leishmanicides were carried out against trypanosomes (*T. equiperdum*), but the discovery that the Chinese hamster could be infected with *L. donovani* (281) resulted in a more rational approach to the evaluation of compounds. Golden hamsters infected with *L. donovani* are now generally used for screening purposes (278). This has led to the discovery of a series of quinquevalent antimony derivatives that have laboratory and clinical efficacy. In addition, quinquevalent antimony derivatives are less toxic and better tolerated than tartar emetic, which is now rarely used in the therapy of leishmaniasis. Sodium stibogluconate (20.**113**) (282) has become one of the drugs of choice for the treatment of the disease, as has meglumine (20.**114**, glucantime) (283).

Urea stibamine, a complex of ill-defined structure derived from urea and *p*-aminophenylstibonic acid, and ethyl stibamine, a substance obtained from *p*-acetamidophenylstibonic acid, antimonic acid, and diethylamine, have been employed clinically (57). The preparation of these antimony complexes is reminiscent of alchemy, and the reader is referred to review articles (57, 277), for more detail on their preparation and use in therapy.

$$\left[\begin{array}{ccc} CH_2OH & & HOCH_2 \\ CHOH & & HOCH \\ CHO \quad OH & {}^-O & OCH \\ CHO-Sb-O-Sb-OCH & & \\ CHO & & OCH \\ COO^{\ominus} & & COO^- \end{array}\right] 3Na^+.9H_2O$$

20.**113**

$$\begin{array}{c} CH_2\overset{+}{N}HCH_3 \\ H-C-OH \\ HOC-H \\ H-C-OH \\ H-C-OH \\ CH_2OH \end{array} \qquad (HO)_2Sb(=O)O^-$$

20.**114**

5.2 Miscellaneous Compounds

Despite the investigation of a wide range of chemical types, few compounds other than the antimonials possess useful activity against laboratory or clinical leishmanial infections. The trypanocidal diamidines, stilbamidine (20.**23**), hydroxystilbamidine (20.**27**), diminazene (20.**26**), propamidine (20.**22**), and pentamidine (20.**21**) all possess useful activity (57, 277). (See Section 2.1.3.) In particular, pentamidine has become the agent of choice for the treatment of antimony-resistant leishmanial infections (57).

The repository antimalarial drug cycloguanil pamoate (20.**115**), when injected intramuscularly as an oily suspension, is regarded as the drug of choice for oriental sore (57, 282), but not all forms of *L. tropica* respond equally well.

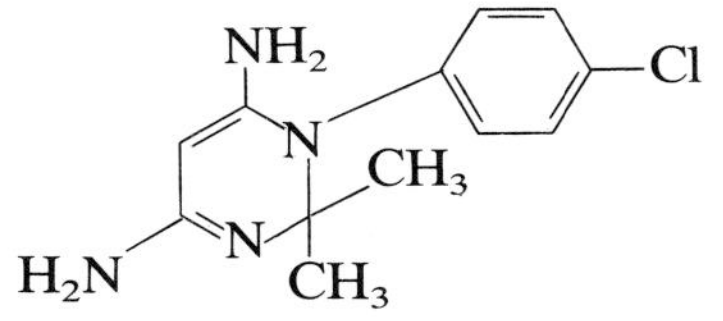

20.**115**

The polyene antibiotics, amphotericin B (20.**59**) and nystatin, both possess antileishmanial activity. The former compound is active against *L. donovani* infections in hamsters and mice (283) and has proved useful in the treatment of mucocutaneous leishmaniasis, particularly cases that have resisted both antimonials and diamidines (57).

Nystatin is active against *L. donovani* infections in laboratory animals (283) and has been used in the treatment of kala-azar (284), but it does not appear to offer any advantage over amphotericin B.

2-Dehydroemetine hydrochloride has produced a good response in cutaneous leishmaniasis (284), as has the alkaloid berberine chloride (57). Various other compounds have been claimed to possess antileishmanial activity; the evidence is not always convincing, however, and the reader is referred to Refs. 57 and 278 for more details.

6 HISTOMONIASIS

6.1 The Disease

Histomoniasis is a disease of poultry, particularly of turkeys and other gallinaceous birds, caused by *Histomonas meleagridis* (285) the only important pathogenic species belonging to the family *Mastigamoebidae.* The parasite is found in lesions of the cecum and liver and sometimes in the cecal contents or feces. The disease is often termed infectious enterohepatitis or "blackhead", and the bird becomes infected by ingesting either the trophozoites or the embryonated eggs of the cecal worm *Heterakis gallinarium* containing *H. meleagridis.* The etiology and dissemination of histomoniasis in turkeys and chickens has been reviewed (286). Young turkeys are the best hosts for chemotherapeutic screening purposes, but it is possible to use young chickens (less than a week old), which are more convenient and economical (287).

6.2 Chemotherapy of Histomoniasis

Until about 1950, acetarsol (20.**116**, stovarsol) (288) and related arsenicals were

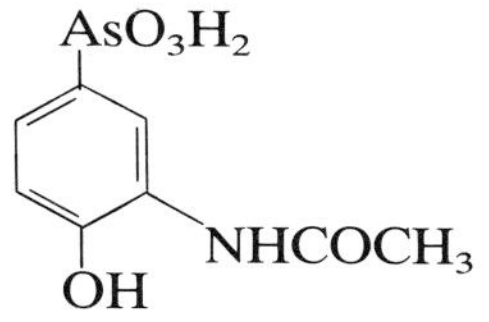

20.**116**

the mainstay in the control of histomonasias in the field, but these have since been superseded by a number of nitroheterocycles.

The first member of the new generation of compounds was 2-amino-5-nitrothiazole (20.**98**), which was the first really effective agent used for the control of *Histomonas* (289). The drug is administered in the diet for manifest infections or as a prophylactic; however it has only a suppressive effect on the parasite unless treatment is begun at the time of infection or shortly thereafter. This compound was superseded by its *N*-acetyl derivative acinitrazole (20.**99**) (290) and the *N*-ethyl urea derivative (20.**100**, nithiazide), which was the most active member of a series of ureas (291).

The discovery of the high prophylactic activity of 1,2-dimethyl-5-nitroimidazole (20.**117**, dimetridazole) against *H. meleagridis* infections in turkeys (292) gave fresh impetus to the study of all aspects of the chemotherapy of the disease.

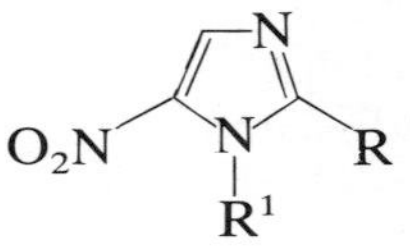

20.**117** R = R^1 = Me
20.**118** R = $CH(CH_3)_2$, R^1 = Me

A detailed study of a wide range of 1-2-disubstituted 5-nitroimidazoles led to the introduction of 1-methyl-2-isopropyl-5-nitro-imidazole (20.**118**, Ipronidazole) as an effective histomonastat (9). This compound is claimed to be twice as effective as dimetridazole and at least 4–8 times more effective than the other related nitroimidazoles tested against *H. meleagridis* in turkeys (293). Ronidazole (20.**49**), 1-methyl-2-carbomoyloxymethyl-5-nitroimidazole is also an effective histomonastat (294, 295). These three drugs, when used at recommended levels, show essentially the same antihistomonal activity in turkey poults (296).

The metabolism of dimetridazole in turkeys has been investigated and a number of metabolites identified (297). The major metabolites were 1-methyl-5-nitroimidazol-2-yl-methyl hydrogen sulfate, 1-methyl-5-nitroimidiazole-2-carboxylic acid, 2-hydroxymethyl-1-methyl-5-nitroimidazole, and the glucuronide of the latter compound. The nitro group appears to resist the reductases of the body, since about 90% of excreted drug comprises various nitroimidazoles.

Other nitrohetercycles have been investigated for antihistomonal activity, the most important being the nitrofurans, furazolidone (20.**119**) (298), the acetylhydrazone (20.**120**) (299), and the important new histomonastat 3,5-dinitrosalicyclic acid (5-nitro-furfurylidene) hydrazide (20.**121**), nifursol (300–302).

Other compounds that have been studied

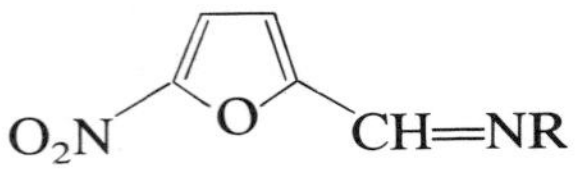

O_2N–(furan)–CH=NR

20.**119** R = (3-oxazolidin-2-one)

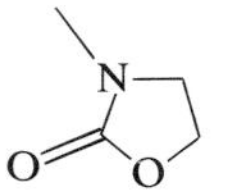

20.**120** R = $NHCOCH_3$

20.**121** R = NHCO–(2-hydroxy-3,5-dinitrophenyl)

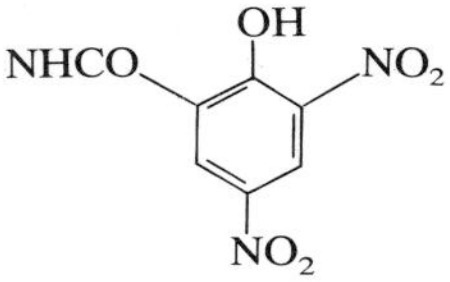

in histomoniasis control include iodochlor hydroxyquinoline (303), tryparsamide (20.**8**) (304), and the antibiotic paromomycin sulfate (305).

7 BABESIASIS

7.1 The Disease

Babesiasis or piroplasmosis is a group of tick-borne diseases caused by various species of *Babesia*, the most important being *B. bigemina*, *B. bovis*, *B. divergens*, *B. caballi*, *B. equini*, and *B. canis*.

Babesiasis is a highly pathogenic disease of animals and may cause high mortality in susceptible species such as cattle, dogs, horses, sheep, and goats. The parasites penetrate, multiply, and ultimately destroy the erythrocytes of various mammals or birds, causing fever, anemia, anorexia, malaise, and hemoglobinuria and, in some cases, death. The disease is more prevalent in the tropics than in the temperate zones, but where a combination of susceptible animals and the appropriate tick vector occurs, the disease can cause severe economic loss (306). Cases of human babesiasis are reported occasionally (307).

Screening of compounds for babesicidal activity can be carried out in laboratory white mice using infections of *B. rodhaini* (306, 308), a parasite originally isolated from a wild rodent in the Congo region.

However screening can also be performed using splenectomized calves infected with *B. divergens* (309) or splenectomized dogs infected with *B. canis* (310). The subject has been reviewed in depth (306, 311, 312).

7.2 Chemotherapy of Babesiasis

The chemotherapy of babesiasis parallels that of trypanosomiasis insofar as most compounds found to possess babesicidal activity were originally used as trypanocides. A close correlation appears to exist between trypanocidal and babesicidal activity, but this probably reflects the empirical development of babesicides (313).

One of the first drugs used to control the disease was trypan blue (20.**3**, 17), which is still used in the treatment of *B. canis* infections. Subsequently, the acridine dyes, particularly acriflavine (20.**122**), were used to

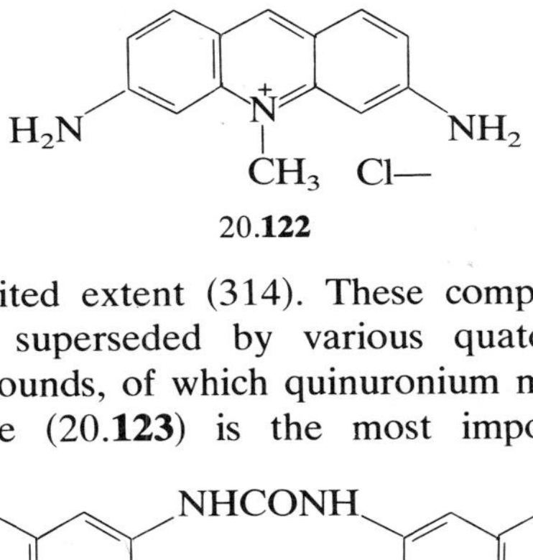

H_2N — acridinium — NH_2; $\overset{+}{N}$–CH_3 Cl^-

20.**122**

a limited extent (314). These compounds were superseded by various quaternary compounds, of which quinuronium methosulfate (20.**123**) is the most important.

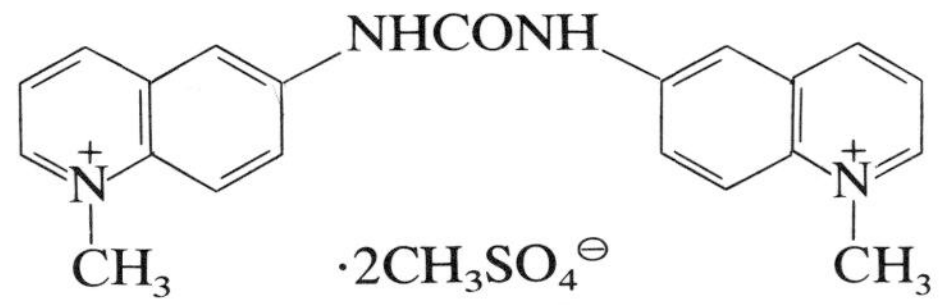

NHCONH; $\overset{+}{N}$–CH_3 $\cdot 2CH_3SO_4^{\ominus}$ $\overset{+}{N}$–CH_3

20.**123**

Until recently the most widely used agent for babesiasis (315), this compound is now being displaced by superior drugs (*vide infra*). The compound has severe toxic reactions at or near therapeutic levels (316).

Nearly all the aromatic diamidines that possess trypanocidal properties have an affect on *B. canis* infections, and three of the older compounds, phenamidine (20.**20**), propamidine (20.**22**), and stilbamidine (20.**23**), are curative (317) (see Section 2).

One of the more recently introduced compounds, diminazene (20.**26**, 4,4′-diamidinodiazoaminobenzene aceturate), has been used successfully in *Babesia* infections in cattle (318), sheep (319), horses (320), and dogs (321).

By incorporating the urea function present in quinuronium and the amidine moiety of the diamidines, a new group of potent babesicidal compounds, exemplified by amicarbalide (20.**124**, 3,3′-diamidinocarbanilide) (322) and imidocarb, (3,3′-bis(2-imidazolin-2-yl)carbanilide) (20.**125**) (323) were discovered.

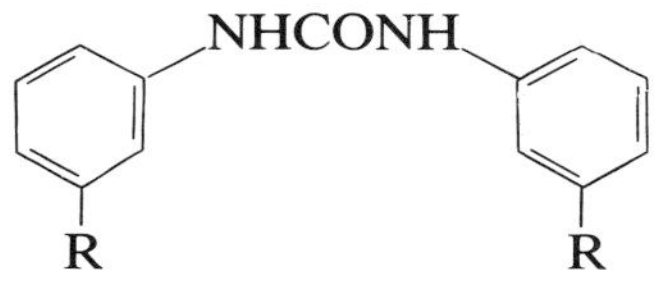

NHCONH; R R

20.**124** R = —C(=NH)NH_2

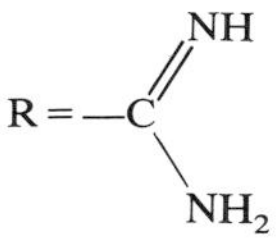

20.**125** R = 2-imidazolinyl (N, N ring)

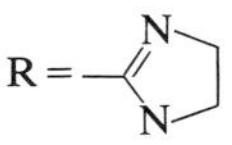

Amicarbalide has been shown to be active against *B. divergens* (324), the cause of redwater in British cattle, and is considered to be the drug of choice for treatment of babesiasis in horses (325). Imidocarb is active against *B. bigemina* (326) and *B. divergens* (327) in cattle and *B. caballi* and *B. equini* in horses (328). Amicarbalide and imidocarb (329) also possess prophylactic activity in tests with *B. rodhaini* in rats.

Homidium bromide (2,7-diamino-10-ethyl-9-phenylphenanthridinium bromide) (see Table 20.1) has activity against *B. rodhaini* infections in mice (330) and some effect on *B. bigemina* (331), but it does not appear to be used in the field. The series of

2-dithiosemicarbazones mentioned in the coccidiosis section are also claimed to have activity against *B. rodhaini* infections in mice (223). The antibiotics chlortetracycline (Aureomycin) (332) and puromycin (333) exhibited some babesicidal activity against experimental infections (333).

8 ANAPLASMOSIS

8.1 The Disease

Anaplasmosis is a tick-borne disease of cattle and sheep caused by *Anaplasma marginale* and *A. ovis*, respectively. *A. marginale* is the more pathogenic species and causes infectious anemia in cattle and other ruminants, often leading to heavy mortality. The disease occurs in many parts of the world including Asia, parts of Africa, and the southern United States.

The nature of the *Anaplasma* is little known, but it is usually grouped with the *Babesia* and *Theileria* because they are transmitted by ticks and all are found in cattle. However recent research suggests that the *Anaplasma* belong to the order Rickettsiales and should not be considered with the Protozoa at all (334).

Detailed reviews on anaplasmosis and its treatment have been published (335–337).

8.2 Chemotherapy of Anaplasmosis

Anaplasmosis has proved to be a most intractable disease, and it is only in recent years that effective therapy has become available. Many compounds, including the standard antimalarials and arsenicals (338), have been investigated in an effort to prevent or cure anaplasmosis. Until recently, however, only the tetracyclines (chlortetracycline, tetracycline, and oxytetracycline) have been effective in curing clinical cases of bovine anaplasmosis (338, 339) and eliminating the carrier state (340).

An extensive series of α-dithiosemicarbazones, mentioned earlier as having babesicidal and anticoccidial activity, also showed activity against *A. marginale* (223). The most promising member of the series, α-ethoxyethylglyoxal dithiosemicarbazone (20.**126**, gloxazone), was selected for detailed study.

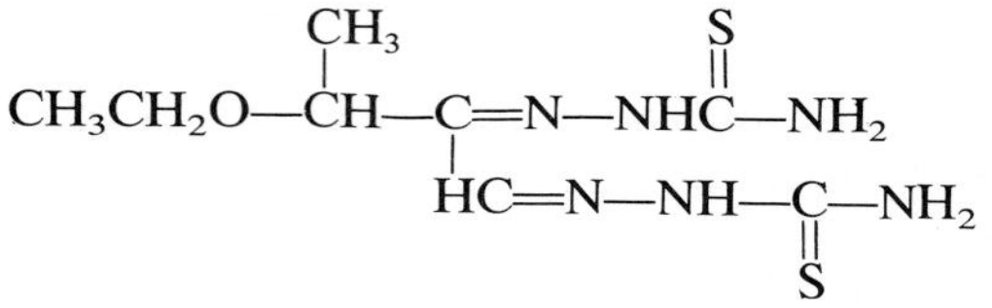

$$CH_3CH_2O{-}CH(CH_3){-}C({=}N{-}NHC({=}S){-}NH_2){-}HC{=}N{-}NH{-}C({=}S){-}NH_2$$

20.**126**

This compound was shown to be effective in experimental infections of *A. marginale* in splenectomized calves (341, 342) but proved to be rather toxic (343) in later experiments. However a combination of gloxazone and oxytetracycline was more efficacious than either drug alone (344).

Another babesicide, imidocarb (20.**125**), has also been shown to possess anaplasmacidal activity in experimental infections of *A. marginale.* The compound was effective when dosed subcutaneously to splenectomized calves infected with a virulent Virginian strain of *A. marginale*, but it was inactive when administered orally (345).

9 TOXOPLASMOSIS

9.1 The Disease

Toxoplasmosis is a poorly defined disease caused by *Toxoplasma gondii*, an organism first isolated from a North African rodent, the gondi (346). The disease is essentially global and affects most warm-blooded animals. In general, the infection is latent, but occasionally acute or chronic illness is produced. It has been claimed that in most areas of the world approximately one-third of the population is infected with *T. gondii* (347). Toxoplasmosis may be congenital or acquired, and transmission of the disease from infected mothers through the placenta to the fetus has been established. However other modes of transmission are possible (348), and until very recently, the question of how man initially acquired the infection was one of the great unsolved mysteries of parasitology. Since all warm-blooded animals carry the infection, the eating of inadequately cooked beef, pork, or chicken may lead to infection. However vegetarians display an incidence of toxoplasmosis similar to that observed among omnivores, and it was only through the work of Hutchison and his associates (349) and Frenkel (350) that the true source of infection became apparent. These workers have established that *T. gondii* is a specific coccidian of cats and other felines, and man and other mammals become infected when in close contact with cats. Acquired lymphatic toxoplasmosis manifests itself in humans by fever, general malaise, myalgia, and posterior cervical adenopathy and may spontaneously disappear or linger for long periods. Congenital toxoplasmosis may cause hydrocephalus, microcephalus, carditis, retinochoroiditis, and hepatitis in newborn children (347). The field of toxoplasmosis has been reviewed in some detail (347, 350–352).

Chemotherapeutic screening of compounds against acute toxoplasmosis can be readily carried out using mice infected with *T. gondii* (350). Toxoplasma may be grown in tissue culture, and this offers an *in vitro* technique for the evaluation of drugs (353, 355).

9.2 Chemotherapy of Toxoplasmosis

The first group of compounds to show definite activity against experimental *T. gondii* infections were the sulfonamides (351). These compounds are active through interference with the PAB-folic acid sequence in the parasite (357). Of the many sulfonamides tested, sulfapyrazine (20.**127**)

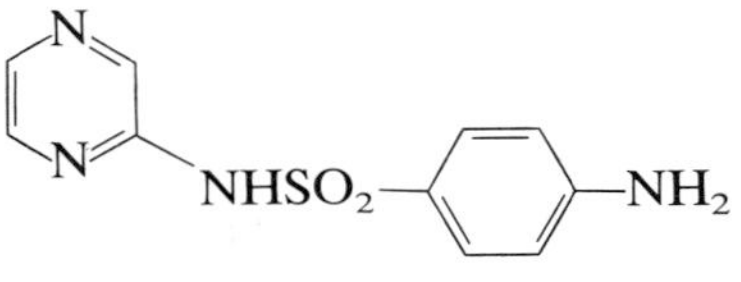

[pyrazinyl]—$NHSO_2$—[p-phenylene]—NH_2

20.**127**

appeared to be the most active. A useful review has been published (358).

Investigation of other PAB–folic acid antagonists led to the discovery of the marked activity of pyrimethamine (20.**64**) (358, 359) against experimental toxoplasmosis in mice. However curative action occurs only near the maximum tolerated dose (359). Fortunately synergism is observed between pyrimethamine and the sulfonamides (359), resulting in the use of nontoxic doses. Such a combination is regarded as the treatment of choice in human toxoplasmosis (360).

The diarylsulfones, particularly 4,4′-diaminodiphenylsulfone (dapsone), possess activity against toxoplasmosis (361, 362). The sulfones, which appear to be folic acid antagonists, act synergistically with pyrimethamine (362).

The wide range of compounds investigated for antitoxoplasmosis activity includes the antibiotics tetracycline, chlortetracycline, oxytetracycline, and demethylchlortetracycline, all of which possess varying degrees of activity (363–365). Spiramycin (366) and trypacidin (367) are also claimed to have significant activity, and clindamycin and its *N*-demethyl-4′-pentyl derivative were found to be active against *T. gondii* in mice (368).

10 BALANTIDIASIS

Balantidiasis is a rarely studied human and porcine disease caused by *Balantidium coli*. Human infection is worldwide, but it is rare where hygienic conditions are good and contact with pigs, the natural host, limited. Balantidial infections have been found in monkeys, ruminants, and rodents, as well as pigs (369). Although guinea pigs (370) and rats (371) have been artificially infected with *B. coli*, most compounds studied clinically have previously shown other antibacterial or antiprotozoal activity. The amebicides, emetine (372), *N*-(2-4-dichlorobenzyl)-*N*-(2-hydroxyethyl)-dichloroacetamide (mantomide) (373), and dichloroacet-4-(2-furoyloxy)-*N*-methylanilide (374) are claimed to be clinically effective. Niridazole (20.**102**) and furazolidone (20.**119**) have been shown to be efficacious in porcine balantidiasis (375). Antibiotics of the tetracycline family have good clinical efficacy (376, 377), and oxytetracycline is the drug of choice in human infections (378).

11 GIARDIASIS

Giardiasis (lambliasis) is an infection of the intestinal tract of man caused by a protozoan flagellate, *Giardia lamblia.* This parasite is considered to be one of the most common parasites found in the intestine of man, where it mainly infects the duodenum and jejunum. Until recently, *G. lamblia* was regarded as nonpathogenic in man, but there is sufficient evidence to indicate that the parasite interferes with absorption of fat-soluble vitamins and fats from the diet (379, 380). The disease causes diarrhea and anorexia in children and diarrhea, flatulence, nausea, and epigastric discomfort in adults (381).

Therapy of giardiasis in the past has generally been a matter of trial and error, utilizing drugs found to be effective in other protozoal diseases. In this manner it was learned that quinacrine (mepacrine) (see Chapter 18) and amodiaquin (20.**128**) (382, 383) are effective antigiardial agents.

However no definitive chemotherapeutic studies on series of compounds active against *G. lamblia* have been reported as a result of this empirical approach. The introduction of *G. muris* infections in mice for screening purposes has greatly facilitated laboratory studies of the disease (384, 385).

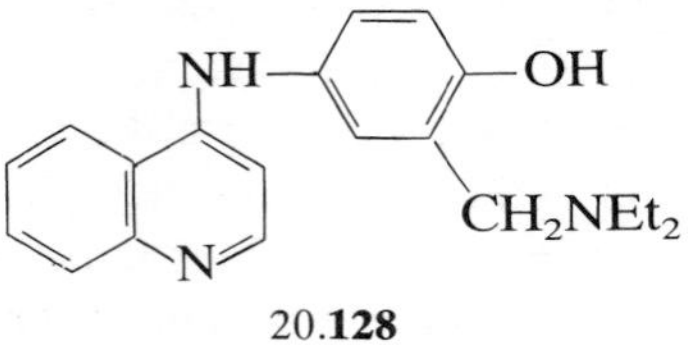

20.**128**

The demonstration of the clinical effectiveness of metronidazole (20.**104**) (381, 386–389), furazolidone (20.**119**) (387), and nitrimidazine (20.**108**) (390) without the distressing side effects of quinacrine therapy presages their replacement of quinacrine as the drugs of choice in giardiasis therapy.

Many compounds, particularly those with antiamebic activity, possess some laboratory or clinical activity in giardiasis (391). Of the new agents, 1-(2-hydroxyethyl)-5-nitropyrrole-2-carboxamide and 2,4-dichlorophenyliodonium chloride (chlodophene) show promise in therapeutic work (392, 393).

12 THEILERIASIS

Theileriasis is a disease of cattle and other ungulates caused by protozoan parasites belonging to the genus *Theileria.* The disease is transmitted by ticks belonging to the family Ixodidae. *Theileria parva* is the most important pathogenic species; it is responsible for East Coast fever of cattle in East Africa and is considered to be an important factor in restraining the development of the livestock industry in that area (394). *T. annulata* causes a milder form of the disease in cattle in North Africa, the Middle East, India, and parts of the Soviet Union. *T. hirci* and *T. ovis* cause the disease in sheep and goats in Africa, Europe, and India.

The theileriae are host specific, and infection of laboratory animals has not yet been achieved. However it has been found possible to culture *T. parva* in bovine lymphocytic cells (395), and this makes available an *in vitro* technique for chemotherapeutic screening purposes.

In vivo testing has been carried out using calves naturally or artificially infected with various species of *Theileria* (396), but such investigations are expensive and necessarily have been limited. Despite the investigation of more than 170 compounds belonging to various chemotherapeutic classes, no useful agent of proved clinical efficacy has emerged (397). Consequently control of the disease is by eradication of the tick vectors. Thus theileriasis remains one of the few protozoal diseases for which there is no definitive treatment. The subject has been comprehensively reviewed by several authors (394, 396, 398).

REFERENCES

1. World Health Organization, *Chronicle*, **30,** 41 (1976).
2. *African Trypanosomiasis*, World Health Organization Technical Report Series No. 434, Geneva, 1969.
3. D. Weinman, in *Infectious Blood Diseases of Man and Animals*, Vol. 2, D. Weinman and M. Ristic, Eds., Academic Press, New York, 1968, Ch. 17, pp. 97–173.
4. D. Scott, in *The African Trypanosomiases*, H. W. Mulligan, Ed., Allen & Unwin, London, 1970, Ch. 33, pp. 614–660.
5. F. I. C. Apted, in *The African Trypanosomiases*, H. W. Mulligan, Ed., Allen & Unwin, London, 1970, Ch. 35, pp. 661–683.
6. World Health Organization Technical Report Series No. 411, Geneva, 1969.
7. F. Köberle, in *Advances in Parasitology*, B. Dawes, Ed., Academic Press, New York, 1968, pp. 63–116.
8. R. S. Desowitz and H. J. C. Watson, *Ann. Trop. Med. Parasitol.*, **49,** 92–100 (1952).
9. R. S. Desowitz and H. J. C. Watson, *Ann. Trop. Med. Parasitol.*, **47,** 324–334 (1953).
10. F. Hawking, in *Experimental Chemotherapy*, Vol. 1, R. J. Schnitzer and F. Hawking, Eds., Academic Press, New York, 1963, pp. 129–256.
11. R. I. Hewitt, J. Entwistle, and E. Gill, *J. Parasitol.*, **49,** 22 (1963).
12. P. Guttmann and P. Ehrlich, *Berlin Klin. Wochenschr.*, **28,** 953 (1891).
13. P. Ehrlich and K. Shiga, *Berlin Klin. Wochenschr.*, **41,** 329–332, 362–365 (1904).
14. P. Ehrlich and A. Bertheim, *Chem. Ber.*, **40,** 3292–3297 (1907).
15. H. W. Thomas, *Brit. Med. J.*, 1140–1143 (I, 1905).
17. G. H. F. Nuttall and S. Hadwen, *Parasitology*, **2,** 156–191, 229–235, 236–266 (1909).
18. M. Nicolle and F. Mesnil, *Ann. Inst. Pasteur*, **20,** 417 (1906).
19. F. K. Kleine and W. Fischer, *Deut. Med. Wochenschr.*, **48,** 1693–1969 (1923).
20. J. Schneider, *Bull. W. Hlth. Org.*, **78,** 763 (1963).
21. M. Mayer and H. Zeiss, *Arch. Schiffs-u. Tropen-Hyg.*, **24,** 257–294 (1920).
22. A. Spinks, *Biochem. J.*, **42,** 109 (1948).
23. A. Adams, J. N. Ashley, and H. Bader, *J. Chem. Soc.*, 3739–344 (1956).
24. J. L. Guinmares and E. M. Lourie, *Brit. J. Pharmacol.*, **6,** 514–530 (1951).
25. J. Williamson and R. S. Desowitz, *Nature*, **177,** 1074–1075 (1956).
26. H. G. Plimmer and N. R. Bateson, *Proc. Roy. Soc.* (London), *Ser.* B. **80,** 477 (1908).
27. W. A. Jacobs and M. Heidelberger, *J. Am. Chem. Soc.*, **41,** 1810 (1919).
28. E. Fourneau, A. M. Navarro-Martin, and M. Tréfonël, *Ann. Inst. Pasteur*, **37,** 551–617 (1923).
29. R. J. Schnitzer and E. Gunberg, in *Drug Resistance of Microorganisms*, Academic Press, New York, 1957, pp. 1–395.
30. H. Eagle and G. O. Doak, *Pharmacol. Rev.*, **3,** 107 (1951).
31. P. Ehrlich, *Chem. Ber.*, **42,** 17 (1909).
32. W. Yorke and F. Murgatroyd, *Ann. Trop. Med.*, **24,** 449 (1930).
33. H. Eagle, *Science*, **101,** 69–71 (1945).
34. J. Williamson, *Exp. Parasitol.*, **12,** 274–322 (1962).
35. E. A. H. Friedheim, *Ann. Inst. Pasteur*, **65,** 108 (1940).
36. E. A. H. Friedheim and R. T. DeJongh, *Trans. Roy. Soc. Trop. Med. Hyg.*, **53,** 262–269 (1959).
37. G. C. Butler, A. J. Duggan, and M. P. Hutchinson, *Trans. Roy. Soc. Trop. Med. Hyg.*, **51,** 69–74 (1957).
38. F. I. C. Apted, *Trans. Roy. Soc. Trop. Med. Hyg.*, **47,** 387–398 (1953).
39. F. I. C. Apted, *Trans. Roy. Soc. Trop. Med. Hyg.*, **51,** 75–86 (1957).

40. H. King and W. I. Strangeways, *Ann. Trop. Med. Parasitol.*, **36,** 47–53 (1942).
41. H. Eagle and G. O. Doak, *Pharmacol Rev.*, **3,** 107–143 (1951).
42. R. L. Mayer and D. Brousseau, *Proc. Soc. Exp. Biol. Med.*, **62,** 238–240 (1946).
43. I. M. Rollo, J. Williamson, and E. M. Lourie, *Ann. Trop. Med. Parasitol.*, **43,** 194–208 (1949).
44. E. A. H. Friedheim, *Ann. Trop. Med. Parasitol.*, **47,** 350–360 (1953).
45. H. A. Poindexter, *J. Parasitol.*, **21,** 292–301 (1935).
46. N. von Jancsó and H. von Jancsó, *Z. Immunitätsforsch.* **86,** 1–30 (1935).
47. E. M. Lourie and W. Yorke, *Ann. Trop. Med. Parasitol.*, **31,** 435–446 (1937).
48. H. King, E. M. Lourie, and W. Yorke, *Lancet*, **2,** 1360–1363 (1937).
49. H. King, E. M. Lourie, and W. Yorke, *Ann. Trop. Med. Parasitol.*, **32,** 177–180 (1938).
50. E. M. Lourie and W. Yorke, *Ann. Trop. Med. Parasitol.*, **33,** 289 (1939).
51. J. N. Ashley, H. J. Barber, A. J. Ewins, G. Newberry, and A. D. H. Self, *J. Chem. Soc.*, 103–116 (1942).
52. D. Gall, *Ann. Trop. Med. Parasitol.*, **48,** 242–258 (1954).
53. J. D. Fulton and W. Yorke, *Ann. Trop. Med. Parasitol.*, **36,** 131 (1942).
54. J. D. Fulton, *Brit. J. Pharmacol.*, **3,** 75–79 (1948).
55. J. N. Ashley and R. Harris, *J. Chem. Soc.*, 1946, 567.
56. F. N. Fastier, *Pharmacol. Rev.*, **14,** 37 (1962).
57. E. A. Steck, *The Chemotherapy of Protozoan Diseases*, Vol. 2, Walter Reed Army Institute of Research, Washington, D.C., 1972.
58. J. N. Ashley, S. S. Berg, and R. D. MacDonald, *J. Chem. Soc.*, 4525–4532 (1960).
59. H. Jensch, *Arzneim.-Forsch.*, **5,** 634 (1955).
60. H. Jensch, *Med. Chem.*, **6,** 134 (1958).
61. R. Fussgänger and R. Baner, *Med. Chem.*, **6,** 504 (1958).
62. O. Dann, E. Hieke, H. Hahn, H.-H. Miserre, G. Lürding, and R. Rössler, *Justus Liebigs Ann. Chem.*, **734,** 23–45 (1970).
63. O. Dann, H. Fick, B. Pietzner, E. Walkenhorst, R. Fernbach, and D. Zeh, *Justus Liebigs Ann. Chem.*, 60–194 (1975).
64. W. Raether and H. Seidenath, *Tropenmed. Parasitol.*, **27,** 238–244 (1976).
65. R. Ogada, E. Fink, and D. Mbwabi, *Trans. Roy. Trop. Med. Hyg.*, **67,** 280–281 (1973).
66. L. Banda, *Chem. Ber.*, **45,** 1787 (1912).
67. A. Albert, *The Acridines*, Arnold, London, 1951.
68. W. Yorke and F. Murgatroyd. *Ann. Trop. Med. Parasitol.*, **24,** 449–476 (1930).
69. C. H. Browning, J. B. Cohen, S. Ellingworth, and R. Gulbransen, *Proc. Roy. Soc.* (London), **113,** 293, 300 (1933), and references cited therein.
70. H. Jensch, *Angew. Chem.*, **50,** 891–895 (1957).
71. P. A. Barrett, F. H. S. Curd, and W. Hepworth, *J. Chem. Soc.*, 50–58 (1953).
72. A. D. Ainley, F. H. S. Curd, W. Hepworth, A. G. Murray, and C. H. Vašey, *J. Chem. Soc.*, 59 (1953).
73. F. H. S. Curd and D. G. Davey, *Nature* (London), **163,** 89 (1949).
74. F. H. S. Curd and D. G. Davey, *Brit. J. Pharmacol.*, **5,** 25 (1950).
75. E. M. Lourie, J. S. Morley, J. C. E. Simpson, and J. M. Walker, *Brit. J. Pharmacol.*, **6,** 643–646 (1951).
76. R. L. Chandler, *Brit, J. Pharmacol.*, **12,** 44–46 (1957).
77. W. C. Austin, M. D. Potter, and E. P. Taylor, *J. Chem. Soc.*, 1489–1498 (1958).
78. J. N. Ashley and M. Davis, *J. Chem. Soc.*, 812–819 (1957).
79. R. V. Schock, *J. Am. Chem. Soc.*, **79,** 1672–1675 (1957).
80. F. C. Goble, *J. Pharmacol. Exp. Ther.*, **98,** 49 (1950).
81. See Ref. 10, p. 195.
82. G. T. Morgan and L. P. Walls, *J. Chem. Soc.*, 2447 (1931).
83. C. H. Browning, G. T. Morgan, J. V. M. Robb, and L. P. Walls, *J. Pathol. Bacteriol.*, **46,** 203–204 (1938).
84. D. G. Davey, *Vet. Rev.*, **3,** 15–36 (1957).
85. G. Brownlee, M. D. Goss, L. G. Goodwin, M. Woodbine, and L. P. Wallis, *Brit. J. Pharmacol. Chemother.*, **5,** 261–276 (1950).
86. L. P. Walls and N. Whittaker, *J. Chem. Soc.*, 41–47 (1950).
87. L. P. Walls and N. Whittaker, *J. Chem. Soc.*, 311–317 (1950).
88. T. I. Watkins and G. Woolfe, *Nature*, **169,** 506 (1952).
89. G. Woolfe, *Ann. Trop. Med. Parasitol.*, **46,** 285–288 (1952).
90. G. Woolfe, *Brit. J. Pharmacol. Chemother.*, **11,** 330–333 (1956); **11,** 334–338 (1956).

91. T. I. Watkins and G. Woolfe, *Nature*, **178,** 368 (1956).

92. T. I. Watkins, *J. Chem. Soc.*, 1443–1450 (1958).

93. W. R. Wragg, K. Washbourn, K. N. Brown, and J. Hill, *Nature*, **182,** 1005–1006 (1958).

94. B. A. Newton, *Advan. Chemother.*, **1,** 36 (1964).

95. M. C. Dodd W. B. Stillman, *J. Pharmacol. Exp. Ther.*, **82,** 11–18 (1944).

96. M. C. Dodd, *J. Pharmacol. Exp. Ther.*, **86,** 311–323 (1946).

97. N. J. Giarman, *J. Pharmacol. Exp. Ther.*, **102,** 185–195 (1951).

98. A. Packchanian, *Am. J. Trop. Med. Hyg.*, **4,** 705–711 (1955).

99. F. Evens, K. N. Niemeegers, and A. Packchanian, *Am. J. Trop. Med. Hyg.*, **6,** 658–664 (1957).

100. F. Evens, K. N. Niemeegers, and A. Packchanian, *Am. J. Trop. Med. Hyg.*, **6,** 665–678 (1957).

101. F. I. C. Apted, *Trans. Roy. Soc. Trop. Med. Hyg.*, **54,** 225–228 (1960).

102. A. Packchanian, *Antibiot. Chemother.*, **7,** 13–23 (1957).

103. B. Cole, L. P. Frick, E. P. Hodges, and R. E. Duxburg, *Antibiot. Chemother.*, **3,** 429–433 (1953).

104. R. Foster, G. Pringle, D. F. King, and J. Paris, *Ann. Trop. Med. Parasitol.*, **63,** 95–107 (1969).

105. K. Adriaenssens, *Ann. Soc. Belg. Med. Trop.*, **40,** 715–723 (1960).

106. M. Bock, A. Haberkorn, H. Herlinger, K. H. Mayer, and S. Petersen, *Arzneim.-Forsch.*, **22,** 1564–1569 (1972).

107. A. Haberkorn and R. Gönnert, *Arzneim.-Forschung.*, **22,** 1570–1582 (1972).

108. R. Gönnert and M. Bock, *Arzneim.-Forsch.* **22,** 1582–1586 (1972).

109. W.-H. Voigt, M. Bock, and R. Gönnert, *Arzneim.-Forsch.*, **22,** 1586–1589 (1972).

110. B. Duhm, W. Maul, H. Medenwald, K. Patzsckke, and L. A. Wegner, *Arzneim.-Forsch.*, **22,** 1617–1624 (1972).

111. D. H. G. Wegner and R. W. Rohwedder, *Arzneim.-Forsch.*, **22,** 1624–1635 (1972).

112. D. H. G. Wegner and R. W. Rohwedder, *Arzneim.-Forsch.*, **22,** 1635–1642 (1972).

113. T. Novinson, B. Bhooshan, T. Okabe, G. P. Revankar, R. K. Robins, K. Sengo, and H. R. Wilson, *J. Med. Chem.* **19,** 512–516 (1976).

114. M. C. Neville and J. P. Verge, *J. Med. Chem.*, **20,** (1977) *in press.*

115. D. H. Chatfield, *Xenobiotica*, **6,** 509–520 (1976).

116. J. P. Verge and P. Roffey, *J. Med. Chem.*, **18,** 794–797 (1975).

117. J. J. Jaffe and E. Meymarian, *Exp. Parasitol.*, **34,** 242–250 (1973).

118. W. E. Gutteridge, B. Cover, and M. Gaborak, *Trans. Roy. Soc. Trop. Med. Hyg.*, **68,** 160–161 (1974).

119. A. C. Cuckler, C. M. Malanga, and J. Conroy, *Am. J. Trop. Med. Hyg.*, **19,** 916–925 (1970).

120. W. J. Ross, W. B. Jamieson, and M. C. McCowen, *J. Med. Chem.*, **15,** 1035–1040 (1972).

121. W. J. Ross, W. B. Jamieson, and M. C. McCowen, *J. Med. Chem.*, **16,** 347–352 (1973); **18,** 158, 430 (1975).

122. D. M. Morton, D. M. Fuller, and J. N. Green, *Xenobiotica*, **3,** 257–266 (1973).

123. M. E. Tarrant, S. Wedley, T. J. Woodage, and J. N. Green, *Biochem. Pharmacol.*, **22,** 639–649 (1973).

124. E. J. Burden and E. Racette, *Antimicrob. Agents Chemother.*, 545–547 (1969).

125. J. N. Porter, R. I. Hewitt C. W. Hesseltine, G. Krupka, J. A. Lowery, W. S. Wallace, N. Bohonos, and J. H. Williams, *Antibiot. Chemother.*, **2,** 409 (1952).

126. B. R. Baker, R. E. Schaub, J. P. Joseph, and J. H. Williams, *J. Am. Chem. Soc.*, **76,** 4044 (1954).

127. R. I. Hewitt, W. S. Wallace, A. R. Gumble, E. R. Gill, and J. H. Williams, *Am. J. Trop. Med. Hyg.*, **2,** 241–249 (1953).

128. E. J. Tobie, *Am. J. Trop. Med. Hyg.*, **3,** 852–859 (1954).

129. J. Heuls, J. Orio, J. Ceccaldi, and P. Merveille, *Bull. Soc. Pathol. Exot.*, **51,** 108–113 (1958).

130. R. J. Hewitt, A. R. Gumble, W. S. Wallace, and J. H. Williams, *Antibiot. Chemother.*, **4,** 1222–1227 1954).

131. M. Agosin and T. von Brand, *Antibiot. Chemother.*, **4,** 624–632 (1954).

132. L. Goldman, J. W. Marsico, and R. B. Angier, *J. Am. Chem. Soc.*, **78,** 4173–4175 (1956).

133. G. O. Morton, J. E. Lancaster, G. E. van Lear, W. Fulmore, and W. E. Meyer, *J. Am. Chem. Soc.*, **91,** 1535–1537 (1969).

134. E. J. Tobie, *J. Parasitol.*, **43,** 291 (1957).

135. R. I. Hewitt, A. R. Gumble, L. H. Taylor, and W. S. Wallace, *Antibiot. Ann.* 1956–1957, 722 (1957).

136. L. E. Stephen and A. R. Gray, *Vet. Rec.*, **73,** 563 (1961).

137. L. E. Stephen and A. R. Gray, *J. Parasitol.*, **46,** 509 (1960).

138. K. G. Cunningham, S. A. Hutchinson, W. Manson, and F. S. Spring, *J. Chem. Soc.*, 2299 (1951).
139. J. Williamson, *Trans. Roy. Soc. Trop. Med. Hyg.*, **60,** 8 (1966).
140. W. T. Butler, *J. Am. Med. Assoc.*, **195,** 371 (1966).
141. A. E. Horvath and C. H. Zierdt, *J. Trop. Med. Hyg.*, **77,** 144–149 (1974).
142. A. B. Clarkson and F. H. Brohn, *Science*, **194,** 204–206 (1976).
143. A. O. Foster, *Ann. N.Y. Acad. Sci.*, **52,** 434 (1949).
144. *Losses in Agriculture*, Agricultural Handbook 291, Agricultural Research Service, US Department of Agriculture, Washington, D.C., 1965.
145. J. F. Ryley and M. J. Betts, in *Advances in Pharmacology and Chemotherapy*, Vol. 2, S. Garattini, A. Goldin, F. Hawking, and I. J. Kopin, Eds., Academic Press, New York, 1973, pp. 221–293.
146. W. C. Marquardt, in *The Coccidia*, D. Hammond, Ed., with P. L. Long, University Park Press, Baltimore, 1973, pp. 21–43.
147. E. F. Rogers, *Ann. N.Y. Acad. Sci.*, **98,** 412–429 (1962).
148. W. M. Read, L. M. Kowalski, E. M. Taylor, and J. Johnson, *Avian Dis.*, **14,** 788–796 (1970).
149. P. L. Long, in *The Coccidia*, D. Hammond, Ed., with P. L. Long, University Park Press, Baltimore, 1973, pp. 263–265.
150. P. L. Long, *Vet. Rec.*, **80,** VIII–XII (1967).
151. L. P. Joyner, S. F. M. Davies, and S. B. Kendall, in *Experimental Chemotherapy*, Vol. 1, R. J. Schnitzer and F. Hawking, Eds., Academic Press, New York, 1963, pp. 455–486.
152. R. C. Bergstrom and L. R. Maki, *J. Am. Vet. Med. Assoc.*, **165,** 288–289 (1974).
153. P. P. Levine, *Cornell Vet.*, **29,** 309 (1939).
154. P. P. Levine, *J. Parasitol.*, **26,** 233 (1940).
155. M. Mitrovic and J. C. Bauernfriend, *Poult. Sci.*, **46,** 402 (1967).
156. P. Yvore, *Recl. Med. Vet.*, **144,** 1059–1973 (1968).
157. C. Horton–Smith and E. L. Taylor, *Vet. Rec.*, **57,** 35 (1945).
158. M. Mitrovic, E. G. Schildknecht, and G. Fusiek, *Poult. Sci.*, **48,** 210–216 (1969).
159. E. F. Rogers, R. L. Clark, H. J. Becker, A. A. Pessoano, W. J. Leanza, E. C. McManus, A. J. Andruili, and A. C. Cuckler, *Proc. Soc. Exp. Biol. Med.*, **117,** 488 (1964).
160. E. C. McManus, M. T. Oberdick, and A. C. Cuckler, *J. Protozool.*, **14,** 379–381 (1967).
161. See Ref. 147.
162. A. C. Cuckler, M. Garzillo, C. Malanger, and E. C. McManus, *Poult. Sci.*, **39,** 1241 (1960).
163. J. Enzeby and C. Garan, *Bull. Soc. Sci. Vet. Lyon*, **71,** 235–239 (1969).
164. H. Oikawa, H. Kawaguchi, E. Yoshida, A. Takami-Bawa, K. Hiroi, T. Ishiba, and T. Misesita, *Ann. Rep. Shionogi Res. Lab.*, **21,** 27–31 (1971).
165. T. Matsuyawa, *Ann. Rep. Sankyo Res. Lab.*, **23,** 192–200 (1970).
166. K. Hirota, Y. Nishibe, Y. Matsuo, H. Oikawa, H. Kawaguchi, and T. Minesita, *Ann. Rep. Shionogi Res. Lab.*, **21,** 40–47 (1971).
167. Merck, US Patent, 3510480 (1970).
168. Tanake, Japanese Patent 70-34585.
169. A. Engle, *Poult. Sci.*, **46,** 810–818 (1967).
170. C. F. Spencer, A. Engle, C.-N. Yu, R. C. Finch, E. J. Watson, F. F. Ebetino, and C. A. Johnson, *J. Med. Chem.*, **9,** 934 (1966).
171. R. A. Bowie, J. P. Cairns, M. S. Grant, A. Hayes, W. G. M. Jones, and J. F. Ryley, *Nature* (London), **214,** 1349 (1967).
172. J. F. Ryley and R. G. Wilson, *J. Parasitol.*, **58,** 664–668 (1968).
173. S. J. Ball, M. Davis, J. N. Hodgson, J. M. S. Lucas, E. W. Parnell, B. W. Sharp, and D. Warburton, *Soc. Chem. Ind.* (London), 56–57 (1968).
174. R. H. Mizzoni, F. Goble, T. Szanto, D. C. Maplesden, J. E. Brown, J. Boxer, and G. de Stevens, *Experientia*, **24,** 1188–1189 (1968).
175. E. C. McManus, W. C. Campbell, and A. C. Cuckler, *J. Parasitol.*, **54,** 1190–1193 (1968).
176. M. Davis and E. W. Parnell, *Soc. Chem. Ind.* (London), Monograph, **33,** 129–134 (1969).
177. R. A. Bowie, J. P. Cairns, M. S. Grant, and W. G. M. Jones, *Soc. Chem. Ind.* (London), Monograph, **33,** 145–155 (1969).
178. B. K. F. Hermans, A. A. C. Janssen, H. L. E. Verhoeven, A. G. Knaeps, T. J. M. van Offenwert, J. F. Mostmans, J. J. M. Willems, B. Maes, and O. Vanparijs, *J. Med. Chem.*, **16,** 1047–1050 (1973).
179. J. N. Hodgson, *Soc. Chem. Ind.* (London), Monograph, **33,** 139–143 (1969).
180. H. D. Chapman, *J. Parasitol.*, **71,** 41–49 (1975).
181. T. K. Jeffers, J. R. Challey, and W. J. Despain, *Poult. Sci.*, **50,** 1588 (1971).
182. J. R. Challey and T. K. Jeffers, *J. Parasitol.*, **59,** 502 (1973).
183. W. M. Reid, E. M. Taylor, and J. Johnson, *Trans. Am. Microsc. Soc.*, **88,** 148–159 (1969).

184. E. Grenel, *Tieraerztl. Umsch.*, **22,** 25–26, 31–33 (1967); *Chem. Abs.*, **65,** 1743d (1966).

185. V. B. Piskov, L. K. Osanova, and I. A. Koblova, *Z. Org. Khim.*, **5,** 1642–1648 (1969).

186. S. J. Ball and E. W. Parnell, *Nature* (London), **199,** 612 (1963).

187 D. E. Welch, R. B. Baron, and B. A. Burton, *J. Med. Chem.*, **12,** 299–301 (1969).

188. D. E. Welch and R. B. Baron, *J. Med. Chem.*, **12,** 957 (1969).

189. V. B. Piskov, L. K. Osanova, and I. A. Koblova, *J. Org. Chem.* (USSR), **5,** 1596–1600 (1969).

190. V. B. Piskov, L. K. Osanova, and I. A. Koblova, *J. Org. Chem.* (USSR), **6,** 556–561 (1970).

191. S. Kantor, R. L. Kennett, Jr., E. Waletzky, and A. S. Tomcufcik, *Science*, **168,** 373–374 (1970).

192. W. M. Reid, L. M. Kowalski, E. M. Taylor, and J. Johnson, *Avian Dis.* **14,** 788–796 (1970).

193. J. Zulalian and P. E. Gotterdam, *J. Agr. Food Chem.*, **21,** 794 (1973).

194. P. L. Long and Mullard, *Avian Pathol.*, **2,** 111 (1973).

195. M. E. Haney, Jr., and M. M. Hoehn, *Antimicrob. Agents Chemother.*,

196. J. Berger, A. I. Rachlin, W. E. Scott, L. H. Sternbach, and M. W. Boldberg, *J. Am. Chem. Soc.*, **73,** 5295 (1951).

197. R. L. Harned, P. H. Kidy, C. J. Corum, and K. L. Jones, *Antibiot. Chemother.*, **1,** 594 (1951).

198. H. Lardy, *Fed. Proc.*, **27,** 1278 (1968).

199. B. C. Pressmann, *Fed. Proc.*, **27,** 1283 (1968).

200. B. C. Pressmann, *Fed. Proc.*, **27,** 1283 (1968).

201. A. Agtarap, J. W. Chamberlin, M. Pinkerton, and L. Steinrauf, *J. Am. Chem. Soc.*, **89,** 5737 (1967).

202. R. F. Shumard and M. E. Callender, *Antimicrob. Agents Chemother.*, 369–377 (1967).

203. M. Gorman, J. W. Chamberlin, and R. L. Hamill, *Antimicrob. Agents Chemother.*, 363–369 (1967).

204. W. M. Reid, J. Johnson, and J. Dick, *Avian Dis.*, **19,** 12–16 (1975).

205. H. Kinashi, M. Otake, H. Yonehara, S. Sato, and Y. Saito, *Tetrahedron Lett.*, 4955–4958 (1973).

206. R. F. Shumard, M. E. Callender, and W. M. Reid, *14th World's Poultry Congress*, Madrid, 421–427 (1970).

207. W. M. Reid, L. Kowalski, and J. Rice, *Poult. Sci.*, **51,** 139–146 (1972).

208. M. L. Clarke, M. Diaz, B. Guilloteau, D. L. Hudd, and J. W. Stoker, *Avian Pathol.*, **3,** 23–55 (1974).

209. P. R. Fitzgerald and M. E. Mansfield, *J. Protozool.*, **20,** 121–126 (1973).

210. R. C. Bergstrom and L. R. Maki, *J. Am. Vet. Med. Assoc.*, **165,** 288–289 (1974).

211. R. L. Hamill, M. M. Hoehn, G. W. Pittenger, J. Chamberlin, and M. Gorman, *J. Antibiot.* (Tokyo), **22,** 161 (1969).

212. M. Gorman and R. L. Hamill, US Patent 3, 555, 150 (1971).

213. E. Ebata, H. Kashara, K. Sekine, and Y. Inone, *J. Antibiot.* (Tokyo), **28,** 118 (1975).

214. N. Otake, M. Koenuma, H. Kinashi, S. Sato, and Y. Saito, *Chem. Commun*, 92 (1975).

215. F. Kitane, K. Ususchikawa, T. Kohama, T. Saito, M. Kikuchi, and N. Ishida, *J. Antibiot. (Tokyo)*, **27,** 884 (1974).

216. N. F. Morehouse and O. J. Mayfield, *J. Parasitol.*, **32,** 20–24 (1946).

217. N. F. Morehouse and O. J. Mayfield, *J. Parasitol.*, **30,** Suppl. 6, (1944).

218. F. C. Goble, *Ann. N.Y. Acad. Sci.*, **52,** 533 (1949).

219. C. Johnson and R. J. Van Ryzin, *Poult. Sci.*, **41,** 1918–1924 (1962).

220. P. L. Long, *Vet. Rec.*, **80,** VIII–XII (1967).

221. A. C. Cuckler, C. M. Malanga, A. J. Basso, and R. C. O'Neill, *Science*, **122,** 244 (1955).

222. R. C. O'Neill and A. J. Basso, US Patent 2, 823, 162 (1958).

223. R. A. Barrett, E. Bereridge, P. L. Bradley, C. G. D. Brown, S. R. M. Bushby, M. L. Clark, R. A. Neal, R. Smith, and J. K. H. Wilde, *Nature* (London), **206,** 1340–1341 (1965).

224. F. J. Bullock, *J. Med. Chem.*, **11,** 419–424 (1968).

225. E. Waletzky, C. O. Huges, and M. C. Brandt, *Ann. N.Y. Acad. Sci.*, **52,** 543 (1949).

226. R. G. Parish, V. J. Theodorides, D. W. Kunble, E. M. Dietz, and E. A. Shultis, *J. Med. Chem.*, **15,** 1324 (1972).

227. M. P. Georgiadis, *J. Med. Chem.*, **19,** 346–349 (1976).

228. J. F. Ryley and G. J. Stacey, *Parasitology*, **53,** 303 (1963).

229. R. J. Schnitzer, in *Experimental Chemotherapy*, Vol. 1, R. J. Schnitzer and F. Hawking, Eds., Academic Press, New York, 1963, pp. 289–331; Vol. 4, 1966, pp. 420–424.

230. O. Jirovec and M. Petru, in *Advances in Parasitology*, Vol. 6, B. Dawes, Ed., Academic Press, New York, 1968, pp. 117–188.

231. S. R. M. Bushby and F. C. Copp, *J. Pharm. Pharmacol.*, **7,** 112–117 (1955).

232. A. C. Cuckler, A. B. Kupferberg, and N. Millman, *Antibiot. Chemother.*, **5,** 540–555 (1955).
233. J. Barnes, A. Boutwood, E. Haines, W. Lewington, E. Lister, and B. J. Haram, *Brit. Med. J.*, **7,** 1160 (1957).
234. A. A. Plentl, M. J. Gracy, E. D. Nelsen, and S. J. Dalali, *Am. J. Obstetr. Gynecol.*, **71,** 116 (1956).
235. E. Kutter, H. Machleidt, W. Reuter, R. Sauter, and A. Wildfeuer, in *Advances in Chemistry* Series No. 114, American Chemical Society, Washington, D.C., 1972, pp. 92113.
236. F. Kradolfer, R. Jurumilinta, and W. Sackmann, *Ann. N.Y. Acad. Sci.*, **160,** 740–748 (1969).
237. R. M. Michaels and R. E. Strube, *J. Pharm. Pharmacol.*, **13,** 601–610 (1961).
238. S. Nakamura and H. Umezawa, *J. Antibiot. (Tokyo), Ser. A.*, **9,** 66 (1955).
239. R. Despois, S. Pinnert-Sindico, L. Ninet, and J. Preud'Homme, *G. Microbiol.*, **2,** 76 (1956).
240. C. Cosar and F. Julon, *Ann. Inst. Pasteur* (Paris), **96,** 238 (1959).
241. M. Moffett and M. I. McGill, *Brit. Med. J.*, **2,** 910 (1960).
242. E. F. Elslager and P. E. Thompson, *Ann. Rev. Pharmacol.*, **2,** 193–214 (1962).
243. F. Davidson, *J. Obstetr. Gynecol. Brit. Commonw.*, **80,** 368 (1973).
244. C. Cosar, C. Crisan, R. Horclois, R. M. Jacob, J. Robert, S. Tchelitcheff, and R. Vaupre, *Arzneim.-Forsch.*, **16,** 23–29 (1966).
245. A. C. Cuckler, L. R. Chapin, C. M. Malanga, E. F. Rogers, H. J. Becker, R. L. Clark, W. J. Leanzer, A. A. Pessolano, T. Y. Shen, and L. H. Sarett, *Proc. Soc. Exp. Biol. Med.*, **98,** 167 (1958).
246. E. F. Rogers and A. A. Pessolano, US Patent 3, 037,909 (1962).
247. R. Leichti, *Schweiz. Med. Wochenschr.*, **100,** 2117 (1970).
248. W. Chari and B. N. Gadiyar, *Am. J. Trop. Hyg.*, 26 (1970).
249. D. R. Hoff, *Proc. Int. Symp. Drug Res., Montreal,* 100 (June 1967).
250. G. N. Perschin, *Pure Appl. Chem.*, **19,** 153–169 (1969).
251. R. M. Ings, G. L. Law, and E. W. Parnell, *Biochem. Pharmacol.*, **15,** 515 (1966).
252. J. E. Stambough, L. G. Feo, and R. W. Manthei, *Life Sci.*, **6,** 1811 (1967).
253. I. de Carneri, *Second International Congress of Parasitology, Washington,* D.C., September 1970.
254. K. Butler, H. L. Howes, J. E. Lynch, and D. K. Pirie, *J. Med. Chem.*, **10,** 891–897 (1967).
255. H. L. Howes, J. E. Lynch, and J. L. Kolvin, *Antimicrob. Agents Chemother.* 261 (1970).
256. P. N. Giraldi, V. Mariothi, G. Nannini, G. P. Tosolini, E. Drachi, W. Logemann, I. de Carneri, nd G. Monti, *Arzneim.-Forsch.*, **20,** 52–54 (1970).
257. S. S. Park, B. S. Ka, S. B. Hong, and S. C. Lee, *New Engl. Med. J.*, **17,** 127 (1974).
258. S. M. Ross, *Brit. J. Vener Dis.*, **49,** 475–477 (1973).
259. B. A. Wood, D. Rycroft, and A. M. Monro, *Xenobiotica*, **3,** 801–812 (1973).
260. P. N. Giraldi, G. P. Tosolini, E. Drachi, G. Nannini, R. Longo, G. Meinardi, G. Monti, and I. de Carneri, *Biochem. Pharmacol.*, **20,** 339–349 (1971).
261. B. A. Wood and A. M. Monro, *Brit. J. Vener Dis.*, **51,** 51–53 (1975).
262. M. W. Miller, H. L. Howes, and A. R. English, *Antimicrob. Agents Chemother.* 257–260 (1970).
263. P. R. Sawyer, R. N. Brogden, R. M. Pinder, T. M. Speight, and G. S. Avery, Drugs, **11,** 423–440 1976).
264. J. Heeres, J. H. Mostmans, B. Meas, and L. J. Backx, *Eur. J. Med. Chem.*, **11,** 237–239 (1976).
265. J. Heindl, E. Schröder, and H.-W. Kelm, *Eur. J. Med. Chem.*, **10,** 121–124 (1975), and references cited therein.
266. C. Rufer, H.-J. Kessler, and E. Schröder, *J. Med. Chem.*, **14,** 94 (1971).
267. H.-J. Kessler, C. Rufer, and K. Schwarz, *Eur. J. Med. Chem.*, **11,** 19–23 (1976).
268. R. G. Micetich, *J. Med. Chem.*, **12,** 611 (1969).
269. P. J. Islip and M. R. Johnson, *J. Med. Chem.*, **16,** 1308–1310 (1973).
270. O. Albert and M. Aurousseau, *Ann. Pharm. Fr.*, **31,** 57–62 (1973).
271. G. L. Dunn, P. Actor, and V. J. di Pasquo, *J. Med. Chem.*, **9,** 751 (1966).
272. J. F. Ryley and M. Stacey, *Parasitology*, **53,** 303 (1963).
273. G. W. Brown, Jr., R. Wellerson, Jr., and A. B. Kupferberg, *J. Pharm. Pharmacol.*, **17,** 747 (1965).
274. F. Benazet, C. Cosar, P. Ganter, L. Julon, P. Populaire, and L. Guillaume, *Compt. Rend.*, **263,** 609 (1966).
275. A. J. Lipenko, *Bull. W.H.O.*, **44,** 515–520 (1971).
276. P.C.C. Garnham, *Bull. W.H.O.*, **44,** 521–527 (1971).
277. E. A. Steck, in *Progress in Drug Research*, Vol. 18, E. Jucker, Ed., Birkhäuser-Verlag, Basel, (1974), pp. 289–351.

278. E. Beveridge, in *Experimental Chemotherapy*, Vol. 1, R. J. Schnitzer and F. Hawking, Eds., Academic ress, New York, 1963, pp. 257–287.

279. G. Vianna, *Arch. Brasil. Med.*, **2,** 426 (1912).

280. H. G. Plimma and N. R. Bateson, *Proc. Roy. Soc.* (London), *Ser. B*, **80,** 477 (1908).

281. H. G. Smyly and C. W. Young, *Proc. Soc. Exp. Biol. Med.*, **21,** 354–356 (1924).

282. M. Ardehali, *Int. J. Dermatol.*, **13,** 26–28 (1974).

283. E. F. Cappucino and R. A. Stauber, *Proc. Soc. Exp. Biol. Med.*, **101,** 742 (1959).

284. H. Abd-Rabbo, *J. Trop. Med. Hyg.*, **69,** 171 (1966).

285. E. E. Tyzzer, *J. Parasitol.*, **6,** 124–131 (1920).

286. W. M. Reid, *Exp. Parasitol.*, **21,** 249–275 (1967).

287. J. M. S. Lucas and J. Goose, *Brit. Vet. J.*, **121,** 65 (1965).

288. R. K. Farmer, *J. Comp. Pathol. Ther.*, **60,** 294–310 (1950).

289. E. Walelzky, J. H. Clark, and H. W. Marson, *Science*, **111,** 720 (1950).

290. G. C. Branden and J. C. Wood, *Vet. Rec.*, **67,** 326 (1955).

291. A. C. Cuckler and C. M. Malanga, *Proc. Soc. Exp. Biol. Med.*, **92,** 483–485 (1956).

292. J. M. S. Lucas, *Vet. Rec.*, **73,** 465–467 (1961).

293. M. Mitrovic, M. Hoffer, and E. G. Schildknecht, *Antimicrob. Agents Chemother.*, 445–448 (1969).

294. E. H. Peterson, *Poult. Sci.*, **47,** 1245–1250 (1968).

295. G. C. Shelton and H. C. McDougle, *Poult. Sci.*, **49,** 1077–1081 (1970).

296. T. W. Sullivan, O. D. Grace, and R. J. Mitchell, *Poult. Sci.*, **52,** 1287–1291 (1973).

297. G. L. Law, G. P. Mansfield, D. F. Muggleton, and E. W. Parnell, *Nature* (London), **197,** 1024 (1963).

298. J. K. McGregor, *Can. J. Comp. Med. Vet. Sci.*, **18,** 397 (1954).

299. C. F. Hall, A. I. Flowers, and L. C. Grumbles, *Avian Dis.*, **9,** 400 (1965).

300. E. W. Berndt, H. Van Essen, B. G. Held, and R. D. Vatne, *J. Med. Chem.*, **12,** 371–374 (1969).

301. R. D. Vatne, R. R. Baron, and N. F. Morehouse, *Poult. Sci.*, **48,** 2157–2160 (1969).

302. R. D. Vatne, R. R. Baron, and N. F. Morehouse, *Poult. Sci.*, **48,** 590–596 (1969).

303. H. M. DeVolt and A. P. Holst, *Poult. Sci.*, **28,** 641–643 (1948).

304. E. E. Tyzzer, *J. Med. Res.*, **44,** 109–111 (1923).

305. W. D. Lindquist, *Am. J. Vet. Res.*, **23,** 1053 (1962).

306. L. P. Joyner, S. F. M. Davies, and S. B. Kendall, in *Experimental Chemotherapy*, Vol. 1, R. J. Schnitzer and F. Hawking, Eds., Academic Press, New York, 1963, pp. 603–624.

307. A. Spielman and N. Gleason, *Science*, **192,** 479–480 (1976).

308. J. M. S. Lucas, *Res. Vet. Sci.*, **1,** 218–225 (1960).

309. S. F. M. Davies, L. P. Joyner, and S. B. Kendall, *Ann. Trop. Med. Parasitol.*, **52,** 206–215 (1958).

310. J. F. Ryley, *Ann. Trop. Med. Parasitol.*, **51,** 38–49 (1957).

311. L. P. Joyner, S. F. M. Davies, and S. B. Kendall, in *Experimental Chemotherapy*, Vol. 4, R. J. Schnitzer and F. Hawking, Eds., Academic Press, New York, 1966, pp. 463–466.

312. L. P. Joyner and D. W. Brocklesby, in *Advances in Pharmacology and Chemotherapy*, Vol. 11, S. Garrattini, A. Goldin, F. Hawking, and I. J. Kopin, Eds., Academic Press, New York, 1973, pp. 328–341.

313. A. E. R. Taylor, R. J. Terry, and D. G. Godfrey, *Brit. J. Pharmacol.*, **11,** 71 (1956).

314. G. Domagk and W. Kikuth, *Zbl. Bakteriol. Parasitenk.*, Abt. 1 (orig.), **118,** 401–406 (1930).

315. W. Kikuth, *Zbl. Bakteriol. Parasitenk.*, Abt. 1 (orig.), **135,** 135 (1935).

316. P. Eyre, *J. Pharm. Pharmacol.*, **19,** 509 (1967).

317. E. M. Lourie and W. Yorke, *Ann. Trop. Med. Parasitol.*, **33,** 305–312 (1939).

318. S. F. Barnett, *Res. Vet. Sci.*, **6,** 397 (1965).

319. K. Enigk and U. Reusse, *Z. Tropenmed. Parasitol.*, **6,** 141 (1957).

320. J. E. Bryant, J. B. Anderson, and K. H. Willers, *J. Am. Vet. Med. Assoc.*, **154,** 1034 (1969).

321. F. Brauer, *Z. Tropenmed. Parasitol.*, **17,** 390 (1966).

322. J. N. Ashley, S. S. Berg, and J. M. S. Lucas, *Nature* (London), **185,** 461 (1960).

323. G. Schmidt, R. Hirt, and R. Fischer, *Res. Vet. Sci.*, **10,** 530–533 (1969).

324. C. G. L. Beveridge, J. W. Thwaite, and G. Shepherd, *Vet. Rec.*, **72,** 383–385 (1960).

325. G. W. Taylor, J. E. Bryant, J. B. Anderson, and K. H. Willers, *J. Am. Vet. Med. Assoc.*, **155,** 915 (1969).

326. L. L. Callow and W. McGregor, *Aust. Vet. J.*, **46,** 195–200 (1970).

327. J. C. Wood, *Ir. Vet. J.*, **25,** 254 (1971).

328. W. W. Kirkham, *J. Am. Vet. Med. Assoc.*, **155,** 457–459 (1969).

329. E. Beveridge, *Res. Vet. Sci.*, **10,** 534 (1969).

330. J. F. Ryley, *Ann. Trop. Med. Parasitol.*, **51,** 38 (1957).

331. S. F. Barnett and D. W. Brocklesby, *Brit. Vet. J.*, **122,** 361 (1966).
332. B. C. Jansen, *Cenderstepoort J. Vet. Res.*, **26,** 175–182 (1953).
333. A. E. R. Taylor, R. J. Terry, and D. G. Godfrey, *Brit. J. Pharmacol.*, **11,** 71 (1956).
334. M. Ristic and A. M. Watrach, *Am. J. Vet. Res.*, **22,** 109–116 (1961).
335. M. Ristic, *Advan. Vet. Sci.*, **6,** 111–192 (1960).
336. M. Ristic, in *Infectious Blood Diseases of Man and Animals*, Vol. 2, D. Weinman and M. Ristic, Eds., Academic Press, New York, 1968, pp. 473–542.
337. L. P. Joyner and D. W. Brocklesby, in *Advances in Pharmacology and Chemotherapy*, Vol. 11, S. Garrattini, A. Goldin, F. Hawking, and I. J. Kopin, Eds., Academic Press, 1973, pp. 322–328.
338. J. F. Christensen, in *Diseases of Cattle*, 2nd ed. American Veterinary Publishers, Santa Barbara, Calif., 1963, pp. 655–665.
339. J. G. Miller, *Ann. N.Y. Acad. Sci.*, **64,** 49 (1956).
340. T. E. Granklin, R. W. Cook, D. J. Anderson, and K. L. Kultler, *Southwest Vet.*, **20,** 101 (1967).
341. C. G. D. Brown, J. K. H. Wilde, and J. Berger, *Brit. Vet. J.*, **124,** 325 (1968).
342. T. O. Roby, T. E. Amerault, and L. A. Spindler, *Res. Vet. Sci.*, **9,** 494–497 (1968).
343. K. L. Kuttler and L. G. Adams, *Res. Vet. Sci.*, **11,** 339 (1970).
344. K. L. Kuttler, *Am. J. Vet. Res.*, **32,** 1349 (1971).
345. T. O. Roby, *Res. Vet. Sci.*, **13,** 519 (1972).
346. E. Chatton and G. Blanc, *Arch. Inst. Pasteur* (Paris), **10,** 1–41 (1917).
347. B. H. Kean, in *Progress in Drug Research*, Vol. 18, E. Jucker, Ed., Birkhäuser-Verlag, Basel, 1974, pp. 205–210.
348. L. Jacobs, *Advan. Parasitol.*, **5,** 1 (1968).
349. W. M. Hutchison, J. F. Dunachie, K. Work, and J. C. Sim, *Trans. Roy. Soc. Trop. Med. Hyg.*, **65,** 380–399 (1971).
350. D. E. Eyles, in *Experimental Chemotherapy*, Vol. 1, R. J. Schnitzer and F. Hawking, Eds., Academic Press, 1963, pp. 641–655.
351. F. Hawking, in *Experimental Chemotherapy*, Vol. 4, R. J. Schnitzer and F. Hawking, Eds., Academic Press, 1966, pp. 467ff.
352. J. K. Frenkel, in *The Coccidia*, D. M. Hammond, Ed., with P. L. Long, University Park Press, Baltimore, 1973, pp. 343-410.
353. M. K. Cook and L. Jacobs, *J. Parasitol.*, **44,** 172–182 (1958).
354. M. K. Cook and L. Jacobs, *J. Parasitol.*, **44,** 280–288 (1958).
355. M. K. Cook, *J. Parasitol.*, **44,** 274–279 (1958).
356. A. B. Sabin and J. Warren, *J. Bacteriol.*, **41,** 80 (1941).
357. W. A. Summers, *Proc. Soc. Exp. Biol. Med.*, **66,** 509 (1947).
358. W. A. Summers, *Am. J. Trop. Med. Hyg.*, **2,** 1037–1044 (1953).
359. D. E. Eyles and N. Coleman, *Antibiot. Chemother.*, **5,** 529–539 (1955).
360. Anonymous, *Med. Lett.*, **11,** · *no.* 6 (1969) (*published by Drug and Therapeutic Information, Inc., New York*).
361. E. Biocca, *Arq. Biol.* (São Paulo), **27,** 7 (1943).
362. D. E. Eyles and N. Coleman, *Antibiot. Chemother.*, 7 (1943).
363. D. E. Eyles and N. Coleman, *Am. J. Trop. Med. Hyg.*, **2,** 64 (1953).
364. W. A. Summers, *Am. J. Trop. Med.*, **29,** 889 (1949).
365. J. P. Garin, M. Perrin–Fayolle, and P. Paliard, *Presse Med.*, **73,** 531 (1965).
366. H. Werner and R. Dannemann, *Z. Tropemed. Parasitol.*, **23,** 63 (1972).
367. J. Balarr, L. Ebringer, and P. Nemec, *Naturwissenschaften*, **9,** 227 (1964).
368. P. R. B. McMaster, K. G. Powers, J. F. Finerty, and N. M. Lunde, *Am. J. Trop. Med. Hyg.*, **22,** 14 (1973).
369. V. M. Arean and E. Koppisch, *Am. J. Pathol.*, **32,** 1089–1115 (1956).
370. A. Westphal, *Z. Tropenmed. Parasitol.*, **8,** 288–294 (1957).
371. G. Woolfe, in *Experimental Chemotherapy*, Vol. 1, R. J. Schitzer and F. Hawking, Eds., Academic Press, New York, 1963, pp. 657–659.
372. L. A. DeLanney and E. H. Beahm, *J. Am. Med. Assoc.*, **123,** 549 (1943).
373. V. D. Nosina, V. F. Gladkich, and O. I. Kellina, *Chem. Abstr.*, **51,** 5297*b* (1957).
374. R. M. D'Offay, *J. Trop. Med. Hyg.*, **63,** 321 (1962).
375. A. Verhulst and R. R. Shukla, in *20th World Veterinarians' Congress, Summaries*, Vol. 2, Thessaloniki, Greece, 1975, pp. 1005–1006.
376. R. B. Burrows and W. G. Hahmes, *Am. J. Trop. Med. Hyg.*, **1,** 626 (1952).
377. P. P. Weinstein, B. T. Garfunkel, and M. M Miller, *Am. J. Trop. Med. Hyg.*, **1,** 980 (1952).
378. Anonymous, *Med. Lett.*, **11,** no. 6 (1969) (published by Drug and Therapeutic Information, Inc., New York).

379. F. J. Payne, F. O. Atchley, M. A. Wasley, and M. E. Wenning, *J. Parasitol.*, **46,** 742 (1960).

380. F. Amini, *J. Trop. Med. Hyg.*, **66,** 190 (1963).

381. H. M. Selzer, *Med. Today*, **3,** 110 (1969).

382. F. Coutelen, A. Bretorr, J. Biquet, S. Deblock, S. Mullet, and J. M. Doby, *Bull. Soc. Pathol. Exot.*, **48,** 529 (1955).

383. A. K. Gupta, B. N. Tanden, and H. S. Mital, *J. Indian Med. Assoc.*, **49,** 117 (1967).

384. C. C. Schneider, *Z. Tropenmed. Parasitol.*, **12,** 276 (1961).

385. W. J. Bemrick, *J. Parasitol.*, **49,** 819 (1963).

386. M. E. Ament and C. E. Rubin, *Gastroenterology*, **62,** 716 (1972).

387. S. Bassily, Z. Farid, J. W. Mikhail, D. C. Kent, and J. S. Lehman, *J. Trop. Med. Hyg.*, **73,** 15 (1970).

388. J. Schneider, *Bull. Soc. Pathol. Exot. Fil.*, **54,** 84–95 (1961).

389. R. B. K. Lambatta, *Ann. Trop. Med. Parasitol.*, **65,** 487 (1971).

390. V. P. Pai, F. F. Wadia, M. Darge, C. R. Sule, and S. S. Kale, *J. Assoc. Phys. Ind.*, **22,** 531–533 (1974).

391. G. Woolfe, in *Experimental Chemotherapy*, Vol. 1, R. J. Schnitzer and F. Hawking, Eds., Academic Press, New York, pp. 351–353, 1963; Vol. 4, 1966, pp. 429–431.

392. F. Benazet, C. Cosar, P. Ganter, L. Julon, P. Populaire, and L. Guillaume, *Compt. Rend.*, **263,** 609 (1966).

393. G. N. Perschin, N. A. Novitskaya, S. N. Milovanova, and T. N. Zykova, *Med. Parazitol. Parazit. Bolezn.*, **40,** 78–81 (1971); *Chem. Abstr.*, **75,** 61988y.

394. L. P. Joyner and D. W. Brocklesby, in *Advances in Pharmacology and Chemotherapy*, Vol. 11, S. Garrattini, A. Goldin, F. Hawking, and I. J. Kopin, Eds., Academic Press, New York, 1973, pp. 341–354.

395. L. Hulliger, J. K. H. Wilde, C. G. D. Brown, and L. Turner, *Nature* (London), **203,** 728–730 (1964).

396. F. Hawking, in *Experimental Chemotherapy*, Vol. 1, R. J. Schnitzer and F. Hawking, Eds., Academic Press, New York, 1963, pp. 625–632; Vol. 4., 1966, pp. 566–467.

397. J. K. H. Wilde, *Advan. Vet. Sci.*, **11,** 224 (1967).

398. S. F. Barnett, in *Infectious Blood Diseases of Man and Animals*, Vol. 2, D. Weinman and M. Ristic, Eds., Academic Press, New York, 1968, pp. 269–328.

CHAPTER TWENTY-ONE

Anthelmintic Agents

PETER J. ISLIP

Chemical Research Laboratory
The Wellcome Research Laboratories
Langley Court
Beckenham, Kent
England

CONTENTS

1 INTRODUCTION

Helminth infections present a prevalence rate in man and animals far greater than that for any other disease, although their importance frequently goes unrecognized. Helminth diseases and primitive treatments were described in some detail in ancient Chinese and Egyptian writings, but it must be emphasized that even now, 3500 years after their first recorded incidence, the treatment of some of these worm infestations is far from satisfactory.

There is no evidence that the worldwide incidence of parasitic infestation has diminished since Stoll presented his estimates of global prevalence in his presidential address to the American Society of Parasitologists in 1946 (1). On the basis of updated values for prevalence rates (2, 3), it can be calculated that the 1 billion or so people afflicted with the roundworm *Ascaris lumbricoides* excrete some 58,000 *tons* of ascaris eggs per annum, and the total *daily* blood consumption of the hookworms *Ancylostoma duodenale* and *Necator americanus*, which parasitize at least 800 million humans, is equivalent to the total exsanguination of some 2 million people.

Regrettably, man's interference with nature, as reflected by grandiose engineering schemes and by rapidly increasing urban pollution, has contributed to the spread of some of the major parasitic infections. Thus there is evidence (4) that the building of the Aswan High Dam—essential for land reclamation and continuous controlled irrigation in Egypt as opposed to annual flooding of the Nile Valley—has led to the spread of schistosomiasis by virtue of the elimination of the "winter closure" period (the time during which the irrigation canals were closed, dried up, and dredged clear of silt and aquatic weeds, and with them both bulinid and *Biomphalaria* snail intermediate hosts of the disease). Population movements in certain parts of the Far East have created urban shanty towns with inadequate housing and no means of disposing of sewage effluent. In turn, this has given rise to the creation of breeding grounds for culicine mosquitoes, with the result that the transmission of Bancroftian and Malaysian filariasis in these areas is becoming an urban rather than a rural problem.

In some quarters the importance of helminth infection is still not properly realized, perhaps because few of these diseases are truly life threatening: centuries of coexistence have led to a host-parasite relationship that generally avoids death of the host. However, human nematode and trematode infections are particularly prevalent in tropical and subtropical regions; and any additional factor aggravating, for example, the malnutrition already present in the undeveloped countries of the Third World must be regarded with the utmost concern. Children too, in all parts of the world, are susceptible to the toxic effects of worm infections, while each year there are immense economic losses in terms of milk and meat production from domestic and farm animals—again, particularly in areas that can least afford such misfortunes.

Moreover, in the last decade or so many of the major pharmaceutical companies (where most of the effective experimental chemotherapy of parasitic infections has been carried out) have closed down their research programs in tropical medicine. This is not surprising, since the spectacular failure rate of experimental lead compounds and the escalating costs of industrial research and development, combined with the ever-increasing stringency of regulatory requirements, are compelling companies to concentrate their resources in the fields of research where there is the greatest likelihood of high returns on investment. Naturally these areas of research focus on the so-called "diseases of civilization" rather than on pathological states occurring mainly in the less developed countries.

Recently, increasing international concern at the lack of suitable drugs for the treatment of parasitic infections in rural populations in particular has led to the creation by the World Health Organization of a "Special Programme for Research and Training in Tropical Diseases". One of the defined objectives of this program is to find economically practical control measures for the major communicable diseases, especially parasitic infections, in the developing countries. In particular, the program, which will be funded by the World Bank and by various government agencies, will be directed toward the control of six specific tropical infections—with schistosomiasis and filariasis representing the helminth diseases.

It is to be hoped that the creation of this program represents, at long last, a real determination to come to grips with the tropical infections that have remained major scourges for far too long.

2 BIOLOGY OF HELMINTHS

Helminths that parasitize humans and animals are derived from two phyla, Platyhelminthes and Nemathelminthes. The phylum Platyhelminthes contains three classes: Turbellaria or eddyworms, which are mainly free living and are not parasitic in man; Trematoda or flukes; and Cestoidea or tapeworms. The phylum Nemathelminthes, or true roundworms, includes many species, some of them free living and some parasitic.

2.1 Trematodes

Trematodes or flukes have nonsegmented bodies that incorporate a mouth, a blind alimentary tract without an anal opening, and an excretory system; each worm has one or more suckers for attachment. The flukes have an external cuticular layer that is often wholly or partly covered with spines, tubercles, or ridges.

Trematodes may be divided into two groups according to their developmental patterns. The monogenetic trematodes (Monogenea) have a direct life cycle in one single host and do not parasitize man.

Digenetic trematodes (Digenea) possess complicated life cycles and require one or more intermediate hosts to complete their life cycles. As the name implies, digenetic trematodes have two generations, sexual and asexual—asexual multiplication taking place in specific snail hosts.

Digenetic trematodes are characteristically flat and leaflike or sometimes globular hermaphrodite organisms. Schistosomes are an exception to this morphology in that adult worms exists normally as pairs in which the male is folded about its long axis (producing the so-called gynecophoric canal), enveloping the cylindrical female worm. (It has been stated that schistosomes lead an idyllic existence—they live for some 20–30 years lapped by a warm nutrient medium, the bloodstream, and remain permanently *in copula*!)

Digenetic trematodes of medical and veterinary significance are listed in Table 21.1. The species mentioned are normal parasites of man except *Fasciola hepatica*. Man is an accidental host for this species and is not involved in its transmission cycle.

Almost certainly, schistosomiasis is the major human helminth disease in terms of morbidity. Although adult schistosomes (and all trematodes) are unable to multiply within the definitive host, and indeed may coexist with the host quite happily for 20–30 years, it is the passage of eggs through tissues and the presence of the parasite (or eggs) in abnormal (ectopic) sites that give rise to the serious pathological lesions associated with the disease process.

2.2 Cestodes

Cestodes are flat tapelike worms (i.e., tapeworms), which vary in length from 1 mm to a frightening 12 m. The worm typically consists of a scolex or head (which may be furnished with suckers and sometimes hooks), joined by a short neck to the strobila, which usually consists of a chain of segments or proglottids that are produced by growth and division of the neck.

In tapeworms of the order Cyclophyllidea (which includes all adult cestodes that are parasitic in man except *Diphyllobothrium* spp.), the proglottids become more mature the further they are from the scolex. Gravid proglottids full of eggs become detached, and pass out in the feces. All tapeworms infecting humans are hermaphroditic, and copulation may take place between different proglottids of the same strobila or even between proglottids of different strobila, if two worms of the same species are present in the one host.

Tapeworms of the order Pseudophyllidea (e.g., *Diphyllobothrium latum*, the broad fish tapeworm) possess a uterine pore through which up to 1 million eggs per day are discharged.

The typical cestode life cycle involves one or more intermediate hosts in which the infective egg develops to become a procercoid, plerocercoid, cysticercoid, or cysticercus larva. The definitive host is infected by consuming infected tissues of an intermediate host. In cases of hydatid infection or cysticercosis, man is seen in the role of an accidental intermediate host. *Hymenolepis nana* is unusual in possessing the capacity to pass through the cysticercoid stage in the intestinal villus of the definitive host, although it may still utilize the more conventional cycle involving an arthropod intermediate.

Table 21.2 lists the main tapeworms parasitizing man, but it should be noted that in most cases no serious pathology is associated with their presence. However,

Table 21.1 Trematodes Found in Man

Species	Site of Adult	Mode of Egg Transmission	Intermediate Host(s)	Definitive Host	Distribution
Schistosoma mansoni	Mesenteric vein	Feces	Snail	Man[a]	Africa, Central and South America
S. japonicum	Mesenteric vein	Feces	Snail	Man[a]	Far East
S. haematobium	Vesicular veins	Urine	Snail	Man[a]	Africa, Middle East
Paragonimus westermani	Cysts in lungs	Sputum and feces	Snail, then fresh-water crustaceans	Man, various carnivores	Far East[b]
Fasciola hepatica	Bile ducts	Feces	Snail, then meta-cercariae encysted on plants	Sheep, cattle, pig, rabbit, man, etc.	Temperate areas
Clonorchis (Opisthorchis) sinensis	Bile and pancreatic ducts	Feces	Snail, then fresh-water fish	Man, dog, cat, pig	Far East
Opisthorchis felineus	Bile and pancreatic ducts	Feces	Snail, then fresh-water fish	Man, dog, cat	Eastern Europe, USSR
Fasciolopsis buski	Small intestine	Feces	Snail, then meta-cercariae encysted on plants	Man, pig	Far East
Metagonimus yokogawai	Small intestine	Feces	Snail, then fresh-water fish	Man, various carnivores	Far East
Heterophyes heterophyes	Small intestine	Feces	Snail, then fresh-water fish	Man, various carnivores	Egypt, Far East

[a] Man is infected by penetration of the cercarial form through unbroken skin.
[b] There are also foci of infection in West Africa, and South America.

Table 21.2 Cestodes Found in Man

Tapeworm[b]	Common Name	Habitat	Infective Stage
Diphyllobothrium latum	Broad fish tapeworm	Small intestine	Plerocercoid in freshwater fish
Taenia saginata	Beef tapeworm	Small intestine	Cysticercus in cattle muscle
T. solium	Pork tapeworm	Small intestine	Cysticercus in pig muscle
Dipylidium caninum	Dog tapeworm	Small intestine	Cysticercoid in dog flea
Hymenolepis nana[a]	Dwarf tapeworm	Small intestine	Egg in human or rodent feces; cysticercoid in various insect species
Echinococcus granulosus larva[a]	Hydatid cyst	All tissues, but predominantly liver and lungs	Egg in dog feces
T. solium larva[a]	*Cysticercus cellulosae*	All tissues	Egg in human feces

[a] The host of a larva becomes infected by virtue of swallowing the egg; from the egg only the larval (cystic) stage can develop, not the adult worm.
[b] The distribution of these tapeworms is cosmopolitan, except that *D. latum* tends to be restricted to areas of the world where raw freshwater fish are eaten.

certain larval (cystic) forms (e.g., *Echinococcus granulosus*, which is essentially a parasite in farm livestock, or cysticercosis due to *Taenia solium* larvae) may cause serious and sometimes fatal parasitic disease in humans.

2.3 Nematodes

Nematodes (roundworms) of the class Nematoda and the phylum Nemathelminthes are generally of a higher zoological organization than cestodes or trematodes. Typical nematodes possess a tough impermeable cuticle that encloses longitudinal muscles, nerve fibers, and a complete digestive system with mouth and anus. The sexes are separate in most nematode species, although it is believed that only parthenogenetic females are present in the parasitic stages of one or two species (particularly *Strongyloides*).

Although nematode infections of dogs, cows, and horses were recognized and adequately described by Hippocrates, Aristotle, and other early writers, the true significance of the damage caused by these parasites in farm animals has been properly appreciated only relatively recently. Early writers were also able to discuss human nematode infections with some accuracy. Thus hookworms were mentioned in the Ebers Papyrus of *ca.* 1550 BC, and Lucretius in the first half of the first century BC referred to the pale skin of miners (presumably due to the anemia associated with hookworm infection).

Nematodes are conveniently divided into intestinal species, lungworms, and filarial or tissue forms. Some of the species infecting man are listed in Table 21.3.

3 ANTHELMINTIC SCREENING METHODS

Detailed descriptions of the various *in vivo* and *in vitro* screening methods available for the detection of potential anthelmintic agents are not listed here, since adequate reviews are available that afford considerable information on this subject (5–11).

Although in recent years much interest has been expressed in the development of a variety of *in vitro* test systems and enzyme assays, nevertheless it is probably still true that no major anthelmintic agent of novel chemical type has emerged from such an approach. Indeed, the nature of *in vitro* test systems is probably such as to preclude development of all except analogs of known anthelmintic agents.

4 TREMATODE DISEASES AND DRUGS ACTIVE AGAINST THEM

The major human trematode (fluke) disease is schistosomiasis, which has been estimated to infect some 200 million–300 million persons in the tropics and subtropics. This disease is considered separately from the other fluke infections, since as a general rule schistosomicidal agents have little activity against other trematodes, and compounds active against *Fasciola*, *Opisthorchis*, and other flukes frequently lack activity against schistosomes.

4.1 Schistosomiasis

The Ebers Papyrus, one of the ancient Egyptian medical texts, described the hematuria generally associated with urinary schistosomiasis (*Schistosoma haematobium*) about 3000 years ago, yet it was not until 1851 that Theodore Bilharz isolated one of the three species of human schistosome (*S. haematobium*) from an Egyptian peasant.

4.1.1 LIFE CYCLE. Since schistosomiasis is the major helminth infection, it is worth describing the complicated life cycle of this parasite in some detail. Adult schistosomes live as pairs in the visceral veins; *S. mansoni* (intestinal schistosomiasis) mainly in

Table 21.3 Nematodes Found in Man

Species	Habitat	Infective Stage	Distribution
Ascaris lumbricoides (roundworm)	Small intestine	Embryonated eggs in soil and water	Cosmopolitan
Trichuris trichiura (whipworm)	Cecum and colon	Embryonated eggs in soil, and water	Cosmopolitan
Enterobius vermicularis (pinworm)	Cecum and colon	Embryonated eggs in soil, water, house dust, etc.	Cosmopolitan
Strongyloides stercoralis	Small intestine	Infective larvae on ground[a]	Cosmopolitan, but mainly in warm climates
Ancylostoma duodenale (hookworm)	Small intestine	Infective larvae on ground[a]	Cosmopolitan, but mainly in warm climates
Necator americanus (hookworm)	Small intestine	Infective larvae on ground[a]	Cosmopolitan, but mainly in warm climates
Trichinella spiralis	Small intestine[b]	Encysted larvae in pork	Cosmopolitan
Dracunculus medinensis (Guinea-worm)	Subcutaneous and intermuscular connective tissue[c]	Infective larvae in (ingested) *Cyclops*	Africa, India
Wuchereria bancrofti	Lymphatic glands or vessels	Infective larvae in various (biting) mosquitoes	Tropics and subtropics
Brugia malayi	Lymphatic vessels	Infective larvae in various (biting) mosquitoes	Far East, India, Sri Lanka
Loa loa	Connective tissue, mesentery, and parietal peritoneum	Infective larvae in (biting) *Chrysops* species	West and Central Africa
Onchocerca volvulus	Subcutaneous nodules and lymph spaces	Infective larvae in (biting) *Simulium* species	West and Central Africa, Central and South America

[a] Active penetration of unbroken skin.
[b] Larvae carried by the circulation to skeletal muscle, where encystment occurs.
[c] Female only.

the inferior mesenteric vein and its tributaries, *S. haematobium* in the veins of the vesical plexus, and *S. japonicum* (which causes the Far Eastern version of the disease) primarily in the superior mesenteric vein and its tributaries.

During oviposition, the female may leave the male and swim against the blood flow to reach the capillaries and venules in either the intestine and rectum (*S. mansoni* and *S. japonicum*) or the wall of the bladder (*S. haematobium*). Eggs migrate into the lumen of the intestine or bladder and are passed out of the body in the feces or urine. In fresh water (less than 0.7% sodium chloride), eggs hatch within several hours to miracidia. The miracidium, a relatively short-lived, free-swimming stage, readily penetrates and infects a variety of aquatic snail intermediate hosts. Within the snail, development and multiplication take place, until finally the minute, forked-tail cercariae emerge from the snail (approximately 100,000 from a single miracidium). Man becomes infected by penetration of the unbroken skin by the actively swimming cercariae. In this process the cercariae lose their tails, and the resulting schistosomules migrate by way of the circulatory system to the liver. There the young worms mature; then they (*S. mansoni*) return to the portal vein and its tributaries where pairing takes place, and the cycle is complete.

Since the disease is transmitted through contact of humans with water containing the infective cercariae, it is hardly surprising that the new irrigation schemes in Africa and the Middle East have led to a considerable spread of the disease. For instance, in the Gezira area of Sudan, between the Blue Nile and the White Nile, nearly 1 million hectares have been irrigated in a bold attempt to make the Sudan a major exporter of agricultural produce. Unfortunately, recent surveys of the area indicate that 60% of 7-year-olds now have schistosomiasis. Regrettably, little serious work appears to have been done to develop irrigation schemes designed to be inimical to the vector molluscs.

4.1.2 PATHOLOGY. Although schistosomiasis in general is not a life-threatening disease, the pathology associated with the condition does include pipestem fibrosis of the liver, pulmonary arteritis, transverse myelitis and other central nervous system lesions, colonic polyposis, schistosomal neuropathy, and obstructive uropathy leading to renal failure with or without associated bacterial pyelonephritis. In addition, in some areas there appears to be a significant association between urinary schistosomiasis and carcinoma of the bladder.

4.1.3 CONTROL MEASURES. Schistosomiasis control depends on (1) preventing the contamination of natural waters by reducing the number of schistosome eggs in human excreta (i.e., chemotherapy), (2) destroying snail intermediate hosts with molluscicides or by biological means, and (3) reducing human contact with infected waters.

It is this first control method that concerns the medicinal chemist, and the others are not discussed further. In fact, several difficulties exist in the design of potential schistosomicidal agents. First, any successful therapeutic agent must have a toxicity low enough to allow mass treatment of rural populations by paramedical personnel. Second, the ideal drug should be active against both urinary and intestinal forms of the disease (activity against the somewhat refractory *S. japonicum* being an added bonus). Third, the drug should be inexpensive. Finally, the formulated drug should possess reasonable stability under field conditions. It is clear that using these criteria, the ideal schistosomicide has yet to be found. Indeed, at an international conference on schistosomiasis in Cairo in October 1975, one of the conclusions was that despite the availability of four or five separate chemical types of schistosomicidal agent, all these compounds, in one way or another, were far from ideal. Since no fully effective, safe drug was available, however, the only recommendation the conference could give to clinicians was to "continue to use existing drugs, but [to] exercise care"!

4.1.4 CHEMOTHERAPY OF SCHISTOSOMIASIS. Several reviews describe the chemotherapy of schistosomiasis (5, 12–18). This section is intended to be selective rather than exhaustive, and describes currently used drugs and structure-activity patterns associated with them.

4.1.4.1 Antimony Compounds. The use of antimony in medicine has roots buried in the distant past. It was introduced to therapy by Paracelsus early in the sixteenth century and was used as a general panacea. One interesting application was the so-called perpetual pill, a pill formulated of the metal that could be used as an emetic, then recovered intact ready for the next patient—a conservationist's dream!

Trivalent antimonials were introduced into schistosomiasis therapy in 1918 by Christopherson (19). Today the use of antimony is limited, since all compounds investigated so far possess major shortcomings, including uncertain toxicity (cardiotoxicity and certain fatal cardiovascular syndromes), difficulty of administration and considerable length of treatment needed (up to 4 weeks of intermittent intravenous injections in some cases), and low, variable efficacy.

Of the antimonial compounds used, potassium antimony tartrate (21.**1**, tartar emetic) or sodium antimony tartrate are

CO—O
CH—O—Sb.$\frac{1}{2}H_2O$
CH—O
CO_2K

21.**1**

effective against all species of human schistosome, but treatment must be on an individual basis, and the drugs cannot be used in mass chemotherapy campaigns. Antimony dimercaptosuccinate (21.**2**, stibo-

CO_2K — CH—S — Sb—S — CH—CH — S—Sb — S—CH — CO_2K
CO_2H — CH—S / HO_2C / CO_2K / S—CH — CO_2H

21.**2**

captate, astiban) is effective intramuscularly against all three species of human schistosome. Other antimonials that have been used in humans include sodium antimony bis(pyrocatechol-3,5-disulfonate) (stibophen, Fuadin) and lithium antimony thiomalate (anthiomaline) (20). Structure-activity relationships among antimony compounds and factors involved in the clinical efficacy of some of these drugs have been reviewed by Friedheim (14).

Since the toxic symptoms produced by organic antimony compounds resemble those caused by inorganic (ionic) antimony, attempts have been made to improve the therapeutic index of the antimonials by chelation (e.g., with penicillamine). Thus in clinical evaluation, a much improved therapeutic index has been claimed for a complex of penicillamine and sodium antimony tartrate (21).

Although research is still being carried out into the preparation of further antimony derivatives as potential schistosomicides, it is likely that the toxicity inherently associated with the metal will preclude clinical use of any of these congeners for the mass chemotherapy of schistosomiasis.

4.1.4.2 Thioxanthenone Derivatives. a. Lucanthone Analogs. The first real advance in the chemotherapy of schistosomiasis came in the 1930s with the recognition by Kikuth and Gönnert at the

Bayer laboratories that certain thioxanthenones possessed efficacy against experimental *S. mansoni* infections in mice (22). The active series (21.**3**–21.**6**), known as the

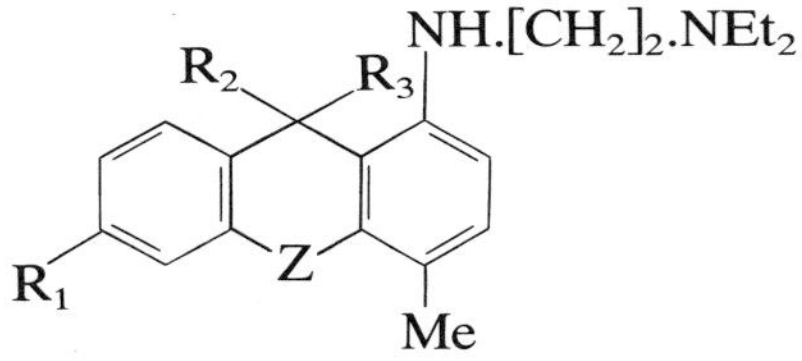

21.**3** $R_1 = H, R_2R_3 = O, Z = O$ (Miracil A)
21.**4** $R_1 = Cl, R_2R_3 = O, Z = O$ (Miracil B)
21.**5** $R_1 = H, R_2R_3 = H, OH, Z = O$ (Miracil C)
21.**6** $R_1 = H, R_2R_3 = O, Z = S$ (Miracil D, lucanthone)

Miracils, was prepared by Mauss (23), and from it lucanthone (21.**6**, Nilodin, Miracil D) emerged in clinical use in 1946 as the first nonmetallic, orally administered schistosomicide. Although the drug had moderate efficacy against *S. haematobium* and *S. mansoni*, the frequency and severity of the side effects (severe gastrointestinal upset, confusional states, mania, and occasional deaths) limited its general acceptance.

b. Mirasans. A wide variety of analogs of the Miracils have been prepared (see, e.g., Refs. 5, 12, 16–18, 24) including the so-called mirasan series (25), the most active of which was *N'*-(3-chloro-*p*-tolyl)-*N,N*-diethylethylenediamine (21.**7**). Although this series, in particular 21.**7**, was

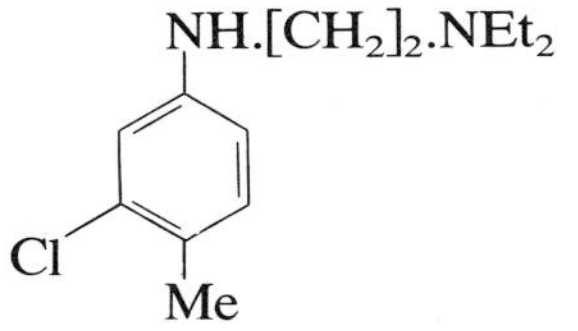

Mirasan
21.**7**

more active against *S. mansoni* in mice than were the Miracils, in general all compounds tested in experimentally infected monkeys appeared to lack activity.

c. Hycanthone. Early experiences with lucanthone in mice, monkeys, and humans led many laboratories to postulate the existence of an active metabolite for this compound (16). Although the absolute requirement in Miracil and mirasan analogs for a *p*-toluidine system containing a basic side chain on the nitrogen had been recognized, all attempts to isolate active metabolites had failed. In addition, extensive modification of the molecular configuration had also failed to produce a variant with an acceptable therapeutic index.

While investigating the action of molds on a variety of medicinal agents, however, workers at the Sterling Winthrop Laboratories cultured lucanthone with the fungus *Aspergillus sclerotiorum* (26, 27). Of the three interrelated products formed (21.**8**–21.**10**), one, designated hycanthone (21.**8**), was subsequently shown to be the active metabolite of lucanthone (16).

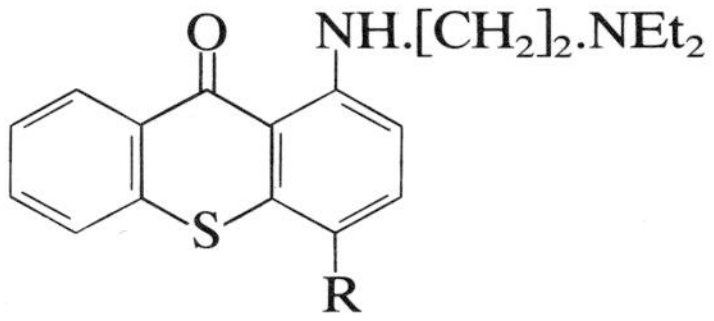

21.**8** $R = CH_2OH$ (hycanthone)
21.**9** $R = CHO$
21.**10** $R = CO_2H$

Hycanthone has been shown to be more potent as a schistosomicidal agent than the parent lucanthone. Thus against *S. mansoni* in hamsters, hycanthone was some 9 times more effective than lucanthone when given orally for 5 days or as a single intraperitoneal injection (28). In addition, in mice the drug was 3 times more active than lucanthone, and in the cebus monkey, Pellegrino and his co-workers discovered (29) that hycanthone was curative at oral doses of 5 or 10 mg/kg, daily for 5 days.

Hycanthone has been found to be very sensitive to acid, and with hindsight it is easy to see why early investigators did not identify the drug in the urine of animals dosed with lucanthone. Isolation methods all appeared to involve treatment of the urine with acid. When the urine extracts were incubated with glucuronidase, however, hycanthone (which is excreted as the glucuronide) was a major component of the mixture.

Administered to humans as the methanesulfonate salt (Etrenol), hycanthone has good efficacy against *S. mansoni* and *S. haematobium* infections at single intramuscular injections of about 3 mg/kg. Side effects are not infrequent at this dose level, however, and these include vomiting (in more than 50% of patients in some trials), nausea, abdominal pain, headache, and dizziness. More serious are isolated examples of acute liver damage (rare fatalities have occurred) and jaundice.

Of more potential concern are the reports from a variety of laboratories indicating that hycanthone is mutagenic and teratogenic, and that it induces prophage, mitotic crossing-over, cytogenic changes, and malignant transformations (for reviews, see Refs. 30 and 31). In addition, the drug has been shown to be carcinogenic in *S. mansoni*-infected mice (32), although these findings were not confirmed in a study that admittedly used a very small number of animals (33).

Another interesting finding with hycanthone was the discovery by Rogers and Bueding (34) that administration of relatively high doses of the drug to mice infected with *S. mansoni* led to the development in the second-generation worms of resistance that was stable for several further generations. These worms were also cross-resistant to lucanthone and the tetrahydroquinoline oxamniquine (21.**46**).

In considering the mode of action of hycanthone, although the drug has been shown to interfere with neuromuscular coordination, it has not been established whether this effect is due to stimulation of low affinity uptake mechanisms for 5-hydroxytryptamine in schistosomes (35), or to competition with acetylcholine (Ach) for the Ach-receptor site (36). Certainly, the last authors believe that an earlier suggestion (16) that hycanthone-treated schistosomes starve to death corroborates their findings.

Following the discovery of the enhanced antischistosome activity of the hydroxymethyl compound hycanthone over the parent methyl congener lucanthone, a wide variety of hydroxymethyl "metabolites" of *p*-toluidine-type experimental schistosomicides have been prepared, although to date no drug of this class has emerged that is better than hycanthone. This subject has been comprehensively reviewed by Archer and Yarinsky (16).

d. Benzothiopyrano[4,3,2-cd]indazoles. As part of a program to investigate whether the adverse toxicological properties of hycanthone could be dissociated from its good antischistosome activity, workers at the Parke, Davis laboratories prepared a series of benzothiopyrano[4,3,2-*cd*]indazoles (37). These compounds (21.**11**–21.**14**)

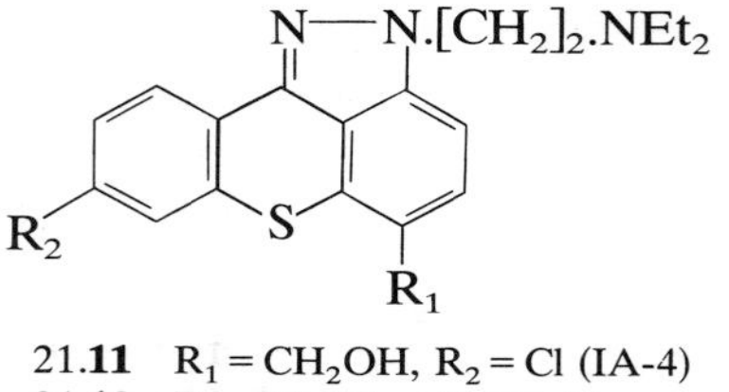

N—N.$[CH_2]_2$.NEt_2 S R_2 R_1

21.**11** $R_1 = CH_2OH$, $R_2 = Cl$ (IA-4)
21.**12** $R_1 = Me$, $R_2 = Cl$ (IA-3)
21.**13** $R_1 = CH_2OH$, $R_2 = H$
21.**14** $R_1 = Me$, $R_2 = H$

were similar in potency to hycanthone against *S. mansoni* in mice on oral administration and by single intramuscular doses in mice and hamsters; however, the 8-chloro compound 21.**11** (IA-4) had an acute toxicity in mice (i.m.) some 5 times less than that of hycanthone. In addition IA-4 and the 5-methyl analog IA-3 were found to have little or no hepatotoxic, mutagenic, teratogenic, or malignant cell transforming properties, although they intercalated well into DNA, and they retained substantial mutagenic activity for

Salmonella, T4 phage, and mouse cells (30, and references therein). In addition, hycanthone-resistant schistosomes were cross-resistant to at least one of the benzothiopyranoindazoles (IA-4) (38).

Preparation of the *N*-oxides of the terminal side chain amine of the benzothiopyranoindazoles afforded congeners that had antischistosome activity greater than that of hycanthone, whether by oral or intramuscular administration, but had considerably reduced mutagenic potential. Thus the *N*-oxide of the 5-methyl derivative IA-3 had mutagenic activity less than 1% of that of hycanthone, but it showed a marked increase in antischistosome effect (39).

In this interesting series of compounds it has been possible, in part at least, to dissociate the long-term toxic potential of hycanthone from its schistosomicidal activity. It remains to be seen, however, whether further structural modification of this series can afford a clinically useful analog. Indeed, it is possible that the genetic activity seemingly inherent in hycanthone-type compounds will prevent any related derivative from coming into large-scale clinical use.

4.1.4.3 Nitro Compounds. This chemical group has provided several interesting schistosomicidal agents, and one in particular (niridazole) has come to be regarded by many clinicians as the drug of choice for the oral treatment of urinary schistosomiasis.

a. Nitrothiazoles. Although 2-acetamido-5-nitrothiazole (21.**15**) was shown in

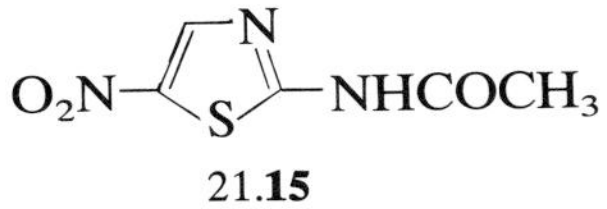

21.**15**

1955 to possess some slight activity against *S. mansoni* in mice at high dose levels (40), it was not until 1964 that workers at the Ciba laboratories announced (41–45) the discovery of niridazole (21.**16**, Ciba 32644-Ba, Ambilhar). This novel schistosomicide, which also possesses amebicidal and trichomonicidal properties, was synthesized as part of a systematic investigation of heterocyclic nitro compounds as potential antiparasitic agents.

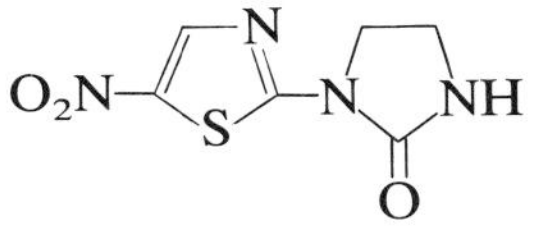

niridazole

21.**16**

Niridazole is highly effective for the treatment of *S. haematobium*, but is somewhat less active against *S. mansoni.* The drug is administered orally at 25 mg/kg per day (as two divided doses) for 5–10 days, and is usually well tolerated, especially by children. Side effects are generally mild and include nausea, vomiting, and anorexia. More serious are certain neuropsychiatric reactions (mania, mental disorientation, generalized convulsions, etc.), and changes in the electroencephalogram pattern.

The utility of the drug in mass chemotherapy appears to depend on the ability of each individual patient to metabolize it. There is good evidence (46) that unchanged drug is not only the active entity *per se*, but is also responsible for the toxicity. In particular, since the drug is normally largely metabolized by the liver on the first passage, it is clear that certain types of damage to the liver can alter the rate of metabolism to a degree that makes the drug unsafe in use. With *S. mansoni* infections, the probability of liver function impairment is significant, thus rendering the drug too dangerous to use for mass chemotherapy.

Of potential concern are the recent findings that considerable genetic activity is associated with niridazole. Thus it has been established that the drug is a direct-acting frameshift mutagen in a host-mediated assay (47), and mutagenic entities have been detected in the blood and urine of rats and humans after administration of the drug (48). In addition, niridazole has recently been shown to be carcinogenic to mice (49). The relevance of the carcinogenicity test (where massive doses of drug were fed daily to mice for their entire lifetimes) to the human clinical situation (where low doses are given for not more than 10 days) has yet to be established. Nevertheless the findings that niridazole has a more selective mechanism of action and a greater potential as an immunosuppressive agent than most cytotoxic compounds currently available (50) should be exploited with some caution.

At an early stage in the determination of structure-activity relationships associated with niridazole it was determined that relatively minor modifications tended to eliminate activity (12, 51). Although several variants containing a modified imidazolidine ring (e.g., 21.**17** and 21.**18**) possessed quite good schistosomicidal properties in experimental animals (52), and in particular the imidazolidinethione 21.**19** was reported

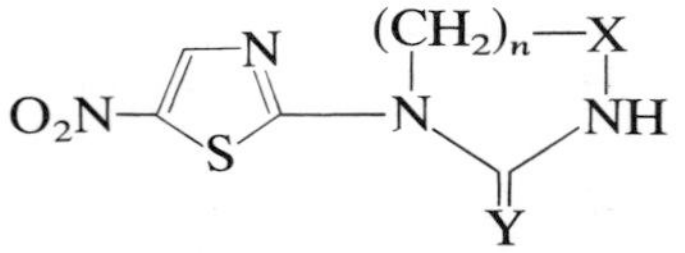

21.**17** Y = O, X = CO, $n = 1$
21.**18** Y = O, X = CO, $n = 2$
21.**19** Y = S, X = CH_2, $n = 1$

to be less toxic than niridazole in a limited number of patients (53), one requirement for activity in all niridazole congeners appeared to be the presence of the 5-nitro group (54).

In this connection, although the internal Bunte salt *S*-2-{[2-(2-thiazolylcarbamoyl)-ethyl]amino}ethyl hydrogen thiosulfate (21.**20**) lacks a 5-nitro group, it is highly active when administered orally to *S. mansoni*-infected mice and is curative in rhesus monkeys at high dose levels (55). There appears to be no evidence, however, that this drug has the same mode of action as niridazole. It is interesting to note with this compound that activity is extremely structure specific. Most structural modifications eliminate or drastically reduce activity: in fact, the corresponding 5-nitro congener is much less active as a schistosomicide than the parent desnitro compound. The thiol 21.**21** is essentially as active as the parent 21.**20**, as is the corresponding disulfide.

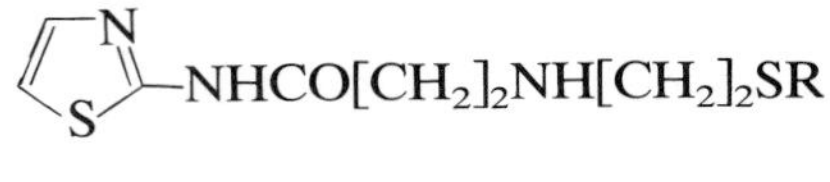

$-NHCO[CH_2]_2NH[CH_2]_2SR$

21.**20** R = SO_3H
21.**21** R = H

Although early investigations had established that analogs of niridazole in which the imidazolidinone ring had been opened [e.g., 1-ethyl-3-(5-nitro-2-thiazolyl)urea] were completely inactive as schistosomicides, work in the Parke, Davis laboratories showed that radical structural alterations could in fact be made to niridazole without drastically diminishing the antischistosome activity. The [(5-nitro-2-thiazolyl)amino]-propionamides 21.**22** and 21.**23** were found to possess good activity against *S. mansoni* in mice, although the propionyl and chloroacetyl analogs 21.**24** and 21.**25** lacked activity in the mouse primary screen. Again, although nitrile 21.**26** also possessed potent schistosomicidal properties, the corresponding amide 21.**27** was inactive (56). Further significant antischistosome activity was found in the nitrothiazolylformamides 21.**28** and 21.**29** (57).

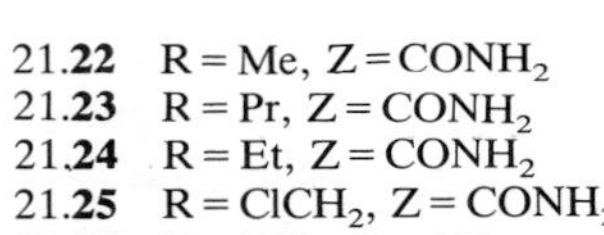

O_2N- thiazolyl $-N[CH_2]_2Z$, N–COR

21.**22** R = Me, Z = $CONH_2$
21.**23** R = Pr, Z = $CONH_2$
21.**24** R = Et, Z = $CONH_2$
21.**25** R = $ClCH_2$, Z = $CONH_2$
21.**26** R = NH_2, Z = CN
21.**27** R = NH_2, Z = $CONH_2$

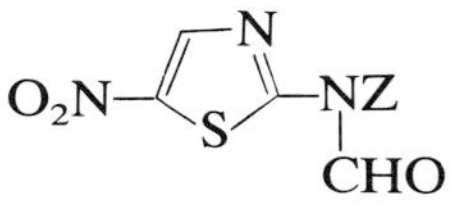

O_2N–(thiazole)–NZ(CHO)

21.**28** $Z = CH_2CONHCO_2Me$
21.**29** $Z = CH_2CON(Me)CO_2Et$

An extension of this work in the same laboratories led to the discovery of extremely high antischistosome activity in a wide range of 5-nitro-4-thiazolines of two general types—thiazoline-3-acetamides (21.**30**) (58, 59), and 3-alkylthiazolines (21.**31**) (60, 61). Interestingly, thiazolyl-3-propionamides and -butyramides were inactive, even though in the corresponding

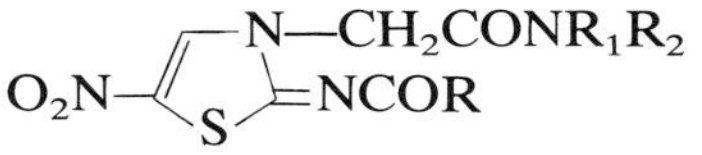

O_2N–(thiazoline)–N—$CH_2CONR_1R_2$, =NCOR

21.**30** R = alkyl, alkoxy, alkylamino, aryl, heterocyclic

O_2N–(thiazoline)–N—R_1, =NCOR

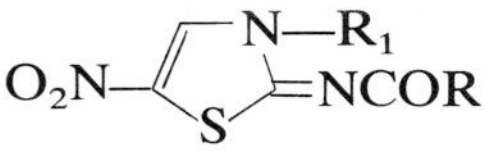

21.**31** R = alkyl, alkoxy, alkylamino, aryl, heterocyclic

3-alkyl series (21.**31**) no such restriction in alkyl chain length applied: good activity was recorded for 21.**31**, where R varied from methyl to heptyl. In addition, although primary acetamides (21.**30**, $NR_1R_2 = NH_2$) and the *N,N*-disubstituted congeners (e.g., 21.**30**, $NR_1R_2 = NMe_2$) were active, the secondary *N*-monosubstituted amides (e.g., 21.**30**, $NR_1R_2 = NHMe$) in general lacked activity (except the *N*-benzyl analogs).

One interesting compound (20.**31**, $R_1 = CH_2CH_2OMe$, R = *t*-Bu) was shown to be more active than niridazole in mice, hamsters, and rhesus monkeys, but to produce fewer side effects in the central nervous system of the dog. In addition, the compound was considerably less potent than niridazole as a mutagen against *Salmonella typhimurium* strains TA-100 and TA-1535 (38).

Bueding and Fisher (62) have shown that on administration to *S. mansoni*-infected mice, niridazole causes a progressive reduction of schistosome phosphorylase phosphatase activity. This is followed by a decrease in glycogen levels and an activation of glycogen phosphorylase. This effect is not selective, however, and therapeutic dose levels of the drug appear to decrease the rate of glycogen phosphorylase inactivation in the skeletal muscle of the host. Other studies have indicated that in mice niridazole possibly acts as a thiamine antagonist, although this work, carried out in a limited number of animals and based on increases in blood pyruvate levels (which could have been stress induced), has yet to be confirmed (63). To date it is not clear whether the nitrothiazolines have a mode of action similar to that of niridazole.

b. Nitrofurans. Although many nitrofurans are active against bacteria and protozoa, only certain derivatives possess schistosomicidal properties. One early clinical candidate was the isopropylamide (21.**32**, Furapromidium, F-30066), which

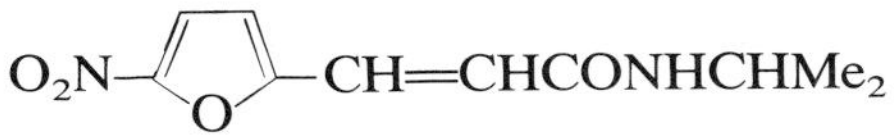

O_2N–(furan)–CH=CHCONHCHMe$_2$

F-30066
21.**32**

was developed by Chinese workers as a therapeutic agent for the treatment of human and animal *S. japonicum* infections (for reviews, see Refs. 16 and 17). Although the drug was effective, the incidence of side effects was high. In addition, activity against intestinal schistosomiasis was at best marginal.

One of the newer, more interesting experimental compounds is *trans*-5-amino-3-[2-(5-nitro-2-furyl)vinyl]-1,2,4-oxadiazole (21.**33**, SQ 18506), which has been thoroughly investigated as a schistosomicide by Bueding and his colleagues (64–66).

The compound was consistently active at high dose levels against both *S. mansoni* and *S. japonicum* in mice and in monkeys, and also (surprisingly) possessed activity against immature *S. mansoni* in mice. Although not unexpectedly, the nonnitrated furan 21.**34** lacked activity (and indeed was toxic), the desamino compound 21.**35** was active against *S. mansoni* in mice, although it was much more toxic than SQ 18506.

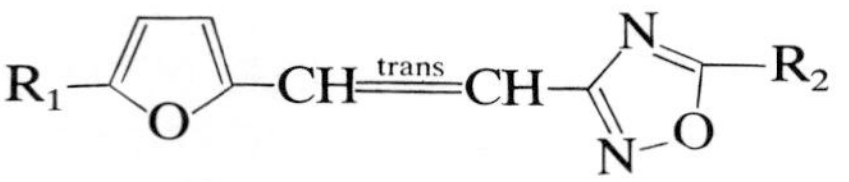

21.**33** $R_1 = NO_2$, $R_2 = NH_2$ (SQ 18506)
21.**34** $R_1 = H$, $R_2 = NH_2$
21.**35** $R_1 = NO_2$, $R_2 = H$

SQ 18506 was shown (65) to inhibit glycogen phosphorylase phosphatase in schistosomes in a similar manner to that of niridazole. However unlike niridazole, the drug had little effect on the isofunctional enzyme in the skeletal muscle of the host. It is interesting that comparison of space-filling models of niridazole and SQ 18506 (in the planar, fully *transoid* conformation, with maximum overlap of the π-electrons of the unsaturated side chain, maximum charge separation, and minimal nonbonded interactions) has indicated that there is a reasonable spatial similarity between the two molecules (64).

Initial tests indicated that unlike many nitrofurans, SQ 18506 appeared to possess minimal genetic activity. However the compound has since been shown to be mutagenic in yeast (67), and carcinogenic as well (38). Further work by Bueding and his colleagues has indicated that other selected nitrofurans do possess antischistosome activity, but that this is not a general property of this molecular species. One interesting finding, from a therapeutic point of view, was that in many cases the activity of nitroheterocyclic compounds, and nitrofurans in particular, could be increased by up to 40% by administration of the drug as a suspension in the emulsifying agent "Cremophor EL" (68).

In spite of the potent antischistosome activity shown by some nitrofurans, the unpleasant side effects associated with this general class make it unlikely that any drug suitable for use in mass chemotherapeutic programs will emerge from this chemical type.

c. Nitrothiophenes. Activity in the remaining nitroheterocyclic series is far less widespread than in the nitrothiazoles and nitrofurans, and this has been attributed to among other structural prerequisites, the absence of a nitrogen-containing substituent attached directly or by way of a rigid side chain to the 2-position of a heterocyclic ring (64, 69, 70). Nevertheless moderate antichistosome activity has recently been detected (71) in certain nitrothiophenes (21.**36**). The most active compound appeared to be 1-[(5-nitro-2-thienylidene)amino]tetrahydro-2(1*H*)pyrimidinone (21.**37**), but one interesting finding

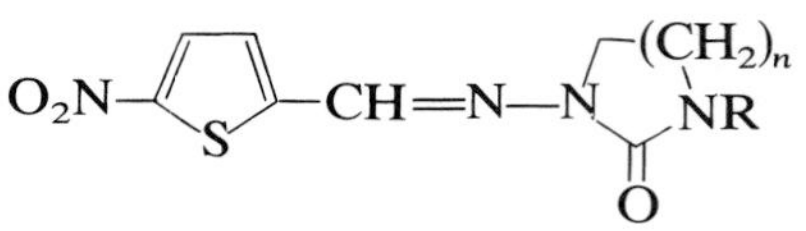

21.**36** R = H or alkyl, *n* = 1 or 2
21.**37** R = H, *n* = 2

to arise from this work was that in general the prepared nitrothiophenes were more potent as schistosomicides than the corresponding nitrofurans.

Reports from Hoffman-La Roche have indicated that 3-(3,5-dinitro-2-thienyl)thiazolidine (21.**38**), one of a series of schistosomicidal nitrothienylamines, is more active than niridazole both *in vitro* and in animals. In addition, somewhat surprisingly, the compound appeared to have little

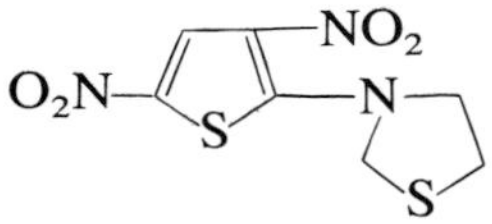

21.**38**

toxicity in the rat, dog, or cebus monkey (72).

d. Nitroimidazoles. No nitroimidazoles appear to have been reported to have significant antischistosome properties, although certain derivatives (21.**39**) affect egg laying in mice (73), and some niridazole analogs (e.g., 21.**40**) are claimed to possess schistosomicidal activity (74, 75).

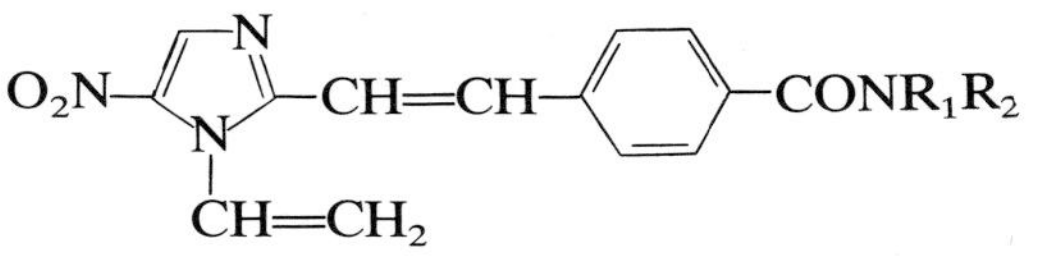

O_2N–(imidazole, N-vinyl)–CH=CH–C_6H_4–$CONR_1R_2$

21.**39**

O_2N–(imidazole, N–R_1)–N(imidazolidinone, C=O)–NR_2

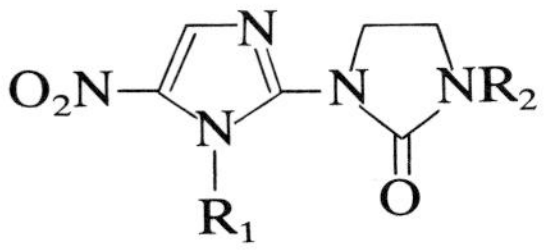

21.**40**

e. Nitrobenzene Derivatives. A novel schistosomicide described recently by Striebel (76) is 21.**41**: 4-isothiocyanato-4′-nitrodiphenylamine (amoscanate, C 9333-Go/CGP 4540). This compound appears to

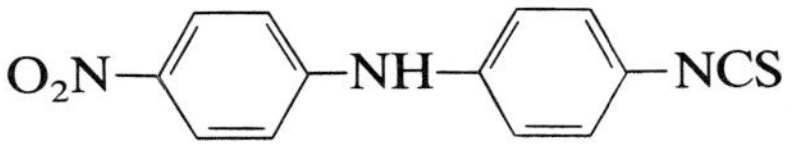

O_2N–C_6H_4–NH–C_6H_4–NCS

amoscanate

21.**41**

be well tolerated in acute toxicity studies in a variety of species, and it is almost equiactive by single oral dose against the three main species of schistosome. It is noteworthy that the antischistosome activity of this drug is greatly enhanced when the particle size has been reduced to about 0.5 μm by the somewhat impractical (from a commercial viewpoint) ball mill treatment of a suspension of the compound in 1% "Cremophor EL" and 25% glycerol for 14 days (77). The drug has been shown to be free from mutagenic activity in several bacterial systems, unlike niridazole (21.**16**), hycanthone (21.**8**), and the nitrofuran Furapromidium (21.**32**), although it appears that the intestinal bacteria of mice afforded a metabolite that was mutagenic to *Salmonella* strain TA-100 (77). The drug also appears to be active against both intestinal and tissue nematodes, in particular the hookworms *Necator americanus* and *Ancylostoma duodenale* (see Section 6.2.2.6).

4.1.4.4 Organophosphorus Compounds. Although various classical cholinesterase inhibitors are known (78) to be inactive as schistosomicides, the organophosphorus anticholinesterase insecticide *O,O*-dimethyl-1-hydroxy-2,2,2-trichloroethylphosphonate (21.**42,** metrifonate, trichlorfon,

$$CCl_3.CH(OH)P(O)(OMe)_2$$

metrifonate

21.**42**

Dipterex) is an interesting addition to the small selection of clinically useful schistosomicides. Metrifonate has been found to be highly effective in the treatment of *S. haematobium* infections at oral dose levels of 7.5 mg/kg repeated at 14 day intervals (to a total of 3 doses). At this level tolerance is good, and the only side effect is the expected depression of plasma cholinesterase values. (Regardless of dose, plasma cholinesterase is almost completely inhibited a few hours after dosing; erythrocyte cholinesterase is almost completely inhibited a few hours after dosing; erythrocyte has indicated that the drug is not teratogenic or carcinogenic in long-term experiments in healthy rats and dogs (20), although it does possess fairly high host-mediated mutagenic activity in *Salmonella typhimurium* strain TA-100 (79).

Unexpectedly, the drug has no effect on *S. mansoni* either in humans or in experimental animals: to date the reasons for this specificity of action are unclear, although

Bueding and his co-workers have established (80) that the difference in chemotherapeutic activity of metrifonate against the two schistosome species in humans could not be accounted for by differences in the inhibitory potency of the drug on the enzymes catalyzing the hydrolysis of acetylcholine. In another connection, it is interesting to note that the compound is active against human hookworms.

On the basis of efficacy, tolerance, ease of administration and, particularly important, cost, metrifonate has been considered to be superior to both niridazole and hycanthone in the treatment of mature *S. haematobium* infections (81). By similar criteria, the drug also fulfils the requirements for a prophylactic against *S. haematobium* (82).

In summary, the potential usefulness of metrifonate must be limited by its narrow spectrum of activity. In addition, the drug should perhaps be distributed with caution in areas where the general population has been exposed to organophosphorus pesticides.

4.1.4.5 Tetrahydroquinolines. a. Oxamniquine. As part of the development of the structure-activity relationships existing in the Miracil D series, a variety of fused ring analogs of Mirasan (21.**7**) were prepared by workers at the Bayer laboratories (83). Although these compounds (e.g., 21.**43**) were effective in mice and, to some

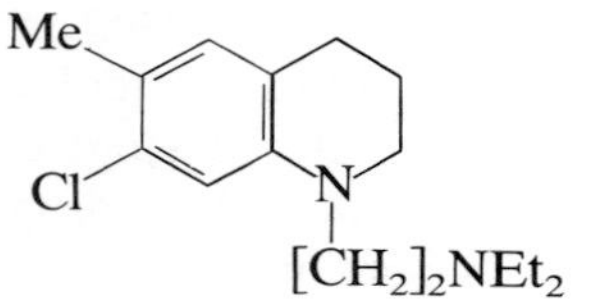

Me
Cl
N
$[CH_2]_2NEt_2$

21.**43**

extent, in monkeys, they lacked convincing activity in humans. In contrast to these Mirasan congeners, a novel series of tetrahydroquinolines (21.**44**) involving an alternative conformationally constrained ring system was developed at Pfizer.

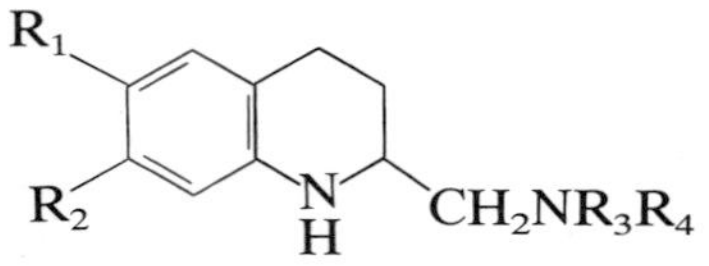

R_1
R_2
N
H
$CH_2NR_3R_4$

21.**44** $R_1 = Me$, $R_2 = NO_2$, halo, CN
21.**45** $R_1 = Me$, $R_2 = NO_2$, $R_3 = H$, $R_4 = i\text{-Pr}$ (UK 3883)
21.**46** $R_1 = CH_2OH$, $R_2 = NO_2$, $R_3 = H$, $R_4 =$ *i*-Pr (oxamniquine, UK 4271)

At a relatively early stage it was established for the 6-methyl series (21.**44**) that greatest activity was obtained when R_2 was NO_2, and that the potency fell off in the order $NO_2 > CN >$ halogen (the reverse of that which applies in the Mirasan series). The most active derivative to emerge initially (84, 85) was 2-[(isopropylamino)-methyl]-6-methyl-7-nitro-1,2,3,4-tetrahydroquinoline (21.**45**, UK 3883).

Further work indicated (86) that *in vivo* UK 3883 was metabolized, as expected, to the corresponding hydroxymethyl analog UK 4271 (21.**46**), which itself was an extremely potent schistosomicide in both rodents (87) and primates (88) infected with *S. mansoni.* The latter drug (which is synthesized microbiologically from UK 3883 using *Aspergillus sclerotiorum*) was subsequently introduced to clinical medicine as oxamniquine (Mansil). It is interesting to note that unlike the Mirasans, which are not particularly active in primates, the parent unmetabolized 6-methyl congener UK 3883 had good efficacy in monkeys, indicating that the stereochemical orientation of the molecule allowed a ready hydroxylation (to the active entity oxamniquine) by these animals.

Originally introduced as a parenteral drug, oxamniquine was found to produce severe pain at the site of the injection, and has been reformulated for oral administration.

In clinical use the drug demonstrated effectiveness in the treatment of *S. mansoni* infections, although it has little activity against *S. haematobium* and is of no value for the treatment of *S. japonicum.* In South

America, at the recommended single oral dose of 12–12.5 mg/kg (for patients over 40 kg) or 15 mg/kg (for those less than 40 kg), the drug is well tolerated, although some dizziness, nausea, and vomiting occur transiently, as does an increase in serum transaminase levels (89). In trials in Rhodesia, however, it has been shown that the drug must be administered at a total dose of 60 mg/kg (given in 4 equal doses over 2 days) to achieve satisfactory cure rates (90). It is not known at present if this disparity in dose levels merely represents differing strain sensitivities to the drug or whether some other factor is involved.

Although oxamniquine is obviously a promising new drug for the treatment of schistosomiasis mansoni, the fact that it is active against only one schistosome species must limit its potential usefulness. In addition, since a fermentation stage is needed in its manufacture, the finished drug is likely to be expensive.

Finally, the drug has been shown to possess fairly high host-mediated mutagenic properties in *Salmonella typhimurium* strain TA-100 (79), but it is far from clear how this finding, or indeed the discovery that hycanthone-resistant worms are cross-resistant to oxamniquine (34), should be applied to the human clinical situation.

b. Hexahydropyrazinoquinolines. In an extension of the oxamniquine work, Richards and his colleagues prepared a variety of 8-methylpyrazinoquinolines, some of which were more active than oxamniquine. A detailed examination of the structure-activity relationships existing in this series of compounds disclosed (91) that the 9-chloro analogs (21.**47**, $R_2 = Cl$, $R_3 = H$) were more active than the corresponding 9-nitro compounds, in direct contrast to the results obtained for the tetrahydroquinolines (21.**44**). In turn, the 9-chloro-10-methyl derivatives (21.**47**, $R_2 = Cl$, $R_3 = Me$) were even more active than the desmethyl compounds, and this was considered to be due to the favorable influence on the stereochemistry of the fused piperazine ring of the 10-methyl group (partial structures 21.**48** and the twist configuration 21.**49** for the 9-chloro and 9-chloro-10-methyl derivatives, respectively) (91).

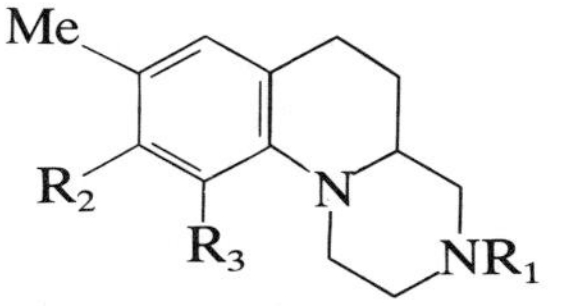

21.**47** $R_1R_3 = H$, alkyl, $R_2 = Cl$, NO_2

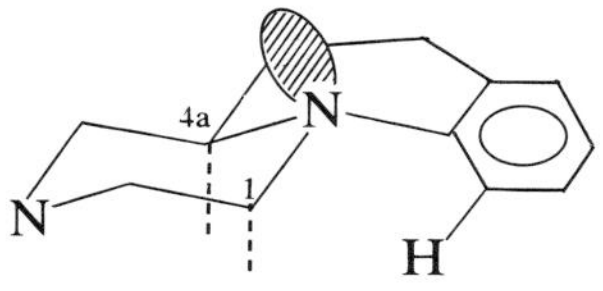

21.**48**

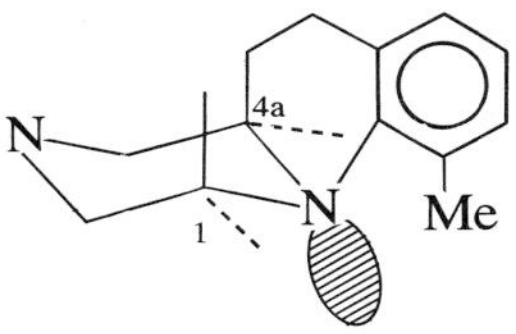

21.**49**

Microbiological hydroxylation of selected pyrazinoquinolines with *Aspergillus sclerotiorum* afforded the corresponding 8-hydroxymethyl analogs. In particular 9-chloro-8-hydroxymethyl-10-methyl-2,3,4,4*a*,5,6-hexahydro-1*H*-pyrazino[1,2-*a*]-quinoline (21.**50**) was twice as potent as oxamniquine in both mice and monkeys (91).

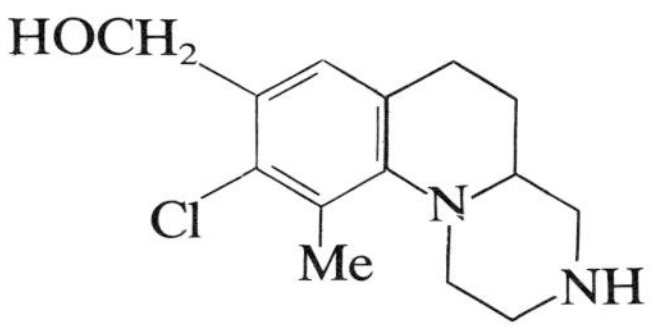

21.**50**

Interestingly, selected members of the tetrahydroquinolines and hexahydropyrazinoquinolines are effective against early developing forms of *S. mansoni*, and indeed possess prophylactic activity against this species (92, 93).

4.1.4.6 Miscellaneous Schistosomicides. In recent years several separate chemical entities have been shown to possess schistosomicidal properties, but so far, for a variety of reasons (efficacy, toxicity, etc.), none has proved to be suitable for use in humans.

The known dependence of schistosomes for preformed purines has been exploited by the use of tubercidin (7-deazaadenosine; 21.**51**) as a schistosomicidal agent. Although the drug is toxic to mice, it is less so

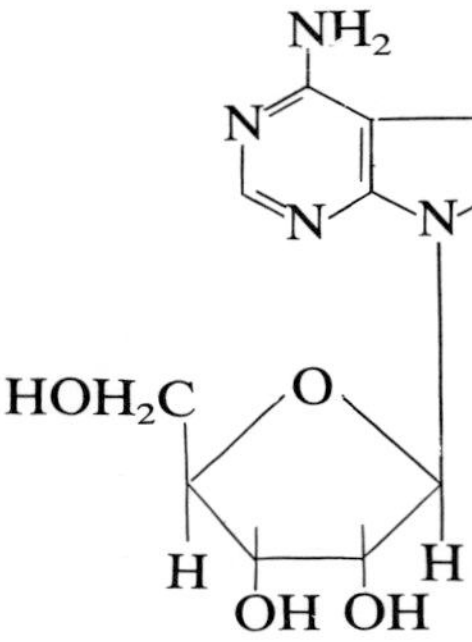

tubercidin
21.**51**

when it has been sequestered into red blood cells and reinjected into the donor animals. The procedure has been used to demonstrate efficacy against both *S. mansoni* and *S. japonicum* in primates, with the female worms being preferentially killed (94, 95). Administered intravenously to baboons, the compound was effective but produced reversible mild to moderate kidney damage at therapeutic dose levels (96). Although this compound is clearly of considerable theoretical interest, it is to be doubted whether any drug of practical use will emerge from these findings.

As part of a systematic investigation into the synthesis of potential schistosomicidal agents, Elslager and his colleagues prepared a large number of interrelated naphthalenediamine derivatives (reviewed in Refs. 12 and 17). One of the most interesting compounds to emerge was 5-[4-[[2-

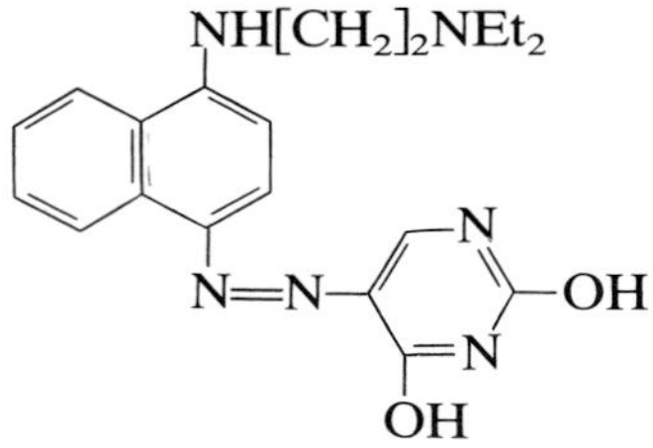

21.**52**

(diethylamino)ethyl]amino]-1-naphthylazo]-uracil (21.**52**). Although this drug had moderate activity against *S. mansoni* and *S. haematobium* in clinical trials, it also produced a high incidence of gastrointestinal side effects (97).

For many years investigations proceeded independently at May and Baker and at the Wellcome Research Laboratories into the synthesis of *p*-aminophenoxyalkane derivatives. Although many of these compounds showed potent schistosomicidal properties in the primary rodent screens, this activity was, in general, much reduced in primates. In addition, many of these compounds exhibited retinotoxic properties. Thus one of the more interesting congeners, amphotalide (21.**53**, Schistomide), had significant therapeutic effect against clinical *S.*

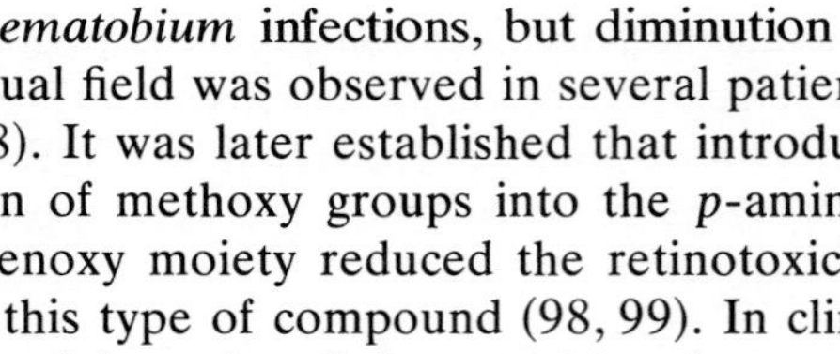

amphotalide
21.**53**

haematobium infections, but diminution of visual field was observed in several patients (98). It was later established that introduction of methoxy groups into the *p*-aminophenoxy moiety reduced the retinotoxicity of this type of compound (98, 99). In clinical trials against *S. haematobium* in a small number of children, one of these methoxy-substituted congeners (21.**54**, M & B 3838A) produced no diminution of visual field but did cause severe vomiting (99).

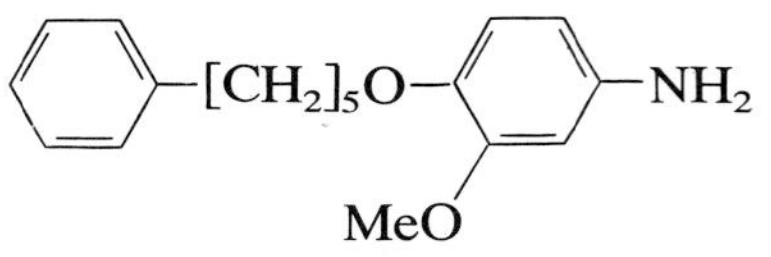

M & B 3838A

21.**54**

Further work leading to the introduction of a phenoxyalkane-type fasciolicide (diamphenethide), in which activity was finally dissociated from retinotoxicity at therapeutic levels, is discussed in Section 4.2.2.4.

Although the antischistosome activity of tris(*p*-aminophenyl)carbonium (TAC) salts has been known for some years (for reviews, see Refs. 17 and 18), the compound is of sufficient interest to warrant mention here. In particular, the pamoate salt 21.**55**

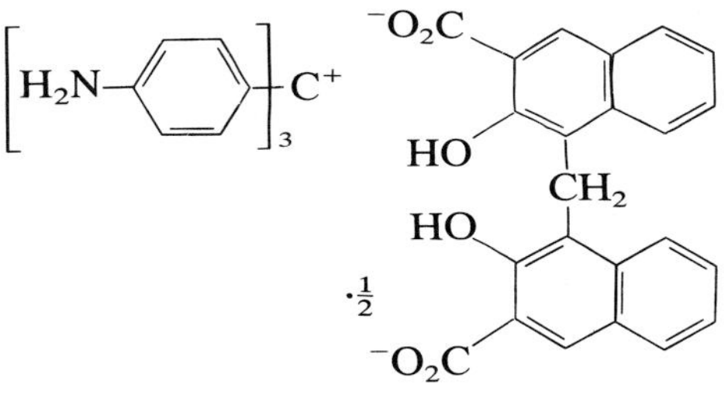

21.**55**

(developed to overcome the emesis and gastritis noted in dogs with the more soluble chloride) was a potent albeit slow-acting schistosomicide active in man against the refractory *S. japonicum*. The drug was shown to inhibit acetylcholinesterase in the nervous system of the worms, giving rise to a paralysis of the adhesive organs that was reversed immediately on *in vitro* exposure of the worms to cholinergic blocking agents (100). In extended administration of TAC pamoate to rats, an increased incidence of skin tumors in female animals was noted, although this effect does not appear in other laboratory species or in man. These toxicity findings, together with the need for prolonged administration of the drug (orally once a week for 16–24 weeks), have prevented its acceptance into clinical medicine.

Finally, a very recent report emanating jointly from the Bayer and E. Merck laboratories has indicated that the veterinary taenicide praziquantel (21.**56**, Droncit, Embay 8440) is also a very potent

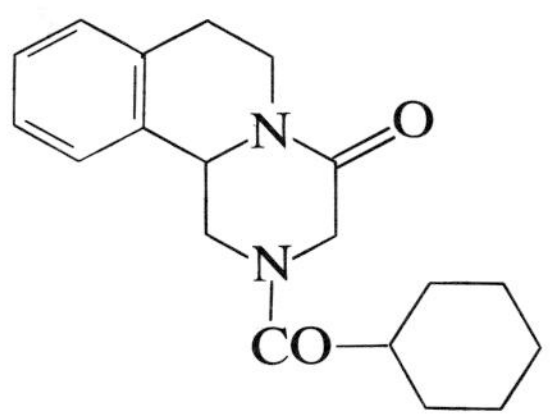

praziquantel

21.**56**

schistosomicide. In preliminary clinical trials the drug appears to be effective against all three human schistosome species at single doses of 20 mg/kg (101). At this early stage the compound looks very promising, although information on cost factors and side effects (if any) has yet to be revealed.

4.1.4.7 Egg Suppressants and Chemosterilants. It is considered that the presence of schistosomes *per se* causes no tissue damage; rather, the passage of eggs through the tissues is thought to be responsible for the pathology of the disease. Since it is also known that infection with living schistosomes tends to prevent reinfection, a variety of compounds have been examined as egg suppressants. This interesting approach to the problem perhaps deserves further investigation. For example, nicarbazin (21.**57**) (an equimolecular complex of 4,4′-dinitrocarbanilide and 2-hydroxy-4,6-dimethylpyrimidine) and allylthiourea (thiosinamine) both suppress egg production: in each case, however, a resumption of oviposition occurs when the drug is withdrawn.

Finally, treatment of *S. mansoni*-infected mice with various conventional chemosterilants (ethylene-1,2-dimethanesulfonate,

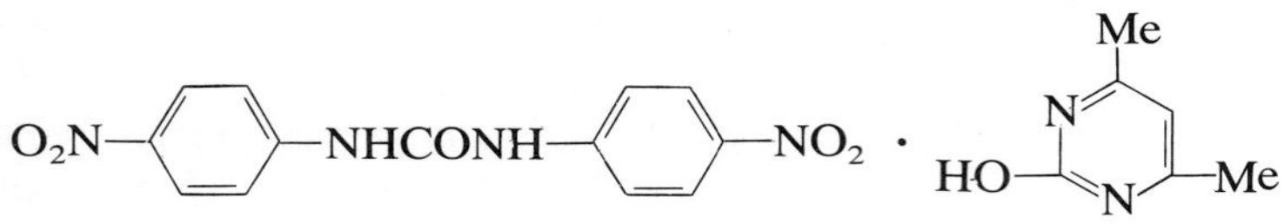

nicarbazin

21.**57**

hexamethylphosphoramide, etc.) has been shown to induce a temporary inhibition of schistosome oviposition.

4.1.4.8 Summary. In spite of the considerable effort that has been expended (mainly by the pharmaceutical industry) in schistosomiasis chemotherapy, no broad spectrum, effective, safe, inexpensive schistosomicide has emerged that is suitable for use in mass eradication schemes. Although the incidence of the disease is certainly on the increase, it appears that pharmaceutical companies, not unnaturally, are tending to concentrate resources on disease areas where return on capital is more certain, and where any novel product developed would receive adequate patent protection.

Finally, it must be emphasized that too little is known of the biochemistry of the schistosome; further advances must be made in this area before systematic investigations into the chemotherapy of the disease can begin.

4.2 Fascioliasis, Clonorchiasis, Dicrocoeliasis, and Opisthorchiasis

Liver fluke infections in humans are caused by *Opisthorchis felineus* (cat liver fluke), and *Clonorchis* (*Opisthorchis*) *sinensis* (Chinese liver fluke), while *Fasciola hepatica* (sheep liver fluke) and *Dicrocoelium dendriticum* (lancet fluke) occur mainly in animals, causing considerable economic losses on a worldwide basis. Thus in 1972 in the United Kingdom the overall loss in cattle and sheep due to fascioliasis was conservatively estimated to be some £50 million (*ca.* $100 million) per annum (102).

Significant research in the chemotherapy of trematode infections has been confined to two genera—*Fasciola* and *Schistosoma*—and the general lack of nontoxic, active compounds merely reflects the biochemical similarity between the host and the parasite.

In considering the chemotherapy of fasciolicides, it must be borne in mind that in the past most of the flukicides developed had a therapeutic index that would not be tolerated in compounds intended for use in man (provided of course that mortality rates or reduced growth rates produced by treatment were minimal compared with losses due to the untreated disease).

4.2.1 LIFE CYCLES. *Fasciola hepatica,* a parasite of sheep and cattle that also occasionally infects man, is transmitted by ingestion of encysted metacercariae on wet grass or (particularly in humans) on watercress. The larvae excyst in the duodenum, migrate through the intestinal wall, and reach the bile ducts after 9–10 weeks by eating their way through the hepatic parenchyma. Eggs (in the feces) that are deposited in fresh water hatch, and the resulting miracidia penetrate an amphibious snail, usually a species of *Lymnaea.* Several developmental stages occur within the snail, followed by emergence of the cercariae, which then encyst, completing the cycle.

Dicrocoelium dendriticum is one of the few trematodes that utilizes a terrestrial snail as intermediate host; ants are the secondary hosts, and it is the consumption of ants infected with metacercariae of *D. dendriticum* that produces infection in sheep.

The life cycles of *Clonorchis sinensis*, *Opisthorchis felineus*, and *O. viverrini*, liver flukes that occur in man in the Far East, are essentially similar; all involve snails as the primary hosts and freshwater fish for the secondary hosts. Man acquires these infections by consuming raw and under-cooked infected fish.

4.2.2 CHEMOTHERAPY. The chemotherapy of liver fluke infections has been reviewed in recent years (12, 103, 104).

4.2.2.1 Halogenated Hydrocarbons. The drug used for many years on a massive scale for the treatment of fascioliasis in sheep is carbon tetrachloride. This compound, apart from diamphenethide (21.**74**), is the only fasciolicide that appears not to be an uncoupler of oxidative phosphorylation. Instead, it is believed to act by blocking cholesterol biosynthesis in the host (105), a finding that correlates with the postulate that *F. hepatica* is probably fully dependent on the host for supplies of cholesterol (106). It has also been suggested that spasmogenic activity induced by carbon tetrachloride and its metabolite chloroform may also contribute to the flukicidal activity of the drug (107).

The other halogenated aliphatic hydrocarbon in general use (in fact, the only fasciolicide available in the United States) is hexachloroethane. Although this drug is not spasmogenic *per se*, its main metabolites pentachloroethane and tetrachloroethylene have potent activity in the *in vitro F. hepatica* preparation (107): in this, pentachloroethane is approximately twice as potent as carbon tetrachloride.

In general, aliphatic halogenated hydrocarbons are only active against *F. hepatica*. In contrast, halogenated aromatic hydrocarbons are broad spectrum antitrematode agents. Thus 1,4-bis(trichloromethyl)benzene (21.**58**, Hetol, chloxyle) is effective against *F. hepatica*, *D. dendriticum*, *O. felineus*, and *C. sinensis*, and also *Fasciolopsis buski* and *Paragonimus* species.

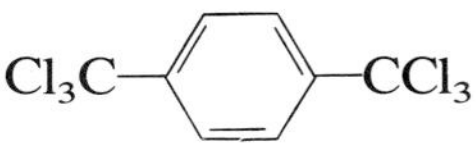

$Cl_3C-C_6H_4-CCl_3$

Hetol

21.**58**

In common with most fasciolicides, Hetol has been shown to be an uncoupler of oxidative phosphorylation, at least in rat mitochondria (108). The drug has been used for the treatment of human *C. sinensis* or *Opisthorchis* species infections and is well tolerated; however it has been withdrawn from use because of the hypochromic anemia that is produced in dogs, and consequently there is no good therapeutic agent available for the treatment of these infections (89).

4.2.2.2 Halogenated Phenols and Bisphenols. 4-Cyano-2-iodo-6-nitrophenol (21.**59**, nitroxynil, Trodax), which was developed from the moderately active adult flukicide disophenol (21.**60**) by workers at May and Baker (109, 110; reviewed in Ref. 12), is one of the most widely used flukicides. It has the advantage (in agricultural terms) of being administered parenterally, and it is active against flukes more than 6 weeks old. However the drug has

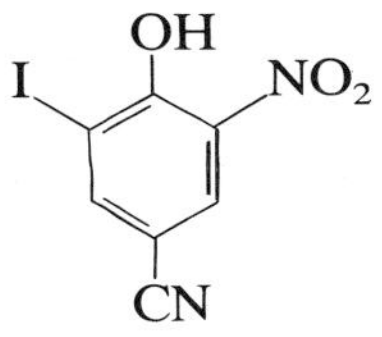

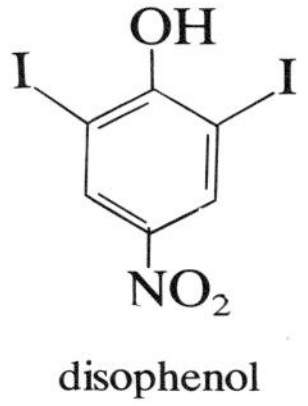

OH, I, NO_2, CN

nitroxynil

21.**59**

OH, I, I, NO_2

disophenol

21.**60**

the drawback of staining badly, and it persists too long to allow it to be used in milking cattle.

A group of fasciolicides that is employed to a greater or lesser degree in veterinary medicine includes bisphenolic compounds that may contain various halogen and/or nitro substituents and may have the aromatic rings linked through a methylene group or sulfur atom, etc. In this category must be included bithionol (21.**61**) and its sulfoxide Bitin-S (21.**62**), hexachlorophene (21.**63**),

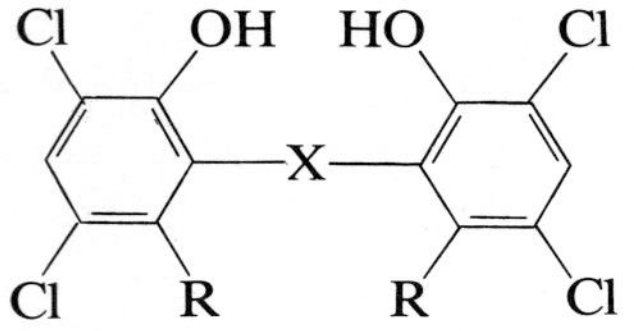

21.**61** R = H, X = S (bithionol)
21.**62** R = H, X = SO (Bitin-S)
21.**63** R = Cl, X = CH_2 (hexachlorophene)

the most active of the cheaper drugs, and bromofenfos (21.**64**, Ph 1882, Acedist), whose popularity is almost exclusively limited to the Netherlands. Hexachlorophene is inexpensive and works well on flukes more than 7–8 weeks old, but it has a relatively poor therapeutic index.

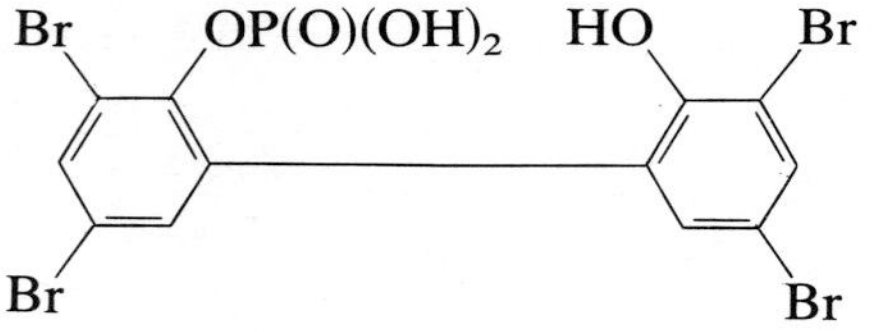

bromofenfos

21.**64**

A fivefold increase in activity over the classical flukicides hexachlorophene and bithionol was achieved (111) by workers from Bayer in their bisphenol derivative menichlopholan (21.**65**, Bayer 9015, niclofolan, Bilevon-M). For the treatment of cattle, a special formulation was developed (Bilevon-R) that prevented metabolism of the drug in the rumen. This drug is not

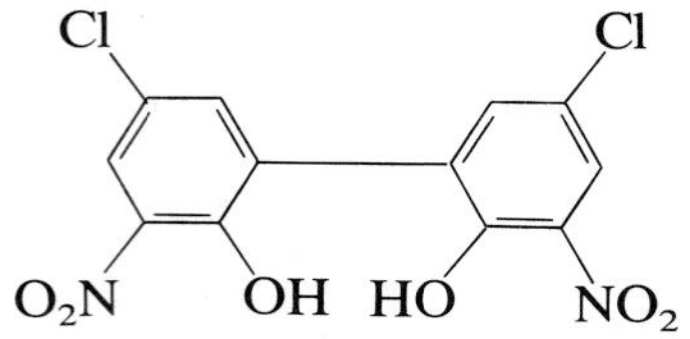

menichlopholan

21.**65**

particularly active against immature flukes and is not regarded as being outstandingly safe, even though therapeutic dose levels are low.

Bithionol is of interest in that it is probably the drug of choice for human *F. hepatica* infections (112).

4.2.2.3 Halogenated Salicylanilides. Halogenated salicylanilides represent another group of active flukicides, although it is not clear whether these are merely extensions to the bisphenol compounds (e.g., 21.**61**–21.**63**) in which the bridging link is —CONH— rather than —CH_2— or —S—, etc. In this group the more active and useful compounds are oxyclozanide (21.**66**, Zanil) (113), clioxanide (21.**67**, Tremerad, SYD-230) (114), rafoxanide

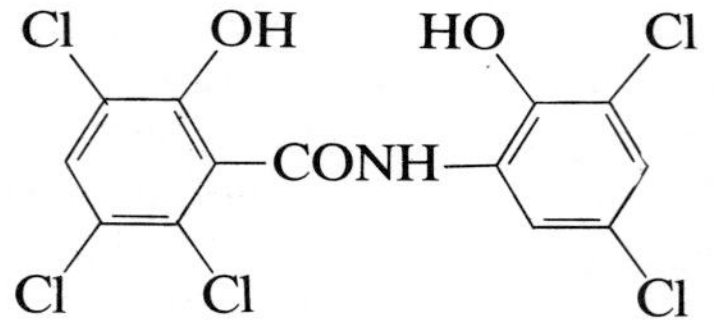

oxyclozanide

21.**66**

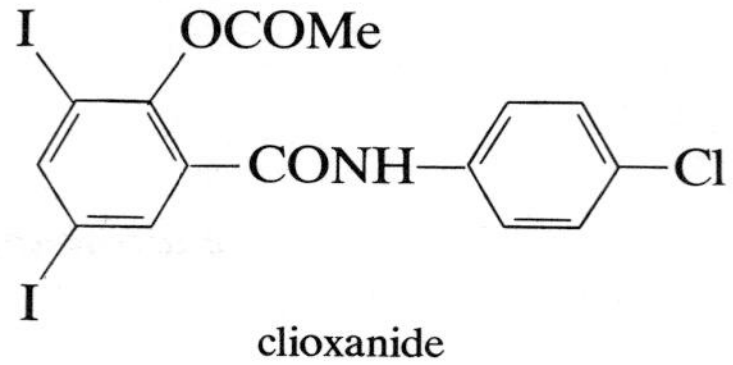

clioxanide

21.**67**

(21.**68**, Ranide, Flukanide) (115), and the new thiosalicylanilide brotianide (21.**70**, Bayer 4059, Dirian) (116). These compounds are all uncouplers of oxidative

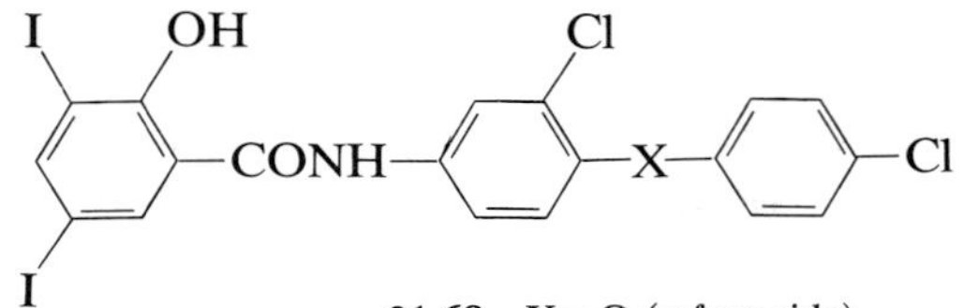

21.**68** X = O (rafoxanide)
21.**69** X = CO (salantel)

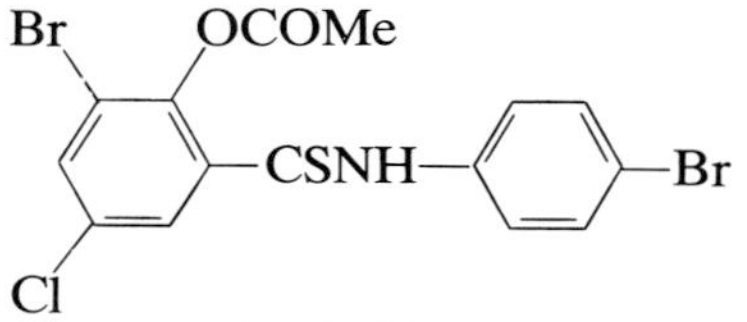

brotianide

21.**70**

phosphorylation, and, with the exception of rafoxanide, are active against adult flukes only (i.e., flukes older than 9–10 weeks situated in the bile ducts). Although rafoxanide cannot be used in dairy cattle, it does have the advantage of possessing a rather broader spectrum of activity than other fasciolicides in this group; in addition to activity against *F. hepatica*, it is effective against the nematode *Haemonchus contortus* and the sheep nostril fly *Oestrus ovis*. An interesting new experimental analog of rafoxanide is salantel (21.**69**). In this compound, prepared by the Janssen Group (117), the *p*-chlorophenoxy moiety of rafoxanide (21.**68**) is replaced by *p*-chlorobenzoyl: the relationship that exists between the two compounds thus bears some resemblance to that between fenbendazole (21.**110**) and mebendazole (21.**108**). In these two antinematode drugs, however, the benzoyl moiety of mebendazole (on the 5-position of the benzimidazole ring) is replaced in fenbendazole by phenylthio rather than substituted phenoxy.

Detailed structure-activity studies (113) on oxyclozanide have been reviewed (12). In essence, these suggested that the antifluke activity of the drug was a function of the ability of the compound (and also of the distantly related hexachlorophene) to form oxidation-reduction systems. Unpublished work (118) has also indicated that the primary mode of action of oxyclozanide could be a direct or indirect action on the nervous system of the flukes, possibly by interference with nerve energy metabolism.

An interesting new salicylanilide that is effective at low dosage against both *F. hepatica* at least 6 weeks old, and the nematode *Haemonchus contortus*, is bromoxanide (21.**71**) (119). Workers from Hoechst

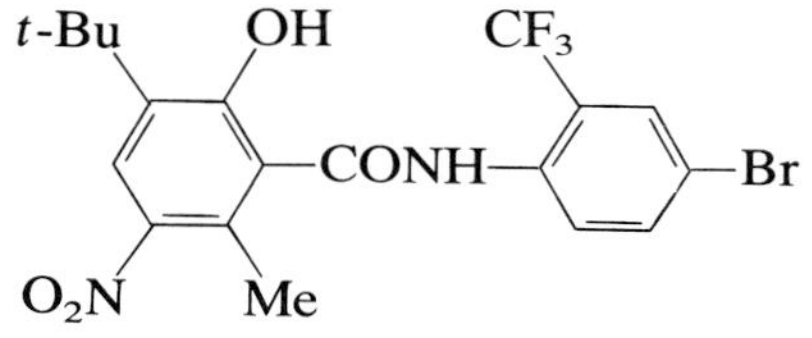

bromoxanide

21.**71**

have published detailed structure–activity relationships for a wide range of 2,6-dihydroxybenzanilides (21.**72**, γ-resorcylanilides) (120–122). In these studies activities against the fluke enzyme succinate dehydrogenase were determined, and with the aid of Hansch analysis, quantitative structure-activity relationships were established between the anilides and their activities (121). It was found that potent, selective inhibitors were obtained only when R_1 was very lipophilic and R_2 was hydrophilic or only very slightly lipophilic. This work was extended (123) to one of the most potent analogs, 2,6-dihydroxy-3,4′,5-trichlorobenzanilide (21.**73**), which was compared with various commercially available salicylanilides. The uncoupling activity

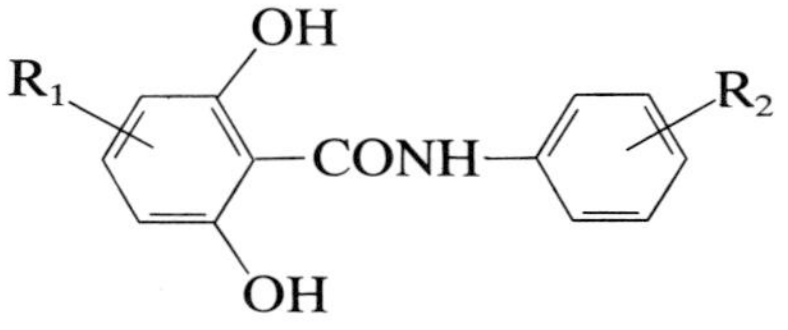

21.**72** R_1 = acyl, halogen, NO_2, etc.
R_2 = halogen, OH, etc.
21.**73** R_1 = 3,5-Cl_2; R_2 = 4-Cl

of other oxidative phosphorylation uncouplers (2-trifluoromethylbenzimidazoles and phenols, as well as salicylanilides) has also been correlated by means of Hansch free energy relationships (124).

None of the salicylanilides or halogenated phenols mentioned so far has much effect on *F. hepatica* in their 10-week development phase, although rafoxanide made some progress in overcoming this defect. In addition, it has not been possible to date to prepare fasciolicides of this type in which the biological effect is specific for the parasite alone.

4.2.2.4 Phenoxyalkanes. Diamphenethide (21.**74**, Coriban), a novel fasciolicide, is the result of a systematic search in the Wellcome Research Laboratories for a fasciolicide effective against immature flukes, using as the biological test system immature *F. gigantica* in mice. (Acute fascioliasis, caused by migration of immature *F. hepatica* in the liver of sheep, is responsible for high mortality and great economic loss.) The events leading up to the introduction of diamphenethide to veterinary medicine and the structure-activity relationships existing in this series of compounds have been reviewed by Harfenist (125).

It was soon established (126, 127) that the compound was unique in sheep in that it was more active against all stages of *F. hepatica* up to 6 weeks of age than it was against mature flukes. In addition, although all phenoxyalkanes examined as schistosomicides had considerable retinotoxic potential (see Section 4.1.4.6), with diamphenethide at therapeutic dose levels, activity appeared to have been dissociated from retinotoxicity.

Although the deacetylated compound 21.**75** is effective against *F. hepatica* in the rat, diamphenethide lacks activity in this species. It has been postulated that this lack of activity is due to the failure of the rat to deacetylate the parent drug (125), although this hypothesis does not explain why diamphenethide is less effective in the cow, and inactive in the rabbit. Since these species are able to metabolize the drug to 21.**75**, it has been suggested that high rates of breakdown and excretion of the active moiety may occur, or rates of deacetylation and acetylation may be such that little free amine is ever present (128).

In any event, diamphenethide does present a unique lead in the search for fully effective fasciolicides.

4.2.2.5 Miscellaneous Flukicides. Lämmler (129) has reviewed the development of 1-methyl-4-[3,3,3-tris(*p*-chlorophenyl)propionyl]piperazine hydrochloride (21.**76**, Hetolin) as a flukicide for the control of *Dicrocoelium dendriticum*. Interestingly, this compound appears to be much less effective against other liver flukes.

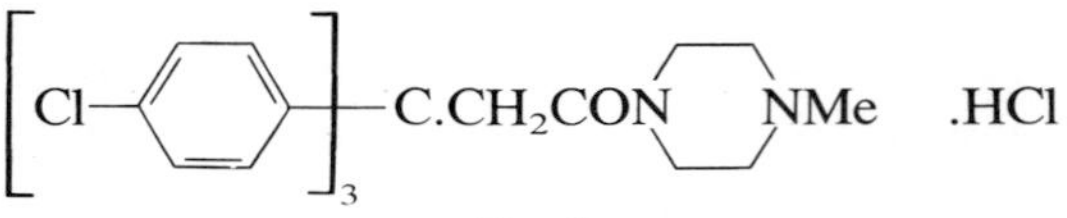

$$[Cl-C_6H_4]_3-C.CH_2CON\langle\rangle NMe \quad .HCl$$

Hetolin

21.**76**

Thiabendazole (21.**102**) has little flukicidal activity, but certain of the newer benzimidazole nematocides [e.g., albendazole, 21.**112** (130)] do possess activity against mature *F. hepatica*, although this is generally at higher dose levels than those used for the treatment of roundworm infections (see Section 6.2.2.1).

Finally, although few compounds are known to be effective against *Clonorchis sinensis* and *Opisthorchis* species, the

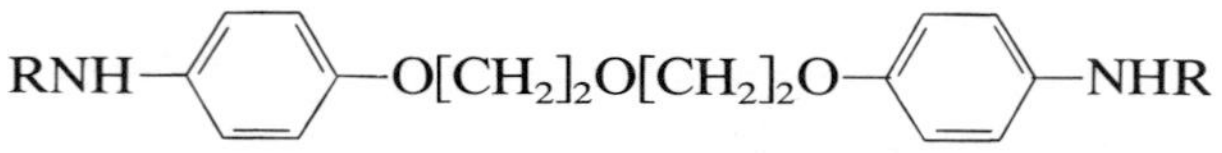

$$RNH-C_6H_4-O[CH_2]_2O[CH_2]_2O-C_6H_4-NHR$$

21.**74** R = MeCO (diamphenethide)
21.**75** R = H

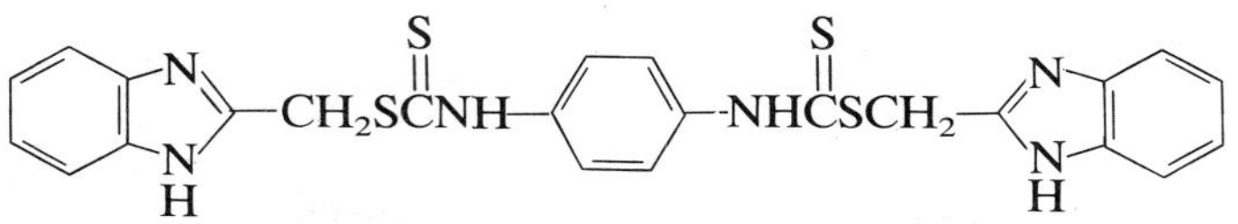

21.**77**

dithiocarbamate 21.**77** (131) and the cyclic congener 21.**78** (132) are members of series that do possess pronounced activity against these species in experimental animals.

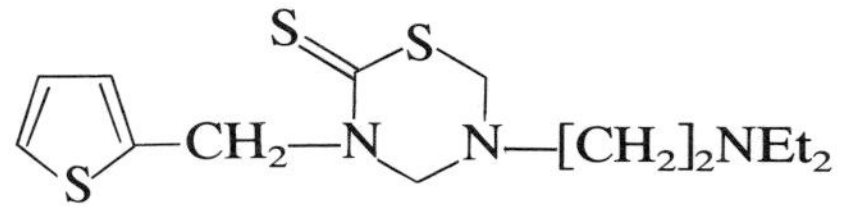

21.**78**

4.3 Paragonimiasis and Other Trematode Infections

Few anthelmintic agents are active against *Paragonimus westermani* (lung fluke disease) (133), although bithionol (21.**61**) is well established as the drug of choice for this infection (89); it is well tolerated, and side effects are mild.

Finally, tetrachloroethylene is the drug mainly used for treating the intestinal fluke *Fasciolopsis buski* (89), although bithionol may well prove to be more effective.

5 CESTODE DISEASES AND DRUGS ACTIVE AGAINST THEM

Although some 150 million persons in the world are estimated (2) to be infected with cestodes (tapeworms), the medical and economic significance of these parasites is considerably less than that of the nematodes or trematodes. In consequence, this class of helminth has received little attention in the past; in recent years, however, it has been recognized that larval cestode infections have a significant role to play in many areas of the world, including the developing countries. In man, larval infections often present a grave prognosis, particularly infection with the larval stages of *Echinococcus granulosus*, which may occur whenever man and dog live in close proximity.

5.1 Adult Cestode Infections

5.1.1 CHEMOTHERAPY OF TAPEWORM INFECTIONS. Certain traditional remedies have been employed for many years in the treatment of human and animal tapeworm infections, including extract of male fern (*Aspidium oleoresin*), arecoline, arsenic compounds, mepacrine, and a plethora of tin and lead organometallic derivatives. However all these have poor therapeutic indices, or variable activities or toxicities. Consequently, with the advent of modern, safe, effective taenicides, there is no place for these older drugs in modern therapy, and they are not considered here.

The chemotherapy of tapeworm infections has been reviewed in recent years, and the reader is referred to these works for details of experimental compounds (7, 12), and for detailed clinical observations (13, 89, 134).

5.1.1.1 Halogenated Bisphenols. Both bithionol (21.**61**) and dichlorophen (21.**79**) come into this chemical class. Dichlorophen was introduced into human medicine in 1956 after many years' use as a veterinary

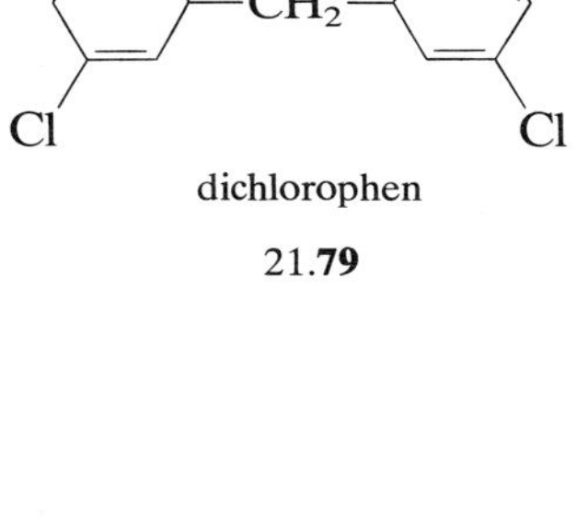

dichlorophen

21.**79**

taenicide. The drug is effective in the treatment of *Taenia* species and fish tapeworms: cure rates are high, and side effects are relatively mild. After treatment with dichlorophen, the worm usually disintegrates; concomitant induced peristalsis aids in removal of the worm fragments.

Although a variety of halogenated bisphenolic compounds are potentially useful as taenicides (for review, see Ref. 12), in general this class of compound has been replaced, in human infections, by niclosamide (21.**80**).

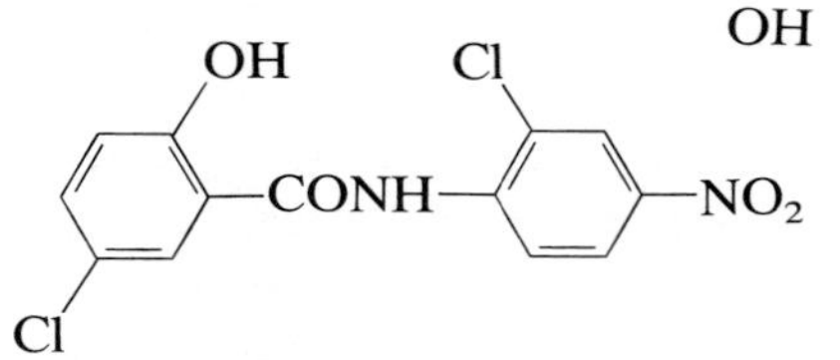

niclosamide

21.**80**

Bithionol does possess activity against most of the important cestode species found in man. Although the drug has been used in the treatment of these parasites in Japan, in particular, it has been replaced by newer, safer taenicides.

5.1.1.2 Halogenated Salicylanilides. Introduced into human medicine some years ago, 2′,5-dichloro-4′-nitrosalicylanilide (21.**80**, niclosamide, Yomesan, Mansonil) is recognized by most authorities to be the drug of choice for the treatment of all species of tapeworms (89, 112). In animals, too, at present the drug appears to be the most favored remedy for cestode infections.

Interestingly, niclosamide is also a potent molluscicide (as the ethanolamine salt, Bayluscid). In this connection the drug is particularly effective against *Biomphalaria glabrata*, one of the snail intermediate hosts in the transmission of schistosomiasis.

Although structure-activity studies on niclosamide analogs (135) had established that the hydroxy group in the benzoic acid moiety had to be in the 2-position, workers at Hoechst extended their investigations into the synthesis of potential anthelmintic agents to include 2,6-dihydroxybenzanilides (e.g., 21.**72**) (122), some of which have already been discussed in relation to their fasciolicidal properties. Optimum anticestode activity was observed for 4′-bromo-2,6-dihydroxybenzanilide (21.**81**), and this

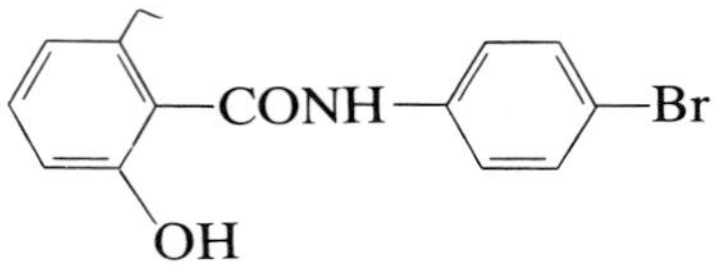

resorantel

21.**81**

drug entered into veterinary medicine (136, 137) as resorantel (Terenol). The drug is also of interest in that unlike niclosamide, it is active against *Paramphistomum* species (138), flukes that predominantly infest cattle in warmer climates.

It is interesting to note that the halogenated bisphenols and salicylanilides are active against both cestodes and certain species of trematodes, although the spectrum of activity does not normally extend to include schistosomes, the major human flukes.

5.1.1.3 Naphthamidines. The development of bunamidine (21.**82**, Scolaban) as a veterinary taenicide for use in dogs, sheep, and poultry was the culmination of an extensive investigation into the synthesis of a variety of naphthamidines (21.**83**) in the Wellcome Research Laboratories (139, 140).

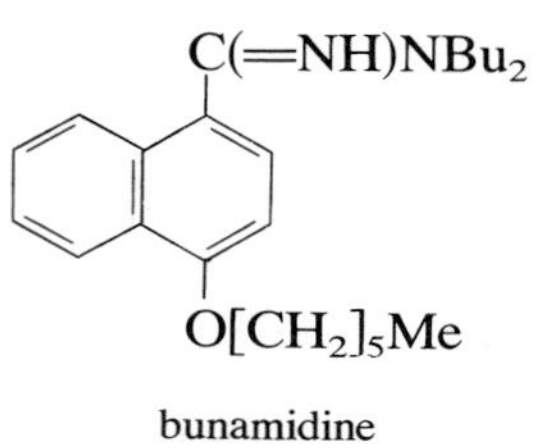

bunamidine

21.**82**

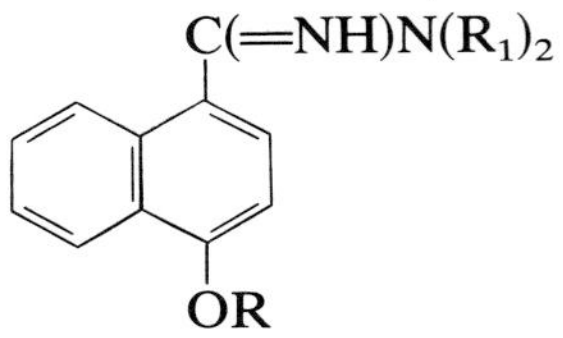

C(=NH)N(R_1)$_2$ [naphthalene] OR

21.**83**

In a detailed evaluation of the amidines (21.**83**) in cats and dogs, maximum activity appeared to reside in the compounds where R contained at least four carbon atoms, and R_1 moieties consisted of not more than four carbon atoms, although this pattern of activity differed markedly from that observed in the primary mouse screens.

Unfortunately, bunamidine is too toxic for use in human medicine. It has, however, proved of benefit in the past in that unlike many taenicides it shows good control of adult *Echinococcus granulosus* in dogs. [This parasite in its larval (cystic) stage can cause a serious and sometimes fatal disease in humans, although normally it is parasitic only in farm livestock.]

In its mode of action, bunamidine has been shown to inhibit cholinesterase activity, producing an irreversible neuromuscular block (141).

5.1.1.4 Isothiocyanates. 1,4-Phenylenediisothiocyanate (21.**84**, bitoscanate, Jonit),

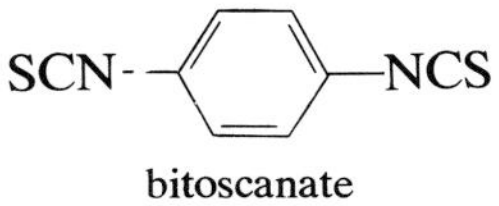

SCN–C_6H_4–NCS

bitoscanate

21.**84**

a drug noted for its pronounced antihookworm properties, is also known to be effective against veterinary (142) and human (143) tapeworms.

Another aryl isothiocyanate that has interesting broad spectrum anthelmintic properties is nitroscanate (21.**85**, cantrodifene, Lopatol), which is clearly closely related to the schistosomicide 4-isothiocyanato-4′-nitrodiphenylamine (21.**41**) mentioned earlier Section 4.1.4.3*e*).

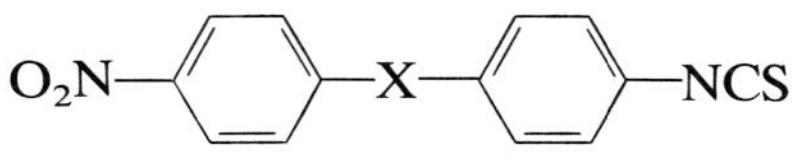

O_2N–C_6H_4–X–C_6H_4–NCS

21.**85** X = O (nitroscanate)
21.**41** X = NH (amoscanate)

Nitroscanate has a wide spectrum of activity against cestode and nematode infections in dogs (including the refractory *E. granulosus* at higher dose levels), but it appears to have only a moderate therapeutic index (144).

5.1.1.5 Miscellaneous Taenicides. Paromomycin (Humatin), the aminoglycoside antibiotic, is effective for treating all species of human tapeworm (89)—by single oral dose for *Taenia* species and *Diphyllobothrium latum*, but by single doses repeated for 5–7 days for infestation with the dwarf tapeworm *Hymenolepis nana.*

Several newer organophosphorus compounds have been shown to be interesting as broad spectrum anthelmintic agents for the treatment of a variety of veterinary cestodes and nematodes. These drugs include diuredosan (21.**86**, Sansalid) (145),

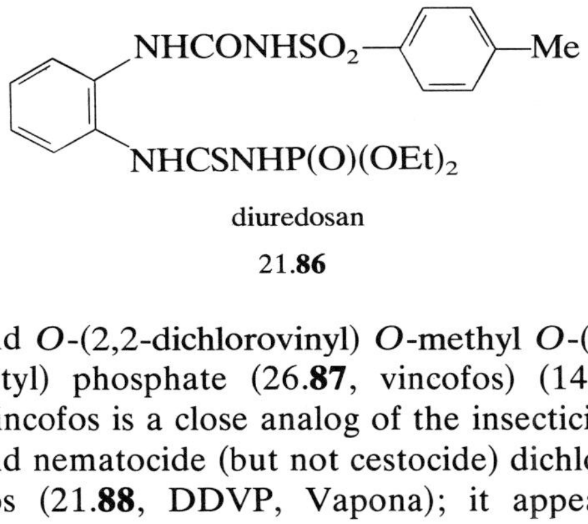

[benzene]–NHCONHSO$_2$–C_6H_4–Me; –NHCSNHP(O)(OEt)$_2$

diuredosan

21.**86**

and *O*-(2,2-dichlorovinyl) *O*-methyl *O*-(*n*-octyl) phosphate (26.**87**, vincofos) (146). Vincofos is a close analog of the insecticide and nematocide (but not cestocide) dichlorvos (21.**88**, DDVP, Vapona); it appears

CCl_2=CH.O—P(O)(OMe)(OR)

21.**87** R = *n*-C_8H_{17} (vincofos)
21.**88** R = Me (dichlorvos)

that the increased lipophilicity of vincofos is responsible for the appearance of anticestode activity (146). Certainly this hypothesis is in accord with the findings of Saz and Lescure (147), who have shown that certain anticestode drugs (which are uncouplers of oxidative phosphorylation) have no chemotherapeutic activity against the nematode *Ascaris lumbricoides*, even though the drugs interrupt oxidative phosphorylation in both tapeworm and ascarid mitochondria. This selectivity of action is attributed to differences in permeability between the two groups of helminths. With regard to vincofos, it remains to be seen whether increased lipophilicity also increases toxicity.

In addition to pronounced nematocidal properties, selected benzimidazoles also have taenicidal activity: these include mebendazole (21.**108**) in man (89), and albendazole (21.**112**) (130) in experimental animals.

Finally, one of the most exciting compounds to emerge as a broad spectrum taenicide (and schistosomicide) is praziquantel (21.**56**, Embay 8440, Droncit). This drug was extremely active against a very wide range of tapeworms in cats, dogs (including *Echinococcus granulosus* and *E. multilocularis*), and sheep at remarkably low single oral dose levels (148, 149).

Initial investigations into the mode of action of this drug against *Hymenolepis diminuta* have revealed (148) that it depletes the glycogen content of the worm and renders the tegument permeable to glucose—an effect that is reversible (*in vitro* only) by placing treated worms in a drug-free medium. The further usefulness of praziquantel in treating infectious larval stages of tapeworms is discussed in Section 5.2.

5.2 Larval Cestode Infections

The therapy of larval cestode infections in the past has been unsatisfactory. However certain benzimidazoles have been shown to be active against larval stages of tapeworms in various experimental animals. In particular, mebendazole (21.**108**) appears to have the broadest spectrum of activity, and this compound is effective against larval stages of *Taenia* and *Echinococcus* species in a variety of experimental animals when administered over a prolonged period. The drug is, however, more active when administered parenterally (150).

Striking results have been obtained with the taenicide praziquantel, which when given as several low oral doses was fully effective against larval stages of *Cysticercus fasciolaris* in mice, *C. pisiformis* in rabbits, *C. tenuicollis* in sheep, and *C. bovis* in cattle. In addition, single, slightly higher doses of the drug were sufficient to sterilize larval *C. pisiformis* in rabbits (the larvae showed no morphological changes, but had lost the ability to infect dogs) (148).

6 NEMATODE DISEASES AND DRUGS ACTIVE AGAINST THEM

As mentioned earlier, nematodes are conveniently divided into intestinal species, lungworms, and filaria or tissue forms.

Intestinal roundworms include all nematodes with their adult stage in the intestinal tract, even though larval stages are sometimes to be found elsewhere in the body. The main species affecting man are the so-called hookworms (*Ancylostoma duodenale* and *Necator americanus*), which must be regarded as the most damaging of the intestinal forms. These parasites occur predominantly in the tropics and subtropics, although *A. duodenale* has been reported in more northerly mining areas of Europe. Infection is usually by penetration of the skin by filariform larvae. The mature forms of the parasites attach themselves to the wall of the intestine and suck blood for the rest of their lifetime—some 5 years or so. Other nematodes commonly parasitizing man include roundworms (*Ascaris lumbricoides*), pinworms (*Enterobius vermicularis*). and whipworms (*Trichuris trichiura*). *Trichinella spiralis*, whose larvae become encysted in the skeletal muscles, causes trichinosis (a disease for which control measures are extremely simple, since it is perpetuated in pigs by the feeding of uncooked garbage, and is transmitted to humans by the ingestion of infected, inadequately cooked pork). Finally *Strongyloides stercoralis*, a parasite of world wide distribution, invades the skin and oral mucosa in an infective larval stage.

Nematodes dwelling in the gut of ruminants are of two main families—the strongyles and the ascarids. Species found in the stomach include *Haemonchus*, *Ostertagia*, and *Trichostrongylus*, while *Nematodirus*, *Bunostomum*, *Cooperia*, and *Trichostrongylus* species are to be found in the small intestine. Finally *Chabertia* and *Oesophagostomum* species reside in the large intestine.

Although of little significance in man, a variety of lungworm species parasitize cattle, sheep, and pigs, causing significant annual economic losses. In the United Kingdom the biggest problem occurs with *Dictyocaulus viviparus*, which as maturing larvae and adults live in the bronchial tree of cattle, causing parasitic bronchitis (husk). Other nematodes causing losses to farm stock include *Syngamus* species (gapeworms), which are normally parasitic in the respiratory tract of poultry, *Metastrongylus* species, which infect swine, and *Dictyocaulus filaria* and other species that parasitize sheep.

The tissue-inhabiting nematodes or filaria are found in a wide variety of organs, tissues, and body cavities, and although producing more striking and bizarre clinical symptoms than the gastrointestinal nematodes, are less widespread (some 500 million cases) than the latter parasites. Six species of filaria are regularly parasitic in man, viz., *Wuchereria bancrofti*, *Brugia malayi*, *Loa loa*, *Dipetalonema perstans*, *Mansonella ozzardi*, and *Onchocerca volvulus*. Onchocerciasis (river blindness), caused by *O. volvulus*, ranks as one of the world's most formidable infectious diseases, affects some 30 million people, and is responsible for blindness rates of more than 20% of the adult population in some African communities. Another tissue nematode affecting man is *Dracunculus medinensis* or Guinea-worm. This parasite has probably been endemic in a wide belt running through Africa and Asia since the beginning of recorded history. Guinea-worms are believed to be the "fiery serpents" referred to in the old Testament (151), and Plutarch mentioned that the worms occurred commonly among populations on the shores of the Red Sea.

Bancroftian and Malayan filariasis (*W. bancrofti* and *B. malayi*) are both diseases of urban areas, since transmission is by culicine mosquitoes that breed in the squalid surroundings associated with developing shanty towns. The industrialization in certain parts of Southeast Asia, for example, will inevitably lead to an increase in these filarias unless drastic measures are taken to remove the breeding grounds of the relevant mosquitoes.

Finally, the most important veterinary tissue nematode is possibly the canine heartworm *Dirofilaria immitis*, which is also transmitted by mosquitoes.

Chemotherapy of tissue nematode infections (human and veterinary) is, in general, rather unsatisfactory. In fact, in parts of the United States surgery is resorted to as the best means of treating favored canine pets and hunting dogs infected with *D. immitis*!

6.1 Filarial Infections

Tissue filarial infections are considered separately from other nematode diseases, since the chemotherapeutic agents used are generally of a different chemical type. (The pharmacokinetics and bioavailability of a successful filaricide must of necessity differ from those of a drug for use in the treatment of gastrointestinal parasites.)

6.1.1 LIFE CYCLES. Adult filarial worms take some 3–15 months to mature, and may then live for up to 15 years or so. Filarial worms are viviparous, and fertile females produce large numbers of larvae—the so-called microfilariae. With some filarias, the disease pathology is produced by blockage of lymphatic vessels by adult worms (*Wuchereria* and *Brugia* spp.), and with others the millions of microfilariae released are responsible for the ultimate pathology; thus it is the microfilariae of *Onchocerca volvulus* that by their entry to the eye, destroy ocular tissue, giving rise to the so-called river blindness.

Microfilariae can develop only if they are ingested by the appropriate insect vector (mosquitoes for *W. bancrofti*, or *Simulium* flies for *O. volvulus*, etc.). In the correct insect host, the larvae develop, and usually reach the infective stage within 7–14 days. At this point the larvae may be transmitted to the normal host by the bite of the infected insect. Once in the host, the larvae migrate to the lymphatics, where sexual maturity occurs and the cycle is complete.

One of the filarias in particular—onchocerciasis—has brought about the desertion by humans of some of the most fertile lands in certain savanna areas of West Africa. This disease is closely associated with the fast-flowing rivers that afford the essential breeding sites for *Simulium* flies, which are the vectors for the disease.

6.1.2 CHEMOTHERAPY OF FILARIASIS. The most striking feature of the reviews of the chemotherapy of filariasis that have appeared in recent years (9, 10, 152, 153) is the general paucity of chemical leads against these infections. This is partly a reflection of the refractory nature of the parasites and partly an indication of the somewhat uncertain relevance of the animal models available for screening purposes. In fact, in spite of research extending over some 30 years (dating essentially from the time that US servicemen were exposed to filarias in the South Pacific), only three filaricides are in general use: diethylcarbamazine, or DEC (21.**93**) and suramin (21.**98**), which are the drugs of choice for treating human infections, and DEC and arsenamide (21.**89**), which are the preferred therapeutic agents for dog filarias.

6.1.2.1 Organic Arsenic Compounds. Although the arsenic derivative arsenamide (21.**89**) is too toxic for normal use in humans, it is recommended as one of the

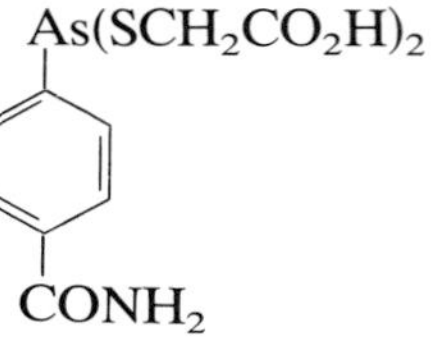

$As(SCH_2CO_2H)_2$ — p-phenylene — $CONH_2$

arsenamide

21.**89**

drugs of choice for the treatment of *Dirofilaria immitis* (hearthworm) in dogs, in which the drug is a highly active macrofilaricide at relatively low levels. Arsenamide is, however, less suitable for use in animals bearing heavy worm burdens.

Another arsenic compound, Mel W (21.**90**, melarsonyl potassium), one of the Melarsen series developed by Friedheim, has been shown to be effective against various filarial infections (including *W. bancrofti* and *O. volvulus* in man) when given as a single intramuscular injection (9, 10). However there appears to be an unacceptably high risk of arsenical encephalopathy associated with the use of this drug.

A new filaricide F 151 (21.**91**), which

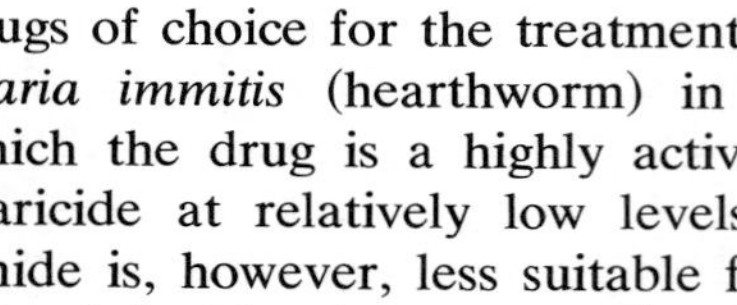

N, N, N (triazine ring) — NH — (benzene ring) — R; H_2N

21.**90** R = 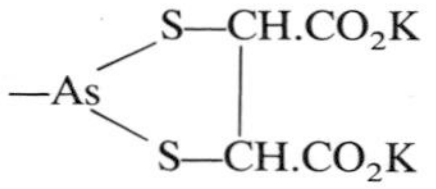 —As(S—CH.CO_2K)(S—CH.CO_2K) (Mel W)

21.**91** —As[SC(Me)$_2$CH(NH_2)CO_2H]$_2$ (F 151)

also possesses trypanocidal activity, apparently has macrofilaricidal properties against *Litomosoides carinii* infections in cotton rats (*Sigmodon hispidus*: one of the most useful animal models for the primary screening of potential filaricides) (154). Friedheim has further established that F 151 has synergistic filaricidal properties when used in combination with the benzimidazolylbenzimidazole HOE 33258 (21.**99**), a known microfilaricide. Thus in field trials in dogs naturally infected with *D. immitis* the combination product appeared to be an effective, well-tolerated, macro- and microfilaricidal agent when administered by single subcutaneous injection (155).

With the advent of more active, nonmetallic drugs, the use of arsenical compounds in the therapy of filariasis has diminished considerably.

6.1.2.2 Piperazines. In 1948 in the Lederle laboratories of American Cyanamid, the ethyl ester (21.**92**) of 4-methyl-1-piperazinecarboxylic acid was shown to be a potent filaricide. Extended investigations, using as the screening model *L. carinii* infections in cotton rats, revealed that the most potent member of the series apparently was the *N,N*-diethylamide (21.**93**). This compound subsequently entered clinical medicine as diethylcarbamazine (DEC) (Banocide, Hetrazan) (156, 157). The drug is currently the primary therapeutic agent for the treatment of Bancroftian and Malayan filariasis, and loaiasis, but it is essentially active against microfilariae only. In onchocerciasis, DEC is also highly effective against the microfilariae, but ensuing anaphylactic reactions are of sufficient frequency to make it potentially dangerous to use the drug in treating this disease (158). Diethylcarbamazine is also used in veterinary medicine for the treatment of lungworm infections in sheep (*Dictyocaulus filaria*) and cattle (*D. viviparus*).

The mode of action of DEC has yet to be revealed, although recent ultrastructural studies (159) have indicated that the drug affects the cuticle of *O. volvulus* microfilariae so that they are recognized as foreign bodies by the host and rejected. Certainly these findings are in accord with earlier work, in which *in vitro* DEC appeared to have little or no activity against microfilariae and adult worms (160).

A wide variety of analogs of DEC have been prepared over the last 30 years, including the related piperazines HOE 28637a (21.**94**) and HOE 29691a (21.**95**)

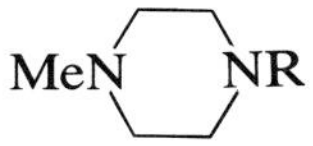

MeN NR

21.**92** R = CO_2Et
21.**93** R = $CONEt_2$ (diethylcarbamazine)

21.**94** 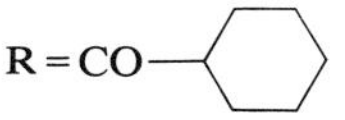 R = CO— (HOE 28637a)

21.**95** 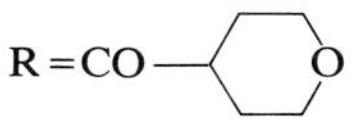 R = CO— O (HOE 29691a)

(161), and various conformationally constrained congeners such as the 3,8-diazabicyclo[3.2.1.]octane (21.**96**) (162) and the 1,3,8-triaza[4.4.0]decane (21.**97**) (163). However none of these compounds appears to possess obvious superiority over DEC.

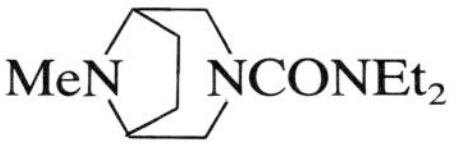

MeN $NCONEt_2$

21.**96**

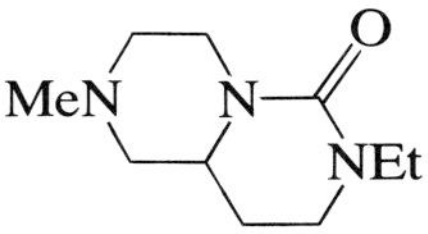

O
MeN N
NEt

21.**97**

6.1.2.3 Suramin. In 1921, suramin (21.**98**, Antrypol, Bayer 205) was introduced into human medicine for the treatment of trypanosomiasis. Subsequently, the drug

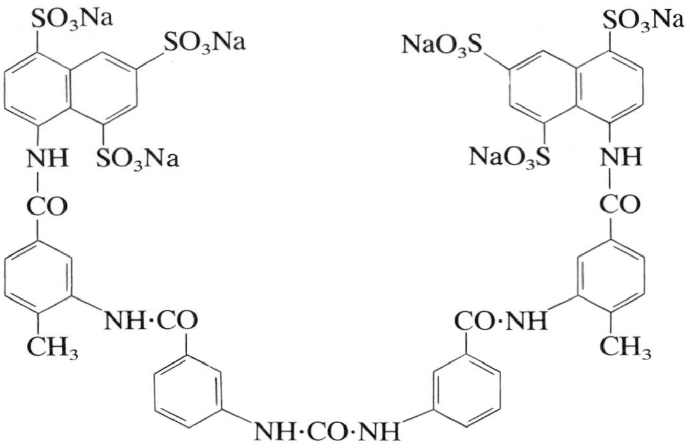

suramin

21.**98**

was shown to be highly effective against adult *O. volvulus* in humans when administered intravenously or by deep intramuscular injection (suramin appears to lack activity against other filarias). Interestingly the drug seems to affect adult female worms initially, while adult males and microfilariae remain alive much longer. Side effects tend to occur relatively frequently, and there is always the possibility of irreversible nephrotoxicity.

Finally, suramin is basically too toxic for use in mass eradication campaigns, and there remains a great need for a safe, effective, readily administered drug for the treatment of onchocerciasis.

6.1.2.4 Miscellaneous Compounds. One interesting filaricide to emerge (164) from the Hoechst laboratories is the benzimidazolylbenzimidazole (21.**99**, HOE 33258), which by single subcutaneous injection is extremely potent against the microfilariae of *L. carinii* in cotton rats, and *D. immitis* in dogs. In the latter trials most adult worms were killed as well (10). Another benzimidazole to possess activity against filarias is the anthelmintic mebendazole (21.**108**). This drug is active against microfilariae of *Dipetalonema perstans* in humans (165) and *Brugia malayi* (166), but it lacks efficacy against human *O. volvulus* infections (165). Mebendazole also appears to be effective as a prophylactic against *D. immitis* in dogs when administered for prolonged periods (167). At present it is not known whether these structurally dissimilar benzimidazoles have a similar mode of action against filarias.

It is unfortunate that the known delayed neurotoxicity of haloxon (21.**135**) prevents the use of this drug in man, since it has been shown to possess pronounced microfilaricidal properties against *L. carinii* in the multimammate rat (*Mastomys natalensis*) (168). In this connection, haloxon is

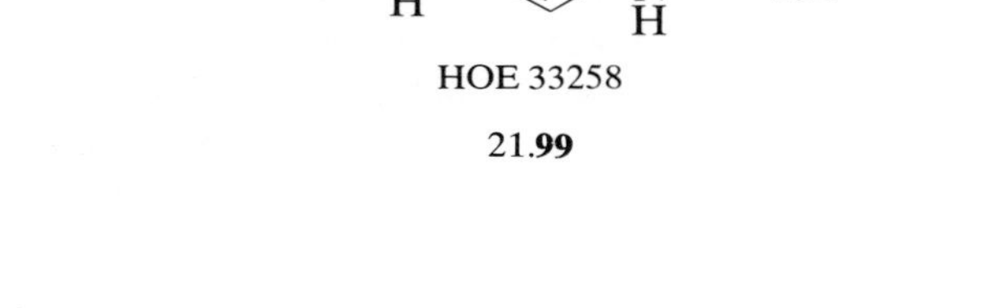

HOE 33258

21.**99**

more active and has a better therapeutic index than the known filaricide metrifonate (21.**42**).

4-Isothiocyanato-4′-nitrodiphenylamine (21.**41**, amoscanate), the novel broad spectrum anthelmintic agent from Ciba-Geigy, appears to include in its spectrum of activity good efficacy against two filarial species (adults as well as microfilariae) in the Mongolian jird after oral administration for 2–5 days; this is in addition to its activity against schistosome species and several gastrointestinal nematodes (76).

Both tetramisole (21.**118**) and its levorotatory isomer levamisole (21.**116**) have high filaricidal activity, including efficacy against adult *L. carinii* at higher dose levels as well as the circulating microfilariae. The present evidence (10) indicates that levamisole has good activity against a range of filarial infections, although the value of its use in humans for this purpose may be in doubt because of the relatively poor therapeutic index, and limited and short duration of action against microfilariae.

Finally, in a review of experimental antifilarial drugs, Elslager (152) indicates that the quinazoline (21.**100**, CI-679), one of a

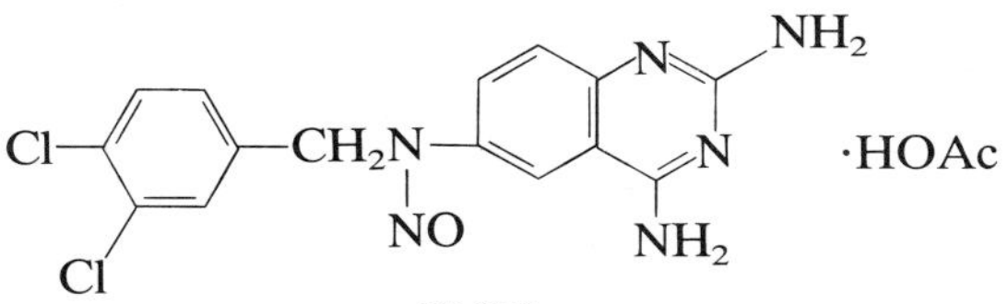

Cl, Cl, CH_2N, NO, NH_2, N, N, NH_2 ·HOAc

CI-679

21.**100**

series of 2,4-diaminoquinazoline antifolates prepared at Parke, Davis, had potent activity against microfilariae and adult *L. carinii* in gerbils, although full details do not appear to have been published to date.

6.1.3 DRACONTIASIS. A parasite that is biologically closely related to the filarias but differs in several ways is the Guinea-worm *Dracunculus medinensis.* Man becomes infected by drinking water containing an infected arthropod host, in this case a crustacean, *Cyclops.* Having penetrated the intestinal wall, the larvae become adult, and the female worms, after fertilization, migrate to the extremities. About 1 year after the ingestion of the infectious larvae, the mature female (up to a horrifying 1 m in length) appears at the skin surface, and a blister forms over the worm. Soon after this the blister bursts, a loop of the uterus prolapses through the anterior end of the worm, and this ruptures, discharging larvae intermittently on contact with water over several weeks.

The traditional treatment of the disease involves the gradual winding of the Guinea-worm onto a stick over 3–4 weeks, although severe anaphylactic reactions may occur if the worm is broken during this process.

Therapy of the disease is unsatisfactory. Niridazole (21.**16**) (169), mebendazole (21.**108**) at higher dose levels (170), and the trichomonicide metronidazole (21.**101**, Flagyl) (171) have been used with varying

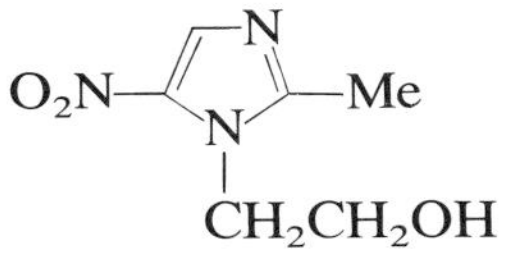

O_2N, N, N, Me, CH_2CH_2OH

metronidazole

21.**101**

degrees of success. Although it has been claimed (172) that the mode of action of niridazole and metronidazole is due to an anti-inflammatory rather than a direct anthelmintic effect, there is some evidence that mebendazole causes a spontaneous extrusion of fragmented, dead worms, and that mechanical removal of the worms is not necessary.

6.2 Gastrointestinal Nematode Infections

As has already been noted, the prevalence of parasitic diseases (especially nematode infections such as ascariasis and hookworm infection) is high, although the exact figures are not readily assessed with any degree of accuracy. However, in terms of human suffering, is it important whether the estimate (2) that 750 million people are infested with the hookworms *Ancylostoma duodenale* and *Necator americanus* is correct or whether it is an under- or overestimate by even as much as 20%?

6.2.1 LIFE CYCLES. The nematodes are the second largest class in the animal kingdom, comprising at least 500,000 species, and it is not surprising that a diversity of life cycles exists for these worms. Thus the life cycle of the pinworm *Enterobius vermicularis* is one of the simplest of the human helminths; it merely involves the migration of gravid female worms toward the anus, and their emergence at night to extrude some 10,000 eggs each on the perianal skin. Within 6 hr these become infective for the same or other persons: additionally, retroinfection may occur when hatched larvae reenter the gastrointestinal tract through the anal route.

The hookworm *A. duodenale* has a more complicated life cycle, in which adult worms in the small intestine lay eggs that pass out in the feces and hatch in suitable soil within about 5 days. The hatched larvae feed, and molt twice, becoming slender, nonfeeding filariform larvae that are infective for the definitive host within another 5 days. The filariform larvae climb up on moist dirt or vegetable particles, wave in the breeze, and (even after several weeks) wait until they are contacted by a suitable host—usually the skin of a bare foot! The larvae penetrate the skin, are carried by the circulation to the lungs, where they emerge into the air sacs, pass up the bronchial tubes and the trachea into the pharynx, and migrate to the intestine.

6.2.2 CHEMOTHERAPY OF NEMATODE INFECTIONS. Over the last 25 years or so, the chemotherapy of intestinal helminthiases has been revolutionized, and now, with the possible exception of trichuriasis, there are drugs of real value for most infections. Therefore the older, less satisfactory remedies are not described here, and attention is concentrated on the new generation of anthelmintic agents.

Several reviews are available on the chemotherapy of nematode infections, and these should be consulted for details of some of the older drugs (5, 8, 13, 173, 174).

6.2.2.1 Benzimidazoles. The year 1961 saw the introduction (175) by workers from the Merck laboratories of 2-(4-thiazolyl)-benzimidazole (21.**102**, thiabendazole,

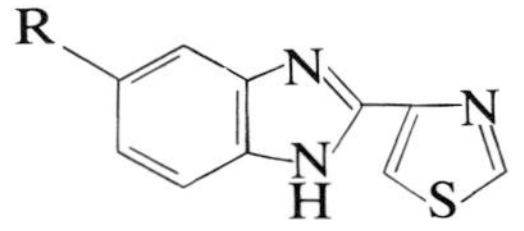

21.**102** R = H (thiabendazole)
21.**103** R = NO_2
21.**104** R = NH_2
21.**105** R = *i*-PrO.CONH (cambendazole)

Thibenzole, Mintezol) as the first of the modern, truly broad spectrum gastrointestinal nematocides, useful for the eradication of most intestinal nematodes with the possible exception of the whipworm *Trichuris trichiura*. Since this date numerous papers have been published on the drug, and no attempt is made to detail them here (e.g., 173, 174).

In vitro, thiabendazole appears to inhibit the fumarate reductase system of susceptible *Haemonchus contortus* nematodes, whereas in resistant worms no inhibition was observed (176). *In vivo*, the drug has a clearly defined anti-inflammatory action, and it has been postulated that this may contribute favorably to the clinical response in man, seen after use of the drug in cases of trichinosis, cutaneous larva migrans (caused by various skin-penetrating larvae that continue to wander in the superficial layers of the body), and visceral larva migrans (caused when ingestion of eggs or larvae leads to the presence of wandering larvae in deep organs) (177).

Various analogs of thiabendazole in which the benzimidazole moiety is substituted in the 2-position by an aromatic or heteroaromatic ring have also been shown to have anthelmintic properties (175). Indeed, one of these derivatives, 2-phenylbenzimidazole, was marketed for a time but was later withdrawn because of nephrotoxicity associated with the production of a very insoluble metabolite—the glucuronide of 5-hydroxy-2-phenylbenzimidazole (178). Thiabendazole congeners in which the benzimidazole moiety has been replaced by other heterocyclic ring systems, including imidazo[1,2-*a*]pyridines (179) and various azaindoles (180), are in general less active than the parent drug.

Although thiabendazole was shown to have an extremely broad spectrum of activity, and its therapeutic index was high, it nevertheless had the disadvantage of apparently being inactivated rapidly in, for example, sheep, by hydroxylation in the 5-position (181).

As part of an extensive program investigating structural modifications of thiabendazole, workers at Merck examined the effect of introducing various substituents into the 5-position of the molecule. It was found that 5-substitution *per se* did not necessarily increase potency: thus the 5-nitro compound 21.**103** had a relative anthelmintic potency of 0.2 compared with that of thiabendazole, while the 5-amino-derivative 21.**104** was approximately 0.8 times as active as the parent drug in the *in vivo* screen. (Interestingly 21.**104** is inactive in the *in vitro* screen; presumably acylation is required to afford the active species.)

The most active compound to emerge (182) from the study was the 5-*i*-propoxycarbonylamino derivative (21.**105**, cambendazole, Cambenzole, Equiben). As one of the second-generation benzimidazole anthelmintics, cambendazole is of low toxicity, has a spectrum of activity similar to that of thiabendazole, but is several times more potent than the latter compound. It is also effective in preventing the development of helminth eggs or larvae.

Cambendazole appears to have a similar mode of action to thiabendazole, although it does retain some inhibitory effects on fumarate reductase obtained from thiabendazole-resistant *H. contortus* (176).

The discovery of thiabendazole stimulated research in a variety of pharmaceutical companies into fresh areas of benzimidazole chemistry, with the result that workers at Smith, Kline and French were able to announce the introduction of parbendazole (21.**106**, Helmatac, Verminum)

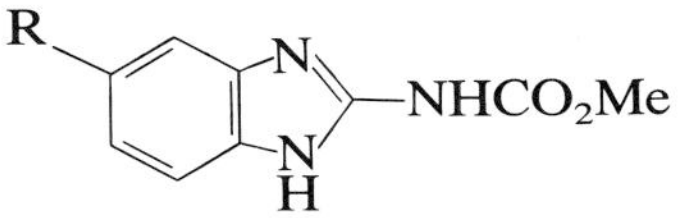

R (5-position of benzimidazole ring, N-H) —$NHCO_2Me$

21.**106** R = *n*-Bu (parbendazole)
21.**107** R = H
21.**108** R = PhCO (mebendazole)
21.**109** R = *n*-PrO (oxibendazole)
21.**110** R = PhS (fenbendazole)
21.**111** R = PhSO (oxfendazole)
21.**112** R = *n*-PrS (albendazole)
21.**113** R = $PhSO_2$

as a potent, broad spectrum anthelmintic agent (183). Interestingly, in this compound the basic thiabendazole moiety has been altered by the replacement of the 4-thiazolyl ring system by a methyl carbamate grouping. In a similar manner to thiabendazole, the presence of the 5-substituent appears to prevent metabolic inactivation—certainly although the corresponding desalkyl derivative 21.**107** is active, parbendazole is an even more potent drug.

Although at high dose levels parbendazole also has useful activity against *Moniezia* species (tapeworms), it does possess slight teratogenic properties when administered to sheep in early pregnancy (184).

Parbendazole represents the first of the benzimidazole anthelmintic agents to contain the methyl carbamate moiety in the 2-position. Following the introduction of this compound, however, Janssen Pharmaceutica produced (185) mebendazole (21.**108**, Pantelmin, Telmin, Vermox), which has been confirmed as a remarkably safe, broad spectrum anthelmintic that is especially useful in the treatment of human whipworm (*Trichuris trichiura*) and pinworm (*Enterobius vermicularis*) infections (186, 187). The drug is also effective against many other nematodes and cestodes as well. At present mebendazole is believed to act by irreversibly blocking glucose uptake by nematodes in the colon (185).

Following the discovery of mebendazole, the development of several other benzimidazole veterinary anthelmintic agents was announced. These included oxibendazole (21.**109**) in which the 5-butyl group of parbendazole had been replaced by *n*-propoxy (188); the 5-phenylthio analog fenbendazole (21.**110**, Panacur, HOE 881) from Hoechst (189); oxfendazole (21.**111**, Systemax, Synanthic) (190), which is the sulfoxide of fenbendazole; and albendazole (21.**112**), the *n*-propylthio congener of oxibendazole (130).

These last three benzimidazoles in particular are characterized by their potent, broad spectrum anthelmintic activity. Thus oxfendazole, fenbendazole, and albendazole are active not only against gastrointestinal helminths, but also against the lungworm *Dictyocaulus viviparus*. In addition albendazole is effective against the liver fluke *Fasciola hepatica* and tapeworms of the genus *Moniezia*. Oxfendazole appears to be much more active than the corresponding sulfide fenbendazole in mice and cattle, but it shows comparable efficacy in sheep: interestingly in the mouse primary screen sulfone 21.**113** appears to be much less active than either the sulfide (fenbendazole or sulfoxide (oxfendazole) (190).

Obviously the benzimidazoles represent an extremely interesting group of anthelmintic agents. Their potential in future years must, however, depend to a degree on the ability of the newer derivatives to maintain full efficacy against benzimidazole-resistant nematode species, which are appearing in various parts of the world. In this connection the synthesis by workers at Hoechst of hexahydrotriazines (21.**114**)

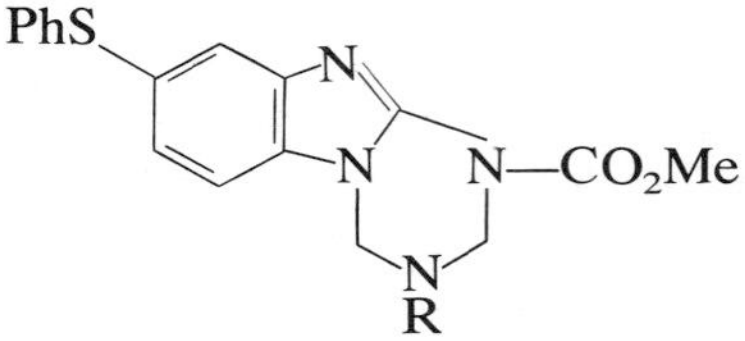

PhS, N, N, N—CO_2Me, N, R

21.**114**

from fenbendazole is of interest (191). Although these compounds appear to have a spectrum of activity different from that of the parent fenbendazole (192), it is not known yet whether they are active against benzimidazole-resistant nematodes.

An open-chain congener of the benzimidazoles, thiophanate (21.**115**, Nemafax), is active against a broad range of

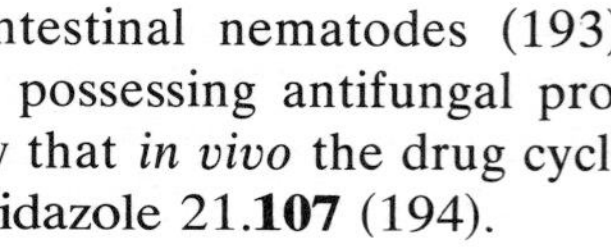

$NHCSNHCO_2Et$

$NHCSNHCO_2Et$

thiophanate

21.**115**

gastrointestinal nematodes (193) in addition to possessing antifungal properties. It is likely that *in vivo* the drug cyclizes to the benzimidazole 21.**107** (194).

6.2.2.2 Tetramisole and Levamisole. In 1966 the second modern broad spectrum anthelmintic agent, tetramisole (21.**118**, Ripercol, Nilverm) was introduced by Janssen Pharmaceutica. The original publications (195, 196) indicated that the drug was fully effective against a wide range of gastrointestinal nematodes in many species of

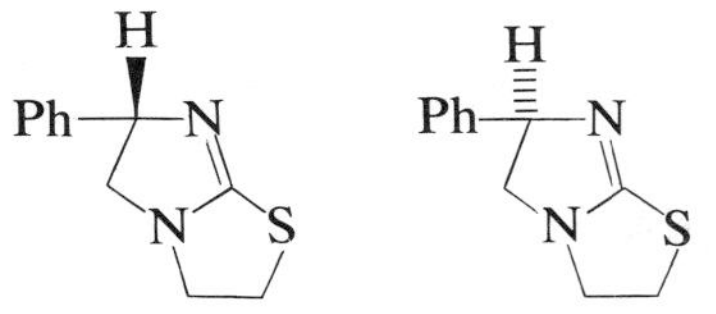

$S(-)$ 21.**116** (levamisole) $R(+)$ 21.**117** (dextramisole)

tetramisole

21.**118**

animals and birds, including tigers! The discovery of tetramisole, which illustrates some of the necessary qualities of a successful pharmaceutical company, viz. serendipity, keen observation, and the ability or desire to follow an interesting lead to the limit, has been reviewed admirably by Janssen (197).

Briefly, in the primary screen in *chickens*, thiazothienol (21.**119**) was shown to possess good nematocidal properties; in mice

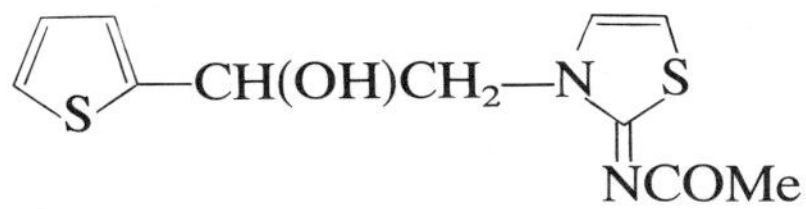

thiazothienol

21.**119**

and rats, however, the compound lacked activity. All the metabolites of thiazothienol that were isolated and synthesized were inactive against nematodes except thiazothielite (21.**120**). This drug was much

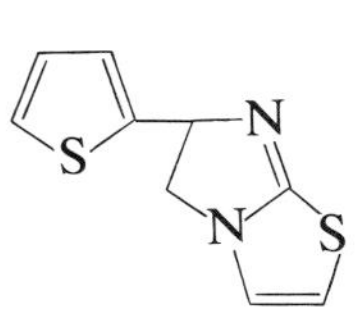

thiazothielite

21.**120**

more potent than its precursor and was also active in rodents. Although this particular compound was expensive and had limited solubility in water, a close analog, *dl*-2,3,5,6-tetrahydro-6-phenylimidazo(2,1-*b*)-thiazole (21.**118**, tetramisole), was developed from a large series of related imidazo(2,1-*b*)thiazoles. Further investigations showed that most of the anthelmintic activity of the racemic tetramisole resided in the levorotatory isomer levamisole (21.**116**, Nemicide, Tramisol), which was several times more potent but no more toxic than the dextrorotatory isomer dextramisole (21.**117**). Since their introduction, tetramisole and levamisole have become probably the most widely used anthelmintic agents for use against a broad range of nematodes in man, cattle, pigs, sheep, and poultry (197).

In addition to its main mode of action as a potent stereospecific inhibitor of fumarate reductase in various nematodes, including thiabendazole-resistant *Haemonchus contortus* (198, 199), levamisole also has other interesting biochemical properties: at low concentrations the drug inhibits mammalian alkaline phosphatases (200). More interestingly, although not within the scope of this review, levamisole has been found to restore host defense mechanisms, and it has a potential therapeutic value as an immunostimulant for a variety of clinical conditions in man and animals (reviewed in Ref. 197). In addition, the dextrorotatory isomer dextramisole, of no value as an anthelmintic agent, has undergone clinical trial as an antidepressant.

Although a variety of tetramisole analogs have been prepared—including, for instance, the imidazo(1,2-*a*)imidazole (21.**121**) (201)—to date none appears to

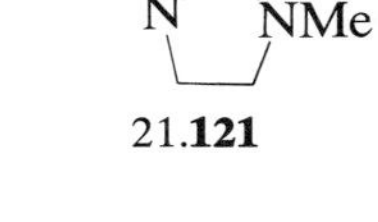

21.**121**

have an anthelmintic potency of the same order as tetramisole.

6.2.2.3 Pyrantel, Morantel, and Oxantel. The discovery of anthelmintic activity in

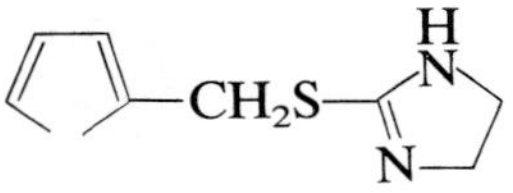

21.**122**

the isothiouronium salt (21.**122**) (202) initiated a program of work in the Pfizer laboratories into the synthesis of analogs of this compound. Although 21.**122** was active against experimental *Nematospiroides dubius* infections in the rodent primary screen, it possessed little activity when administered to sheep. This lack of activity was ascribed to a rapid hydrolysis of the compound to inactive products (2-thenylthiol and 2-imidazolidinone) in this species. Further studies based on attempts to prevent this ready hydrolysis led to the discovery of good anthelmintic activity in cyclic amidines of general formula 21.**123**,

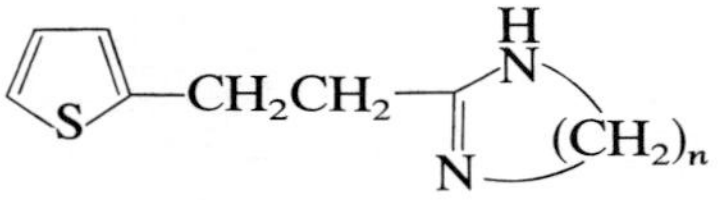

21.**123** $n = 2$ or 3

and this work culminated in the introduction of pyrantel (21.**124**, Banminth, Strongid, Combantrin) and morantel (21.**125**) as

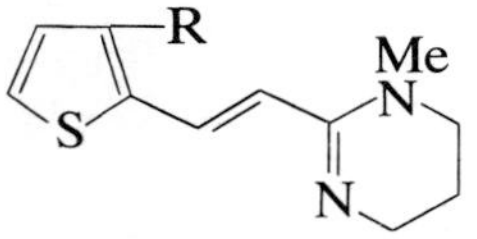

21.**124** R = H (pyrantel)
21.**125** R = Me (morantel)

broad spectrum anthelmintic agents (203, 204). In human medicine pyrantel is used as the very insoluble pamoate salt, whereas for veterinary use it is normally employed as the water-soluble tartrate.

Pyrantel is effective against a wide range of gastrointestinal nematodes and is certainly one of the drugs of choice for the treatment of human pinworm, hookworm, and *Ascaris* infections (89, 173, 174).

Structure-activity studies on pyrantel analogs indicated that in compounds of general formula 21.**126**, anthelmintic activ-

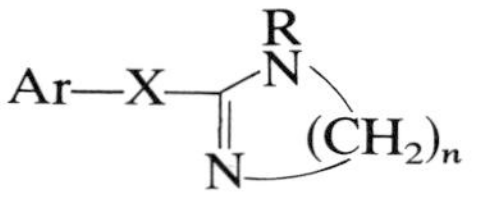

21.**126**

ity for different values of Ar was of the order 2-thienyl > 3-thienyl > phenyl > 2-furyl; maximum activity occurred in tetrahydropyrimidine derivatives ($n = 3$). Except for introduction of groups into the ortho position of the Ar moiety, and *N*-methyl substitution (R) in the cyclic amidine system, the introduction of groups into other parts of the molecule eliminated activity. In addition, maximum efficacy was established for compounds in which X was *trans*—CH=CH—. Analogs where X was CH_2CH_2 or *cis*—CH=CH— were less active in that order (204). In these studies a quantitative Hansch analysis of activity and structure revealed good correlation between lipophilicity and activity.

Further work in the same laboratories uncovered interesting anthelmintic properties in related 1-(2-arylvinyl)pyridinium salts (21.**127**) (205), certain noncyclic amidines (21.**128**) (206), and some dihydrothiazines (21.**129**) (207). However no

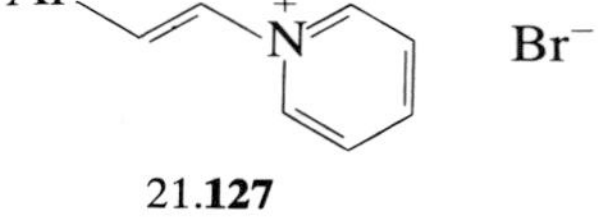

21.**127**

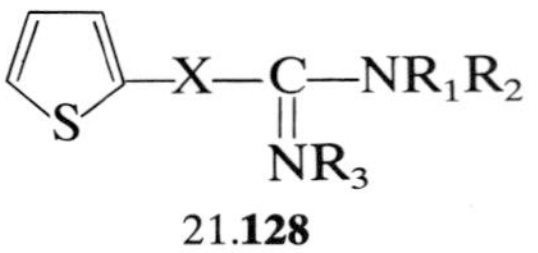

21.**128**

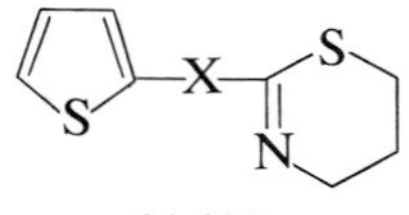

21.**129**

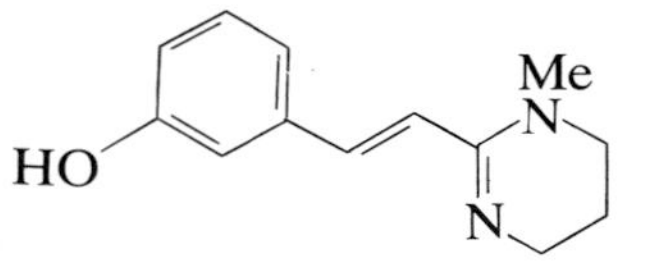

HO–C₆H₄–CH=CH–(1-methyl-tetrahydropyrimidin-2-yl)

oxantel

21.**130**

$$PhOCH_2CH_2.\overset{+}{N}(Me)_2.CH_2R \quad X^-$$

21.**131** R = Ph, X = 3-hydroxy-2-naphthoate anion (bephenium hydroxynaphthoate)
21.**132** R = 2-thienyl, X = *p*-chlorobenzenesulfonate anion (thenium closylate)
21.**133** R = 3-acetyl-5-chloro-2-hydroxyphenyl, X = 3-hydroxy-2-naphthoate anion (diphezyl hydroxynaphthoate)

analog emerged as clearly superior to pyrantel or morantel, particularly when a selection of all these compounds was evaluated further in sheep naturally infected with a wide variety of gastrointestinal nematodes (208).

A further interesting development was the discovery (209) of antiwhipworm activity in some *m*-hydroxyphenyl congeners of pyrantel, although the parent drug itself lacks activity against the adult worms (*Trichuris* spp.). The most active analog was 21.**130** (oxantel, CP-14,445) which was shown to have a different spectrum of activity from other pyrantel derivatives. In humans, oxantel has recently been reported to be a safe and effective anthelmintic for use in severe clinical trichuriasis (210).

Both pyrantel (211, 212) and morantel (213) are depolarizing neuromuscular blocking agents that stimulate ganglia and also possess acetylcholine-like actions on smooth muscle.

6.2.2.4 Bephenium and Thenium. Although bephenium hydroxynaphthoate (21.**131**, Alcopar) was introduced to human clinical medicine nearly 20 years ago (5, 214), it remains one of the drugs of choice for the treatment of hookworm infections (*Ancylostoma duodenale* and *Necator americanus*) (5, 89, 173). It has the added advantage that it is effective against the roundworm *Ascaris lumbricoides*, and against *Trichostrongylus* species when administered as a single oral dose. Structure-activity relationships existing in this series of compounds are not dealt with here, but another drug to emerge from the work was the veterinary anthelmintic agent thenium closylate (21.**132**, Canopar) (215), for use against hookworms in dogs. In combination with piperazine (as Ancaris) the drug appeared to be very effective against both canine hookworms and roundworms (216).

An analog of bephenium developed later by Soviet workers is diphezyl (21.**133**), which has a spectrum of activity slightly different from that of the parent drug in that it appears to be effective in human trichuriasis but is less active against pinworms, hookworms, and *Ascaris* species (217).

6.2.2.5 Piperazine. The development of piperazine (21.**134**, Antepar, Entacyl) as an

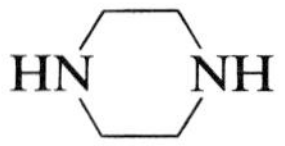

HN NH (piperazine ring)

21.**134**

anthelmintic agent for the treatment of nematode infections, and clinical trials associated with this compound and its many salts and derivatives, have been well documented by Cavier (8), Davis (173), and Standen (5), among others.

Piperazine appears to be nearly the ideal anthelmintic agent. Certainly it is nontoxic at therapeutic dose levels, it is economical and nonstaining, and it is palatable in conventional formulations. Consequently, even after many years, it remains one of the drugs of choice for the therapy of pinworm (*Enterobius vermicularis*) and *Ascaris* infections.

Piperazine has been shown to block neuromuscular transmission in *Ascaris* by means of an anticholinergic action at the myoneural junction (218, 219), although this effect is reversed if treated worms are removed to a piperazine-free medium. Paralyzed worms are unable to resist peristalsis of the small intestine and are carried down the gastrointestinal tract and excreted in the feces. Further work has established that the drug also inhibits certain glycolytic enzymes in *Ascaris* species (220), and very recently it has been shown to decrease phospholipid levels in human *A. lumbricoides* (221).

A wide variety of piperazine derivatives and salts have been prepared since the original discovery of the anthelmintic properties of this simple compound. To date, however, no derivative that appears to be superior to piperazine has been reported.

6.2.2.6 Isothiocyanates. 1,4-Phenylenediisothiocyanate (21.**84**, bitoscanate, Jonit) is a potent antihookworm agent for use in humans, and it has been used in India, for example, on a relatively large scale with varying degrees of success (222). The drug appears to be active against both *Ancylostoma duodenale* and *Necator americanus* but has little effect on *Ascaris* species. Side effects are not infrequently associated with the use of the drug, and although these are usually mild to moderate and transient, bitoscanate is not now regarded as one of the drugs of choice for hookworm infestations.

Another isothiocyanate that is of potential interest is the diphenylamine derivative amoscanate (21.**41**). In addition to its schistosomicidal and filaricidal properties in experimental animals, the drug is also effective against various intestinal nematodes (76). It has also been shown in preliminary trials to be effective in man against both *A. duodenale* and *N. americanus* (223), although no details are available at present.

6.2.2.7 Organophosphorus Compounds. Organophosphorus anthelmintic agents are all potent inhibitors of cholinesterases; consequently they depend for their safety on a selective action on the enzyme of the parasite. Hence although many organophosphorus compounds do possess efficacy *in vivo* against intestinal nematodes, most cannot be used for therapy, either because the spectrum of activity is too narrow or because the therapeutic index is too low. Nevertheless one useful nematocide that has entered veterinary medicine is the insecticide dichlorvos (21.**88**, DDVP, Atgard, Vapona) (224). Advantage is taken of the known ability of organic phosphorus compounds to act as excellent plasticizers for vinyl resins by incorporating dichlorvos into a plastic vehicle that affords a continuous controlled release of low levels of the otherwise volatile active material. Detailed structure-activity relationships of dichlorvos analogs (including phosphonates and phosphinates) have appeared in recent years in several publications emanating from the Shell laboratories (225–227).

Although haloxon (21.**135**, Loxon) is unsuitable for administration to humans because a certain degree of delayed neurotoxicity has been associated with its use, nevertheless, in animals, it is an extremely useful, inexpensive drug. It is especially

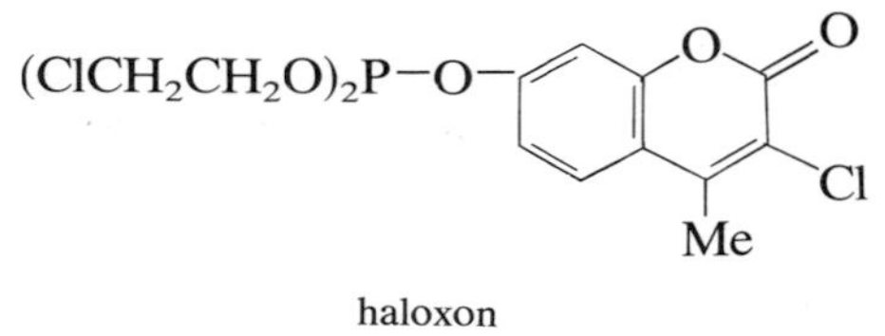

$(ClCH_2CH_2O)_2P{-}O{-}$ [coumarin ring with O, =O, Cl, Me]

haloxon
21.**135**

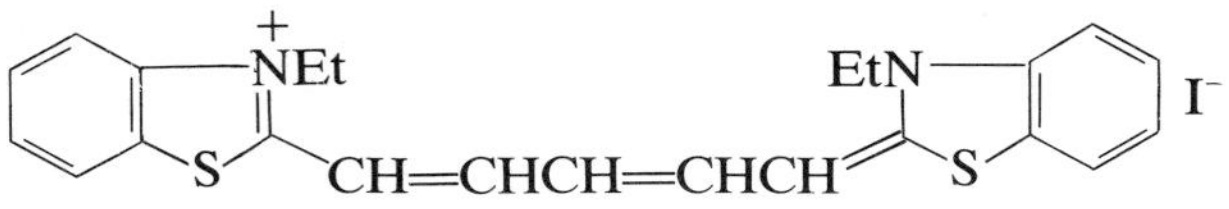

dithiazanine iodide

21.**136**

suitable for the treatment of ascariasis in young puppies, and in cattle, for instance, it is certainly one of the safest and most effective of the currently available veterinary anthelmintic agents (228).

Other organophosphorus compounds with nematocidal properties include the dichlorvos congener vincofos (21.**87**) (146), while diuredosan (21.**86**, Sansalid) (145) is a recently announced broad spectrum anthelmintic agent that is active against a variety of intestinal nematodes and cestodes in dogs and cats.

6.2.2.8 Cyanine Derivatives. The cyanine dye dithiazanine iodide (21.**136**, Telmid) has good activity (229) against pinworm and *Ascaris* infections, and also against the refractory whipworm and *Strongyloides stercoralis* in humans. However, the drug has been withdrawn from general use because of the severe gastrointestinal side effects produced on occasion.

Pyrvinium pamoate (21.**137**, Povan, Vanquin), an unsymmetrical cyanine dye, possesses potent activity against *Enterobius vermicularis* (230) and is generally accepted as one of the drugs of choice for the single dose treatment of pinworm infestations, despite its post treatment stool-staining propensities and its narrow spectrum of activity. The drug is almost insoluble and is not absorbed from the gastrointestinal tract to any significant degree. It is consequently more palatable than the chloride, which is more soluble and has marked nauseating properties.

Finally, a combination product containing haloxon (21.**135**) and a new drug bidimazium iodide (21.**138**) has been described (231) as providing a safe, efficacious treatment of hookworm and roundworm infections in dogs of all ages (infestation with the roundworm *Toxocara canis* represents a potential hazard to man as being the cause of the visceral larva migrans syndrome).

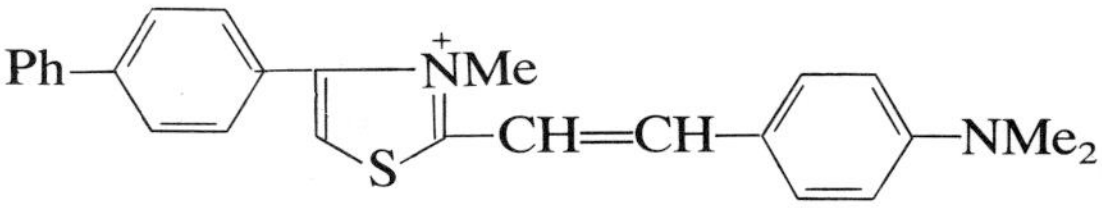

bidimazium iodide

21.**138**

6.2.2.9 Miscellaneous Nematocides. Methyridine (21.**139**) was introduced as a veterinary anthelmintic agent by ICI in 1961

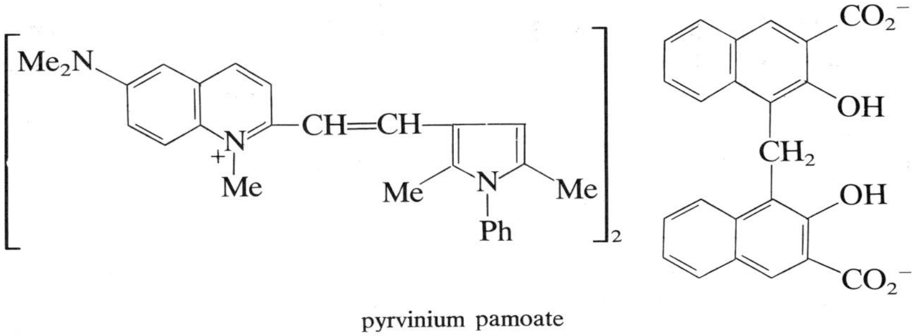

pyrvinium pamoate

21.**137**

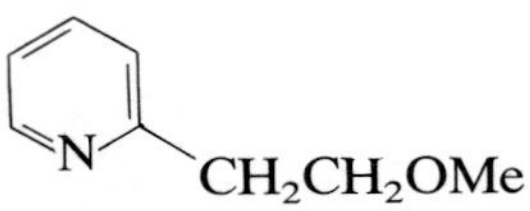

$\text{2-pyridyl}-CH_2CH_2OMe$

methyridine

21.**139**

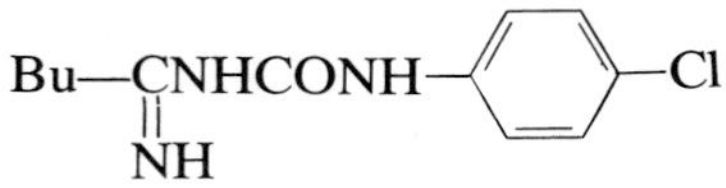

(232, 233). Although the drug has a relatively low toxicity, it is neither as active as the newer anthelmintic agents, nor does it have such a broad spectrum of activity. It appears to be a weak depolarizing blocker of neuromuscular transmission, in addition to being a somewhat weak cholinesterase inhibitor (211).

An interesting new experimental anthelmintic to emerge from the Upjohn Laboratories is *p*-toluoyl chloride phenylhydrazone (21.**140**). This compound, of unusual

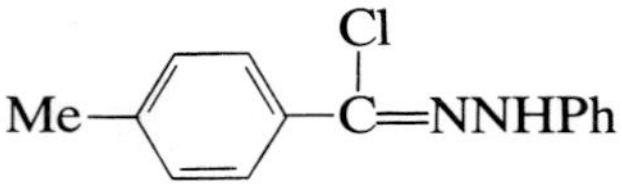

$Me-C_6H_4-C(Cl)=NNHPh$

21.**140**

structure, appears to be active against a wide range of mature and immature gastrointestinal nematodes and cestodes in sheep (234). Metabolic studies (235) have indicated that not surprisingly, the main metabolite is *p*-toluic acid phenylhydrazide (21.**141**). It is not known whether this drug

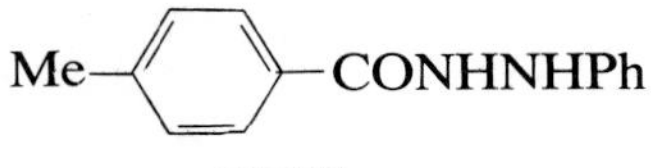

$Me-C_6H_4-CONHNHPh$

21.**141**

is of sufficiently low toxicity to be acceptable for general use as a veterinary anthelmintic.

Potent antihookworm activity in dogs was discovered in a series of imidoylureas developed by Diana and his co-workers (236). The most active analog appeared to be 1-(*p*-chlorophenyl)-3-pentanimidoylurea (21.**142**, carbantel), and this drug was also active against naturally occurring dog tapeworm infections at higher dose levels.

$Bu-C(=NH)NHCONH-C_6H_4-Cl$

carbantel

21.**142**

Finally, antinematode properties have been established for a variety of structural types as diverse as *N,N*-dimethyloctadecylamine (21.**143**, dymanthine, Thelmesan)

$Me[CH_2]_{17}NMe_2$

dymanthine

21.**143**

(237), tetrachloroethylene (particularly for human hookworm infestations) (173), and certain phenols (reviewed in Ref. 5). In addition, the flukicides rafoxanide (21.**68**) (115) and clioxanide (21.**67**) (114) are both quite effective against the nematode *Haemonchus contortus* in sheep.

6.3 Lungworm Infections

Parasitic bronchitis (husk) is an important animal infection caused by *Dictyocaulus filaria* (sheep) or *D. viviparus* (cattle) in which the late larval or early adult stages of the worm break out of the bloodstream into the air spaces of the lungs.

This disease is the one major helminth infection for which a prophylactic vaccine (prepared from X-irradiated third-stage larvae) is available. Nevertheless, diethylcarbamazine (21.**93**) is still used for the treatment of immature worms, and levamisole (21.**116**) (197) is probably the main therapeutic agent in use today. Certain of the newer benzimidazoles [e.g., fenbendazole (21.**110**) (189) and oxfendazole (21.**111**) (190)] also possess pronounced activity against *Dictyocaulus* species in addition to broad spectrum gastrointestinal nematocidal properties.

7 CONCLUSIONS

Since World War II the pharmaceutical industry has invested massive sums of money in the search for therapeutic and prophylactic agents for a very wide range of diseases of man and animals. In this time, considerable advances have been made in, for instance, the development of psychotropic agents and other drugs for the treatment of the so-called diseases of civilization.

The last decade has seen a progressive withdrawal by the pharmaceutical industry from the less profitable area of tropical parasitic diseases. Consequently, research into the great vector-borne infections such as schistosomiasis (where no drug yet exists for the mass treatment of rural populations) and filariasis (where no new clinical agent has been introduced for 30 years) is now at a scale that is causing concern at the international level.

It is essential that in the future more effort be expended on the development of safe, effective remedies for the treatment of the diseases that have remained for far too long scourges of mankind.

REFERENCES

1. N. R. Stoll, *J. Parasitol.*, **33,** 1 (1947).
2. O. D. Standen, *Fortschr. Arzneimittelforsch.*, **19,** 158 (1975).
3. P. A. J. Janssen, *Fortschr. Arzneimittelforsch.*, **18,** 191 (1974).
4. E. A. Malek, *Trop. Geogr. Med.*, **27,** 359 (1975).
5. O. D. Standen, in *Experimental Chemotherapy*, Vol. 1, R. J. Schnitzer and F. Hawking, Eds., Academic Press, New York, 1963, p. 701.
6. R. Cavier and A. Erhardt, in *International Encyclopedia of Pharmacology and Therapeutics*, Section 64, Vol. 1, R. Cavier and F. Hawking, Eds., Pergamon Press, Oxford, 1973, p. 4.
7. I. de Carneri and G. Vita, in *International Encyclopedia of Pharmacology and Therapeutics*, Section 64, Vol. 1, R. Cavier and F. Hawking, Eds., Pergamon Press, Oxford, 1973, p. 145.
8. R. Cavier, in *International Encyclopedia of Pharmacology and Therapeutics*, Section 64, Vol. 1, R. Cavier and F. Hawking, Eds., Pergamon Press, Oxford, 1973, p. 215.
9. F. Hawking, in *International Encyclopedia of Pharmacology and Therapeutics*, Section 64, Vol. 1, R. Cavier and F. Hawking, Eds., Pergamon Press, Oxford, 1973, p. 437.
10. G. Lämmler, H. Herzog, and D. Grüner, *Development of Chemotherapeutic Agents for Parasitic Diseases*, in M. Marois, Ed., North-Holland, Amsterdam, 1975, p. 157.
11. D. Düwel, *Fortschr. Arzneimittelforsch.*, **19,** 48 (1975).
12. P. J. Islip, *Fortschr. Arzneimittelforsch.*, **17,** 241 (1973).
13. R. B. Burrows, *Fortschr. Arzneimittelforsch.*, **17,** 108 (1973).
14. E. A. H. Friedheim, in *International Encyclopedia of Pharmacology and Therapeutics*, Section 64, Vol. 1, R. Cavier and F. Hawking, Eds., Pergamon Press, Oxford, 1973, p. 29.
15. N. Katz and J. Pellegrino, *Advan. Parasitol.*, **12,** 369 (1974).
16. S. Archer and A. Yarinsky, *Fortschr. Arzneimittelforsch.*, **16,** 11 (1972).
17. L. M. Werbel, *Top. Med. Chem.*, **3,** 125 (1970).
18. G. Lämmler, *Advan. Chemother.*, **3,** 155 (1968).
19. J. B. Christopherson, *Lancet*, 325 (1918).
20. A. Davis, *J. Toxicol. Environ. Health*, **1,** 191 (1975).
21. M. Ron Pedrique and N. Ercoli, *Bull. W.H.O.*, **45,** 411 (1971).
22. W. Kikuth and R. Gönnert, *Ann. Trop. Med. Parasitol.*, **42,** 256 (1948).
23. H. Mauss, *Chem. Ber.*, **81,** 19 (1948).
24. R. Gönnert, *Bull. W.H.O.*, **25,** 702 (1961).
25. H. Mauss, H. Kölling, and R. Gönnert, *Med. Chem. Abhandl. Med.-Chem. Forschungsstätten Farbenfabriken Bayer A. G.*, **5,** 185 (1956).
26. D. Rosi, G. Peruzzotti, E. W. Dennis, D. A. Berberian, H. Freele, and S. Archer, *Nature*, **208,** 1005 (1965).
27. D. Rosi, E. W. Dennis, D. A. Berberian, H. Freele, B. F. Tullar, and S. Archer, *J. Med. Chem.*, **10,** 867 (1967).
28. D. A. Berberian, H. Freele, D. Rosi, E. W. Dennis, and S. Archer, *J. Parasitol.*, **53,** 306 (1967).
29. J. Pellegrino, N. Katz, and J. F. Scherrer, *J. Parasitol.*, **53,** 55 (1967).
30. P. E. Hartman and P. B. Hulbert, *J. Toxicol. Environ. Health*, **1,** 243 (1975).
31. E. Bueding, *J. Toxicol. Environ. Health*, **1,** 329 (1975).

32. W. H. Haese, D. L. Smith, and E. Bueding, *J. Pharmacol. Exp. Ther.*, **186,** 430 (1973).
33. A. Yarinsky, H. P. Drobeck, H. Freele, J. Wiland, and K. I. Gumner, *Toxicol. Appl. Pharmacol.*, **27,** 169 (1974).
34. S. H. Rogers and E. Bueding, *Science*, **172,** 1057 (1971).
35. T. T. Chou, J. L. Bennett, C. Pert, and E. Bueding, *J. Pharmacol. Exp. Ther.*, **186,** 408 (1973).
36. A. W. Senft, D. G. Senft, G. R. Hillman, D. Polk, and S. Kryger, *Am. J. Trop. Med. Hyg.*, **25,** 832 (1976).
37. E. F. Elslager, D. F. Worth, and J. D. Howells, German Patent 1,876,086 (1969).
38. L. M. Werbel, *Israel J. Chem.*, **14,** 185 (1975).
39. P. B. Hulbert, E. Bueding, and P. E. Hartman, *Science*, **186,** 647 (1974).
40. A. C. Cuckler, A. B. Kupferberg, and N. Millman, *Antibiot. Chemother.*, **5,** 540 (1955).
41. C. R. Lambert, M. Wilhelm, H. Striebel, F. Kradolfer, and P. Schmidt, *Experientia*, **20,** 452 (1964).
42. P. Schmidt and M. Wilhelm, *Angew. Chem., Int. Ed. Engl.*, **5,** 857 (1966).
43. M. Wilhelm, F. H. Marquardt, K. Meier, and P. Schmidt, *Helv. Chim. Acta*, **49,** 2443 (1966).
44. Conference Report, Lisbon, June 1955, *Acta Trop., Suppl.*, **9,** (1966).
45. Conference Report, New York, October 1967, *Ann. N.Y. Acad. Sci.*, **160,** Art. 2, 423–946 (1969).
46. J. W. Faigle and H. Keberle, *Ann. N.Y. Acad. Sci.*, Art. 2, 544 (1969).
47. T. Connor, M. Stoeckel, and M. S. Legator, *Mutat. Res.*, **26,** 456 (1974).
48. M. S. Legator, T. H. Connor, and M. Stoeckel, *Science*, **188,** 1118 (1975).
49. H. K. Urman, O. Bulay, D. B. Clayson, and P. Shubik, *Cancer Lett.*, **1,** 69 (1975).
50. L. T. Webster, Jr., A. E. Butterworth, A. A. F. Mahmoud, E. N. Mngola, and K. S. Warren, *N. Engl. J. Med.*, **292,** 1144 (1975).
51. L. M. Werbel and J. R. Battaglia, *J. Med. Chem.*, **14,** 10 (1971).
52. P. J. Islip, British Patent 1,070,675 (1966). Activities reported by E. F. Elslager, 12th National Medicinal Chemistry Symposium of the American Chemical Society, Seattle, Wash., 1970.
53. M. Gentilini, M. Danis, G. Niel, and G. Charmot, *Bull. Soc. Pathol. Exot.*, **67,** 516 (1974).
54. P. J. Islip, M. D. Closier, M. R. Johnson, and M. C. Neville, *J. Med. Chem.*, **15,** 101 (1972).
55. R. D. Westland, L. M. Werbel, J. R. Dice, J. L. Holmes, and B. G. Zahm, *J. Med. Chem.*, **14,** 916 (1971).
56. P. J. Islip, M. D. Closier, and J. E. Weale, *J. Med. Chem.*, **16,** 1027 (1973).
57. P. J. Islip, M. D. Closier, and M. C. Neville, *J. Med. Chem.*, **16,** 1030 (1973).
58. P. J. Islip, M. D. Closier, M. C. Neville, L. M. Werbel, and D. B. Capps, *J. Med. Chem.*, **15,** 951 (1972).
59. P. J. Islip, M. D. Closier, and M. C. Neville, *J. Med. Chem.*, **17,** 207 (1974).
60. L. M. Werbel, M. B. Degnan, G. F. Harger, D. B. Capps, P. J. Islip, and M. D. Closier, *J. Med. Chem.*, **15,** 955 (1972).
61. D. B. Capps, German Patent 1,911,256 (1969).
62. E. Bueding and J. Fisher, *Mol. Pharmacol.*, **6,** 532 (1970).
63. I. Nabih, F. El-Hawary, and H. Zoorob, *J. Pharm. Sci.*, **61,** 1327 (1972).
64. C. H. Robinson, E. Bueding, and J. Fisher, *Mol. Pharmacol.*, **6,** 604 (1970).
65. E. Bueding, C. Náquira, S. Bouwman, and G. Rose, *J. Pharmacol. Exp. Ther.*, **178,** 402 (1971).
66. D. G. Erickson, J. G. Bourgeois, E. H. Sadun, and E. Bueding, *J. Pharmacol. Exp. Ther.*, **178,** 411 (1971).
67. M. M. Shahin and B. J. Kilbey, *Mutat. Res.*, **26,** 193 (1973).
68. Y. Lin, P. B. Hulbert, E. Bueding, and C. H. Robinson, *J. Med. Chem.*, **17,** 835 (1974).
69. D. W. Henry, V. H. Brown, M. Cory, J. G. Johansson, and E. Bueding, *J. Med. Chem.*, **16,** 1287 (1973).
70. P. B. Hulbert, E. Bueding, and C. H. Robinson, *J. Med. Chem.*, **16,** 72 (1973).
71. R. M. Lee, M. W. Mills, and G. S. Sach, *Experientia*, **33,** 198 (1977).
72. H. R. Stohler and A. Szente, Third International Congress of Parasitology, Munich, 1974 [Abstract E3(11), p. 1330].
73. W. J. Ross, W. B. Jamieson, and M. C. McCowen, *J. Med. Chem.*, **16,** 347 (1973).
74. J. Hellerbach and A. Szente, German Patent 2,342,931 (1974).
75. A. Ilvespää, South African Patent 72/2846 (1972).
76. H. P. Striebel, *Experientia*, **32,** 457 (1976).
77. E. Bueding, R. Batzinger, and G. Petterson, *Experientia*, **32,** 604 (1976).
78. L. M. Werbel and P. E. Thompson, *J. Med. Chem.*, **10,** 32 (1967).

79. R. P. Batzinger and E. Bueding, *J. Pharmacol. Exp. Ther.*, **200,** 1 (1977).

80. E. Bueding, C. L. Liu, and S. H. Rogers, *Brit. J. Pharmacol.*, **46,** 480 (1972).

81. World Health Organization Technical Report Series, No. 515, WHO, Geneva, 1973.

82. J. M. Jewsbury, M. J. Cooke, and M. C. Weber, *Ann. Trop. Med. Parasitol.*, **71,** 67 (1977).

83. R. Gönnert, *Bull. W.H.O.*, **25,** 702 (1961).

84. H. C. Richards and R. Foster, *Nature*, **222,** 581 (1969).

85. C. A. R. Baxter and H. C. Richards, *J. Med. Chem.*, **14,** 1033 (1971).

86. B. Kaye and N. M. Woolhouse, *Xenobiotica*, **2,** 169 (1972).

87. R. Foster and B. L. Cheetham, *Trans. Roy. Soc. Trop. Med. Hyg.*, **67,** 674 (1973).

88. R. Foster, B. L. Cheetham, and D. F. King, *Trans. Roy. Soc. Trop. Med. Hyg.*, **67,** 685 (1973).

89. Reviewed by M. J. Miller, *Fortschr. Arzneimittelforsch.*, **20,** 449 (1976).

90. V. de V. Clarke, D. M. Blair, M. C. Weber, and P. A. Garnett, *S. Afr. Med. J.*, **50,** 1867 (1976).

91. C. A. R. Baxter and H. C. Richards, *J. Med. Chem.*, **15,** 351 (1972).

92. J. Pellegrino, L. H. Pereira, and R. T. Mello, *J. Parasitol.*, **60,** 723 (1974).

93. J. Pellegrino, R. T. Mello, and L. H. Pereira, *Rev. Inst. Med. Trop. (São Paulo)*, **18,** 149 (1976).

94. J. J. Jaffe, H. M. Doremus, H. A. Dunsford, and E. Meymarian, *Am. J. Trop. Med. Hyg.*, **23,** 65 (1974).

95. J. J. Jaffe, H. M. Doremus, H. A. Dunsford, and E. Meymarian, *Am. J. Trop. Med. Hyg.*, **24,** 289 (1975).

96. J. J. Jaffe, H. M. Doremus, H. A. Dunsford, and E. Meymarian, *Am. J. Trop. Med. Hyg.*, **24,** 835 (1975).

97. E. F. Elslager, D. B. Capps, L. M. Werbel, D. F. Worth, J. E. Meisenhelder, H. Najarian, and P. E. Thompson, *J. Med. Chem.*, **6,** 217 (1963).

98. R. F. Collins, V. A. Cox, M. Davis, N. D. Edge, J. Hill, K. F. Rivett, and M. A. Rust, *Brit. J. Pharmacol.*, **29,** 248 (1967).

99. R. F. Collins and M. Davis, *J. Chem. Soc.*, 366, 873, 2196 (1966).

100. E. Bueding, E. L. Schiller, and J. G. Bourgeois, *Am. J. Trop. Med. Hyg.*, **16,** 500 (1967).

101. P. Andrews, British Society for Parasitology Meeting, Dundee, Scotland, April 1977.

102. Anonymous, *Fluke Disease*, ICI Alderley Park; quoted by G. C. Coles, *Helminthol. Abstr.*, **44,** 147 (1975).

103. G. Lämmler, *Advan. Chemother.*, **3,** 185 (1968).

104. R. Cavier and A. Erhardt, in *International Encylopedia of Pharmacology and Therapeutics*, Section 64, Vol. 1, R. Cavier and F. Hawking, Eds., Pergamon Press, Oxford, 1973, p. 1.

105. D. Posthuma and W. J. Vaatstra, *Biochem. Pharmacol.*, **20,** 1133 (1971).

106. F. Meyer and H. Meyer, in *Comparative Biochemistry of Parasites*, H. Van den Bossche, Ed., Academic Press, New York, 1972, Ch. 26.

107. A. L. Bartlet, *Brit. J. Pharmacol.*, **58,** 395 (1976).

108. H.-Y. Chang and C.-T. Yuan, *Shen Wu Hua Hsueh Yu Sheng Wu Wu Li Hsueh Pao*, **6,** 273 (1966); through *Chem. Abstr.*, **66,** 1240 (1967).

109. M. Davis and D. E. Wright, in *Veterinary Pesticides*, SCI Monograph No. 33, Society of Chemical Industry, London, 1969, p. 25.

110. J. M. S. Lucas, in *Veterinary Pesticides*, SCI Monograph No. 33, Society of Chemical Industry, London, 1969, p. 34.

111. W. Flucke, S. Wirtz, and H. Feltkamp, in *Veterinary Pesticides*, SCI Monograph No. 33, Society of Chemical Industry, London, 1969, p. 12.

112. Anonymous, *Drug Ther. Bull.*, **13,** 69 (1975).

113. A. W. J. Broome, J. P. Cairns, N. S. Crossley, W. G. M. Jones, and M. A. Stevens, *Ind. Chim. Belg.*, **32** (Spec. No.), 204 (1967).

114. A. Campbell, M. K. Martin, K. J. Farrington, A. Erdelyi, R. Johnston, P. Sorby, H. V. Whitlock, I. G. Pearson, R. C. Jones, J. A. Haigh, and C. P. DeGoosh, *Experientia*, **23,** 992 (1967).

115. H. Mrozik, H. Jones, J. Friedman, G. Schwartzkopf, R. A. Schardt, A. A. Patchett, D. R. Hoff, J. J. Yakstis, R. F. Riek, D. A. Ostlind, G. A. Plishker, R. W. Butler, A. C. Cuckler, and W. C. Campbell, *Experientia*, **25,** 883 (1969).

116. H. Koelling and I. Kurz, *Adv. Antimicrob. Antineoplast. Chemother.*, **1,** 445 (1971).

117. M. A. C. Janssen, T. T. J. M. van Offenwert, and S. Sanczuk, German Patent 2,311,229 (1973).

118. G. C. Coles and J. M. East, unpublished observations; described by G. C. Coles, *Helminthol. Abstr.*, **44,** 147 (1975).

119. V. J. Theodorides, R. C. Parish, C. H. Fuchsman, and R. M. Lee, *Vet. Rec.*, **95,** 84 (1974).

120. D. Düwel and H. Metzger, *J. Med. Chem.*, **16,** 433 (1973).

121. E. Druckrey and H. Metzger, *J. Med. Chem.*, **16,** 436 (1973).

122. Von H. Ruschig, J. König, D. Düwel, and H. Loewe, *Arzneim.-Forsch.*, **23,** 1745 (1973).
123. H. Metzger and D. Düwel, *Int. J. Biochem.*, **4,** 133 (1973).
124. J. P. Tollenaere, *J. Med. Chem.*, **16,** 791 (1973).
125. M. Harfenist, *Pestic. Sci.*, **4,** 871 (1973).
126. P. A. Kingsbury and D. ap T. Rowlands, *Brit. Vet. J.*, **128,** 235 (1972).
127. D. ap T. Rowlands, *Pestic. Sci.*, **4,** 883 (1973).
128. G. C. Coles, *Res. Vet. Sci.*, **20,** 110 (1976).
129. G. Lämmler, *Advan. Chemother.*, **3,** 207 (1968).
130. V. J. Theodorides, R. J. Gyurik, W. D. Kingsbury, and R. C. Parish, *Experientia*, **32,** 702 (1976).
131. D. Düwel, W. Dürckheimer, and M. Schorr, *Z. Tropenmed. Parasitol.*, **21,** 77 (1970).
132. M. Schorr, W. Dürckheimer, P. Klatt, G. Lämmler, G. Nesemann, and E. Schrinner, *Arzneim.-Forsch.*, **19,** 1807 (1969).
133. G. Lämmler, *Advan. Chemother.*, **3,** 223 (1968).
134. A. Davis, *Drug Treatment in Intestinal Helminthiases*, World Health Organization, Geneva, 1973, p. 93.
135. R. Gönnert, J. Johannis, E. Schraufstaetter, and R. Strufe, *Med. Chem. (Leverkusen, Ger.)*, **7,** 540 (1963).
136. D. Düwel, *Deut. Tieraeztl. Wochenschr.*, **77,** 97 (1970).
137. O. Christ, D. Düwel, P. Hajdu, H. M. Kellner, G. Kloepffer, and E. Schuetz, *Berl. Münch. Tieraeztl. Wochenschr.*, **83,** 61 (1970).
138. J. G. Gaenssler and R. K. Reinecke, *J. S. Afr. Vet. Med. Assoc.*, **41,** 211 (1970).
139. R. B. Burrows, C. J. Hatton, W. G. Lillis, and G. R. Hunt, *J. Med. Chem.*, **14,** 87 (1971).
140. M. Harfenist, R. B. Burrows, R. Baltzly, E. Pedersen, G. R. Hunt, S. Gurbaxani, J. E. D. Keeling, and O. D. Standen, *J. Med. Chem.*, **14,** 97 (1971).
141. P. Eyre, *Vet. Rec.*, **83,** 605 (1968).
142. G. Lämmler and E. Saupe, *Z. Tropenmed. Parasitol.*, **20,** 346 (1969).
143. G. S. Mutalik, R. B. Gulati, and A. K. Iqbal, *Fortschr. Arzneimittelforsch.*, **19,** 81 (1975).
144. M. A. Gemmell and G. Oudemans, *Res. Vet. Sci.*, **19,** 217 (1975).
145. M. C. Seidel, E. E. Kilbourn, D. L. Peardon, R. D. Tetzlaff, E. D. Weiler, and W. D. Weir, in *20th World Veterinary Congress Summaries*, Vol. 2, Thessalonki, Greece, 1975, p. 805; through *Vet. Bull.* (London), **45,** 904 (1975).
146. D. K. Hass and J. A. Collins, *Am. J. Vet. Res.*, **35,** 103 (1974).
147. H. J. Saz and O. L. Lescure, *Mol. Pharmacol.*, **4,** 402 (1968).
148. H. Thomas and P. Andrews, *Pestic. Sci.*, **8,** 556 (1977).
149. H. Thomas and R. Gönnert, *Res. Vet. Sci.*, **24,** 20 (1978).
150. W. C. Campbell, R. O. McCracken, and L. S. Blair, *J. Parasitol.*, **61,** 844 (1975).
151. Numbers, 21–6.
152. E. F. Elslager, *Forschr. Arzneimittelforsch.*, **18,** 142 (1974).
153. G. Lämmler, *Pestic. Sci.*, **8,** 563 (1977).
154. E. A. H. Friedheim and R. Cavier, *Bull. Soc. Pathol. Exot.*, **66,** 531 (1973).
155. E. A. H. Friedheim, *Bull. W.H.O.*, **50,** 572 (1974).
156. S. Kushner, L. M. Brancone, R. I. Hewitt, W. L. McEwen, Y. Subbarow, H. W. Stewart, R. J. Turner, and J. J. Denton, *J. Org. Chem.*, **13,** 144 (1948).
157. S. Kushner, L. M. Brancone, R. I. Hewitt, W. L. McEwen, Y. Subbarow, H. W. Stewart, R. J. Turner, and J. J. Denton, *Ann. N.Y. Acad. Sci.*, **50,** 120 (1948).
158. A. D. M. Bryceson, D. A. Warrell, and H. M. Pope, *Brit. Med. J.*, **1,** 742 (1977).
159. D. W. Gibson, D. H. Connor, H. L. Brown, H. Fuglsang, J. Anderson, B. O. L. Duke, and A. A. Buck, *Am. J. Trop. Med. Hyg.*, **25,** 74 (1976).
160. P. N. Natarajan, V. Zaman, and T. S. Yeoh, *Int. J. Parasitol.*, **3,** 803 (1973).
161. G. Lämmler, H. Herzog, and H. R. Schütze, *Bull. W.H.O.*, **44,** 757 (1971).
162. P. A. Sturm, D. W. Henry, P. E. Thompson, J. B. Zeigler, and J. W. McCall, *J. Med. Chem.*, **17,** 481 (1974).
163. R. Saxena, R. N. Iyer, N. Anand, R. K. Chatterjee, and A. B. Sen, *J. Pharm. Pharmacol.*, **22,** 307 (1970).
164. W. Raether and G. Lämmler, *Ann. Trop. Med. Parasitol.*, **65,** 107 (1971).
165. K. Maertens and M. Wery, *Trans. Roy. Soc. Trop. Med. Hyg.*, **69,** 359 (1975).
166. A. Suardi, unpublished observations; quoted in Ref. 167.
167. J. W. McCall and H. H. Crouthamel, *J. Parasitol.*, **62,** 844 (1976).
168. G. Lämmler and D. Grüner, *Tropenmed. Parasitol.*, **26,** 359 (1975).
169. A. O. Lucas, S. O. Oduntan, and H. M. Gilles, *Ann. N.Y. Acad. Sci.*, **160,** 729 (1969).
170. A. Z. Shafei, *J. Trop. Med. Hyg.*, **79,** 197 (1976).
171. D. S. Pardanani, V. D. Trivedi, L. G. Joshi, J.

Daulatram, and J. S. Nandi, *Ann. Trop. Med. Parasitol.*, **71,** 49 (1977).

172. R. Muller, *Trans. Roy. Soc. Trop. Med. Hyg.*, **65,** 843 (1971).

173. A. Davis, *Drug Treatment in Intestinal Helminthiases*, World Health Organization, Geneva, 1973, p. 13.

174. J. W. McFarland, *Fortschr. Arzneimittelforsch.*, **16,** 157 (1972).

175. H. D. Brown, A. R. Matzuk, I. R. Ilves, L. H. Peterson, S. A. Harris, L. H. Sarett, J. R. Egerton, J. J. Yakstis, W. C. Campbell, and A. C. Cuckler, *J. Am. Chem. Soc.*, **83,** 1764 (1961).

176. R. K. Prichard, *Int. J. Parasitol.*, **3,** 409 (1973).

177. G. G. Van Arman and W. C. Campbell, *Tex. Rep. Biol. Med.*, **33,** 303 (1975).

178. L. H. P. Jones, D. D. Leaver, and A. A. Milne, *Res. Vet. Sci.*, **6,** 316 (1965).

179. M. H. Fisher and A. Lusi, *J. Med. Chem.*, **15,** 982 (1972).

180. M. H. Fisher, G. Schwartzkopf, Jr., and D. R. Hoff, *J. Med. Chem.*, **15,** 1168 (1972).

181. D. J. Tocco, R. P. Buhs, H. D. Brown, A. R. Matzuk, H. E. Mertel, R. E. Harman, and N. R. Trenner, *J. Med. Chem.*, **7,** 399 (1964).

182. D. R. Hoff, M. H. Fisher, R. J. Bochis, A. Lusi, F. Waksmunski, J. R. Egerton, J. J. Yakstis, A. C. Cuckler, and W. C. Campbell, *Experientia*, **26,** 550 (1970).

183. P. Actor, E. L. Anderson, C. J. DiCuollo, R. J. Ferlauto, J. R. E. Hoover, J. F. Pagano, L. R. Ravin, S. F. Scheidy, R. J. Stedman, and V. J. Theodorides, *Nature*, **215,** 321 (1967).

184. M. Lapras, G. Lourge, J. Gastellu, B. Regnier, P. Delatour, J. P. Deschanel, and M. Lombard, *Cornell Vet.*, **64,** 457 (1974).

185. J. P. Brugmans, D. C. Thienpont, I. van Wijngaarden, O. F. J. Vanparijs, V. L. Schuermans, and H. L. Lauwers, *J. Am. Med. Assoc.*, **217,** 313 (1971).

186. M. S. Wolfe and J. M. Wershing, *J. Am. Med. Assoc.*, **230,** 1408 (1974).

187. M. J. Miller, I. M. Krupp, M. D. Little, and C. Santos, *J. Am. Med. Assoc.*, **230,** 1412 (1974).

188. V. J. Theodorides, J. Chang, C. J. DiCuollo, G. M. Grass, R. C. Parish, and G. C. Scott, *Brit. Vet. J.*, **129,** xcvii (1973).

189. C. Baeder, H. Bähr, O. Christ, D. Düwel, H.-M. Kellner, R. Kirsch, H. Loewe, E. Schultes, E. Schütz, and H. Westen, *Experientia*, **30,** 753 (1974).

90. E. A. Averkin, C. C. Beard, C. A. Dvorak, J. A. Edwards, J. H. Fried, J. G. Kilian, R. A. Schiltz, T. P. Kistner, J. H. Drudge, E. T. Lyons, M. L. Sharp, and R. M. Corwin, *J. Med. Chem.*, **18,** 1164 (1975).

191. Hoechst AG, German Patent 2,356,258 (1975).

192. H. Loewe and J. Urbanietz, *Pestic. Sci.*, **8,** 544 (1977).

193. D. A. Eichler, *Brit. Vet. J.*, **129,** 533 (1973).

194. H. A. Selling, J. M. Vonk, and A. K. Sijpesteijn, *Chem. Ind.* (London), 1625 (1970).

195. D. Thienpont, O. F. J. Vanparijs, A. H. M. Raeymaekers, J. Vandenberk, P. J. A. Demoen, F. T. N. Allewijn, R. P. H. Marsboom, C. J. E. Niemegeers, K. H. L. Schellekens, and P. A. J. Janssen, *Nature*, **209,** 1084 (1966).

196. A. H. M. Raeymaekers, F. T. N. Allewijn, J. Vandenberk, P. J. A. Demoen, T. T. T. Van Offenwert, and P. A. J. Janssen, *J. Med. Chem.*, **9,** 545 (1966).

197. P. A. J. Janssen, *Fortschr. Arzneimittelforsch.*, **20,** 347 (1976).

198. H. Van den Bossche and P. A. J. Janssen, *Life Sci.*, **6,** 1781 (1967).

199. H. Van den Bossche and P. A. J. Janssen, *Biochem. Pharmacol.*, **18,** 35 (1969).

200. H. Van Belle, *Biochim. Biophys. Acta*, **289,** 158 (1972).

201. L. F. Miller and R. E. Bambury, *J. Med. Chem.*, **15,** 415 (1972).

202. J. E. Lynch and B. Nelson, *J. Parasitol.*, **45,** 659 (1959).

203. W. C. Austin, W. Courtney, J. C. Danilewicz, D. H. Morgan, L. H. Conover, H. L. Howes, Jr., J. E. Lynch, J. W. McFarland, R. L. Cornwell, and V. J. Theodorides, *Nature*, **212,** 1273 (1966).

204. J. W. McFarland, L. H. Conover, H. L. Howes, Jr., J. E. Lynch, D. R. Chisholm, W. C. Austin, R. L. Cornwell, J. C. Danilewicz, W. Courtney, and D. H. Morgan, *J. Med. Chem.*, **12,** 1066 (1969).

205. J. W. McFarland and H. L. Howes, Jr., *J. Med. Chem.*, **12,** 1079 (1969).

206. J. W. McFarland and H. L. Howes, Jr., *J. Med. Chem.*, **13,** 109 (1970).

207. J. W. McFarland, H. L. Howes, Jr., L. H. Conover, J. E. Lynch, W. C. Austin, and D. H. Morgan, *J. Med. Chem.*, **13,** 113 (1970).

208. W. C. Austin, R. L. Cornwell, R. M. Jones, and M. Robinson, *J. Med. Chem.*, **15,** 281 (1972).

209. J. W. McFarland and H. L. Howes, Jr., *J. Med. Chem.*, **15,** 365 (1972).

210. E.-L. Lee, N. Iyngkaran, A. W. Grieve, M. J. Robinson, and A. S. Dissanaike, *Am. J. Trop. Med. Hyg.*, **25,** 563 (1976).

211. P. Eyre, *J. Pharm. Pharmacol.*, **22,** 26 (1970).
212. M. L. Aubry, P. Cowell, M. J. Davey, and S. Shevde, *Brit. J. Pharmacol.*, **38,** 332 (1970).
213. S. O. A. Bamgbose, V. O. Marquis, and L. A. Salako, *Brit. J. Pharmacol.*, **47,** 117 (1973).
214. F. C. Copp, O. D. Standen, J. Scarnell, D. A. Rawes, and R. B. Burrows, *Nature*, **181,** 183 (1958).
215. D. A. Rawes and P. A. Clapham, *Vet. Rec.*, **73,** 1755 (1961).
216. D. A. Rawes and P. A. Clapham, *Vet. Rec.*, **74,** 383 (1962).
217. A. I. Krotov, T. K. Konopleva, M. B. Braude, and A. F. Bekhli, *Med. Parazitol. Parazit. Bolezn.*, **38,** 80 (1969); through *Helminthol. Abstr. Ser. A*, **39,** 3443 (1970).
218. J. Del Castillo, T. A. Morales, and V. Sanchez, *Nature*, **200,** 706 (1963).
219. J. Del Castillo, W. C. De Mello, and T. Morales, *Brit. J. Pharmacol. Chemother.*, **22,** 463 (1964).
220. H. J. Saz and E. Bueding, *Pharmacol. Rev.*, **18,** 871 (1966).
221. P. K. Sasi and R. K. Raj, *Experientia*, **31,** 1261 (1975).
222. Various authors in E. Jucker, Ed., *Fortschr. Arzneimittelforsch.*, **19** 2–175 (1975).
223. H. G. Sen, *Acta Trop.*, **33,** 101 (1976).
224. D. K. Hass, *Top. Med. Chem.*, **3,** 171 (1970).
225. J. G. Morales, R. R. Whetstone, D. W. Stoutamire, and D. K. Hass, *J. Med. Chem.*, **15,** 1225 (1972).
226. J. B. Carr, P. Kirby, M. H. Goodrow, H. G. Durham, D. K. Hass, and J. J. Boudreau, *J. Med. Chem.*, **15,** 1231 (1972).
227. K. Pilgram and D. K. Hass, *J. Med. Chem.*, **18,** 1204 (1975).
228. R. J. Hart and R. M. Lee, *Exp. Parasitol.*, **18,** 332 (1966).
229. M. C. MacCowen, M. E. Callender, and M. C. Brandt, *Am. J. Trop. Med. Hyg.*, **6,** 894 (1957).
230. J. K. Weston, P. E. Thompson, J. W. Reinertson, R. A. Fisken, and T. F. Reutner, *J. Pharmacol. Exp. Ther.*, **107,** 315 (1953).
231. J. Berger, M. H. Biggs, R. B. Burrows, J. E. D. Keeling, P. A. Kingsbury, and A. P. Phillips, Third International Congress of Parasitology, Munich, 1974 [Abstract E7(46), p. 1428].
232. A. W. J. Broome and N. Greenhalgh, *Nature*, **189,** 59 (1961).
233. A. W. J. Broome and N. Greenhalgh, *Brit. J. Pharmacol.*, **17,** 321 (1961).
234. S. D. Folz, D. L. Rector, and S. Geng, *J. Parasitol.*, **62,** 281 (1976).
235. P. S. Jaglan, R. E. Gosline, and A. W. Neff, *J. Agr. Food Chem.*, **24,** 659 (1976).
236. G. D. Diana, A. Yarinsky, E. S. Zalay, D. A. Berberian, and S. Schalit, *J. Med. Chem.*, **12,** 791 (1969).
237. R. Cavier and Y. Piton, *Thérapie*, **19,** 265, 947 (1964).

CHAPTER TWENTY-TWO

Antifungal Agents

EUGENE D. WEINBERG

Department of Biology and Program in Medical Sciences,
Indiana University
Bloomington, Indiana 47401, USA

CONTENTS

1 INTRODUCTION

Fungi are heterotrophic microorganisms that are distinguished from algae by lack of photosynthetic ability. They differ from protozoa by lack of motility, possession of chitinous cell walls, and ease of culture on simple media, and from bacteria by greater size and possession of such intracellular structures as nuclear membranes and mitochondria. As with bacteria, fungi occupy an amazing variety and number of ecological niches. They fulfill a critical function in nature by converting such polymers as lignin, chitin, and cellulose into humus. But this "destructive" function is quite undesirable when the substrates

Table 22.1 Pathogenic Fungi of Humans

Group	Etiologic Agent	Disease Produced	Useful Drugs
1	Dermatophytes (*Epidermophyton* spp. *Microsporum* spp., *Trichophyton* spp.	Athlete's foot; ringworm of skin, hair, nails; tinea	Clotrimazole, griseofulvin, haloprogin, miconazole, thiabendazole, tolnaftate
2	*Candida albicans* and related species	Candidiasis (candidosis) of skin, nails, mucous membranes	Clotrimazole, gentian violet, haloprogin, miconazole, nystatin
3	*Aspergillus* spp.	Aspergillosis	Amphotericin B
	Blastomyces brasiliensis	South American blastomycosis	Amphotericin B
	B. dermatitidis	North American blastomycosis	Amphotericin B, 2-hydroxystilbamidine
	Candida albicans and related species	Candidiasis (candidosis)	Amphotericin B
	Cladosporium spp., *Fonsecea* spp., *Phialophora* spp.	Chromoblastomycosis	Amphotericin B (remove infected tissue)
	Coccidioides immitis	Coccidioidomycosis	Amphotericin B (use no drug in primary infection)
	Cryptococcus neoformans	Cryptococcosis	Amphotericin B, 5-fluorocytosine
	Histoplasma capsulatum	Histoplasmosis	Amphotericin B (use no drug in primary infection)
	Mucor spp., *Rhizopus* spp.	Mucormycosis	Amphotericin B (remove infected tissue)
	Prototheca spp.	Protothecosis	Amphotericin B
	Rhinosporidium seeberi	Rhinosporidiosis	Amphotericin B (remove infected tissue)
	Sporotrichum schenkii	Sporotrichosis	Amphotericin B (in disseminated disease), potassium iodide (in localized skin lesions)

under attack are contained in fabrics, electrical insulation, leather, wooden posts, or foodstuffs. Fortunately, relatively few fungi cause infectious disease in animals or humans; pathogens of the humans are listed in Table 22.1.

The word *fungi* is a general term that includes both yeasts and molds. The former are spherical, oval, or elongated cells that usually reproduce by budding and form mucoid colonies on agar media. The latter consist of elongated branching cells or *hyphae*, tangled masses of hyphae constitute *mycelia*, and these appear as dry colonies on agar surfaces or in natural habitats. Some yeastlike fungi can be induced, by environmental or nutritional factors, to grow in a filamentous manner; conversely, some molds may be stimulated to grow in a yeastlike manner.

The true fungi are grouped into four classes: Phycomycetes (algalike), Ascomycetes (sac-fungi), Basidiomycetes (mushrooms), and Dueteromycetes (imperfect fungi). The fourth class contains many of the 50,000–100,000 fungal species; when a sexual reproductive stage is demonstrated for a species in this group, the organism is reassigned to its proper class.

In addition to true fungi, an order of bacteria termed Actinomycetales is sometimes included in the science of mycology. Cells of species in this order can grow into branching filaments and produce on agar surfaces dry colonies that superficially resemble mold colonies. However the dimensions of the cells are similar to those of bacteria rather than fungi, the cells contain neither nuclear membranes nor mitochondria, and the "hyphae" tend to fragment into bacillary elements. Moreover, strains of Actinomycetales are susceptible to antibacterial rather than to antifungal chemotherapeutic agents. Members of the order are important in humus formation, and a number of clinically useful antibiotics are produced by specific strains of these bacteria.

2 FUNGAL DISEASES

Many infections of plants are caused by fungi; the lesions produced include various types of blights, mildews, leafspots, and galls, and such systemic diseases as rusts and smuts. In contrast to plants, far fewer infectious diseases of animals and humans are caused by fungi than are initiated by bacteria or viruses. Mycotic infections of humans are conveniently divided into three groups (Table 22.1). (1) The dermatophytoses consist of contagious superficial skin infections that are limited to the epidermal region. (2) Candidiasis (candidosis, moniliasis) can affect the skin and mucous membranes, and occasionally becomes systemic; the disease is not contagious except in the case of neonates who have acquired the fungus from their mother or other attendants. (3) The subcutaneous, pulmonary, lymphatic, and systemic mycoses are not contagious; they are caused by free-living saprophytes that invade the skin, lungs, lymphatic tissue, and various organs of susceptible hosts who have accidentally been in contact with the fungal environment. The actinomycoses resemble the third group of mycotic diseases in that they are not contagious and cause subcutaneous, pulmonary, lymphatic, and systemic infections.

Severe toxic and hemorrhagic diseases can occur in animals and humans after ingestion of grains and nuts in which *saprophytic* fungi have grown and produced toxins; likewise, hemolytic, neurotoxic, and gastrotoxic diseases are associated with ingestion of certain types of *saprophytic* mushrooms. Fortunately, the pathogenic fungi listed in Table 22.1 produce no known toxins in infected hosts. Often, however, a marked hypersensitivity to chemical components of the invading organism is induced. The lesions caused by dermatophytes that utilize dead cornified hair, skin, and nails are essentially allergic reactions to the fungi and their metabolites.

The typical tissue reaction in the systemic mycotic and actinomycotic diseases is a chronic granuloma with necrosis and abscess formation.

The discovery that specific fungi are the etiological agents of specific infectious diseases preceded by three decades the work of Pasteur and Koch on pathogenic bacteria. Nevertheless, medical mycology has not received as much attention as have other areas of medical microbiology, and at present there exist neither clinically available vaccines nor useful antisera for mycotic diseases. Moreover, in the case of diseases of group (3), there is not presently a sufficiently diverse selection of safe and effective chemotherapeutic agents (Table 22.1).

The need for more and better antifungal agents is becoming more critical because of the increasing detection of systemic mycoses in patients suffering from debilitating diseases such as neoplasias and in persons on long-term total parenteral nutrition. Additionally, conditions that depress cell-mediated immunity, such as the latter half of pregnancy, excessive use of corticosteroids, carcinostats, or immunosuppressives, or defects in thymus gland tissue, result in marked enhancement of susceptibility to serious fungal disease. For example, systemic mycoses have been found in 61% of patients dying with acute leukemia and in 45% of deaths in renal transplant recipients (1).

3 ANTIFUNGAL SUBSTANCES

The screening tests for *in vitro* and *in vivo* antifungal action are quite similar to those employed for antibacterial potency. It is not difficult in the *in vitro* procedures to discover a reasonable number and variety of synthetic and natural compounds that are active in small quantities. But many of the substances detected by such screening must be eliminated from practical consideration after examination in systems *in vivo.* In the case of prospective plant fungistats, such factors as particle size, combination with suitable wetting agents, and resistance to weathering and to microbial deterioration are of great importance (2). In the case of both plant and animal fungistats, toxicity as well as inability to penetrate to the site of fungal invasion can cause new candidates to be eliminated.

With animal or human infections, the test substance may appear to be inactive because the hosts are unable to provide sufficient natural defense factors to prevent relapses after the substance has been metabolized. The route of introduction of the test substance can also be critical; for

Table 22.2 Examples of Trade Names of Antifungal Drugs

Generic Name	Trade Names
Amphotericin B	Fungizone
Clotrimazole	Canesten, Lotrimin
5-Fluorocytosine	Ancobon, Flucytosine
Griseofulvin	Fulcin, Fulvicin, Grifulvin, Grisactin, Grisovin, Gris-Peg, Lamoryl, Likuden, Poncyl, Spirofulvin, Sporostatin
Haloprogin	Halotex, Polik
Miconazole	Micatin, Monistat
Nystatin	Fungicidin, Moronal, Mycostatin, Nystan, Nilstat, O-V Statin
Pimaricin	Myprozine, Natamycin, Pimifucin, Tennecetin
Thiabendazole	Mintezol
Tolnaftate	Focusan, Hi-Alazin, Sporiline, Tinactin, Tinaderm, Tonoftal

example, griseofulvin is active against dermatophytes in systemic, but not topical, administration. Each of the numerous polyene antibiotics has high *in vitro* activity against both dermatophytes and systemic fungal pathogens. Despite structural similarity, however, they vary widely in effectiveness *in vivo*, presumably because of differences in solubility, diffusability, toxicity for host cells, and inactivation by serum components.

3.1 Synthetic Compounds

3.1.1 METAL-CONTAINING MOLECULES, CHELATING AGENTS, AND ANILINE DYES. Such heavy metal ions as Ag^{+}, Hg^{2+}, Cu^{2+}, and Zn^{2+} have long been used as fungitoxicants in agriculture and also in topical ointments for dermatophytoses (2). Most of the toxic metals are contained in groups IB, IIB, and VIII of the periodic table of the elements; it is assumed that these metals combine with functional groups on the surface of enzymes and, in high concentrations, may actually precipitate proteins. A combination of a heavy metal atom with an organic molecule sometimes increases the antifungal action and, more important, the selective toxicity of the metal (2). Examples of antifungal compounds that are combined with an atom of a heavy metal include zinc (or iron) dimethyldithiocarbamate (22.**1**), 5-chloro,7-iodo,8-hydroxyquinoline (22.**2**), chloroiodoquin), sodium ethylmercurithiosalicylate (22.**3**), zinc caprylate (22.**4**), zinc (or copper) 10-undecylenate (22.**5**), and pyrithione (22.**6**). The thiocarbamates are employed against plant fungal pathogens and the others in animal and

$((CH_3)_2NCS_2)_2Zn$

22.**1**

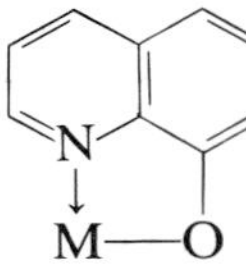

22.**2**

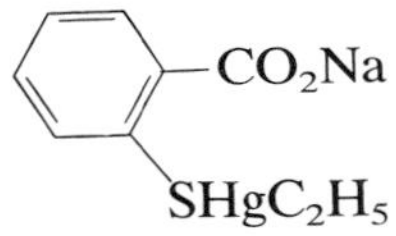

22.**3**

$(CH_3(CH_2)_6CO_2)_2Zn$

22.**4**

$(CH_2{=}CH(CH_2)_8CO_2)_2Zn$

22.**5**

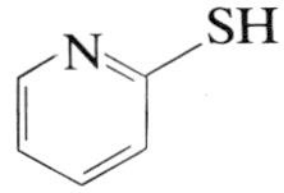

22.**6**

human dermatophytoses. Although no specific metal is included in the chloroiodoquin structure, it is generally believed that one atom of copper is required per molecule of ligand for maximum fungitoxicity. The atoms of heavy metals needed for activity of 8-hydroxyquinolines are obtained from the environment; in metal-free media, the compounds are inactive (3). In the case of pyrithione, two molecules are combined with one atom of zinc.

Among chelating agents with considerable *in vitro* antifungal potency are such substituted biguanides as N^1N^5-di(3,4-dichlorobenzyl)biguanide (22.**7**) and N^1-γ-lauroxypropyl biguanide (22.**8**) (4). 1,1′-Hexamethylene bis (5-[*p*]chlorophenyl]-biguanide) (22.**9**) is employed as a topical antiseptic. Such triphenylmethane dyes as malachite green (22.**10**), gentian violet (22.**11**), methylrosaniline chloride), and basic fuchsin (pararosaniline chloride) have been employed in topical therapy of dermatophytoses as well as of candidiasis of the skin and mucous membranes.

3.1.2 PHENOLICS AND DIAMIDINES. Many phenols and compounds with phenolic groups have antifungal potency. In the treatment of superficial mycoses, the simple phenols are employed for their keratolytic as well as fungistatic action. Among the numerous compounds that have been used externally for mycotic infections are phenol, phenylmercuric nitrate, cresol, *m*-cresyl acetate, benzoic acid, *p*-hydroxybenzoic acid, salicyclic acid, salicylanilide (22.**13**), 5-chlorosalicylanilide, 5,5′-dibromosalicil, 3,5-dibromosalicylaldehyde (22.**14**), ethyl vanillate

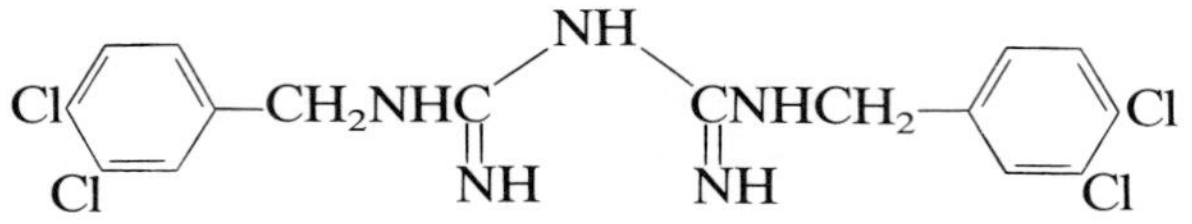

22.7

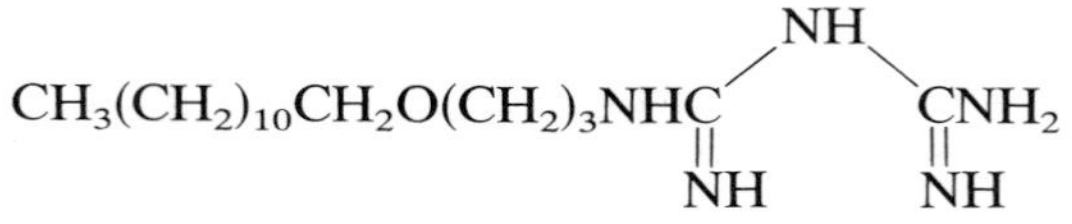

$CH_3(CH_2)_{10}CH_2O(CH_2)_3NHC(=NH)NHC(=NH)NH_2$

22.8

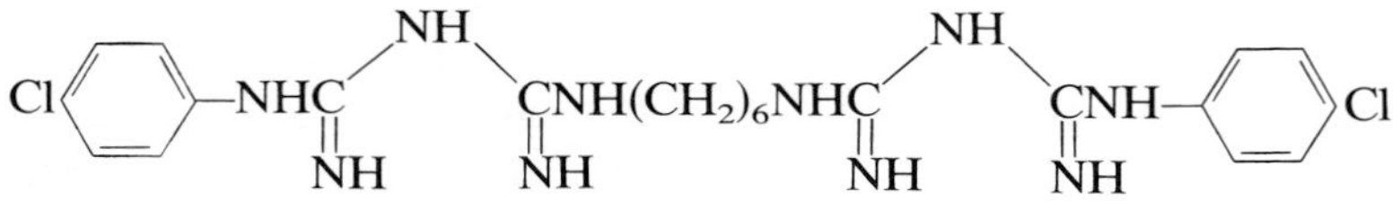

22.9

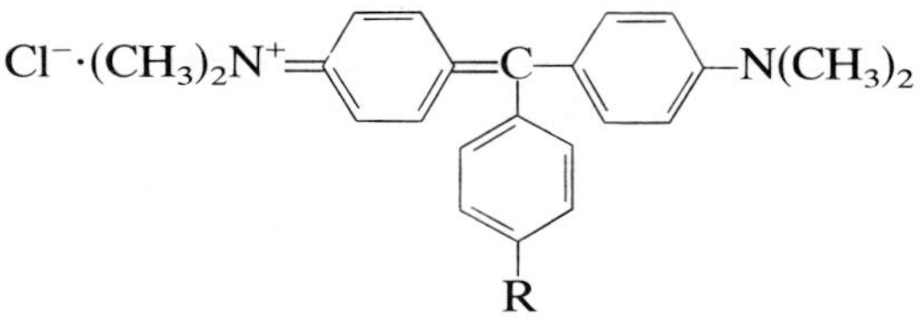

22.10 R = H
22.11 R = $N(CH_3)_2$

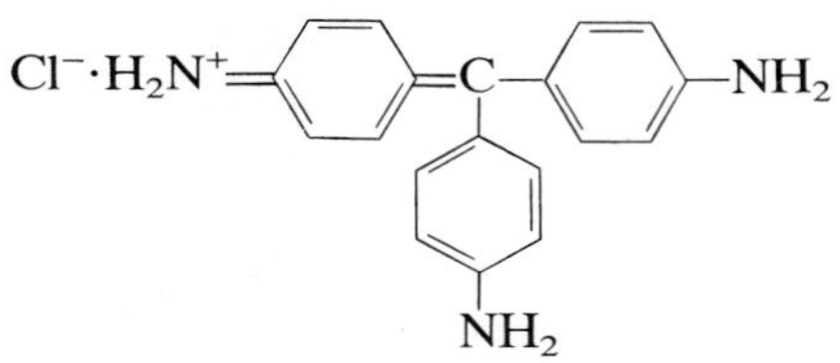

22.12

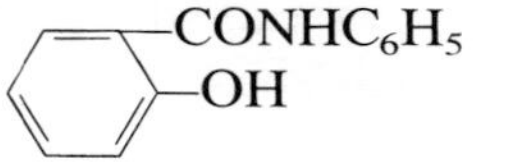

22.13

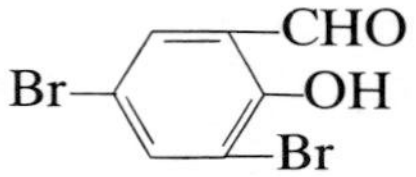

22.14

(22.**15**), pyrogallol triacetate (22.**16**), 3-iodo-2-propynyl-2,4,5-trichlorophenylether (22.**17**), haloprogin, 1,8-dihydroxyanthranol (22.**18**), and tetrachlorobenzoquinone (22.**19**). Various bisphenols and thiobisphenols are also effective fungistats in preparations for topical use.

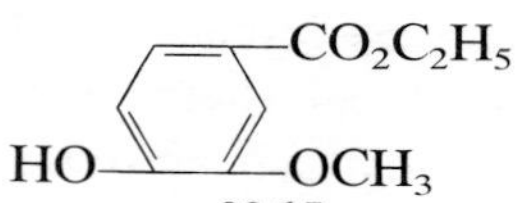

22.15

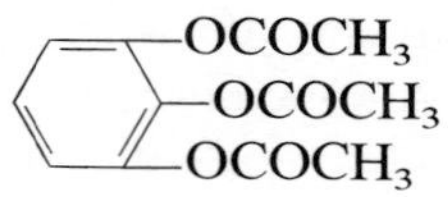

22.16

Several bisamidines (e.g., stilbamidine, propamidine, pentamidine) are antifungal *in vitro*; the isoethionate of 2-hydroxystilbamidine (22.**20**) has been successfully employed in patients with North

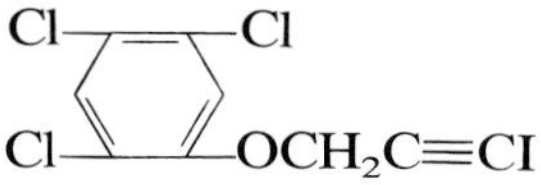

22.17

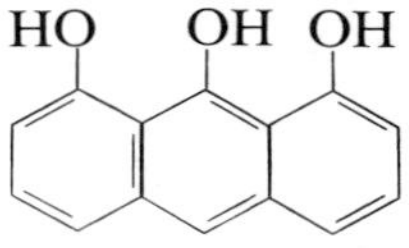

22.18

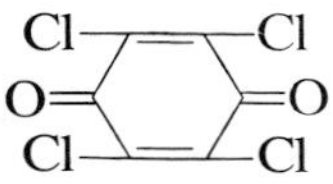

22.19

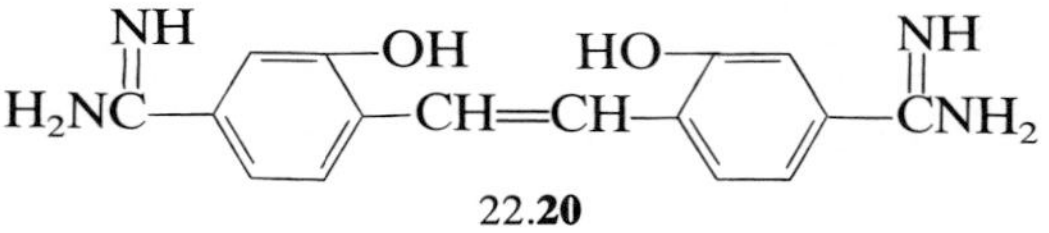

22.20

American blastomycosis (5). It is less toxic than amphotericin B but does not have the consistent therapeutic effectiveness of the latter.

3.1.3 SULFUR-CONTAINING MOLECULES. A variety of organic compounds that contain divalent sulfur attached to carbon atoms have *in vitro* fungistatic action, and many of these have been employed in topical therapy of dermatophytoses. Among these are dithiocarbamates such as the dimethyl derivative (22.**1**), thiurams such as tetraethylthiuram disulfide (22.**21**), and benzothiazoles such as the 6-(β-diethylaminoethoxy-2-dimethylamino derivative (22.**22**) (6, 7).

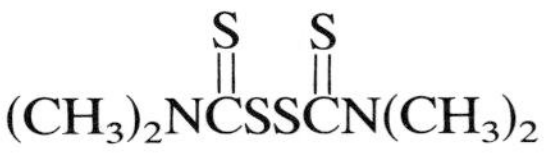

$$(CH_3)_2NC(=S)SSC(=S)N(CH_3)_2$$

22.**21**

$$(C_2H_5)_2NCH_2CH_2O\text{–[benzothiazole]–}N(CH_3)_2$$

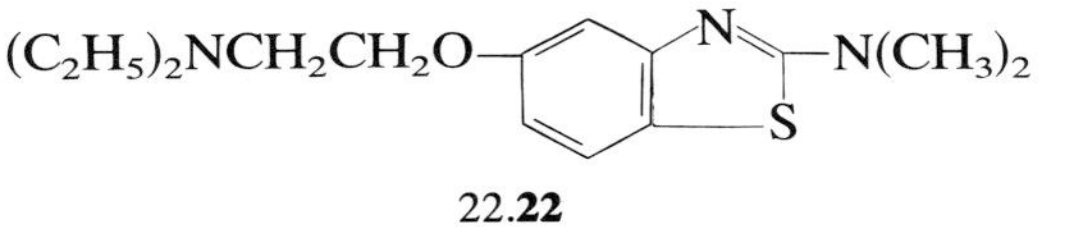

22.**22**

A widely used compound with unusually high *in vitro* and *in vivo* activity against the dermatophytes (but essentially no action against most other fungi or bacteria) is the *O*-2-naphthyl ester of *N*-dimethylthiocarbanilic acid ((22.**23**) (tolnaftate). Good potency is maintained if the aromatic methyl

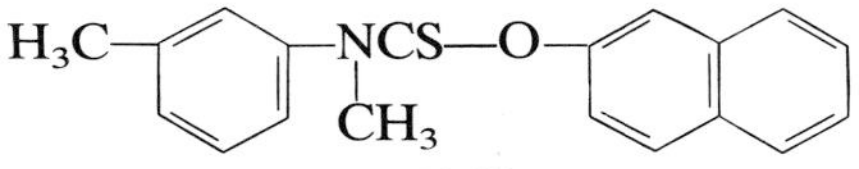

$$H_3C\text{–}C_6H_4\text{–}N(CH_3)CS\text{–}O\text{–}C_{10}H_7$$

22.**23**

group is removed or replaced by hydroxy or methoxy, or if the entire tolyl group is replaced by an α- or β-naphthyl substituent. Activity is lost if the aromatic methyl group is replaced by halogen, or by a carboxyl or nitro group (8). In clinical practice, the efficacy of tolnaftate is comparable to that of haloprogin; however the latter has the advantage of being effective also against candidal lesions (9).

3.1.4 IMIDAZOLES AND PYRIMIDINES. Imidazoles with good clinical activity in dermatophytoses and nonsystemic candidiasis include 2,4-dichloro-β(2,4-dichlorobenzyloxyphenethyl)imidazole (22.**24**) miconazole and bisphenyl (2-chlorophenyl)-1-imidazole methane (22.**25**), (clotrimazole) (9,10,11). A third imidazole with good clinical efficacy in topical therapy of dermatophytic infections is 2-(4-thiazolyl)benzimadazole (22.**26**), (thiabendazole) (12). Miconazole and clotrimazole also have been administered to a limited number of patients with systemic mycotic infection. Unfortunately, systemic use of miconazole has been accompanied by reversible thrombocytosis and anemia (13) and of clotrimazole by severe gastrointestinal disturbances (14). Inasmuch as miconazole impairs membrane functions (15), such side effects on the host are not surprising.

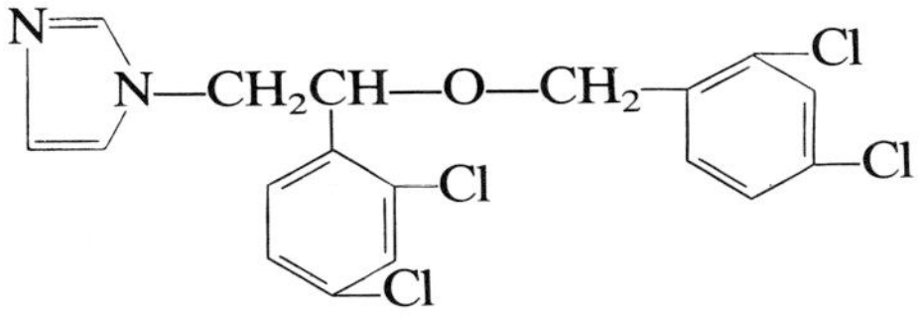

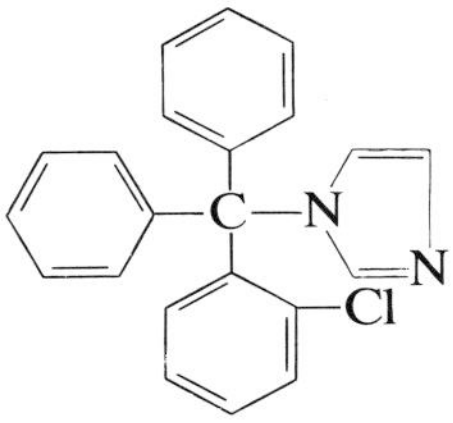

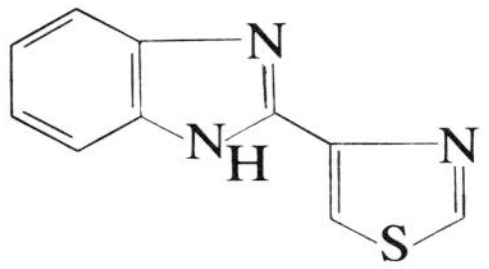

$$\text{Imidazolyl–}N\text{–}CH_2CH(C_6H_3Cl_2)\text{–}O\text{–}CH_2\text{–}C_6H_3Cl_2$$

22.**24**

22.**25**

22.**26**

The pyrimidine 5-fluorocytosine (22.**27**) is effective in some cases of systemic candidiasis and cryptococcosis (9). The drug is particularly useful in urinary tract candidiasis because it can be given orally, has few side effects, and it is excreted in urine at high levels (16). However, as many as 85% of yeast strains are resistant to the compound (17). The culture medium employed to determine minimal inhibitory concentrations must be free of complex ingredients that might contain cytosine of uridine; such pyrimidines will interfere with activity of the drug (9). Combinations of 5-fluorocytosine and amphotericin B are

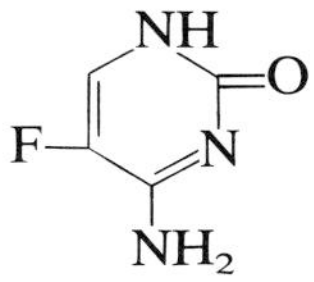

22.**27**

synergistic in both *in vitro* and *in vivo* systems (16).

3.2 Natural Products

3.2.1 ANTIBACTERIAL ANTIBIOTICS. The antibiotics that have significant *in vitro* and *in vivo* antibacterial potency are not usually active against true fungi. Indeed, by supressing indigenous bacterial flora, these compounds have sometimes permitted excess growth of *Candida* with the subsequent development of intestinal or vaginal candidiasis. As expected, the antibacterial antibiotics are effective in the "mycotic" diseases caused by strains of Actinomycetales. Curiously, streptomycin is active also against a group of plant fungal pathogens contained in Oomycetes; the hyphal walls of these organisms are cellulosic and are permeable to the antiobiotic, whereas other fungi possess chitinous cell walls that do not absorb the compound (18).

3.2.2 GRISEOFULVIN (22.**28**) Although this antibiotic, a product of *Penicillium*

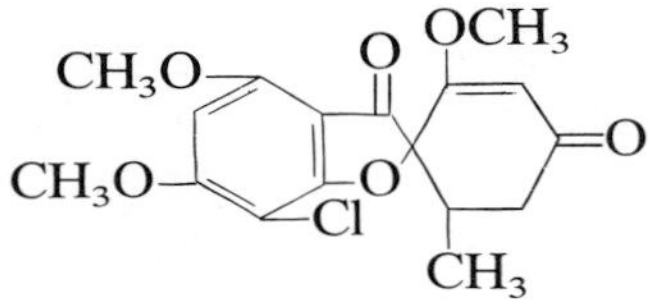

CH_3O OCH_3 O CH_3O O Cl O CH_3

22.**28**

griseofulvum was discovered in 1939, its antifungal activity was not utilized until 1951. At that time the compound was shown to be active against plant pathogenic fungi on systemic as well as topical administration (9). Of the four stereoisomers, only griseolfulvin itself is active (19). The fluoro analog retains the potency of the original drug, but the bromo and dechloro analogs are ineffective. Neither the methoxy group on ring A nor the keto group on ring C is required for potency. Replacement of the methoxy substituent in ring C with either propoxy or butoxy increases activity twenty- to fifty fold (19). The molecular site of action apparently is associated with DNA replication. In addition to causing the formation of abnormal fungal cells, the drug inhibits mitosis of animal and plant cells, causes multipolar mitosis, and produces abnormal nuclei (20).

Griseofulvin has no action against bacteria, yeasts, or fungi that cause systemic disease (9, 20). Moreover, when used topically, the drug is inactive in dermatophytic infections. In 1958 the antibiotic was found to be effective against dermatophytes when administered orally. Apparently a small amount of the drug can diffuse from the blood to the site of fungal multiplication in the skin and hair. This low concentration sufficiently slows the rate of hyphal penetration so that the outward thrust of keratinized host cells is able to deprive the fungus of access to nutrients. Because of low toxicity, the antibiotic can be given to most patients for a period of many weeks. However griseofulvin induces hepatic microsomal enzymes that decrease the activity of warfarin-type oral anticoagulants (21). Moreover, it has demonstrated teratogenic and carcinogenic activities in experimental animals (21). Thus the drug should be reserved for treatment of dermatophytes that are known to be resistant to each of the five topical therapeutic agents listed in group A of Table 22.1.

3.2.3 POLYENE ANTIBIOTICS. The polyene antibiotics, produced by actinomycetes, contain a large lactone ring with four to seven unsubstituted, conjugated double bonds. The conjugated systems are usually in an all-trans configuration, so that the ring contains a planar lipophilic segment and a less rigid hydrophilic portion (22). Each substance generally contains a carbohydrate moiety; in amphotericin B (22.**29**), nystatin (22.**30**), and pimaricin (22.**31**) this is D-mycosamine.

Polyenes are essentially insoluble in water and, because of extensive unsaturation, are rather unstable. They act against

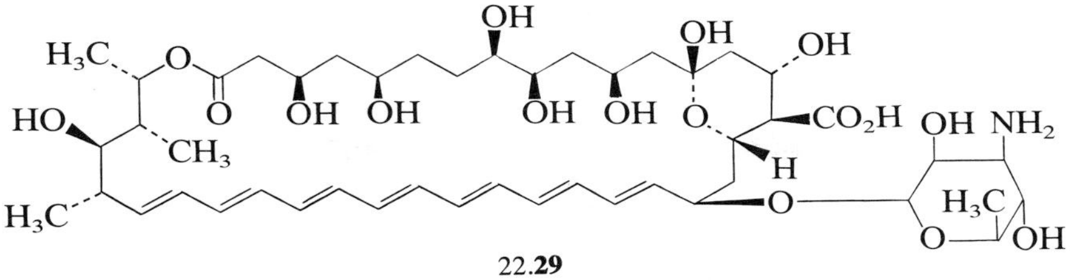

22.**29**

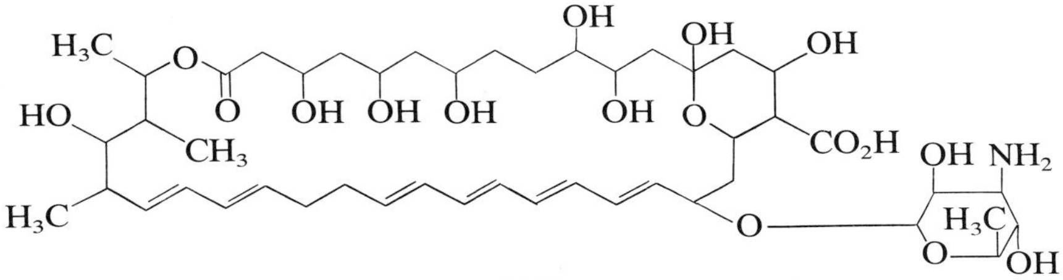

22.**30**

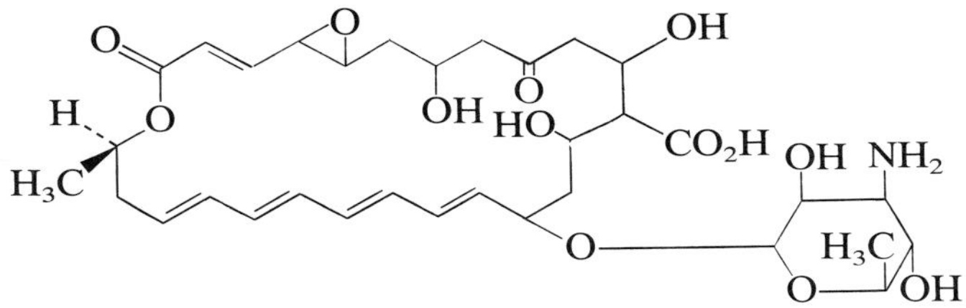

22.**31**

sensitive fungal, algal, and animal cells by combining with sterols in the membranes, with a resulting alteration in permeability and loss of essential organic and inorganic cell constituents; most bacteria lack sterols in their cell membranes, thus are resistant to the polyenes (23).

Of numerous polyene antibiotics, the three listed above have received most attention as useful anti-infectives (9). Amphotericin B is administered intravenously or intrathecally as a colloidal dispersion in aqueous sodium deoxycholate solution in patients with systemic mycoses (Table 22.1). The drug is also useful in treatment of mucocutaneous and visceral leishmaniasis. Nystatin is employed as a cutaneous, vaginal, or oral preparation for therapy of nonsystemic candidiasis. Pimaricin is recommended as the drug of choice for mycotic keratosis, irrespective of specific etiology (9).

Because of their insolubility in host fluids and tissues, local or topical use of the polyenes rarely causes side effects. However systemic administration of amphotericin B frequently results in some degree of nausea, anoxeria, chills, fever, headache, hemolytic anemia, phlebitis, hypokalemia, and azotemia (9). Despite its dangerous nature, amphotericin B is the only proved standardized agent for treatment of the systemic mycoses; thus numerous attempts continue to be made to reduce its toxicity.

Permanent kidney damage has been avoided by reducing the dose to a quantity that enables attainment of a peak serum level that is not more than twice the *in vitro* fungistatic concentration (4). Alternate-day double dose therapy may increase patient tolerance (9), and the addition of mannitol has mitigated the renal damage (16). Laboratory studies have indicated some amount of synergy of amphotericin B with

5-fluorocytosine and rifampin (25, 26), and a combination of the first two in patients has given encouraging results (16). Simultaneous administration of diethylstilbestrol with amphotericin B appears to enhance the antifungal activity of the drug in some mycotic diseases (16). The methyl ester of the antibiotic is water soluble and less toxic than amphotericin B (9). Unfortunately, it also is substantially less efficacious (27).

4 NOVEL APPROACHES TO ANTIFUNGAL THERAPY

4.1 Transfer Factor

Persons who develop opportunistic mycoses because of defects in cell-mediated immunity have been aided by leucocyte transfusion therapy. To eliminate problems of immunological incompatibility, transfer factor has been recommended for use in place of leucocytes. The factor is a dialyzable extract of T lymphocytes that can convert patient macrophages to a specific antigen-responsive state. It is obtained by repeated freezing and thawing of donor peripheral leucocytes and has a molecular weight of about 5000 daltons. In patients with candidiasis, the factor has been found to prolong remissions induced by amphotericin B or clotrimazole (28).

4.2 Iron-Binding Agents

An important component of human and animal defense against microbial invasion is a group of phenomena termed "nutritional immunity" (29). By a variety of means, normal hosts are capable of withholding growth-essential iron from most strains of fungi and bacteria; such hosts are far more resistant to microbial infection than are hyperferremic or hypotransferrinemic persons or animals. The serum dermatophyte-inhibitory -component has now been definitely identified as unsaturated transferrin (30). Studies are presently in progress to determine whether low molecular weight synthetic or natural product iron-binding agents can be used as therapeutic adjuncts in fungal infections.

5 CONCLUSIONS

As with other kinds of anti-infectives, a variety of useful antifungal drugs have been developed in the last three decades from screening programs. The diversity of active structures and of their antifungal mechanisms of action sheds little light on the kinds of molecules that should be tested in future screens. Moreover, no single type of structure thus far discovered possesses useful broad spectrum activity. Antifungal drugs with the remarkable selective toxicity of such antibacterial substances as the sulfonamides, β-lactams, or tetracyclines are not yet available for systemic mycoses. Thus the search for novel, effective and less toxic antifungal drugs must continue. Additionally, development of immunological aspects of prevention and therapy should be expanded. Successful eradication and treatment of human fungal diseases may well require appropriate combinations of vaccines, transfer factor, antifungal drugs, and iron-binding agents.

REFERENCES

1. J. E. Bennett, *Prevent. Med.*, **3,** 515 (1974).
2. S. Rich, in *Plant Pathology, an Advanced Treatise*, Vol. 2, J. G. Horsfall and A. E. Diamond, Eds., Academic Press, New York, 1960, p. 553.
3. E. D. Weinberg, *Bacteriol. Rev.*, **21,** 46 (1957).
4. E. D. Weinberg, *Ann. N.Y. Acad. Sci.*, **148,** 587 (1968).
5. U. W. Leavell, Jr., in *The Diagnosis and Treatment of Fungal Infections*, H. M. Robinson, Ed., Thomas, Springfield, I11., 1974, p. 89.
6. A. H. Campbell, in *Experimental Chemotherapy*, Vol. 3, R. J. Schnitzer and F. Hawking, Eds., Academic Press, New York, 1964, p. 461.

7. R. Brown, in *Experimental Chemotherapy*, Vol. 3, R. J. Schnitzer and F. Hawking, Eds., Academic Press, New York, 1964, p. 418.
8. T. Noguchi, A. Kaji, Y. Igarashi, A. Shigematsu, and K. Taniguchi, *Antimicrob. Agents Chemother.*, 259 (1963).
9. J. W. Rippon, *Medical Mycology*, Saunders, Philadelphia, 1974, p. 531.
10. E. B. Smith, *Cutis*, **17,** 54 (1976).
11. H. Brincker, Scand. J. Infect. Dis., **8,** 117 (1976).
12. F. Bottistini, N. Zaias, R. Sierra, and G. Rebell, *Arch. Dermatol.* **109,** 695 (1974).
13. L. C. Marmion, K. B. Desser, R. B. Lilly, and D. A. Stevens, *Antimicrob. Agents Chemother.*, **10,** 447 (1976).
14. W. H. Beggs, G. A. Sarosi, and N. M. Steele, *Antimicrob. Agents Chemother.*, **9,** 863 (1976).
15. K. H. S. Swamy, A. Joshi, and G. R. Rao, *Antimicrob. Agents Chemother.*, **9,** 903 (1976).
16. S. D. Codish and J. S. Tobias, *J. Am. Med. Assoc.*, **235,** 2132 (1976).
17. S. Montplaisir, B. Nabarra, and E. Drouhet, *Antimicrob. Agents Chemother.*, **9,** 1028 (1976).
18. R. N. Goodman, *Antimicrob. Agents Chemother.*, **749** (1967).
19. K. J. Bent and R. H. Moore, *Symp. Soc. Gen. Microbiol.*, **16,** 82 (1966).
20. F. M. Huber, in *Antibiotics. Mechanism of Action of Antimicrobial and Antitumor Agents*, J. W. Corcoran and F. E. Hahn, Springer, Berlin, 1975, p. 606.
21. Anonymous, *Med. Lett.*, **18,** 17 (1976).
22. J. O. Lampen, *Symp. Soc. Gen. Microbiol.*, **16,** 111 (1966).
23. S. C. Kinsky, in *Antibiotics*, Vol. 1, *Mechanism of Action*, D. Gottlieb and P. D. Shaw, Eds., Springer, Berlin, 1967, p. 122.
24. D. J. Drutz, A. Spickard, and M. G. Koenig, *Antimicrob. Agents Chemother.*, 202 (1967).
25. M. Kitahara, V. K. Seth, G. Medoff, and G. S. Kobayashi, *Antimicrob. Agents Chemother.*, **9,** 915 (1976).
26. M. Kitahara, G. S. Kobayashi, and G. Medoff, *J. Infect. Dis.*, **133,** 663 (1976).
27. H. Gadebusch, F. Pansy, C. Klepner, and R. Schwind, *J. Infect. Dis.*, **134,** 423 (1976).
28. C. H. Kirkpatrick and J. I. Gallin, *Oncology*, **29,** 46 (1974).
29. E. D. Weinberg, *Microbiol. Revs.*, **42,** 45 (1978).
30. R. D. King, H. A. Khan, J. C. Foye, J. H. Greenberg, and H. E. Jones, *J. Lab. Clin. Med.*, **86,** 204 (1975).

GENERAL REFERENCE

C. W. Emmons, C. H. Binford, J. P. Utz, and K. J. Kwon-Chung, *Medical Mycology*, 3rd ed., Lea & Febiger, Philadelphia, 1977.

CHAPTER TWENTY–THREE

Antiviral Agents

ROBERT W. SIDWELL

Department of Biology
Utah State University,
Logan, Utah 84322, USA

and

JOSEPH T. WITKOWSKI

Schering Corporation
60 Orange Street
Bloomfield, New Jersey 07003, USA

CONTENTS

1 INTRODUCTION

Virus infections exceed all other categories of disease in terms of frequency and disability, and perhaps 60% of all episodes of human illness result from viral infections (1). For example, the influenza virus, during the pandemic year of 1968–1969, caused more than 51 million reported cases of influenza in the United States, and more than 80,000 deaths (2). similar high virus infection rates occur among pets, livestock, and plants.

The high morbidity and the resulting economic loss caused by these diseases have stimulated efforts in recent years to develop means to control virus infections using antiviral agents. Whereas earlier such research efforts were considered to be in their infancy, today we may be justified in saying the state of the art has progressed to "midadolescence." In the past decade, many compounds were synthesized and evaluated as antiviral agents. Thus chemicals are now known that have significant antiviral activity and are potentially usable as clinically effective agents. A number, indeed, have exhibited positive clinical antiviral activity. Marked progress in viral molecular biology has substantially aided in elucidating the mechanism of action of these antiviral drugs, while pointing to biochemical sites of importance as we seek to develop other agents.

This chapter reviews the progress made in antiviral chemotherapy and emphasizes the significant structure–antiviral activity relationships that have been established in the various categories of the more important antiviral substances. Since it would be desirable to associate the mechanism by which compounds exert their antiviral effect with the structure-activity relationships, we briefly review the mechanism of action, where known, of each class of substances.

As a means of introduction, an overview is presented of the properties and classifications of viruses and of systems utilized for testing antiviral substances. Some steps in viral replication that may be amenable to chemotherapy are suggested to the medicinal chemist who attempts to design new antiviral drugs. Consideration must also be given to the failure of many substances in animal or human trials, in spite of definite activity in enzyme studies or in cellular antiviral systems. Because of the considerable progress in developing clinically effective antiviral agents, the most important substances are discussed initially; structure-activity relationships and mechanisms of action are described in Section 5.

2 VIRUSES: PROPERTIES AND CLASSIFICATION

Viruses constitute a separate and unique class of infectious agents that differ from other disease agents on the basis of their smaller size, simpler chemical composition, lack of enzymes that function in energy metabolism, lack of protein synthetic machinery, and cell-dependent mechanism of multiplication. These properties result in the important characteristic that viruses can replicate only within the most cell. Different viruses are known to attack bacteria, insects, plants, animals, or man, although here we limit our discussion to the important viruses of vertebrates.

Viruses contain either RNA or DNA, and it is this nucleic acid composition that forms the initial basis for their classification. An International Committee on Taxonomy of Viruses has recently published an extensive revision of the overall classification and nomenclature of viruses (3); the viruses that are considered relevant to this review of antiviral agents are summarized in Table 23.1, using the nomenclature and taxonomy recommended by that committee. It is important to consider the taxonomic families in which the various viruses are categorized, for the antiviral activity of various compounds is often specific for viruses within such a family.

The nucleic acid of the complete virus particle is surrounded by a protein coat, which in turn may be covered by an outer envelope that contains lipoprotein. The nucleic acid core, which can be single or double stranded, represents the genetic material of the particle and differs from the host cell nucleic acid. The protein coat is antigenic. Since it differs from the protein in the host cell, the coat is responsible for the majority of the immunologic reactions that viruses induce in the host. The viral protein serves principally a structural role, protecting the viral genome from degradation; certain viral-associated proteins act to lend specificity to the virus for purposes of adsorption to the cell. They may also act catalytically, creating ideal conditions for replication of the virus, or they may act as inhibitors of specific host cell functions (4).

Certain viruses contain enzymes or contain genetic code for synthesis of enzymes not normally found in cells (Table 23.2), a fact of considerable importance because theoretically these enzymes could be specific targets for antiviral substances. Virus-associated enzymes are extensively reviewed by Mitchell (4) and by McAuslan (5).

The viral replicative process within the cell is quite complex and varies according to the virus. Reviews of the sequential molecular events provide specific detail (6). Basically, however, a number of key steps in the infection process (Fig. 23.1) should be considered in the development of an antiviral drug (7). The first steps involve the attachment and adsorption of the virus to the host cell's plasma membrane, often requiring proper positioning of complementary receptors of the virus to those of the cell. This is followed by penetration of the virus through the membrane into the cell. At this point, at varying sites in the cell depending on the virus, the envelope and the protein coat are removed from the viral nucleic acid core. From this viral nucleic acid, especially in the DNA viruses and also with double-stranded RNA viruses, transcription of messenger RNA (mRNA) occurs. Virion-associated polymerase or cellular transcriptase is involved in this step. Certain single-stranded RNA viruses (e.g., Enteroviruses and Alphaviruses) act as their own messengers. Oncovirus single-stranded RNA acts as a template for RNA-dependent DNA polymerase to synthesize proviral DNA, which in turn acts as templates for the eventual synthesis of viral RNA and mRNA. Translation of the viral mRNA leads to replication of new viral nucleic acid and also to synthesis of viral peptides; the latter coat the viral nucleic acid later in the encapsulation process. Envelopment, if necessary for a particular virus, is accomplished with cellular membrane components, after which the mature virus particle is released from the cell.

Usually infected cells eventually degenerate and die; the disease state in the host is caused when sufficient numbers of cell deaths occur. Certain viruses, however, can cause the cells to transform to a neoplastic state; others may not noticeably affect the cell, but the presence of one or more viral

Table 23.1 Important[a] Viruses of Vertebrates

Nucleic Acid Type	Family	Genus	Virus	Type of Infection Induced
DNA	Adenoviridae	*Mastadenovirus*	Numerous adeno types	Respiratory and ophthalmic
DNA	Herpetoviridae	*Herpesvirus*	Herpes types 1 and 2	Ophthalmic, central nervous system, genital, cutaneous, oral, upper respiratory
			Cytomegalo	Generalized of infant, respiratory, glandular
			Varicella (herpes zoster)	Nervous, cutaneous
			Pseudorabies	Central nervous system of livestock
			Infectious rhinotracheitis	Respiratory of livestock, fowl
DNA	Poxviridae	*Orthopoxvirus*	Variola (smallpox)	Generalized
			Vaccinia	Cutaneous
DNA	Papovaviridae	*Polyomavirus*	Polyoma, SV40	Tumors of rodents
RNA	Orthomyxoviridae	*Influenzavirus*	Influenza	Respiratory
RNA	Paramyxoviridae	*Paramyxovirus*	Parainfluenza	Respiratory
			Mumps	Glandular
			Newcastle disease	Respiratory and nervous of fowl
		Morbillivirus	Measles	Generalized
			Canine distemper	Generalized in dogs
		Pneumovirus	Respiratory syncytial	Respiratory
RNA	Piconaviridae	*Enterovirus*	Polio	Nervous
			Coxsackie	Respiratory, nervous, cardiovascular
			Echo	Nervous, intestinal
		Rhinovirus	Numerous rhino types	Respiratory
			Foot and mouth disease	Generalized of livestock
		Calicivirus	Feline calici	Respiratory of cats
			Vesicular exanthema	Generalized of swine
RNA	Rhabdoviridae	*Vesiculovirus*	Vesicular stomatitis	Generalized of livestock
		Lyssavirus	Rabies	Nervous
RNA	Coronaviridae	*Coronavirus*	Corona	Respiratory
			Infectious bronchitis	Respiratory of fowl
RNA	Togaviridae	*Alphavirus*	Eastern, Western, Venezuelan equine encephalomyelitis	Nervous, respiratory
			Semliki forest	Nervous
		Flavivirus	Yellow Fever	Nervous
			Numerous encephalitides, including Japanese B, St. Louis, Russian spring-summer	Nervous
			Dengue	Joints, cutaneous
		Rubivirus	Rubella	Skin, generalized, nervous
RNA	Bunyaviridae	*Bunyavirus*	Numerous encephalitides, including Bunyamwera and California	Nervous
RNA	Arenaviridae	*Arenavirus*	Lymphocytic choriomeningitis	Nervous
			Lassa	Generalized
RNA	Retroviridae	Types B and C *Oncovirus*	Numerous leukemias, including Friend, Gross, Moloney, Rauscher	Oncogenic of lower animals
			Rous sarcoma	Oncogenic of fowl

[a] Based on disease incidence or severity or on previous use in antiviral testing.

Table 23.2 Virus-Associated Enzymes

Activity	Viruses
Neuraminidase	Influenza virus, paramyxovirus
Protein kinase	Orthopoxvirus, herpes virus, oncovirus
Nucleases	Mastadenovirus, orthopoxvirus, oncovirus
Nucleotide phosphohydrolases	Orthopoxvirus
DNA-dependent RNA polymerase	Orthopoxvirus
RNA-dependent RNA polymerase	Influenza virus, paramyxovirus, vesiculovirus
RNA-dependent DNA polymerase (reverse transcriptase)	Oncovirus

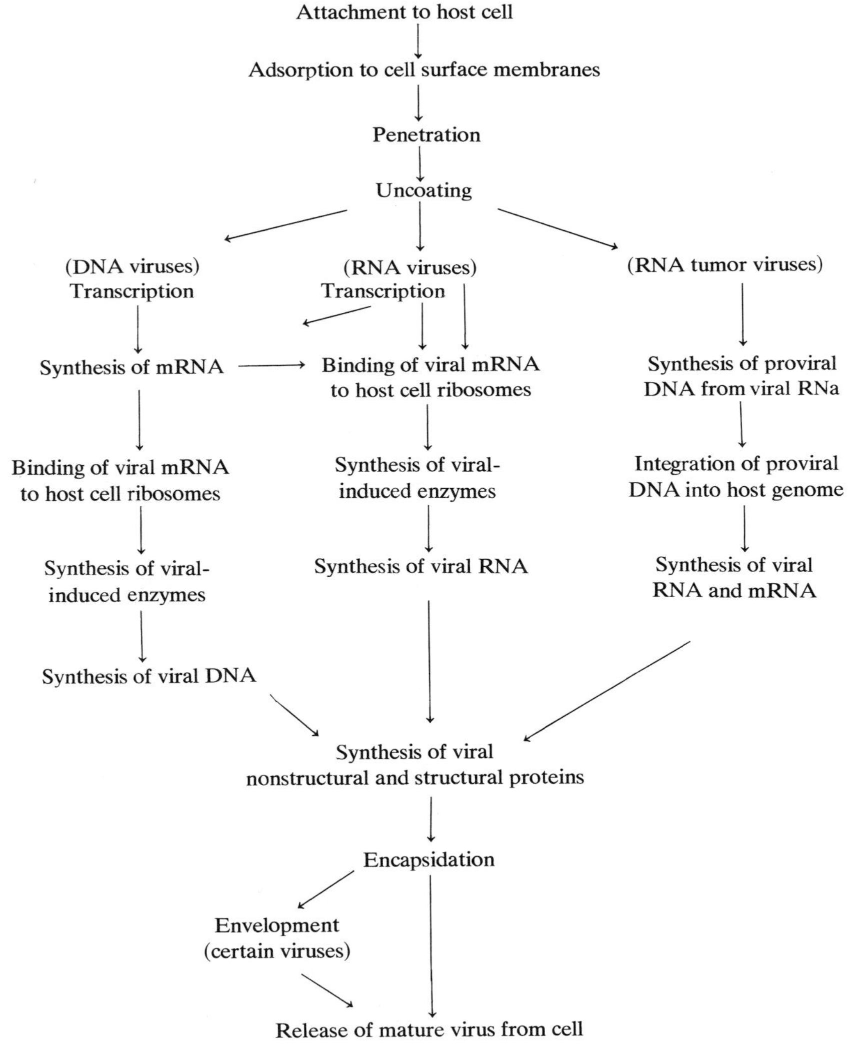

Fig. 23.1 Key steps in the viral replicative process.

components can be detected in the apparently unaltered cell.

3 ANTIVIRAL TESTING SYSTEMS

A serious problem in the development of significant antiviral drugs has been an apparent lack of predictability in the most commonly utilized antiviral chemotherapy testing systems; initial positive screening results in cell systems that do not always relate to later activity in use against animal or human viral disease. Therefore, we briefly consider the more commonly accepted screening procedures and the factors that may influence later correlation in tests against animal or human infections. This topic has been the subject of a recent review (8). Careful selection of the proper screening systems plays a most meaningful role in the eventual evaluation of newly synthesized compounds. Antiviral screening systems usually utilized include cell culture procedures, embryonated egg tests, and occasionally actual animal infections. Not yet widely utilized, yet worthy of serious consideration, are assays using inhibition of viral-specific enzymes.

3.1 *In Vitro* Antiviral Screens

Cells susceptible to a particular virus can be cultured in an artificial medium and allowed to divide until a confluent layer is established. When the virus is introduced into the medium, it enters the cell, and in time (the period varying from a few hours to days) the cells are altered. This alteration can be observed as holes or plaques appearing in the cell layer, as individual cell destruction or cytopathogenic effect (CPE) viewed under the microscope, as color change due to the pH alteration of the medium caused by less metabolism of the cell, or occasionally as inhibition of the uptake of labeled metabolites such as thymidine or uridine into viral nucleic acid. When added to the medium, the test compound will, if effective, inhibit these parameters of viral replication. The degree of viral inhibition can be expressed as the minimum inhibitory concentration (MIC), which is the least amount of test compound that will still cause viral inhibition, or numerically as a virus rating (VR), wherein the degree of inhibition of viral CPE and the toxicity of the compound for the host cell are considered (8). A therapeutic index (TI), defined as the maximum noncytotoxic concentration divided by the minimum antiviral effective concentration, may be used in place of a VR.

Although widely used, cell culture screening systems often fail to predict accurately a test compound's *in vivo* antiviral efficacy. Numerous factors affect these systems and should be considered in the evaluation of the results of every test. One important factor is the action of metabolizing enzymes that may be absent in the cell but in animal systems seriously alter the structure of the compound. Aqueous insolubility will limit a compound's cell culture antiviral efficacy, although an animal host may still be able to assimilate it. Cell culture systems will lack most of the natural immunity factors that may play a vital role in aiding a drug's battle against a viral infection in animals. Some compounds, for reasons not fully known, will exert an antiviral activity that is very dependent on the type of cell used, indicating a need for the use of more than one cell type in a screening system. Factors in the test itself, such as the parameter used to measure antiviral activity, incubation time of the cell-virus-compound combination, concentration of virus, and the period that elapses between the times virus and the compound are added to the cell, often have a profound effect on the outcome of the test. Contaminants, such as mycoplasma, may also affect a test by enzymatically altering the compound.

Despite these difficulties, the cell culture system can be very useful as a primary screen, especially when only small quantities of the test chemical are available. One should insist on as uniform a test as possible with regard to concentration of virus, cell number, timing, etc., and there should be at least one known active drug run in parallel to compare as a standard.

3.2 Embryonated Egg Antiviral Systems

Before cell culturing procedures became the refined tools they are today, the antiviral chemotherapist often utilized the embryonated egg as an initial screen. In this system, various parts of the developing egg are exposed to specific viruses, which either kill the embryo or cause in the egg certain disease manifestations that are typical of the virus. Active test chemicals, when injected into the same area of the egg, prevent these manifestations. Thus the influenza virus can be injected into the allantoic cavity or the amniotic sac, with death of the embryo or virus multiplication, as measured by hemagglutinin, used as an end point. The Alpha- and Flaviviruses, (e.g., eastern equine encephalomyelitis, St. Louis encephalitis), produce death in the embryo. Herpes and vaccinia viruses induce pocks on chorioallantoic membranes. Several of the Enteroviruses (e.g., polio, coxsackie) grow in the yolk sac or allantoic membrane, with eventual death of the embryo caused by nervous system disease. The factors of cost, complexities of handling, and evaluation of tests performed in embryonated eggs, as will as the increasing efficiency of cell culture procedures, have led to the decline in the use of this system as an antiviral testing tool.

3.3 *In Vivo* Antiviral Tests

In vivo antiviral systems vary widely depending on the virus to be used, the degree of infection to be evaluated, and the type of animal host selected. Ideally, if the animal system is to be predictive of efficacy against human disease, it should mimic as closely as possible the infection seen in man. For example, if one were to seek a drug for treating human respiratory infections, it would be best to avoid the highly lethal influenza-induced pneumonia in mice, using instead inhibition of abnormal respiratory sounds (rales) and changes in weight and water intake in more mildly infected mice. Alternatively, one could utilize another host such as ferrets, hamsters, or squirrel monkeys, in which the manifested infection more nearly resembles the human disease.

A virus that is a natural parasite of the experimental animal is often better for antiviral testing than a human virus that has been markedly altered in adapting it to cause a discernible disease in the animal. A truly acceptable antiviral test system is uniform with regard to animal size, sex, and species, amount of virus inoculated, mode of inoculation, handling of the animal, and final measurement of antiviral activity. Sham-infected animals treated with the test compound should always be included as toxicity controls. As a standard, a known positive antiviral drug should be included in such *in vivo* tests.

3.4 Inhibition of Viral-Specific Enzymes

Listed in Table 23.2 are the known viral-associated enzymes that conceivably could be used for antiviral testing. A few laboratories have actually used such tests to date, with efforts concentrated predominantly on the influenza virus–associated enzymes (9–13). Few compounds inhibitory to such virus-associated enzymes have shown efficacy in human studies, but this concept of antiviral screening, still in its infancy, should be considered if an attempt is being made to relate chemical structure to antiviral activity.

4 CLINICALLY ACTIVE ANTIVIRAL DRUGS

An increasing number of substances that are significantly active in cell and animal systems have been evaluated for efficacy against virus diseases in humans; many have been found to have antiviral activity sufficient to lead to their being registered as antiviral drugs in several major countries. It is appropriate to discuss briefly the efficacy of each, as well as the problems known to have been encountered that may curtail their widespread use.

1-Methylisatin-3-thiosemicarbazone (methisazone, 23.**1**), one of the more active

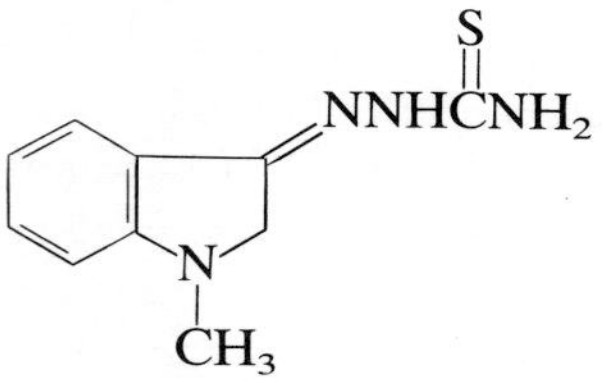

23.**1**

in the isatin-3-thiosemicarbazone series, has been used in the prevention and treatment of smallpox and alastrim (a mild form of smallpox). It has also had limited use in the treatment of vaccinia infections that develop as complications of smallpox vaccination (14–16). The drug is limited by its overall prophylactic mode of action and the relatively few viral infections susceptible to it (15). Certain side effects associated with use of methisazone have been noted (15).

5-Iodo-2′-deoxyuridine (iododeoxyuridine, IdU, 23.**2**) has been extensively

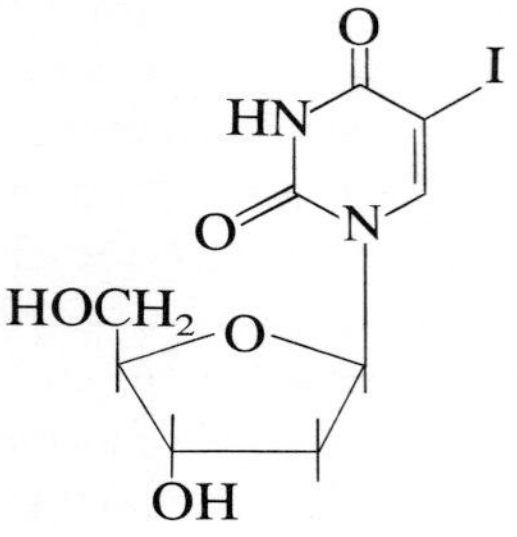

23.**2**

utilized for the topical therapy of herpes virus ocular diseases (17). Less frequent use has also been reported for cutaneous herpes and vaccinia infections (17). Mixed results have been reported when the drug was used in treating patients with herpes brain infections, congenital cytomegalovirus disease, and smallpox (17–19). Therapy with IdU can result in viruses that are resistant to the drug (18), posing a significant problem to clinicians. A variety of side effects have been seen in patients treated with IdU, especially when the drug is administered systemically. An important problem is the apparent inhibition of healing, particularly in certain cells of the eye damaged by herpes virus infection (18). Another possible side effect mentioned in the recent reports is that IdU induces or enhances the replication of both DNA and RNA viruses when it is incorporated into cellular DNA *in vitro* (20, 21).

5-Trifluoromethyl-2′-deoxyuridine (trifluorothymidine, F_3TdR, 23.**3**) is a more

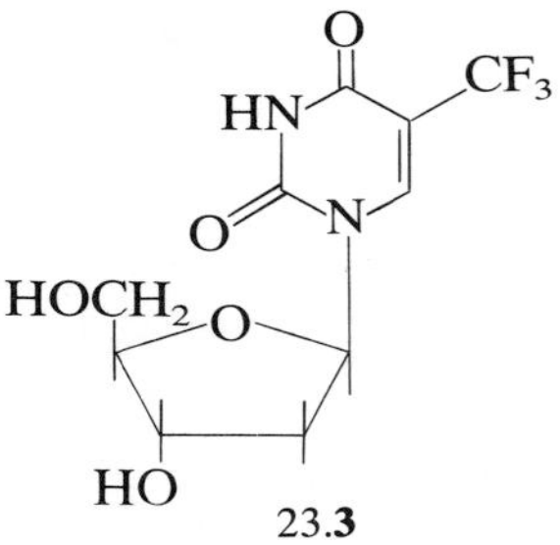

23.**3**

recently introduced drug that, like IdU, is used particularly for topical therapy of herpes virus-infected eyes (17, 18). It has been found especially useful for treating infections that are resistant to IdU therapy. The markedly improved aqueous solubility compared to IdU is also an advantage. The drug apparently is less toxic than IdU.

1-Adamantanamine hydrochloride (amantadine HCl, 23.**4**) is indicated for the prophylactic treatment of influenza A virus infections (22). The drug is also utilized for the totally unrelated Parkinson's Disease

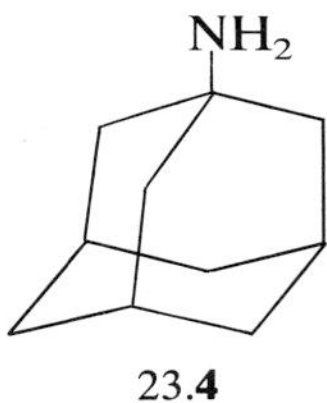

23.4

(23), which is not virus associated. Although side effects, chiefly instability of the nervous system, have been noted, the drug is generally considered reasonably safe to use in human patients and has been recommended for use over relatively long periods of time for the prevention of influenza A (24). Although marketed in the United States, the drug has not yet found wide acceptance, possibly because of its prophylactic action and the limited spectrum of influenza viruses it inhibits.

α-Methyl-1-adamantanemethylamine hydrochloride (rimantadine HCl, 23.**5**) is

$NH_2 \cdot HCl$

$HC—CH_3$

23.**5**

closely related to amantadine HCl, with similar antiviral activity. Experimental studies indicate that rimantadine HCl may be somewhat more potent as an antiviral agent than amantadine HCl. Clinical trials show this drug to be well tolerated and to have significant chemoprophylactic activity against human influenza A_2 infections (22).

The *N*-dimethylaminoethoxyacetyl analog of amantadine, tromantadine HCl (23.**6**), reportedly is effective against clinical herpes labialis, herpes genitalis, and generalized herpes infections when administered topically (25). Little has yet been published on the efficacy or side effects of this drug.

$NHC(=O)CH_2OCH_2CH_2N(CH_3)_2 \cdot HCl$

23.**6**

1-β-D-Arabinofuranosylcytosine (cytarabine, ara-C, 23.**7**) reportedly has had significant therapeutic effects in patients with

NH_2, N, O, N, $HOCH_2$, O, HO, OH

23.**7**

localized herpes zoster, herpes eye infections, severe generalized herpes virus infection, and herpes encephalitis (26, 27), although several negative results have also been reported (28–30). It is chiefly used as an anticancer agent. The drug is quite toxic and is usually only recommended for very severe viral infections. Ara-C is rapidly deaminated in man to the inactive uracil derivative, lessening the drug's antiviral potency.

9-β-D-Arabinofuranosyladenine (vidarabine, ara-A, 23.**8**) is a relatively new antiviral drug, effective against herpes eye, cutaneous, and brain infections. It has

NH_2, N, N, N, N, $HOCH_2$, O, HO, HO

23.**8**

proved to be especially useful for treating infections of IdU-resistant herpes virus. Relatively recent reviews of the drug are available (26, 31). Ara-A is relatively insoluble in aqueous solution, which has caused difficulties when ophthalmic or intravenous solutions are needed. Although a number of potential toxicological problems exist with ara-A (32), the drug has recently received acceptance to be marketed as an ophthalmic ointment in the United States. Ara-A is deaminated to 9-β-D-arabinofuranosylhypoxanthine, which also has antiviral properties, thus extending the duration of this drug's antiviral effect.

1-β-D-Ribofuranosyl-1,2,4-triazole-3-carboxamide (ribavirin, 23.**9**) is also a new entry to the antiviral field, having efficacy against type A (infectious) hepatitis (33), influenza A (34, 35) and B (36), measles (36a), and possibly cutaneous infections caused by the herpes viruses (37, 37a). The mode of action of ribavirin appears to be more therapeutic than prophylactic. Toxicology studies indicate an adequate tolerance to the drug, although teratogenicity seen in rodents may limit its human use.

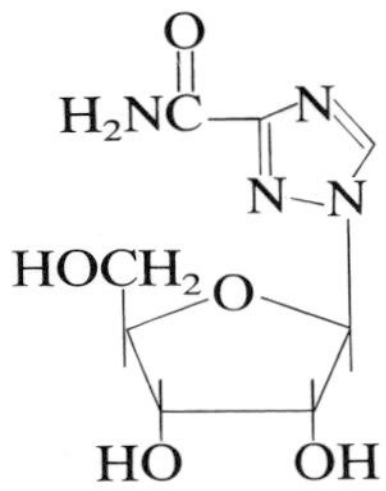

23.**9**

Inosiplex (23.**10**), an adduct consisting of inosine and the 1-(dimethylamino)-2-propanol salt of 4-acetaminobenzoic acid in a 1:3 ratio, has had mixed reports of antiviral efficacy in humans, apparently acting as a stimulator of cell-mediated immunity. Against human rhino virus infections, two tests indicated no significant effect (38, 39), but in a third test, definite suppression of disease symptoms was seen (40). The latter test had been reported elsewhere (orange juice and inosiplex were studied together), and equal efficacy was seen with the two substances (41). A preliminary report indicates possible efficacy against human herpes cutaneous infections (42). Activity against human influenza has also very recently been described (42a, 42b).

Levamisole, the levoisomer of tetramisole (6-phenyl-2,3,5,6-tetrahydroimidazo[2,1-*b*]thiazole, 23.**11**) was initially developed as an antihelmintic agent but has also been found effective against herpes virus infections in man (43, 44). The compound, like inosiplex, apparently acts as a modulator of host resistance mechanisms, especially as an enhancer of cellular immunity.

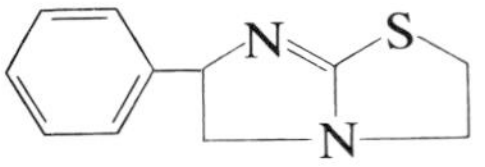

23.**11**

Heterotricyclic dyes such as neutral red (23.**12**), acridine orange, and proflavine, which act by binding to viral nucleic acid, absorbing visible light, and inactivating the virus by oxidation, have demonstrated considerable clinical antiviral activity. These

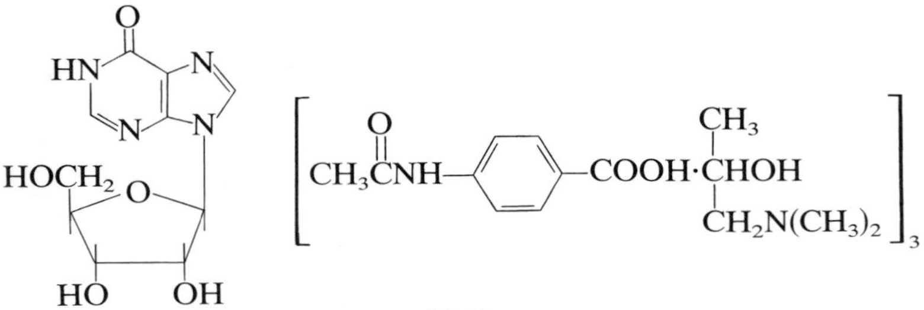

$$\left[CH_3\overset{O}{\overset{\|}{C}}NH-C_6H_4-COOH\cdot\underset{CH_2N(CH_3)_2}{\overset{CH_3}{CHOH}} \right]_3$$

23.**10**

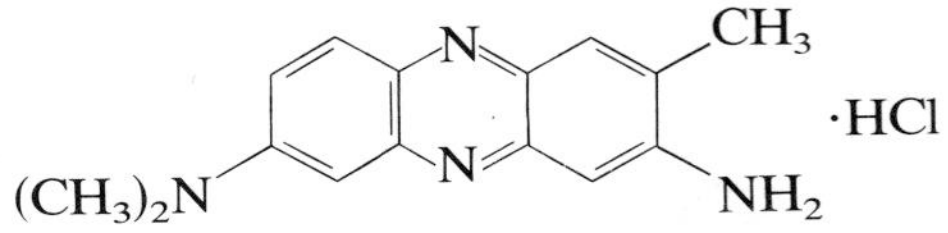

23.12

light-sensitive dyes have been found to be effective in treating cutaneous herpes virus infections (45–48). Concern has been expressed that photoinactivation of herpes viruses may be clinically hazardous because the inactivated virus is capable of transforming normal cells to a malignant state (49). The dyes also have a strong affinity for the nuclei of cells and may damage their genetic makeup (50, 51). These dyes, though publicly accessible, are not registered specifically as antiviral drugs.

Several compounds have been reported by Soviet scientists to be effective against certain virus infections in human patients, and they are being utilized in the USSR. These are 6-bromonaphthoquinone (bonaphton, 23.**13**), used against influenza virus infections (52); the substituted biphenyl compound tebrophen (23.**14**), which is used in an ointment for influenza, herpes, adeno, and possibly other viral diseases (53, 54); and florenal (23.**15**), which

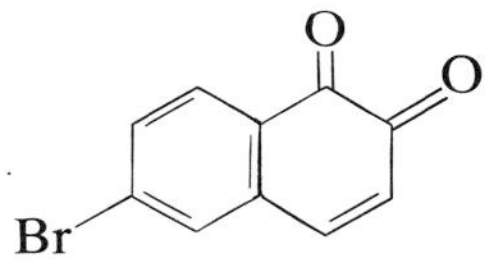

23.13

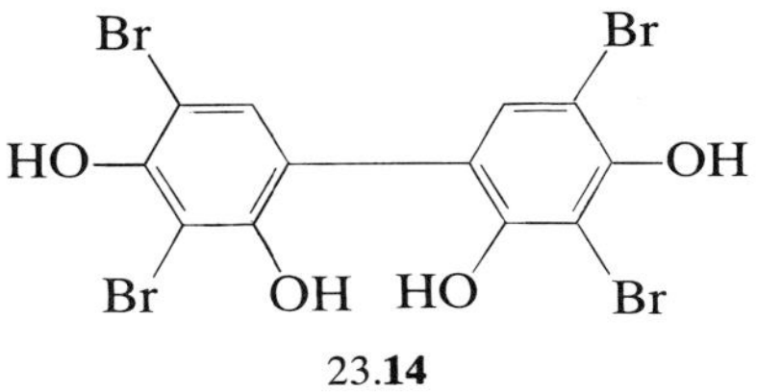

23.14

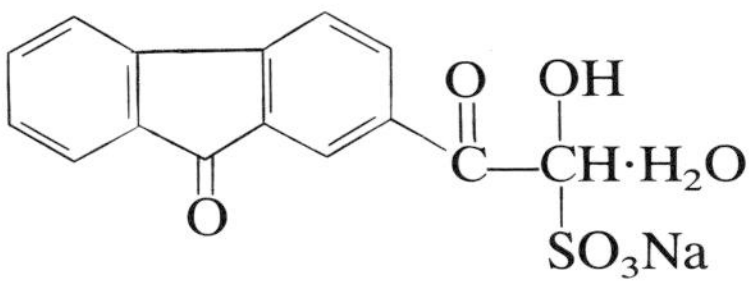

23.15

is also used against herpes infections in man (53, 55). A cooperative antiviral testing group sponsored by the US National Institute for Allergy and Infectious Diseases has been unable to confirm the antiviral activity of these compounds in animal studies to date (56).

5 MECHANISM OF ACTION AND STRUCTURE–ACTIVITY RELATIONSHIPS

5.1 Thiosemicarbazones

The clinically active drug 1-methylisatin-3-thiosemicarbazone (methisazone, 23.**1**) and related compounds, including isatin-3-thiosemicarbazone (23.**16**), have shown activity against DNA viruses, principally the

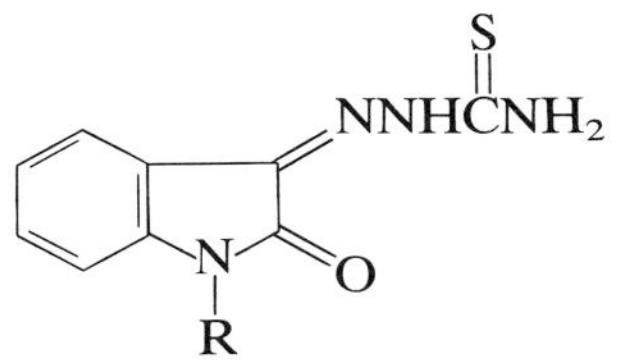

23.**1** $R = CH_3$
23.**16** $R = H$
23.**17** $R = CH_3CH_2$
23.**18** $R = HOCH_2CH_2$

Orthopoxviruses, both *in vitro* and *in vivo.* Limited *in vitro* studies also indicate a moderate inhibitory effect against some RNA viruses (57). Benzaldehyde thiosemicarbazone and several derivatives were effective in early studies against vaccinia virus infections in eggs and mice (58).

Methisazone has no significant effect on vaccinia virus DNA synthesis (59) but does appear to inhibit late protein synthesis by a mechanism that remains to be defined. Though unclear, the antiviral action of the thiosemicarbazones appears to relate to their ability to form coordination compounds with metal ions including copper, zinc, cobalt, nickel, and manganese (60–62). Complexes of methisazone and copper have been shown to interact with nucleic acids (62); indeed, certain non-Orthopoxviruses (RNA tumor viruses, herpes viruses) are inactivated by direct contact with methisazone, which may be a function of the chelating ability of the drug (63). The RNA-dependent DNA polymerase of RNA tumor viruses is also inhibited by methisazone (61, 63). A potential side effect of methisazone is a suppression of the host immune system (61).

Structure-activity relationship studies have shown (64) that in addition to methisazone, the most active compounds in this series are 1-ethyl (23.**17**) and 1-(2-hydroxyethyl) (23.**18**) derivatives of isatin-3-thiosemicarbazone (23.**16**). Modifications of the thiosemicarbazone moiety generally resulted in loss of antiviral activity, although, interestingly, 1-methyl-4′,4′-dibutylisatin-3-thiosemicarbazone has activity *in vitro* against the RNA-containing polio virus (65). Isatin-3-semicarbazone does not exhibit antiviral activity, indicating that the thio group is essential for activity (15). A number of benzaldehyde thiosemicarbazones have been evaluated for their antiviral activity (58, 66, 67). Of these, benzaldehyde thiosemicarbazone (23.**19**) itself and derivatives 23.**20** and 23.**21** were

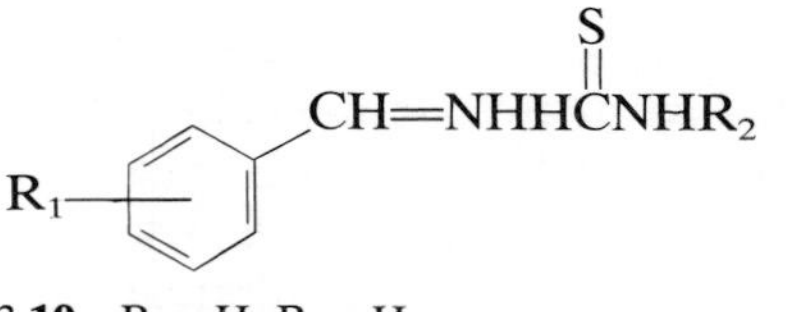

R_1–C_6H_4–CH=NNHC(=S)NHR$_2$

23.**19** $R_1 = H$, $R_2 = H$
23.**20** $R_1 = NH_2$, $R_2 = H$
23.**21** $R_1 = CH_3CONH$, $R_2 = (CH_3)_2CHCH_2$

most inhibitory to Orthopoxviruses. Substitutions on the benzene ring generally reduced the antiviral activity of these compounds. Incorporation of the thiosemicarbazone group into a cyclic system appears to increase the spectrum of antiviral activity of these compounds. 3-(4-Bromophenyl)-5-carboxymethylthiazolidine-2,4-dione-2-benzylidenehydrazone (23.**22**) of

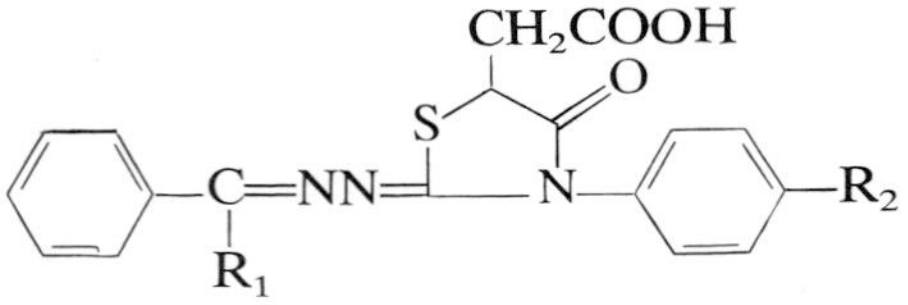

CH_2COOH, O, S, C_6H_5–C(R_1)=NN=, N–C_6H_4–R_2

23.**22** $R_1 = H$, $R_2 = Br$
23.**23** $R_1 = CH_3$, $R_2 = CH_3$

this series had an especially significant *in vitro* effect on herpes and polio viruses (68), and several related compounds were similarly inhibitory to herpes, vaccinia, polio types 1 and 2, and influenza viruses (69). 5-Carboxymethyl-3-(*p*-tolyl)thiazolidine-2,4-dione-2-acetophenonehydrazone (23.**23**) was effective when used as an ointment on herpetic dermal lesions in human volunteers (70).

5.2 Benzimidazoles

A number of benzimidazole derivatives have been investigated as antiviral agents. The most extensively studied of these is 2-(α-hydroxybenzylbenzimidazole) (HBB, 23.**24**), which is a selective inhibitor of the

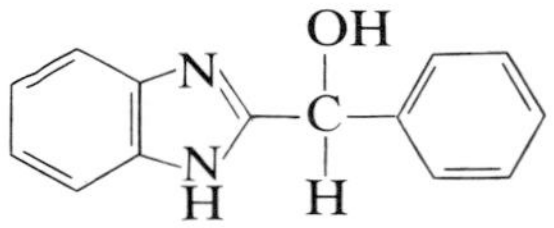

OH, N, C, N, H, H

23.**24**

RNA-containing Enteroviruses, although lymphocytic choriomeningitis virus, an Arenavirus, is also inhibited to a degree (71, 72). Another significant substance in this class of chemicals is 5,6-dichloro-1-β-D-ribofuranosylbenzimidazole (23.**25**),

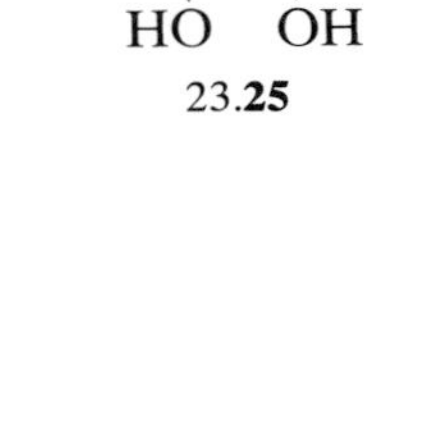

Cl, Cl, N, N, $HOCH_2$, O, HO, OH

23.**25**

which, together with the corresponding trichloro derivative, is inhibitory *in vitro* to both RNA viruses (influenza, parainfluenza, mumps, polio, encephalomyocarditis) and DNA viruses (vaccinia, adeno) (71, 73).

Mechanism of action studies indicate that HBB has no effect on virus adsorption, penetration, and uncoating (72). The primary site of action of this antiviral agent appears to be inhibition of viral RNA synthesis (71, 72), although the precise mechanism of this inhibition is still unclear. The halogenated benzimidazole nucleosides are rather potent inhibitors of cell RNA synthesis (72); they have had little value as antiviral agents. It is interesting that 5,6-dichloro-1-β-D-ribofuranosylbenzimidazole is an enhancer of interferon induction, a possible result of inhibition of interferon RNA synthesis and of the shutoff of interferon production (73). The benzimidazoles have varying degrees of immunosuppressive activity, which is thought to be the reason for their protective effect against lymphocytic choriomeningitis virus infections in mice (74).

Extensive structure-activity studies on benzimidazoles as antiviral agents have shown that the virus-inhibitory activity and the cytotoxicity of these derivatives can vary independently (71, 75–80). Of the 2-benzylbenzimidazoles, HBB has been the most extensively studied and is among the most active. These compounds have not been reported to have significant *in vivo* antiviral activity. A series of 1-(benzimidazol-2-yl)-3-substituted ureas has been studied by Paget et al. (77), using a coxsackie virus *in vivo* antiviral assay system. No toxicologic studies on these substances were reported, except for their relative potency as immunosuppressive agents. Only the 3-cyclohexyl derivative (23.**26**)

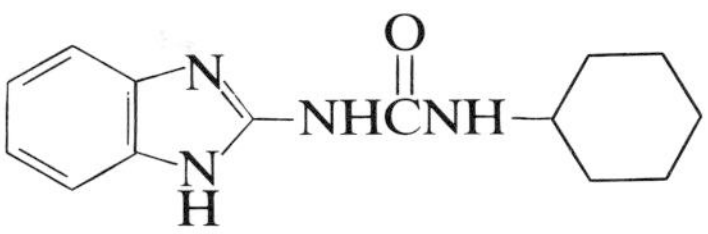

23.**26**

had potent antiviral activity without a concomitant immunosuppressive effect. A regression analysis of this structure-activity study has been described, with the general conclusion that the activity seems to depend on the gross shape of the molecule rather than on fine adjustments of structure (81).

Among a series of bisbenzimidazoles evaluated as antiviral agents, only 1,2-bis(5-methoxy-2-benzimidazol-2-yl)-1,2-ethanediol (23.**27**) has been shown to have antiviral activity *in vitro* (78) and *in vivo*, the animal test being a rhino virus infection experimentally induced in chimpanzees (79). The *in vivo* antiviral efficacy was accompanied by signs of toxicity, however. In reviewing the overall structure-activity relationships of the bisbenzimidazoles, only compounds with a two-carbon chain connecting the benzimidazoles appeared to have significant antiviral activity (78). It is of interest that related monobenzimidazoles tested *in vitro* against rhino viruses in a manner similar to that used for the bisbenzimidazoles were uniformly ineffective (78). The bisbenzimidazoles are especially important in that certain of these antiviral agents have been found to be highly inhibitory to all serotypes of Rhinovirus *in vitro* (78); such broad spectrum efficacy is important if ultimate control of the common cold is to be achieved.

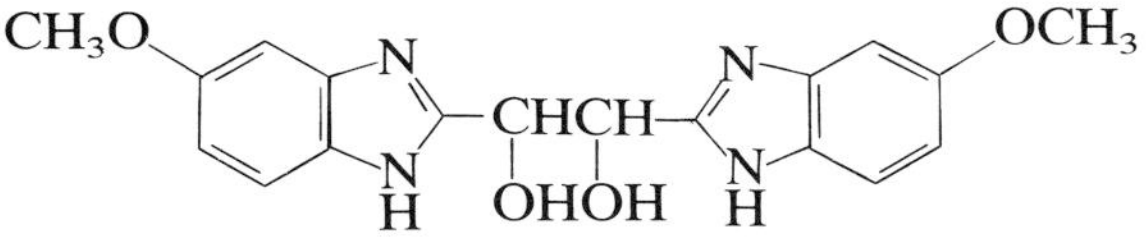

23.**27**

5.3 Ureas and Thioureas

An interesting class of compounds reported in a single study (82) to have *in vivo* Enterovirus-inhibitory activity is the 1-(benzothiazol-2-yl)-3-substituted ureas (23.**28**, 23.**29**). These compounds had activity similar to the benzimidazole ureas discussed in Section 5.2; but the significant protective effect against coxsackie virus infections in mice exhibited by these substituted ureas was usually associated with a marked immunosuppression. A group of 1-(2-naphtho[1,2-*d*]thiazolyl)-3-substituted ureas and 1-(2-naphtho[2,1-d]thiazolyl)-3-substituted ureas had similar significant *in vivo* antiviral activity that could not be separated from potent immunosuppression (82). Of a series of 2-pyrimidyl ureas, the derivatives 23.**30** through 23.**34** were active against coxsackie virus infections of mice, with no associated immunosuppression, indicating the antiviral activity may be quite specific (83).

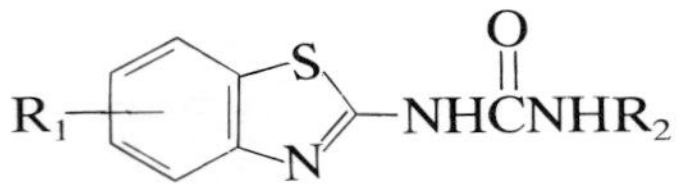

23.**28** $R_1 = H$, $R_2 = 4\text{-}NO_2C_6H_4$
23.**29** $R_1 = 5,6\text{-diCH}_3$, $R_2 = 1\text{-}C_{10}H_7$

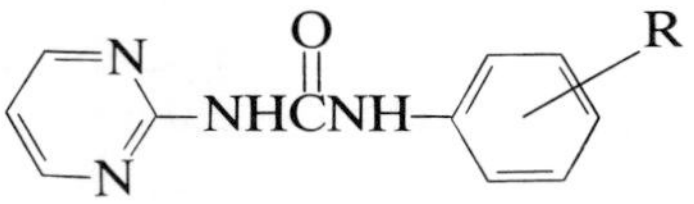

23.**30** R = 3,4-diCl
23.**31** R = 2,5-diCl
23.**32** R = 3-Cl
23.**33** $R = 3\text{-}NO_2$
23.**34** $R = 2\text{-}CH_3CH_2O$

An extensive series of thioureas has been examined for antiviral activity (84, 85); of these, 1-phenyl-3-(3-hydroxyphenyl)thiourea (23.**35**) had the greatest efficacy, inhibiting Enteroviruses (polio, coxsackie, ECHO) *in vitro* and also exhibiting a pronounced effect on coxsackie virus infections of mice (85).

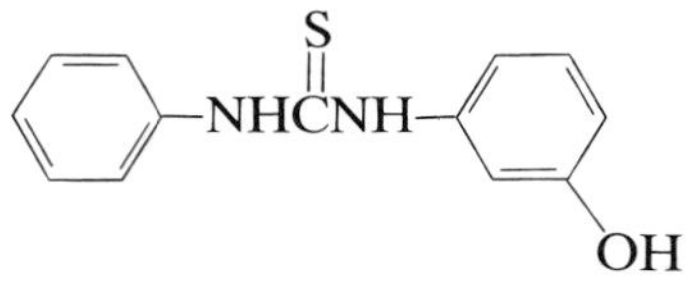

23.**35**

5.4 Guanidines and Biguanides

Guanidine hydrochloride (23.**36**) has been recognized for many years as a rather selective inhibitor in cell culture systems of the Enteroviruses, especially polio virus, although in animal systems it is virtually ineffective (72). The lack of activity *in vivo* apparently results from rapid renal excretion from the host (86), making the maintenance of adequate blood levels difficult. In addition, drug-resistant mutants are rapidly developed in animals (87). Guanidine has served a useful role as a tool for further elucidating the features of the Enteroviruses. The mode of action of guanidine involves inhibition of viral RNA synthesis. The initiation of viral RNA chains is blocked by the compound, possibly by interaction between viral RNA polymerase and guanidine. The compound is a specific inhibitor of the synthesis of viral RNA polymerase (88).

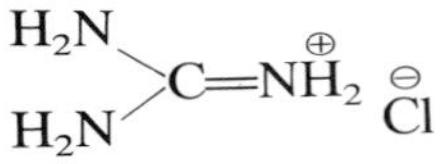

$$(H_2N)_2C{=}NH_2^{\oplus}\ Cl^{\ominus}$$

23.**36**

Structural alteration of guanidine generally reduces the antiviral activity. Simple salts (e.g., hydrochloride, nitrate, hydrosulfate) have approximately equal antiviral effects. Methylglyoxal-bis(guanylhydrazone) (23.**37**) possesses a selectivity of

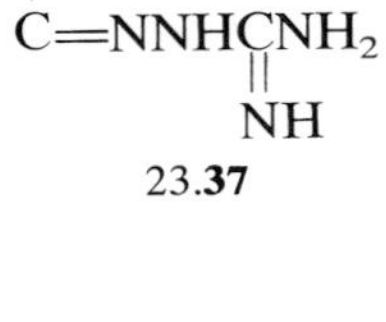

23.**37**

effect similar to that of guanidine HCl. Canavanine (23.**38**), an arginine analog, is

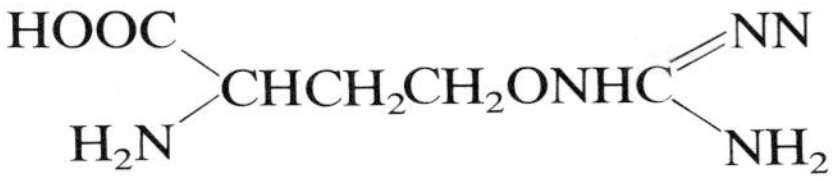

$$\mathrm{HOOC(H_2N)CHCH_2CH_2ONHC({=}NN)NH_2}$$

23.**38**

a mild inhibitor of the RNA-containing Semliki Forest virus (89). Some aromatic derivatives (23.**39**–23.41) of guanidine are

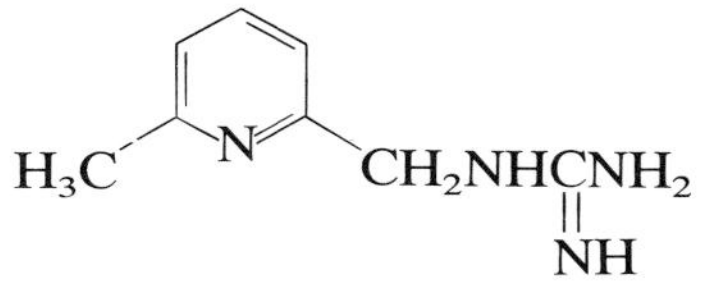

23.**39**

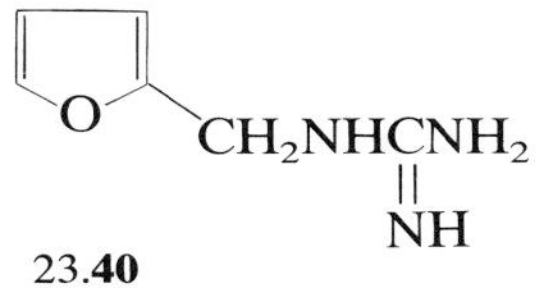

23.**40**

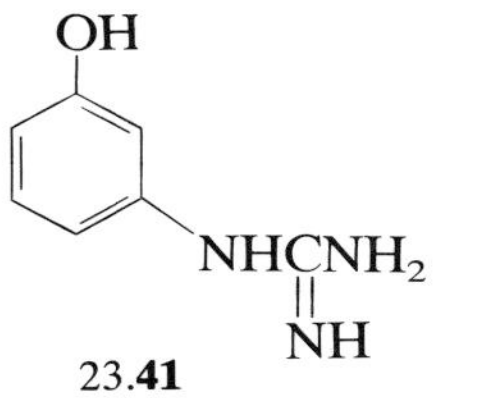

23.**41**

moderately effective against influenza and parainfluenza viruses *in vitro* (90). Recent reports show that 1-(4-chlorophenyl)-3-(3-isobutylguanidinophenyl)urea hydrochloride (23.**42**) is quite active against several rhino viruses, although this activity was dependent on the cells used in the studies (91, 92). The compound appears to act by affecting a late stage in viral replication, possibly at the point of assembly of viral nucleic acid and coat protein (92). Investigations of the antiviral activity of a number of derivatives of 23.**42** failed to demonstrate a definite structure-activity relationship (92).

The biguanides are another group of compounds that have received little attention in recent years. Probably most controversial of these compounds was *N*-amidino-4-morpholine carboxamidine hydrochloride (23.**43**), which had conflicting claims for activity in man (93). Numerous other biguanide derivatives have reportedly had moderate *in vitro* and *in vivo* activity against RNA viruses. Alkyl biguanides are inhibitory to parainfluenza virus *in vitro*; carbamoyl and sulfamoyl derivatives of phenyl- and benzylbiguanides are effective against polio virus; certain derivatives of benzenesulfonylbiguanide have been shown to have *in vivo* efficacy against polio virus (94). *N*-Furfuryl biguanide hydrochloride (23,**44**) has a relatively broader

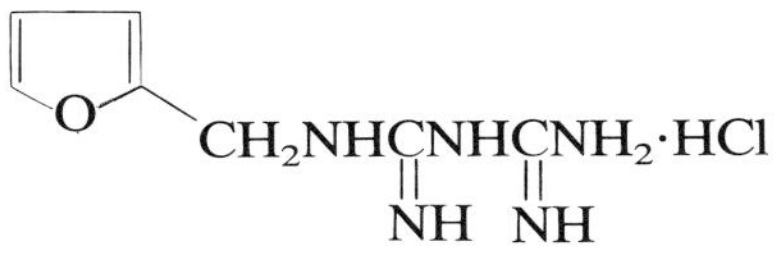

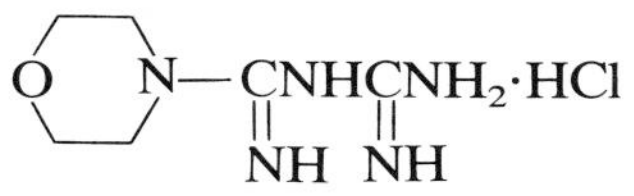

23.**43**

23.**44**

spectrum of antiviral activity, being inhibitory *in vitro* to influenza A, vesicular stomatitis, polio, and Newcastle disease viruses (95).

5.5 Adamantane Amines and Related Compounds

Amantadine HCl (23.**4**), a clinically active antiviral drug, is active against a number of RNA and DNA viruses *in vitro*; its major effectiveness is against influenza A group viruses. Similar anti influenza virus activity has also been seen in embryonated egg

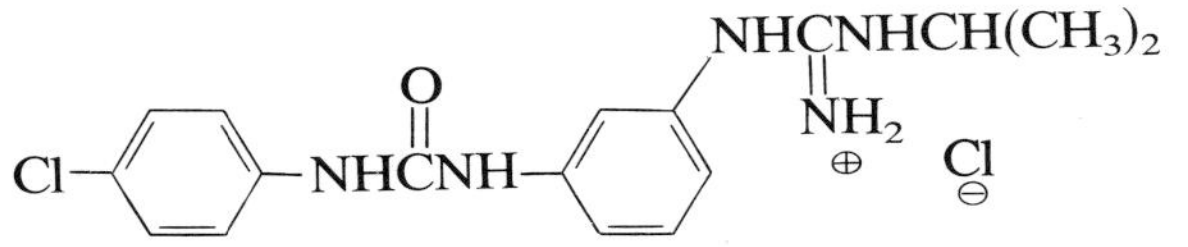

23.**42**

tests and in animals (96). The relatively strong prophylactic antiviral efficacy exhibited by this compound has incited a great deal of work with it and related derivatives. The closely related rimantadine HCl (23.**5**) has proved to have somewhat more antiviral activity than amantadine HCl in experimental systems and in man (96).

The exact mechanism of action of amantadine HCl is still unclear. This antiviral agent does not inactivate virus, interfere with attachment of the virus to the cell, or affect release of virus from cells. Studies indicate that it and related compounds prevent the viral nucleic acid from initiating new viral growth by preventing penetration of sensitive strains of influenza virus into the cell or by inhibiting the uncoating of the virus particle (96–101). Rimantadine HCl is thought to act in the same manner as amantadine HCl (102).

A number of compounds related to amantadine HCl have been investigated as antiviral agents. *N*-Alkyl and *N,N*-dialkyl derivatives of amantadine exhibit antiviral activity similar to that of amantadine HCl. In parallel experiments with amantadine HCl 23.**45**–23.**55** caused half-log decreases in the infectivity of influenza A virus to mice at doses of <10 mg/kg. Adamantane

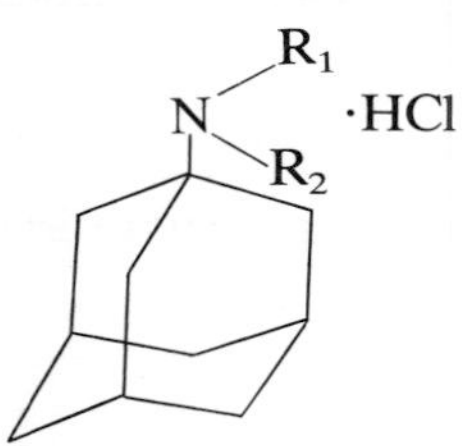

23.**4** $R_1 = H, R_2 = H$
23.**45** $R_1 = H, R_2 = CH_3$
23.**46** $R_1 = H, R_2 = CH_3CH_2$
23.**47** $R_1 = H, R_2 = CH_3CH_3CH_2$
23.**48** $R_1 = H, R_2 = (CH_3)_2CH$
23.**49** $R_1 = H, R_2 = CH_2{=}CHCH_2$
23.**50** $R_1 = CH_3, R_2 = CH_3$
23.**51** $R_1 = CH_3CH_2, R_2 = CH_3CH_2$
23.**52** $R_1 = CH_3, R_2 = CH_2{=}CHCH_2$
23.**53** $R_1 = CH_2{=}CHCH_2, R_2 = CH_2{=}CHCH_2$
23.**54** $R_1 = C_6H_5CH{=}$(not an HCl salt)
23.**55** $R_1 = H, R_2 = NH_2CH_2CO$

compounds with a hydroxyl, thiol, halogen, or cyano group in place of the amino group were inactive (103). With the possible exception of the glycyl derivative (23.**55**), *N*-acyl derivatives of amantadine generally show reduced antiviral activity (103). A number of substituted acetyl derivatives of amantadine have been evaluated for activity against a wide variety of viruses (104). Of these, tromantadine HCl (23.**6**) has been reported to have strong efficacy, especially against herpes viruses (25).

Derivatives of rimantadine having significant *in vivo* influenza virus activity include 23.**56**–23.**65** (103). Treatment of

23.**5** $R_1 = H, R_2 = CH_3, R_3 = H, R_4 = H$
23.**56** $R_1 = H, R_2 = H, R_3 = H, R_4 = CH_3$
23.**57** $R_1 = H, R_2 = H, R_3 = CH_3, R_4 = CH_3$
23.**58** $R_1 = H, R_2 = H_3, R_3 = H, R_4 = H$
23.**59** $R_1 = H, R_2 = CH_3CH_2, R_3 = H, R_4 = H$
23.**60** $R_1 = H, R_2 = CH_3, R_3 = H, R_4 = CH_3$
23.**61** $R_1 = H, R_2 = CH_3, R_3 = CH_3, R_4 = CH_3$
23.**62** $R_1 = CH_3, R_2 = CH_3, R_3 = H, R_4 = H$
23.**63** $R_1 = CH_3, R_2 = CH_3, R_3 = H, R_4 = CH_3$
23.**64** $R_1 = CH_3, R_2 = CH_3, R_3 = H, R_4 = CH_3CH_2$
23.**65** $R_1 = CH_3, R_2 = CH_3, R_3 = CH_3, R_4 = CH_3$

mice with $\leqq 10$ mg/kg of these compounds caused at least a half-log decrease in influenza A virus infectivity. Rimantadine exerted similar activity. As in the case of the amantadine derivatives, *N*-alkyl and *N,N*-dialkyl derivatives also exhibit potent antiviral effect. Both optical isomers and the racemic mixture of rimantadine show essentially equivalent potency to influenza viruses. A DARC/PELCO computer analysis of a number of amantadine and rimantadine derivatives has shown a close correlation of predicted activity with experimentally observed activity (105).

Adamantanespiro-3′-pyrrolidine (23.**66**) and the *N*-methyl (23.**67**) and *N*-ethyl (23.**68**) derivatives have activity equal to or

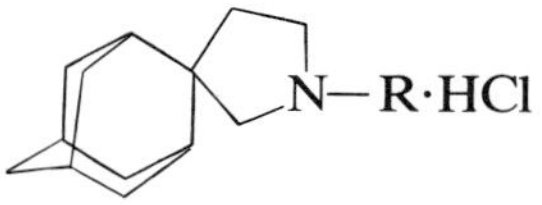

N—R·HCl

23.**66** R = H
23.**67** R = CH_3(Hydromaleate salt)
23.**68** R = CH_3CH_2

greater than that of amantadine HCl against influenza A_2 virus *in vivo*; significantly, they also have *in vitro* activity against other unrelated RNA viruses (106–108), suggesting possible greater utility than amantadine due to an increased spectrum of virus-inhibitory effect. Indeed, 23.**67** has been proved to be active in a clinical trial against influenza A_2 (109), but failed in a study using volunteers challenged with rhino viruses 2 and 9 (108). Other spiro amines reportedly also show similar influenza virus-inhibiting effects (110). Among these *N*-methylbornane-2-spiro-3′-pyrrolidine hydrochloride (23.**69**) has special interest because it also inhibits rhino, coxsackie, and parainfluenza viruses.

3-Amino- and 3-methylaminohomoadamantane derivatives (23.**70**–23.**73**) were

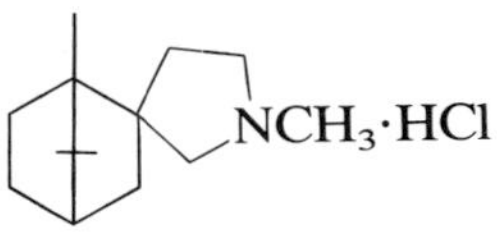

NCH_3·HCl

23.**69**

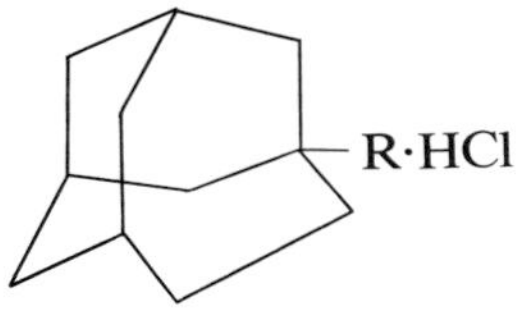

R·HCl

23.**70** R = NH_2
23.**71** R = CH_2NH_2
23.**72** R = $CH(CH_3)NH_2$
23.**73** R = $C(CH_3)_2NH_2$

found to be inhibitory to influenza A (Swine) virus infections in mice at dosages of <10 mg/kg; this efficacy appeared similar to or greater than that of amantadine HCl, which was tested in the same system (103).

The recently described homoisotwistane derivatives (23.**74**, 23.**75**) appear to have

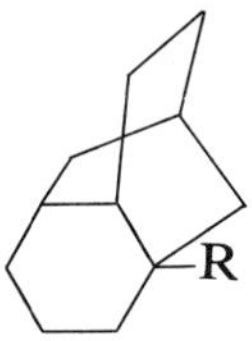

R

23.**74** R = NH_2 · HCl
23.**75** R = CH_2NH_2·HCl

good potential as antiviral agents, although in the studies reported to date, they have been subjected only to *in vitro* evaluations using a Paramyxovirus, Newcastle disease virus, as the assay agent, with activity exceeding that of amantadine HCl (111). A number of cage amines have been explored with regard to their usefulness as antiviral agents. Several amine and methylamine derivatives of bicyclo[2.2.2]octane have shown activity against influenza virus similar to that of amantadine HCl. Among the more active of these derivatives are 23.**76** and 23.**77** (112).

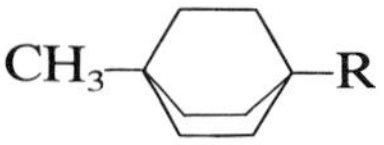

CH_3—R

23.**76** R = NH_2
23.**77** R = CH_2NH_2·HCl

Another antiviral amine compound of interest is cyclooctylamine hydrochloride (23.**78**). This compound inhibits influenza,

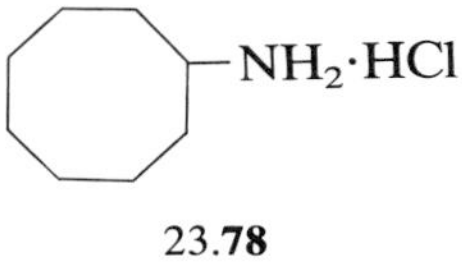

NH_2·HCl

23.**78**

parainfluenza, herpes, and vaccinia viruses *in vitro* (113), with a mode of action similar to that of amantadine. The activity against influenza viruses has also been seen in several animal systems (96), and a definite but incomplete protective effect has been seen in a clinical study using volunteers challenged with influenza A_2 virus and treated with drops of cyclooctylamine administered intranasally (114).

5.6 Pyrimidine Nucleosides and Nucleotides

Numerous pyrimidine nucleosides have exhibited highly significant antiviral activity, and several have found some clinical utility. Because extensive studies have been conducted on structure-activity correlations, on mechanism of action, and on experimental and clinical antiviral activity, reference is made primarily to the major published reviews, with emphasis on the antiviral nucleosides having the greatest significance.

5.6.1 HALOGENATED 2′-DEOXYPYRIMIDINE NUCLEOSIDES. The more important of the halogenated 2′-deoxypyrimidine nucleosides include IdU (23.**2**), F_3TdR (23.**3**), and 5-iodo-2′-deoxycytidine (IdC, 23.**79**). Repeated efforts have been directed toward

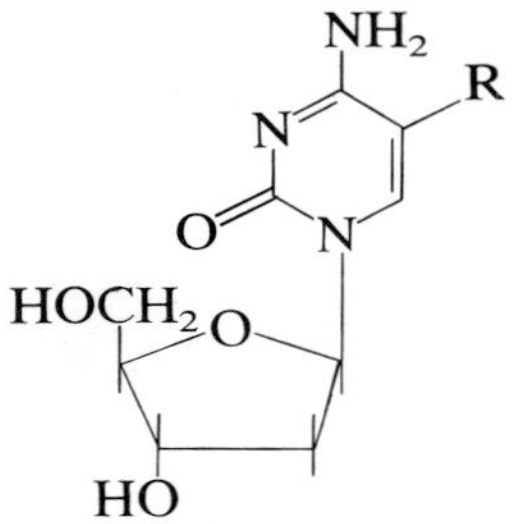

NH2 R N O N HOCH2 O HO

23.**79** R = I
23.**80** R = Br

the synthesis of modified pyrimidine nucleosides, that have a more selective virus inhibitory effect. Representative of such efforts are the 5′-amino-2′,5′-dideoxypyrimidine nucleosides, some of which may hold promise as future antiviral drugs. IdU is one of the first synthetic nucleosides found to be effective as an antiviral agent (115, 116). This nucleoside is active against a number of DNA viruses, including herpes types 1 and 2 and vaccinia, and it has been used extensively in topical form as a clinically effective agent. The other halogenated 2′-deoxyuridines have had mixed reports of activity in experimental systems and have not found clinical usefulness as antiviral agents (17, 18).

Detailed studies have been reported on the mechanism of action of IdU, 5-bromo-2′-deoxyuridine (BdU), and 5-fluoro-2′-deoxyuridine (FdU), as reviewed by others (18, 117). IdU and BdU are sterically very similar to thymidine, as shown by comparison of the effective size of the 5-substituents of these nucleosides. The Van der Waals radius of the methyl group is 2.00 Å, compared to 1.95 Å for the bromo group and 2.15 Å for the iodo group. It is therefore not surprising that these nucleosides enter into, and subsequently affect, a number of biochemical reactions. In both virus-infected and uninfected cells, they are phosphorylated to their mono, di-, and triphosphate forms, and they interact with thymidine kinase, thymidylate kinase, and DNA polymerase. No significant differences were found in inhibition of these enzymes in virus-infected cells compared to uninfected cells (117). The principal basis for antiviral activity of IdU is incorporation into viral DNA. Unfortunately, the drug is also incorporated into the DNA of normal, uninfected cells, which is probably the primary reason for the toxicity it exhibits (117). The abnormal viral DNA formed in cells treated with IdU results in viral subunits that do not function correctly in the viral replicative process. It has also been shown that replacement of DNA thymidine by IdU results in the formation of either no protein coat or an inadequate one (118).

F_3TdR (23.**3**) inhibits the replication of adeno, herpes, and vaccinia viruses *in vitro* and has strong *in vivo* activity against rabbit corneal infections and mouse encephalitis caused by herpes and vaccinia viruses (119, 120). It is apparently more effective than IdU in treating herpes keratitis in humans. The mechanism of action of F_3TdR has been extensively reviewed (121). The compound is phosphorylated by thymidine kinase to the 5′-phosphate, which is a potent inhibitor of thymidylate synthetase. It is unclear, however, whether this inhibition is related to antiviral activity. A significantly greater incorporation of F_3TdR into virion DNA than into cellular DNA has been seen. The resultant viral DNA is too small and is not completely transcribed into late RNA, which probably leads to defective proteins. Overall, an abnormal, defective virus is produced. Comparison tests with F_3TdR, F_3TdR-5′-monophosphate, 5-trifluoromethyluracil, and F_3TdR-5′-methylphosphonate showed F_3TdR and its 5′-phosphate to be the most potent inhibitors of vaccinia virus replication (122).

IdC and 5-bromo-2′-deoxycytidine (BdC, 23.**80**) exhibit antiviral activity against Herpesviruses similar to that of the corresponding 5-halogenated analogs of 2′-deoxyuridine, apparently with a more selective inhibition of virus replication, since less cytotoxicity is seen (123, 124). In a limited number of tests, IdC has had possible activity against vaccinia and herpes zoster infections in humans (18). The basis for the antiviral selectivity seen appears to be a virus-induced nucleoside kinase that phosphorylates these nucleosides, whereas in uninfected cells this phosphorylation does not readily occur (125).

In view of the significant antiviral activity of several thymidine analogs, a number of related 5′-amino-2′,5′-dideoxypyrimidine nucleosides were synthesized and evaluated as antiviral agents, and significant inhibitory effects were observed, especially against herpes viruses (126–130). 5′-Amino-5-iodo-2′,5′-dideoxyuridine (23.**81**) has generally exhibited the greatest degree of antiviral activity and also was effective against herpes keratitis in rabbits (311). It is very significant that this compound is markedly less cytotoxic than IdU, indicating that it has a more specific mode of antiviral activity and possibly greater safety. A potential drawback to these nucleosides is their very specificity, for they fail to inhibit all strains of herpes viruses. The specific antiviral activity of 23.**81** is considered to be a result

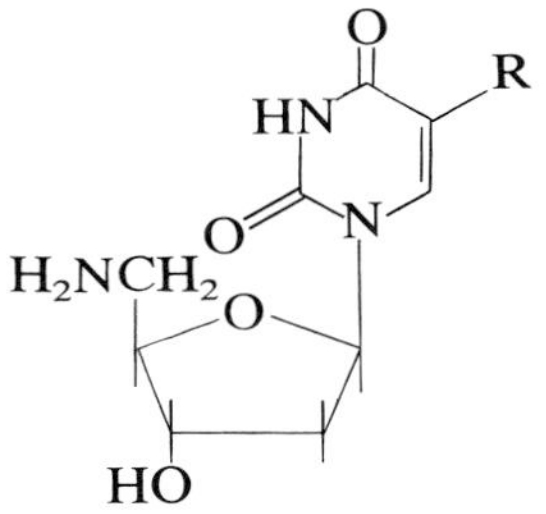

O, R, HN, O, N, H_2NCH_2, O, HO

23.**81** R = I
23.**82** R = Br
23.**83** R = Cl
23.**84** R = CF_3

of the incorporation of the 5′-*N*-phosphate into both viral and host DNA in infected cells, but not into the DNA of normal cells. Phosphorylation of this 5′-aminonucleoside occurs only in herpes virus-infected cells, brought about by a virus-induced thymidine kinase (127).

Other derivatives of 5′-amino-2′,5′-dideoxyuridine that exhibit significant antiviral activity include those containing the 5-bromo- (23.**82**), 5-chloro- (23.**83**), and 5-trifluoromethyl (23.**84**) substituents (130).

5.6.2. 5-ALKYL AND OTHER 5-SUBSTITUTED 2′-DEOXYPYRIMIDINE NUCLEOSIDES. Most significant among this class of nucleosides is 5-ethyl-2′-deoxyuridine (23.**85**), which is markedly inhibitory to herpes and vaccinia

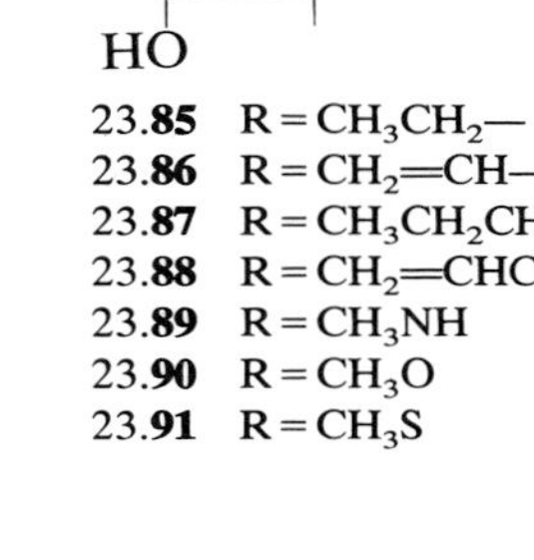

O, R, HN, O, N, $HOCH_2$, O, HO

23.**85** R = CH_3CH_2—
23.**86** R = $CH_2{=}CH$—
23.**87** R = $CH_3CH_2CH_2$—
23.**88** R = $CH_2{=}CHCH_2$—
23.**89** R = CH_3NH
23.**90** R = CH_3O
23.**91** R = CH_3S

viruses in cell culture and animal systems and also exhibits positive therapeutic effects against herpetic keratitis in man (117, 119). It is important that no inhibition of regeneration of damaged corneas occurred under the same conditions at which IdU was markedly inhibitory (132). 5-Methylamino-2′-deoxyuridine has been shown to be at least equivalent to IdU against herpes keratitis and possibly less toxic (133).

The mode of action of 5-ethyl-2′-deoxyuridine is not clearly established, but reportedly it is converted to the 5′-triphosphate, then incorporated into DNA (134). The compound is an inhibitor of DNA synthesis but at concentrations well above those that are virus inhibitory (135). In a study with herpes virus-induced thymidine kinases, this nucleoside was found to have a much higher affinity for the virus-induced enzymes than for normal cellular thymidine kinase (136).

Other 5-alkyl derivatives of 2′-deoxyuridine having significant antiherpes virus inhibitory effects include those with 5-vinyl (23.**86**), 5-propyl (23.**87**), and 5-allyl (23.**88**) substituents (137). Certain other 5-substituted 2′-deoxyuridines, including the methylamino (23.**89**), methoxy (23.**90**), and methylthio (23.**91**) derivatives, have shown moderate *in vitro* antiherpes virus activity (138–140).

5.6.3 PYRIMIDINE ARABINONUCLEOSIDES. The anti-cancer drug ara-C (23.**7**) has a strong inhibitory effect on a number of DNA viruses *in vitro* and *in vivo* (119), being limited in human antiviral use primarily because of toxicological manifestations and its rapid deamination to the relatively inactive 1-β-D-arabinofuranosyluracil in man. The mechanism of action of this nucleoside has been reviewed (26, 117). Ara-C is involved in several biochemical processes, although much of the work reported has been with nonviral systems. The nucleoside is converted in the cell to the 5′-monophosphate by deoxycytidine kinase, followed by formation of the di- and triphosphate; this may be a key step in the antiviral action of ara-C, since cell and virus resistance to it is observed in cells that are deficient in deoxycytidine kinase or in a mutant herpes virus that does not induce this kinase activity in cells. The nucleoside is a strong inhibitor of the synthesis of both DNA and RNA, and the triphosphate has been shown to inhibit both DNA and RNA polymerases (141). Incorporation of ara-C into both DNA and RNA has also been observed. These biochemical actions imply a lack of virus-specific inhibitory action.

An enormous number of derivatives of ara-C have been investigated in an effort to improve the activity of this nucleoside. The primary biological evaluations of these compounds have been for antitumor and immunosuppressive activity. Montgomery et al. (142), in their chapter on antitumor drugs included in this volume, have extensively reviewed this structure-activity relationship, and only a brief mention of those having striking activity or rather novel structure appears here. Acyl derivatives of ara-C that have been studied include numerous mono-, di-, or triesters of the nucleoside hydroxyl groups (143–145). These derivatives are resistant to cytidine deaminase. Enzymatic hydrolysis of the acyl groups results in slow release of ara-C. Most of these derivatives have a significant degree of *in vitro* activity against herpes and vaccinia viruses, although usually no greater than that of ara-C itself. Reduced activity has generally been seen with the addition of substituents on the cytosine ring (147, 148), and by addition of biologically irreversible modifications such as methyl esters (149, 150) on the sugar moiety.

A novel cyclonucleoside, 2,2′-anhydro-1-β-D-arabinofuranosylcytosine hydrochloride (23.**92**), is resistant to cytidine deaminase and is slowly hydrolyzed to ara-C (151–155). This cyclonucleoside and a number of

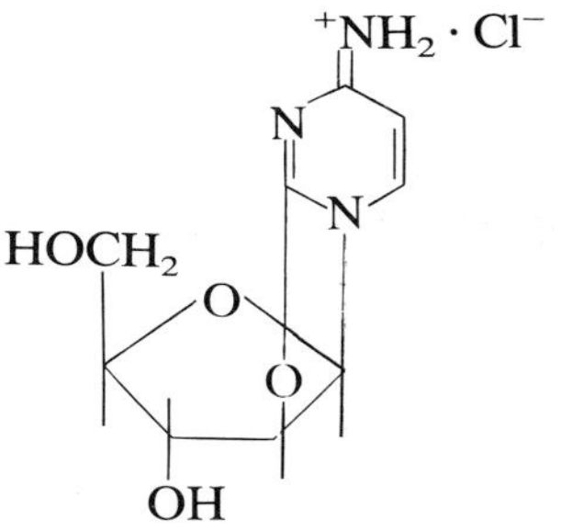

$^{+}NH_2 \cdot Cl^-$ ... $HOCH_2$ ... OH

23.**92**

O-acyl derivatives show significant activity against several DNA viruses (156, 157). The 3′,5′-cyclic phosphate of ara-C (23.**93**)

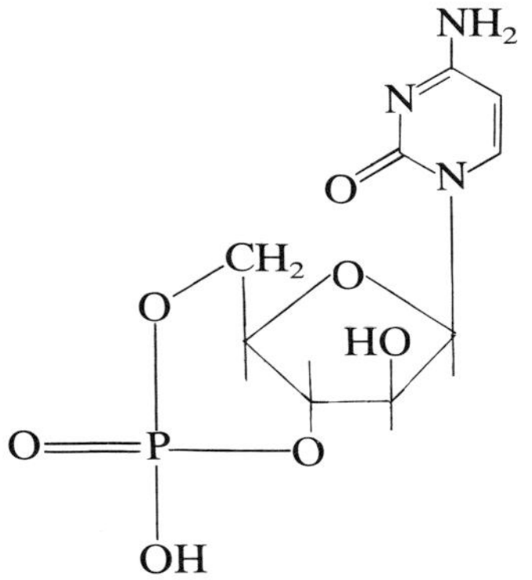

NH_2 ... CH_2 ... HO ... O=P ... OH

23.**93**

has also shown significant antiviral activity both *in vitro* and *in vivo*, its efficacy being greater than that exhibited by ara-C itself (158, 159). It was speculated that the 3′,5′-cyclic phosphate moiety may inhibit the deamination of ara-C, thus causing the increased *in vivo* potency (159).

An interesting pyrimidine arabinonucleoside recently reported to have significant antiherpes virus activity *in vitro*, but weak effects in animal systems, is 1-β-D-arabinofuranosylthymine (ara-T, 23.**94**), which inhibits DNA synthesis only in virus-infected cells (160–162). It was suggested that ara-T may be phosphorylated only by a virus-induced enzyme, but not by the normal cellular enzymes. The weak *in vivo* antiviral activity was probably due to rapid urinary excretion of ara-T. 1-β-D-Arabinofuranosyl-5-methylcytosine (5-methyl-ara-C, 23.**95**), which is deaminated to ara-T, also had strong anti-herpes virus activity *in vitro* but only in cells with high levels of deoxycytidine deaminase (162). 5-Methyl ara-C (23.**95**) is an example of a pyrimidine nucleoside analog in which the deaminated product retains antiviral activity, in contrast to ara-C, which is deaminated to a relatively inactive nucleoside. Thorough *in vivo* antiviral studies on 5-methyl ara-C have not yet been reported, however.

5.6.4 AZAPYRIMIDINE NUCLEOSIDES. A compound in this class of nucleosides that is currently considered to be of significance as an antiviral agent is 6-azuridine (23.**96**), which inhibits several DNA and RNA viruses in cell culture (119, 163). This compound has also exhibited activity *in vivo* against vaccinia and herpes virus infections (164, 165) and has been reported to be effective against herpes simplex and smallpox infections in man, although side effects have curtailed the use of the drug (17, 166). 6-Azacytidine reportedly inhibits

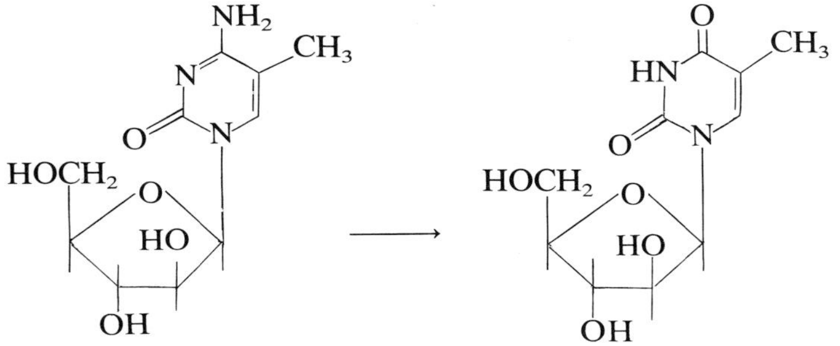

NH_2, CH_3, $HOCH_2$, HO, OH → O, CH_3, HN, $HOCH_2$, HO, OH

23.**94** 23.**95**

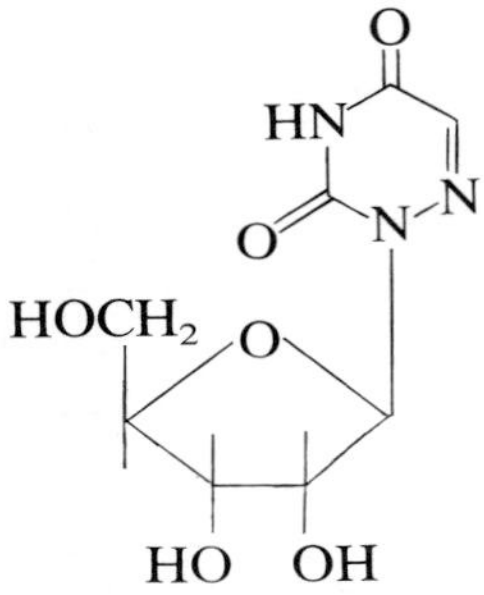

HN, O, N, HOCH$_2$, HO, OH

23.**96**

DNA viruses *in vitro* (167) but failed to be active in *in vivo* systems (168).

The basis for the antiviral activity of 6-azauridine has appeared to be conversion of this nucleoside to the 5′-monophosphate, which inhibits orotidylic acid decarboxylase (169). Inhibition of this route of biosynthesis of uridine-5′-monophosphate presumably interferes with formation of viral RNA during the replicative cycle of sensitive viruses. In support of this postulated mechanism of action, uridine and cytidine have been shown to reverse the inhibition caused by 6-azauridine (170, 171). Recent studies have demonstrated, however, that no differences in orotic acid pathways exist between 6-azauridine-sensitive and -resistant viruses (vaccinia, Newcastle disease, vesicular stomatitis), with the drug strongly inhibiting ^{14}C-orotic acid incorporation into both viral and cellular RNA (163). This suggests that 6-azauridine may also act on some other site of action in exerting its antiviral effect.

In addition to the 6-azapyrimidine nucleosides, certain 6-azapyrimidine heterocycles showing antiviral activity include 6-azauracil (23.**97**), which has a mild *in vivo* vaccinia virus-inhibitory effect (168), as

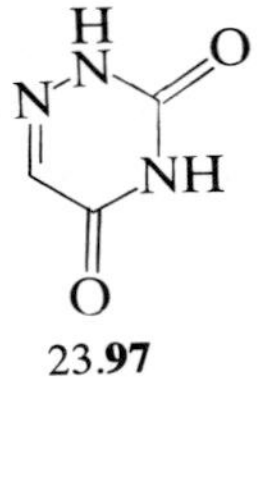

H, N, O, NH, O

23.**97**

well as a number of alkyl derivatives of 2-thio- and 4-thio-6-azauracil, which inhibit DNA viruses *in vitro* (172).

Another active azapyrimidine nucleoside is 5,6-dihydro-5-azathymidine (23.**97a**),

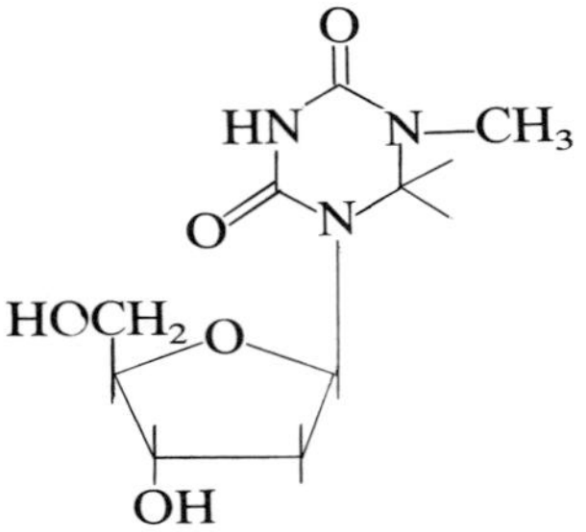

O, HN, N—CH$_3$, N, HOCH$_2$, O, OH

23.**97a**

which appears to have strong antiherpes virus activity *in vitro* and *in vivo* (172a, 172b). This nucleoside was discovered in a fermentation broth from *Streptomyces platensis* var *clarensis* (172c). The activity of this compound may be due to inhibition of thymidine phosphorylation in the infected cell (172a).

5.6.5 DEAZAPYRIMIDINE NUCLEOSIDES. 3-Deazauridine (23.**98**) and 3-deazacytidine (23.**99**) inhibit *in vitro* replication of several

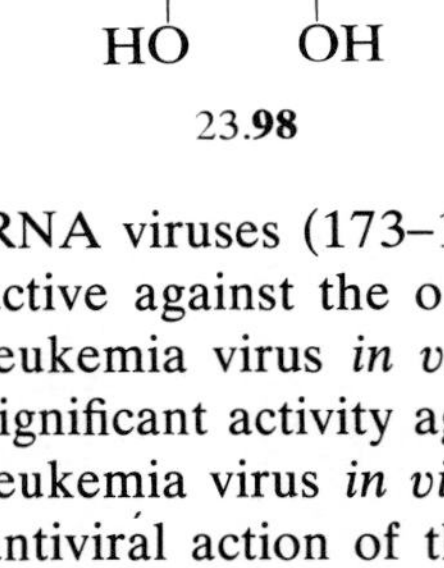

OH, O, N, HOCH$_2$, HO, OH

23.**98**

NH$_2$, O, N, HOCH$_2$, HO, OH

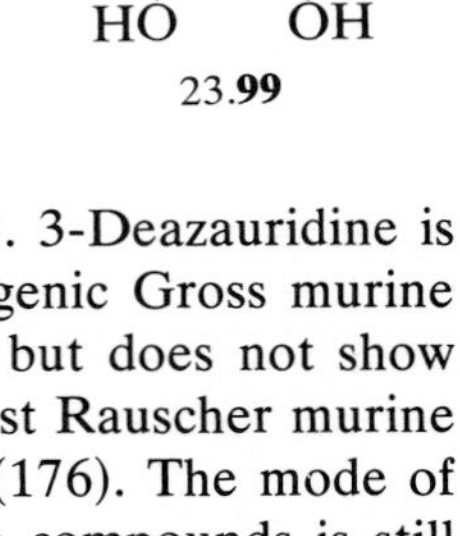

23.**99**

RNA viruses (173–176). 3-Deazauridine is active against the oncogenic Gross murine leukemia virus *in vitro* but does not show significant activity against Rauscher murine leukemia virus *in vivo* (176). The mode of antiviral action of these compounds is still obscure, although their activity can be reversed by addition of their corresponding naturally occurring pyrimidine nucleosides, indicating a competitive inhibition of viral and possibly cellular processes (173). In studies with tumor cells, both 3-deazauridine and 3-deazacytidine are converted to their 5′-triphosphates, which interfere with pyrimidine nucleotide biosynthesis (177).

5.7 Pyrimidine Heterocycles

Dichloropyrimidines exhibit significant *in vitro* activity against unrelated DNA and RNA viruses, including polio, coxsakie, vaccinia, and herpes viruses; the most active compound seen in these cell culture systems, 2-amino-4,6-dichloropyrimidine (23.**100**), has also exhibited protective

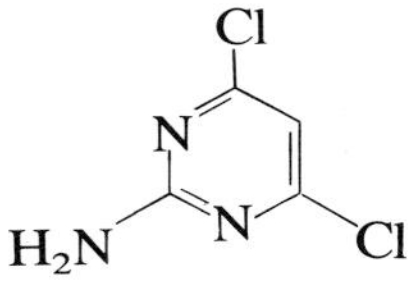

Cl
N
H_2N N Cl

23.**100**

effect in rabbits infected with herpetic keratitis (178). An important aspect of the activity of these compounds is the observation that they are still active late in the viral replicative cycle. Studies into the mechanism of action of these compounds suggest their activity against RNA and DNA viruses (polio and vaccinia were investigated) to be similar; 23.**100**, especially, inhibits assembly of poliovirus proteins into procapsides, subsequently preventing coating of available infectious viral nucleic acid to form mature virus particles (178). The exact mechanism by which this occurs is still unclear.

Early studies with a series of substituted 5-phenoxy-2-thiouracils indicated that several have a protective effect on mice infected with vaccinia virus. 5-(2,4-Dichlorophenoxy)-2-thiouracil (23.**101**) was the most effective of this group (179). Other

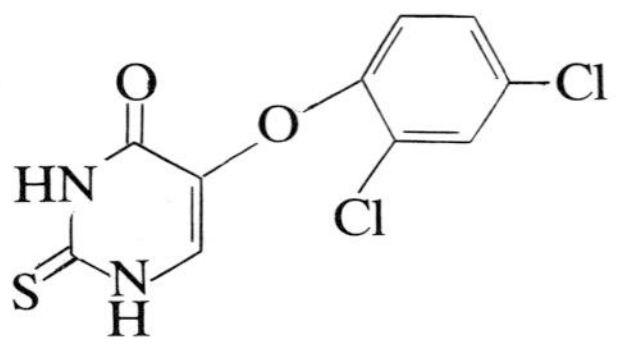

O
HN O Cl
Cl
S N
H

23.**101**

uracil derivatives exhibiting a moderate degree of vaccinia virus inhibitory activity *in vivo* include 3-(Mercaptomethyl)uracil (168), 5-amino-6-methyluracil, 5-hydroxy-6-methyluracil, and 5-formamidouracil (180). 1-Allyl-6-chloro-3,5-diethyluracil (23.**102**) was shown to significantly inhibit

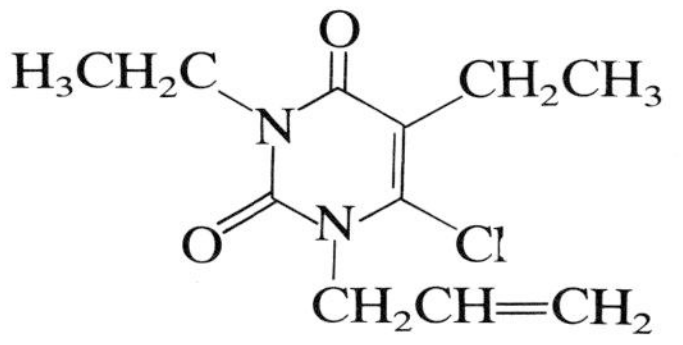

O
H_3CH_2C CH_2CH_3
N
O N Cl
$CH_2CH{=}CH_2$

23.**102**
23.**103**
23.**104** see Figure 23.1
23.**105**

herpes virus-induced keratitis in rabbits and to be efficacious in treating herpetic skin and mucus diseases in man (181). The latter compound was the most effective of a series of alkylated pyrimidines (182).

5.8 Purine Nucleosides and Nucleotides

5.8.1 PURINE ARABINONUCLEOSIDES AND ARABINONUCLEOTIDES. The clinically active antiviral drug ara-A (23.**8**) is active *in vitro* and *in vivo* against a number of DNA viruses and also inhibits certain RNA tumor viruses which replicate through a DNA intermediate (119, 183–185). The antiviral mechanism of action of ara-A is difficult to define, since the metabolism of the compound in the host is still unclear; as a result, the actual compound exerting the antiviral effect in the cell is not fully identified (186). The possible metabolic pathways for ara-A are summarized in Fig. 23.2. Ara-A may be acting, as originally

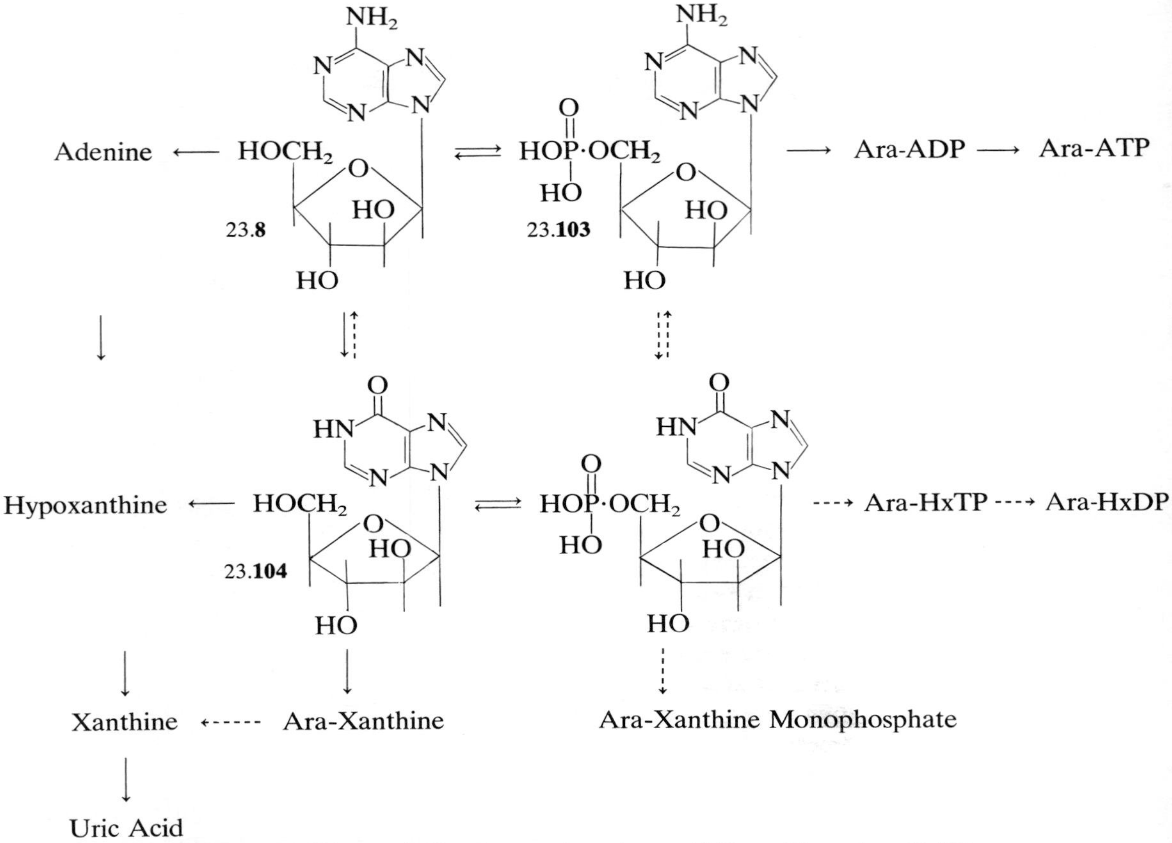

Fig. 23.2 Possible metabolic pathways of ara-A, ara-AMP, ara-Hx, and ara-HxMP.

speculated (187, 188), as its monophosphate (9-β-D-arabinofuranosyladenine monophosphate, ara-AMP, 23.**103**), diphosphate (ara-ADP), or triphosphate (ara-ATP), but more evidence is accumulating to indicate the compound is being deaminated to its hypoxanthine form (9-β-D-arabinofuranosylhypoxanthine, ara-Hx, 23.**104**) (189, 190). Studies have also shown ara-A to be converted to adenine ribonucleotides (191). The hypoxanthine arabino nucleoside (23.**104**) may be exerting antiviral action in that form, or as the monophosphate (9-β-D-arabinofuranosylhypoxanthine 5′-monophosphate, ara-HxMP, 23.**105**), diphosphate, or triphosphate; ara-Hx may itself be broken down to the inactive hypoxanthine. Ara-Hx does apparently retain a degree of antiviral activity, but higher concentrations are necessary for effective inhibition compared to ara-A (192, 193). Inhibition of ribonucleotide reductase and herpes virus-specific DNA polymerase by ara-ATP has been observed (194). Ara-A is incorporated into the DNA of types 1 and 2 herpes viruses, possibly acting as a chain terminator (194). A selective inhibition of viral DNA synthesis by ara-A has been demonstrated; it was speculated that this selective inhibition may be due to the increased sensitivity to ara-A of one of the enzymes, either on the pathway of DNA synthesis in the infected cell or leading to it, compared to the corresponding enzyme in the uninfected host cell.

Adenosine deaminase converts ara-A to the less active ara-Hx; studies with combinations of ara-A and inhibitors of adenosine deaminase ([*R*]-3-β-D-ribofuranosyl-3,6,7,8-tetrahydroimidazol[4,5-*d*][1, 3]-diazapin-8-ol, coformycin, 23.**106**, 2′-deoxy coformycin, 23.**107**), and *erythro*-9-(2-hydroxy-3-nonyl)adenine hydrochloride, 23.**108**) have displayed enhanced antiviral

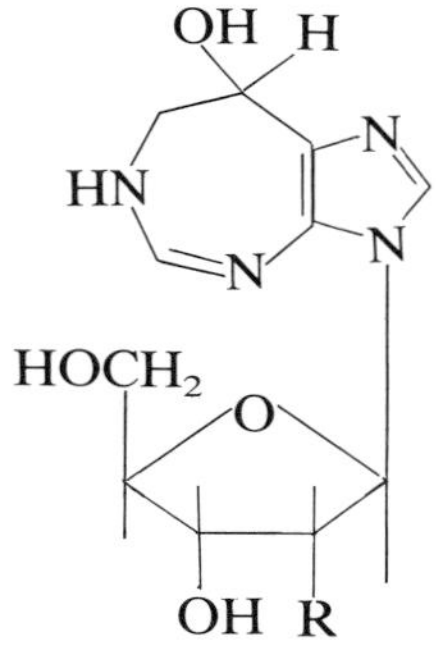

23.**106** R = OH
23.**107** R = H

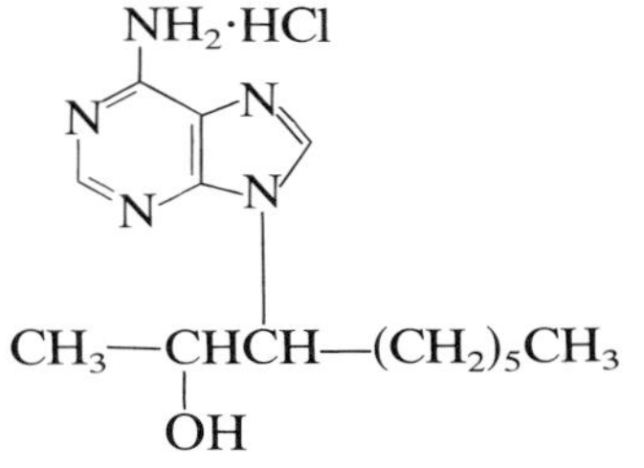

23.**108**

activity compared to the ara-A alone (195, 196), although careful study shows the toxic effects of ara-A usually are increased concomitantly (197, 198). The 5′-monophosphates (23.**103**, 23.**105**) and the 3′,5′-cyclic nucleotides (23.**109**, 23.**110**) of ara-

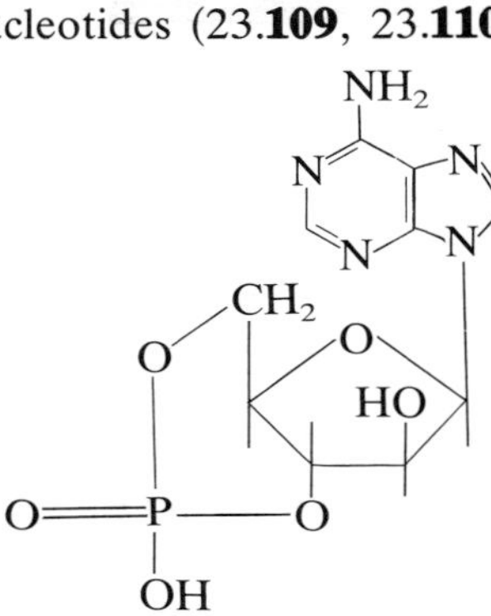

23.**109**

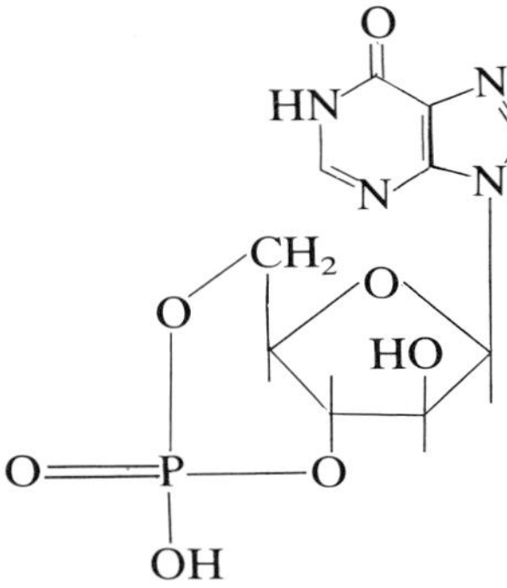

23.**110**

A and ara-Hx offer soluble forms of these antiviral nucleosides. Each of these nucleotides significantly inhibits a number of DNA viruses *in vitro* and *in vivo* (186, 199–203), with a greater effect than ara-A seen in *in vivo* systems using topical application of each. It was thought that the latter improved result might be due to the increased solubility of the nucleotides (186, 199). Of significance is a study disclosing that ara-AMP is not readily deaminated and slowly penetrates cells in its intact form (197), suggesting a useful sustained release form of ara-A. Indeed, a marked prolongation of blood levels of the nucleotide has been demonstrated in human patients (196, 204). The monophosphate and cyclic phosphate forms of ara-A also apparently produce a sustained cytotoxic effect, however (197, 198). The 5′-*O*-methylphosphates of ara-A and ara-Hx also exhibit significant antiviral activity (200).

Structure-activity relationship studies on ara-A indicate that substitution with alkyl groups at the N^1 and N^6 positions results. in a reduction or loss of antiviral activity (205). The N^6-hydroxy analog (23.**111**) had strong antiherpes virus activity *in vitro* and *in vivo*, although some immunosuppression, especially using *in vitro* assays, was also seen (206). Certain 2,6-disubstituted 9-β-D-arabinofuranosylpurines also exhibited significant antiviral activity (23.**112**–23–**119**). Of these, the 2,6-diamino derivative (23.**113**) was especially active, and its

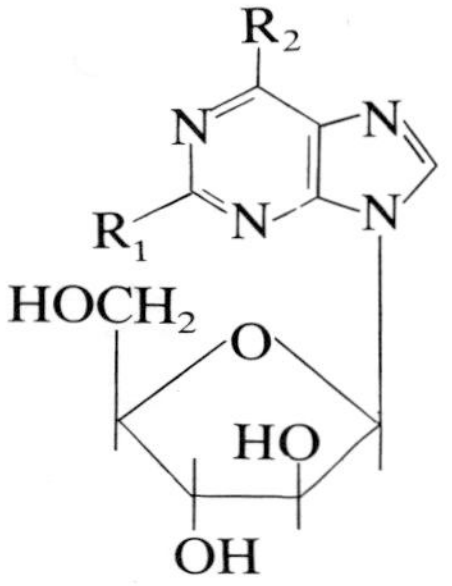

23.**111** $R_1 = H, R_2 = NHOH$
23.**112** $R_1 = Cl, R_2 = NH_2$
23.**113** $R_1 = NH_2, R_2 = NH_2$
23.**114** $R_1 = NH_2, R_2 = OH$
23.**115** $R_1 = NH_2, R_2 = NHCH_3$
23.**116** $R_1 = NHCH_3, R_2 = NH_2$
23.**117** $R_1 = OH, R_2 = NH_2$
23.**118** $R_1 = NHCH_3, R_2 = NHCH_3$
23.**119** $R_1 = NH_2 R_2 = SH$

deamination product, 9-β-D-arabinofuranosylguanine (23.**114**) similarly exerted potent *in vivo* antiviral activity (207).

An isomer of ara-A, 3-β-D-arabinofuranosyladenine (23.**120**) displayed activity approximately equivalent to that of ara-A (186). 5′-Deoxy-5′-substituted arabinonucleosides were inactive as antiviral agents (205). Prodrug forms of ara-A such as

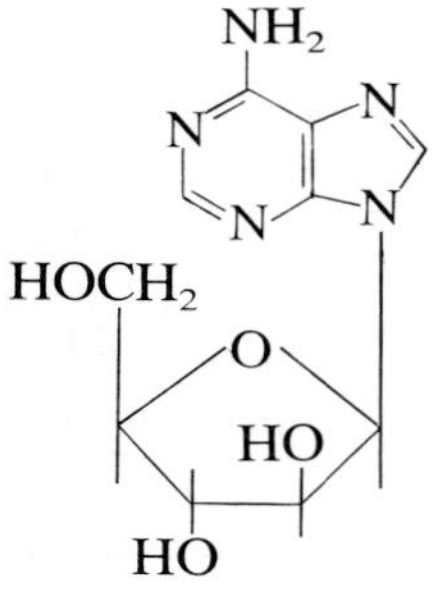

23.**120**

the 5′-*O*-acyl and 2′,3′,5′-tri-*O*-acyl derivatives retain significant *in vitro* activity consistent with their ease of aqueous or enzymatic hydrolysis to the parent nucleoside (205). It is of interest that two α-D-arabinonucleosides, 9-α-D-arabinofuranosyladenine (23.**121**) and 9-α-D-arabinofuranosyl-8-azaadenine (23.**122**), as well as the α-arabinonucleotide, 9-α-D-arabinofuranosyladenine-5′-monophosphate (23.**123**), have a significant degree of antiviral activity (186, 191, 208, 209). These α-nucleosides apparently are not readily deaminated (191).

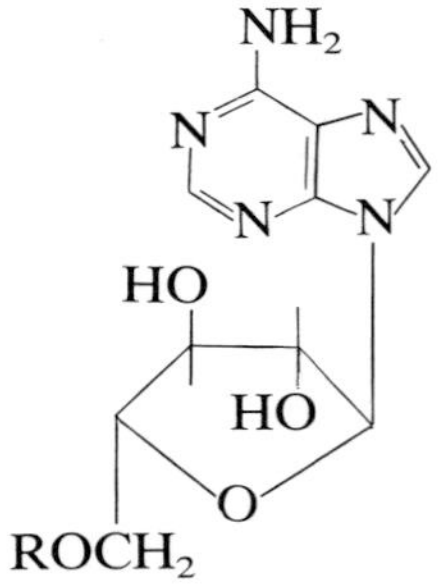

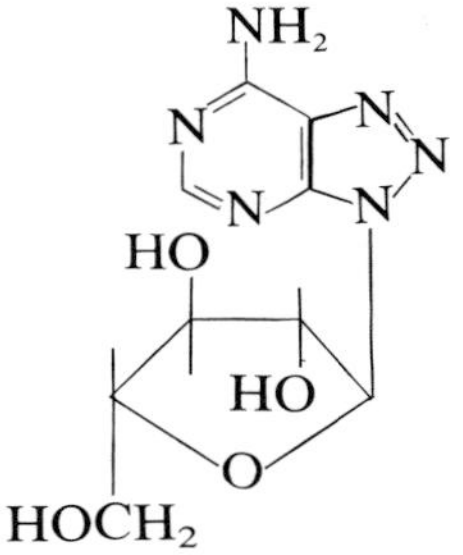

23.**121** R = H
23.**123** $R = PO_3H_2$

23.**122**

5.8.2 PURINE RIBO- AND XYLONUCLEOSIDES AND XYLONUCLEOTIDES. A number of purine nucleosides other than the ara-A derivatives have also been reported to have antiviral activity. Both 2′- and 3′-*C*-methyladenosine (23.**124**, 23.**125**) are active

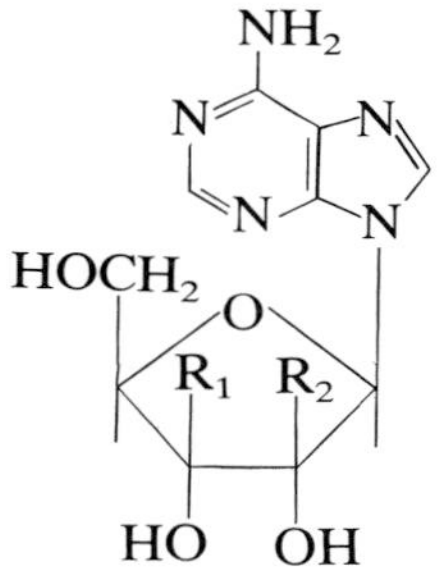

23.**124** $R_1 = H, R_2 = CH_3$
23.**125** $R_1 = CH_3, R_2 = H$

against *in vivo* vaccinia virus infections (210); 1-benzyloxyadenosine (23.**126**), 1-(3-methylbenzyloxy)adenosine (23.**127**), and 1-(4-Fluorobenzyloxy)adenosine (23.**128**) have had significant *in vitro* antiherpes virus activity, with the fluoro derivative (23.**128**) having the greatest relative effect (211). The latter derivatives had little cytotoxic effect (191). A series of carbocyclic analogs (23.**129**–23.**134**) of some purine and 8-azapurine nucleosides have exhibited substantial *in vitro* activity, with little accompanying cytotoxicity, against herpes and vaccinia viruses (191). This antiviral activity was similar to that exerted by ara-A. In contrast to the significant antiviral activity seen using the carbocyclic

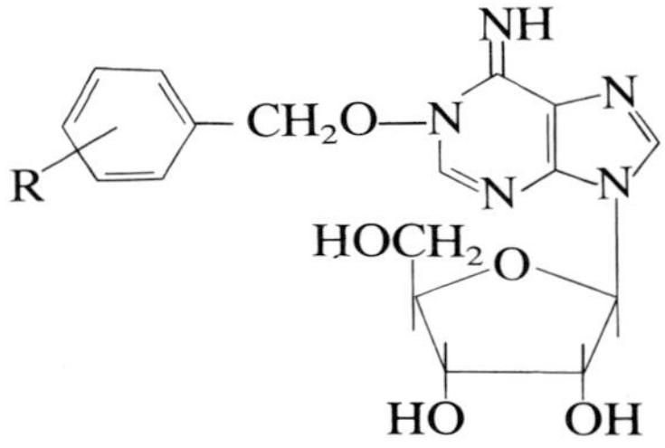

23.**126** R = H
23.**127** R = 3-CH_3
23.**128** R = 4-F

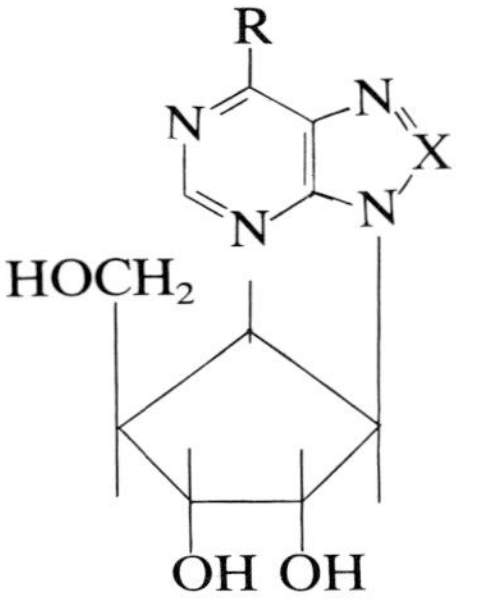

23.**129** R = SCH_3, X = CH
23.**130** R = OCH_3, X = CH
23.**131** R = NHOH, X = CH
23.**132** R = Cl, X = CH
23.**133** R = OH, X = CH
23.**134** R = OH, X = N

analog of 8-azainosine (23.**134**), the carbocyclic analog of 8-azaadenosine did not exhibit an antiviral effect. Moderate *in vivo* anti-herpes virus activity was demonstrated by 9-β-D-xylofuranosylguanine (23.**135**) and the 5′-mono- and 3′,5′-cyclic phosphates of 23.**135**, although none was as active as ara-A (212).

It is apparent that 3′,5′-cyclic phosphate derivatives of 9-β-D-ribofuranosylpurine have an interesting spectrum of antiviral activity, although their practical usefulness is yet to be defined. N^6,2′-*O*-Dibutyryladenosine-3′,5′-cyclic phosphate (23.**136**) markedly inhibits the induction *in vitro* of DNA synthesis by adeno virus (213); the

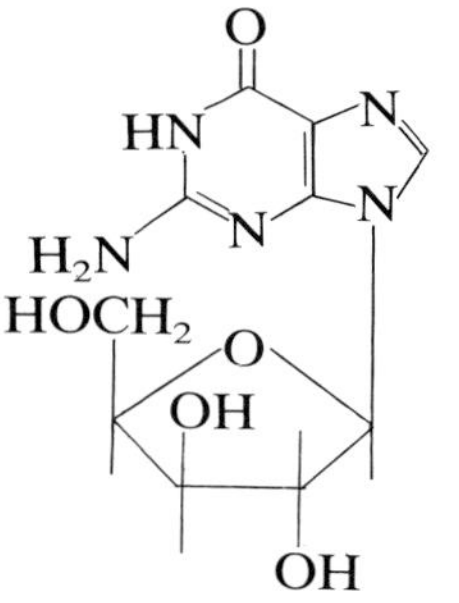

23.**135**

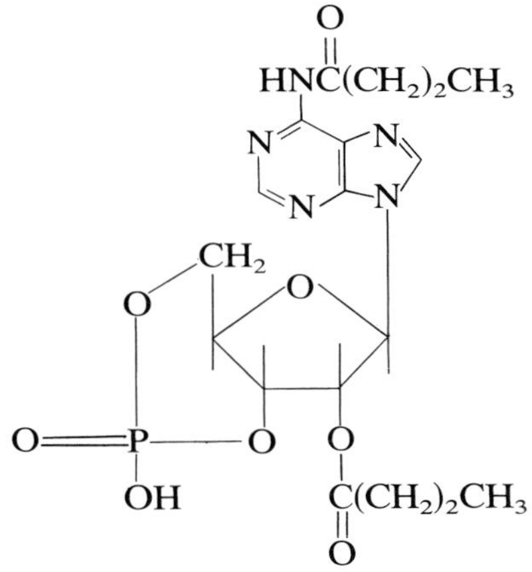

23.**136**

natural metabolite, adenosine 3′,5′-cyclic phosphate (23.**137**), which plays a key role in many cellular functions, and its 8-bromo (23.**138**), 8-methylthio (23.**139**), and 1-*N*-oxide derivatives have exhibited *in vitro*

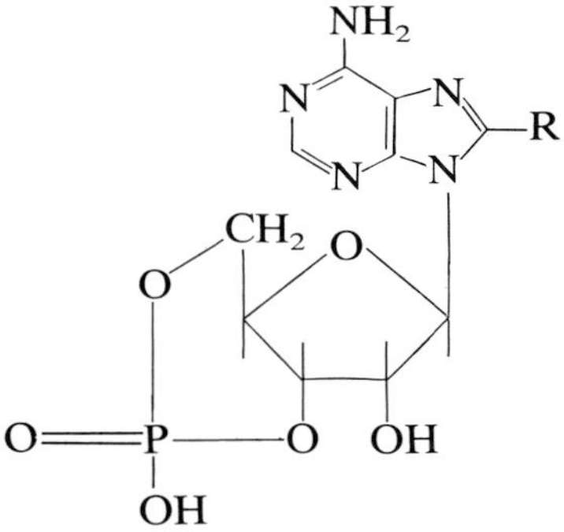

23.**137** R = H
23.**138** R = Br
23.**139** R = SCH_3

activity against the DNA-containing herpes virus and the RNA-containing rhino virus; moderate inhibitory effects on herpes virus-induced lesions in mice were also observed following topical administration of these compounds (214). Among a series of 6-substituted derivatives of 9-β-D-ribofuranosylpurine-3′,5′-cyclic phosphate evaluated for *in vitro* activity against a variety of DNA and RNA viruses, the 6-methylthio (23.**139**) derivative was most effective, inhibiting types 1 and 2 herpes, cytomegalo, vaccinia, and several rhino viruses (215). This compound has also demonstrated an interesting ability to enhance 16- to 32-fold the *in vitro* antiviral action of interferon (216).

An aliphatic nucleoside analog, (S)-9-(2,3-dihydroxypropyl)adenine (23.**139a**)

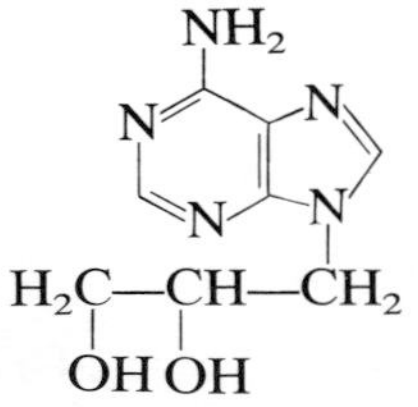

23.**139a**

has recently been shown to exert a broad-spectrum antiviral effect, inhibiting vaccinia, herpes, vesicular stomatitis, and measles viruses *in vitro* and vesicular stomatitis infections *in vivo* (216a). This compound, in its "D-glycero", or (S)-enantiomeric form, apparently imitates the conformation of the β-D-ribonucleosides (216b). The mechanism of antiviral action is yet to be elucidated; but, significantly, it apparently does not affect DNA, RNA, or protein synthesis (216a), suggesting its potential to have a low toxicity, but full toxicity studies are yet to be reported.

An interesting new guanosine analog with significant and apparently specific antiherpes virus activity *in vitro* and *in vivo* is 9(2-hydroxyethoxymethyl)guanine, or acycloguanosine (23.**139b**). Studies have shown that the intact cyclic carbohydrate moiety is

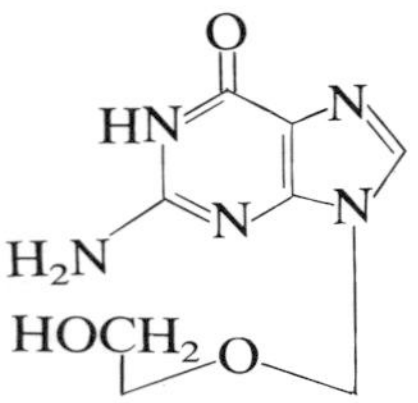

23.**139b**

not necessary to mimic nucleoside binding to enzymes (216c); this observation prompted the synthesis of acycloguanosine (216d). The compound is phosphorylated by herpes virus-specified thymidine kinase and thus converted to the triphosphate in cells infected with the herpesvirus to a much greater extent than in uninfected cells (216d). In addition, the triphosphate is more inhibitory to the viral DNA polymerase than to the α-DNA polymerase in the cell (216e). Thus, acycloguanosine has a very low toxicity in studies to date, and is not readily degraded metabolically when administered systemically.

5.8.3 DEAZAPURINE NUCLEOSIDES. 6-Amino-1-β-D-ribofuranosylimidazo[4,5-*c*]-pyridin-4(5*H*)-one (3-deazaguanosine, 23.**140**) has been reported to have significant antiviral activity (217, 218). This compound, together with its precursor, 3-deazaguanine, and corresponding 5′-nucleotide, 3-deazaguanylic acid, are

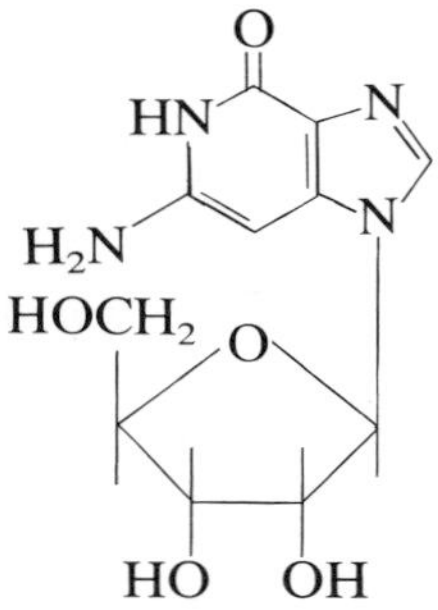

23.**140**

strongly inhibitory to a variety of DNA and RNA viruses *in vitro* and were similarly active against influenza A and B, parainfluenza, herpes, and Friend leukemia virus infections of laboratory animals. 3-Deazaguanine also possesses significant activity against non-viral-induced solid tumors in animals (219). These compounds are inhibitory to hypoxanthine guanine phosphoribosyl transferase and inosine monophosphate dehydrogenase (220), with the antiviral activity thought to be associated especially with the inhibition of the latter enzyme that results in inhibition of viral nucleic acid (218). Another deazapurine ribonucleoside, 3-β-D-ribofuranosylimidazole[4,5-*b*]pyridine (23.**141**),

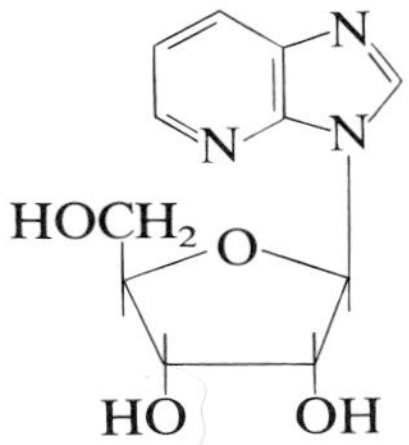

23.**141**

was reported some years ago to have activity against a parainfluenza virus *in vitro* and in embryonated eggs (221, 222).

5.9 Azole Nucleosides and Related Compounds

Most significant of the azole nucleosides is ribavirin (23.**9**), which was discussed under Clinically Active Drugs (Section 4). Ribavirin has *in vitro* inhibitory activity against a variety of viruses, the most sensitive being herpes types 1 and 2 and vaccinia among the DNA viruses, and influenza, parainfluenza, measles, rhino, and certain tumor viruses of the RNA viruses (176, 223–225). The compound also significantly inhibits a similar spectrum of virus infections *in vivo* (224, 225).

The exact mechanism by which ribavirin exerts its antiviral effect is not fully elucidated, but the extensive studies reported to date indicate a possible multifaceted effect, depending on the virus inhibited. The drug appears to exert a virustatic effect that can be reversed by its removal from the cell or by addition of the naturally occurring nucleosides guanosine or xanthosine, and to a lesser extent, inosine (226, 227). This suggests ribavirin may interfere with the conversion of inosine 5′-monophosphate (IMP) to xanthosine-5′-monophosphate on the pathway to nucleic acid. Ribavirin does not inhibit IMP dehydrogenase, but its 5′-monophosphate (23.**142**), which is readily

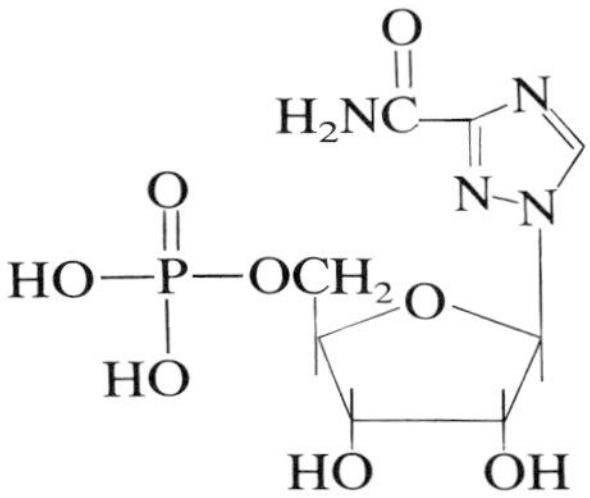

23.**142**

formed in cells (228, 229), is a potent inhibitor of this enzyme (226). Several studies indicate ribavirin may have quite a virus-specific mechanism of action. Scholtissek (230) has shown it to inhibit the virion and complementary RNA synthesis of an influenza A virus, while virtually not affecting cellular RNA synthesis and not interfering with the synthesis of guanosine triphosphate from guanosine. Ribavirin also apparently specifically inhibits synthesis of virus-induced polypeptides, while not inhibiting normal cellular polypeptide synthesis at doses up to 10 times higher (231, 232). Of great significance, Eriksson et al. (233) have demonstrated that ribavirin-5′-triphosphate, a cellular metabolic product of ribavirin, can selectively inhibit influenza virus RNA polymerase in a cell-free assay. Neither ribavirin nor its mono-, di-, or triphosphates apparently inhibits cellular RNA polymerase (233, 234). Against the DNA-containing vaccinia virus, ribavirin's action seems to prevent the formed virus polypeptides from coating the viral DNA, although it is not clear whether this is due to the production of a non-fuctional viral DNA or to a defective viral protein in the presence of the drug (235).

A number of nucleosides structurally related to ribavirin have been synthesized and evaluated as antiviral agents (185, 236–240). The structural features of ribavirin that appear to be necessary for antiviral activity are the carboxamide groups, the 1,2,4-triazole ring, and β-D-ribofuranose as the glycosyl moiety. Changes in the glycosyl portion of the nucleoside to 2′-deoxy-β-D-erythropentofuranosyl, β-D-arabinofuranosyl, β-D-xylofuranosyl, and 5′-deoxy-5′-substituted β-D-ribofuranosyl derivatives resulted in loss of antiviral activity. 1-β-D-Ribofuranosyl-1,2,4-triazole-3-carboxamidine hydrochloride (23.**143**) is active

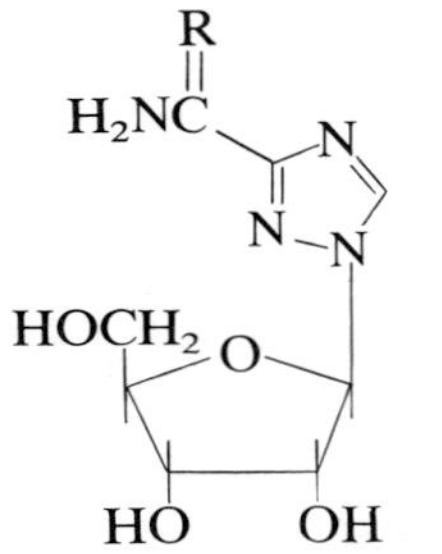

23.**9** R=O
23.**143** R=NH·HCl
23.**144** R=S

against both DNA and RNA viruses. The corresponding 1,2,4-triazole-3-thiocarboxamide nucleoside (23.**144**) is active only against DNA viruses. The 5′-phosphate (23.**142**), 3′,5′-cyclic phosphate (23.**145**), and 2′,3′,5′-tri-*O*-acetyl derivatives of ribavirin also exhibit *in vivo* antiviral activity. The heterocycle, 1,2,4-triazole-3-carboxamide, is effective as an antiviral agent, apparently by enzymatic conversion to the ribonucleoside (225, 229). This heterocycle, in contrast to the freely soluble ribavirin, is only slightly soluble in water.

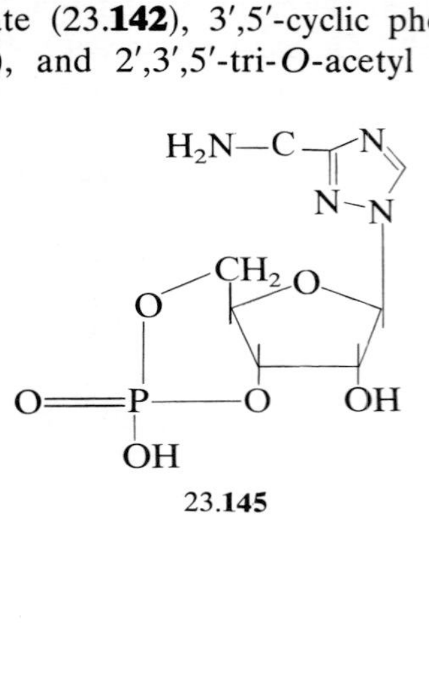

23.**145**

Fluoroimidazoles have also exhibited significant broad spectrum antiviral activity. Of several of these derivatives investigated, 5-fluoro-1-β-D-ribofuranosylimidazole-4-carboxamide (23.**146**) had the greatest antiviral activity, inhibiting the replication of

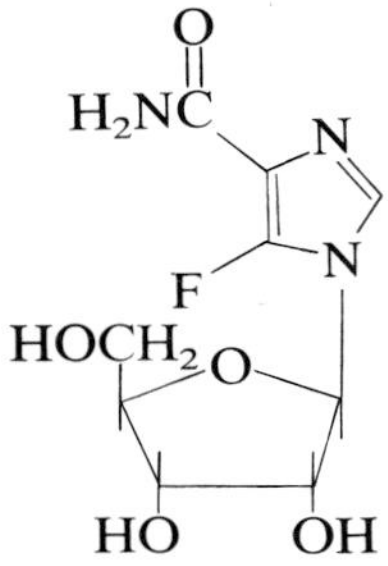

23.**146**

herpes, vesicular stomatitis, coxsackie, Newcastle disease, Sindbis, and measles viruses *in vitro* (241). The activity was somewhat less than that of ribavirin, which was run in parallel in the same study. Other 5-halogenated imidazole-4-carboxamide nucleosides showed similar activity (242). Each of the above named azole nucleosides contains a primary carboxamide group in the same relative position on the azole heterocycle. This suggests that hydrogen bonding properties may be important in the mechanism of action of these antiviral agents by allowing them to interact with the enzymes involved in viral nucleic acid synthesis in a manner paralleling that of similar naturally occurring nucleosides (227). Figure 23.3 gives a proposed hydrogen bonding scheme for ribavirin 5′-phosphate (23.**142**) compared to inosine 5′-monophosphate (23.**147**) (243).

An azole nucleoside also reported to

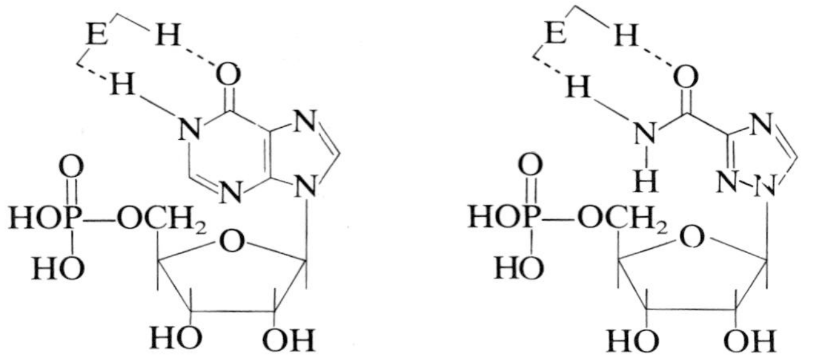

23.147

23.142

Fig. 23.3 Proposed hydrogen bonding scheme for inosine-5′-monophosphate and ribavirin-5′-monophosphate.

have broad spectrum antiviral activity, although with greater cytotoxicity, is 4-hydroxy-3-β-D-ribofuranosylpyrazolo-5-carboxamide (pyrazofurin, 23.**148**). Pyrazofurin is a C-nucleoside that was isolated

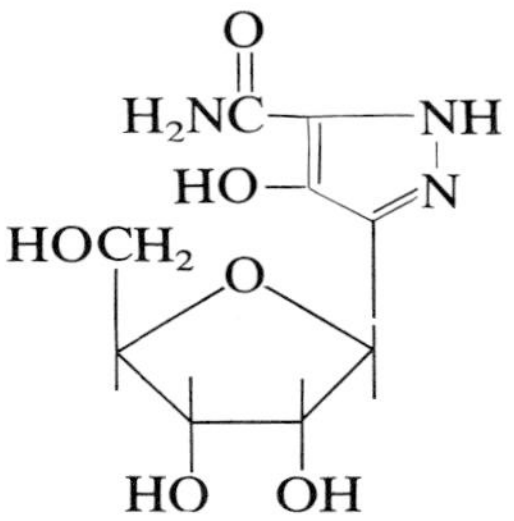

23.**148**

from the fermentation broth of *Streptomyces candidus.* This nucleoside inhibits replication of vaccinia, herpes, measles, rhino, and influenza viruses *in vitro* (244). Pyrazofurin is active against vaccinia virus, and certain RNA tumor virus infections in mice, although it is being considered more as an anticancer agent and has undergone limited human trials for such activity (176, 244).

The antiviral activity of pyrazofurin is reversed by uridine and uridine 5′-monophosphate; pyrazofurin 5′-monophosphate, an apparent metabolite, inhibits orotidylic acid decarboxylase. Similar enzymatic inhibition has been observed with 6-azauridine-5′-phosphate at higher concentrations. Pyrazofurin is slowly converted to the inactive α-anomer in aqueous solutions. Acyl derivatives of pyrazofurin are active against Friend leukemia virus infections in mice and were less toxic that pyrazofurin (176, 244).

5.10 Bisbasic Substituted Polycyclic Aromatic Compounds

2,7-Bis(2-diethylaminoethoxy)-9-fluorenone dihydrochloride (tilorone HCl, 23.**149**) is an oral inducer of interferon production, effective against DNA and RNA virus infections *in vivo* (245–247); but like many interferon inducers, it has a rather species-specific interferon-inducing capability (248). Tilorone HCl was not able to induce interferon in man with even high doses (249), thus is not yet of practical antiviral usefulness. The compound also has a slow rate of clearance from certain host cells, which may cause eventual unfavorable toxic reactions (249). Tilorone and related compounds are also active against RNA tumor virus infections in animals (250).

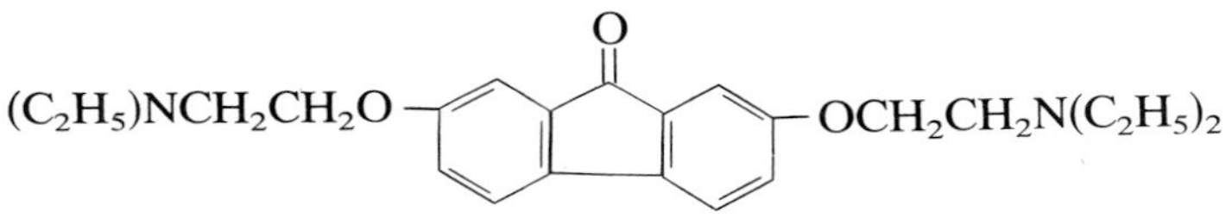

23.**149**

Although tilorone and related compounds have been shown to be effective interferon inducers in mice, the antiviral activity does not always correlate with the levels of circulating interferon detected (251), suggesting that the mechanism of antiviral action may not be due entirely to interferon induction. Studies on the mode of action of tilorone have shown that this compound changes the physicochemical properties of DNA. The interaction of tilorone with DNA stabilizes the double-helical structure, indicating the possibility of intercalation as the mode of binding of tilorone (248, 250, 252). The complex of tilorone with double-stranded DNA may result in a modified nucleic acid that acts as an interferon inducer. In addition, tilorone has been shown to inhibit the DNA template functions in DNA and RNA polymerase reactions (250). A correlation of antiviral activity with inhibition of the DNA-polymerase reaction by tilorone and related compounds has been demonstrated in a leukemia virus system (250). A fluorene derivative with only one basic group, 2-diethylaminoacetylfluorene, was not active against this virus and did not inhibit DNA-polymerase activity.

The interesting interferon-inducing capability of tilorone HCl has stimulated extensive structure-activity studies with bisbasic substituted polycyclic aromatic compounds. Ester (23.**150**) and amide (23.**151**) derivatives of fluorenone, and ketone derivatives (23.**152**) of fluorene-containing bis(dialkylaminoalkyl) groups, exhibit interferon-inducing activity similar to that of tilorone HCl (253–256). Certain derivatives of fluoranthene (23.**153**, 23.**154**), anthraquinone (23.**155**), xanthene (23.**156**), xanthenone (23.**157**), dibenzofuran (23.**158**), and dibenzothiophene (23.**159**), containing two basic groups, are also strong interferon inducers (255, 257–260). Two basic groups appear to be essential for antiviral activity in this class of compound. This is illustrated by the inactivity of the monoether [2-(2-diethylaminoethoxy)-fluoren-9-one (245)] related to tilorone, and dialkylaminoalkyl esters of fluorene monocarboxylic acid (253). It should be pointed out that the route of administration of these compounds to the interferon-producing host may have a pronounced effect on the activity obtained. For example, certain bis(dialkylaminoalkoxy)-fluorenones were highly effective when injected subcutaneously into mice but were ineffective antiviral agents when administered orally (245).

Another group of interferon inducers of

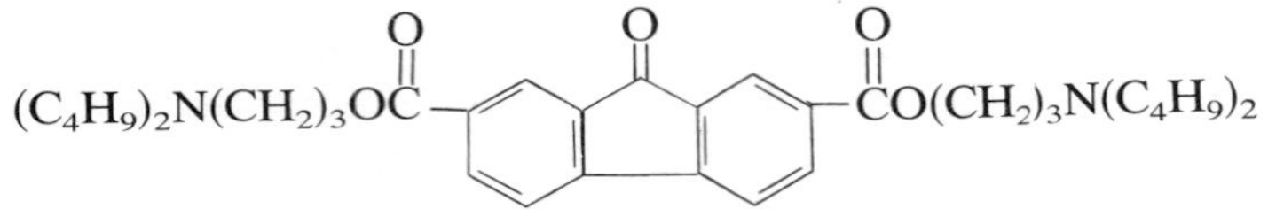

23.**150**

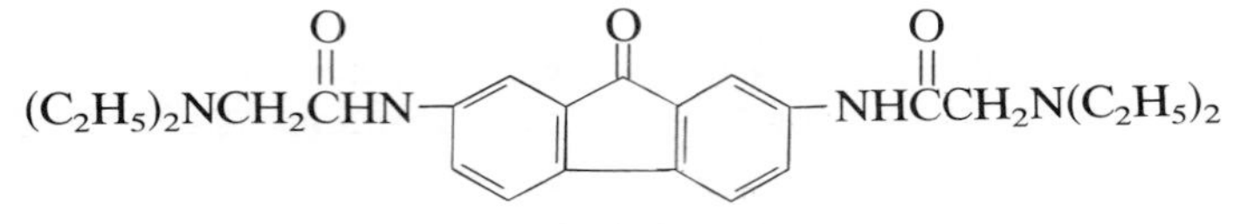

23.**151**

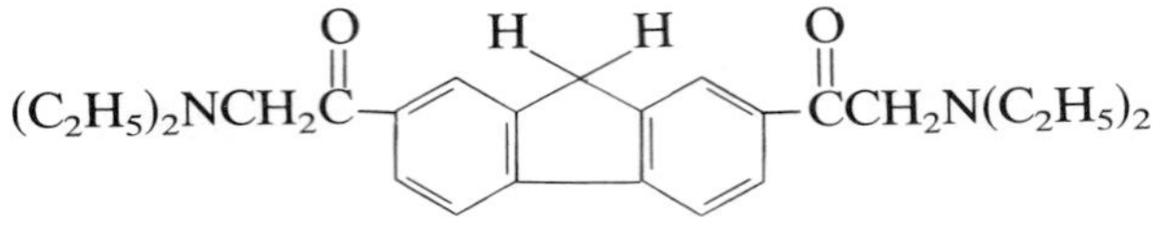

23.**152**

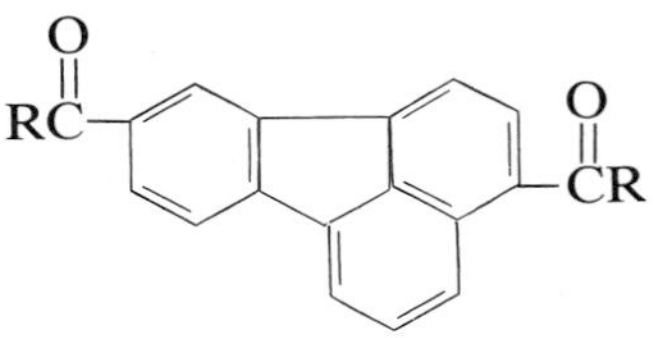

23.**153** R = $O(CH_2)_3N(C_2H_5)_2$
23.**154** R = $CH_2N(CH_3)_2$

rather different structure type from the tilorone derivatives is the pyrazolo[3,4-*b*]-quinolines (261). Of these, 4-(3-dimethylaminopropylamino)-1,3-dimethyl-1*H*-pyrazolo[3,4-*b*]quinoline dihydrochloride (23.**160**) and the 7-methyl derivative (23.**161**) have undergone considerable experimental evaluation. Each demonstrates interferon induction approximately equivalent to that of tilorone, and each protects mice infected with vaccinia, herpes type 2, Semliki forest, and encephalomyocarditis viruses (261–265). It has been observed that these compounds appear to offer an advantage over other reputed interferon inducers by delaying the onset of a hyporesponsive interferon-inductive state in the host after multiple dosing. In a structure-activity study, the 5,7-dimethoxy derivative (23.**162**) was among the most active.

5.11 Polynucleotides and Other Polymers

A number of polynucleotides have demonstrated considerable antiviral activity against a wide variety of viruses in cell culture and in animals, which usually is correlated with stimulation of interferon production. An enormous amount of research into the synthetic interferon inducers has been reported, but space does not permit an elaborate discussion in this survey. Several recent reviews have been published on the subject (266–268). Work in

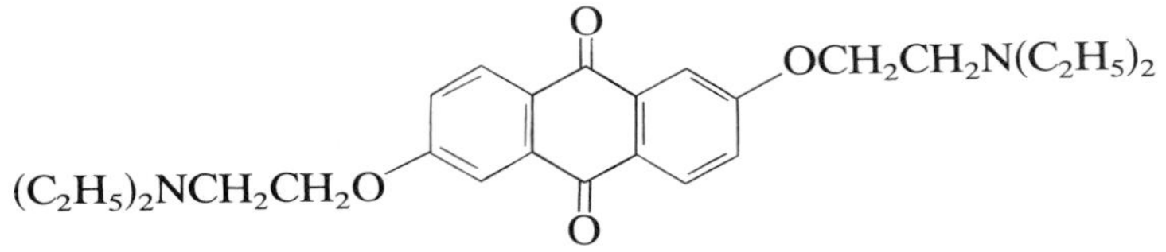

23.**155**

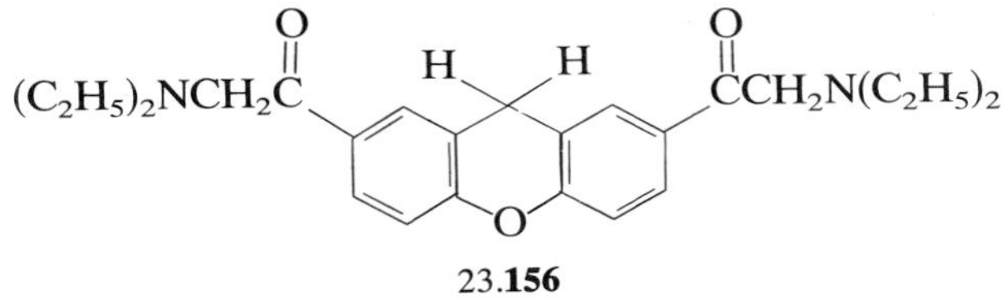

23.**156**

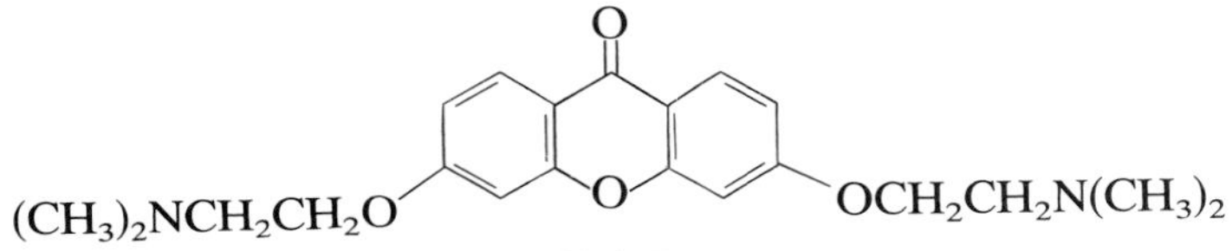

23.**157**

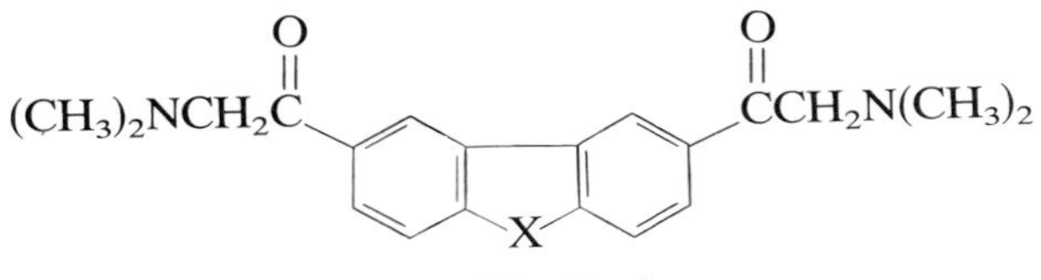

23.**158** X = O
23.**159** X = S

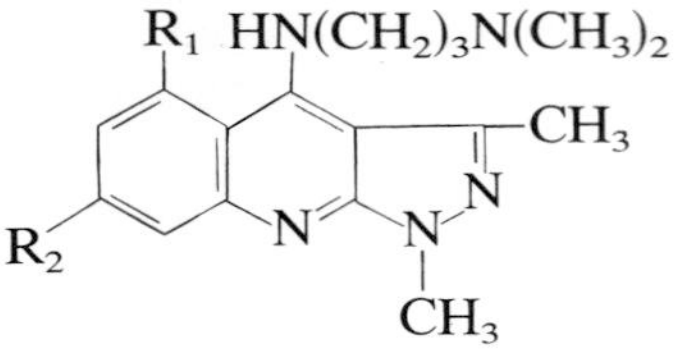

R_1 $HN(CH_2)_3N(CH_3)_2$, CH_3, R_2, CH_3

23.**160** $R_1 = H, R_2 = H$
23.**161** $R_1 = CH_3, R_2 = H$
23.**162** $R_1 = CH_3O, R_2 = CH_3O$

the field was stimulated when studies on extracts of bacteria led to the observation that a double-stranded RNA was effective as an interferon inducer. Such results prompted the investigation of synthetic polynucleotides as possible inducers of interferon, and it was found that certain double-stranded ribonucleotides were especially effective. Single-stranded polyribonucleotides, and both single-stranded and double-stranded polydeoxyribonucleotides are not significantly active as interferon inducers. Several combinations of polyribonucleotides have been studied for their interferon-inducing properties. Effective double-stranded homopolymers include polyinosinic acid·polycytidylic acid (poly I·poly C) and polyguanylic acid·polycytidylic acid (poly G·poly C). Alternating copolymers such as poly(inosinic acid·cytidylic acid) and poly(adenylic acid·uridyclic acid) also induce interferon formation.

The activity of polyribonucleotides as interferon inducers generally increases with the thermal stability and resistance to ribonuclease of the double-stranded helix. The presence of the 2′-hydroxyl groups in polynucleotides appears to be essential for activity. Double-stranded polynucleotides in which one of the polymers consists of 2′-deoxynucleotides or nucleotides with a halogen or methoxy group at the 2′ position show greatly diminished effectiveness. The double-stranded complex of poly I·poly C is the most effective of the polynucleotides as an interferon inducer, with strong activity seen both *in vitro* and *in vivo*. In man, this complex has been a rather poor interferon inducer; however it provided significant, though not clinically useful, protection against respiratory infections and herpes eye infections (269–271). The poor interferon induction seen in man may be due to degradation of the polynucleotides by serum nucleases (272). A complex of poly I·poly C with poly-L-lysine and carboxymethylcellulose has proved to be partially resistant to enzymatic degradation and, in contrast to poly I·poly C alone, is an effective interferon inducer in subhuman primates (273). In monkeys, this complex provided marked protection against a usually lethal simian hemorrhagic fever (274). Toxicity studies of poly I·poly C in animals have indicated the possibility of a number of serious toxic effects, although in man few side effects have been observed to date (56).

Other significant interferon inducers include polyacrylic acid, polymethacrylic acid, maleic anhydride–divinyl ether (pyran) copolymer, and chlorite-oxidized oxyamylose, which have had demonstrable efficacy when used prophylactically against both DNA and RNA virus infections in animals (275–278). These polymers induce interferon, although antiviral activity has also been observed with their use in animals when interferon production was not detected (279). Structure-activity relationship studies with polycarboxylates indicate that a high molecular weight (10^4–10^6) and a polyanionic character of the polymer are necessary for antiviral activity (279).

5.12 Antibiotics

A number of antibiotics, many structures of which have been well defined, have exhibited considerable antiviral activity, although many have not been extensively studied. Among the more recent and significant of this group of antiviral agents are the rifamycins, the streptovaricins, the gliotoxins, distamycin A, 9-methylstreptimidone, and the bleomycins.

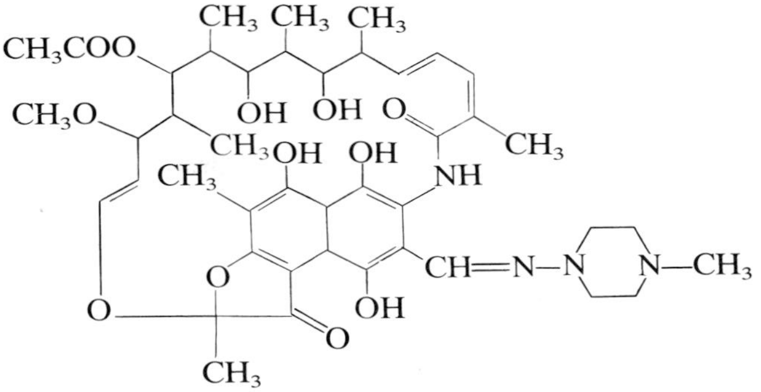

23.**163**

5.12.1 RIFAMYCINS. Rifamycin refers to a class of antibiotics isolated from the fermentation broth of *Streptomyces mediterranei.* In addition to the naturally occurring substances, a number of semisynthetic derivatives have been investigated as antibacterial and antiviral agents (280). One of these semisynthetic derivatives selected for use as an antibacterial drug, rifampin (23.**163**), inhibits replication *in vitro* of certain DNA viruses, including Orthopoxviruses and Herpesviruses (281, 282). Some rifamycin derivatives are effective inhibitors of the RNA-dependent DNA polymerase of RNA and DNA tumor viruses (280). Cell transformation by the viruses and consequent tumor induction is inhibited, as well as virus multiplication itself (280).

The mode of antiviral action of the rifamycin derivatives has not been fully determined. Studies indicate that these antibiotics bind to the polymerase molecule in the RNA leukemia viruses, as well as to the nucleic acid template, inhibiting DNA synthesis of the DNA tumor virus (280). The nonpolar side chains of these antibiotics may impart a detergent quality (283). Rifampin appears to interfere with assembly of viral components, resulting in formation of abnormal virus particles. Many derivatives of rifamycin have been synthesized and studied, primarily for their ability to inhibit the RNA-dependent DNA polymerase of RNA tumor viruses (284, 285). The macrocyclic ring structure of rifamycin with large side chain substitutions in position 3 seems to impart the greatest degree of polymerase-inhibitory activity. Whether such polymerase-inhibitory compounds will have practical antiviral usefulness remains to be seen.

5.12.2 STREPTOVARICINS. The streptovaricins (23.**164**) are other members of the ansamycin antibiotics, obtained from fermentation of a strain of *Streptomyces spectabilis.* These substances have properties similar to those of the rifamycins and are more recognized for their antibacterial effects (286). They inhibit the *in vitro* replication of Orthopoxviruses, as well as of certain RNA tumor viruses (286). Streptovaricin inhibits DNA-dependent RNA polymerase; but because of the formation of unstable complexes with RNA polymerase, it has lower efficacy than is seen with the rifamycins (287).

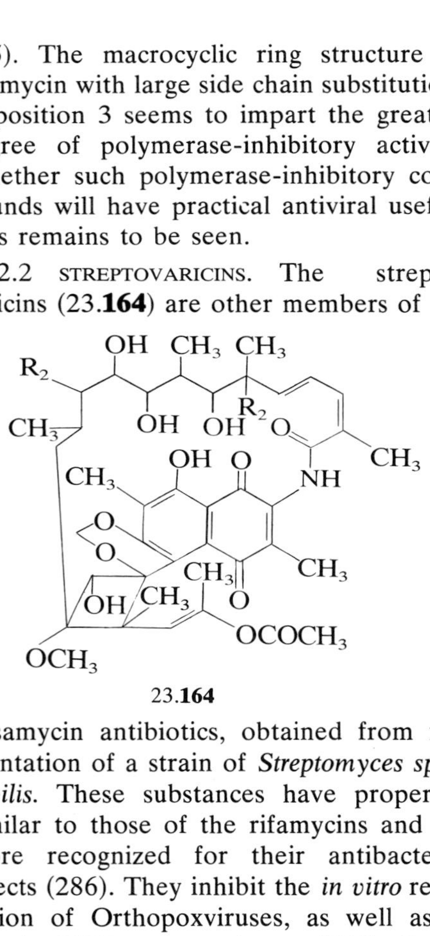

23.**164**

5.12.3 GLIOTOXIN AND ANALOGS. Gliotoxin (23.**165**), a fungal metabolic product,

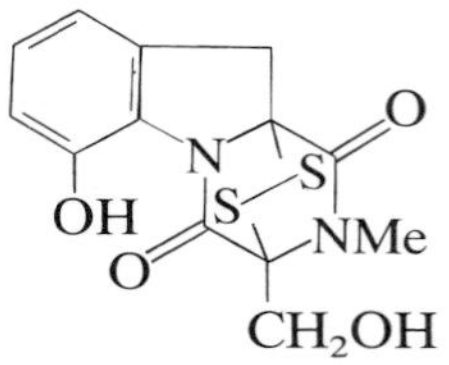

23.**165**

has significant activity *in vitro* against polio, herpes, and influenza viruses (288, 289). The compound is thought to inhibit viral RNA-dependent RNA polymerase (290). It has been shown to specifically inhibit the synthesis of viral RNA (289). Related compounds exhibiting similar activity all contained the epidithia-diketopiperazine ring system seen in the gliotoxin structure (291).

5.12.4 DISTAMYCINS. Distamycin A (23.**166**) and its derivatives or analogs are antibiotics that are active *in vitro* and *in vivo* against DNA viruses and RNA tumor viruses (292–294). The mode of action of distamycin A involves its interactions with viral DNA. Binding of distamycin A to DNA has been demonstrated by changes in ultraviolet spectra and thermal stability of DNA in its presence. The antibiotic also inhibits the RNA-dependent DNA polymerase of RNA tumor viruses (295, 296). The antiviral activity of distamycin A derivatives containing from two to five substituted pyrrole subunits was compared with that of distamycin, which contains three pyrrole groups. Analogs with four and five pyrrole groups were more active than distamycin A against vaccinia virus. The extent of binding of distamycin analogs with DNA increases with the number of pyrrole subunits in the compound. Also, inhibition of DNA-dependent RNA synthesis by distamycin and derivatives appears to increase with the number of pyrrole rings in the molecule (295–297).

5.12.5 9-METHYLSTREPTIMIDONE. 9-Methylstreptimidone (23.**167**) is an isolate

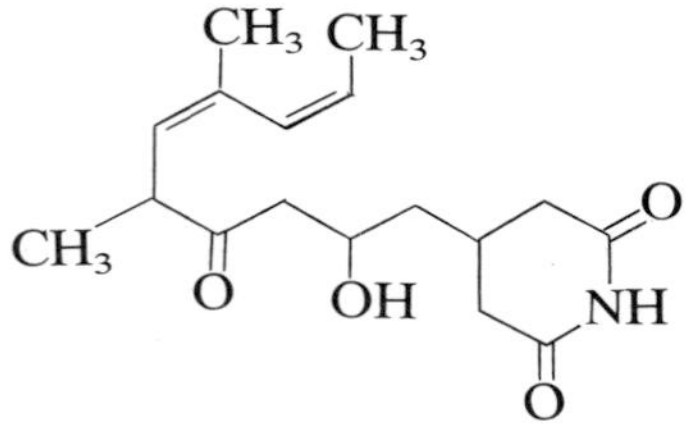

23.**167**

from a culture filtrate of a *Streptomyces* species that inhibits the growth of Enteroviruses *in vitro* and protects mice infected with influenza virus (298). The compound appears to be an inducer of interferon, which is probably its primary mode of action.

5.12.6 BLEOMYCINS. Bleomycin A2 (23.**168**) is one of a group of glycopeptide antibiotics especially known for their efficacy in treatment of cancer (299). The bleomycins recently have also been shown to exhibit significant inhibition of vaccinia virus *in vitro* and *in vivo* (300, 301). The antibiotic seems to inhibit the synthesis of viral nucleic acid (300, 301), although it also causes breaks in cellular DNA (302).

Its structure has recently been revised (see Chapter 16).

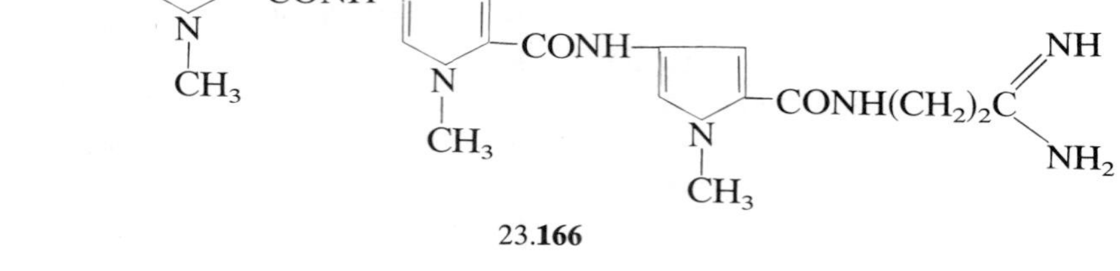

23.**166**

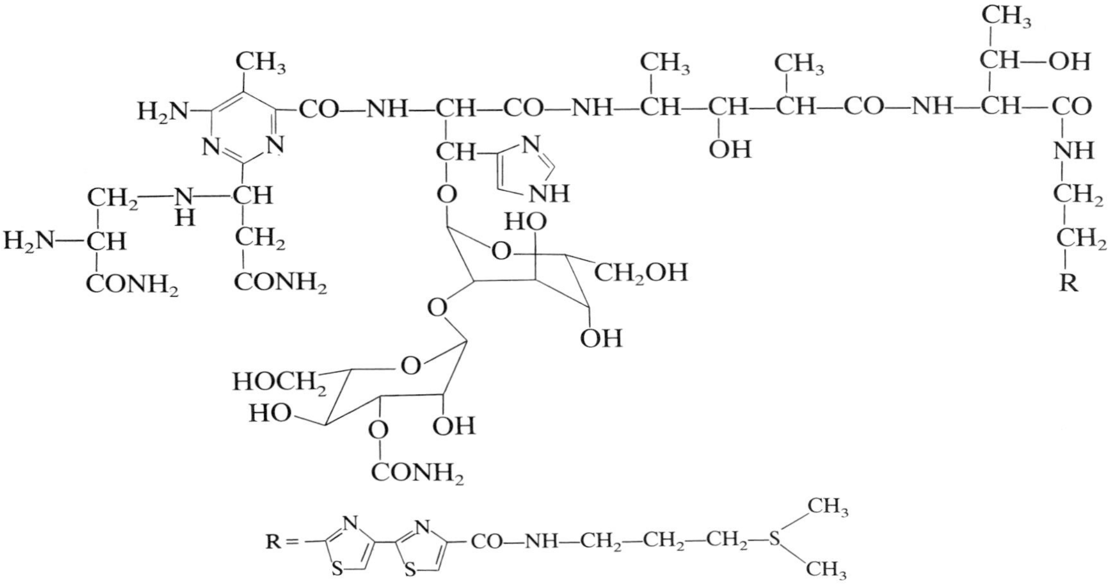

R = thiazole–thiazole–CO—NH—CH_2—CH_2—CH_2—$S(CH_3)_2$

23.**168**

5.13 Miscellaneous Compounds

5.13.1 PHOSPHONOACETIC ACID. Phosphonoacetic acid (23.**169**) is active against several

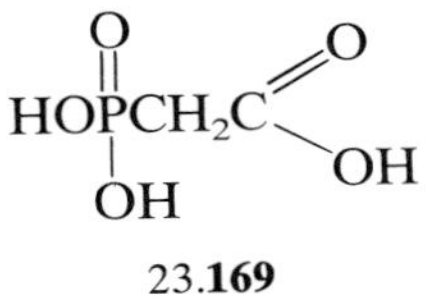

$$HOP(=O)(OH)CH_2C(=O)OH$$

23.**169**

viruses *in vitro* and *in vivo*, including herpes types 1 and 2, cytomegalo, and Gross murine leukemia viruses (176, 303–305). As the disodium salt, phosphonoacetic acid is effective in animal systems in treatment of herpes keratitis (303, 306, 307), including infections of herpes virus resistant to 5-iodo-2′-deoxyuridine (307). Resistance to phosphonoacetic acid developed, however, after repeated passage of herpes virus in the presence of this inhibitor (308).

Studies on the mode of action of phosphonoacetic acid indicate that it selectively inhibits viral DNA synthesis and is a specific inhibitor of DNA polymerase induced by herpes and cytomegalo viruses (305, 309–311). The inhibition of virus-induced DNA polymerase activity by phosphonoacetic acid involves interaction with the enzyme, not with the DNA template (310).

Recently synthesized analogs of phosphonoacetic acid that have substantial antiherpes virus activity include the propyl ester (23.**169a**) and the hexyl ester (23.**169b**) (311a).

A pyrophosphate analog synthesized in 1924 (311b), trisodium phosphoroformate (23.**169c**), has very recently been shown to have a strong antiviral effect on the Herpesvirus *in vitro* and *in vivo* (311c). Little

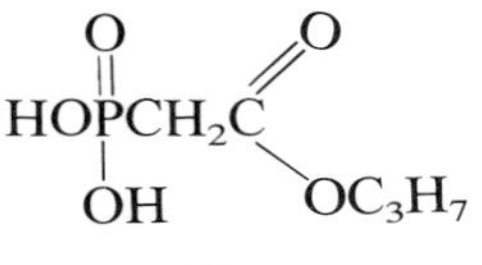

$$HOP(=O)(OH)CH_2C(=O)OC_3H_7$$

23.**169a**

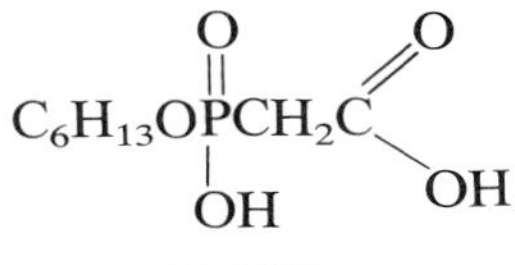

$$C_6H_{13}OP(=O)(OH)CH_2C(=O)OH$$

23.**169b**

$$Na_3^{\oplus}\left[{}^{\ominus}O{-}P(=O)(O^{\ominus}){-}C(=O)O^{\ominus}\right]$$

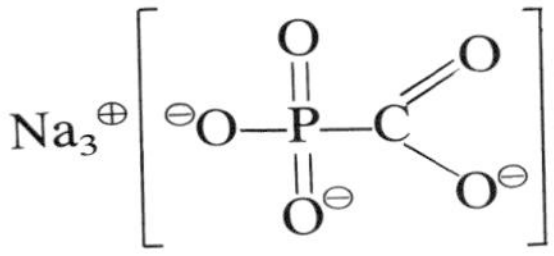

23.**169c**

toxicity has yet been demonstrated. This compound appears to inhibit herpes virus DNA polymerase while not having a demonstrable effect on various cellular DNA polymerases (311c).

5.13.2 KETHOXAL. 3-Ethoxy-2-oxobutyraldehyde hydrate (kethoxal, 23.**170**)

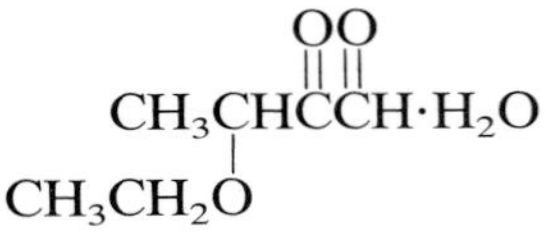

$$\begin{array}{c} \quad OO \\ \quad \| \; \| \\ CH_3CHCCH \cdot H_2O \\ | \\ CH_3CH_2O \end{array}$$

23.**170**

has *in vitro* antiviral effect against a variety of DNA and RNA viruses, including herpes, vaccinia, influenza A, and parainfluenza (312–314). Topical application of kethoxal significantly affects upper respiratory parainfluenza virus infections in hamsters (313) and cutaneous herpes virus infections in mice (315). The compound is a potent inactivator of extracellular virus, but also exhibits an inhibition of intracellular virus multiplication (314). Dicarbonyl compounds can be structurally modified to a considerable degree and still retain antiviral activity, provided a terminal α-ketoaldehyde or α-hydroxyaldehyde group is present in the molecule (312).

5.13.3 DECALIN DERIVATIVES. Several compounds having structures based on the *trans*-decalin nucleus are inhibitory to certain selected influenza viruses *in vitro* (316–318). They appear to act by blocking penetration of the virus into the cell (317). Significant antiviral activity with little associated cytotoxicity has been seen with certain vinyl ether decalins (23.**171**–23.**173**), 4*a*-acetyl-*trans*-decalins (23.**174**, 23.**175**), 4*a*-alkanoyl-1-β-hydroxy-*trans*-decalins (23.**176**–23.**179**) and *trans*-4*a*-decalylamides (23.**180**–23.**186**) (317). Among those evaluated for *in vivo* influenza virus activity, none had significant inhibitory effect, possibly because of rapid metabolism or inactivation of the compounds in the animal (317).

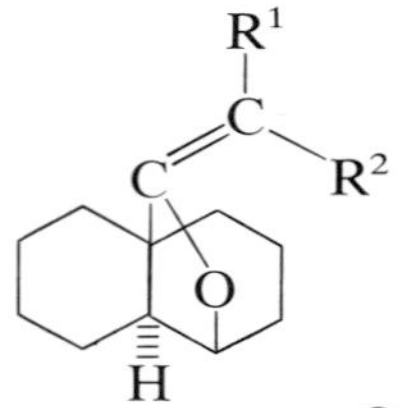

23.**171** $R_1 = H, R_2 = \overset{O}{\overset{\|}{C}}NH_2$

23.**172** $R_1 = H, R_2 = \overset{O}{\overset{\|}{C}}CH_3$

23.**173** $R_1 = Br, R_2 = Br$

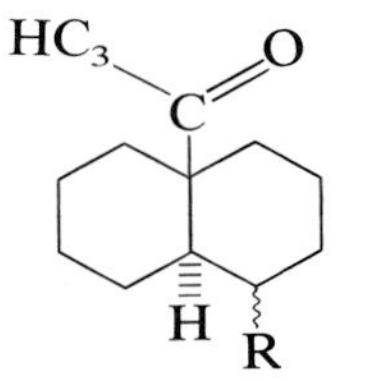

23.**174** $R = \alpha\text{-}OCH_3$

23.**175** $R = \alpha\text{-}OC_2H_5$

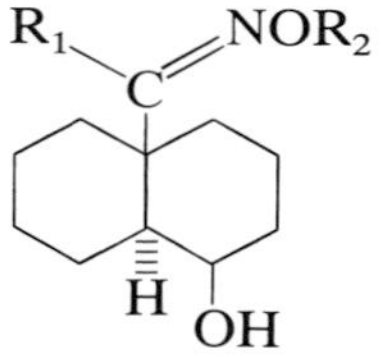

23.**176** $R_1 = CH_3, R_2 = H$

23.**177** $R_1 = CH_3CH_2, R_2 = H$

23.**178** $R_1 = CH_3CH_2CH_2, R_2 = H$

23.**179** $R_1 = CH_3, R_2 = CH_3$

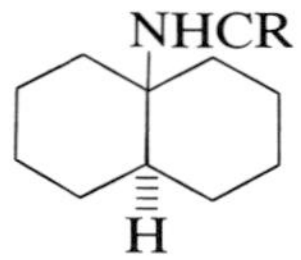

NHCR

23.**180** $R = \overset{O}{\overset{\|}{C}}CH_2$–phenyl

23.**181** $R = \overset{O}{\overset{\|}{C}}CH_2$–C₆H₄–Cl

23.**182** $R = \overset{O}{\overset{\|}{C}}CH_2S$–phenyl

23.**183** $R = \overset{O}{\overset{\|}{C}}CH_2S$–C₆H₄–Cl

23.**184** $R = \overset{O}{\overset{\|}{C}}CF_2$–phenyl

23.**185** $R = \overset{O}{\overset{\|}{C}}CH_2O$–phenyl

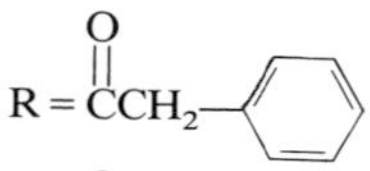

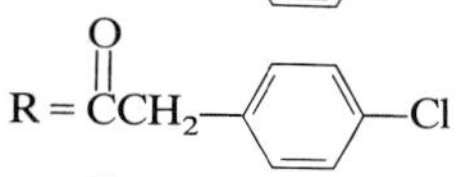

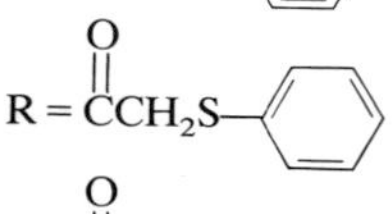

23.**186** $R = \overset{O}{\overset{\|}{C}}CH_2$–N(indolyl)

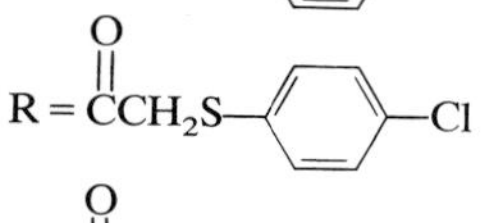

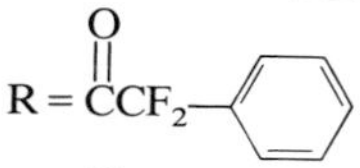

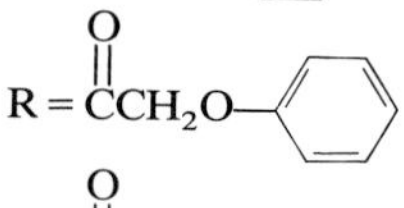

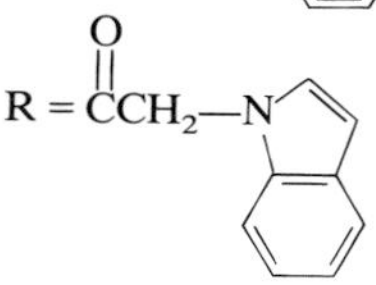

5.13.4 DIHYDROISOQUINOLINES. Certain dihydroisoquinolines have been strongly considered as potential antiviral agents because of initial observations that they markedly inhibit influenza A_2 virus neuraminidase (319, 320), although later studies could not confirm this enzyme-inhibitory effect (321, 322). Of a series of these compounds studied, 1-(4-chlorophenoxymethyl)-3,4- dihydroisoquinoline hydrochloride (23.**187**) and 1-(4-methoxyphenoxymethyl)-3,4-dihydroisoquinoline hydrochloride (23.**188**) have exhibited an

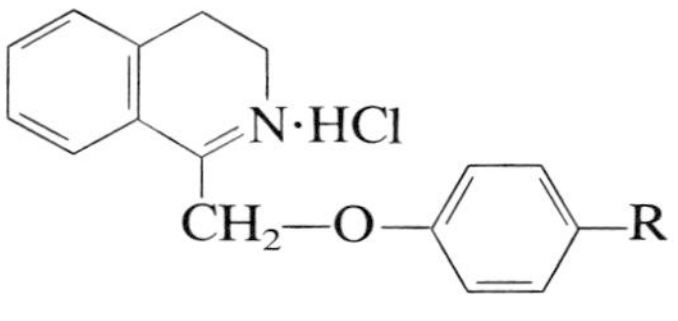

N·HCl

CH_2—O—⟨ ⟩—R

23.**187** R = Cl
23.**188** R = OCH_3

inactivating effect on influenza A and B viruses and on some Paramyxoviruses *in vitro*; a moderate activity was seen in mice and dogs against influenza, and subsequent activity was also demonstrated in human volunteers when each compound was used prophylactically against a challenge of influenza virus (319, 323–326). No side effects were observed. A later study using 23.**188** against a natural influenza A_2 infection in patients failed to demonstrate efficacy, and it was suggested that a difference in susceptibility of different viruses to the compounds may exist (327). Another compound in this class, 3,4-dihydro-1-isoquinolineacetamide hydrochloride (23.**189**) has

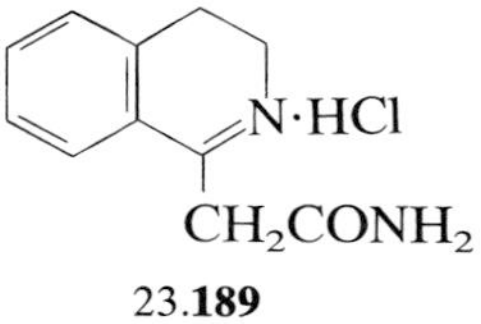

N·HCl

CH_2CONH_2

23.**189**

strong *in vivo* activity against influenza A, ECHO, Columbia SK, and herpes viruses, although *in vitro* antiviral activity is apparently slight (328, 329). The antiviral activity has been attributed to a delay of penetration of virus into the cells (330).

5.13.5 *N,N*-DIOCTADECYL-*N′,N′*-BIS(2-HYDROXYMETHYL)-1,3-PROPANEDIAMINE. One of the most significant inducers of interferon is the long chain alkyl propanediamine, *N,N*-dioctadecyl-*N′,N′*-bis(2-hydroxyethyl)-1,3-propanediamine (23.**190**). This compound induces strong protection to both

$$[CH_3(CH_2)_{17}]_2NCH_2CH_2CH_2N(CH_2CH_2OH)_2$$

23.**190**

DNA and RNA viruses *in vivo* (331). It has been tested in humans, and results against rhino virus infections have been positive (332–334). The human studies yielded conflicting results on the effect of this compound on virus shedding (332, 333).

5.13.6 GLUCOSE DERIVATIVES. Significant inhibition of viruses has been exhibited by glucosamine, *N*-fluoroacetylglucosamine, and 2-deoxy-D-glucose (335–337). The viruses inhibited *in vitro* are primarily those containing envelopes, including influenza, respiratory syncytial, parainfluenza, measles, Semliki Forest, herpes, and avian sarcoma viruses. *In vivo* activity has also been demonstrated (337). These glucose derivatives inhibit production of viral glycopeptides, resulting in interference with the formation of the virus-specific membranes of the viral envelope. Thus infectious viral progeny are inhibited from being formed in the cells (338–340).

5.13.7 2-DEOXY-2,3-DEHYDRO-*N*-TRIFLUOROACETYLNEURAMIC ACID. A synthetic analog of *N*-acetylneuramic acid, 2-deoxy-2,3-dehydro-*N*-trifluoroacetylneuramic acid (23.**191**), is a strong *in vitro* inhibitor of Influenzaviruses and Paramyxoviruses (341). This activity was directly associated with the ability of 23.**191** to inhibit the neuraminidase activity of these viruses (342, 343). The compound does not affect viruses that do not contain neuraminidase.

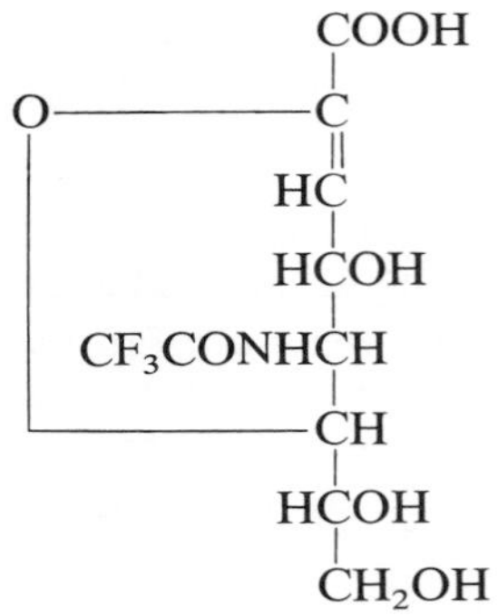

$$\begin{array}{c} COOH \\ | \\ O\text{—}C \\ \| \\ HC \\ | \\ HCOH \\ | \\ CF_3CONHCH \\ | \\ \text{—}CH \\ | \\ HCOH \\ | \\ CH_2OH \end{array}$$

23.**191**

The inhibition of neuraminidase of susceptible viruses prevents the enzymatic removal of neuraminic acid from the virus envelope, resulting in extensive aggregation of virus particles and subsequent inhibition of virus replication (342–344). The compound 23.**191** is the most active of a number of derivatives of *N*-acetylneuramic acid (345).

5.13.8 TRIAZINOINDOLES. Several *as*-triazino[5,6-*b*]indole-3-thiols (23.**192**–23.**195**) have been strongly considered as

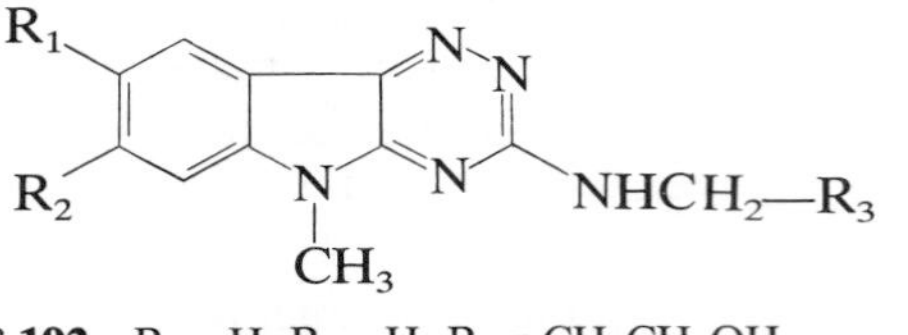

23.**192** $R_1 = H, R_2 = H, R_3 = CH_2CH_2OH$
23.**193** $R_1 = H, R_2 = H, R_3 = CH_2C(CH_3)_2OH$
23.**194** $R_1 = H, R_2 = H, R_3 = C(CH_3)_2CH_2OH$
23.**195** $R_1 = NH_2, R_2 = Cl, R_3 = CH_2C(CH_3)_2OH$

potential drugs for treating common cold infections caused by rhino viruses, with strong *in vitro* activity observed against many rhino virus strains (346–349), and moderate effect reported following administration to experimentally infected chimpanzees (347). One of the more effective of these compounds, 2-[(5-methyl-5*H*-*as*-triazino[5,6-*b*]indole-3-yl)amino]-1-propanol (23.**192**), was evaluated in humans, but if failed to prevent rhino virus-induced respiratory illness in the trial reported (350). Another, 23.**195**, has a positive effect both in chimpanzees (351) and in humans (91). These compounds also reportedly have activity *in vitro* against a number of other RNA and DNA viruses, as well as inhibiting vaccinia virus infections in mice (347). The mechanism of antiviral action of these compounds has not been described.

5.13.9 FLAVONES. Several flavones have exhibited interesting antiviral activity against a variety of viruses, primarily in cell culture systems. The best studied of these is 3,3′,4′,5,7-*penta*hydroxyflavone (quercetin, 23.**196**), which significantly affects herpes

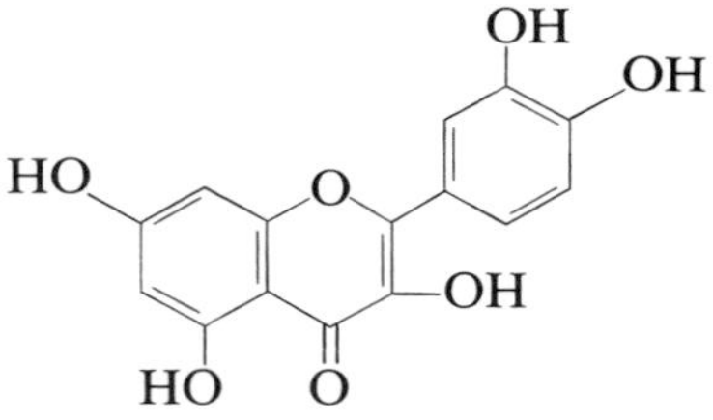

23.**196**

and parainfluenza viruses *in vitro* (352) and has prophylactic activity against rabies virus in mice (353). The *in vitro* activity was due to virus-inactivation action of the flavones. 4′-Hydroxy-5,6,7,8-tetramethoxyflavone (23.**197**), unlike the quercetin flavones, has

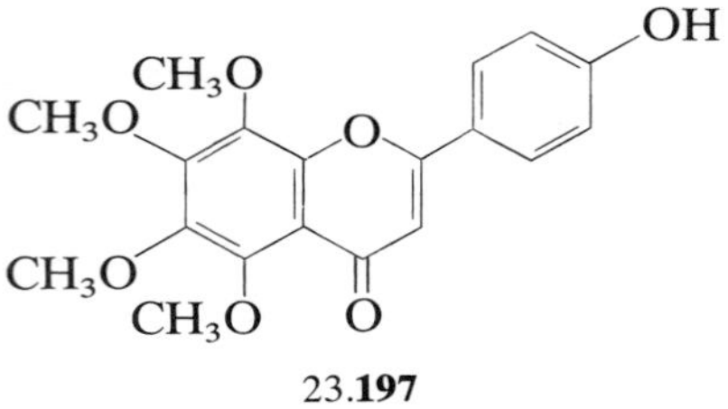

23.**197**

a more virus-inhibitory effect, with activity limited to rhino viruses (354).

5.13.10 CALCIUM ELENOLATE. The monoterpene calcium elenolate (23.**198**), obtained from acid-hydrolyzed aqueous extracts of various parts of the olive plant (*Olea europa*), is virucidal *in vitro* for a variety of RNA and DNA viruses (355). The compound, when applied intranasally, reduced parainfluenza virus yields (356) but

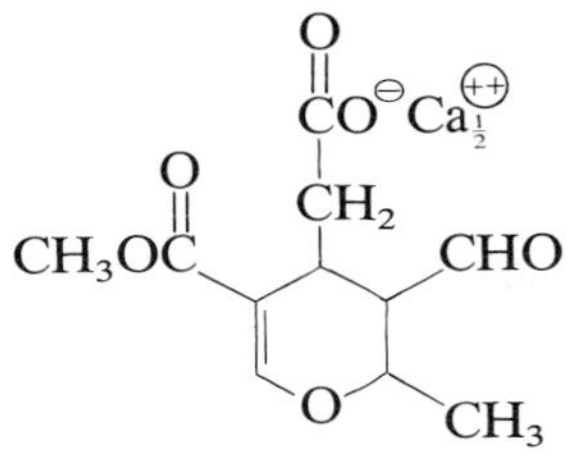

$$\begin{array}{c} CH_3O_2C-\text{(dihydropyran ring)}-CH_2CO_2^{\ominus}Ca^{++}_{1/2} \\ \text{with CHO and } CH_3 \end{array}$$

23.**198**

did not demonstrate significant toxicity (357). The viral inactivation appears to be a result of interaction of calcium elenolate with the protein coat of the virus particle (355).

6 CONCLUSIONS

The amount of chemical synthesis oriented toward the development of effective, safe antiviral agents has been overwhelming in recent years, and it is frustrating to be required to summarize such extensive studies in a few pages. It is gratifying to see such efforts yielding significantly positive efficacy in clinical studies. Antiviral drugs now do exist, although considerable improvement can still be made. It becomes obvious that to achieve greater efficacy and safety, we must move to more studies involving the coordinated efforts of chemist, biochemist, pharmacologist, and clinician, if we are to overcome such obstacles as metabolic breakdown of the drug, lack of adsorption in the host, rapid excretion, toxicity, interactions with other drugs, and natural host barriers. One has the feeling that basically good antiviral substances now exist but that formulation into better vehicles or preparation of improved depot forms is needed. Increased knowledge of the pharmacokinetics of the more active substances is definitely required, if more adequate treatment regimens are to be used. We look with optimism toward a time when the major viral diseases of the world will be controlled through the use of effective antiviral agents.

REFERENCES

1. F. L. Horsfall, Jr., "General Principles and Historical Aspects", in *Viral and Rickettsial Infections of Man*, 4th ed., F. L. Horsfall, Jr., and I. Tamm, Eds., Lippincott, Philadelphia, 1965, p. 1.
2. E. D. Kilbourne, "Epidemiology of Influenza," in *The Influenza Viruses and Influenza*, Academic Press, New York, 1975, p. 483.
3. F. Fenner, *Intervirology*, **7,** 4 (1976).
4. W. M. Mitchell, "Active Sites of the Animal Viruses: Potential Sites of Specific Chemotherapeutic Attack", in *Selective Inhibitors of Viral Functions*, W. A. Carter, Ed., CRC Press, Cleveland, 1973, p. 51.
5. B. R. McAuslan, *Life Sci.*, **14,** 2085 (1974).
6. F. Fenner, B. R. McAuslan, C. A. Mims, J. Sambrook, and D. O. White, *The Biology of Animal Viruses*, 2nd ed., Academic Press, New York, 1974, p. 1.
7. F. Fenner and D. O. White, "Chemotherapy of Viral Diseases", in *Medical Virology*, Academic Press, New York, 1976, p. 241.
8. R. W. Sidwell, "Viral Diseases: A Review of Chemotherapy Systems", in *Chemotherapy of Infectious Disease*, H. H. Gadebusch, Ed., CRC Press, Cleveland, 1976, p. 31.
9. E. D. Kilbourne, P. Palese, and J. L. Schulman, "Inhibition of Viral Neuraminidase as an Approach to the Prevention of Influenza", in *Perspectives in Virology*, Vol. 9, M. Pollard, Ed., Academic Press, New York, 1975, p. 99.
10. P. P. K. Ho and C. P. Walters, *Ann. N.Y. Acad. Sci.*, **173,** 438 (1970).
11. J. S. Oxford, *J. Gen. Virol.*, **18,** 11 (1973).
12. W. Billard and E. Peets, *Antimicrob. Agents Chemother.*, **5,** 19 (1974).
13. J. S. Oxford and D. D. Perrin, *Ann. N.Y. Acad. Sci.*, **284,** 613 (1977).
14. D. M. McLean, *Ann. N.Y. Acad. Sci.*, **284,** 118 (1977).
15. D. J. Bauer, "Thiosemicarbazones", in *Chemotherapy of Virus Diseases* Vol. 1, *International Encyclopedia of Pharmacology*, D. J. Bauer, Ed., Pergamon Press, Oxford, 1972, p. 35.
16. W. Levinson, "Inhibition of Viruses, Tumors, and Pathogenic Microorganisms by Isatin-β-Thiosemicarbazone, and Other Thiosemicarbazones", in *Selective Inhibitors of Viral Functions*, W. A. Carter, Ed., CRC Press, Cleveland, 1973, p. 213.
17. W. H. Prusoff and D. C. Ward, *Biochem. Pharmacol.*, **25,** 1233 (1976).

18. J. Sugar and H. E. Kaufman, "Halogenated Pyrimidines in Antiviral Therapy", in *Selective Inhibitors of Viral Functions,* W. A. Carter, Ed., CRC Press, Cleveland, 1973, p. 295.
19. E. Jawetz, "Chemotherapy of Herpesviruses—Clinical Aspects", in *The Herpesviruses,* A. S. Kaplan, Ed., Academic Press, New York, 1973, p. 665.
20. N. Teich, D. R. Lowy, J. W. Hartley, and W. P. Rowe, *Virology,* **51,** 163 (1973).
21. S. St. Jeor and F. Rapp, *Science,* **181,** 1060 (1973).
22. C. E. Hoffman, "Amantadine HCl and Related Compounds", in *Selective Inhibitors of Viral Functions,* W. A. Carter, Ed., CRC Press, Cleveland, 1973, p. 199.
23. D. B. Calne, *Parkinsonism: Physiology, Pharmacology and Treatment,* Edward Arnold., London, 1970, p. 109.
24. L. Weinstein and T. W. Chang, *New Engl. J. Med.,* **289,** 725 (1973).
25. J. Berger–Roscher and T. Meyer–Rohn, *Med. Welt,* **26,** 897 (1975).
26. L. T. Ch'ien, F. M. Schabel, Jr., and C. A. Alford, "Arabinosyl Nucleosides and Nucleotides", in *Selective Inhibitors of Viral Functions,* W. A. Carter, Ed., CRC Press, Cleveland, 1973, 227.
27. B. E. Juel–Jensen, *Brit. Med. J.,* **1,** 406 (1973).
28. D. A. Stevens, G. W. Jordan, T. F. Waddell, and T. C. Merigan, *N. Engl. J. Med.,* **289,** 873 (1973).
29. S. C. Schimpff, C. L. Fortner, W. H. Green, and P. H. Wiernik, *J. Infect. Dis.,* **130,** 673 (1974).
30. C. B. Lauter, C. J. Bailey, and A. M. Lerner, *Antimicrob. Agents Chemother.,* **6,** 598 (1974).
31. D. Pavan–Langston, R. Buchanan, and C. A. Alford, Jr., Eds., *Adenine Arabinoside: An Antiviral Agent,* Raven Press, New York, 1975.
32. S. Kurtz, "Toxicology of Adenine Arabinoside", in *Adenine Arabinoside: An Antiviral Agent,* D. Pavan–Langston, R., Buchanan, and C. A. Alford, Jr., Eds, Raven Press, New York, 1975, p. 145.
33. P. A. A. Galvao and I. O. Castro, *Ann. N.Y. Acad. Sci.,* **284,** 278 (1977).
34. F. Salido–Rengell, H. Nasser–Quinones, and B. Briseno–Garcia, *Ann. N.Y. Acad. Sci.,* **284,** 272 (1977).
35. C. R. Magnussen, R. G. Douglas, Jr., R. F. Betts, F. K. Roth, and M. P. Meagher, *Antimicrob. Agents Chemother.,* **12,** 498 (1977).
36. Y. Togo and E. A. McCracken, *J. Infect. Dis.,* **133,** (Suppl.), A109 (1976).
36a. J. Hernandez-Manon and C. A. Arroyo, *Sem. Med. Mexico,* **92,** 171 (1977).
37. H. Fernandez Zertuche, and R. Diaz Perches, *Ann. N.Y. Acad. Sci.,* **284,** 284 (1977).
37a. O. Esper Dib, L. Scholz, and P. Arroyo, *Sem. Med. Mexico,* **92,** 245 (1977).
38. D. M. Pachuta, T. Yasushi, R. B. Hornick, A. R. Schwartz, and S. Tominago, *Antimicrob. Agents Chemother.,* **5,** 403 (1974).
39. A. J. Soto, T. S. Hall, and S. E. Reed, *Antimicrob. Agents Chemother.,* **3,** 332 (1973).
40. R. H. Waldman and R. Ganguly, *Ann. N.Y. Acad. Sci.,* **284,** 153 (1977).
41. R. H. Waldman, E. Galleher, M. F. Durieux, and R. Ganguly, *Symposium on Antivirals with Clinical Potential,* T. Merigan, Chairman, Stanford University, Stanford, Abstr. V-D, August 26–29, 1975.
42. L. J. Bradshaw, *Abstr. Am. Soc. Microbiol.,* 78 (1976).
42a. G. M. Schiff, G. Roselle, B. Young, D. May, T. Rotte, and A. J. Glasky, *Abstr. Am. Soc. Microbiol.,* 13 (1978).
42b. R. F. Betts, R. G. Douglas, Jr., S. D. George, and C. J. Rinehart, *Abstr. Am. Soc. Microbiol.,* 13 (1978).
43. R. J. O'Reilly, A. Chibbaro, R. Wilmot, and C. Lopez, *Ann. N.Y. Acad. Sci.,* **284,** 161 (1977).
44. A. Kint and L. Verlinden, *N. Engl. J. Med.,* **291,** 308 (1974).
45. T. D. Felber, E. B. Smith, J. M. Knox, C. Wallis, W. E. Rawls, and J. L. Melnick, *J. Am. Med. Assoc.,* **223,** 289 (1973).
46. R. H. Kaufman, H. L. Gardner, D. Brown, C. Wallis, W. E. Rawls, and J. L. Melnick, *Am. J. Obstetr. Gynecol.,* **117,** 1114 (1973).
47. J. D. Lanier, *Antimicrob. Agents Chemother.,* **6,** 613 (1974).
48. J. L. Melnick and C. Wallis, *Ann. N.Y. Acad. Sci.,* **284,** 171 (1977).
49. F. Rapp, *J. Am. Med. Assoc.,* **225,** 456 (1973).
50. L. Weinstein and T. Chang, *N. Engl. J. Med.,* **289,** 725 (1973).
51. E. G. Friedrick, *J. Obstetr. Gynecol.,* **43,** 304 (1974).
52. G. N. Pershin, N. S. Bogdanova, L. S. Nikolaeva, A. N. Grinev, G. Y. Uretskaya, and N. V. Arkhangel'skaya, *Farmakol. Toksikol.* (Moscow), **38,** 69 (1975).
53. Y. Maichuk, "New Drugs in Chemotherapy of Herpesvirus and Adenovirus Ocular Infections", in *Progress in Chemotherapy* Vol. 2, G. K. Daikos, Ed., Hellenic Society of Chemotherapy, Athens, 1974, p. 968.

54. G. A. Galegov, *Mendelev. Chem. J.*, **18,** 200 (1973).
55. N. S. Bogdanova, G. N. Pershin, and I. S. Nikolayeva, "The Antiviral Drug Florenal", *Progress in Chemotherapy*, Vol. 2, G. K. Daikos, Ed., Hellenic Society of Chemotherapy, Athens, 1974, p. 963.
56. S. Baron and G. Galasso, *Ann. Rep. Med. Chem.*, **10,** 161 (1975).
57. D. J. Bauer, K. Apostolov, and I. W. T. Selway, *Ann. N.Y. Acad. Sci.*, **173,** 314 (1970).
58. D. A. Hamre, K. A. Brownlee, and R. J. Donovick, *J. Immunol.*, **67,** 304 (1951).
59. K. Easterbrook, *Virology*, **17,** 245, (1962).
60. J. S. Oxford and D. D. Perrin, *J. Gen. Virol.*, **23,** 59 (1974).
61. J. A. Levy, S. B. Levy, and W. Levinson, *Virology*, **74,** 426 (1976).
62. P. E. Mikelens, B. A. Woodson, and W. E. Levinson, *Biochem. Pharmacol.*, **25,** 821 (1976).
63. W. E. Levinson, A. Faras, R. Morris, P. Mikelens, G. Ringold, S. Kass, B. Levinson, and J. Jackson, in *Virus Research* (*ICN–UCLA Symposium*), F. Fox and W. Robinson, Eds., Academic Press, New York, 1973, p. 403.
64. D. J. Bauer and P. W. Sadler, *Brit. J. Pharm. Chemother.*, **15,** 101 (1960).
65. G. Pearson and E. Zimmerman, *Virology*, **38,** 641 (1969).
66. R. L. Thompson, M. L. Price, and S. A. Minton, *Proc. Soc. Exp. Biol. Med.*, **78,** 11 (1951).
67. R. L. Thompson, J. Davis, P. B. Russell, and G. H. Hitchings, *Proc. Soc. Exp. Biol. Med.*, **84,** 496 (1953).
68. P. Schauer, M. Likar, M. Tisler, A. Krbavcic, and A. Pollak, *Pathol-Microb.*, **28,** 382 (1965).
69. P. Schauer, A. Krbavcic, M. Tisler, and M. Likar, *Experimentia*, **22,** 304 (1966).
70. P. Schauer, M. Likar, and S. Klement–Vebek, *Ann. N.Y. Acad. Sci.*, **173,** 603 (1970).
71. I. Tamm and L. A. Caliguiri, "2-(α-Hydroxybenzyl)benzimidazole and Related Compounds", in *Chemotherapy of Virus Diseases*, Vol. 1, (*International Encyclopedia of Pharmacology and Therapeutics*, D. J. Bauer, Ed., Pergamon Press, Oxford, 1972, p. 115.
72. L. A. Caliguiri and I. Tamm, "Guanidine and 2-(α-Hydroxybenzyl)benzimidazole (HBB): Selective Inhibitors of Picornavirus Multiplication", in *Selective Inhibitors of Viral Functions*, W. A. Carter, Ed., CRC Press, Cleveland, 1973, p. 257.
73. P. B. Sehgal, I. Tamm, and J. Vilcek, *Virology*, **70,** 532 (1976).
74. J. P. Stella, J. Michaelson, S. L. Dorfman, J. H. Morgan, and C. J. Pfau, *Antimicrob. Agents Chemother.*, **6,** 754 (1974).
75. F. Gaultieri, G. Brody, A. H. Fieldsteel, and W. A. Skinner, *J. Med. Chem.*, **15,** 420 (1972).
76. D. G. O'Sullivan and A. K. Wallis, *J. Med. Chem.*, **15,** 103 (1972).
77. C. J. Paget, K. Kisner, R. L. Stone, and D. C. DeLong, *J. Med. Chem.*, **12,** 1010 (1969).
78. W. R. Roderick, C. W. Nordeen, A. M. Von Esch, and R. N. Appel, *J. Med. Chem.*, **15,** 655 (1972).
79. N. L. Shipkowitz, R. R. Bower, J. B. Schleicher, F. Aquino, R. N. Appell, and R. R. Roderick, *Appl. Microbiol.*, **23,** 117 (1972).
80. S. Akihama, M. Okude, K. Sata, and S. Iwabuchii, *Nature* (London), **217,** 562 (1968).
81. B. Tinland, *Res. Commun. Chem. Pathol. Pharmacol.*, **8,** 571 (1974).
82. C. J. Paget, K. Kisner, R. L. Stone, and D. C. DeLong, *J. Med. Chem.*, **12,** 1016 (1969).
83. C. J. Paget, C. W. Ashbrook, R. L. Stone, and D. C. DeLong, *J. Med. Chem.*, **12,** 1097 (1969).
84. L. Shindarov, A. Galabov, N. Neykova, D. Simov, K. Davidkov, and V. Kalcheva, *Acta Virol.*, **15,** 404 (1971).
85. A. Galabov, "*N*-Phenyl-*N'*-Aryl- or Alkylthiourea Derivatives: Inhibitors of Picornavirus Multiplication", in *Progress in Chemotherapy*, Vol. 2, G. K. Daikos, Ed., Hellenic Society of Chemotherapy, Athens, 1974, p. 981.
86. J. G. Barrera–Oro and J. L. Melnick, *Tex. Rep. Biol. Med.*, **19,** 529 (1961).
87. J. L. Melnick, D. Crowther, and J. Barrera-Oro, *Science*, **134,** 557 (1961).
88. D. Baltimore, H. J. Eggers, R. M. Franklin, and I. Tamm, *Proc. Nat. Acad. Sci., US*, **49,** 843 (1963).
89. M. Ranki and L. Kaariainen, *Ann. Med. Exp. Biol. Fenn*, **47,** 69 (1969).
90. L. Vaczi, D. Hankovszky, K. Hideg, L. Gergely, and G. Hadhazy, *Acta Microbiol. Acad. Sci. Hung.*, **16,** 171 (1969).
91. S. A. Reed, J. W. Craig, and D. A. J. Tyrell, *J. Infect. Dis.*, **133,** (*Suppl.*), A128 (1976).
92. D. L. Swallow, R. A. Bucknall, W. E. Stainer, A. Hutchison, and H. Gaskin, *Ann. N.Y. Acad. Sci.*, **284,** 305 (1977).
93. E. D. Stanley, R. E. Muldoon, L. W. Akers, and G. G. Jackson, *Ann. N.Y. Acad. Sci.*, **130,** 44 (1965).
94. N. Ishida, *Ann. N.Y. Acad. Sci.*, **130,** 460 (1965).

95. Y. Schimizu, A. Tsunoda, and N. Ishida, *Proc. Soc. Exp. Biol. Med.*, **123,** 488 (1966).
96. C. E. Hoffman, "Amantadine HCl and Related Compounds", in *Selective Inhibitors of Viral Functions*, W. A. Carter, Ed., CRC Press, Cleveland, 1973, p. 199.
97. N. Kato and H. J. Eggers, *Virology*, **37,** 632 (1969).
98. C. E. Hoffman, E. M. Neumayer, R. F. Haff, and R. A. Goldsby, *J. Bacteriol.*, **90,** 623 (1965).
99. W. T. Goedermans and A. Peters, *Proc. Fifth Int. Congr. Chemother.*, **2,** 1 (1967).
100. J. S. Oxford and G. S. Schild, *Brit. J. Exp. Pathol.*, **48,** 235 (1967).
101. R. D. Fletcher and A. Yusa, *Virology*, **31,** 382 (1967).
102. A. Tsunoda, H. H. Maasab, K. W. Cochran, and W. C. Eveland, "Antiviral Activity of α-Methyl-1-adamantanemethylamine Hydrochloride", in *Antimicrobial Agents and Chemotherapy*—1965, G. L. Hobby, Ed., American Society for Microbiology, Ann Arbor, Mich., 1966, p. 553.
103. D. E. Aldrich, E. C. Herrmann, Jr., W. E. Meier, M. Paulshock, W. W. Pritchard, J. A. Snyder, and J. C. Watts, *J. Med. Chem.*, **14,** 535 (1971).
104. V. G. May and D. Peteri, *Arzneim.-Forsch. (Drug Res.)*, **23,** 718 (1973).
105. J. E. Dubois, D. Laurent, P. Bost, S. Chambaud, and C. Mercier, *Eu. J. Med. Chem.—Chem. Ther.*, **11,** 225 (1976).
106. K. Lundahl, J. Schut, J. L. M. A. Schatmann, G. B. Paerels, and A. Peters, *J. Med. Chem.*, **15,** 129 (1973).
107. A. Peters, C. A. De Bock, G. B. Paerels, and J. L. M. A. Schlatmann, "Antiviral Activity of a New Derivative, Adamantane *N*-Methyl-Adamantane-2-Spiro-3′-Pyrrolidine", in *Progress in Antimicrobial and Anticancer Chemotherapy*, Vol. 2, University of Tokyo, Tokyo, 1970, p. 71.
108. A. Mathur, A. S. Beare, and S. A. Reed, *Antimicrob. Agents Chemother.*, **4,** 421 (1973).
109. A. S. Beare, T. S. Hall, and D. A. J. Tyrell, *Lancet*, **1,** 1039 (1972).
110. R. Van Hes, A. Smit, and A. Peters, *J. Med. Chem.*, **15,** 132 (1972).
111. A. Takatsuki and G. Tamura, *J. Med. Chem.*, **19,** 536 (1972).
112. J. G. Whitney, W. A. Gregory, J. C. Kaner, J. R. Roland, J. A. Snyder, R. E. Benson, and E. C. Herrmann, Jr., *J. Med. Chem.*, **13,** 254 (1970).
113. W. B. Flagg, F. J. Stanfield, R. F. Haff, R. C. Stewart, R. J. Stedman, J. Gold, and R. J. Ferlauto, "Antiviral Activity of Cyclooctylamine Hydrochloride in Cell Culture and Mouse Systems", in *Antimicrobial Agents and Chemotherapy*—1968, G. L. Hobby, Ed., American Society for Microbiology, Ann Arbor, Mich., 1969, p. 194.
114. Y. Togo, A. R. Schwartz, S. Tominaga, and R. B. Hornick, *J. Am. Med. Assoc.*, **220,** 837 (1972).
115. E. C. Herrmann, Jr., *Proc. Soc. Exp. Biol. Med.*, **107,** 142 (1961).
116. H. E. Kaufman, *Proc. Soc. Exp. Biol. Med.*, **109,** 251, (1962).
117. W. H. Prusoff and B. Goz, "Chemotherapy—Molecular Aspects", in *The Herpesviruses*, A. S. Kaplan, Ed., Academic Press, New York, 1973, p. 641.
118. A. S. Kaplan and T. Ben–Porat, *J. Mol. Biol.*, **19,** 320 (1966).
119. F. M. Schabel, Jr., and J. A. Montgomery, "Purines and Pyrimidines", in *Chemotherapy of Virus Diseases*, Vol. I, *International Encyclopedia of Pharmacology and Therapeutics*, D. J. Bauer, Ed., Pergamon Press, Oxford, 1972, p. 231.
120. L. B. Allen and R. W. Sidwell, *Antimicrob. Agents Chemother.*, **2,** 229 (1972).
121. C. Heidelberger, *Ann. N.Y. Acad. Sci.*, **225,** 317 (1975).
122. J. R. Parkhurst, P. V. Danenberg, and C. Heidelberger, *Chemotherapy*, **22,** 221 (1976).
123. I. Schildkraut, G. M. Cooper, and S. Greer, *Mol. Pharmacol.*, **11,** 153 (1975).
124. R. W. Sidwell, G. Arnett, and H. W. Brockman, *Ann. N.Y. Acad. Sci.*, **173,** 592 (1970).
125. M. J. Doberson, M. Jerkofsky, and S. Greer, *J. Virol.*, **20,** 478 (1976).
126. Y. C. Cheng, B. Goz, J. P. Neenan, D. C. Ward, and W. H. Prusoff, *J. Virol.*, **15,** 1284 (1975).
127. M. S. Chen, D. C. Ward, and W. H. Prusoff, *J. Biol. Chem.*, **251,** 4833 (1976).
128. M. S. Chen, D. C. Ward, and W. H. Prusoff, *J. Biol. Chem.*, **251,** 4839 (1976).
129. T. S. Lin, C. Chai, and W. H. Prusoff, *J. Med. Chem.*, **19,** 915 (1976).
130. T. S. Lin, J. P. Neenan, Y. C. Cheng, W. H. Prusoff, and D. C. Ward, *J. Med. Chem.*, **19,** 495 (1976).
131. D. M. Albert, M. Lahav, P. N. Bhatt, T. W. Reid, R. E. Ward, R. C. Cykiert, T. S. Lin, D. C. Ward, and W. H. Prusoff, *J. Invest. Ophthalmol.*, **15,** 470 (1976).
132. K. K. Gauri, G. Malorny, and E. Riehm, *Arch. Klin. Exp. Ophthalmol. Albrecht von Gractes*, **179,** 287 (1970).

133. M. M. Nemes and M. R. Hilleman, *Proc. Soc. Exp. Biol. Med.*, **119,** 515 (1965).

134. D. Shugar, "Alkylated Pyrimidine Nucleosides and (Poly)nucleotides as Potential Antiviral Agents", in *Virus-Cell Interactions and Viral Antimetabolites,* D. Shugar, Ed., Academic Press, London, 1972, p. 193.

135. E. DeClerq and D. Shugar, *Biochem. Pharmacol.*, **24,** 1073 (1975).

136. Y. C. Cheng, *Ann. N.Y. Acad. Sci.*, **284,** 594 (1977).

137. Y. C. Cheng, B. A. Domin, R. A. Sharma, and M. Bobek, *Antimicrob. Agents Chemother.*, **10,** 119 (1976).

138. M. G. Stout and R. K. Robins, *J. Hetercycl. Chem.*, **913,** 545 (1972).

139. L. A. Babiuk, B. Meldrum, V. A. Gupta, and B. T. Rouse, Antimicrob. Agents Chemother., **8,** 643 (1975).

140. R. Hardi, R. G. Hughes, Jr., Y. K. Ho, K. C. Chadha, and T. J. Bardos, *Antimicrob. Agents Chemother.*, **10,** 682 (1976).

141. R. Y. Chuang and L. F. Chuang, *Nature,* **260,** 549 (1976).

142. J. A. Montgomery, T. P. Johnson, and Y. F. Shealy, "Antineoplastic Agents", in *Medicinal Chemistry,* M. E. Wolff, Ed., Wiley-Interscience, New York, 1979, Ch. 24.

143. W. J. Wechter, M. A. Johnson, C. M. Hall, D. T. Warner A. E. Berger, A. H. Wenzil, D. T. Gish, and G. L. Neil, *J. Med. Chem.*, **18,** 339 (1975).

144. E. K. Hamamura, M. Prystasz, J. P. H. Verheyden, J. G. Moffatt, K. Yamaguchi, N. Uchida, K. Sato, A. Normura, O. Shiratori, S. Takase, and K. Katagiri, *J. Med. Chem.*, **19,** 667 (1976).

145. J. A. Montgomery and H. J. Thomas, *J. Med. Chem.*, **15,** 116 (1972).

146. H. E. Renis, G. E. Underwood, and J. H. Hunter, in *Antimicrobial Agents and Chemotherapy*—1976, G. Hobby, Ed., American Society for Microbiology, Ann Arbor, Mich., 1968, p. 675.

147. R. P. Panzica, R. K. Robins, and L. B. Townsend, *J. Med. Chem.*, **14,** 259 (1971).

148. W. V. Ruyle and T. Y. Shea, *J. Med. Chem.*, **10,** 331 (1967).

149. E. DeClerq, E. Darzyukiewicz, and D. Shugar, *Biochem. Pharmacol.*, **24,** 523 (1975).

150. J. A. Montgomery and A. G. Laseter, *J. Med. Chem.*, **17,** 360 (1974).

151. E. R. Walwick, W. R. Roberts, and C. A. Dekker, *Proc. Chem. Soc.* (London), 84 (1959) through Ch'ien et al. in *Selective Inhibitors of Viral Functions,* W. A. Carter, Ed., CRC Press, Cleveland, 973, p. 227.

152. K. Kikugawa and M. Ichino, *J. Org. Chem.*, **37,** 284 (1972).

153. D. H. Shaunahoff and R. A. Sanchez, *J. Org. Chem.*, **38,** 593 (1973).

154. A. F. Russell, M. Prystasz, E. K. Hamamura, J. P. H. Verheyden, and J. G. Moffatt. *J. Org. Chem.*, **39,** 2182 (1974).

155. A. Hoshi, M. Iigo, M. Saneyoshi, and K. Kuretani, *Chem. Pharm. Bull.* (Tokyo), **21,** 1535 (1973).

156. E. K. Hamamura, M. Prystasz, J. P. H. Verheyden, J. G. Moffatt, K. Yamaguchi, N. Uchida, K. Sato, A. Nomura, O. Shiratori, S. Takase, and K. Katagiri, *J. Med. Chem.*, **19,** 654 (1976).

157. E. K. Hamamura, M. Prystasz, J. P. H. Verheyden, J. G. Moffatt, K. Yamaguchi, N. Uchida, K. Sato, A. Nomura, O. Shiratori, S. Takase, and K. Katagiri, *J. Med. Chem.*, **19,** 663 (1976).

158. R. A. Long, G. L. Skeres, T. A. Khwaja, R. W. Sidwell, L. N. Simon, and R. K. Robins, *J. Med. Chem.* **15,** 1215 (1972).

159. R. W. Sidwell, L. N. Simon, J. H. Huffman, L. B. Allen, R. A. Long, and R. K. Robins, *Nature New Biol.*, **242,** 204 (1973).

160. G. E. Underwood, "Chemotherapy of Herpes Keratitis in Rabbits," in *Third International Congress of Chemotherapy,* Vol. 1, H. P. Kuemmerle and P. Preziosi, Eds., Hafner, New York, 1964, p. 858.

161. G. A. Gentry and J. F. Aswell, *Virology,* **65,** 294 (1975).

162. J. G. Aswell and G. A. Gentry, *Ann. N.Y. Acad. Sci.*, **284,** 342 (1977).

163. B. Rada and M. Dragun, *Ann. N.Y. Acad. Sci.*, **284,** 410 (1977).

164. S. Jasinska, F. Link̆, D. Blaškovič, and B. Rada, *Acta Virol.*, **6,** 17 (1962).

165. G. A. Galegov, R. M. Bikbulatov, K. A. Vanag, and R. M. Shen, *Vop. Virusol.*, **13,** 18 (1968).

166. J. Elis and N. Raškova, *Eur. J. Clin. Pharm.*, **4,** 77 (1972).

167. A. P. Starcheus and V. P. Chernetskii, *Mykrobiol. Zh.* (Kiev), **29,** 157 (1967).

168. R. W. Sidwell, G. J. Dixon, S. M. Sellers, and F. M. Schabel, Jr., *Appl. Microbiol.*, **16,** 370 (1968).

169. R. E. Handschumaker and C. A. Pasternak, *Biochem. Biophys. Acta,* **30,** 451 (1958).

170. J. Skoda, *Progr. Nucleic Acid Res. Mol. Biol.*, **2,** 197 (1963).

171. B. Rada and V. Altanerova, *Acta Virol.*, **14,** 425 (1970).

172. F. Smejkal, J. Gut, and F. Šorm, *Acta Virol.*, **6,** 364 (1962).

172a. H. E. Renis, *Antimicrob. Agents Chemother.*, **13,** 613 (1978).

172b. G. E. Underwood and S. D. Weed, *Antimicrob. Agents Chemother.*, **11,** 765 (1977).

172c. C. De Boer, B. Bannister, A. Dietz, C. Lewis, and J. E. Gray, *Abst. Ann. Mtg. Am. Soc. Microbiol.*, 185 (1976).

173. G. P. Khare, R. W. Sidwell, J. H. Huffman, R. L. Tolman, and R. K. Robins, *Proc. Soc. Exp. Biol. Med.*, **140,** 880 (1972).

174. W. M. Shannon, G. Arnett, and F. M. Schabel, Jr., *Antimicrob. Agents Chemother.*, **2,** 159 (1972).

175. W. M. Shannon, R. W. Brockman, L. Westbrook, S. Shaddix, and F. M. Schabel, Jr., *J. Nat. Cancer Inst.*, **52,** 199 (1974).

176. W. M. Shannon, *Ann. N.Y. Acad. Sci.*, **284,** 472 (1977).

177. M. C. Wang and A. Bloch, *Biochem. Pharmacol.*, **21,** 1063 (1972).

178. P. La Colla, M. A. Marcialis, O. Flore, M. Sau, A. Garzia, and B. Loddo, *Ann. N.Y. Acad. Sci.*, **284,** 294 (1977).

179. R. L. Thompson, M. Price, S. A. Minton, E. A. Falco, and G. M. Hitchings, *J. Immunol.*, **67,** 483 (1951).

180. R. H. Dreisbach, B. J. Neff, M. Azima, V. P. Tiffany, and W. C. Cutting, *Stanford Med. Bull.*, **7,** 193 (1949).

181. K. K. Gauri and B. Rohde, *Klin.-Ther. Wochenschr.*, **47,** 375 (1969).

182. K. K. Gauri and H. Kohlhage, *Chemotherapy*, **14,** 158 (1969).

183. F. M. Schabel, Jr., *Chemotherapy*, **13,** 321 (1968).

184. W. M. Shannon, "Adenine Arabinoside: Antiviral Activity *in Vitro*," in *Adenine Arabinoside: An Antiviral Agent*, D. Pavan-Langston, R. A. Buchanan, and C. A. Alford, Jr., Eds., Raven Press, New York, 1975, p. 1.

185. B. J. Sloan, "Adenine Arabinoside: Chemotherapy Studies in Animals," in *Adenine Arabinoside: An Antiviral Agent*, D. Pavan-Langston, R. A. Buchanan and C. A. Alford, Jr., Eds., Raven Press, New York, 1975, p. 45.

186. R. W. Sidwell, L. B. Allen, J. H. Huffman, J. T. Witkowski, P. D. Cook, R. L. Tolman, G. R. Revankar, L. N. Simon, and R. K. Robins, "The Potential of Nucleosides as Antiviral Agents," in *Chemotherapy* (*Proceedings of the Ninth International Congress of Chemotherapy*), Vol. 6, J. D. Williams and A. M. Geddes, Eds, Plenum Press, New York, 1976, p. 279.

187. J. L. York and G. A. LePage, *Can. J. Biochem.*, **44,** 19 (1966).

188. J. J. Furth and S. S. Cohen, *Cancer Res.*, **27,** 1528 (1967).

189. L. Sweetman, J. D. Connor, R. Seshamani, M. A. Stuckey, S. Carey, and R. Buchanan, "Deamination of Adenine Arabinoside in Cell Culture for *in Vitro* Viral Inhibition Studies," in *Adenine Arabinoside: An Antiviral Agent*, D. Pavan-Langston, R. A. Buchanan, and C. A. Alford, Jr., Eds., Raven Press, New York, 1975, p. 135.

190. A. J. Glazko, T. Chang, J. C. Drach, D. R. Mourer, P. E. Barondy, H. Schneider, L. Croskey, and E. Maschewske, "Species Differences in the Metabolic Distribution of Adenine Arabinoside," in *Adenine Arabinoside: An Antiviral Agent*, D. Pavan-Langston, Raven Press, New York, 1975, p. 111.

191. L. L. Bennett, Jr., W. M. Shannon, P. W. Allan, and G. Arnett, *Ann. N.Y. Acad. Sci.*, **255,** 342 (1975).

192. F. A. Miller, G. J. Dixon, J. Ehrlich, B. J. Sloan, and I. W. McLean, Jr., in, *Antimicrobial Agents and Chemotherapy*—1968, American Society for Microbiology, Ann Arbor; Mich., 1969, p. 136.

193. D. Pavan-Langston, R. H. S. Langston, and P. A. Geary, *Arch. Ophthalmol.*, **92,** 417 (1974).

194. W. E. G. Müller, R. K. Zahn, K. Bittlingmaier, and D. Falke, *Ann. N.Y. Acad. Sci.*, **284,** 34 (1977).

195. P. M. Schwartz, C. Shipman, Jr., and J. C. Drach, *Antimicrob. Agents Chemother.*, **10,** 64 (1976).

196. P. E. Borondy, T. Chang, E. Maschewske, and A. J. Glazko, *Ann. N.Y. Acad. Sci.*, **284,** 9 (1977).

197. W. Plunkett and S. Cohen, *Cancer Res.*, **35,** 1547 (1975).

198. W. Plunkett and S. Cohen, *Ann. N.Y. Acad. Sci.*, **284,** 91 (1977).

199. R. W. Sidwell, L. B. Allen, J. H. Huffman, T. A. Khwaja, R. L. Tolman, and R. K. Robins, *Chemotherapy*, **19,** 325 (1973).

200. G. R. Revankar, J. H. Huffman, L. B. Allen, R. W. Sidwell, R. K. Robins, and R. L. Tolman, *J. Med. Chem.*, **18,** 721 (1975).

201. R. W. Sidwell, L. B. Allen, J. H. Huffman, G. R. Revankar, R. K. Robins, and R. L. Tolman, *Antimicrob. Agents Chemother.*, **8,** 463 (1975).

202. L. B. Allen, J. M. Thompson, J. H. Huffman, G. R. Revankar, R. L. Tolman, L. N. Simon, R. K.

Robins, and R. W. Sidwell, *Antimicrob. Agents Chemother.*, **8,** 474 (1975).

203. A. M. Mian, R. Harris, R. W. Sidwell, R. K. Robins, and T. A. Khwaja, *J. Med. Chem.*, **17,** 259 (1974).

204. G. A. LePage, Y. T. Lin, R. E. Orth, and J. A. Gottleid, *Cancer Res.*, **32,** 2441 (1972).

205. T. H. Haskell, *Ann. N.Y. Acad. Sci.*, **284,** 81 (1977).

206. C. Lopez and A. Giner-Sorolla, *Ann. N.Y. Acad. Sci.*, **284,** 351 (1977).

207. G. B. Elion, J. L. Rideout, P. de Miranda, P. Collins, and D. J. Bauer, *Ann. N.Y. Acad. Sci.*, **255,** 468 (1975).

208. C. W. Smith, R. W. Sidwell, R. K. Robins, and R. L. Tolman, *J. Med. Chem.*, **15,** 883 (1972).

209. J. A. Montgomery and H. J. Thomas, *J. Med. Chem.*, **15,** 305 (1972).

210. E. Walton, S. R. Jenkins, R. F. Nutt, and F. W. Holly, *J. Med. Chem.*, **12,** 306 (1969).

211. W. M. Shannon, A. Shortnacy, G. Arnett, and J. A. Montgomery, *J. Med. Chem.*, **17,** 361 (1974).

212. G. R. Revankar, J. H. Huffman, R. W. Sidwell, R. L. Tolman, R. K. Robins, and L. B. Allen, *J. Med. Chem.*, **19,** 1026 (1976).

213. J. E. Zimmerman, Jr., and K. Raska, Jr., *Nature New Biol.*, **239,** 145 (1972).

214. R. W. Sidwell, J. H. Huffman, D. Shuman, K. Muneyama, and R. K. Robins, "Cyclic AMP Derivatives as Antiviral Agents," in *Advances in Antimicrobial and Antineoplastic Chemotherapy* Vol. 1, M. Hejzlar, M. Semonsky, and S. Masak, Eds., University Park Press, Baltimore, 1972, p. 313.

215. R. W. Sidwell, J. H. Huffman, L. B. Allen, R. B. Meyer, Jr., D. A. Shuman, L. N. Simon, and R. K. Robins, *Antimicrob. Agents Chemother.*, **5,** 652 (1974).

216. L. B. Allen, N. C. Eagle, J. H. Huffman, D. A. Shuman, R. B. Meyer, Jr., and R. W. Sidwell, *Proc. Soc. Exp. Biol. Med.*, **146,** 580 (1974).

216a. E. DeClercq, J. Descamps, P. Desomer, and A. Holy, *Science*, **200,** 563 (1978).

216b. A. Holy, *Collect. Czech Chem. Commun.*, **40,** 187 (1975).

216c. H. J. Schaeffler, S. Gurwara, R. Vince, and S. Bittner, *J. Med. Chem.*, **14,** 367 (1971).

216d. H. J. Schaeffer, L. Beauchamp, P. de Miranda, G. B. Elion, D. J. Bauer, and P. Collins, *Nature*, **272,** 583 (1978).

216e. G. B. Elion, P. A. Furman, J. A. Fyfe, P. de Miranda, L. Beauchamp, and H. J. Schaeffer, *Proc. Nat. Acad. Sci. U.S.*, **74,** 5716 (1977).

217. P. D. Cook, R. J. Rousseau, A. M. Mian, R. B. Meyer, Jr., P. Dea, G. Ivanovics, D. G. Streeter, J. T. Witkowski, M. G. Stout, L. N. Simon, R. W. Sidwell, and R. K. Robins, *J. Am. Chem. Soc.*, **97,** 2916 (1975).

218. L. B. Allen, J. H. Huffman, P. D. Cook, R. B. Meyer, Jr., R. K. Robins, and R. W. Sidwell, *Antimicrob. Agents Chemother.*, **12,** 114 (1977).

219. T. A. Khwaja, L. Kigwana, R. B. Meyer, Jr., and R. K. Robins, *Proc. Am. Assoc. Cancer Res.*, **16,** 162 (1975).

220. D. G. Streeter and H. H. P. Koyama, *Biochem. Pharmacol.*, **25,** 2413 (1976).

221. O. P. Babbar, *J. Sci. In. Res.*, **20C,** 216 (1961).

222. O. P. Babbar and B. L. Chowdhury, *J. Sci. In. Res.*, **21C,** 312 (1962).

223. J. T. Witkowski, R. K. Robins, R. W. Sidwell, and L. N. Simon, *J. Med. Chem.*, **15,** 1150 (1972).

224. R. W. Sidwell, J. H. Huffman, G. P. Khare, L. B. Allen, J. T. Witkowski, and R. K. Robins, *Science*, **177,** 705 (1972).

225. R. W. Sidwell, L. N. Simon, J. T. Witkowski, and R. K. Robins, "Antiviral Activity of Virazole: Review and Structure-Activity Relationships," in *Progress in Chemotherapy*, Vol. 2, G. K. Daikos, Ed., Hellenic Society of Chemotherapy Athens, 1974, p. 889.

226. D. G. Streeter, J. T. Witkowski, G. P. Khare, R. W. Sidwell, R. J. Bauer, R. K. Robins, and L. N. Simon, *Proc. Nat. Acad Sci., US*, **70,** 1174 (1973).

227. L. N. Simon, R. W. Sidwell, G. P. Khare, D. G. Streeter, J. P. Miller, J. T. Witkowski, J. H. Huffman, and R. K. Robins, "Molecular Basis of Antiviral Chemotherapy: Virazole, A New Broad Spectrum Antiviral Agent", in *Virus Research, Second ICN–UCLA Symposium on Molecular Biology*, C. F. Fox and W. S. Robinson, Eds., Academic Press, New York, 1973, p. 415.

228. D. G. Streeter, J. P. Miller, R. K. Robins, and L. N. Simon, *Ann. N.Y. Acad. Sci.*, **284,** 201 (1977).

229. J. P. Miller, L. J. Kigwana, D. G. Streeter, R. K. Robins, L. N. Simon, and J. Roboz, *Ann. N.Y. Acad. Sci.*, **284,** 211 (1977).

230. C. Scholtissek, *Arch. Virol.*, **50,** 349 (1976).

231. J. S. Oxford, *J. Gen. Virol.*, **28,** 409 (1975).

232. J. S. Oxford, *Antimicrob. Agents Chemother.*, **1,** 7 (1975).

233. B. Eriksson, E. Helgstrand, K. N. G. Johansson, A. Larsson, A. Misiorny, J. O. Norén, L. Philipson, K. Stenburg, G. Stening, S. Stridh, and B.

Öberg, *Antimicrob. Agents Chemother.*, **11,** 946 (1977).
234. W. E. G. Müller, A. Maidhof, H. Taschner, and R. K. Zahn, *Biochem. Pharmacol.*, **26,** 1071 (1977).
235. E. Katz, E. Margalith, and B. Winer, *J. Gen. Virol.*, **32,** 327 (1976).
236. J. T. Witkowski, R. K. Robins, G. P. Khare, and R. W. Sidwell, *J. Med. Chem.*, **16,** 935 (1973).
237. M. Fuertes, J. T. Witkowski, D. G. Streeter, and R. K. Robins, *J. Med. Chem.*, **17,** 642 (1974).
238. J. T. Witkowski, M. Fuertes, P. D. Cook, and R. K. Robins, *J. Carbohyd. Nucl.*, **2,** 1 (1975).
239. M. S. Poonian, E. F. Nowoswiat, J. F. Blount, T. H. Williams, R. G. Pitcher, and M. J. Kramer, *J. Med. Chem.*, **19,** 286 (1976).
240. M. V. Pickering, J. T. Witkowski, and R. K. Robins, *J. Med. Chem.*, **19,** 841 (1976).
241. E. DeClerq and M. Luczak, *Life Sci.*, **17,** 187 (1975).
242. P. C. Strivastava, D. G. Streeter, T. R. Matthews, L. B. Allen, R. W. Sidwell, and R. K. Robins, *J. Med. Chem.*, **19,** 1020 (1976).
243. A. Hampton, *J. Biol. Chem.*, **238,** 3068 (1963).
244. G. E. Gutowski, M. J. Sweeney, D. C. DeLong, R. L. Hamill, K. Gazon, and R. W. Dyer, *Ann. N.Y. Acad. Sci.*, **255,** 544 (1975).
245. E. R. Andrews, R. W. Fleming, J. M. Grisar, J. C. Kihm, D. L. Wenstrup, and G. D. Mayer, *J. Med. Chem.*, **17,** 882 (1974).
246. R. F. Krueger and G. D. Mayer, *Science*, **169,** 1213 (1970).
247. G. D. Mayer and R. F. Krueger, *Science*, **169,** 1214 (1970).
248. E. DeClerq, "Nonpolynucleotide Interferon Inducers," in *Selective Inhibitors of Viral Functions*, W. A. Carter, Ed., CRC Press, Cleveland, 1973, p. 177.
249. H. E. Kaufman, Y. M. Centifanto, E. D. Ellison, and D. C. Brown, *Proc. Soc. Exp. Biol. Med.*, **137,** 357 (1971).
250. P. Chandra, G. Will, D. Gericke, and A. Götz, *Biochem. Pharmacol.*, **23,** 3259 (1974).
251. D. J. Giron, J. P. Schmidt, and F. F. Pindak, *Antimicrob. Agents Chemother.*, **1,** 78 (1972).
252. P. Chandra, *Top. Curr. Chem.*, **52,** 99 (1974).
253. W. L. Albrecht, R. W. Fleming, S. W. Horgan, J. C. Kihm, and G. D. Mayer, *J. Med. Chem.*, **17,** 886 (1974).
254. V. P. Meindl, G. Bodo, and H. Tuppy, *Arzneim.-Forsch.*, **26,** 312 (1976).
255. J. M. Gisar, K. R. Hickey, R. W. Fleming, and G. D. Mayer, *J. Med. Chem.*, **17,** 890 (1974).
256. A. D. Sill, W. L. Albrecht, E. R. Andrews, R. W. Fleming, S. W. Horgan, E. M. Roberts, and F. W. Sweet, *J. Med. Chem.*, **16,** 240 (1973).
257. A. D. Sill, E. R. Andrews, F. W. Sweet, J. W. Hoffman, P. L. Tiernan, J. M. Grisar, R. W. Fleming, and G. D. Mayer, *J. Med. Chem.*, **17,** 965 (1974).
258. W. L. Albrecht, R. W. Fleming, S. W. Horgan, B. A. Deck, J. W. Hoffman, and G. D. Mayer, *J. Med. Chem.*, **17,** 1150 (1974).
259. W. L. Albrecht, R. W. Fleming, S. W. Horgan, and G. D. Mayer, *J. Med. Chem.*, **20,** 364 (1977).
260. A. A. Carr, J. F. Grunwell, A. D. Sill, D. R. Meyer, F. W. Sweet, B. J. Scheue, J. M. Grisar, R. W. Fleming, and G. D. Mayer, *J. Med. Chem.*, **19,** 1142 (1976).
261. R. R. Crenshaw, G. M. Luke, and P. Simonoff, *J. Med. Chem.*, **19,** 262 (1976).
262. P. Simonoff, A. M. Bernard, V. S. Hursky, and K. E. Price, *Antimicrob. Agents Chemother.*, **3,** 742 (1973).
263. P. Simonoff, *Infect. Immun.* **12,** 1051 (1975).
264. P. Simonoff, *J. Infect. Dis.*, **133** (Suppl.), A37 (1976).
265. E. R. Kern, J. R. Hamilton, J. C. Overall, Jr., and L. A. Glasgow, *Antimicrob. Agents Chemother.*, **10,** 691 (1976).
266. D. H. Metz, *Advan. Drug Res.*, **10,** 101 (1975).
267. E. DeClerq, *Top. Curr. Chem.* **52,** 173 (1974).
268. A. K. Field, "Interferon Induction by Polynucleotides," in *Selective Inhibitors of Viral Functions*, W. A. Carter, Ed., CRC Press, Cleveland, 1973, p. 149.
269. D. A. Hill, S. Baron, H. B. Levy, J. Bellanti, C. E. Buckler, G. Cannellos, P. Carbone, R. M. Chanock, V. De Vita, M. A. Guggenheim, E. Homan, A. Z. Kapikian, R. L. Kirchstein, J. Mills, J. C. Perkins, J. E. Van Kirk, and M. Worthington, *Perspect. Virol.*, **7,** 197 (1971).
270. R. Guerra, R. Frezzoti, R. Bonani, F. Dianzani, and G. Rita, *Ann. N.Y. Acad. Sci.*, **173,** 823 (1970).
271. V. De Vita, G. Cannellos, P. Carbone, S. Baron, H. Levy, and H. Gralnick, *Proc. Am. Assoc. Cancer Res.*, **11,** 21 (1970).
272. J. J. Nordlund, S. M. Wolfe, and H. B. Levy, *Proc. Soc. Exp. Biol. Med.*, **133,** 439 (1970).
273. H. B. Levy, G. Baer, S. Baron, C. Buckler, C. J. Gibbs, M. J. Iadarola, W. T. London, and J. A. Rice, *J. Infect. Dis.*, **132,** 434 (1975).
274. H. B. Levy, W. London, D. A. Fuccillo, S. Baron, and J. Rice, *J. Infect. Dis.*, **133** (Suppl.), A256 (1976).

275. W. Regelson, *J. Am. Med. Assoc.*, **201,** 27 (1967).
276. T. C. Merigan and M. S. Finkelstein, *Virology,* **35,** 363 (1968).
277. P. De Somer, E. DeClerq, A. Billiau, E. Schoune, and M. Claeson, *J. Virol.*, **2,** 886 (1968).
278. A. Billiau, J. Desmyter, and P. De Somer, *J. Virol.*, **5,** 321 (1970).
279. E. DeClerq, "Nonpolynucleotide Interferon Inducers," in *Selective Inhibitors of Viral Functions,* W. A. Carter, Ed., CRC Press, Cleveland, 1973, p. 177.
280. B. Moss, "Ansamycins: (A) Rifamycin SV Derivatives," in *Selective Inhibitors of Viral Functions,* W. A. Carter, Ed., CRC Press, Cleveland, 1973, p. 313.
281. E. Heller, "The Antiviral Effect of Rifampicin," in *RNA Polymerase and Transcription, Proceedings of the First International Lepetit Colloquium,* L. Silvestri, Ed., Amsterdam, North Holland, 1969, p. 287.
282. J. H. Subak-Sharpe, T. H. Pennington, T. F. Szilagyi, M. C. Timbury, and J. F. Williams, "The Effect of Rifamycin on Mammalian Viruses and Cells," in *RNA Polymerase and Transcription, Proceedings of the First International Lepetit Colloquium,* L. Silvestei, Ed., Amsterdam, North Holland, 1969, p. 739.
283. S. Barlati, A. Brega, and L. G. Silvestri, *Intervirology,* **2,** 33 (1973/4).
284. C. Gurgo, R. K. Ray, and M. Green, *J. Nat. Cancer Inst.*, **49,** 61 (1972).
285. T. E. O'Connor, C. D. Aldrich, and V. S. Sethi, *Ann. N.Y. Acad. Sci.*, **284,** 544 (1977).
286. D. M. Byrd and W. A. Carter, "Ansamycins: (B) Streptovaricins," in *Selective Inhibitors of Viral Functions,* W. A. Carter, Ed., CRC Press, Cleveland, 1973, p. 329.
287. W. Wehrli and M. Staehelin, *Bacteriol. Rev.*, **35,** 290 (1971).
288. W. A. Rightsel, H. G. Schneider, B. J. Sloan, P. R. Graf, F. A. Miller, Q. R. Bartz, and J. Ehrlich, *Nature,* **204,** 1333 (1964).
289. P. A. Miller, K. P. Milstrey, and P. W. Trown, *Science,* **159,** 431 (1968).
290. P. W. Trown and J. A. Bilello, *Antimicrob. Agents Chemother.*, **2,** 261 (1972).
291. N. Neuss, L. D. Boeck, D. R. Brannon, J. C. Cline, D. C. De Long, M. Gorman, L. L. Huckstep, D. H. Lively, J. Mabe, M. M. Marsh, B. B. Molloy, R. Nagarajan, J. D. Nelson, and W. M. Stark, in *Antimicrob. Agents and Chemotherapy—1968,* G. Hobby, Ed., American Society for Microbiology, Ann Arbor, Mich., 1969, p. 213.
292. F. M. Schabel, Jr., W. R. Laster, R. W. Brockman, and H. E. Skipper, *Proc. Soc. Exp. Biol. Med.*, **83,** 1 (1953).
293. Y. Becker, Y. Asher, and Z. Zakay-Rones, *Antimicrob. Agents Chemother.*, **1,** 483 (1972).
294. Y. De Ratuld and G. H. Werner, "*In Vitro* and *In Vivo* Studies on the Inhibitory Activity of Distamycin A on DNA Viruses," in *Progress in Antimicrobial and Anticancer Chemotherapy* Vol. 2, University of Tokyo Press, Tokyo, 1970, p. 14.
295. R. M. Ruprecht, N. C. Goodman, and S. Spiegelman, *Biochim. Biophys. Acta,* **294,** 192 (1973).
296. P. Chandra, F. Zunino, A. Götz, A. Wacker, D. Gericke, A. Di Marco, A. Casazza, and F. Giuliani, *FEBS Lett.*, **21,** 154 (1972).
297. M. Kotler and Y. Becker, *J. Israel Med. Assoc.*, **81,** 412 (1971).
298. F. Suzuki, N. Saito, and N. Ishida, *Ann. N.Y. Acad. Sci.*, **284,** 667 (1977).
299. H. Umezawa, "Bleomycin," in *Antibiotics,* Vol. 3, J. W. Corcoran and F. E. Hahn, Eds., Springer-Verlag, New York, 1975, p. 21.
300. M. Takeshita, A. P. Grollman, and S. B. Horowitz, *Virology,* **69,** 453 (1976).
301. M. S. Takeshita, S. B. Horowitz, and A. P. Grollman, *Virology,* **60,** 455 (1974).
302. W. E. G. Müller, Z. Yomazaki, J. H. Bretter, and R. K. Zahn, *Eur. J. Biochem.*, **31,** 518 (1972).
303. N. L. Shipkowitz, R. Bower, R. N. Appell, C. W. Nordeen, L. R. Overby, W. R. Roderick, J. B. Schleicher, and A. M. Von Esch, *Appl. Microbiol.*, **26,** 264 (1973).
304. L. R. Overby, E. E. Robishaw, J. B. Schleicher, A. Rueter, N. L. Shipkowitz, and J. C.-h. Mao, *Antimicrob. Agents Chemother.*, **6,** 360 (1974).
305. E.-s. Huang, *J. Virol.*, **16,** 1560 (1975).
306. D. D. Gerstein, C. R. Dawson, and J. O. Oh, *Antimicrob. Agents Chemother.*, **7,** 285 (1975).
307. R. F. Meyer, E. D. Varnell, and H. E. Kaufman, *Antimicrob. Agents Chemother.*, **9,** 308 (1976).
308. R. J. Klein and A. E. Friedman-Kien, *Antimicrob. Agents Chemother.*, **7,** 289 (1975).
309. J. C.-h. Mao, E. E. Robishaw, and L. R. Overby, *J. Virology,* **15,** 1281 (1975).
310. J. C.-h. Mao and E. E. Robishaw, *Biochemistry,* **14,** 5475 (1975).
311. L. R. Overby, R. G. Duff, and J. C.-h. Mao, *Ann. N.Y. Acad. Sci.*, **284,** 310 (1977).

311a. T. R. Herrin, J. S. Fairgreave, R. R. Bower, N. L. Shipkowitz, and J. C.-h. Mao, *J. Med. Chem.*, **20,** 660 (1977).

311b. P. Nylén, *Chem. Ber.*, **57B,** 1023 (1924).

311c. E. Helgstrand, B. Eriksson, N. G. Johansson, B. Lannerö, A. Larsson, A. Misiorny, J. O. Norén, B. Sjöberg, K. Stenberg, G. Stening, S. Stridh, B. Öberg, S. Alenius, and L. Philipson, *Science*, **201,** 820 (1978).

312. W. F. McLimans, G. E. Underwood, E. A. Slater, E. V. Davis, and R. A. Siem, *J. Immunol.*, **78,** 104 (1957).

313. G. E. Underwood and S. D. Weed, *Virology*, **13,** 138 (1961).

314. H. E. Renis, *Ann. N.Y. Acad. Sci.*, **173,** 527 (1970).

315. G. E. Underwood. *Proc. Soc. Exp. Biol. Med.*, **129,** 235 (1968).

316. N. B. Finter, *Ann. N.Y. Acad. Sci.*, **173,** 131 (1970).

317. D. L. Swallow, P. N. Edwards, and N. B. Finter, *Ann. N.Y. Acad. Sci.*, **173,** 292 (1970).

318. D. L. Swallow, "Antiviral Agents," in *Progress in Medicinal Chemistry*, Vol. 8, G. P. Ellis and G. B. West, Eds., Appleton, New York, 1971, p. 119.

319. K. W. Brammer, C. R. McDonald, and M. S. Tute, *Nature*, **219,** 515 (1968).

320. M. S. Tute, K. W. Brammer, B. Kaye, and R. W. Broadbent, *J. Med. Chem.*, **13,** 44 (1970).

321. T. H. Haskell, F. E. Peterson, D. Watson, N. R. Plessas, and T. Culbertson, *J. Med. Chem.*, **13,** 697 (1970).

322. K. Shinkai and T. Nishimura, *J. Gen. Virol.*, **16,** 227 (1972).

323. J. D. Coombes, K. W. Brammer, R. H. Herbst-Laier, N. M. Larin, C. R. McDonald, M. S. Tute, E. A. Wickham, and G. M. Williamson, *Ann. N.Y. Acad. Sci.*, **173,** 462 (1970).

324. A. S. Beare, M. L. Bynoe, and D. A. J. Tyrell, *Lancet*, **1,** 843 (1968).

325. P. N. Mienan and I. B. Hillary, *Lancet*, **2,** 614 (1969).

326. S. E. Reed and M. L. Bynoe, *J. Med. Microbiol.*, **3,** 346 (1970).

327. J. E. Stark, R. B. Heath, N. C. Oswald, V. Booth, R. Tall, W. Fox, K. O. Moynagh, and J. M. Inglis, *Thorax*, **25,** 649 (1970).

328. E. Grunberg and H. N. Prince, *Proc. Soc. Exp. Biol. Med.*, **129,** 422 (1968).

329. E. Grunberg and H. N. Prince, *Ann. N.Y. Acad. Sci.*, **173,** 122 (1970).

330. B. R. Murphy and L. A. Glasgow, *Ann. N.Y. Acad. Sci.*, **173,** 255 (1970).

331. W. W. Hoffman, J. J. Korst, J. F. Niblack, and T. H. Cronin, *Antimicrob. Agents Chemother.*, **3,** 498 (1973).

332. R. G. Douglas, Jr., and R. F. Betts, *Infect. Immunol.*, **9,** 506 (1974).

333. E. D. Stanley, G. G. Jackson, V. A. Dirda, and M. M. Rubenis, *J. Infect. Dis.*, **133** (Suppl.), A121 (1976).

334. C. Panusarn, E. D. Stanley, V. Dirda, M. Rubenis, and G. G. Jackson, *N. Engl. J. Med.*, **291,** 57 (1974).

335. C. Scholtissek, *Curr. Top. Microbiol Immunol.*, **70,** 101 (1975).

336. D. S. Hodes, T. J. Schnitzer, A. R. Kalica, E. Camargo, and R. M. Chanock, *Virology*, **63,** 201 (1975).

337. F. Floch and G. H. Werner, *Arch. Virol.*, **52,** 169 (1976).

338. H. D. Klemk, C. Scholtissek, and R. Rott, *Virology*, **49,** 723 (1972).

339. R. J. Courtney, S. M. Steiner, and M. Benyesh-Melnick, *Virology*, **52,** 447 (1973).

340. S. Steiner, R. J. Courtney, and J. L. Melnick, *Cancer Res.*, **33,** 2402 (1973).

341. P. Palase, J. L. Schulman, G. Bodo, and P. Meindl, *Virology*, **59,** 490 (1974).

342. J. L. Schulman and P. Palase, *Virology*, **63,** 98 (1975).

343. P. Palase and R. W. Compans, *J. Gen. Virol.*, **33,** 159 (1976).

344. D. Bucher and P. Palase, "The Biologically Active Proteins of Influenza Virus: Neuraminidase," in *The Influenza viruses and Influenza*, E. D. Kilbourne, Ed., Academic Press, New York, 1975, p. 84.

345. P. Meindl, G. Bodo, P. Palase, J. Schulman, and H. Tuppy, *Virology*, **58,** 457 (1974).

346. J. M. Z. Gladych, J. H. Hunt, D. Jack, R. F. Haff, J. J. Boyle, R. C. Stewart, and R. J. Ferlauto, *Nature*, **221,** 286 (1969).

347. J. J. Boyle, W. G. Raupp, F. J. Stanfield, R. F. Haff, E. C. Dick, D. D'Allessio, and C. R. Dick, *Ann. N.Y. Acad. Sci.*, **173,** 477 (1970).

348. J. M. Gwaltney, *Proc. Soc. Exp. Biol. Med.*, **133,** 1148 (1970).

349. R. F. Haff, W. B. Flagg, J. J. Gallo, J. R. E. Hoover, J. A. Miller, C. A. Pinto, and J. F. Pegano, *Proc. Soc. Exp. Biol. Med.*, **141,** 475 (1972).

350. Y. Togo, A. R. Schwartz, and R. B. Hornick, *Chemotherapy*, **18,** 17 (1973).

351. C. A. Pinto, H. P. Bahnsen, L. J. Ravin, R. F. Haff, and J. F. Pagano, *Proc. Soc. Exp. Biol. Med.*, **141,** 467 (1972).

352. I. Beladi, R. Pusztai, I. Mucsi, M. Bakay, and M. Gabor, *Ann. N.Y. Acad. Sci.*, **284,** 358 (1977).

353. W. C. Cutting, R. H. Dreisbach, and F. Matsushima, *Stanford Med. Bull.*, **11,** 227 (1953).

354. W. S. Burnham, R. W. Sidwell, R. L. Tolman, and M. G. Stout, *J. Med. Chem.*, **15,** 1075 (1972).

355. H. E. Renis, in *Antimicrobial Agents and Chemotherapy—1969,* G. L. Hobby, Ed., American Society for Microbiology, Ann Arbor, Mich. 1970, p. 167.

356. M. G. Soret, in *Antimicrobial Agents and Chemotherapy*–1969, G. L. Hobby, Ed., American Society for Microbiology, Ann Arbor, Mich., 1970, for p. 160.

357. G. A. Elliott, D. A. Buthala, and E. N. De Young, *Antimicrobial Agents and Chemotherapy–1969;* G. L. Hobby, Ed., American Society for Microbiology, Ann Arbor, Mich., 1970, p. 173.

CHAPTER TWENTY–FOUR

Drugs for Neoplastic Diseases

JOHN A. MONTGOMERY
THOMAS P. JOHNSTON
and
Y. FULMER SHEALY

Kettering-Meyer Laboratory
Southern Research Institute
Birmingham, Alabama 35205, USA

CONTENTS

1 INTRODUCTION

Cancer is not one disease, but a group of diseases affecting different organs and systems of the body. Although there are a number of known causes of cancer, such as exposure to carcinogenic hydrocarbons or to excessive radiation, cellular mutation of unknown origin may be important in many cases. The numerous different forms of cancer possess certain common features: it is a disease typified by abnormal and uncontrolled cell division, frequently at a rate greater than that of most normal body cells. Neither the etiology of cancer nor the manner in which it causes death (in the vast majority of cases) is understood, despite the effort that has been devoted over the years to studies of these phenomena. The incidence of and mortality from cancer have risen steadily ever since reliable statistics on the subject have been available. Although it is obviously preferable to prevent rather than cure any disease, current efforts to provide preventive measures that undoubtedly will be rewarding in the long run seem unlikely to reduce the incidence of human cancer significantly in the foreseeable future, particularly since the median age of the human population continues to increase. It appears that more effective methods of treatment are unlikely to result from further improvements in surgery or radiotherapy alone. At the same time, chemotherapy is today providing increasing cure rates in 10–15 forms of human cancer (1–3); and recent developments, particularly in surgical adjuvant therapy in the management of breast cancer and osteogenic sarcoma, indicate that new neoplastic diseases will be added to the list. The events leading to the current successes in chemotherapy have resulted from the development of a greater variety of agents, including superior agents, and from the improved use of both old and new agents, thanks to our better understanding of the effects of drugs on cells, both normal and cancerous. Although we can expect continued improvements in the use of available agents (such as earlier treatment of refractory tumors that today are treated only terminally, in desperation, when failure is thus assured), it is clear that there are limits to this approach. For the immediate future, the use of combination chemotherapy and combined modalities—surgical adjuvant therapy, radiation, and chemotherapy—seems sure to provide better responses and response rates; but again there are limits to reasonable expectations. It is undeniable that more effective agents are needed for continued advances.

Much discussion of the rational design of drugs has taken place over the past few years, and a six-volume treatise on the subject has appeared (4). Despite the enormous body of written material contained in that treatise and in many other places, the question "Is there such a thing as rational drug design?" is quite appropriate, even if attempts to answer it have been less than satisfactory. The rational design of an agent with specific activity toward a selected target requires that this target be so precisely defined that it can be hit selectively in the presence of other targets to which it is identical or similar in almost all respects (5). The target of anticancer drugs is obviously the cancer cell, but there is little information on unique characteristics of cancer cells that might be exploitable in the pursuit of new agents. Despite this lack of any well-defined metabolic basis for design, however, useful new agents are being produced, most of them related in some way to active agents that have been conceived or discovered empirically. This situation has led some to label the discovery of new anticancer drugs as "serendipity"; others, with perhaps more wisdom and understanding, refer to the findings as resulting from "enlightened empiricism". Certainly no case comes to mind in which an investigator set as his goal the development of an anticancer agent by, for example, the inhibition of a certain enzyme, and the inhibition of that enzyme did, in fact, result in useful anticancer activity. Attempts to correlate physicochemical parameters (4) of anticancer agents to activity have, as yet, failed to benefit the frustrated medicinal chemist in his prospective search for better agents.

About the best the chemist can do, even today, is search blindly through random synthetics, antibiotic beers, and plant and animal extracts—or examine past successes for clues to the future. Although the mechanism by which even such early drugs as nitrogen mustard and methotrexate selectively kill cancer cells has not been clearly established, and although results of studies of some of the new agents are still ambiguous, the overwhelming weight of evidence points to interference with the synthesis or function of nucleic acids, or with the mitotic process itself, as the ultimate mechanism by which most, if not all, agents kill cells. Indeed, such a statement may be almost self-evident, since cancer is clearly a disease caused by uncontrolled proliferation of cells that have mutated from normal body cells.

At this point, most of our progress in cancer chemotherapy has been in the treatment of leukemias and lymphomas and certain other virulent diseases like choriocarcinoma in women, because these forms of cancer tend to be more sensitive to drugs (1–3). The most logical explanation for this greater sensitivity is that in such cases most of the cells in the cancer population are in cycle—i.e., continuously undergoing mitosis—and cells in cycle are more sensitive to all types of anticancer agents than are resting cells. On the other hand, most of the cells of the slower growing solid tumors that resist therapy are in the so-called G_0 or resting state and are less sensitive to all agents (6). Generally speaking, however, chemically reactive compounds such as the nitrogen mustards, and DNA complexors such as actinomycin D and adriamycin, are much more effective against resting cells than are the antimetabolites, which inhibit specific enzymatic transformations or are incorporated into macromolecules (7). Nevertheless, antimetabolites do have activity against solid tumors, particularly when used in conjunction with agents of other types (8).

In the sections that follow, we discuss the status of the various classes of therapeutic agents, with particular emphasis on the agents that are in clinical use today. Wherever possible, the anticancer activity of these agents is related to their chemical structure, and the mechanisms underlying their biologic activity are discussed. Much of the material presented is based on experimental animal therapy, for it is only in animals that we have meaningful comparative data on many agents and their congeners. One should be aware, however, of the difficulties involved in relating animal and clinical data. Among the reasons for this difficulty are the scarcity of quantitative clinical data already mentioned and the variation in individual response, but there are other problems also. For example, drug metabolism and, consequently, toxicity and effectiveness may vary widely from species to species. Toxicity that is not important, or not even detected, in rodent test systems may be so serious in man that the drug cannot be used effectively clinically. Despite these problems, most if not all of the drugs used clinically today, with the exception of the hormones, were introduced to the clinic because of demonstrated activity in some animal tumor system. Therefore, relating drugs through their activity against animal tumors seems to be a valid and, in fact, a necessary approach.

An attempt has been made to consider topics of major interest to the medicinal chemist; no attempt has been made at comprehensive coverage of the literature. Review articles by the authors (5, 9, 10) and others (1–3, 11–13) have been relied on heavily and are recommended to the reader interested in more detailed accounts of the various topics discussed herein. Particularly valuable and timely are the reviews contained in *Cancer Medicine* (2) and Parts 1 and 2 of *Antineoplastic and Immunosuppressive Agents* (3) to be found in the *Handbook of Experimental Pharmacology.*

2 CHEMOTHERAPEUTIC AGENTS

2.1 Antimetabolites

An antimetabolite interferes with the formation or utilization of a normal cellular metabolite. This interference may result from the inhibition of an enzyme or enzymes (see Chapter 9) or from incorporation, as a fradulent building unit, into macromolecules such as proteins or nucleic acids.

Most antimetabolites have resulted from one or in some cases two bioisosteric or other *small* changes in the structure of a metabolite (e.g., F for H, S or CH_2 for O, NH_2 for OH, S for —CH=CH—), although the result of such a change cannot be predicted accurately. Furthermore, it is now recognized that the position of change is as important as the *size* or *nature* of the change. Thus a large change on a metabolite's back side, which does not fit the surface of the enzyme closely, may result in an inhibitor, which in turn may exhibit antimetabolite properties. A compound may be an excellent enzyme inhibitor *in vitro*, however, and not possess significant antimetabolite activity *in vivo*, since many additional factors come into play in *in vivo* systems.

An antimetabolite that functions as an enzyme inhibitor may do so by combining with the enzyme active site in the position normally occupied by the substrate or by the cofactor, if the enzyme utilizes one. It may, if it resembles the end product of a biosynthetic pathway under feedback control, inhibit the enzyme allosterically—that is, at a site apart from the active site. In either case the antimetabolite must be structured to fit and bind to the enzyme in the manner of the normal metabolite, otherwise it will not inhibit or it will lack specificity for the enzyme in question. In some cases the antimetabolite must be metabolized to the active inhibitor, and thus must serve as a substrate for the appropriate enzymes. Metabolism is, of course, also necessary for incorporation into macromolecules.

Many metabolites are substrates or cofactors for more than one enzyme, and a structurally related antimetabolite may be an inhibitor of any or all of these enzymes (6-mercaptopurine and its metabolites, e.g., are known to interact with more than 20 enzymes). In addition, certain antimetabolites also act as feedback inhibitors and others are also incorporated into macromolecules. Because of this multiplicity of function, the antimetabolites discussed in this chapter are classified according to the metabolites with whose metabolism they interfere rather than according to the enzyme or enzymes whose catalytic action they block.

Essentially all known antimetabolite types have been investigated for anticancer activity, and many have been found to have some effect on neoplasms. Unfortunately the observed anticancer effects are quite often accompanied by prohibitive host toxicity. The greatest success in the development of antimetabolites with useful anticancer activity has occurred with analogs of the metabolites involved in the biosynthesis of nucleic acids and the purine- and pyrimidine-containing cofactors. That this should be the case is not surprising, since cancer is a disease of abnormal cellular metabolism and mitosis, and mitosis is controlled by the nucleic acids. Specific interference with the *de novo* nucleic acid pathways in cancer cells and not in normal cells is probably impossible, however, since the same biosynthetic pathways are used by both types of cell. In fact, only one qualitative anabolic difference, such as those that exist between mammalian and bacterial cells, has been found to exist between normal and neoplastic cells—the L-asparagine requirement of some neoplasms. Nevertheless, compounds such as 6-mercaptopurine, 5-fluorouracil, and methotrexate are remarkably effective, albeit in many cases temporarily, against some human cancers.

Where appropriate in the discussions that follow, emphasis is placed on the biochemical interactions that in our opinion are primarily responsible for the cytotoxicity of the various antimetabolites. Possible reasons for the cytotoxic specificity exhibited by these agents are also discussed.

Figures 24.1 and 24.2 depict the biosynthetic pathways to purine and pyrimidine nucleotides and purine- and pyrimidine-containing cofactors. The enzymic conversions known to be inhibited by the various clinically used antimetabolites are marked on these charts. The details of these enzyme inhibitions and the anticancer activity of the antimetabolites are discussed in the following sections.

2.1.1 GLUTAMINE ANTAGONISTS. Azaserine (*O*-diazoacetyl-L-serine, 24.**34**) (14) and DON (6-diazo-5-oxo-L-norleucine, 24.**35**) (15), two carcinolytic compounds first isolated from culture broths of *Streptomyces* and later synthesized (16, 17), derive their biologic activity from interference with the various metabolic processes in which glutamine is involved as a cofactor. They inhibit the conversion of 5-phosphoribosylpyrophosphate (24.**19**) to 5-phosphoribosylamine (24.**20**) (18, 19), the formation of guanylic acid (24, **30**) from xanthylic acid (24.**31**) (20), the synthesis of cytidine triphosphate (24.**12**) from uridine triphosphate (24.**9**) (21), the amination of nicotinic acid–adenine dinucleotide to NAD (22, 23), and the formation of *p*-aminobenzoic acid (24) and anthranilic acid (25) from shikimic acid-5-phosphate. The reaction most sensitive to both azaserine and DON, however, is the conversion of formylglycinamide ribonucleotide (24.**22**) to formylglycinamidine ribonucleotide (24.**26**) (18, 19, 26). Azaserine combines with the enzyme that catalyzes this reaction (phosphoribosylformylglycinamidine synthetase) in a reversibly competitive manner initially. This reversible attachment through the binding points normally utilized by the cofactor glutamine allows the diazomethyl group of azaserine to be positioned for a finite length of time near the sulfhydryl group of a cysteine residue in the active site of the enzyme. Under these conditions the alkylation of the sulfhydryl group by the diazomethyl group occurs, and the inhibitor becomes irreversibly bound to the enzyme by a covalent bond (27–29). The alkylation is specific for this enzyme and does not occur with proteins in general. DON is a more potent inhibitor than azaserine (27, 30, 31), presumably because it is a better reversible inhibitor, since it resembles the normal cofactor L-glutamine more closely than does azaserine. Compounds less closely related to L-glutamine, such as alanylserine diazoacetic ester (24.**36**) and 5-diazo-4-oxonorvaline (24.**37**) are much less effective inhibitors of phosphoribosylformylglycinamidine synthetase (32), since the diazomethyl group of these compounds is not properly positioned for accelerated reaction with the enzyme sulfhydryl group.

Since Skipper et al. (33) originally observed that azaserine inhibited formate incorporation into the tissues of tumor-bearing mice and Bennett et al. (34) demonstrated its inhibition of *de novo* purine

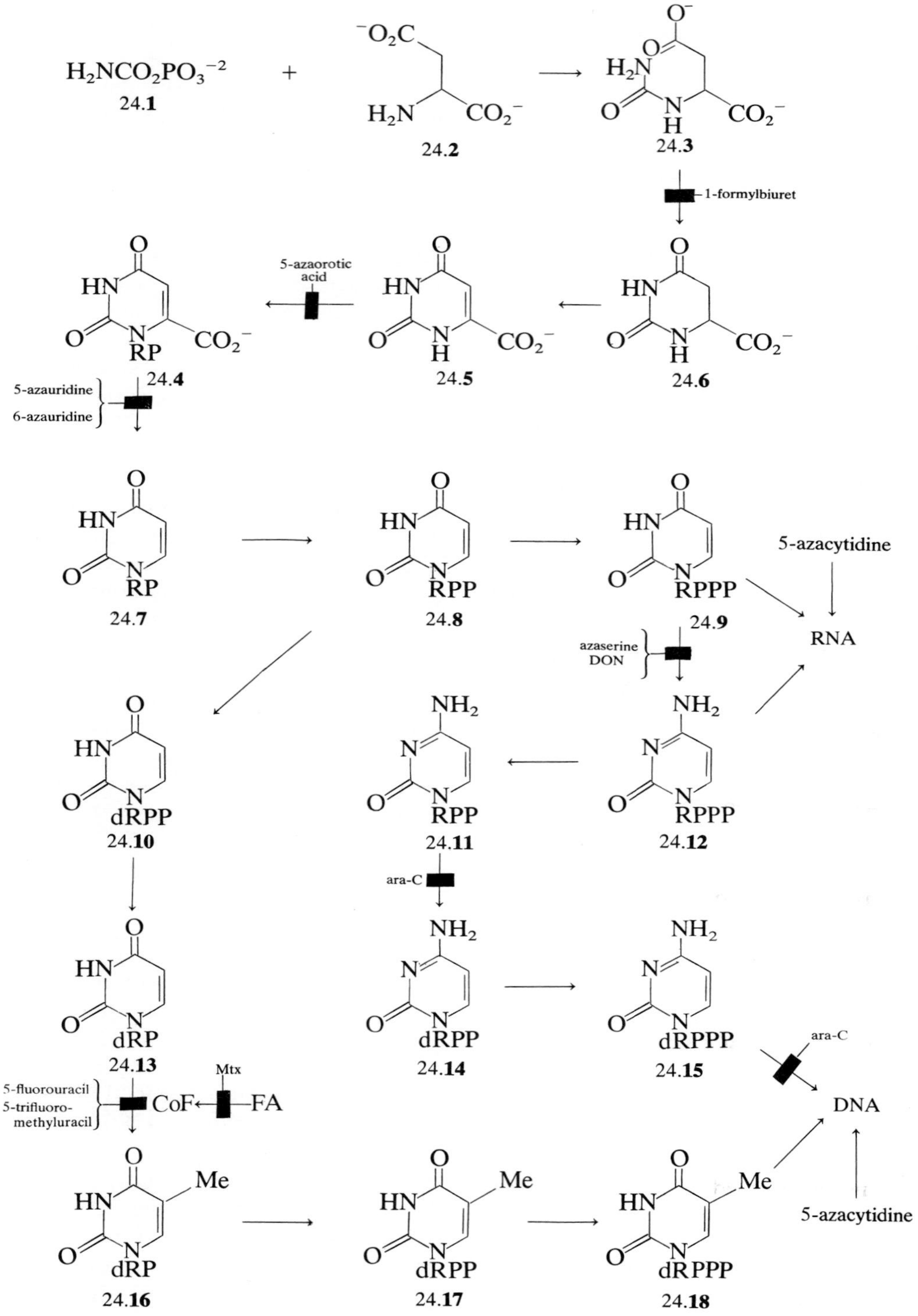

$H_2NCO_2PO_3^{-2}$ 24.**1** + 24.**2** → 24.**3**

24.**3** → (1-formylbiuret) → 24.**6** → 24.**5** → (5-azaorotic acid) → 24.**4**

24.**4** → (5-azauridine, 6-azauridine) → 24.**7** → 24.**8** → 24.**9** → RNA

24.**9** → (azaserine, DON) → 24.**12** → RNA

5-azacytidine → RNA

24.**12** → 24.**11** → (ara-C) → 24.**14** → 24.**15** → (ara-C) → DNA

24.**8** → 24.**10** → 24.**13** → (5-fluorouracil, 5-trifluoro-methyluracil; CoF ← Mtx — FA) → 24.**16** → 24.**17** → 24.**18** → DNA

5-azacytidine → DNA

R = β-D-ribofuranose

dR = 2′-deoxy-β-D-ribofuranose

P = phosphate

Fig. 24.1 Biosynthetic pathway to pyrimidine nucleotides and nucleic acids showing enzymatic blockades.

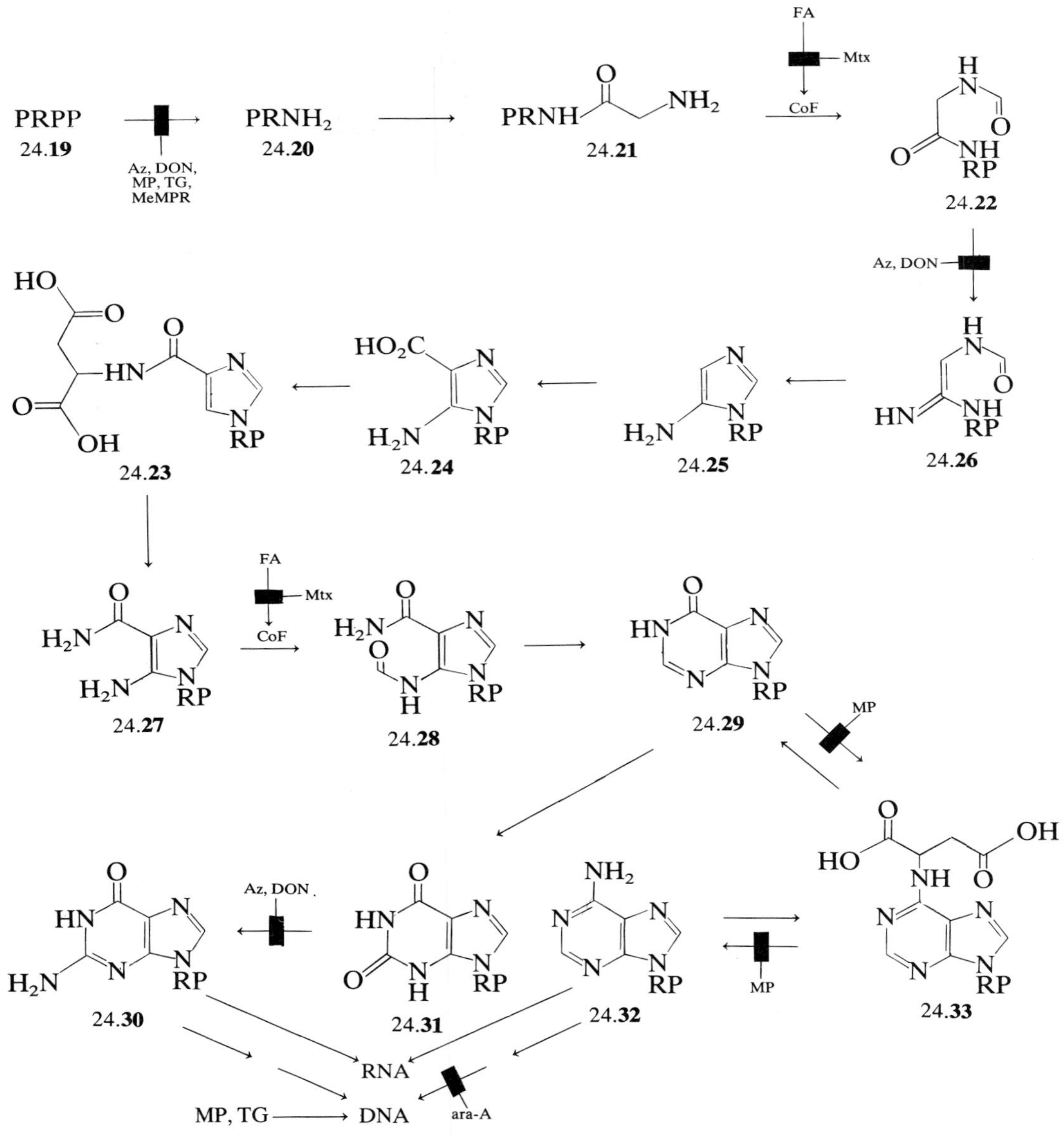

R = β-D-ribofuranose
P = phosphate

Fig. 24.2 Biosynthetic pathway to purine nucleotides and nucleic acids showing enzymatic blockades.

nucleotide synthesis at a stage prior to the formation of 5-aminoimidazole-4-carboxamide ribonucleotide (24.**21**), both *in vitro* and *in vivo*, it appears that the anticancer activity (35) of azaserine and DON is due primarily to the enzymic block described above. [In contrast, the *de novo* purine nucleotide pathway is unimportant to *Trypanosoma equiperdum*; thus inhibition of this organism by azaserine seems to

$$\underset{\displaystyle NH_2}{HO_2C\overset{|}{C}HCH_2XCOCHN_2}$$

24.**34** X = O
24.**35** X = CH_2

$$HO_2CCHCH_2O_2CCHN_2$$
$$MeCHCONH$$
$$NH_2$$

24.**36**

$$\underset{\displaystyle NH_2}{HO_2C\overset{|}{C}HCH_2COCHN_2}$$

24.**37**

be due to interference with pyrimidine biosynthesis—the conversion of uridine triphosphate to cytidine triphosphate (36).]

A secondary effect of azaserine resulting from depletion of the adenine nucleotide pool by the *de novo* purine biosynthetic block has been observed—the depression of thymidine kinase and thymidine monophosphate kinase levels in sarcoma 180 cells. Depression of these enzymes, particularly the latter, could contribute to the inhibition of cell growth (37).

Azaserine, like DON, is actively concentrated in tumor cells by the amino acid transport mechanism, for which competition by glycine, glutamine, and tryptophan was noted (38, 39).

Azaserine disappears from the blood of mice much more rapidly than from the blood of man (40) because of enzymic destruction by tissues such as kidney, spleen, and particularly liver (41). The compound was degraded stoichiometrically to pyruvic acid and ammonia, presumably by α,β-elimination of ammonia and diazoacetate (42). DON is not attacked, but *O*-acetyl-L-serine (24.**38**) is and can protect azaserine from destruction, resulting in an increase,

$$\underset{\displaystyle NH_2}{HO_2C\overset{|}{C}HCH_2O_2CMe}$$

24.**38**

on a weight basis, of the effectiveness of the drug (43).

Duazomycin A has been identified as the *N*-acetyl derivative of DON (44), and alazopeptin is thought to contain 1 mole of alanine linked through peptide bonds to 2 moles of DON or a closely related diazo amino acid (45). It remains to be established whether these compounds are active *per se* or by *in vivo* conversion to DON, although it is known that duazomycin A is deacetylated by mouse kidney (46).

Azaserine and DON have shown activity against sarcoma 180 (47) and other mouse tumors (48) and leukemias (49), but many animal neoplasms are inhibited only at the expense of considerable toxicity. Clinic trials have shown that these drugs are ineffective or have slight transitory effectiveness against a variety of human cancers at tolerated doses (35, 50, 51), although excellent remissions of choriocarcinoma with DON have been reported (52).

2.1.2 FOLIC ACID ANTAGONISTS. Folic acid (*N*-[*p*-[[(2-amino-4-hydroxy-6-pteridinyl)-methyl]amino]benzoyl]-L-glutamic acid) (24.**39**) must be reduced to *l*,L-tetrahydrofolic acid (24.**44**) (53) before it can serve as a coenzyme. The reduction takes place stepwise by way of dihydrofolic acid (24.**40**, 24.**41**), and both steps are generally thought to be carried out by the same enzyme (54), called both folic reductase and dihydrofolic reductase; in one instance, however, separation of the two enzymic activities has been reported (55). That the reduction of dihydrofolate is much more rapid than is the reduction of folate (56) may be related to the critical nature of the former transformation to the participation of N^5,N^{10}-methylenetetrahydrofolate (24.**45**) as the cofactor for thymidylate synthetase (*vide infra*). Tetrahydrofolic acid (24.**44**) is then formylated and converted to its other cofactor forms (see Fig. 24.3).

The folic acid coenzymes participate at three places in the nucleic acid biosynthetic

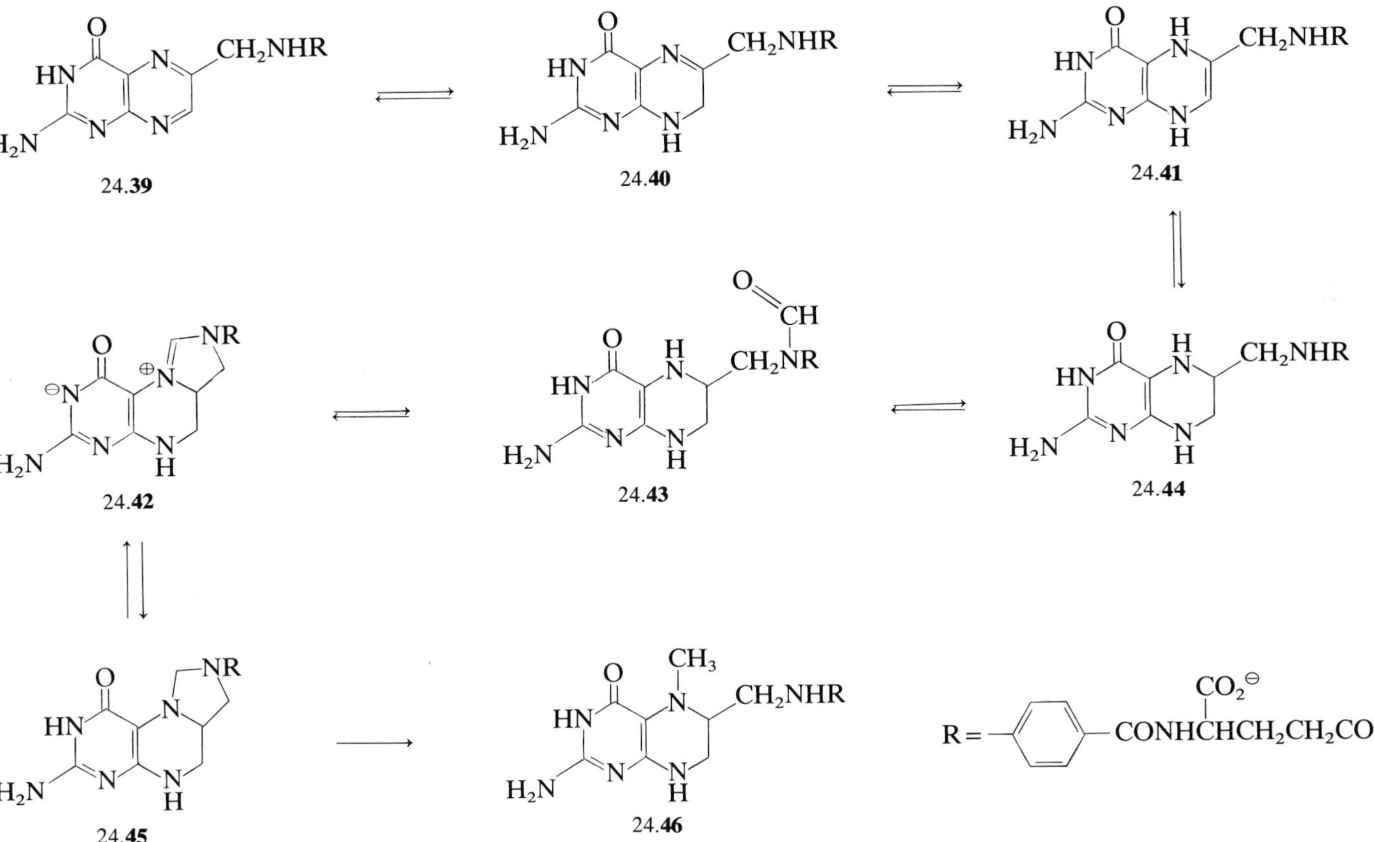

Fig. 24.3 The interconversion of the cofactor forms of folic acid.

pathway (see Fig. 24.1 and 24.2). N^5,N^{10}-Methenyltetrahydrofolic acid (24.**42**) supplies the formyl group for the conversion of glycinamide ribonucleotide (24.**21**) to formylglycinamide ribonucleotide (24.**22**); N^{10}-formyltetrahydrofolic acid (24.**43**) provides a formyl group to 5-aminoimidazole-4-carboxamide ribonucleotide (24.**27**); finally, N^5,N^{10}-methylenetetrahydrofolic acid (24.**45**) donates the methyl group necessary for the conversion of 2′-deoxyuridylic acid (24.**13**) to thymidylic acid (24.**16**) (57–60). There is evidence that the last mentioned conversion is the one most sensitive to the inhibitory action of folic acid antagonists (59), very likely because in this reaction the tetrahydrofolic acid (24.**45**) is oxidized to dihydrofolic acid (24.**40**), which must be reduced to tetrahydrofolic acid (24.**44**) again to regain its cofactor activity (61–64). (In the other one-carbon transfers, oxidation of the cofactor does not occur.) The idea has been advanced that inhibition of thymidylate synthesis, therefore DNA synthesis, is important to action not only of the antifolates but other anticancer agents as well (65). There are indications, however, that the action of folic acid antagonists is directed chiefly against rapidly proliferating tissues, not specifically against neoplasms (66, 67).

A number of alterations were made in the structure of folic acid before the synthesis of the 4-amino-4-deoxy derivatives aminopterin, *N*-[*p*-[[2,4-diamino-6-pteridinyl)methyl]amino]benzoyl]-L-glutamic acid (24.**47**), and its N^{10}-methyl derivative, methotrexate (Mtx, amethopterin, 24.**48**) (68), two potent antifolates with a high degree of anticancer activity.

An investigation into the action of aminopterin showed that it had a strong affinity for the enzyme system postulated to form citrovorum factor (69). Several studies with purified dihydrofolic reductase have since shown that the pH-dependent binding of aminopterin and methotrexate is stoichiometric with excess enzyme, but reversible with equivalent or excess amounts of the inhibitors (70–74). Thus although the binding is in fact reversible and dependent on the conditions under which it is measured, it is extremely tight and so has been termed "pseudoirreversible" (71).

Two hypotheses have been put forth to explain why these 4-amino analogs of folic acid bind more tightly to dihydrofolic reductase than folic acid itself. Zakrzewski has proposed that four hydrogen bonds are formed between the enzyme and the 2,4-diaminopyrimidine portion of the inhibitors. He further concluded from thermodynamic studies that folic acid, which normally exists in the keto form, must tautomerize to the enol form to bind to the enzyme, and this event is associated with an increase in entropy (75, 76). [Matthews and Huennekens proposed that aminopterin was more tightly bound to the enzyme because of an additional hydrogen bond afforded by its 4-amino group (77).] According to Baker, this tight binding is a result of the increased basicity of aminopterin or methotrexate (78), which results in their protonation (at physiological pH); then the protonated inhibitor binds to

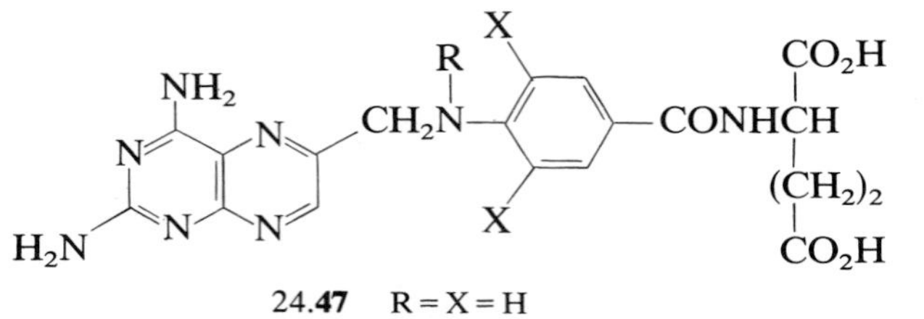

24.**47** R = X = H
24.**48** R = Me, X = H
24.**49** R = Me, X = Cl

anionic groups in the active site of the enzyme (79). In any event, alkyl groups on the 2- and 4-amino groups of aminopterin destroy biologic activity (80, 81), undoubtedly because they interfere with binding to dihydrofolic reductase.

Whatever the true nature of the binding is, it seems certain that the biologic activity of these compounds is due principally to their ability to prevent cells from reducing folic and dihydrofolic acid to tetrahydrofolic acid, although they may also interfere with one-carbon transfers (69, 82, 83).

A number of aminopterin and methotrexate derivatives halogenated in the benzene ring have been prepared (84–86), and a few of these are significantly less toxic and more effective than the parent compounds against leukemia L1210 (87), although this therapeutic advantage has not been realized clinically (88). The most active of these compounds, 3′,5′-dichloromethotrexate (24.**49**), is readily metabolized by man and some rodents to 3′,5′-dichloro-7-hydroxymethotrexate (24.**50**) (89), and the enzyme responsible for this oxidation is a hepatic aldehyde oxidase. The ease of this metabolism, relative to methotrexate, to an inactive compound probably explains the lower toxicity of 3′,5′-dichloromethotrexate, since it is equally effective in the inhibition of dihydrofolic reductase (71). The resistance of the rabbit to methotrexate has now been explained by the ability of its liver aldehyde oxidase to inactivate the drug; and evidence has been presented that the metabolite is the 7-hydroxy derivative of methotrexate (24.**51**) (90), although the 4,7-dihydroxy structure has also been suggested (91). Mouse and rat liver oxidases are unable to catalyze the oxidation of aminopterin (92), which may explain the greater toxicity of this substance in many species, including man. On the other hand, guinea pig liver oxidase readily oxidizes aminopterin, a property which correlates well with the resistance of the guinea pig to aminopterin toxicity (92).

Recently the di- and triglutamates of 4-amino-4-deoxypteroic acid have been identified as metabolites of methotrexate in rats (93, 94). Methotrexate polyglutamates comprised 47 ± 20% of the Mtx in L1210 cells in leukemic mice treated with the drug (94). The significance of this metabolism is not known, but it has been established that 4-amino-4-deoxypteroyl diglutamate is as effective an inhibitor of dihydrofolic reductase as Mtx itself. It is also known that the diglutamate is as effective in the treatment of leukemia L1210 as Mtx (95), although this could be explained by *in vivo* cleavage back to Mtx.

Other diaminoheterocycles such as diaminopteridines (76, 96), diaminopyridopyrimidines (97), diaminoquinazolines (97), diamino-8-azapurines (98), diaminopyrimidines (99–101), and diaminodihydrotriazines (102, 103) all have a structural feature in common with aminopterin and methotrexate and inhibit dihydrofolic reductase to significant but varying degrees. Some of these small molecule inhibitors are

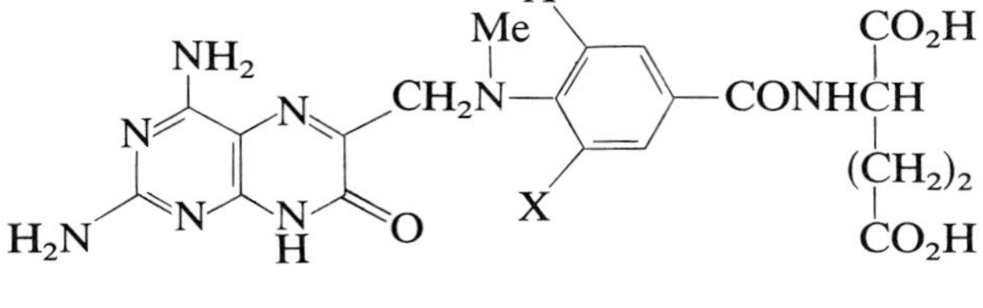

24.**50** X = Cl
24.**51** X = H

useful in the chemotherapy of a variety of microbial infections, but have not yet found a place in the treatment of cancer. Nevertheless, recent developments are encouraging: a strain of Walker carcinosarcoma 256 that is naturally resistant to aminopterin and methotrexate, apparently because of failure of this cell line to take up enough of these drugs by active transport (104, 105), responds to certain diaminopyrimidines, which can enter cells by passive diffusion (106). The implications of this observation are great, since in 11 clinical cases of leukemia the susceptibility of the leukemia to methotrexate was related to the relative ability of the leukemic cells to take up tritiated methotrexate—the unresponsive cases showed almost no uptake of drug (107, 108). Such cases might well respond to diaminopyrimidines, particularly with simultaneous administration of citrovorum factor to protect normal cells having a good active transport mechanism (109). In this connection, it has been demonstrated that citrovorum factor (CF) administered on the proper schedule enhances the effectiveness of methotrexate against leukemia L1210 (110, 111) and, more recently, that CF improves the therapeutic index of 2,4-diamino-5-(3,4-dichlorophenyl)-6-methylpyrimidine (DDMP) in the treatment of an ascitic form of sarcoma 180 in mice (112).

Intensive therapy with methotrexate of choriocarcinoma in women has resulted in an apparent cure rate of 70% or greater, the most successful chemotherapeutic treatment of a human cancer thus far reported (113, 114). Of the other diseases reported to respond to this antifolate, acute childhood leukemia is probably the most sensitive, remissions being obtained in 30–50% of the cases treated (115). Aminopterin was used in much of the early clinical work with antifolates (116), but it has largely been displaced by methotrexate because the latter appears to be somewhat less toxic at effective dose levels (115). Clinical comparisons between methotrexate and 3′,5′-dichloromethotrexate have shown that the latter is not significantly better (88, 117, 118).

2.1.3 PYRIMIDINE ANTAGONISTS

2.1.3.1 Azapyrimidines. 5-Azauracil (1,3,5-triazine-2,4(1*H*, 3*H*)dione, 24.**54**) and 5-azaorotic acid (4,6-dioxy-1,2,3,4-tetrahydro-1,3,5-triazine-2-carboxylic acid, 24.**55**) have shown the ability to inhibit adenocarcinoma 755 (119), but not leukemia L1210 (120). They both are competitive inhibitors of orotidylate pyrophosphorylase, which converts orotic acid (24.**5**) to orotidylic acid (24.**4**), although azaorotate (24.**55**) is unable to enter many cells because it exists as an anion at physiological pH (121). In addition to being metabolized by *E. coli* and cell-free extracts therefrom to 5-azauridine (24.**61**) and 5-azauridylic acid (24.**59**), 5-azauracil (24.**54**) also decomposes to 1-formylbiuret (24.**53**) and other products (Fig. 24.4) (122–124). 1-Formylbiuret inhibits the cyclization of ureidosuccinic acid (24.**3**) to dihydroorotic acid (24.**6**) catalyzed by dihydroorotase and has shown bactericidal action (125). It has been suggested that both 1-formylbiuret and 5-azauridylic acid, after *in situ* formation, may contribute to the anticancer activity of 5-azauracil (126).

The most active of these azapyrimidines, 5-azacytidine (2-amino-1-β-D-ribofuranosyl-1,3,5-triazin-4-one, 24.**62**) (127), was found to be quite effective against leukemia in AKR mice (128), producing some cures (129). Ehrlich ascites cells phosphorylate 5-azacytidine to the mono-, di-, and triphosphate levels (24.**64a**–24.**66a**) and incorporate it *in vivo* into RNA (130). Since no significant interference with *de novo* pyrimidine biosynthesis has been observed with 5-azacytidine, this incorporation, together with the pronounced inhibition of RNA synthesis in isolated nuclei of calf thymus (131), indicates that its biological effects can be explained on the basis of interference with higher phases of nucleic

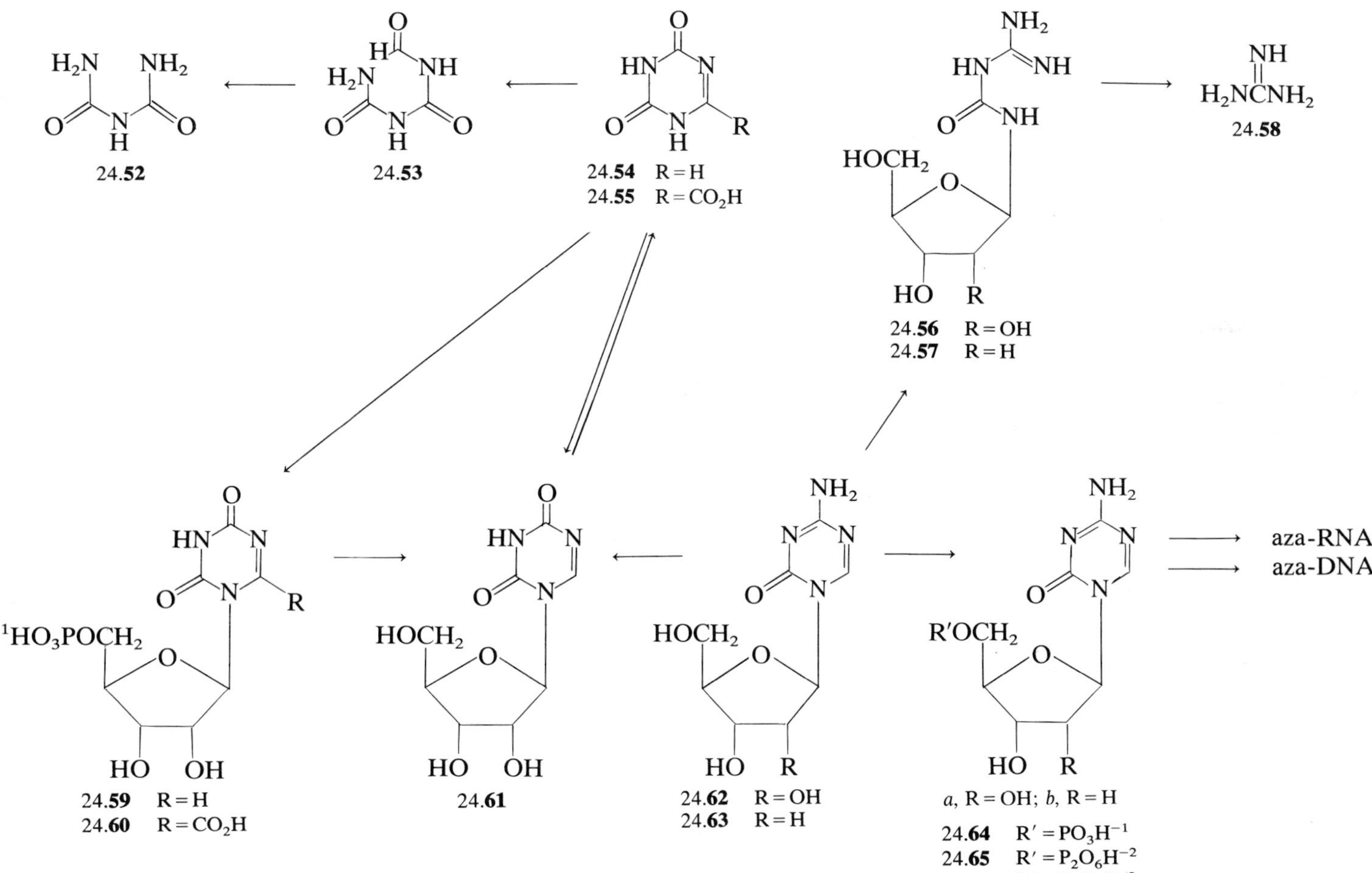

Fig. 24.4 Metabolism and decomposition of 5-azauracil (24.**54**) and its nucleosides.

acid synthesis. It has also been observed that 5-azacytidine inhibits protein synthesis by incorporation into soluble RNA, which results in a strikingly decreased acceptor activity for all amino acids except leucine (132), as well as by the inhibition of the synthesis of messenger RNA (131). The chemical instability of 5-azacytidine (133) and its observed incorporation into DNA of *E. coli* by way of 24.**65b**–24.**66b** (134) have led to the proposition that its biologic and mutagenic activity results from its decomposition after incorporation into the polynucleotide.

5-Azacytidine has shown considerable activity in the treatment of human leukemias, but its activity against solid tumors has been disappointing in the limited studies that have been carried out (11).

A number of the isomeric 1,2,4-triazines have been prepared and evaluated as anticancer agents (135–139), but despite the considerable effort devoted to these compounds, particularly 6-azauridine and its derivatives, they have not proven to have any clinical utility.

2.1.3.2 Fluoropyrimidines. Most of the possible halogenated pyrimidines have been prepared, but only the fluorinated pyrimidines and their nucleosides—which are, for the most part, readily metabolized by enzymes that normally metabolize uracil, cytosine, and their nucleosides—have significant anticancer activity. Since this subject has been reviewed in depth by Heidelberger (140, 141) recently, it is discussed only briefly here. Of these compounds, the most active are 5-fluorouracil (FU, 24.**71**) and its 2′-deoxyribonucleoside (FUdR, 24.**73**), both of which are metabolized to 5-fluoro-2′-deoxyuridylic acid (FUdRP, 24.**76**) (Fig. 24.5), a potent competitive inhibitor of thymidylate synthetase (140, 141), the enzyme that normally converts 2′-deoxyuridylic acid (24.**13**) to thymidylic acid (24.**16**) for DNA synthesis.

Although FU and its anabolites are known to cause a large number of other biological effects (140, 141), its anticancer activity is probably due to this enzymatic blockade, causing "thymineless death" of neoplastic cells. A significant correlation between the extent of conversion of FU to FUdRP in cancer cells *in vitro* and their response *in vivo* has been noted (142). Its effect on pyrimidine nucleotide biosynthesis is, then, largely the same as that of methotrexate. 5-Chloro-2′-deoxyuridine and 5-bromo-2′-deoxyuridine (after conversion to the nucleotides) are less effective inhibitors, whereas 5-iodo-2′-deoxyuridine is inactive (143). The remarkably effective inhibition of this enzyme by the fluoro compound results from the unique nature of the fluorine atom, which has a van der Waals radius of 1.35 Å, compared to hydrogen, which has a radius of 1.2 Å. Also, the introduction into the molecule of fluorine, the most electronegative element, has a great effect on the electron distribution in the molecule. Thus the acidic strength of FU is 30 times that of uracil. Thus FUdRP should fit quite well the active site of an enzyme that normally accepts 2′-deoxyuridylic acid as a substrate, but at the same time its affinity for the active site should be quite different from that of 2′-deoxyuridylic acid, as in fact it is. Recent evidence indicates that FUdRP combines covalently with enzyme through a sulfide linkage, indicating that a sulfhydryl group is the nucleophilic species that initiates the enzymic reaction (144). In contrast, the other halogens are much larger than fluorine and less electronegative; consequently analogs containing them might be expected to behave quite differently.

5-Fluorouridine (FUR, 24.**74**), an anabolic product of FU (see Fig. 24.5), is relatively ineffective against tumors because of its greater toxicity, perhaps resulting from the inability of normal cells to catabolize it as effectively as they do FU. [The consequences of the incorporation of FUR into ribosomal and transfer RNA are

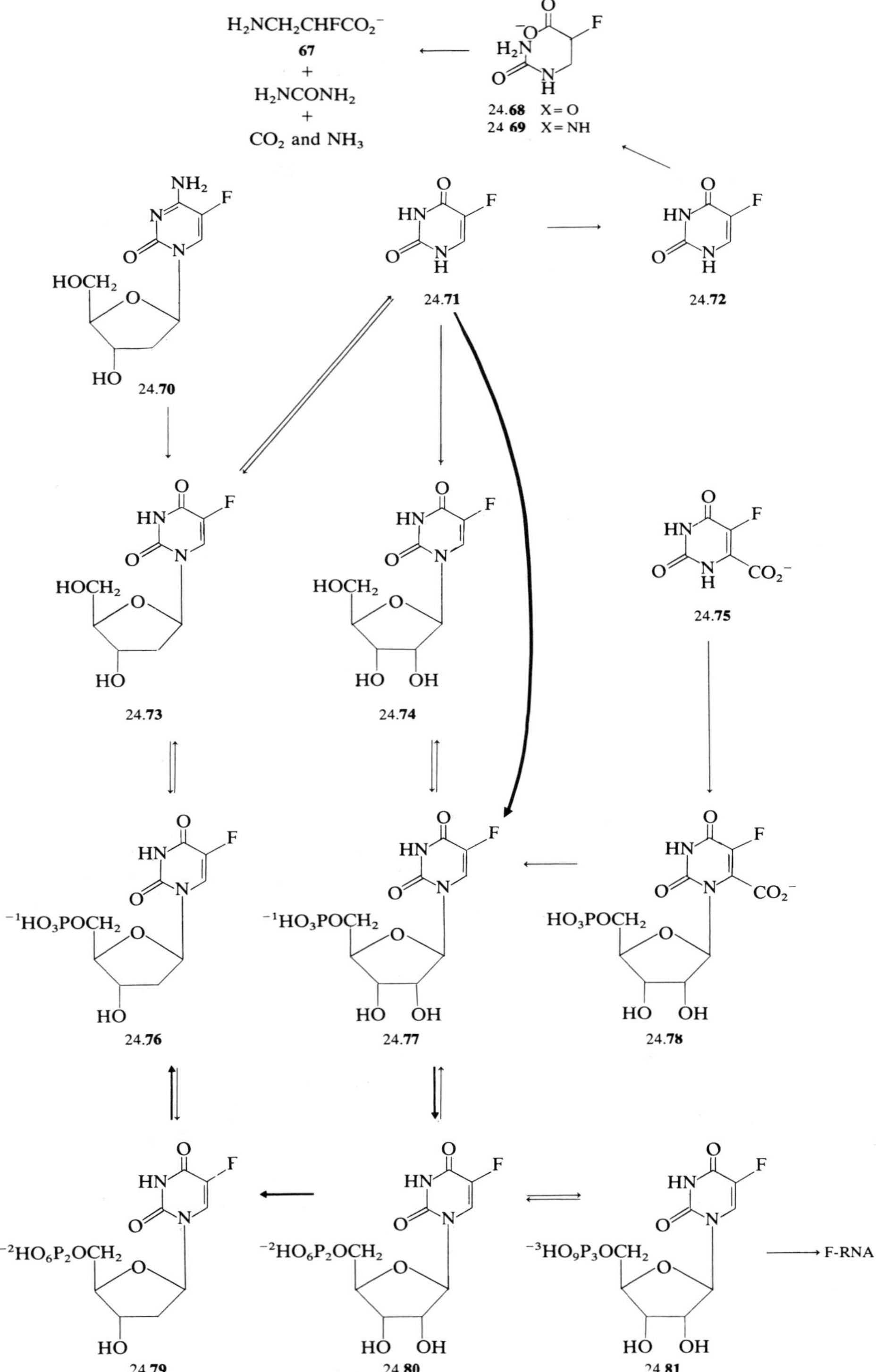

Fig. 24.5 Metabolism of FU (24.**71**) and FUdRP (24.**73**); heavy arrows indicate probable principal pathway.

not known at this time (145).] 5-Fluorocytosine is inactive in many systems (146–148), apparently because of lack of cytidine phosphorylase activity (149), whereas 5-fluoro-2′-deoxycytidine (24.**70**), 5-fluorocytidine, and 5-fluoroorotic acid (24.**75**) all probably owe their anticancer activity to their *in vivo* conversion to FUdRP (150, 151) (see Fig. 24.5) (this statement does not imply that all the biologic activity of these compounds is explainable on this basis). 1-(2-Deoxy-β-D-lyxofuranosyl)-5-fluorouracil (152) and 2′-deoxy-2′,5-difluorouridine (153) are inactive, whereas 1-β-D-arabinofuranosyl-5-fluorouracil (154) is one-fourth as potent as FUdR. These results may be related to the ability of these compounds to serve as substrates for 2′-deoxyuridine kinase. In contrast, 1-β-D-arabinofuranosyl-5-fluorocytosine is highly active against mouse leukemias (155), but since its activity is reversed by 2′-deoxycytidine and not by thymidine, it is probably interfering with the reduction of cytidine diphosphate (24.**11**) to 2′-deoxycytidine diphosphate (24.**14**) (156) (*vide infra*), not thymidylate synthesis. This may mean that the fluorocytosine arabinonucleoside is a substrate for a kinase, whereas the fluorouracil arabinonucleoside is not. 2′,3′-Dihydro-5-fluoro-2′-deoxyuridine is active against sarcoma 180, leukemia L1210, and leukemia L5178BF (resistant to 5-fluoro-2′-deoxyuridine), but its mechanism of action has not been established (157).

The enzymes that metabolize uracil readily degrade 5-fluorouracil to the corresponding fluorine-containing degradation products (24.**67**–24.**69**, 24.**72**) (Fig. 24.5) (158, 159). That this process takes place in normal cells but not in cancer cells such as Ehrlich ascites and sarcoma 180 cells may be the key to the anticancer activity of this compound (140, 158, 159). On the other hand, although in general the anticancer activity of FUdR appears to be somewhat superior to that of FU, the full advantage of FUdR over FU is not always apparent because of its facile cleavage *in vivo* back to FU. Attempts to overcome this limitation by the use of 3′-mono- and 3′,5′-diacyl derivatives of FUdR (160), which might not undergo glycosyl cleavage but might be slowly converted back to FUdR by esterases, or by the use of inhibitors of the phosphorylase that cleaves FUdR (160), so far have not improved the carcinolytic effectiveness of this nucleoside. In a related approach, that of selective toxicity reversal, a combination of FUdR and 3′,5′-di-*O*-acetylthymidine was evaluated for enhanced anticancer activity (161, 162). If the esterase content of normal cells is significantly greater than that of cancer cells, this combination should show enhancement, for more thymidine would be released in normal cells to reverse the action of FUdR. If cancer cells contain more esterase activity than normal cells, 3′,5′-di-*O*-acyl-5-fluoro-2′-deoxyuridines should show better activity than FUdR. Selective inhibition of esterase activity in either type of cell could also be utilized to accentuate any selective cytotoxicity of these derivatives of FUdR. Studies based on these ideas have not led to a significant improvement in activity and, in fact, an increase in toxicity by combination of FUdR and esters of thymine was observed (161).

A number of 5,6-substituted 5-fluorodihydropyrimidines and their 2′-deoxyribonucleosides were prepared as latent forms (*vide supra*) of FU and FUdR. On a molar basis, the releasers of FU were less potent than FU, and the releasers of FUdR were more potent. Thus these compounds mimic, somewhat, the effects reported for slow infusion of FU and FUdR in humans (163). The most potent compound of this group, 5-bromo-6-methoxydihydro-5-fluoro-2′-deoxyuridine, was 2–4 times as effective as FUdR in the test system employed.

5-Fluoropyrimidin-4(1*H*)-one has demonstrated anticancer activity against experimental animal tumors (164, 165), and its conversion to FU in man has been demonstrated (166). It is a poor substrate for rabbit liver aldehyde oxidase, which converts the isomeric 5-fluoropyrimidin-2(1*H*)-one to FU, but it is oxidized by xanthine oxidase (166). Presumably the latter conversion is responsible for its activity.

A report on the biologic activity of bis(thioinosine 5′,5‴-phosphate (167) provoked an investigation of similar nucleotide derivatives of FU, but none of the compounds reported exhibited any activity above that which can be attributed to extracellular cleavage back to FU (168–170).

5 - Trifluoromethyl - 2′ - deoxyuridine (F_3TDR) (171), which has a better therapeutic index against adenocarcinoma 755 in mice than FUdR (172), is incorporated into DNA, but only to a very small extent *in vivo* (173), and it inhibits thymidylate synthetase (174). This inhibition is initially competitive, but after incubation it becomes noncompetitive and probably irreversible. It has been proposed that this compound, after its reversible attachment to the active site of the enzyme, may form a covalent bond to it (174).

Not only are the fluorinated pyrimidines active against a wide spectrum of animal tumors, but some of them, particularly 5-fluorouracil, are useful clinically, being employed primarily against solid tumors such as tumors of the gastrointestinal tract, breast, and female genital tract; oddly, they are not useful against leukemias and lymphomas (11).

2.1.3.3 1-β-D-Arabinofuranosylcytosine and Its Derivatives. 1-β-DArabinofuranosylcytosine (ara-C, 24.**83**: see Fig. 24.6) is active against both rodent (175–177) and human neoplasms (178). It inhibits the conversion of uridine to 2′-deoxycytidylic acid but not to cytidylic acid, and this effect can be reversed by 2′-deoxycytidine *in vitro* (179) and *in vivo* (180). These results have been interpreted to indicate that ara-C blocks the conversion of cytidine diphosphate (24.**11**) to 2′-deoxycytidine diphosphate (24.**14**) (179), although studies of the inhibitory activity of ara-C diphosphate (24.**85**) on this reduction by a purified reductase from mammalian tumor cells disclose that it is only slightly more effective than 2′-deoxycytidine triphosphate (181), whereas ara-C triphosphate (24.**86**) is an effective inhibitor of mammalian DNA polymerase

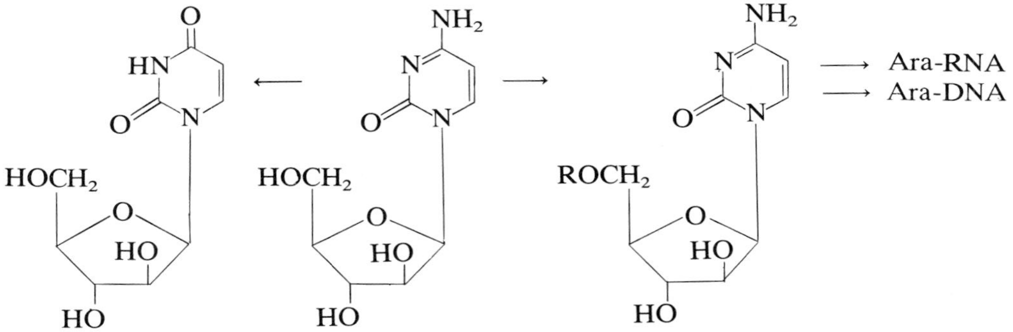

24.**82** ⟵ 24.**83** ⟶ 24.**84**–24.**86** ⟶ Ara-RNA, ⟶ Ara-DNA

24.**84** $R = PO_3H^{-1}$
24.**85** $R = P_2O_6H^{-2}$
24.**86** $R = P_3O_9H^{-3}$

Fig. 24.6 Metabolism of Ara-C (24.**83**).

(182). Thus it appears that the phosphorylated forms of ara-C are the active forms of the drug, and the capacity of leukemic cells for nucleotide formation has been correlated with the *in vivo*-response of these leukemias to ara-C (183). At the same time, human leukemic leukocytes incorporate the analog to a small but significant degree into their DNA and RNA, but the consequences of this incorporation have not been established.

The observation that ara-C is deaminated to the biologically inactive 1-β-D-arabinofuranosyluracil (24.**82**) much more rapidly in humans than in rodents (184, 185) led to a search for pyrimidine nucleoside deaminase inhibitors, which if used in conjunction with ara-C might increase its clinical utility. Two totally different inhibitors of this enzyme, 9-[*p*-(2-amino-1-hydroxyethyl)anilino]-6-chloro-2-methoxyacridine and tetrahydrouridine (186) have been found (187, 188), and the latter compound is effective in reducing the deamination of ara-C in monkeys and dogs (189).

A number of 5′-*O*-acyl derivatives of ara-C serve as effective repository forms, which are not deaminated but slowly dissolve and are then cleaved by esterases to give sustained low blood levels of ara-C (190). 2′,3′,5′-Tri-*O*-acyl derivatives can also act as effective repository forms of the drug (191). 2,2′-Anhydro-1-β-D-arabinofuranosylcytosine (anhydroara-C) is another latent form of ara-C that is slowly, nonenzymatically hydrolyzed back to ara-C *in vivo* (192). Unexpected side effects with both the 5′-*O*-acyl derivative of ara-C and cyclocytidine have precluded so far their acceptance for clinical use. Nucleotide derivatives of ara-C have shown no advantage over the nucleoside and, in fact, probably owe their activity to cleavage back to ara-C, since they are not active against kinase-deficient leukemia L1210 resistant to ara-C (193, 194).

Ara-C seems to be unique among antileukemic agents in that it is more effective against acute myelocytic and monocytic leukemia than it is against acute lymphocytic and undifferentiated leukemias. It showed no activity against four types of solid tumor in humans (11).

2.1.4 PURINE ANTAGONISTS

2.1.4.1 Thiopurines. Of the unnatural purines that have been evaluated for anticancer activity, 6-mercaptopurine [purine-6(1*H*)-thione, MP, 24.**94**] and 6-thioguanine [2-aminopurine-6(1*H*)-thione, TG, 24.**117**] are by far the most active against a variety of experimental neoplasms (195) and in treatment of the human disease. The remission rate of acute childhood leukemias treated with MP is about 50%, and chronic myelocytic leukemia responds to it about as well as to the alkylating agent busulfan (196). TG is more effective on a milligram per kilogram basis, but it is also more toxic and, as a single agent, does not show any particular advantage over MP.

Although MP itself is known to inhibit a number of enzyme systems (197), these inhibitions are not important to its anticancer activity, since neoplasms sensitive to MP convert it to the nucleotide (MPRP, 24.**96**) and lines that have become resistant to it do not (198). The extent of this conversion, which results from the reaction of MP with 5-phosphoribosylpyrophosphate catalyzed by hypoxanthine–guanine phosphoribosyltransferase (199–209)—an enzyme it also competitively inhibits (203, 209)—has been correlated with tumor response (210, 211) and is schedule dependent (212), partially because prior doses of MP enhance the ability of cells to convert MP to its ribonucleotide (213, 214). Although MPRP inhibits several reactions on the biosynthetic pathway to purine nucleotides (see Fig. 24.2), the most sensitive site appears to be an early *de novo* reaction (215–217), presumably the conversion of phosphoribosylpyroposphate (24.**19**) to phosphoribosylamine (24.**20**) by phosphoribosylpyrophosphate amidotransferase (218, 219). Evaluation of the significance of the isolated enzyme data is complicated, however, by the observation that MPRP is methylated intracellularly (220) to 6-(methylthio)-purine ribonucleotide (MeMPRP, 24.**90**), which inhibits the enzymatic formation of 5-phosphoribosylamine at less than 10% of the effective concentration of 6-thioinosinic acid (221). The cytotoxic effects of both MP (222) and 6-(methylthio)purine ribonucleoside (MeMPR, 24.**89**) (*vide infra*) can be reversed by 5-aminoimidazole-4-carboxamide (223), presumably the result of circumvention of the blockade of the amidotransferase by MPRP and MeMPRP. The *in vitro* enzymatic methylation of MP, MPR (24.**95**) and MPRP (24.**96**) (see Fig. 24.7) has been observed (224, 225), and *in vivo* MPR, as well as MP, is converted to MeMPRP. Although several routes for these conversions are conceivable, it would appear that MPRP is the principal, if not the exclusive, intermediate in the formation of MeMPRP. 6-(Methylthio)purine (MeMP, 24.**88**), which is formed *in vivo* by the methylation of MP (226), is not a substrate for the purine phosphoribosyltransferases (227); and MPR is rapidly cleaved to MP by inosine phosphorylase (228, 229). Furthermore, cells resistant to MP lacking hypoxanthine–guanine phosphoribosyltransferase are also resistant to MPR and form only a very small amount of MeMPRP from MPRP (220).

Since MeMP is not activated by cultured cells, its *in vivo* anticancer activity must be a result of *S*-demethylation to MP, which does occur in the rat (226) and is carried out by an enzyme found exclusively in the liver (230–232). A number of other *S*-alkyl and *S*-substituted alkyl derivatives of MP also exhibit *in vivo* activity (233), presumably by conversion back to MP. In contrast to the purine base, MeMPR, an excellent substrate for adenosine kinase (234, 235), is highly cytotoxic to cultured cells—even MP-resistant cells, which have lost hypoxanthine–guanine phosphoribosyltransferase activity (227). It is readily phosphorylated by H.Ep.-2 cells *in vitro* (227) and by Ehrlich cells *in vivo* (236) and is cleaved only very slowly by nucleoside phosphorylase (237), although it may be demethylated to some extent. As a result of its conversion to the monophosphate, it accumulates and persists in human erythrocytes (238). Studies on the uptake of MeMPRP by sensitive and resistant Ehrlich cells, however, indicate that, in keeping with earlier observations (239), MeMPRP must be dephosphorylated by extracellular phosphatases before entry into cells (240). Resistance to MeMPR results from a loss of adenosine kinase activity (241, 242). The therapeutic potentiation observed with a combination of MP and MeMPR (243–246) has been attributed to the greater production of MPRP in cells treated with the combination, resulting from an increase in the phosphoribosylpyrophosphate pool caused by the inhibition of *de novo* purine nucleotide biosynthesis by MeMPRP (247–249). This explanation, however, can be valid for *therapeutic potentiation* only if increased biosynthesis of MPRP occurs in cancer cells alone, and this does not appear to be the case (248). Since synergism is not observed in resistant cell lines that do not produce both nucleotides (24.**90** and 24.**96**) (243, 246), it seems likely that therapeutic potentiation is a result of the combined action of the two agents against heterogenous cell populations containing mutants resistant to the single agents. Also, the effect of increased 6-thioxanthylic acid (24.**101**) production (248, 249), which could result in increased incorporation of MP into DNA, has not been determined (*vide infra*).

Although MPR, which is less toxic to rodents than the purine base (233), is phosphorylated in some cell lines by inosine kinase (250, 251), the activity of this enzyme in mammalian cells is normally low; and in view of the ease with which it is cleaved back to MP by inosine phosphorylase (229, 237, 252), it is doubtful that the conversion of MPR to MPRP is normally of any consequence to the activity of MPR. More likely, MPR is usually

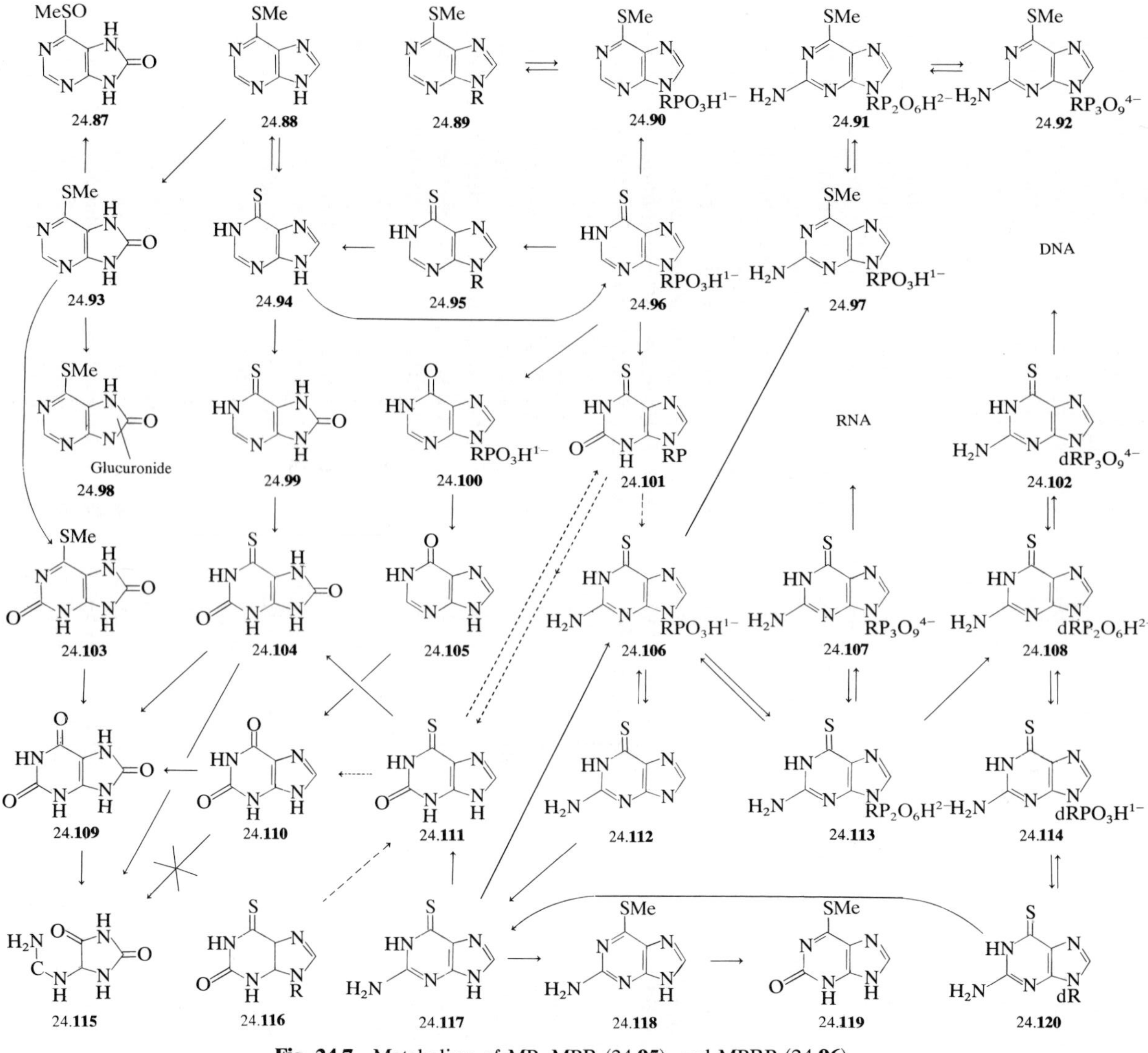

Fig. 24.7 Metabolism of MP, MPR (24.**95**), and MPRP (24.**96**).

metabolized by way of the above-mentioned cleavage to MP, which is then converted to MPRP by hypoxanthine–guanine phosphoribosyltransferase, as evidenced by the observation that, in contrast to MeMPR, MPR is not active against cell lines resistant to MP (198).

In addition to its metabolism to MeMPRP and MPRP, MP is converted to 6-thioxanthylic acid (24.**101**) as are 6-thioxanthine (24.**111**) and its ribonucleoside (24.**116**) in the presence of allopurinol (*vide infra*) (253). The incorporation of MP into DNA (254) as 2′-deoxy-6-thioguanylic acid (24.**114**) may proceed by way of 24.**101** through 24.**106**, 24.**113**, 24.**108**, and 24.**102**, but this pathway has not been established. Nor has the incorporation of MP into RNA been established; in fact, there is no evidence for the phosphorylation of MPRP to the di- and triphosphates, requisites for the polymerization.

MPRP is degraded to inosinic acid by *E. coli*/MP (255) and by both MP-sensitive and MP-resistant human leukocytes (256), and this detoxification has been proposed as a mechanism of resistance to MP. The main degradative pathway of MPRP, however, is dephosphorylation, followed by cleavage of MPR to MP, which can then be methylated to MeMP (24.**88**) (226) or oxidized by xanthine oxidase to 8-oxy-6-mercaptopurine (24.**99**) and further to 6-thiouric acid (24.**104**) (257). Whether *in vivo* methylation of the oxo derivatives 24.**99** and 24.**104** occurs is not known, but 6-(methylsulfinyl)-8-oxopurine (24.**87**), *S*-methylthiouric acid (24.**103**), and the N_7- or N_9-glucuronide of 6-(methylthio)-8-oxypurine (24.**98**) have been isolated from the urine of patients receiving MP or MeMP (257). MeMP and 6-(methylsulfinyl)purine are oxidized to 6-(methylthio)-8-oxopurine (24.**93**) (258, 259) and 6-(methylsulfinyl)-8-oxopurine (24.**87**) (259), respectively, not by xanthine oxidase but by hepatic aldehyde oxidase. The thiopurines give rise to considerable inorganic sulfate. In man, this desulfurization appears to occur by way of the (methylthio)purines, presumably through oxidation of the methylthio group to the more easily displaced methylsulfinyl or methylsulfonyl groups; this formation of sulfate is not affected by the inhibition of xanthine oxidase, in keeping with the observation that MeMP and its *S*-oxide are oxidized by hepatic aldehyde oxidase. In the mouse, sulfate is formed from MP by way of thiouric acid (24.**104**) through the action of uricase to give allantoin (24.**115**), and its formation can be inhibited with allopurinol, which reduces the formation of thiouric acid from MP (260, 261) by the inhibition of xanthine oxidase (261, 262). The combination of allopurinol with MP, 6-(alkylthio)purines, and 6-chloropurine resulted in slightly greater effectiveness against adenocarcinoma 755 in mice (261); but allopurinol, 6-mercaptopurine, and prednisone were not therapeutically potentiating in the treatment of acute childhood leukemia. Although both the effectiveness and the toxicity of MP were increased by the sparing action of allopurinol (263), there was no observable effect on the pharmacokinetics of MP in humans (264).

The heterocyclic derivatives of 6-mercaptopurine (Imuran) and of 6-thioguanine (Guaneran) were designed to afford protection from the usual processes of oxidation and methylation, and thus to assist in delivery of the active compounds to tumors (257, 265); they are cleaved to the thiopurines (MP and TG) *in vitro* and *in vivo* by sulfhydryl compounds (257). Imuran has shown an advantage over MP as an immunosuppressive agent at least in some cases (257), but neither derivative of these thiopurines has been more effective than the parent as anticancer agents.

The metabolism of TG (24.**117**) is similar to that of MP, but there are important differences. TG, like MP, is a good substrate for hypoxanthine–guanine phosphoribosyltransferase, which metabolizes it to 6-thioguanylic acid (TGRP, 24.**106**) (266). In contrast to MPRP, TGRP is further phosphorylated to the di- and triphosphates (24.**113** and 24.**107**), which are incorporated into RNA (266, 267). TG is also incorporated into DNA as 2′-deoxy-6-thioguanylic acid (TGdRP, 24.**114**); and a correlation between its antitumor activity and the extent of this latter incorporation has been noted (266–268), although incorporation into DNA does not explain all of its metabolic effects in bacteria (269), and some investigators feel that the metabolic effects of TGRP may be more universally important to the activity of TG than its incorporation (270, 271). More recent results, however, clearly indicate that the cytotoxicity of both MP and TG, at least to the cell lines studied, is due to incorporation into DNA (272).

The high incorporation of TG into the DNA of bone marrow cells of humans after five daily doses (273) may be responsible for toxicity, since the potentiation observed in both the mouse (274) and man (275) between ara-C (24.**81**) and TG appears to be due at least in part to subadditive toxicity (274) resulting from decreased incorporation of TG into DNA (276) caused by the inhibition of DNA polymerase by ara-C. In any event, the conversion of TG to nucleotides is much more extensive than is that of MP, and the development of resistance by a tumor to TG has been attributed to enhanced nucleotide breakdown by alkaline phosphohydrolase (277, 278). The biosynthetic pathway by which TG is incorporated into DNA has not been elucidated. The diphosphate (24.**113**) may be reduced by nucleoside diphosphate reductase to 24.**108**, which is the normal pathway for guanine incorporation or, less likely, TG may be converted by a deoxyribosyltransferase to the 2′-deoxyribonucleoside (24.**120**) (279) followed by phosphorylation to 24.**114**, 24.**108**, and 24.**102**, since 2′-deoxy-6-thioguanosine (TGdR, 24.**120**) itself is phosphorylated and incorporated into DNA, but TGdR is also phosphorolyzed to TG (252). Somewhat surprisingly, the α-anomer of TGdR is also phosphorylated and incorporated into DNA (and RNA) but is not cleaved to TG (279–284). The usefulness of 6-thioguanosine (TGR, 24.**112**) is doubtful because of its easy phosphorolysis to TG and because of the very limited guanosine kinase activity in mammalian cells (252, 285). The mono-, di-, and triphosphates (24.**97**, 24.**91**, 24.**92**) of *S*-methyl-6-thioguanosine (MeTGR), identified as metabolites of TG, probably result *in vivo* from the methylation of TGRP; but in contrast to the situation with MP, little is known about the contribution of these *S*-methylated compounds to the biologic activity of TG (286). Methylation of TG itself to 24.**118** (224), followed by deamination to 24.**119**, is more extensive in man than in the mouse, whereas deamination of TG to thioxanthine (24.**111**) and subsequent oxidation to 6-thiouric acid (24.**104**) occur only to a small extent in man but is the main degradative pathway in the mouse (257). Sulfate is a major end product of the catabolism of TG, but the exact route of its formation is not known. The differential sensitivity of intestinal mucosa and bone marrow to TG has been attributed to the relative rates of metabolic conversions of the drug in these tissues (287). The synergism observed with MP and MeMPR (24.**89**) also occurs with TG, but in this case an increase in the half-life of TGRP, perhaps due to competition by MeMPRP for the phosphohydrolase that cleaves TGRP, was also noted (288).

Thus studies of the metabolism of the thiopurines, although still incomplete, have been extensive and have revealed an extremely complex picture that in general follows the normal metabolism of the naturally occurring oxopurines hypoxanthine and guanine. The most notable deviations result from *S*-methylation, which, for example, changes MPR (24.**95**) from an inosine analog to MeMPR (24.**89**), an adenosine analog (in terms of enzyme specificities), and has no counterpart with the oxopurines. The metabolism of the thiopurines is partially responsible for an equally complex pattern of enzyme inhibitions, most of which probably contribute to the biologic activity of these compounds.

In contrast to the behavior of the parent purines MP and TG and their ribo- or 2-deoxyribonucleosides, the arabino- or xylonucleosides are not metabolized *in vivo* or *in vitro* (289–292). 9-Alkyl derivatives are metabolized only to a small extent to *S*-glucuronides (293–296), and this is probably unrelated to their activity. Furthermore, the effects of these derivatives on cellular metabolism are quite different from those of MP, TG, and their metabolites (9). Since MP arabinonucleotide is water soluble and is slowly dephosphorylated in humans, providing sustained blood plasma levels of the nucleoside, it appears to have potential advantages (297).

2.1.4.2 9-β-D-Arabinofuranosyladenine. A number of adenine nucleosides are cytotoxic and exhibit varying degrees of inhibitory action against rodent neoplasms (298, 299). Of these, only 9-β-D-arabinofuranosyladenine (ara-A, 24.**122**) (300, 301) appears to be of interest for the treatment of human cancer. It inhibited the growth of ascites tumors TA3 and 6C3HED, and although essentially inactive against L1210 and solid tumors (302), it was active against leukemias in humans (303). Despite being a relatively poor substrate for adenosine kinase (234), ara-A is metabolized *in vivo* to the triphosphate (24.**125**) (304), which is a noncompetitive inhibitor of DNA polymerase in TA3 cells (305). This effect is thought to account for the compound's growth inhibitory properties, although other sites of action may also be important (306). Ara-A is extensively deaminated to 24.**121** *in vivo* to the inactive inosine analog, but this deamination can be inhibited by 2′-deoxycoformycin (24.**126**) (see Fig. 24.8) (307, 308). The combination of 2′-deoxycoformycin with ara-A, on the optimal dose schedule, has resulted in high cure rates of both the L1210 and P388 leukemias in mice (309). Apparently deamination in the absence of inhibitor is so rapid and the phosphorylation so slow that effective intracellular ara-ATP levels cannot be achieved. Substitution at the 2-position of ara-A by a fluorine atom (310) prevents deamination, and the resulting compound, 9-β-D-arabinofuranosyl-2-fluoroadenine (24.**127**), is active against the L1210 leukemia (309).

2.1.5 RIBONUCLEOSIDE DIPHOSPHATE REDUCTASE INHIBITORS. Hydroxyurea (24.**128**) has shown activity against a number of

$$\mathrm{HONHCONH_2}$$

24.**128**

animal neoplasms (311) and some activity against human cancers (312, 313). It interferes with the synthesis of DNA in intact animals (314, 315) and in mammalian cells *in vitro* (316, 317); this interference is a result of decreased conversion of ribonucleotides to 2′-deoxyribonucleotides (312, 318), caused primarily by the inhibition of nucleoside diphosphate reductase (319, 320), although multiple sites may be involved (318). Inhibition of the reductase may result from the binding of free ferrous ions by hydroxyurea. Since such binding has not been demonstrated experimentally (320), metabolic activation of hydroxyurea may be necessary, but this has not been established. Acetohydroxamic acid has been found in the blood of three patients on hydroxyurea therapy, suggesting that the drug is hydrolyzed to hydroxylamine (321), which then cleaves acetyl–coenzyme A. The other product of this hydrolysis must be isocyanate, but additional studies indicate that isocyanate ions cannot account for the activity of hydroxyurea (322). The biologic activity of a number of other

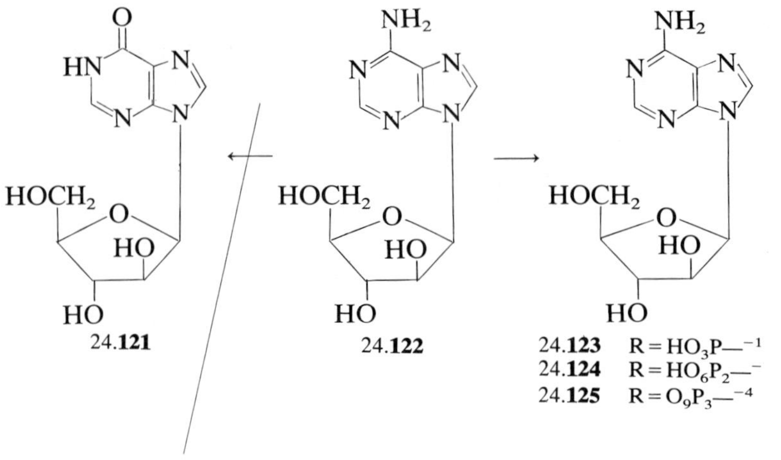

24.121 24.122 24.123 $R = HO_3P—^{-1}$ 24.124 $R = HO_6P_2—^{-}$ 24.125 $R = O_9P_3—^{-4}$

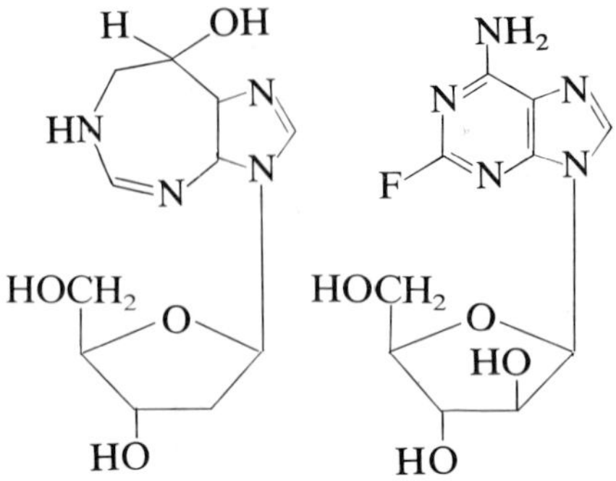

24.126 24.127

Fig. 24.8 Metabolism of ara-A (24.**122**).

proposed active intermediates of hydroxyurea has been investigated, but none of these compounds has been identified *in vivo* (323–325).

Guanazole (24.**129**) also inhibits nucleoside diphosphate reductase, and this inhibition is thought to be responsible for activity it has shown in experimental animal tumor systems (326).

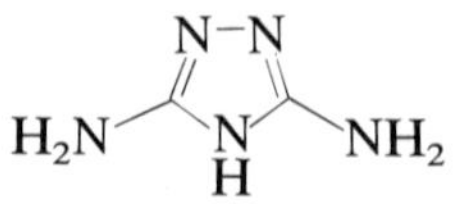

24.**129**

The initial observation (327) of the antileukemic activity of picolinaldehyde thiosemicarbazone (24.**130**) has been extended to a number of related heterocyclic thiosemicarbazones, all of which appear to owe their activity to coordinate iron that is involved in the enzymic reduction of the ribonucleoside diphosphates (328–333).

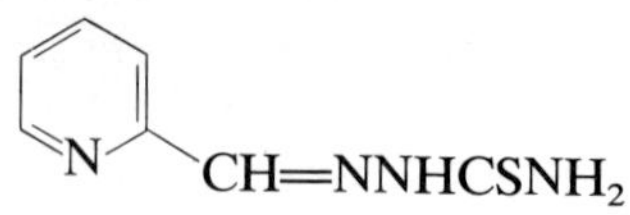

CH=NNHCSNH$_2$

24.**130**

Although the thiosemicarbazones are much better inhibitors of the enzyme than hydroxyurea or guanazole, clinical results with these compounds have been disappointing, probably because of their toxicity, which may be an inherent result of their effectiveness as inhibitors of the enzyme.

2.2 Chemically Reactive Drugs Having Nonspecific Action

Modern cancer chemotherapy was inaugurated with the discovery of the clinical activity of selected nitrogen mustards against lymphoid neoplasms as revealed in a classic summation of confidential observations made during World War II on the biological effects and therapeutic applications of certain chemical warfare agents (334). Since that time thousands of chemically reactive compounds classified as alkylating agents have been synthesized, most on a seemingly random basis, and tested for antineoplastic activity in various animal test systems. The value of unabated synthesis was challenged by the findings of a prodigious comparison of the activity of more than a hundred representative alkylating agents and 12 nonalkylating reference compounds against some or all of 18 rat and 7 mouse neoplasms (335). This study indicated an almost general lack of tumor specificity among the classes of alkylating agents examined and offered, superficially at least, little hope that any alkylating agent would exhibit unique antitumor activity or toxicological characteristics. Restriction of the synthesis of new alkylating agents to those based on rational design has been advocated (336, 337) and reiterated with emphasis on a narrow cytotoxic spectrum for increased specificity (338). The number of clinically useful alkylating agents has expanded from one to possibly a dozen, most of them products of empiricism, enlightened empiricism, or serendipity (339) and each is yet to be displaced by a superior rationally designed agent.

Alkylating agents are chemically reactive compounds that combine covalently with nucleophilic centers, a fully saturated carbon atom of the alkylating group becoming attached to the nucleophile. Alkylations of biological interest involve attack at the nitrogen, sulfur, or oxygen atoms of biologically important functional groups, such as amino groups, thiolate anions of proteins, and ring nitrogen atoms and phosphate anions of nucleic acids. The mechanisms by which alkylations can occur are classified by the extreme cases of first-order (S_N1) and second-order (S_N2) nucleophilic substitutions, although in practice division between the two is usually not distinct. The rate-controlling step of the S_N1 alkylation is a solvent-assisted ionization of the alkylating agent to give a solvated carbocation. The rate-controlling step of the S_N2 alkylation involves simultaneous bond-forming and bond-breaking interaction of the alkylating agent and the nucleophile, the rate of alkylation being dependent on the concentrations of both. An important modification of the S_N2 reaction applies to a number of alkylating agents in which neighboring group participation results in an internal displacement, which forms a solvent-stabilized, but strained and reactive, three-membered cyclic cation; with difunctional agents, the process is repeatable after one arm reacts. The relative rates of the successive formation and opening of the cyclic ion determine the apparent order of the overall reaction. Thus alkylations with the aliphatic nitrogen mustards resemble an S_N2 process because the rate-controlling step is the reaction with an available nucleophile of the readily formed, yet relatively stable aziridinium ion. A polar solvent (water in the case of biological fluids) stabilizes the ions formed. Such cyclizations do not occur in nonpolar solvents (and presumably not in body lipids) (340). Biological alkylations with conventional alkylating agents are generally of the S_N2 type, involving either the original molecule or a cyclic ion derived from it.

Nitrogen mustards, aziridines, esters of sulfonic acids, nitrosoureas, and triazenes are the principal types of biological alkylating agent in current clinical use. The high chemical reactivity of these agents and the high probability of nonselective reaction with diverse nucleophilic centers available *in vivo* not only result in numerous toxic side effects, but magnify the problem of defining the exact nature of the event responsible for the anticancer activity of these agents. It was, in fact, the damaging effects to bone marrow and other proliferating normal cells that first suggested that the mustards might also affect the growth of lymphoid tumors (334). A cogent body of evidence indicates that DNA is the critical target of the biological alkylating agents and that the 7-position of guanine is the primary site of attack. The principal biological effects of alkylation are cytotoxicity, which is requisite for anticancer activity, mutagenesis, and also carcinogenesis and teratogenesis.

Although bifunctionality is not a prerequisite for significant anticancer activity, the most active agents are usually bifunctional. The greater cytotoxicity of bifunctional agents has been attributed to interstrand cross-linking of DNA, which results in impaired template function for further replication (341). Resistant cells repair the damaged portion of DNA by enzymatic excision of alkylated bases and restoration. Intrastrand cross-linking of DNA can occur, and also the linking of DNA to protein (342, 343). It has been suggested that rapidly proliferating cells are more sensitive to cross-linking than resting cells because the former fail to repair damaged DNA before the damage becomes irreversible during the next DNA synthesis cycle. This conclusion was based on studies of the action of typical bifunctional alkylating agents on resting and rapidly proliferating spleen clonogenic cells (344). Although DNA remains the likely critical target of biological alkylation, and cross-linking is more cytotoxic than monofunctional alkylation, there exists no general explanation of the basic mechanism of action of alkylating agents as anticancer agents (345).

The following discussions of individual classes of chemically reactive drugs are, in general, limited to clinically useful agents.

2.2.1 NITROGEN MUSTARDS

2.2.1.1 Mechlorethamine. The prototype of nitrogen mustards and the original anticancer agent (334) is nitrogen mustard itself [24.**131**, 2-chloro-*N*-(2-chloroethyl)-*N*-methylethanamine, mechlorethamine, chloromethine, HN2], which was first synthesized in 1935 (346) and appears to remain the alkylating agent of choice in the treatment of advanced Hodgkin's disease (11), although current practice favors its use in combination with other agents (347). Mechlorethamine and other aliphatic nitrogen mustards are toxic, vesicant, unstable compounds, which are best handled as the crystalline water-soluble hydrochlorides. Mechlorethamine is the fastest acting clinical alkylating agent, being usually administered intravenously immediately after solubilizing in saline or water; topical applications have been developed in the treatment of mycosis fungoides (348).

At physiological pH mechlorethamine hydrochloride is readily and unimolecularly converted by way of the free base to a relatively stable aziridinium ion, which in turn reacts bimolecularly with available nucleophilic centers. The second chloroethyl arm may then react by repetition of the cyclization process (Fig. 24.9), thus enabling cross-linking of DNA strands as depicted in Fig. 24.10 with guanyl units. This illustration with mechlorethamine is typical of bifunctional alkylating agents in that *in vivo* alkylation of guanine occurs mainly at the N-7 position. The scission of a DNA strand by depurination (349) is illustrated in Fig. 24.10 as one of the damaging effects of cross-linking. A possible consequence of monoalkylation is the mispairing of bases in DNA: for example, hydrogen bonding of the keto form of guanine with cytosine is normal, but after N-7 alkylation, the enol form of guanine is favored and can pair atypically with thymine (350). Such mispairing could lead

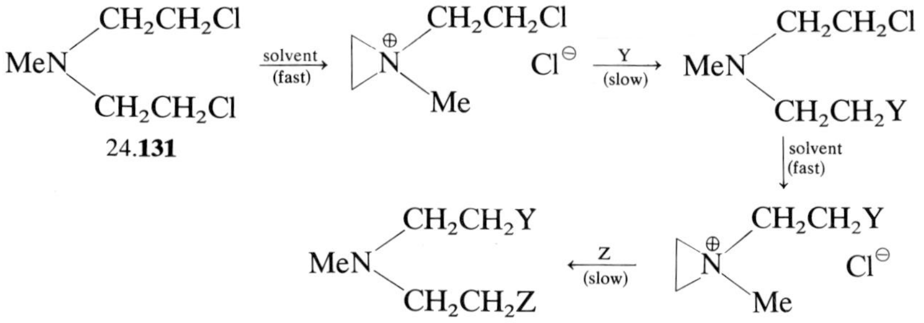

Y and Z = nucleophiles such as $RS^{\ominus}$, RNH_2, =N—, =O

Fig. 24.9 Bifunctional alkylation with mechlorethamine.

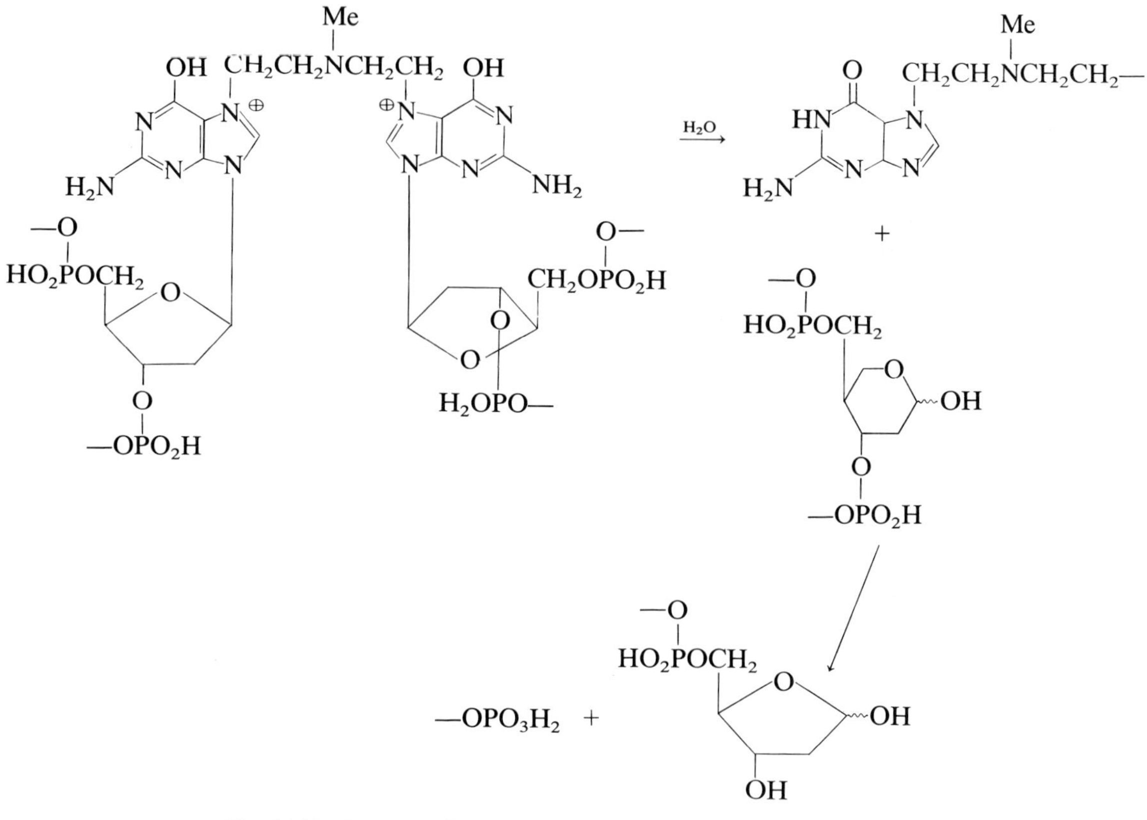

Fig. 24.10 Deguanylation of DNA strands cross-linked with mechlorethamine.

to miscoding and mutation, but on a theoretical basis, alkylations at O-6 and N-3 may be more effective in mispairing than at N-7 (351).

2.2.1.2 Aromatic Nitrogen Mustards. Replacement of the methyl group of mechlorethamine by groups that markedly alter basicity affects both chemical reactivity and biological activity, as revealed in a study of aromatic nitrogen mustards (352). The less reactive compounds of this class—those having electron-withdrawing substituents—apparently do not alkylate under physiological conditions. Aromatic nitrogen mustards have been reported to react by an S_N1 mechanism (352), but further kinetic studies indicated that they react by a two-step process involving the formation of a cyclic intermediate similar to that described for the aliphatic nitrogen mustards (353). Such alkylations would simulate the S_N1 type when cyclization is the slower step. Interstrand cross-linking of the DNA of sensitive cells with aromatic nitrogen mustards was observed to be considerably delayed, an effect not seen with mechlorethamine (354).

Although the goal of highly selective cytotoxic action against malignant cells by structural modifications of aromatic nitrogen mustards has not been achieved, pharmacological differences were noted among congeners, two of which, chlorambucil [24.**132**, 4-[bis(2-chloroethyl)-

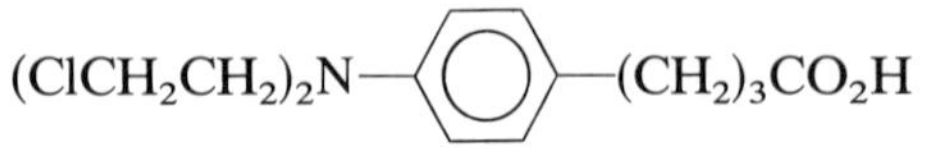

$(ClCH_2CH_2)_2N-C_6H_4-(CH_2)_3CO_2H$

24.**132**

amino]benzenebutanoic acid] and melphalan [24.**133**, 4-[bis(2-chloroethyl)amino]-L-phenylalanine, L-sarcolysin, L-phenylalanine mustard, L-PAM], have had longstanding clinical utility. These agents have

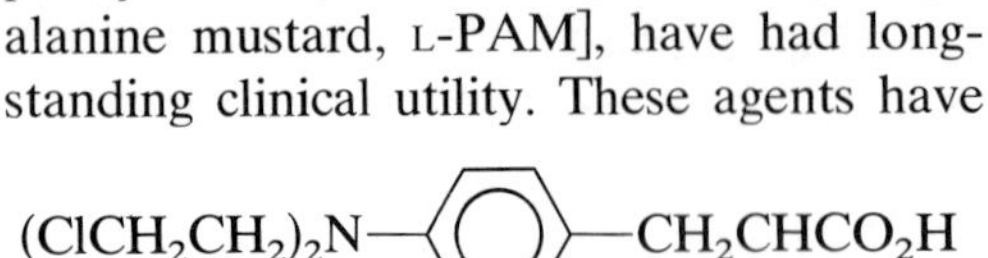

$(ClCH_2CH_2)_2N-C_6H_4-CH_2CH(NH_2)CO_2H$

24.**133**

the same general spectrum of action as other nitrogen mustards; however they are not nearly so highly reactive as mechlorethamine, may be administered orally, and are safer and more convenient in multidose therapy.

Chloroambucil, whose synthesis was reported in 1953 (355), was designed as a water-soluble agent advantageous for intravenous injection (338), but has since emerged as a standard orally administered agent. For the treatment of chronic lymphocytic leukemia, it is probably the most effective agent yet brought to the clinic; its other primary uses have been in the treatment of ovarian carcinoma and lymphomas (11).

The synthesis of melphalan (356, 357) was inspired by the possibility that a nitrogen mustard derivative of a natural amino acid might be directed to a metabolic site critical to neoplastic cells; for example, a nitrogen mustard derivative of L-phenylalanine, a precursor of melanin, might effect selective action against malignant melanoma (11, 347). No compelling evidence, however, has come forth to verify an improvement in the selective action of these agents by facilitated transport. The D-form of melphalan appeared to be much less active against Walker carcinosarcoma 256 than the L-form, an observation that led to the conclusion that sarcolysin, the independently developed DL-form of melphalan (358), owed its high activity to the presence of the L-isomer (349). The subsequent comprehensive comparison of the phenylalanine mustards (D-, L-, DL-; *ortho*-, *meta*-, *para*-) against a variety of animal tumors, including three strains of Walker carcinosarcoma 256, revealed no significant differences attributable to optical configuration (335). Nevertheless, this approach has provided the clinic with potent anticancer agents. An effective oral alkylating agent similar in its time-dose action to chlorambucil (348), melphalan is widely considered to be the drug of choice in the treatment of multiple myeloma (11). Its use in the surgical adjuvant chemotherapy of breast cancer has resulted in marked increases in the disease-free interval after surgery (359), which hold promise for significantly improved long-term cure rates.

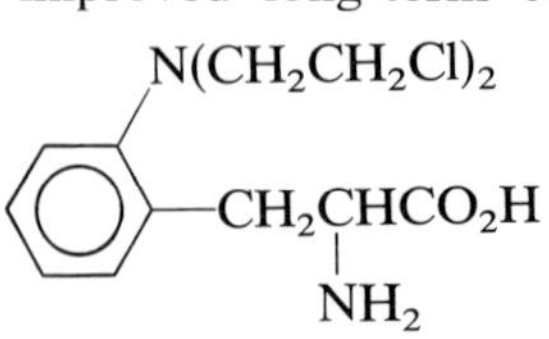

$N(CH_2CH_2Cl)_2$ (ortho) $-C_6H_4-CH_2CH(NH_2)CO_2H$

24.**134**

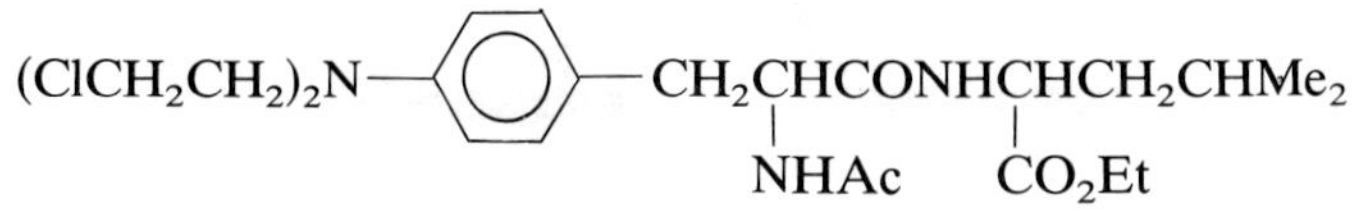

$$(ClCH_2CH_2)_2N-C_6H_4-CH_2CH(NHAc)CONHCH(CO_2Et)CH_2CHMe_2$$

24.**135**

The DL-form of *ortho*-phenylalanine mustard (24.**134**) (360) has been termed the agent of choice against Burkitt's lymphoma (361). Asaley [24.**135**, ethyl *N*-[*N*-acetyl-4-[bis(2-chloroethyl)amino]-DL-phenylalanyl]-L-leucinate], a peptide derivative of sarcolysin, is being clinically investigated in the United States as part of an exchange program with the Soviet Union (362).

2.2.1.3 Cyclophosphamide. The concept of latentiation—the *in vivo* release of a biologically active compound from a suitably derivatized form (363)—has been invoked to explain the action of certain nitrogen mustards and has influenced the design of others. An early example of such a modification was the oxidation of mechlorethamine to a less basic, therefore less reactive, form, which was obtained as the hydrochloride 24.**136** [2-chloro-*N*-(2-chloroethyl)-*N*-methylethanamine-*N*-oxide

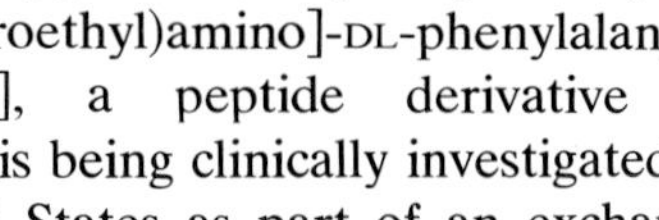

$$MeN(\rightarrow O)(CH_2CH_2Cl)_2 \cdot HCl$$

24.**136**

hydrochloride, mechlorethamine oxide hydrochloride, nitromin] (364, 365). The oxide was reported to be less toxic and more active in certain tumor systems than the parent (365, 366), and it may be a latent form that is activated by *in vivo* reduction (367, 368).

The search for suitable substrates for the phosphoramidases that were reportedly more abundant in neoplastic cells than in normal cells (369) resulted in the synthesis of numerous acyclic and cyclic phosphorylated nitrogen mustard derivatives (370–372), which showed a high degree of activity against animal tumors (371, 373, 374). The most successful latentiation of this type is exemplified by the development of cyclophosphamide [24.**137**, *N,N*-bis-(2-chloroethyl)tetrahydro-2*H*-1,3,2-oxazaphosphorin-2-amine 2-oxide] as a widely used clinical alkylating agent. Proposed as a potentially latent form of nornitrogen mustard [24.**144**, 2-chloro-*N*-(2-chloroethyl)-ethanamine, nor-HN2], cyclophosphamide emerged from the synthesis of more than 500 phosphamides (375–377) as the most effective congener in evaluations against Yoshida ascitic sarcoma of the rat. Cyclophosphamide was definitely superior to nornitrogen mustard (335) and other nitrogen mustards (378, 379) in a number of animal tumor systems. Cyclophosphamide, which is itself nontoxic—even at high concentrations—to tumor cells growing in culture (376), is converted to a highly cytotoxic form by prior incubation with liver homogenate (380). The original concept of an activation of the inert transport form by hydrolytic enzymes inside the tumor cell (370, 377) thus could not account for the observed biological effects and eventually proved to be untenable. This dilemma engendered persistent efforts in several laboratories, which have come far in clarifying the metabolism of cyclophosphamide and identifying the active metabolite. These efforts have been reviewed (10, 381, 382) and provide a basis for the metabolic scheme that appears in Fig. 24.11.

Cyclophosphamide is metabolized in the liver at a species-dependent rate, fast in rodents, but slower in man; the resulting 4-hydroxycyclophosphamide (24.**138**) tautomerizes to unstable aldophosphamide (24.**140**), which spontaneously loses acrolein (24.**142**) to form phosphoramide mustard [24.**143**, *N,N*-bis(2-chloroethyl)-phosphorodiamidic acid]. Phosphoramide

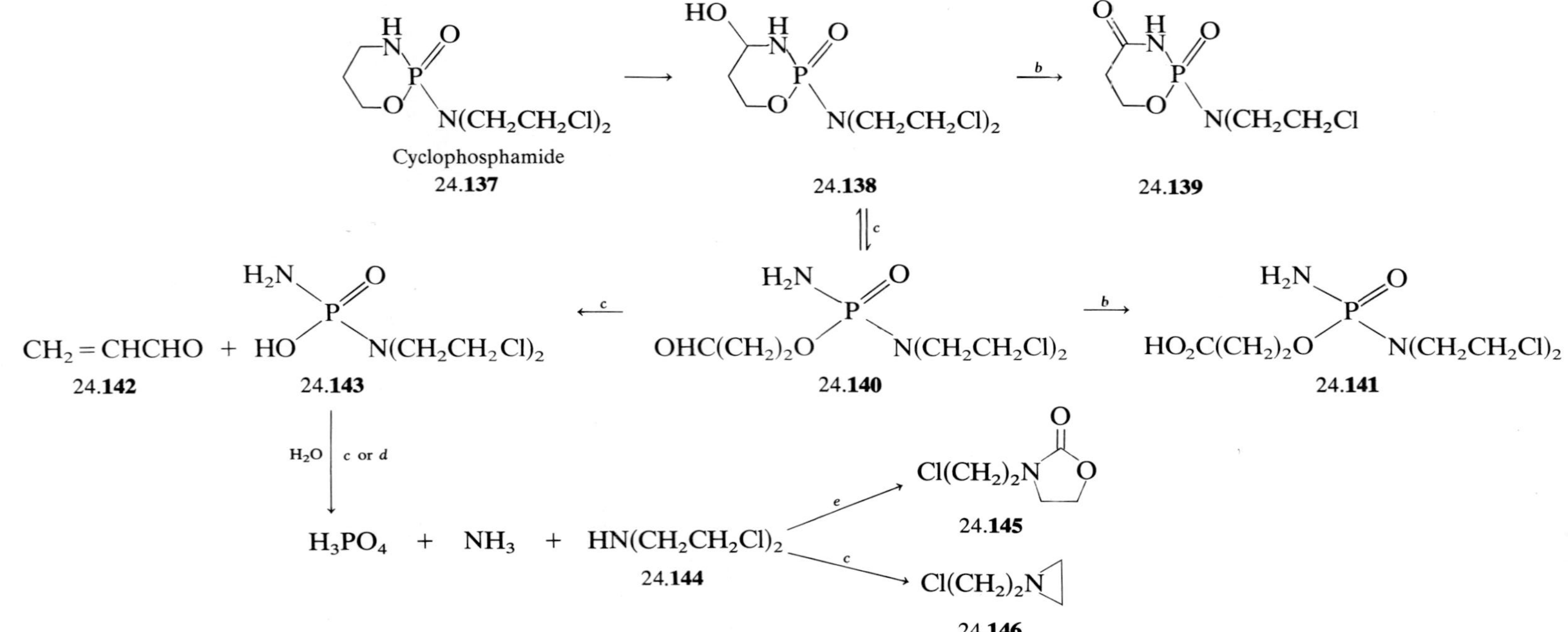

Fig. 24.11 Metabolism of cyclophosphamide. (*a*) Liver microsomes, O_2, NADPH. (*b*) Aldehyde oxidase, O_2. (*c*) Spontaneous. (*d*) Phosphoramidase. (*e*) Carbon dioxide in blood.

mustard, also unstable, decomposes to nornitrogen mustard (24.**144**), which cyclizes to 1-(2-chloroethyl)aziridine (24.**146**) or is detoxified in the blood (383) as 3-(2-chloroethyl)-2-oxazolidinone (24.**145**). The alkylating form [24.**146**, 1-(2-chloroethyl)-aziridine] of nornitrogen mustard is uncharged at physiological pH (349) and thus differs from the aziridinium ion formed from mechlorethamine. Phosphoramide mustard, as its cyclohexanamine salt, was among the synthetic congeners mentioned earlier (371) and has had clinical trial (348). The essentially inactive urinary metabolites, 4-ketocyclophosphamide (24.**139**) and carboxyphosphamide (24.**141**), are detoxification products, but among the other metabolites (24.**138** ⇌ 24.**140**, 24.**143**, 24.**144**), the alkylating species ultimately responsible for the anticancer activity of cyclophosphamide may not be unequivocally decided. If 24.**138** ⇌ 24.**140** is the important transport form that enters tumor cells, as is widely speculated, then detoxification by cellular aldehyde oxidase in resistant cells must be considered.

The slower rate of hydroxylation in man mentioned earlier suggested syntheses of 4-hydroxycyclophosphamide (24.**138**) and stabilized derivatives thereof, 4-hydroperoxycyclophosphamide (24.**147**) and 4-

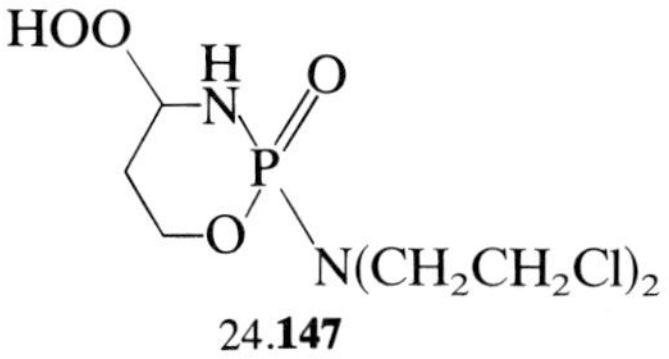

HOO, H, N, O, P, O, $N(CH_2CH_2Cl)_2$

24.**147**

peroxycyclophosphamide (24.**148**) (385, 386); these compounds, which spontaneously yield 24.**138** under physiological conditions (387), were at least as active as

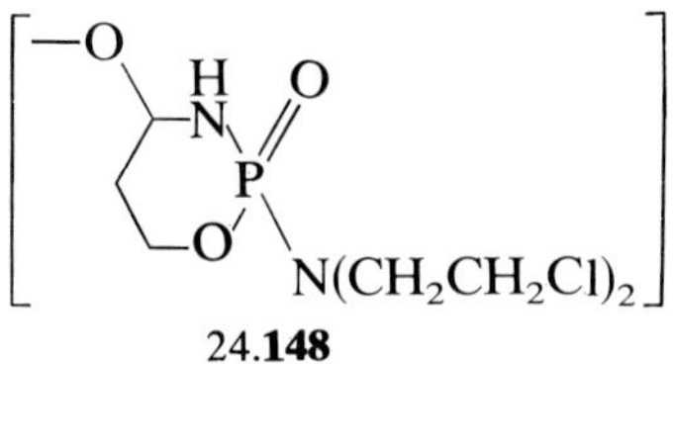

—O, H, N, O, P, O, $N(CH_2CH_2Cl)_2$

24.**148**

cyclophosphamide in animal tumor systems. The 4-hydroperoxy derivative (24.**149**) of isophosphamide [*N*,3-bis(2-chloroethyl)-tetrahydro-2*H*-1,3,2-oxazaphosphorin-2-amine 2-oxide, ifosfamide], an investigational analog of cyclophosphamide (362,

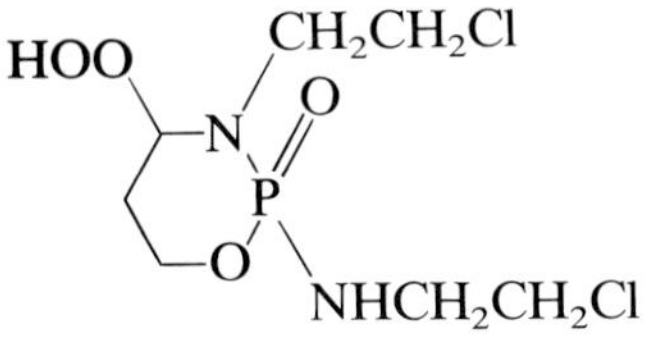

HOO, CH_2CH_2Cl, N, O, P, O, $NHCH_2CH_2Cl$

24.**149**

388), appeared to have superior activity in the leukemia L1210 system in a comparison with phosphoramide mustard, the parent compounds, and other peroxidized derivatives, and is undergoing clinical trials in Japan (389).

Clinically, cyclophosphamide is the most widely useful alkylating agent, effectively inhibiting a variety of human carcinomas and sarcomas as well as leukemias and lymphomas. It can be effectively administered in a number of ways and used in combination with a number of agents (11, 348, 390). Its principal side effects are leukopenia, alopecia, and cystitis, the latter being produced by a urinary metabolite. Its range of therapeutic applications has widened steadily to include its present use as an immunosuppressive agent (391).

2.2.2 AZIRIDINES. The development of aziridines as biological alkylating agents was a logical outgrowth of the *in vivo* correspondence of nitrogen mustards to aziridinium ions and nornitrogen mustard to uncharged 1-(2-chloroethyl)aziridine already mentioned. Ring-opening reactions of unprotonated aziridines with nucleophiles are slower than those of their aziridinium counterparts; the reactivity of aziridines is due to ring strain and is enhanced in the quaternized form and by protonation, which is not likely to occur at physiological pH with carcinolytic aziridines of reduced basicity. The reactivity of 1-phenylaziridine, unlike that of aromatic nitrogen mustards, is augmented by electron-withdrawing substitution on the phenyl group: the monofunctional 1-(2,4-dinitrophenyl)aziridine (24.**150**), in contrast to the corresponding bifunctional nitrogen

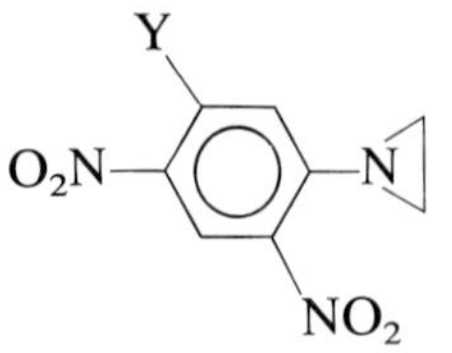

24.**150** Y = H
24.**151** Y = $CONH_2$

mustard, is both chemically reactive and inhibitory to Walker carcinosarcoma 256 (352). Among compounds of this type, the carbamoyl derivative [24.**151**, 5-(1-aziridinyl)-2,4-dinitrobenzamide] (392) showed exceptional activity against the Walker tumor, yet was inactive against a number of other tumors, many of which are highly sensitive to bifunctional alkylating agents (393).

As alkylating agents that are slower acting than mechlorethamine, a few aziridines—notably triethylenemelamin [24.**152**, 2,4,6-tris(1-aziridinyl)-1,3,5-triazine, TEM], the first alkylating agent

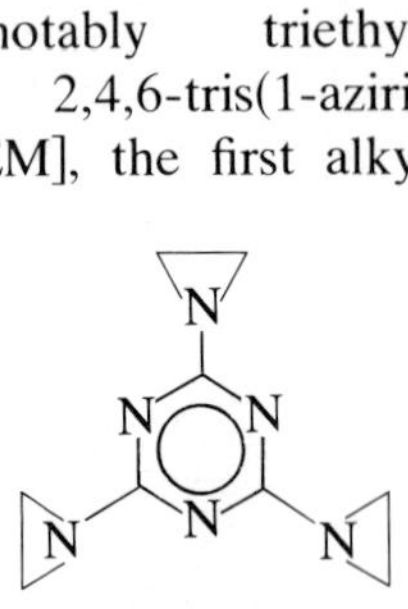

24.**152**

found to be suitable for oral administration; thio-TEPA [24.**153**, 1,1′,1″-phosphinothioylidynetrisaziridine, triethylenethiophosphoramide], preferred over triethylenephoramide (24.**154**, TEPA) because of its greater stability; and triaziquone [24.**155**, 2,3,5-tris(1-aziridinyl)-2,5-cyclohexadiene-1,4-dione, trenimon], a European development—have had exten-

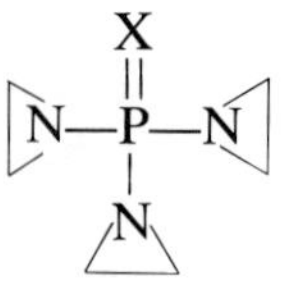

24.**153** X = S
24.**154** X = O

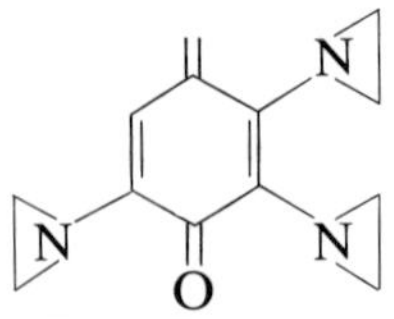

24.**155**

sive clinical use, but are of limited clinical interest today.

The first examples of naturally occurring aziridines and a special class of alkylating agents are the mitomycins, a group of closely related antibiotics produced by several strains of *Streptomyces.* The anticancer activity of mitomycin C (24.**156**) was discovered and developed in Japan, where this drug has been widely used clinically, mainly in combination with other agents (394); elsewhere its use has been infrequent owing to its severe toxic potential (11). Mitomycin C appears to effect interstrand cross-linking of DNA after being metabolically reduced to the active form 24.**157**; the aziridine ring and the methylene-oxygen linkage are the likely reactive centers (Fig. 24.12), and the amino groups of adenine or cytosine and the oxygen atom of guanine are the postulated cross-linking sites (395, 396).

Piperidinedione [24.**158**, 3,6-bis(5-chloro-2-piperidyl)-2,5-piperidinedione dihydrochloride], another antibiotic obtained from a strain of *Streptomyces* (397) and an anticancer agent of clinical interest (362), has been shown to act as an alkylating agent (398, 399). It is more cytotoxic

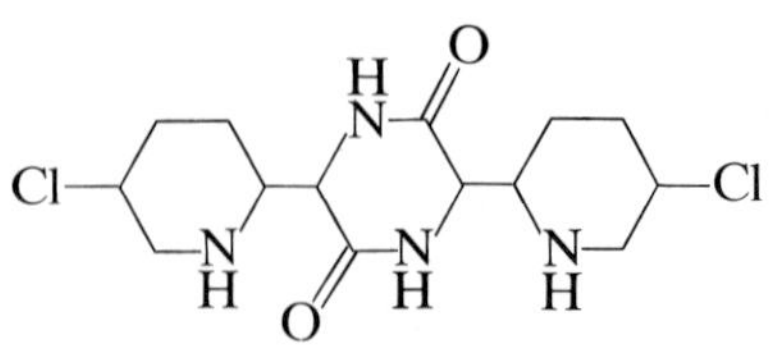

24.**158**

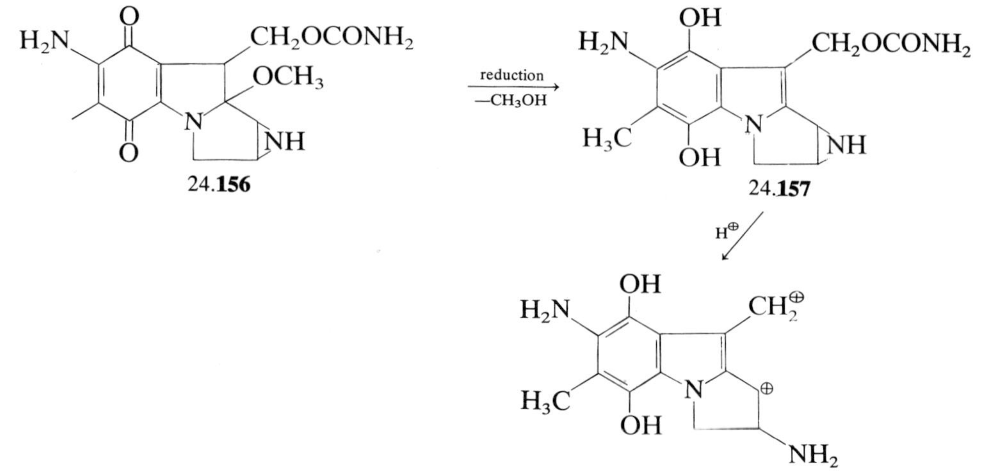

Fig. 24.12 Metabolism of mitomycin C (24.**157**).

than the chemically derived bisaziridine 24.**159** [3,6-bis(1-azabicyclo[3.1.0]hex-2-yl)-2,5-piperazinedione], hence probably does not alkylate through an aziridinyl intermediate (399).

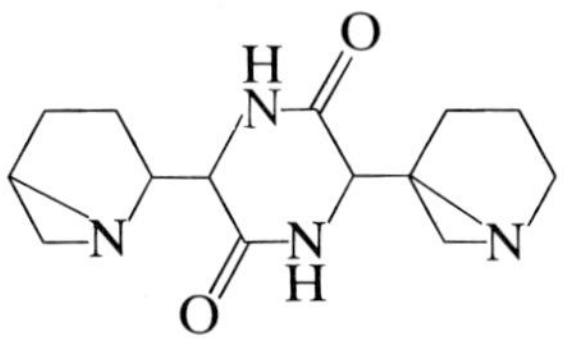

24.**159**

2.2.3 METHANESULFONIC ESTERS. Symmetrical bifunctionality characterizes the methanesulfonic esters of major interest as anticancer agents. On the other hand, the monofunctional methyl methanesulfonate (24.**160**) and 2-chloroethyl methanesulfonate (24.**161**), which has potential

$MeSO_2OR$

24.**160** R = Me
24.**161** $R = CH_2CH_2Cl$

bifunctional character (400), showed uniquely specific activity against lymphoma 8, a tumor that is relatively resistant to other alkylating agents (335). 1,4-Butanediol dimethanesulfonate (24.**162**, busulfan) (401) evolved as the most active member of a homologous series of dimethanesulfonates (402) and the only one that has had sustained clinical use. The clinical effectiveness of busulfan, however, is limited

$MeSO_2O(CH_2)_4OSO_2Me$

24.**162**

to the treatment of chronic myelogenous leukemia for which it is the most commonly used therapeutic agent, affording remission of clinical evidence of this disease in almost all patients who receive it as primary therapy (11). The identification of tetrahydrothiophene-3-ol 1,1-dioxide (24.**163**) as the major urinary metabolite of busulfan

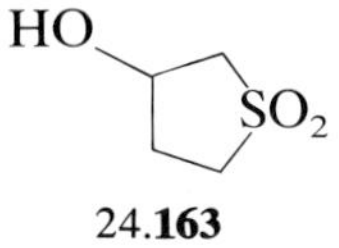

24.**163**

implicates the cycloalkylation of cysteinyl units in protein (403) as a factor in the biological activity of this drug, but the relevance of proteinaceous sulfur extraction to anticancer activity has not been established (404). Busulfan, which reacts by a typical S_N2 mechanism, is unusual among clinical alkylating agents in that its pharmacological action is limited to myelosuppression, apparently having little effect on lymphoid tissue or intestinal mucosa (347).

Other carcinolytic methanesulfonates of special interest are nitrogen mustard analogs, among which are the dimethanesulfonates of 3,3′-(methylimino)bis-1-propanol (24.**164**, Yoshi-864), the most effective of such compounds against Yoshida sarcoma (405) and leukemia L1210 (406) and an investigational drug of clinical interest (362); and of 3,3′-iminobis-1-propanol (24.**165**), an agent uniquely effective

$$RN(CH_2CH_2CH_2OSO_2Me)_2$$

24.**164** R = Me
24.**165** R = H

against two rat tumors resistant to other alkylating agents tried (407). Structure-activity relationships among 277 methanesulfonates against experimental animal tumors indicated that the presence of nitrogen, though not an absolute requirement,

2.2.4 1,2-EPOXIDES. The 1,2-epoxides, whose evaluation as antineoplastic agents was suggested by their use in textile technology as cross-linking agents (408), have not, as a group, proved to be as effective as other types of biological alkylating agents. Structure-activity studies established bifunctionality, a minimum level of reactivity, and appreciable solubility as requirements for anticancer activity in this class of chemically reactive compounds (409). These agents have not achieved clinical status; but on the other hand, hexitol derivatives of clinical interest, such as dibromomannitol (24.**166**, 1,6-dibromo-1,6-dideoxy-D-mannitol) (11) and dibromodulcitol (24.**169**, 1,6-dibromo-1,6-dideoxygalactitol), are reportedly converted *in vivo* to, among other things, the corresponding diepoxides, dianhydromannitol (24.**168**, 1,2:5,6-dianhydro-D-mannitol) and dianhydrogalactitol [24.**170**, 1,2:5,6-dianhydrogalactitol, galactitol, an investigational drug (362)], which may be the cytotoxic agents effecting cross-linking of DNA (410, 411). The *in vitro* formation of 24.**168** from 24.**166** and from mannitol myleran (24.**167**, D-mannitol 1,6-dimethanesulfonate) under slightly alkaline conditions has been demonstrated (412), and dianhydrohexitols have been found to exert a far greater cytostatic action than the parent compounds (413). These transformations are depicted in Fig. 24.13.

The hexitol family of agents grew from mannomustine [24.**171**, 1,6-bis(2-chloro-

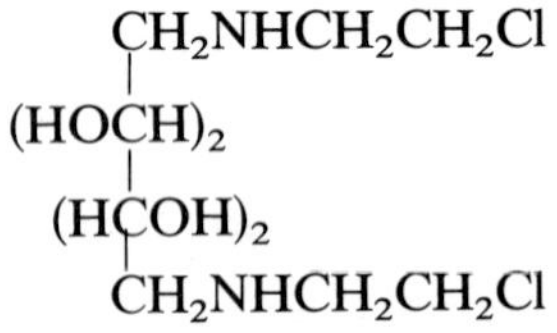

$CH_2NHCH_2CH_2Cl$
$(HOCH)_2$
$(HCOH)_2$
$CH_2NHCH_2CH_2Cl$
24.**171**

ethylamino)-1,6-dideoxy-D-mannitol, degranol], a nitrogen mustard analog whose antitumor activity was reportedly due to a stereospecific carrier group (414). In view

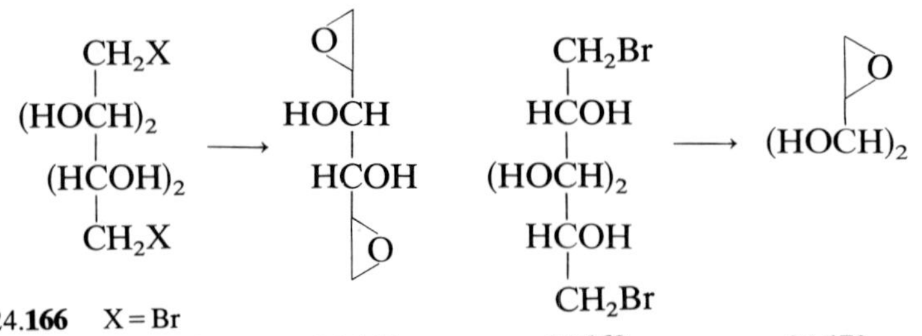

CH_2X / $(HOCH)_2$ / $(HCOH)_2$ / CH_2X ⟶ (epoxide) / $HOCH$ / $HCOH$ / (epoxide)

CH_2Br / $HCOH$ / $(HOCH)_2$ / $HCOH$ / CH_2Br ⟶ (epoxide) / $(HOCH)_2$ / (epoxide)

24.**166** X = Br
24.**167** X = OSO_2Me
24.**168**
24.**169**
24.**170**

Fig. 24.13 Transformation of hexitol derivatives to the corresponding diepoxides.

of the clinical limitations of hexitol derivatives owing to characteristic and undesirable effects on blood elements, the tetrafunctional dimesyldianhydroiditol (24.**172**,

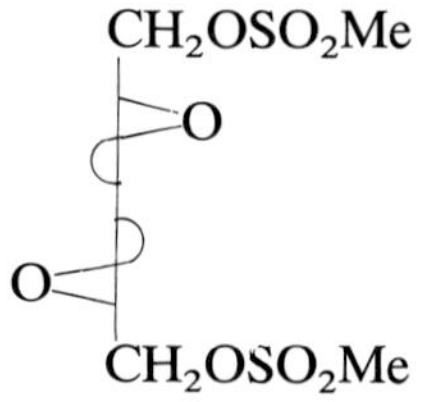

CH_2OSO_2Me ... CH_2OSO_2Me

24.**172**

2,3:4,5-dianhydro-L-iditol 1,6-dimethanesulfonate) has warranted attention because of its strong anticancer activity, yet reportedly mild effect on the hematopoietic system (415, 416).

2.2.5 NITROSOUREAS Among the newer types of chemically reactive anticancer agents that have risen to clinical prominence are the nitrosoureas. Extensive synthesis (417–421) and evaluation against experimental animal tumors (417–422) established a structure-activity pattern (423, 424) that led to successive clinical trials of BCNU [24.**173**, *N,N'*-bis(2-chloroethyl)-*N*-nitrosourea, carmustine] and orally administered CCNU [24.**174**, *N*-(2-chloroethyl)-*N'*-cyclohexyl-*N*-nitrosourea, lomustine], and MeCCNU [24.**175**, *N*-(2-chloroethyl)-*N'*-(*trans*-4-methylcyclohexyl)-*N*-nitrosourea, semustine] (425–427). An *N*-(2-chloroethyl)-*N*-nitrosoureido or *N*-(2-fluoroethyl)-*N*-nitrosoureido group proved

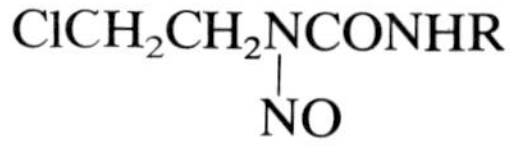

$ClCH_2CH_2N(NO)CONHR$

24.**173** R = CH_2CH_2Cl

24.**174** R = cyclohexyl

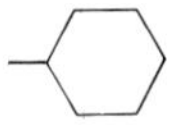

24.**175** R = 4-methylcyclohexyl

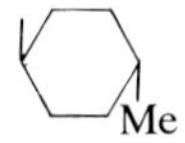

24.**179** R = 2,6-dioxo-3-piperidyl

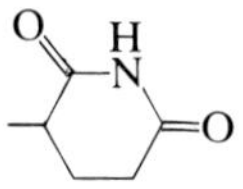

to be a structural requirement for optimal activity (cures) of leukemia L1210 implanted both intraperitoneally and intracerebrally. CCNU showed improved activity against the intracerebrally implanted tumor; MeCCNU showed superior activity against Lewis lung carcinoma (424, 428) and other experimental solid tumors. These agents are clinically active against a variety of solid neoplasms as well as Hodgkin's disease, but they appear to be most promising in the treatment of certain brain tumors (429, 430) and, particularly in combination with 5-fluorouracil, certain colon tumors (431, 432). In addition, MNU (24.**176**, *N*-methyl-*N*-nitrosourea) has undergone clinical trial in the Soviet Union,

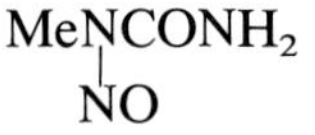

$MeN(NO)CONH_2$

24.**176**

where good activity in lung cancer and Hodgkin's disease was reported (433), and streptozotocin [24.**177**, 2-deoxy-2-[[(methylnitrosoamino)carbonyl]amino]-D-glucose], a natural nitrosourea (434) and broad spectrum antibiotic (435), has shown

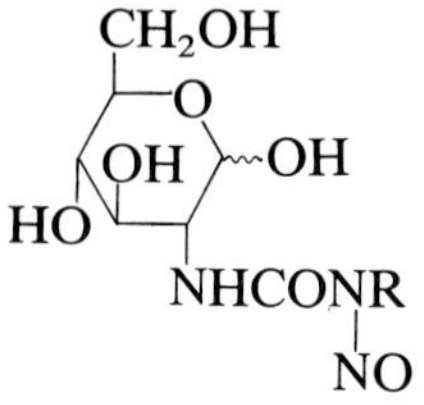

CH_2OH, O, OH, OH, HO, $NHCON(NO)R$

24.**177** R = Me
24.**178** R = CH_2CH_2Cl

clinical activity against functional pancreatic islet cell cancers (11, 436). Other congeners that are in preclinical study and may find clinical application are chlorozotocin [24.**178**, 2-[[[(2-chloroethyl)nitrosoamino]-carbonyl]amino]-2-deoxy-D-glucose], which was much more active against leukemia L1210 than streptozotocin (437) and showed reduced bone marrow toxicity in mice (438); and PCNU [24.**179**, *N*-(2-chloroethyl) *N'*-3-(2,6-dioxo-3-piperidyl-*N*-nitrosourea], which was exceptionally active against intracerebrally implanted leukemia L1210 (418) and rat sarcoma 9L (439).

Although the mechanism of action has not been established amid a multitude of chemical activities and biological effects (440), numerous studies on the behavior of nitrosoureas indicate that chemically reactive entities are produced under physiological conditions (441–446). The normal decomposition of an *N,N′*-disubstituted *N*-nitrosourea in phosphate buffer at pH 7.4 produces an alcohol, nitrogen, and an isocyanate, whose fate depends on the conditions under which it is generated:

$$F(CH_2)_2N(NO)CONHR \rightarrow F(CH_2)_2OH + N_2 + [RNCO]$$

Both *N,N′*-dicyclohexylurea and cyclohexylamine were identified as urinary metabolites of CCNU in mice, attesting to the intermediacy of cyclohexyl isocyanate (447). The aqueous decomposition of *N*-(2-chloroethyl)-*N*-nitrosoureas at pH 7.4, however, is complicated by the lability of the carbon–chlorine bond, both acetaldehyde and 2-chloroethanol being produced; two pathways for the formation of acetaldehyde have been proposed (Fig. 24.14). The reaction of one or more of these reactive species with biologic macromolecules is undoubtedly responsible for both anticancer activity and toxicity of the nitrosoureas, which provide a unique latentiation of carbocations and isocyanates. Results of *in vitro* and *in vivo* studies with different ^{14}C-labeled samples of CCNU were interpreted as a demonstration of the dual capacity of CCNU to alkylate nucleic acids and carbamoylate proteins (448, 449). The carbamoylation of lysine moieties of histone was similarly observed with BCNU (450). The nitrosoureas are monofunctional in regard to direct alkylation as exemplified by the active *N*-methyl-*N*-nitrosoureas, but *N*-(2-chloroethyl)-*N*-nitrosoureas appear to cross-link DNA by a two-step process involving transfer of a 2-chloroethyl cation to a nucleophilic site followed by displacement of chloride ion and suggesting a latent bifunctionality (451). One effect of protein carbamoylation appears to be interference with the repair of damaged DNA (452, 453). An attempted assessment of the relative importance of lipophilicity (partition

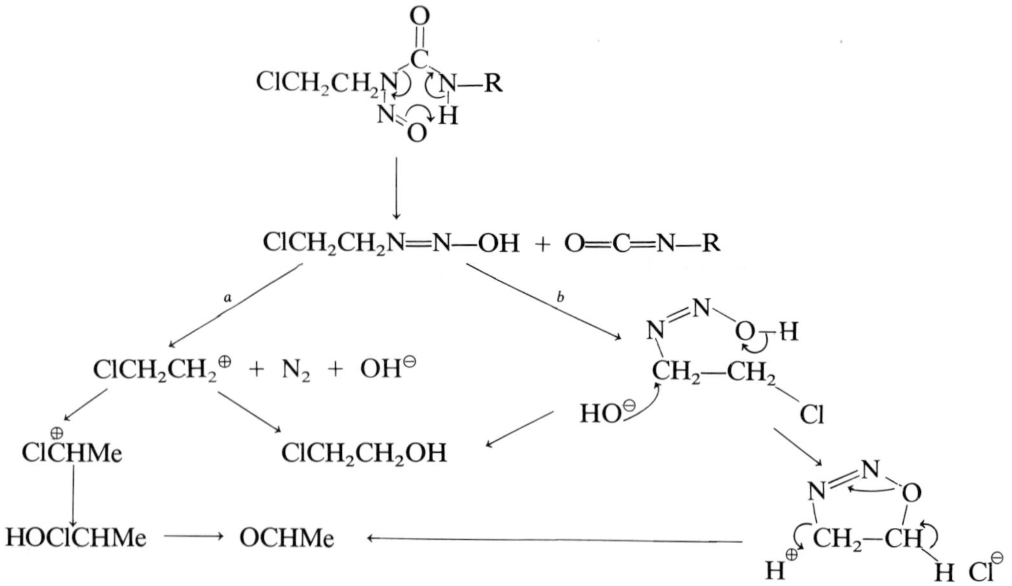

$ClCH_2CH_2N(NO)C(=O)NHR$

$\downarrow$

$ClCH_2CH_2N{=}N{-}OH + O{=}C{=}N{-}R$

a: $ClCH_2CH_2^{\oplus} + N_2 + OH^{\ominus}$ → $Cl\overset{\oplus}{C}HMe$ → $HOClCHMe$ → $OCHMe$; $ClCH_2CH_2^{\oplus}$ → $ClCH_2CH_2OH$

b: cyclic N=N–O–H / $CH_2{-}CH_2$ / Cl, $HO^{\ominus}$ → $ClCH_2CH_2OH$; → cyclic N=N–O / $CH_2{-}CH$, $H^{\oplus}$, H $Cl^{\ominus}$ → $OCHMe$

Fig. 24.14 Proposed pathways for the formation of acetaldehyde in the decomposition of *N*-(2-chloroethyl)-*N*-nitrosoureas at pH 7.4.

coefficient), alkylating activity, and carbamoylating activity to therapeutic activity against leukemia L1210 led to the conclusion that all three are important: lipophilicity as a major factor in transport, alkylating activity as a major determinant of therapeutic index, and carbamoylating activity as a contributing factor to whole animal toxicity (454).

The rapid hydroxylation of the cyclohexyl ring of CCNU by liver microsomes (455, 456) raised the possibility that the anticancer activity of CCNU is due primarily to its metabolites. The activity of CCNU in rats produced varying ratios of possibly all six of the ring-monohydroxylated derivatives (457–460), but only the *cis*-4 and *trans*-4 isomers were found (in about equal amounts) in human plasma following the intravenous administration of CCNU (460). Synthetic samples of the six hydroxy isomers (461, 462) showed better therapeutic indexes than CCNU in evaluations against both intraperitoneally and intracerebrally implanted leukemia L1210, but the alkylating and carbamoylating activities of individual isomers were markedly affected by the position and steric configuration of the hydroxy substituent (462). On the other hand, liver microsomes denitrosate BCNU, converting it into *N,N'*-bis(2-chloroethyl)-urea (456), which is inactive against leukemia L1210. The rates of microsomal metabolism of BCNU, CCNU, and MeCCNU are fast enough to allow metabolism of large portions of administered doses before chemical decomposition occurs (456). Fully substituted nitrosoureas having a suitably positioned methyl group as in *N*-(2-chloroethyl)-*N'*-methyl-*N*-nitroso-*N'*-propylurea (24.**180**) were shown to be relatively stable in aqueous solution and active against leukemia L1210 only *in vivo*, an observation indicative of enzymatic demethylation (463).

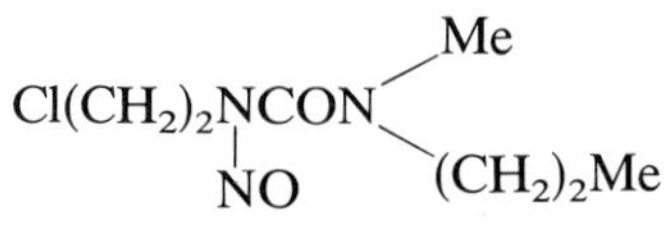

$Cl(CH_2)_2N(NO)CON(Me)(CH_2)_2Me$

24.**180**

2.2.6 TRIAZENOIMIDAZOLES. The triazenes first reported to inhibit mouse neoplasms were 3,3-dimethyl-1-phenyltriazene (24.**181**) and derivatives thereof (464, 465). The carcinogenicity of triazenes prompted studies of the action of liver microsomes on

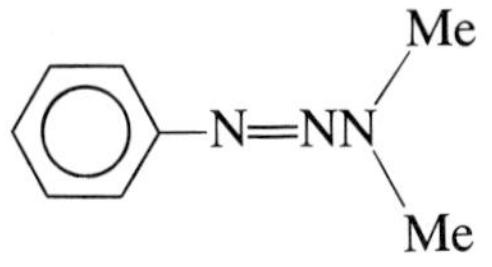

$C_6H_5{-}N{=}NN(Me)_2$

24.**181**

24.**181**, which revealed extensive demethylation and provided the basis for a proposed metabolic pathway involving the generation of methyl cations as the reactive species responsible for activity (466). This type of mechanism, supported by enzymatic, metabolic, biological, and chemical studies, was later validated for the triazenoimidazoles (467, 468), which, by virtue of their activation by enzymatic *N*-dealkylation, represent a new type of clinical alkylating agent.

Interest in the triazenoimidazoles began with the synthesis (469) of a series of dialkyl derivatives as latentiated forms of 5-diazoimidazole-4-carboxamide, a precursor of 2-azahypoxanthine and an unstable compound that had shown some activity against experimental tumors (470). The most promising member of the series was the dimethyl derivative 24.**182** [5-(3,3-dimethyl-1-triazenyl)-1*H*-imidazole-4-carboxamide, dacarbazine, DTIC], which was active against leukemia L1210 and two solid tumors, sarcoma 180 and adenocarcinoma 755 (471, 472). It was this broad spectrum of activity that engendered clinical trials of DTIC, which emerged as a drug of choice in the treatment of melanotic melanoma (473, 474) and has shown synergistic activity with adriamycin in the treatment of soft tissue sarcomas (475).

Structure-activity relationships of several

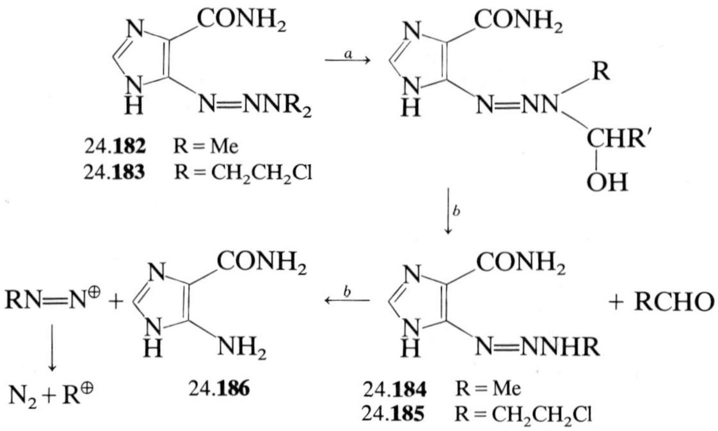

24.**182** R = Me
24.**183** R = CH_2CH_2Cl

24.**186**

24.**184** R = Me
24.**185** R = CH_2CH_2Cl

Fig. 24.15 Metabolism of DTIC (24.**182**) and BTIC (24.**183**). (*a*) Microsomal oxidases, NADPH, O_2. (*b*) Spontaneous.

series of structural variants of DTIC (476–479) revealed a number of congeners having activity against leukemia L1210, but none was significantly better than DTIC. The unstable monomethyl analog (24.**184**, MIC), which rapidly decomposes in solution, even in the absence of light, to form 5 - amino - 1*H* - imidazole - 4 - carboxamide (24.**186**, AIC) and a short-lived methyldiazonium ion (Fig. 24.15) was about as active as DTIC in animal tumor systems (480); in aqueous media, the methyldiazonium ion reacts primarily with water to form methanol (481). The activities of DTIC and MIC were eventually exceeded, however, by those of the corresponding 2-chloroethyl derivatives 24.**183** [5-[3,3-bis(2-chloroethyl)-1-triazenyl]-1*H*-imidazole-4-carboxamide, BTIC] (482) and 24.**185** [5-[3-(2-chloroethyl)-1-triazenyl]-1*H*-imidazole-4-carboxamide] (467). As an anticancer agent, BTIC has been much more effective in mice than in man (483); the disappointing clinical trials of BTIC were perhaps due to formulation difficulties arising from facile transformation to the inactive triazolinium chloride 24.**187** (468).

Enzymatic conversions of ^{14}C-labeled DTIC to AIC (24.**186**), formaldehyde, and nucleic acids containing radioactive 7-methylguanine were demonstrated with microsomal preparations (484, 485), showing demethylation by microsomal oxidases and the generation of a methylating agent. Like the monomethyltriazene 24.**184** (480), the mono(2-chloroethyl)triazene 24.**185**

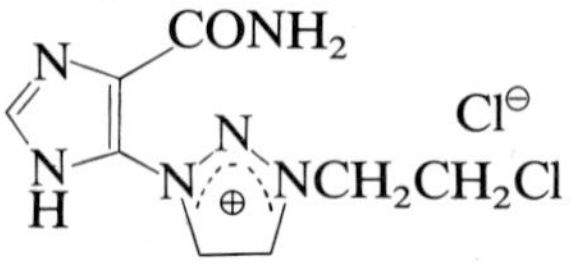

24.**187**

also dissociated in water to AIC; the accompanying generation of the 2-chloroethyl cation was evidenced by the formation of 2-chloroethanol in high yield (467). [Here the 2-chloroethyl cation was not a major precursor of acetaldehyde, as has been postulated for the (2-chloroethyl)-nitrosoureas (446).] Moreover, the microsomal oxidation of BTIC to form AIC has been demonstrated (486). Thus microsomal activation relates the biological activities of corresponding mono- and disubstituted triazenes (Fig. 24.15).

Investigations of the elevated urinary excretion of AIC in patients given DTIC suggested a direct biotransformation rather than interference with the metabolism of AIC (487, 488). The primary urinary metabolite of BTIC was found to be the ionic transformation product 24.**187** (489), which was previously observed to form readily *in vitro* and was inactive against leukemia L1210 (482).

2.2.7 PROCARBAZINE. Several methylhydrazine derivatives, originally prepared as monoamine oxidase inhibitors (490), were reported to have activity against experimental animal tumors (491). The most promising of these was procarbazine [24.**188**, *N*-(1-methylethyl)-4-[(2-methylhydrazino)methyl]benzamide], which received extensive animal and clinical trials as a new type of agent (11, 492).

Procarbazine is rapidly and extensively metabolized *in vivo*, and since freshly prepared solutions of procarbazine do not inhibit tumor cells *in vitro* (493, 494), it seems probable that the metabolites are involved in its biologic activity (492, 495). Azoprocarbazine [24.**189**, 4-[(methylazo)methyl]-*N*-(1-methylethyl)benzamide], which is also cytotoxic (496), is the initial product of *in vivo* oxidation of procarbazine (497), and 4-[[(1-methylethyl)amino]-carbonyl]benzoic acid (24.**191**) is the major urinary metabolite (498). The formation of a methylating agent is supported by the identification of 7-methylguanine in the urine of mice given procarbazine (499), yet the active intermediate and the metabolic pathway leading to it are undecided. The ratios of methane and carbon dioxide metabolically derived from the *N*-methyl group suggest multiple metabolic pathways, and a possibly minor pathway (Fig. 24.16) postulating the formation of methyldiazene (24.**190**), an oxygen-mediated source of methyl radicals (500) and a potentially proximate methylating agent (10), may be the key to the cytotoxic action of procarbazine (492). The importance of the methylation of nucleic acids to the biologic activity of procarbazine is still unclear because the low level of methylation observed would not be expected to produce significant cell toxicity (501), and the role of free radicals derivable *in vivo* is still equivocal (492).

Procarbazine proved to be useful in the treatment of advanced Hodgkin's disease (11) and is being used in combination with nitrosoureas in the therapy of brain tumors (430).

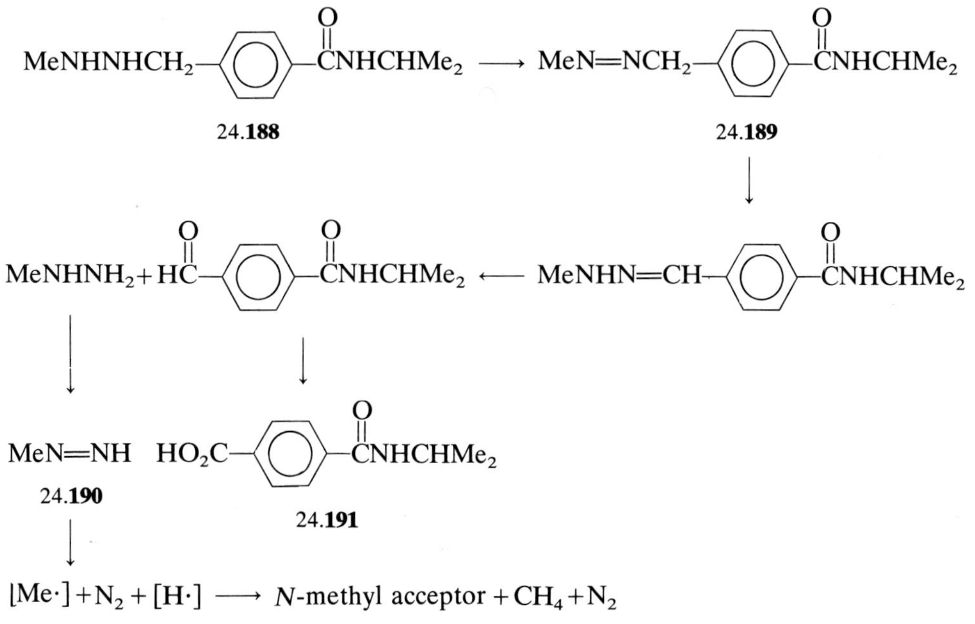

$MeNHNHCH_2-C_6H_4-C(=O)NHCHMe_2$ (24.**188**) ⟶ $MeN{=}NCH_2-C_6H_4-C(=O)NHCHMe_2$ (24.**189**)

↓

$MeNHN{=}CH-C_6H_4-C(=O)NHCHMe_2$ ⟶ $MeNHNH_2 + HC(=O)-C_6H_4-C(=O)NHCHMe_2$

↓ ↓

$MeN{=}NH$ (24.**190**) $HO_2C-C_6H_4-C(=O)NHCHMe_2$ (24.**191**)

↓

$[Me\cdot] + N_2 + [H\cdot]$ ⟶ *N*-methyl acceptor $+ CH_4 + N_2$

Fig. 24.16 A proposed pathway in the metabolism of procarbazine.

2.3 DNA Complexors

2.3.1 THE ACTINOMYCINS. The first actinomycins were isolated from *Actinomycetes* in 1940 (502), and since that time a number of structural variants have been reported (503). These bright red materials are powerful bacteriostatic agents and are extremely toxic (504, 505). Their cytostatic properties aroused interest in their potential anticancer activity (506).

All the actinomycins contain the same 2-amino-4,6-dimethylphenoxaz-3-one-4,5-dicarboxylic acid chromophore with a varicty of polypeptide side chains attached by way of the carboxyl functions (503). The lactone rings and polypeptide chains, although variable, are absolutely required for biologic activity, since the free chromophore is not active (507). Also essential are the amino group function at C-2 and the carbonyl function at C-3 (507).

Actinomycin D (24.**192**), one of the most potent of these agents, complexes with DNA and selectively inhibits RNA synthesis, the synthesis of ribosomal RNA being preferentially affected. In a model for the

```
        O                    O
        ‖                    ‖
        C——┐            ┌——C
(Me)2CHCH   |            |   CHCH(Me)2
        |   |            |   |
   Me—N     O    O     N—Me
        |                     |
   Sarcosine          Sarcosine
        |                     |
   L-Proline           L-Proline
        |                     |
   D-Valine            D-Valine
        |                     |
       CO                    CO
        |                     |
       NH—CH  CH—NH
        |     |     |     |
       CO   Me   Me   CO
               N              NH2
                              
               O              O
      Me                  Me
```

24.**192**

actinomycin-DNA complex based on X-ray data obtained from a crystalline complex of actinomycin and 2′-deoxyguanosine, the phenoxazine ring system intercalates between adjacent G—C base pairs of DNA, where the guanine moieties are on opposite DNA strands, and the 2-amino groups of the guanines interact with both cyclic peptides through specific hydrogen bonds. As in other models, the cyclic peptides lie in the minor groove of helical DNA (508).

Used alone for the treatment of disseminated cancers, actinomycin D has proved to be of value against Wilms' tumor, soft tissue sarcomas, trophoblastic malignancies, and testicular tumors. Its usefulness in the treatment of malignant melanoma is controversial, and it appears to be without activity against breast, lung, and colorectal cancer (11).

2.3.2 MITHRAMYCIN. Mithramycin (24.**193**), another *Streptomyces* antibiotic with antitumor properties, is thought to stabilize the secondary structure of DNA by forming bridges between complementary strands of the helix, but the precise geometry of its binding is not known. Mithramycin's inhibition of protein and DNA synthesis was not dose related, indicating that the primary effect of its DNA binding is on RNA synthesis (509). Mithramycin produced a 32% response rate in patients with testicular cancer, but because of its toxicity, it has received only limited clinical trials (11). Olivomycin and chromomycin A_3 are close structural relatives of mithramycin.

2.3.3 THE BLEOMYCINS. The bleomycins are relatively high molecular weight peptide antibiotics (394, 510) (see Chapter 16). Of the two antibiotic complexes that have been described, bleomycin A was superior to bleomycin B in antitumor activity, inhibiting Ehrlich carcinoma, sarcoma 180, and Yoshida sarcoma cells in culture. From the bleomycin A complex, bleomycin A_2 has been isolated and partially characterized. The bleomycins bind to DNA and

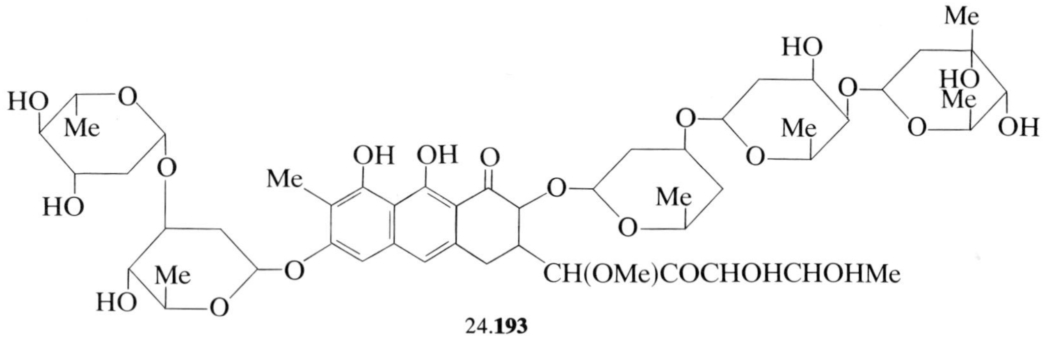

CH(OMe)COCHOHCHOHMe

24.**193**

cause cleavage of the macromolecule. It has been suggested that the drug establishes a span, reinforced by sulfur linkages, across diester bonds in the sugar phosphate skeleton. A consideration of the entropy involved in preventing free rotation around the 3′- or 5′-linkage indicates that chain rupture would occur, satisfactorily explaining the observed effects of the complexes. Bleomycin has produced objective tumor response in 30–60% of patients with lymphoma, in 40–70% of patients with testicular tumors, and in 20–40% of patients with squamous cell carcinomas of various primary sites (11).

2.3.4 THE ANTHRACYCLINES. Of the various antibiotics that owe their activity to binding to DNA, the anthracyclines duanomycin (24.**194**) and adriamycin (24.**195**) appear to be the most promising for clinical applications (511, 512). Adriamycin seems to be somewhat more active, since it is effective against a number of solid tumors as well as against the lymphomas and acute leukemias. Despite this broad spectrum of activity, the duration of drug response is often disappointingly short, leading to the use of adriamycin in combination with other drugs. Minor toxic effects of the drug include alopecia and nausea. More serious is the dose-related and irreversible cardiac myopathy that often leads to congestive heart failure.

Both duanomycin and adriamycin are extensively metabolized *in vivo*, the main metabolites resulting from reduction of the carbonyl function to an alcohol (see Fig. 24.17) (10, 511, 512). Since these alcohols seem to be as biologically active as the parent drugs, this enzymatic reduction may be important to their activity.

The anthracyclines are thought to intercalate into DNA, and the consequent alteration in stereochemical configuration to cause steric hindrance to the formation of the hypothetical DNA:DNA polymerase complex. The same mechanism should be operative for both DNA polymerase and DNA-dependent RNA polymerase, since duanomycin, unlike actinomycin D, inhibits both polymerizations nearly equally (511, 512).

Recently a number of chemical modifications of adriamycin and duanomycin have been made. One of the most promising of these, AD 32 (513), is an *N,O*-diacyl derivative that appears to be *O*-deacylated *in vivo*.

2.4 The Mitotic Inhibitors

The vinca alkaloids, colchicine derivatives, the podophyllotoxins, and griseofulvin may be considered to constitute a single class of agents in view of the many similarities in their biological actions, most notably their ability to produce metaphase arrest, probably through microtubule interactions that cause spindle dissolution, interference with some phases of phagacytosis, and changes in morphology and motility. Although a number of other effects of these compounds have been observed, such as the

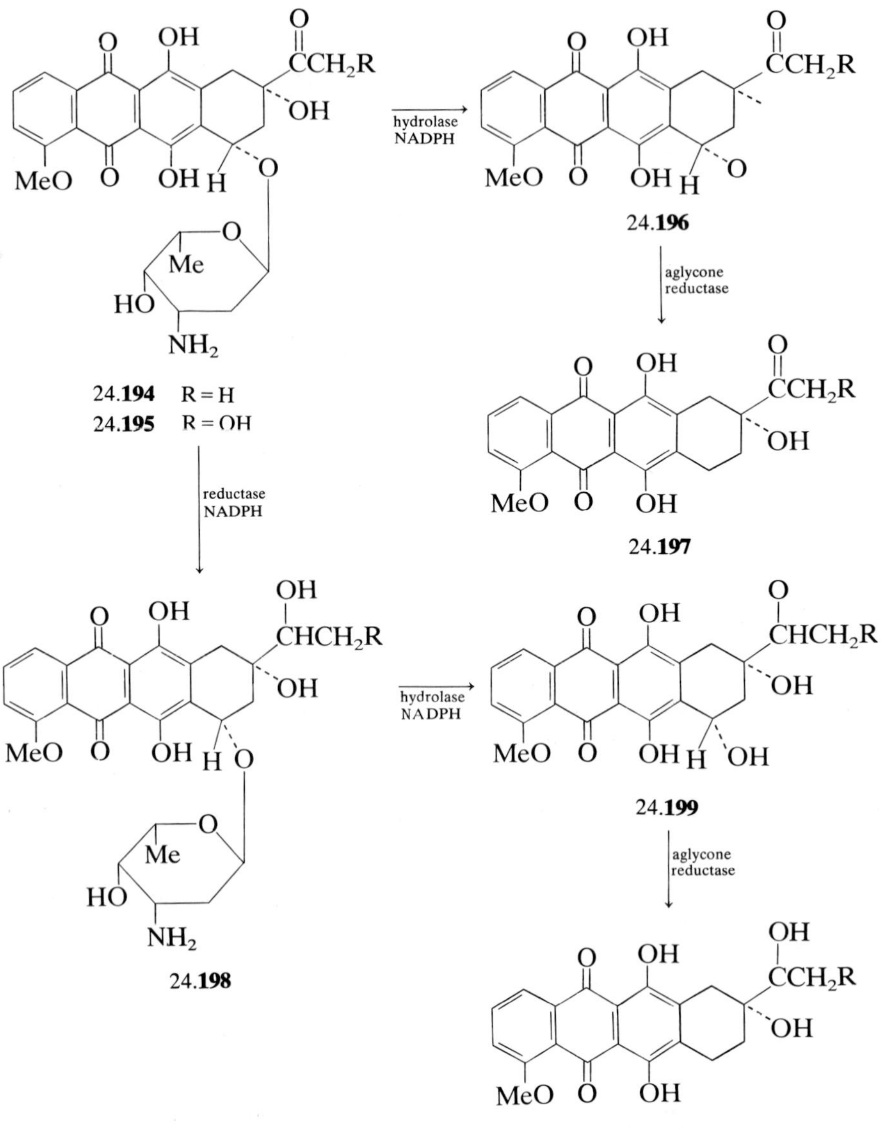

24.**194** R = H
24.**195** R = OH

reductase NADPH

hydrolase NADPH

24.**196**

aglycone reductase

24.**197**

24.**198**

hydrolase NADPH

24.**199**

aglycone reductase

24.**200**

Fig. 24.17 Metabolism of duanomycin (24.**194**) and adriamycin (24.**195**).

inhibition of RNA synthesis, mitotic arrest is probably the most important to their cytotoxicity and antitumor activity (514, 515).

In cancer chemotherapy, the vinca alkaloids are the only antimitotic agents to be recognized as truly important and valuable drugs. Although the more recent podophyllum derivatives, VM-26 and podophyllic acid ethyl hydrazide, are currently of interest and are receiving clinical trials of some promise, in the past agents of this class have not proved to be of any real value. The vinca alkaloids are effective in the treatment of the leukemias, lymphomas, choriocarcinoma, Wilms' tumor, neuroblastoma, rhabdomyosarcoma, and carcinoma of the testis and are less effective in the treatment of a variety of other solid tumors, such as breast and lung. There are significant differences in the spectra of activity of vinblastine (24.**201**) and vincristine (24.**202**), with vincristine appearing to be the more effective of the two overall (11).

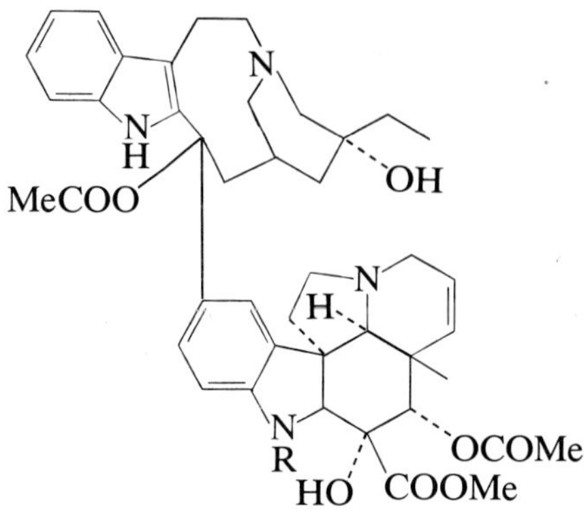

24.**201** R = Me
24.**202** R = CHO

Certain chemical modifications have produced compounds that may be superior to the natural products (516).

2.5 Hormones

Cancer of certain organs that are normally subject to hormonal regulation may respond favorably to hormonal therapy. The first effective chemotherapy of human cancer with structurally defined entities was the treatment of cancer of the breast (517, 518) and of the prostate (519) with hormonal agents. Hormonal therapy is based on the concept that neoplastic cells derived from a hormone-responsive organ may likewise be subject to hormonal control, at least during some part of the life of the neoplasm. Hormonal therapy of these kinds of cancer may sometimes produce dramatic results (520), but not all tumors of a hormone-responsive organ are hormone responsive, and most of the hormone-responsive tumors eventually become reactivated and refractory. Alteration of the hormonal milieu causes remissions of some cases of cancer of the breast, prostate, and endometrium, and hormonal therapy of tumors of other organs, such as the kidney, may also produce favorable results. In addition, malignant lymphomas and leukemias may be suppressed by administered hormones.

Cancer of the breast is one of the most prevalent forms of human cancer and is the leading cause of cancer deaths among women in the United States (521). The conventional initial treatment of primary breast cancer is mastectomy, frequently followed by postoperative irradiation of surrounding areas as adjuvant therapy (e.g., 522–528). Until recently, treatment of advanced inoperable mammary cancer, disseminated cancer beyond the reach of surgical or radiological treatment, or recurrent mammary cancer (already treated by surgery or radiation) was based on alteration of the hormonal status of the patient (e.g., 529–534). Hormonal alteration, which sometimes produces profoundly favorable results, is accomplished either by endocrine gland ablation (surgical or radiological) or by administration of exogenous hormones or hormone analogs. Therapy by hormonal deprivation began in 1896 with the report by Beatson (535) of regression of inoperable breast cancer following ovariectomy (castration, oophorectomy). Data accumulated over many years show that castration induces remissions in about one-third of premenopausal patients (529–532, 536–538), and this type of therapy is still considered (538–541) to be the most effective method of hormonal treatment of advanced breast cancer in premenopausal women and may also be of value in postmenopausal women with some residual ovarian function. Bilateral adrenalectomy is an endocrine ablative measure introduced originally (542, 543) for the purpose of removing another source of endogenous estrogenic hormones, and it likewise induces temporary remissions in a significant percentage of patients so treated (529–532, 537, 538, 544, 545). Hypophysectomy (546, 547) (pituitary ablation) has also been found to produce objective regressions of metastatic breast cancer (529–532, 538, 545–548) by removing hormones that act on the breast directly and by way of steroids (533). In general, adrenalectomy and hypophysectomy are not undertaken until castration and hormone administration have been tried (541).

A few years after testosterone (24.**203**) had been isolated, it (or its esters) was

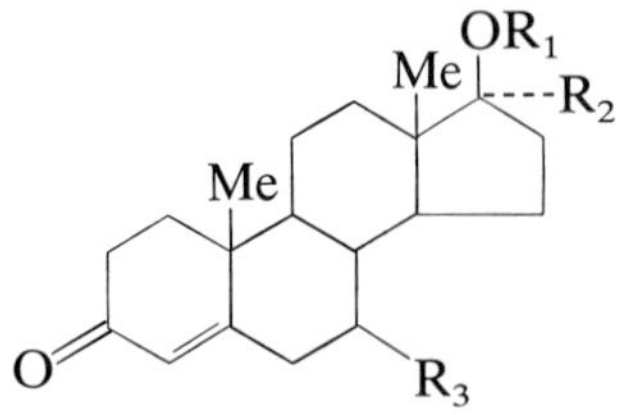

24.**203** $R_1 = R_2 = R_3 = H$
24.**204** $R_1 = COC_2H_5$, $R_2 = R_3 = H$
24.**205** $R_1 = H$, $R_2 = R_3 = Me$

reported to be beneficial to patients with recurrent breast cancer (517, 518, 549–552), and these reports included evidence of some objective regressions. The assumption of an estrogenic induction or sustenance of breast cancer, combined with the antagonistic action of testosterone on the physiological effects of estrogens, motivated these early investigations. Soon after the introduction of androgen therapy, favorable responses of some cases of breast cancer in postmenopausal women to treatment with the estrogens diethylstilbestrol (α,α'-diethyl-4,4′-stilbenediol, 24.**206**) (553, 554) and 17α-ethynylestradiol (24.**207**) (555) were reported. The effectiveness of both androgens and estrogens

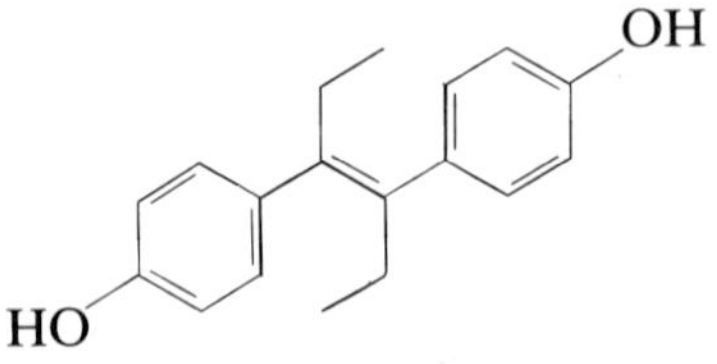

24.**206**

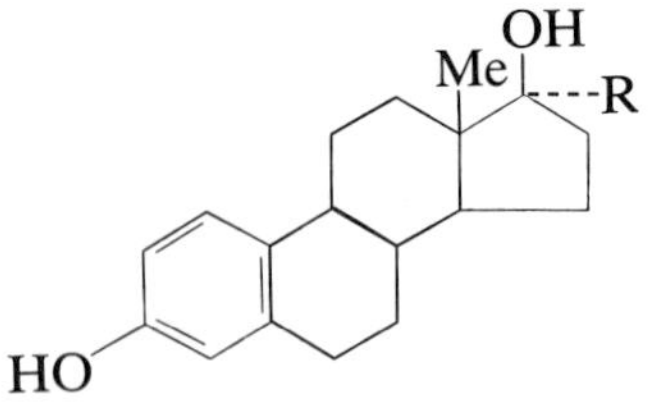

24.**207** R = —C≡CH
24.**208** R = H

was confirmed in subsequent clinical studies (e.g., 556, 557).

The classical androgen for the treatment of advanced, metastatic breast cancer is testosterone propionate (24.**204**). Data generated by numerous clinical evaluations have led to a generally accepted objective regression rate for testosterone propionate (and other androgens) of about 20–25% (529–534, 541, 556, 558–562). A cooperative clinical study that included a large number of androgens, estrogens, progestogens, and corticosteroids was carried out by the Cooperative Breast Cancer Group under the auspices of the National Cancer Institute (559–565). Among the many androgens or androgen analogs evaluated in small groups of patients by the Cooperative Breast Cancer Group, a substantial number were as effective as testosterone propionate; but none—except, possibly, calusterone (564, 565)—was significantly better. Although strong androgens generally produced some objective regressions (566, 567), certain other compounds with little, or no, androgenic activity or with differing anabolic-androgenic ratios gave similar regression rates (558, 566, 567). There was a similar lack of parallelism between antitumor activity and the capacity of a steroid to depress urinary gonadotropin excretion (558, 566, 567).

As a result of these clinical studies (559–565), and others, the androgens most commonly used (539–541, 558, 568–571) in the treatment of human breast cancer are testosterone propionate (24.**204**) and other testosterone esters, 2α-methyldihydrotestosterone propionate (dromostanolone propionate, 2α-methyl-17β-hydroxy-5α-androstan-3-one propionate), fluoxymesterone (11β,17β-dihydroxy-9α-fluoro-17α-methylandrost-4-en-3-one), 1-dehydrotestololactone (testolactone, 17α-oxa-D-homoandrosta-1,4-dien-3,17-dione), and calusterone (24.**205**, 7β,17α-dimethyltestosterone). 2α-Methyldihydrotestosterone, a potent anabolic agent, is less virilizing than testosterone propionate at equally effective doses (539, 572). Fluoxymesterone, a strongly androgenic and anabolic agent (573, 574), is similar in clinical effectiveness to testosterone propionate, but it is an orally active androgen showing less virilization than comparably effective oral androgens (539). 1-Dehydrotestololactone is devoid of hormonal activity in routine bioassays (575) and is not virilizing in patients (576). Calusterone (24.**205**) (577) is a weakly androgenic, orally active steroid that was introduced more recently than the other commonly employed androgen analogs. It is said to be the most effective steroid for primary or secondary hormonal therapy of breast cancer patients (564, 565, 578).

Estrogens, administered in high doses, are generally considered (529–532, 534, 541, 556, 569, 579) to be superior to androgens for hormonal therapy of breast cancer in postmenopausal women, with objective responses being observed in about one-third of the treated patients. Estrogens manifest a biphasic effect on mammary tumor growth; small doses may accelerate tumor growth, whereas large (pharmacologic) doses may cause regression (558). There is little, or no, difference in effectiveness among different estrogens (541); the estrogens used clinically against breast cancer are diethylstilbestrol (24.**206**), 17α-ethynylestradiol (24.**207**), and esters of 17β-estradiol (24.**208**) (541, 558, 569–571).

Recently, investigations of the therapy of breast cancer have focused on the role of estrogen receptors in predicting responses to hormonal therapy, the clinical use of nonsteroidal antiestrogens, and the employment of cytotoxic chemotherapeutic agents. Intracellular receptor proteins for the various classes of steroid hormones (estrogens, androgens, progestogens, and corticosteroids) have been detected and characterized. Among these classes, intracellular receptors for estrogens in target tissues, as well as the presence or absence of these receptors in relation to breast cancer, have been most extensively studied and widely reviewed (580–593). An essential characteristic of an estrogen target cell is the capacity to bind estradiol specifically and with great affinity. The following sequence of events is now considered to comprise the mechanism of estrogen action (580–582, 584, 589, 590). After the hormone has entered the target cell, apparently by passive diffusion, it binds to the cytoplasmic form of the receptor protein, which is specific for each target tissue. The estrogen-receptor complex undergoes an activation step. The transformed complex is then translocated to the nucleus, where it binds to an acceptor site on the chromatin. In the nucleus, the estrogen-receptor complex stimulates RNA synthesis (transcription) and subsequent formation of cellular proteins (translation).

Studies of estrogen receptors in both animal and human breast tumor tissue have shown that hormone-responsive breast cancers contain significant amounts of estrogen receptors, whereas tumors that are not hormone-responsive are deficient in estrogen receptors (582–590, 592). This correlation between the presence of estrogen receptors and hormone-responsiveness is the basis for the use of estrogen-receptor measurements to select patients on a logical basis for hormonal therapy. About 55–60% of receptor-positive patients will respond to hormonal additive therapy or to endocrine ablative therapy (593–595). Equally important, accumulated data indicate that the absence of measurable receptors negates the usefulness of hormonal manipulations. Receptor-negative patients may thus be spared major surgical procedures or ineffective hormonal treatment and its accompanying side effects; furthermore, cytotoxic chemotherapy may be started earlier in such patients.

Inhibition of the uptake of estrogens by antiestrogens has been a valuable tool in the study of estrogen receptors. Antiestrogens antagonize estrogen-induced responses of one or more target organs (e.g., uterus, breast, vagina, pituitary), but most antiestrogens are also weakly estrogenic (596–598). Several well-known antiestrogens are related structurally to the strong estrogen chlorotrianisene (24.**209**). The mechanism of action of antiestrogens is generally considered to involve the complex between estradiol and cytoplasmic protein receptors (598, 599). Competitive binding of antiestrogens to cytoplasmic estrogen receptors (600–603), allosteric inhibition (binding at a second site) of the receptors (604), failure of antiestrogens to stimulate replenishment of receptor proteins (605), and inhibition of translocation of the estrogen-receptor complex to the nucleus (606) have all been proposed as the mode of interference with receptor function by antiestrogens. The antiestrogens clomiphene (24.**210**), nafoxidene, and tamoxifen (24.**211**) have been evaluated in a substantial number of breast cancer patients and have elicited response rates of about 30% (599). [Tamoxifen is the trans isomer, as represented by 24.**211**. Clomiphene is a mixture of cis and trans isomers. The original assignment of structures to the separate isomers has recently been reversed (599, 607), and the antiestrogen, formerly considered to be the cis isomer, is the trans isomer (24.**210**.] These response rates indicate that antiestrogens are comparable in effectiveness to estrogens and may be somewhat superior to androgens. They offer advantages over both of these types of additive hormonal therapy because the side effects of antiestrogens are milder.

R_1 R_2 R_2 R_3

24.**209** $R_1 = R_2 = MeO$, $R_3 = Cl$
24.**210** $R_1 = O(CH_2)_2NEt_2$, $R_2 = H$, $R_3 = Cl$
24.**211** $R_1 = O(CH_2)_2NMe_2$, $R_2 = H$, $R_3 = Et$

Estrogens are also used in the treatment of prostatic cancer, one of the most prevalent forms of malignancy in men. Since the growth and function of the prostate are under the regulation of androgens, the principal goal of hormonal therapy of advanced prostatic cancer is the suppression of androgenic stimuli. Beginning in 1941, Huggins and co-workers introduced orchiectomy (castration) and estrogen administration, to counteract androgenic stimulation of the prostate, as methods of controlling human prostatic cancer (519, 608, 609). Tumor regression and depression of the serum acid phosphatase concentration, which frequently is elevated in advanced prostatic cancer (610–613), occurred in most of the patients treated by orchiectomy or with diethylstilbestrol. Since the pioneering work of Huggins and Hodges (519), the various methods of endocrine therapy employed in the treatment of advanced prostatic cancer have included orchiectomy, estrogen administration, adrenalectomy, hypophysectomy, corticosteroid administration, and (more recently) administration of antiandrogens (538, 614–618); but adrenalectomy and hypophysectomy, which remove extratesticular stimuli of prostatic tissue—androgens (testosterone precursors) produced by the adrenal gland and prolactin and LH by the pituitary (618)—are now infrequently used (538, 616).

Estrogens are potent inhibitors of

gonadotropin secretion, and it is believed that they exert their major effect on prostatic cancer by suppressing LH release by the pituitary, thereby inhibiting testicular testosterone production (615, 616, 618). Estrogens may also have a direct effect on testicular steroidogenesis and on the prostate (616, 618). Estrogens employed (558, 570, 571, 616, 619, 620) in the clinical treatment of prostatic cancer are diethylstilbestrol (24.**206**), ethynylestradiol (24.**207**), chlorotrianisene (24.**209**), diethylstilbestrol diphosphate, and polyestradiol phosphate. About 60–80% of patients with disseminated prostatic cancer are benefited temporarily by diethylstilbestrol (558, 613), the estrogen that is probably most widely used to treat prostatic cancer. Survival of 40% of patients with metastatic disease for more than 5 years after initiation of therapy with polyestradiol phosphate (620, 621) and an increase in this survival rate to 62% by treatment with both estradiol polyphosphate, a fairly weak gonadotopin inhibitor, and ethynylestradiol, a stronger gonadotropin inhibitor, have been reported (621). Regardless of the type of estrogen treatment given, most patients with prostatic cancer eventually relapse (613, 621).

Recently, estramustine phosphate, an estradiol derivative containing a deactivated bis(2-chloroethyl) group, has shown considerable promise against prostatic cancer (621–624), and side effects are minimal (621). This compound may have a role in the primary treatment of prostatic carcinoma (625), since the response rate was greater in previously untreated patients (621, 623).

Antiandrogens interfere with the action of androgens at the target organ. The antiandrogen cyproterone acetate (24.**212**) has elicited symptomatic improvement and objective regressions in a considerable number of patients with advanced prostatic carcinoma (626, 627). The side effects are less serious than those produced by estrogens;

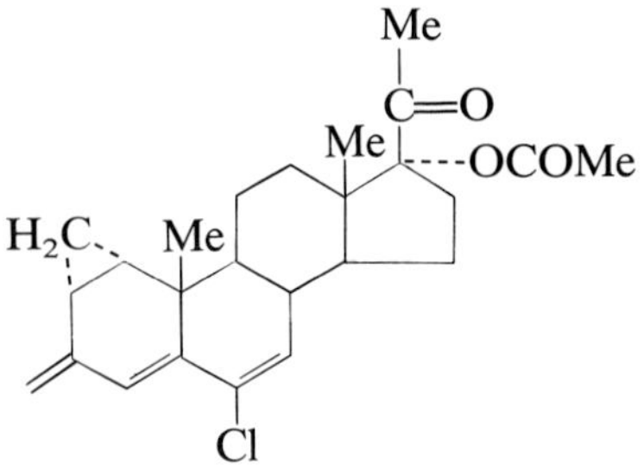

Me C=O Me OCOMe H_2C Me Cl

24.**212**

and, as with estramustine phosphate, the response rate was greater in patients who had not previously received conventional therapy. Like anticstrogens, antiandrogens apparently act at the level of the intracellular hormone-receptor complex (628, 629). In prostate cells, testosterone is first reduced to dihydrotestosterone (17β-hydroxy-5α-androst-4-en-3-one), which binds to a cytoplasmic receptor protein; then the sequence of events is similar to that described for estrogen receptors. The potential of the hormone-receptor area and of antiandrogens for further development is illustrated by the nonsteroidal antiandrogen flutamide [24.**213**, 4′-nitro-3′-(trifluoro-

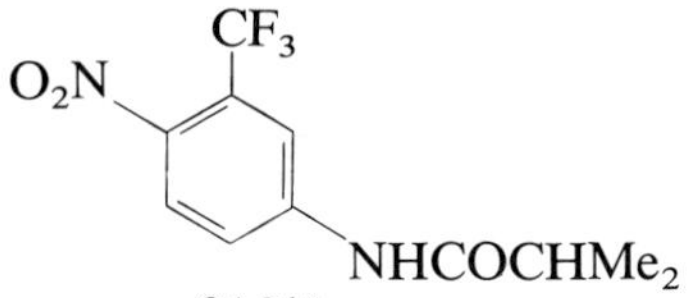

CF_3 O_2N $NHCOCHMe_2$

24.**213**

methyl)isobutyranilide], a potent antiandrogen that may have considerable utility in the treatment of prostatic cancer (625, 629).

Progestogens (compounds related in structure or in biological effects to progesterone) have been employed for the hormonal therapy of several kinds of cancer. Although certain progestogens included in the clinical evaluations of the Cooperative Breast Cancer Group (560, 561) produced some regressions, the effectiveness of progestogens in breast cancer is controversial (558, 569, 630). Advanced, primary carcinoma of the uterus (endometrium) or disseminated endometrial cancer recurrent after surgery (hysterectomy), radiation therapy, or a combination of these procedures may respond to progestational agents. Objective remissions occur in 30–35% of patients treated with 17α-hydroxyprogesterone hexanoate (24.**214**, delalutin) or medroxyprogesterone acetate (24.**215**) (558, 630–635). Treatment of metastatic cancer of the kidney with medroxyprogesterone acetate has induced remission in about 20% of the patients in some, but apparently not all, clinical studies (558,

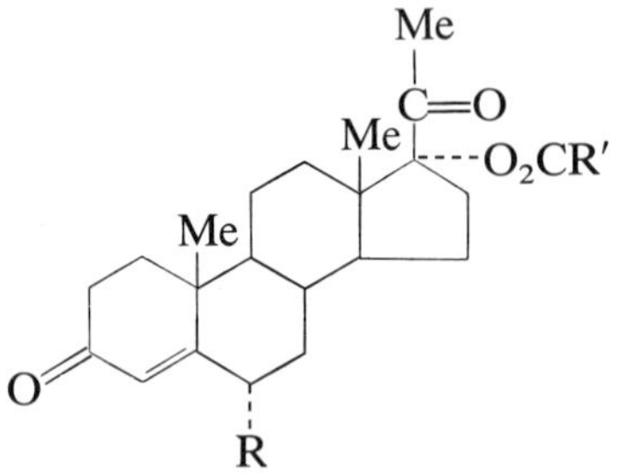

24.**214** R = H, R′ = —$(CH_2)_4Me$
24.**215** R = R′ = Me

636–638). The effectiveness in prostatic cancer of the antiandrogen cyproterone acetate (24.**212**), a progesterone derivative, was mentioned previously.

Corticosteroids comprise one of several types of agent used in the treatment of leukemias and lymphomas; in fact, the major role of corticosteroids in cancer therapy is in the treatment of these forms of human neoplasia. The natural corticosteroids cortisone and cortisol (hydrocortisone), as well as ACTH, were employed in the early clinical applications of corticosteroids to neoplastic diseases; but these hormones have been largely replaced by synthetic glucocorticoids such as prednisone (24.**216**), prednisolone, triamcinolone, dexamethasone, and 6α-methylprednisolone. The glucocorticoid activity of these synthetic compounds is enhanced in comparison with the natural corticosteroids, and mineralocorticoid activity is absent or diminished (639). The result is that side effects (e.g., electrolyte

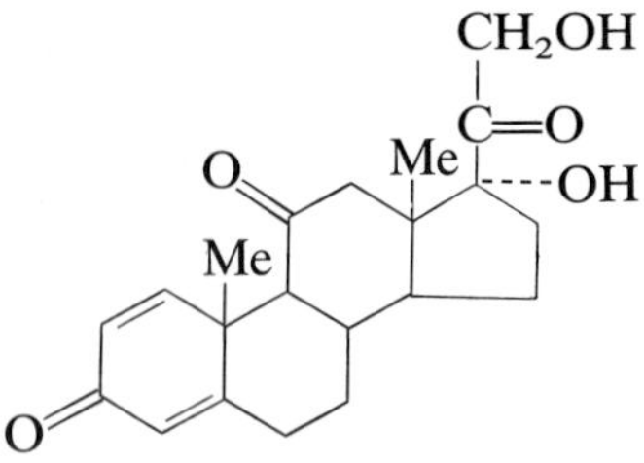

24.**216**

imbalance and water retention) are less severe. There appears to be no definite advantage in the use, at comparably effective doses, of any of these glucocorticoids over the others (639); prednisone and prednisolone, especially the former, are the glucocorticoids generally specified in clinical reports of the use of glucocorticoids for the treatment of neoplasias (639, 640).

Prednisone (or an equivalent glucocorticoid) is a major drug in the treatment of acute lymphoblastic leukemia (639–642) and is the basis for most drug combinations used in treating this kind of leukemia (641, 642). It is effective in inducing objective responses in chronic lymphocytic leukemia (639, 640, 643), Hodgkin's disease (639, 644), malignant lymphomas (lymphosarcoma and reticulum cell sarcoma) (639, 645, 646), and multiple myeloma (639, 647); but its usual role now is in combination chemotherapy of these diseases. Prednisone is also used in combination chemotherapy of acute (648) and chronic (649) myelocytic leukemias, but the role of glucocorticoid therapy of these kinds of leukemia is controversial (640).

Glucocorticoids have been used for many years to treat metastatic breast cancer, since they suppress the functioning of the adrenal and pituitary glands (540, 639); they are effective in producing subjective and objective responses, but the objective response rate is only about 10% (541, 639).

Glucocorticoids are useful in the palliative management of two major complications of cancer: (1) hypercalcemia frequently associated with breast cancer and sometimes with other kinds of cancer and (2) brain edema resulting from intracranial metastases from other sites or from primary brain tumors.

As outlined earlier, the major applications of hormonal therapy of cancer are in treating breast cancer, prostatic cancer, and leukemias and lymphomas. Cytotoxic agents have been important in the therapy of the leukemias and lymphomas since the inception of cytotoxic cancer chemotherapy, and such agents have become more prominent in recent years in the treatment of breast cancer (528, 533, 650) and prostatic cancer (651). The relative importance of hormonal manipulation of breast cancer has declined as cytotoxic chemotherapy has come increasingly into use (534). Paradoxically, the relative decline of hormonal therapy has occurred during the period in which investigations of steroid hormone receptors indicate that hormonal therapy may be more logically and effectively used. There is ample evidence that androgens (e.g., 589, 628, 629, 652), progestogens (589, 629, 653), and glucocorticoids (589, 629, 654, 655), as well as estrogens, act on target tissues and cells by binding to specific cytoplasmic receptors and that the hormone-receptor complexes are then transferred to the nucleus. Knowledge gained from these studies may elucidate the problems of hormone-responsive and hormone-independent tumors, permit a logical application of hormonal therapy in relation to cytotoxic chemotherapy, and provide the rationale for the design of new hormone antagonists.

2.6 Other Agents

L-Asparaginase is unique among anticancer agents, since it is an enzyme and since early results indicated that it exploits probably the only known qualitative difference between certain cancer cells and normal host cells (656, 657). That this is not a general qualitative difference between cancer and normal cells is indicated by the narrow spectrum of neoplasms inhibited by this drug. Also, the failure of larger doses of enzyme to give better results, coupled with increased toxicity therefrom and the rapid development of resistance to the agent, suggest that the difference in the requirement for L-asparagine between sensitive neoplastic cells and some normal tissues may be quantitative rather than qualitative—that is, most normal cells can adapt faster and better than sensitive cancer cells to L-asparagine deficiency. At present, the enzyme is often used as a temporarily effective agent in the treatment of acute lymphoblastic and myeloblastic leukemia and rarely in the treatment of other types of cancer (11).

Hexamethylmelamine (24.**217**), originally suggested as an anticancer agent in

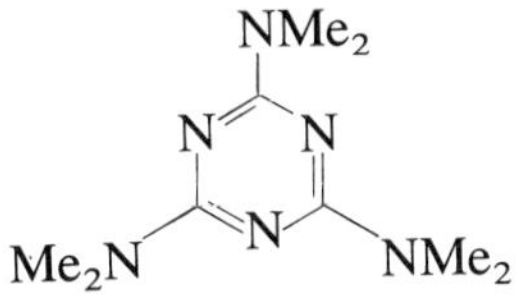

24.**217**

1950 (658), has only recently been shown to possess clinical activity, giving a greater than 70% response rate in carcinoma of the lung, ovarian adenocarcinoma, lymphoma, and breast cancer (659). The drug is rapidly demethylated by way of the corresponding methylol compounds, which could be the active agents, since such structures are active against Walker carcinosarcoma in rats. Other similarities in the biologic activity of hexamethylmelamine and the conventional alkylating agents support the idea that reaction with macromolecules, such as DNA, could be responsible for the activity of this compound.

In studies utilizing mouse embryo fibroblasts *in vitro*, 1,2-bis(3,5-dioxopiperazin-1-yl)propane (ICRF 159, 24.**218**), a nonpolar derivative of EDTA, was shown to be a potent inhibitor of DNA synthesis but had

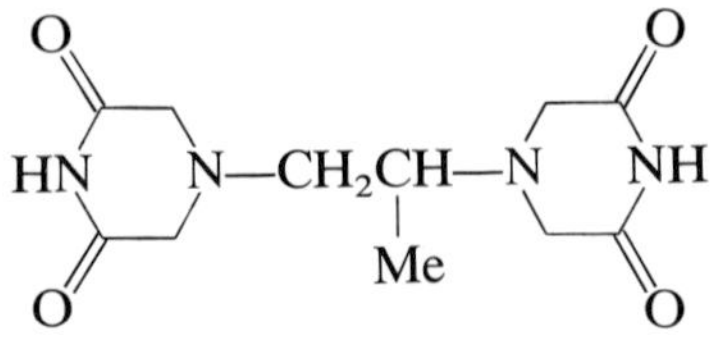

O O
HN N—CH_2CH—N NH
Me
O O

24.**218**

little effect on RNA or protein synthesis. The time course for the inhibition of tritiated thymidine uptake was similar to that for ionizing radiation and chemically reactive compounds. Therefore ICRF 159 may be acting as a mono- or bifunctional acylating agent. ICRF 159 has shown activity in acute lymphocytic leukemia and lymphoma, but further clinical trials are necessary before the value of this drug in clinical chemotherapy can be assessed (388).

The discovery of the effects of *cis*-dichlorodiammineplatinum(II) (24.**219**) on

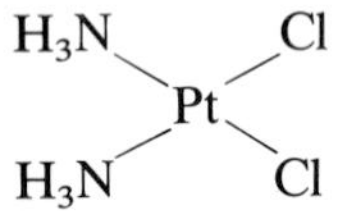

H_3N Cl
Pt
H_3N Cl

24.**219**

E. coli (660) led to its evaluation as an anticancer agent in experimental animals (661). The activity observed with this compound against animal tumors has been attributed to its binding to cellular DNA (662). It has been proposed that two types of bidentate bonds are formed—bidentate to one strand and bidentate between strands—and that it binds to all the bases in DNA except thymine (663). It would appear then that *cis*-dichlorodiammineplatinum(II) is similar in its action to the alkylating agents such as nitrogen mustard. Many variations of the structure of the *cis*-dichlorodiammineplatinum(II) have not yet provided a compound clearly superior to it.

This compound has shown an overall 19% response rate against solid tumors in man. Five major types of toxicity were encountered; a dose-related, cumulative, and only partially reversible, renal toxicity appeared to be the most serious (664).

Although a number of plant products, such as maytansine, have attracted much attention recently and have shown some activity in experimental animal tumor systems (665), the vinca alkaloids remain the only plant products that have been shown to have clinical activity.

3 DRUG METABOLISM

From the discussions above it is clear that most antimetabolites, specifically the purines and pyrimidines, must be metabolized to inhibit cell growth, because the important reactions with which they interfere occur at the nucleotide or di- and triphosphate levels in cells; or because they must be incorporated into nucleic acids at the nucleoside triphosphate level. Since nucleotides are readily dephosphorylated extracellularly and normally cannot penetrate cell membranes to any significant extent, these agents must be administered as free bases or their nucleosides. There are exceptions to this broad generalization: some antimetabolites such as psicofuranine, certain 9-substituted-6-thiopurines, and methotrexate are not metabolically activated but themselves inhibit specific enzymatic reactions. In contrast to the general rule for antimetabolites, however, the other types of agent—chemically reactive compounds, DNA complexors, mitotic inhibitors, and hormones—are generally not activated metabolically and do not function by the inhibition of specific enzymes by binding to the active or allosteric sites. Rather, the chemically reactive compounds and the DNA complexors combine with macromolecules, the most important of which is undoubtedly DNA. Interference with the function of DNA by this binding is probably the cause of cell death in mitotically active cells. Less is known about the specific action of the mitotic inhibitors and the hormones, but most of them are not metabolically activated either. Again, however, there are important exceptions to the generalization: cyclophosphamide, procarbazine, and prednisone are among these. It is significant that the latter agents are all activated in the liver primarily, then transported to the target—cancer cells, whereas the antimetabolites are activated in cancer cells and also, unfortunately, in metabolically active normal cells. Cellular metabolic activity is necessary for both activation of the antimetabolites and, in most cases, for effective inhibition of cellular growth by the active agents thus formed. On the other hand, although proliferating cells are more sensitive than resting cells to other drugs such as the chemically reactive compounds, resting cells are also killed quite effectively.

Drug inactivation by metabolic processes may also be important to the anticancer activity of the drug. There is evidence that 5-fluorouracil is more effectively metabolized by normal mouse cells than cancer cells, and this difference has been offered as the explanation of the selective cytotoxicity of 5-FU for cancer cells *in vivo* (*vide supra*). Since many neoplastic cells are low in xanthine oxidase, the same type of metabolic difference may explain, at least in part, the selectivity of action of 6-mercaptopurine. Indeed, such differences argue against the possibility of enhancement of the selective action of a drug by agents that inhibit its metabolism. 6-Mercaptopurine is more effective at lower doses when administered with allopurinol, an inhibitor of xanthine oxidase, but only questionable enhancement of its chemotherapeutic index was noted in rodent neoplasms, and no clinical advantage was evident. It is clear that the inhibition of guanase by 5-aminoimidazole-4-carboxamide enhances both the toxicity and antitumor effect of 8-azaguanine in experimental animal systems, with no net gain in therapeutic index. Much work has been done on tetrahydrouridine, an effective *in vivo* inhibitor of the deamination of ara-C, but the critical experiments that would reveal whether the combination is therapeutically synergistic have not been described. In fact, tetrahydrouridine had little effect on the activity of ara-C against L1210 leukemia when the drug was administered intraperitoneally. Attempts to improve the therapeutic effects of cyclophosphamide against L1210 leukemia by combination with substrates or inhibitors of aldehyde oxidase or aldehyde dehydrogenase to block the catabolism of aldophosphamide, the activated form of the drug, met with little or no success. Neither toxicity nor antileukemic activity was significantly increased, even though metabolism was affected. This rather discouraging picture of failure of rational attempts to enhance drug effects by the suppression of drug metabolism has been ameliorated, somewhat, by the recent finding that the therapeutic activity of 9-β-D-arabinofuranosyladenine (ara-A) against murine neoplasms is increased when it is given in combination with an adenosine deaminase inhibitor (307, 309). Whether the observed clinical activity of ara-A can be enhanced in the same manner remains to be demonstrated.

The modification of antineoplastic drugs to protect them against metabolism has also had only limited success. Immuran appears to be superior to 6-mercaptopurine in some instances as an immunosuppressive agent, but not as an anticancer agent (666). In fact, the importance of metabolic inactivation to the maximum effectiveness of drugs converted to inactive forms is questionable for those cases in which the products are nontoxic, since, in principle, it could be overcome by administration of higher levels of drug and/or by proper scheduling. Substitution of ara-A at the 2-position by fluorine prevents its deamination (*vide supra*) and appears to enhance its antitumor activity.

Other attempts to alter the pharmacokinetics of drugs by structural modification have also met with only limited success. Acylation of nucleosides affects their absorption and distribution, but there is no indication that it has a profound effect on antitumor activity or on metabolism—other than necessitating esterase activity (10). The triacetate of 6-azauridine is better absorbed orally than 6-azauridine itself, but it does not have a greater therapeutic index. The 5′-adamantoate of ara-C is an effective repository form of this agent that protects it from deamination and obviates the need for repetitive injections or continuous infusion for maximum activity; but again the therapeutic index of ara-C against animal neoplasms is not improved by this modification, which caused complications when its use was attempted clinically. Studies on acyl derivatives of 5-fluorouracil and its reversal agent thymidine and/or a combination of these agents with esterase inhibitors resulted only in enhanced toxicity.

Cyclophosphamide remains the best, if not the only, example of successful drug latentiation, in which a nitrogen mustard has been modified so that it is unreactive and, consequently, biologically inactive under physiological conditions until it is metabolized. Evidence of the superiority of cyclophosphamide to nitrogen mustard as a clinical agent continues to accumulate (11). Recently a latent form of an *N*-(2-chloroethyl)-*N*-nitrosourea that must be metabolically activated has been reported (667), but its utility has not yet been established.

It is obvious that metabolism is unimportant to the anticancer activity of certain agents, but essential to the activity of others. The many attempts to alter metabolism of these latter agents favorably have largely been unsuccessful, and these failures may be related to the quantitative aspects of the problem, at least in some cases. Still it must be recognized that searches for agents, or structural modifications, that many favorably affect the activity of an anticancer agent by altering its metabolism face the same obstacle that the searches for new and better agents themselves face: obtaining selective action—either in cancer cells or in normal cells, depending on the particular approach. At the same time, the relationship of metabolic activation, as well as drug action, to the metabolic activity of the target cancer cells is important, yet often overlooked.

4 TOXICITY

Interference with cell division is responsible for the effectiveness of most anticancer agents; hence the toxicity associated with their use is usually encountered in parts of the body where rapid cell proliferation takes place, such as bone marrow and the gastrointestinal tract. In addition to marrow and gastrointestinal disturbances, the most frequently encountered side reactions are nausea and vomiting, probably resulting from disturbances to the central nervous system. Other toxic symptoms observed with various drugs are alopecia, anorexia, hepatotoxicity, renal toxicity, cystitis, and thrombophlebitis. Despite these and other unusual disturbances such as the cardiac myopathy caused by adriamycin (511, 512), the dose-limiting toxicity of most of the best anticancer agents is directed toward bone marrow stem cells and intestinal crypt cells (1–3, 9, 668). Onset of toxicity from damage to the intestinal stem cells is usually rapid, and recovery is also rapid (exceptions, such as the slow recovery from damage by adriamycin, are known), whereas toxicity from marrow stem cell death develops more slowly and recovery from it is slower. In both cases, increased mitotic activity resulting from initial injury causes these tissues to become more susceptible to damage from intensive, multiple-dose therapy, and this problem as well as the temporal relationships must be given careful consideration in designing clinical schedules, particularly on combination chemotherapy regimens (669, 670).

These toxic effects prevent more effective therapy with the drugs that are available today. The problem, of course, is lack of specificity of these agents for cancer cells, which is a result of the close metabolic resemblance of cancer cells to the normal tissue from which they derive. The extensive, largely futile search for exploitable differences between normal and neoplastic cells serves to emphasize the similarity of the two types of cells. Because most of the metabolic differences that do exist are quantitative and kinetic in origin and are not readily exploitable, it is usually necessary to push drugs into their toxic ranges to obtain therapeutic effects.

Several attempts to improve the utilization of presently available drugs by toxicity reversal have met with limited success. For example, local thrombophlebitis resulting from the injection of nitrogen mustard was reduced by cooling the affected area or by the promotion of diffusion by the use of hyaluronidase (5, 9). Administration of L-cysteine before injection of nitrogen mustard decreased or modified the leukopenia, thrombocytopenia, and nausea and vomiting usually caused by this drug (5, 9). More recently, reduced toxicity and improved therapeutic effects of isophosphamide in experimental animals treated with *N*-acetylcysteine have been reported (671), but whether clinical advantage can be obtained in this manner remains to be demonstrated.

Enhancement of the activity of methotrexate against cancers of the head and neck has been sought by intraarterial perfusion of large, virtually toxic doses of the drug while affording systemic protection to the body by means of intramuscular administration of citrovorum factor, a specific antidote for methotrexate (5). More recently, success has been achieved in the treatment of osteogenic sarcoma after surgery with massive doses of methotrexate followed a short time later by citrovorum factor (672).

A different approach to the problem, which is only beginning to be explored with any degree of success, is the structural modification of drugs to alter toxicity. The observation of the low bone marrow toxicity of streptozotocin (673) led to renewed and successful efforts to prepare its 2-chloroethyl analog, chlorozotocin, since it was predicted that chlorozotocin would be more efficacious than streptozotocin against leukemia, while retaining relatively low bone marrow toxicity (438). The correctness of these predictions has led to preclinical studies in large animals that verified the different dose-limiting toxicity, which in dogs appears to be renal (674). It seems reasonable to hope that this approach may lead to a modification of adriamycin that is less damaging to muscle tissue, therefore to the heart, while retaining its effectiveness as an anticancer agent. At least it is a goal worthy of pursuit.

5 RESISTANCE

As with microorganisms, resistance of a neoplasm to a drug, whether natural or acquired, can arise in a number of ways, and in the past, confusion has resulted from failure to establish the true cause of resistance in particular cases. For example, mice inoculated with relatively small numbers of leukemia L1210 cells (10^3) can be cured by treatment with methotrexate, but mice with 10^5 cells can never be cured, i.e., "resistance" develops. But if cells from these mice that are dying in the face of treatment are injected in other nonleukemic mice, the disease again responds to treatment (675). Thus resistance in this case is due to the body burden and can be explained by cell kinetics. That is, although the leukemic cells individually are sensitive to the drug and are killed by it, the rate of cell division and repopulation exceeds that of cell killing. In the past, this type of "resistance" has probably been the most common cause of clinical failure in the treatment of cancer. Now that more effective drugs and treatment schedules have been developed, other causes of drug failure are undoubtedly becoming more and more important.

Three types of drug resistance have been identified (676).

Type I. Permanently resistant variant tumor cells, e.g., 1 in 10^6–10^7 tumor cells resistant to a specific drug or class of drugs. This type of resistance is usually called biochemical resistance.

Type II. Temporarily resistant resting tumor cells, e.g., cells with unusually long residence times in the G_1 phase of the cell cycle, sometimes called G_0 cells.

Type III. Tumor cells that because of their anatomical site(s), such as the central nervous system, receive less than average exposure to drug.

Obviously, different approaches must be taken to circumvent these three different types of resistance. Type I or biochemical resistance can be caused by a variety of factors (677–679). Lack of uptake or decreased rates of drug entry have been associated with resistance to nitrogen mustard, actinomycin D, methotrexate, and 6-mercaptopurine. Lack of activating enzyme activity such as phosphoribosyltransferase activity or kinase activity resulted in resistance to the purine and pyrimidine antimetabolites, such as 6-mercaptopurine, 5-azacytidine, ara-C, and 5-fluorouracil. Increased catabolism such as the deamination of ara-C or the dephosphorylation of the 6-thiopurines has also been associated with resistance to these agents. Evidence that inactivation of other drugs such as the alkylating agents and methotrexate causes resistance is less convincing. Altered enzyme affinity has been held responsible for resistance to methotrexate and to 5-fluorouracil. The rate of repair of damage or of recovery from the initial effects of a drug is a factor that may modify its activity. For example, resistance to nitrogen mustard has been attributed in some instances to accelerated removal of bound drug from DNA, presumably the result of increased activities of the enzymes involved in DNA repair. The observed increase in asparagine synthetase activity, which accompanies resistance to L-asparaginase in some tumors, appears to be causitive. It is well known that treatment with methotrexate often leads to elevated cellular concentrations of dihydrofolate reductase and that high levels of this enzyme are sometimes associated with resistance to this drug. Approaches to the circumvention of biochemical resistance such as congeners that are anabolized by alternative pathways or that take advantage of elevated enzyme levels, have met with some success at least in animal systems (10, 680).

Type II resistance, due to cell kinetics, has been attacked by the optimal use of cycle-nonspecific agents and by combination chemotherapy, and the results are discussed in the next section.

The primary approach to sanctuary problems (type III resistance) has been the use of drugs known to have advantageous transport characteristics such as streptozotocin in the treatment of pancreatic cancer and other nitrosoureas that readily cross the blood-brain barrier, such as BCNU and CCNU, in the treatment of brain tumors. Alternatively, the intrathecal administration of methotrexate has been used to advantage (681, 682). Thus an understanding of the mechanisms of resistance has led to some progress in overcoming this problem, which promises to become more serious as chemotherapy progresses. Perhaps the most promising approach altogether is to avoid or delay the development of resistance by means of combination chemotherapy (*vide supra*), but this has its limitations also.

6 CELL POPULATION KINETICS

Since the toxicity of a drug is the result of the combination of the drug with a constituent of the cell, cytotoxicity is dependent not only on drug concentration and duration of exposure of the cell, but also on the state of the cellular receptors (6, 7, 683). The sensitivity of the receptors to the drug, or their availability for binding to the drug, varies with the phase of the cell cycle, which is generally considered to consist of four phases: a mitotic phase (M), a postmitotic phase (G_1), a synthetic phase (S), and a postsynthetic phase (G_2). Protein and RNA are synthesized in all phases of the cycle but more rapidly during the S-phase, whereas synthesis of DNA is confined largely to the S-phase; the duration of the cycle and the phases varies widely in cells of different types.

Compounds such as ara-C that inhibit the synthesis of DNA, i.e., the polymerization of the deoxyribonucleotides, are effective only against cells in the S-phase, as would be expected, and are totally ineffective against cells not in cycle. Compounds such as methotrexate, 6-mercaptopurine, and 5-fluorodeoxyuridine, which act principally by inhibition of the synthesis of DNA precursors, are also usually regarded as S-phase inhibitors, but because of their other effects, are self-limiting in their action. The alkylating agents and the DNA complexors are cycle-phase nonspecific but are usually more lethal to cells in cycle than to resting cells. The mitotic inhibitors are obviously toxic only to cells in cycle, i.e., cells attempting to divide.

The pertinence of these observations to anticancer activity is readily apparent if the case of an agent known to act only on cells in S-phase is considered. If the metabolism of the drug is the same in normal cells and in cancer cells, the percentages of the cell populations, both normal and neoplastic, that will be damaged by the drug will be determined by the percentages of the cells that are in S-phase during exposure to an effective concentration of the drug. Therefore the relative toxicity of the drug to normal and neoplastic cells will depend on the percentages of cells in cycle and on differences in the duration of their cycles or of the S-phases of the cycles. Information on the cycle of various types of neoplasms and on drug actions is necessary for optimal use of anticancer agents of various types.

Basic studies during the past few years on the kinetics of cell proliferation in experimental tumor systems and the effects of drugs thereon have led to results indicating the possibility that presently known agents may be administered on a schedule that will provide sufficient selective toxicity for the cure of some neoplastic diseases. These studies have emphasized that (1) the kill of experimental tumor cells *in vivo* by drugs follows pseudo-first-order kinetics, (2) cells surviving kill by drug probably continue dividing with the normal doubling time (unless only one or a "few" cells survive; then mutant slow-growing populations can develop), (3) one cancer cell surviving can proliferate to a lethal number, and (4) as a consequence of these facts, the fewer cells that are present when treatment is begun, the better the chances of cure. Conversely, if the cancer cell population is large enough when treatment is begun, the number of cells resulting from proliferation of surviving cells will, in time, become greater than the number of cells killed by the drug. The implications for the chemotherapy of tumors are quite plain: if the aim is cure rather than prolongation of life, the optimum regimen is one or a small number of doses of drug at the highest tolerated concentrations at the earliest possible time. Particular attention must be given to the scheduling of S-phase specific agents that must be maintained above their minimum effective concentrations for a sufficient period to expose all cancer cells during their S-phase.

To this point attention has been directed to the response of cells in cycle to the various agents, and resting or nonproliferating cells have only been mentioned, since they compose but a small percentage of the neoplasms most responsive to chemotherapy, such as the leukemias and lymphomas. The kinetics of cell proliferation of most solid tumors, which are less responsive to therapy, is quite different because the mass doubling time increases as the tumor increases in size, according to the Gompertz equation. This increase is due primarily to a progressively increasing portion of the viable cell population entering a nonproliferative (metabolically resting) state sometimes referred to as the G_0 state and to a progressively increasing cell loss from the tumor by exfoliation, metastasis, and cell death. This increase in resting cells, which are not responsive to cycle-phase specific agents such as most of the antimetabolites and are less responsive to cycle-phase nonspecific agents such as the chemically reactive compounds and the DNA complexors, is one of the major limitations in solid tumor chemotherapy. One approach to this problem is the sequential use of a cycle-nonspecific agent followed by a phase-specific agent, as illustrated by cures of solid tumors in animals by the use of cyclophosphamide followed in one case by ara-C and in another by 6-mercaptopurine (8, 684).

Equally important to successful therapy is the recovery of host tissue, since the cells of certain host organs such as bone marrow and intestinal epithelia are quite sensitive to almost all anticancer agents (*vide supra*). Differences in recovery times of these or other normal host cells and cancer cells can permit the proper spacing of drug doses that are effective in reducing tumor mass, while permitting host organs to maintain at least minimal essential function. Complications arise, however, from the increased sensitivity of proliferating host cells to further drug insult, particularly in the case of bone marrow stem cells.

7 COMBINATION CHEMOTHERAPY AND COMBINED TREATMENT MODALITIES

Since no single anticancer agent has been effective in curing the more common forms of neoplastic disease (1), and since in other areas of modern medicine drug combinations have provided therapeutic advantage, it is quite logical that a good deal of effort has been devoted to the evaluation of many combinations of agents in many different experimental animal systems and in man.

Drugs in combination can be antagonistic, subadditive, additive, or synergistic, depending on the relative effects of the combination on normal and neoplastic cells; but the goal of most investigations has been "therapeutic synergism"—resulting from combinations of agents that have greater than additive anticancer effects without causing a corresponding increase in host toxicity. A large number of drug combinations have been evaluated by many different protocols; but even though these varied approaches make it difficult to compare results, it is obvious that the experimental design of many investigations in which synergism was reportedly observed does not permit a proper evaluation of the toxic effects of the combinations on the host. In many instances enhancement of antitumor effect could be obtained only at the expense of increased host toxicity, with no net therapeutic gain. Moreover, a real synergistic effect observed in animals may be too small for practical clinical exploitation, which probably explains a number of early clinical failures.

Whether one can logically expect synergistic effects from sequential blocks of a metabolic pathway has been questioned, but it seems obvious, at least theoretically, that concurrent blockades of more than one metabolic pathway can give potentiation. In fact, it seems likely that the efficacy of many antimetabolites as cytotoxic agents, used singly, may depend on concurrent blockades. Such potentiation, however, does not necessarily result in therapeutic synergism. The basic problem is still one of differential action or selective toxicity, and there is no fundamental biochemical reason, other than the circumvention of resistance, for most of the reported antimetabolite combinations to exhibit true therapeutic synergism. On the other hand, combinations of antimetabolites and agents of other types, such as chemically reactive compounds, DNA complexors, or mitotic inhibitors, might display therapeutic advantage because of the difference in response to these agents depending on the metabolic state of exposed cells.

A recently reported method for quantitatively examining the lethal toxicity of combinations of drugs in mice (685) has shown that although subadditive toxicity is not essential for therapeutic synergism against rodent tumors, it is predictive in a high percentage of cases, since 13 or 16 therapeutically synergistic combinations showed significant subadditive toxicity (686). In the case of ara-C plus the 6-thiopurines, a clinically useful combination, ara-C clearly reduces the toxicity of the 6-thiopurines (670), apparently by blocking their incorporation (after appropriate metabolic transformations) into DNA. Since this block is not operative in cells resistant to ara-C, TG is lethal to such cells, and the combination is synergistic against a heterogeneous cell population containing them (274, 664).

The major advances in the treatment of acute leukemia in children have resulted from the use of four-drug combinations such as prednisone, vincristine, methotrexate, and 6-mercaptopurine, which are active alone against the disease and have qualitatively different toxicities and mechanisms of action that result in increased activity when used in combination (669). Such drug regimens have resulted in an ever-increasing 5 year survival rate, with 5 year survival predicting normal life expectancy in at least 50% of the cases. These results are matched by the response of Hodgkin's disease to another four-drug combination—nitrogen mustard, vincristine, procarbazine, and prednisone—that also promises to produce long-term survivors and normal life expectancy in an increasing number of cases. Less impressive but continued improvement is also being experienced in multiple drug therapy of acute myelogenous leukemia in adults, of non-Hodgkin's lymphoma, and of multiple myeloma (669).

The results in the treatment of the leukemias and lymphomas have overshadowed those obtained with solid tumors, but recently increases in response are being obtained in breast cancer with a five-drug regimen of vincristine, methotrexate, 5-fluorouracil, cyclophosphamide, and prednisone and a number of modifications thereof (669), in soft tissue sarcomas with adriamycin and DIC (475), and in colorectal cancer with 5-fluorouracil and MeCCNU (431, 432).

Combined modalities appear to offer even more promise in the treatment of solid tumors than does combination chemotherapy. The former approach is a logical outgrowth of our understanding of the needs to lower the burden of cancer cells before beginning chemotherapy and to institute *early* chemotherapy of metastatic lesions that cannot be eradicated by surgery or ionizing radiation. Results of studies on the effect of cyclophosphamide (687) and later of melphalan (359) on the recurrence of breast cancer after surgery in women with positive axillary nodes are so dramatic that the melphalan protocol has been dropped and a new study begun comparing melphalan with 5-fluorouracil. In the ensuing months there has been no recurrence in either group. Another study employing combination chemotherapy (cyclophosphamide, methotrexate, and 5-fluorouracil) after surgery looks even more promising (688).

Osteogenic sarcoma, one of the major forms of bone cancer, is usually treated by surgical amputation of the primary tumor, but the development of pulmonary metastases leading to death within a year has held the cure rate by surgery to about 20%. Treatment of patients after surgery with massive doses of methotrexate followed by citrovorum factor for toxicity reversal has reduced the incidence of metastasis to about 10% in patients who have been observed for up to 22 months (672). Similar results have been obtained with surgery followed by adriamycin (689). Other groups of investigators have begun to combine high dose methotrexate and adriamycin with other drugs, and early reports from these combination studies have indicated a similar lengthening of the disease-free period after surgery (690).

Marked improvement in the treatment of Ewing's sarcoma has resulted from irradiation of the primary tumor site combined with intensive combination chemotherapy and preventive irradiation of the central nervous system, a frequent site of recurrence. Drugs used include cyclophosphamide, vincristine, and adriamycin. Similar results have been obtained with primary radiotherapy followed by a four-drug combination of cyclophosphamide, vincristine, adriamycin, and actinomycin D (669).

These encouraging results using combined modalities follow the results obtained several years ago in the treatment of Wilms' tumor by surgery followed by irradiation and chemotherapy with actinomycin D, a protocol that gave an 89% survival rate (690). It is hoped that combination chemotherapy, which is now being tried in this disease also, will give further improvement.

8 SUMMARY AND CONCLUSIONS

It seems clear that the likelihood of finding a universal cure for cancer in the form of a single drug or mode of therapy is too slim to consider seriously. It is doubtful that new drugs quite superior to those we now have will be found. At the same time, new and useful drugs will be found (although they will probably belong to one of the broad classes discussed in Section 2); and a drug capable of killing another decade of cancer cells at tolerated doses could, in combination with other drugs and modalities, provide cures of neoplasms that are now almost always fatal. Still, the lack of a "wonder drug" has caused progress against cancer to be stepwise, and it is this lack that will cause it to remain stepwise. It seems likely that progress may be speeded by the increasing use of combination chemotherapy and combined modalities and, ideally, *early* treatment by these means of large numbers of cancer victims. But the immediate hope for many is still dim. Furthermore, the carcinogenicity to rodents of most, if not all, of the clinically useful anticancer agents, when given at high levels for long periods, may indicate a future problem in the treatment of the human disease, now that long-term survivors resulting from chemotherapy are not uncommon. Other developments should be mentioned because they offer promise for the future, but they must be viewed in that light.

Biochemical markers—substances that correlate with tumor cell burden—may provide a valuable means for monitoring the response of patients to treatment (a large factor in the successful treatment of choriocarcinoma) and perhaps in some cases for earlier detection, a long sought and potentially invaluable aid. Ideally, blood or urinary levels of these substances would be elevated in patients with otherwise undetectable cancer cells, and these levels would decrease with response to therapy. Already six or more such substances with varying degrees of utility have been identified (12).

As stated at the onset of this chapter, the prevention of cancer, or any other disease, is much better than treatment of the established disease. In the future there may be hope of preventing some cancers by vaccination with tumor viruses or by immunization with tumor antigens, but today we cannot think practically about preventing human cancer by immunologic methods.

With the single exception of Marck's lymphomatosis in the chicken, known to be caused by a herpes virus, this has not been accomplished in naturally occurring animal tumors either. Methods that have been used in attempts to treat established tumors in animals are (1) active immunization with tumor cells or their extracts, (2) treatment with agents that stimulate general immunologic response, (3) transfer of immunity with lymphocytes or lymphocyte extracts from immunized donors, and (4) transfer of immunity with serum (691). Because of the generally disappointing results with active immunization, attempts have been made to increase the antigenicity of the tumor cells. Recent reports indicate that the inoculation of cancer cells treated *in vitro* with neuraminidase is effective both in animal systems (692, 693) and in man (693).

Another aspect of active immunization that is under intensive investigation is the use of certain microorganisms or their products to raise the general level of immune responsiveness. A variety of agents, including Bacillus Calmette Guérin (BCG), *Corynebacterium parvum*, and zymosan, are known to increase the resistance of animals to infections and histoincompatible skin grafts, and to be effective against certain experimental tumors. The activity of *C. parvum* against an established fibrosarcoma in mice is particularly encouraging (694). But because of the proved effectiveness of chemotherapy, however limited, and because immunologic cell kill is of zero order, therefore usually effective only against a low body burden of neoplastic cells, clinical investigations have been limited primarily to chemoimmunotherapy—chiefly with BCG and, more recently, with MER, a methanol extract residue from BCG (695, 696). One exception is the regression of malignant melanomas injected with BCG (691), although more recently treatment of this disease with DIC and BCG has also shown promise (697).

Most cancer scientists accept the basic premise that many (if not all) human cancers are virally induced, even if arguments over details remain serious and incontrovertible evidence is lacking. This has led to efforts, albeit less long range than those to produce a cancer vaccine (698), to use viral chemotherapy to prevent induction or reinduction of cancer eradicated by means of cellular chemotherapy. Approaches include attempts to inhibit reverse transcriptase from RNA oncorna viruses (699) and to use known antiviral agents such as ara-A and virazole in combination with anticancer agents in attempts to cure animal neoplasms that are virally transmitted (700, 701). A phase I study of virazole, preparatory to its use in an attempt to prevent reinduction of human tumors thought to be of viral etiology, has been reported (702).

Thus it appears that for the foreseeable future, even the recently flowering fields of immunotherapy and viral chemotherapy are destined to be used as adjuvants to the proven, though limited, treatments of cancer with cytotoxic agents.

ACKNOWLEDGMENTS

We gratefully acknowledge the outstanding work of Mrs. Joan Whitworth in the preparation of this manuscript. Thanks are also due to Mrs. Catherine Brown and Mrs. Shelia Bruce for their assistance in manuscript preparation.

REFERENCES

1. C. G. Zubrod, *Life Sci.*, **14,** 809 (1974).
2. J. F. Holland and E. Frei, III, *Cancer Medicine*, Lea & Febiger, Philadelphia, 1973.
3. A. C. Sartorelli and D. G. Johns, *Antineoplastic and Immunosuppressive Agents*, Parts 1 and 2, Springer-Verlag, Heidelberg, 1974 and 1975.
4. E. J. Ariens, *Drug Design*, Academic Press, New York, 1971–1975.

5. L. L. Bennett, Jr., and J. A. Montgomery, in *Methods in Cancer Research*, Vol. 3, H. Busch, Ed., Academic Press, New York, 1967, p. 549.
6. H. E. Skipper, in *The Cell Cycle and Cancer*, R. Baserga, Ed., Dekker, New York, 1971, p. 358.
7. H. E. Skipper, F. M. Schabel, Jr., L. B. Mellett, J. A. Montgomery, L. J. Wilkoff, H. A. Lloyd, and R. W. Brockman, *Cancer Chemother. Rep.*, **54,** 431 (1970).
8. F. M. Schabel, Jr., *Cancer*, **35,** 15 (1975).
9. J. A. Montgomery, T. P. Johnston, and Y. F. Shealy, in *Medicinal Chemistry*, 3rd ed., Part 1, A. Burger, Ed., Wiley-Interscience, New York, 1970, p. 680.
10. J. A. Montgomery and R. F. Struck, in *Progress in Drug Research*, Vol. 17, E. Jucker, Ed., Birkhäuser-Verlag, Basel, 1973, p. 320.
11. R. B. Livingston and S. K. Carter, *Single Agents in Cancer Chemotherapy*, IFI/Plenum, New York, 1970.
12. P. S. Schein, in *Current Research in Oncology, 1972*, C. B. Anfinsen, Ed., Academic Press, New York, 1973, p. 167.
13. Proceedings of the American Cancer Society–National Cancer Institute National Conference on Advances in Cancer Management, Part I, Treatment and Rehabilitation, *Cancer* (Suppl.), **36,** 623–824 (1975).
14. S. A. Fusari, T. H. Haskell, R. P. Frohardt, and Q. R. Bartz, *J. Am. Chem. Soc.*, **76,** 2881 (1954).
15. H. W. Dion, S. A. Fusari, Z. L. Jakubowski, J. G. Zora, and Q. R. Bartz, *J. Am. Chem. Soc.*, **78,** 3075 (1956).
16. J. A. Moore, J. R. Dice, E. D. Nicolaides, R. D. Westland, and E. L. Wittle, *J. Am. Chem. Soc.*, **76,** 2884 (1954).
17. H. A. DeWald and A. M. Moore, *J. Am. Chem. Soc.*, **80,** 3941 (1958).
18. D. A. Goldthwait, *J. Biol. Chem.*, **222,** 1051 (1956).
19. E. C. Moore and G. A. LePage, *Cancer Res.*, **17,** 804 (1957).
20. R. Abrams and M. Bentley, *Arch. Biochem. Biophys.*, **79,** 91 (1959).
21. M. L. Eidinoff, J. E. Knoll, B. Marano, and L. Cheong, *Cancer Res.*, **18,** 105 (1958).
22. J. Preiss and P. Handler, *J. Biol. Chem.*, **233,** 493 (1958).
23. T. A. Langan, Jr., N. O. Kaplan, and L. Shuster, *J. Biol. Chem.*, **234,** 2161 (1959).
24. P. R. Srinivasan and B. Weiss, *Biochim. Biophys. Acta*, **51,** 597 (1961).
25. P. R. Srinivasan, *J. Am. Chem. Soc.*, **81,** 1772 (1959).
26. A. J. Tomisek, H. J. Kelly, and H. E. Skipper, *Arch. Biochem. Biophys.*, **64,** 437 (1956).
27. T. C. French, I. B. Dawid, R. A. Day, and J. M. Buchanan, *J. Biol. Chem.*, **238,** 2171 (1963).
28. T. C. French, I. B. Dawid, and J. M. Buchanan, *J. Biol. Chem.*, **238,** 2186 (1963).
29. I. B. Dawid, T. C. French, and J. M. Buchanan, *J. Biol. Chem.*, **238,** 2178 (1963).
30. B. Levenberg, I. Melnick, and J. M. Buchanan, *J. Biol. Chem.*, **225,** 163 (1957).
31. A. J. Tomisek and M. R. Reid, *J. Biol. Chem.*, **237,** 807 (1962).
32. J. M. Buchanan, in *Amino Acids and Peptides with Antimetabolite Activity* (Ciba Foundation Symposium), G. E. W. Wolstenholme and C. M. O'Connor, Eds., Churchill, London, 1958, p. 75.
33. H. E. Skipper, L. L. Bennett, Jr., and F. M. Schabel, Jr., *Fed. Proc.*, **13,** 298 (1954).
34. L. L. Bennett, Jr., F. M. Schabel, Jr., and H. E. Skipper, *Arch. Biochem. Biophys.*, **64,** 423 (1956).
35. L. R. Duvall, *Cancer Chemother. Rep.*, **7,** 65 (1960).
36. R. L. Momparler and J. J. Jaffe, *Biochem. Pharmacol.*, **14,** 255 (1965).
37. A. C. Sartorelli and B. A. Booth, *Mol. Pharmacol.*, **3,** 71 (1967).
38. J. A. Jacquez, *Cancer Res.*, **17,** 890 (1957).
39. J. A. Jacquez, *Proc. Soc. Exp. Biol. Med.*, **99,** 611 (1958).
40. J. F. Henderson, G. A. LePage, and F. McIver, *Cancer Res.*, **17,** 609 (1957).
41. H. C. Reilly, *Bacteriol. Proc.*, **79** (1954); *Fed. Proc.*, **13,** 279 (1954).
42. J. A. Jacquez and J. H. Sherman, *Cancer Res.*, **22,** 56 (1962).
43. H. C. Reilly, *Proc. Am. Assoc. Cancer Res.*, **2,** 41 (1955).
44. K. V. Rao, in *Antimicrobial Agents and Chemotherapy—1961*, M. Findland and G. M. Savage, Eds., American Society for Microbiology, Ann Arbor, Mich. 1962, p. 178.
45. S. E. DeVoe, N. E. Rigler, A. J. Shay, J. H. Martin, T. C. Boyd, E. J. Backus, J. H. Mowat, and N. Bohonos, *Antibiot. Ann., 1956–1957*, 730 (1954).
46. E. P. Anderson and R. W. Brockman, *Biochem. Pharmacol.*, **12,** 1335 (1963).
47. C. C. Stock, H. C. Reilly, S. M. Buckley, D. A. Clarke, and C. P. Rhoads, *Nature*, **173,** 71 (1954).

48. D. A. Clarke, H. C. Reilly, and C. C. Stock, *Antibiot. Chemother.*, **7,** 653 (1957).
49. K. Sugiura and C. C. Stock, *Proc. Soc. Exp. Biol. Med.*, **88,** 127 (1955).
50. J. H. Burchenal, *Curr. Res. Cancer Chemother.*, **4,** 3 (1956).
51. H. C. Reilly, in *Amino Acids and Peptides with Antimetabolic Activity* (Ciba Foundation Symposium), G. E. W. Wolstenholme and C. M. O'Connor, Eds., Churchill, London, 1958, p. 62.
52. D. A. Karnofsky, R. B. Golbey, and M. C. Li, *Proc. Am. Assoc. Cancer Res.*, **5,** 33 (1964).
53. C. K. Mathews and F. M. Huennekens, *J. Biol. Chem.*, **235,** 3304 (1960).
54. S. F. Zakrzewski and C. A. Nichol, *J. Biol. Chem.*, **235,** 2984 (1960).
55. U. W. Kenkare and B. M. Braganca, *Biochem. J.*, **86,** 160 (1963).
56. S. F. Zakrzewski, M. T. Hakala, and C. A. Nichol, *Mol. Pharmacol.*, **2,** 423 (1966).
57. F. M. Huennekens and M. J. Osborn, *Advan. Enzymol.*, **21,** 369 (1959).
58. J. C. Rabinowitz, in *The Enzymes*, 2nd ed., Vol. 2, Part A, P. D. Boyer, H. Lardy, and K. Myrbäck, Eds., Academic Press, New York, 1960, p. 185.
59. J. S. O'Brien, *Cancer Res.*, **22,** 267 (1962).
60. M. Friedkin, *Ann. Rev. Biochem.*, **32,** 185 (1963).
61. G. K. Humphreys and D. M. Greenberg, *Arch. Biochem. Biophys.*, **78,** 275 (1958).
62. A. J. Walba and M. Friedkin, *J. Biol. Chem.*, **236,** PC11 (1961).
63. B. M. McDougall and R. L. Blakley, *J. Biol. Chem.*, **236,** 832 (1961).
64. E. J. Pastore and M. Friedkin, *J. Biol. Chem.*, **237,** 3802 (1962).
65. S. S. Cohen, in *Essays in Biochemistry*, S. Graff, Ed., Wiley, New York, 1956, p. 77.
66. A. D. Barton and A. K. Laird, *J. Biol. Chem.*, **227,** 795 (1957).
67. A. Baserga, *Minerva Med.*, **50,** 4186 (1959).
68. D. R. Seeger, D. B. Cosulich, J. M. Smith, Jr., and M. E. Hultquist, *J. Am. Chem. Soc.*, **71,** 1753 (1949).
69. C. A. Nichol and A. D. Welch, *Proc. Soc. Exp. Biol. Med.*, **74,** 403 (1950).
70. J. R. Bertino, J. P. Perkins, and D. G. Johns, *Biochemistry*, **4,** 839 (1965).
71. W. C. Werkheiser, *J. Biol. Chem.*, **236,** 888 (1961).
72. W. C. Werkheiser, *Cancer Res.*, **25,** 1608 (1965).
73. J. R. Bertino, B. A. Booth, A. L. Bieber, A. Cashmore, and A. C. Sartorelli, *J. Biol. Chem.*, **239,** 479 (1964).
74. A. W. Schrecker and F. M. Huennekens, *Biochem. Pharmacol.*, **13,** 731 (1964).
75. S. F. Zakrzewski, *J. Biol. Chem.*, **238,** 1485 (1963).
76. S. F. Zakrzewski, *J. Biol. Chem.*, **238,** 4002 (1963).
77. C. K. Mathews and F. M. Huennekens, *J. Biol. Chem.*, **238,** 3436 (1963).
78. B. R. Baker, *Cancer Chemother. Rep.*, **4,** 1 (1959).
79. B. R. Baker and J. H. Jordaan, *J. Pharm. Sci.*, **54,** 1740 (1965).
80. B. Roth, J. M. Smith, Jr., and M. E. Hultquist, *J. Am. Chem. Soc.*, **72,** 1914 (1950).
81. B. Roth, J. M. Smith, Jr., and M. E. Hultquist, *J. Am. Chem. Soc.*, **73,** 2864 (1951).
82. T. H. Jukes and H. P. Broquist, in *Metabolic Inhibitors*, Vol. 1, R. M. Hochester and J. H. Quastel, Eds., Academic Press, New York, 1963, pp. 481–534.
83. G. H. Hitchings and J. J. Burchall, in *Advances in Enzymology*, Vol. 27, F. F. Nord, Ed., Wiley-Interscience, New York, 1965, pp. 417–468.
84. D. B. Cosulich, D. R. Seeger, M. J. Fahrenbach, B. Roth, J. H. Mowat, J. M. Smith, Jr., and M. E. Hultquist, *J. Am. Chem. Soc.*, **73,** 2554 (1951).
85. A. S. Tomcufcik and D. R. Seeger, *J. Org. Chem.*, **26,** 3351 (1961).
86. T. L. Loo, R. L. Dion, R. H. Adamson, M. A. Chirigos, and R. L. Kisliuk, *J. Med. Chem.*, **8,** 713 (1965).
87. A. Goldin, S. R. Humphreys, J. M. Venditti, and N. Mantel, *J. Nat. Cancer Inst.*, **22,** 811 (1959).
88. L. R. Schroeder, *Proc. Am. Assoc. Cancer Res.*, **3,** 267 (1961).
89. T. L. Loo and R. H. Adamson, *J. Med. Chem.*, **8,** 513 (1965).
90. D. G. Johns and T. L. Loo, *J. Pharm. Sci.*, **56,** 356 (1967).
91. H. M. Redetzki, J. E. Redetzki, and A. L. Elias, *Biochem. Pharmacol.*, **15,** 425 (1966).
92. D. G. Johns, A. T. Iannotti, A. C. Sartorelli, and J. R. Bertino, *Biochem. Pharmacol.*, **15,** 555 (1966).
93. C. M. Baugh, C. L. Krumdieck, and M. G. Nair, *Biochem. Biophys. Res. Commun.*, **52,** 27 (1973).
94. V. M. Whitehead, *Cancer Res.*, **37,** 408 (1977).
95. S. A. Jacobs, R. H. Adamson, B. A. Chabner, C.

J. Derr, and D. G. Johns, *Biochem. Biophys. Res. Commun.*, **63,** 692 (1975).

96. B. R. Baker and B.-T. Ho, *J. Pharm. Sci.*, **54,** 1261 (1965).
97. J. J. Burchall and G. H. Hitchings, *Mol. Pharmacol.*, **1,** 126 (1965).
98. G. M. Timmis, D. G. I. Felton, H. O. J. Collier, and P. L. Huskinson, *J. Pharm. Pharmacol.*, **9,** 46 (1957).
99. G. H. Hitchings, G. B. Elion, E. A. Falco, P. B. Russell, and H. Vander Werff, *Ann. N.Y. Acad. Sci.*, **52,** 1318 (1950).
100. E. A. Falco, S. DuBreuil, and G. H. Hitchings, *J. Am. Chem. Soc.*, **73,** 3758 (1951).
101. B. Roth, E. A. Falco, G. H. Hitchings, and S. R. M. Bushby, *J. Med. Pharm. Chem.*, **5,** 1103 (1962).
102. H. C. Carrington, A. F. Crowther, D. G. Davey, A. A. Elvi, and F. L. Rose, *Nature*, **168,** 1080 (1951).
103. E. J. Modest, G. E. Foley, M. M. Pechet, and S. Farber, *J. Am. Chem. Soc.*, **74,** 855 (1952).
104. F. Rosen and C. A. Nichol, *Cancer Res.*, **22,** 495 (1962).
105. W. C. Werkheiser, *Cancer Res.*, **23,** 1277 (1963).
106. W. C. Werkheiser, unpublished observations.
107. G. A. Fischer, J. R. Bertino, P. Calabresi, D. H. Clement, R. P. Zanes, M. S. Lyman, J. H. Burchenal, and A. D. Welch, *Blood*, **22,** 819 (1963).
108. J. R. Bertino, *Cancer Res.*, **25,** 1614 (1965).
109. B. R. Baker, *Design of Active-Site-Directed Irreversible Enzyme Inhibitors*, Wiley, New York, 1967.
110. J. A. R. Mead, J. M. Venditti, A. W. Schrecker, A. Goldin, and J. C. Keresztesy, *Biochem. Pharmacol.*, **12,** 371 (1963).
111. A. Goldin, J. M. Venditti, I. Kline, and N. Mantel, *Nature*, **212,** 1548 (1966).
112. F. M. Sirotnak, D. M. Dorick, and D. M. Moccio, *Cancer Treat. Rep.*, **60,** 547 (1976).
113. R. Hertz, D. M. Bergenstal, M. B. Lipsett, E. B. Price, and T. F. Hilbish, *J. Am. Med. Assoc.*, **168,** 845 (1958).
114. D. A. Karnofsky, *Cancer*, **18,** 1517 (1965).
115. C. G. Zubrod, *Arch. Intern. Med.*, **106,** 663 (1960).
116. S. Farber, K. L. Diamond, R. D. Mercer, R. F. Sylvester, and Y. A. Wolff, *New Engl. J. Med.*, **238,** 787 (1948).
117. J. A. Wolff, C. L. Brubaker, M. L. Murphy, M. I. Pierce, and N. Severo, *Proc. Am. Assoc. Cancer Res.*, **4,** 73 (1963).
118. J. A. Wolff, C. L. Brubaker, M. L. Murphy, M. I. Pierce, and N. Severo, *Cancer Chemother. Rep.*, **30,** 63 (1963).
119. G. B. Elion, S. Bieber, H. Nathan, and G. H. Hitchings, *Cancer Res.*, **18,** 802 (1958).
120. M. T. Hakala, L. W. Law, and A. D. Welch, *Proc. Am. Assoc. Cancer Res.*, **2,** 113 (1956).
121. R. E. Handschumacher, *Cancer Res.*, **23,** 634 (1963).
122. A. Cihak, J. Škoda, and F. Šorm, *Collect. Czech. Chem. Commun.*, **28,** 3297 (1963).
123. A. Cihak, J. Škoda, and F. Šorm, *Collect. Czech. Chem. Commun.*, **29,** 300 (1964).
124. A. Cihak, J. Škoda, and F. Šorm, *Collect. Czech. Chem. Commun.*, **29,** 814 (1964).
125. A. Cihak, J. Škoda, and F. Šorm, *Collect. Czech. Chem. Commun.*, **29,** 1322 (1964).
126. J. Škoda, in *Progress in Nucleic Acid Research and Molecular Biology*, Vol. 2, J. N. Davidson and W. E. Cohn, Eds., Academic Press, New York, 1963, pp. 197–221.
127. A. Piskala and F. Šorm, *Collect. Czech. Chem. Commun.*, **29,** 2060 (1964).
128. F. Šorm, A. Piskala, A. Cihak, and J. Veselý, *Experientia*, **20,** 202 (1964).
129. F. Šorm and J. Veselý, *Neoplasma*, **11,** 123 (1964).
130. M. Jurovcik, K. Raska, Jr., Z. Sormova, and F. Šorm, *Collect. Czech. Chem. Commun.*, **30,** 3370 (1965).
131. K. Raska, Jr., M. Jurovcik, Z. Sormova, and F. Šorm, *Collect. Czech. Chem. Commun.*, **30,** 3215 (1965).
132. F. Kalousek, K. Raska, Jr., M. Jurovcik, and F. Šorm, *Collect. Czech. Chem. Commun.*, **31,** 1421 (1966).
133. P. Pithova, A. Piskala, J. Pitha, and F. Šorm, *Collect. Czech. Chem. Commun.*, **30,** 2801 (1965).
134. S. Zadrazil, V. Fucik, P. Bartl, Z. Sormova, and F. Šorm, *Biochim. Biophys. Acta*, **108,** 701 (1965).
135. E. A. Falco, E. Pappas, and G. H. Hitchings, *J. Am. Chem. Soc.*, **78,** 1938 (1956).
136. R. B. Barlow and A. D. Welch, *J. Am. Chem. Soc.*, **78,** 1258 (1956).
137. R. Schindler and A. D. Welch, *Science*, **125,** 548 (1957).
138. R. Schindler and A. D. Welch, *Biochem. Pharmacol.*, **1,** 132 (1958).
139. R. E. Handschumacher, *J. Biol. Chem.*, **235,** 764 (1960).

140. C. Heidelberger, in *Cancer Medicine*, J. F. Holland and E. Frei, III, Eds., Lea & Febiger, Philadelphia, 1973, p. 768.

141. C. Heidelberger, in *Antineoplastic and Immunosuppressive Agents*, Part 2, A. C. Sartorelli and D. G. Johns, Eds., Springer-Verlag, Heidelberg, 1975, p. 193.

142. D. Kessel, T. C. Hall, and I. Wodinsky, *Science*, **154,** 911 (1966).

143. K.-U. Hartmann and C. Heidelberger, *J. Biol. Chem.*, **236,** 3006 (1961).

144. P. V. Danenberg and C. Heidelberger, *Biochemistry*, **15,** 1331 (1976).

145. H. Bujard and C. Heidelberger, *Biochemistry*, **5,** 3339 (1966).

146. C. Heidelberger, L. Griesbach, O. Cruz, R. J. Schnitzer, and E. Grunberg, *Proc. Soc. Exp. Biol. Med.*, **97,** 470 (1958).

147. M. L. Eidinoff, M. A. Rich, and A. G. Perez, *Cancer Res.*, **19,** 638 (1959).

148. R. W. Brockman, J. M. Davis, and P. Stutts, *Biochim. Biophys. Acta*, **40,** 22 (1960).

149. B. A. Koechlin, F. Rubio, S. Palmer, T. Gabriel, and R. Duschinsky, *Biochem. Pharmacol.*, **15,** 435 (1966).

150. N. K. Chaudhuri, B. J. Montag, and C. Heidelberger, *Cancer Res.*, **18,** 318 (1958).

151. J. Lichenstein, H. D. Barner, and S. S. Cohen, *J. Biol. Chem.*, **235,** 457 (1960).

152. J. J. Fox and N. C. Miller, *J. Org. Chem.*, **28,** 936 (1963).

153. J. F. Codington, I. L. Doerr, and J. J. Fox, *J. Org. Chem.*, **29,** 558 (1964).

154. N. C. Yung, J. H. Burchenal, R. Fecher, R. Duschinsky, and J. J. Fox, *J. Am. Chem. Soc.*, **83,** 4060 (1961).

155. J. H. Burchenal, H. H. Adams, N. S. Newell, and J. J. Fox, *Cancer Res.*, **26,** 370 (1966).

156. J. H. Kim, M. L. Eidinoff, and J. J. Fox, *Cancer Res.*, **26,** 1661 (1966).

157. T. A. Khwaja and C. Heidelberger, *J. Med. Chem.*, **10,** 1066 (1967).

158. N. K. Chaudhuri, K. L. Mukherjee, and C. Heidelberger, *Biochem. Pharmacol.*, **1,** 328 (1958).

159. K. L. Mukherjee and C. Heidelberger, *J. Biol. Chem.*, **235,** 433 (1960).

160. G. D. Birnie, H. Kroeger, and C. Heidelberger, *Biochemistry*, **2,** 566 (1963).

161. Y. Nishizawa, J. E. Casida, S. W. Anderson, and C. Heidelberger, *Biochem. Pharmacol.*, **14,** 1605 (1965).

162. J. E. Casida, J. L. Engel, and Y. Nishizawa, *Biochem. Pharmacol.*, **15,** 627 (1966).

163. R. Duschinsky, T. Gabriel, W. Tautz, A. Nussbaum, M. Hoffer, E. Grunberg, J. H. Burchenal, and J. J. Fox, *J. Med. Chem.*, **10,** 47 (1967).

164. Z. Buděšínský, V̌. Jellínek, and J. Přikryl, *Collect. Czech. Chem. Commun.*, **27,** 2550 (1962).

165. V. Pujman, J. Sandberg, L. Howsden, and A. Goldin, *Neoplasma*, **17,** 133 (1970).

166. D. G. Johns, A. C. Sartorelli, J. R. Bertino, A. T. Iannotti, B. A. Booth, and A. D. Welch, *Biochem. Pharmacol.*, **15,** 400 (1966).

167. J. A. Montgomery, G. J. Dixon, E. A. Dulmadge, H. J. Thomas, R. W. Brockman, and H. E. Skipper, *Nature*, **199,** 769 (1963).

168. C. Heidelberger, J. Boohar, and G. D. Birnie, *Biochim. Biophys. Acta*, **91,** 636 (1964).

169. A. Bloch, M. H. Fleysher, R. Thedford, R. J. Maue, and R. H. Hall, *J. Med. Chem.*, **9,** 886 (1966).

170. J. A. Montgomery and H. J. Thomas, *J. Med. Chem.*, **10,** 1163 (1967).

171. C. Heidelberger, D. G. Parsons, and D. C. Remy, *J. Med. Chem.*, **7,** 1 (1964).

172. C. Heidelberger and S. W. Anderson, *Cancer Res.*, **24,** 1979 (1964).

173. C. Heidelberger, J. Boohar, and B. Kampschroer, *Cancer Res.*, **25,** 377 (1965).

174. P. Reyes and C. Heidelberger, *Mol. Pharmacol.*, **1,** 14 (1965).

175. J. S. Evans, E. A. Musser, G. D. Mengel, K. R. Forsblad, and J. H. Hunter, *Proc. Soc. Exp. Biol. Med.*, **106,** 350 (1961).

176. J. S. Evans, E. A. Musser, L. Bostwick, and G. D. Mengel, *Cancer Res.*, **24,** 1285 (1964).

177. R. L. Dixon and R. H. Adamson, *Cancer Chemother. Rep.*, **48,** 11 (1965).

178. R. W. Talley and V. K. Vaitkevicius, *Blood*, **21,** 352 (1963).

179. M. Y. Chu and G. A. Fischer, *Biochem. Pharmacol.*, **11,** 423 (1962).

180. J. S. Evans and G. D. Mengel, *Biochem. Pharmacol.*, **13,** 989 (1964).

181. S. S. Cohen, in *Progress in Nucleic Acid Research and Molecular Biology*, Vol. 5, J. N. Davidson and W. E. Cohn, Eds., Academic Press, New York, 1966, pp. 1–88.

182. J. J. Furth and S. S. Cohen, *Cancer Res.*, **28,** 2061 (1968).

183. D. Kessel, T. C. Hall, and I. Wodinsky, *Science*, **156,** 1240 (1967).

184. W. A. Creasey, R. J. Papac, M. E. Markiw, P.

Calabresi, and A. D. Welch, *Biochem. Pharmacol.*, **15,** 1417 (1966).

185. G. W. Camiener and C. G. Smith, *Biochem. Pharmacol.*, **14,** 1405 (1965).
186. A. R. Hanze, *J. Am. Chem. Soc.*, **89,** 6720 (1967).
187. G. W. Camiener, Abstracts P32, 154th American Chemical Society Meeting, September 1967.
188. G. W. Camiener, Abstracts P33, 154th American Chemical Society Meeting, September 1967.
189. L. T. Mulligan, Jr., and L. B. Mellett, *Pharmacologist*, **10,** 167 (1968).
190. W. J. Wechter, M. A. Johnson, C. M. Hall, D. T. Warner, A. E. Berger, A. H. Wenzel, D. T. Gish, and G. L. Weil, *J. Med. Chem.*, **18,** 339 (1975).
191. J. A. Montgomery and H. J. Thomas, *J. Med. Chem.*, **15,** 116 (1972).
192. A. Hoshi, F. Kanzawa, K. Kuretani, M. Sanoyoshi, and Y. Arai, *Gann*, **62,** 145 (1971).
193. C. G. Smith, H. H. Buskirk, and W. L. Lummis, *J. Med. Chem.*, **10,** 774 (1967).
194. A. W. Schrecker and A. Goldin, *Cancer Res.*, **28,** 802 (1968).
195. J. A. Stock, in *Experimental Chemotherapy*, Vol. 4, R. J. Schnitzer and F. Hawking, Eds., Academic Press, New York, 1966, p. 80.
196. M. S. Lyman and J. H. Burchenal, *Am. J. Nursing*, **63,** 82 (1963).
197. G. B. Elion and G. H. Hitchings, in *Advances in Chemotherapy*, Vol. 2, A. Goldin, F. Hawking, and R. J. Schnitzer, Eds., Academic Press, New York, 1965, p. 91.
198. R. W. Brockman, in *Advances in Cancer Research*, Vol. 7, A. Haddow and S. Weinhouse, Eds., Academic Press, New York, 1963, p. 129.
199. L. N. Lukens and K. A. Herrington, *Biochim. Biophys. Acta*, **24,** 432 (1957).
200. C. E. Carter, *Biochem. Pharmacol.*, **2,** 105 (1959).
201. R. W. Brockman, *Clin. Pharmacol. Ther.*, **2,** 237 (1961).
202. R. W. Brockman, *Cancer Res.*, **23,** 1191 (1963).
203. M. R. Atkinson and A. W. Murray, *Biochem. J.*, **94,** 71 (1965).
204. T. A. Krenitsky, R. Papaioannou, and G. B. Elion, *J. Biol. Chem.*, **244,** 1263 (1969).
205. T. A. Krenitsky and R. Papaioannou, *J. Biol. Chem.*, **244,** 1271 (1969).
206. T. A. Krenitsky, *Biochim. Biophys. Acta*, **179,** 506 (1969).
207. J. F. Henderson, L. W. Brox, W. N. Kelley, F. M. Rosenbloom, and J. E. Seegmiller, *J. Biol. Chem.*, **243,** 2514 (1968).
208. J. F. Henderson, *Can. J. Biochem.*, **47,** 69 (1969).
209. D. L. Hill, *Biochem. Pharmacol.*, **19,** 545 (1970).
210. M. L. Meloni and W. I. Rogers, *Proc. Am. Assoc. Cancer Res.*, **9,** 47 (1968).
211. D. Kessel and T. C. Hall, *Cancer Res.*, **29,** 2116 (1969).
212. W. I. Rogers, M. L. Meloni, I. Wodinsky, and C. J. Kensler, *Proc. Am. Assoc. Cancer Res.*, **10,** 74 (1969).
213. A. R. P. Paterson, *Can. J. Biochem. Physiol.*, **37,** 1011 (1959).
214. M. L. Meloni and W. I. Rogers, *Biochem. Pharmacol.*, **18,** 413 (1969).
215. J. S. Gots and E. G. Gollub, *Proc. Soc. Exp. Biol. Med.*, **101,** 641 (1959).
216. G. A. LePage and M. Jones, *Cancer Res.*, **21,** 642 (1961).
217. J. F. Henderson and M. K. Y. Khoo, *J. Biol. Chem.*, **240,** 3104 (1965).
218. R. J. McCollister, W. R. Gilbert, Jr., D. M. Ashton, and J. B. Wyngaarden, *J. Biol. Chem.*, **239,** 1560 (1964).
219. C. T. Caskey, D. M. Ashton, and J. B. Wyngaarden, *J. Biol. Chem.*, **239,** 2570 (1964).
220. L. L. Bennett, Jr., and P. W. Allan, *Cancer Res.*, **31,** 152 (1971).
221. D. L. Hill and L. L. Bennett, Jr., *Biochemistry*, **8,** 122 (1969).
222. M. T. Hakala and C. A. Nichol, *Biochim. Biophys. Acta*, **80,** 665 (1964).
223. L. L. Bennett, Jr., and D. J. Adamson, *Biochem. Pharmacol.*, **19,** 2172 (1970).
224. C. N. Remy, *J. Biol. Chem.*, **238,** 1078 (1963).
225. C. N. Remy, *Biochim. Biophys. Acta*, **138,** 258 (1967).
226. E. J. Sarcione and L. Stutzman, *Cancer Res.*, **20,** 387 (1960).
227. L. L. Bennett, Jr., R. W. Brockman, H. P. Schnebli, S. Chumley, G. J. Dixon, F. M. Schabel, Jr., E. A. Dulmadge, H. E. Skipper, J. A. Montgomery, and H. J. Thomas, *Nature*, **205,** 1276 (1965).
228. R. E. Parks, Jr., and R. P. Agarwal, in *The Enzymes*, Vol. 7, P. D. Boyer, Ed., Academic Press, New York, 1972, p. 483.
229. A. R. P. Paterson and A. Sutherland, *Can. J. Biochem.*, **42,** 1415 (1964).
230. P. Mazel, J. F. Henderson, and J. Axelrod, *J. Pharmacol. Exp. Ther.*, **143,** 1 (1964).

231. J. F. Henderson and P. Mazel, *Biochem. Pharmacol.*, **13,** 207 (1964).

232. J. F. Henderson and P. Mazel, *Biochem. Pharmacol.*, **13,** 1471 (1964).

233. F. M. Schabel, Jr., J. A. Montgomery, H. E. Skipper, W. R. Laster, Jr., and J. R. Thomson, *Cancer Res.*, **21,** 690 (1961).

234. H. P. Schnebli, D. L. Hill, and L. L. Bennett, Jr., *J. Biol. Chem.*, **243,** 1997 (1967).

235. D. H. W. Ho, J. K. Luce, and E. Frei, III, *Biochem. Pharmacol.*, **17,** 1925 (1968).

236. I. C. Caldwell, J. F. Henderson, and A. R. P. Paterson, *Can. J. Biochem.*, **44,** 229 (1966).

237. T. A. Krenitsky, G. B. Elion, A. M. Henderson, and G. H. Hitchings, *J. Biol. Chem.*, **243,** 2876 (1968).

238. T. L. Loo, D. H. W. Ho, D. R. Blossom, B. J. Shepard, and E. Frei, III, *Biochem. Pharmacol.*, **18,** 1711 (1969).

239. P. M. Roll, H. Weinfeld, E. Carroll, and G. B. Brown, *J. Biol. Chem.*, **220,** 439 (1956).

240. D. H. W. Ho, *Biochem. Pharmacol.*, **20,** 3538 (1971).

241. L. L. Bennett, Jr., H. P. Schnebli, M. H. Vail, P. W. Allan, and J. A. Montgomery, *Mol. Pharmacol.*, **2,** 432 (1966).

242. I. C. Caldwell, J. F. Henderson, and A. R. P. Paterson, *Can. J. Biochem.*, **45,** 735 (1967).

243. F. M. Schabel, Jr., W. R. Laster, Jr., and H. E. Skipper, *Cancer Chemother. Rep.*, **51,** 111 (1967).

244. M. C. Wang, A. I. Simpson, and A. R. P. Paterson, *Cancer Chemother. Rep.*, **51,** 101 (1967).

245. G. P. Bodey, H. S. Brodovsky, A. A. Isassi, M. L. Samuels, and E. J. Freireich, *Cancer Chemother. Rep.*, **52,** 315 (1968).

246. A. R. P. Paterson and M. C. Wang, *Can. J. Biochem.*, **48,** 79 (1970).

247. A. R. P. Paterson and A. Moriwaki, *Cancer Res.*, **29,** 681 (1969).

248. A. R. P. Paterson and M. C. Wang, *Cancer Res.*, **30,** 2379 (1970).

249. E. M. Scholar, P. R. Brown, and R. E. Parks, Jr., *Cancer Res.*, **32,** 259 (1972).

250. K. J. Pierre, A. P. Kimball, and G. A. LePage, *Can. J. Biochem.*, **45,** 1619 (1967).

251. K. J. Pierre and G. A. LePage, *Proc. Soc. Exp. Biol. Med.*, **127,** 432 (1968).

252. G. A. LePage and I. G. Junga, *Cancer Res.*, **25,** 46 (1965).

253. M. R. Atkinson, G. Eckermann, and J. Stephenson, *Biochim. Biophys. Acta*, **108,** 320 (1965).

254. J. P. Scannell and G. H. Hitchings, *Proc. Soc. Exp. Biol. Med.*, **122,** 627 (1966).

255. J. H. Coggin, M. Loosemore, and W. R. Martin, *J. Bacteriol.*, **92,** 446 (1966).

256. W. R. Martin, I. K. Crichton, R. C. Yang, and A. E. Evans, *Proc. Soc. Exp. Biol. Med.*, **140,** 423 (1972).

257. G. B. Elion, *Fed. Proc.*, **26,** 898 (1967).

258. T. L. Loo, C. Lim, and D. G. Johns, *Biochim. Biophys. Acta*, **134,** 467 (1967).

259. T. A. Krenitsky, S. M. Neil, G. B. Elion, and G. H. Hitchings, *Arch. Biochem. Biophys.*, **150,** 585 (1972).

260. F. Bergmann, H. Burger-Rachamimov, and M. Tamari, *Biochem. Biophys. Res. Commun.*, **12,** 284 (1963).

261. G. B. Elion, S. Callahan, H. Nathan, S. Bieber, R. W. Rundles, and G. H. Hitchings, *Biochem. Pharmacol.*, **12,** 85 (1963).

262. P. Feigelson, J. D. Davidson, and R. K. Robins, *J. Biol. Chem.*, **226,** 993 (1957).

263. A. S. Levine, H. L. Sharp, J. Mitchell, W. Krivit, and M. E. Nesbit, *Cancer Chemother. Rep.*, **53,** 53 (1969).

264. J. J. Coffey, C. A. White, A. B. Lesk, W. I. Rogers, and A. A. Serpick, *Cancer Res.*, **32,** 1283 (1972).

265. G. B. Elion, S. Bieber, and G. H. Hitchings, *Cancer Chemother. Rep.*, **8,** 36 (1960).

266. G. A. LePage, *Cancer Res.*, **23,** 1202 (1963).

267. G. A. LePage and M. Jones, *Cancer Res.*, **21,** 1590 (1961).

268. G. A. LePage, *Cancer Res.*, **20,** 403 (1960).

269. H. B. Mandel, R. G. Latimer, and M. Riis, *Biochem. Pharmacol.*, **14,** 661 (1965).

270. R. P. Miech, R. E. Parks, Jr., J. H. Anderson, Jr., and A. C. Sartorelli, *Biochem. Pharmacol.*, **16,** 2222 (1967).

271. R. P. Miech, R. York, and R. E. Parks, Jr., *Mol. Pharmacol.*, **5,** 30 (1969).

272. J. A. Nelson, J. W. Carpenter, L. M. Rose, and D. J. Adamson, *Cancer Res.*, **35,** 2872 (1975).

273. G. A. LePage and J. P. Whitecar, Jr., *Cancer Res.*, **31,** 1627 (1971).

274. L. H. Schmidt, J. A. Montgomery, W. R. Laster, Jr., and F. M. Schabel, Jr., *Proc. Am. Assoc. Cancer Res.*, **11,** 70 (1970).

275. T. S. Gee, K.-P. Yu, and B. D. Clarkson, *Cancer*, **23,** 1019 (1969).

276. G. A. LePage and T. Kaneko, *Cancer Res.*, **29,** 2314 (1969).

277. A. L. Bieber and A. C. Sartorelli, *Cancer Res.*, **24,** 1210 (1964).

278. M. K. Wolpert, S. P. Damale, J. E. Brown, E. Sznycer, K. C. Agrawal, and A. C. Sartorelli, *Cancer Res.*, **31,** 1620 (1971).

279. A. L. Bieber and A. C. Sartorelli, *Nature*, **201,** 624 (1964).

280. G. A. LePage, I. G. Junga, and B. Bowman, *Cancer Res.*, **24,** 835 (1964).

281. G. A. LePage and I. G. Junga, *Mol. Pharmacol.*, **3,** 37 (1967).

282. G. A. LePage, *Can. J. Biochem.*, **46,** 655 (1968).

283. A. Peery and G. A. LePage, *Cancer Res.*, **29,** 617 (1969).

284. Y. Nakai and G. A. LePage, *Cancer Res.*, **32,** 2445 (1972).

285. G. A. LePage and I. G. Junga, *Cancer Res.*, **23,** 739 (1963).

286. P. W. Allan and L. L. Bennett, Jr., *Biochem. Pharmacol.*, **20,** 847 (1971).

287. S. L. Marchesi and A. C. Sartorelli, *Cancer Res.*, **23,** 1769 (1963).

288. J. A. Nelson and R. E. Parks, Jr., *Cancer Res.*, **32,** 2034 (1972).

289. A. P. Kimball, G. A. LePage, and B. Bowman, *Can. J. Biochem.*, **42,** 1753 (1964).

290. E. M. Hersh and G. A. LePage, *Biochem. Pharmacol.*, **20,** 2459 (1971).

291. K. Sato, G. A. LePage, and A. P. Kimball, *Cancer Res.*, **26,** 741 (1966).

292. T. Kaneko and G. A. LePage, *Cancer Res.*, **30,** 699 (1970).

293. H. J. Hansen, W. G. Giles, and S. B. Nadler, *Cancer Res.*, **22,** 761 (1962).

294. H. J. Hansen, W. G. Giles, and S. B. Nadler, *Proc. Soc. Exp. Biol. Med.*, **113,** 163 (1963).

295. H. J. Hansen, J. P. Vandevoorde, W. G. Giles, and S. B. Nadler, *Proc. Soc. Exp. Biol. Med.*, **115,** 713 (1964).

296. A. P. Kimball and G. A. LePage, *Cancer Res.*, **22,** 1301 (1962).

297. G. A. LePage, Y.-T. Lin, R. E. Orth, and J. A. Gottlieb, *Cancer Res.*, **32,** 2441 (1972).

298. J. A. Montgomery, in *Progress in Medicinal Chemistry*, Vol. 7, Part 1, G. P. Ellis and G. B. West, Eds., Butterworths, London, 1970, p. 69.

299. R. J. Suhadolnik, *Nucleoside Antibiotics*, Wiley-Interscience, New York, 1970.

300. W. W. Lee, A. Benitez, L. Goodman, and B. R. Baker, *J. Am. Chem. Soc.*, **82,** 2648 (1960).

301. C. P. J. Glaudemans and H. G. Fletcher, Jr., *J. Org. Chem.*, **29,** 3286 (1964).

302. J. J. Brink and G. A. LePage, *Cancer Res.*, **24,** 312 (1964).

303. G. P. Bodey, J. Gottlieb, K. B. McCredie, and E. J. Freireich, *Proc. Am. Assoc. Cancer Res.*, **15,** 129 (1974).

304. J. J. Brink and G. A. LePage, *Cancer Res.*, **24,** 1042 (1964).

305. J. L. York and G. A. LePage, *Can. J. Biochem.*, **44,** 19 (1966).

306. A. J. Guarino and N. M. Kredich, *Biochim. Biophys. Acta*, **68,** 317 (1963).

307. G. A. LePage, L. S. Worth, and A. P. Kimball, *Cancer Res.*, **36,** 1481 (1976).

308. C. E. Cass and T. H. Au-Yeung, *Cancer Res.*, **36,** 1486 (1976).

309. R. W. Brockman, F. M. Schabel, Jr., and J. A. Montgomery, *Biochem. Pharmacol.*, **26,** 2193 (1977).

310. J. A. Montgomery and K. Hewson, *J. Med. Chem.*, **12,** 498 (1969).

311. J. A. Stock, in *Experimental Chemotherapy*, Vol. 5, R. J. Schnitzer and F. Hawking, Eds., Academic Press, New York, 1967, p. 333.

312. Symposium on Hydroxyurea, *Cancer Chemother. Rep.*, **40** (1964).

313. W. A. Creasey, R. L. Capizzi, and R. C. Deconti, *Cancer Chemother. Rep.*, **54,** 191 (1970).

314. H. S. Schwartz, M. Garofalo, S. S. Sternberg, and F. S. Phillips, *Cancer Res.*, **25,** 1867 (1965).

315. J. W. Yarbro, W. G. Niehaus, and C. P. Barnum, *Biochem. Biophys. Res. Commun.*, **19,** 592 (1965).

316. C. W. Young and S. Hodas, *Science*, **146,** 1172 (1964).

317. G. R. Gale, *Biochem. Pharmacol.*, **13,** 1377 (1964).

318. C. W. Young, G. Schochetman, and D. A. Karnofsky, *Cancer Res.*, **27,** 526 (1967).

319. I. H. Krakoff, N. C. Brown, and P. Reichard, *Cancer Res.*, **28,** 1559 (1968).

320. E. C. Moore, *Cancer Res.*, **29,** 291 (1969).

321. W. N. Fishbein and P. P. Carbone, *Science*, **142,** 1069 (1963).

322. V. H. Bono, Jr., and R. L. Dion, *Proc. Am. Assoc. Cancer Res.*, **10,** 8 (1969).

323. H. S. Rosenkranz, R. D. Pollak, and R. M. Schmidt, *Cancer Res.*, **29,** 209 (1969).

324. H. S. Rosenkranz and S. Rosenkranz, *Biochim. Biophys. Acta*, **195,** 266 (1969).

325. H. S. Rosenkranz, R. Hjorth, and H. S. Carr, *Biochim. Biophys. Acta*, **232,** 48 (1971).

326. R. W. Brockman, S. Shaddix, W. R. Laster, Jr., and F. M. Schabel, Jr., *Cancer Res.*, **30,** 2358 (1970).

327. R. W. Brockman, J. R. Thomson, M. J. Bell, and H. E. Skipper, *Cancer Res.*, **16,** 167 (1956).

328. F. A. French and E. J. Blanz, Jr., *Cancer Res.*, **26,** 1638 (1966).

329. E. J. Blanz, Jr., and F. A. French, *Cancer Res.*, **28,** 2419 (1968).

330. F. A. French and E. J. Blanz, Jr., *Cancer Res.*, **25,** 1454 (1965).

331. F. A. French and E. J. Blanz, Jr., *J. Med. Chem.*, **9,** 585 (1966).

332. E. C. Moore, M. S. Zedeck, K. C. Agrawal, and A. C. Sartorelli, *Biochemistry*, **9,** 4492 (1970).

333. A. C. Sartorelli, M. S. Zedeck, K. C. Agrawal, and E. C. Moore, *Fed. Proc.*, **27,** 650 (1968).

334. A. Gilman and F. S. Philips, *Science*, **103,** 409 (1946).

335. L. H. Schmidt, R. Fradkin, R. Sullivan, and A. Flowers, *Cancer Chemother. Rep.*, Suppl. 2, Parts 1–3, pp. 1–1528 (1965).

336. C. Heidelberger, *Cancer Res.*, **29,** 2435 (1969).

337. T. A. Conners, *Cancer Res.*, **29,** 2443 (1969).

338. W. C. J. Ross, in *Antineoplastic and Immunosuppressive Agents*, Part I, A. C. Sartorelli and D. G. Johns, Eds., Springer-Verlag, Heidelberg, 1974, Ch. 3.

339. J. A. Montgomery, in *Progress in Drug Research*, Vol. 20, E. Jucker, Ed., Birkhäuser-Verlag, Basel, 1976, pp. 465–490.

340. C. C. Price, in *Antineoplastic and Immunosuppressive Agents*, Part II, A. C. Sartorelli and D. G. Johns, Eds., Springer-Verlag, Heidelberg, 1975, Ch. 30.

341. P. D. Lawley and P. Brookes, *Nature*, **260,** 480 (1965).

342. O. Klatt, J. S. Stehlin, Jr., C. McBride, and A. C. Griffin, *Cancer Res.*, **29,** 286 (1969).

343. B. Puschendorf, H. Wolf, and H. Grunicke, *Biochem. Pharmacol.*, **20,** 3039 (1971).

344. L. M. van Putten and P. Lelieveld, *Eur. J. Cancer*, **7,** 11 (1971).

345. T. A. Connors, in *Antineoplastic and Immunosuppressive Agents*, Part II, A. C. Sartorelli and D. G. Johns, Eds., Springer-Verlag, Heidelberg, 1975, Ch. 32.

346. V. Prelog and V. Stepan, *Collect. Czech. Chem. Commun.*, **7,** 93 (1935).

347. P. Calabresi and R. E. Parks, Jr., in *The Pharmacological Basis of Therapeutics*, 5th ed., L. S. Goodman and A. Gilman, Eds., Macmillan, New York, 1975, Ch. 62.

348. E. M. Greenspan and H. W. Bruckner, in *Clinical Cancer Chemotherapy*, E. M. Greenspan, Ed., Raven Press, New York, 1975, Ch. 3.

349. W. C. J. Ross, *Biological Alkylating Agents*, Butterworths, London, 1962.

350. R. Shapiro, in *Progress in Nucleic Acid Research and Molecular Biology*, Vol. 8, J. N. Davidson and W. E. Cohn, Eds., Academic Press, New York, 1968, pp. 73–112.

351. S. F. Abdulnur and R. L. Flurry, Jr., *Nature*, **264,** 369 (1976).

352. W. C. J. Ross, in *Advances in Cancer Research*, Vol. 1, J. P. Greenstein and A. Haddow, Eds., Academic Press, New York, 1953, pp. 397–449.

353. C. E. Williamson and B. Witten, *Cancer Res.*, **27,** 33 (1967).

354. K. R. Harrap and E. W. Gascoigne, *Eur. J. Cancer*, **12,** 53 (1976).

355. J. L. Everett, J. J. Roberts, and W. C. J. Ross, *J. Chem. Soc.*, 2386 (1953).

356. F. Bergel and J. A. Stock, *J. Chem. Soc.*, 2409 (1954).

357. F. Bergel, V. C. E. Burnop, and J. A. Stock, *J. Chem. Soc.*, 1223 (1955).

358. L. F. Larionov, A. S. Khokhlov, E. N. Shkodinskaja, O. S. Vasina, V. I. Troosheikina, and M. A. Novikova, *Lancet*, **269,** 169 (1955).

359. B. Fisher, P. Carbone, S. G. Economou, R. Frelick, A. Glass, H. Lerner, C. Redmond, M. Zelen, P. Band, D. L. Katrych, N. Wolmark, and E. R. Fisher, *N. Engl. J. Med.*, **292,** 117 (1975).

360. T. A. Connors and W. C. J. Ross, *Chem. Ind.* (London), 492 (1960).

361. P. Clifford, in *Burkitt's Lymphoma*, D. P. Burkitt and D. H. Wright, Eds., Livingstone, Edinburgh, 1970, pp. 52–63.

362. S. K. Carter and M. Slavik, *Cancer Treat. Rev.*, **3,** 43 (1976).

363. N. J. Harper, *J. Med. Pharm. Chem.*, **1,** 467 (1959).

364. M. A. Stahmann and M. Bergmann, *J. Org. Chem.*, **11,** 586 (1946).

365. I. Aiko, S. Owari, and M. Torigoe, *J. Pharm. Soc. Japan*, **72,** 1297 (1952); through *Chem. Abstr.*, **47,** 1289 (1953).

366. S. Farber, R. Toch, E. M. Sears, and D. Pinkel, in *Advances in Cancer Research*, Vol. 4, J. P. Greenstein and A. Haddow, Eds., Academic Press, New York, 1956, pp. 1–71.

367. M. Ishidate, *Acta Unio Int. Cancrum*, **15,** 139 (1959).

368. H. Imamura, *Chem. Pharm. Bull.* (Tokyo), **8,** 449 (1960).

369. G. Gomori, *Proc. Soc. Exp. Biol. Med.*, **69,** 407 (1948).

370. O. M. Friedman and A. M. Seligman, *J. Am. Chem. Soc.*, **76,** 655 (1954).
371. O. M. Friedman, E. Boger, V. Grubliauskas, and H. Sommer, *J. Med. Chem.*, **6,** 50 (1963).
372. O. M. Friedman, Z. B. Papanastassiou, R. S. Levi, H. R. Till, Jr., and W. M. Whaley, *J. Med. Chem.*, **6,** 82 (1963).
373. C. L. Maddock, A. H. Handler, O. M. Friedman, G. E. Foley, and S. Farber, *Cancer Chemother. Rep.*, **50,** 629 (1966).
374. O. M. Friedman, *Cancer Chemother. Rep.*, **51,** 347 (1967).
375. H. Arnold and F. Bourseaux, *Angew. Chem.*, **70,** 539 (1958).
376. H. Arnold, F. Bourseaux, and N. Brock, *Naturwissenschaften*, **45,** 64 (1958).
377. H. Arnold, F. Bourseaux, and N. Brock, *Arzneim.-Forsch.*, **11,** 143 (1961).
378. K. Sugiura, F. Schmid, and M. Schmid, *Proc. Am. Assoc. Cancer Res.*, **3,** 271 (1961).
379. N. Brock, *Cancer Chemother. Rep.*, **51,** 315 (1967).
380. G. E. Foley, O. M. Friedman, and B. P. Drolet, *Cancer Res.*, **21,** 57 (1961).
381. D. L. Hill, *A Review of Cyclophosphamide*, Thomas, Springfield, Ill., 1975, Ch. 3.
382. P. J. Cox, P. B. Farmer, and M. Jarman., Eds., *Proceedings of the Symposium on the Metabolism and Mechanism of Action of Cyclophosphamide*, July 10–12, 1975, London, *Cancer Treat. Rep.*, **60,** 299–525 (1976).
383. C. E. Williamson, J. G. Kirby, J. I. Miller, S. Sass, S. P. Kramer, A. M. Seligman, and B. Witten, *Cancer Res.*, **26,** 323 (1966).
384. L. Nathanson, T. C. Hall, A. Rutenberg, and R. K. Shadduck, *Cancer Chemother. Rep.*, **51,** 35 (1967).
385. A. Takamizawa, S. Matsumoto, T. Iwata, Y. Tochino, K. Katagiri, K. Yamaguchi, and O. Shiratori, *J. Med. Chem.*, **18,** 376 (1975).
386. J. A. Montgomery and R. F. Struck, *Cancer Treat. Rep.*, **60,** 381 (1976).
387. J. van der Steen, E. C. Timmer, J. G. Westra, and C. Benckhuysen, *J. Am. Chem. Soc.*, **95,** 7535 (1973).
388. R. H. Adamson, in *Antineoplastic and Immunosuppressive Agents*, Part II, A. C. Sartorelli and D. G. Johns, Eds., Springer-Verlag, Heidelberg, 1975, Ch. 79.
389. H.-J. Hohorst, G. Peter, and R. F. Struck, *Cancer Res.*, **36,** 2278 (1976).
390. S. K. Carter and R. B. Livingston, *Cancer Treat. Rev.*, **2,** 295 (1975).
391. B. A. Chabner, C. E. Myers, C. N. Coleman, and D. G. Johns, *N. Engl. J. Med.*, **292,** 1159 (1975).
392. A. H. Khan and W. C. J. Ross, *Chem. Biol. Interact.*, **1,** 27 (1969/70).
393. T. A. Connors and D. H. Melzack, *Int. J. Cancer*, **7,** 86 (1971).
394. H. Umezawa, in *Cancer Medicine*, J. F. Holland and E. Frei, III, Eds., Lea & Febiger, Philadelphia, 1973, Sect. XIII-6.
395. W. Szybalski and V. N. Iyer, *Fed. Proc., Fed. Am. Soc. Exp. Biol.*, **23,** 946 (1964).
396. W. Szybalski and V. N. Iyer, in *Antibiotics*, Vol. 1, D. Gottlieb and P. D. Shaw, Eds., Springer-Verlag, New York, 1967, pp. 211–245.
397. C. O. Gitterman, E. L. Rickes, D. E. Wolf, J. Madas, S. B. Zimmerman, T. H. Stoudt, and T. C. Demny, *J. Antibiot.* (Tokyo), **23,** 305 (1970).
398. G. P. Wheeler, V. H. Bono, B. J. Bowdon, D. J. Adamson, and R. W. Brockman, *Cancer Treat. Rep.*, **60,** 1307 (1976).
399. R. W. Brockman, S. C. Shaddix, M. Williams, and R. F. Struck, *Cancer Treat. Rep.*, **60,** 1317 (1976).
400. T. A. Connors and W. C. J. Ross, *Chem. Ind.* (London), 366 (1958).
401. A. Haddow and G. M. Timmis, *Lancet*, **264,** 207 (1953).
402. G. M. Timmis and R. F. Hudson, *Ann N.Y. Acad. Sci.*, **68,** 727 (1958).
403. J. J. Roberts and G. P. Warwick, *Nature*, **184,** 1288 (1959).
404. G. P. Warwick, *Cancer Res.*, **23,** 1315 (1963).
405. Y. Sakurai and M. M. El-Merzabani, *Chem. Pharm. Bull.* (Tokyo), **12,** 954 (1964).
406. J. S. Sandberg, H. B. Wood, Jr., R. R. Engle, J. M. Venditti, and A. Goldin, *Cancer Chemother. Rep.*, Part 2, **3,** 137 (1972).
407. M. M. El-Merzabani and Y. Sakurai, *Gann*, **56,** 589 (1965).
408. J. A. Hendry, R. F. Homer, F. L. Rose, and A. L. Walpole, *Brit. J. Pharmacol.*, **6,** 235 (1951).
409. W. C. J. Ross, *Ann. N.Y. Acad. Sci.*, **68,** 669 (1958).
410. I. P. Horvath, J. Kralovanszky, I. Elekes, S. Eckhardt, and C. Sellai, in *Advances in Antimicrobial and Antineoplastic Chemotherapy* (*Proceedings of the 7th International Congress of Chemotherapy*, 1971, Vol. 2), M. Hejzler, Ed., University Park Press, Baltimore, 1972, pp. 27–29.
411. I. P. Horvath, J. Csetenyi, S. Eckhardt, M. Fuzi, and Z. Karika, in *Progress in Chemotherapy*, Vol. 3, *Antineoplastic Chemotherapy* (*Proceedings of*

the 8th International Congress of Chemotherapy, Athens, 1973), G. K. Daikos, Ed., Hellenic Society for Chemotherapy, Athens, 1974, pp. 718–723.

412. M. Jarman and W. C. J. Ross, *Chem. Ind.* (London), 1789 (1967).
413. L. A. Elson, M. Jarman, and W. C. J. Ross, *Eur. J. Cancer,* **4,** 617 (1968).
414. L. Vargha, L. Toldy, O. Feher, and S. Lendvai, *J. Chem. Soc.*, 805 (1957).
415. E. Csanyi and M. Halasz, *Arzneim.-Forsch.*, **23,** 961 (1973).
416. M. Fuzy, P. Lelieveld, and L. M. van Putten, *Eur. J. Cancer,* **11,** 169 (1975).
417. T. P. Johnston, G. S. McCaleb, and J. A. Montgomery, *J. Med. Chem.*, **6,** 669 (1963).
418. T. P. Johnston, G. S. McCaleb, P. S. Opliger, and J. A. Montgomery, *J. Med. Chem.*, **9,** 892 (1966).
419. T. P. Johnston and P. S. Opliger, *J. Med. Chem.*, **10,** 675 (1967).
420. T. P. Johnston, G. S. McCaleb, P. S. Opliger, W. R. Laster, Jr., and J. A. Montgomery, *J. Med. Chem.*, **14,** 600 (1971).
421. T. P. Johnston, G. S. McCaleb, S. D. Clayton, J. L. Frye, C. A. Krauth, and J. A. Montgomery, *J. Med. Chem.*, **20,** 279 (1977).
422. F. M. Schabel, Jr., *Cancer Treat. Rep.*, **60,** 665 (1976).
423. J. A. Montgomery, *Cancer Treat. Rep.*, **60,** 651 (1976).
424. J. A. Montgomery, G. S. McCaleb, T. P. Johnston, J. G. Mayo, and W. R. Laster, Jr., *J. Med. Chem.*, **20,** 291 (1977).
425. S. K. Carter, F. M. Schabel, Jr., L. E. Broder, and T. P. Johnston, in *Advances in Cancer Research*, Vol. 16, G. Klein and S. Weinhouse, Eds., Academic Press, New York, 1972, pp. 273–332.
426. T. H. Wasserman, M. Slavik, and S. K. Carter, *Cancer Treat. Rev.*, **1,** 131 (1974).
427. T. H. Wasserman, M. Slavik, and S. K. Carter, *Cancer,* **36,** 1258 (1975).
428. J. G. Mayo, W. R. Laster, Jr., C. M. Andrews, and F. M. Schabel, Jr., *Cancer Chemother. Rep.*, Part 1, **56,** 183 (1972).
429. M. D. Walker, *Cancer Chemother. Rep.*, Part 3, **4** (No. 3), 21 (1973).
430. D. Fewer, C. B. Wilson, and V. A. Levin, *Brain Tumor Chemotherapy*, Thomas, Springfield, Ill., 1976.
431. C. G. Moertel, A. J. Schutt, R. G. Hahn, and R. J. Reitemeier, *J. Nat. Cancer Inst.*, **54,** 69 (1975).
432. C. G. Moertel, *Cancer,* **36,** 675 (1975).
433. N. M. Emanuel, E. M. Vermel, L. A. Ostrovskaya, and N. P. Korman, *Cancer Chemother. Rep.*, Part 1, **58,** 135 (1974).
434. R. R. Herr, H. K. Jahnke, and A. G. Argoudelis, *J. Am. Chem. Soc.*, **89,** 4808 (1967).
435. J. J. Vavra, C. DeBoer, A. Dietz, L. J. Hanka, and W. T. Sokolski, *Antibiot. Ann.*, 1959–1960, 230 (1960).
436. S. K. Carter and R. L. Comis, *Cancer Treat. Rev.*, **2,** 193 (1975).
437. T. P. Johnston, G. S. McCaleb, and J. A. Montgomery, *J. Med. Chem.*, **18,** 104 (1975).
438. T. Anderson, M. G. McMenamin, and P. S. Schein, *Cancer Res.*, **35,** 761 (1975).
439. V. A. Levin and P. Kabra, *Cancer Chemother. Rep.*, **58,** 787 (1974).
440. G. P. Wheeler, in *Cancer Chemotherapy* (*ACS Symposium Series No. 30*), A. C. Sartorelli, Ed., American Chemical Society, Washington, D.C., 1976, pp. 87–119.
441. J. A. Montgomery, R. James, G. S. McCaleb, and T. P. Johnston, *J. Med. Chem.*, **10,** 668 (1967).
442. M. Colvin, J. W. Cowens, R. B. Brundrett, B. S. Kramer, and D. B. Ludlum, *Biochem. Biophys. Res. Commun.*, **60,** 515 (1974).
443. D. J. Reed, H. E. May, R. B. Boose, K. M. Gregory, and M. A. Beilstein, *Cancer Res.*, **35,** 568 (1975).
444. J. A. Montgomery, R. James, G. S. McCaleb, M. C. Kirk, and T. P. Johnston, *J. Med. Chem.*, **18,** 568 (1975).
445. D. B. Ludlum, B. S. Kramer, J. Wang, and C. Fenselau, *Biochemistry,* **14,** 5480 (1975).
446. M. Colvin, R. B. Brundrett, W. Cowens, I. Jardine, and D. B. Ludlum, *Biochem. Pharmacol.*, **25,** 695 (1976).
447. V. T. Oliverio, *Cancer Chemother. Rep.*, Part 3, **4** (No. 3), 13 (1973).
448. C. J. Cheng, S. Fujimura, D. Grunberger, and I. B. Weinstein, *Cancer Res.*, **32,** 22 (1972).
449. B. Schmall, C. J. Cheng, S. Fujimura, N. Gersten, D. Grunberger, and I. B. Weinstein, *Cancer Res.*, **33,** 1921 (1973).
450. B. J. Bowdon and G. P. Wheeler, *Proc. Am. Assoc. Cancer Res.*, **12,** 67 (1971).
451. K. W. Kohn, *Cancer Res.*, **37,** 1450 (1977).
452. H. E. Kann, Jr., K. W. Kohn, and J. M. Lyles, *Cancer Res.*, **34,** 398 (1974).
453. A. J. Fornace, Jr., K. W. Kohn, and H. E. Kann,

Jr., *Proc. Am. Assoc. Cancer Res. Am. Soc. Clin. Oncol.*, **16,** 128 (1975).
454. G. P. Wheeler, B. J. Bowdon, J. A. Grimsley, and H. H. Lloyd, *Cancer Res.*, **34,** 194 (1974).
455. H. E. May, R. Boose, and D. J. Reed, *Biochem. Biophys. Res. Commun.*, **57,** 426 (1974).
456. D. L. Hill, M. C. Kirk, and R. F. Struck, *Cancer Res.*, **35,** 296 (1975).
457. D. J. Reed and H. E. May, *Life Sci.*, **16,** 1263 (1975).
458. D. J. Reed, *Proc. Am. Assoc. Cancer Res. Am. Soc. Clin. Oncol.*, **16,** 92 (1975).
459. J. Hilton and M. D. Walker, *Biochem. Pharmacol.*, **24,** 2153 (1975).
460. J. Hilton and M. D. Walker, *Proc. Am. Assoc. Cancer Res. Am. Soc. Clin. Oncol.*, **16,** 103 (1975).
461. T. P. Johnston, G. S. McCaleb, and J. A. Montgomery, *J. Med. Chem.*, **18,** 634 (1975).
462. G. P. Wheeler, T. P. Johnston, B. J. Bowden, G. S. McCaleb, D. L. Hill, and J. A. Montgomery, *Biochem. Pharmacol.*, **26,** 2331 (1977).
463. R. B. Brundrett, J. W. Cowens, and M. Colvin, *Proc. Am. Assoc. Cancer Res. Am. Soc. Clin. Oncol.*, **17,** 102 (1976).
464. D. A. Clarke, R. K. Barclay, C. C. Stock, and C. S. Rondestvedt, Jr., *Proc. Soc. Exp. Biol. Med.*, **90,** 484 (1955).
465. J. H. Burchenal, M. K. Dagg, M. Beyer, and C. C. Stock, *Proc. Soc. Exp. Biol. Med.*, **91,** 398 (1956).
466. R. Preussmann, H. Druckrey, S. Ivankovik, and O. von Hodenberg, *Ann. N.Y. Acad. Sci.*, **163,** 697 (1969).
467. Y. F. Shealy, C. A. O'Dell, and C. A. Krauth, *J. Pharm. Sci.*, **64,** 177 (1975).
468. J. A. Montgomery, *Cancer Treat. Rep.*, **60,** 125 (1976).
469. Y. F. Shealy, C. A. Krauth, and J. A. Montgomery, *J. Org. Chem.*, **27,** 2150 (1962).
470. Y. F. Shealy, R. F. Struck, L. B. Holum, and J. A. Montgomery, *J. Org. Chem.*, **26,** 2396 (1961).
471. Y. F. Shealy, J. A. Montgomery, and W. R. Laster, Jr., *Biochem. Pharmacol.*, **11,** 674 (1962).
472. J. M. Venditti, *Cancer Treat. Rep.*, **60,** 135 (1976).
473. S. K. Carter and M. A. Friedman, *Eur. J. Cancer*, **8,** 85 (1972).
474. R. L. Comis, *Cancer Treat. Rep.*, **60,** 165 (1976).
475. J. R. Wilbur, W. W. Sutow, M. P. Sullivan, and J. A. Gottlieb, *Cancer*, **36,** 765 (1975).
476. Y. F. Shealy, *J. Pharm. Sci.*, **59,** 1533 (1970).
477. Y. F. Shealy, C. A. O'Dell, J. D. Clayton, and C. A. Krauth, *J. Pharm. Sci.*, **60,** 1426 (1971).
478. Y. F. Shealy and C. A. O'Dell, *J. Pharm. Sci.*, **60,** 554 (1971).
479. Y. F. Shealy, C. A. Krauth, C. E. Opliger, H. W. Guin, and W. R. Laster, Jr., *J. Pharm. Sci.*, **60,** 1192 (1971).
480. Y. F. Shealy and C. A. Krauth, *J. Med. Chem.*, **9,** 34 (1966).
481. H. T. Nagasawa, F. N. Shirota, and N. S. Mizuno, *Chem. Biol. Interact.*, **8,** 403 (1974).
482. Y. F. Shealy and C. A. Krauth, *Nature*, **210,** 208 (1966).
483. T. L. Loo, in *Antineoplastic and Immunosuppressive Agents*, Part II, A. C. Sartorelli and D. G. Johns, Eds., Springer-Verlag, Heidelberg, 1975, Ch. 56.
484. J. L. Skibba, G. Ramirez, D. D. Beal, and G. T. Bryan, *Biochem. Pharmacol.*, **19,** 2043 (1970).
485. N. S. Mizuno and E. W. Humphrey, *Cancer Chemother. Rep.*, Part 1, **56,** 465 (1972).
486. D. L. Hill, *Proc. Am. Assoc. Cancer Res. Am. Soc. Clin. Oncol.*, **16,** 38 (1975).
487. G. E. Housholder and T. L. Loo, *Life Sci.*, **8,** 533 (1969).
488. J. L. Skibba, G. Ramirez, D. D. Beal, and G. T. Bryan, *Cancer Res.*, **29,** 1944 (1969).
489. C. L. Vogel, V. T. DeVita, C. Denham, H. T. Foley, R. B. Field, and P. P. Carbone, *Cancer Chemother. Rep.*, Part 1, **55,** 159 (1971).
490. P. Zeller, H. Gutmann, B. Hegedüs, A. Kaiser, A. Langemann, and M. Müller, *Experientia*, **19,** 129 (1963).
491. W. Bollag and E. Grunberg, *Experientia*, **19,** 130 (1963).
492. D. J. Reed, in *Antineoplastic and Immunosuppressive Agents*, Part II, A. C. Sartorelli and D. G. Johns, Eds., Springer-Verlag, Heidelberg, 1975, Ch. 70.
493. G. R. Gale, J. G. Simpson, and A. B. Smith, *Cancer Res.*, **27,** 1186 (1967).
494. A. T. Huang and W. B. Kremer, *Proc. Am. Assoc. Cancer Res.*, **10,** 41 (1969).
495. V. T. Oliverio, in *Cancer Medicine*, J. F. Holland and E. Frei, III, Eds., Lea & Febiger, Philadelphia, 1973, Sect. XIII-5.
496. W. Bollag, A. Kaiser, A. Langemann, and P. Zeller, *Experientia*, **20,** 503 (1964).
497. J. Raaflaub and D. E. Schwartz, *Experientia*, **21,** 44 (1965).
498. V. T. Oliverio, C. Denham, V. T. DeVita, and

M. G. Kelly, *Cancer Chemother. Rep.*, **42,** 1 (1964).

499. W. Kreis, S. B. Piepho, and H. V. Bernhard, *Experientia*, **22,** 431 (1966).
500. T. Tsuji and E. M. Kosower, *J. Am. Chem. Soc.*, **93,** 1992 (1971).
501. P. Brookes, in *Report of the Proceedings of the Symposium, Downing College, Cambridge, June 22, 1965, Sponsored by Roche Products, Limited; Natulan (Ibenzmethyzin)*, A. M. Jellife and J. Marks, Eds., John Wright & Sons, Bristol, 1965, pp. 9–12.
502. S. A. Waksman and H. B. Woodruff, *Proc. Soc. Exp. Biol. Med.*, **45,** 609 (1940).
503. H. Brockmann, G. Bohnsack, B. Franck, H. Grone, H. Muxfeldt, and C. Suling, *Angew. Chem.*, **68,** 70 (1956).
504. G. E. Foley, in *Antibiotics Annual, 1955–1956*, H. Welch and F. Marti-Ibañez, Eds., Medical Encyclopedia, New York, 1956, p. 432.
505. I. J. Slotnick, *Antibiot. Chemother.*, **7,** 387 (1957); **8,** 476 (1958).
506. J. P. Cobb and D. G. Walker, *J. Nat. Cancer Inst.*, **21,** 263 (1958).
507. W. Muller, *Naturwissenschaften*, **49,** 156 (1962).
508. H. M. Sobell, in *Progress in Nucleic Acid Research and Molecular Biology*, Vol. 13A, Academic Press, New York, 1972.
509. G. F. Gause, in *Antineoplastic and Immunosuppressive Agents*, Part II, A. C. Sartorelli and D. G. Johns, Eds., Springer-Verlag, Heidelberg, 1975, p. 615.
510. P. Pietsch, in *Antineoplastic and Immunosuppressive Agents*, Part II, A. C. Sartorelli and D. G. Johns, Eds., Springer-Verlag, Heidelberg, 1975, p. 850.
511. A. DiMarco and L. Lenaz, in *Cancer Medicine*, J. F. Holland and E. Frei, III, Eds., Lea & Febiger, Philadelphia, 1973, p. 826.
512. A. DiMarco, in *Antineoplastic and Immunosuppressive Agents*, Part II, A. C. Sartorelli and D. G. Johns, Eds., Springer-Verlag, Heidelberg, 1975, p. 593.
513. M. Israel, E. J. Modest, and E. Frei, III, *Cancer Res.*, **35,** 1365 (1975).
514. I. S. Johnson, in *Cancer Medicine*, J. F. Holland and E. Frei, III, Eds., Lea & Febiger, Philadelphia, 1973, p. 840.
515. W. A. Creasey, in *Antineoplastic and Immunosuppressive Agents*, Part II, A. C. Sartorelli and D. G. Johns, Eds., Springer-Verlag, Heidelberg, 1975, p. 760.
516. G. P. Bodey and E. J. Freireich, *Abstr. Am. Assoc. Cancer Res.*, **17,** 128 (1976).
517. P. Ulrich, *Acta Unio Int. Contra Cancrum*, **4,** 377 (1939).
518. A. A. Loeser, *Acta Unio Int. Contra Cancrum*, **4,** 375 (1939).
519. C. Huggins and C. V. Hodges, *Cancer Res.*, **1,** 293 (1941).
520. C. Huggins, Nobel Prize Lecture, *Cancer Res.*, Part 1, **27,** 1925 (1967).
521. H. Seidman, *Cancer*, **24,** 1355 (1969).
522. G. M. Bonser, J. A. Dossett, and J. W. Jull, *Human and Experimental Breast Cancer*, Thomas, Springfield, Ill., 1961, pp. 411–434.
523. M. Cutler, *Tumors of the Breast*, Lippincott, Philadelphia, 1962, pp. 256–297.
524. L. H. Garland, in *Breast Cancer*, A. Segaloff, Ed., Mosby, St. Louis, 1958, pp. 114–122.
525. S. J. Cutler and H. W. Heise, *Cancer*, **24,** 1117 (1969).
526. J. Bruce, *Cancer*, **28,** 1443 (1971).
527. J. A. Urban and E. B. Castro, *Cancer*, **28,** 1615 (1971).
528. S. K. Carter, *Cancer Treat. Rev.*, **3,** 141–174 (1976).
529. B. J. Kennedy, in *Treatment of Cancer and Allied Diseases: Tumors of the Breast, Chest, and Esophagus*, Vol. 4, 2nd ed., G. T. Pack and I. M. Ariel, Eds., Hoeber, New York, 1960, pp. 178–204.
530. G. M. Bonser, J. A. Dossett, and J. W. Jull, *Human and Experimental Breast Cancer*, Thomas, Springfield, Ill., 1961, pp. 435–463.
531. M. Cutler, *Tumors of the Breast*, Lippincott, Philadelphia, 1962, pp. 316–334.
532. B. J. Kennedy, *Cancer*, **18,** 1551 (1965).
533. D. C. Tormey and P. P. Carbone, in *Methods in Cancer Research*, Vol. 13, H. Busch, Ed., Academic Press, New York, 1976, Ch. 1.
534. H. J. Tagnon, in *Breast Cancer: A Multidisciplinary Approach*, G. St. Arneault, P. Band, and L. Israël, Eds., Springer-Verlag, New York, 1976, Ch. 16.
535. G. T. Beatson, *Lancet*, **2,** 104, 162 (1896).
536. E. F. Lewiston, *Cancer*, **24,** 1297 (1969).
537. A. A. Fracchia, *Cancer*, **28,** 1699 (1971).
538. B. J. Kennedy, in *Cancer Medicine*, J. F. Holland and E. Frei, III, Eds., Lea & Febiger, Philadelphia, 1973, Ch. XIV-10.
539. A. Segaloff, *Cancer*, **30,** 1541 (1972).
540. A. Segaloff, *Cancer Treat. Rev.*, **2,** 129 (1975).
541. M. J. Brennan, in *Cancer Medicine*, J. F. Holland and E. Frei, III, Eds., Lea & Febiger, Philadelphia, 1973, Ch. 27, pp. 1769–1788.

542. C. Huggins and D. M. Bergenstall, *Cancer Res.*, **12,** 134 (1952).
543. C. Huggins and T. L.-Y. Dao, *J. Am. Med. Assoc.*, **151,** 1388 (1953).
544. A. A. Fracchia, A. I. Holleb, J. H. Farrow, N. E. Treves, H. T. Randall, J. A. Finkbeiner, and W. F. Whitmore, Jr., *Cancer*, **12,** 58 (1959).
545. R. E. Wilson, A. J. Piro, M. A. Aliapoulios, and F. D. Moore, *Cancer*, **24,** 1322 (1969).
546. R. Luft and H. Olivecrona, *J. Neurosurg.*, **10,** 301 (1953).
547. R. Luft and H. Olivecrona, *Cancer*, **8,** 261 (1955).
548. O. H. Pearson and B. S. Ray, *Cancer*, **12,** 85 (1959).
549. A. A. Loeser, *Brit. Med. J.*, **1,** 479 (1940).
550. A. A. Loeser, *Lancet*, **2,** 698 (1941).
551. E. Fels, *J. Clin. Endocrinol.*, **4,** 121 (1944).
552. F. E. Adair and J. B. Herrmann, *Ann. Surg.*, **123,** 1023 (1946).
553. A. Haddow, J. M. Watkinson, and E. Paterson, *Brit. Med. J.*, **2,** 393 (1944).
554. F. Ellis, S. B. Adams, G. W. Blomfield, A. Haddow, W. M. Levitt, R. McWhirter, E. Paterson, C. J. L. Thurgar, J. Z. Walker, and B. W. Windeyer, *Brit. Med. J.*, **2,** 20 (1944); *Proc. Roy. Soc. Med.*, **37,** 731 (1944).
555. J. B. Herrmann, F. E. Adair, and H. Q. Woodward, *Arch. Surg.*, **54,** 1 (1947).
556. Subcommittee on Breast and Genital Cancer, Committee on Research, Am. Med. Assoc., I. T. Nathanson, E. T. Engle, and I. Macdonald, Chairmen, *J. Am. Med. Assoc.*, **172,** 1271 (1960).
557. I. T. Nathanson, *Cancer*, **5,** 754 (1952).
558. T. L. Dao, in *Antineoplastic and Immunosuppressive Agents*, Part II, A. C. Sartorelli and D. G. Johns, Eds., Springer-Verlag, Heidelberg, 1975, Ch. 40.
559. I. S. Goldenberg, for the Cooperative Breast Cancer Group, *J. Am. Med. Assoc.*, **188,** 1069 (1964).
560. Cooperative Breast Cancer Group, A. Segaloff, Chairman, *Cancer Chemother. Rep.*, **11,** 109 (1961).
561. Cooperative Breast Cancer Group, A. Segaloff, Chairman, *Cancer Chemother. Rep.*, **41,** Suppl. 1, 1 (1964).
562. A. Segaloff, in *Methods in Hormone Research*, Vol. 5, R. I. Dorfman, Ed., Academic Press, New York, 1966, Ch. 5.
563. A. Segaloff, *Rec. Progr. Hormone Res.*, **22,** 351 (1966).
564. G. S. Gordan, A. Halden, Y. Horn, J. J. Fuery, R. J. Parsons, and R. M. Walter, *Oncology*, **28,** 138 (1973).
565. I. S. Goldenberg, M. N. Waters, R. S. Ravdin, F. J. Ansfield, and A. Segaloff, *J. Am. Med. Assoc.*, **223,** 1267 (1973).
566. A. Segaloff, in *Methods in Hormone Research*, Vol. 5, R. I. Dorfman, Ed., Academic Press, New York, 1966, Ch. 4.
567. A. Segaloff, in *Cancer Medicine*, J. F. Holland and E. Frei, III, Eds., Lea & Febiger, Philadelphia, 1973, Ch. XIV-3, pp. 896–899.
568. I. S. Goldenberg and A. Segaloff, in *Cancer Medicine*, J. F. Holland and E. Frei, III, Eds., Lea & Febiger, Philadelphia, 1973, Ch. XIV-8, pp. 929–933.
569. R. M. Kelley, *Cancer*, **28,** 1686 (1971).
570. S. K. Carter and L. M. Kershner, *Pharm. Times*, 56–66 (August 1975).
571. H. B. Wood, Jr., "Chemical Structures of Current Interest to the Division of Cancer Treatment, Drugs with Clinical Activity", National Cancer Institute, p. 14 (January 1977).
572. C. M. Blackburn, *Cancer Chemother. Rep.*, **16,** 279 (1962).
573. M. E. Herr, J. A. Hogg, and R. H. Levin, *J. Am. Chem. Soc.*, **78,** 500 (1956).
574. S. C. Lyster, G. H. Lund, and R. O. Stafford, *Endocrinology*, **58,** 781 (1956).
575. L. J. Lerner, A. Bianchi, and A. Borman, *Cancer*, **13,** 1201 (1960).
576. European Breast Cancer Group (E. Anglesio, A. Calciati, M. Margottini, G. Jacobelli, G. Martz, K. Brunner, A. Netter, A. Gorins, H. Nowakowski, J. Dittert, H. Tagnon, M. Van Rymenant, H. Van Gilse, and J. Scheltema), *Cancer Chemother. Rep.*, **27,** 79 (1963).
577. J. A. Campbell and J. C. Babcock, *J. Am. Chem. Soc.*, **81,** 4069 (1959).
578. R. Rosso, G. Porcile, and F. Brema, *Cancer Chemother. Rep.*, Part 1, **59,** 890 (1975).
579. B. J. Kennedy, *Cancer*, **24,** 1345 (1969).
580. E. V. Jensen, M. Numata, P. I. Brecher, and E. R. DeSombre, in *The Biochemistry of Steroid Hormone Action*, R. M. S. Smellie, Ed., Academic Press, New York, 1971, pp. 133–159.
581. E. V. Jensen and E. R. DeSombre, *Ann. Rev. Biochem.*, **41,** 203 (1972).
582. E. V. Jensen, in *Cancer Medicine*, J. F. Holland and E. Frei, III, Eds., Lea & Febiger, Philadelphia, 1973, Ch. XIV-4.
583. E. V. Jensen, G. E. Block, S. Smith, and E. R. DeSombre, in *Breast Cancer: A Challenging*

Problem, M. L. Griem, E. V. Jensen, J. E. Ultmann, and R. W. Wissler, Eds., Springer-Verlag, New York, 1973, pp. 55–62.

584. R. Hilf and J. L. Wittliff, in *Hormones and Cancer*, K. W. McKerns, Ed., Academic Press, New York, 1974, Ch. 4.

585. W. L. McGuire, G. C. Chamness, M. E. Costlow, and R. E. Shepherd, in *Hormones and Cancer*, K. W. McKerns, Ed., Academic Press, New York, 1974, Ch. 3.

586. W. L. McGuire, G. C. Chamness, and R. E. Shepherd, *Life Sci.*, **14,** 19 (1974).

587. W. L. McGuire, *Ann. Rev. Med.*, **26,** 353 (1975).

588. W. L. McGuire, P. P. Carbone, and E. P. Vollmer, *Estrogen Receptors in Breast Cancer*, Raven Press, New York, 1975.

589. J. L. Wittliff, in *Methods in Cancer Research*, Vol. 11, H. Busch, Ed., Academic Press, New York, 1975, Ch. 7.

590. J. L. Wittliff, B. W. Beatty, E. D. Savlov, W. B. Patterson, and R. A. Cooper, Jr., in *Breast Cancer: A Multidisciplinary Approach*, G. St. Arneault, P. Band, and L. Israël, Eds., Springer-Verlag, New York, 1976, Ch. 7.

591. N. Bruchovsky and E. Van Doorn, in *Breast Cancer: A Multidisciplinary Approach*, G. St. Arneault, P. Band, and L. Israël, Eds., Springer-Verlag, New York, 1976, Ch. 11.

592. E. E. Baulieu, in *Breast Cancer: Trends in Research and Treatment*, J. C. Heuson, W. H. Mattheiem, and M. Rozencweig, Eds., Raven Press, New York, 1976, pp. 165–176.

593. W. L. McGuire, K. B. Horwitz, and M. DeLa Garza, in *Breast Cancer: Trends in Research and Treatment*, J. C. Heuson, W. H. Mattheiem, and M. Rozencweig, Eds., Raven Press, New York, 1976, pp. 177–184.

594. W. L. McGuire, P. P. Carbone, M. E. Sears, and G. C. Escher, in *Estrogen Receptors in Human Breast Cancer*, W. L. McGuire, P. P. Carbone, and E. P. Vollmer, Eds., Raven Press, New York, 1975, Ch. 1.

595. E. V. Jensen, T. Z. Polley, S. Smith, G. E. Block, D. J. Ferguson, and E. R. DeSombre, in *Estrogen Receptors in Human Breast Cancer*, W. L. McGuire, P. P. Carbone, and E. P. Vollmer, Eds., Raven Press, New York, 1975, Ch. 5.

596. R. L. Hilf and J. L. Wittliff, in *Antineoplastic and Immunosuppressive Agents*, Part II, A. C. Sartorelli and D. G. Johns, Eds., Springer-Verlag, Heidelberg, 1975, Ch. 37.

597. L. J. Lerner, *Rec. Progr. Hormone Res.*, **20,** 435 (1964).

598. L. Terenius, *Acta Endocrinol.*, **66,** 431 (1971).

599. S. S. Legha and S. K. Carter, *Cancer Treat. Rev.*, **3,** 205 (1976).

600. L. Terenius, *Eur. J. Cancer*, **7,** 57 (1971).

601. H. Rochefort and F. Capony, *FEBS Lett.*, **20,** 11 (1972).

602. V. C. Jordan and S. Koerner, *Eur. J. Cancer*, **11,** 205 (1975).

603. V. C. Jordan and L. J. Dowse, *J. Endocrinol.*, **68,** 297 (1976).

604. R. Hähnel, E. Twaddle, and T. Ratajczak, *J. Steroid Biochem.*, **4,** 687 (1973).

605. J. H. Clark, E. J. Peck, Jr., and J. N. Anderson, *Nature*, **251,** 446 (1974).

606. T. S. Ruh and M. F. Ruh, *Steroids*, **24,** 209 (1974).

607. S. Ernst, G. Hite, J. S. Cantrell, A. Richardson, Jr., and H. D. Benson, *J. Pharm. Sci.*, **65,** 148 (1976).

608. C. Huggins, R. E. Stevens, Jr., and C. V. Hodges, *Arch. Surg.*, **43,** 209 (1941).

609. C. Huggins, *J. Am. Med. Assoc.*, **131,** 576 (1946).

610. A. B. Gutman and E. B. Gutman, *J. Clin. Invest.*, **17,** 473 (1938).

611. J. B. Goetsch, *J. Urol.*, **84,** 636 (1960).

612. H. Brendler and G. Prout, Jr., *Cancer Chemother. Rep.*, **16,** 323 (1962).

613. G. R. Prout, Jr., in *Cancer Medicine*, J. F. Holland and E. Frei, III, Eds., Lea & Febiger, Philadelphia, 1973, Ch. XXV-4.

614. R. M. Nesbit and W. C. Baum, *J. Am. Med. Assoc.*, **143,** 1317 (1950).

615. C. V. Hodges and D. Kirchheim, in *Recent Results in Cancer Research*, Vol. 8, L. Manuila, S. Moles, and P. Rentchnick, Eds., Springer-Verlag, New York, 1967, pp. 133–142.

616. G. D. Chisholm and E. P. N. O'Donoghue, *Vitam. Hormones*, **33,** 377 (1975).

617. G. P. Murphy, *Vitam. Hormones*, **33,** 399 (1975).

618. P. C. Walsh, *Urolog. Clin. N. Am.*, **2,** 125 (1975).

619. H. M. Lemon, in *Cancer Medicine*, J. F. Holland and E. Frei, III, Eds., Lea & Febiger, Philadelphia, 1973, Ch. XIV-6.

620. G. Jönsson, E. Diczfalusy, L.-O. Plantin, L. Röhl, and G. Birke, *Acta Endocrinol.*, **Suppl. 83,** 3 (1963).

621. G. Jönsson, A. M. Olsson, W. Luttrop, Z. Cekan, K. Purvis, and E. Diczfalusy, *Vitam. Hormones*, **33,** 351 (1975).

622. T. Nilsson and G. Jönsson, *Cancer Chemother. Rep.*, Part 1, **59,** 229 (1975).

623. R. Nagel and C.-P. Kölln, in *Prostatic Disease*, H. Marberger, H. Haschek, H. K. A. Schirmer, J. A. C. Colston, and E. Witkin, Eds., Alan R. Liss, New York, 1976, pp. 267–284.

624. A. Mittelman, R. Catane, and G. P. Murphy, *Cancer Treat. Rep.*, **61,** 307 (1977).

625. G. P. Murphy and C. E. Merrin, in *Prostatic Disease*, H. Marberger, H. Haschek, H. K. A. Schirmer, J. A. C. Colston, and E. Witkin, Eds., Alan R. Liss, New York, 1976, pp. 285–299.

626. W. W. Scott and H. K. A. Schirmer, *Trans. Am. Assoc. Genitourin. Surg.*, **58,** 54 (1966).

627. F. Neumann, B. Schenck, T. Senge, and K.-D. Richter, in *Prostatic Disease*, H. Marberger, H. Haschek, H. K. A. Schirmer, J. A. C. Colston, and E. Witkin, Eds., Alan R. Liss, New York, 1976, pp. 169–188.

628. S. Liao and T. Liang, in *Hormones and Cancer*, K. W. McKerns, Ed., Academic Press, New York, 1974, Ch. 8.

629. W. I. P. Mainwaring, *Vitam. Hormones*, **33,** 223 (1975).

630. R. M. Kelley, in *Cancer Medicine*, J. F. Holland and E. Frei, III, Eds., Lea & Febiger, Philadelphia, 1973, Ch. XIV-7.

631. S. B. Gusberg, in *Cancer Medicine*, J. F. Holland and E. Frei, III, Eds., Lea & Febiger, Philadelphia, 1973, Ch. XXVI-3.

632. R. M. Kelley and W. H. Baker, *New Engl. J. Med.*, **264,** 216 (1961).

633. B. J. Kennedy, *J. Am. Med. Assoc.*, **184,** 758 (1963).

634. R. M. Kelley and W. H. Baker, *Cancer Res.*, **25,** 1190 (1965).

635. R. W. Kistner, C. T. Griffiths, and J. M. Craig, *Cancer*, **18,** 1563 (1965).

636. H. J. G. Bloom and D. M. Wallace, *Brit. J. Med.*, **2,** 476 (1964).

637. H. J. G. Bloom, *Brit. J. Cancer*, **25,** 250 (1971).

638. G. R. Pout, Jr., in *Cancer Medicine*, J. F. Holland and E. Frei, III, Eds., Lea & Febiger, Philadelphia, 1973, Ch. XXV-2.

639. R. W. Talley, in *Cancer Medicine*, J. F. Holland and E. Frei, III, Eds., Lea & Febiger, Philadelphia, 1973, Ch. XIV-9.

640. R. B. Livingston and S. K. Carter, *Single Agents in Cancer Chemotherapy*, IFI/Plenum, New York, 1970, pp. 337–358.

641. E. S. Henderson, in *Cancer Medicine*, J. F. Holland and E. Frei, III, Eds., Lea & Febiger, Philadelphia, 1973, Ch. XIX-2.

642. A. M. Mauer and J. V. Simone, *Cancer Treat. Rev.*, **3,** 17 (1976).

643. F. W. Gunz, in *Cancer Medicine*, J. F. Holland and E. Frei, III, Eds., Lea & Febiger, Philadelphia, 1973, Ch. XIX-5.

644. S. A. Rosenberg, in *Cancer Medicine*, J. F. Holland and E. Frei, III, Eds., Lea & Febiger, Philadelphia, 1973, Ch. XIX-6.

645. P. P. Carbone and V. T. DeVita, in *Cancer Medicine*, J. F. Holland and E. Frei, III, Eds., Lea & Febiger, Philadelphia, 1973, Ch. XIX-7.

646. R. E. Lenhard, Jr., R. L. Prentice, A. H. Owens, Jr., R. Bakemeier, J. H. Horton, B. I. Shnider, L. Stolbach, C. W. Berard, and P. P. Carbone, *Cancer*, **38,** 1052 (1976).

647. S. E. Salmon, R. K. Shadduck, and A. Schilling, *Cancer Chemother. Rep.*, **51,** 179 (1967).

648. R. R. Ellison, in *Cancer Medicine*, J. F. Holland and E. Frei, III, Eds., Lea & Febiger, Philadelphia, 1973, Ch. XIX-3.

649. J. Bernard and J. Tanzer, in *Cancer Medicine*, J. F. Holland and E. Frei, III, Eds., Lea & Febiger, Philadelphia, 1973, Ch. XIX-4.

650. S. K. Carter, *Cancer*, **30,** 1543 (1972).

651. D. E. Johnson, W. W. Scott, R. P. Gibbons, G. R. Prout, J. D. Schmidt, T. M. Chu, J. Gaeta, J. Saroff, and G. P. Murphy, *Cancer Treat. Rep.*, **61,** 317 (1977).

652. S. Liao, J. L. Tymoczko, E. Castaneda, and T. Liang, *Vitam. Hormones*, **33,** 297 (1975).

653. J. H. Clark, E. J. Peck, Jr., W. T. Schrader, and B. W. O'Malley, in *Methods in Cancer Research*, Vol. 12, H. Busch, Ed., Academic Press, New York, 1976, Ch. 7.

654. F. Rosen, N. Kaiser, M. Mayer, and R. J. Milholland, in *Methods in Cancer Research*, Vol. 13, H. Busch, Ed., Academic Press, New York, 1976, Ch. 3.

655. D. Feldman, *Ann. Rev. Med.*, **26,** 83 (1975).

656. R. L. Capizzi and R. E. Handschumacher, in *Cancer Medicine*, J. F. Holland and E. Frei, III, Eds., Lea & Febiger, Philadelphia, 1973, p. 850.

657. H. F. Oettgen, in *Antineoplastic and Immunosuppressive Agents*, Part 2, A. C. Sartorelli and D. G. Johns, Eds., Springer-Verlag, Heidelberg, 1975, p. 723.

658. S. M. Buckley, C. C. Stock, M. L. Crossley, and C. P. Rhoads, *Cancer Res.*, **10,** 207 (1950).

659. R. H. Blum, R. B. Livingston, and S. K. Carter, *Eur. J. Cancer*, **9,** 195 (1973).

660. B. Rosenberg, E. Reushaw, L. Van Camp, T. Hartwick, and J. Drobnik, *J. Bacteriol.*, **93,** 716 (1967).

661. B. Rosenberg and L. Van Camp, *Cancer Res.*, **30,** 1799 (1970).

662. H. C. Harder and B. Rosenberg, *Int. J. Cancer*, **6,** 707 (1970).

663. L. L. Munchausen and R. O. Rahn, *Cancer Chemother. Rep.*, Part 1, **59,** 643 (1975).

664. J. M. Hill, E. Loeb, R. J. Speer, A. MacLellan, and N. O. Hill, *Proc. Am. Assoc. Cancer Res.*, **13,** 20 (1972).

665. Proceedings of the 16th Annual Meeting of the Society for Economic Botany: "Plants and Cancer", *Cancer Treat. Rep.*, **60,** 973 (1976).

666. G. B. Elion and G. H. Hitchings, in *Antineoplastic and Immunosuppressive Agents*, Part 2, A. C. Sartorelli and D. G. Johns, Eds., Springer-Verlag, Heidelberg, 1975, p. 404.

667. W. Cowens, R. Brundrett, and M. Colvin, *Proc. Am. Assoc. Cancer Res. Am. Soc. Clin. Oncol.*, **16,** 100 (1975).

668. D. P. Rall, in *Cancer Medicine*, J. F. Holland and E. Frei, III, Eds., Lea & Febiger, Philadelphia, 1973, p. 675.

669. E. Frei, III, and J. A. Gottlieb, in *Antineoplastic and Immunosuppressive Agents*, Part 1, A. C. Sartorelli and D. G. Johns, Eds., Springer-Verlag, Heidelberg, 1974, p. 449.

670. B. Clarkson, in *Antineoplastic and Immunosuppressive Agents*, Part 1, A. C. Sartorelli and D. G. Johns, Eds., Springer-Verlag, Heidelberg, 1974, p. 156.

671. I. Kline, M. Gang, R. J. Woodman, R. L. Cysyk, and J. M. Venditti, *Cancer Chemother. Rep.*, **57,** 299 (1973).

672. Proceedings of High-Dose Methotrexate Therapy Meeting: December 19, 1974, *Cancer Chemother. Rep.*, Part 3, **6** (No. 1), 1 (1975).

673. P. S. Schein and S. Loftus, *Cancer Res.*, **28,** 1501 (1968).

674. P. S. Schein, personal communication.

675. H. E. Skipper, F. M. Schabel, Jr., M. Bell, J. R. Thomson, and S. Johnson, *Cancer Res.*, **17,** 717 (1957).

676. H. E. Skipper, unpublished observations.

677. J. F. Henderson and R. W. Brockman, in *Pharmacological Basis of Cancer Chemotherapy*, Williams & Wilkins, Baltimore, 1975, p. 629.

678. R. W. Brockman, in *Pharmacological Basis of Cancer Chemotherapy*, Williams & Wilkins, Baltimore, 1975, p. 671.

679. R. W. Brockman, in *Antineoplastic and Immunosuppressive Agents*, Part 1, A. C. Sartorelli and D. G. Johns, Eds., Springer-Verlag, Heidelberg, 1974, p. 352.

680. J. A. Montgomery, in *Antineoplastic and Immunosuppressive Agents*, Part 1, A. C. Sartorelli and D. G. Johns, Eds., Springer-Verlag, Heidelberg, 1974, p. 76.

681. J. R. Bertino, in *Antineoplastic and Immunosuppressive Agents*, Part 2, A. C. Sartorelli and D. G. Johns, Eds., Springer-Verlag, Heidelberg, 1975, p. 468.

682. D. G. Johns and J. R. Bertino, in *Cancer Medicine*, J. F. Holland and E. Frei, III, Eds., Lea & Febiger, Philadelphia, 1973, p. 739.

683. H. E. Skipper and F. M. Schabel, Jr., in *Cancer Medicine*, J. F. Holland and E. Frei, III, Eds., Lea & Febiger, Philadelphia, 1973, p. 629.

684. F. M. Schabel, Jr., *Cancer Res.*, **29,** 2384 (1967).

685. H. E. Skipper, *Cancer Chemother. Rep.*, Part 2, **4** (No. 1), 137 (1974).

686. F. M. Schabel, Jr., in *Pharmacological Basis of Cancer Chemotherapy*, Williams & Wilkins, Baltimore, 1975, p. 596.

687. R. Nissen-Meyer, K. Kjellgren, and B. Mansson, *Cancer Chemother. Rep.*, **55,** 561 (1971).

688. G. Bonadonna, E. Brusamolino, P. Valagussa, A. Rossi, L. Brugnatelli, C. Brambilla, M. Delena, G. Taneini, E. Bajetta, R. Musumeci, and V. Veronesi, *New Engl. J. Med.*, **294,** 405 (1976).

689. E. P. Cortes, J. F. Holland, J. J. Wang, L. F. Sinks, J. Blom, H. Senn, A. Bank, and O. Glidewell, *New Engl. J. Med.*, **291,** 998 (1974).

690. F. H. Kung and W. L. Nyhan, in *Cancer Medicine*, J. F. Holland and E. Frei, III, Eds., Lea & Febiger, Philadelphia, 1973, p. 1881.

691. H. F. Oettgen and K. E. Hellström, in *Cancer Medicine*, J. F. Holland and E. Frei, III, Eds., Lea & Febiger, Philadelphia, 1973, p. 951.

692. R. L. Simmons, A. Rios, G. Lundgren, P. K. Ray, C. F. McKhann, and G. Haywood, *Surgery*, **70,** 38 (1971).

693. J. G. Bekesi, J. F. Holland, J. W. Yates, E. Henderson, and R. Fleminger, *Proc. Am. Assoc. Cancer Res. Am. Soc. Clin. Oncol.*, **16,** 121 (1975).

694. H. D. Suit, R. Sedlacek, M. Wagner, L. Orsi, V. Silobrcic, and K. J. Rothman, *Cancer Res.*, **36,** 1305 (1976).

695. *Proc. Am. Assoc. Cancer Res. Am. Soc. Clin. Oncology*, **16,** (1975).

696. W. D. Terry, *Cancer*, **25,** 198 (1975).

697. J. U. Gutterman, G. Mavligit, J. A. Gottlieb, M. A. Burgess, C. E. McBride, L. Einhorn, E. J. Freireich, and E. N. Hersh, *New Engl. J. Med.*, **291,** 592 (1972).

698. M. R. Hilleman, *Cancer,* **34,** 1439 (1974).

699. R. C. Gallo, *Am. J. Clin. Pathol.*, **60,** 80 (1973).

700. J. F. Holland, J. Roboz, N. Wald, and J. G. Bekes, *Proc. Am. Assoc. Cancer Res. Am. Soc. Clin. Oncol.*, **15,** 117 (1974).

701. F. M. Schabel, Jr., *Cancer Chemother. Rep.*, **59,** 261 (1975).

702. M. Perloff, J. Roboz, and J. F. Holland, *Proc. Am. Assoc. Cancer Res. Am. Soc. Clin. Oncol.*, **16,** 142 (1975).

CHAPTER TWENTY-FIVE

Agents Affecting the Immune Response

FRITZ K. HESS

and

KURT R. FRETER

Pharma-Research Canada Ltd.,
Pointe Claire, Quebec H9R 1G8, Canada

CONTENTS

1 THE IMMUNE RESPONSE

1.1 General

It has been known for a long time that survivors of diseases such as smallpox usually resist a second infection; such "immune" people were often the only ones to care for the sick during severe epidemics.

The discovery that microorganisms are the causative agents of infectious diseases became the scientific basis of the vaccination procedures in today's health care. What began nearly 100 years ago as a study of resistance to infection by the invasion of foreign structures (antigens), has developed into a major field of modern medicochemical science. During the past 20 years we have seen an unprecedented proliferation of discoveries in immunology which has increased our understanding of some of the basic mechanisms underlying the initiation and regulation of the immune response.

The normal and beneficial immune reaction, elicited by foreign agents, can become perverted and directed against the individual's own products, resulting in a variety of undesirable consequences, as in the so-called autoimmune diseases. These comprise a large and heterogeneous group of clinical conditions, the most important ones being rheumatoid arthritis, hemolytic anemia, lupus erythematosus, and scleroderma. They may result from aberrations in the immune defense system with the formation of antibodies against the host's own cells, or they may derive from tissue damage, with the immunological system treating the altered tissues as foreign. Allergic reactions are also consequences of a malfunctioning immune response; this aspect is treated in another chapter. Therefore the ability to control the immune response would enable us to deal with a number of serious diseases; the transplantations of tissue and organ allografts (from another individual of the same species) and their maintenance has created a further need for immunosuppressive therapy.

Immunosuppressive agents may be defined as substances that are able to prevent or reduce the immune response; a considerable number of materials are available to abate its humoral and cellular manifestations (1–3). Most of the compounds known today are related in some way to active agents from the field of cancer research. Ideally, suppression of the immune response should be specific; because of the complexity of the immune system and because of the multiple sites of action of these drugs, however, our ability to suppress selectively different parts of the immune response without directly affecting others is still limited. Although chemical immunosuppression has not achieved full immunological specificity, appropriate regimens of drug administration have been very useful for therapeutic purposes in many instances.

There are essentially two main types of immunity, humoral and cellular; humoral responses result in antibody production, whereas cell-mediated responses become manifest in delayed hypersensitivity, graft-versus-host reaction, graft rejection, and protection against infection.

All immune responses undergo the same general pattern: the primary response follows first exposure to the antigen of the animal or the individual; it reaches its peak after 8–10 days. The secondary response, obtained after a second challenge, is accelerated and more intense (Fig. 25.1). In general, immunoreductive agents suppress the primary response with greater facility than the secondary immune response or an established antibody production.

The actual mechanism of initiation of an immune response is difficult to determine

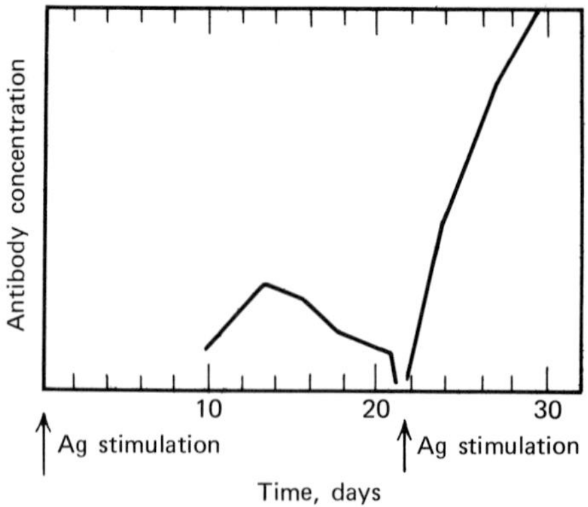

Fig. 25.1 Primary versus secondary antibody response.

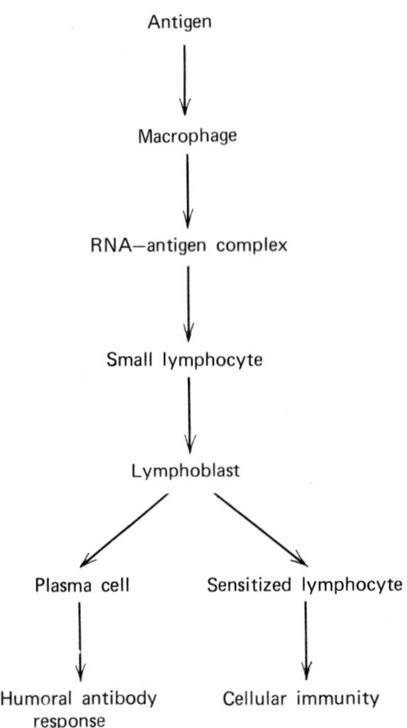

Fig. 25.2 Schematic representation of the immune response.

and is not understood in full detail. It may be represented by a number of processes, shown schematically in Fig. 25.2. Immunosuppressive agents can have as their target one or more steps in the sequence of these cellular events.

To assess the effect of immunosuppressive drugs, models *in vivo* as well as *in vitro* have been employed; Table 25.1 lists some of the parameters most frequently used in the study of these drugs. Despite the availability of an extensive literature, it is difficult to evaluate comparatively the effect of immunosuppressive drugs. The degree of immunosuppression caused by a drug depends on a number of factors, and very different results can be obtained depending on dosage, dosage schedule, time of antigen administration, and effects of single and multiple doses (4–6). With almost every immunosuppressive drug there is a period, relative to antigen stimulation, in which therapy may result in an enhanced immune response (7).

Although corticosteroids have proved to be most useful in multiple drug regimens for the treatment of immunological disorders and in facilitating homograft acceptance, there is no valid evidence that they are immunosuppressive in man. Thus they have not been included in this chapter.

1.2 T- and B-Cells

The idea of a "two-component concept", that thymus cells and marrow cells in combination have antibody-forming properties

Table 25.1 Biological Tests for Immunosuppressive Agents

In Vivo Assays	*In Vitro* Assays[a]
1. Humoral antibody (SRBC; heterologous proteins)	1. Plaque forming cell test (PFC)
2. Allografts (skin, kidney, bone marrow)	2. Tissue culture of lymph node or spleen cells for antibody production
3. Graft vs. host reaction (GVH)	3. Blastogenesis:
4. Experimental allergic encephalomyelitis (EAE)	3.1. After antigen challenge
	3.2. Nonspecific (PHA, ConA)
	4. Migration inhibition factor (MIF)
	5. Cell-mediated cytotoxicity
	6. T- and B-Cell function (rosette formation; fluorescent antibody)

[a] Tests done with cells taken from either drug-treated animals or with the drug added to the *in vitro* system.

not possessed by either population alone, was presaged more than 50 years ago by Alexis Carrel (8). He found that when cultivated together *in vitro*, guinea pig bone marrow and lymph glands generated a substance that "has acquired the power to hemolyse markedly goat red blood corpuscles, while the serum of the control cultures remained nonhemolytic". From this he concluded "that tissues living outside of the organism react against an antigen by the production of antibodies".

Today it is generally accepted that there are at least two distinct and interacting cell types and that one of these cell lines is derived from the thymus (9, 10). The cells that play a pivotal role in immune reactions are the small lymphocytes; they are the major cellular constituents of lymphoid tissues and are widely distributed throughout the body (11). Two broad subclasses of lymphocytes have been identified, and their involvement in the development and manifestations of both humoral and cellular immunity has been demonstrated (12–14): the T-cells deriving from the thymus and the B-cells—(bursa)—not quite correctly said to be derived from bone marrow, since the exact origin in mammals is not quite clear. Both subclasses arise from stem cells that are found first in the yolk sac of the embryo, later in the fetal liver, and finally in the bone marrow.

The need for cooperation of both cell lines could be demonstrated by suppressing the immune competence in mice using neonatal or adult thymectomy (15) and restoration of the response by reconstitution with thymus cells alone or together with bone marrow cells (9, 10, 16).

Cooperation between T- and B-cells is not always necessary in the elaboration of B-cells; certain antigens can bypass the T-cell system and stimulate B-cells directly without the need for binding to "helper" T-cells (17). These so called T-cell-independent antigens are high molecular weight materials with a large number of repeating identical determinants [e.g., polyvinylpyrrolidone, polyfructose (levan), and polysaccharides].

The T- and B-cells differ in origin, function, fate, and life span. T-Cells make up 70% of the peripheral circulating lymphocyte population; they are long-lived and slowly replicating. T-cells not only modulate B-lymphocyte function, but also play a crucial role in cell-mediated immune responses, such as delayed hypersensitivity, graft-versus-host reaction, and graft rejection, as well as host resistance to bacterial, viral, and parasite infections. It has been suggested (18) that T-cells of different types participate in cellular and humoral immune reactions. Preliminary treatment of mice with hydrocortisone inhibited T-cell function in humoral immunity, while enhancing the graft-versus-host reactivity of the same population of spleen cells.

The regulatory role of T-cells for the development of an antibody response is not always positive; there is another type of T-cell, the "suppressor" T-cell (19), which can inhibit antibody production. This suppression might be essential for the normal control of immune responses. A malfunction could lead either to an excess or lack of antibodies or to the production of aberrant cells.

Humoral immunity is mediated by circulating antibodies secreted by lymphoid cells that are not derived from the thymus. In chickens these lymphocytes are derived from a central lymphoid organ, the bursa of Fabricius (20), (named after the sixteenth century Paduan anatomist Hieronymus Fabricius ab Aquapendente) and probably from bone marrow in rodents. The main immunological function is the synthesis and secretion of antibody. A reduced antibody-producing capacity occurs in children with agammaglobulinemia, and in chickens after bursectomy (21) or by suppression of bursa development with 19-nortestosterone (22).

In contrast to T-cells, B-lymphocytes are short-lived, relatively small cells and are found in blood, lymph, and connective tissues. The precise mechanism of B-lymphocyte stimulation is largely unknown; model systems have been used to unravel the involvement of T-cells in antibody formation. Using haptens coupled to carrier molecules, it has been suggested, that T-lymphocytes concentrate antigen to the B-cell surface by an antigen-bridging mechanism and that T- and B-cells recognize and combine with different determinants on the hapten-carrier molecule (23, 24).

A third type of cell involved in the induction of an antibody response is the macrophage; in this scheme, T-cells may produce a specific soluble factor that is cytophilic for macrophages. The macrophage then presents the antigen to the B-cells (25–28).

The developments in this field of immunobiology have been eloquently described as follows:

1. *The Age of Innocence.* Immune induction follows simple contact between antigen and a precursor cell.
2. *The Coming of Cooperation.* Synergistic inductive effects between thymus and bone marrow cells and between carrier- and hapten-reactive lymphocytes play a role.
3. *The Age of Complex Regulation.* Tolerance, like induction, may depend on cell interaction; the lymphocyte population is richly interconnected: any one immune response may affect the whole network; the control of specific immune responses may be immensely complex.*

1.3 Structure of Antibodies

One of the most exciting developments in the field of immunology was the elucidation of the structural framework of the immunoglobulin molecule and the unraveling of the intricate relationship of antigen-antibody interactions (30–32).

The early observation by von Behring and Kitasato (33) that immunity to tetanus and diphtheria is associated with protective substances—"antitoxins"—in the serum, was instrumental in the development of the practical treatment of many infectious diseases. The antitoxins (antibodies) that are elicited by foreign substances such as bacteria, viruses, polysaccharides, and killed microorganisms have a specific affinity for the invading agents and trigger the events leading to their elimination.

Many theories have been advanced for the mechanism of antibody formation, but frequent reexamination was needed as our knowledge of the molecular basis of antibody formation evolved. Ehrlich (34) proposed that cells with appropriate side chain groups interract with the toxin, causing the release of receptors into the circulation. This selective theory was superseded by the work of Landsteiner (35), who demonstrated that antibodies are very sensitive to minor structural changes. Simple chemical substances (haptens), which by themselves do not stimulate antibody production, become immunogenic when attached to a macromolecule such as a protein. Using a series of such conjugates, Landsteiner was able to show that the antibodies formed were specific for the group(s) attached as well as to subtle structural changes within the determinant group(s).

The template theory of Pauling (36) represents an attempt to reduce the problem of antibody formation to a molecular level. Pauling hypothesized that the antigen influences the folding of the antibody chain in a complementary fashion specific for a given antigen. However certain crucial questions such as immunological memory, recognition, and tolerance remained unanswered. In their selective theory, Jerne and Burnet (37, 38) postulated that the body

* From Ref. 29.

Table 25.2 Some Characteristics of the Major Immunoglobulin Classes

	Immunoglobulin Class				
Property	IgM	IgG	IgA	IgD	IgE
Molecular weight $\times 10^{-3}$	$\geqq$800	150	150–600	175	190
Sedimentation coefficients (S)	19–32	7	7–13	7	8
Light chains	κ or λ	κ or λ	κ or λ	κ or λ	κ or λ
Heavy chains	μ	γ	α	δ	ε
Serum level, mg/ml	1	12	3	0.03	0.001
Half-life, days	5	23	6	3	2.3

had all the information for making antibody of all potential specificities before they encountered antigen.

Antibodies belong to a very heterogeneous group of serum proteins known as immunoglobulins; on the basis of their electrophoretic migration pattern they were classified as γ-globulins (39). Table 25.2 summarizes the five major classes of immunoglobulins and their main characteristics. Each major class of immunoglobulins (IgM, IgG, IgA, IgD, and IgE) has a heavy chain that differs from that of other class structurally and antigenically, whereas they all share in common two light chains, either λ or κ. The heavy chains are called μ, γ, α, δ, and ε.

Immunoglobulin M is the first class of antibodies to appear in the serum, and immunoglobulin G is the principal antibody; the majority of antibacterial, antiviral, and antitoxic antibodies belongs to this class of immunoglobulins. Immunoglobulin A is present mainly in external secretions (saliva, tears, bronchial mucus, gastrointestinal fluids, milk, etc.). The physiological functions of IgD have not yet been elucidated. IgE is responsible for mediating allergic reactions.

Immunoglobulins may appear as monomers (IgG), in polymeric form (IgM), or in both forms (IgA). The difficulties in the elucidation of the structure of the antibody molecule were due to a large measure to their complex nature (e.g., size and amino acid sequence). Immunoglobulins of apparently a single variety are made in patients with multiple myeloma. Some myeloma tumors secrete homogeneous light chains, called Bence–Jones proteins. The nature of these proteins, and their chemical similarity to polypeptide chains of myeloma globulins as well as to normal γ-globulins, was determined (40). These and related studies led ultimately to the elucidation of the entire amino acid sequence of a whole immunoglobulin molecule (41).

In spite of the complexity of these molecules, structural studies have revealed a simple underlying pattern: all immunoglobulins have fundamentally the same structure and consist of two symmetrical polypeptide chains, two identical "light" chains and two identical "heavy" chains, which are at least twice as large. The chains are linked by a number of disulfide bonds.

Papain cleavage of IgG (42) results in two functionally different fragments, F_{ab} and F_c : F_{ab} has the ability to bind antigen, whereas the other fragment F_c (easily crystallizable) mediates several effector functions (e.g., fixing of complement). The variable region of the light chain V_L is homologous with the variable region of the heavy chain V_H. The constant region of the heavy chain consists of equal parts, C_H1, C_H2, C_H3, which are similar in sequence. Furthermore, the constant region of the light chain is homologous with the three parts of the heavy chain. The F_c and two

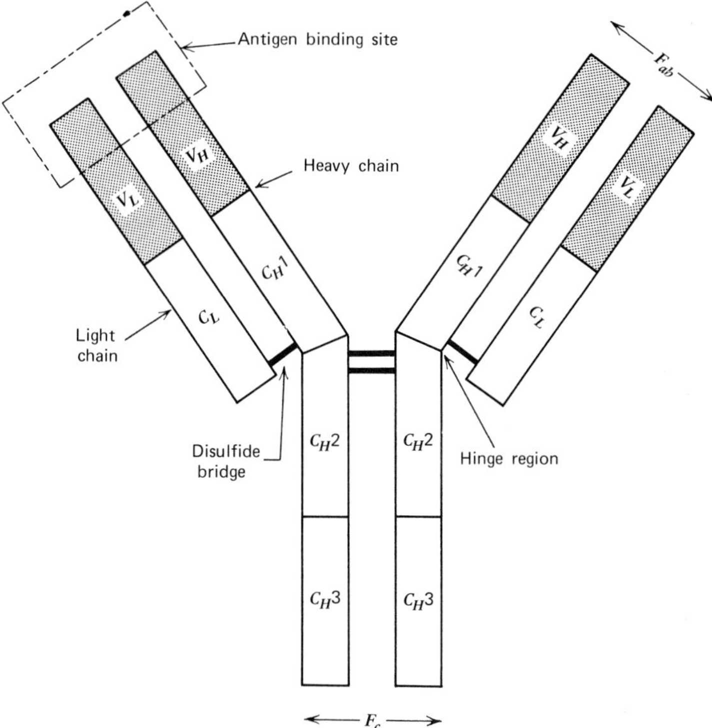

Fig. 25.3 Schematic diagram of the four peptide chains of an immunoglobulin molecule.

F_{ab} units of the molecule are joined by a "hinge" region in the heavy chain. This endows the immunoglobulin with a great degree of flexibility; it facilitates the formation of antibody-antigen complexes by permitting variations in the angle between the F_{ab} units, according to the distance between antigenic determinants.

Several crystal structures of immunoglobulin fragments have been analyzed in recent years (32); these studies verified earlier proposals that immunoglobulins are composed of globular domains formed by the variable and constant segments. Electron microscopic studies revealed that the antibody molecule diverges out in Y fashion when combined with a divalent hapten (43), as shown in Fig. 25.3.

2 IMMUNOSUPPRESSIVE DRUGS

2.1 Alkylating Agents

The observation by Meyer (44) and Ehrlich (45) that certain chemical agents are able to alkylate biological material, was followed some 40 years later by the finding of Gilman and Philips (46) that aliphatic nitrogen mustards have a specific effect on lymphoid tissue (spleen, bone marrow, thymus, and lymph nodes). Once it was appreciated that similar compounds might be useful in the treatment of lymphomas, many variants of the nitrogen mustards were prepared.

Alkylating agents were among the first classes of chemical substances to be evaluated for their immunosuppressive properties. Hektoen and Corper (47) showed that the formation of agglutinin and hemolysin to sheep red blood cells (SRBC) could be inhibited in both rabbits and dogs after the administration of sulfur mustard. Later it was found that alkylating agents effectively suppress the immune response and interfere with antibody formation in several animal species when given at the very beginning or 1–2 days before antigen stimulus (48).

It became soon very clear, however, as more experimental details became available, that the efficacy of alkylating agents varies considerably, qualitatively and quantitatively, depending on the agent used, the nature of the antigenic stimulus, and the time relationship between drug treatment and immunization (1, 49, 50). The more potent alkylating agents are active against the primary and secondary immune response; both the cellular and humoral antibody responses can be affected in animals and man.

The class of alkylating agents comprises a variety of functional groupings:

1. Mustards, e.g., HN2 (25.**1**), mannomustine (25.**2**), melphalan (25.**3**), chlorambucil (5.**4**), cyclophosphamide (25.**5**).

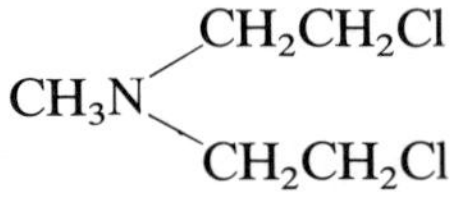

$CH_3N(CH_2CH_2Cl)_2$

25.**1**

$CH_2NHCH_2CH_2Cl$–HOCH–HOCH–HCOH–HCOH–$CH_2NHCH_2CH_2Cl$

25.**2**

$(ClCH_2CH_2)_2N–C_6H_4–CH_2CH(NH_2)–COOH$

25.**3**

$(ClCH_2CH_2)_2N–C_6H_4–CH_2CH_2CH_2COOH$

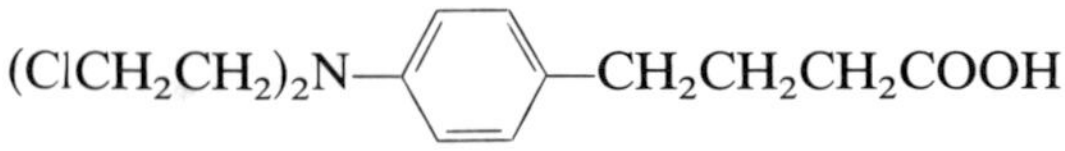

25.**4**

$N(CH_2CH_2Cl)_2$ on P of cyclic NH–P(→O)–O ring

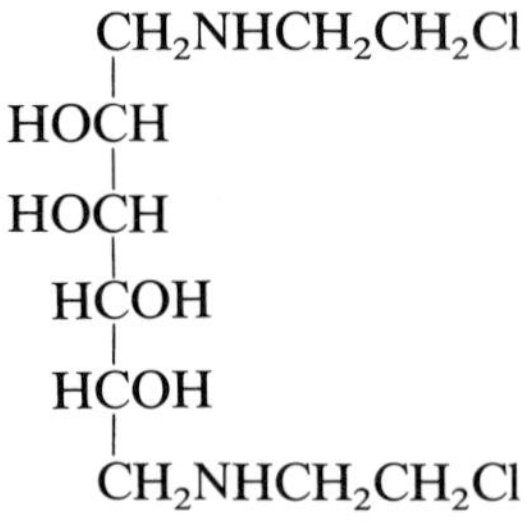

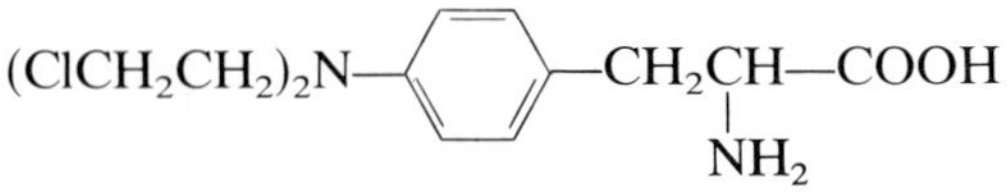

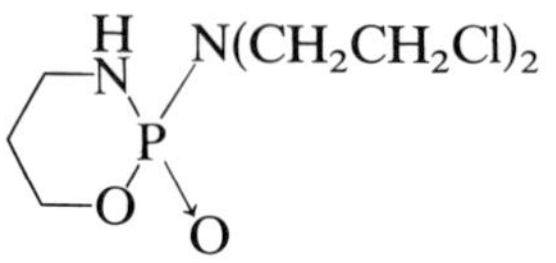

25.**5**

2. Sulfonic acid esters, e.g., busulfan (25.**6**).

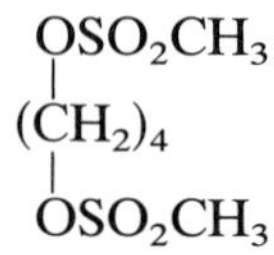

OSO_2CH_3–$(CH_2)_4$–OSO_2CH_3

25.**6**

3. Epoxides, e.g., 1.2.3.4.-diepoxybutane (25.**7**).
4. Ethyleneimines, e.g., TEPA (25.**8**).

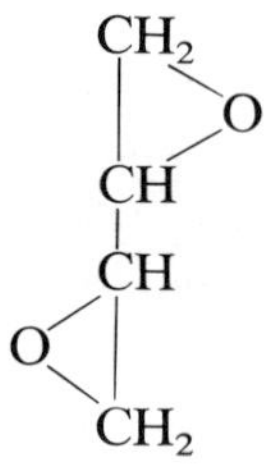

CH_2(–O–)CH–CH(–O–)CH_2

25.**7**

Tris(aziridinyl) N–P=O

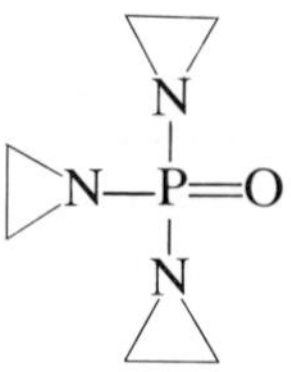

25.**8**

Their biological activity is influenced to a large measure by the nature of the carrier; a variety of chemical substances— amino acids, carbohydrates, steroids, and various heterocyclic molecules—have been employed for this purpose.

In vitro, alkylation proceeds through a second-order nucleophilic substitution:

$$R{-}N\!\!\lhd \;+\; A^{\ominus} \xrightarrow{H_2O} RNHCH_2CH_2A \;+\; OH^{\ominus}$$

$$R{-}\underset{\diagdown O \diagup}{CH{-}CH_2} \;+\; A^{\ominus} \xrightarrow{H_2O} RCH(OH)CH_2A + OH^{\ominus}$$

Aliphatic nitrogen mustards act similarly after formation of a cyclic immonium ion; the unimolecular conversion to the immonium ion is relatively fast, and once formed, it reacts by an SN_2 mechanism.

$$R_2NCH_2CH_2CP \rightleftharpoons R_2\overset{\oplus}{N}\!\!\lhd \;+\; CP^{\ominus}$$

$$\downarrow$$

$$R_2NCH_2CH_2A$$

A proposal by Ross (51) that aromatic nitrogen mustards proceed through a carbonium ion, followed by first-order kinetics in the alkylation reaction, was later questioned (52–54). There is agreement that the action of such compounds is similar to that of other alkylating agents and that the mechanism of alkylation superficially resembles that of an SN_1 nucleophilic substitution.

Many proposals have been advanced to explain the gross biological effect of alkylating agents. It is generally accepted that they react with functionally important cellular macromolecules. Compounds like the nitrogen mustards can form covalent linkages with a number of functional groups (amines, carboxylic acids, thiol-, and phosphate groups, or compounds with tertiary nitrogen in heterocyclic systems), which are common structural features of most biomolecules; action seems to occur principally on proteins and nucleic acids (55–57). It is unlikely that one specific reaction is responsible for the observed biological effects. The mechanism of alkylation has been studied in greatest detail for nitrogen mustards: alkylation of guanine at C-7 leads to a weakening of the glycosidic linkage and excision of alkylated base; this labilizes the sugar-phosphate bond, and chain scission is likely to occur. In addition, intra- and interstrand cross-linking of DNA is another possible mode of impairment, leading to errors in base pairing, nucleic acid transcription, replication, and protein synthesis (58).

The most widely used alkylating agent is cyclophosphamide (25.**5**), which has a broad spectrum of activity in animal and human malignancies. It was first synthesized in 1958 by Arnold and Bourseaux (59), together with a number of related *N*-phosphorylated derivatives of nitrogen mustard. The drug is now increasingly studied in various immunological disorders. In comparison with other alkylating agents, it interferes with cell growth only after activation in tissues. It is capable of inhibiting both the humoral (60) and cell-mediated immune responses (61). Unlike many other cytostatic agents used as immunosuppressants, cyclophosphamide also prevents the development of cell-mediated autoimmune diseases in animals (62, 63).

When equitoxic dosages of cyclophosphamide and a recent cyclophosphamide analog, ASTA 5122 (25.**9**) were compared with 6-mercaptopurine (25.**16**), and azathioprine (25.**17**) for their immunosuppressive potency on the early primary and secondary immune responses in mice, only

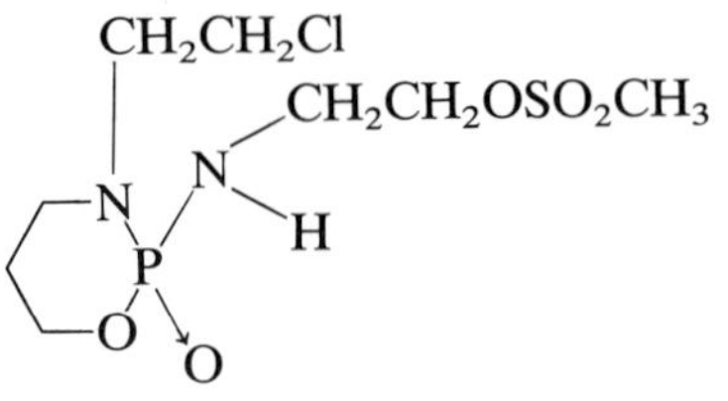

CH_2CH_2Cl ... $CH_2CH_2OSO_2CH_3$ ... N ... N ... H ... P ... O ... O

25.**9**

the two alkylating agents gave complete suppression (64).

Cyclophosphamide failed to prolong renal homograft survival in dogs, and it did not add to the effectiveness of azathioprine (25.**17**). However a significant prolongation of rabbit renal allograft was observed when cyclophosphamide was given in conjunction with azathioprine and prednisolone (65).

Several severe side effects accompany the use of cyclophosphamide: alopecia, hemorrhagic cystitis, and infertility due to testicular and ovarian destruction.

Cyclophosphamide is initially converted by hepatic microsomal enzymes to 4-hydroxycyclophosphamide (25.**10**) (66–68); upon further oxidation carboxyphosphamide (25.**12**) is formed, which is the principal alkylating metabolite of cyclophosphamide in dog urine (66) and a major urinary metabolite in rabbits (67), rats (67, 68), and man (68) (see Fig. 25.4).

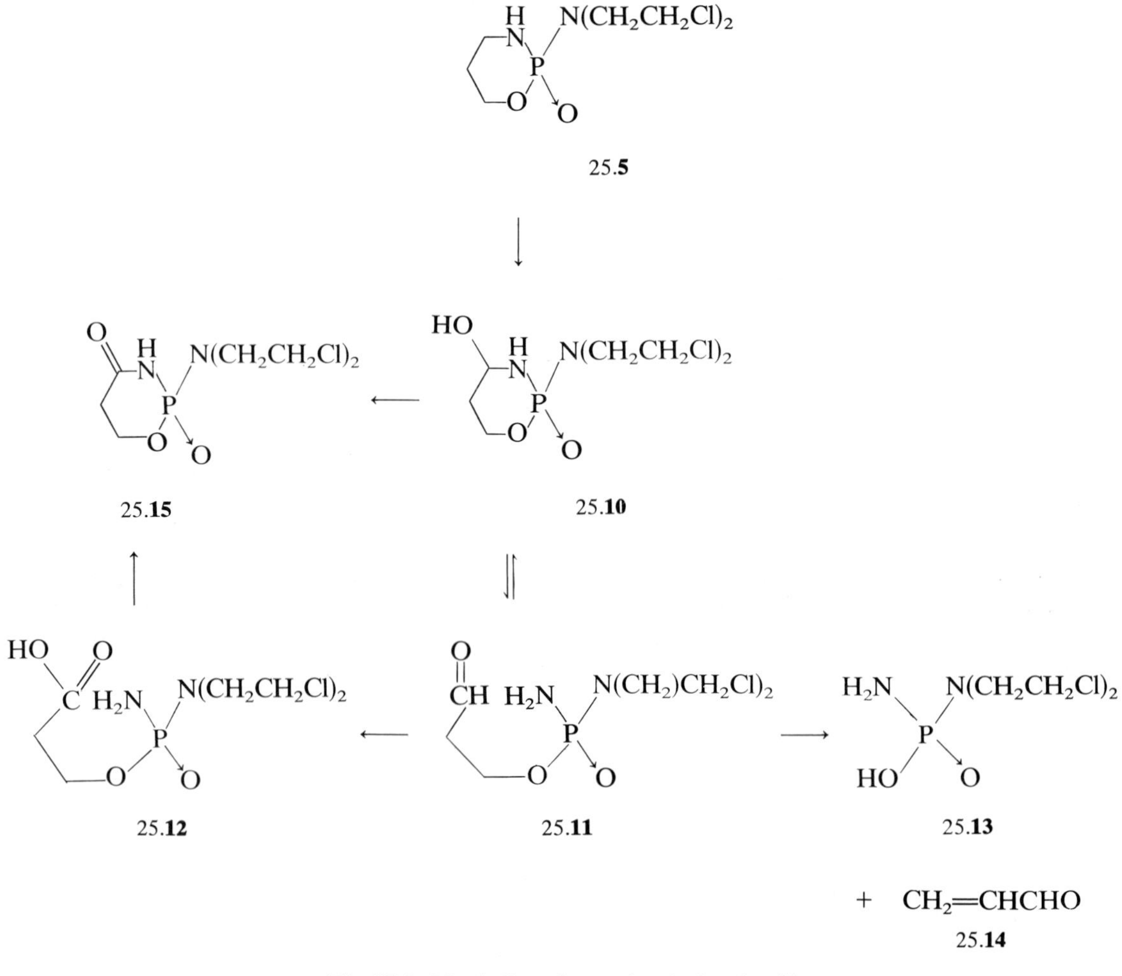

H $N(CH_2CH_2Cl)_2$ N P O O

25.**5**

↓

O H $N(CH_2CH_2Cl)_2$ N P O O ← HO H $N(CH_2CH_2Cl)_2$ N P O O

25.**15** 25.**10**

↑ ⇅

HO O C H_2N $N(CH_2CH_2Cl)_2$ P O O ← O CH H_2N $N(CH_2)CH_2Cl)_2$ P O O → H_2N $N(CH_2CH_2Cl)_2$ P HO O

25.**12** 25.**11** 25.**13**

+ $CH_2{=}CHCHO$

25.**14**

Fig. 25.4 Metabolic pathway of cyclophosphamide.

The acyclic form of 4-hydroxycyclophosphamide, aldophosphamide (25.**11**), decomposes to give phosphoramide mustard (25.**13**), and acrolein (25.**14**) (69).

From dog urine another metabolite, 4-oxocyclophosphamide (25.**15**), was isolated and identified by independent synthesis. It is probably derived from 25.**10** or 25.**12**. The 4-oxo compound is very active as an inhibitor of cell growth and is considered to be the activated form of cyclophosphamide or one of a number of such forms (70).

Because of its severe toxicity, the drug is used only as adjunct therapy in kidney transplantations and in very few cases of otherwise therapy-resistant rheumatoid arthritis.

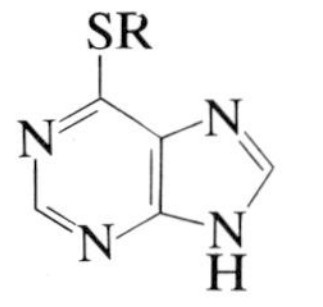

SR

25.**16** R = H

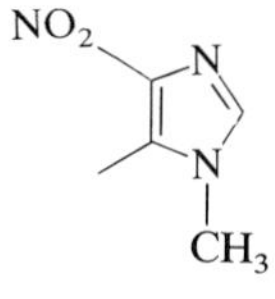

R =

25.**17**

2.2 Purines

The purine antagonists are the classical immunosuppressant drugs: designed for this purpose and extensively studied in many animal models, they remain the accepted treatment in organ transplantation in man.

In 1959 Schwartz and Dameshek could demonstrate that when given at the time of stimulation, the antileukemic agent 6-mercaptopurine (6-MP, 25.**16**) suppressed the immune response to human serum albumin in rabbits, (71). Since then, considerable efforts were made to improve the therapeutic profile of this drug. One derivative, 6-(1-methyl-4-nitro-5-imidazolyl)thiopurine, (25.**17**), azathioprine), which was designed as a transport form for 25.**16** (72), is now the drug of choice in clinical immunosuppression, particularly for kidney transplants.

Azathioprine (25.**17**) can be cleaved *in vitro* by hydrogen sulfide or mercaptans to 6-mercaptopurine; this reaction also occurs *in vivo* using various sulfhydryl compounds or amines, with the release of the bioactive molecule. The imidazolyl moiety was found in the urine of patients treated with 25.**17** as 1-methyl-4-nitro-5-mercaptoimidazole (25.**18**). It appears that at least two pathways for the cleavage of 25.**17** are possible. Chalmers has shown that the sulfur in 25.**18** can originate from glutathion (73). It is still an open question whether azathioprine owes its effectiveness to the release of

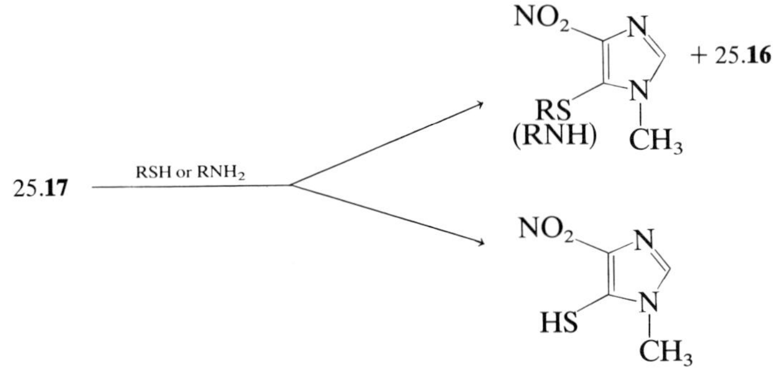

25.**17** —RSH or RNH_2→ [RS (RNH) imidazole] + 25.**16**; [HS imidazole]

25.**18**

25.**16**, or whether it has a preferential activity of its own (74). Indeed, it has not been clearly established whether azathioprine has advantages over 6-mercaptopurine as an immunosuppressant (75, 76).

6-Mercaptopurine (25.**16**) interferes in various ways with purine metabolism, therefore ultimately with protein synthesis. It is a competitive inhibitor of hypoxanthine phosphoribosyltransferase. Furthermore, it can be transformed into thioinosinic acid (25.**19**); this in turn will inhibit the enzymatic sequences leading to guanosylic and adenylic acid. Thioinosinic acid (25.**19**) is also enzymatically aminated to thioguanylic acid (25.**20**), which again is an inhibitor of enzymes of the purine anabolism.

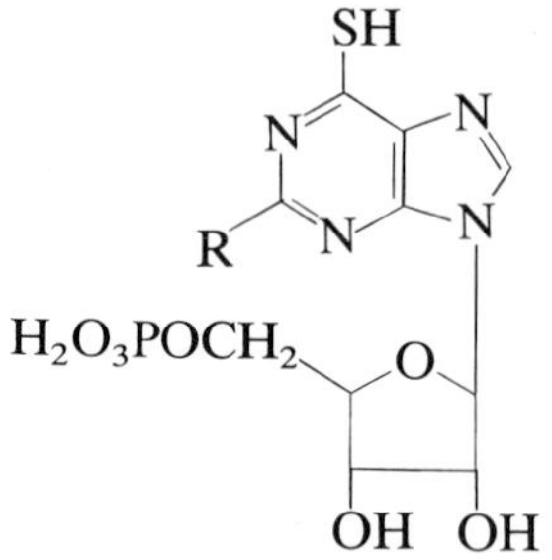

SH
N N
R N N
$H_2O_3POCH_2$ O
OH OH

25.**19** R = H
25.**20** $R = NH_2$

In contrast to our understanding of the biochemical transformations, little is known to explain the relative specificity this drug displays toward antibody synthesis, while leaving other protein syntheses intact. Since 6-mercaptopurine and 25.**17** are most effective when given at the time of antigen stimulation, it is likely that they interfere at the sensitization stage of lymphocytes.

Paradoxically, under certain conditions the opposite effect can be demonstrated: when a 1 week course of 6-MP (25.**16**) is given to rabbits before antigen stimulation, an increase in the primary antibody response is observed. This immunostimulating effect is largest when a small dose of antigen is injected 5 days after the last drug treatment. Similar results can be obtained with other immunosuppressants, which may be of consequence for their clinical use. An explanation for this paradox may be the following: destruction of cells through the cytotoxic agents leads to a release of cell constituents, which could act as immunostimulants; it is known, for instance, that nucleic acids have the property of enhancing antibody formation as well as stimulating cell division (7).

Reports are conflicting with regard to whether these agents influence predominantly the T- or B-cell system (3, 77, 78); in animal studies, either effect can be demonstrated, depending on the species. In man, where effectiveness has been established in many kidney transplantations, a suppression of (T-) cell-mediated immunity must be assumed; but in view of the complexity of feedback mechanisms between B- and T-cells, a direct influence on B-cells cannot be excluded.

Most of the very large number of successful kidney transplantations were done with the standard treatment of steroids and azathioprine. The use of these drugs in grafting other organs like heart or liver was less successful, because of additional inherent difficulties.

In recent years azathioprine (25.**17**) has been tried for the treatment of a number of diseases associated with the immune response, including hepatitis (3, 79) and rheumatoid arthritis (3, 80). Clinicians, naturally, are hesitant to employ these drugs, which so dramatically interfere with purine and protein synthesis at an early stage. Consequently these compounds are often selected and are expected to show results when the disease has progressed to a degree where the underlying immunological cause is overshadowed by secondary, often irreversible changes. Thus the efficacy of azathioprine and other immunosuppressants used for similar purposes is not clear-cut and is still controversial.

Many attempts have been made to obtain purine antagonists with improved properties. Replacing the nitromethylimidazolyl moiety in mercaptopurines and in thioguanines (25.**21**) by alkyl, substituted

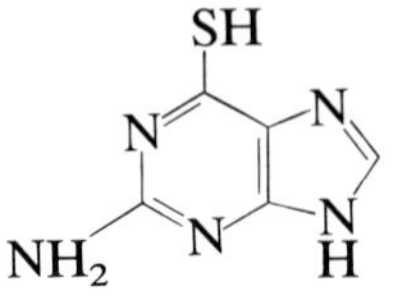

25.**21**

benzyl, or cyano groups does not lead to significantly improved therapeutic ratios (81). Substitution in the 8-position by a phenyl group abolishes immunosuppressive activity (82).

A study by Kimball and co-workers indicated that specificity with regard to suppression of cellular versus humoral immunity can be achieved in 6-mercaptopurines: β-L-ribosyl-6-mercaptopurine (25.**22**) and β-D-arabinosyl-6-mercaptopurine (25.**23**) prolong skin graft survival times in mice without interfering with hemagglutinating antibodies, whereas α-D-2′-deoxythioguanosine (25.**24**) was found to inhibit both responses (83). No clinical applications of these findings became known.

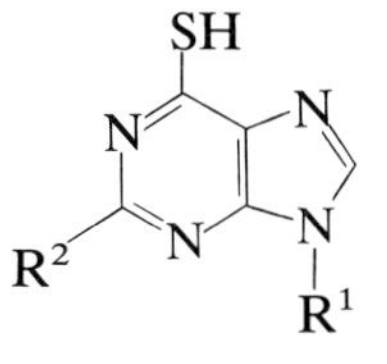

25.**22** R^1 = [ribosyl] $R^2 = H$

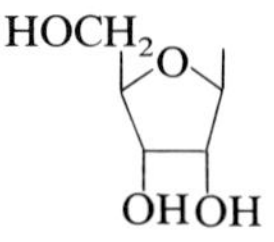

25.**23** R^1 = [arabinosyl] $R^2 = H$

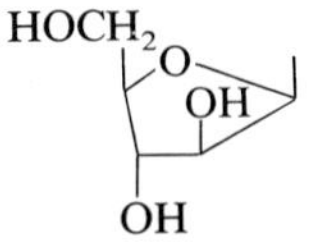

25.**24** R^1 = [2′-deoxyribosyl] $R^2 = NH_2$

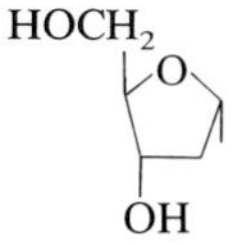

25.**25** $R^1 = C_4H_9$ $R^2 = NH_2$

Here again, the species differences must not be overlooked.

9-Alkyl derivatives are interesting compounds, since they probably are not transformed into nucleotide analogs metabolically. In mice, 9-butyl-6-thioguanine (25.**25**) showed potency comparable to that of 6-thioguanine (25.**21**) against circulating antibody formation (84).

2.3 Pyrimidines

The pyrimidine group of antimetabolites has been studied extensively in animals and man, and some compounds have found an established place in antiviral therapy or in the treatment of neoplasms. But they are of secondary importance as immunosuppressants, and none has undergone extended clinical studies in immune related diseases.

Best known in this group are the halogenated uracils, in which the hydrogen on C-5 of the pyrimidine ring has been replaced by a halogen atom, e.g., 25.**26**, 6-azauracil (25.**27**), and their arabinosides (25.**28**, 25.**29**) or ribosides (25.**30**, 25.**31**), as well as the corresponding glycosides (25.**34**–25.**36**) of cytidine (25.**32**) and 5-azacytidine

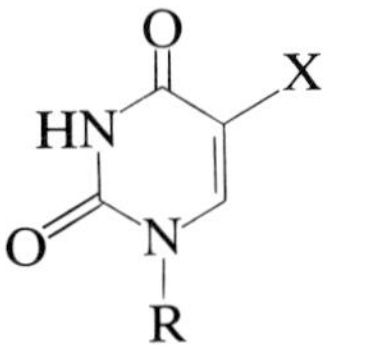

X = F, Br, I

25.**26** R = H
25.**28** R = arabinosyl
25.**30** R = riboxyl

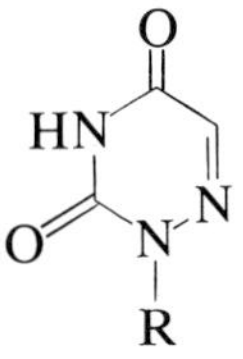

25.**27** R = H
25.**29** R = arabinosyl
25.**31** R = ribosyl

(25.**33**). All are inhibitors of DNA and RNA synthesis, and it is not surprising, therefore, that they exhibit immunosuppressant activity in a number of animal models: hemagglutination, plaque forming, and skin grafting (3).

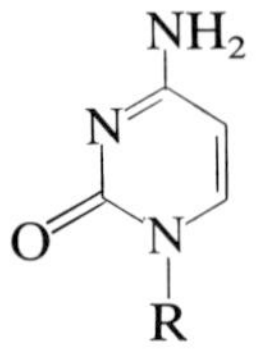

25.**32** R = H
25.**34** R = arabinosyl

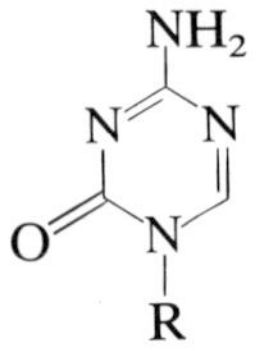

25.**33** R = H
25.**35** R = arabinosyl
25.**36** R = ribosyl

The biochemistry and pharmacology of arabinosyl-cytidine (ara-C, 25.**34**) has been particularly well studied (85). The drug is phosphorylated and as such inhibits DNA synthesis, interfering with cell replication during the phase of immunogen stimulation. Consequently 25.**34** is most active when given at the time of antigen administration. The half-life is very short, making several daily injections necessary.

To overcome the short duration of action of ara-C, a number of acyl derivatives as pro-drugs have been synthesized, which are slowly hydrolyzed with the release of the active molecule. The 5′-adamantoyl (25.**37**) and 5′-benzoyl (25.**38**) esters are the most active members of this series (86).

Depending on the dose and time of administration, either the B-cells can be suppressed selectively or both B- and T-cells can be suppressed together. As a consequence, either accelerated or inhibited tumor growth may be observed in immunological

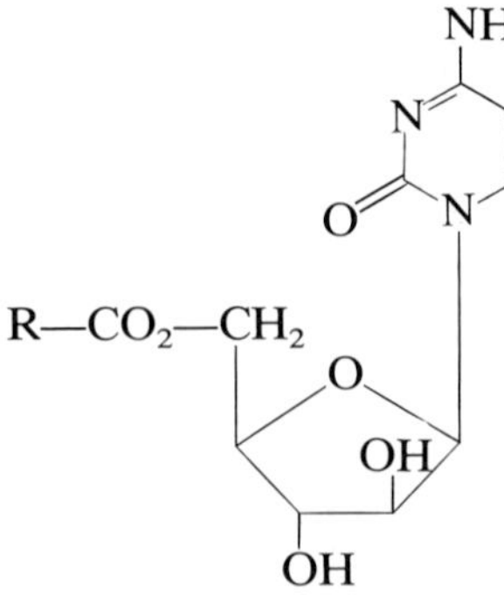

$R-CO_2-CH_2$

25.**37** R = adamantyl
25.**38** R = C_6H_5

tumor models (87), which again illustrates the interrelationship between the two types of lymphocyte discussed above.

2.4 Folic Acid Antagonists

The mechanism of action of the folic acid antagonists is fairly well understood (88). Folic acid (25.**39**) is enzymatically converted to tetrahydrofolic acid (25.**40**), which plays an important role in the synthesis of purines by transferring one-carbon fragments ("activated formaldehyde") (89).

Didhydrofolate reductase, one of the enzymes responsible for the conversion of 25.**39** to 25.**40**, can be inhibited by synthetic analogs (90), among which aminopterin (25.**41**) and methotrexate (25.**42**) are the most important. These compounds indirectly suppress the synthesis of purine and are particularly effective in rapidly proliferating cell populations. Both compounds have been extensively studied for their immunosuppressive properties (1, 91); 25.**42** markedly depresses the primary and secondary antibody response, the homograft reaction, the graft-versus-host response,

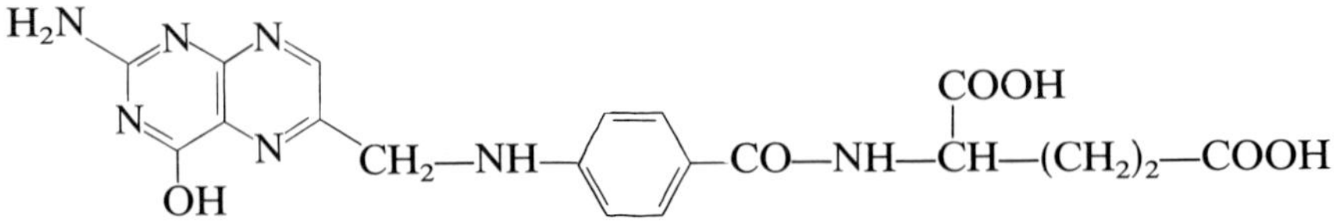

25.**39**

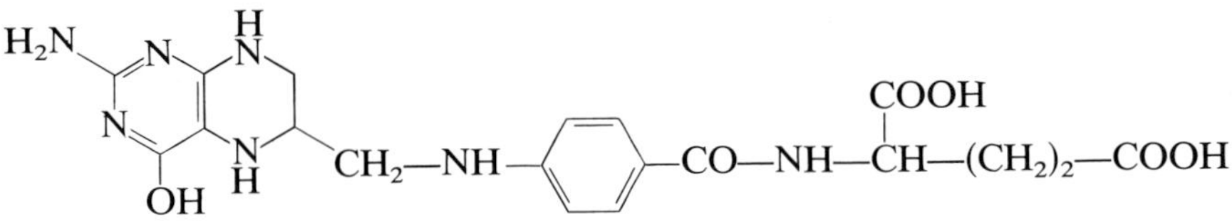

25.**40**

and the development of hypersensitivity. Its activity is somewhat variable, depending on the species, the test systems used, and the timing of administration.

Methotrexate is slightly less toxic than aminopterin and is more widely studied in such autoimmune diseases as lupus erythematosus and particularly in psoriasis (92). The latter widespread disease becomes crippling in some cases and is successfully treated with methotrexate. The drug must be used with great caution, however, because it is severely toxic in long-term use, especially toward the liver (93).

The toxic effects of methotrexate can be reversed if the immunosuppressive dose of 25.**42** is followed by folinic acid (5-formyltetrahydrofolic acid), leaving the immunosuppressive capacity unaltered (94). This finding led to the discovery of the "rescue technique" in therapy: through sequential administration of 25.**42** and folinic acid, one attempts to kill most of the rapidly dividing cells and to save the others by supplying the necessary one-carbon fragments (95).

2.5 L-Asparaginase

A new area in the field of immunosuppression has developed as a result of the discovery that the enzyme L-asparaginase has immunosuppressive properties. This enzyme catalyzes the hydrolysis of asparagine to aspartic acid. When asparagine is lacking, protein synthesis comes to a halt. The reverse process, the synthesis of asparagine from aspartate, is catalyzed by asparagine synthetase. Lymphoid tissue in man is deficient in asparagine synthetase, consequently is susceptible to the depletion of asparagine by L-asparaginase. Thus the enzyme affects the lymphoid tissues directly; it induces lymphopenia and reduces the size of lymph nodes, thymus, and spleen. This explains the specificity of this enzyme toward lymphoid malignancies.

It is not surprising, therefore, that an agent specifically blocking protein synthesis in lymphoid cells is also a potent immunosuppressant. This could be demonstrated in the usual tests for humoral and cell-mediated immunity: suppression of circulating antibodies and plaque-forming cells, as well as the development of delayed hypersensitivity and graft-versus-host disease; skin graft survival in mice even across strong histocompatibility barriers, and increased survival times of organ allografts in several animal species have also been observed.

The enzyme, generally prepared from *E. coli* cultures, is of course a protein, and its

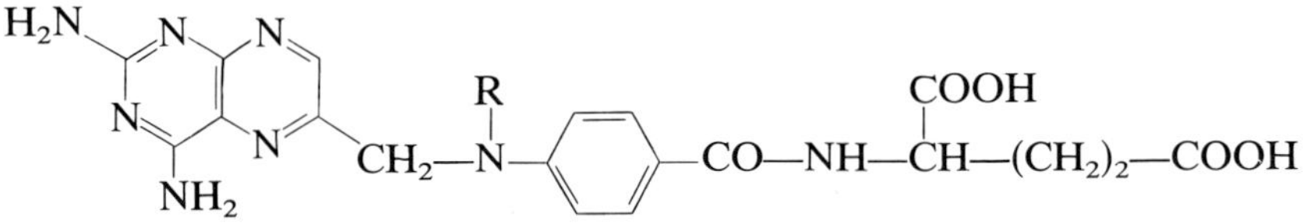

25.**41** R = H
25.**42** R = CH_3

use in man is limited by the expected side effects such as symptoms resembling those of serum sickness. After a prolonged period of application, in spite of the suppression of the recipient's immune system, antibodies are formed against it. Nevertheless, L-asparaginase can be tolerated in many cases for several weeks, and its successful employment in the treatment of lymphocytic leukemia allows the prediction that this enzyme will play a role in adjunctive therapy, where immunosuppression is indicated (96, 97).

2.6 Penicillamine

β,β-Dimethylcysteine or penicillamine (25.**43**) is quite distinct in structure and biological effects from the other groups of immunosuppressants discussed here. Originally introduced into therapy because of its

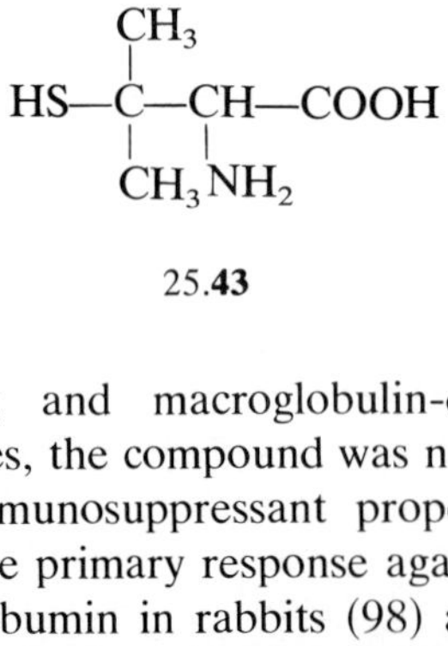

$$HS\text{—}\underset{CH_3}{\overset{CH_3}{\underset{|}{\overset{|}{C}}}}\text{—}\underset{NH_2}{\underset{|}{CH}}\text{—}COOH$$

25.**43**

chelating and macroglobulin-dissociating properties, the compound was not found to have immunosuppressant properties until later. The primary response against human serum albumin in rabbits (98) and against typhoid H antigen in mice (99) can be suppressed. On the other hand, acceleration of antibody formation in rabbits against human serum albumin is observed when the drug is given 28 days before immunization (100). In mice, enhancement of antibody formation against SRBC could be demonstrated (101). The drug was found to be inactive in the polyarthritis model in rats (102).

In spite of contradicting pharmacological results and toxicity, the drug enjoys increasing use in severe chronic rheumatoid arthritis, and several controlled studies confirm its effectiveness (103–106). Penicillamine most likely exerts its effect on the membranes of proliferating immunocompetent cells in the early stages of the response; it inhibits predominantly the T-lymphocytes (107). A study to improve the therapeutic qualities through structural modifications using rat skin tensile strength as a screening test (for lack of any better model) failed to uncover significant improvements (108).

Only very recently, a study employing the Pertussis vaccine oedema test supported the view that 25.**43**, like levamisole (25.**80**), can act as an immunostimulant (109). It is hoped that this new test will facilitate the search for improved penicillaminelike agents.

2.7 Procarbazine

Procarbazine (25.**44**) has been selected from a large group of methylhydrazines that were originally tested as monoamine oxidase inhibitors; it was subsequently found to possess antitumor activity (110) and is now clinically used for the palliative treatment of Hodgkin's disease.

It was soon discovered that 25.**44** is a strong inhibitor of the immune response. Procarbazine prolongs the survival of skin allografts across a strong histocompatibility barrier (H-2) in mice (111) and produces

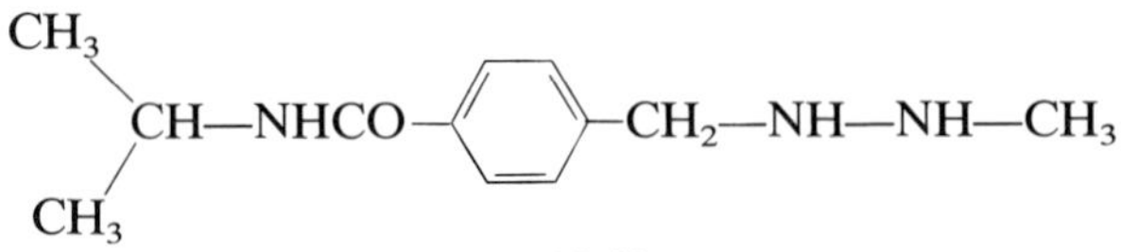

$$(CH_3)_2CH\text{—}NHCO\text{—}C_6H_4\text{—}CH_2\text{—}NH\text{—}NH\text{—}CH_3$$

25.**44**

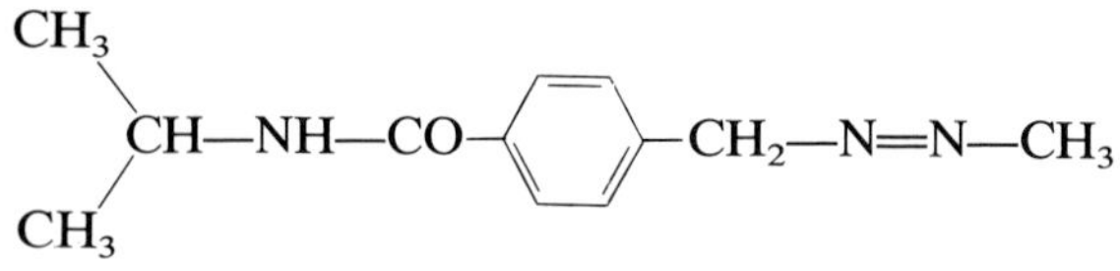

$$(CH_3)_2CH\text{—NH—CO—}C_6H_4\text{—}CH_2\text{—N=N—}CH_3$$

25.**45**

potent suppression of the circulating antibody response (112). Furthermore, the drug is active in the adjuvant-induced arthritis model in rats (113). Nevertheless, procarbazine has not been tested clinically in rheumatoid arthritis, probably because of the threat of carcinogenicity (114). Recently the drug found renewed interest through studies by Floersheim (115): procarbazine and ALS (Section 2.11) combined resulted in longer skin survival times in mice than either treatment alone. This synergistic effect may be the result of suppression of antibody formation against ALS. The ALS-sparing effect of 25.**44** and probably of similar chemical immunosuppressants will certainly be put to the clinical test in the near future.

The mode of action of 25.**44** is dependent on the methyl group (116). In rat liver, 25.**44** is oxidized to the equally potent but less stable azo compound 25.**45**, further to the inactive aldehyde 25.**46** and a nitrogen fragment, possibly the unstable methyldiimine 25.**47**.

2.8 Antibiotics

A large variety of antibiotics have been tested for their immunosuppressive properties, but only a few have shown any significant effects. In most cases these compounds were investigated because of their established antitumor activity in animal models or in man. Except for the actinomycins and thiamphenicol, none of the compounds discussed below has been studied clinically in immune-related diseases.

The actinomycins differ from one another by the peptide side chains, which are attached to the 4- and 5-positions of the chromophore (117). Actinomycin D (25.**48**), the most widely investigated representative of this group, inhibits DNA

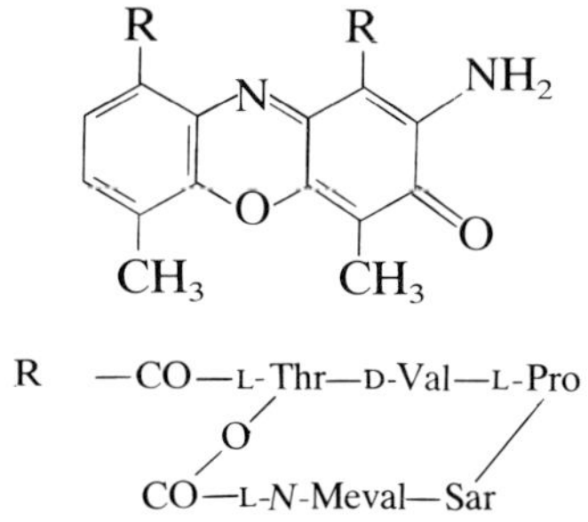

R R NH$_2$ N O O CH$_3$ CH$_3$

R —CO—L-Thr—D-Val—L-Pro
O
CO—L-*N*-Meval—Sar

25.**48**

transcriptase activity. The drug suppresses predominantly the production of 19*S* antibodies (118). Actinomycin has found only limited clinical application because of its poor therapeutic ratio.

Because of their powerful antimicrobial and antitumor activity, the group of mitomycins has been extensively studied (119). Their alkylating properties, which

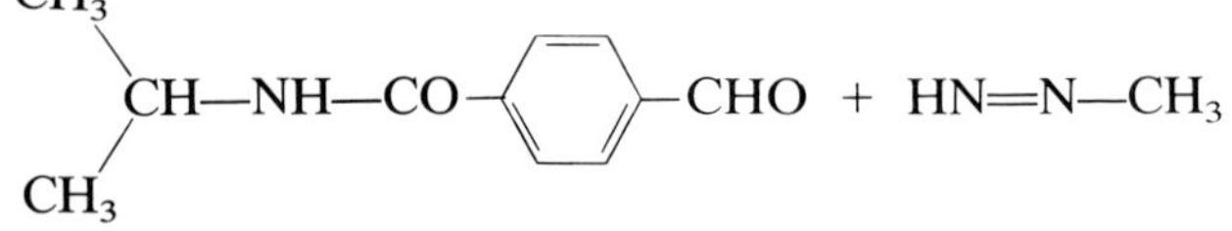

$$(CH_3)_2CH\text{—NH—CO—}C_6H_4\text{—CHO} + HN\text{=N—}CH_3$$

25.**46** 25.**47**

cause cross-linking of DNA strands (120), render the mitomycins cytostatic. Mitomycin C (25.**49**) is in clinical use as an anticancer agent (121). The immunosuppressive activity of 25.**49** has been demonstrated in mice through the prolongation of skin graft survival and suppression of the graft-versus-host reaction (122).

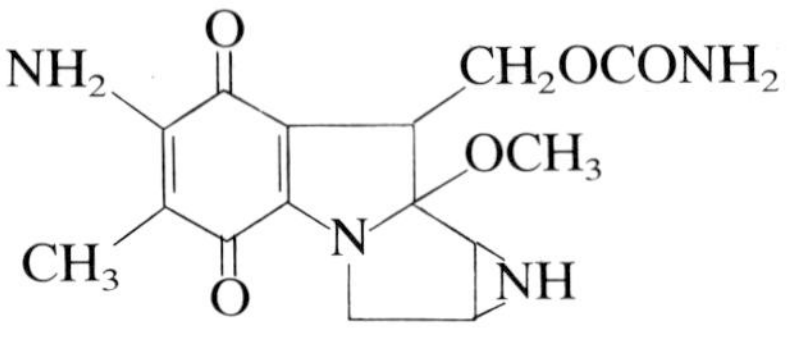

25.**49**

Chloramphenicol (25.**50**), one of the better known and more widely used antibiotics, is synthetically more easily accessible. A number of analogs have been tested in immunological systems and have been found—like 25.**50** itself—to be active: thiamphenicol (25.**51**) is superior to 25.**50**

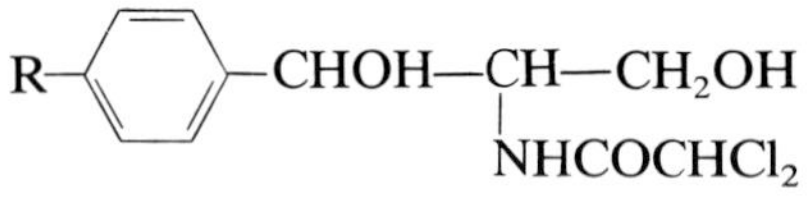

25.**50** R = NO_2
25.**51** R = CH_3SO_2

in prolonging skin grafts in mice (123) and in rabbits (124). The figures are impressive, however, only when weak histocompatibility barriers are considered: when grafting is studied across the more difficult H-2 histocompatibility locus, the graft survival times differ little from those of the controls; 25.**51** has been evaluated in patients with lupus glomerulonephritis (125).

Two antibiotics extracted from *Streptomyces peucetius*, adriamycin (25.**52**) and daunomycin (25.**53**) have been investigated in immunological systems because of their activity in a wide range of human cancers (126). Although 25.**52** differs from 25.**53** only by one hydroxyl group, the effect on the immune system is quite distinct: When 25.**52** was injected at the optimal time—2

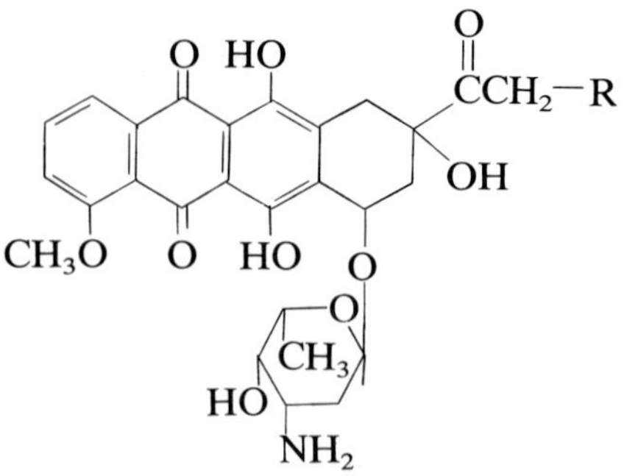

25.**52** R = OH
25.**53** R = H

days after SRBC in mice—it suppressed the primary response better than 25.**53**. In contrast, 25.**53** had a more pronounced influence on the secondary response (127). This reversal in activity toward different stages of the immune response became manifest in other tests as well and may have a bearing on the relative antitumor activities of the two drugs.

Puromycin (25.**54**) suppresses circulating antibodies in mice, probably by way of inhibition of protein synthesis (128). From the structure, one might suspect that the action of 25.**54** is similar to that of the purine antagonists.

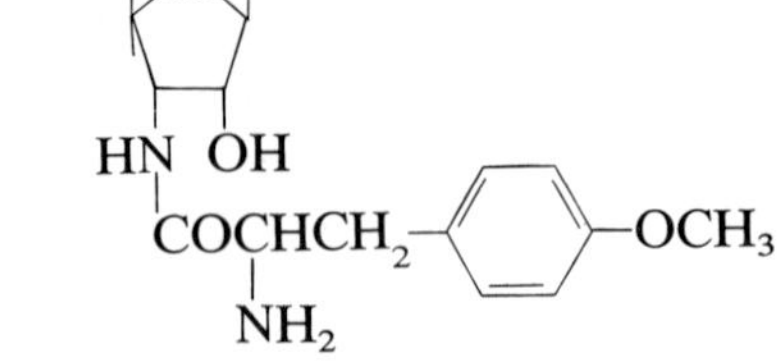

25.**54**

Studies of other antibiotics with immunosuppressive activity have appeared, but it is impossible to discuss even a fraction of this rather interesting field within this chapter. A selection of structures may illustrate this untapped wealth of chemical leads: alanosine, a nitrosohydroxylaminoamino acid (129); lankacidins (130) and rifampicin (131), macrolide antibiotics; azaserin (132) and duazomycin (133), diazoamino acids; trimethoprim, a synthetic antibacterial diaminopyrimidine (134) as well as chromomycin A3, a complicated glycoside antibiotic (135).

2.9 Alkaloids

Several classes of alkaloids have been tested in immunological systems, a development that resembles the studies with antibiotics. Here again, the incentive for biological evaluation came from alleged or established anticancer activities.

The best known group in this respect are the vinca alkaloids; which have found their place in the treatment of neoplastic diseases, particularly Hodgkin's disease and lymphosarcoma (see Chapter 24). In animal systems, immunosuppressive properties were demonstrated when the drugs were administered daily during the proliferative phase of the immune response (136).

Ellipticine (25.**55**) and 9-methoxyellipticine (25.**56**) have attracted some interest recently. As suggested by structural similarity to that of the "classical" intercalating drugs (e.g., 25.**63**), 25.**56** was shown to bind to nucleic acid helices by

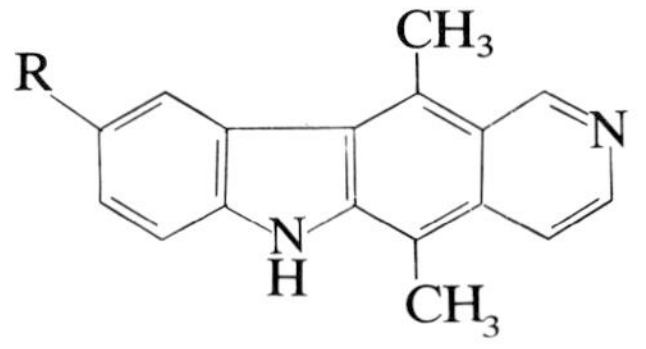

R, CH_3, N, N H, CH_3

25.**55** R = H
25.**56** R = OCH_3

intercalation (137). When administered after antigen, 25.**56** suppresses antibody formation against SRBC in mice (138).

One representative of the well-known group of pyrrolizidine alkaloids, dehydroheliotridine (25.**57**), suppresses the primary response to SRBC in mice when given before or with the antigen (139).

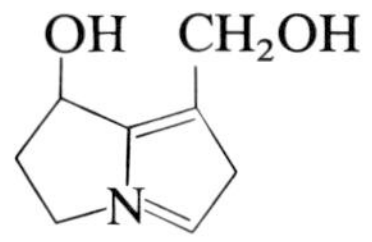

OH CH_2OH, N

25.**57**

2.10 Oxisuran

In contrast to most immunosuppressive agents including 6-mercaptopurine (25.**16**), oxisuran (25.**58**) inhibits cell-mediated immunity in the mouse, rat, and dog at readily tolerated doses without lowering the antibody response to sheep erythrocytes. When mice, which differed at the H-2 histocompatibility locus, were treated daily from day 7 until graft rejection occurred, allograft survival was significantly enhanced over that of untreated controls (17.2 days vs. 7.4 days) (140). The 3- and 4-positional isomers did not show the differential biological activity of the 2-isomer.

The half-life of oxisuran in man is relatively long (55 hr) (141), compared to 10 hr in the rat (142) and 12 hr in the dog (143). Four metabolites have been identified: the diastereomeric alcohols (25.**59**), which still possess the differential immunosuppressive activity of the parent compound, the sulfone (25.**60**), and the alcohol sulfone (25.**61**). Several major differences in the metabolisms of man, dog, and rat may be related to the differences of the immunosuppressive activity in these species. In man and to a somewhat lesser degree in the rat, reduction is the major pathway; but it is only a minor pathway in the dog, and this may account for its lower potency in this species. In addition, rodents and dogs oxidize the drug to oxisuran sulfone (142, 143), a metabolite not found in the urine or plasma of man.

$$R\text{—}CH(OH)CH_2\overset{O}{\overset{\|}{S}}CH_3 \quad 25.\mathbf{59}$$

$$\underset{25.\mathbf{58}}{C_5H_4N\text{—}\overset{O}{\overset{\|}{C}}\text{—}CH_2\text{—}\overset{\|}{S}\text{—}CH_3} \longrightarrow R\text{—}COCH_2\overset{O}{\underset{O}{\overset{\|}{\underset{\|}{S}}}}CH_3 \quad 25.\mathbf{60}$$

$$R\text{—}CH(OH)CH_2\overset{O}{\underset{O}{\overset{\|}{\underset{\|}{S}}}}CH_3 \quad 25.\mathbf{61}$$

R = 2-pyridyl

It seems rather probable that oxisuran acts preferentially on the thymus-derived lymphocytes and only insignificantly on the B-cells (144, 145). This property, combined with low toxicity, makes the compound an interesting candidate for future research.

2.11 Antilymphocyte Serum

Antilymphocyte serum (ALS) is not exactly within the domain of the medicinal chemist. However, this agent clearly belongs in a chapter on immunosuppressants for two reasons. First, it offers some insight into the mechanism of the immune response and is therefore of great theoretical importance. Second, ALS has found wide application in human organ transplantations and is one of the most potent and effective agents (146).

The rationale of ALS is simple: when animals are immunized with lymphocytes (or thymocytes or membranes from these cells) from another species, a serum is obtained that contains antibodies against these lymphoid cells—cells that are known to participate in reactions against organ transplants. Depending on the degree of impurity of the immunogen, antibodies against these impurities are also present. Antibodies against erythrocytes, for instance, can be removed by treatment with red blood cell suspensions, on which the antibodies are absorbed.

When such a serum is injected into the "donor" of the lymphoid cells, it agglutinates and lyses them. Several points are of interest here. Small doses of ALS reduce the number of lymphocytes only slightly; they cause, however, complete reduction of cell-mediated immunity. Larger and repeated doses cause severe leukopenia. Lance (147) has studied and reviewed the many theories that explain the different facets of ALS actions. It seems clear that ALS acts primarily against thymus-derived cells (T-cells). Consequently, in animal studies, the effects of cell-mediated immunity are primarily influenced by ALS: skin graft survival, experimental encephalomyelitis, tuberculin reaction. Humoral immunity is affected only when ALS is given before the antigen. This explains also why animals treated with ALS have not lost their resistance to infections.

Although ALS seems to have advantages over the agents mentioned earlier by virtue of its specific mechanism, it has two decisive drawbacks: one is the difficulty in standardizing the sera. Only biological tests are available, and the results of immunosuppression in smaller animals do not necessarily reflect the potency of the substance for use in man. The second problem is inherent in the nature of the agent. On prolonged use, the recipient of ALS begins to form antibodies against the globulins of ALS, that is, against the very agent itself. This not only renders it ineffective but engenders risks such as anaphylactic shock or serum sickness, and the treatment must be discontinued.

In spite of this, ALS has been successfully employed in conjunction with azathioprine (25.**17**) and steroids in human organ transplants, particularly kidneys (148). It is more and more used, however, to overcome acute rejection crises, while the long-term treatment is left to the chemical agents discussed previously.

2.12 Miscellaneous Agents

A large number of substances of natural or synthetic origin have been reported to possess immunosuppressive properties. This is not surprising, since the immune response can be interfered with in many ways and the primary screening tests are fairly simple. Without enumerating every study that claims immunosuppressive properties for an old or new compound, this section briefly mentions those that either survived somewhat extended pharmacological testing or appear to be promising leads for future development.

Cinaserin (25.**62**) is a potent serotonin antagonist. It was found to suppress the

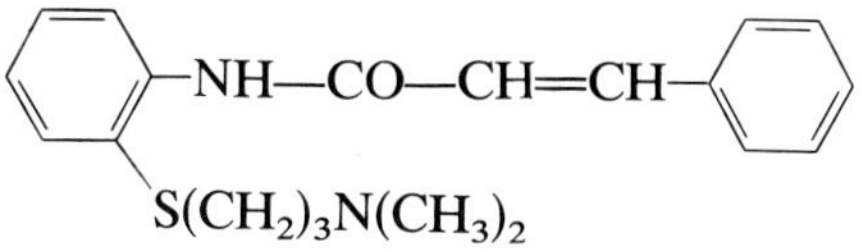

NH—CO—CH=CH—
$S(CH_2)_3N(CH_3)_2$

25.**62**

formation of circulating antibodies, prolong mouse skin homografts, and exhibit activity in the EAE test as well as in adjuvant-induced arthritis (149).

Other drugs, which like cinaserin influence the metabolism of biogenic amines, have long been recognized as being immunosuppressive in animal models. Reserpine and some phenothiazines (150), particularly promethazine (151), also 5-hydroxytryptophan but not iproniazide (152), have been found to be active in skin graft prolongation or against circulating antibodies.

NH_2 $N^{\oplus}$ CH_3 $Cl^{\ominus}$ NH_2

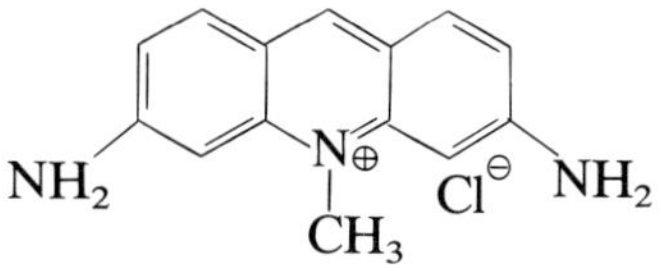

25.**63**

Acriflavine (25.**63**), an antibacterial agent, inhibits the primary immune response and prolongs skin allograft survival in rabbits (153). It was suggested that the ability of 25.**63** and related compounds to intercalate between adjacent base pairs of the double helix of DNA (154) is responsible for the immunosuppression. The experimental antitumor compound 4′-[(9-acridinyl)amino]methanesulfon-*m*-anisidide (25.**64**), has immunosuppressant properties

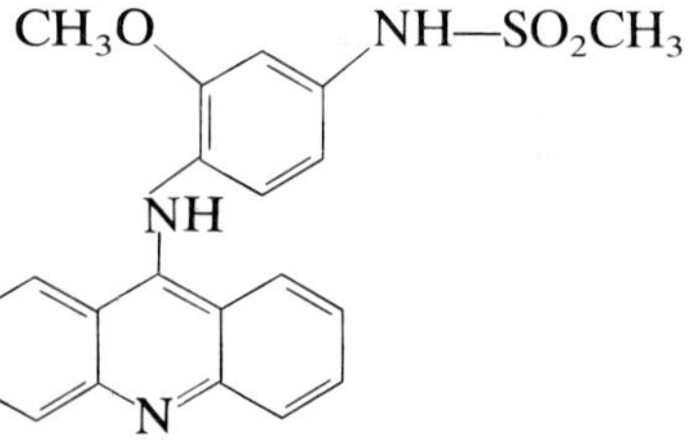

CH_3O NH—SO_2CH_3
NH
N

25.**64**

(155), most likely through a similar mechanism. In the same category falls a very potent inhibitor reported recently: 4,5-bis(aminomethyl)acridine (25.**65**) (156).

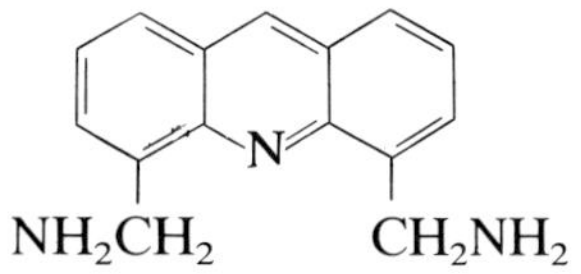

N
NH_2CH_2 CH_2NH_2

25.**65**

The infamous sedative thalidomide (25.**66**) and closely related derivatives (157) were found to be immunosuppressive; 25.**66** prolonged the skin graft

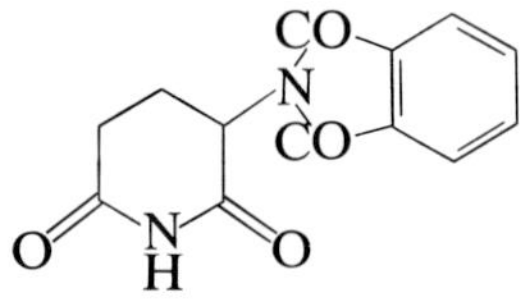

25.**66**

survival time in mice to some extent in the weak histocompatibility model (158), leading to an interesting theory with regard to the occurrence of malformations. Assuming that spontaneous abortions of malformed fetuses are the result of an immune response, the drug may have allowed such fetuses to develop by suppressing the normal immune mechanism.

Aryltriazenes resemble to a certain degree the benzylhydrazines (e.g., 25.**44**) and most likely act by a similar mechanism. The best-known compound from this group, dimethyltriazenoimidazole carboxamide (25.**67**), which is clinically useful in the

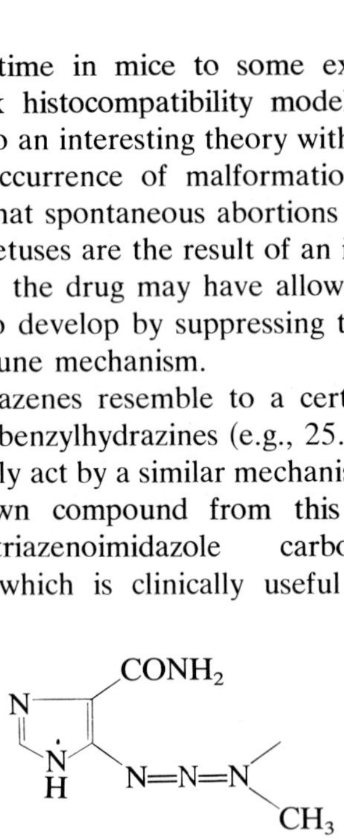

25.**67**

treatment of melanoma (159), was highly suppressive against humoral and cell-mediated immunity (160). The 3-hydroxytriazene 25.**68** was effective in prolonging skin graft survival from 10 days in

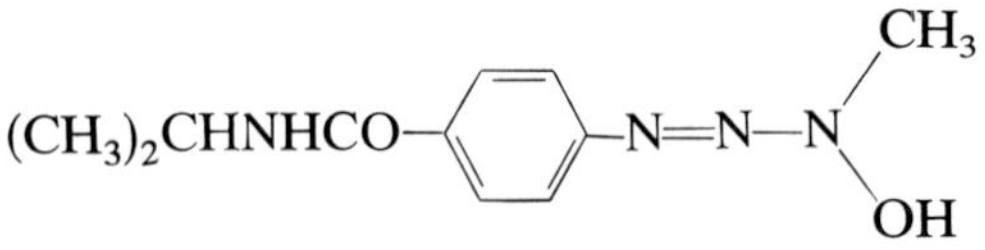

25.**68**

controls to 22.5 days when given daily orally, starting 7 days before grafting (161).

From a large series of benzimidazoyl (25.**69**), benzthiazolyl (25.**70**), and benzoxazolyl (25.**71**) ureas, which suppressed antibody formation against SRBC in mice (162, 163)—compound 25.**72,** for instance,

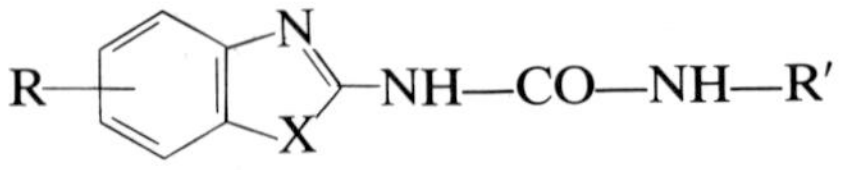

25.**69** X = NH
25.**70** X = S
25.**71** X = O
25.**73** X = S, R = 6-OCH_3, R′ = C_6H_5

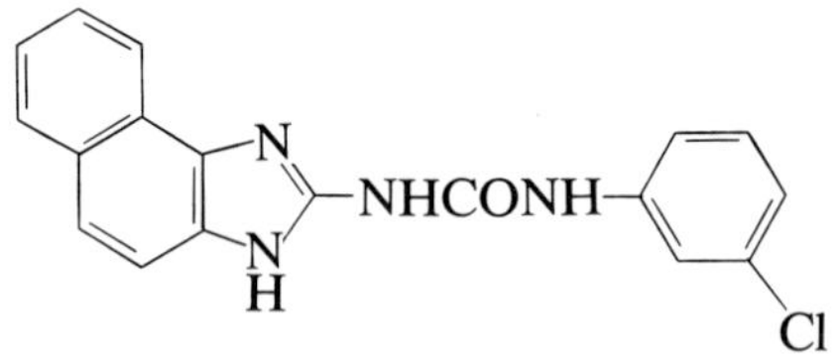

25.**72**

was more potent than azathioprine—one candidate, Frenazole (25.**73**), was selected for extended studies (164). It had a better therapeutic index than azathioprine (25.**17**), cyclophosphamide (25.**5**), cortisone, and methotrexate (25.**42**) in the standard tests for immunosuppression, and it improved the symptoms of NZ mice autoimmune disease.

The anthelmintic drug niridazole (25.**74**) has recently been found to prolong the

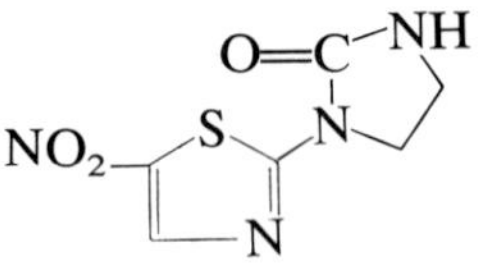

25.**74**

survival time of mouse skin grafts in the same range as antilymphocyte serum across a strong histocompatibility locus (165, 166).

A number of "unnatural" amino acids have been tested in animal experiments. The rationale for their synthesis and screening was, of course, to interfere with protein synthesis through incorporation of "false" and possibly nondegradable amino acids.

The most widely studied compound of this group is 1-aminocyclopentanecarboxylic acid (25.**75**). It cannot be metabolized and remains essentially unchanged within the cell (167). When 25.**75**

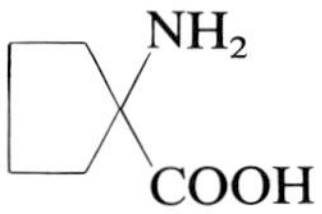

NH_2

COOH

25.**75**

was given before the administration of antigen, it prevented the formation of hemagglutinins and hemolysins but did not inhibit the secondary immune response. The compound was ineffective in prolonging graft survival in mice, but it suppressed experimental allergic encephalomyelitis in a dose-dependent manner (168).

$$NH_2—(CH_2)_5—COOH$$

25.**76**

ε-Aminocaproic acid (25.**76**) has received some attention as a possible immunosuppressive agent (169, 170), but its clinical use would seem to be impractical because of the large dose requirements and toxic effects. The immunosuppressive properties of β-3-thienylalanine (25.**77**) were restricted to the inhibition of antibody response in rats (171).

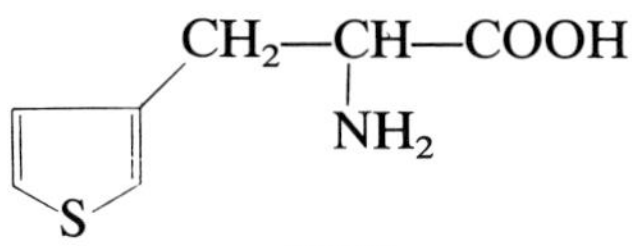

CH_2—CH—COOH

NH_2

S

25.**77**

None of these compounds has been subjected to extended clinical studies, and this approach appears to have lost its attraction.

Many efforts have been made to find a naturally occurring factor believed to be part of the regulatory mechanism of the immune response. Particularly, serum of human, cattle, or rat blood has been fractionated with a variety of physicochemical techniques, and the fractions have been subjected to the established models of immunosuppression. Indeed, it is now possible to dissociate a dialyzable peptide fraction from an active human globulin fraction, and the peptide has been shown to suppress the plaque-forming cells in mice after immunization with SRBC (172).

The concept of chalones, which one day undoubtedly will influence the thinking of medicinal chemists, defines these substances as specific and endogenous negative feedback inhibitors of mitosis. A fraction of calf lymphoid tissue with a molecular weight range of 30,000–50,000, which inhibited the thymidine uptake in cultured human lymphocytes, was consequently tested in the mouse skin homograft test. An impressive 2.5-fold prolongation of survival time was reported (173).

Less convincing were the results obtained with concanavalin A, a protein derived from the jack bean and associated with a variety of biological activities (174). In the rat adjuvant arthritis model, however, doses between 1 and 5 mg/kg daily produced good results, in the developing as well as in the developed symptoms (175).

The parade of so many diversified products from nature or the chemist's retort may be concluded with a product from a fungus *Trichoderma polysporum* (176): cyclosporine A (25.**78**) is a cyclic peptide of 11 amino acids, including some unusual *N*-methylamino acids and one D-alanine. This combination renders the product stable to gastric peptidases; thus it is active by the oral route. The results in suppression of humoral and cell-mediated immunity are very impressive, as well as its activity in both models of adjuvant arthritis (177).

25.**78**

3 IMMUNOSTIMULANTS

In contrast to the well-recognized field of immunosuppression, stimulation of the immune response received less attention in the past; it was limited to the application of specific antisera and immunopotentiation with classical adjuvants. Yet the restoration of an impaired immune response and the enhancement of existing immune mechanisms should be potentially useful in a variety of diseases.

During recent years a number of unrelated substances with immunopotentiating properties have come into focus, and more attention is given to the use of adjuvants, their nature, and the concepts underlying immunostimulation (178, 179).

Adjuvants (Latin, *adjuvare*—to assist) are substances that aid in the development and manifestation of the immune system: when injected with an antigen, they enhance the antigenic properties of a weak antigen or convert a nonantigenic substance to an effective antigen. They lead to increased antibody production and to induction of delayed hypersensitivity.

3.1 Water-in-Oil Emulsions

It was shown by Freund (180) that incorporation of an antigen into water-in-mineral oil emulsions (Freund's incomplete adjuvant) leads to an enhanced and prolonged period of antibody production; the complete adjuvant is similar in composition but includes killed *Mycobacterium tuberculosis.* As a possible mechanism, it was suggested that destruction and elimination of the antigen may be retarded, resulting in a slow release from the depot. Granulomatous lesions resulted when Freund's adjuvant preparations were used in animals, and this side effect has discouraged their use in man.

3.2 Aluminum Salts

Absorption of antigens to precipitated aluminum hydroxide or phosphate gels markedly increases the humoral antibody response. Retention and wider dissemination may account for the increase. Toxicity and side reactions are low. Aluminum salts are useful adjuvants for immunization against diphtheria and tetanus. Aluminum salts preferentially enhance the humoral antibody response, whereas Freund's adjuvant can stimulate both cell-mediated and humoral antibody responses.

3.3 Substances of Bacterial Origin

The discovery by Freund, just outlined, and an earlier observation by Lewis and Loomis (181) that higher hemolysin titers are produced in tuberculous than in normal guinea pigs, alluded to the role of mycobacteria as potential adjuvants.

Several immunostimulants in this category—for instance, *Bacillus Calmette Guérin* (BCG), *Corynebacterium parvum*, and *Bordella pertussis*—are increasingly being tried in the control of cancer (178).

Extensive studies on various fractions derived from mycobacterial cells established the active components (182). A wax fraction, called Wax D, was isolated from human strains of *M. tuberculosis*; it exhibited adjuvant activity in both the humoral and cellular immune response (183, 184). The main constituents of Wax D are macromolecular lipids, consisting of various esters of mycolic acid, a polysaccharide moiety, and a small peptide fragment linked to amino sugars.

A nontoxic and nonpyrogenic water soluble fraction (mol wt ~20,000) with marked adjuvant properties was obtained after lyophilization of delipidated cell walls of *Mycobacterium smegmatis* (185). Several hydrosoluble compounds of low molecular weight still exhibited a strong adjuvant effect when injected with mineral oil (186). The smallest active fragments of bacterial origin seem to be *N*-acetylmuramyltripeptides (187).

3.4 Mitogens

Certain plant proteins that react specifically with various sugars of glycoproteines on lymphocyte surfaces can induce differentiation into blast cells. Mitogens have been successfully used as analogs for antigens in studies of lymphocyte activation, providing insight into the mechanism of cell activation for T- and B-cells (188).

Most soluble plant mitogens such as concanavalin A (isolated from the jack bean) and phytohemagglutinin (obtained from the bean *Phaseolus vulgaris*) require the presence of thymus-dependent lymphocytes (189). Extracts of *Phytolacca americana* (pokeweed) are reported to have mitogenic activities directed toward both T- and B-lymphoid cells (190). Differences in mitogenic specificity of proteins isolated from *P. americana* were shown to be related to their physicochemical properties (191).

3.5 Polynucleotides

Complementary copolymers, such as double-stranded polyadenylic acid:polyuridylic acid (poly A:U) and polyinosinic acid:polycytidylic acid (poly I:C), enhance the formation of antibodies in mice immunized with SRBC (192); they appear to act directly on host cells rather than in a special complex with antigen. Poly I:C also reduced the survival time of isografts in mice from 23 days for controls to 10 days for treated animals (193), indicating that a polynucleotide copolymer is capable of stimulating both humoral and cellular immune responses. In contrast, single-stranded polynucleotides enhance the immune response *in vitro* but not *in vivo*. The adjuvant effect of these polynucleotide complexes has been extended to many antigens in several animal species (194).

3.6 Polyanions

Polyanions, for example, alginic acid and pentosan sulfate, are also known to augment the immune response. Alginic acid, obtained from seaweed, is a hydrophilic, colloidal carbohydrate acid and contains varying proportions of D-mannuronic and L-guluronic acids. At doses of 4 mg/mouse it enhances the immune response of 19*S* plaque-forming cells 44-fold, 4 days after inoculation with suboptimal doses of SRBC (195).

The smallest polyanion oligomer capable of stimulating the antigen response was a pentosan sulfate SP 54, composed of 6–12 sugar units (196).

Synthetic polymers with carboxy groups ("Pyrancopolymer") have also been shown to potentiate the immune response in mice (197).

3.7 Miscellaneous Compounds

Recently a number of small and chemically well-defined molecules (tilorone, levamisole, vitamin A, and vitamin A acid), devoid of antigenicity and free of the undesirable attributes of some adjuvants, have been shown to have a modulatory effect on the immune response in experimental models and in clinical trials.

Tilorone (25.**79**) is an orally and parenterally active broad spectrum antiviral substance and interferon inducer. It is also capable of stimulating the immune response to SRBC in mice (198). The increase was more pronounced at suboptimal antigen dose when given 2 hr or less before antigen inoculation.

Additional properties of tilorone indicating contrasting effects in humoral and cell-mediated immunity were reported (199). Administration of tilorone resulted in a twofold increase in the immune response to both thymus-dependent (SRBC) and thymus-independent (*E. coli* endotoxin) antigens. Stimulation of the secondary immune response to SRBC was observed, as well as a threefold increase in IgE-like antibody.

Contrary to its effect on humoral antibody production, tilorone suppressed cell-mediated immune responses as demonstrated by a decrease in paralysis in experimentally induced allergic encephalomyelitis in rats, the inhibition of the tuberculin skin reaction, and a reduction in the secondary swelling in adjuvant arthritis.

Another synthetic substance that shows great promise as an agent to restore an impaired immune response is levamisole (25.**80**), which has been used successfully as

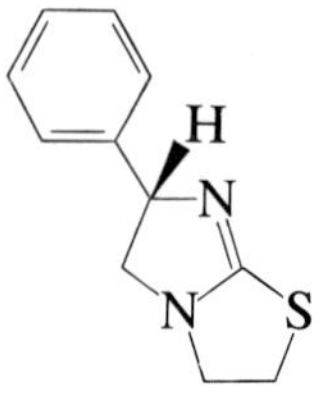

H N N S

25.**80**

a potent anthelmintic in humans and animals against a wide range of nematodal infections (215).

The capacity of levamisole to stimulate aspects of cell-mediated immunity was first demonstrated by Renoux and Renoux

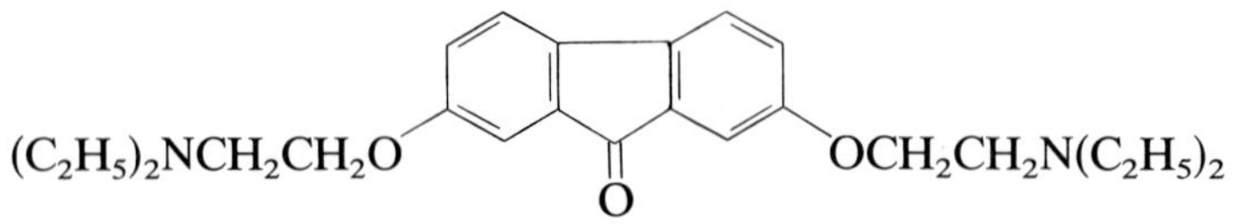

$(C_2H_5)_2NCH_2CH_2O$ O $OCH_2CH_2N(C_2H_5)_2$

25.**79**

(200). Levamisole affects primarily cellular immunity rather than the humoral response. Under certain conditions, levamisole leads to a two- to threefold increase in the number of plaque-forming cells (201, 202). When given before cell transfer, it has an effect on the graft-versus-host reaction (203). Renoux et al. (204) determined the effectiveness of levamisole in modifying cellular responses, using the rejection of skin grafts and the induction of a delayed type of hypersensitivity as an assay system. Their results confirmed previous reports that levamisole stimulates cell-mediated immunity, as evidenced by increased and sustained delayed-type hypersensitivity levels and accelerated rejection of skin isografts in mice.

The restorative capacity by levamisole of E-rosette forming cells in patients suffering from various clinical conditions, where underlying immunologic disturbances were thought to play a major role, has been demonstrated (205). Furthermore, the increase in the number of E-rosettes was associated with an improvement of symptoms.

Clinically promising results have also been described with levamisole in recurrent aphtous stomatitis (206), herpes infection (207), and persistent skin infections (208). The drug also has a beneficial effect on recurrent upper respiratory tract infections in about two-thirds of the children who received the treatment (209). Highly encouraging results were obtained in some patients with systemic lupus erythematosus (210).

The use of levamisole in rheumatic diseases is still experimental. Several reports of studies with levamisole in patients with rheumatoid arthritis have appeared, citing generally beneficial effects. In a placebo-controlled study, levamisole was shown to be as effective as D-penicillamine in the treatment of rheumatoid arthritis. It produced relief of pain and reduction in the duration of morning stiffness, accompanied by changes in the erythrocyte sedimentation rate and the rheumatoid factor (211).

In another study, the drug was administered either continuously or intermittently in a daily dose of 150 mg over several months (212). Significant improvement was noted in about half the rheumatic arthritic patients.

It was found that several agents known to labilize lysosomal membranes, such as vitamin A (retinol, 25.**81**), have adjuvant effects (213). The observation that vitamin A acid (25.**82**) causes a regression of chemically induced carcinomas of the skin led to

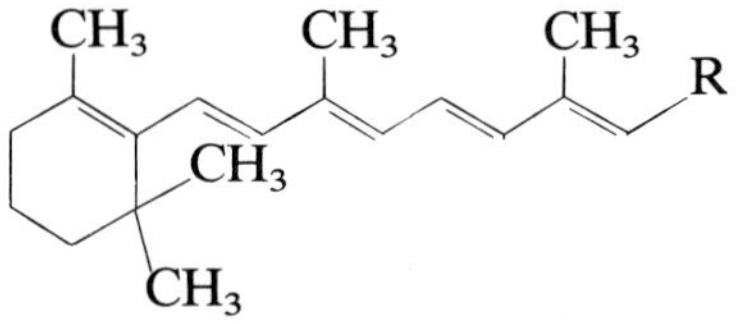

CH_3 CH_3 CH_3 R CH_3 CH_3

25.**81** R = CH_2OH
25.**82** R = COOH

a trial of this compound to investigate its immunopotentiating properties (214). Both substances displayed a pronounced effect on immunological responses in animals. Skin grafts were rejected more expeditiously when mice were treated with either of these compounds. In addition, daily vitamin A injections preceding or following sensitization with SRBC led to a large increase in the production of hemagglutinin antibodies.

We are far from understanding why diseases with obvious immune deficiency, like lupus erythematosus, are successfully treated either with immunosuppressants or with immunostimulants. The complex interplay between T- and B-cells, the specific suppression of the suppressor cells, resulting in an overall increased response, and similar matters, certainly need more understanding. Until then, the obvious dilemma for the drug researcher persists.

4 OUTLOOK

Serendipity, vision, scientific inquisitiveness, and ancient practice all contributed to pave the long, often arduous, and seemingly hopeless road to the first successful human heart transplant at the Groote Schuur Hospital at the Cape of Good Hope on December 3, 1967.

Already in 1912 Carrel had pointed out "that the idea of replacing diseased organs with sound ones, of putting back an amputated limb or even grafting a new limb onto a patient who has undergone an amputation, is far from being original". Indeed, the replacement of injured or diseased organs has stimulated the imagination of man for many centuries, but a scientific approach to transplantation research did not begin until the 1800s. Initial attempts at organ transplantation were described by Emerich Ullmann in 1902 (216). The first reported performance of organ grafting was by Carrel and Charles Guthrie in 1905 (217), who transplanted the heart of one dog into the neck of a larger dog.

Although the precise mechanism of graft rejection was far from clear at the time, experiments several years later by Emile Holman (218) on skin transplant studies led him to conclude that the rejection of grafts was due to a type-specific antibody.

New vistas to transplant science were opened by the pioneering work of Sir Macfarlane Burnet and Peter Medawar, followed by many brilliant discoveries in clinics and laboratories throughout the world. In 1959 began the age of chemical immunosuppression, with the demonstration by Schwartz and Dameshek that the immunological response of rabbits could be successfully modified by treatment with 6-mercaptopurine (71); other drugs were rapidly added to the armamentarium of immunosuppressants. The success of renal homografts had created renewed interest in the entire problem of organ transplantation.

Aside from their use in organ grafting, a wide range of compounds as well as some biological agents have served in a variety of immune-oriented diseases. The precise site of action is incompletely understood for most of the immunosuppressants in clinical use; no drug is yet available to interfere with a particular step.

The bulk of the data on the immunosuppressive potency of these agents has evolved from studies in animals; therefore caution and skepticism must be exercised in extrapolating the results to human therapy, especially for inflammatory diseases of unknown etiology. The issue is further complicated by the lack of information regarding the principal mechanisms of immunological processes that are abnormal in different diseases, the fact that these drugs are often applied at an advanced disease state, the nonspecific nature of the therapy, and the observation that a remission in many cases does not last indefinitely after drug withdrawal.

There are many reports on the use of immunosuppressive drugs; but most studies deal with single or a limited number of cases. Only a few long-term, carefully designed and controlled studies have been done for the drugs currently in use, and many more are needed to ensure a more rational and consistent approach, to evaluate risk versus benefit, and to establish the therapeutic efficacy of these agents. Some general principles in immunosuppressive therapy (220) and guidelines for the use of cytotoxic drugs in rheumatoid arthritis (221) have been outlined.

The drugs most widely used in a variety of immune-oriented diseases or transplant situations are listed in Table 25.3. Many of the treatments include steroids in their drug regimen.

Immunosuppressants affect both wanted and unwanted immunological parameters; thus they impede both normal and abnormal responses, leading to several potential complications. One of the greatest single hazards of immunosuppressive therapy is predisposition to infection associated with a diminution of immune surveillance; this property is shared by all the drugs now in

Table 25.3

Name	Structure	Clinical Use as Immunosuppressant
Alkylating agents Cyclophosphamide (Endoxan)	Cyclic phosphamide ring (O–P–NH) with P=O and $N(CH_2CH_2Cl)_2$	Kidney transplantations, severe rheumatoid arthritis
Chlorambucil (Leukeran)	$(ClCH_2CH_2)_2N-C_6H_4-(CH_2)_3COOH$	Severe rheumatoid arthritis
Antimetabolites 6-Mercaptopurine	R=H— ; R—S on purine ring	Organ transplantations, autoimmune diseases, including rheumatoid arthritis
Azathioprine (Imuran)	R = 1-Methyl-4-nitro-5-imidazolyl	
Methotrexate	2,4-diamino-pteridinyl–CH_2–N(CH_3)–C_6H_4–CO—NH—CH(COOH)$(CH_2)_2$COOH	Lupus erythematosus, psoriatic arthritis
D-Penicillamine (Cuprimine)	$HS-C(CH_3)_2-CH(NH_2)-COOH$	Rheumatoid arthritis, various autoimmune diseases
Antilymphocyte serum		Organ transplantations

use. Furthermore, these agents may lead to malignancies in the patient. Other side effects such as alopecia, bone marrow depression, hemorrhagic cystitis, and gastrointestinal ulceritis are reversible if recognized in time.

Although our present knowledge of chemical immunosuppression is still limited and imperfect, dramatic advances and definite inroads are made each year in our understanding of the factors that control the immune response and its role in the development of disease, raising hope that a more effective and specific therapy may some day become available.

REFERENCES

1. A. E. Gabrielsen and R. A. Good, *Advan. Immunol,* **6,** 91 (1967).
2. T. Makinodan, G. W. Santos, and R. P. Quinn, *Pharmacol. Rev.,* **22,** 189 (1970).
3. G. W. Camiener and W. J. Wechter, in *Progress in Drug Research,* Vol. 16, E. Jucker, Ed., Birkhäuser-Verlag, Basel, 1972, p. 67.
4. M. C. Berenbaum, *Biochem. Pharmacol.,* **11,** 29 (1962).
5. A. W. Frisch and G. H. Davies, *Proc. Soc. Exp. Biol. Med.* **110,** 444 (1962).
6. G. W. Santos, *Fed. Proc.,* **26,** 907 (1967).
7. D. Chanmougan and R. S. Schwartz, *J. Exp. Med.,* **124,** 363 (1966).

8. A. Carrel and R. Ingebrigtsen, *J. Exp. Med.*, **15,** 287 (1912).
9. H. N. Claman, E. A. Chaperon, and R. F. Triplett, *J. Immunol.*, **97,** 828 (1966).
10. J. F. A. P. Miller and G. F. Mitchell, *J. Exp. Med.*, **128,** 801 (1968).
11. J. L. Gowans, in *Immunobiology*, R. A. Good and D. W. Fisher, Eds., Sinauer, Stamford, Conn., 1971, p. 18.
12. H. N. Claman and E. A. Chaperon, *Transplant. Rev.*, **1,** 92 (1969).
13. D. H. Katz and B. Benacerraf, *Advan. Immunol.*, **15,** 1 (1972).
14. J. F. A. P. Miller and G. F. Mitchell, *Transplant. Rev.*, **1,** 3 (1969).
15. J. F. A. P. Miller and D. Osoba, *Physiol. Rev.*, **47,** 437 (1967).
16. G. F. Mitchell and J. F. A. P. Miller, *J. Exp. Med.*, **128,** 821 (1968).
17. J. F. A. P. Miller, A. Basten, J. Sprent, and C. Cheers, *Cell. Immunol.*, **2,** 469 (1971).
18. S. Segal, J. R. Cohen, and M. Feldmann, *Science*, **175,** 1126 (1972).
19. Special issue on T- and B-cells, *Transplant Rev.*, **26,** (1975).
20. B. Glick, T. S. Chang, and R. G. Jaap, *Poult. Sci.*, **35,** 224 (1956).
21. M. D. Cooper, W. A. Cain, P. J. Van Alten, and R. A. Good, *Int. Arch. Allergy Appl. Immunol.*, **35,** 242 (1969).
22. R. K. Meyer, M. A. Rao, and R. L. Aspinall, *Endocrinology*, **64,** 890 (1959).
23. K. Rajewski, V. Schirrmacher, S. Nase, and N. K. Jerne, *J. Exp. Med.*, **129,** 1131 (1969).
24. N. A. Mitchison, *Eur. J. Immunol.*, **1,** 10 (1971).
25. E. R. Unanue, *Advan. Immunol.*, **15,** 95 (1972).
26. M. Feldmann, *J. Exp. Med.*, **136,** 737 (1972).
27. M. Feldmann and G. J. V. Nossal, *Transplant. Rev.*, **13,** 3 (1972).
28. M. Feldmann and A. Basten, *J. Exp. Med.*, **136,** 49 (1972).
29. A. J. Cunningham, *Transplant Rev.*, **31,** 23 (1976).
30. G. M. Edelman and W. E. Gall, *Ann. Rev. Biochem.*, **38,** 415 (1969).
31. *L. Hood and J. Prahl, Advan. Immunol.*, **14,** 291 (1971).
32. R. J. Poljak, *Advan. Immunol.*, **21,** 1 (1975).
33. E. von Behring and S. Kitasato, *Deut. Med. Wochenschr.*, **49,** 1113 (1890).
34. P. Ehrlich, *Proc. Roy. Soc., Ser. B*, **66,** 424 (1900).
35. K. Landsteiner, *The Specificity of Serological Reactions*, 2nd ed., Harvard University Press, Cambridge, Mass., 1945.
36. L. Pauling, *J. Am. Chem. Soc.*, **62,** 2643 (1940).
37. N. K. Jerne, *Proc. Nat. Acad. Sci., US*, **41,** 849 (1955).
38. F. M. Burnet, *The Clonal Selection Theory of Acquired Immunity*, Cambridge University Press, Cambridge, 1959.
39. A. Tiselius and E. A. Kabat, *Science*, **87,** 416 (1938).
40. G. M. Edelman and J. A. Gally, *J. Exp. Med.* **116,** 207 (1962).
41. G. M. Edelman, *Biochemistry*, **9,** 3197 (1970).
42. R. R. Porter, *Biochem. J.*, **73,** 119 (1959).
43. R. C. Valentine and N. M. Green, *J. Mol. Biol.*, **27,** 615 (1967).
44. V. Meyer, *Ber. Deut. Chem. Ges.*, **1,** 1725 (1887).
45. P. Ehrlich, *Collected Papers of Paul Ehrlich*, Vol. 1, F. Himmelweit, Ed., Pergamon Press, London 1956, p. 596.
46. A. Gilman and F. S. Philips, *Science*, 103, 409 (1946).
47. L. Hektoen and H. J. Corper, *J. Infect. Dis.*, **28,** 279 (1921).
48. C. L. Spur, *Proc. Soc. Exp. Biol. Med.*, **64,** 259 (1947).
49. M. C. Berenbaum and I. N. Brown, *Immunology*, **7,** 65 (1964).
50. E. M. Hersh, in *Handbook of Experimental Pharmacology*, Vol. 28, Springer-Verlag, New York, 1974, p. 577.
51. W. C. J. Ross, *Biological Alkylating Agents*, Butterworths, London, 1962.
52. D. Triggle, *J. Theor. Biol.*, **7,** 241 (1964).
53. C. C. Price, G. M. Gaucher, P. Koneru, R. Shibakawa, J. R. Sowa, and M. Yamaguchi, *Ann. N.Y. Acad. Sci.*, **163,** 593 (1969).
54. T. J. Bardos, Z. F. Chmielewicz, and P. Hebborn, *Ann. N.Y. Acad. Sci.*, **163,** 1006 (1969).
55. M. Ochoa, Jr., and E. Hirschberg, *Exp. Chemother.*, **5,** 1 (1967).
56. G. P. Wheeler, *Fed. Proc.*, **26,** 885 (1967).
57. M. C. Berenbaum, *Pharmacol. J.*, **203,** 671 (1969).
58. M. E. Balis, *Antagonists and Nucleic Acids*, American Elsevier Publishing, New York, 1968, p. 177.
59. H. Arnold and F. Bourseaux, *Angew. Chem.*, **70,** 539 (1958).
60. E. M. Uyeki, *Biochem. Pharmacol.*, **16,** 53 (1967).

61. J. L. Turk, *Int. Arch. Allergy Appl. Immunol.*, **24,** 191 (1964).

62. M. E. Rosenthale, L. J. Datko, J. Kassarich, and F. Schneider, *Arch. Int. Pharmacodyn. Ther.*, **179,** 251 (1969).

63. B. H. Hahn, L. Knotts, M. Ng, and T. R. Hamilton, *Arthritis Rheum.*, **18,** 145 (1975).

64. U. Botzenhardt and E. M. Lemmel, *Agents Actions*, **6,** 596 (1976).

65. E. A. Friedman, A. Ueno, M. M. Beyer, and A. D. Nicastri, *Transplantation*, **15,** 619 (1973).

66. R. F. Struck, M. C. Kirk, L. B. Mellet, S. El Dareer, and D. L. Hill, *Mol. Pharmacol.*, **7,** 519 (1971).

67. A. Takamizawa, Y. Tochino, Y. Hamashima, and T. Iwata, *Chem. Pharm. Bull.* (Tokyo), **20,** 1612 (1972).

68. N. E. Sladek, *Cancer Res.*, **33,** 651 (1973).

69. R. A. Alarcon and J. Meienhofer, *Nature* (*New Biol.*), **233,** 250 (1971).

70. D. L. Hill, M. C. Kirk, and R. F. Struck, *J. Am. Chem. Soc.*, **92,** 3207 (1970).

71. R. Schwartz and W. Dameshek, *Nature*, **183,** 1682 (1959).

72. G. H. Hitchings and G. B. Elion. *Acc. Chem. Res.*, **2,** 202 (1969).

73. A. H. Chalmers, *Biochem. Pharmacol.*, **23,** 1891 (1974).

74. G. B. Elion, *Proc. Roy. Soc. Med.*, **65,** 257 (1972).

75. I. R. Mackay, S. Weiden, and B. Ungar, *Lancet*, **1,** 899 (1964).

76. M. C. Berenbaum, *Clin. Exp. Immunol.* **8,** 1 (1971).

77. J. F. Bach, *Drugs*, **11,** 1 (1976).

78. G. H. Heppner and P. Calabresi, *Ann. Rev. Pharm. Tox.*, **16,** 367 (1976).

79. G. Whelan and S. Sherlock, *Gut*, 13, 907 (1972).

80. E. M. Lemmel and U. Botzenhardt, *Arzneim.-Forsch.*, **26,** 1281 (1976).

81. T. Sekine, Y. Arai, and M. Saneyoshi, *Japan, J. Exp. Med.*, **43,** 369 (1973).

82. S.-c. J. Fu, B. J. Hargis, E. Chinoporos, and S. Malkiel, *J. Med. Chem.*, **10,** 109 (1967).

83. A. P. Kimball, S. J. Herriot, and P. S. Allinson, *Proc. Soc. Exp. Biol. Med.*, **126,** 181 (1967).

84. A. H. Chalmers, T. Burdorf, and A. W. Murray, *Biochem. Pharmacol.*, **21,** 2662 (1972).

85. G. D. Gray, *Transplant. Proc.*, **5,** 1203 (1973).

86. G. D. Gray, F. R. Nichol, M. M. Mickelson, G. W. Camiener, D. T. Gish, R. C. Kelly, W. J. Wechter, T. E. Moxley, and G. L. Neil, *Biochem. Pharmacol.*, **21,** 465 (1972).

87. G. H. Heppner and P. Calabresi, *J. Nat. Cancer Inst.*, **48,** 1161 (1972).

88. J. R. Bertino, B. L. Hillcoat, and D. G. Johns, *Fed. Proc.*, **26,** 893 (1967).

89. L. Jaenicke, *Angew. Chem.*, **73,** 449 (1961).

90. D. R. Seeger, D. B. Cosulich, J. M. Smith, Jr., and M. E. Hultquist, *J. Am. Chem. Soc.*, **71,** 1753 (1949).

91. G. H. Hitchings and G. B. Elion, *Pharmacol. Rev.*, **15,** 365 (1963).

92. R. L. Black, W. M. O'Brien, E. J. Van Scott, R. Auerbach, A. Z. Eisen, and J. J. Bunim. *J. Am. Med. Assoc.*, **189,** 743 (1964).

93. H. H. Roenigk, H. J. Maibach, and G. D. Weinstein, *Arch. Dermatol.*, **105,** 363 (1972).

94. M. C. Berenbaum, *Lancet*, **2,** 1363 (1964).

95. M. C. Berenbaum and I. N. Brown, *Immunology*, **8,** 251 (1965).

96. E. M. Hersh, *Transplantation*, **12,** 368 (1971).

97. M. D. Prager and J. M. Mehta, *Transplant. Proc.*, **5,** 1171 (1973).

98. K. Altman and M. S. Tobin, *Proc. Soc. Exp. Biol. Med.*, **118,** 554 (1965).

99. K. F. Hübner and N. Gengozian, *Proc. Soc. Exp. Biol. Med.*, **118,** 561 (1965).

100. M. S. Tobin and K. Altman, *Proc. Soc. Exp. Biol. Med.*, **115,** 225 (1964).

101. O. J. Mellbye, *Scand. J. Rheumatol.* **4,** 115 (1975).

102. S. P. Liyanage and H. L. F. Currey, *Ann. Rheum. Dis.*, **31,** 521 (1972).

103. J. Zuckner, R. H. Ramsey, R. W. Dorner, and G. E. Gantner, *Arthritis Rheum.*, **13,** 131 (1970).

104. K. Miehlke, J. Kohlhardt, B. Wirth, and U. Kafaenik, *Ther. Gegenw.*, **109,** 1714 (1970).

105. Multicentre Trial Group, *Lancet*, **1,** 275 (1973).

106. H. Berry, S. P. Liyanage, R. A. Durance, C. G. Barnes, L. A. Berger, and S. Evans, *Brit. Med. J.*, **1,** 1052 (1976).

107. K. Schumacher, *Internist*, **16,** 460 (1975).

108. B. J. Sweetman, M. M. Vestling, S. T. Ticaric, P. L. Kelly, L. Field, P. Merryman, and I. A. Jaffe, *J. Med. Chem.*, **14,** 868 (1971).

109. E. Arrigoni-Martelli, E. Bramm, E. C. Huskisson, D. A. Willoughby, and P. A. Dieppe, *Agents Actions*, **6,** 613 (1976).

110. P. Zeller, H. Gutmann, B. Hegeolus, A. Kaiser, A. Langemann, and M. Müller, *Experientia*, **19,** 129 (1963).

111. W. Bollag, *Experientia*, **19,** 304 (1963).

112. P. B. Stewart and V. Cohen, *Science*, **164,** 1082 (1969).
113. G. J. Possanza and P. B. Stewart, *Clin. Exp. Immunol.*, **6,** 291 (1970).
114. E. Grunberg and H. N. Prince, *Chemotherapy*, **14,** 65 (1969).
115. G. L. Floersheim, *Transplantation*, **15,** 195 (1973).
116. M. Baggiolini, B. Dewald, and H. Aebi, *Biochem. Pharmacol.*, **18,** 2187 (1969).
117. H. Brockmann, *Angew. Chem.*, **72,** 939 (1960).
118. M. Fishman, J. J. van Rood, and F. L. Adler, in *Molecular and Cellular Basis of Antibody Formation*, J. Sterzl et al. Eds., Acadmic Press, New York, 1965, p. 491.
119. M. J. Weiss, G. S. Redin, G. R. Allen, Jr., A. C. Dornbush, H. L. Lindsay, J. F. Poletto, W. A. Remers, R. H. Roth, and A. E. Sloboda, *J. Med. Chem.*, **11,** 742 (1968).
120. V. N. Iyer and W. Szybalski, *Proc. Nat. Acad. Sci., US*, **50,** 355 (1963).
121. L. H. Manheimer and J. Vital, *Cancer*, **19,** 207 (1966).
122. E. M. Lemmel and R. A. Good, *Int. Arch. Allergy Appl. Immunol.*, **36,** 554 (1969).
123. K. Nouza and M. Nemec, *Fol. Biol.*, **19,** 144 (1973).
124. A. S. Weisberger and T. M. Daniel, *Proc. Soc. Exp. Biol. Med.*, **131,** 570 (1969).
125. K. H. Svec, A. S. Weisberger, R. S. Post, and G. B. Naff, *J. Lab. Clin. Med.*, **72,** 1023 (1968).
126. R. H. Blum and S. K. Karter, *Ann. Intern. Med.*, **80,** 249 (1974).
127. A. Vecchi, A. Mantovani, A. Tagliabue, and F. Spreafico, *Cancer Res.*, **36,** 1222 (1976).
128. J. S. Ingraham and A. Bussard, *J. Exp. Med.*, **119,** 667 (1964).
129. D. Fumarola, *Pharmacology*, **2,** 107 (1970).
130. K. Ootsu, T. Matsumoto, S. Harada, and T. Kishi, *Cancer Chemother. Rep.*, **59,** 919 (1975).
131. L. Bassi, L. Di Beradino, V. Arioli, L. G. Silvestri, and E. L. C. Lignière, *J. Infect. Dis.*, **128,** 736 (1973).
132. G. P. J. Alexander, J. E. Murray, G. J. Dammin, and B. Nolan, *Transplantation*, **1,** 432 (1963).
133. S. R. Kaplan, J. P. Hayslett, and P. Calabresi, *New Engl. J. Med.*, **278,** 239 (1968).
134. M. W. Ghilchik, A. S. Morris, and D. S. Reeves, *Nature*, **227,** 393 (1970).
135. R. Nayak, K. S. Prasat, and M. Sirsi, *Infect. Immun.*, **12,** 943 (1975), from *Chem. Abstr.*, **84,** 69515y (1976).
136. A. C. Aisenberg, *Nature*, **200,** 484 (1963).
137. B. Festy, J. Poisson, and C. Paoletty, *FEBS Lett.*, **17,** 321 (1971).
138. J. LeMen, M. Hayat, G. Mathé, J. C. Guillon, E. Chenu, M. Humblot, and Y. Masson, *Rev. Eu. Etud. Clin. Biol.*, **15,** 534 (1970).
139. J. J. Percy and A. E. Pierce, *Immunology*, **21,** 273 (1971).
140. H. H. Freedman, A. E. Fox, J. Shavel, Jr., and G. C. Morrison, *Proc. Soc. Exp. Biol. Med.*, **139,** 909 (1972).
141. M. C. Crew, E. S. Vesell, G. T. Passananti, R. L. Gala, and F. J. Di Carlo, *Clin. Pharmacol. Ther.*, **14,** 1013 (1973).
142. F. J. Di Carlo, M. C. Crew, L. J. Haynes, and R. L. Gala, *Xenobiotica*, **2,** 159 (1972), from *Chem. Abstr.*, **77,** 109249d (1972).
143. M. C. Crew, M. D. Melgar, L. J. Haynes, R. L. Gala, and F. J. Di Carlo, *Xenobiotica*, **2,** 431 (1972), from *Chem. Abstr.*, **78,** 119056y (1973).
144. A. E. Fox, D. L. Gawlak, D. L. Ballantyne, Jr., and H. H. Freedman, *Transplantation*, **15,** 389 (1973).
145. M. Tan, T. Nishihira, H. Tsutsumi, M. Kasai, M. Sato, and T. Kato, *Igaku No Ayumi*, **90,** 30 (1974), from *Chem., Abstr.*, **81,** 163353d (1974).
146. R. N. Taub, *Progr. Allergy*, **14,** 208 (1970).
147. E. M. Lance, *Clin. Exp. Immunol.* **6,** 789 (1970).
148. A. G. R. Sheil, G. E. Kelly, B. G. Storey, J. May, S. Kalowski, D. Mears, J. H. Rogers, J. R. Johnson, J. Charlesworth, and J. H. Stewart, *Lancet*, **1,** 359 (1971).
149. R. C. Millonig, B. J. Amrein, J. Kirschbaum, and S. M. Hess, *J. Med. Chem.*, **17,** 772 (1974).
150. Z. Eyal, W. J. Warwick, C. H. Mayo, and R. C. Lillehei, *Science*, **148,** 1468 (1965).
151. J. P. Gusdon, V. L. Moore, Q. N. Myrvik, and P. A. Holyfield, *J. Immunol.*, **108,** 1340 (1972).
152. L. V. Devoino, L. S. Korovina, and R. Y. Ilyutchenok, *Eur. J. Pharmacol.*, **4,** 441 (1968).
153. R. S. Farr, J. S. Samuelson, and P. B. Stewart, *J. Immunol.*, **94,** 682 (1965).
154. M. J. Waring, *Nature*, **219,** 1320 (1968).
155. B. C. Baguley, E. M. Falkenhaug, J. M. Rastrick, and M. Marbrook, *Eur. J. Cancer*, **10,** 169 (1974).
156. F. K. Hess and P. B. Stewart, *J. Med. Chem.*, **18,** 320 (1975).
157. M. Ellenrieder, E. Frankus, and D. Krüpe, *Klin. Wochenschr*; **45,** 1159 (1967).
158. K. Hellmann, D. I. Duke, and D. F. Tucker, *Brit. Med. J.*, **2,** 687 (1965).
159. J. K. Luce, W. G. Thurman, B. L. Issacs, and R.

W. Talley, *Cancer Chemother, Rep.*, **54,** 119 (1970).

160. A. Vecchi, M. C. Fioretti, A. Mantovani, A. Barzi, and F. Spreafico, *Transplantation*, **22,** 619 (1976).
161. P. B. Stewart, G. J. Possanza, and F. K. Hess, *J. Immunol.*, **110,** 1180 (1973).
162. C. J. Paget, K. Kisner, R. L. Stone, and D. C. DeLong, *J. Med. Chem.*, **12,** 1010 (1969).
163. C. J. Paget, K. Kisner, R. L. Stone, and D. C. DeLong, *J. Med. Chem.*, **12,** 1016 (1969).
164. R. L. Stone, R. N. Wolfe, C. G. Culbertson, and C. J. Paget, *Fed. Proc.*, **35,** 333 (1976).
165. M. A. Mandel, A. A. F. Mahmoud, and K. S. Warren, *Plast. Reconstr. Surg.*, **55,** 76 (1975).
166. A. A. F. Mahmoud, M. A. Mandel, K. S. Warren, and L. T. Webster, Jr., *J. Immunol.*, **114,** 279 (1975).
167. H. N. Christensen and J. C. Jones, *J. biol. Chem.*, **237,** 1203 (1962).
168. M. E. Rosenthale and M. I. Gluckman, *Experientia*, **24,** 1229 (1968).
169. W. A. Atchley and N. V. Bhagavan, *Science*, **138,** 528 (1962).
170. R. Wüthrich, H. P. Rieder, and G. Ritzel, *Experientia*, **19,** 421 (1963).
171. M. F. LaVia, *Proc. Soc. Exp. biol. Med.*, **114,** 133 (1963).
172. J. C. Occhino, A. H. Glasgow, L. R. Cooperbrand, J. A. Mannick, and Karl Schmid, *J. Immunol.*, **110,** 685 (1973).
173. J. C. Houck, A. M. Attallah, and J. R. Lilly, *Nature*, **245,** 149 (1973).
174. H. Markowitz, D. A. Person, G. L. Gitnick, and R. E. Ritts, Jr., *Science*, **163,** 476 (1969).
175. A. K. Delitheos and G. B. West, *Int. Arch. Allergy Appl. Immunol.*, **50,** 282 (1976).
176. R. Rüegger, M. Kuhn, H. Lichti, H. R. Loosli, R. Huguenin, C. Quiquerez, and A. von Wartburg, *Helv. Chim. Acta*, **59,** 1075 (1976).
177. J. F. Borel, C. Feurer, H. V. Gubler, and H. Stähelin, *Agents Actions*, **6,** 468 (1976).
178. *International Symposium on Adjuvants of Immunity*, R. H. Regamey et al., Eds., Karger, Basel, 1967.
179. *Immunopotentiation* (Ciba Foundation Symposium 18), G. E. W. Wolstenholme and J. Knight, Eds., Elsevier–Excerpta Medica–North Holland, Amsterdam, 1973.
180. J. Freund, J. Casals, and E. P. Hosmer, *Proc. Soc. Exp. Biol. Med.*, **37,** 509 (1937).
181. P. A. Lewis and D. Loomis, *J. Exp. Med.*, **40,** 503 1924).
182. P. Jollès, *Experientia*, **32,** 677 (1976).
183. R. G. White, L. Bernstock, R. G. S. Johns, and E. Lederer, *Immunology*, **1,** 54 (1958).
184. R. G. White, P. Jollès, D. Samour, and E. Lederer, *Immunology*, **7,** 158 (1964).
185. L. Chedid, M. Parant, F. Parant, R. H. Gustafson, and F. M. Berger, *Proc. Nat. Acad. Sci., US*, **69,** 855 (1972).
186. D. Migliore-Samour and P. Jollès, *FEBS Lett.*, **35,** 317 (1973).
187. F. Ellouz, A. Adam, R. Ciorbaru, and E. Lederer, *Biochem. Biophys. Res. Commun.*, **59,** 1317 (1974).
188. J. Andersson, O. Sjörberg, and G. Möller, *Transplant. Rev.*, **11,** 131 (1972).
189. G. Janossy and M. F. Greaves, *Clin. Exp. Immunol.*, **9,** 483 (1971).
190. M. F. Greaves, S. Bauminger, and G. Janossy, *Clin. Exp. Immunol.*, **10,** 537 (1972).
191. M. J. Waxdal and T. Y. Basham, *Nature* (London), **251,** 163 (1974).
192. W. Braun and M. Nakano, *Science*, **157,** 819 (1967).
193. W. Turner, S. P. Chan, and M. A. Chirigos, *Proc. Soc. Exp. Biol. Med.*, **133,** 334 (1970).
194. A. G. Johnson, *J. Reticuloendothel. Soc.*, **14,** 441 (1973).
195. T. Diamantstein, G. Odenwald, and D. Odenwald, *Experientia*, **27,** 953 (1971).
196. T. Diamantstein, C. Stork, and R. Malchus, *Experientia*, **29,** 214 (1973).
197. W. Braun, W. Regelson, Y. Yajima, and M. Ishizuka, *Proc. Soc. Exp. Biol. Med.*, **133,** 171 (1970).
198. T. Diamantstein, *Immunology*, **24,** 771 (1973).
199. H. Megel, A. Raychaudhuri, S. Goldstein, C. R. Kinsolving, I. Shemano, and J. G. Michael, *Proc. Soc. Exp. Biol. Med.*, **145,** 513 (1974).
200. G. Renoux and M. Renoux, *C.R. Acad. Sci., Paris, Ser. D*, **272,** 349 (1971).
201. A. Mantovani and F. Spreafico, *Eur. J. Cancer*, **11,** 537 (1975).
202. F. Spreafico, A. Vecchi, A. Mantovani, A. Poggi, G. Franchi, A. Anaclerio, and S. Garattini, *Eur. J. Cancer*, **11,** 555 (1975).
203. G. Renoux and M. Renoux, *C.R. Acad. Sci., Paris, Ser. D*, **274,** 3320 (1972).
204. G. Renoux, M. Renoux, M. N. Teller, S. McMahon, and J. M. Guillaumin, *Clin. Exp. Immunol.*, **25,** 288 (1976).
205. H. Verhaegen, J. De Cree, W. De Cock, and F. Verbruggen, *Clin. Exp. Immunol.*, **27,** 313 (1977).

206. J. Symoens and J. Brugmans, *Brit. Med. J.*, **4,** 592 (1974).

207. A. Kint and L. Verlinden, *New Engl. J. Med.*, **291,** 308 (1974).

208. H. Ippen and S. A. Qadripur, Deut. Med. *Wochemschr.*, **100,** 1710 (1975).

209. M. van Eygen, P. Y. Znamensky, E. Heck, and I. Raymaekers, *Lancet*, **1,** 382 (1976).

210. B. L. Gordon and J. P. Keenan, *Ann. Allergy*, **35,** 343 (1975).

211. E. C. Huskisson, J. Scott, H. W. Balme, P. A. Dieppe, J. Trapnell, and D. A. Willoughby, *Lancet*, **1,** 393 (1976).

212. U. Trabert, M. Rosenthal, and W. Müller, *Schweiz, Med. Wochenschr.*, **106,** 1293 (1976).

213. M. Jurin and I. F. Tannock, *Immunology*, **23,** 283 (1972).

214. G. L. Floersheim and W. Bollag, *Transplantation*, **14,** 564 (1972).

215. P. A. Janssen, in Progress in Drug Research; Vol. 20, E. Jucker, Ed., Birkhäuser-Verlag, Basel, 1976, p. 347.

216. E. Ullmann, *Wien, Klin. Wochenschr.*, **15,** 281 (1902).

217. A. Carrel and C. C. Guthrie, *Am. Med.*, **10,** 1101 (1905).

218. E. Holman, *Surg. Gynecol. Obstetr.*, **38,** 100 (1924).

219. N. L. Gerber and A. D. Steinberg, *Drugs*, **11,** 14 (1976); **11,** 90 (1976).

220. I. J. Forbes, *Med. J. Aust.*, **1,** 749 (1973).

221. R. S. Schwartz and J. D. C. Gowans, *Arthritis Rheum.*, **14,** 134 (1971).

CHAPTER TWENTY-SIX

Blood Calcium Regulators

JOSEPH L. NAPOLI

and

HECTOR F. DELUCA

Department of Biochemistry
College of Agricultural and Life Sciences
University of Wisconsin
Madison, Wisconsin 53706, USA

CONTENTS

1 INTRODUCTION

Plasma and extracellular fluid (ECF) concentrations of calcium in higher animals are tightly regulated (1–5). In normal man and in normal animals, serum calcium concentration is quite constant at about 10 mg/100 ml or approximately 2.5 mM (6).

Deviations from normal occur only under certain pathological conditions. This tight regulation of ECF calcium concentration is necessitated by the complex and extensive role calcium plays in life processes. Calcium and phosphate are the major structural components of animal skeleton. Moreover, normal excitation and relaxation of neuromuscular junctions are crucially sensitive to the calcium concentration in ECF. Furthermore, calcium is required for blood clotting, nerve conduction, fertilization, intercellular adhesion, muscle contraction, cell membrane integrity, certain enzymic reactions, and probably other subcellular functions.

The most critical of all calcium functions is at the neuromuscular junction. In the absence of adequate calcium, the neuromuscular junction ceases to function appropriately and instead institutes a condition of incessant excitation, which results in continuous muscle contraction. The resulting state of convulsion is known as tetany. Thus an adequate supply of calcium is imperative to neurotransmission. On the other hand, excessive amounts of calcium are harmful. Neurological damage and soft tissue calcification are consequences of hypercalcemia. Particularly susceptible tissues are kidney tubules, aorta, heart, and dermis. Noteworthy is the role of calcium in the development of atherosclerotic lesions. In light of these considerations, it is understandable that an organism sacrifices all other calcium components, including the skeleton, to maintain the serum calcium concentration at normality. Consequently the central concept in understanding calcium homeostasis is that blood calcium levels have priority over the skeleton, and that blood calcium is tightly and acutely regulated at the expense of the skeleton.

It is instructive to note total flux of calcium into and out of the adult human to illustrate the task of concentrating calcium and regulating serum calcium concentration. Although a 70 kg adult body contains roughly one kilogram of calcium, an average diet delivers only about 500 mg/day. Of this about 40% is absorbed, mainly by the duodenum and the upper jejunum. About 250 mg of calcium is secreted into the gastrointestinal tract per day, of which less than 40% is reabsorbed. The balance of calcium left in the gastrointestinal tract from both sources is excreted. Other avenues of excretion are breast milk and sweat glands. Sweat accounts for a loss of 15 mg/day. Kidneys filter approximately 10 g/day, of which 99% is reabsorbed, leaving only 100 mg excreted in urine. Significantly, the concentration of calcium in freshly filtered urine is only about one-half the concentration found in the ECF. The adult, consequently, has a balanced calcium intake and efflux.

Skeleton contains 99% of body calcium, whereas the remaining 1% is distributed between ECF and soft tissues. The major portion of skeletal calcium is in a stable, crystalline hydroxyapatite structure (7). However there is a small portion (0.5%) on the crystal surface that is exchanged with calcium in ECF. A flux of about 0.5 g/day between bone and ECF results. Bone mineral is entirely membrane encased, hence is not readily accessible to ECF. This barrier is necessary because the ECF level of calcium is 3 times greater than in the fluid surrounding the bone mineral. Without the barrier, living organisms would not be able to maintain the supersaturating calcium concentration in the ECF.

Since the high calcium concentration in the ECF is in sharp contrast to calcium levels in urine, bone fluid, and intestinal contents, it is apparent that physiological pumps must exist in the kidney, bone, and intestine to concentrate calcium in the ECF. It is now known that regulation and concentration of calcium in blood are controlled by an endocrine system consisting of parathyroid hormone (PTH) (8–16), 1,25-dihydroxyvitamin D_3 (1,25-$(OH)_2D_3$), (10–12, 17–26), and to a lesser extent calcitonin

(CT) (9, 13, 15, 16, 27–31). Bone and kidney cellular calcium control mechanisms are managed by the two peptide hormones, parathyroid hormone and calcitonin, and the steroid hormone 1,25-$(OH)_2D_3$. Intestinal calcium control is apparently governed by 1,25-$(OH)_2D_3$ alone.

2 CALCITONIN

2.1 Historical Background

In 1925 Zondrek and Veko observed a 30% decrease in the serum calcium concentration of rabbits dosed with a bovine parathyroid gland extract. Unfortunately their paper was withdrawn after it had been accepted for publication and was not published until 1966 (32). Meanwhile, in 1957, Marnay and Prelot (33) reported that some bovine parathyroid extracts were hypocalcemic in dogs and rabbits. These were probably the first modern indications of a possible humoral hypocalcemic agent in mammals.

The idea remained dormant until renewed interest in the probability of a hypocalcemic factor was aroused by Copp and Cameron in 1961 (34). They demonstrated that commercial parathyroid extracts produced a transitory hypocalcemia in dogs before the appearance of the customary hypercalcemia. The following year Copp and associates (35, 36) provided further evidence for the existence of this newly postulated hypocalcemic hormone. They perfused the isolated thyroid-parathyroid gland complex of dogs intraarterially with blood varying in calcium concentration. It was noted that when the perfusate was low in calcium, the systemic calcium concentration became relatively high. This, of course, was the result of increased parathyroid hormone secretion. Conversely, when the perfusate was high in calcium, there was a significant decrease in the systemic calcium concentration. Most important, the rate of systemic calcium concentration drop was faster during perfusion with high calcium blood than the rate of decrease after thyroparathyroidectomy. Consequently Copp et al. correctly reasoned that a simple inhibition of parathyroid hormone release was not responsible and that the release of a separate hypocalcemic agent, which they called calcitonin, must have been stimulated by high blood calcium concentration. At this time, the parathyroid glands were incorrectly pinpointed as the source of CT (34–37). A year later, the existence of CT was confirmed (38–40).

A discrepancy in the serum calcium levels of rats whose parathyroid tissue was destroyed by two different methods led to the study that first suggested thyroid gland as the source of CT. Rats whose parathyroids were removed by surgery manifested a serum calcium drop to 7.6 mg/100 ml. In contrast, after destruction of the glands by hot wire cautery, the serum calcium value fell to 5.5 mg/100 ml (39). The parathyroid glands of rats are located on a lobe of the thyroid. Because of this, Hirsch et al. (40) reasoned that cautery of the parathyroids must have caused the release of a hypocalcemic substance from the thyroids. Thus they demonstrated that cautery of rat thyroid glands at sites distant from the parathyroids caused release of a powerful hypocalcemic substance. To differentiate it from the substance CT released by the parathyroids, they named it thyrocalcitonin. They further demonstrated the presence of thyrocalcitonin in aqueous extracts of thyroid glands. Additional work proved that thyroid extracts of many mammalian species possessed hypocalcemic properties in the rat (41, 42). Later Talmage et al. (43, 44) resolved the apparent difference between CT and thyrocalcitonin, when they demonstrated that thyroid, not parathyroids, is the source of the hypocalcemic factor. Their work was soon confirmed (45, 46). Currently, either CT or thyrocalcitonin is used to name the hypocalcemic hormone secreted from thyroid.

Subsequent work from many laboratories has shown that mammalian CT is secreted by small groups of interstitial cells embedded throughout the thyroid glands. In some cases, these parafollicular or "C" cells can also be found in thymus or parathyroid tissue. In contrast, in submammalian vertebrates, such as birds, reptiles, amphibians, and fish, CT-secreting "C" cells remain as discrete glands known as the ultimobranchial bodies (29, 31, 47, 48).

2.2 Control of Calcitonin Secretion

Although knowledge about CT has been increasing, the importance of the hormone remains an enigma. It is usually undetectable in unconcentrated human plasma by radioimmunoassays specifically sensitive to human calcitonin (hTC) at concentrations of 50–300 pg/ml (49–51). However within minutes of hypercalcemic challenge, either by direct infusion (52) or by ingestion of calcium (53, 54), the rate of CT secretion increases. As opposed to this, EDTA infusion decreases CT output (52). In both these circumstances CT concentrations are directly proportional to plasma calcium levels. Thus blood calcium levels are commonly accepted as the most important factor in controlling rate of CT secretion (9, 27, 28, 55). Magnesium also can change rate of CT secretion, albeit at high, nonphysiological doses (56).

In addition, physiological changes associated with eating also stimulate CT secretion. The cause is not limited to the rise in blood calcium resulting from increased intestinal calcium absorption, since the digestive hormones gastrin, pentagastrin, pancreazymin, and cholecystokinin, act to augment CT secretion (57, 58). This has been demonstrated under experimental conditions by the measurement of CT levels *in vivo* after injections of digestive hormones. Other factors also have been demonstrated to affect CT secretion *in vivo*. Glucagon, catecholamines, and theophylline (58, 59), as well as dibutyryl cyclic AMP (60), heighten CT release in pigs. The latter results have been interpreted as indications that CT secretion is cyclic-AMP mediated (28, 60).

2.3 Biosynthesis

The biogenesis of CT, the factors affecting its rate of synthesis, and the mechanisms involved in its storage, all remain a mystery. In 1975 Moya and co-workers (61) isolated a pro-CT from incubation of chick ultimobranchial bodies with tritiated amino acids. They were able to purify pro-CT by polyacrylamide gel electrophoresis, and demonstrated a molecular weight of about 13,000, compared to 3500 for CT. The biological activity of pro-CT was shown to be only 9% of calcitonin in the rat assay. Pro-Ct is probably distinct from the CT dimer found in human blood (62), since the former does not dissociate on gel electrophoresis nor on performic acid oxidation (Fig. 26.1).

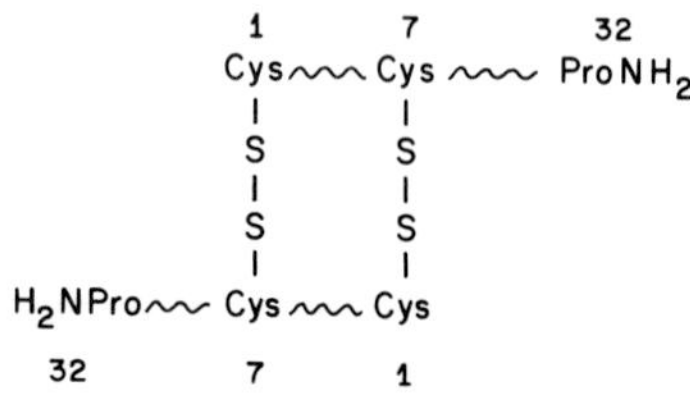

Fig. 26.1 The structure of an antiparallel dimer of CT found in human blood.

Further studies have been hampered because CT-producing cells are dispersed. Furthermore, the rate of CT synthesis is poorly coupled to the rate of its secretion. For instance, the thyroidal concentration of CT in rats is significantly increased by parathyroidectomy-induced hypocalcemia, whereas it is depleted by calcium (59). Moreover, hypocalcemic patients treated with calcium and pentagastrin had increased serum CT levels (63).

2.4 Calcitonin Function

Fortunately, mechanisms of CT-induced hypocalcemia are understood more clearly than is control of CT secretion. It has been well established that CT decreases calcium mobilization from deep bone (64–70). There the hormone binds to receptors (71, 72) and acts through the intermediacy of cyclic-AMP (73). CT increases the membrane potential of osteoclasts, the bone resorbing cells (74). Losses in resorptive activity are accompanied by morphological changes in osteoclasts. The ruffled border area of these cells, which is considered to be the intracellular calcium resorbing system, is reduced by CT (75–77). In all these respects, CT functions in opposition to PTH. The main consequence of CT action, therefore, is to arrest bone resorption, and possibly to augment the rate of new bone formation.

CT also acts on kidney to stimulate increased urinary calcium and phosphate clearance (13, 78–84). In the case of phosphate, CT and PTH behave synergistically; whereas with calcium, the two have antagonistic effects. However, paralleling the situation in bone, CT and PTH act at different receptors in kidney, even though both hormones exert their actions through cyclic-AMP (81, 85, 86). Possibly a further effect of CT on kidney cells is sequestering of calcium in mitochondria. This inhibits cellular calcium efflux and effectively lowers extracellular fluid calcium concentration (87).

Although the movement of water and electrolytes across intestine may also be influenced by CT (88, 89), in comparison to bone and kidney, intestinal CT actions are minor.

The role of digestive hormones as CT secretagogues and the rapid release of CT in response to blood calcium elevations together suggest that the main purpose of CT is to protect higher animals from acute hypercalcemic episodes. Particularly, the control of postprandial hypercalcemia has been proposed as the special duty of CT (53, 90, 91). However effects of CT in the young are much more significant than in mature higher animals. Indeed, CT secretion in adults is virtually undetectable (92). Although postprandial hypercalcemia is prevented in most mammals, such a role has not been demonstrated in man. More pointedly, thyroidectomized patients, supplemented only with thyroid hormone, manifest no detectable abnormalities in calcium and skeletal metabolism. Moreover, individuals with thyroidal medullary carcinoma, who frequently manifest CT levels as much as thousands of times higher than normal, are not hypocalcemic and apparently have normal calcium metabolism (93). Consequently, the importance of CT to adult man must be questioned. Perhaps CT is important only during embryonic development, or perhaps CT is a vestigial hormone.

Nevertheless, a lively interest in CT currently remains. Radioimmunoassays for CT have been developed and are continually undergoing improvement (49–51). They are important to the study of CT *in vivo*, and are sensitive to increased CT output, which occurs in medullary carcinoma of the thyroid. These assays are able to aid in the diagnosis of neoplasia, even when there are no visible signs of a tumor. CT is also undergoing testing in the control of Paget's disease. Because this condition is basically a problem of accelerated bone remodeling, it seems to be tractable to CT treatment. Practically, headway has been made in the suppression of Paget's disease by CT, particularly with salmon calcitonin (sCT) (94–96). Consequently, an understanding of the structure-activity relationship of CT is important as a practical matter, as well as desirable academically.

2.5 Chemistry

As a result of the research just described, CT from ovine (97), porcine (98–102), bovine (103–105), salmon (106–109), eel (110–112), rat (113–116), and human (62, 117, 118) sources has been purified, characterized, and even synthesized in some cases. All these substances were isolated from normal organs except hCT, which was isolated from thyroidal medullary carcinoma because of its exceedingly low concentration in normal tissue. Rat calcitonin (rCT) isolated from medullary carcinoma (114, 116) was identical to rCT from normal glands (113). Presumably, therefore, hCT from medullary carcinoma is the same as hCT from normal thyroid. Figure 26.2 gives the amino acid sequences of nine calcitonins. These hormones naturally fall into three groups because of similarities in sequence, immunological properties, and biological activity. Porcine, ovine, and bovine CT constitute one group. Eel CT and the three salmon isohormones form another; possibly chicken CT can be included in this group on the basis of its biological potency (119). Finally, rat and human CT are similar. Piscine calcitonins are about 30–70 times more active in mammals than hCT. Bovine, ovine, and porcine are 1–2 times as active as hCT (109, 120, 121). With sCT in particular, the increased activity is a reflection of both greater affinity for binding to receptors in bone and kidney, and longer serum half-life (120, 121). For instance, sCT is approximately 5 times longer in duration of action than hCT. Table 26.1 compares the biological potency of several calcitonins.

Species differences in amino acid sequences of CT reflect conservation of chemical properties at the *N*-terminus and *C*-terminus of the molecule; whereas differences in the middle portion of the polypeptide are often without regard to chemical similarities. All contain a disulfide bridge between a pair of cysteine residues at positions 1 and 7. Indeed, the first nine amino acids in all are virtually unchanged, with

	N-Terminus 1	2	3	4	5	6	7	8	9	10	11	12	13	14	15	16
Human	H_2N–Cys	Gly	Asn	Leu	Ser	Thr	Cys	Met	Leu	Gly	Thr	Thy	Thr	Gln	Asp	Phe
Rat																Leu
Salmon$_3$		Ser									Lys	Leu	Ser			Leu
Salmon$_2$		Ser						Val			Lys	Leu	Ser			Leu
Salmon$_1$		Ser						Val			Lys	Leu	Ser			Leu
Eel		Ser						Val			Lys	Leu	Ser			Leu
Bovine		Ser						Val		Ser	Ala		Trp	Lys		Leu
Porcine		Ser						Val		Ser	Ala		Trp	Arg	Asn	Leu
Ovine		Ser						Val		Ser	Ala		Trp	Lys		Leu

	17	18	19	20	21	22	23	24	25	26	27	28	29	30	31	C-Terminus 32
Human	Asn	Lys	Phe	His	Thr	Phe	Pro	Gln	Thr	Ala	Ile	Gly	Val	Gly	Ala	Pro–$CONH_2$
Rat										Ser						
Salmon$_3$	His		Leu	Gln				Arg		Asn	Thr		Ala		Val	
Salmon$_2$	His		Leu	Gln				Arg		Asn	Thr		Ala		Val	
Salmon$_1$	His		Leu	Gln		Tyr		Arg		Asn	Thr		Ser		Thr	
Eel	His	Lys	Leu	Gln	Thr	Tyr	Pro	Arg	Thr	Asp	Val		Ala	Gly	Thr	
Bovine		Asn	Tyr		Arg		Ser	Gly	Met	Gly	Phe		Pro	Glu	Thr	
Porcine		Asn			Arg		Ser	Gly	Met	Gly	Phe		Pro	Glu	Thr	
Ovine		Asn	Tyr		Arg	Tyr	Ser	Gly	Met	Gly	Phe		Pro	Glu	Thr	

Fig. 26.2 A comparison of the CT amino acid sequence of different species. Hormones are listed in order of their similarity to human CT. Blanks represent positions identical to human CT.

Table 26.1 Relative Activities of Calcitonins from Different Species

Calcitonin	MRC Units/ Microgram (Reference)	Relative Activity[a]
$Salmon_1$	2300–3200 (109)	30–46
	3500 (108)	50
	5000 (107)	70
$Salmon_2$	2400 (109)	34
$Salmon_3$	— (127)	10–20
Eel	3500–5000 (112)	50–70
Porcine	120 (109)	2
Human	70 (109)	1
Ovine	60 (109)	1
Bovine	50 (109)	1

[a] Activity is determined by measuring inorganic calcium (atomic absorption) in rat plasma after dosing with individual compounds (122).

the exception of glycine at position 2 in rCT and hCT as opposed to serine in the others. The exchange of methionine for valine at position 8 is more apparent than real, since both are nonpolar, hydrophobic amino acids, likely to be found on the interior of a folded polypeptide. The only other amino acids similar throughout are the glycine at position 28 and the terminal prolinamide.

2.6 Structure-Activity Relationships

Among calcitonins of various species, large differences in primary amino acid sequence can be tolerated with no detectable qualitative effects on immunological-biological response. On the other hand, studies with both porcine calcitonin (pCT) (123, 124) and hCT (125) have show that the entire chain of a particular CT must be present for appreciable activity. Figure 26.3 compares biological potencies of sections of the porcine molecule, determined in the rat bioassay (122). Drastic reductions in activity are evident when only fragments of the molecule are available. This rule extends to the elimination of one or two of the terminal amino acids. The compound that ends with prolinamide at position 29, in the cases of pCT and hCT, is as inactive as all other fragments. The pCT and hCT analogs with *C*-terminus threoninamides at positions 31 are only 1–2% as active as the complete hormones. Simple hydrolysis of *C*-terminus prolinamides, in the two normal hormones, decreases activity by at least 97%. Consequently, a prolinamide at the *C*-terminus is necessary for activity but is not sufficient in itself to confer activity. Esterification of the *C*-terminal acid does not restore activity.

The disulfide bridge of calcitonin is necessary to establish the proper conformation for activity, but apparently it does not interact with the receptor itself. An analog of hCT in which the twin cysteines at positions 1 and 7 have been replaced by two methionines is essentially inactive (125). In contrast to this, replacement of the disulfide bridge in eel calcitonin (eCT) with a hydrocarbon bridge (Fig. 26.4) results in an

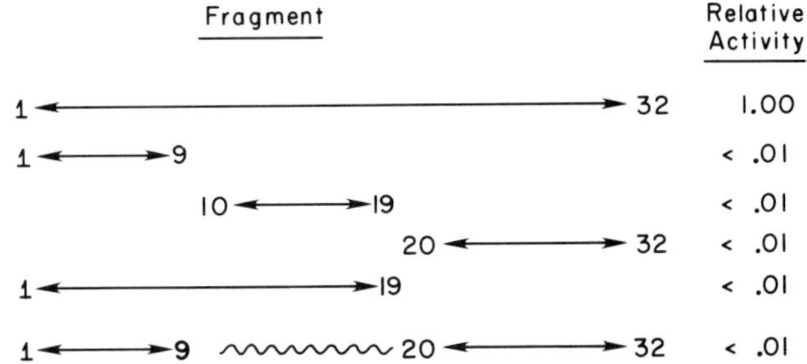

Fig. 26.3 The relative activities of synthetic fragments of porcine CT.

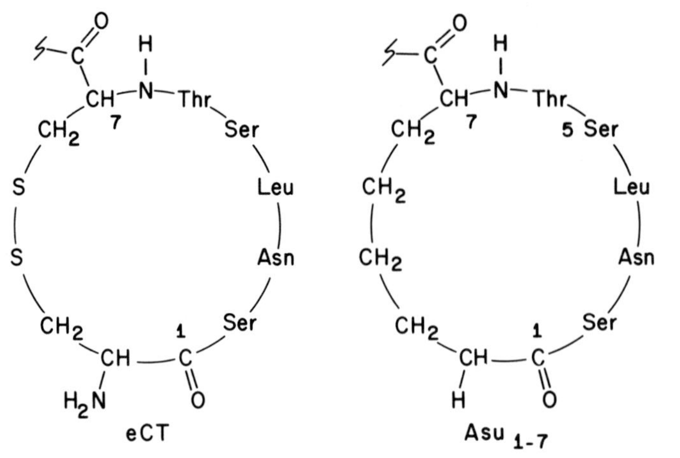

Fig. 26.4 Amino acids 1 to 7 in eCT (left) and an analog (right) in which aminosuberic acid (Asu) substitutes for cysteines 1 and 7 in eCT. The Asu_{1-7} compound, which is a deamino, hydrocarbon-bridged analog, is 80% as active as eCT in the rat bioassay (112).

analog 80% as active as natural eCT (112). Thus electronic and steric characteristics inherent to the sulfur atoms in the disulfide bridge are probably far less important than the conformation enforced by the bridge. Additionally, plasma breakdown of natural calcitonins may result from reduction of the disulfide bridge. This may be inferred from observed breakdown of natural eCT during isolation and purification—a process that does not occur with the hydrocarbon bridged analog.

Advantageous substitutions of amino acids frequently can be made (Table 26.2).

Table 26.2a Amino Acid Substituted Analogs of hCT: Blank Spaces Represent Amino Acids that Do Not Deviate from the Parent Hormone

	1	8	12	16	19	22	29	31	Relative Activity[a]
hCT	Cys	Met	Tyr	Phe	Phe	Phe	Val	Ala	1.0
1	Bmp[b]								1.2
2	Ac-Cys								1.5
3		Val							4–5
4			Leu						4–5
5				Leu					1.0
6					Leu				1.0
7						Tyr			4–5
8	Bmp		Leu						10
9		Val				Tyr			4–5
10							Ser	Thr	5
11							Ala	Val	0.06
12			Leu	Leu	Leu				10
13		Val	Leu	Leu	Leu				10
14			Leu	Leu	Leu	Tyr			15–20

[a] Activity relative to assigned hCT activity of 1.
[b] Bmp = β-mercaptopropionate.

Table 26.2b Amino Acid Substituted Analogs of sCT_2: Blank Spaces Represent Amino Acids that Do Not Deviate from the Parent Hormone

	15	22	29	31	Relative Activity[a]
SCT_2	Asp	Phe	Ala	Val	30
15			Val	Ala	30
16	Glu	Tyr			15
17	Glu	Tyr	Val	Ala	15
18			Ser	Thr	30

[a] Activity relative to assigned sCT_1 activity of 30.

The greater activity of the three salmon isocalcitonins in comparison to hCT led to the synthesis of hCT analogs with sCT amino acids in select locations (125–128). Amino acid residues that remained similar in each of the sCT's, but differed from those in hCT were generally chosen for study. For example, the two most active salmon isohormones, salmon calcitonin$_1$ (sCT_1) and salmon calcitonin$_2$ (sCT_2) have a valine at position 8. In both hCT and the least active salmon isohormone$_3$ (sCT_3), this position is occupied by methionine. As might be expected, substitution of valine for methionine at position 8 in hCT increases activity (analog 3). Similar situations exist further down the chain. In all three sCT's, the aliphatic residue leucine occurs in positions 12, 16, and 19, whereas in hCT these positions are occupied by aromatic amino acids. In only one instance, however—exchange of leucine for tyrosine at position 12 in hCT (analog 4)—does substitution with an sCT amino acid improve the activity of the hCT analog. Substitutions at positions 16 and 19 (analogs 5 and 6) did not alter activity. A single substitution is beneficial in one other known case. Position 22 in sCT_1 is occupied by the polar amino acid tyrosine; but in hCT a phenylalanine occurs. Placing tyrosine at 22 improves activity by a factor of 4–5 (analog 7).

Altering the number 1 cysteine either by deamination (analog 1) or by acetylation (analog 2) improve activity only slightly. However deamination of cysteine 1 with concomitant substitution by leucine at position 12 results in a tenfold increase in potency. Unfortunately dual substitution does not always offer greater improvements. Although analogs 3 and 6 each resulted in a four- to fivefold increase in activity, their two substitutions occurring together (analog 5) gave no further improvement in potency. In contrast, replacement of amino acids 29 and 31 in hCT by those occurring in sCT_1 (analog 10) promoted activity fivefold. Analogous substitution of amino acids 29 and 31 from sCT_2 and sCT_3 in hCT (analog 11) drastically decreased activity.

More than two substitutions in one analog often produce unexpected results. Analog 12, in which leucines have been placed at positions 12, 16, and 19, is more potent than the singly leucine 12 substituted analog 4. This is surprising, since single leucine substitutions at positions 16 or 19 failed to alter activity. There is no further gain from the next analog (number 13), in which valine is substituted at position 8 in addition to the triple replacements by leucine. In contrast, the tyrosine-22 substitution, coupled with three replacements by leucine, does potentiate response.

Similar manipulations were performed with sCT_2 (129). In this case, exchange between valine and analine at positions 29 and 31 to mimic the sequence in hCT (analog 15) causes no loss of potency. Interestingly, substitution of sCT_1's glutamic acid at 15 and tyrosine at 22 for the amino acids found in sCT_2 force a diminution of response (analog 16). This is not corrected by further exchange of the alanine and valine at positions 29 and 31 (analog 17). Replacement of amino acids 29 and 31 with serine and threonine, respectively, as found in sCT_1, was not more advantageous (analog 18). Incidentally, no change in activity is noticed upon oxidation of methionine at position 25 in pCT (130). Contrast this with the result of oxidizing methionine at position 8 in hCT, which causes a precipitous fall in activity (131).

Generally, an analog of increased potency is also longer acting. This direct proportion between activity and biological half-life also exists with the naturally occurring hormones. Apparently the structural features that determine the quality of the hormone-receptor interaction and those that influence biodegradation are linked. It remains to be seen whether this is a consequence of the three-dimensional protein structure or a matter of increased affinity for the receptor on one hand, and decreased affinity for degradative enzymes on the other, or both. Further analogs should help to clarify the structure-function relationship of CT. In particular, compounds in which positions 11, 26, and 27 of hCT are substituted with the appropriate sCT amino acids should be most interesting.

2.7 Summary

Although CT definitely has a hypocalcemic effect in experimental animals, and in man, the question of its importance in the adult remains unanswered. CT is not yet universally accepted as an important facet of the endocrine system, responsible for blood calcium homeostasis in mature higher animals. It may offer therapeutic benefits in Paget's disease, but probably will not aid in the treatment of osteoporosis.

3 PARATHYROID HORMONE

3.1 Historical Background

The significance of parathyroid glands in calcium metabolism was first demonstrated by MacCallum and Voegtlin (132) in 1909. They related tetany to parathyroid glands and blood calcium concentrations. Two years later, Greenwald (133) discovered a second physiological role of the glands when he noticed that parathyroidectomized dogs had decreased urinary phosphate clearance. Unfortunately, in the following years only sporadic success was achieved in obtaining biologically active extracts of the glands, and at one point the physiological role of parathyroids in calcium and phosphate metabolism was questioned. In 1925, however, Collip (134) obtained an extract of PTH from bovine parathyroid glands with hot hydrochloric acid. He demonstrated that crude hormone prevented or controlled tetany in parathyroidectomized dogs and also regulated blood calcium concentration. Patt and Luckhardt (135), 17 years after Collip's experiment, showed that PTH secretion is inversely dependent on the blood calcium concentration. Subsequently research in this area turned toward obtaining purified hormone. Finally, in 1959, the isolation of material several thousand times more potent than crude gland powders was reported by two laboratories (136, 137). Both groups had replaced hot hydrochloric acid as extractant. This precluded peptide hydrolysis, which was the cause of the highly variable results obtained by previous investigators. Second, countercurrent distribution was used to further purify the extract. Additional gains were made in the isolation and purification of PTH. Chromatography of crude extracts by gel filtration (138–140) and ion exchange resins (141) allowed purification of increasingly greater amounts. Undoubtedly, advances in understanding PTH metabolism and actions were catalyzed by increased availability of purified PTH in reasonable quantities. Current interest in this vital hormone focuses on its biosynthesis and metabolism, in addition to exact mechanisms by which it instills phosphaturia and helps increase plasma calcium concentration.

3.2 Control of PTH Secretion

Calcium is the single most important governor of PTH secretion known (135, 142–148). Variations in blood calcium concentrations have a rapid, inverse effect on the rate of PTH secretion. Phosphate levels also affect PTH secretion, but only indirectly by affecting ECF calcium concentration (144). On the other hand, magnesium can apparently alter PTH secretion directly, but only at levels several times greater than normally occur in ECF (145–150). On a molar basis, magnesium is 2–3 times less effective than calcium in controlling hormone secretion (151, 152). Calcium concentration is the primary determinate of PTH blood levels under physiological conditions.

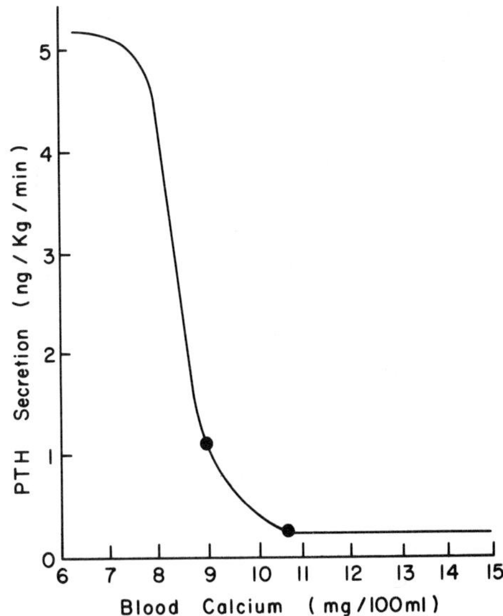

Fig. 26.5 The relationship between blood calcium concentration and PTH secretion *in vivo*. The portion of the curve between the large dots represents physiological range of blood calcium concentration and normal PTH secretion rate. After Ref. 154.

The relationship between PTH secretion and blood calcium levels was once considered to be proportional over a wide calcium concentration range (144, 145). Recently a more sophisticated picture emerged (8, 153, 154). Anesthetized calves were challenged by intrajugular infusions of either calcium chloride or disodium EDTA. Their parathyroid gland effluent blood was analyzed for changes in hormone secretory rate. A near-linear relationship between the rate of PTH secretion and blood calcium concentration was found only in the normal physiological concentration range of 9.5–10.5 mg of calcium per 100 ml of plasma (Fig. 26.5). Above 10.5 mg/100 ml, PTH secretion declined to a basal rate of about 0.3 ng/(kg)(min) despite increases in calcium concentration to 15 mg/100 ml. Between 9.5 and about 8 mg/100 ml, there was a magnified increase in PTH secretory rate in response to small decreases in blood calcium concentration. The disproportionate response to falling blood calcium levels gradually subsided, so that below 7 mg/100 ml, PTH secretion rate stabilized to roughly 5 ng/(kg)(min). Measured rates of PTH secretion, in the limited range of physiological blood calcium concentration, contrast sharply with exaggerated rates during hypocalcemic stress. However an amplified response to pressure is appropriate in a homeostatic system charged with regulating concentrations of a crucial hormone.

Experimentally induced hypocalcemia stimulates PTH secretion within minutes, indicating a direct calcium interaction with parathyroid glands (155). Accordingly, evidence suggests that the membrane-bound enzyme adenylate cyclase mediates calcium modulation of PTH secretion. A calcium-sensitive adenylate cyclase has been found in dog parathyroids (156); and release of cyclic-AMP, the product of adenylate cyclase, can be correlated with PTH secretion at several calcium concentrations *in vitro*. Furthermore, either theophylline or dibutyryl–cyclic AMP causes stimulation of PTH secretion *in vitro*, regardless of calcium concentration (157). Therefore calcium interaction with parathyroid gland membranes, resulting in stimulation of cyclic-AMP synthesis, represents a plausible model for regulation of PTH release by fluctuating blood calcium concentration.

The rapid increases in PTH secretion caused by hypocalcemia invite one other conclusion; namely, that in response to decreasing ECF calcium concentrations, stores of preformed PTH are secreted. Initially at least, parathyroid glands probably do not react to hypocalcemia by accelerating hormone synthesis (8). Bovine parathyroid glands contain about 200 μg of preformed PTH, enough to maintain a basal secretion rate for 7 hr. Even a fivefold increase in secretion brought on by moderate hypocalcemia could be tolerated for 1.5 hr by utilizing pools of preformed PTH. Thus the judgment that low calcium concentrations directly affect parathyroid glands by inducing release of preformed PTH is apparently sustained.

3.3 PTH Function

Once released, PTH acts directly on kidney and bone to raise the concentration of calcium in ECF. In kidney, PTH binds to receptors on cell membranes and causes a rise in cellular cyclic-AMP concentrations (158–160). One result is increased renal tubular reabsorption of calcium (160–162). All but 1–2% of the calcium filtered is routinely reabsorbed, without PTH, however (1–5). Although total amount of calcium reclaimed by this PTH action is relatively small in a brief period, it is significant nonetheless.

Besides its effect on calcium, PTH decreases reabsorption of phosphate (85, 160, 163, 164) by the proximal convoluted renal tubule (165). A relationship between PTH and renal tubular hydrogen ion concentration has long been known (166–169). Recent clarification of this intereaction has shown that PTH may increase phosphate clearance by raising the kidney intraluminal pH (170). Since divalent phosphate is less readily reabsorbed than monovalent phosphate, changes in the divalent/monovalent ratio caused by pH changes could account for PTH effects on renal phosphate clearance. PTH has another effect in kidney; it stimulates production of 1,25-$(OH)_2D_3$, a hormone important to intestine, bone, and kidney calcium metabolism. This extremely important function of PTH is discussed more thoroughly in the vitamin D section.

In bone, PTH action may also be mediated through cyclic-AMP. Several groups have shown that cyclic-AMP levels are greater in bone after PTH stimulation (171–173). Likewise, dibutyryl cyclic-AMP mimics some of the actions of PTH in bone (174–178). But recently two different investigations found no increase in cyclic-AMP levels in tissue-cultured calvaria after adding PTH to the media, although both experiments demonstrated an increased release of calcium (179, 180). This may result from failure to detect small increases in cyclic-AMP concentration; or it may indicate that PTH works through two second messengers—cyclic-AMP and perhaps calcium. Nevertheless, PTH has two distinct functions in bone. It controls bone remodeling, and it promotes entry of calcium into ECF from membrane-encased bone compartmental fluid (BCF). These two actions are not necessarily related, especially in acute blood calcium regulation and the precise role of cyclic-AMP in each is obscure.

The role of PTH in bone remodeling is well documented (181–184). PTH increases activation of macrophages to osteoclasts. Significant increases in the number of bone macrophages are noted after dosage of test animals with PTH or after stimulation of endogenous PTH secretion (184–186). Microradiography and scanning electron microscopy have shown that change occurs in extent, not in character of resorbing surfaces (184). Besides this, PTH activates resting osteoclasts (185). Thus PTH-promoted bone resorption occurs because new osteoclasts are generated and existing cells are activated. It has been estimated that each mode of action accounts for 50% of new osteoclastic activity (184, 187). An immediate result of augmented osteoclastic activity is increased calcium concentration in the bone compartmental fluid (BCF). This effect is transient, and in the short-term probably is not significant in blood calcium regulation.

Concomitant with an increase in the number of osteoclasts, is an increase in the number of osteoblasts, the bone forming cells. But whereas PTH activates resting osteoclasts, it decreases the rate of bone formation by osteoblasts (188). Consequently, at low levels of PTH a balance between bone resorption and bone formation results; that is, bone remodeling occurs. At higher levels of PTH, the balance is upset, and exaggerated osteoclastic activity overshadows repressed osteoblastic activity. Serious losses of bone tissue are minifested when the imbalance is not corrected (189).

Osteoclastic cell proliferation requires about 18 hr (190, 191) and even then, the accompanying rise in BCF calcium is soon depleted by osteoblastic action. Minute-to-minute ECF calcium needs, which are to be satisfied by BCF calcium, must therefore be independent of bone remodeling.

A model of PTH action on bone in correcting short-term ECF calcium losses has been advocated by Talmage (192). In this formalization (Fig. 26.6), PTH initially acts by switching on a transcellular pumping mechanism in surface osteoblasts. This action is coupled with a PTH-directed increase of calcium permeability into the same cells. Together these mechanisms work to pump calcium against a gradient into blood from BCF. The model, consequently, differentiates between PTH assisted bone remodeling on one hand, and the contribution of PTH to acute blood calcium homeostasis on the other hand. The fact that initial calcium release after PTH administration occurs in a section of

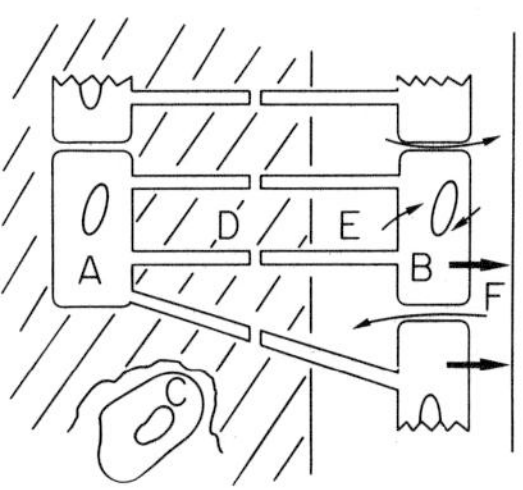

Fig. 26.6 Simplified model of PTH action on bone. Small arrows indicate calcium diffusion between BCF and blood. Large arrows indicate PTH-mediated transport of calcium from BCF into blood: *A*, osteoblast; *B*, surface osteoblast; *C*, osteocyte; *D*, deep bone; *E*, BCF; *F*, blood. After Ref. 184.

bone that is morphologically distinct from the osteoclast proliferation section, supports at least part of the theory (193). More support is provided by the realization that the rapid increase of ECF calcium concentration after PTH stimulation is undisturbed, even when osteoclast proliferation is experimentally impaired by radiation (194). Furthermore, outward calcium flux has actually been pinpointed in the surface osteoblasts (192). Additionally, the existence of an active transport mechanism has been supported by the discovery of just such a mechanism in chick calvaria (195).

Experiments using ^{45}Ca provide further support for the model. Rats dosed with PTH after administration of ^{45}Ca for 1–2 weeks, demonstrated no initial change in specific activity of blood calcium, indicating that the calcium source had the same specific activity as blood calcium (196). This source would be BCF, not deep bone. Calcium from the latter arises from osteoclastic resorption. However after prolonged dosage with PTH, blood calcium specific activity began to rise, indicating that ^{45}Ca incorporated within deep bone was undergoing resorption. In Japanese quail coadministration of PTH and ^{45}Ca results in higher blood ^{45}Ca levels than does ^{45}Ca dosage alone (197). This further indicates that PTH causes a rapid recycling of calcium from surface osteoblasts. In case of no PTH-stimulated active transport, calcium diffuses past surface osteoblasts into BCF. The equilibrium between BCF and blood results in a lowered blood calcium specific activity.

Consequently, in acute control of blood calcium concentration, PTH has two well-documented target tissues. It acts on kidney to augment calcium reabsorption, a function that may be its most important direct action. Also in kidney, it causes increased urinary phosphate excretion. Finally, it controls the renal synthesis of $1,25(OH)_2D_3$, the only known hormonal mediator of intestinal calcium absorption. The second target tissue, bone, is affected by PTH in two ways. In an action dependent on $1,25\text{-}(OH)_2D_3$, PTH promotes increased pumping of calcium from BCF to blood, to aid in the acute control of blood calcium concentration. Second, PTH mediates bone remodeling, which affects blood calcium levels chronically.

3.4 Chemistry

Parathyroid hormones have been isolated from bovine (198), porcine (199), and human (200, 201) sources. All are single-chain polypeptides, 84 amino acids long, devoid of cysteine. There are three bovine isohormones, but there is no evidence of more than one porcine hormone. Complete amino acid sequences of the major form of bovine PTH (bPTH) (202, 203), and of porcine PTH (pPTH) (204) have been determined. The entire amino acid sequence of hPTH is unknown. Only residues 1–34 (205–207) and 44–68 (208) have been identified. In the case of hPTH, there is a disagreement between Niall et al. (206) and Brewer et al. (205) about amino acid composition in three positions. The former investigators found that like pPTH and bPTH, hPTH contains glutamic acid, leucine, and aspartic acid at positions 22, 28, and 30, respectively. In contrast, Brewer and co-workers report that these positions are occupied by glutamine, lysine, and leucine, respectively. Reinvestigations by both groups (209, 210) did not resolve the discrepancies, since the results of each team confirmed its own earlier findings. Immunological studies (211) and biological evaluation (212) of synthetic analogs of

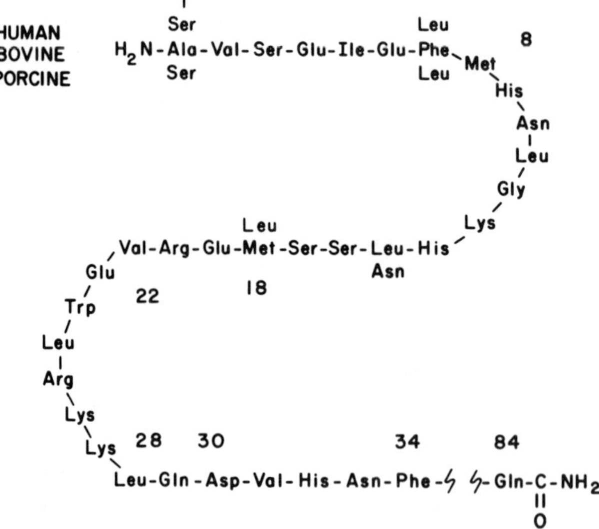

Fig. 26.7 A comparison of the amino acid sequences of bovine, human, and porcine PTH. Residues 22, 28, and 30 in hPTH are disputed. Niall et al. (206) report that hPTH is like bPTH and pPTH in these positions, whereas Brewer et al. (205) report positions 22, 28, and 30 in hPTH to be occupied by glutamine, lysine, and leucine, respectively.

both sequences are inconclusive. It is not clear why the differences exist; but they do not appear to result from each group's isolation of different isohormones, since neither laboratory can demonstrate heterogeneity in its hPTH samples. A systematic error in either lab may be involved.

Figure 26.7 diagrams the sequences of the biologically important 34 *N*-terminal amino acids of bovine, porcine, and human PTH. On the whole, disregarding the disputed residues, there is close interspecific conservation of amino acids in corresponding positions. Most differences, with the exception of the serine-alanine contrast at position 1, involve exchanges of amino acids that are similar in polarity.

3.5 Biosynthesis

The chemistry of PTH has not been investigated quite as comprehensively as that of CT. Possibly the larger structure of PTH has complicated examination. More likely, however, was the realization that unlike mammalian CT, PTH is synthesized in discrete, localized tissue, rendering its intracellular biochemistry accessible to thorough probing. As a result, much research has been directed toward understanding and relating biosynthesis and metabolism of PTH to its mechanism of action.

Despite these efforts, it was recognized only recently that PTH is not the initial product of translation, but rather arises from two successive proteolytic cleavages of a larger polypeptide (8, 213). The direct ribosomal product, designated Pre-proPTH, was obtained by translation of bovine (214, 215) and human (216) parathyroid mRNA fractions in heterologous cell-free systems derived from wheat germ (214, 216) and Krebs II ascites tumor cells (215). Related work with the mRNA itself supports the view that Pre-proPTH is a faithful product of an intact mRNA (217, 218). Finally, the detection of Pre-proPTH in intact bPTH gland cells provided further evidence that Pre-proPTH is a true biosynthetic precursor of PTH (219).

Part of the amino acid sequence of bovine Pre-proPTH has been determined (220, 221). Pre-proPTH comprises 31 additional amino acids attached to the amino terminus of PTH, for a total of 115 residues. It is unlikely that this peptide contributes to the physiological actions of PTH, since it is rapidly cleaved to a smaller protein, possibly while still attached to the ribosomes. Within 1–2 min after biosynthesis, Pre-proPTH loses 25 of its *N*-terminal residues, giving rise to the 90 amino acid polypeptide ProPTH (219).

The existence of ProPTH was first suggested by Hamilton, Cohn, and coworkers (222, 223). Subsequently Hamilton and Cohn (224), as well as others (225, 226), provided final proof for ProPTH well before Pre-proPTH had been discovered. Consequently, for a while it appeared possible that proPTH might represent the mRNA translation product (154). Thus ProPTH had already been chemically characterized and studied when evidence for Pre-proPTH began to emerge.

ProPTH has been detected in human (226, 227), chicken (228), rat (229), and porcine (230), besides bovine (226) parathyroid glands. The prohormone appears to be similar in these species, indicating that ProPTH is part of a general pathway of PTH biosynthesis in higher animals (Fig. 26.8). As such, control of its metabolism and its biological role are important topics. It is now understood that ProPTH itself is not secreted from parathyroid glands, with the exception of some human adenomas (231–233). For example, no ProPTH was found in calf or human plasma with radioimmunoassays 5000 times more sensitive to ProPTH than PTH (234). Additionally, ProPTH itself possesses only a fraction of the biological activity of PTH *in vitro* (235). ProPTH is active *in vivo* (222,

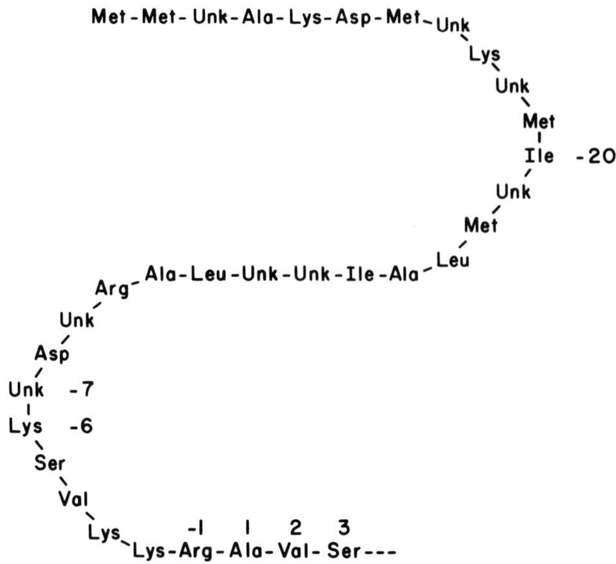

Fig. 26.8 Bovine Pre-ProPTH consists of 31 amino acids attached to the *N*-terminus of PTH. After biosynthesis, Pre-ProPTH is cleaved by an endopeptidase between residues −7 and −6 to yield ProPTH. ProPTH undergoes proteolysis between residues −1 and 1 to produce PTH.

235), but this has been attributed to the formation of PTH. Its slight activity *in vitro* most likely results from partial cleavage to PTH, since ProPTH is extremely labile to proteolytic enzymes (154). A sustaining consideration is provided by analog work, which has indicated that PTH-like compounds with *N*-terminus additions are virtually inactive (235, 236). These facts position ProPTH as an intermediate in PTH biosynthesis, not as a polypeptide involved in the direct manifestation of PTH action.

The role of ProPTH synthesis and cleavage in PTH secretion could be a more important factor than any inherent activity ProPTH might have. Although it has been well established that ECF calcium concentration directly affects preformed PTH release in short-term demand, it is possible that in chronic need, the rate of PTH release is determined by the availability of prohormone and the kinetics of its cleavage to the hormone. There is indeed evidence that ECF calcium levels affect intracellular parathyroid gland amino acid availability (237), indicating that chronic PTH release may be dependent on the rate of ProPTH synthesis. It must be understood, however, that research in this area is dynamic, and formalized views of PTH synthesis and secretion must be amenable to absorbing new evidence.

In the context of this warning, a simplified model of PTH biosynthesis and secretion is pictured in Fig. 26.9 (154, 219). After cleavage of Pre-proPTH to ProPTH, the newly formed prohormone is translocated to the Golgi apparatus within 10–20 min. Subcellular fractionation of tissues incubated with radiolabeled amino acids support the interpretation that most newly synthesized ProPTH and PTH can be found associated with the endoplasmic reticulum (ER) and the Golgi apparatus (238, 239). In the Golgi, the six *N*-terminal amino acids of ProPTH are removed to yield PTH by an enzyme with trypsinlike specificity that has not yet been isolated (240, 241). This conversion can be inhibited by agents that disrupt the Golgi apparatus, such as biogenic amines (242). The cleavage of ProPTH to PTH is efficient, and only about

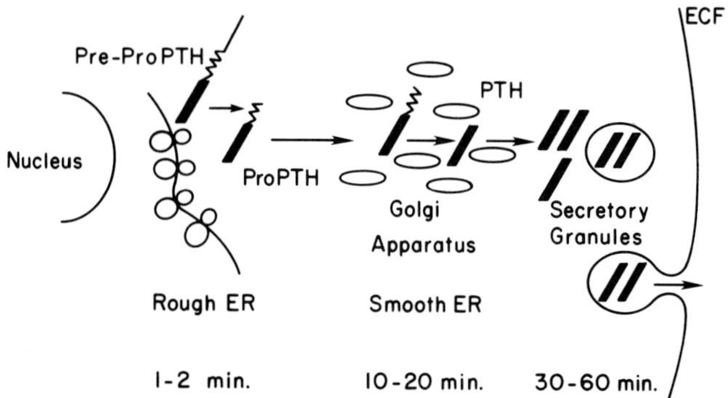

Fig. 26.9 The biosynthesis and packaging of PTH in the parathyroid gland cell. Pre-ProPTH, the direct ribosomal product, is hydrolyzed to proPTH soon after synthesis. ProPTH translocates to the Golgi apparatus, where it is cleaved to PTH. PTH is stored in secretory granules that merge with the cell membrane to release PTH during calcium need. After Ref. 219.

7% of total PTH metabolic intermediates are present as ProPTH (234, 240, 243). Once PTH has been produced, it is packaged in secretory granules in a process that spans about one hour. One fractional centrifugation experiment also demonstrated that in incubations lasting up to 6 hr, about 75% of hormone was from existing pools (239). The secretory granules in which these pools are incorporated are visible under the electron microscope and can be isolated by centrifugation. Under the influence of low ECF calcium concentrations, storage vesicles merge with the cytoplasmic membrane to release PTH into blood. There are speculative aspects to this model, but the formalization is encouraged by the knowledge that other peptide hormone producing tissues, such as pancreas, operate in a similar manner (244).

3.6 Metabolism

PTH released into blood does not remain intact, but undergoes further metabolism to produce a variety of immunoreactive PTH fragments in circulation (232, 233, 245, 246). This important fact was first suggested by Berson and Yalow (247), who demonstrated that circulating "PTH" was immunologically distinct from PTH present in parathyroid glands. Cleavage occurs after PTH is secreted into circulation, since the weight of evidence demonstrates that direct gland effluent is almost exclusively polypeptides of the same size as PTH. Both parathyroid cell cultures (248) and slices of parathyroid glands incubated for 6 hr *in vitro* (249) secrete polypeptides at least as large as gland-extracted material. Furthermore, gel-permeation analysis of immunoreactive hormone obtained by thyroid vein catheterizations of patients with primary hyperparathyroidism demonstrated largely intact PTH (250). Similar experiments done with samples of peripheral blood showed as little as 2% the concentration of intact hormone found in thyroid effluent blood. Thus with the available information, it seems reasonable that the entire 84 amino acid polypeptide sequence of PTH enters the blood only to be subsequently metabolized. Indeed, much data have accumulated to show that after PTH is secreted, it is short-lived, having a serum half-life of less than 20 min (144, 251–254).

Both kidney and liver, but not plasma, can metabolize PTH. Incubation of PTH in plasma results in no cleavage of PTH to smaller forms (255), which indicates that the metabolism probably occurs in specific organs. Accordingly, there is a 20–30% difference in immunoreactive PTH concentration between arterial and venous blood across dog kidney and liver, but not across lung or hind limb (254, 256). Perfusion of rat liver produced a similar result (257). Since one target tissue (kidney) and one nontarget tissue (liver) are involved, there is no immediate indication that peripheral cleavage is exclusively degradative metabolism.

The cleavage position has been established by amino acid analysis of recovered radioiodinated PTH fragments (255). Primary cleavage is endopeptidase and occurs between residues 33 and 34. Then exopeptidase reactions produce fragments with sequences of 37–84, 41–84, and 43–84, in addition to the 34–84 segment. It is known that biological activity of PTH is manifested by the 1–27 fragment (258), but not by carboxyl-end fragments with residue 34 as the initial amino acid (259). Therefore the 6000–7000 dalton carboxyl terminal segments, which are the known major circulating forms of PTH, must be biologically inactive, even though they are immunoreactive. Unfortunately, attempts to identify the biologically active 1–33 fragment in blood that should be produced by this cleavage have had variable results. Two laboratories (246, 260) have reported smaller fragments of molecular weight in the 2000–4000 dalton range, but no data on biological activity accompany the findings. Other investigators simply have not found smaller fragments.

It is unlikely that the fragmentation pathway is a way to release the biologically active initial 33 amino acid sequence for function at target sites. This was demonstrated by the finding that intact bovine PTH was as active *in vitro* as the 1–34 fragment of bovine PTH (261). There was no evidence of proteolysis, and both fragments manifested similar rates of action. Therefore intact hormone must possess inherent activity.

3.7 Structure-Activity Relationships

Despite the limited number of analogs of PTH synthesized and tested, much valuable information has been gathered concerning PTH structure-activity relationships. It was mentioned previously that peripheral PTH metabolism must produce active PTH fragments as well as the inactive fragments, which have already been characterized. This reasoning is based on synthetic work that verified that the entire polypeptide chain of PTH is not mandatory for biological activity. Early observers had reported that bPTH fragments obtained during hydrochloric acid extraction were biologically active (199, 262). This led to the testing, in 1971, of a synthetic fragment of bovine PTH consisting of the first 34 amino terminal residues ($bPTH_{1-34}$) (263). The tetratriacontapeptide possessed the exact physiological properties of authentic bPTH. In sharp contrast, a fragment of bPTH consisting of residues 53–84 was shown to be inactive (259). Consequently, the first studies relating PTH function and structure provided information essential to understanding the ramifications of PTH metabolism.

More systematic structure-activity relationship studies followed. The effect of polypeptide chain length on physiological activity of bPTH was thoroughly investigated by Tregear and colleagues (258). They tested each analog *in vitro* with the rat kidney adenylate cyclase assay developed by Marcus and Aurbach (264). The *in vitro* results were compared with *in vivo* results obtained from the chick hypercalcemia assay reported by Parsons, Reit, and Robinson (265). Test results appear in Table 26.3. The response of native $bPTH_{1-84}$ (fragment 1–84) was considered to be 100% in both assays. Synthetic compound responses were then compared to that of $bPTH_{1-84}$ on a molar basis. These results reaffirm the well-known fact that the entire sequence of $bPTH_{1-84}$ is not needed for

Table 26.3 Effect of Polypeptide Chain Length on Activity of Bovine PTH[a]

Fragment (bPTH)	Activity per Molar Equivalent, %[b]	
	In Vitro	*In Vivo*
1–84	100	100
1–34	77	132
1–31	10	62
1–28	5	<0.3
1–27	2	<0.2
1–26	<0.3	<0.2
2–34	3	64
3–34	<0.3	<0.2

[a] A series of chain-shortened analogs was synthesized and tested (139) *in vitro* in the rat adenylate cyclase assay (68) and *in vivo* in the chick hypercalcemia assay (90).

[b] Activities are given as percentage response caused by equimolar doses relative to fragment 1–84, which represents the major isohormonal form of bovine PTH ($bPTH_{1-84}$).

activity. The shortened hormone $bPTH_{1-34}$ compares well in degree of activity to native $bPTH_{1-84}$. Differences between rat and chick data most likely represent species variance rather than metabolic events occurring during *in vivo* assay. Further chain-shortening causes additional potency losses, and $bPTH_{1-26}$ can be considered to be inactive. Although these data do not fix the exact number of residues necessary for efficacious PTH, they do suggest that at least 27 residues are needed for minimal function and that 34 residues are sufficient. Furthermore, the amino-terminal end of the molecule is more sensitive to deletions than is carboxyterminal. Deletion of the alanine at position 1 is tolerated ($bPTH_{2-34}$), but deletion of alanine plus the valine at position 2 ($bPTH_{3-34}$) destroys efficacy.

Further studies by Tregear et al. (266, 267) elaborated structural tolerances at the amino terminus. Various position 1 substituted analogs of $bPTH_{1-34}$ and $hPTH_{1-34}$ were synthesized and tested in the rat adenylate cyclase assay (Table 26.4). The standard, $bPTH_{1-34}$, was assigned 100% activity (entry 1). A switch of D-alanine for L-alanine in $bPTH_{1-34}$ (entry 2) was tolerated better than substituting the first residue (serine) of hPTH in $bPTH_{1-34}$ (entry 3). Thus, as might be expected, the activity of $hPTH_{1-34}$ (entry 7) could be increased substantially by placing alanine at position 1 rather than serine (entry 8). Since serine is actually hydroxymethylalanine, the increased polarity and bulk of the hydroxy group must be responsible for loss of activity. No alanine analog is available with a small, nonpolar substituent; but either larger polar substitutions (entry 4) or deletions (entry 6) on the alanine α-carbon cause significant loss of activity. Therefore there is apparently a very specific structural requirement for a methyl or similar group on the α-carbon of the first amino acid in PTH. The remainder of analogs demonstrate that an unaltered amine in the first residue is also necessary for appreciable activity (entries 6 and 11). Note that additions to the terminal amine (entries 5 and 10) dramatically reduce potency.

Other work by Rosenblatt et al. (268) has shown that replacement of the methionines at positions 8 and 18 with isosteric norleucine residues preserves activity. Conversely, oxidation of the two methionines eliminates activity.

Also, substitution of tyrosine or radioiodinated tyrosine for the phenylalanine at position 34 in $bPTH_{1-34}$ increases potency by about 30% as measured in the rat adenylate cyclase assay. Substituting norleucine at positions 8 and 18 and tyrosine at 34 yields a compound about 80% as active as $bPTH_{1-34}$. Since bPTH and hPTH are similar in amino acid sequence, these conclusions probably can be applied safely to hPTH as well.

At least two synthetic polypeptides are antagonists of PTH. Both $bPTH_{3-34}$ and desaminoalanine$_1$-PTH_{1-34} (entry 6, Table 26.4) lack agonist activity but prevent

Table 26.4 Effect of Position-1 Substitution in Human and Bovine PTH Sequences 1–34[a]

	$bPTH_{1-34}$			$hPTH_{1-34}$	
Entry	Structure	Activity, %[b]	Entry	Structure	Activity, %[b]
1[c]	(L) $H_2N—CH—CO—$ | CH_3	100	7[d]	$H_2N—CH—CO—$ | CH_2 | OH	32
2	(D) $H_3C—CH—CO—$ | NH_2	61	8	$H_2N—CH—CO–$ | CH_3	80
3	$H_2N—CH—CO$ | CH_2 | OH	23	9	$H_2N—CH_2—CO—$	6
4	$H_2N—CH—CO—$ | ⌬ | OH	10	10	$HN—CH—CO—$ | | OC CH_2 | | H_3C OH	0.9
5	$HN—CH—CO—$ | CH_3	9	11	$CH_2—CO—$ | CH_2 | OH	<0.7
6	$H—CH—CO—$ | CH_3	<0.2			

[a] Several different amino acids were substituted for the serine and alanine that are native to the human and bovine tetratriacontapeptides, respectively. Analogs were evaluated *in vitro* with the rat adenylate cyclase assay (68).
[b] Activities are expressed as percentage potency with respect to bovine PTH_{1-34}.
[c] Authentic bovine PTH_{1-34}.
[d] Authentic human PTH_{1-34}.

expression of bPTH activity *in vitro* (269). The inhibition exhibited was proportional to dose, reversed by addition of excess bPTH, and specific for PTH renal adenyl cyclase. Under these circumstances $bPTH_{1-26}$ and $bPTH_{13-34}$ possessed neither agonist nor antagonist activity. This introduces another dimension in PTH analog evaluation. For data to be complete, investigators should recognized the potential of PTH analogs as antagonists of hormone action.

These investigations have provided several important conclusions. The minimum polypeptide chain of an active PTH analog must consist of an amino acid sequence of at least 2–27. Further addition, deletion, or alteration at the amino terminal end severely diminishes activity. The sulfur atoms of PTH probably play no role in activity—methionine can be replaced successfully by the isosteric norleucine. Also, carboxyl terminus residue substitution can frequently increase activity (154), perhaps reflecting resistance to proteolytic breakdown. Generally such observations have proved to be useful to investigations of PTH biosynthesis and metabolism and should provide further insight into the receptor-site active form of PTH. More potent analogs of PTH should also result.

3.8 Summary

In the last several years significant gains have been made in understanding the biosynthesis, secretion, and metabolism of PTH. This knowledge should aid in understanding and perhaps controlling the several diseases associated with abnormal PTH secretion. Indeed, realization that many immunoreactive but biologically inactive PTH fragments circulate in blood precipitated a reevaluation of PTH-associated disease symptoms and provoked a more sophisticated appraisal of immunoreactive PTH blood concentrations.

4 VITAMIN D

4.1 Historical Background

Although there is some evidence that rickets was known in ancient civilizations (270), the first well-defined description of the disease was provided by Whistler in 1645 (271). For nearly three centuries after, rickets was frequently treated by nonphysicians with home remedies such as cod liver oil. But these cures were not widely accepted as valid by the medical community. In 1919 Sir Edward Mellanby provided sound scientific footing for the largely ignored observations of laypersons when he demonstrated that rickets could be produced in experimental animals by dietary manipulation (272, 273). He further demonstrated that administration of cod liver oil could prevent or cure rickets. Unfortunately, Mellanby incorrectly concluded that the dietary antirachitic factor was vitamin A, which had been discovered by McCollum in the mid-1910s (274, 275).

Subsequently, McCollum reported that passing oxygen through hot cod liver oil destroyed the antixerophthalmic properties of the oil, but not the antirachitic properties (276). McCollum also observed that low calcium and phosphate levels in experimental diets are important in the causation of rickets. These experiments established the existence of a new substance important to the growth and maintenance of healthy bone, named vitamin D by McCollum. During the same period, Huldshinsky (277) discovered that rickets can also be prevented or cured by sunlight or by artificial UV light.

Potential confusion over these seemingly unrelated facts was averted in part when Goldblatt and Soames (278) reported that livers from rachitic rats irradiated with UV light cured rickets when ingested, but livers from nonirradiated rats did not. This concept led Steenbock (279, 280), and later Hess and Weinstock (281), to show that irradiation of diets could prevent or cure rickets. Steenbock (282) and Hess (283) had demonstrated that a provitamin D exists in certain foodstuffs which on UV irradiation chemically converts to vitamin D. These observations led to the eradication of rickets as a major medical problem. Additional investigations also showed that the nonsaponifiable fraction converted to vitamin D upon irradiation.

Soon after, Windaus and collaborators (284), and Rosenheim and Webster (285) concluded that provitamin D was either ergosterol or a very closely related steroid. The next several years were occupied with determining the structure of ergosterol and with studying the irradiation products of that sterol. Finally in the 1930s Askew and co-workers (286) and Windaus and co-workers (287) isolated pure vitamin D_2, obtained from the irradiation of ergosterol. This area of research culminated in the late 1930s with the elucidation of the structures of vitamin D_2 by Windaus and Thiel (288) and of vitamin D_3 by Windaus and co-workers (289).

The physiological actions of the D vitamins had also been undergoing examination throughout this period. Howland and Kramer (290) had noted in 1921 that blood is undersaturated with the calcium-times-phosphate product in vitamin D deficiency. These data were overlooked despite Shipley's reports (291, 292) that rickets is characterized by calcification sites in bone that are inadequately supplied with calcium and phosphate. Furthermore, even though the low calcium-times-phosphate product was used to diagnose rickets in early clinical work, the relationship between amount of calcium and phosphate in blood and rickets was unappreciated until much later, when Neuman and Neuman (293) advanced the concept that blood is normally supersaturated with calcium and phosphate. Thereafter Neuman (294) confirmed Howland and Kramer's (290) earlier report that blood from rachitic subjects contained undersaturating concentrations of calcium and phosphate.

Related developments include the observation by Orr in 1923 (295) of high fecal calcium losses in rachitic children. Orr suggested that UV light cured rickets by stimulating intestinal calcium absorption. This was confirmed by Nicolaysen in 1937 (296–299) when he demonstrated that vitamin D actually increases intestinal calcium absorption. Moreover, Carlsson and colleagues (300, 301) showed that even at physiological levels, vitamin D causes decalcification of bone rather than mineralization. Therefore even though vitamin D had been associated initially with the maintenance of healthy bone, early evidence suggested that this was a collateral function. In fact, bone mineralization occurs because blood is supersaturated with calcium and phosphate. When the calcium-times-phosphate product concentration in blood decreases, vitamin D acts on intestine to stimulate calcium and phosphate absorption and on bone to mobilize calcium and phosphorus from previously formed bone. Both actions serve to increase blood calcium and phosphate concentrations necessary for mineralization of new bone. Furthermore, these basic functions also result in the prevention of hypocalcemia tetany.

However the role of vitamin D in regulating blood calcium concentration was not fully illuminated until vitamin D's functional metabolism was understood. After early work, it had been assumed that vitamin D functioned directly without metabolic activation. In the 1950s Kodicek and co-workers (302–305) considered the possibility that vitamin D must be metabolized before function. Massive doses were administered, but only 20% of active material could be accounted for by biological assay. In other experiments, Kodicek (306) dosed with biosynthetically radiolabeled vitamin D_2 of low specific activity. Once again pharmacological doses were used. In neither case were any biologically active metabolites of D found, which seemed to sustain the conclusion that the vitamin acts directly. Certainly, Kodicek's experiments correctly demonstrated that vitamin D is metabolized to inactive products.

The chemical synthesis of vitamin D_3 of high specific activity (307), and the adaptation of powerful chromatographic systems to the separation of vitamin D and its metabolites by DeLuca and colleagues (308, 309), paved the way for investigation of the metabolism of this vitamin at physiological levels. These tools were used to isolate from the plasma of pigs the major circulating metabolite of D_3, which was identified as 25-hydroxyvitamin D_3 (25-OH-D_3) in 1968 (310). Subsequent work demonstrated that 25-OH-D_3 acts more rapidly than D_3 and is approximately 2–5 times more active than D_3 in all D-responsive systems (311, 312). During the work on 25-OH-D_3, even more polar metabolites were detected by DeLuca and co-workers (310). At the same time, Haussler, Myrtle, and Norman (313) reported the existence in intestine of a biologically active metabolite more polar than 25-OH-D_3. Shortly afterward Kodicek and co-workers (314) found that the metabolite lost tritium at position 1 and that the transformation occurred in the kidney (315). In 1971 DeLuca and co-workers (316, 317) isolated 2 μg of pure metabolite from the intestines of 1500 rachitic chickens dosed with radioactive vitamin D_3. Through chemical reactivity, mass spectroscopy, and UV spectrophotometry they unequivocally identified the metabolite as 1,25-dihydroxyvitamin D_3. Independent evidence was presented for the structure by Lawson et al. (318), who obtained several micrograms of 1,25-$(OH)_2D_3$ about 30% pure from incubations of 25-OH-D_3 with kidney homogenates. Further work established that 1,25-$(OH)_2D_3$ acts more rapidly than either D_3 or 25-OH-D_3. Additionally, 1,25-$(OH)_2D_3$ is 5–10 times more potent than D_3 and about 2–5 times more potent than 25-OH-D_3 *in vivo*, provided it is dosed parenterally and daily (312, 319–321). The discovery of active vitamin D metabolites provided for the ultimate understanding of D_3 as a prohormone giving rise to the hormone 1,25-$(OH)_2D_3$ under specific physiological circumstances.

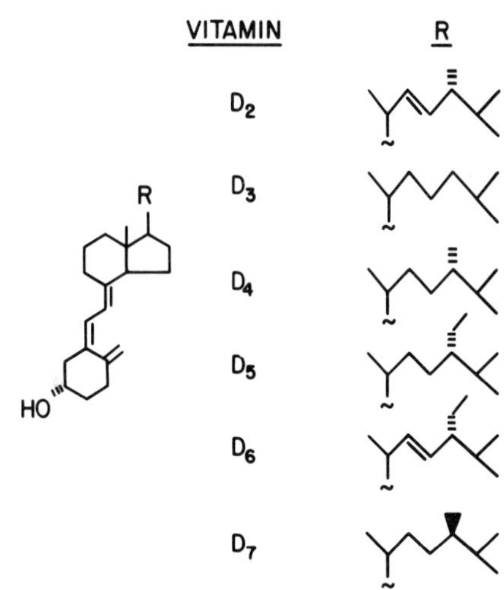

Fig. 26.10 Structures of the several forms of vitamin D. D_1 is a mixture of lumisterol$_2$ and D_2 (287). Only D_2 and D_3 are commercially and physiologically important. Except for D_4, the others have been poorly characterized, chemically and biologically (322).

4.2 Biosynthesis

Vitamin D can accumulate *in vivo* as a result of intestinal absorption from diet or by UV irradiation of precursors in skin. Since 7-dehydrocholesterol—the precursor or provitamin of D_3—is the only known provitamin found in skin, D_3 is the form of D that is naturally endogenous to animal organisms. Other forms are known; but these are commercially and physiologically inconsequential except for D_2, which has the ergosterol side chain (Fig. 26.10). Vitamin D_2 has been used extensively as an additive for animal and human food, and clinically as treatment for vitamin D deficiency.

Hess and Weinstock (323) first demonstrated that irradiation of rat skin conferred antirachitic properties. Until recently, no further work had been undertaken in this area. It has been assumed that sunlight that penetrates the skin causes the transformation to vitamin D_3 of 7-dehydrocholesterol, an abundant skin sterol, much as it generally occurs *in vitro*. The *in vitro* reactions have been well studied (324). Upon UV excitation, 7-dehydrocholesterol opens to previtamin D_3, which is in photoequilibrium with two reverse reaction closure products, lumisterol$_3$ and 7-dehydrocholesterol (Fig. 26.11). Further photoexcitation of previtamin causes an isomerization to tachysterol$_3$. The equilibrium constant for the latter reaction favors formation of tachysterol$_3$. Thus prolonged irradiation of previtamin *in vitro* ultimately produces mostly tachysterol$_3$. On the other hand, thermal treatment of previtamin converts it to vitamin in a temperature-dependent process. The reaction is slow at 37° with a half-life of at least 14 hr.

Very recently vitamin D has actually been isolated from irradiated rachitic rat skin (325). UV and mass spectra firmly identified the product, which was present in

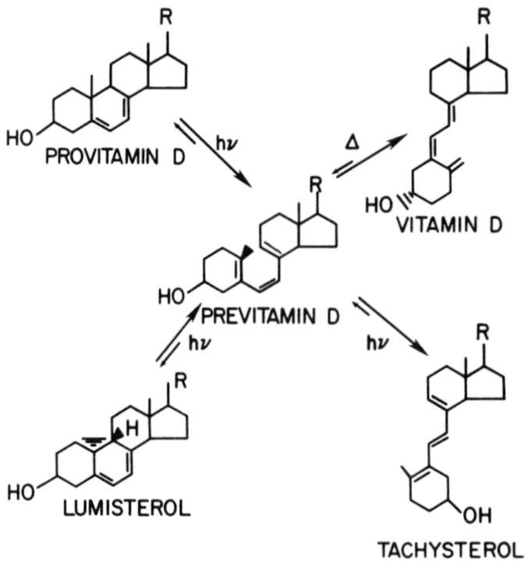

Fig. 26.11 Photoreactions of provitamin D *in vitro*. Upon photolysis with 254 to 313 nm light, provitamin undergoes ring opening through the first excited singlet state to previtamin. Previtamin is in photoequilibrium with provitamin and lumisterol. Each is obtained by conrotatory ring closure of previtamin. In both cases the equilibrium favors formation of previtamin. By photo Z to E isomerization, previtamin can be converted to tachysterol. In this case equilibrium favors formation of tachysterol. By a thermally induced antarafacial 1,7-sigmatropic shift, previtamin is converted to vitamin. The equilibrium, which favors formation of vitamin, is controlled through conformational strain induced by the five-membered D-ring (313).

concentrations of 320 ng/g tissue compared to nonirradiated control values no greater than 40 ng/g. No tachysterol$_3$ was isolated, but this could be the result of many factors, including the inherent instability of tachysterol$_3$. Consequently failure to isolate tachysterol$_3$ should be viewed with caution. These investigations gave no evidence of protein involvement in the conversion of 7-dehydrocholesterol to vitamin D_3 in skin. However since it is known that previtamin D is only slowly converted to vitamin D, even at physiological temperatures, it is likely that once previtamin is formed in the skin, it slowly converts to vitamin D, providing a steady supply of vitamin to the organism.

4.3 Functional Metabolism

Once formed, vitamin D_3 circulates in the blood bound to a specific carrier protein or on a β-lipoprotein (326–328). But its half-life in blood is brief, inasmuch as 60–80% of administered radiolabeled D_3 accumulates in the liver within an hour after intravenous administration (329, 330). In liver, D_3 undergoes hydroxylation by an enzyme in the endoplasmic reticulum. The hydroxylase requires molecular oxygen, NADPH, and magnesium (331–334). Hydroxylation is also facilitated by a cytosolic protein, which may protect the substrate from degradation (332). Since the enzyme is insensitive to cytochrome P-450 inhibitors such as carbon monoxide and is not induced by *in vivo* phenobarbital administration, it may not be dependent on cytochrome P-450 (332, 333). The enzyme is affected by its product, however. High levels of intrahepatic 25-OH-D_3, but not circulating 25-OH-D_3, decrease the rate of 25-hydroxylation (332, 335, 336). The regulation can be overcome at very high circulating vitamin D_3 levels, but it is not understood how this occurs (335, 337). Possibly a second nonspecific 25-hydroxylase begins to function on large amounts of vitamin D_3. The existence of such an enzyme is suggested by the unregulated 25-hydroxylation of tachysterol (338). Yet under normal physiological conditions, the regulated 25-hydroxylase provides a steady level of about 30 ng/ml of 25-OH-D_3 in blood (339).

Though 25-OH-D_3 is more active than vitamin D_3 *in vivo*, its activity, as well as the activity of vitamin D_3, can be eliminated by nephrectomy. *In vitro*, 25-OH-D_3 stimulates bone (340, 341) and intestine cells (342, 343) only at superphysiological concentrations. Therefore in the functional metabolism of vitamin D_3, 25-OH-D_3 can be considered to be an obligatory intermediate without a direct physiological effect at normal circulating levels. Ex-

Fig. 26.12 The functional metabolism of vitamin D_3.

tremely high plasma concentrations do cause toxicity because of direct effects, which indicates that the feedback control of 25-hydroxylase is a regulatory process important to preventing vitamin D toxicity.

The 25-OH-D_3 is transported to the kidney, where it undergoes further metabolism to either 24*R*,25-dihydroxyvitamin D_3 [24,25-$(OH)_2D_3$] or 1α,25-$(OH)_2D_3$ (Fig. 26.12). The amount of each product formed depends on blood calcium and phosphate concentrations (344–346). When calcium and phosphate levels fall below the normal physiological range, the 1α-hydroxylase responds producing 1,25-$(OH)_2D_3$. Conversely, normal to high blood mineral concentrations stimulate the 24-hydroxylase, resulting in increased levels of 24,25-$(OH)_2D_3$ (Fig. 26.13).

Much attention has been drawn to the renal 25-OH-D_3-1α-hydroxylase, since it is the enzyme that produces the hormonal

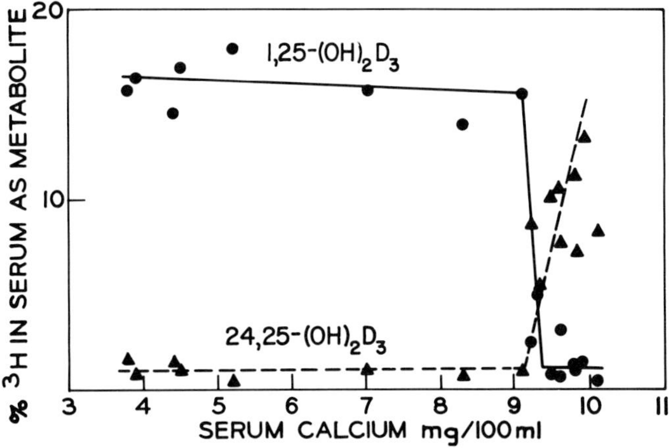

Fig. 26.13 Relation of serum calcium to accumulation of 1,25-$(OH)_2D_3$ or 24,25-$(OH)_2D_3$ in blood of rats (10).

form of vitamin D_3. This enzyme is located in the heavy mitochondria and utilizes both molecular oxygen and NADPH (315, 347–349). It is a cytochrome P-450, and it has a supporting renal electron transport system that is closely analogous to the adrenal mitochrondrial cytochrome P-450 oxidase system (350, 351). Thus the 1α-hydroxylase reaction involves the sequential reduction of a flavoprotein, a nonheme iron protein (renal ferredoxin), and cytochrome P-450. Since nephrectomy abolishes all 1α-hydroxylation in mammals, kidney is the exclusive site of 25-OH-D_2-1α-hydroxylase (315, 352).

As expected of an enzyme that produces a hormone, 25-OH-D_3-1α-hydroxylase is closely regulated. Blood levels of calcium, phosphate, PTH, and 1,25-$(OH)_2D_3$ control the production of 1,25-$(OH)_2D_3$ (344–346, 353–355). In times of low blood calcium, the synthesis of 1,25-$(OH)_2D_3$ is increased. During normal calcium states, 1,25-$(OH)_2D_3$ production is precluded (356, 357). However low blood calcium levels do not directly affect the 1α-hydroxylase; rather, they act through PTH. Parathyroidectomy abolishes the hypocalcemic stimulation of 1α-hydroxylation, but it can be restored by PTH administration (346, 354). Results of *in vitro* studies are conflicting, but they tend to indicate that calcium ions have no direct inhibitory effect on the enzyme (358–361). In light of these experiments, PTH must be viewed as calcium's messenger to the 1α-hydroxylase. Besides low blood calcium, phosphate deprivation also stimulates 1,25-$(OH)_2D_3$ production, even in parathyroidectomized animals (345, 362). In these experimental models, an inverse relationship between blood phosphate levels and 1,25-$(OH)_2D_3$ production has been established (Fig. 26.14). One of the actions of PTH is to promote excretion of phosphate from kidney. This may be the mechanism by which PTH augments 1,25-$(OH)_2D_3$ production, but that is not certain.

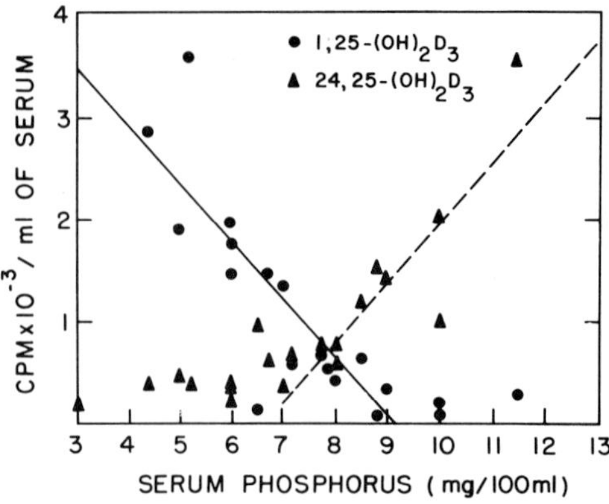

Fig. 26.14 Relation between serum phosphate levels and accumulation of 1,25-$(OH)_2D_3$ and 24,25-$(OH)_2D_3$ in serum of parathyroidectomized rats (11).

High blood calcium concentrations also act indirectly to regulate the 1α-hydroxylase. In vitamin D deficiency calcium does not have an inhibitory effect on the enzyme. But dosage of 1,25-$(OH)_2D_3$ to D-deficient animals suppresses the 1α-hydroxylase and causes a concomitant rise in the 24-hydroxylase (Fig. 26.15) (355, 363, 364). It is not known whether this represents enzyme induction or activation

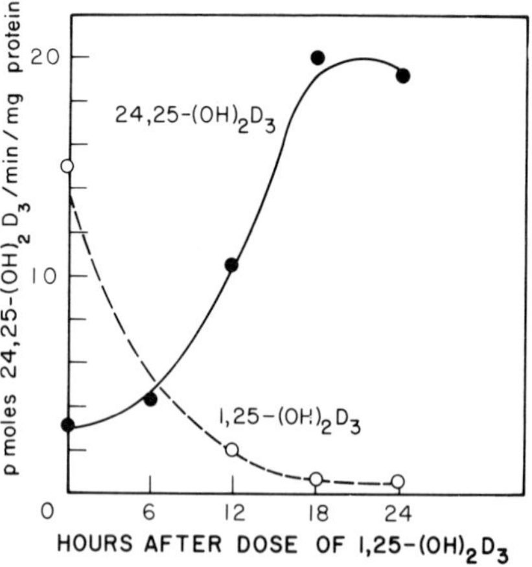

Fig. 26.15 Repression of 25-OH-D_2-1α-hydroxylase and the stimulation of 25-OH-D_3-24-hydroxylase by administration of 650 pmol of 1,25-$(OH)_2D_3$ to rachitic chicks (11).

of a preexisting enzyme. However it is certain that 1,25-$(OH)_2D_3$ stimulates mRNA synthesis in kidney tissue (364, 365); but no connection between the mRNA and the 24-hydroxylase has been made. The entire regulatory process mediated by calcium through PTH and by phosphate takes several hours (346, 354). In this time, the gross observable change is a stimulation of the 1α-hydroxylase and a retardation of the 24-hydroxylase by low blood calcium and phosphate levels, whereas the converse is true when blood calcium and phsophate concentrations exceed physiological levels.

The renal 25-OH-D_3-24-hydroxylase is also a mitochondrial enzyme and requires an electron transport system and reducing equivalents similar to those of the 1α-hydroxylase (366). In contrast to the 1α-hydroxylase, however, the 24-hydroxylase is insensitive to cytochrome P-450 inhibitors. Though the latter is inconclusive evidence, more detailed information is unavailable. However substrate specificity is well defined. Besides 25-OH-D_3, renal 24-hydroxylase metabolizes 1,25-$(OH)_2D_3$ *in vitro*, giving 1,24*R*,25-trihydroxyvitamin D_3 [1,24,25-$(OH)_3D_3$]. Among the several D_3 metabolites, apparently only 25-hydroxy compounds can serve as substrates for this hydroxylase (367–369).

A second 24-hydroxylase exists in intestine. This enzyme prefers 1,25-$(OH)_2D_3$ as substrate but can also metabolize 25-OH-D_3, albeit much less efficiently (370). Since nephrectomy significantly decreases circulating 24,25-$(OH)_2D_3$, but not 1,24,25-$(OH)_3D_3$, it seems plausible that *in vivo* the renal 24-hydroxylase preferentially metabolizes 25-OH-D_3, whereas the intestinal 24-hydroxylase preferentially metabolizes 1,25-$(OH)_2D_3$ (370, 371).

Like the enzymes that produce them, the 24-hydroxylated metabolites of vitamin D_3 remain an enigma. It is known that 24,25-$(OH)_2D_3$ is about as potent as 25-OH-D_3 but shorter acting (372); 1,24,25-$(OH)_3D_3$ is both shorter acting and less potent than 1,25-$(OH)_2D_3$ (373). Since vicinal alcohols are generally easily oxidized, it is tempting to suggest that 24,25-dihydroxylated D_3-like compounds have been set up for oxidative degradation. This coupled with the decrease in biological half-life seems to indicate that 24-hydroxylation represents the first step in metabolic inactivation and excretion of vitamin D_3 metabolites. Solid evidence for this is lacking, however. It is still possible, therefore, that 24-hydroxylation confers on vitamin D_3 metabolites biological activity, that is not yet recognized. This appears more probable, since the 24*R*-hydroxyl group is produced exclusively *in vivo* and 24*R*- but not 24*S*-hydroxy compounds can undergo further metabolism (374).

There is one further characterized metabolite of 25-OH-D_3. This is 25,26-dihydroxyvitamin D_3 [25,26-$(OH)_2D_3$], which was first isolated from the plasma of pigs (375). It is produced in the kidney, but little else has been established (376). Nevertheless, it is intriguing to consider that each metabolite might have a selective role in calcium or phosphate metabolism in different target tissues.

When 1,25-$(OH)_2D_3$ is labeled in the 25,26-carbons with ^{14}C, it undergoes side chain oxidation *in vivo* to produce $^{14}CO_2$ and an unknown metabolite. Nephrectomy abolishes a similar response from 25-OH-D_3, showing that this is a significant occurance only in 1α-hydroxylated metabolites (377–379). Removal of the jejunum, ileum, and colon reduces response, suggesting intestine as the site of metabolism, at least in part. Additionally, since "germ-free" animals also produced the response, intestinal flora can be excluded as the cause of metabolism (380). Currently the significance of further metabolism of 1,25-$(OH)_2D_3$ is obscure. Because the $^{14}CO_2$ evolution occurs within 4 hr after 1,25-$(OH)_2$[26,27^{14}C]D_3 administration, this may be a functional rather than a degradative pathway; but that possibility remains to be demonstrated.

4.4 1,25-$(OH)_2D_3$ Function

The 1,25-$(OH)_2D_3$ produced by the kidney when blood calcium or phosphate concentrations fall below normal levels works in several organs to reestablish physiological blood calcium levels. Kidney, bone, and intestine are primary target tissues for the hormone. The kidney action of 1,25-$(OH)_2D_3$ in feedback inhibition of the 25-OH-D_3-1α-hydroxylase is well known (10–12, 17–26). But less understood is the effect of 1,25-$(OH)_2D_3$ on renal tubular reabsorption of calcium and phosphate. Older experiments did show increased renal tubular resorption of calcium on administration of vitamin D to deficient animals (381, 382). But they were done on animals with intact parathyroid glands. Therefore the effects of vitamin D could not be dissociated from those of PTH. More recent experiments done with parathyroidectomized animals do implicate 1,25-$(OH)_2D_3$ in the improvement of renal calcium reabsorption (383). This likelihood is strengthened by the discovery of a calcium-binding protein in kidney that is suppressed in vitamin D deficiency but is augmented by vitamin D administration (384). On the other hand, past experiments have implicated 1,25-$(OH)_2D_3$ in an improvement of phosphate resorbtion (385), although recent experiments gave no such results (386).

Effects of 1,25-$(OH)_2D_3$ on bone are well established, but the mechanisms are poorly understood. In physiological amounts vitamin D (300, 301, 311, 387), acting through 1,25-$(OH)_2D_3$ (388–390), causes resorption of bone. Radioisotopic methods were first used to demonstrate this effect. Later experiments revealed that vitamin D deficient rats fed a low calcium diet respond to vitamin D administration by increasing blood calcium concentration. Even though D stimulates the intestine to absorb calcium, this source of calcium can be ruled out with a low calcium diet. Therefore the source of blood calcium in these rats must be bone. Currently this experimental protocol is used to evaluate the bone calcium mobilizing ability of newly discovered D metabolites and analogs. *In vivo*, bone calcium mobilization stimulated by 1,25-$(OH)_2D_3$ requires the presence of PTH (391). PTH-stimulated bone calcium mobilization *in vivo* does not occur in the absence of 1,25-$(OH)_2D_3$; from this it appears that the steroidlike hormone facilitates the action of the peptide hormone. On the other hand, quite a different situation exists in organ culture (389, 392), where 1,25-$(OH)_2D_3$ functions well in the absence of PTH. No explanation has been afforded for this discrepancy, and no satisfactory explanation is likely until the molecular mechanisms of the two hormones are defined. Presently one clue to the puzzle is provided by actinomycin D. Prior administration of the antibiotic blocks bone calcium mobilization after dosage with 1,25-$(OH)_2D_3$, whereas if 1,25-$(OH)_2D_3$ is dosed first, no inhibition results (393). Though this indicates that transcription may precede bone calcium mobilization, it by no means satisfies the quest for information.

Phosphate is also mobilized from bone by 1,25-$(OH)_2D_3$ in a PTH-independent process. Significant increases in serum phosphate concentrations result when rats on a rachitogenic diet (low phosphate, high calcium) are administered 1,25-$(OH)_2D_3$ (394). This effect occurs equally well in parathyroidectomized animals (395). Increased intestinal absorption is precluded as the source of phosphate by the low phosphorus diet. More directly, ^{32}P experiments pinpointed bone as the source (395). A dramatic testament to increased serum phosphate concentrations occurring in rats on the rachitogenic diet after dosage with vitamin D is provided by the degree of new bone mineralization. This can be measured by staining radii and ulnae with silver nitrate solution. The epiphyseal plate remains colorless in control animals, indicating a lack of endochondrial mineralization. In animals dosed with active D compounds, the epiphyseal plate stains in intensity proportional to the degree of endochondrial mineralization. This protocol is known as the "line test", since a mineralized episphyseal plate forms a dark line across the radius and ulna. Formal standards for the "line test" are encoded in the US Pharmacopoeia and are precise enough to allow quantitation of D-like activity (396). The "line test" is a fairly good way to measure activity of D-like compounds, but it is limited because it measures only phosphate response and gives no indication of ability to stimulate intestinal calcium transport.

Perhaps the most important immediate action of 1,25-$(OH)_2D_3$ in regulating blood calcium occurs in the intestine. There 1,25-$(OH)_2D_3$ alone acts to increase the transport rate of dietary calcium across intestinal mucosa (397). Experiments done with the everted gut sac technique demonstrated that intestinal calcium transport is an active process in which calcium is moved against a concentration gradient (398–400). Transport occurs throughout the intestine but is optimal in the duodenum. The overall process is saturable, which indicates involvement of a carrier. Moreover, sodium is required for expulsion of calcium from the intestinal cell into ECF (401). Furthermore, the same studies established the dependency of intestinal calcium transport on vitamin D (299, 387, 400, 402).

Yet the mechanism by which 1,25-$(OH)_2D_3$ increases rate of intestinal calcium transport is only partially understood. Much work has suggested, but not definitively established, that 1,25-$(OH)_2D_3$ acts as a typical steroid hormone. Both chick and rat intestinal cytosol contain a binding protein, which has high affinity and low capacity for 1,25-$(OH)_2D_3$ (403–408). This protein, 1,25-$(OH)_2D_3$ intestinal cytosol binding protein, is specific for 1,25-$(OH)_2D_3$ or 1,25-$(OH)_2D_2$ and discriminates against all other vitamin D analogs and metabolites by substantial margins (409, 410). It migrates in the 3.7*S* (chick) or 3.2*S* (rat) region on sucrose density gradients and is not a plasma contaminant. Some evidence suggests that this protein bound to 1,25-$(OH)_2D_3$ translocates to intestinal nuclei (404). Other work has shown that depending on experimental rigors, about 40–80% of 1,25-$(OH)_2D_3$ that accumulates in the intestine localizes in the nuclei and associates with chromatin (411–415). Most recently, autoradiography has shown an accumulation of 1,25-$(OH)_2D_3$ in intestinal villus cell nuclei (416). An increase in chromatin template activity of intestinal tissue has also been suggested (417). Furthermore, evidence for enhancement of DNA-dependent RNA polymerase activity (418) and initiation of new RNA synthesis in intestinal cells has been presented (419). Some of these experiments were performed in crude systems, wherein observations are not necessarily clear, but purification of experimental systems, particularly the cytosolic binding protein, will help establish rigorous evidence. Additionally, direct experimental evidence for nuclear events is missing. Specifically, gene products produced in response to 1,25-$(OH)_2D_3$ have not yet been demonstrated.

A calcium binding protein (CaBP) has been detected in intestine after dosage of deplete animals with vitamin D (26). Mammalian intestinal CaBP is in the molecular weight range of 8000–12,000 daltons and binds 4 calcium ions per mole protein. It is not found in D-deplete animals but is present in D-replete animals. Additionally, CaBP concentration and rate of intestinal calcum absorption roughly correlate. Nevertheless, no direct role of CaBP in intestinal calcium transport has been established. Indeed, several observations suggest that CaBP may be only a secondary aspect of intestinal calcium transport. For example, the time course of CaBP appearance and disappearance is out of sequence with intestinal calcium transport appearance and disappearance. In the rat, increased intestinal calcium transport occurs before appearance of CaBP and continues after disappearance of CaBP (420). In the chick, after intestinal calcium transport decays, CaBP concentration remains high (421). Oddly, cortisone diminishes rate of intestinal calcium transport but augments production of CaBP (422). Therefore despite appearance of CaBP during intestinal response to vitamin D administration, and despite its calcium binding capacity, much work remains to be done before it can be accepted that CaBP mediates the function of 1,25-$(OH)_2D_3$ in intestinal calcium transport.

4.5 Structure-Activity Relationships

Thorough evaluation of vitamin D metabolites and analogs comprises an assay of biological potency in all systems responsive to D-like compounds. Tests should include evaluation of ability to mobilize both bone calcium and phosphate (antirachitic or "line test"), as well as ability to stimulate the intestinal transport of calcium and of phosphate. These *in vivo* tests provide a general picture of compound activity in provoking several distinct and potentially differentiable responses. Inappropriately, many analogs have been assayed for antirachitic activity only; thus the possibility that the compounds might be capable of initiating selective response has been overlooked. Exclusive assay of 1,25-$(OH)_2D_3$-like compounds with the "line test" virtually ignores their potential in regulating blood calcium homeostasis. Discovery of hormone analogs that demonstrate selective activity with respect to parent hormone is not only academically satisfying, but may be of tremendous therapeutic importance.

As an adjunct to *in vivo* test systems, several *in vitro* test systems are available. These include the competitive binding protein assay (423, 424) and detection of bone resorption in cultured embryonic bone (425, 426). The former measures concentration of analog [or unlabeled (1,25-$(OH)_2D_3$] needed to displace radiolabeled 1,25-$(OH)_2D_3$ from a binding protein prepared from chick intestinal cytosol. The latter measures ability of analog to stimulate bone calcium mobilization in cultured fetal rat bone. These systems can be useful in establishing relative orders of activity, or in studying specific effects associated with certain compounds. They are perhaps most useful when used in conjunction with *in vivo* assays. However often the *in vitro* assays produce quantitative results discordant with the *in vivo* assays. Therefore caution is advised in their use. Figure 26.16

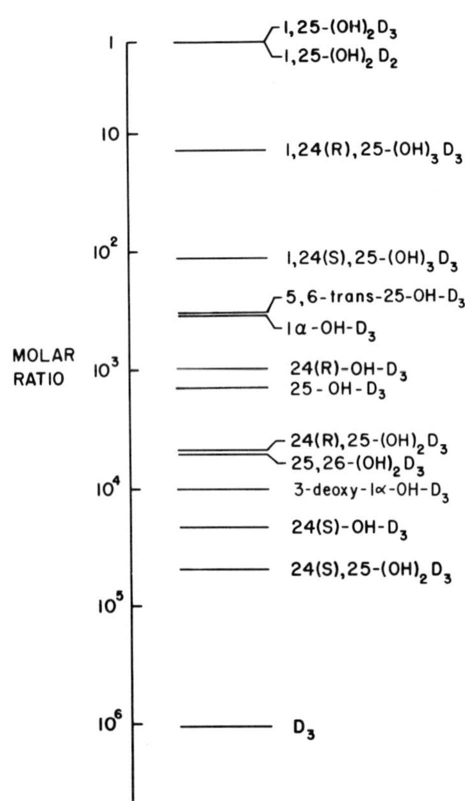

Fig. 26.16 Ability of vitamin D-like compounds to compete with radiolabeled 1,25-$(OH)_2D_3$ for chick intestinal binding protein. The log molar ratio of analog compared to 1,25-$(OH)_2D_3$ required to cause 50% displacement of radiolabeled 1,25-$(OH)_2D_3$ from the protein is plotted.

presents the relative binding order of several vitamin D metabolites in the competitive binding protein assay (409).

Considerable effort has been devoted to understanding the relative importance of 1,25-$(OH)_2D_3$'s three hydroxyl groups at target sites. *In vivo*, 1,25-$(OH)_2D_3$ is 2–5 times more potent than 25-OH-D_3, which is in turn 2–5 times more potent than D_3 itself (311, 312, 319–321). However nephrectomy abolishes activity of 25-OH-D_3 and D_3, but not 1,25-$(OH)_2D_3$. Similarly, hepatectomy diminishes activity of D_3, but not 25-OH-D_3 or 1,25-$(OH)_2D_3$ (315). Clearly the relative order established depends on normal metabolism and gives no indication of each hydroxyl's inherent importance in initiating subcellular events, except for the 1α-hydroxyl. One plausible hypothesis is that the 3-hydroxyl and the 25-hydroxyl are important only during intermediary metabolism, and the 1α-hydroxyl is important solely in triggering conformational changes in target tissue receptors. In any case, analog evaluations (Fig. 26.17) suggest that each hydroxyl influences target tissue response. For example, the entries in Fig. 26.16 demonstrate that all three hydroxyls are necessary for maximum displacement of 1,25-$(OH)_2D_3$ from the chick intestinal binding protein. 1α-Hydroxylated analogs, 3-deoxy-1,25-$(OH)_2D_3$ (not shown) 3-deoxy-1α-OH-D_3, and 1α-OH-D_3, all bind considerably less effectively than 1,25-$(OH)_2D_3$. This suggests active roles for the 3- and 25-hydroxyl groups in final manifestation of biological response. 3-Deoxy-1α-OH-D_3 is also less active than 1α-OH-D_3 *in vivo*, but only by a factor of about 30–50 (427–431). Since 3-deoxy-1,25-$(OH)_2D_3$ was unsuitably tested at saturating doses, no conclusions about its activity relative to 1,25-$(OH)_2D_3$ *in vivo* can be drawn (432). The cumulative evidence does tend to indicate that although the 3-hydroxyl may be the least important hydroxyl, it still facilitates maximum response of 1,25-$(OH)_2D_3$ *in vivo* and *in vitro*.

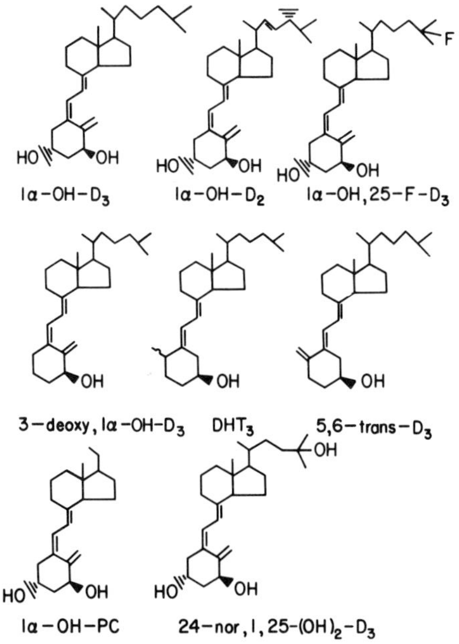

Fig. 26.17 Vitamin D analogs.

The finding that 1α-OH-D_3 is about 50% as active as 1,25-$(OH)_2D_3$ in the rat and equal in strength in the chick (433–435) does not contradict the idea that the 25-hydroxyl group is important in ultimate expression of activity, since 1α-OH-D_3 is rapidly metabolized to 1,25-$(OH)_2D_3$ in both rat and chick (436–438). Further light was shed on this question with the synthesis and evaluation of 1α-hydroxy-25-fluorovitamin D_3 (1α-OH-25-F-D_3) (439). This analog binds nearly equipotently with 1α-OH-D_3 in the competitive binding protein assay, which shows that the fluorine in the 25-position mimics a proton, at least with the intestinal binding protein. But *in vivo*, 1α-OH-25-F-D_3 is approximately 50 times less active than 1,25-$(OH)_2D_3$ in calcification, bone calcium mobilization, and intestinal calcium transport. Consequently, like the 3-hydroxyl, the 25-hydroxyl is not obligatory for physiological activity, but rather potentiates compound response and helps impose maximum activity. Practically, this demonstrates that metabolism of 1α-OH-D_3 to 1,25-$(OH)_2D_3$ is not obligatory prior to expression of activity by 1α-OH-D_3. Thus 1α-OH-D_3 may cause toxicity directly, as well as through its metabolic product 1,25-$(OH)_2D_3$.

Although the biological significance of 24-hydroxylation is not understood, its effect on activity of D compounds has been thoroughly studied. In the rat, both 24*R*- and 24*S*-OH-D_3 (Fig. 26.18) stimulate intestinal calcium transport roughly 50–70% as effectively as 25-OH-D_3 (374, 440). Only 24*R*-OH-D_3 approaches 25-OH-D_3 in bone calcium mobilization response; 24*S*-OH-D_3 lags behind in intensity and rate of response. In healing rachitic lesions ("line test"), 25-OH-D_3 and 24*R*-OH-D_3 appear to be equipotent, whereas 24*S*-OH-D_3 demonstrates no activity (Table 26.5). These data seem to indicate that 24*S*-OH-D_3-like compounds might be preferentially active in stimulation of intestinal calcium transport.

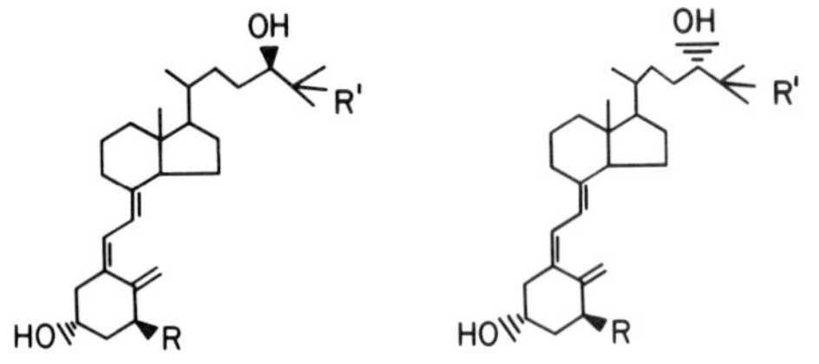

OH R' HO R 24R – OH

OH R' HO R 24S – OH

24 – OH – D_3 : R = R' = H

24,25–$(OH)_2$ –D_3 : R = H, R' = OH

1,24–$(OH)_2$ –D_3 : R = OH, R' = H

1,24,25 – $(OH)_3$ –D_3 : R = R' = OH

Fig. 26.18 The *R* and *S* forms of 24-hydroxylated vitamin D_3 metabolites.

Studies with 24*S*- and 24*R*-1,24-$(OH)_2D_3$ have shown that neither epimer manifests discretionary activity (441). At equivalent doses, 1,24*R*-OH-D_3 is somewhat more active than 1α-OH-D_3 in intestinal calcium transport and bone calcium mobilization in the rat. In bone mobilization and intestinal response, 1,24*S*-OH-D_3 is about equal in potency to 1α-OH-D_3. In antirachitic activity, 1,24*S*-$(OH)_2D_3$ is only 70% as active as 1α-OH-D_3 and 1,24*R*-OH-D_3, which are equipotent. Furthermore, the *S*-epimer has a considerably shorter duration of action. Similar results were obtained with 24*S*- and 24*R*-1,24,25-$(OH)_3D_3$ (373). Neither of the latter two compounds demonstrates differential activity with respect to the other or to 1,25-$(OH)_2D_3$. Both are less active and shorter acting than 1,25-$(OH)_2D_3$. These results

Table 26.5 Biological Activity of 24-Hydroxyvitamin D_3 Compounds in Rats[a]

	Activity, units/μg[b]		
Compound	Calcium Transport in Intestine	Mobilization of Bone Calcium	Calcification
Vitamin D_3	40	40	40
25-OH-D_3	150	150	150
24*R*-OH-D_3	150	150	150
24*S*-OH-D_3	120	<1	<1
24*R*-25-$(OH)_2D_3$	140	140	140
24*S*-25-$(OH)_2D_3$	120	<1	<1

[a] Log dose curves were determined for each compound in each system.

[b] The activity of vitamin D_3 was arbitrarily set at 40 units/μg and used as a basis for calculation of units of activity for the other compounds (11).

demonstrate quite clearly that the apparent selectivity seen with 24*S*-OH-D_3 is a result of its failure to undergo 1α-hydroxylation as well as the 24*R*-epimer *in vivo.*

It is well known that the dose required to stimulate intestinal calcium transport is 2–10 times less than the dose that is effective in causing bone calcium mobilization or in mobilizing phosphate. In the case of an analog undergoing 1α-hydroxylation only poorly, the 1α-hydroxylated metabolite could circulate in concentrations still sufficient to stimulate intestinal calcium transport. But the same concentrations might be insufficient to promote bone calcium mobilization or phosphate mobilization. Investigation with radiolabeled 24*S*- and 24*R*,25-OH-D_3 has shown that the renal 1α-hydroxylase does indeed discriminate against 24*S*,25-$(OH)_2D_3$, and selectively converts 24*R*,25-$(OH)_2D_3$ to 1,24*R*,25-$(OH)_3D_3$ (374). This is not true of the 25-hydroxylase, which accepts either 24*S*- or 24*R*-24-OH-D_3 with equal facility as substrate to produce 24,25-$(OH)_2D_3$. Therefore the data indicate that the 1α-hydroxylase is probably the most particular protein in the entire D system. Certainly the 25-hydroxylase grants more leeway in substrate differences than the 1α-hydroxylase. Moreover, intestinal calcium transport, bone calcium mobilization, and phosphate mobilization respond to either 24*S*- or 24*R*-24-hydroxylated D compounds.

Because the 1α-hydroxylase may be more exclusive than the tissue receptors, prudence is necessary in deducing structure-activity relationships from *in vivo* intestinal transport or bone mobilization responses to analogs that are not 1α-hydroxylated. For instance, if a certain non-1α-hydroxylated side chain analog demonstrates no activity *in vivo*, does this mean that intestinal and bone receptors are not responding or that the compound fails to undergo 1α-hydroxylation?

Vitamin D_2 and its metabolites can be considered to be side chain analogs of vitamin D_3. In the rat, both activity and metabolism of vitamin D_2 parallel those of D_3. The normal metabolic sequence D_2, 25-OH-D_2, and 1,25-$(OH)_2D_2$ occurs, and each metabolite mimics its corresponding D_3 metabolite in overall activity (442, 443). Even the analog 1α-OH-D_2 closely corresponds to the analog 1α-OH-D_3 in stimulating the several D responsive systems (444). Vitamin D_4, which is side chain saturated D_2, approximates D_2 in potency (332). These results indicate that neither a 22, 23 double bond, nor a 24-methyl group in the natural D_2 configuration (24*S*-methyl in D_2, 24*R*-methyl in D_4) disrupts D activity in the rat. The 24-methyl epimer of 25-OH-D_2 is essentially inactive. But there is no way of telling whether this represents discrimination by the 1α-hydroxylase or by intestinal and bone receptors.

Vitamin D_2 activity takes an entirely different course in the chick. The chick discriminates against D_2 (445, 446) such that generally vitamin D_2 and its metabolites are about 0.2–0.1 as active as D_3 and its metabolites (443). Discrimination does not occur in the functional metabolism of D_2 (442), nor at the intestinal receptor (409). It might represent an acceleration of metabolic inactivation with respect to the D_3 family (447, 448). Curiously, the 24-hydroxylated D_3 analogs also have shorter half-lives in chick than in rat (372). It is hardly likely that the 24-hydroxyl is mimicking a 24-methyl group, especially since the 24*R*-hydroxyl is in the opposite configuration compared to 24-methyl D_2. The fact remains that 24-substituted D analogs are considerably less active in chicken than in rat, and this probably represents contrasts between chick and rat metabolic deactivation and excretion. In testing D analogs, one must bear these species differences in mind.

Additional side chain analogs that are noteworthy, since they are 1α-hydroxylated, include 1α-hydroxypregcalciferol

(1α-OH-PC) (449) and 1α-nor-1,25-$(OH)_2D_3$ (450). In the rat, the former compound evokes no response in bone calcium mobilization and intestinal calcium transport. Nor does it possess antirachitic activity. Oddly, it causes ^{45}Ca release from cultured fetal rat bones at 10 times the concentration of 1α-OH-D_3. 24-Nor-1,25-$(OH)_2D_3$ is similar to 1α-OH-PC, in that it is inactive *in vivo* but does stimulate ^{45}Ca release from rat bone *in vivo.*

Other analogs of vitamin D_3 that are of interest include 5,6-*trans*-D_3 and dihydrotachysterol$_3$ (DHT_3). Each compound has been known to the medical world for some time, and each is efficacious in treating D-related diseases such as hypoparathyroidism or D-resistant rickets (20). Both analogs are converted *in vivo* to their 25-hydroxylated metabolites (451, 452). Unlike the 25-hydroxylation of D_3, 25-hydroxylations of 5,6-*trans*-D_3 and DHT_3 are unregulated, which allows accumulation of high blood levels of 25-OH-5,6-*trans*-D_3 and 25-OH-DHT_3 (453). This property, together with the substitute 1α-OH group each possesses, probably explains activity. But each is 1000–5000 times less active than 1,25-$(OH)_2D_3$. Given all the structural changes in the analogs—lack of a 3-hydroxyl group, disrupted triene system, different A-ring stereochemistry, and a hydroxyl group that only approximates the position of a 1α-hydroxyl group—it is difficult to draw structure-activity relationship inferences from these examples.

Certain conclusions concerning the structure-activity relationship of D-like compounds now seem to be apparent. All three hydroxyls of 1,25-$(OH)_2D_3$ contribute to physiological activity and are necessary for optimal dose/response ratios. However analog studies (3-deoxy compounds and 1α-OH-25-fluoro-D_3) indicate that at least the 3- and 25-hydroxyls are not obligatory for some expression of *in vivo* activity. Satisfactory responses and presumably vitamin D toxicity can be obtained with 3-deoxy or 25-fluorinated compounds. Even more flexibility is manifested by the side chain. Introduction of a double bond (Δ22), 24-methyl, or 24-hydroxyl does not eradicate activity in the rat. Stereochemistry at the 24-position does have serious effects on 1α-hydroxylase, though. On the other hand, shortening of the side chain precludes significant activity *in vivo.* More detailed knowledge must await the synthesis and evaluation of appropriate compounds.

4.6 Summary

Vitamin D_3 is rapidly converted to 25-OH-D_3 in the liver. In response to hypocalcemia, 25-OH-D_3, the major circulating metabolite of the vitamin, undergoes further metabolism in the kidney to 1,25-$(OH)_2D_3$. Then 1,25-$(OH)_2D_3$ acts on target tissues (intestine, kidney, and bone) to increase blood calcium concentration. When blood calcium concentrations rise, the synthesis of 1,25-$(OH)_2D_3$ is inhibited. Also, 1,25-$(OH)_2D_3$ inhibits its own synthesis. Hence 1,25-$(OH)_2D_3$ is actually a hormone, since it is made in one organ in response to specific stimuli, then translocates to several target organs. In true hormonal fashion, its biosynthesis is highly regulated. This understanding of the functional metabolism of vitamin D has already produced tremendous practical benefits in the treatment of some diseases. Certain complications inherent in several hyper- and hypoparathyroid diseases, as well as in chronic renal disease, are now understood in terms of disrupted or accelerated vitamin D metabolism. Indeed patients with renal disease who formerly suffered the consequences of renal osteodystrophy now can be satisfactorily treated with 1α-OH-D_3 or 1,25-$(OH)_2D_3$. In the future, it is likely that serious bone diseases besides osteomalacia will prove to involve complications of D metabolism.

5 BLOOD CALCIUM REGULATION

Current knowledge of the endocrine system controlling blood calcium concentration is summarized in Fig. 26.19. When blood calcium concentrations are in the normal physiological range, there is only a basal secretion rate of PTH, which mediates bone remodeling. Likewise, 1,25-$(OH)_2D_3$ levels in blood are minimal, since the renal 25-hydroxyvitamin D_3-1α-hydroxylase is suppressed. Vitamin D_3 ingested or synthesized during this time is metabolized in the liver to 25-$(OH)_2D_3$, which undergoes further hydroxylation in the kidney to 24,25-$(OH)_2D_3$. These two forms of the vitamin represent the major circulating metabolites of vitamin D_3 during states of normal blood calcium concentrations. In the adult mammal, CT is undetectable when blood calcium levels are normal.

When blood calcium levels fall below the normal physiological range of about 10 mg/100 ml plasma, preformed PTH is secreted from the parathyroid glands. The mechanism of PTH secretion involves calcium interaction with parathyroid gland cell membranes and a stimulation of adenyl cyclase. In response to increased cellular cyclic-AMP levels, PTH is released from secretory granules. PTH then acts at two different sites to facilitate an increase in

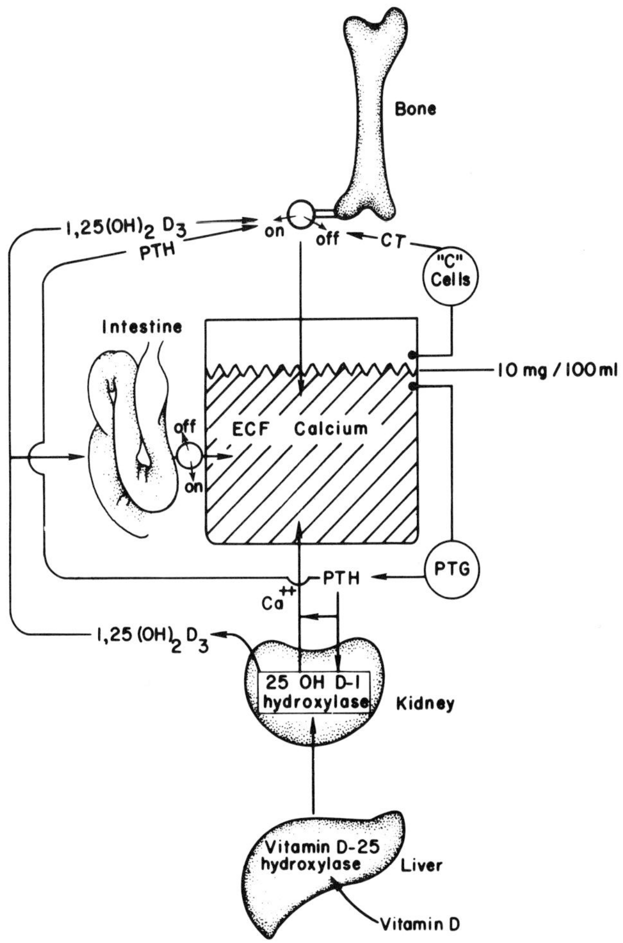

Fig. 26.19 Formalization of the blood calcium regulatory system.

blood calcium concentration. In the kidney, PTH increases renal tubular reabsorption of calcium, sparing loss of calcium in urine. A further action of PTH is the promotion of renal phosphate excretion, possibly by altering pH of intratubular fluid. Both decreased kidney cellular phosphate and PTH act to stimulate 25-hydroxyvitamin D_3-1α-hydroxylase. This enzyme draws on the relatively large circulating supply of 25-OH-D_3 to produce 1,25-$(OH)_2D_3$.

PTH also acts on bone, in concert with 1,25-$(OH)_2D_3$, to mobilize calcium from the bone fluid compartment. This action taps an organism's largest store of calcium to supply blood needs.

The 1,25-$(OH)_2D_3$ formed in response to PTH secretion promotes an increase in blood calcium concentration by working in three organs. In combination with PTH, it augments calcium mobilization from bone. Most important, however, 1,25-$(OH)_2D_3$ accumulates in the intestine. There, the D metabolite is the sole known hormone responsible for stimulating active transport of calcium from the mucosal side of intestine against a concentration gradient, into the intestinal cell, with ultimate delivery of calcium to ECF. It is probable but not firmly established that 1,25-$(OH)_2D_3$ exercises its ability to stimulate intestinal calcium transport by a classical steroid hormone mechanism. With high affinity, 1,25-$(OH)_2D_3$ binds to a specific intestinal cytosol receptor protein and translocates to the nucleus, with a resultant increase in mRNA synthesis. Actual transcription products subsequent to 1,25-$(OH)_2D_3$ accumulation have yet to be found. Nevertheless, the intestinal action of 1,25-$(OH)_2D_3$ results in accumulation of calcium from diet in the organism.

In the kidney, where 1,25-$(OH)_2D_3$ also functions, it promotes calcium conservation by promoting renal tubular reabsorption of calcium. Finally, it inhibits its own synthesis in feedback regulation and switches on the renal 24-hydroxylase, which reestablishes vitamin D_3 metabolism as it was prior to calcium need. Blood calcium concentration, now returned to normal by the actions of PTH and 1,25-$(OH)_2D_3$ jointly on bone and kidney, and by 1,25-$(OH)_2D_3$ alone on intestine, inhibits the secretion of PTH. Thus with the feedback inhibition of 1,25-$(OH)_2D_3$ synthesis by 1,25-$(OH)_2D_3$ itself, and the repression of PTH secretion by blood calcium, the hormonal loop is complete.

It has not been proved that CT functions routinely in maintaining calcium homeostastis. CT certainly can decrease blood calcium levels by operating in opposition to PTH in bone and kidney. Whether it does so in adults remains to be seen. However it can be speculated that, CT may control postprandial hypercalcemia and electrolyte balance, particularly in the young.

Primarily two hormones monitor blood calcium and maintain homeostasis. The peptide hormone PTH controls kidney and bone calcium metabolism and controls synthesis of the steroid hormone 1,25-$(OH)_2D_3$. The steroid hormone 1,25-$(OH)_2D_3$ also manages kidney and bone calcium metabolism, but additionally is responsible for promoting calcium intake through the gut. The members of the triumverate of blood calcium, PTH, and 1,25-$(OH)_2D_3$ are locked in concert, each responding to changes in the other, in a balanced system that regulates blood calcium. Perhaps CT is also part of this order.

REFERENCES

1. A. Cuthbert, Ed., *Calcium and Cellular Function*, Macmillan, London, 1970.
2. H. Rasmussen, *Textbook of Endocrinology*, 5th ed., Saunders, Philadelphia, 1974, Ch. 11.
3. H. Rasmussen and P. Bordier, *Bone Cells, Mineral Homeostasis and Skeletal Remodeling*, Williams & Wilkin, Baltimore, 1973.
4. R. V. Talmage and P. L. Munson, Eds., *Calcium, Parathyroid Hormone and the Calcitonins*, Excerpta Medica, Amsterdam, 1972.

5. G. Nichols, Jr., and R. H. Wasserman, Eds., *Cellular Mechanisms for Calcium Transfer and Homeostasis*, Academic Press, New York, 1971.
6. B. S. Roof, C. F. Piel, J. Hansen, and H. H. Fudenberg, *Mech. Aging Develop.*, **5,** 289 (1976).
7. A. S. Posner and F. Betts, *Acc. Chem. Res.*, **8,** 273 (1975).
8. J. F. Habener, in *Polypeptide Hormones: Molecular and Cellular Aspects*, Elsevier, New York, 1976, p. 197.
9. J. T. Potts, Jr., in *Peptide Hormones*, J. A. Parsons, Ed., University Park Press, Baltimore, 1976, Ch. 8.
10. H. F. DeLuca, *Ann. Intern. Med.*, **85,** 367 (1976).
11. H. F. DeLuca, *J. Lab. Clin. Med.*, **87,** 7 (1976).
12. H. F. DeLuca, *Clin. Endocrinol.*, **5,** Suppl. 97S (1976).
13. A. B. Borle, *Ann. Rev. Physiol.*, **36,** 361 (1974).
14. G. D. Aurbach, H. T. Keutmann, H. D. Niall, G. W. Tregear, J. L. O'Riordan, R. Marcus, S. J. Marc, and J. T. Potts, Jr., *Rec. Progr. Hormone Res.*, **28,** 353 (1972).
15. J. T. Potts, Jr., H. T. Keutmann, H. D. Niall, and G. W. Tregear, *Vitam. Horm.*, **29,** 41 (1971).
16. D. H. Copp, *Ann. Rev. Physiol.*, **32,** 61 (1970).
17. H. F. DeLuca and H. K. Schnoes, *Ann. Rev. Biochem.*, **45,** 631 (1976).
18. H. F. DeLuca, *Am. J. Clin. Nutr.*, **29,** 1258 (1976).
19. H. F. DeLuca, *Acta Orthopaed. Scand.*, **46,** 286 (1975).
20. H. K. Schnoes and H. F. DeLuca, *Vitam. Horm.*, **32,** 385 (1974).
21. J. L. Napoli, *Ann. Rep. Med. Chem.*, **10,** 295 (1975).
22. H. F. DeLuca, *Fed. Proc.*, **33,** 2211 (1974).
23. M. F. Holick and H. F. DeLuca, *Ann. Rev. Med.*, **25,** 349 (1974).
24. A. W. Norman and H. Henry, *Rec. Prog. Hormone Res.*, **30,** 431 (1974).
25. E. Kodicek, *Lancet*, **1,** 325 (1974).
26. R. H. Wasserman and R. A. Corradino, *Ann. Rev. Biochem.*, **40,** 501 (1971).
27. C. W. Cooper, *Ann. Clin. Lab. Sci.*, **6,** 119 (1976).
28. S. F. Queener and N. H. Bell, *Metabolism*, **24,** 555 (1975).
29. P. F. Hirsch and P. L. Munson, *Physiol. Rev.*, **49,** 548 (1969).
30. R. H. Savage, *Guys Hosp. Rep.*, **118,** 433 (1969).
31. J. T. Potts, Jr., H. D. Niall, and L. J. Deftos, *Curr. Top. Exp. Endocrinol.*, **1,** 151 (1971).
32. H. Zondeck, *Klin. Wochenschr.*, **44,** 528 (1966).
33. C. Marnay and M. Prelot, *Arch. Sci. Physiol.*, **11,** 77 (1957).
34. D. H. Copp and E. C. Cameron, *Science*, **134,** 2038 (1961).
35. D. H. Copp, E. C. Cameron, B. A. Cheney, A. G. F. Davidson, and K. G. Henze, *Endocrinology*, **70,** 638 (1962).
36. D. H. Copp, A. G. F. Davidson, and B. L. Henry, *Proc. Can. Fed. Biol. Soc.*, **4,** 17 (1961).
37. D. H. Copp, *Rec. Prog. Hormone Res.*, **20,** 59 (1964).
38. M. A. Kumar, G. V. Foster, and I. MacIntyre, *Lancet*, **2,** 480 (1963).
39. P. L. Munson, in *The Parathyroids*, R. O. Green and R. V. Talmage, Eds., Thomas, Springfield, Ill., 1971, p. 94.
40. P. F. Hirsch, G. F. Gauthier, and P. L. Munson, *Endocrinology*, **73,** 244 (1963).
41. P. F. Hirsch, E. F. Voelkel, and P. L. Munson, *Science*, **146,** 412 (1964).
42. P. L. Munson, P. F. Hirsch, H. B. Brewer, R. A. Reisfeld, C. W. Cooper, A. B. Wasthed, H. Orino, and J. T. Potts, Jr., *Rec. Prog. Hormone Res.*, **24,** 589 (1968).
43. R. V. Talmage, J. Neuenschwander, and L. Kraintz, *Fed. Proc.*, **23,** 204 (1964).
44. R. V. Talmage, J. Neunschwander, and L. Kraintz, *Endocrinology*, **76,** 103 (1965).
45. G. V. Foster, A. Baghdiantz, M. A. Kumar, E. Slack, H. A. Soliman, and I. MacIntyre, *Nature*, **202,** 1303 (1964).
46. A. D. Care, *Nature*, **205,** 1289 (1965).
47. D. H. Copp, *Ann. Rev. Pharmacol.*, **9,** 327 (1969).
48. J. T. Potts, Jr., *Fed. Proc.*, **29,** 1200 (1970).
49. M. B. Clark, G. W. Boyd, P. G. H. Byfield, and G. V. Foster, *Lancet*, **2,** 74 (1969).
50. A. H. Tashjian, Jr., B. G. Howland, K. E. W. Melvin, and C. S. Hill, Jr., *New Engl. J. Med.*, **283,** 890 (1970).
51. L. T. Deftos, *Metabolism*, **20,** 1122 (1971).
52. L. J. Deftos, E. G. Watts, D. L. Copp, and J. T. Potts, Jr., *Endocrinology*, **94,** 155 (1974).
53. T. K. Gray and P. L. Munson, *Science*, **166,** 512 (1969).
54. P. F. Hirsch, *J. Exp. Zool.*, **178,** 139 (1971).
55. A. D. Care, R. F. L. Bates, R. Swaminathan, C. G. Scanes, M. Peacock, E. B. Mawer, C. M. Taylor, H. F. DeLuca, S. Tomlinson, and J. L. H. O'Riordan, in *Calcium Regulating Hormones*,

R. V. Talmage, M. Owen, and T. A. Parsons, Eds., American Elsevier, New York, 1975, p. 100.

56. A. D. Care, N. H. Bell, and R. F. L. Bates, *J. Endocrinol.*, **51,** 381 (1971).
57. C. W. Cooper, J. E. McGwigan, W. H. Schweisinger, R. L. Brubaker, and P. L. Munson, *Endocrinology*, **89,** 262 (1971).
58. A. D. Care, J. B. Bruce, J. Boelkins, A. D. Kenny, H. Conaway, and C. S. Anast, *Endocrinology*, **89,** 262 (1971).
59. R. F. Gittes, S. V. Toverud, and C. W. Cooper, *Endocrinology*, **82,** 83 (1968).
60. A. D. Care, R. F. C. Bates, and H. J. Gitelman, *J. Endocrinol.*, **48,** 1 (1970).
61. F. Moya, A. Nieto, and J. L. R. Candela, *Eur. J. Biochem.*, **55,** 407 (1975).
62. R. Neher, B. Riniker, W. Rittal, and H. Zuber, *Helv. Chim. Acta*, **51,** 1900 (1968).
63. L. J. Deftos, D. Powell, J. G. Parthemore, and J. T. Potts, Jr., *J. Clin. Invest.*, **52,** 3109 (1973).
64. M. A. Aliapoulios, P. Goldhaber, and P. L. Munson, *Science*, **151,** 330 (1966).
65. J. L. H. O'Riordan and G. D. Aurbach, *Endocrinology*, **82,** 377 (1968).
66. J. Friedman, W. Y. W. Au, and L. G. Raisz, *Endocrinology*, **82,** 149 (1968).
67. D. N. Kaln, A. Hadji-Georgopoulos, and G. V. Foster, *Endocrinology*, **98,** 534 (1976).
68. C. C. Johnston and W. P. Deiss, *Endocrinology*, **78,** 1139 (1960).
69. D. C. Klein, H. Morii, and R. V. Talmage, *Proc. Soc. Exp. Biol. Med.*, **124,** 627 (1967).
70. J. Friedman and L. G. Raisz, *Science*, **150,** 1465 (1965).
71. S. J. Marx, C. Woodward, and G. D. Aurback, *Science*, **178,** 999 (1972).
72. S. J. Marx and G. D. Aurbach, in *Calcium Regulating Hormones*, R. V. Talmage, M. Owen, and J. A. Parsons, Eds., American Elsevier, New York, 1975, p. 163.
73. N. H. Bell and P. H. Stern, *Am. J. Physiol*, **218,** 64 (1970).
74. D. C. Sears, *Endocrinology*, **88,** 1021 (1971).
75. L. Zichner, *Res. Exp. Med.*, **157,** 95 (1970).
76. D. M. Kallio, P. R. Garant, and C. Minking, *J. Ultrastruct. Res.*, **39,** 205 (1972).
77. M. E. Holtrop, L. G. Raisz, and H. A. Simmons, *J. Cell Biol.*, **60,** 346 (1974).
78. A. D. Kenny and C. A. Heiskell, *Proc. Soc. Exp. Biol. Med.*, **125,** 269 (1965).
79. T. J. Martin, C. J. Robinson, and I. MacIntyre, *Lancet*, **1,** 876 (1968).
80. C. J. Robinson, T. J. Martin, and I. MacIntyre, *Lancet*, **2,** 83 (1966).
81. O. L. M. Bigvuet, J. van der Sluys Veer, and A. P. Jansen, *Lancet*, **1,** 876 (1968).
82. F. R. Singer, N. J. Y. Woodhouse, O. K. Parkinson, and G. F. Joplin, *Clin. Sci.*, **37,** 181 (1969).
83. M. Cochran, M. Peacock, C. Sachs, and B. E. C. Nordin, *Brit. Med. J.*, **1,** 135 (1970).
84. H. G. Haas, M. A. Dambacher, J. Gunvaga, and T. Lauffenburger, *J. Clin. Invest.*, **50,** 2709 (1971).
85. N. Loreau, C. Lepreux, and R. Ardaillon, *Biochem. J.*, **150,** 305 (1975).
86. G. L. Nielson, L. R. Chase, and G. D. Aurbach, *Endocrinology*, **86,** 511 (1970).
78. A. B. Borle, *J. Membrane. Biol.*, **21,** 125 (1975).
88. E. B. Olson, H. F. DeLuca, and J. T. Potts, Jr., *Endocrinology*, **90,** 151 (1972).
89. T. K. Gray, F. A. Bieberdorf, S. Morwaski, and J. S. Fordtran, *J. Clin. Invest.*, **52,** 3084 (1973).
90. C. W. Cooper, P. F. Hirsch, and P. L. Munson, *Endocrinology*, **86,** 406 (1970).
91. G. Milhand, A. M. Perault-Staub, and J. F. Staub, *J. Physiol.* (London), **222,** 559 (1972).
92. A. H. Tashjian, Jr., H. J. Wolfe, and E. F. Voelkel, *Am. J. Med.*, **56,** 840 (1974).
93. J. T. Potts, Jr., and L. J. Deftos, in *Duncan's Diseases of Metabolism*, 7th ed., P. K. Bondy and L. E. Rosenburg, Eds., Saunders, Philadelphia, 1974, p. 1225.
94. M. C. Chapuy, P. Meunier, M. Terrier, L. David, and G. Vignon, *Pathol. Biol.*, **23,** 349 (1975).
95. G. Coutris, J. Cayla, J. Rondier, J. N. Talbot, J. P. Bonvarot, and G. Milhand, *Rev. Rhumatol. Mal. Osteoartic.*, **42,** 759 (1975).
96. A. Avramides, R. F. Baker, and S. Wallach, *Metabolism*, **23,** 1037 (1974).
97. R. Sauer, H. D. Niall, and J. T. Potts, Jr., *Fed. Proc.*, **29,** 728 (1970).
98. R. Neher, B. Riniker, H. Zuber, W. Rittel, and F. W. Kahnt, *Helv. Chim. Acta*, **51,** 917 (1968).
99. J. T. Potts, Jr., H. D. Niall, H. T. Keutmann, H. B. Brewer, and L. J. Deftos, *Proc. Nat. Acad. Sci., USA*, **59,** 1321 (1968).
100. D. H. Bell, W. F. Barg, Jr., D. F. Colucci, M. C. Davies, C. Dziobkowski, M. E. Englert, E. Heyder, R. Paul, and E. H. Sredeker, *J. Am. Chem. Soc.*, **90,** 2704 (1968).
101. N. Rittel, M. Brugger, B. Kamber, B. Riniker, and P. Sieber, *Helv. Chim. Acta*, **51,** 924 (1968).
102. H. B. Brewer, Jr., H. T. Keutmann, J. T. Potts, Jr., R. A. Reisfield, R. Schlueter, and P. L. Munson, *J. Biol. Chem.*, **243,** 5739 (1968).

103. H. D. Niall, H. Pehasi, P. Gilbert, R. C. Meyers, F. G. Williams, and J. T. Potts, Jr., *Fed. Proc.*, **28,** 661 (1969).

104. H. B. Brewer and R. Roman, *Proc. Nat. Acad. Sci., USA*, **63,** 940 (1969).

105. J. T. Potts, Jr., *Fed. Proc.*, **29,** 1200 (1970).

106. H. D. Niall, H. T. Keutmann, D. H. Copp, and J. T. Potts, Jr., *Proc. Nat. Acad. Sci., USA*, **64,** 771 (1969).

107. R. K. O'Dor, C. O. Parkes, and D. H. Copp, *Can. J. Biochem.*, **47,** 823 (1969).

108. S. Guttmann, J. Pless, R. L. Huguenin, E. Sandrin, H. Bossert, and K. Zehnder, *Helv. Chim. Acta*, **52,** 1789 (1969).

109. H. T. Keutmann, J. A. Parsons, J. T. Potts, Jr., and R. J. Schlueter, *J. Biol. Chem.*, **245,** 1491 (1970).

110. M. Otani, H. Yamauchi, T. Meguro, S. Kitazawa, S. Watanabe, and H. Orimo, *J. Biochem.*, **79,** 345 (1976).

111. T. Noda and K. Narita, *J. Biochem.*, **79,** 353 (1976).

112. T. Morikawa, E. Munekata, S. Sakakibara, T. Noda, and M. Otani, *Experientia*, **32,** 1104 (1976).

113. H. J. Burford, D. A. Ontjes, C. W. Cooper, A. F. Parlon, and P. F. Hirsch, *Endocrinology*, **96,** 340 (1975).

114. P. G. H. Byfield, E. W. Matthews, J. N. M. Heersche, G. A. Boorman, S. I. Girgis, and I. MacIntyre, *FEBS Lett.*, **65,** 238 (1976).

115. D. Raulais, J. Hogaman, D. A. Ontjes, R. L. Lundblad, and H. S. Kingdon, *Eur. J. Biochem.*, **64,** 607 (1976).

116. P. G. H. Byfield, J. L. McLoughlin, E. W. Matthews, and I. MacIntyre, *FEBS Lett.*, **65,** 242 (1976).

117. R. Neher, B. Riniker, R. Maier, P. G. H. Byfield, T. V. Gudmundsson, and I. MacIntyre, *Nature* (London), **220,** 984 (1968).

118. B. Riniker, R. Neher, R. Maier, F. W. Kahnt, P. G. H. Byfield, T. V. Gudmundsson, L. Galante, and I. MacIntyre, *Helv. Chim. Acta*, **51,** 1738 (1968).

119. A. Nieto, F. Moya, and J. C. R. Candela, *Biochim. Biophys. Acta*, **322,** 383 (1973).

120. S. J. Marx, C. Woodward, G. D. Aurbach, H. Glossman, and H. T. Keutmann, *J. Biol. Chem.*, **248,** 4797 (1973).

121. S. J. Marx, C. Woodward, and G. D. Aurbach, *Science*, **178,** 999 (1972).

122. M. A. Kumar, E. Slack, A. Edwards, H. A. Soliman, A. Baghdiantz, G. V. Foster, and I. MacIntyre, *J. Endocrinol.*, **33,** 469 (1965).

123. S. Guttmann, J. Pless, R. Huguenin, E. Sandrin, and K. Zehnder, *Helv. Chim. Acta*, **52,** 1789 (1969).

124. P. Sieber, M. Brugger, B. Kamber, B. Riniker, W. Rittel, R. Maier, and M. Staehelin, in *Calcitonin 1969; Proceedings of the Second International Symposium*, S. F. Taylor and G. V. Foster, Eds., Springer-Verlag, New York, 1969, p. 28.

125. W. Rittel, R. Maier, M. Bruegger, B. Kamber, B. Riniker, and P. Siebe, *Experientia*, **32,** 246 (1976).

126. R. Maier, B. Kambler, B. Riniker, and W. Rittel, *Horm. Metab. Res.*, **2,** 511 (1975).

127. R. Maier, in *Calcified Tissues 1975*, S. Pors Nielson and E. Hjørsting-Hansen, Eds., Fadl, Copenhagen, 1975, p. 317.

128. R. Maier, B. Kamber, B. Riniker, and W. Rittel, *Clin. Endocrinol.*, **5,** 3275 (1976).

129. J. Pless, W. Bauer, H. Bosserts, K. Zehnder, and S. Guttman, in *Endocrinology 1971; Proceedings of the Third International Symposium*, S. Taylor, Ed., Heineman, London, 1972, p. 67.

130. H. B. Brewer, Jr., H. T. Keutmann, R. A. Reisfield, P. C. Munson, R. J. Schlueter, and J. T. Potts, Jr., *Fed. Proc.*, **27,** 690 (1968).

131. R. Neher, B. Riniker, P. G. H. Byfield, T. V. Gudmundsson, and I. MacIntyre, *Nature* (London), **220,** 984 (1968).

132. W. G. MacCallum and C. Voegtlin, *J. Exp. Med.*, **11,** 118 (1909).

133. J. Greenwald, *Am. J. Med.*, **28,** 103 (1911).

134. J. B. Collip, *J. Biol. Chem.*, **73,** 395 (1925).

135. H. M. Patt and A. B. Luckhardt, *Endocrinology*, **31,** 384 (1942).

136. G. D. Aurbach, *J. Biol. Chem.*, **234,** 3179 (1959).

137. H. Rasmussen and L. C. Craig, *J. Am. Chem. Soc.*, **81,** 5003 (1959).

138. H. Rasmussen and L. C. Craig, *Biochim. Biophys. Acta*, **56,** 332 (1962).

139. G. D. Aurbach and J. T. Potts, Jr., *Endocrinology*, **75,** 290 (1964).

140. H. Rasmussen, Y. L. Sze, and R. Young, *J. Biol. Chem.*, **239,** 2852 (1964).

141. J. T. Potts, Jr., and G. D. Aurbach, in *The Parathyroid Glands*, P. J. Gaillard, R. V. Talmage, and A. M. Budy, Eds., University of Chicago Press, Chicago, 1975, p. 53.

142. D. H. Copp and A. G. F. Davidson, *Proc. Soc. Exp. Biol. Med.*, **107,** 342 (1961).

143. W. Y. W. Au, A. P. Poland, P. H. Stern, and L. G. Raisz, *J. Clin. Invest.*, **49,** 1039 (1970).

144. L. M. Sherwood, G. P. Mayer, C. F. Ramberg, D. S. Kronfeld, G. D. Aurbach, and J. T. Potts, Jr., *Endocrinology*, **83,** 1043 (1968).
145. L. M. Sherwood, J. T. Potts, Jr., A. D. Care, G. P. Mayer, and G. D. Aurbach, *Nature*, **209,** 52 (1966).
146. L. M. Sherwood, W. B. Lundberg, Jr., J. H. Targovnik, J. S. Rodman, and A. Seyfer, *Am. J. Med.*, **50,** 658 (1971).
147. J. H. Targovnik, J. S. Rodman, and L. M. Sherwood, *Endocrinology*, **88,** 1477 (1971).
148. S. B. Oldham, J. A. Kischer, C. C. Capen, G. W. Sizemore, and C. D. Arnaud, *Am. J. Med.*, **50,** 560 (1971).
149. P. J. Gaillard, *Develop. Biol.*, **1,** 152 (1959).
150. R. M. Buckle, *J. Endocrinol.*, **42,** 529 (1968).
151. G. P. Mayer, *Endocrinology*, **94** (Suppl.), A-181 (1974).
152. J. F. Habener and J. T. Potts, Jr., *Endocrinology*, **98,** 209 (1976).
153. G. P. Mayer, *Endocrinology*, **92** (Suppl.), A-160 (1973).
154. J. F. Habener and J. T. Potts, Jr., in *Handbook of Physiology*, Vol. 7, G. D. Aurbach, Ed., American Physiology Society, Washington, D.C., 1976, Ch. 13.
155. A. D. Care, L. M. Sherwood, J. T. Potts, Jr., and G. D. Aurbach, *Nature*, **209,** 55 (1966).
156. L. R. Dufresne, R. Anderson, and H. J. Gietelman, *Clin. Res.*, **19,** 529 (1971).
157. M. Abe and L. M. Sherwood, *Biochem. Biophys. Res. Commun.*, **48,** 396 (1972).
158. G. L. Melson, L. R. Chase, and G. D. Aurbach, *Endocrinology*, **86,** 511 (1970).
159. R. Marcus and G. D. Aurbach, *Biochim. Biophys. Acta*, **242,** 410 (1971).
160. D. Butler and S. Jard, *Pfluegers Arch.*, **331,** 172 (1972).
161. R. V. Talmage and F. W. Kraintz, *Proc. Soc. Exp. Biol. Med.*, **85,** 416 (1954).
162. B. R. Edwards, R. A. C. Sutten, and J. H. Dirks, *Clin. Res*, **20,** 592 (1972).
163. Z. S. Agus, J. B. Puschett, D. Senesky, and M. Goldberg, *J. Clin. Invest.*, **50,** 617 (1971).
164. J. P. Barlet, and A. D. Care, *Horm. Metab. Res.*, **4,** 315 (1972).
165. M. G. Brunette, L. Taleb, and S. Cannier, *Am. J. Physiol.*, **225,** 1076 (1973).
166. J. B. Puschett and M. Goldberg, *J. Lab. Clin. Med.*, **73,** 956 (1969).
167. R. C. Morris, Jr., and E. McSherry, *J. Clin. Invest.*, **50,** 67a (1971).
168. U. S. Barzel, *Lancet*, **1,** 1329 (1971).
169. F. P. Muldowney, D. V. Carroll, J. F. Donohue, and R. Freaney, *Quart. J. Med.*, **40,** 487 (1971).
170. T. Uchikawa, A. B. Borle, and R. J. Midgett, in *Calcified Tissues, 1975*, S. Pors Nielson and E. Hjørsting-Hansen, Eds., Fadl, Copenhagen, 1975, p. 284.
171. L. R. Chase and G. D. Aurbach, *J. Biol. Chem.*, **245,** 1520 (1970).
172. W. A. Peck, J. Carpenter, K. Messinger, and D. DeBra, *Endocrinology*, **92,** 692 (1973).
173. S. Rodan and G. Rodan, *J. Biol. Chem.*, **249,** 3068 (1974).
174. G. Vaes, *Nature*, **219,** 939 (1968).
175. H. Rasmussen, M. Pechet, and D. Fast, *J. Clin. Invest.*, **47,** 1843 (1968).
176. D. G. Klein and L. G. Raisz, *Endocrinology*, **89,** 819 (1971).
177. A. Delong, J. Klinblatt, and H. Rasmussen, *Calc. Tiss. Res.*, **47,** 1843 (1968).
178. M. P. M. Hermann-Erlee and J. M. van den Meer, *Endocrinology*, **94,** 424 (1974).
179. D. Dziak and P. Stern, *Endocrinology*, **97,** 1281 (1975).
180. N. Nagata, M. Sasaki, N. Kimura, and K. Nakane, *Endocrinology*, **96,** 725 (1975).
181. L. G. Raisz, *J. Clin. Invest.*, **44,** 103 (1965).
182. L. G. Raisz, *N. Engl. J. Med.*, **282,** 909 (1970).
183. H. B. Brewer, *N. Engl. J. Med.*, **291,** 1081 (1974).
184. A. M. Parfitt, *Metabolism*, **25,** 909 (1976).
185. H. Rohr, *Klin. Wochenschr.*, **42,** 1209 (1964).
186. S. E. Weisbrode, C. C. Capen, and L. A. Nagode, *Am. J. Pathol.*, **75,** 529 (1974).
187. M. E. Holtrop, L. G. Raisz, and H. A. Simmons, *J. Cell. Biol.*, **60,** 346 (1974).
188. C. L. Johnston, Jr., W. P. Deiss, and E. G. Miner, *J. Biol. Chem.*, **237,** 3560 (1962).
189. R. V. Talmage and R. A. Meyer, Jr., in *Handbook of Physiology*, Vol. 7, G. D. Aurbach, Ed., American Physiological Society, Washington, D.C., 1976, Ch. 14.
190. W. E. Roberts, *Am. J. Anat.*, **143,** 363 (1975).
191. W. E. Roberts, *Arch. Oral Bio.*, **29,** 465 (1975).
192. R. V. Talmage, *Clin. Orthopaed.*, **67,** 210 (1969).
193. C. W. Cooper, C. W. Yates, and R. V. Talmage, *Proc. Soc. Exp. Biol. Med.*, **119,** 81 (1965).
194. S. B. Doty, C. W. Yates, W. E. Cotz, W. Kisecleski, and R. V. Talmage, *Proc. Soc. Exp. Biol. Med.*, **114,** 77 (1965).
195. W. F. Neuman, B. J. Muliyan, M. W. Neumann, and K. Lane, *Am. J. Physiol.*, **224,** 600 (1973).
196. R. V. Talmage, *Calc. Tiss. Res.*, **17,** 103 (1975).

197. A. D. Kenny and C. D. Dache, *J. Endocrinol.*, **62,** 15 (1974).

198. H. T. Keutmann, P. M. Barling, G. N. Hendy, G. V. Segre, H. D. Niall, G. D. Aurbach, J. T. Potts, Jr., and J. L. H. O'Riordon, *Biochemistry*, **10,** 2779 (1971).

199. J. S. Woodhead, J. L. H. O'Riordon, H. T. Keutmann, M. L. Stoltz, B. F. Dawson, H. D. Niall, C. J. Robinson, and J. T. Potts, Jr., *Biochemistry*, **10,** 2787 (1971).

200. H. T. Keutmann, P. M. Barling, G. N. Hendy, G. V. Segre, H. D. Niall, G. D. Aurbach, J. T. Potts, Jr., and J. L. H. O'Riordan, *Biochemistry*, **13,** 1646 (1974).

201. J. L. H. O'Riordan, J. T. Potts, Jr., and G. D. Aurbach, *Endocrinology*, **89,** 234 (1971).

202. H. B. Brewer, Jr., and R. Ronan, *Proc. Nat. Acad. Sci. USA*, **67,** 1862 (1970).

203. H. D. Niall, H. J. Keutmann, R. Sauer, M. L. Hogan, B. F. Dawson, G. D. Aurbach, and J. T. Potts, Jr., Hoppe-Seyler's *Z. Physiol. Chem.*, **351,** 1586 (1970).

204. R. T. Sauer, H. D. Niall, M. L. Hogan, H. T. Keutmann, J. L. H. O'Riordan, and J. T. Potts, Jr., *Biochemistry*, **13,** 1994 (1974).

205. H. B. Brewer, Jr., T. Fairwell, R. Ronan, G. W. Sizemore, and C. D. Arnaud, *Proc. Nat. Acad. Sci, USA*, **69,** 3585 (1972).

206. H. D. Niall, R. T. Sauer, J. W. Jacobs, H. T. Keutmann, G. V. Segre, J. L. H. O'Riordan, G. D. Aurbach, and J. T. Potts, Jr., *Proc. Nat. Acad. Sci. USA*, **71,** 384 (1974).

207. R. M. Andreatta, A. Hartmann, A. Jöhl, B. Kamber, R. Maier, B. Riniker, W. Rittel, and P. Sieber, *Helv. Chim. Acta*, **56,** 470 (1973).

208. H. T. Keutmann, H. D. Niall, J. W. Jacobs, P. M. Barling, G. N. Hendy, J. L. H. O'Riordan, and J. T. Potts, Jr., in *Calcium Regulating Hormones*, R. V. Talmage, M. Owen, and T. A. Parsons, Eds., American Elsevier, New York, 1975, p. 9.

209. H. T. Keutmann, H. D. Niall, J. L. H. O'Riordan, and J. T. Potts, Jr., *Biochemistry*, **14,** 1842 (1975).

210. H. B. Brewer, Jr., T. Fairwell, R. Ronan, W. Rittel, and C. Arnaud, in *Calcium Regulating Hormones*, R. V. Talmage, M. Owen, and T. A. Parsons, Eds., American Elsevier, New York, 1975, p. 23.

211. G. V. Segre and J. T. Potts, Jr., *Endocrinology*, **98,** 1294 (1976).

212. C. A. Bader, J. D. Monet, P. Rivaille, C. M. Gaubert, M. S. Moukhtar, and J. L. Funck-Brentano, *Endocrinol. Res. Commun.*, **3,** 167 (1976).

213. J. T. Potts, Jr., *Clin. Endocrinol.*, **5,** 307s (1976).

214. B. Kemper, J. F. Habener, R. C. Mulligan, J. T. Potts, Jr., and A. Rich, *Proc. Nat. Acad. Sci. USA*, **71,** 3731 (1974).

215. J. F. Habener, B. Kemper, J. T. Potts, Jr., and A. Rich, *Biochem. Biophys. Res. Commun.*, **67,** 1114 (1975).

216. J. F. Habener, B. Kemper, J. T. Potts, Jr., and A. Rich, *J. Clin. Invest.*, **56,** 1378 (1975).

217. B. Kemper, *Nature*, **262,** 321 (1976).

218. B. Kemper, J. F. Habener, J. T. Potts, Jr., and A. Rich, *Biochemistry*, **15,** 15 (1976).

219. J. F. Habener, J. T. Potts, Jr., and A. Rich, *J. Biol. Chem.*, **251,** 3893 (1976).

220. J. F. Habener, B. Kemper, M. Ernst, A. Rich, and J. T. Potts, Jr., *Clin. Res.*, **23,** 321A (1975).

221. B. Kemper, J. F. Habener, J. T. Potts, Jr., and A. Rich, *Biochemistry*, **15,** 15 (1976).

222. J. W. Hamilton, R. R. MacGregor, L. L. H. Chu, and D. V. Cohn, *Endocrinology*, **89,** 1440 (1971).

223. J. W. Hamilton, F. W. Spierto, R. R. MacGregor, and D. V. Cohn, *J. Biol. Chem.*, **246,** 3224 (1971).

224. D. V. Cohn, R. R. MacGregor, L. L. H. Chu, J. R. Kimmel, and J. W. Hamilton, *Proc. Nat. Acad. Sci. USA*, **69,** 1521 (1972).

225. J. F. Habener, B. Kemper, J. T. Potts, Jr., and A. Rich, *Science*, **178,** 630 (1972).

226. B. Kemper, J. F. Mabener, J. T. Potts, Jr., and A. Rich, *Proc. Nat. Acad. Sci. USA*, **69,** 643 (1972).

227. L. L. H. Chu, R. R. MacGregor, P. I. Liu, J. W. Hamilton, and D. V. Cohn, *J. Clin. Invest.*, **52,** 3089 (1973).

228. R. R. MacGregor, L. L. H. Chu, J. W. Hamilton, and D. V. Cohn, *Endocrinology*, **92,** 1312 (1973).

229. L. L. H. Chu, R. R. MacGregor, C. S. Anast, J. W. Hamilton, and D. V. Cohn, *Endocrinology*, **93,** 915 (1973).

230. L. K. Chu, W. Y. Huang, E. T. Littledike, J. W. Hamilton, and D. V. Cohn, *Biochemistry*, **14,** 3631 (1975).

231. J. M. Canterbury, G. S. Levy, and E. Reiss, *J. Clin. Invest.*, **52,** 524 (1973).

232. C. D. Arnaud, G. W. Sizemore, S. B. Oldham, J. A. Fischer, H. S. Tsao, and E. T. Littledike, *Am. J. Med.*, **50,** 630 (1971).

233. J. F. Habener, D. Powell, T. M. Murray, G. P. Mayer, and J. T. Potts, Jr., *Proc. Nat. Acad. Sci. USA*, **68,** 2986 (1971).

234. J. F. Habener, T. D. Stevens, G. W. Tregear,

and J. T. Potts, Jr., *J. Clin. Endocrinol. Metab.*, **42,** 520 (1976).

235. J. F. Habener, G. W. Tregear, J. Van Rietschoten, J. W. Hamilton, D. V. Cohn, and J. T. Potts, Jr., *Clin. Res.*, **21,** 493 (1973).
236. J. A. Parsons and J. T. Potts, Jr., *Clin. Endocrinol. Metab.*, **1,** 33 (1972).
237. L. G. Raisz and J. E. O'Brien, *Am. J. Physiol.*, **205,** 816 (1963).
238. M. V. L'Henreux and P. Meilus, *Biochem. Biophys. Acta*, **20,** 447 (1956).
239. R. R. MacGregor, L. L. H. Chu, J. W. Hamilton, and D. V. Cohn, *Endocrinology*, **93,** 1387 (1973).
240. J. F. Habener, G. W. Tregear, T. D. Stevens, P. C. Dee, and J. T. Potts, Jr., *Endocrinol. Res. Commun.*, **1,** 1 (1974).
241. D. Goltzman, A. Peytremann, E. Callahan, G. W. Tregear, and J. T. Potts, Jr., *Endocrinology*, **76,** A-000 (1975).
242. L. L. H. Chu, R. R. MacGregor, J. W. Hamilton, and D. V. Cohn, *Endocrinology*, **95,** 1431 (1974).
243. A. Peytremann, D. Goltzmann, E. N. Callahan, G. W. Tregear, and J. T. Potts, Jr., *Endocrinology*, **97,** 1270 (1975).
244. C. M. Redman, P. Siehevitz, and G. E. Palade, *J. Biol. Chem.*, **241,** 1150 (1966).
245. L. M. Sherwood, J. S. Rodman, and W. B. Lundberg, *Proc. Nat. Acad. Sci. USA*, **67,** 1631 (1970).
246. R. Silverman and R. S. Yalow, *J. Clin. Invest.*, **28,** 1958 (1973).
247. S. A. Berson and R. S. Yalow, *J. Clin. Invest.*, **28,** 1037 (1968).
248. T. J. Martin, P. B. Greenberg, and R. A. Milik, *J. Clin. Endocrinol. Metab.*, **34,** 437 (1972).
249. B. Kemper, J. F. Habener, A. Rich, and J. T. Potts, Jr., *Science*, **184,** 167 (1974).
250. D. Powell, M. Shimkin, J. L. Doppman, S. Wells, G. D. Aurbach, S. J. Marx, A. S. Ketcham, and J. T. Potts, Jr., *New Engl. J. Med.*, **286,** 1169 (1972).
251. S. A. Berson and R. S. Yalow, *J. Clin. Endocrinol.*, **28,** 1037 (1968).
252. J. L. O'Riordan, J. Page, D. N. S. Kerr, J. Walls, J. Moorhead, R. E. Crockett, H. Franz, and E. Ritz, *Quartz. J. Med.*, **39,** 359 (1970).
253. J. T. Potts, Jr., T. M. Murray, M. Peacock, H. D. Niall, G. W. Tregear, H. T. Keutmann, D. Powell, and L. J. Deftos, *Am. J. Med.*, **50,** 639 (1971).
254. J. F. Habener, G. P. Mayer, G. V. Segre, D. Dee, and J. T. Potts, Jr., *Clin. Res.*, **20,** 864 (1972).
255. G. V. Segre, H. D. Niall, J. W. Jacobs, R. T. Sauer, K. G. Swenson, and J. T. Potts, Jr., *Endocrinology*, **92,** A-158 (1973).
256. F. R. Singer, G. V. Segre, J. F. Habener, and J. T. Potts, Jr., *Metabolism*, **24,** 139 (1975).
257. J. M. Canterbury, L. A. Brickler, P. L. Koslouskis, and E. Reiss, *Endocrinology*, **74,** A-203 (1974).
258. G. W. Tregear, J. van Rietschoten, E. Greene, H. T. Keutmann, H. D. Niall, B. Reit, J. A. Parsons, and J. T. Potts, Jr., *Endocrinology*, **93,** 1349 (1973).
259. J. T. Potts, Jr., H. T. Keutmann, H. D. Niall, G. W. Tregear, J. F. Habener, J. L. H. O'Riordan, T. M. Murray, D. Powell, and G. D. Aurbach, in *Endocrinology 1971: Proceedings of the Third International Symposium*, S. Taylor, Ed., Heinemann, London, 1972, p. 333.
260. J. M. Canterbury, G. S. Lavey, and E. Reiss, *J. Clin. Invest.*, **52,** 524 (1973).
261. D. Goltzmann, A. Peytremann, E. N. Callahan, G. V. Segre, and J. T. Potts, Jr., *J. Clin. Invest.*, **57,** 8 (1976).
262. H. Rasmussen and L. C. Craig, *Biochim. Biophys. Acta*, **56,** 332 (1962).
263. J. T. Potts, Jr., G. W. Tregear, H. T. Keutmann, H. D. Niall, R. Sauer, L. J. Deftos, B. F. Dawson, and G. D. Aurbach, *Proc. Nat. Acad. Sci. USA*, **68,** 63 (1971).
264. R. Marcus and G. D. Aurbach, *Endocrinology*, **85,** 801 (1969).
265. J. A. Parsons, B. Reit, and C. J. Robinson, *Endocrinology*, **92,** 454 (1973).
266. G. W. Tregear and J. T. Potts, Jr., *Endocrine Res. Commun.*, **2,** 501 (1975).
267. G. W. Tregear, J. van Rietschoten, E. Greene, H. D. Niall, H. T. Keutmann, J. A. Parsons, and J. L. H. O'Riordan, Hoppe-Seyler's *Z. Physiol. Chem.*, **355,** 415 (1974).
268. M. Rosenblatt, D. Goltsmann, H. T. Keutmann, G. W. Tregear, and J. T. Potts, Jr., *J. Biol. Chem.*, **251,** 159 (1976).
269. D. Goltzmann, A. Peytremann, E. Callahan, G. W. Tregear, and J. T. Potts, Jr., *J. Biol. Chem.*, **250,** 3199 (1975).
270. G. Griffenhagen, *Kokuritsu Eiyo Kenkyusho Kenkyu Hokoku*, 2: *Bull.*, **9,** 8 (1952).
271. D. Whistler, cited by G. T. Smerdon in *J. Hist. Med.*, **5,** 397 (1950).
272. E. Mellanby, *Lancet*, **1,** 407 (1919).

273. E. Mellanby, *J. Physiol.* (London), **52,** liii, (1919).

274. E. V. McCollum and M. Davis, *J. Biol. Chem.*, **15,** 167 (1913).

275. E. V. McCollum, N. Simmonds, and W. Pitz, *J. Biol. Chem.*, **27,** 33 (1916).

276. E. V. McCollum, N. Simmonds, J. E. Becker, and P. G. Shipley, *J. Biol. Chem.*, **53,** 293 (1922).

277. K. Huldsinsky, *Deut. Med. Wochenschr.*, **45,** 712 (1919).

278. H. Goldblatt and K. M. Soames, *Biochem. J.*, **17,** 446 (1923).

279. H. Steenbock, *Science*, **60,** 224 (1924).

280. H. Steenbock and A. Black, *J. Biol. Chem.*, **61,** 405 (1924).

281. A. F. Hess and M. Weinstock, *Proc. Soc. Exp. Biol. Med.*, **22,** 5 (1924).

282. H. Steenbock and A. Black, *J. Biol. Chem.*, **64,** 263 (1925).

283. A. F. Hess, M. Weinstock, and E. Sherman, *J. Biol. Chem.*, **67,** 413 (1926).

284. A. Windaus, A. Hess, O. Rosenheim, R. Pohl, and T. A. Webster, *Chem.-Ztg., Chem. Appl.*, **51,** 113 (1927).

285. O. Rosenheim and T. A. Webster, *Biochem. J.*, **21,** 389 (1927).

286. F. A. Askew, R. B. Bourdillon, H. M. Bruce, R. K. Callow, J. St. L. Philpot, and T. A. Webster, *Proc. Roy. Soc.* (London), **B109,** 488 (1932).

287. A. Windaus, O. Linsert, A. Lüttringhaus, and G. Weidlich, *Justus Liebigs Ann. Chem.*, **492,** 226 (1932).

288. A. Windaus and W. Thiel, *Justus Liebigs Ann. Chem.*, **521,** 160 (1936).

289. A. Windaus, H. Lettre, and F. Schenck, *Justus Liebigs Ann. Chem.*, **520,** 98 (1935).

290. J. Howland and B. Kramer, *Am. J. Dis. Child.*, **22,** 105 (1921).

291. P. G. Shipley, B. Kramer, and J. Howland, *Am. J. Dis. Child.*, **30,** 37 (1925).

292. P. G. Shipley, B. Kramer, and J. Howland, *Biochem. J.*, **20,** 379 (1926).

293. W. F. Neuman and M. W. Neuman, *The Chemical Dynamics of Bone Disease*, University of Chicago Press, Chicago, 1958.

294. W. F. Newman, *Am. Med. Assoc. Arch. Pathol.*, **66,** 204 (1948).

295. W. J. Orr, L. E. Holt, Jr., L. Wilkens, and F. H. Boone, *Am. J. Dis. Child.*, **26,** 362 (1923).

296. R. Nicolaysen, *Biochem. J.*, **31,** 107 (1937).

297. R. Nicolaysen, *Biochem. J.*, **31,** 122 (1937).

298. R. Nicolaysen, *Biochem. J.*, **31,** 323 (1938).

299. R. Nicolaysen, *Acta Physiol. Scand.*, **6,** 201 (1943).

300. A. Carlsson, *Acta, Physiol. Scand.*, **26,** 212 (1952).

301. A. Carlsson and B. Lindquist, *Acta Paediatr. Stockholm*, **44,** 548 (1955).

302. E. M. Cruickshank and E. Kodicek, *Biochem. J.*, **54,** 337 (1953).

303. E. M. Cruickshank, E. Kodicek, and P. Armitage, *Biochem. J.*, **58,** 172 (1954).

304. E. Kodicek, in *Ciba Foundation Symposium on Bone Structure and Metabolism*, G. W. E. Wolstenholme and C. M. O'Connor, Eds., Little-Brown, Boston, 1956, p. 161.

305. E. Kodicek, in *Fourth International Congress on Biochemistry and Vitamin Metabolism*, Vol. 11, Pergamon Press, London, 1960, p. 198.

306. E. Kodicek, *Biochem. J.*, **60,** XXV (1955).

307. P. F. Neville and H. F. DeLuca, *Biochemistry*, **5,** 2201 (1966).

308. A. W. Norman and H. F. DeLuca, *Anal. Chem.*, **35,** 1247 (1963).

309. M. F. Holick and H. F. DeLuca, *J. Lipid Res.*, **12,** 460 (1971).

310. J. W. Blunt, H. F. DeLuca, and H. K. Schnoes, *Biochemistry*, **7,** 3317 (1968).

311. J. W. Blunt, Y. Tanaka, and H. F. DeLuca, *Proc. Nat. Acad. Sci. USA*, **61,** 1503 (1968).

312. Y. Tanaka, H. Frank, and H. F. DeLuca, *Endocrinology*, **92,** 417 (1973).

313. M. R. Haussler, J. F. Myrtle, and A. W. Norman, *J. Biol. Chem.*, **243,** 4055 (1968).

314. D. E. M. Lawson, P. W. Wilson, and E. Kodicek, *Biochem. J.*, **115,** 269 (1969).

315. D. R. Fraser and E. Kodicek, *Nature*, **228,** 764 (1970).

316. M. F. Holick, H. K. Schnoes, and H. F. DeLuca, *Proc. Nat. Acad. Sci. USA*, **68,** 803 (1971).

317. M. F. Holick, H. K. Schnoes, H. F. DeLuca, T. Suda, and R. J. Cousins, *Biochemistry*, **10,** 2799 (1971).

318. D. E. M. Lawson, D. R. Fraser, E. Kodicek, H. R. Morris, and D. H. Williams, *Nature*, **230,** 228 (1971).

319. Y. Tanaka, H. Frank, and H. F. DeLuca, *J. Nutr.*, **102,** 1509 (1972).

320. A. W. Norman and R. G. Wong, *J. Nutr.*, **102,** 1709 (1972).

321. A. Boris, J. F. Hurley, and T. Timal, *J. Nutr.*, **107,** 194 (1977).

322. H. F. DeLuca, M. Weller, J. W. Blunt, and P. F.

Neville, *Arch. Biochem. Biophys.*, **124,** 122 (1968).

323. A. F. Hess and M. Weinstock, *J. Biol. Chem.*, **64,** 181 193 (1925).

324. E. Havinga, *Experientia*, **29,** 1181 (1973).

325. R. Esvelt, H. K. Schnoes, and H. F. DeLuca, *Proceedings of the Sixth Parathyroid Conference*, University of British Columbia, Vancouver, B.C., June 12–17, 1977.

326. H. Rikkers and H. F. DeLuca, *Am. J. Physiol.*, **213,** 380 (1967).

327. S. Edelstein, D. E. M. Lawson, and E. Kodicek, *Biochem. J.*, **135,** 417 (1973).

328. R. Belsey, M. B. Clark, M. Bernat, J. Glowacki, M. F. Holick, H. F. DeLuca, and J. T. Potts, Jr., *Am. J. Med.*, **57,** 50 (1974).

329. P. F. Neville and H. F. DeLuca, *Biochemistry*, **5,** 2201 (1966).

330. G. Ponchon and H. F. DeLuca, *J. Clin. Invest.*, **48,** 1273 (1969).

331. E. B. Olson, Jr., J. C. Knutson, and M. H. Bhattacharyya, *J. Clin. Invest.*, **56,** 1213 (1976).

332. M. H. Bhattacharyya and H. F. DeLuca, *Arch. Biochem. Biophys.*, **160,** 58 (1973).

333. M. H. Bhattacharyya and H. F. DeLuca, *J. Biol. Chem.*, **248,** 2969 (1973).

334. G. Ponchon, A. L. Kennan, and H. F. DeLuca, *J. Clin. Invest.*, **48,** 2032 (1969).

335. M. H. Bhattacharyya and H. F. DeLuca, *J. Biol. Chem.*, **248,** 2974 (1973).

336. G. Ponchon, H. F. DeLuca, and T. Suda, *Arch. Biochem. Biophys.*, **141,** 397 (1970).

327. A. W. Norman, *Am. J. Med.*, **57,** 21 (1974).

338. R. B. Hallick and H. F. DeLuca, *J. Biol. Chem.*, **246,** 5733 (1971).

339. J. A. Eisman, R. M. Shepard, and H. F. DeLuca, *Anal. Biochem.*, **80,** 298 (1977).

340. R. V. Talmage, *Clin. Orthopaed.*, **67,** 210 (1969).

341. C. L. Trummel, L. G. Raisz, J. W. Blunt, and H. F. DeLuca, *Science*, **163,** 1450 (1969).

342. R. A. Corradino, *Science*, **179,** 402 (1973).

343. E. B. Olson and H. F. DeLuca, *Science*, **165,** 405 (1969).

344. I. T. Boyle, R. W. Gray, J. L. Omdahl, and H. F. DeLuca, in *Endocrinology 1971*, Heinemann Medibooks, London, 1972, p. 468.

345. Y. Tanaka and H. F. DeLuca, *Arch. Biochem. Biophys.* **154,** 566 (1973).

346. M. Garabedian, M. F. Holick, H. F. DeLuca, and I. T. Boyle, *Proc. Nat. Acad. Sci. USA*, **69,** 1673 (1973).

347. R. W. Gray, J. L. Omdahl, J. G. Ghazarian, and H. F. DeLuca, *J. Biol. Chem.*, **247,** 7528 (1972).

348. J. G. Ghazarian, H. K. Schnoes, and H. F. DeLuca, *Biochemistry*, **12,** 2555 (1973).

349. J. G. Ghazarian and H. F. DeLuca, *Arch. Biochem. Biophys.*, **160,** 63 (1974).

350. J. G. Ghazarian, C. R. Jefcoate, J. C. Knutson, W. H. Orme-Johnson, and H. F. DeLuca, *J. Biol. Chem.*, **249,** 3026 (1974).

351. J. Pederson, J. G. Ghazarian, N. Orme-Johnson, and H. F. DeLuca, *J. Biol. Chem.*, **251,** 3933 (1976).

352. R. Gray, I. T. Boyle, and H. F. DeLuca, *Science*, **172,** 1232 (1971).

353. I. T. Boyle, R. Gray, and H. F. DeLuca, *Proc. Nat. Acad. Sci. USA*, **68,** 2131 (1971).

354. D. R. Fraser and E. Kodicek, *Nature New Biol.*, **241,** 163 (1973).

355. Y. Tanaka, R. S. Lorenc, and H. F. DeLuca, *Arch. Biochem. Biophys.*, **171,** 521 (1975).

356. J. L. Omdahl, R. W. Gray, I. T. Boyle, J. Knutson, and H. F. DeLuca, *Nature New Biol.*, **237,** 63 (1972).

357. H. L. Henry, R. J. Midgett, and A. W. Norman, *J. Biol. Chem.*, **249,** 7584 (1974).

358. K. W. Colston, I. M. A. Evans, L. Galante, I. MacIntyre, and D. W. Moss, *Biochem. J.*, **134,** 817 (1973).

359. D. D. Bikle and H. Rasmussen, *J. Clin. Invest.*, **55,** 292 (1975).

360. D. D. Bikle, E. W. Murphy, and H. Rasmussen, *J. Clin. Invest.*, **55,** 299 (1975).

361. N. Horiuchi, T. Suda, S. Sasaki, I. Tzawa, Y. Sano,and E. Ogata, *Fed. Eur. Biochem. Soc. Lett.*, **43,** 353 (1974).

362. L. A. Baxter and H. F. DeLuca, *J. Biol. Chem.*, **251,** 3158 (1976).

363. Y. Tanaka and H. F. DeLuca, *Science*, **183,** 1198 (1974).

364. R. G. Larkins, S. J. MacAuleyard, and I. MacIntyre, *Nature*, **252,** 412 (1972).

365. T. C. Chen and H. F. DeLuca, *Arch. Biochem. Biophys.*, **156,** 321 (1973).

366. J. C. Knutson and H. F. DeLuca, *Biochemistry*, **13,** 1543 (1974).

367. A. Kleiner-Bossaller and H. F. DeLuca, *Biochim. Biophys. Acta*, **338,** 489 (1974).

368. Y. Tanaka, H. F. DeLuca, N. Ikekawa, M. Morisaki, and N. Koizumi, *Arch. Biochem. Biophys.*, **170,** 620 (1975).

369. Y. Tanaka, L. Castillo, H. F. DeLuca, and N. Ikekawa, *J. Biol. Chem.*, **252,** 1421 (1977).

370. R. Kumar, H. K. Schnoes, and H. F. DeLuca, unpublished results.

371. M. Garabedian, H. Pavlovitch, C. Fellot, and S.

Balsan, *Proc. Nat. Acad., Sci. USA*, **71,** 554 (1974).

372. M. F. Holick, L. A. Baxter, P. K. Schraufrogel, T. E. Tavela, and H. F. DeLuca, *J. Biol. Chem.*, **251,** 397 (1976).
373. Y. Tanaka and H. F. DeLuca, unpublished results.
374. Y. Tanaka, H. F. DeLuca, A. Akaiwa, M. Morisaki, and N. Ikekawa, *Arch. Biochem. Biophys.*, **177,** 615 (1976).
375. T. Suda, H. F. DeLuca, H. K. Schnoes, Y. Tanaka, and M. F. Holick, *Biochemistry*, **9,** 4776 (1970).
376. Y. Tanaka and H. F. DeLuca, unpublished results.
377. D. Harnden, R. Kumar, M. F. Holick, and H. F. DeLuca, *Science*, **193,** 493 (1976).
378. R. Kumar, D. Harnden, and H. F. DeLuca, *Biochemistry*, **15,** 2420 (1976).
379. R. Kumar and H. F. DeLuca, *Biochem. Biophys. Res. Commun.*, **69,** 197 (1976).
380. R. Kumar and H. F. DeLuca, *Biochem. Biophys. Res. Commun.*, **76,** 253 (1977).
381. H. E. Harrison and H. C. Harrison, *J. Clin. Invest.*, **20,** 27 (1941).
382. F. Gran, *Acta Physiol. Scand.*, **50,** 132 (1960).
383. T. H. Steele, J. E. Engle, Y. Tanaka, R. S. Lorenc, K. L. Dudgeon, and H. F. DeLuca, *Am. J. Physiol.*, **229,** 489 (1975).
384. A. N. Taylor and R. H. Wasserman, *Am. J. Physiol.*, **223,** 110 (1972).
385. J. B. Puschett, J. Moranz, and W. S. Kurnick, *J. Clin. Invest.*, **51,** 373 (1972).
386. J. Brodehl, W. P. Kaas, and H.-P. Weber, *Pediatr. Res.*, **5,** 591 (1971).
387. R. Nicolaysen and N. Eeg-Larsen, in *Ciba Foundations Symposium on Bone Structure and Metabolism*, G. W. E. Wolstenholme and C. M. O'Connor, Eds., Little, Brown, Boston, 1956, p. 171.
388. M. F. Holick, M. Garabedian, and H. F. DeLuca, *Science*, **176,** 1146 (1972).
389. J. J. Reynolds, M. F. Holick, and H. F. DeLuca, *Calc. Tiss. Res.*, **12,** 295 (1973).
390. L. G. Raisz, C. L. Trummel, M. F. Holick, and H. F. DeLuca, *Science*, **175,** 768 (1972).
391. M. Garabedian, Y. Tanaka, M. F. Holick, and H. F. DeLuca, *Endocrinology*, **94,** 1022 (1974).
392. C. L. Trummel, L. G. Raisz, J. W. Blunt, and H. F. deLuca, *Science*, **163,** 1450 (1969).
393. Y. Tanaka and H. F. DeLuca, *Arch. Biochem. Biophys.*, **146,** 574 (1971).
394. Y. Tanaka and H. F. DeLuca, *Proc. Nat. Acad. Sci. USA*, **71,** 1040 (1974).
395. L. Castillo, Y. Tanaka, and H. F. DeLuca, *Endocrinology*, **97,** 995 (1975).
396. US Pharmacopoeia, 15th revision, Mack Publishing Co., Easton, Pa., 1955, p. 889.
397. H. F. DeLuca, in *Handbook of Physiology*, Vol. 7, G. D. Aurbach, Ed., American Physiological Society, Washington, D.C., 1976, Ch. 11.
398. D. Schachter and S. M. Rosen, *Am. J. Physiol.*, **196,** 357 (1959).
399. D. Schachter, in *The Transfer of Calcium and Stronium Across Biological Membranes*, R. H. Wasserman, Ed., Academic Press, New York, 1963, p. 197.
400. D. L. Martin and H. F. DeLuca, *Arch. Biochem. Biophys.*, **134,** 139 (1969).
401. D. L. Martin and H. F. DeLuca, *Am. J. Physiol.*, **216,** 1351 (1969).
402. R. Nicolaysen and N. Eeg-Larsen, *Vitam. Horm.*, **11,** 29 (1953).
403. D. E. M. Lawson and P. W. Wilson, *Biochem. J.*, **144,** 573 (1974).
404. P. F. Brumbaugh and M. R. Haussler, *J. Biol. Chem.*, **349,** 1258 (1974).
405. P. F. Brumbaugh and M. R. Haussler, *J. Biol. Chem.*, **250,** 1588 (1975).
406. P. F. Brumbuagh and M. R. Haussler, *Life Sci.*, **16,** 353 (1975).
407. B. E. Kream, R. D. Reynolds, J. C. Knutson, A. A. Eisman, and H. F. DeLuca, *Arch. Biochem. Biophys.*, **176,** 770 (1976).
408. B. E. Kream, S. Yamada, H. K. Schnoes, and H. F. DeLuca, *J. Biol. Chem.*, **252,** 4501 (1977).
409. J. Eisman and H. F. DeLuca, unpublished results.
410. B. E. Kream, J. J. L. Jose, and H. F. DeLuca, *Arch. Biochem. Biophys.*, **179,** 462 (1977).
411. M. R. Haussler, J. F. Myrtle, and A. W. Norman, *J. Biol. Chem.*, **243,** 4055 (1968).
412. D. E. M. Lawson, P. W. Wilson, and E. Kodicek, *Biochem. J.*, **115,** 269 (1969).
413. T. C. Chen, J. C. Weber, and H. F. DeLuca, *J. Biol. Chem.*, **245,** 3776 (1970).
414. T. C. Chen and H. F. DeLuca, *J. Biol. Chem.*, **248,** 4890 (1973).
415. P. F. Brumbaugh and M. R. Haussler, *J. Biol. Chem.*, **249,** 1251 (1974).
416. H. F. DeLuca and H. K. Schnoes, *Proceedings of the Sixth Parathyroid Conference*, University of British Columbia, Vancouver, B.C., June 12–17, 1977.
417. J. E. Zerwekl, T. J. Lindell, and M. R. Haussler, *J. Biol. Chem.*, **251,** 2388 (1976).
418. J. E. Zerwekh, M. R. Haussler, and T. J. Lindell, *Proc. Nat. Acad. Sci. USA*, **71,** 2337 (1974).

419. H. C. Tsai and A. W. Norman, *Biochem. Biophys. Res. Commun.*, **54,** 622 (1973).
420. J. Harmeyer and H. F. DeLuca, *Arch. Biochem. Biophys.*, **133,** 247 (1969).
421. R. H. Wasserman, A. N. Taylor, and C. S. Fullmer, *Biochem. Soc. Spec. Publ.*, **3,** 55 (1974).
422. G. Ellon, E. Mor, H. Karaman, and J. Menczel, in *Cellular Mechanisms for Calcium Transfer and Homeostatis*, Academic Press, New York, 1971, p. 501.
423. J. A. Eisman, A. J. Hamstra, B. E. Kream, and H. F. DeLuca, *Science*, **193,** 1021 (1976).
424. J. A. Eisman, A. J. Hamstra, B. E. Kream, and H. F. DeLuca, *Arch. Biochem. Biophys.*, **176,** 235 (1976).
425. L. G. Raisz, *J. Clin. Invest.*, **44,** 103 (1965).
426. P. H. Stern, *J. Pharm. Exp. Ther.*, **168,** 211 (1969).
427. H.-y. Lam, B. L. Onisko, H. K. Schnoes, and H. F. DeLuca, *Biochem. Biophys. Res. Commun.*, **59,** 845 (1974).
428. W. H. Okamura, M. N. Mitra, R. M. Wing, and A. W. Norman, *Biochem. Biophys. Res. Commun.*, **60,** 179 (1974).
429. M. N. Mitra, A. W. Norman, and W. H. Okamura, *J. Org. Chem.*, **39,** 2931 (1974).
430. B. Onisko, L. Reeve, H. K. Schnoes, and H. F. DeLuca, *Bioorg. Chem.*, **6,** 203 (1977).
431. A. W. Norman, M. N. Mitra, W. H. Okamura, and R. M. Wing, *Science*, **188,** 1013 (1975).
432. W. H. Okamura, M. N. Mitra, D. A. Proscal. and A. W. Norman, *Biochem. Biophys. Res. Commun.*, **65,** 24 (1975).
433. M. F. Holick, E. J. Semmler, H. K. Schnoes, and H. F. DeLuca, *Science*, **180,** 190 (1973).
434. M. R. Haussler, J. E. Zerwekh, R. H. Hess, E. Rizzardo, and M. M. Pecket, *Proc. Nat. Acad. Sci. USA*, **70,** 2248 (1973).
435. M. F. Holick, P. Kasten-Schraufrogel, T. Tavela, and H. F. DeLuca, *Arch. Biochem. Biophys.*, **166,** 63 (1975).
436. M. F. Holick, T. E. Tavela, S. A. Holick, H. K. Schnoes, H. F. DeLuca, and B. M. Gallagher, *J. Biol. Chem.*, **251,** 1020 (1976).
437. S. A. Holick, M. F. Holick, T. E. Tavela, H. K. Schnoes, and H. F. DeLuca, *J. Biol. Chem.*, **251,** 1025 (1976).
438. M. Fukishima, Y. Suzuki, Y. Tohira, I. Matsunga, K. Ochi, H. Nagano, Y. Nishii, and T. Suda, *Biochem. Biophys. Res. Commun.*, **66,** 632 (1975).
439. J. L. Napoli, M. A. Fivizzani, H. K. Schnoes, and H. F. DeLuca, *Proceedings of the Sixth Parathyroid Conference*, University of British Columbia, Vancouver, B.C., June 12–17, 1977.
440. Y. Tanaka, H. Frank, H. F. DeLuca, N. Koizumi, and N. Ikekawa, *Biochemistry*, **14,** 3293 (1975).
441. H. Kawashima, K. Hoshina, Y. Hashimoto, T. Takeshita, S. Ishimoto, T. Noguchi, N. Ikekawa, M. Morisaki, and H. Orimo, *Fed. Eur. Biochem. Soc., Lett.*, **76,** 177 (1977).
442. G. Jones, H. K. Schnoes, and H. F. DeLuca, *J. Biol. Chem.*, **251,** 24 (1976).
443. G. Jones, L. A. Baxter, H. F. DeLuca, and H. K. Schnoes, *Biochemistry*, **15,** 713 (1976).
444. H.-y. Lam, H. K. Schnoes, and H. F. DeLuca, *Science*, **186,** 1038 (1974).
445. H. Steenbock, S. W. F. Kletzien, and J. G. Halpin, *J. Biol. Chem.* **97,** 249 (1932).
446. P. S. Chen and H. B. Busmann, *J. Nutr.*, **83,** 133 (1964).
447. M. H. Imrie, P. F. Neville, A. W. Snellgrove, and H. F. DeLuca, *Arch. Biochem. Biophys.*, **120,** 525 (1967).
448. D. Dresscher, H. F. DeLuca, and M. H. Imrie, *Arch, Biochem. Biophys.*, **130,** 657 (1969).
449. H.-y. Lam, H. K. Schnoes, H. F. DeLuca, L. Reeve, and P. H. Stern, *Steroids*, **26,** 422 (1976).
450. H.-y. Lam, H. K. Schnoes, P. H. Stern, A. F. Chen, and H. F. DeLuca, unpublished results.
451. R. B. Hallick and H. F. DeLuca, *J. Biol. Chem.*, **246,** 5733 (1971).
452. M. F. Holick, M. Garabedian, and H. F. DeLuca, *Biochemistry*, **11,** 2715 (1972).
453. M. H. Bhattacharyya and H. F. DeLuca, *J. Biol. Chem.*, **248,** 2974 (1973).

CHAPTER TWENTY–SEVEN

Peptide and Protein Hormones

JOHANNES MEIENHOFER

Chemical Research Department
Hoffmann–La Roche, Inc.
Nutley, New Jersey, 07110,
USA

CONTENTS

1 INTRODUCTION

The field of peptide and protein hormones has kept growing exponentially for nearly 20 years. Refined laboratory techniques and instrumentation have led to successful isolation, structure elucidation, and synthesis of many new individual hormones and even entire new classes, such as endogenous opioid agonists or thymic immunostimulatory factors. The study of these hormones in turn stimulates further refinement in methodology. Advanced synthetic methods have permitted synthesis of numerous analogs for structure-activity studies. Close to 500 analogs of oxytocin and vasopressin and more than 100 of so formidable a molecule as insulin have been synthesized. Increasingly rapid and sensitive bioassays allow for the deduction of ever more meaningful structure-activity relationships. Knowledge is gained of the three-dimensional structure or solution conformation of hormone molecules by X-ray crystal structure analysis (e.g., of insulin) or by NMR, ORD, and CD spectroscopy (e.g., of oxytocin). These growing insights permit the study of conformation-activity relationships and allow for novel rationales in predictive analog design. All these efforts lead, naturally, to an explosive increase in literature. Consequently this chapter is severely selective, but an attempt is made to emphasize different aspects of the total spectrum of research accomplishments during the description of the various individual hormones. Only chemically and structurally identified hormones are discussed.

A cardinal question concerns the impact on human medicine of the enormous progress in peptide and protein hormone research. Insulin still remains as the single stalwart, with synthetic ACTH a distant runner-up. The main obstacle preventing peptides and proteins from becoming useful therapeutic agents is the mandatory intravenous route of administration. This is acceptable for insulin in averting acutely life-threatening diabetic ketoacidosis, but not for other peptides in treating less severe diseases. Development of vehicles for noninvasive peptide administration or of carriers permitting oral use should receive high priority. Encouraging progress has already been made in increasing the frequently very short half-life of peptide hormones by designing analogs of higher metabolic stability.

The prospects for peptide hormones becoming clinically useful therapeutic agents will depend directly on progress in noninvasive administration and metabolic stabilization. Production costs should be readily competitive, even for larger peptides, since dosage will be quite low because of the extraordinary potency of many peptide hormones that are active at picomolar or femtomolar levels.

1.1 Nomenclature, Abbreviations and Chapter Disposition

The nomenclature of peptide hormones recommended by the IUPAC-IUB Commission on Biochemical Nomenclature (1a) is followed in most cases. Table 27.1 lists relatively novel terms; traditional names that were not changed (e.g., insulin, glucagon) do not appear. In abbreviations, lowercase prefix letters indicate species origin: b, bovine; h, human; o, ovine; p, porcine. Abbreviations for amino acids, symbols for peptide structures and side chain abbreviations, and rules for naming synthetic analogs are generally those recommended by the IUPAC–IUB Commission (1b). Other abbreviations are listed in alphabetical order in Table 27.2.

The chapter disposition follows that of Berson and Yalow (2), which distinguishes between glandular hormones, classified by their gland of origin, and tissue hormones, classified by their biological effects. Although several hormones are now known to be secreted at different sites (e.g., somatostatin in the hypothalamus and in the pancreas), this disposition still appears to be the most practical one.

1.2 Methodology and Laboratory Techniques

Progress in the peptide hormone field depends on methodological advances in analysis, isolation and purification, bioassay, structure analysis, synthesis, and conformational analysis, to name but a few of the most essential techniques.

In *analysis*, modern high pressure liquid chromatographic instruments permit rapid amino acid analysis of nano- and picomolar quantities. The precision and sensitivity of these techniques has been authoritatively reviewed by Moore (3). In a fluorometric method for the quantitative assay of peptide hormones in individual glands (e.g., a

Table 27.1 Recommended IUPAC–IUB Nomenclature for Peptide Hormones

Recommended Name	Other Names	Current Abbreviation
	Hypothalamic Hormones (Factors)	
Gonadoliberin	Gonadotropin-releasing hormone	GnRH
Melanoliberin	Melanotropin-releasing factor	MRF
Melanostatin	Melanotropin release-inhibiting factor	MIF
Somatostatin	Somatotropin release-inhibiting hormone	SS
Thyroliberin	Thyrotropin-releasing hormone	TRH
	Adenohypophyseal Hormones	
Choriogonadotropin	Chorionic gonadotropin	CG
Choriomammotropin	Chorionic somatomammotropin	CS
Corticotropin	Adrenocorticotropic hormone	ACTH
Follitropin	Follicle-stimulating hormone	FSH
Gonadotropin	Gonadotropic hormone	
Lipotropin	Lipotropic hormone	LPH
Lutropin	Luteinizing hormone; interstitial cell-stimulating hormone (ICSH)	LH
Melanotropin	Melanocyte-stimulating hormone	MSH
Prolactin	Lactogenic hormone; lactotropin; mammatropin	PRL
Somatotropin	Growth hormone; somatotropic hormone	GH
Thyrotropin	Thyroid-stimulating hormone	TSH
	Other Hormones	
Calcitonin	Thyrocalcitonin	CT
Endorphin	C-Peptide	EP
Leucine-enkephalin		Leu-EK
Methionine-enkephalin		Met-EK
Parathyrin	Parathyroid hormone	PTH

Neurohypophyseal hormones, see Table 27.27

rat pituitary) Udenfriend et al. (4) are able to separate picomolar amounts by reverse phase column chromatography. Each eluted hormone is characterized by amino acid analysis and bioassay. This unprecedented ultramicroscale level opens exciting new potentials and enhances versatility in hormone *isolation*. The amounts of peptides obtained in this manner require microsequencing techniques (5a) for *structure analysis*. The use of ^{35}S-phenylisothiocyanate (5b), *in vitro* culture labeling techniques (5c), or solid phase work (5d) permits sequencing of 1–10 nmol of protein. Peptide *synthesis* permits preparation of peptides with up to 50 or 60 residues both by solution methods (for reviews, see Refs. 6, 7) or by the Merrifield solid phase method (for reviews, see Refs. 8, 9) but further improvements in methodology will be required for routine protein synthesis (>100 amino acid residues).

Knowledge of the *conformation* of peptide hormones contributes not only to a better understanding of the mechanism of action but also to increasing sophistication

Table 27.2 Abbreviations

γAbu	γ-Aminobutyric acid	Met(O)	Methionine sulfoxide
Acm	Acetamidomethyl	Mpr	β-Mercaptopropionic acid
Asu	Aminosuberic acid	Msc	Methylsulfonylethyloxycarbonyl
b	Bovine (species)	N^{τ}	tele His imidazole position
Boc	*tert*-Butyloxycarbonyl	N^{π}	pros His imidazole position
Bpoc	2-(*p*-Biphenylyl)isopropyloxycarbonyl	NMR	Nuclear magnetic resonance
Bu^t	*tert*-Butyl (ether)	o	Ovine
Bzl	Benzyl	OBu^t	*tert*-Butyl ester
c	Canine	OBzl	Benzyl ester
CCK	Cholecystokinin	OMe	Methyl ester
CD	Circular dichroism	ONp	*p*-Nitrophenyl ester
Dbu	α,γ-Diaminobutyric acid	ORD	Optical rotatory dispersion
DCC	Dicyclohexylcarbodiimid	OSu	*N*-Hydroxysuccinimide ester
DMSO	Dimethylsulfoxide	OTcp	2,4,5-Trichlorophenyl ester
DOPA	3,4-Dihydroxyphenylalanine	p	Porcine
DTγE	(des-Tyr^1)γ-endorphin	pGlu	Pyroglutamic acid
Et	Ethyl	Ptc	Phenylthiocarbamoyl
GI	Gastrointestinal	TFA	Trifluoroacetic acid
GIP	Gastric inhibitory polypeptide	Tfa	Trifluoroacetyl
h	Human	TFE	Trifluoroethanol
HOBt	1-Hydroxybenzotriazole	3D	three-dimensional
HOSu	*N*-Hydroxysuccinimide	Thr(Me)	Threonine methyl ether
i.c.v.	Intracerebroventricular	Thz	Thiazolidine carboxylic acid
*i*Noc	Isonicotinyloxycarbonyl	Tos	*p*-Toluenesulfonyl
m	Murine	Trt	Triphenylmethyl
MeOH	Methanol	VIP	Vasointestinal polypeptide
MePhe	*N*-Methylphenylalanine	Z	Benzyloxycarbonyl

in analog design. Great progress has been made in the efficiency of X-ray crystal structure analysis (10) and determination of solution conformation (11) by ORD, CD, and NMR spectroscopy.

Entire important areas in peptide hormone research have not been covered here, since each would easily fill separate chapters. Prominent among these is the radioimmunoassay technique, introduced in 1960 by Yalow and Berson (12) for plasma insulin measurement. It has become the predominant assay method for most peptide hormones and has served in the discovery of a sometimes confusing multitude of circulating forms (see books and reviews, Refs. 2 and 13). The continuing progress in the study of hormone-receptor interactions is impressive, especially with respect to the development of highly sensitive radioreceptor assays capable of measuring femtomolar amounts (for reviews, see Refs. 14 and 15). At the same time, pharmacological assay techniques have been greatly refined, permitting more sophisticated evaluation of structure-activity relationships. Phylogenetic traits of many hormones have been examined in search for a potential common ancestral protein (16).

1.3 Literature Resources

Several books (2, 18, 19), special volumes (20–24), and series of collective volumes (25–27) provide comprehensive and/or continuing coverage of the peptide and protein hormone field.

H–Tyr–Gly–Gly–Phe–Met–OH	H–Tyr–Gly–Gly–Phe–Leu–OH
1 2 3 4 5	1 2 3 4 5
Met-EK	Leu-EK
(*a*)	(*b*)

Fig. 27.1 Structure of methionine enkephalin (*a*) and leucine enkephalin (*b*). Hughes et al. (28).

2 ENDOGENOUS OPIOID* AGONISTS

In December 1975, J. Hughes, H. W. Kosterlitz, and collaborators (28) reported the isolation, structure determination, and synthesis of two similar pentapeptides from porcine brain with potent *in vitro* opiate agonist activity. The peptides, named methionine enkephalin (Met–EK) and leucine enkephalin (Leu–EK) differ in their COOH-terminal residues (Fig. 27.1). The existence of endogenous opioid agonists in brain had been predicted for some time from the highly selective properties of opiate receptors located in nerve endings in brain and spinal cord (for reviews, see Ref. 29). Hughes et al. (28) noted that the sequence of Met–EK is contained as residues 61–65 in the sequence (30) of the known pituitary hormone β-lipotropin (β-LPH). The COOH-terminal (61–91)-untriacontapeptide (31), which was named β-endorphin (β-EP) by C. H. Li, was soon found to possess more potent and long-lasting activity *in vitro* than enkephalin and to elicit strong analgesic effects *in vivo* (31b, 32). Several smaller fragments of β-LPH, e.g., α-, γ-endorphins of considerably lower *in vitro* opioid activity than β-EP, have also been isolated from hypothalamic and pituitary gland extracts (32a, 34).

Profound behavioral effects of β-EP, by intracerebroventricular (i.c.v.) administration into rats, were observed in several laboratories in 1976 (35a–c) and implications in mental illness were suggested. While the interest in endorphins remains focused on their effects on behavior, the enkephalins are receiving broad attention as potential analgesics. Extensive analog synthesis in many laboratories is aiming at analgesics of high potency, long duration, and, perhaps, lack of addiction liability.

Several reviews have appeared on the overall progress (36), on enkephalins (37), and on endorphins (38).

* Opioid = opiatelike, resembling opiate.

2.1 Enkephalins (EK)

2.1.1 BIOLOGICAL ACTIVITY AND DISTRIBUTION. Highly specific *in vitro* assays (29), based on the ability of morphine and related drugs to block electrically stimulated contractions of mouse vas deferens or of guinea pig ileum, were essential for the discovery and isolation of opioid peptides. These effects must be reversible by low doses of naloxone, a known specific morphine antagonist. Opiate receptor binding assays are frequently used (29b, 39).

Met–EK is 20 times, Leu–EK 10 times more potent than normorphine in the mouse vas deferens assay (28). In contrast, the *in vivo* analgesic effects of Met–EK and Leu–EK are extremely weak and of very short duration (few minutes) even after intraventricular administration (40, 41). The short duration of these activities may be a consequence of rapid enzymatic degradation, primarily, by cleavage of the Tyr^1–Gly^2 peptide bond (42). Synthetic analogs with D-amino acid residues in position 2 exhibit prolonged activity and increased potency (43, 44).

The *in vivo* bioactivity spectrum of the enkephalins resembles phenomenologically that of morphine and includes mixed agonist–antagonist type analgesic effects in tail flick (40b) and hot plate assays (45a), induction of fatigue in gut (45b), opiate receptor-mediated inhibition of adenylate cyclase activity in neuroblastoma *x* glioma cells (36b), release of prolactin and somatotropin from the anterior pituitary gland (46a, 52c), inhibition of morphine abstinence syndrome (46b), a high degree of dependence liability (46c, d) and a variety of behavioral effects, e.g., DOPA potentiation (47a) and learning enhancement in rats (47b), euphorigenic or rewarding properties (49c), increased locomotor activity (49d), and epileptic properties (49e). A variety of criteria (37a, 50c) indicate a neurotransmitter role for these peptides in both brain and peripheral tissues in which Met–EK and Leu–EK may subserve separate neuronal functions.

Opiate receptors and the enkephalins occur in all vertebrate species examined (48) but not in invertebrates (48b). The regional distribution of total enkephalin, determined by immunofluorescence histochemistry with antiserum to enkephalin (49a), parallels that of the opiate receptor distribution with highest concentrations of both in the striatum, anterior hypothalamus, mesencephalic central gray, and amygdala (49a–d). This shows no fixed relationship to the regional distribution of β-endorphin in rat brain (49e) and many areas rich in enkephalin immunoreactivity are devoid of detectable β-endorphin. Evidence is mounting that the biosynthesis of the enkephalins, e.g., within the striatum, is independent and different from that of β-EP and does not involve intermediate β-lipotropin. Outside the brain, enkephalin has been detected in human cerebrospinal fluid (50a) and throughout the gastrointestinal tract (50b, c) of many species but not in other tissues.

2.1.2 SYNTHESIS.

With two adjacent glycine residues posing no danger of racemization, enkephalins may be synthesized in many different ways. Synthetic Met–EK and Leu–EK became available from numerous peptide laboratories within a few weeks of the publication of their structure. Figure 27.2 shows one of the approaches that appeared in the literature (51).

2.1.3 STRUCTURE-ACTIVITY RELATIONSHIPS.

Over 1000 analogs of EK have been synthesized, predominantly by the solid phase method (8), in the hope of obtaining a potent analgesic that would not lead to dependence or tolerance. Only a few of these studies have as yet been published (e.g., 37, 43, 44, 52, 53). Remarkable increases in potency, duration of action, and metabolic stability, compared to native EK, have been obtained by selective multiple amino acid substitutions, and several of these analogs are orally active in laboratory animals.

Examples of the most potent analogs include:

[D-Ala^2]Met–EK-amide (43a)
[D-Ala^2, D-Leu^5]EK (43b)
[D-Met^2, Pro^5]EK-amide (44a)
[D-Ala^2, MePhe^4, Met(O)ol^5]EK (44b)
[D-Thr^2, Thz^5]EK-amide (44c)

H-Tyr-DAla-Gly-Phe-Met-NH_2
H-Tyr-DAla-Gly-Phe-DMet-OH
H-Tyr-DMet-Gly-Phe-Pro-NH_2
H-Tyr-DAla-Gly-MePhe-Met(O)-ol
H-Tyr-DThr-Gly-Phe-Thz-NH_2

Structure-activity relations emerging from these studies (43, 44, 52, 53) may be summarized as follows. Replacement of glycine in position 2 by D-amino acids results in two- to three-fold potency increases

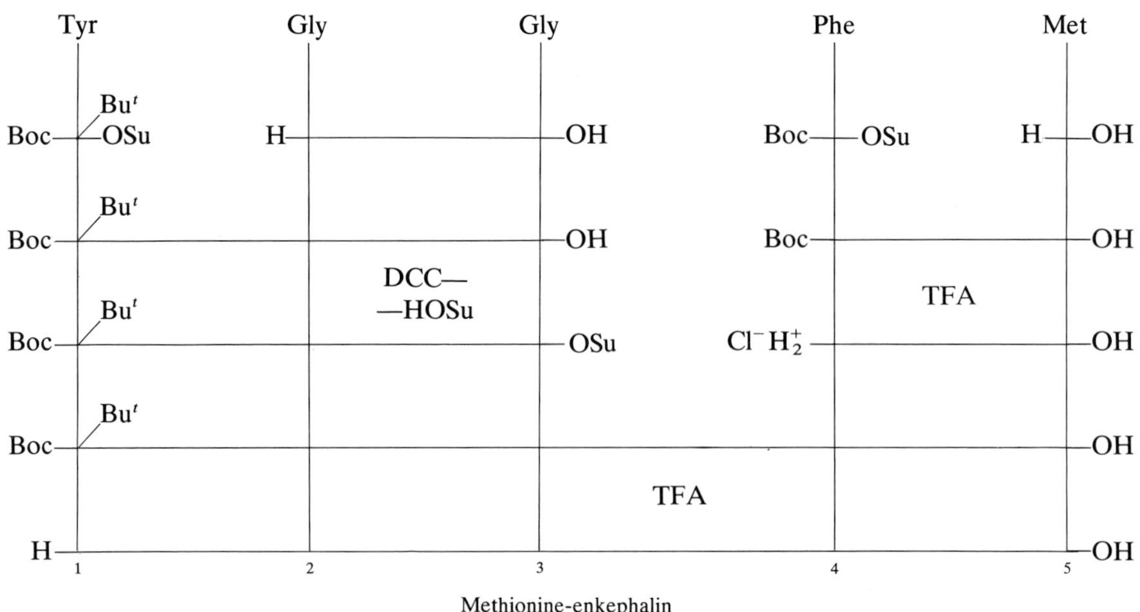

Fig. 27.2 A synthesis of methionine-enkephalin (51).

(in the guinea pig ileum assay) and in *ca.* ten-fold prolongation of *in vivo* analgesic effects (2–3 hr, i.c.v., rat tail flick test), and is most likely due to protection from enzymatic degradation. This 2-position substitution has become a basic feature of most analog work. Substitutions by D-amino acids in positions 1, 3, and 4 results in drastic loss of activity. The amino acid side chains in these same positions, i.e., those of Tyr^1, Gly^3, and Phe^4, are essential for potent activity. The distance between Tyr^1 and Phe^4 is important (37), and Tyr^1 and Phe^4 cannot be mutually exchanged, but both do tolerate minor amino group modification (e.g., *N*-alkylation) (52b, f). COOH-terminal modification (e.g., by amide, ester, decarboxy, carbinol residues) leads frequently, but not always, to potency increases. Chain elongation at either terminus results, with a few exceptions (52c, 53b), in decreasing activity. From the sum of these observations it appears that only the 2- and 5-positions may be safely modified to obtain analogs with high activity, and that simultaneous changes in these positions may increase analgesic activity dramatically.

One of the most noted of the "superactive" analogs, [D-Ala^2,$MePhe^4$,Met(O)ol^5]-EK, developed by Römer et al. (44b), exhibited a remarkable thirty-fold increase in opiate receptor binding affinity compared to Met–EK. Yet this was dwarfed by dramatic increases of the *in vivo* analgesic potency which was 30,000 times that of Met–EK, 1000 times that of morphine, and 23 times that of endorphin in the mouse tail flick test, (i.c.v.). This analog was orally active in animals, including monkeys, and showed many of the biological properties exhibited by β-EP. Its long-lasting analgesic effect after systematic administration was superior to that of β-EP.

It was, therefore, quite unexpected that the analog produced effects in clinical trials in man that were not morphinelike but rather of an anaphylactoid vascular and gastrointestinal nature (54). These trials had to be terminated and it remains to be seen whether (1) the observed lack of correlation between the effects of extensively

β-LPH-(1–60)
~~~~~~61— — — — —65— — — — — — — —70— — — — — — —75— — — — — — — —80— — — — — — —85— — — — — — — —90—91—OH

β-Endorphin, potent analgesia — H–Tyr–Gly–Gly–Phe–Met–Thr–Ser–Glu–Lys–Ser–Gln–Thr–Pro–Leu–Val–Thr–Leu–Phe–Lys–Asn–Ala–Ile–Ile–Lys–Asn–Ala–His–Lys–Lys–Gly–Gln–OH (residues numbered 1, 5, 10, 15, 20, 25, 30)

δ-Endorphin, mild analgesia — H–Tyr–Gly–Gly–Phe–Met–Thr–Ser–Glu–Lys–Ser–Gln–Thr–Pro–Leu–Val–Thr–Leu–Phe–Lys–OH

γ-Endorphin, violent behavior — H–Tyr–Gly–Gly–Phe–Met–Thr–Ser–Glu–Lys–Ser–Gln–Thr–Pro–Leu–Val–Thr–Leu–OH

α-Endorphin, mild analgesia — H–Tyr–Gly–Gly–Phe–Met–Thr–Ser–Glu–Lys–Ser–Gln–Thr–Pro–Leu–Val–Thr–OH

β-EP-(1–9), mild analgesia — H–Tyr–Gly–Gly–Phe–Met–Thr–Ser–Glu–Lys–OH

Fig. 27.3 The structures of camel, sheep β-endorphin (31a, b) and peptides derived from it, i.e., α- and γ-endorphin (33a), δ-endorphin (33b), and β-LPH-(61–69)-nonapeptide (33a, b). Different behavior-modifying effects are elicited by γ-endorphin [in rats] (33a).
~~~~~~

modified peptide agonists in animals and in the clinic as well as (2) the undesired side effects in man will remain a curiosity confined to [D-Ala^2,MePhe^4,Met(O)ol^5]EK or whether they will be of a more general significance for peptide analog design.

2.2 Endorphins (EP)

2.2.1 ISOLATION, STRUCTURE, BIOLOGICAL ACTIVITY. β-Endorphin was first isolated by Li and Chung from camel pituitary (55a). It is identical with the COOH-terminal sequence 61–91 of ovine lipotropin [β_s-LPH-(61–91)] (30a); see Figs. 27.3 and 27.4. β-EP possesses very low lipotropic activity, but strong opioid activity (55b). Similar 31-residue peptides were obtained from porcine (31b, 55c) and ovine (55d) pituitary glands. Human β-endorphin (β_h-EP) was recently isolated [3 mg from 1000 glands] (56a, b) and its sequence shown to differ in positions 27 (His → Tyr) and 31 (Gln → Glu) from the ovine peptide.

The β-endorphins are potent analgesic agents (32) by both i.c.v. and i.v. administration. When injected directly into the brain of rats or mice, β_h-EP is 33 to 48 times more potent than morphine on a molar basis (56a), and its actions are blocked by the specific opiate antagonist naloxone (32). Intravenous administration of β-EP into mice [9.4 and 19 mg/kg] (57) produced 3–4 times more potent effects than morphine in the tail flick and hot plate tests with parallel dose–response curves (Fig. 27.5). These effects lasted 30 to 60 min, depending on the dose used. Similar

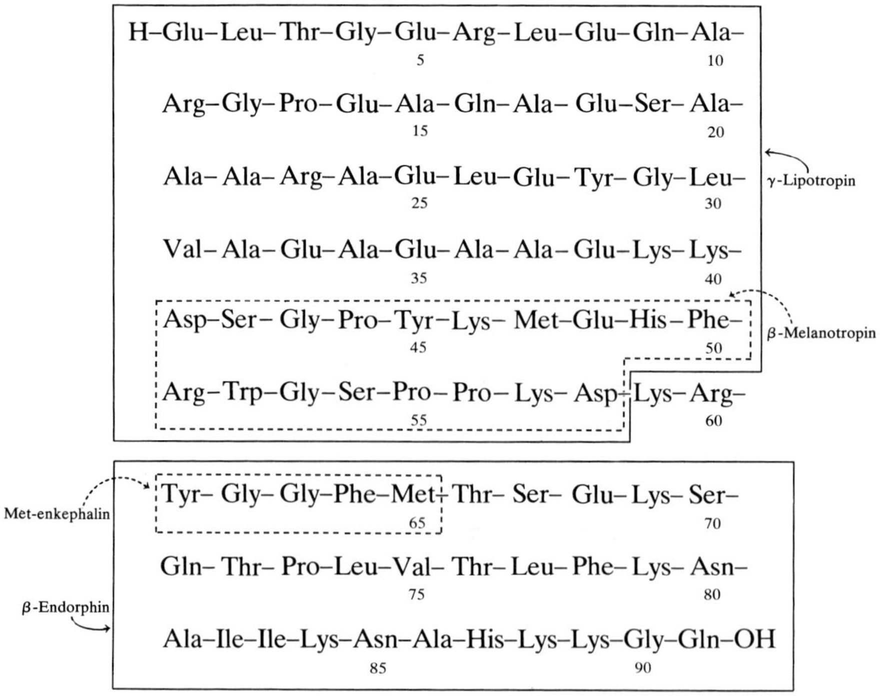

H–Glu–Leu–Thr–Gly–Glu–Arg–Leu–Glu–Gln–Ala– (5, 10)
Arg–Gly–Pro–Glu–Ala–Gln–Ala–Glu–Ser–Ala– (15, 20)
Ala–Ala–Arg–Ala–Glu–Leu–Glu–Tyr–Gly–Leu– (25, 30) γ-Lipotropin
Val–Ala–Glu–Ala–Glu–Ala–Ala–Glu–Lys–Lys– (35, 40)
Asp–Ser–Gly–Pro–Tyr–Lys–Met–Glu–His–Phe– (45, 50) β-Melanotropin
Arg–Trp–Gly–Ser–Pro–Pro–Lys–Asp–Lys–Arg– (55, 60)

Met-enkephalin
Tyr–Gly–Gly–Phe–Met–Thr–Ser–Glu–Lys–Ser– (65, 70)
Gln–Thr–Pro–Leu–Val–Thr–Leu–Phe–Lys–Asn– (75, 80)
β-Endorphin
Ala–Ile–Ile–Lys–Asn–Ala–His–Lys–Lys–Gly–Gln–OH (85, 90)

Amino acid sequence of ovine β-lipotropin

Fig. 27.4 Schematic of ovine β-lipotropin (β-LPH) showing proposed precursor relationship to β-melanotropin (β-MSH), sequence region 41–58, and β-endorphin, sequence region 61–91. In human β-LPH residues 87 and 91 Tyr are Tyr and Glu, respectively. From Li (38a). Reprinted with permission of Academic Press, Inc.

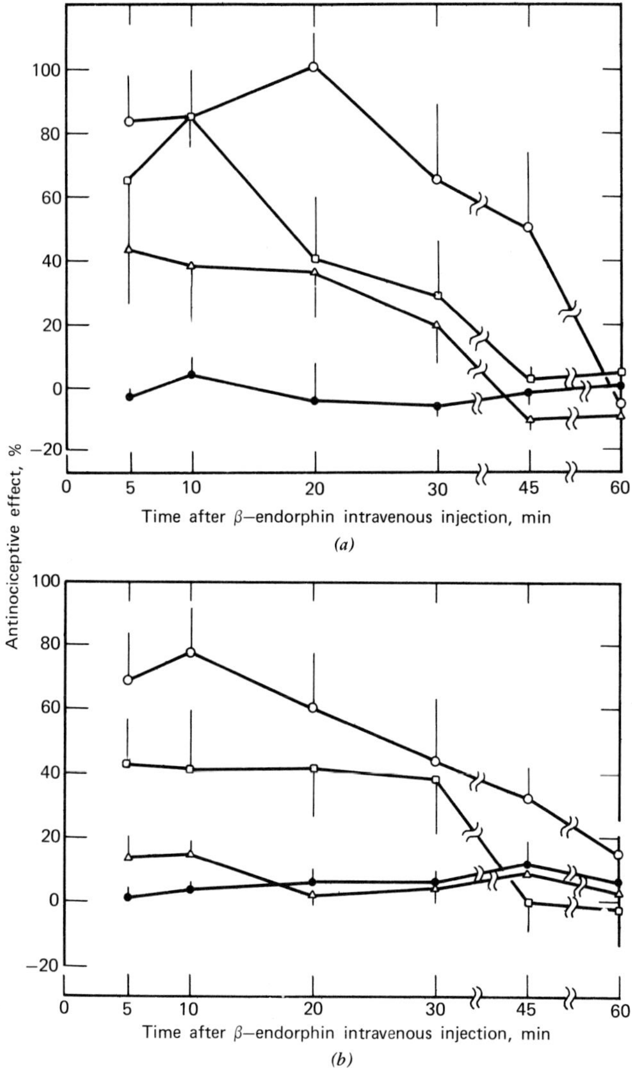

Fig. 27.5 Antinociceptive effects following the intravenous injection of β-endorphin in (a) the tail flick test and (b) the hot plate test, and its blockage by naloxone. Mice, 6 or 7 per group, were injected intravenously with 8.2 (△), 14.5 (□), and 20.1 (○) mg/kg of β-endorphin at time 0. Naloxone·HCl (1 mg/kg) (●) was injected subcutaneously 5 min before the intravenous injection of β-endorphin. The vertical bars indicate the standard error of the mean. From Tseng et al. (57). Reprinted with permission of Macmillan Journals, Ltd.

to enkephalin, β_h-EP induces cross-tolerance to and cross-physical dependence on morphine in animals (58). Like morphine, β-EP stimulates the release of somatotropin and prolactin in rats (52c, 59a, b).

Certain behavioral effects of β-EP in rats attracted wide attention. Jacquet et al. (35b) and Bloom et al. (35a) observed pronounced and prolonged sedation and a state of immobility (catatonia) without motor paralysis after i.c.v. injection of β-EP. This state was instantaneously reversed by naloxone. Both groups agreed that these findings may have mental health implications. Other behavioral activities of β-EP include excessive grooming (35c), influence on male sexual behavior (60a), profound hypothermia (58a), and a salivation effect (60b) not elicited by morphine.

Several smaller peptide segments of β-LPH (Fig. 27.3) have been isolated from brain and pituitary extracts, including α- and γ-EP, which exhibit 5–15% the morphinomimetic activity of β-EP in the guinea pig ileum assay (33a). Whereas α-EP [β-LPH-(61–76)] produces hypothermia and mild sedation on i.c.v. injection into rats, γ-EP [β-LPH-(61–71)], containing one additional leucine residue, causes hyperthermia and excited behavior (33a, 72).

2.2.2 BIOSYNTHESIS AND DISTRIBUTION. Biosynthesis of β-EP takes place in the pituitary and was shown to be linked to that of corticotropin (61a–c). A common precursor, for which the name proopiocortin has been proposed (61d), gives rise to β-lipotropin and corticotropin (61a, b). β-lipotropin and corticotropin (61a, b) β-LPH in turn serves as intermediate precursor for β-EP (34). Steps involved in the processing of several differently glycosylated forms of proopiocortin have recently been delineated (61c) and several of the subsequent intermediates, e.g., β-LPH, α-, β-, and γ-EP, have been isolated by high performance liquid chromatography and characterized chemically and biologically (34).

While the small amount of Met-EK in the pituitary is probably derived from β-EP, the main biosynthetic pathway of Met–EK and Leu–EK in the brain is distinctly different from that of β-EP and does not appear to involve intermediate β-LPH (61f). Two large proteins (>40,000 and >100,000 daltons) that appear to be precursors of the enkephalins have been found in extracts of the striatum of cattle, pigs, and rats.

Immunocytochemical studies on the distribution in rat brain show that the neurons containing β-EP exist separately (49e) from those containing enkephalin (49a–d) and are localized in the basal tuberal hypothalamus, in the diencephalon, and in the anterior pons. These β-EP containing neurons and nerve fibers within the brain are also anatomically separable from those pituitary cells that contain the same peptide. The pituitary is the primary site of β-lipotropin but small amounts have also been detected in the brain (62b, c). The localization of β-EP and the enkephalin pentapeptides in apparently separate cellular systems in brain (62a) may indicate quite diverse functional roles of these peptides.

2.2.3 SYNTHESIS. The first synthetic β-endorphin of camel (sheep) sequence was prepared by C. H. Li et al. (63), who also synthesized the human 31-peptide (64a). Using improved solid phase procedures (64b) synthetic β_h-EP was obtained in *ca.* 30% overall yield. Several solid phase syntheses of β_h-EP have since been reported (64c–f). Total syntheses of β_h-EP by conventional methods in solution via segment condensation have recently been reported by two groups (65a, b). In one of these syntheses (65a) the fractionation power of preparative high performance liquid chromatography was utilized for purification of the final crude product to homogeneity by single reversed phase chromatographic runs each of 100 mg batches.

2.2.4 STRUCTURE-ACTIVITY RELATIONSHIPS. Approximately 50 analogs of β-EP have been prepared as yet (66–73). Most of these exhibited lower biological activity and only one or two were more potent than native β-EP. The analog [Phe^{27}, Gly^{31}]β_h-EP (69) was 50% more active in the tail flick assay by i.v. injection. Several other substitutions in positions 27 and 31 resulted in decreased potency, i.e., in [$Ala^{6,7}$, Phe^{27}, Gly^{31}]β_h-EP, [Nle^5, Phe^{27}, Gly^{31}]β_h-EP, and [D-Thr^2,

Phe^{27}, Gly^{31}]β_h-EP (69). The analog [D-Ala^2]β_h-EP was found by Walker et al. (71) to be of somewhat higher activity than β_h-EP (i.c.v., tail flick assay), whereas Yamashiro et al. (66) reported this analog to be equipotent with β_h-EP. In contrast to the large potency increase obtained with [D-Ala^2]EK-amide (43a), the same substitution did not lead to any significant further stabilization of β-EP, presumably because it is already quite stable to exopeptidase degradation (66). As in the enkephalin series, substitution by D-amino acid residues in positions 1, 4, and 5 resulted in decreased activity in [D-Tyr^1]β_c-EP, [DPhe^4]β_c-EP, and [D-Met^5]β_c-EP (66). Generally lower activity was also observed with a series of analogs modified in positions 2 and 5 (68). β-EP homologs with shortened peptide chains were generally of lower activity (67, 70) up to a chain length of 29 residues. Interestingly, the homolog β_c-EP-(1–5)-(16–31) in which the sequence segment 6–15 was omitted, was more active than β_c-EP in the *in vitro* guinea pig ileum assay but of very low (0.3%) *in vivo* analgesic activity (67). Lack of correlation between the *in vitro* and *in vivo* assay results has also been observed with other synthetic analogs (66). In sum, these studies indicated that the entire length of the β-EP molecule seem to be required for full *in vivo* analgesic activity and that substitutions that produce high potency increases in the enkaphalins do not produce similar effects in the endorphins.

Removal of Tyr^1 from γ-EP, which in rats elicits behavioral effects opposite to β-EP (33a, 72), abolished its opiatelike activity. The ensuing (des-Tyr^1)γ-endorphin (DTγE) appeared more potent than γ-EP on avoidance behavior (72), and was postulated to be an endogenous neuroleptic.

2.2.5 CLINICAL POTENTIAL. The profound behavioral effects elicited by β-EP in rats (35a–c) led Bloom et al. (35a) to suggest that β_h-EP antagonists may have therapeutic properties in mental disease, whereas Jacquet and Marks (35b) implicated β_h-EP therapy assuming that mental disease may be due to β_h-EP deficiency. Recently, Kline et al. have administered β_h-EP (6–10 mg, i.v.) in uncontrolled studies to patients with several mental disorders, including schizophrenia and depression, and reported apparent improvements (73).

In a different indication, male heroin addict patients suffering from acute abstinence syndrome were treated at peak stage by single β_h-EP injections each (80 μg/kg). Within 30 min suppression of the severe withdrawal effects and impressive improvement was observed, and no adverse side effects were detected. Single injections of β_h-EP proved to be of lasting effect (74). Similar observations have been made with patients undergoing abrupt withdrawal from methadone (75). Exploratory studies on the ability of β_h-EP to relieve intractable pain in man by i.c.v. administration (76, 77) and clinical trials with (des-Tyr^1)-endorphin (DTγE) (78) have also been reported. Extended and carefully controlled studies will be required to verify all of these findings.

3 HYPOTHALAMIC HORMONES

The central nervous system regulates endocrinologic processes in the anterior pituitary gland through hypothalamic factors. These are synthesized in nerve cells of the hypothalamus and accumulate in the median eminence for storage. In response to neural stimuli, these control factors are secreted into the pituitary portal venous system and transported to the anterior hypophysis, where they stimulate or inhibit the release of the pituitary hormones.

The presence of several hypothalamic factors has been detected in extracts of hypothalami by their effects on anterior

Table 27.3 Hypothalamic Factors Regulating the Secretion of Anterior Pituitary Hormones

Anterior Pituitary Hormone	Hypothalamic Factor[a]
Lutropin (LH)	Gonadoliberin (GnRH)
Follitropin (FSH)	Lutropin release-inhibiting factor (LHIF)
Somatotropin (GH)	Somatotropin-releasing factor (GHRF)
	Somatostatin (SS)
Thyrotropin (TSH)	Thyroliberin (TRH)
Prolactin (PRL)	Prolactin-releasing factor (PRF)
	Prolactin release-inhibiting factor (PIF)
Corticotropin (ACTH)	Corticotropin-releasing factor (CRF)
Melanotropin (MSH)	Melanoliberin (MRF)
	Melanostatin (MIF)

[a] Nomenclature for chemically characterized compounds is as recommended by the IUPAC–IUB Commission on Biochemical Nomenclature [*J. Biol. Chem.*, **250,** 3215–3216 (1975)]; for traditional nomenclature, see Table 27.1.

pituitary function. These are listed in Table 27.3. Enormous efforts in the laboratories of R. Guillemin and A. V. Schally succeeded in the isolation of three of these factors from more than a million glands. The structure elucidation and chemical synthesis of thyroliberin (TRH), gonadoliberin (GnRH), and somatostatin (SS) within the period 1969–1972 generated enormous excitement. Expectations were high for arriving at relatively simple clinical controls of pituitary hormone secretion, based on the concept of one chemically distinct hypothalamic control factor for each of seven pituitary hormones, as presented in Table 27.3. However this idea has evaporated in the face of multiple functions, multiple controls, multiple target organs, and multiple sites of origin. These findings are discussed in several recent books (21, 26d, e, 79, 80) and general reviews (81–83).

When the three hypothalamic regulatory hormones of known structure became available in homogeneous synthetic form, they permitted for the first time a direct evaluation of pituitary function. It was then possible to determine the available amounts of a pituitary hormone stored in the gland. Synthesis of radiolabeled analogs allowed the development of sensitive and specific immunoassays for quantitating gonadoliberin, somatostatin, and thyroliberin (84). This led to the unexpected discovery of these molecules in extrahypothalamic loci throughout the central nervous system (84a). No details are known yet about the biosynthesis of hypothalamic hormones. Earlier evidence of a nonribosomal mechanism was not confirmed (82).

In clinical practice the availability of synthetic hypothalamic hormones allowed assessment of changes in pituitary hormone synthesis and secretion, and distinction between diseases of the pituitary and hypothalamus as causes of apparent hypopituitarism. In addition to their diagnostic value, hypothalamic hormones may yet become useful for the treatment of hypothalamic and pituitary disease (85).

This discussion is focused on the three hormones of known structure (i.e., GnRH, SS, and TRH). In addition, the COOH-terminal tripeptide of oxytocin, which has been implicated in control of melanotropin release (MIF), is briefly reviewed, as well as substance P and neurotensin, whose biological activities are attracting increasing attention.

Interesting advances include development of "superactive" and inhibitory analogs of GnRH, the surprising influence pGlu–His–Trp–Ser–Tyr–Gly–Leu–Arg–Pro–Gly–NH_2

Fig. 27.6 The structure of gonadoliberin (GnRH) [gonadotropin-releasing hormone, luteinizing hormone–follicle-stimulating hormone-releasing hormone] as determined by Schally and collaborators (88).

of somatostatin on pancreatic and gastrointestinal hormones, the behavioral effects elicited by TRH and MIF in the central nervous system, and the regulatory effects of neurotensin on liver glycogen metabolism and blood pressure.

3.1 Gonadoliberin (GnRH)*

3.1.1 ISOLATION, STRUCTURE, AND ACTIVITY. Gonadoliberin was isolated from porcine hypothalami and characterized by Schally et al. (86) in 1971 and shortly afterward by Guillemin and co-workers (87), using ovine glands. The porcine and ovine molecules and all other analyzed GnRH from different species are of identical structure, i.e., a linear decapeptide with blocked termini (Fig. 27.6), which was confirmed by synthesis (88). A controversy about the existence of two different releasing hormones for separate physiologic control each of lutropin (LH) and follitropin (FSH) seems to have abated. A consensus appeared in the literature that (1) the decapeptide (Fig. 27.6), controls physiologically the release of both LH and FSH in man and animals, and (2) another hormone that releases only or predominantly FSH might possibly be present in hypothalamic tissue (89, 90). Gonadoliberin does not stimulate secretion of growth hormone, thyrotropin or corticotropin; see Refs. 89 and 90 for reviews.

In man, GnRH releases both gonadotropins in a dose-dependent manner. In the adult, the LH response is much greater than that of FSH, but prepubertally the relative effects are reversed. After intravenous injection, GnRH exhibits a short half-life in animals and in man of 4–7 min, as a consequence of rapid enzymatic degradation (for review, see Ref. 91). The distribution and effects of GnRH (reviewed in Ref. 92) have been investigated recently by immunohistochemical, antibody enzyme, and microdissection techniques (93). GnRH is contained in axons and nerve endings in confined parts of the median eminence. The majority of axons containing the hormone originate in the medial basal hypothalamus.

Clinical studies have clearly indicated the usefulness of GnRH for both diagnostic and therapeutic application, in particular in the treatment of men and women with hypogonadothrophic infertility (81, 83, 85). Since GnRH has such a short half-life in man, however, it is vital to develop compounds with prolonged biological activity.

3.1.2 CONFORMATIONAL STUDIES. Gonadoliberin appears to behave like a random coil polypeptide in aqueous solution devoid of any intrachain residue interaction. Yet when dissolved in trifluoroethanol GnRH seems to form a folded structure with a β-turn at the level of the aromatic residues in positions 3 and 5. This structure might also prevail during receptor interaction. These conclusions were derived from conformational energy analysis and ORD/CD, fluorescence, and ^{13}C-NMR spectroscopy (94). No difference was detectable between the behavior of highly active and inactive analogs in these spectral analyses. A three-dimensional structure analysis will have to await crystallization and X-ray structure analysis of GnRH.

3.1.3 SYNTHESIS. Following the first synthesis and structure confirmation of GnRH in 1971, all investigational and clinical material has been of synthetic origin. More than 20 different approaches by solid phase and solution techniques have been

* Synonyms: gonadotropin-releasing factor, luteinizing hormone-follicle-stimulating hormone releasing hormone (LH/FSH-RH, LHRH).

reported (for a literature compilation, see Ref. 95). Immer et al. (96) have designed an interesting synthetic scheme (Fig. 27.7), which uses a minimal protection strategy (97) and is well suited for large-scale preparation and analog synthesis. The final coupling of fragments 1–6 and 7–10 directly yields GnRH, which required just one gel filtration for purification. This approach is possible because native GnRH has protected α-functions, i.e., an NH_2-terminal pyroglutamic acid residue and a COOH-terminal glycinamide residue.

3.1.4 STRUCTURE-ACTIVITY RELATIONSHIPS. Some of the most remarkable results in peptide hormone analog work have been obtained by modification of the GnRH molecule. "Superactive" analogs have been developed with up to hundred-fold potency increases and with greatly enhanced half-life of action. Moreover, antagonists of considerable activity have been synthesized. Variations in assay procedures among different laboratories make it difficult to correlate the activities of analogs from published assay data. *In vitro* activity of GnRH analogs is generally determined in rat pituitary cell cultures. *In vivo* assays measure induction of ovulation in rats.

More than 400 analogs of gonadoliberin have been reported, but discussion of a few interesting prototypes will amply illustrate the progress made. Potentiation and increased duration of agonist activity was most consistently obtained by modifications at positions Gly^6 and Gly^{10}. Omission of the 10-glycinamide residue and protection of the ensuing Pro^9 carboxyl provided several (1–9)-nonapeptide alkylamides. The most potent of these was des-(Gly–NH_2^{10})–GnRH ethylamide, which exhibited activity three- to sixfold higher than GnRH *in vitro* and *in vivo* assays (98). Replacement of the 6-glycine residue by D-amino acid residues (99–101) effected up to fourteenfold *in vitro* potentiation, e.g., [D-Ala^6]–GnRH was threefold, [D-Lys^6]–GnRH fourfold, [D-Leu^6]–GnRh sevenfold, and [D-Tyr^6]–GnRH 13.5-fold more active than the native hormone. Recently [D-Phe^6]–GnRH and [D-Trp^6]–GnRH were reported to exhibit 90 and 100 times, respectively, the *in vitro* potency, but only 10–13 times the *in vivo* potency of gonadoliberin (102). These results underscore the need of conducting dual bioassays as a tool in developing GnRH analogs.

Combination of the modifications above at positions 6 and 10 often has cumulative effects in providing "superactive" analogs with highly increased potencies and prolonged *in vivo* activities. For example, des-(Gly–NH_2^{10})–[D-Leu^6]–GnRH ethylamide elicited 54- to 82-fold greater *in vivo* effects than GnRH when integrated levels of released LH or FSH were compared over a 6 hr period after injection (103, 104). An even higher (140-fold) potency in the rat ovulation assay was reported (105) for des-(Gly–NH_2^{10})–[6-D-serine butyl ether]–GnRH ethylamide. When tested in normal man (5 μg, *i.v.*), the analog was 20 times more potent than gonadoliberin, and the LH and FSH levels remained elevated for 8–10 hr (106). These results indicate a potential for therapeutic application of this analog.

No potentiating effects, but rather strong losses of activity were obtained with other than the 6-position diastereoisomers. Highly active agonist analogs smaller than nonapeptides have not been found, indicating that most parts of the GnRH molecule are required for high potency.

The search for analogs with antagonistic activity has been prompted by expectations of their potential usefulness as contraceptive agents. Modification of the 2-histidine residue provides antagonists. The first indication was a loss of agonist activity by omission of His^2. Des-His^2–GnRH inhibited *in vitro* LH release by GnRH to 50%, at an agonist-to-inhibitor ratio of about 1:4000 (107). The octapeptide des-(His^2, Gly–NH_2^{10})–GnRH ethylamide (108) and

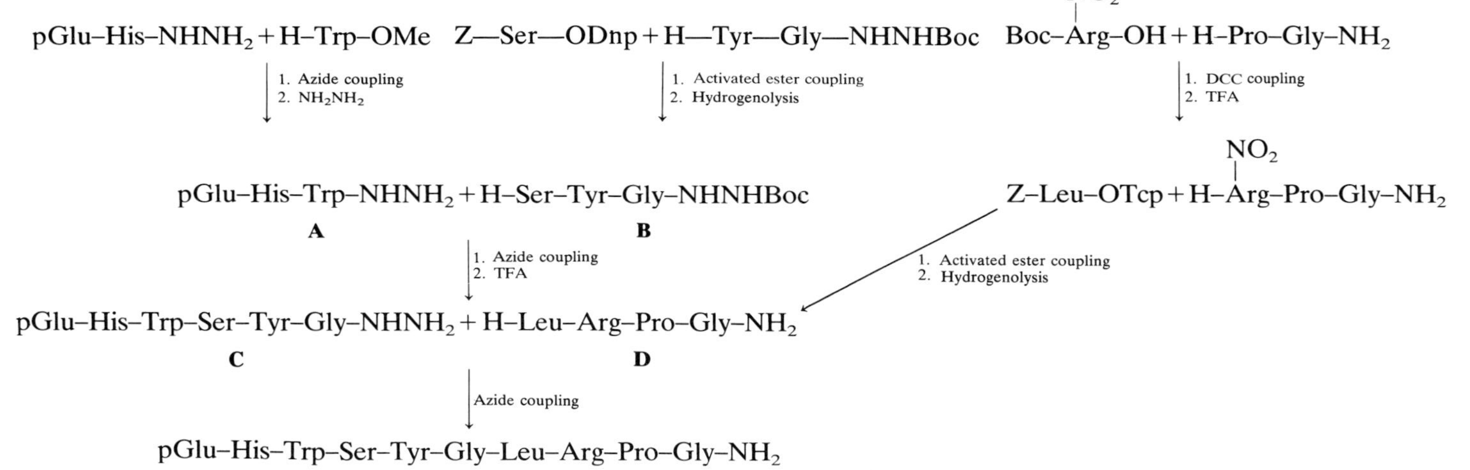

Fig. 27.7 A solution synthesis of gonadoliberin using fragment condensation with minimal side chain protection. ODnp, 2,4-dinitrophenyl ester. From Immer et al. (96).

the analog des-His^2-[D-Ala^6]-GnRH (101) were tenfold and threefold more potent inhibitors than des-His^2–GnRH and were also effective *in vivo*. However the combined 6- and 10-position modifications providing the superactive agonists, discussed previously, did not effect similar antagonist potentiation in des-His^2-analogs (109). Replacement of His^2 by D-amino acid analogs provided a series of inhibitors such as [D-Phe^2]-GnRH (110, 111), which were further potentiated by D-amino acid residues in position 6. For example, [2-D-*p*-fluorophenylalanine, 6-D-alanine]-GnRH, inhibited GnRH-induced (5 μg/rat) ovulation in rats at doses of 6×500 μg/rat, a ratio of about 1:1000 (112). Still higher potency has been obtained by replacement of the Gly^{10} residue by α-azaglycine [H_2N—NH—COOH] (113) and one of the most potent antagonists yet prepared, i.e. [D-pGlu^1, D-Phe^2, D-Trp^{3,6}]GnRH, effected complete inhibition of ovulation in rats at 250 μg and 100 μg doses (113a). Some of the antagonistic analogs are currently being tested in animals, and in man and their importance as contraceptive agents remains to be established. For reviews on structure-activity relations, see Ref. 113b.

3.2 Melanostatin and Melanoliberin*

It has been proposed (114) that the release of pituitary melanotropin (MSH) is regulated by factors that are formed by hypothalamic enzymes using oxytocin as a substrate (Fig. 27.8). Pro–Leu–Gly–NH_2 (peptide **C**) and Pro–His–Phe–Arg–Gly–NH_2 (**D**) both isolated from hypothalamic glands, have been implicated in inhibiting MSH release; peptides **A** and **B** appear to be involved in stimulating it. This hypothesis has been questioned because the MIF or MRF activities of the synthetic peptides remain controversial, partly because of great experimental difficulties associated with *in vivo* bioassays. A recent comparative *in vitro* study of the effects of Pro–Leu–Gly–NH_2 (MIF) and tocinoic acid (Fig. 27.8 peptide **B**) on MSH release in rat pituitary cultures revealed a strong dose dependence of MIF effects (116). At dose levels of 20 ng/ml, MSH release was inhibited, at 1–10 μg no effects were seen, and at

* Synonyms: Melanocyte-stimulating hormone-release inhibiting factor (MIF), melanocyte-stimulating hormone releasing factor (MRF); melanotropin-release inhibiting factor, melanotropin releasing factor.

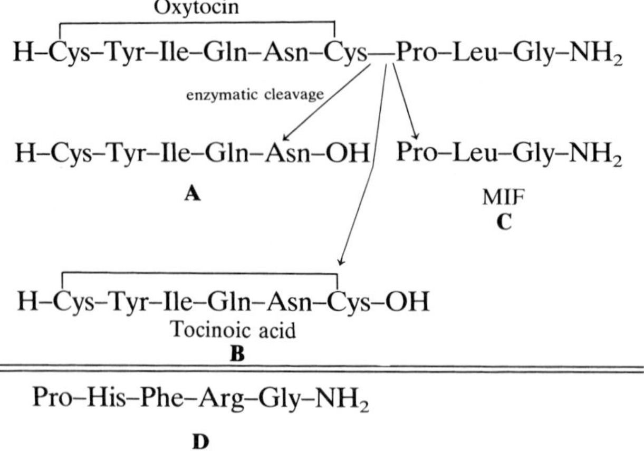

Fig. 27.8 Peptides that have been implicated in the control of melanotropin (MSH) release. Peptides **A**, **B**, and **C** originate from oxytocin (114). Peptides **C** and **D** have been isolated from hypothalamic glands (115). MSH-releasing activity has been reported for peptides **A** and **B**, release-inhibiting activity for **C** and **D**.

100 μg MSH release was stimulated. These results offer an explanation for differences reported in the literature in MIF activity of synthetic peptides in rats. However the endocrinologic significance and physiologic roles of Pro–Leu–Gly–NH_2 and other peptides that elicit MIF or MRF effects remain to be established (for review, see Ref. 83).

In the meantime, the focus of attention on Pro–Leu–Gly–NH_2 has been shifted to its strong behavioral effects in the central nervous system, in particular in the DOPA potentiation and oxytremorin antagonism tests (92, 117). Beneficial effects in patients with Parkinsons's disease have been observed (for review, see Ref. 83). Radioautographic localization of [^{3}H]Pro–Leu–Gly–NH_2 In several brain areas of rats after intracarotid injection suggest that the peptide may cross the blood-brain barrier (118, 119). A high uptake of radioactivity by the pineal gland after intrajugular injection in rats suggests a role for Pro–Leu–Gly–NH_2 in the control of pineal activity (120). A synthetic analog, pGlu–Leu–Gly–NHEt, with fourfold higher potency in the oxytremorin antagonism test, has been described (121).

3.3 Somatostatin*

3.3.1 ISOLATION, STRUCTURE, AND ACTIVITY. While searching in ovine hypothalamic extracts for somatoliberin (still elusive at this time), Guillemin and collaborators isolated in 1972 a peptide from certain chromatographic fractions that consistently inhibited the release of radioimmunoassayable growth hormone in a dose-dependent manner in monolayer rat pituitary cell cultures (122). Sequence analysis by Edman degradation and mass spectrometry showed the hormone, named somatostatin, to be a tetradecapeptide with a 3–14 disulfide bond forming a 38-member heterodetic ring (Fig. 27.9). The structure has been confirmed by synthesis. No species variant has yet been described. Both the oxidized and the "reduced" 3,14-bissulfhydryl forms of the molecule exhibit identical equipotent biological activity in several *in vitro* and *in vivo* assays in various animal species (for reviews, see Refs. 123–125).

It soon became apparent from studies in laboratory animals that somatostatin inhibits not only the secretion of several pituitary hormones but also the secretion of insulin and glucagon and several gastrointestinal hormones. These findings suggest a physiological role for somatostatin in regulating the secretion of these hormones. The presence of somatostatin in locations other than the hypothalamus was detected by radioimmunoassay (126), immunohistochemical techniques, and bioassay. In the rat pancreas somatostatin-secreting cells were identified (D cells) by electron microscopic investigation (127). Somatostatin-containing cells are also present in the duodenum, the fundic and antral mucosa of the stomach, and, in smaller numbers, in the jejunum and ileum of vertebrates. Somatostatin is widely distributed in the central nervous system, with a high level present in the spinal cord. In these locations the hormone is contained in the secretory granules of nerve endings, indicating a possible neurotransmitter function (for reviews, see Refs. 81, 124, 128–130).

Somatostatin is active at nanomolar concentrations both at adenohypophyseal and pancreatic receptor sites, i.e., *in vitro* at 1

* Synonyms: growth-hormone-release-inhibiting hormone (GHRIH, GIF), somatotropin-release-inhibiting hormone (SRIH).

H–Ala–Gly–Cys–Lys–Asn–Phe–Phe–Trp–Lys–Thr–Phe–Thr–Ser–Cys–OH
(disulfide bridge Cys 3 – Cys 14)
1 2 3 4 5 6 7 8 9 10 11 12 13 14

Fig. 27.9 The structure of somatostatin (122).

n*M* and *in vivo* at 200–400 ng/100 g of body weight (123). The *in vivo* biological half-life is very short (2–4 min), which restricts the value of somatostatin as a therapeutic agent. Its inactivation in brain and tissue was shown (131) to result from endopeptidase cleavage, mainly at the Trp^8–Lys^9 peptide bond. Rat serum is two- to fivefold more active than human serum in cleaving somatostatin (132). The synthetic [D-Trp^8]-somatostatin analog is resistant to cleavage at the Trp^8–Lys^9 bond and exhibits approximately eight fold potency in several assays (133). Obviously, knowledge about the mechanisms of action (91) would facilitate rational approaches in analog design.

The multiple biological activities of somatostatin in suppressing the release of peptide hormones are directed at pituitary, pancreatic, and gastrointestinal target sites. Thus affected are growth hormone (GH), thyrotropin responses to TRH, insulin and glucagon (see Section 8.3), and gastrin, pepsin, secretin, and vasoactive intestinal peptide. The secretion of the following hormones does not seem to be affected: ACTH, LH, FSH, PTH (134); reviews are contained in Refs. 81, 82, and 124.

Growth hormone secretion, both basal and stimulated by the normal secretagogs, is suppressed by somatostatin *in vitro* and *in vivo* in man and animals. Constant intravenous infusion (e.g., 0.5–1 mg per adult human over 30–60 min) is required to obtain measurable effects. Rapid rebound of suppressed GH has been observed on terminating infusions. *Thyrotropin secretion* induced by TRH and other stimuli, *in vitro* and *in vivo*, is inhibited in a dose-dependent manner, indicating a potential physiological role in thyroid regulation. Secretions of *insulin* and *glucagon* are affected by pancreatic somatostatin; see Section 8.3. *Gastrin* secretion, both basal and in response to a meal, is partially suppressed by somatostatin in normal man and in patients with pernicious anemia. Gastric acid and pepsin secretion in laboratory animals is inhibited by a direct action of somatostatin on the parietal and peptic cells (135, 126). The *secretin*- and *cholecystokinin*-induced excretory pancreatic response and gall bladder contraction in man are inhibited by somatostatin (137).

Somatostatin has been proposed as a potential *therapeutic agent* (for reviews, see Refs. 124 and 138) for the treatment of acromegaly (for its suppression of GH-release), of diabetes mellitus (for inhibiting glucagon and GH-release, see Section 8.3), of bleeding ulcers in patients [for lowering gastric acid release (139)], and of pancreatitis (for reducing CCK-stimulated pancreatic exocrine secretion). However the diverse effects of somatostatin on the secretion of several hormones and its short duration of action render its clinical use impractical at this time. Its long-term effectiveness and safety have not yet been established. This makes the search for synthetic analogs exhibiting prolonged activity and specificity for single hormones all the more important.

3.3.2 SYNTHESIS. Several syntheses of somatostatin have been reported (literature cited in Ref. 141), and most of the biological and clinical work has been carried out with synthetic preparations. Synthesis by solid phase procedures has typically yielded 15–35% of the linear dithiol form ("dihydrosomatostatin"). Oxidation by air or ferricyanide competes with dimer and oligomer formation. Therefore high dilution conditions must be used to obtain cyclic somatostatin in good yields [>60%, (142)]. For synthesis of somatostatin by solution procedures, various fragment condensation schemes have been followed which were designed to provide flexibility for different programs of analog synthesis (141, 143–145). A methodological study of a synthesis (142) by the stepwise incremental chain elongation strategy (146) is summarized in Fig. 27.10.

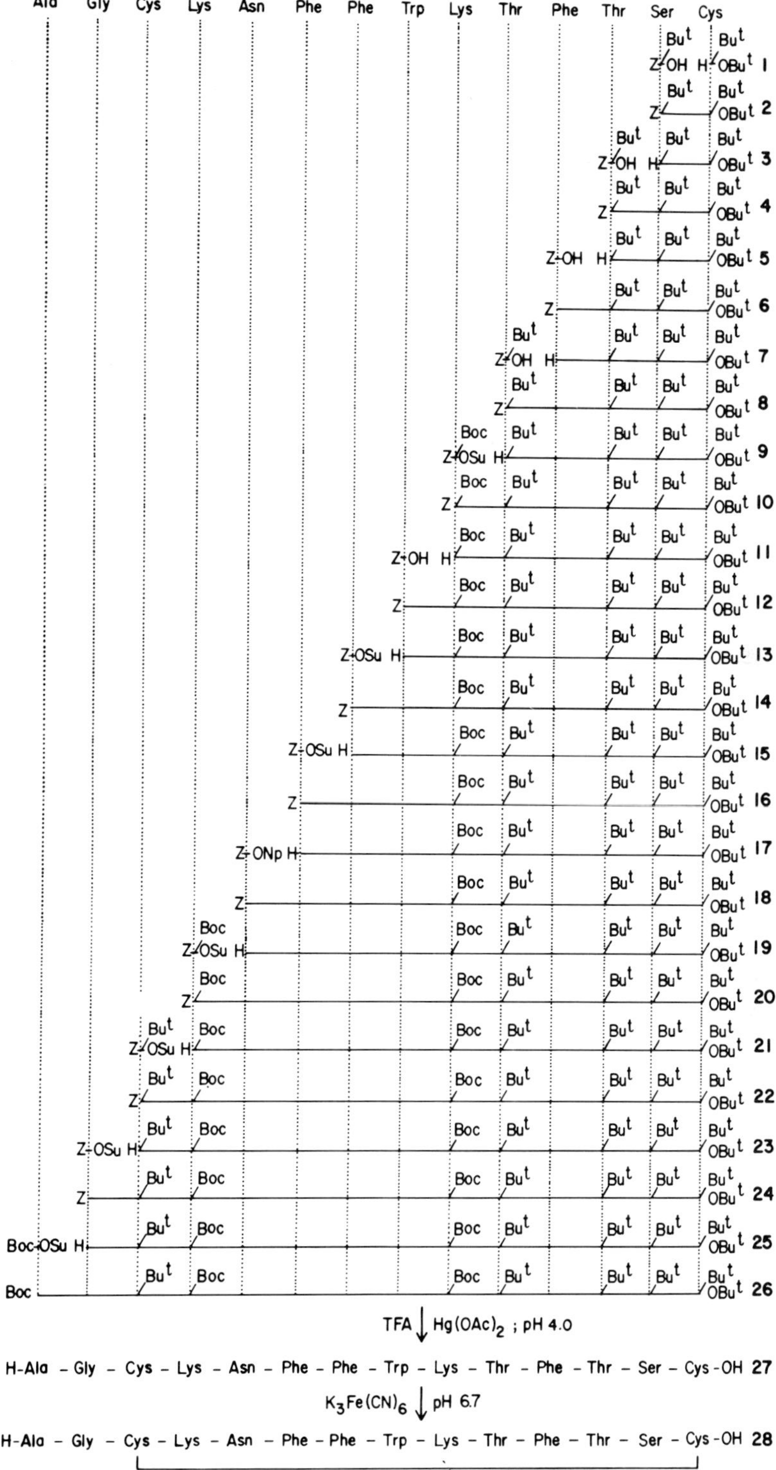

Fig. 27.10 Synthesis of somatostatin by stepwise incremental chain elongation; Z = benzyloxycarbonyl. Each alpha N^{α}-benzyloxycarbonyl group was cleaved by catalytic hydrogenation in liquid ammonia as a solvent, which prevents catalyst poisoning by cysteine residues (147). From Felix et al. (142).

Analog synthesis has been highly motivated by the therapeutic potentials of somatostatin, discussed earlier. Long-acting analogs are desired for all clinical applications. Specificity of action on only one or two targets would be very advantageous for therapeutic use, i.e., selective suppression of glucagon and growth hormone release without causing the suppression of insulin release for treatment of diabetes mellitus, selective suppression of gastrin and gastric acid release for bleeding ulcer treatment, or selective inhibition of growth hormone release for treatment of acromegaly. The majority of analog syntheses (only a small part of the total effort has been published) has been carried out by solid phase procedures or by following the synthetic schemes of solution synthesis used for the native hormone. However somewhat different synthetic schemes were required for the preparation of dicarba (Fig. 27.11) or carbocyclic analogs in which the disulfide has been replaced by ethylene (145) or amide bridges (148).

3.3.3 STRUCTURE-ACTIVITY RELATIONSHIPS. Approximately 150 synthetic analogs of somatostatin had been published as of October 1978. Prolonged activity has been observed with one of these, the des-(Ala[1]-Gly[2])-desaminodicarbasomatostatin (see Fig. 27.11). Its inhibition of pentagastrin-induced gastric acid secretion was prolonged for 30 min after the infusion had stopped (145). Increased potency in several assays has been obtained by each of three amino acid replacements: 1.3-fold with [Ala[5]]-somatostatin (123), 1.9-fold with [Ala[2]]-somatostatin (123), and a dramatic

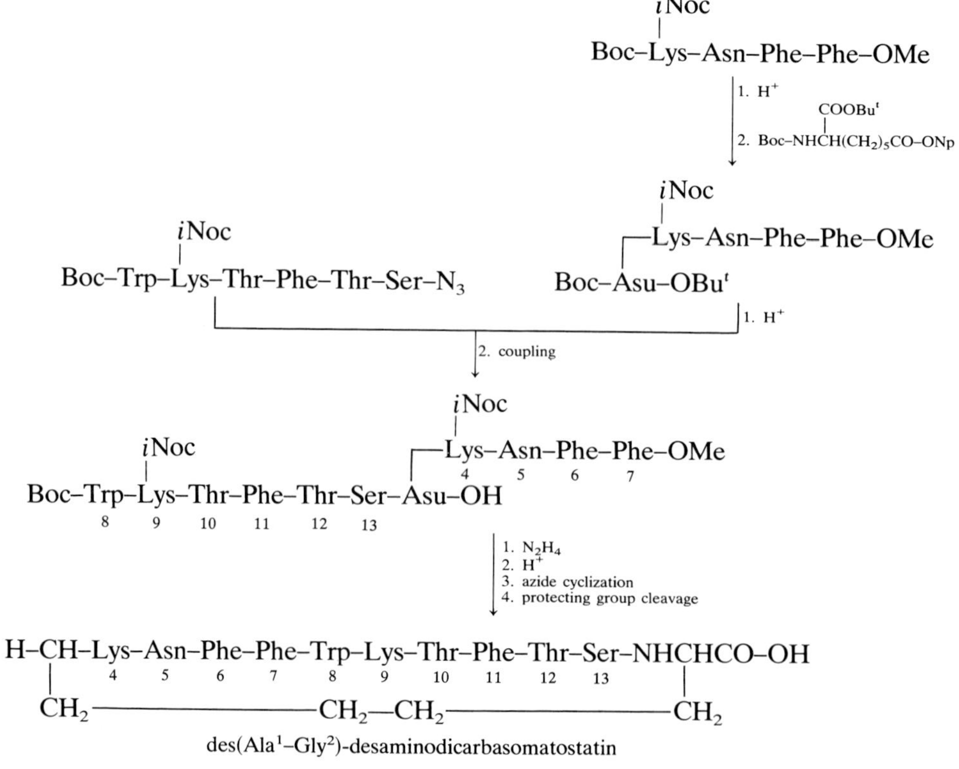

Fig. 27.11 Synthesis of des(Ala[1]-Gly[2])-desaminodicarbasomatostatin by way of azide cyclization between residues 7 and 8. In this nonreducible cyclic analog, the disulfide bond is replaced by an ethylene bridge, i.e., the cystine residue by an aminosuberic acid (Asu) residue; *i*Noc = isonicotinyloxycarbonyl. From Veber et al. (145).

$$\gamma\text{-Abu}^{3}\text{–Lys}^{4}\text{–Asn}^{5}\text{–Phe}^{6}\text{–Phe}^{7}\text{–Trp}^{8}\text{–Lys}^{9}\text{–Thr}^{10}\text{–Phe}^{11}\text{–Thr}^{12}\text{–Ser}^{13}\text{–Asp}^{14}\text{–OH}$$

des-(Ala^1–Gly^2)–[γ-Abu^3, Asp^{14}]-somatostatin lactam (ω-14 → 3)

$$\text{H–Lys}^{4}\text{–Asn}^{5}\text{–Phe}^{6}\text{–Phe}^{7}\text{–Trp}^{8}\text{–Lys}^{9}\text{–Thr}^{10}\text{–Phe}^{11}\text{–Thr}^{12}\text{–Ser}^{13}\text{–Glu}^{14}\text{–OH}$$

des-(Ala^1–Gly^2–Cys^3)–[Glu^{14}]-somatostatin lactam (ω-14→4]

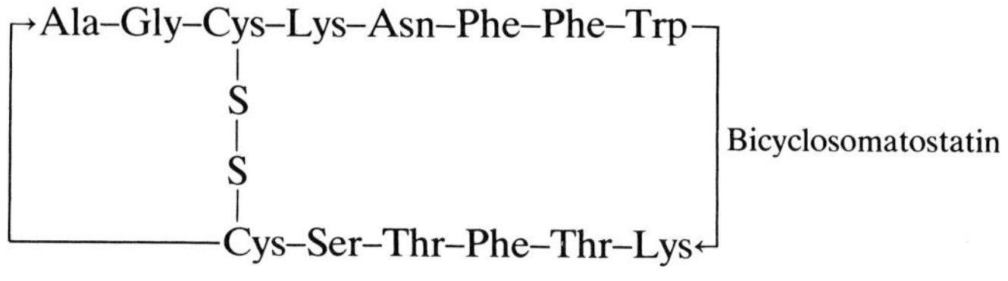

→Ala–Gly–Cys–Lys–Asn–Phe–Phe–Trp
S–S
Cys–Ser–Thr–Phe–Thr–Lys←

Bicyclosomatostatin

Somatostatin-lactam (α-14→1)

Fig. 27.12 Somatostatin lactam analogs that show selective inhibition of growth-hormone release (148, 152, 153).

eightfold potentiation with [D-Trp^8]-somatostatin (133). Changes of the pharmacologic activity profile were accomplished by several modifications. Omission of the Ala^1-Gly^2 "tail" (149, 150) or the 5-asparagine residue (151) and replacement of the 13-serine residue by its D-enantiomer (151) increased the insulin specificity over glucagon and growth hormone. Introduction of lactam rings obtained by peptide cyclization (148, 152, 153), schematized in Fig. 27.12, provided growth hormone selectivity. Replacement of the 14-cysteine residue by its D-enantiomer (151, 154) has been reported to result in glucagon specificity. The potentiating effects just described were also obtained in an additive manner for some of the "specific" analogs by multiple substitution.

From the limited experience in somatostatin analog work, it has already become clear that the molecule is amenable to more extensive modification than oxytocin and vasopressin, which are of similar structural type, i.e., heterodetic cyclic disulfide peptides (see Section 5). The NH_2-terminal linear (tail) part of somatostatin (SS) is not required for high activity. Des-(Ala^1-Gly^2)-SS and its reduced form exhibit 30–100% the potency of native SS (155). The ring size of the molecule is also not critical. Deletions of the 4-lysine, 5-asparagine, or 13-serine residue provide homologs that retain appreciable activity (156).

The role of the disulfide is to maintain the essential cyclic architecture of somatostatin. Thiol methylation (155) and replacement of both cysteine residues by alanine (157) result in drastic loss of activity, but substitution of the disulfide bridge by amide bonds (148, 152, 153) preserves considerable activity, and replacement by ethylene (145) even potentiates and prolongs it. The full bioactivity of the reduced dithiol form ("dihydrosomatostatin") (155) indicates that the cyclic structure may be formed during circulation or receptor binding.

The terminal functions of somatostatin, i.e., its α-amino group and its carboxyl group, are not essential for activity. Desamino^1-descarboxy^{14}-SS exhibits 10% the potency of the native hormone (158), as does the ring-closed bicyclosomatostatin (153). N^{α}-Acetyl- and N^{α}-benzoyl-des-(Ala^1-Gly^2)-SS are equipotent (158) with native SS, but a possible depot effect of these and other N^{α}-acylated derivatives (159) was not confirmed (158).

A systematic study (123) in which all 14 residues of somatostatin were substituted in turn by alanine residues revealed potentiation in positions 2 and 5 but a strong decrease in bioactivity in most other positions. Substitution of the aromatic residues ($Phe^{6,7,11}$, Trp^{8}) by tyrosine (156, 160) resulted in retention of high activity except for the 8-tryptophan replacement, where drastic loss of activity occurred. The impressive eightfold potentiation of somatostatin potency in the [D-Trp^{8}]-SS diastereoisomer is explained by the finding (131) that the Trp^{8}-Lys^{9} peptide bond is a prime enzymatic cleavage site of the hormone. No potentiation resulted from D-enantiomer substitutions in position 1 and 4 (158), but shifts in target specificity, discussed earlier, occurred in the [D-Ser^{13}]- and [D-Cys^{14}]-analogs (151, 154).

The results of these initial somatostatin analog studies are very encouraging. It has been shown that prolongation and potentiation of bioactivity can be obtained. Even more important, shifts in the pharmacological activity profile can be effected that may eventually allow complete separation of activities to provide "single-target" analogs. The promising potential of such analogs for medicine will certainly be a strong incentive for highly intensive work in the future.

3.4 Thyroliberin*

3.4.1 PROPERTIES, DISTRIBUTION, AND ACTIVITY. Thyroliberin (TRH) is a tripeptide, pGlu–His–Pro–NH_2 (Fig. 27.13) that stimulates the release of thyrotropin (TSH) and prolactin (PRL) in experimental animals and in man, and release of somatotropin (GH) in acromegalic but not in normal

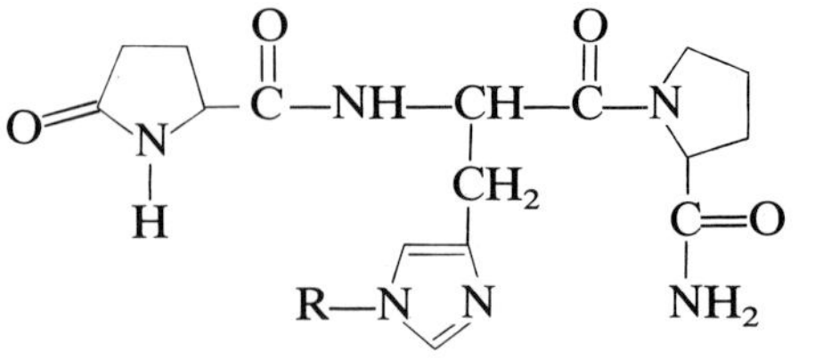

Fig. 27.13 The structure of thyroliberin (R = H), i.e., L-pyroglutamyl-L-histidyl-L-prolinamide, as determined by mass spectrometry with the aid of chemical synthesis (161). The N^{τ}-methylhistidine analog (R = CH_3) exhibits eightfold higher potency (162).

humans. Dosages range from nanogram to microgram quantities by intravenous or peripheral administration. Thyroliberin is active orally (in milligram amounts), an exceptional feature for a peptide hormone. Its plasma half-life in rats is 2–4 min. Plasma enzymes degrade TRH by cleavage of each peptide bond with liberation of histidine. Rat serum is two- to fivefold more active in metabolizing TRH than human serum (91, 132). In rats, exogenous thyroliberin accumulates in kidney, liver, thyroid, and brain, with highest concentrations in the hypothalamus. The thyrotropin response to TRH is inhibited by exogenous administration of either triiodothyronine (T_3) or thyroxine (T_4) in a dose-dependent manner. Since the stimulating effect of TRH is blocked by an increase in circulating thyrotropin level acting at the pituitary, this negative feedback may be the principal regulatory mechanism for TSH secretion (85). Thyroliberin has been reported to accelerate brain norepinephrin turnover in rats (163) for reviews of TRH chemistry and biology see Refs. 90 and 83, respectively).

Thyroliberin has been localized by bioassay and immunoassay in many areas of the central nervous system. With the indirect immunofluorescence technique TRH-containing nerve terminals were found in the median eminence and other areas of the hypothalamus, and in extrahypothalamic nuclei and in several motor nuclei of

* Synonym: thyrotropin-releasing hormone (TRH).

the brain stem and spinal cord. These findings suggest that thyroliberin may act as a hormone, released into the portal vessels, and also as a neurotransmitter or modulator, released at synapses in discrete regions of the brain and spinal cord (164). Thyroliberin has significant central effects, e.g., potentiation of the behavioral excitation induced by L-DOPA in mice, or suppression of the sedation and hypothermia produced by pentobarbital or ethanol (92, 165).

A standard clinical intravenous or oral TRH test has been developed [TRF Roche® (165a)] that differentiates both hyper- and hypothyroidism from the euthyroid state. The test has been found to be valuable in differentiating hypothyroidism due to pituitary dysfunction from that due to hypothalamic dysfunction. Therapeutically, TRH has been used in the treatment of carcinoma of the thyroid. No major toxic side effects have been reported, but some mild and transient symptoms such as nausea were observed. The efficacy of THR in the treatment of mental depression is still subject to controversy (for reviews on clinical neuroendocrinology, see Refs. 81 and 85).

3.4.2 SYNTHESIS. More than a dozen approaches have been used for synthesis of thyroliberin. The unusually high tendency of the 2-histidine residue to racemize has presented considerable difficulties (166a). An improved procedure using carbodiimide in the presence of *N*-hydroxy-5-norbornene-2,3-dicarboximide for coupling provided the first crystalline TRH in the form of a tartrate (166b). Two syntheses by solution methods have been described in which homogeneous TRH is directly obtained from crystalline protected tripeptide intermediates in total yields exceeding 50% (166a, 167). Both syntheses appear to be suitable for large-scale production of highly purified TRH, judging by their high coupling yields and simple final purification step, Fig. 27.14 provides an example.

3.4.3 STRUCTURE-ACTIVITY RELATIONSHIPS. Most chemical modifications in more than 100 analogs were accompanied by a substantial loss of biological activity, with one notable exception: the [2-N^{τ}-methylhistidine]-TRH (162), see Fig. 27.13. This analog exhibits 8 times the potency of the natural hormone, in striking contrast to the dramatic decrease in activity (0.01% of

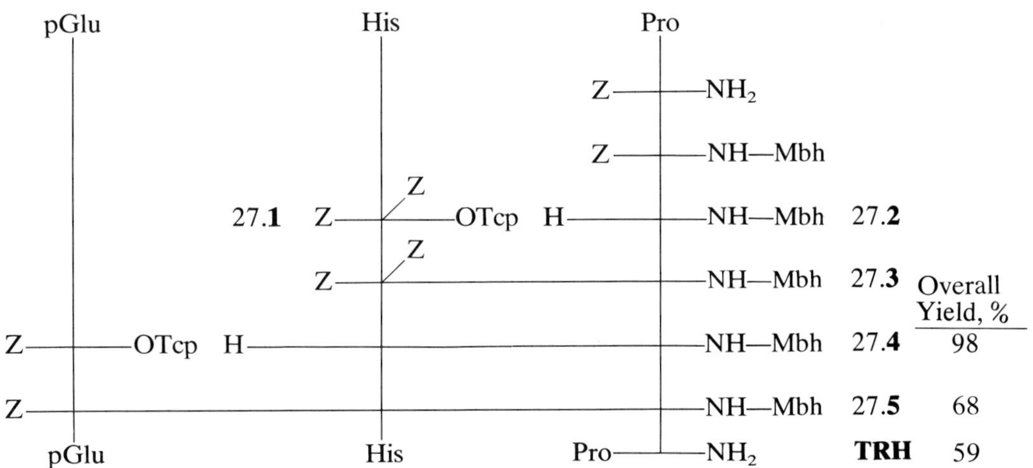

Fig. 27.14 A synthesis of thyroliberin by incremental chain elongation in solution. Protecting group removal from crystallized homogeneous 27.**5** by trifluoroacetic acid provided directly 19 g of homogeneous TRH. Abbreviations: Mbh, *p,p'*-dimethoxybenzhydryl; OTcp, 2,4,5-trichlorophenyl ester. From Bajusz and Fauszt (166a).

TRH) by methylating the N^{π}-nitrogen. The results of all this analog work, conducted in several laboratories, have been summarized by Guillemin et al. (90, 168), who conclude that "the molecule must be hydrophobic; rigid stereochemical or bulk properties must be met for each residue; pGlu may act in a nucleophilic capacity; His may be involved as a general acid; and, amide substitutions retain high potency except for charged groups and groups of large bulk". More definitive conclusions were precluded by the absence of information on TRH conformation. Analog work has largely ceased in the face of failures to find either antagonistic activity, prolonged duration of action, or separation of target specificity for thyrotropin and prolactin release.

In the meantime several three-dimensional models have been proposed for TRH based on semiempirical calculations and spectroscopic studies (literature cited in Refs. 169 and 170). From the results of proton NMR studies it was suggested that TRH is preferentially in an extended conformation in polar solvents (169). Chemical modifications associated with loss of bioactivity do not significantly affect the preferred backbone conformation of the hormone, emphasizing the critical role of each functional group in TRH for optimal binding to the receptor sites. An analog designed on the basis of conformational considerations to further stabilize the molecule in an extended form, i.e., [2-N^{α}-methylhistidine]-TRH, was found to exhibit the full biological activity and potency (115 ±8%) of the native hormone (171)

Although thyrotropin and prolactin-release specificity have not yet been separated, a possibly even more important separation of central nervous system activity from endocrine activity has been obtained with two analogs. Brain responses to [2-β-pyrazolyl(3)alanine]-TRH and to TRH-β-alaninamide are equal to those of TRH, but thyrotropin and prolactin release are greatly reduced (172). It seems that conformation-oriented and target-directed analog programs might yet provide rewarding discoveries.

3.5 Substance P and Neutrotensin

In addition to releasing hormones, other neurosecretory peptides with potent biological activity are present in the hypothalamus. The isolation of neurotensin and substance P (Fig. 27.15) revealed a novel group of peptides that may have important neurotransmitter function (173). Both peptides stimulate the release of prolactin and growth hormone in rats (174). The structures of neurotensin, a tridecapeptide, and of substance P, an undecapeptide, have been confirmed by synthesis (175, 176).

Substance "P" ("pain producing") has long been known as an active principle in extracts of nervous and intestinal tissue (for reviews, see Refs. 177 and 178). In brain, concentrations of substance P are highest in the substantia nigra and hypothalamus, where most of it is located in nerve-ending granules. Substance P depolarizes central neurons of the cat when applied by micro-iontophoresis, and it elicits central depressant effects. It stimulates nerve endings in

H–Arg–Pro–Lys–Pro–Gln–Gln–Phe–Phe–Gly–Leu–Met–NH_2

Substance P

pGlu–Leu–Tyr–Glu–Asn–Lys–Pro–Arg–Arg–Pro–Tyr–Ile–Leu–OH

Neurotensin

Fig. 27.15 The structures of substance P and neurotensin, each confirmed by synthesis (175).

many tissues, including guinea pig vas deferens, and exhibits peripheral kininlike effects. In the whole animal substance P exerts a tranquilizing rather than a stimulatory effect (179). It has been proposed (180) that substance P may be a transmitter of sensory neurons or a modulator of neuronal activity.

Neurotensin may also have a neurotransmitter role in the brain, as indicated by its receptor binding properties (181) as well as its preferential localization in synaptosomal fractions and in specific grey matter areas of the brain. The highest concentrations of neurotensin in rat brain are present in the median eminence. When administered intracisternally, neurotensin induces hypothermia and intolerance to cold, which suggests an involvement in central thermoregulatory processes (182). These central effects cannot be obtained by intravenous administration of neurotensin, but a wide spectrum of other effects is observed. Neurotensin causes hypotension and smooth muscle (gut) contraction, increased vascular permeability, and elevation of plasma glucagon and glucose in the rat. Neurotensin may be involved in liver glycogen metabolism, since intravenous injection into rats was observed to cause hyperglycemia within minutes, accompanied by a fall in liver glycogen and a rise in activity of liver glycogen phosphorylase (183). However a physiological role for neurotensin remains to be identified. For analog synthesis and structure-activity relations, see Ref. 183a.

4 ADENOHYPOPHYSEAL HORMONES

The pituitary gland is a tiny organ located beneath the brain. It weighs only about 0.6 g in man, but it is the central governing organ for many other endocrine glands that regulate vital metabolic processes. The pituitary consists of three lobes. The anterior and intermediate lobes, together, are known as the adenohypophysis, and the posterior lobe is called the neurohypophysis (see Section 5). The adenohypophyseal hormones are either metabolic, regulating body chemistry, or gonadotropic, being concerned with sexual activity. Six major hormones, a prohormone, and the two melanotropins are now known to be secreted by the adenohypophysis (Fig. 27.16). These pituitary hormones regulate the following organs and functions (184):

1. The adrenal cortex, producing more than 30 steroid hormones, by adrenocorticotropin (ACTH).
2. The sex glands, producing male sperm and female ova, and male and female sex hormones, by lutropin (LH) and follitropin (FSH).
3. The thyroid gland, regulating energy exchange, by thyrotropin (TSH).
4. The mammary gland, its growth and initiation of lactation, by prolactin (PRL).
5. The total growth and development of the body, by somatotropin (GH).

The hormonelike β-lipotropin (β-LPH), thought to be primarily involved in fat mobilization, was recently found to be a candidate prohormone for β-endorphin (Fig. 27.17), a potent analgesic agent interacting with opioid receptors (see Section 2). β-LPH may also be a prohormone for β-melanotropin [MSH], which influences skin pigmentation in certain animals.

Some of the pituitary hormones act as tropic hormones in stimulating a specific endocrine gland to secrete its own hormone(s), which then participates in the actual physiological function. The tropic stimulation is delicately balanced by a feedback mechanism (Fig. 27.16). When a certain concentration of adrenal or thyroid or sex hormones is reached in the blood, the pituitary shuts off the supply of the respective tropic hormone allowing it to resume when the concentration of one or more hormones in the blood becomes low.

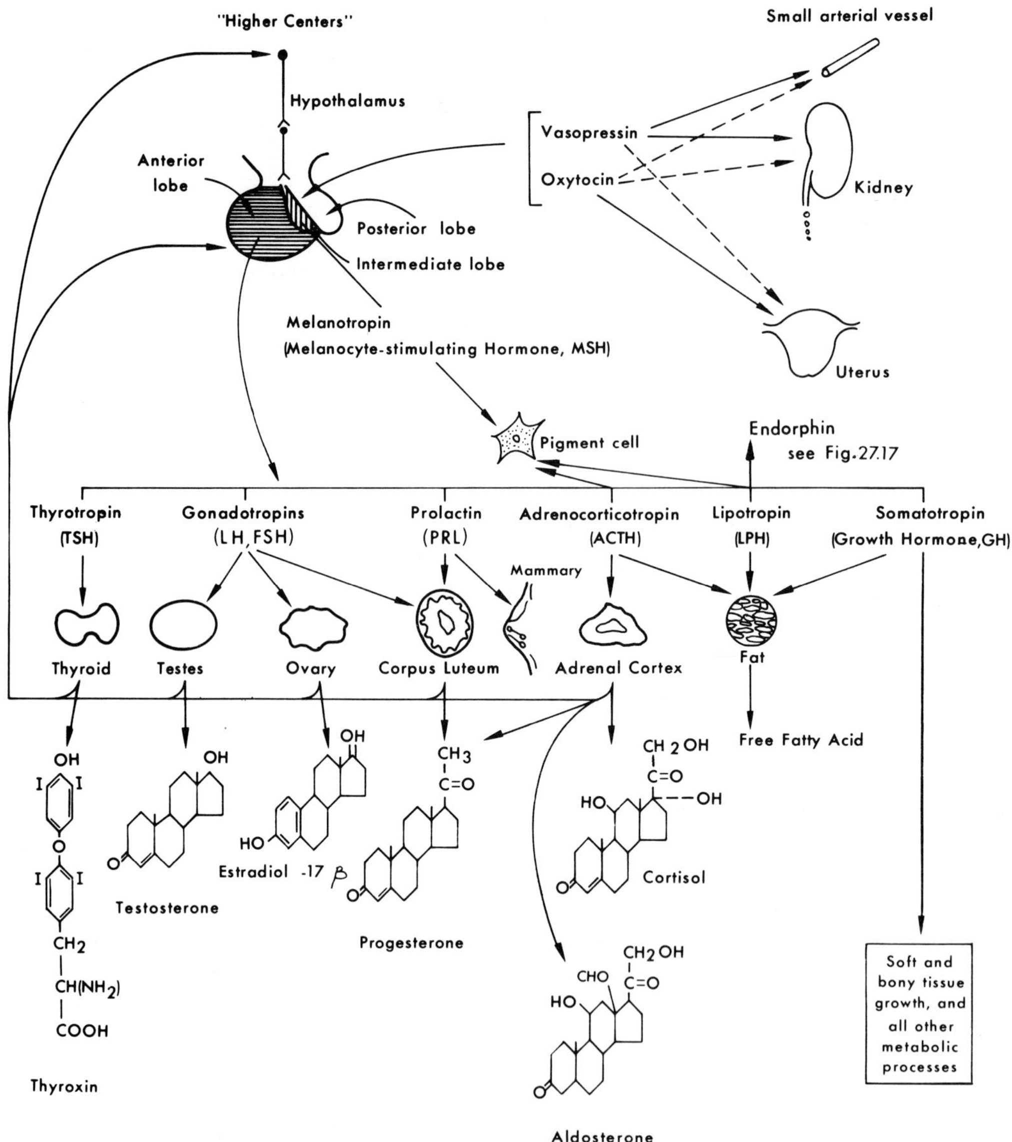

Fig. 27.16 Diagrammatic depiction of biological properties of pituitary hormones. Modified from Li (184).

The α-β-subunit architecture of the glycoprotein hormones LH, FSH, and TSH has been one of the most interesting discoveries of recent years (184), only to be surpassed by the intriguing finding (185) that fragments of human growth hormone will recombine noncovalently to form a "recombinant hormone" that possesses close to full biological activity and conformational properties of native hGH. Other interesting developments include the growing insights into hormone-receptor interactions in general (14, 15, 186) and in specific systems, e.g., for ACTH (187, 188).

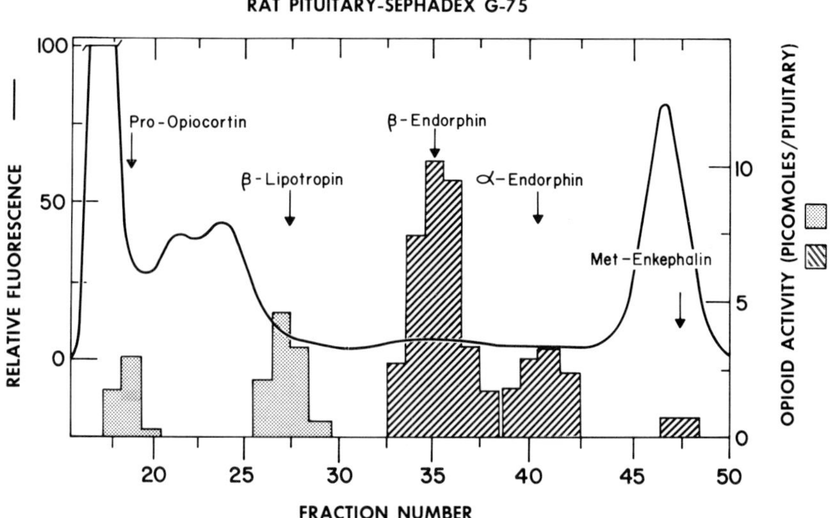

Fig. 27.17 Five areas of opioid activity at marker positions of pro-opiocortin (31 K protein, Refs. 61a, b), β-lipotropin, β-endorphin, α-endorphin, and Met-enkephalin were present in Sephadex G-75 chromatogram of a rat pituitary extract. A biosynthetic precursor relationship of pro-opiocortin to β-lipotropin to β-endorphin has been suggested (61a–f). Aliquots of fractions in the high molecular weight (>4000 daltons) region of the chromatogram (fractions 15–30) were digested with trypsin prior to the radioreceptor assay. Activity units have been converted into picomoles for each opioid peptide. Modified from Udenfriend et al. (184a).

ACTH is the first peptide hormone of which a modified synthetic product has become commercially available. The large increase in recent years in the use of synthetic ACTH-(1-24)-tetracosapeptide (189) (Synacthen®, Ciba-Geigy, Basel) in human medicine underscores the potential for clinical applications of other pituitary hormones and analogs.

4.1 Corticotropin (ACTH)*

4.1.1 CHEMISTRY AND BIOLOGY. Corticotropins have been isolated in pure form from ovine, porcine, bovine, and human pituitaries. The structures of these 39 residue peptides (Fig. 27.18) vary only in positions 31 and 33.

The biological actions of ACTH may be summarized as follows (184): (1) direct effects on the adrenal cortex, including adrenal steroidogenesis, ascorbic acid depletion, and growth processes; and (2) indirect effects (thymus involution, erythropoiesis, galactopoiesis, etc.) which are mediated by the adrenal cortex. In addition to these two main functions, ACTH exhibits *in vivo* and *in vitro* effects in the absence of adrenals, e.g., *in vitro* melanotropic and lipolytic activities (for reviews, see Refs. 193–195).

Most studies of the conformation of ACTH (for review, see Ref. 193) have led to the conclusion that the hormone exists as a highly flexible random coil in solution; recently, however, a preferred conformation containing two helical parts has been proposed (196).

The first total synthesis of porcine ACTH by Schwyzer and Sieber in 1963 (197) constituted a major advance in peptide synthesis, and the 39 residue molecule remained for many years the longest peptide chain synthesized. Following the recent revisions

* Synonym: adrenocorticotropic hormone.

H–Ser–Tyr–Ser–Met–Glu–His–Phe–Arg–Trp–Gly–Lys–Pro–Val–Gly–Lys–Lys–Arg–Arg–Pro–Val–
1 5 10 15 20

Lys–Val–Tyr–Pro–Asn–Gly–Ala–Glu–Asp–Glu–Ser–Ala–Glu–Ala–Phe–Pro–Leu–Glu–Phe–OH
25 30 31 33 35

	Human ACTH
–Ser–Ala–Gln–	Bovine, ovine
–Leu–Ala–Glu–	Porcine
31 33	

Fig. 27.18 Amino acid sequences of the known corticotropins from mammalian species as recently revised (190, 191) from structures originally proposed; see Ref. 192. The continuous chain is that of the human ACTH.

(1971–1974) of the sequences (see Fig. 27.18) the revised molecules have all been resynthesized (literature cited in Ref. 198). There have been several different syntheses of human ACTH by fragment condensation in solution; that of Yajima and collaborators (199) is shown schematically in Fig. 27.19. Improved solid phase synthesis employing symmetrical anhydride coupling (200) provided greatly increased yields of hACTH and analogs (201). Numerous analogs have been prepared for the study of structure-activity relationships.

The clinical use of ACTH comprises diagnostic application (e.g., in Cushing's disease) and therapeutic application in rheumatic disorders, dermatologic diseases, allergic states, and ophthalmic diseases.

4.1.2 STRUCTURE-ACTIVITY RELATIONSHIPS. The entire *length* of the ACTH molecule is not required for bioactivity. Peptides corresponding to the NH_2-terminal half of the hormone e.g., (1–19)-nonadecapeptide amide or (1–24)-tetracosapeptide] exhibit 70–80% of the molar *in vivo* steroidogenic

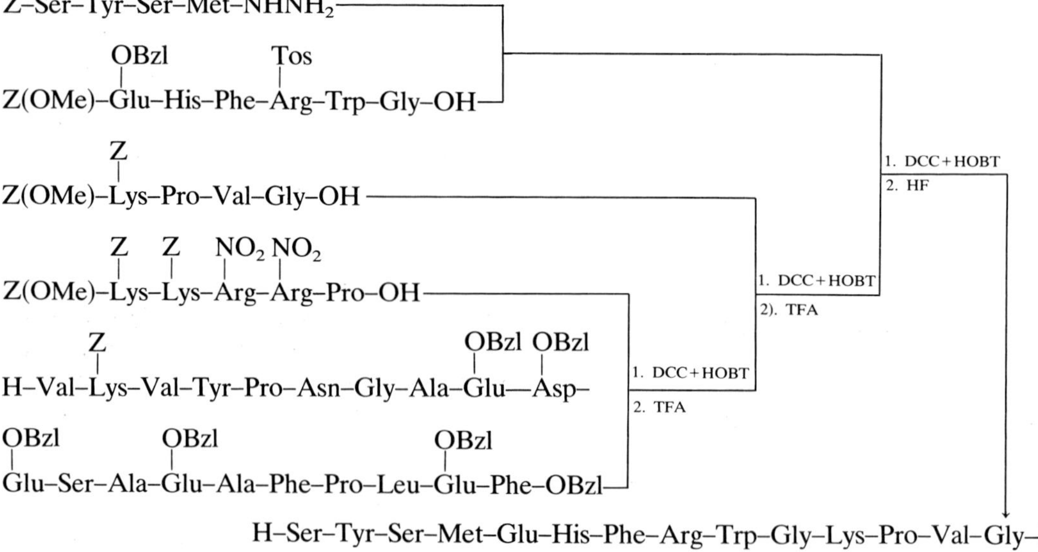

Fig. 27.19 Synthetic route to human corticotropin by Yajima and collaborators (199): DCC/HOBt, dicyclohexylcarbodiimide and 1-hydroxybenzotriazole.

potency of native ACTH. With further decreasing chain length, the activity drops rapidly to zero. It appears that the COOH-terminal part of ACTH has no role in the interaction of the hormone with target cells but may provide metabolic stability (193). Increased resistance to enzymatic degradation has also been achieved for NH_2-terminal ACTH fragment analogs by introducing COOH-terminal amide or alkylamide and NH_2-terminal D-Ser or β-Ala replacements (202–204); see Fig. 27.20. Up to sevenfold potency increases have been obtained in this manner.

That the *basic core*, –Lys–Lys–Arg–Arg–, of ACTH in positions 15–18 serves as a receptor binding site, has been learned from evaluation of various synthetic analogs, modified in these positions (193).

The five *amino-terminal* residues of ACTH are not essential for steroidogenic activity but serve to increase potency, probably through participation in receptor binding. Synthetic efforts in NH_2-terminal modification were successful in achieving potency increases (see Fig. 27.20), but analogs with significantly prolonged duration of action have yet to be found (193).

The *core peptide* 6–13 appears to be essential for the stimulation of steroidogenesis, as deduced from bioassay data of numerous synthetic fragments (205, 206).

From these results it has become clear that ACTH is a molecule in which discrete sequences of adjacent amino acids are responsible for different components of its total biological activity spectrum. The term "sychnologic" has been proposed (207) for this type of molecular organization, as compared to a "rhegnylogic" organization, in which the information for biological activity resides in separate residues of the sequence, which are brought into close proximity by conformational adaptation.

In sum, the COOH-terminal sequence region 20–39 is probably not involved in ACTH receptor interaction but increases metabolic stability. The basic core (residues 15–18) may be the major affinity site attaching the hormone to the adrenal receptor. Residues 1–5 serve as additional attachment sites. The sequence –His–Phe–Arg–Trp–Gly–Lys–Pro–Val– (residues 9–13) triggers changes in the structure of the receptor, which stimulate the enzyme adenylate cyclase, leading to cAMP increase. The action of ACTH on other tissues may proceed in similar fashion.

4.2 Lipotropin (LPH) and Melanotropin (MSH)*

4.2.1 LIPOTROPIN. Lipotropin was discovered fortuitously by C. H. Li and collaborators, during investigation of a simplified isolation procedure for ACTH. Two peptides were obtained from ovine pituitaries, and their structures were determined (208). These peptides exhibited lipolytic activity similar to those of corticotropin and melanotropin and were designated as β-lipotropin (β-LPH) and γ-lipotropin (γ-LPH). β-LPH is a linear polypeptide consisting of 91 amino acid residues. The sequence of human β-LPH has recently been reported (33) (see Fig. 27.4). It contains no half-cystine and no disulfide bonds. The 58 residue γ-LPH is identical with the sequence region 1–58 of β-LPH (Fig. 27.4). The actual physiological role of LPH has remained obscure (for a review, see Ref. 209).

The sequence region 41–58 of LPH is identical with that of β-melanotropin (Fig. 27.21) and is flanked by –Lys–Lys– at its NH_2-terminus and by –Lys–Arg– at its COOH-terminus (Fig. 27.4). Since pairs of basic residues occur at enzymatic cleavage sites of such established prohormones as proinsulin (Section 8.1) or proparathyrine (Section 6.2), and since β-MSH can indeed be released from LPH by trypsin digestion,

* Synonyms: lipotropic hormone; melanocyte-stimulating hormone.

	In vivo Molar steroidogenic Activity, % of Native ACTH	Reference
D-Ser–Tyr–Ser–Nle–Glu–His–Phe–Arg–Trp–Gly–Lys–Pro–Val–Gly–Lys–Lys–Arg–Arg–Pro–Val–Lys–Val–Tyr–Pro–Val–NH_2 (residue numbers 5, 10, 15, 20, 25 printed below)	550	202
[D-Ser^1, Nle^4, Val-$NH2_2^{25}$]-β-corticotropin-(1–25)-pentacosapeptide amide		
D-Ser–Tyr–Ser–Met–Glu–His–Phe–Arg–Trp–Gly–Lys–Pro–Val–Gly–Lys–Lys–Lys–Lys–NH_2 (residue numbers 5, 10, 15 printed below)	700	203
[D-Ser^1, $Lys^{17,18}$]-β-corticotropin—(1—18)—octadecapeptide amide		
β-Ala–Tyr–Ser–Met–Glu–His–Phe–Arg–Trp–Gly–Lys–Pro–Val–Gly–Lys–Lys–Lys–NH–$(CH_2)_4$–NH_2 (residue numbers 5, 10, 15 printed below)	700	204
[β-Ala^1, Lys^{17}]-β-corticotropin-(1–17)-(4-amino-*n*-butylamide)		

Fig. 27.20 Synthetic ACTH analogs of NH_2-terminal parts of the molecule possessing enhanced biological potency.

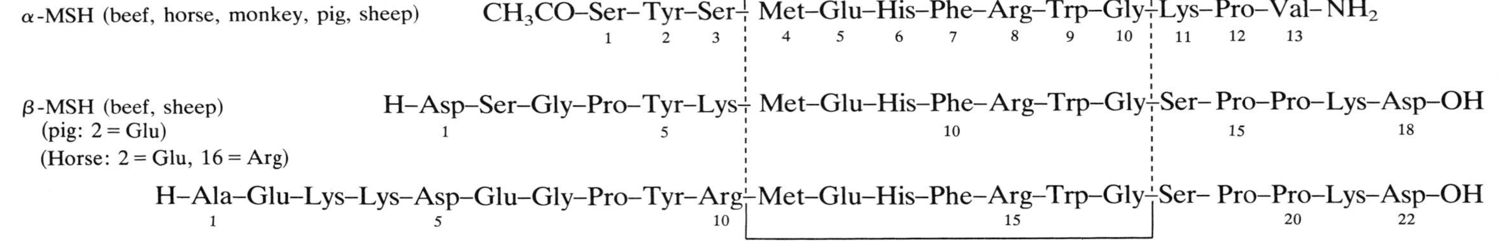

Fig. 27.21 The amino acid sequences of α-melanotropin (α-MSH) and β-melanotropin (β-MSH) from various mammalian species. The heptapeptide sequence –Met–Glu–His–Phe–Arg–TRP–Gly– is invariant in all known melanotropins and occurs as sequence region 4–10 in ACTH.

it has been suggested that β-LPH might be a precursor molecule for β-MSH (69). The recent discovery that β-LPH is also very likely a precursor of β-endorphin, identical with the sequence region 61–91 of β-LPH, strongly indicates that the biological role of β-LPH is that of a prohormone. The high sensitivity of β-LPH to enzymatic cleavage, in part a consequence of the lack of disulfide bridges, is in accord with its suggested prohormone function.

4.2.2 α-MELANOTROPIN AND β-MELANOTROPIN. Among the two melanotropins, α-MSH is the most potent melanocyte-stimulating agent. It has been isolated from pituitaries of several mammalian species and characterized as an N^{α}-acetyltridecapeptide amide (Fig. 27.21). The amino acid sequence of α-MSH is identical with the first 13 residues in ACTH (Fig. 27.18).

The isolation and sequence analysis of several mammalian β-melanotropins showed these to consist of 18 amino acid residues. Species variation exists in positions 2, 10, and 16, but human β-MSH (210) has four additional amino acid residues at the NH_2-terminus (see Fig. 27.21). The sequence of this 22 residue peptide is identical with the sequence region 37–58 of human β-LPH (see Fig. 27.4).

The chemical and biological properties of MSH have been described in detailed texts (211). All natural species analogs have been synthesized. This work and structure-activity relationships based on more than 50 synthetic analogs have been superbly reviewed with a complete bibliography by Yajima and Kiso (212). Analyses of the contributions of individual sequence regions of the sychnologic molecular architecture of MSH to the overall biological activity spectrum have been discussed (213).

There is increasing evidence that the melanocyte-stimulating activity of MSH does not play any role in man. Radioimmunoassay, bioassay, and physicochemical data indicate that the human pituitary does not normally produce α- or β-MSH, and it was suggested that these peptides may be artifacts formed by enzymatic degradation of β-lipotropin during extraction (214). However recent findings might suggest yet unknown roles of MSH in the central nervous system. There have been reports (215) that α-MSH affects behavior and cerebral electric activity in animals and in man (216) by direct (endocrine-independent) action on the CNS, and the related ACTH-(4–10) heptapeptide has been implicated in learning processes (217). Levels of endogenous MSH in human brain might perhaps be below the present limits of detection.

4.3 Lutropin (LH) and Follitropin (FSH)*

Lutropin and follitropin act synergistically to induce ovarian growth and estrogen production and secretion in the female. FSH is primarily responsible for follicular development, and this effect is augmented by both LH and estrogen. LH affects the ovary by inducing a rapid preovulation enlargement of one or more selected follicles, followed by ovulation, transformation of granulosa cells to luteal cells—thus formation of the corpus luteum, maintenance of the corpus luteum, and secretion of progesterone. The ovulatory effect of LH is augmented by FSH. LH also stimulates the morphological development and steroid secretion of ovarian interstitial cells. In the male, FSH is mainly responsible for spermatogenesis in stimulating the germinal epithelium of the testis, an effect augmented by LH and androgen. LH promotes morphological development and stimulation of androgen secretion by the Leydig cell. Human

* Synonyms: luteinizing hormone or interstitial cell-stimulating hormone (ICSH); follicle-stimulating hormone. Collective designation for LH and FSH: gonadotropins.

chorionic gonadotropin (see Section 10.1) shares many of the biological actions of LH but exhibits higher potency because its half-life of circulation is longer (218).

Secretion of pituitary LH and FSH is under hypothalamic control and stimulated by the decapeptide gonadoliberin (GnRH, see Section 3.1). The reader is referred to several texts and reviews for details of gonadotropin bioactivity (19, 219–224).

LH and FSH, as well as TSH and hCG, are glycoproteins having molecular weights between 27,500 and 28,500 daltons. They are the most complex hormonal structures known. Each consists of two subunits (α and β), i.e., peptide chains whose specific noncovalent association is necessary for activity. Each of β-subunits is hormone unique and determines the specificity of action of each α-β complex. The α-subunits are common to all four glycoprotein hormones. Each subunit, α and β, has several branched carbohydrate chains covalently bonded at specific locations (Asn residues)

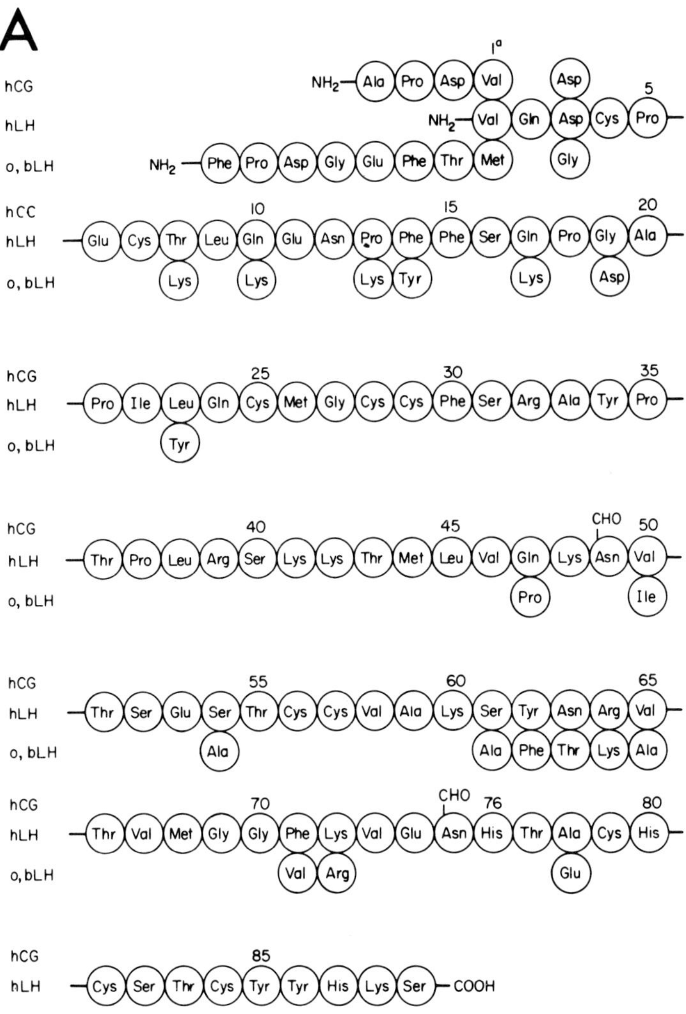

Fig. 27.22 (*a*) Primary structures of the α-subunits of gonadotropins from several mammalian gonadotropins. From Bishop et al. (218) (consult Ref. 219 for references). Reprinted with permission of Macmillan London and Basingstoke.

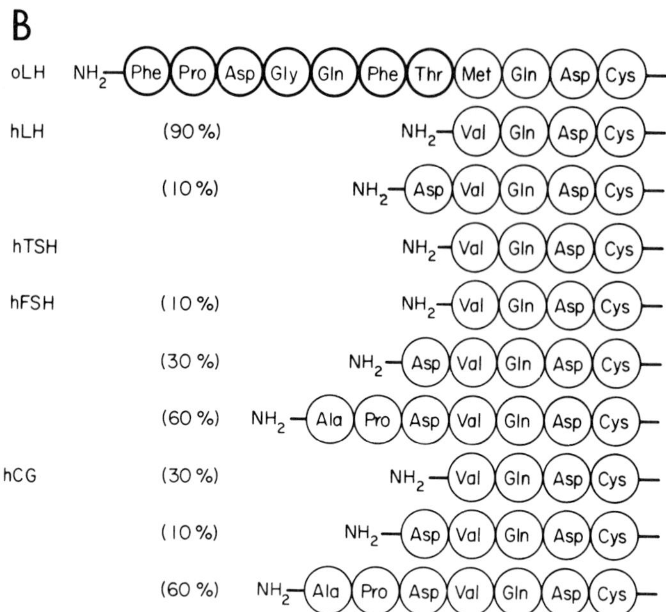

Fig. 27.22 (*Continued*) (*b*) Amino-terminal heterogeneity of the α-subunits. The ovine peptides may be isolated, having any of the residues in a bold ring as NH_2-terminus. From Bishop et al. (218) (consult Ref. 219 for references). Reprinted with permission of Macmillan London and Basingstoke.

in their respective structures. Specific alterations of the carbohydrate portion result in both immunologic and biologic alterations. All four glycoprotein hormones—LH, FSH, TSH, and hCG—share a common quaternary structure composed of identical α-subunits (225). Interestingly, both the pituitary and placenta contain excess of free α-subunits, suggesting that the mechanisms of synthesis and secretion of the glycoprotein hormones from those organs may be quite similar (220). The biochemical properties of LH and FSH have been well reviewed (218, 223, 226).

Lutropin has been isolated in highly purified state from ovine, bovine, porcine, rat, and human glands (184). Under acidic conditions, LH dissociates into its subunits. These have been purified from several species. Figure 27.22*a* shows the sequence of the α-subunits of ovine, bovine, and human LH, and hCG. A high degree of homology exists between these structures, 70% of the residues being identical and an additional 21% highly acceptable replacements (single base mutations in the codon) (184). Considerable heterogeneity in chain length occurs at the amino-termini (Fig. 27.22*b*), with as many as seven residues being absent, which shows that a specific length is not necessary for the α-subunits to function. All 10 half-cystine residues have been conserved, indicating an important role of the disulfides in maintaining the molecular architecture essential for bioactivity. The assignments of the disulfide bond positions is exceedingly difficult because of several adjacent or neighboring half-cystines, and further work is needed to reconcile divergent results (227).

A comparison of the amino acid sequences of the hormone-specific β-subunits of hLH, hFSH, and hCG (Fig. 27.23) shows complete conservation of half-cystine residues. The major differences occur at the COOH-termini and in the location of the carbohydrate side chains. The structures of the carbohydrate chains of LH and FSH, as well as TSH are not yet known.

The primary structure of human *follitropin* needs to be confirmed. Other isolated species variants of FSH include the ovine

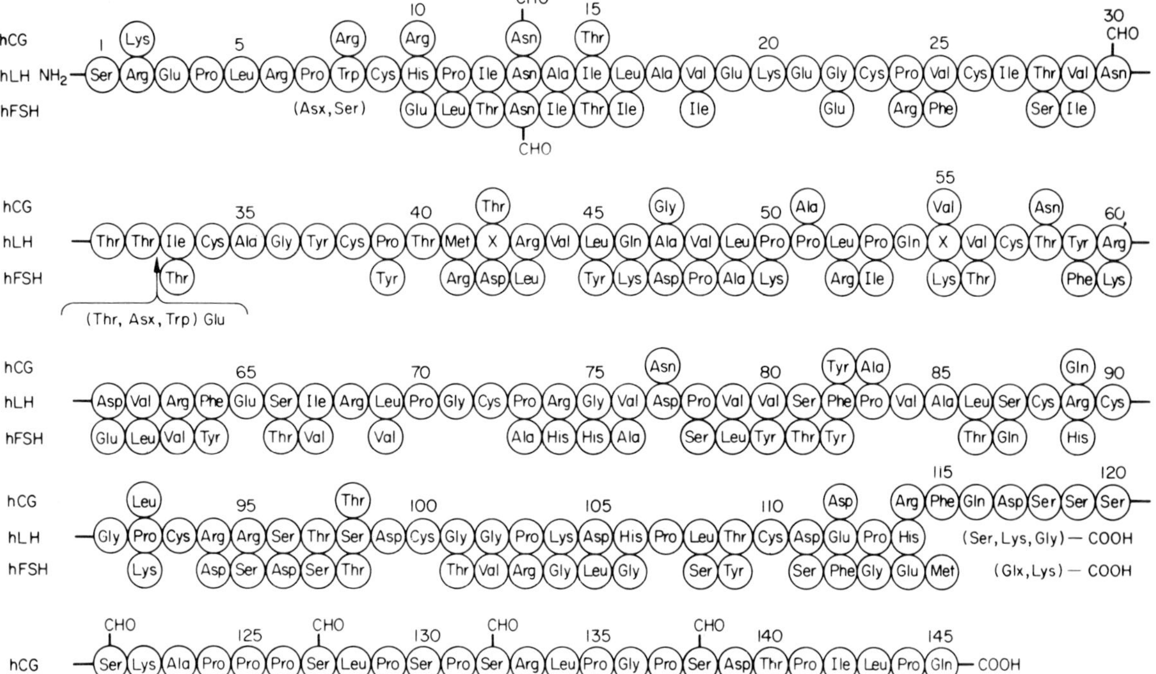

Fig. 27.23 A comparison of the amino acid sequences of the β-subunits of the human gonadotropins. The sequence of hLH is drawn as a continuous chain. Differing residues in hCG appear above the line, those in hFSH, below. Regions of incomplete sequencing information are shown without circles and in parentheses. The far greater homology between hLH and hCG than between hLH and hFSH is obvious. To keep Cys residues in register, a tetrapeptide part of the FHS sequence that normally follows residue 32 is shown in subscript. Similarly, positions 42 and 55 are inserted, marked X. They might represent true deletions or sequencing errors. From Bishop et al. (218) (consult Ref. 219) for references. Reprinted with permission of Macmillan London and Basingstoke.

and equine hormones. Highly purified FSH is more difficult to obtain than LH. FSH seems to be present in smaller quantities in the pituitary and less stable during isolation.

Studies on structure-activity relationships by chemical modification of oLH or bLH indicate that both Tyr residues in LH are masked in the native hormone, and that two Lys ε-amino groups of oLH are involved in receptor binding, two amino groups on α are involved in subunit interaction, and 2–8 amino groups on α are implicated in receptor binding (218, 226).

Clinical uses of gonadotropins include diagnosis of testicular abnormality by radioimmunoassay for LH and FSH and therapeutic application for the induction of ovulation in infertile women; these substances have also been employed successfully in the treatment of certain gonadotropin deficiencies in males.

4.4 Thyrotropin (TSH)*

Thyrotropin stimulates the growth of the thyroid gland and the secretion of the thyroid hormones. The secretion of TSH by specific basophilic cells is under hypothalamic control and is stimulated by thyroliberin and suppressed by somatostatin; for review, see Ref. 227a–d. TSH has been highly purified from bovine and human pituitaries. TSH belongs to the group of glycoproteins discussed in detail in Section 4.3. The α-subunit of hTSH is identical (225) to that of hLH (see Fig. 27.22). The

* Synonym: thyroid-stimulating hormone.

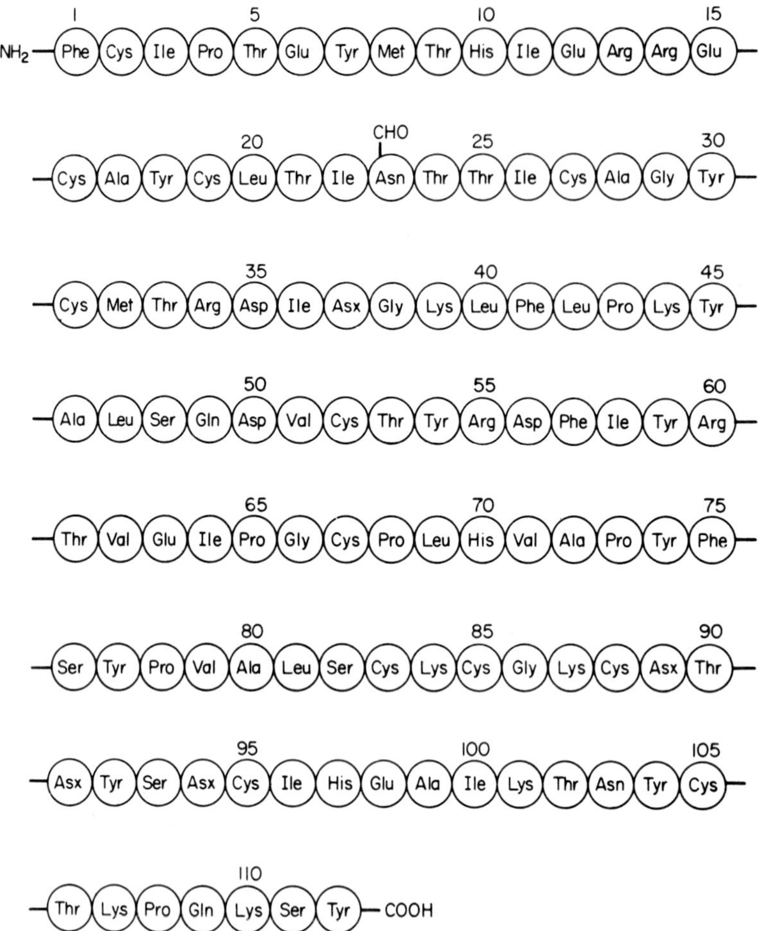

Fig. 27.24 Amino acid sequence of the hormone-specific β-subunit of human thyrotropin as proposed by Sairam and Li (227b). From Smith and Hall (227c). Reprinted with permission of Macmillan London and Basingstoke.

amino acid sequence of the β-subunit (227b) appears in Fig. 27.24. The structure of the single carbohydrate chain in the β-subunit has not yet been determined. Few chemical modification studies have been carried out with TSH. Clinical applications are restricted to the diagnostic use of radioimmunoassay for measuring TSH levels after thyroliberin injection.

4.5 Prolactin (PRL)*

Prolactin is a versatile hormone playing a significant role in various aspects of growth and metabolism. In addition to its function as a stimulator of the growth and development of the mammary gland, PRL influences parental behavior and crop (milk) production, and contributes, along with other hormones, to the initiation and maintenance of lactation. More than 80 different actions attributed to PRL have been listed (228) (see also Ref. 184).

Highly purified PRL has been obtained from human, ovine, bovine, porcine, and rat pituitaries (184). Teleost PRL (229) and canine pituitary PRL (230) have recently been isolated. Prolactins from different mammalian species are single-chain proteins consisting of 199 amino acid residues

* Synonyms: lactogenic hormone, lactotropic hormone, mammatropic hormone.

					5									15					20
Human:	H–Leu	Pro	Ile	Cys	Pro	Gly	Gly	Ala	Ala	Arg	Cys	Gln	Val	Thr	Leu	Arg	Asp	Leu	Phe	Asp
Ovine:	H–Thr		Val			Asn		Pro	Gly	Asp				Ser						
Porcine:	H–					Ser			Val	Asn										

									30					35					40
Human:	Arg	Ala	Val	Val	Leu	Ser	His	Tyr	Ile	His	Asn	Leu	Ser	Ser	Glu	Met	Phe	Ser	Glu	Phe
Ovine:				Met	Val													Asn		
Porcine:				Ile																

									50										60
Human:	Asp	Lys	Arg	Tyr	Thr	His	Gly	Arg	Gly	Phe	Ile	Thr	Lys	Ala	Ile	Asn	Ser	Cys	His	Thr
Ovine:					Ala	Gln		Lys					Met		Leu					
Porcine:																				

					65					70										
Human:	Ser	Ser	Leu	Ala	Thr	Pro	Glu	Asp	Lys	Glu	Gln	Ala	Gln	Gln	Met	Asn	Gln	Lys	Asp	Phe
Ovine:				Pro											Thr	His	His	Glu	Val	Leu
Porcine:				Ser											Ile					

					85					90					95					100
Human:	Leu	Val	Ser	Ile	Leu	Ile	Leu	X	Arg	Ser	Trp	Asn	Glu	Pro	Leu	Tyr	His	Leu	Val	Thr
Ovine:	Met	Ser	Leu			Gly		Leu					Asp							
Porcine:		Asn				Arg	Val													

																			120
Human:	Glu	Val	Arg	Gly	Asx	Gln	Glu	Ala	Pro	Glu	Ala	Ile	Leu	Ser	Lys	Ala	Val	Glu	Ile	Glu
Ovine:					Met	Lys	Gly	Val		Asp					Arg		Ile			
Porcine:																				

					125					130										
Human:	Glu	Gln	Thr	Lys	Arg	Leu	Leu	Glu	Gly	Met	Glu	Leu	Ile	Val	Ser	Gln	Val	His	Pro	Glu
Ovine:		Glu	Asn									Met		Phe	Gly			Ile		Gly
Porcine:												Lys								

					145					150					155					160
Human:	Thr	Lys	Glu	Asp	Glu	Ile	Tyr	Pro	Val	Trp	Ser	Gly	Leu	Pro	Ser	Leu	Gln	Met	Ala	Asp
Ovine:	Ala			Thr		Pro												Thr	Lys	
Porcine:	Ile			Asn		Val	Ser													

										170					175					
Human:	Glu	Ser	Glu	Arg	Leu	Ser	Ala	Tyr	Tyr	Asn	Leu	Leu	His	Cys	Leu	Arg	Arg	Asp	Ser	His
Ovine:		Asp	Ala		His			Phe												Ser
Porcine:			Thr			Phe														

					185														199
Human:	Lys	Ile	Asp	Asn	Tyr	Leu	Lys	Leu	Leu	Lys	Cys	Arg	Ile	Ile	His	Asn	Asn	Asn	Cys–OH
Ovine:				Thr						Asn						Tyr			
Porcine:																	Ser		

Fig. 27.25 Comparison of the structures of human prolactin (continuous chain) and ovine and porcine prolactin (subscript residues). The bovine molecule differs from ovine in residues 108 (Ala instead of Val) and 165 (Tyr instead of His). Data from Li (oPLR, pPLR; Ref. 231) and from Shome and Parlow (hPRL; Ref. 231a).

and cross-linked by three disulfide bonds. Molecular weights range between 22,400 and 23,000 daltons, and isoelectric points lie between pH 5.7 and 5.85. The primary structures of human (231a) ovine, bovine, and porcine PRL (Fig. 27.25) have been determined (231b). The bovine and ovine structures differ in only two positions, but comparison between the ovine and porcine molecules shows 36 replacements, 22 of which are acceptable (single-base mutations), thus amounting to a 94% homology (184). Human PRL has only recently been identified as a molecule distinct from human somatotropin (232). Its biologic actions, control of secretion, and associated pathologic conditions have recently been summarized (233). Reviews on the chemistry and biology of prolactin are available (232, 234–236).

4.6 Somatotropin (GH)*

The most readily observed effect of somatotropin following its administration to either normal or hypophysectomized animals is enhancement of body weight and length. The hormone also influences the growth of bone tissue. In addition, GH accelerates the mobilization and oxidation of depot fat (for reviews, see Refs. 237 and 238). GH biosynthesis appears to proceed via a larger precursor (238a).

Somatotropin has been isolated in highly purified form from bovine, ovine, and human pituitaries. The human hormone is a globular protein (239) with a molecular weight of 22,000 daltons, isoelectric point at pH 4.9, and α-helical content of 55%. It consists of a single polypeptide chain of 191 amino acid residues, cross-linked by two disulfide bonds (Fig. 27.26). A series of physicochemical investigations indicates a high stability of the solution conformation of hGH. Only in strongly acidic solution or in the presence of powerful denaturing agents are conformational changes observed by CD spectroscopy (239). The molecule appears to be unusually resistant to alkaline denaturation, which explains the stability of its bioactivity to extremes of pH and the

* Synonym: growth hormone.

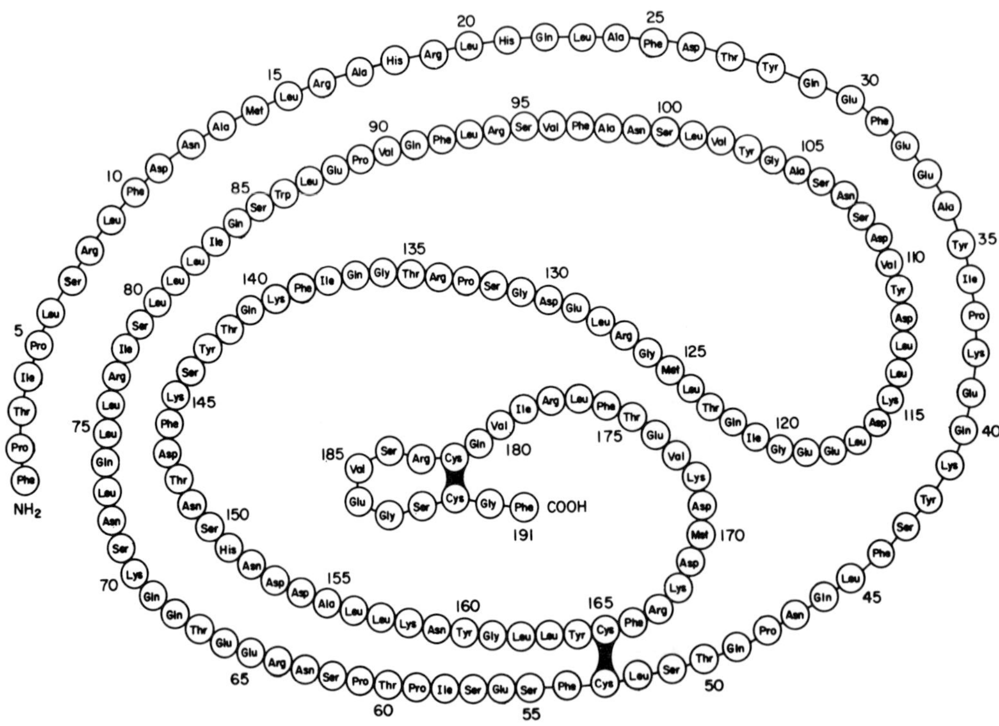

Fig. 27.26 The primary structure of human somatotropin from Li (239). Reprinted with permission of Academic Press, Inc.

action of denaturants (for a review, see Ref. 239).

Comparison of the primary structure of hGH with those of the bovine and ovine hormones shows a close to 90% homology: 123 positions have identical amino acid residues, 34 have highly acceptable replacements, and 13 have acceptable replacements (184). However the animal hormones are inactive in man, which is surprising in view of the high degree of homology; this condition is not readily explained by differences in the primary structures. Moreover, the helic content of 45–55% in both bGH and oGH closely resembles that of hGH. However the strong tendency of the animal somatotropins to dimerize in neutral solution may explain their inactivity in man (239).

There have been many efforts to identify and isolate smaller bioactive parts of the hormone, prompted by the consistent failure of animal GH to exhibit any growth-promoting activity in man (184), along with the limited supply (insufficient for clinical needs) of hormone from human pituitaries and the slim prospects for routine chemical synthesis of a molecule the size of human somatotropin. Partial digestion of hGH with chymotrypsin, trypsin, pepsin, and plasmin indicated that the growth-promoting activity of the hormone does not depend on the integrity of the molecule (239, 240). Recently Li and Gráf (241) succeeded in isolating biologically active fragments from plasmin digests of hGH. The enzyme cleaves a hexapeptide (residues 135–140) from the hGH molecule without changing its biologic activity. Disulfide reduction, *S*-carboxamidomethylation, and chromatographic separation provided two peptide fragments. The larger one, corresponding to sequence regions 1–134, exhibits 5–10% of the potency of hGH in different assays. The smaller 51 residue fragment (sequence 141–191) retained 2–5% activity.

Subsequently, in one of the most exciting recent discoveries in the protein hormone field, Li and Bewley (241a) reported the successful noncovalent recombination of these fragments to regenerate the almost full (97%) biological potency of human somatotropin in the mouse mammary gland and the pigeon crop sac assays. Moreover, the recombinant hormone exhibits complete recovery of immunoreactivity by radioimmunoassay. The CD spectra and the chromatographic elution position are identical to those of the native hormone. This shows that the three-dimensional structure of the hGH molecule can be restored to its original conformation by a noncovalent interaction of the NH_2-terminal 134 residue fragment with the COOH-terminal 51 residue fragment. It is known (242–244) that peptide fragments derived from native *enzymes* can recombine noncovalently to regenerate enzymic activity; yet human somatotropin represents the first *protein hormone* in which two peptide fragments were observed to complement with restoration of full biologic potency.

This work opens the potential for semisynthesis of hGH. In a preliminary announcement (241), recombination of a synthetic 51 residue fragment with natural NH_2-terminal 134 residue material was reported to restore biological activity. Perhaps smaller fragments might still be capable of generating hGH activity by complementation to provide supplies of somatotropin for use in human medicine.

The clinical usefulness of hGH for the successful treatment of hypopituitary children is well established (79, 245, 246). In addition, the hormone exhibits beneficial effects on patients with bleeding ulcers (240, 247) and has potential in the treatment of muscular dystrophy (248).

5 NEUROHYPOPHYSEAL HORMONES

Oxytocin and vasopressin are isolated from the posterior lobe of the pituitary (neurohypophysis), but they originate in the hypothalamus, where they are independently synthesized in cell bodies of neurons located in supraoptic and paraventricular nuclei. From there the hormones are transported through neuronal axons into the posterior pituitary, where they are stored in secretory granules of nerve endings. During transport, the hormones are bound to specific transport proteins, called neurophysins (NP). Oxytocin and vasopressin are produced in different neurons, and each is associated with a separate neurophysin. The binding is specific and requires the intact amino group of the hormone and hydrophobic or aromatic amino acids in positions 2 and 3. The structures and binding characteristics of several neurophysins have been determined (for a review, see Refs. 249 and 250). They are low molecular weight proteins of 97 amino acid residues (bovine NPs). Their possible role as a biosynthetic precursor has not yet been confirmed.

In 1953 du Vigneaud and collaborators announced the structure of oxytocin and disclosed its confirmation by synthesis (251). This created great excitement, not only because oxytocin was the first peptide hormone with known structure, but also because immense opportunities had been opened up for structure-activity studies by analog synthesis. More than 350 analogs of oxytocin and vasopressin have since been synthesized, originally by a trial-and-error approach giving all constituent amino acid residues equal weight. The experience gained from the study of more than 250 analogs prepared in this manner between 1954 and 1970 was superbly reviewed by J. Rudinger in 1971 (252). Rudinger analyzed the evolving structure-activity relationships by comparing the relative effects of substitutions in different residue positions on the ensuing shifts of the pharmacological activity profile. This data base provided empirical rules for more sophisticated analog design [see Manning et al. (253); Zaoral et al. (254)]. At the same time, novel rationales for analog design were proposed by Walter and collaborators (255) based on the developing insights into the solution conformation of the neurohypophyseal hormones. As a consequence, oxytocin and vasopressin analog synthesis was revived dramatically during the past 5 years, leading to a second generation of highly active and selective analogs, including long-acting compounds, highly specific agonists, and potent antagonists. Another area in which sophistication is increasing involves the detailed pharmacological evaluation of neurohypophyseal hormone effects, for example, on vascular smooth muscle (256).

Because of the close structural relationships between oxytocin and vasopressin, along with close resemblance of chemical and conformational properties and the overlap in bioactivity, the hormones are best discussed side by side with respect to their phylogeny, bioactivity, conformation, synthesis, structure-activity relationships, and clinical potentials. A number of reviews are available (24a, 27, 253, 255, 257–262).

5.1 Phylogeny of the Neurohypophyseal Hormones

Nine neurohypophyseal hormones have been characterized, comprising six oxytocinlike hormones with neutral amino acid residues in position 8 and three vasopressinlike hormones with basic residues in position 8 (Fig. 27.27). At present, neurohypophyseal hormones have been identified in about 40 vertebrate species, including examples from all classes. The following general conclusions can be made (16):

1. The neurohypophysis of each species contains generally two hormones (except for cyclostomes with AVT only).

	Oxytocin-like hormone		Vasopressin-like hormone	
	1 2 3 4 5 6 7 8 9		1 2 3 4 5 6 7 8 9	
Mammals (except pig)	Cys–Tyr–Ile–*Gln*–Asn–Cys–Pro–*Leu*–Gly–NH_2 Oxytocin	OT	Cys–Tyr–*Phe*–Gln–Asn–Cys–Pro–*Arg*–Gly–NH_2 Arginine-vasopressin	AVP
Pig	Cys–Tyr–Ile–*Gln*–Asn–Cys–Pro–*Leu*–Gly–NH_2 Oxytocin	OT	Cys–Tyr–*Phe*–Gln–Asn–Cys–Pro–*Lys*–Gly–NH_2 Lysine-vasopressin	LVP
Birds, reptiles, amphibians, lungfishes	Cys–Tyr–Ile–*Gln*–Asn–Cys–Pro–*Ile*– Gly–NH_2 Mesotocin	MT	Cys–Tyr–*Ile*– Gln–Asn–Cys–Pro–*Arg*–Gly–NH_2 Vasotocin	AVT
Bonyfishes (paleopterygians and neopterygians)	Cys–Tyr–Ile–*Ser*– Asn–Cys–Pro–*Ile*– Gly–NH_2 Isotocin	IT	Cys–Tyr–*Ile*– Gln–Asn–Cys–Pro–*Arg*–Gly–NH_2 Vasotocin	
Cartilaginous fishes (rays)	Cys–Tyr–Ile–*Ser*– Asn–Cys–Pro–*Gln*–Gly–NH_2 Glumitocin	GT	Vasotocin (?)	
Cartilaginous fishes (sharks)	Cys–Tyr–Ile–*Gln*–Asn–Cys–Pro–*Val*–Gly–NH_2 Valitocin	VT	Vasotocin (?)	
Holocephali (ratfishes)	Cys–Tyr–Ile–*Asn*–Asn–Cys–Pro–*Leu*–Gly–NH_2 Aspartocin			

Fig. 27.27 Structures and abbreviations of neurohypophyseal hormones of vertebrates. From Acher (259).

2. All these hormones have a common structural pattern of nine amino acid residues with a 1,6-disulfide bridge.
3. The same hormones are generally found in a zoological class.
4. The structure varies by only one or two residues between the hormones of two different classes.
5. The changes of mutations affect particular positions, i.e., 4 and 8, and less frequently position 3 (see Fig. 27.27).

Figure 27.28 depicts the phyletic distribution of neurohypophyseal hormones among the vertebrates (263). Arginine-vasotocin (AVT) is ubiquitous, occurring in pituitary glands from representatives of all the major vertebrate groups. It is probably the ancestral neurohypophyseal hormone. There is more variation among the oxytocinlike than among the vasopressinlike hormones. The manner in which these evolved remains unclear because there is no single genetic mutation that leads from glutamine to serine or asparagine.

AVT stimulates smooth muscles from a wide variety of vertebrate species. It can stimulate contraction of oviducts from many jawed fishes and tetrapods and can regulate water retention. In mammals,

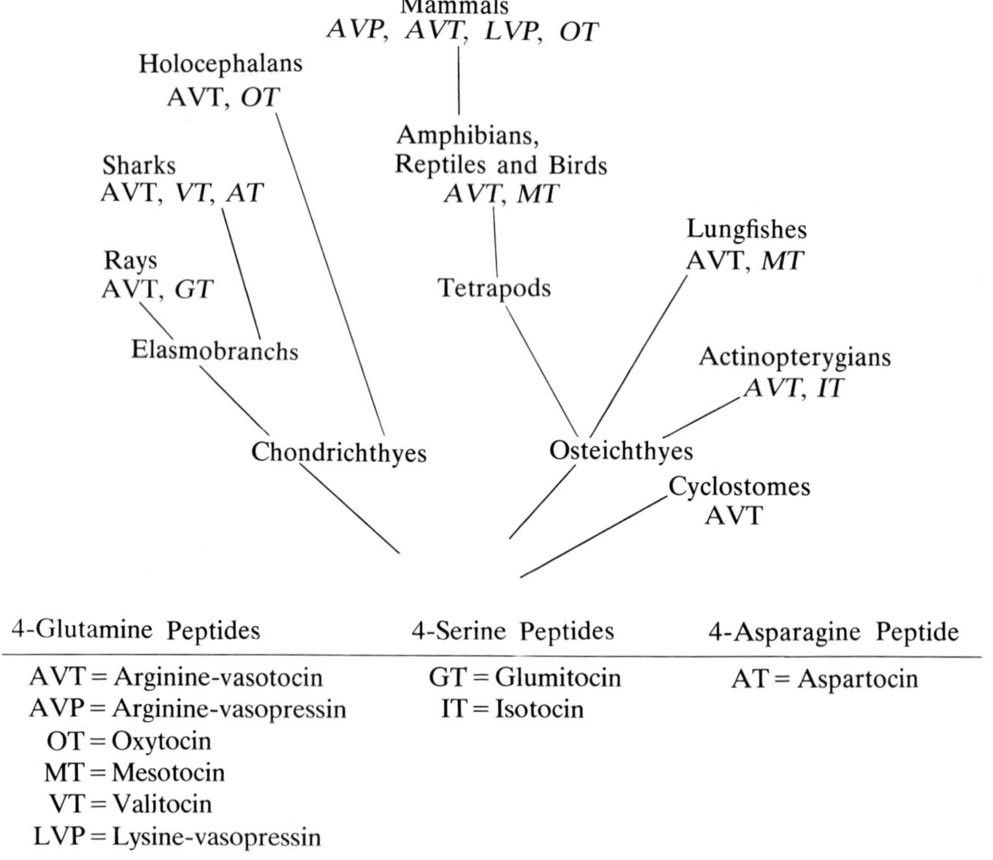

Fig. 27.28 Schematic diagram of the phyletic distribution of neurohypophyseal principles among the vertebrates. Italicized principles have been chemically identified in species representing the indicated groups. From Sawyer (263).

however, oxytocic and antidiuretic function are regulated independently by oxytocin and vasopression. Although AVT and mesotocin occur in nonmammalian tetrapods with great evolutionary stability, oxytocin and argine-vasopressin have been found in echidna (Australian spiney anteater), a monotreme and most primitive known protherian mammal. The double change in neurohypophyseal hormones between mammals and other tetrapods points to a fundamental physiological meaning (264).

5.2 Biological Activity

The neurohypophyseal hormones subserve different physiological functions in an organism. These include antidiuretic, uterotonic, galactobolic, natriuretic, lipolytic, natriferic, and hydrosomatic actions, as well as actions on blood pressure and flow. Thus a number of these effects are exerted on smooth muscle cells of different types (265).

Oxytocin plays an essential role in lactation in most mammalian species. It produces milk ejection by contraction of myoepithelial cells surrounding the alveoli and smaller ducts in the lactating mammary gland. Milk ejection is a process distinct from milk secretion. The latter is controlled by prolactin and other adenohypophyseal hormones. Oxytocin contracts smooth muscle of the uterus, but its role in parturition is unclear.

Vasopressin effects water reabsorption by increasing the permeability of the distal kidney tubules. The important physiological function is the homeostatic control of extracellular fluid volume. In case of insufficient vasopressin levels, water reabsorption declines and large amounts of low concentration urine are excreted (water diuresis, diabetes insipidus). In amphibians, vasopressin regulates the water permeability of the bladder. At high nonphysiological doses of vasopressin, the contraction of the smooth vessels effects constriction of arterioles and capillaries, causing rise in blood pressure. This effect is widely used for bioassay (see Table 27.4), but carefully controlled studies on the actions of vasopressins on vascular smooth muscles reveal a much more complex, pluralistic system of responses (256).

Neurohypophyseal hormones appear to be able to contract and relax vascular smooth

Table 27.4 Biological Activities of Naturally Occurring Neurohypophyseal Hormones in Several Widely Used Bioassay Systems (266)

	Oxytocin Effects, IU/mg			Vasopressin Effects, IU/mg	
Neurohypophyseal Hormone	Uterotonic *in Vitro* (rat)	Vasodepressor *in Vivo* (chicken)	Milk Ejection *in Vivo* (rabbit)	Vaso pressor *in Vivo* (rat)	Antidiuresis *in Vitro* (rat or dog)
Oxytocin (OT)	546	507	440	3.1	2.7
Glumitocin (GT)	9		53	0.4	0.4
Isotocin (IT)	150	380	300	0.06	0.2
Mesotocin (MT)	289	498	328	6	1
Arginine-vasopressin (AVP)	16	100	64	487	503
Lysine-vasopressin (LVP)	5	45	60	270	250
Arginine-vasotocin (AVT)	155	439	210	160	250

muscle, the exact type of response being dependent on species, vascular bed, and region within a vascular bed. Receptors that subserve both contraction and relaxation may exist on different blood vessels in a species, with a preponderance of receptors that subserve contraction being present in most blood vessels. Physiologic concentrations of vasopressin (10^{-13} to 10^{-11} M) can evoke responses on a variety of microscopic as well as large blood vessels (256).

Arginine-vasopressin appears to be, relatively, the most potent contractile substance on rat blood vessels investigated to date. Highly purified oxytocin is a contractile agent on all mammalian arterial and arteriolar vessels so far studied. These effects can be markedly affected by sex, sex hormones, alcohols, Ca^{2+}, Mg^{2+}, oxygen deficit, and glucose deprivation, whereas extracellular Na^+ and K^+ appear to have little influence on vasopressin-induced contractions of rat arterial smooth muscle (256).

The terminal amino group, the phenolic hydroxyl (in position 2), the aromatic ring (in position 3), and the basicity (in position 8) of neurohypophyseal hormones and analogs are important for optimizing hormone-receptor affinity and intrinsic contractile activity on vascular smooth muscle. Basicity in position 8 is not an absolute requirement for contractile activation of these smooth muscles. Alteration in molecular structure can result in neurohypophyseal peptides, with unique and selective microcirculatory effects that may be beneficial in the treatment of low flow states. Thus [Phe^2, Orn^8]vasopressin is 375 times more selective for rat mesenteric venules than for arterioles, and [Orn^8]vasopressin exhibits higher affinity for the vasopressin receptors of isolated rat aortas than arginine- or lysine-vasopressin (256).

Table 27.4 gives the most widely used bioassays and the potencies of seven of the naturally occurring neurohypophyseal hormones.

5.3 Conformation

Based on NMR and CD characteristics of oxytocin, Urry and Walter proposed a solution conformation of the hormone in 1971 (267). The backbone conformation of the 20-membered cyclic moiety of oxytocin in dimethylsulfoxide is characterized by a type II β-turn involving the sequence –Tyr–Ile–Gln–Asn–. Thus the chain is folded back into an antiparallel pleated sheet conformation with the disulfide bridge closing the ring and stabilizing the structure. The backbone NH of the Asn^5 residue is hydrogen-bonded to the C═O of the Tyr^2 residue and provides additional intramolecular stabilization. The $CONH_2$-terminal tail moiety forms a second β-turn (type I) comprising residues –Cys–Pro–Leu–Gly–, which folds the tail over one side of the ring and is stabilized by another hydrogen bond between the NH of Leu^8 and the side chain C═O of the Asn^5 residue (Fig. 27.29*A*). All peptide bonds are of trans configuration, including the Cys–Pro bond. Similar but not identical conformations have been deduced for lysine-vasopressin (Fig. 27.29*B*), arginine-vasopressin, and argine-vasotocin (268). Most likely the overall backbone structure with the two β-turns involving residues 2–5 and 6–9 is a common conformational feature for all nine neurohypophyseal peptides found in nature. However the charged tail portion of lysine-vasopressin seems to possess a *slightly* larger conformational freedom, and those of arginine-vasopressin and arginine-vasotocin appear to have *considerably* larger conformational freedom, compared to oxytocin.

During its interaction with receptors, oxytocin is proposed to assume a somewhat different, so-called cooperative, conformation in which the tyrosine side chain is folded over the 20-membered ring of oxytocin, Fig. 27.29*C*. In this model the tyrosine hydroxy group, acting cooperatively with the asparagine carboxamide group, appears as the predominant active element initiating the oxytocic response (269).

In an aqueous medium conformational averaging increases significantly and the hydrogen bonds may be loosened, but the gross structure is presumed to be conserved (255). With lysine-vasopressin in an aqueous medium a stacking interaction of the two aromatic rings of the neighboring Tyr–Phe residues is observed (Fig. 27.29*D*). These proposed conformations should be viewed as time-averaged, preferred structures of the peptide backbone.

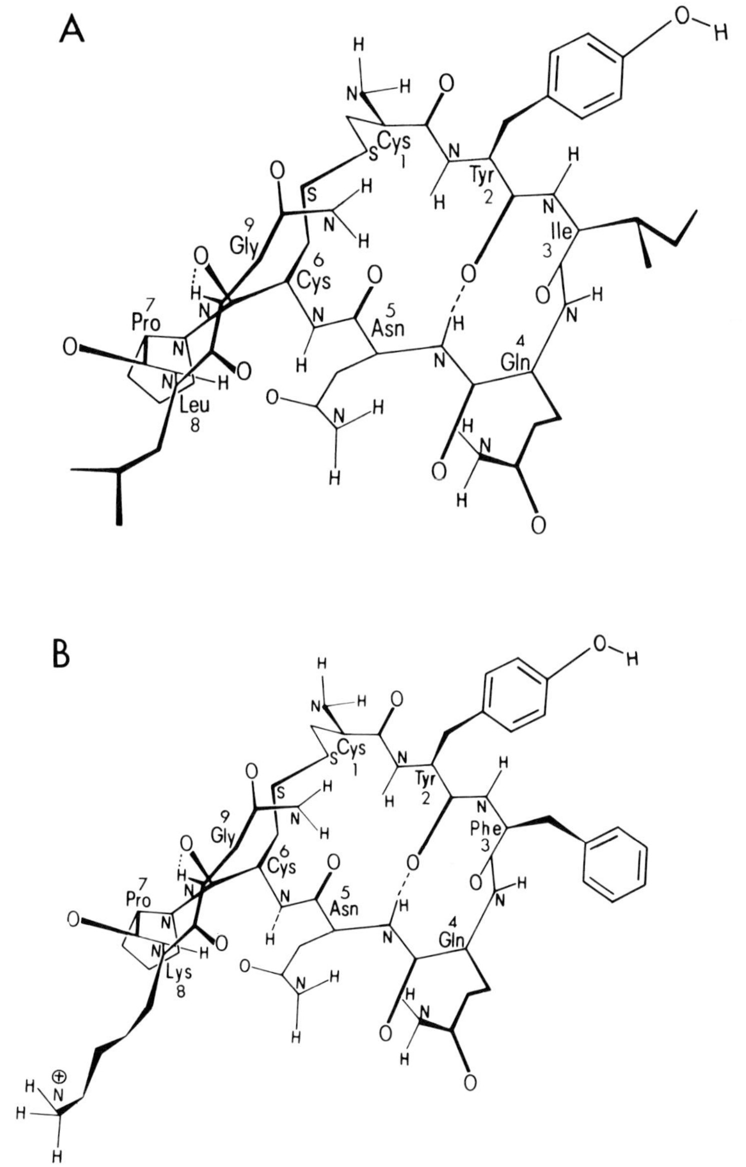

Fig. 27.29 Proposed solution conformations of oxytocin and lysine-vasopressin in dimethylsulfoxide, water, and at receptor sites. (*a*) Ocytocin in DMSO (267). (*b*) Lysine-vasopressin in DMSO (268).

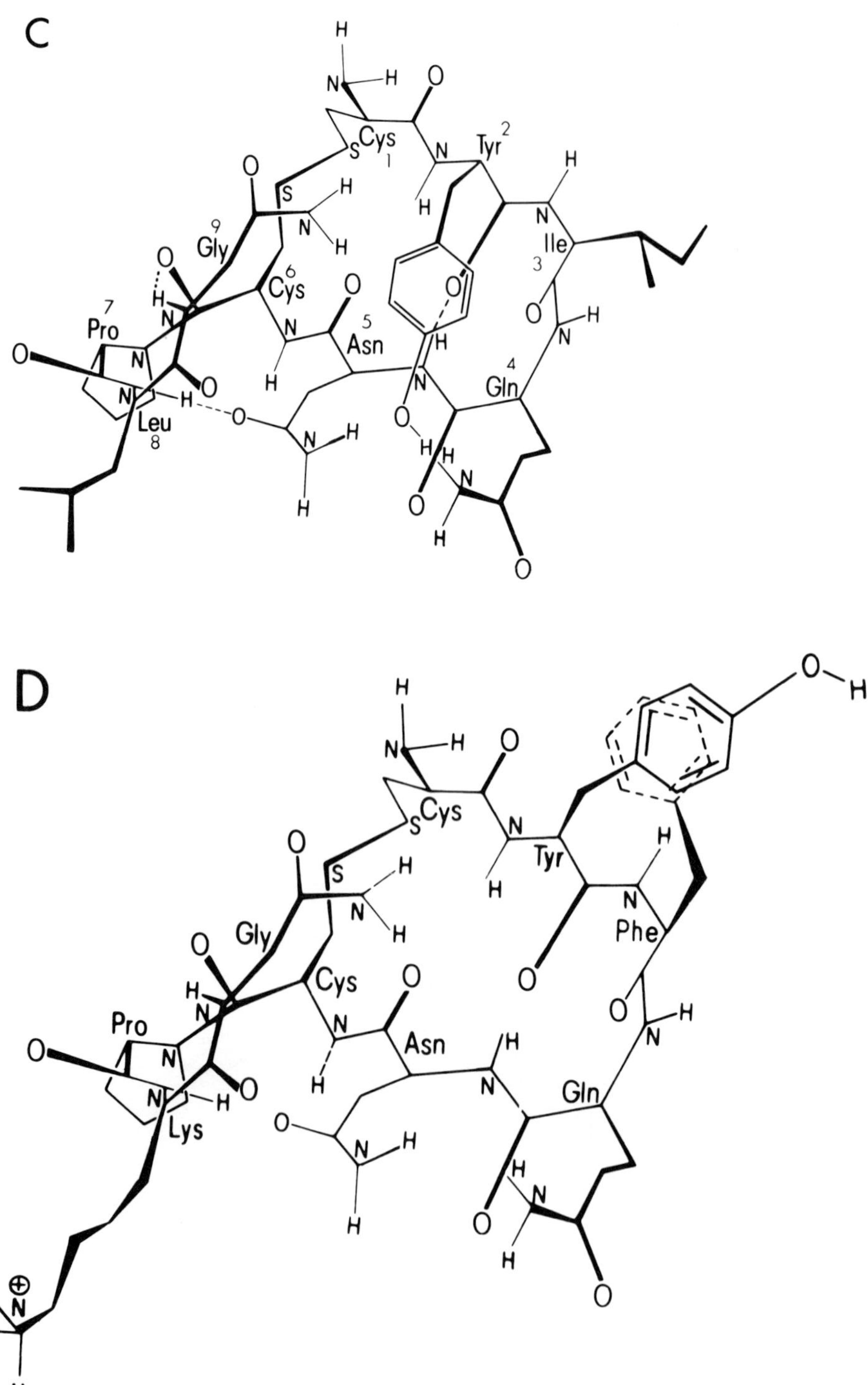

Fig. 27.29 (*Continued*) (*c*) Biologically active conformation of oxytocin at receptor sites (269). (*d*) Lysine-vasopressin in water (255).

The evolving insights into the solution conformation allowed the pursuit of conformation-activity studies. Furthermore, novel rationales for analog design were developed. Analogs with selectively modified activity profiles should result from amino acid substitutions in the corners of the β-turns (positions 3, 4, 7, 8 in Fig. 27.29) that are not primarily involved in the intramolecular stabilization of the peptide backbone and available for interaction with receptor sites; see Section 5.5.

5.4 Synthesis

Numerous syntheses of oxytocin have been described which differ in the choice of protecting groups, coupling agents, and protected intermediates. In the first historic oxytocin synthesis of du Vigneaud et al. (251), which was the first synthesis of a peptide hormone, a tripeptide (sequence 3–5) was coupled with a tetrapeptide (sequence 6–9), and the ensuing heptapeptide was joined with a dipeptide [fragment condensation 2+(3+4)]. This and several other synthetic schemes for preparation of protected nonapeptides are shown in Fig. 27.30. The protecting groups were removed by sodium in liquid ammonia. Disulfide bond formation was carried out at high dilution, but competing dimerization remains a problem with oxytocin and analogs (272), whereas vasopressin and analogs cyclize more readily. Ion exchange or partition chromatography as well as countercurrent distribution are usually required for obtaining homogeneous products.

A large number of analogs have been prepared by the solid phase procedure using the *p*-methoxybenzyl group for thiol protection and either the regular Merrifield resin (8) or the benzhydrylamine resin (273).

5.5 Structure-Activity Relationships

Structure-activity relationships that emanated from the early period (1954–1970) of analog synthesis were summarized in the past (27) in terms of the consequences of amino acid replacements in each individual residue position on the overall bioactivity profile. It is now realized that such a generalized elemental treatment is inadequate, given the effects of targeted multisubstitution. A detailed discussion of the complex structure-activity relationships emerging with the second-generation analogs would go far beyond this space (see Ref. 253–255). However one early rule has withstood the test of time: the essentiality of the 20-membered ring of the neurohypophyseal hormones for bioactivity. Enlargement or contraction is accompanied by loss of activity. Noncyclic structures are inactive. However analogs in which the sulfur atoms of the disulfide bridges are replaced by CH_2 (carba analogs) exhibit high activity, as do those with selenium in place of sulfur.

Several analogs with increased selectivity of action were obtained in the early period. For example, the ratio of milk-ejecting potency to uterotonic potency of [Ala^4]OT is 6:1, versus 1:1 in native oxytocin (274). In the vasopressin series, differentiation of the activity profile has been obtained with modifications at position 8 (Table 27.5). Replacements with various basic amino acids (ornithine or α,γ-diaminobutyric acid) enhance vasopressor activity, whereas the D-enantiomers of these basic amino acids increase the selectivity for antidiuretic action, which is further enhanced in the corresponding deamino analogs. Table 27.5 lists representative results of the early period, i.e. severalfold, but occasionally several hundredfold, selectivity enhancement.

Structure-activity studies gain in practical importance when they lead to rational

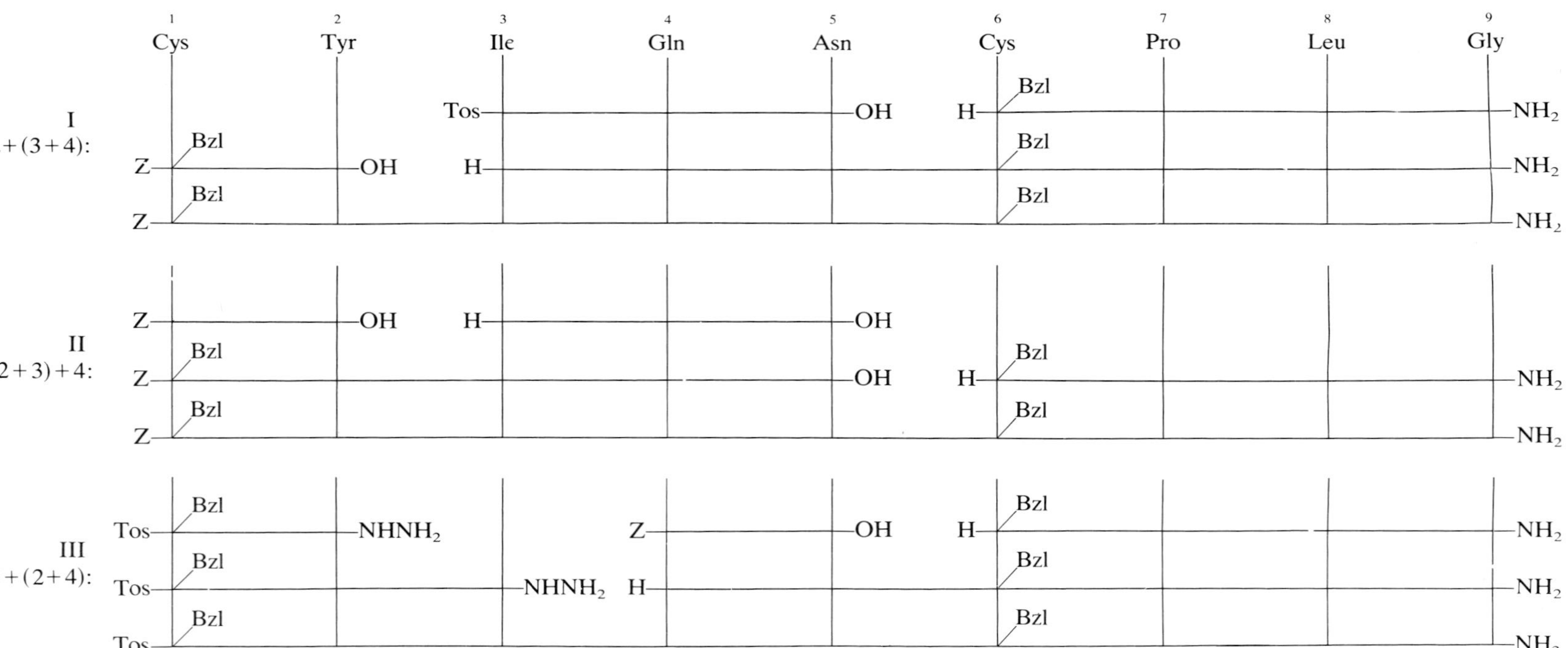

Fig. 27.30 Schemes of different syntheses of oxytocin. (I) du Vigneaud et al. (251). (II) Bodanszky and du Vigneaud (270). (III) Rudinger et al. (271).

Table 27.5 Selectivity of Action (Pressor v. Antidiuretic) Obtained in the "Early Period" of Vasopressin Analog Synthesis[a]

Vasopressins	Vasopressor Activity (rat)	Antidiuretic Activity (rat)	Ratio of Pressor to Antidiuretic Activity
[Arg^8]	400	430	1:1
[D-Arg^8]	4	114	1:28
[Lys^8]	270	250	1:1
[D-Lys^8]	1	20	1:20
[Orn^8]	360	88	4:1
[D-Orn^8]	0.24	60	1:250
[Dbu^8]	240	140	2:1
[D-Dbu^8]	4	120	1:30
[1-Mercaptopropionic acid, Arg^8]	370	1300	1:4
[1-Mercaptopropionic acid, D-Arg^8]	11	870	1:80
[1-Mercaptopropionic acid, Lys^8]	126	300	1:2
[1-Mercaptopropionic acid, D-Lys^8]	1	4	1:4
[1-Mercaptopropionic[b] acid, D-Dbu^8]	2	360	1:180
[Phe^2, Arg^8]	122	350	1:3
[Phe^2, Lys^8]	80	30	3:1
[Phe^2, Orn^8]	120	0.5	240:1
[Ile^3, Arg^8]	245	250	1:1
[Ile^3, Lys^8]	130	24	1:4
[Ile^3, Orn^8]	103	2.5	40:1

[a] Data from Ref. 274.
[b] Dbu = α,γ-Diaminobutyric acid.

guidelines for the development of hormone analogs with selectively enhanced biological activities or favorable activity ratios, or to analogs that competitively inhibit the biological response induced by the natural hormone. These goals have been very successfully pursued in recent years. Two approaches have been taken; (1) analysis of pharmacological data from more than 300 synthetic analogs (252, 274, 275) by Manning et al. (253), and (2) analog design based on the solution conformations of oxytocin and vasopressin by Walter (255).

Manning et al. (253) distinguish patterns of selectivity within the characteristic pharmacologic activities: oxytocic (O), milk-ejecting (ME), antidiuretic (A), pressor (P) of the following types: (1) interpeptidelike, A/O, O/P; (2) intraoxytocinlike O/ME, ME/O; (3) intravasopressinlike A/P, P/A. Consideration of structural modifications that individually or in combination give rise to peptides possessing enhanced selectivity of a given type can provide a rational basis for the design of analogs with even greater agonistic or antagonistic selectivity. The most remarkable example of a super-selective second-generation analog that had been designed in this manner is [1-deamino, 4-D-valine, 8-D-arginine]-vasopressin (DVDAVP), which possesses an antidiuretic-to-pressor activity ratio (A/P) exceeding 125,000:1, compared with a ratio of 1:1 for AVP (276). Similarly, Zaoral and Blaha (277) prepared [1-β-mercaptopropionic acid, 4-asparagine, 8-D-arginine]vasopressin with an antidiuretic potency of 11,000 IU/mg and negligible uterotonic activity. Potent inhibitors, which were developed along similar guidelines, include [1-L-penicillamine]oxytocin (278a), [1-β-mercaptopropionic acid, 2-(3,5-dibromo-L-tyrosine)]oxytocin (278b), and [2-*o*-iodo-L-tyrosine)]oxytocin (279).

Walter (269) gives a different weight to each amino acid residue in the three-dimensional structure (Fig. 27.29). Residues in the corner positions 3, 4, 7, and 8 that are not primarily involved in the intramolecular stabilization of the peptide backbone appear to contain the elements for oxytocic receptor recognition, the *binding element.* The hydroxy group of the tyrosine side chain, folded over the 20-membered ring of oxytocin (Fig. 27.29*c*), acting cooperatively with the asparagine carboxamide group, is considered to be the *active element.* Although modifications of the active element influence potency and/or agonist-antagonist characteristics, substitutions in the corner positions should provide analogs with selectively modified activity profiles. Indeed, the amino acid substitutions that distinguish the naturally occurring neurohypophyseal hormones (Table 27.4) are confined to position 3, 4, and 8. A striking example of a second-generation superselective analog that had been designed from a conformation-activity rationale is [4-L-threonine,7-glycine]oxytocin, exhibiting an oxytocic-to-antidiuretic activity ratio of 135,000:1, compared to a ratio of 200:1 for native oxytocin (280). Interestingly, Manning and collaborators (281) arrived simultaneously at the same analog by their independent rationale for analog design, discussed earlier. An interesting second-generation analog is [1-deamino,7-(3,4-dehydroproline)]arginine-vasopressin, in which a dramatic sevenfold increase of antidiuretic potency compared to AVP was obtained, along with an enhancement of the A/P ratio of 17:1 (282a). In pursuing this lead further, Smith and Walter (282b) developed a vasopressin analog with extraordinarily high antidiuretic potency. [1-Deamino,2-phenylalanine,7-(3,4-dehydroproline)]arginine-vasopressin exhibits a specific antidiuretic activity of 13,000 ± 1250 USP units/mg, thus being the most potent antidiuretic analog yet prepared. Moreover, the A/P ratio was determined to be 30,000:1.

The significance of this new level of sophistication in analog design on a predictable basis goes beyond the preparation of oxytocin or vasopressin analogs with exceptionally high potencies and/or specificity for a given activity. The development of conformation-activity relationships and their application to analog synthesis of other peptide hormones (e.g., insulin, see Section 8) should save some of the enormous expenditure of effort that was required for the synthesis of hundreds of analogs of neurohypophyseal hormones during the earlier, more empirical structure-activity approach to analog design.

5.6 Clinical Potential

Oxytocin is widely used for the induction of labor in the parturition and placenta expulsion periods. A disadvantage of oxytocin is its intrinsic antidiuretic activity, which can induce water retention when the hormone is given in a large volume of fluid by intravenous infusion. Analogs with high uterotonic-to-antidiuretic activity ratios should be superior to oxytocin for the induction of labor. Although by itself ineffective, oxytocin potentiates the action of prostaglandin E_2 in therapeutic abortion (283).

Diabetes insipidus, due to vasopressin deficiency, can now be treated advantageously with a synthetic analog [1-deamino,D-Arg^8]vasopressin, (DDAVP), a highly selective antidiuretic of prolonged action that exhibits extremely low pressor or uterotonic activity (284). A single intranasal dose produces antidiuresis lasting for up to 20 hr. The related analog, [1-deamino,Val^4,D-Arg^8]-vasopressin (DVDAVP) (276), possesses an even more favorable antidiuretic-to-pressor activity ratio exceeding 125,000 : 1, compared with 1 : 1 for arginine-vasopressin. This indicates a high potential usefulness for DVDAVP in the treatment of diabetes insipidus.

6 CALCITROPIC (THYROID) HORMONES

Besides the biologically active amino acid hormones thyroxin and triiodothyronine, the thyroid gland produces two peptide hormones. *Parathyrin* (PTH)* originates from the parathyroid glands, and *calcitonin* (CT)† is secreted from the parafollicular cells (C-cells) of mammalian thyroid glands. Both hormones participate in the regulation of calcium and phosphate metabolism and influence bone metabolism. PTH raises the Ca^{2+} level and decreases the phosphate level in blood. CT, the hypocalcemic, hypophosphatemic hormone, is synergistic with PTH in promoting the increase in urinary clearance of phosphate; but in its actions on bone or on urinary calcium, CT is antagonistic to PTH. Much progress has been made in the isolation, structure elucidation, and synthesis of PTH and CT from various species. On the other hand, radioimmunoassay techniques have revealed unforeseen complexities in the secretion, metabolism, and nature of circulating PTH. The sensitivity of these assays appears to be insufficient to measure circulating levels of CT in a reproducible manner. This has made the assessment of the physiological role of calcitonin in man exceedingly difficult. For details see Refs. 285–287.

* Synonyms: parathyroid hormone, parathormone.
† Synonym: thyreocalcitonin.

6.1 Parathyrin (PTH)

6.1.1 ISOLATION, STRUCTURE, AND BIOLOGICAL ACTIVITY. Although the influence of the parathyroid gland on calcium metabolism was recognized in 1909, highly purified PTH was first obtained by Rasmussen and Craig in 1961 (228). PTH is a linear peptide of 84 amino acid residues. More recently, three "isohormones" of the bovine hormone have been separated chromatographically which differ in one amino acid replacement (Val → Thr) each (289). The complete structures of the human, bovine and porcine hormones have been determined by Potts and collaborators (290), see Fig. 27.31. A review (291) is available.

PTH raises the Ca^{2+} content and lowers the phosphate content of blood by direct action on bone and kidney. In bone tissue, stimulation of osteoclasts (bone-resorbing cells) effects increased solubilization of hydroxylapatite and a rise in blood calcium. In the kidney the inhibition of phosphate resorption in the proximal tubules, and a rise of active phosphate secretion in the distal tubules, serve to lower the blood phosphate level. In hyperparathyroidism withdrawal of calcium from bone produces an excess in the blood. In hypoparathyroidism blood calcium levels fall, through a rise in phosphate levels (reduced phosphate excretion by the kidneys) and deposition of calcium phosphate in skeletal tissue. This causes changes in the ion tonicity of muscle and nerve cells, leading to tetanic convulsion. The level of blood Ca^{2+} is regulated within narrow limits by a negative feedback mechanism; i.e., a fall in calcium stimulates

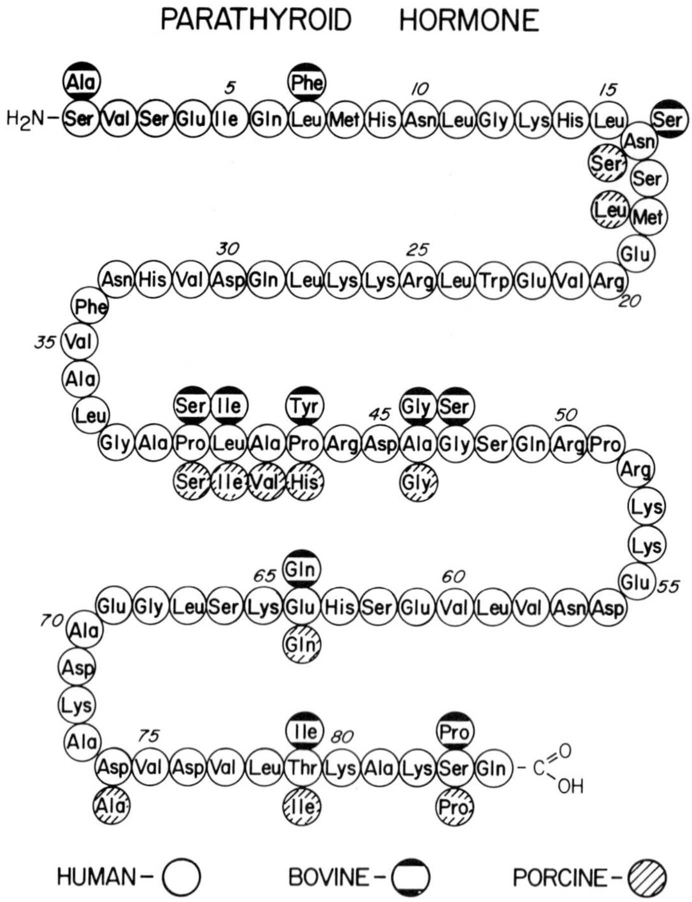

PARATHYROID HORMONE

HUMAN – BOVINE – PORCINE –

Fig. 27.31 Amino acid sequences of human, bovine, and porcine parathyrin. The continuous structure shown in open circles is that of human PTH. The appended residues indicate differences in amino acids in the sequence of bovine and porcine PTH. From Keutmann et al. (290). Reprinted with permission from H. T. Keutmann et al., *Biochemistry*, **17**, (1978). Copyright by the American Chemical Society.

PTH secretion. However the PTH antagonist calcitonin contributes in a major way to blood calcium and phosphate regulation (see Section 6.2), as does vitamin D_3.

PTH appears to activate the adenyl cyclase system during interaction with its receptor sites in kidney cortex tubules (292) and in bone tissue (293). The structural elements essential for the bioactivity are located in the NH_2-terminal part of PTH. Synthetic parathyrin-(1-34)-tetratriacontapeptide elicits in bone and kidney potent effects that are qualitatively identical to those of the native hormone.

Radioimmunoassay shows the presence of multiple immunoreactive forms of PTH in the circulation of man and animals. The predominant form appears to be a large biologically inactive fragment (sequence region *ca.* 30–84). At times, smaller bioactive fragments may also appear in blood. Most circulating fragments of PTH probably arise from peripheral cleavage of the intact secreted hormone in kidney and liver, but some forms of the hormone, including prohormones, may also be secreted from the parathyroid gland. For these reasons, it is still impossible to determine by immunoassay the true concentration of circulating biologically active hormone (291).

6.1.2 BIOSYNTHESIS. Biosynthesis of PTH proceeds by way of large precursor molecules. Bovine PTH prohormone contains a highly basic hexapeptide extension, H–Lys–Ser–Val–Lys–Lys–Arg–, at its NH_2-terminus. In a still larger "preprohormone" the NH_2-terminus is further extended by 25 residues (294) (Fig. 27.32). Preproparathyrin formation in intact parathyroid cells has been established. It is an early biosynthetic precursor that is converted into the prohormone within 1 min on the rough endoplasmic reticulum. The prohormone is converted in the Golgi complex into parathyrin 10–20 min later (Fig. 27.33), then packaged into secretory granules and secreted when calcium levels in the extracellular fluid decrease (287).

6.1.3 SYNTHESIS AND STRUCTURE-ACTIVITY RELATIONSHIPS. Both the bovine and the human PTH-(1–34) active fragments have been synthesized (295) by the solid phase method with the use of modified solid phase supports prepared by graft polymerization (296). The synthetic peptides possess all the specific physiological and biochemical properties associated with native PTH and exhibit approximately 80–120% of the potency of the native hormones on a molar basis in both the *in vitro* rat kidney adenylate cyclase and the *in vivo* chick hypercalcemia assays. Synthesis of smaller fragments showed that a continuous sequence of at least 27 residues from the NH_2-terminus is required for *in vitro* activity; i.e., the PTH-(1–27) peptide exhibits 6%, the

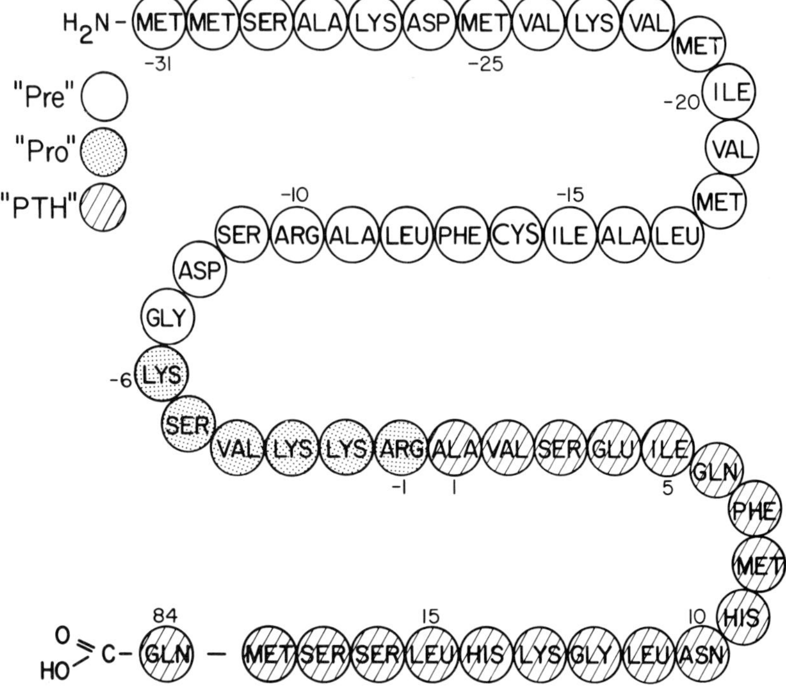

Fig. 27.32 Amino acid sequence of bovine preproparathyrin as determined by microsequencing technique. The radiolabeled prehormone was synthesized in the cell-free extract of wheat germ by addition of parathyroid RNA and radioactive amino acids (294). Stippled circles indicate amino acids in the sequence of ProPTH and shaded circles in that of PTH detected by the microsequence analysis, thus determining the exact length of the sequence of Pre-ProPTH. The NH_2-terminal methionine (residue −31) is the initiator amino acid not removed in the wheat germ system. Modified from Habener, et al. (287a).

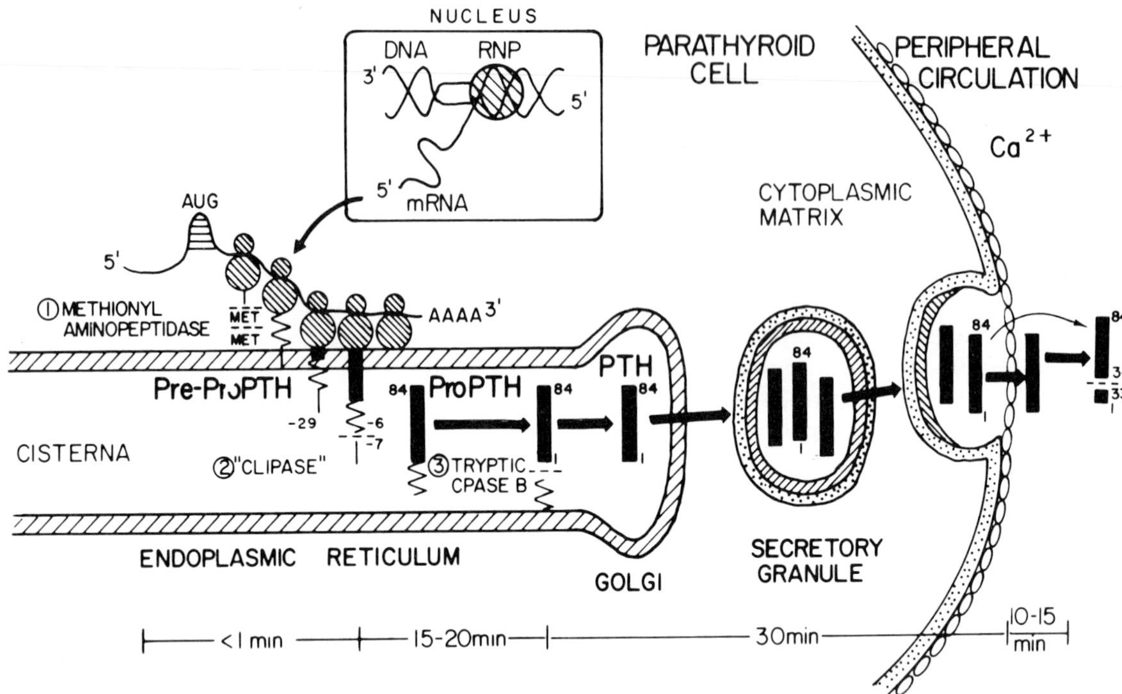

Fig. 27.33 Scheme depicting the proposed intracellular pathway of the biosynthesis of parathyrin. Pre-proparathyrin (Pre-ProPTH), the initial product of synthesis on the ribosomes, is converted into proparathyrin (ProPTH) by removal of (1) the NH_2-terminal methionine residues and (2) the NH_2-terminal sequence (–29 to –7) of 23 amino acids during synthesis and/or within seconds after synthesis, respectively. The conversion of Pre-ProPTH probably occurs during transport of the polypeptide into the cisterna of the rough endoplasmic reticulum. By 20 min after synthesis, ProPTH reaches the Golgi region and is converted into PTH by (3) removal of the NH_2-terminal hexapeptide. PTH is stored in the secretory granule until released into the circulation in response to a fall in the blood concentration of calcium. The time needed for these events is given below the scheme. From Habener, et al. (287). Reprinted with permission of Elsevier/Excerpta Medica.

PTH-(1–26) peptide less than 0.3% activity. For high *in vivo* activity, more than 28 residues are required. Removal of the amino-terminal residue results in drastic loss of activity. Prolongation of the chain beyond the NH_2-terminus also sharply lowers activity. The methionine residues in positions 8 and 18 may be replaced by norleucine with preservation of activity and introduction of a D-Ala in position 1, and an amide at the COOH-terminus increases activity (291).

6.2 Calcitonin (CT)

6.2.1 ISOLATION, STRUCTURE, AND BIOLOGICAL ACTIVITY. Calcitonin was discovered in 1962 by Copp in thyroid gland extracts. Within a few years several mammalian calcitonins, including the human hormone and salmon CT were isolated. Calcitonins are linear peptides consisting of 32 amino acid residues with an amino-terminal disulfide ring between Cys^1 and Cys^7 (Fig. 27.34). Whereas porcine and bovine CT differ in only three amino acid residues, the difference between porcine and human CT is 18 residues, and that between porcine and salmon[1] is 19. The bovine, ovine, porcine, and human hormones are about equipotent (150–200 IU/mg). The salmon and eel hormones, in contrast, exhibit a potency of 4000–5000 IU/mg and a fivefold longer duration of action. The greatly increased

Porcine	H–Cys–Ser–Asn–Leu–Ser–Thr–Cys–Val–Leu–Ser–Ala–Tyr–Trp–Arg–Asn–Leu–Asn–Asn–Phe–His–Arg–Phe–Ser–Gly–Met–Gly–Phe–Gly–Pro–Glu–Thr–Pro–NH_2
Bovine	Lys–Asp Tyr
Ovine	Lys–Asp Tyr Tyr
Salmon	Gly–Lys–Leu–Ser–Gln–Glu His–Lys–Leu–Gln–Thr–Tyr–Pro–Arg–Thr–Asn–Thr Ser–Gly
Eel	Gly–Lys–Leu–Ser–Gln– His–Lys–Leu–Gln–Thr–Thr–Pro–Arg–Thr–Asp–Val Ala–Gly
Human (M)	H–Cys–Gly–Asn–Leu–Ser–Thr–Cys–Met–Leu–Gly–Thr–Tyr–Thr–Gln–Asp–Phe–Asn–Lys–Phe–His–Thr–Phe–Pro–Gln–Thr–Ala–Ile–Gly–Val–Gly–Ala–Pro–NH_2

Fig. 27.34 The structures of calculations from different species. The invarient residues, common to all species, are indicated by broken vertical lines; residues identical to those of porcine are not shown (except in human CT). Two other salmon hormones (sCT_2 and sCT_3) have been identified, and these differ in four and five residues, respectively, from $salmon_1$ (285, 303).

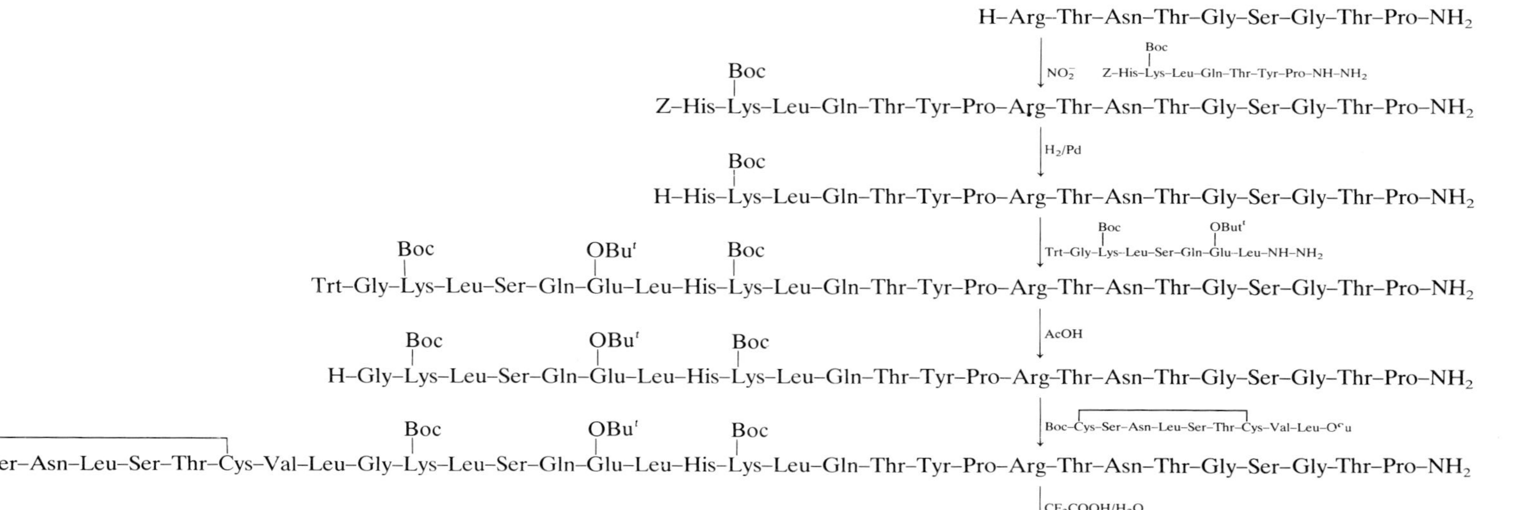

Fig. 27.35 A synthesis of $salmon_1$ calcitonin in which the NH_2-terminal nonapeptide fragment containing the disulfide bond was coupled to the intermediate (10–32)-fragment. From Guttmann et al. (305).

bioactivity of salmon and eel CT is explained by their higher affinity to receptor sites in bone and kidney, as well as their higher resistance to metabolic degradation, compared to the porcine hormone (for a review, see Ref. 285).

CT promotes urinary clearance of calcium and phosphate, but its principal action in mammalian species is inhibition of bone resorption. The hormone effects calcium phosphate deposition in bone by stimulating osteoblasts (bone-forming cells). This activity is also accompanied by a decrease of calcium and phosphate levels in blood. The half-life of circulation ranges from 2 to 20 min, depending on assay and calcitonin species. The effects of calcitonin on skeletal tissue and on cortical tubules of the kidney may be mediated through cyclic AMP (297).

CT also affects gastrointestinal tract function by inhibiting the intestinal absorption of calcium, and one of its main functions may be the prevention of postprandial hypercalcemia (298). The hormone inhibits 1α-hydroxylation of 25-hydroxycholecalciferol in chick kidney (299).

The results of early radioimmunoassay determination of circulating CT levels of 0.1–0.6 ng/ml in normal human subjects have recently been corrected to 100 pg/ml with the use of more highly specific assays (286). Accurate determination of these low levels of CT in blood must await the development of still more sensitive techniques.

CT has found clinical application in diagnosis and as a therapeutic agent. The radioimmunoassay for CT is used in the detection of occult medullary carcinoma of the thyroid (300, 301) and may become useful for diagnosis of oat cell carcinoma of the lung. Both salmon and human CT have been successfully used in the treatment of Paget's disease of bone (302). For reviews, see Refs. 19, 285, 286, 303, and 304.

6.2.2 SYNTHESIS AND STRUCTURE-ACTIVITY RELATIONSHIPS. Conventional fragment condensation in solution has been used for most syntheses of calcitonins and analogs, as illustrated in Fig. 27.35, for a synthesis of ${}_{\text{salm}}\text{CT}_1$ (305). Solid phase procedures have been used in a few instances, e.g., for syntheses of human CT (306). Analog synthesis established that the entire sequence of 32 amino acid residues is required for bioactivity; any shortening of the chain results in severe loss of activity, as does substitution of proline or proline methyl ester for the 32-prolinamide (307). Opening of the disulfide ring by replacement of Cys with *S*-methyl-Cys results in large loss of activity. Increase of *in vivo* activity (20–50%) is obtained by replacement of the α-amino function with hydrogen ("deaminocalcitonin") or by acetylation of the α-amino group of human CT. This increase of hypocalcemic activity in rats, accompanied by prolongation of action, may be a result of increased stability toward degradation by aminopeptidases (307). Preparation of analogs by amino acid replacements in the interior of the molecule have been motivated by the ten- to thirtyfold potency difference between human and salmon CT. Replacement of Met^8 of human CT by Val, or Phe^{22} by Tyr, yielded the analogs $[\text{Val}^8]$hCT and $[\text{Tyr}^{22}]$hCT, which are 4–5 times as potent and nearly twice as long acting as the native hormone. The doubly substituted $[\text{Val}^8, \text{Tyr}^{22}]$hCT closely resembles $[\text{Val}^8]$hCT and $[\text{Tyr}^{22}]$hCT in bioactivity. Desamino-$[\text{Val}^8]$hCT is about 6 times more potent than the native hormone and slightly longer acting than $[\text{Val}^8]$hCT (308). Replacement of the three aromatic amino acids in positions 12, 16, and 19 of human CT by leucine residues that occupy the corresponding positions in salmon and eel CT increased hypocalcemic activity in rats about tenfold (Fig. 27.36). The individual substitutions are not all equally augmentative. Combination of the Leu^{12} substitution with an NH_2-terminal deaminocysteine yields the 10 times more potent deamino-$[\text{Leu}^{12}]$hCT analog. The additional substitution of Tyr for Phe^{22} in

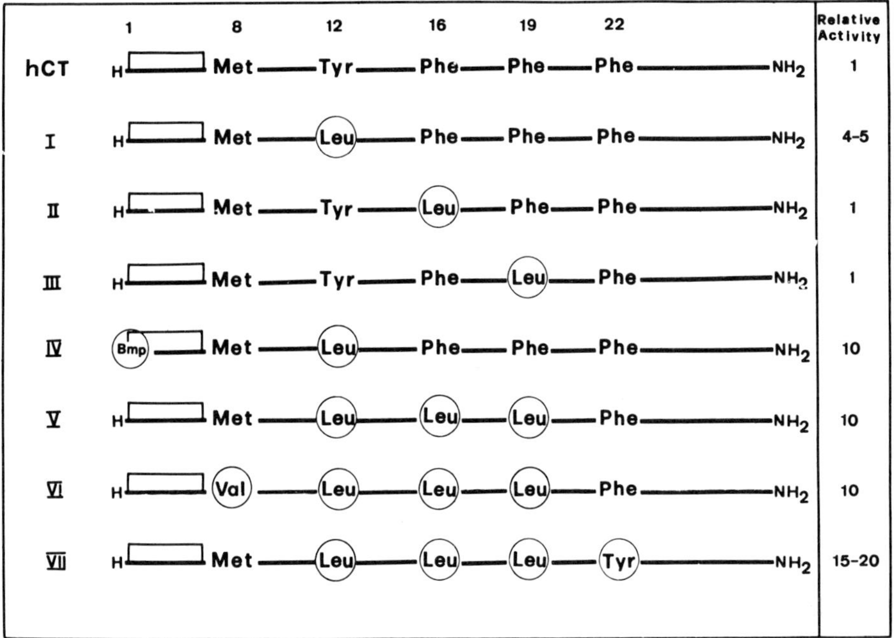

Fig. 27.36 Schematic structures of calcitonin analogs. Circled amino acids except Bmp[1] indicate substitution of those occurring in salmon calcitonin; noncircled residues are those of human calcitonin (hCT); Bmp = β-mercaptopropionic acid. Activities are expressed relative to hCT = 1, as deduced from hypocalcemic assay in rats. From Maier et al. (309). Reprinted with permission of Blackwell Scientific Publ. Ltd.

the trileucine analog provides the [Leu^{12,16,19}, Tyr^{22}]hCT analog possessing fifteen- to twentyfold potency and twofold duration of action of native human CT. This potency equals about half that of salmon CT (309).

In sum promising progress has been made in efforts to unravel the underlying structure-activity relationships responsible for the large potency differences between human and salmon calcitonin. Prospects are excellent for developing analogs for clinical use that may combine the benefits of each of the human and the salmon hormone.

7 THYMIC FACTORS

Recognition in 1963 of the central role of the thymus in immunity (310) and evidence of an endocrine function for the thymus gland have stimulated increasing efforts to identify and isolate the factors responsible for the maturation of thymus-derived cells (T-cells). Three peptides have been isolated, characterized, and sequenced: thymopoietin (311), thymosin α_1 (312), and circulating thymic factor (313). A fourth peptide, thymic humoral factor (314), has been characterized by amino acid composition. Compelling evidence for the thymic hormone concept, details of the biological and chemical properties of the available preparations, their bioactivity, and their as yet unclear roles in T-cell differentiation have been reviewed comprehensively (315–318).

One of the major difficulties in evaluating the bioactivity of thymic factors has been the dearth of relevant and reproducible assay procedures. Indeed, thymic factors have been referred to as "hormones in search of bioassay" (315). Whereas in general the demonstration of the endocrine function of a gland is based on the effects of gland ablation and its correction by injecting gland extracts, this procedure proved to be difficult or inadequate with the thymus. Thymectomy has little or no immediate effects on immune capacity in adult mice, and heterologous bovine thymus extracts may lack specificity (insufficient amounts are available from mouse thymus). However neonatal thymectomy induces characteristic alterations of the immune system, and recent assay procedures aim at restoration of isolated aspects of the immune response. *In vitro* bioassays fall into three main categories: (1) analysis of surface markers, (2) lymphocytic stimulation by lectins or allogeneic cells, and (3) study of functional responses such as cytotoxicity, production and release of lymphokines, and amplification of antibody responses. Very careful controls are needed, since several agents can be active, such as endotoxins, polyribonucleotides, and ubiquitin (318a), or even chemicals such as mercaptoethanol.

The clinical potentials of thymic factors appear to be promising for the treatment of certain primary immunodeficiency diseases. The prospects in the treatment of secondary immunodeficiency diseases seem to be very favorable in initial clinical cancer studies.

7.1 Thymosin

Thymosin is obtained from extracts of calf thymus glands and processed through a five-stage purification procedure, including ultracentrifugation, heat denaturation, acetone precipitation, ammonium sulfate precipitation, hollow fiber ultrafiltration, and final Sephadex G-50 gel filtration [A. L. Goldstein et al. (319)]. The ensuing "thymosin fraction 5" (F-5) consists of more than 50 peptide components ranging in molecular weight from 1000 to 15,000 daltons and in isoelectric points between pI 3 and pI 8 (320). This material has been active in a variety of *in vitro* and *in vivo* assay systems, including the mixed lymphocyte reaction of mouse lympoid cells and immunologic restoration of both thymectomized and athymic nude mice. Figure 27.37 depicts A. L. Goldstein's working hypothesis on the mechanism of action of thymosin (321). It is suggested that thymosin acts on cells that may not necessarily have resided in the thymus but are already genetically programmed to differentiate into T-cells. Phase I clinical trials with thymosin F-5 showed no adverse effects or toxicity at therapeutic doses. Controlled phase II clinical trials are in progress (322a). In a lung cancer study thymosin F-5 ($60\ mg/m^2$, i.v., twice weekly for 6 weeks) prolonged the survival of small cell lung cancer patients treated with intensive combination chemotherapy (322b).

Further chromatographic fractionation led to the isolation of one of the acidic peptide components (pI *ca.* 4.2), named thymosin α_1 (312), which was highly active in mitogen and rosette-forming assays. Sequence analysis of the 28 residue peptide showed it to contain an NH_2-terminal acetyl group (Fig. 27.38). It does not contain aromatic amino acid residues, methionine, histidine, cysteine, proline, and glycine. The clinical effectiveness of thymosin α_1 is being evaluated.

7.2 Thymopoietin

Two closely related peptides have been isolated by Gideon Goldstein (323) from bovine thymus extracts through a seven-stage fractionation procedure including heat denaturation, ultrafiltration, and five

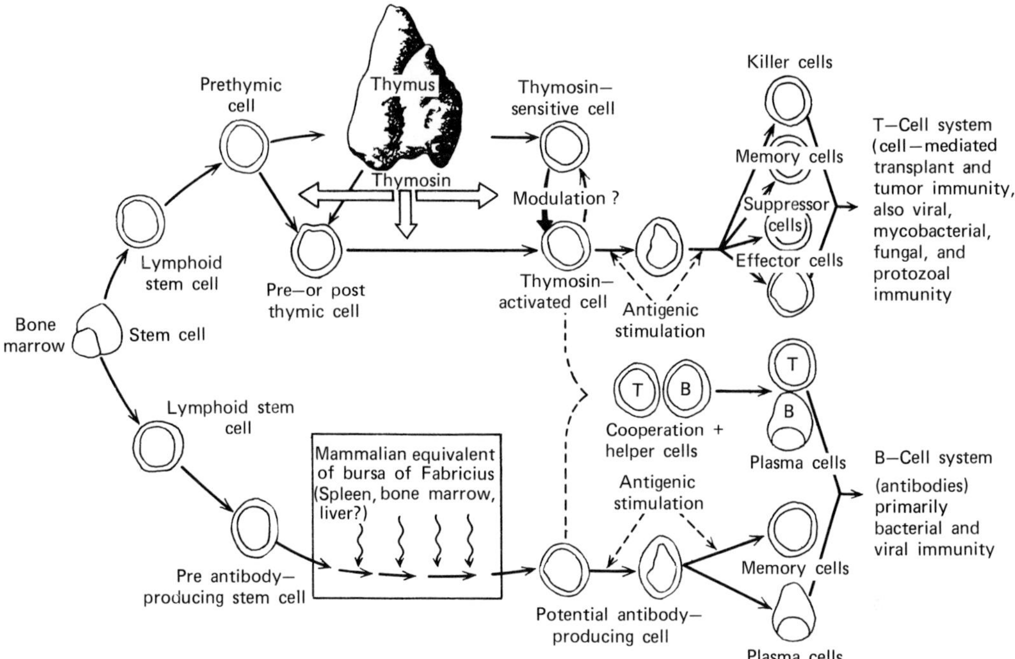

Fig. 27.37 A hypothetical role of thymosin in the maturation of the immune system. From A. L. Goldstein et al. (321). Reprinted from Federation. Proceedings *33*: 2053–2056, 1974.

chromatographic separations. One kilogram of thymus provides about 1 mg each of the peptides. One of these, thymopoietin II, has been sequenced (Fig. 27.39) and shown to be a 49 residue peptide (mol wt 5562) that lacks methionine, cysteine, histidine, tryptophan, and isoleucine (311).

Thymopoietin II induces the differentiation of early T-cells from precursor cells (prothymocytes) found in bone marrow or

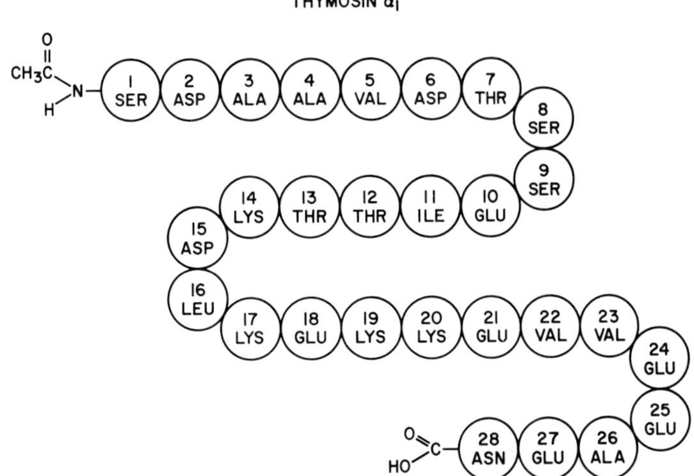

Fig. 27.38 The structure of thymosin α_1 (mol wt 3108 daltons) proposed by A. L. Goldstein et al. (312).

NH_2–Ser[1]–Gln–Phe–Leu–Glu[5]–Asp–Pro–Ser–Val–Leu[10]–Thr–Lys–Glu–Lys–Leu[15]–

Lys–Ser–Glu–Leu–Val[20]–Ala–Asn–Asn–Val–Thr[25]–Leu–Pro–Ala–Gly–Glu[30]–

Gln–Arg–Lys–Asp–Val[35]–Tyr–Val–Gln–Leu–Tyr[40]–Leu–Gln–Thr–Leu–Thr[45]–

Ala–Val–Lys–Arg[49]–COOH

Fig. 27.39 The structure of thymopoietin II as proposed by Schlesinger and G. Goldstein (311).

spleen (324). In bioassay, this activity is measured by the expression of various T-cell alloantigens in mouse bone marrow cells.

A tridecapeptide corresponding to positions 29–41 of thymopoietin II was synthesized by a solid phase technique. It displayed a selectivity of action similar to that of the native factor and exhibited a potency of 3% compared to thymopoietin (325). Clinical evaluation of thymopoietin must await synthesis of large enough quantities.

7.3 Circulating Thymic Factor

Although most thymic factor isolation programs use thymus extracts, J.-F. Bach and collaborators isolated a neutral (pI 7.3) nonapeptide from porcine serum called facteur thymique serique (FTS). The presence of this peptide in the serum is thymus dependent (for a review, see Ref. 315). Isolation involves several stages, as dialysis, ultrafiltration through polyacrylonitrile membranes, gel filtration, and ion exchange chromatography, followed by desalting. The assay procedure used during isolation and purification is based on the capacity of thymic extracts to render spleen rosette-forming cells from adult thymectomized mice sensitive to inhibition by antitheta serum and azathioprine. Sequence analysis has not led to the precise identification of the NH_2-terminal residue of the nonapeptide (Fig. 27.40); it is thought to be a pyroglutamic acid or a glutamine residue (313).

The pyroglutamine-containing peptide has been synthesized by solid phase techniques, and the biological activity was of the same order of magnitude as natural FTS both *in vivo* and *in vitro* assay. Clinical use of FTS has not as yet been reported.

7.4 Thymic Humoral Factor (THF)

Starting from homogenized bovine thymus glands Trainin et al. (314, 316) used repeated ultracentrifugation and filtration, isolate a preparation that has shown activity in a variety of assays. The bioassay used routinely in this work to evaluate the activity of THF is the *in vitro* graft-versus-host (GVH) model. The biological activity of the THF preparation is expressed by its ability to induce competence in spleen cells of neonatally thymectomized mice to react to challenges by parental and syngeneic cells (for reviews, see Refs. 315 and 316).

Further purification of the foregoing preparation by several gel filtration steps and ion exchange chromatography yielded a preparation with an isoelectric point of

pGlu–Ala–Lys–Ser–Gln–Gly–Gly–Ser–Asn–OH
or Gln

Fig. 27.40 The structure of circulating thymic factor (FTS) nonapeptide. Alternatively, the amino-terminal residue may be Gln. From Bach et al. (313).

5.66–5.90. Amino acid analysis indicates the presence of 31 residues with a high proportion of acidic amino acids. The structure of the purified peptide has not yet been reported.

The study of thymic factors and their potential in the clinical treatment of immunodeficiency diseases is still in its infancy. The relevance and correlation of bioassays to immune restoration in animals and in man needs to be improved. Vexing problems will have to be resolved. For example, how do thymic factors control T-cell maturation and immune competence, and which type of signals causes the release of thymic factors into circulation? The site of thymic factor synthesis in the epithelium of the thymus is unknown, or even whether all thymic factor peptides originate from one or several biosynthetic precursors (prohormones). However the potential medical benefit of thymic factor replacement therapy could be enormous.

8 PANCREATIC HORMONES

The two long known pancreatic hormones, insulin and glucagon, have recently been joined by the newcomer somatostatin, which was first discovered in the hypothalamus (see Section 3) and is also present in brain. Insulin (Fig. 27.41) is a polypeptide (mol wt *ca.* 5808) and is produced in the B cells of the islets of Langerhans. Glucagon (Fig. 27.42, mol wt *ca.* 3483) is produced in the A cells, and somatostatin (Fig. 27.43, mol wt *ca.* 1638) is produced in the D cells.

The major role of insulin in the treatment of diabetes was recognized even before the hormone was isolated, but investigations of potential major involvements of both glucagon and somatostatin have begun only recently. The successful treatment with insulin of diabetic ketoacidosis and coma, starting in 1922, led to a steady increase in the life expectancy of diabetic patients (329). However along with increasing duration of diabetes, there occurred a rising frequency (>70%) of cardiovascular-renal disease [including retinopathy, microangiopathy (330), and neuropathy] as a cause of death. Ascertaining the origin, prevention, and treatment of these complications presents the major problem and challenge in diabetes today (329, 331); for a review, see Ref. 332. New leads might develop from a bihormonal imbalance hypothesis (333) of diabetes mellitus according to which a combination of insulin deficiency and glucagon overabundance is responsible for the diabetic syndrome. A combined therapy of stimulating insulin release and inhibiting glucagon secretion might be desirable. Therefore somatostatin, a potent inhibitor of both glucagon and insulin release, might become a useful adjunct to insulin in the treatment of diabetes (for a review, see Ref. 332).

The biochemistry and pharmacology of insulin, glucagon, and somatostatin, their physiological roles in blood sugar regulation and growth, and their medical use are described in detail in Chapter 31 and are mentioned only peripherally here. The emphasis in this chapter is on the chemistry of the pancreatic hormones, especially on structure, conformation, synthesis, and structure-activity relations.

8.1 Insulin

8.1.1 HISTORY. The isolation of insulin from bovine pancreas glands by Banting, MacLeod, Best, and Collip in 1922 was one of the starting points of polypeptide hormone chemistry and biochemistry and of diabetes therapy. The sustained success of insulin therapy in the treatment of diabetes mellitus (329) has been accompanied by intensive research that still continues to grow. Several of the numerous accomplishments were "firsts" in the polypeptide field, and some revolutionized scientific thought.

A. Chain

H–Gly–Ile– Val– Glu–Gln–Cys–Cys–Thr– Ser– Ile– Cys– Ser– Leu–Tyr–Gln– Leu–Glu–Asn–Tyr– Cys–Asn–OH

Ala–Ser–Val (bovine)

H–Phe–Val–Asn–Gln–His– Leu–Cys–Gly– Ser– His– Leu–Val– Glu–Ala–Leu–Tyr–Leu–Val– Cys– Gly–Glu– Arg–Gly–Phe–Phe–Tyr–Thr–Pro–Lys–Thr–OH

B. Chain

Fig. 27.41 Structures of human insulin (326) and bovine insulin. From F. Sanger et al. (336).

H–His– Ser–Gln–Gly–Thr–Phe–Thr–Ser–Asp–Tyr–Ser– Lys– Tyr–Leu–Asp–Ser– Arg–Arg– Ala–Gln–Asp–Phe–Val–Gln–Trp–Leu–Met–Asn–Thr–OH

Fig. 27.42 Structure of human glucagon (327).

H–Ala–Gly–Cys–Lys–Asn–Phe– Phe–Trp–Lys– Thr–Phe– Thr–Ser– Cys–OH

Fig. 27.43 Structure of human somatostatin (122).

These advances in insulin research include: (1) crystallization of the hormone by Abel in 1926 (334), (2) the recognition in 1928–1930 from chemical investigations that biological activity can be elicited by a "plain" polypeptide (335) lacking any "prosthetic group", (3) structure determination by F. Sanger and collaborators (336) in 1955—this was the first demonstration that proteins are defined molecules, not complex mixtures of closely related congeners, (4) discovery of proinsulin, the first polypeptide hormone precursor, by Steiner et al. (337) in 1967, (5) X-ray crystal structure determination by D. Hodgkin and collaborators (10, 338, 339) in 1969—the first molecular interpretation of peptide hormone monomer-dimer-hexamer association, and (6) total synthesis of crystalline human insulin by the Ciba-Geigy peptide group (340) in 1975—the first synthesis of a two-chain peptide by stepwise formation of three disulfide bonds.

8.1.2 PREPARATION, PROPERTIES, AND BIOLOGICAL ACTIVITY. Sources of commercial preparation of insulin are bovine and porcine pancreas glands.* Beef pancreas yields 75 mg/kg of the hormone. The main problem consists of its speedy separation from the proteolytic enzymes (*ca.* 40 g/kg) in pancreatic tissue. This is accomplished by extraction of insulin with 70% ethanol at pH 1–2 (HCl). A five-step purification by fractional precipitation and final crystallization yields insulin with 26–28 IU/mg as assayed (for a review, see Ref. 341) by the *in vivo* rabbit blood glucose depression, the mouse convulsion test, or *in vitro* tests such as rat epididymal glucose oxidation.

Insulin circulates in blood as unbound and, probably, monodisperse molecule with a half-life of about 5 min. It plays the dominant role in maintaining plasma glucose levels in man between 50 and 150 mg/ml and occupies the central control function in the interplay of fuel utilization and mobilization, as described in a recent review (342).

The incidence of allergic reactions of diabetic patients to insulin (343) has been considerably reduced during the past 10 years, following the improvement of the purity of commercial preparations by chromatographic techniques (344–346). Moreover, with the available rapid desensitizing techniques (347), insulin allergy has never been a serious clinical problem (329), although it has been of great interest to immunologists. Contamination of insulin with proinsulin, which exhibits larger species differences, therefore higher antigenicity, appears to have caused most of the allergenic properties of commercial insulins (345). These high molecular weight contaminations can be readily removed by gel filtration.

Reviews and books on biological (10, 19, 344, 348–352) and chemical (19, 353–355) aspects are available.

8.1.3 SEQUENCE AND SPECIES VARIATION. The Sanger structure of insulin (Fig. 27.41) consists of the acidic A chain of 21 amino acid residues and the basic B chain of 30 residues. The chains are linked by two disulfide bonds. A third disulfide forms a 20-membered intrachain ring in the A chain. All known insulin molecules of different animal species (>30 at present) possess the same basic structural framework with variable amino acid substitutions. Closest to human insulin and differing only in one residue (B30 = Ala) is the commercially produced porcine hormone and the identical insulins of dogs and whales. The bovine hormone, which amounts to about 90% of all therapeutically used insulin, differs in three residues (A8 = Ala, A10 = Ile, B30 = Ala).

Four groups of insulins can be distinguished by their degrees of variation from

* The world supply seems to be large enough to permit a severalfold increase of insulin production over present volume, especially if other sources (sheep, fish) were more fully utilized. Nevertheless, a supply crisis could arise, even at this time, in case of international disaster.

Table 27.6 The Known Amino Acid Sequences of Insulin[a]

A CHAIN[b]

	(1)	(2)	3	4	(5)	(6)	(7)	8	9	10	(11)	12	13	14	15	(16)	17	18	(19)	(20)	(21)	22
	Gly	Ile	Val	Glu	Gln	Cys	Cys	Thr	Ser	Ile	Cys	Ser	Leu	Tyr	Gln	Leu	Gln	Asn	Tyr	Cys	Asn	
Mammals				Asp				Ala	Gly	Thr												
										Val												
Birds								His	Asn	Thr												
			Leu					His	His	Pro		Asn	Lys	Phe	Asp		Gln	Ser				
Fishes									Lys			Asp	Ile					Asn				
									Arg													
Guinea pig				Asp				Ala	Gly	Thr		Thr	Arg	His			Gln					
Coypu				Asp				Thr	Asn	Ile			Arg	Asn			Met					Asp

B CHAIN

	0	1	2	3	4	5	(6)	(7)	(8)	9	10	(11)	(12)	13	14	(15)	(16)	17	(18)	(19)	20	21	22	(23)	(24)	25	26	27	28	29	30
		Phe	Val	Asn	Gln	His	Leu	Cys	Gly	Ser	His	Leu	Val	Glu	Ala	Leu	Tyr	Leu	Val	Cys	Gly	Glu	Arg	Gly	Phe	Phe	Tyr	Thr	Pro	Lys	Ala
Mammals				Lys						Pro																				Met	Ser
																															Thr
Birds		Ala	Ala																												
	Met	Ala	Ala	Ala										Asp								Asp						Asn	Ser	Lys	⊖
Fishes	Ala		Pro	Pro																										⊖	
	Val																														
Guinea pig				Ser	Arg						Asn				Thr			Ser			Gln	Asp	Asp					Ile		Lys	Asp
Coypu		Tyr		Ser		Arg					Gln			Asp	Thr			Ser			Arg	His	Arg			Tyr	Arg	Pro	Asn	Asp	⊖

[a] From Blundell et al. (10); reprinted with permission of Academic Press, Inc.
[b] Circled numbers represent invariant residues.
[c] ⊖ Represents deletions.

the porcine species (10), as Table 27.6 illustrates. The mammalian insulins all have very similar sequences, with variations limited to the sequence segments A8–10 and B29, 30, and residue B3, except for the more variant guinea pig and coypu hormones. Bird insulins differ at A8 and B1, 2 but are similar at A9, 10 and B29, 30. Fish insulins vary between A12–15, 17, 18, at both the NH_2- and COOH-termini of the B chain, and are very different at A8–10. Guinea pig and coypu insulins are quite abnormal in having 6 and 8 substitutions, respectively, and in being variable, together, at 10 residues that otherwise remain invariant (A22, B4, 5, 10, 14, 17, 20, 22, 5, 26). With the knowledge of the three-dimensional structure of insulin, the effects of these substitutions on conformation have been correlated with the relatively low bioactivity of guinea pig and coypu insulins and with modified aggregation properties in dimer and hexamer formation (10); *vide infra.* The invariant residues, among the insulin structures known at present, are circled in Table 27.6. They include all cysteine residues.

8.1.4 BIOSYNTHESIS. The biosynthesis of insulin proceeds through larger single-chain precursors. In 1967 Steiner and collaborators (337) discovered proinsulin (for reviews, see Refs. 10 and 356) in which a connecting peptide chain ("C-peptide") of 29–35 residues, in different species, joins the B chain at B30 through two arginine residues with the A chain at A1 through an –Lys–Arg– linkage (Fig. 27.44*a*). The amino acid sequences of 10 different mammalian and avian C-peptides show considerably larger variability than the respective insulins (356), which indicates the absence of vital hormonal functionality in this part of the molecule. The C-peptide serves to control the folding of proinsulin into the conformation exhibited by the A and B chains in insulin, and it assures the correct pairing of the three disulfide bonds that stabilize the structure, i.e., disulfides A6–11, A7–B12, and A20–B19 (Fig. 27.41). Proinsulins display low intrinsic insulinlike activity *in vitro* (3–5%), but *in vivo* the apparent activity may be 20–30%, possibly as a result of prolonged metabolic half-life. Concerning the clinical significance of circulating proinsulin, see Ref. 356a.

Proinsulins have a considerably higher solubility than the corresponding insulins, but they share very similar aggregation behavior. Proinsulin forms stable dimers readily and aggregates in the presence of zinc and above pH 6 to a stable hexamer (10). Enzymatic conversion of proinsulin by cleavage at the basic connecting residues forms active insulin within the β-cell, with liberation of the C-peptide and the four basic amino acids (residues 31, 32, 64, and 65 in Fig. 27.44*a*). Blundell et al. (10) have proposed that the proinsulin hexamer is formed soon after synthesis, transported to the storage granule, and converted to insulin while in the hexameric state. The ensuing zinc-containing crystalline insulin hexamer is resistant to further tryptic and other enzymatic proteolysis and degradation during storage.

Recently a still larger precursor molecule (mol wt *ca.* 11,500), designated preproinsulin, has been discovered (359) when isolated mRNA from rat islets of Langerhans was used to prime cell-free synthesis of protein in a wheat germ ribosomal system. Microsequence determination revealed the presence of 23 additional amino acid residues, NH_2-terminal to the B chain of proinsulin (Fig. 27.44b_2). Twelve of these residues were identified. In another approach (359a) sequencing of DNA copies of isolated rat pre-proinsulin messenger RNA provided almost complete sequence information (Fig. 27.44b_1). This presequence, similar to that of preproparathyrin (287), may play a role in vectorial discharge and sequestration of the nascent peptide chain within the microsomal cisternae and is rapidly cleaved during each cycle of protein synthesis.

The processes in the β-cell leading to secretion of insulin into the bloodstream

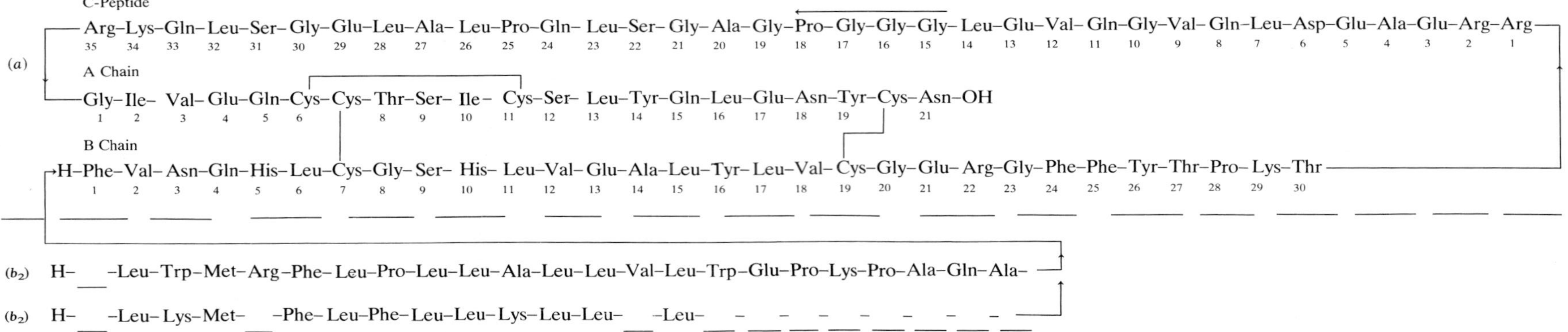

Fig. 27.44 Biosynthetic insulin precursors. (*a*) The structure of human proinsulin (357, 358). (b_1) The preproinsulin extension (sequence of rat species) derived from cell-free protein synthesis in a wheat germ ribosomal system (359); (b_2) derived from DNA sequencing (359a).

have been reviewed (10, 356). Synthesis of preproinsulin at the ribosomes of the endoplasmic reticulum is followed within seconds by conversion to proinsulin through microsomal enzymes and by disulfide bond formation. The proinsulin then aggregates into hexamers and is transported within 10–20 min to the Golgi complex, where the storage granules are formed. At this stage begins the conversion of proinsulin to hexameric insulin, which continues within the storage granules for several hours. In response to stimuli such as increased blood glucose levels, the insulin granules move to the edge of the cell, probably by way of microtubules, and the hormone is secreted into the bloodstream, where it dissolves rapidly at the higher pH.

8.1.5 X-RAY CRYSTAL STRUCTURE. The three-dimensional structure of insulin was determined in 1969 by Hodgkin et al. (338, 339). This achievement represents an outstanding landmark in peptide hormone research and provided the basis for interpretation of many of the chemical and biological properties of insulin on a molecular level. This work has been superbly described by Blundell et al. (10). Several fascinating developments followed this breakthrough, for example, the collaborative efforts in establishing more sophisticated structure-activity relations (360). Thus the low potencies of guinea pig and coypu insulins can now be explained by the profound effects of B10 histidine substitution on the molecular architecture of insulin. Studies of a series of synthetic A1 glycine-acylated derivatives led to the recognition of a receptor binding region of insulin (*vide infra*).

The crystal structure analysis was based on electron density maps first obtained

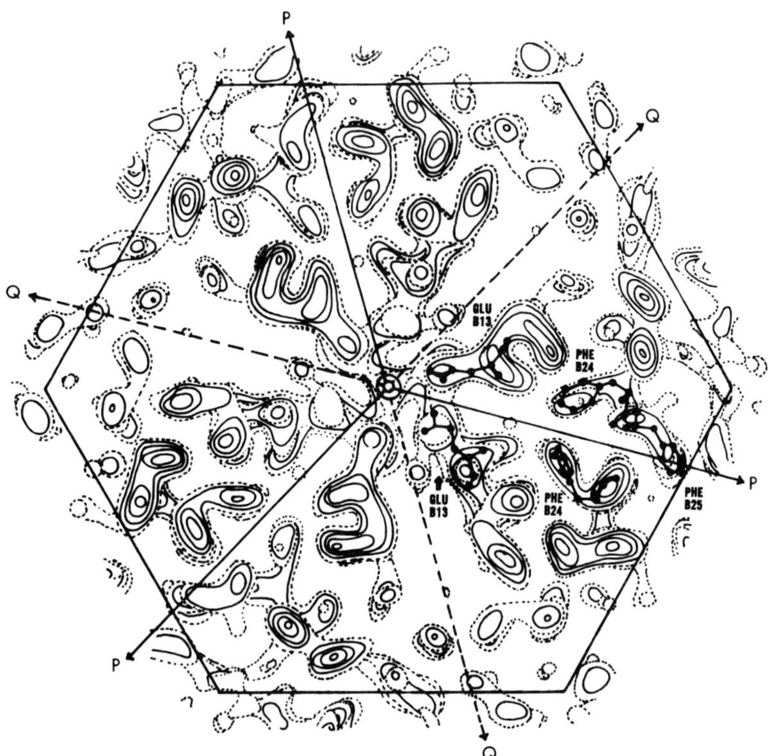

Fig. 27.45 Electron density map of crystalline zinc insulin at 2.8 Å resolution. The unit cell is outlined by the hexagon. The threefold symmetry is clearly visible. From Blundell et al. (10). Reprinted with permission of Academic Press, Inc.

from porcine zinc insulin at 2.8 Å (Fig. 27.45) and followed by 1.9 Å resolution. In the rhombohedral crystal the unit cell consists of six insulin molecules arranged as three equivalent dimers in threefold symmetry (Fig. 27.46*a*). The compact packing of the hexamer produces an oblate spheroid (*ca.* 50 Å wide, 35 Å high), with polar amino acid side chains covering its surface. The two zinc ions are situated, 17 Å apart, on the threefold crystal axis and coordinated to three equivalent B10 histidines. Perpendicular to the threefold crystal axis are noncrystallographic twofold symmetry axes (Fig. 27.46*a*) relating two dimers of the hexamer ($O \rightarrow Q$) and the

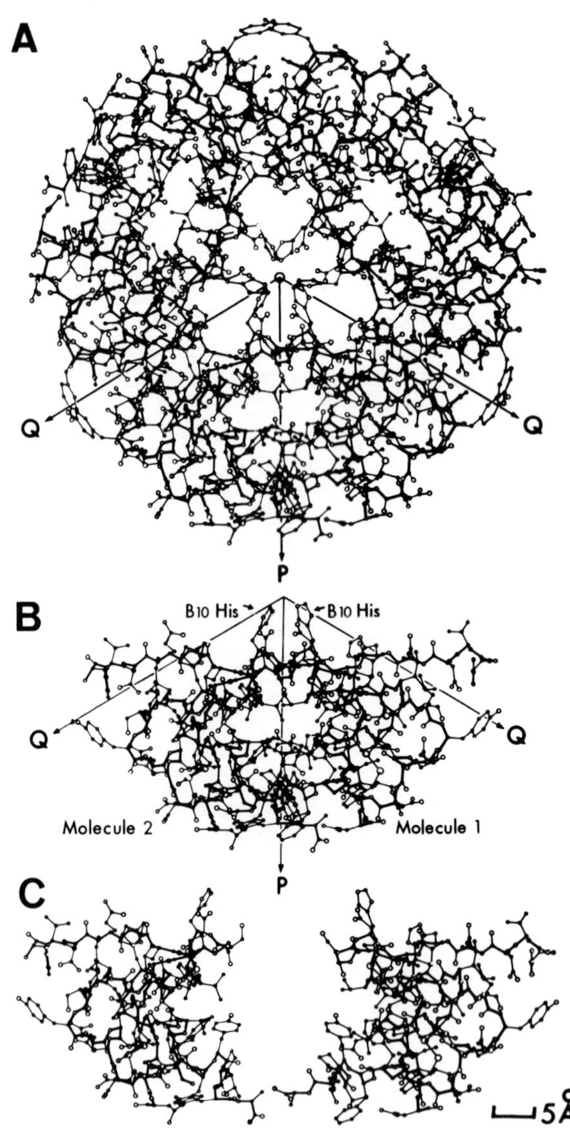

Fig. 27.46 The aggregation of the insulin monomers (*c*) to dimers (*b*) and then hexamers (*a*) in the presence of zinc, viewed along the threefold axis (perpendicular to the view in Fig. 27.47). From Blundell et al. (10). Reprinted with permission of Academic Press, Inc.

two monomers, molecules 1 and 2, of the dimer ($O \rightarrow P$) (Fig. 27.46*b*). The dimers constitute the asymmetric units. In the monomers (Fig. 27.46*c*) the two chains each are arranged almost identically.

The zinc-binding hexamer in the crystal corresponds to the 36,000 dalton molecular weight species in neutral solution, which is composed of three dimers, having a molecular weight of 12,000 daltons. The dimers are also observed in solution under appropriate conditions of pH and dilution.

The detailed three-dimensional structure of the monomeric insulin molecule appears in Fig. 27.47, as viewed perpendicular to the threefold crystal axis. The A chain contains two helical regions, extending from A2 Ile to A8 Thr and from A13 Leu to A20 Cys, which run almost antiparallel, thus bringing the NH_2- and COOH-termini

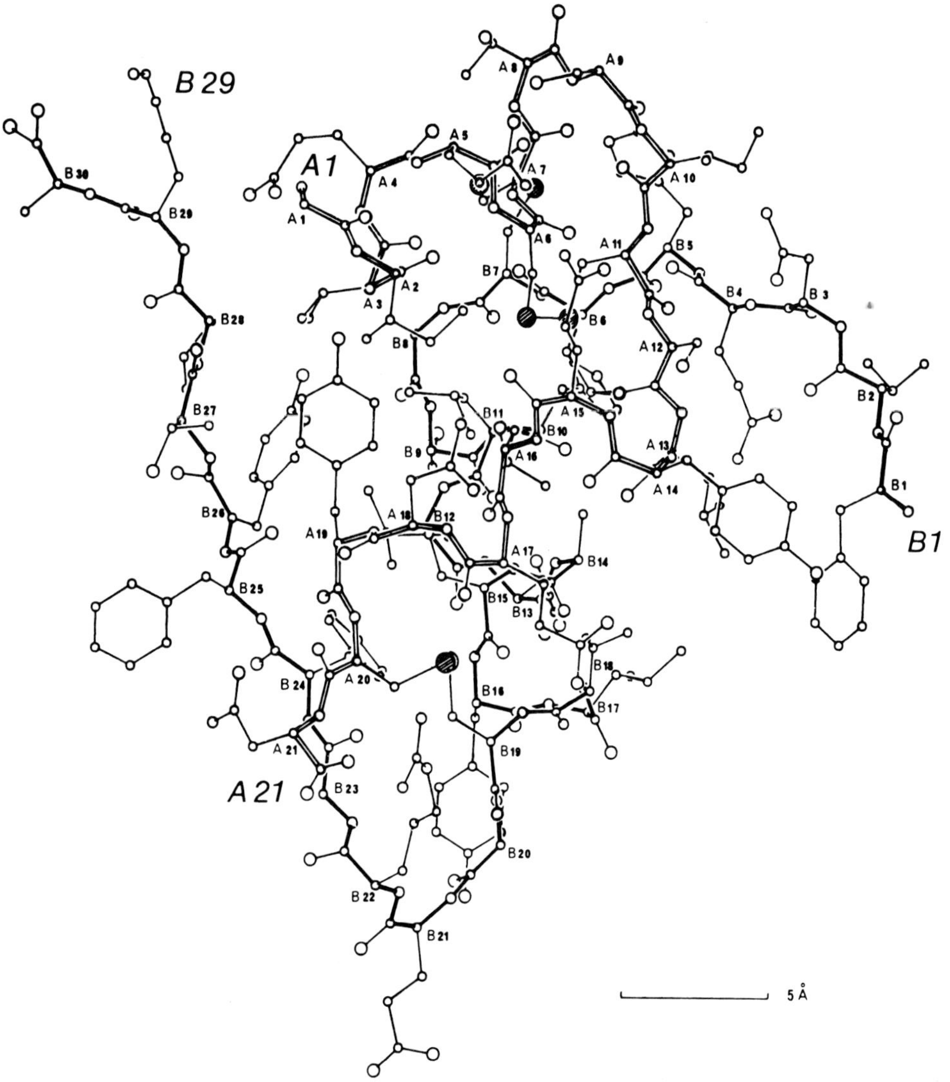

Fig. 27.47 The crystal structure of the insulin monomer (molecule 2, viewed perpendicular to the threefold axis). The backbone of the B chain is indicated by the heavy line, that of the A chain by the double line. See Fig. 27.50 for a schematic drawing. From Blundell et al. (10). Reprinted with permission of Academic Press, Inc.

close together. The side chains of A2 Ile and A19 Tyr are in van der Waals contact. In the B chain an α-helix extends from B9 Ser to B19 Cys. A sharp turn at residues 20–23 brings the side chains of B24 Phe and B26 Tyr into contact with those of B15 Leu and B11 Leu in the helix. The two chains are linked together by disulfides A7–B7 and A20–B19 in a manner that buries several nonpolar residues, i.e., the A6–11 cystine, leucines A16 and B11, and isoleucines B2 and B15. This provides a hydrophobic interior that stabilizes the molecule's structure.

The 23 polar residues of insulin all lie on the surface of the molecule. The NH_2-terminus of the B chain runs antiparallel to the central part of the A chain, which it crosses. At this crossing two hydrogen bonds exist, between A11 Cys and B4 Glu and between B5 His and the carbonyl oxygen of A7 Cys. The COOH-terminal residues lie alongside the A chain NH_2-terminus, giving rise to a charge interaction between B29 Lys and A4 Glu. The A1 Gly residue is in close proximity to the side chain ε-amino group of B29 Lys. This has allowed intramolecular cross-linking of insulin with bifunctional reagents (for reviews, see Refs. 10 and 355). The two surface areas of the insulin molecule at the $O \rightarrow P$ and $O \rightarrow Q$ axes (Fig. 27.46*b*, *c*) are occupied by clusters of nonpolar residues. These surfaces are involved in dimer and hexamer formation, respectively.

The dimeric unit (Fig. 27.48) is held together between the B21–30 sequence regions of the two monomers by an antiparallel β-pleated sheet structure (Fig. 27.49), which results in very strong binding through four hydrogen bonds and hydrophobic interaction between the two B25 Phe residues. Other hydrophobic interactions between molecules 1 and 2 of the

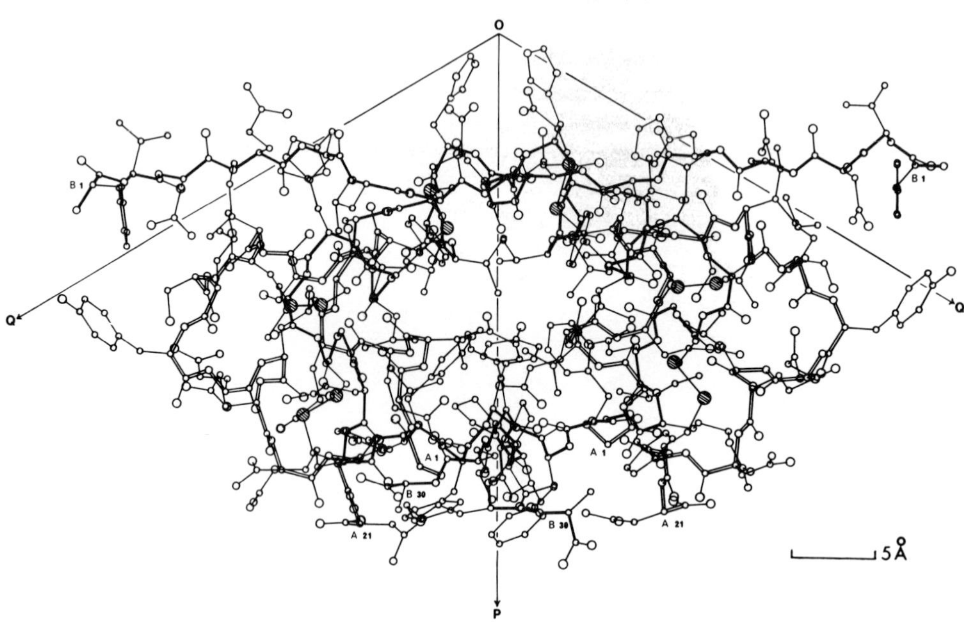

Fig. 27.48 The insulin dimer viewed down the threefold axis. The local axes *OP* and *OQ* are indicated. Molecule 1 is at the right, molecule 2 at the left. From Blundell et al. (10). Reprinted with permission of Academic Press, Inc.

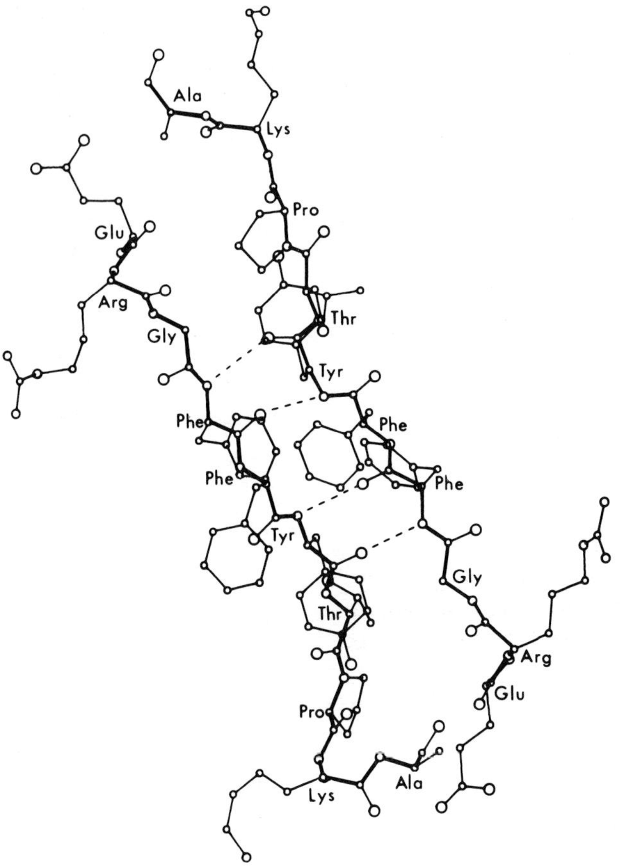

Fig. 27.49 The arrangement of residues B21–B30 in the insulin dimer, viewed in the direction of the local axis. The COOH-terminal chains run antiparallel to each other, forming an antiparallel pleated sheet structure with four hydrogen bonds. From Blundell et al. (10). Reprinted with permission from Academic Press, Inc.

dimer involve the B12 valines, the B24 phenylalanines, and the B16 tyrosine with B26 tyrosine and B12 valine.

The dimers align along *OQ* in approximate twofold symmetry to form the hexamer (Fig. 27.46*a*). Nonpolar interactions between the equivalent B14 alanines, B17 leucines, and B18 valines are the main driving force. The NH_2-termini of the B chains cross over into adjacent molecules and are located in pockets between the respective A13 Leu and A14 Tyr residues. The center of the hexamer contains a hydrophylic core with structural water.

In sum, nonpolar groups on the subunit surfaces are pivotal in the contacts between monomers and dimers, and most of these are from B chain residues. Eight aromatic residues take part in dimer formation, four others in hexamer formation. The progressive shielding of nonpolar residues during aggregation leads to a hexamer whose surface is almost entirely polar. Because of this, insulin resembles in many ways a typical medium-sized, densely packed globular protein. Further association takes place only at comparatively high concentrations.

The knowledge of the three-dimensional

structure of insulin allowed investigators (1) to examine the structural roles of invariant amino acid residues such as the cystines, which are essential for the molecule's architecture, or the nonpolar B chain residues that are important for subunit aggregation (10), (2) to ascertain (10, 360, 361) that high biological activity of insulin depends on the integrity of the overall three-dimensional structure, as previously proposed (362, 363), rather than on a localized active site, (3) to identify a receptor binding region (360, 361, 364) comprising residues A1, 4, 5, 19, 21 and B12, 16, 24–26, i.e., the hydrophobic surface between the two molecules of a dimer (Fig. 27.50; see also Fig. 27.48), and (4) to interpret relationships between three-dimensional structure and function on a molecular basis (10, 360, 361). Indications for the range of flexibility allowable in the three-dimensional structure was obtained by the recent X-ray crystal structure analysis of highly active 4-zinc porcine insulin, which retained the overall molecular architecture of the hexamer while showing considerable variation in molecule I of the dimer but not in molecule II (366).

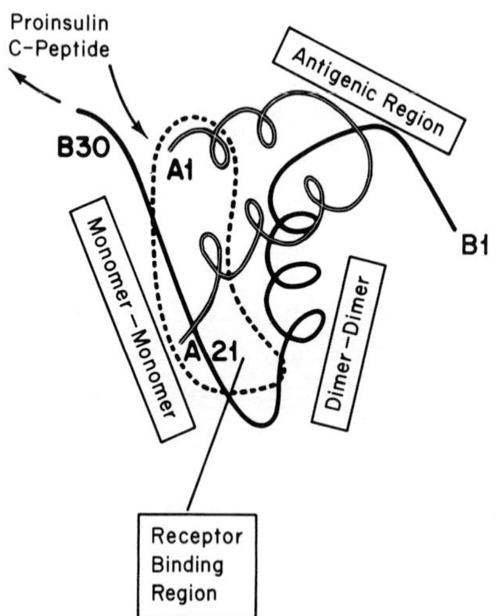

Fig. 27.50 Schematic view of the crystal structure of insulin, indicating the areas of monomer-monomer and dimer-dimer interaction (10), the connecting points of the proinsulin C-peptides (337), an antigenic region (365), and the proposed receptor binding region (broken line) (360, 361).

The foregoing selected examples are meant to show the enormous broadening in the understanding of the chemistry and biology of insulin that has been derived from its crystal structure analysis. Moreover, the crystal structure appears to be conserved in solution (367) and during its receptor interaction (361),* which lends added significance to the data just discussed.

8.1.6 SYNTHESIS. The synthesis of insulin is a laborious and difficult task requiring more than 100 synthetic steps, but there are several important reasons for undertaking such a complex effort: the chemist aims at a confirmation of the chemical structure of insulin (Fig. 27.41), the biochemist is interested in structure-activity relations to obtain insight in the mode of action of the hormone, and the clinician is concerned about future shortages of the natural supply.

The structure of insulin points to an obvious synthesis in three stages: (1) preparation of the A chain, (2) preparation of the B chain, and (3) linking of the two chains through the formation of the disulfide bonds. By the beginning of the 1960s the rapidly developing methodology in peptide synthesis, along with expanding commercial supplies of amino acids and reagents, brought the prospects for synthesis (stages 1 and 2) of the individual insulin chains within potential reach. On the contrary, the protecting group methodology available at that time did not provide for a directed stepwise formation of the correctly paired three disulfides A6–11, A7–B7, and A20–B19 (see Fig. 27.41). However as

* Identity of crystal structure with solution conformation and conformation in the receptor complex has also been indicated for the peptide antibiotic actinomycin D (368, 369).

soon as it was shown in two independent studies (370, 371) that small amounts (1–5%) of insulin could be generated by random cooxidation of natural chains, several attempts at insulin synthesis were initiated. In 1963–1965, after several years of enormous efforts, milligram amounts of synthetic insulin were obtained almost simultaneously in three institutions (372–374). Subsequently, methodological improvements were made, and numerous syntheses of natural insulins and analogs by solution methods and (less suitable for insulin) solid phase techniques have since been reported; for reviews, see Refs. 10, 274, 354, 355, and 375.

Accumulating experience indicated that yields of insulin would probably remain low as long as the two synthetic chains had to be linked by random *interchain* disulfide bond formation. The discovery of proinsulin in 1967 (337) offered an exciting new approach. *Intrachain* oxidation of reduced hexasulfhydryl proinsulin afforded high yields (>70%) of native prohormone (376) from which insulin can be obtained by enzymatic cleavage (356), see Section 8.1.4. Despite many heroic efforts, however, synthesis of a proinsulin consisting of 81–86 amino acid residues in different species, has not yet been achieved, although several C-peptides were prepared (377–379). Problems arising from poor solubility of intermediate protected fragments in suitable solvents have thus far prevented the assembly of a complete proinsulin chain.

Recently an ingenious strategy of using much shorter chain connections, e.g., linking of the A1 Gly and B29 ε-Lys amino groups by α,α'-diaminosuberic acid, allowed intramolecular formation of the correctly paired disulfides in 50–75% yields. Subsequent removal of the cross-links provides insulin (380–382), see Fig. 27.51. The prerequisite close juxtaposition of the two amino groups (A1 and B29) in the three-dimensional structure of the insulin molecule has been shown by the X-ray crystal structure analysis (338), which confirmed earlier indications from cross-linking studies (383).

These approaches have been superseded by a recent genuine total synthesis of crystallized human insulin by the Ciba-Geigy

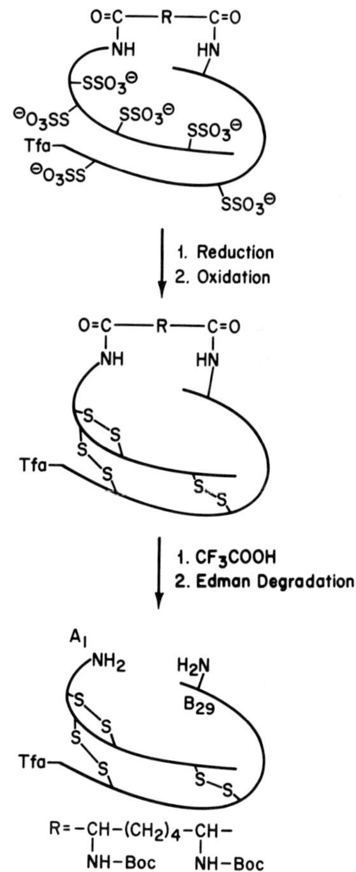

Fig. 27.51 Reversible-link strategy of joining the A and B chains of insulin. Separately prepared thiol-protected chains are linked between the A1 Gly and the B29 N^{ε}-Lys amino groups by bifunctional reagents such as an activated ester of bis-*t*-butyloxycarbonyl-α,α'-diaminosuberic acid. Cleavage of the thiol-protecting groups is followed by oxidative formation of the correctly paired disulfide bonds, which shows that the reversibly linked linear peptide has all the necessary properties for proper folding and forming of the correct disulfide bridges. Cleavage of the auxiliary link (and remaining protecting groups) provides insulin. From Gėiger (355). Reprinted with permission of Dr. Alfred Hüthig Verlag.

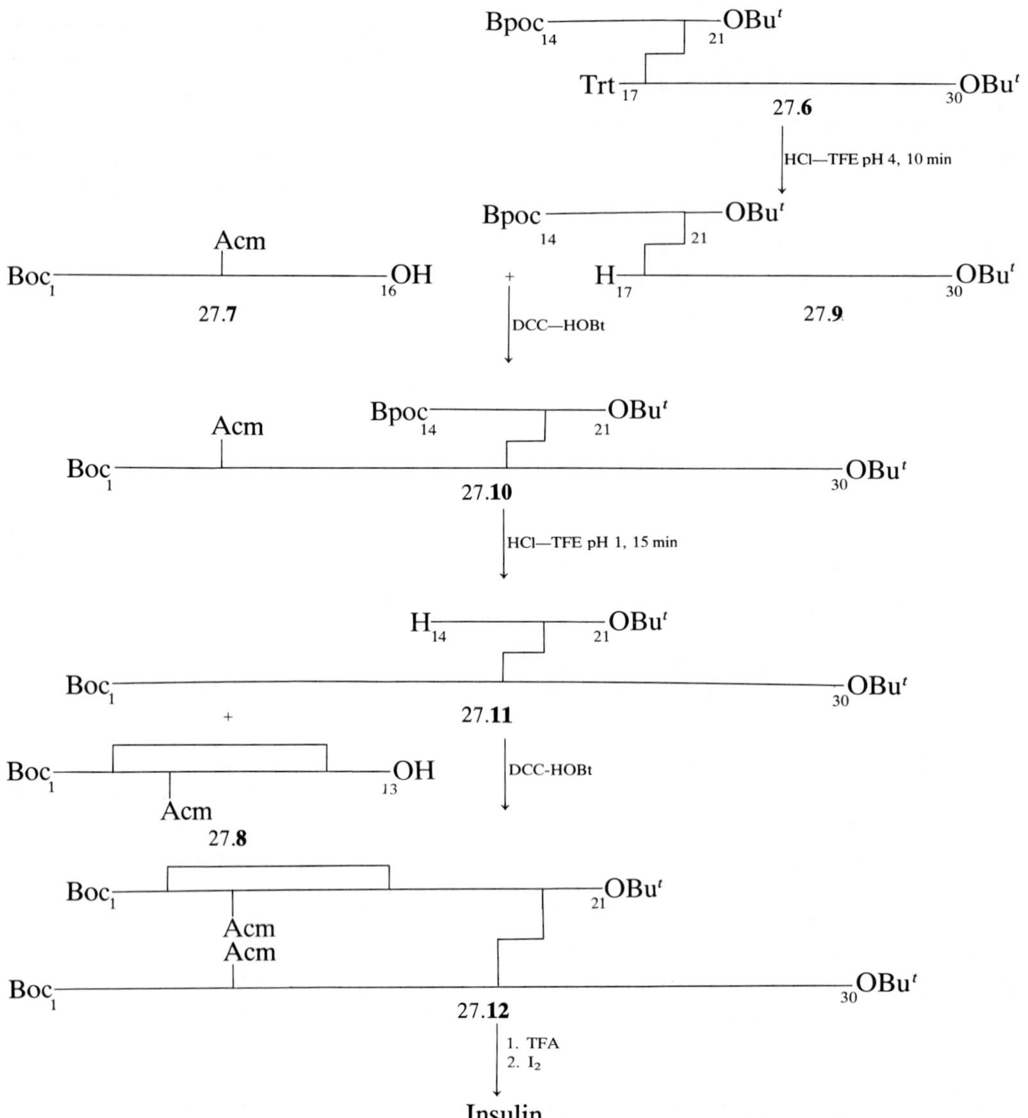

Fig. 27.52 A "total" synthesis of human insulin by way of consecutive formation of the three correctly paired disulfide bonds (340). For abbreviations, see Table 27.2.

peptide group (340) in which the correctly paired disulfide bonds were formed one by one in a stepwise directed manner (Fig. 27.52). Two disulfides, A6–11 in protected fragment 27.**8**, and A20–B19 in fragment 27.**6**, were formed in intermediate stages of the synthesis, and one, A7–B7, was formed after the complete assembly of the two chains. The success of this synthesis reflects the overall progress made in peptide protecting group methodology, yet the contributions of three groups to the development of selectively removable thiol protecting groups deserve special mention: L. Zervas and I. Photaki (384), R. G. Hiskey and collaborators (385, 386), and R. Hirschmann et al. (387), who introduced the acetamidomethyl group. The decisive contribution of the Ciba-Geigy workers was the elaboration of selective cleavage conditions for the trityl and Bpoc* amine protecting groups by pH controlled acidolysis (HCl) in trifluoroethanol as a solvent.

The key fragment for the final stages of the synthesis (Fig. 27.52) was the unsymmetrical cystine derivative 27.**6** consisting of sequences A(14–21) and B(17–30) linked by the disulfide bond A20–B19, which resulted from a reaction of the A20 thiol with the B19 sulfenylthiocarbonate. After selective removal of the N^{α}-trityl group at pH 3.5 from leucine B17, the B chain was completed by dicyclohexylcarbodiimide—hydroxybenzotriazole mediated coupling with fragment 27.**7**, i.e., B(1–16). Selective removal of the N^{α}-2-(*p*-biphenylyl)isopropyloxycarbonyl group at tyrosine A14 by HCl in trifluoroethanol and subsequent coupling with fragment 27.**8** containing the intrachain A6–11 disulfide completed the A chain, giving intermediate 27.**12**. Removal of the acid-labile protecting groups of 27.**12** by 95% trifluoroacetic acid and direct conversion of the *S*-acetamidomethyl groups into disulfide in 70% yield by treatment with iodine in 60% aqueous acetic acid at high dilution provided insulin. The product was purified by a countercurrent distribution of 1000 transfers, then crystallized. Synthetic and natural human insulin were indistinguishable in a series of analytical tests and in several bioassay systems.

The significance of this "total" synthesis lies in the methodological advance paving the way for future syntheses of other multichain molecules such as immunoglobulins, as well as in the confirmation of the disulfide positions in the Sanger structure of insulin (Fig. 27.41). Whether this approach will become the most attractive and practical way for routine synthesis of insulins and analogs remains to be evaluated (355) in comparison with some of the above-described reversible chain linking strategies; for an example (381), see Fig. 27.51.

* 2-(*p*-Biphenylyl)isopropyloxycarbonyl,

$$C_6H_5-C_6H_4-C(CH_3)_2-OCO-$$

8.1.7 CHEMICAL MODIFICATION OF NATURAL INSULIN. Because of the enormous efforts required for total synthesis, and because natural insulins are readily available, semisynthesis or chemical modification has been widely used in obtaining much valuable information, e.g., on structure-activity correlations.

In *semisynthesis* or *partial synthesis*, parts of native insulin are coupled with synthetic peptides. The first reported synthetic preparation of insulin-active material (388) represented a "semisynthesis" insofar as reduced synthetic A chain was cooxidized with reduced natural B chain (389). In recent years several laboratories (355, 390–392) have studied the conversion of porcine (B30 = Ala) to human insulin (B30 = Thr) by enzymatic removal of sequence B23–30 and coupling of the ensuing suitably protected desoctapeptide insulin derivative (362) with synthetic octapeptide of the human sequence.

Chemical modification has aimed at iodination of tyrosine residues for radioimmunoassay development, at esterification of the six carboxyl groups by HCl/MeOH, CH_2N_2, Et_3OBF_4, or BF_3/MeOH (393), and especially at substitution of the three amino groups in positions A1, B1, and B29 (N^{ε}-Lys). Rather selective acylations can be obtained at different controlled pH values. Introduction of reversible protecting groups, such as the acid-labile *t*-butyloxycarbonyl (Boc) and/or the base-labile trifluoroacetyl (Tfa) or methylsulfonylethyloxycarbonyl (Msc) groups provide for reaction schemes (355) as exemplified in Fig. 27.53. Selective derivatization of any one of the three amino groups is accessible by this or other related schemes (355, 394, 395).

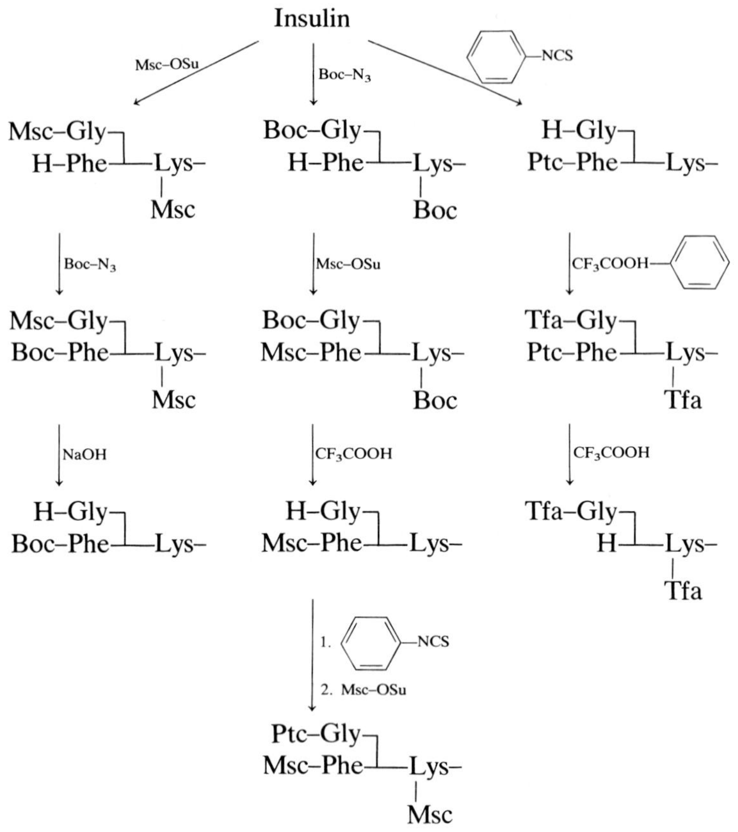

Insulin

Msc–OSu | Boc–N_3 | –NCS

Msc–Gly┐ H–Phe┴–Lys– | Msc

Boc–Gly┐ H–Phe┴–Lys– | Boc

H–Gly┐ Ptc–Phe┴–Lys–

Boc–N_3 | Msc–OSu | CF_3COOH–

Msc–Gly┐ Boc–Phe┴–Lys– | Msc

Boc–Gly┐ Msc–Phe┴–Lys– | Boc

Tfa–Gly┐ Ptc–Phe┴–Lys– | Tfa

NaOH | CF_3COOH | CF_3COOH

H–Gly┐ Boc–Phe┴–Lys–

H–Gly┐ Msc–Phe┴–Lys–

Tfa–Gly┐ H┴–Lys– | Tfa

1. –NCS
2. Msc–OSu

Ptc–Gly┐ Msc–Phe┴–Lys– | Msc

Fig. 27.53 Selective acylation of the amino groups (A1 Gly, B1 Phe, B29 N^{ε} Lys) of insulin. Reaction with methylsulfonylethyl-succinimidoylcarbonate (Msc-OSu) at pH 8.5 affords Gly^{A1}, Lys^{B29}-bis-Msc-insulin. Similarly, reaction with *t*-butyloxycarbonylazide (Boc-N_3) in DMF/H_2O/$NaHCO_3$ yields Gly^{A1}, Lys^{B29}-bis-Boc-insulin. However reaction with phenylisothiocyanate at pH 9.1 provides Phe^{B1}-monophenylthiocarbamoylinsulin (Ptc). For selective B1 Phe, B29 Lys diacylation, see Ref. 395. Combination with other reversible protecting groups offers numerous options of selective insulin modification. From Geiger (355).

8.1.8 STRUCTURE-ACTIVITY RELATIONSHIPS. More than 150 synthetic insulin analogs and derivatives have been prepared (for a review, see Ref. 355), but a more potent one has not yet been discovered, and native crystalline zinc insulins with potencies of 26–28 IU/mg remain the most active preparations. This is presumably a consequence of the high metabolic stability of the native hormone, which is hard to improve by synthetic modifications. The compact three-dimensional structure stabilizes a hydrophobic receptor binding area on the surface of the molecule. Thus the integrity of the overall molecular geometry is vital for bioactivity, whereas the relative importance of sequences or single amino acid residues, which can vary widely, depends on their respective contributions to the stability of the three-dimensional structure. Increasing changes in this overall geometry, which may be monitored by CD spectroscopy (361, 395, 396), are accompanied by progressive loss of activity.

Syntheses of truncated insulins revealed that several residues of the B chain are not required for full bioactivity. The first four to six (397, 398) and the last three residues (B28–30) (399) are dispensable. As further residues from the COOH-terminus (B27,

Table 27.7 Biological Activities of Insulins with COOH-Terminally Truncated B Chains[a]

. . . –Glu–Arg–Gly–Phe–Phe–Tyr–Thr–Pro–Lys–Ala 21 22 23 24 25 26 27 28 29 30	Biological Activity: Insulin = 100	References
————————————	100	400
——————————	100	399
—————————	50	401
————————— Ala	50	402
———————	30	403
——————	25–30	390
————	0	404

[a] Data from Ref. 355.

B26 etc.) are omitted one by one, the biological activity decreases gradually to desheptapeptide-(B26–30)-insulin, which is totally inactive (Table 27.7). These observations can be interpreted rationally from the molecular architecture (Section 8.1.5) in which residues 24–26 occupy important parts of the receptor binding area of insulin. Unlike the B chain, the A chain cannot be shortened. Omission of A1 glycine reduces the hormonal potency to less than 1% (405, 406), and omission of A21 asparagine abolishes all activity. However replacement of A21 Asn by alanine preserves full bioactivity. Table 27.8 gives the effects of various synthetic amino acid replacements in the A chain on the potency of insulin. Modifications in position A1 effect

Table 27.8 Influence of A-Chain Modifications on the Biological Activity of Insulin[a]

Gly–Ile–Val–Glu–Gln– . . . –Tyr–Gln– . . . –Asn–Tyr– . . . –Asn 1 2 3 4 5 14 15 18 19 21	Biological Activity: Insulin = 100	References
————————————————	<1	405, 406
Ala ———————————————	20/10	394, 407
Val ———————————————	2	408
β-Ala ———————————————	50/20/30	408, 409
D-Ala ———————————————	100	394
Sar ———————————————	30	410
—— Ala ——————————————	0	407
—— Val ——————————————	100	411
——— Leu —————————————	0	407
——— Ile —————————————	≪10	409
————— Ala ————————————	40–50	408
—————— Glu ——— Glu ———————	100	411
—————— Ala ———————————	30	409
———————— Ala —————————	100	409
————————— Ala ————————	30	409
——————————— Ala —————	100	407
———————————— Phe ———	100	406
———————————————	0	362, 390, 404
——————————————— Ala	100	409
——————————————— D-Asn	30	412

[a] Data from Ref. 355.

subtle and rather specific conformational changes in the molecule (360, 361). Insulin activity is reduced to 10–20% by replacement of A1 glycine with L-alanine, and full activity is retained by replacement with D-alanine (394). When the bulkier L-valine replaces A1 Gly, the bioactivity decreases to 2% (408). The entire amino-terminal sequence A1–5, which is a part of the proposed receptor binding region (see Fig. 27.50), is very sensitive to change. X-Ray studies showed that distortions of the helical region A1–5 also effect, in turn, shifts of the A19 tyrosine side chain and small displacements of residues B24–28 (361).

Acylation and aminoacylation of the α-amino group of A1 glycine exerts similar structure-activity influences (Table 27.9). These derivatives were recently prepared from native insulin by way of selective amino group modification (395). The A1 guanidinated insulin is the most active (80–90%) derivative, showing a CD spectrum and X-ray diffraction pattern very close to that of the native hormone. Uncharged substituents (e.g., acetyl, trifluoroacetyl, *t*-butyloxycarbonyl, thiozolidyl) reduce potency and cause increasing three-dimensional structural changes with increasing size or bulkiness. The activities of A1 aminoacylated insulins with uncharged side chains range between 25 and 35%, and their X-ray diffraction patterns indicated small shifts in the helical A1–5 region, at A19 and at B24–26. Size or bulkiness seems to have little influence in these derivatives, but a positive charge increases (40–45% for A1 Lys- and A1 Arg-insulins) and a negative charge decreases activities (20% for the A1 Glu derivative).

Table 27.9 Biological Activity of Insulin Derivatives Prepared by Acylation or Aminoacylation of the A Chain's NH_2-Terminal Amino Group[a]

Derivative Prepared by N^{α}-Acylation	Bioactivity *in Vitro:* Fat Cell[b] (rat)	Derivative Prepared by N^{α}-Aminoacylation	Bioactivity *in Vitro:* Fat Cell[b] (rat)
Amidinyl[c]	88±5	H–Gly–	58–78
Acetyl[d]	37.5±2.5	H–Lys–	40–50
Trifluoroacetyl[e]	32±2	H–Arg–	37–43
Carbamoyl	31±2	H–Lys–Arg–	24–28
Methylsulfonyl		H–Arg–Arg–	39–44
ethyloxycarbonyl	26±2	H–Arg–Arg–Arg–	31–33
Methylthioethyl		H–D-Phe–	32–37
oxycarbonyl	22±2	H–L-Phe–	29–35
t-Butyloxycarbonyl[f]	19±1	H–D-Met–	34–40
Thiazolidyl[g]	11–14	H–L-Met–	25–29
		H–Trp–[h]	25–35
		H–Glu–	20–24

[a] Data from Ref. 395.
[b] Conversion of glucose to lipid in isolated rat fat cells according to Moody et al. (413). Insulin = 100.
[c] The derivative is called [guanidoacetyl^{A1}]-insulin.
[d] From Brandenburg et al. (414). See also Lindsay and Shall (415).
[e] See also Levy and Paselk (416).
[f] From Krail (417).
[g] From Pullen et al. (360).
[h] From Brandenburg et al. (418).

For more detailed accounts on structure-activity correlations, see reviews (10, 355, 396). The few selected points discussed above are to draw attention to the beginning development of correlations between chemical structure, biological activity, and molecular architecture which are essential for deriving refined concepts of peptide hormone action. Ultimately a fourth parameter, the receptor surface geometry, must be included, but the current advances represent encouraging departures from simple correlations between structure and bioactivity which have been of very limited use for peptides.

A formidable shortcoming in establishing valid structure-activity relationships in insulins arises from the limited biological data. Many analogs have been tested in one assay system only, either because only small amounts of material were available or because of the complexities of assays. Thus activities obtained in different laboratories from different assays are being compared, and the degree of correlation is not always clear. Because of the enormous effort spent in preparing synthetic or semisynthetic insulins, it is hoped that more comprehensive biological testing will be conducted henceforth.

8.2 Glucagon

8.2.1 HISTORY. Soon after the isolation of insulin, transient hyperglycemic effects were observed in impure preparations. In 1953 Staub, Sinn, and Behrens (419) succeeded in isolating and crystallizing the active principle, named glucagon, from a side fraction of insulin production. This work has been reviewed (420).

8.2.2 STRUCTURE AND PROPERTIES. Glucagon is a linear peptide of neutral character (pI ~7.5) consisting of 29 amino acid residues. The determination of its primary structure (Fig. 27.42) and its chemical and physicochemical properties have been reviewed (420). Porcine, bovine, and human glucagons have identical sequences, and physicochemical comparison suggests identity also with glucagons from camel, rabbit, and rat. Turkey and chicken glucagons differ in position 28 (Asn → Ser), duck glucagon has in addition a second replacement in position 16 (Ser → Thr). The glucagons of anglerfish and spiny dogfish differ considerably more but still have a total of 29 residues, whereas guinea pig glucagon differs profoundly in having 40 amino acid residues (421).

The reactivities of turkey and chicken glucagons to specific antisera are 5% that of pancreatic porcine glucagon. Biologically inactivated glucagon may retain immunoreactivity (422), and this property should be kept in mind because radioimmunoassays are used almost exclusively in glucagon research (423). The molecular nature of "enteroglucagon" or "gut glucagon" in human and animal intestine remains to be elucidated. Secretory granules, indistinguishable from pancreatic α-cells, have been identified in the gastric mucosa of dogs (424), and evidence for their possible existence in the human stomach has been presented (425).

Glucagon elevates blood glucose levels by stimulating both glycogenolysis and gluconeogenesis in the liver. Lowering of blood glucose below normal levels stimulates secretion of glucagon (the plasma half-life is *ca.* 3 min). The hormone is transported through the portal vessel into the liver, where it binds to a plasma membrane receptor site to activate adenyl cyclase and to increase intracellular levels of the second messenger cyclic AMP (426), which sets in motion the chain of enzymatic events of glycolysis. Glucagon behaves like an insulin antagonist in glucose homeostasis. Glucagon may play a fundamental role in maintaining blood glucose levels, whereas insulin is important in minute-to-minute regulation (342). The question of

$\underset{1}{|}$ Glucagon $\underset{29\ 30}{|}$–Lys–Arg–Asn–Asn–Lys–$\underset{35}{\text{Asn}}$–Ile–Ala–OH

Extension?

Fig. 27.54 Schematic representation of the structure of glucagon precursor forms (431). (A definite biosynthetic evidence of a precursor relationship remains to be established.)

whether elevated glucagon levels contribute in a major way to the development of the diabetic syndrome (427) or whether low insulin utilization is solely responsible (428, 429) remains controversial. For reviews, see Refs. 333, 349, 423, and 430; see also Chapter 31.

8.2.3 BIOSYNTHESIS. A form of immunoreactive glucagon that has been shown by radioimmunoassay to be present in the pancreas of man and in the pancreas and plasma of various animals, is believed to be proglucagon. This substance has a molecular weight of 9000 daltons. Tager and Steiner (431) have isolated from crystalline bovine and porcine glucagon a strongly basic 37 residue peptide having a molecular weight of 4500 daltons, and they have determined its structure (Fig. 27.54). The amino acid sequence of the NH_2-terminal 29 residues is identical to that of glucagon. Traces of several other glucagon-immunoreactive peptides (up to mol wt 9000) were also detected, and it was proposed that the 37 residue peptide is a fragment of bovine or porcine proglucagon. Fragments of a putative anglerfish proglucagon have been partially characterized (432, 433). However a definite biosynthetic evidence of a precursor-product relationship is lacking (356).

8.2.4 X-RAY CRYSTAL STRUCTURE. ORD and CD studies indicate that glucagon has little helix content in dilute aqueous solution but becomes helical in certain favorable environments such as lipid micelles or detergents, or on self-association. The three-dimensional structure was determined by Blundell et al. (434) and appears in Fig. 27.55*a*. The molecule is approximately α-helical between residues 6 and 27. As a result, two hydrophobic regions are formed, one of residues 6 Phe, 10 Tyr, 13 Tyr, and 14 Leu, the other of 19 Ala, 22 Phe, 23 Val, 25 Trp, 26 Leu, and 27 Met. Glucagon trimers are formed in the crystal (Fig. 27.55*b*) by interaction of the hydrophobic areas. The trimers are further packed together as oligomers. However residues 1–5 are not constrained by intermolecular interactions and seem to be flexible, even in the crystal. CD data indicate that the trimer is also formed in solution when glucagon aggregates. Moreover, the trimeric form appears to be present in the amorphous α-storage granules of the islet of Langerhans cells. In this form it may be more stable and resistant to enzymatic degradation. Upon release into the bloodstream, glucagon concentrations decrease so much that the trimers dissociate and the hormone circulates as a monomer, assuming random conformations. It seems likely that upon its predominantly hydrophobic interaction with the receptor, the hormone resumes its α-helical conformation (435).

8.2.5 SYNTHESIS AND CHEMICAL MODIFICATION. Glucagon for many years has resisted major attempts at synthesis by solution and by solid phase procedures. The hormone's high content of Ser and Thr, and the presence of Trp and Met residues gave rise to numerous undesired side reactions. Only when Wünsch et al. designed a strategy of global protection of all functional side chains and strictly adhered to it, was a successful synthesis of glucagon

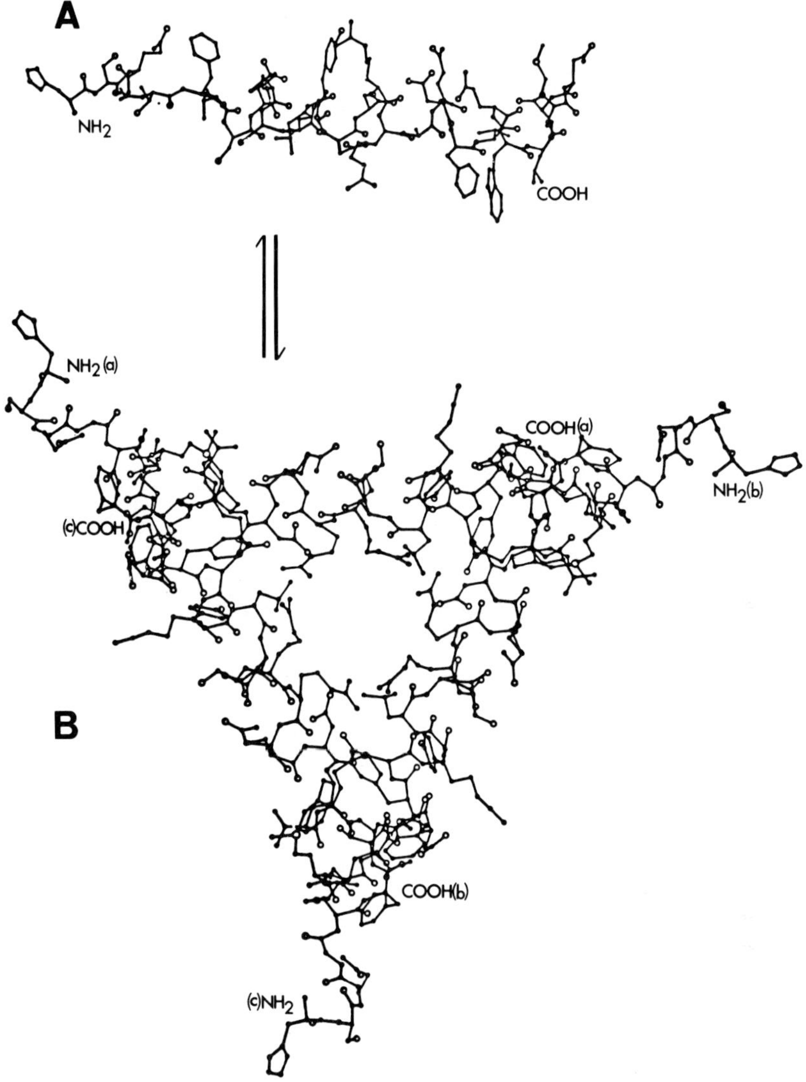

Fig. 27.55 Equilibrium between the unstable helical form of the glucagon monomer (*a*) and the trimer (*b*) in which the helical form is stabilized by hydrophobic interactions. From Sasaki et al. (434).

achieved in 1967 (436). The protected nonacosapeptide (Fig. 27.56) was prepared by segment condensation of five intermediate peptides, starting with the COOH-terminal tripeptide segment. All four couplings were carried out by dicyclohexylcarbodiimide in the presence of *N*-hydroxysuccinimide (437). After mild acidolytic protecting group cleavage, using trifluoroacetic acid, and gel filtration on Sephadex G-50, 5 g of chromatographically homogeneous glucagon was obtained, which crystallized from aqueous solution at pH 9.3. The synthetic hormone was indistinguishable from natural glucagon in biological potency and in physical and chemical properties. This synthesis confirmed the structure (Fig. 27.42) established by Bromer et al. (438) and made glucagon, which is hard to obtain from natural

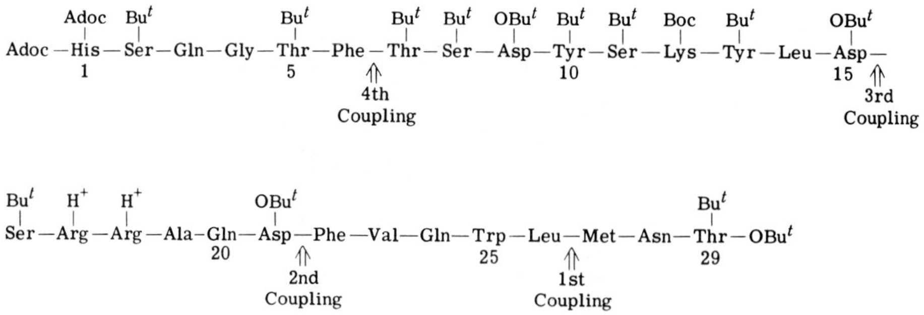

```
       Adoc  Bu^t               Bu^t        Bu^t  Bu^t  OBu^t  Bu^t  Bu^t  Boc   Bu^t          OBu^t
        |     |                  |           |     |     |      |     |     |     |              |
Adoc — His — Ser — Gln — Gly — Thr — Phe — Thr — Ser — Asp — Tyr — Ser — Lys — Tyr — Leu — Asp —
        1                        5      ⇑                        10                           15 ⇑
                                       4th                                                       3rd
                                    Coupling                                                  Coupling

Bu^t   H+    H+                OBu^t                                                Bu^t
 |     |     |                  |                                                    |
Ser — Arg — Arg — Ala — Gln — Asp — Phe — Val — Gln — Trp — Leu — Met — Asn — Thr — OBu^t
                         20      ⇑                      25         ⇑                29
                                2nd                               1st
                             Coupling                          Coupling
```

Fig. 27.56 Protected nonacosapeptide intermediate of a glucagon synthesis by solution methods (436). Arrows indicate points of fragment condensation; Adoc = adamantyloxycarbonyl.

sources, available for biological and clinical studies.

Recently a second synthesis of glucagon was reported by the Shanghai Protein Synthesis Group (439), which employed a solid phase segment condensation procedure. Crystalline glucagon was obtained in a remarkably good overall yield of 17%. Total synthesis has not been used yet for the preparation of analogs.

Chemical modification of glucagon provided: des(Asn^{28},Thr^{29}) [homoserine lactone^{27}]glucagon (27.**14**) by cyanogen bromide cleavage of the native hormone, three derivatives (27.**15**–27.**17**) obtained from 27.**14** by aminolysis of the homoserine lactone, two N^{α},N^{ε}-bisacylated derivatives (27.**13** and 27.**19**) of the native hormone, (des-His^{1})glucagon (27.**20**) by treatment with an insoluble Edman reagent, and monoiodo glucagon (27.**21**) (440); see Table 27.10.

8.2.6 STRUCTURE-ACTIVITY RELATIONSHIPS. The relative potencies of modified glucagon in two *in vitro* assays are listed in Table

Table 27.10 Relative Activity and Binding of Glucagon and Glucagon Derivatives and Analogs with Hepatic Plasma Membranes

Compound[a]		Adenylate Cyclase Activity	Receptor Binding Activity
27.**13**	Glucagon	100	100
27.**14**	CNBr-Glucagon	2–3	2–3
27.**15**	CNBr-Glucagon-$NHNH_2$	3	3
27.**16**	CNBr-Glucagon-$NH(CH_2)_3CH_3$	3	3–4
27.**17**	CNBr-Glucagon-$NH(CH_2)_6NH$-Biotin	0.1–0.2	—
27.**18**	N^{α},N^{ε}-BisBoc-CNBr-Glucagon	None	None
27.**19**	N^{α},N^{ε}-BisIodoacetyl-glucagon	None	None
27.**20**	DH-Glucagon	2	7–10
27.**21**	[^{125}I]Glucagon	90–300[b]	30–300[b]
27.**22**	[des-His^{1}]Glucagon	—	2
27.**23**	[des-Met^{27}-Asn^{28}-Thr^{29}]glucagon	—	0.5

[a] Compounds 27.**13**–27.**21** from Hruby et al. (440); 27.**22** and 27.**23** from Bromer (441).
[b] Activity dependent on pH of assay medium.

27.10. N^{α},N^{ε}-Diacylation abolished all activity. Biological activity was lowered drastically by shortening of glucagon at either end by elimination of the 1-histidine or of two residues at the COOH-terminus. This was confirmed by the low potencies of truncated glucagons (27.**22** and 27.**23**), which were obtained from side fractions during isolation of natural glucagon (441).

8.3 Somatostatin

The chemistry and biochemistry of somatostatin, which was first discovered in the hypothalamus, is described in Section 3.3. This section covers the aspects of somatostatin action and structure-activity relationships that relate to the inhibition of insulin and glucagon release and to diabetes treatment. See also Chapter 31, and reviews (81, 82, 123, 124, 129).

Somatostatin inhibits basal secretion of insulin and glucagon in man, as well as glucose-stimulated insulin secretion and arginine-stimulated glucagon secretion, and the insulin and glucagon responses to a meal and to a variety of secretagogues. The effects of somatostatin on plasma insulin and glucagon result from direct action of the hormone on the α- and β-cells of the pancreas.

These findings suggested the presence of secretory glands for somatostatin in pancreas. Immunoassay, ultrastructural, and immunohistochemical studies identified the pancreatic D-cells as the site of somatostatin secretion (328).

Diabetes mellitus is characterized by both insulin deficiency and glucagon excess. Whereas current treatment of diabetes focuses on insulin deficiency, somatostatin may offer potentials for suppressing glucagon. Infusions of somatostatin in diabetic patients diminish both fasting and postprandial hyperglycemia by suppressing glucagon secretion for several hours but not over longer periods. In other studies the combination of somatostatin and exogenous insulin allowed reductions in insulin dose and appeared to improve diabetic control during long-term (3 day) somatostatin infusion in insulin-dependent diabetics (442). Through inhibition of glucagon and somatotropin secretion, somatostatin might decrease the development of diabetic ketoacidosis and, perhaps, of diabetic retinopathy. However the clinical value of somatostatin in diabetes control (124, 333) is still difficult to assess, and careful long-term studies appear to be necessary (443, 444).

In any event, for practical use in diabetes control, it would appear to be desirable to develop somatostatin analogs that (1) exhibit selectivity in suppressing glucagon but not insulin secretion and (2) possess long-lasting biological activity. Many laboratories are engaged in the search for suitable analogs. Recently [D-Cys^{14}]somatostatin and [D-Trp^{8}, D-Cys^{14}]somatostatin were reported to have some of the desired selectivity of action (154). However long-term studies in diabetic patients must await the development of still longer acting and/or more glucagon-specific preparations, as well as proof of lack of undesirable side effects under these conditions.

9 GASTROINTESTINAL HORMONES

The mucous membrane of the gastrointestinal (GI) tract is the largest endocrine organ of the body (445). Gastrointestinal hormones and related peptides are located in endocrine cells scattered throughout the GI mucosa from the stomach through the colon. At least 11 different types of endocrine cells have been identified by electron microscopy (446, 447). These cells are members of a widely distributed system of "clear cells" (enterochromaffin, argyrophil, argentaffin) that produce peptides and amines. Pearse (448) developed the unifying concept that all peptide hormone-producing cells are embryologically derived from neuroectoderm. Since these cells do not occur in cumulative glandular form but are widely scattered throughout the gut, identification and isolation of their respective hormones is much more difficult than with glandular hormones. Moreover, it is virtually impossible to surgically remove the source of a gastrointestinal hormone and examine the effect of its absence in the classical manner. Of the six gastrointestinal peptides with known structure, it is generally agreed that four qualify as hormones, viz., gastrin, secretin, cholecystokinin (CCK), and gastric inhibitory polypeptide (GIP). In fact, the term "hormone" was first proposed in connection with the discovery of secretin and the postulation of the concept of bloodborne chemical messengers by Bayliss and Starling in 1902 (449). The physiological roles of the other two structurally identified factors, vasointestinal peptide (VIP) and motilin, still need to be unequivocally defined (445).

All known GI hormones are linear peptides that contain no disulfide bonds. They range in size from the 13 residue minigastrin (mol wt 1647 daltons) to the 43 residue gastric inhibitory polypeptide (mol wt 5105 daltons) and encompass very acidic (gastrins), neutral (motilin), and very basic (secretin) peptides. Radioimmunoassays have been developed for each (13). Presumably the biosynthesis of these peptides proceeds by way of larger precursors, but only for gastrin has a candidate prohormone (big gastrin) been identified.

There are similarities of structure and bioactivity between gastrin and cholecystokinin, which have a common COOH-terminal tetrapeptide. Similarly, the secretin family of peptides includes GIP and VIP, as well as glucagon. Evolution from a common ancestral protein has been suggested (450). Considerable overlap in the biological activity of the GI hormones (447, 451) and identical actions are observed. For example, secretin, GIP, and VIP all inhibit gastric acid secretion; gastrin and CCK stimulate gastric acid and pancreatic enzyme production; and motilin and CCK have powerful gut motor activity. Some of the effects may be species dependent. For example (445), in the cat CCK is a full agonist, producing the same rate of gastric acid secretion as gastrin; but in the dog it is a potent competitive inhibitor of gastrin, and its actions in man lie in between. Many of the biological effects of GI hormones recorded in the literature are pharmacological. Those of physiological significance are listed in Table 27.11. Two types of physiological action—the tropic action and the hormone-releasing action—have emerged only recently, when precise endocrine studies became possible with the availability of pure hormones through isolation or synthesis. The tropic action of gastrin and cholecystokinin (i.e., growth promotion of GI tract tissue) appears to be independent of the secretory functions

Table 27.11 Physiological actions[a] of Gastrointestinal Hormones

Hormone	Physiological Action
Gastrin	Gastric acid secretion, gastrointestinal mucosal growth
Secretin	Pancreatic and biliary bicarbonate secretion, potentiation of CCK-stimulated pancreatic enzyme secretion
CCK	Gall bladder contraction, pancreatic enzyme secretion, potentiation of secretin-stimulated pancreatic bicarbonate secretion, inhibition of gastric emptying, growth of exocrine pancreas
GIP	Inhibition of gastric acid secretion, insulin release

[a] Stimulatory unless stated otherwise. From Johnson (445).

(445). For reviews, see Refs. 2b, 19, 352, 445, and 452–455.

9.1 Gastrin

9.1.1 ISOLATION, STRUCTURE, AND ACTIVITY. The most important recent development in the chemistry of gastrin is the isolation and structure elucidation of "big gastrin" by Gregory and Tracy (456, 457). Loosely called a "larger circulating form of gastrin" since its discovery in 1970 by radioimmunoassay (458), this 34 residue peptide (Fig. 27.57*a*) contains, in fact, the entire gastrin molecule as it COOH-terminal half. The structure of the heptadecapeptide gastrin (459, 460) appears in Fig. 27.57*b*. A still smaller form, the tridecapeptide called minigastrin (Fig. 27.57*c*) has recently been isolated from gastrinoma tissue (461). It is identical with the COOH-terminal tridecapeptide region of gastrin. All three forms occur in pairs, unsulfated and sulfated at the single tyrosine residue, which is located in the "sixth" position from the COOH-terminus. Gastrin has been purified from antral mucosa of several species, including man (460), pig, dog, cat, sheep, and cow, which differ by only one or two amino acid substitutions in positions 5, 7, and 8 (Fig. 27.57*b*).

Gastrin is the most potent secretagogue and the predominant agonist in stimulating gastric acid secretion. The potency of big gastrin is 20%, and that of minigastrin 40% of the potency of gastrin (453). The circulation half-lives of gastrin and big gastrin are 3 and 9 min, respectively. Normal (fasting) serum gastrin concentrations in man are approximately 40 pg/ml. The antagonistic effects on gastric acid secretion elicited by secretin, VIP, and GIP are part of the complex and subtle interplay of the GI hormones. The primary function of gastrin may well be its tropic action, i.e., stimulation of cell division and differentiation, which maintains the functional integrity of GI tract tissue. For reviews, see Refs. 445, 452, 457, 462, and 463.

Trypsin digestion converts big gastrin to gastrin by cleavage at the Lys^{16}–Lys^{17} sequence. The NH_2-terminal glutamine residue

(*a*) pGlu–Leu–Gly–Pro–Gln–Gly–His–Pro–Ser–Leu–Val–Ala–Asp–Pro–Ser–Lys–Lys–
1 5 10 15

Human big gastrin Gln–Gly–Pro–Trp–Leu–Glu–Glu–Glu–Glu–Glu–Ala–Tyr(R)–Gly–Trp–Met–Asp–Phe–NH_2
20 25 30 34

(*b*) pGlu–Gly–Pro–Trp–Leu–Glu–Glu–Glu–Glu–Glu–Ala–Tyr(R)–Gly–Trp–Met–Asp–Phe–NH_2
5 10 15 17

Human gastrin

Species	Position 5	Position 7	Position 8
Hog	Met		
Cat			Ala
Dog	Met	Ala	
Cow, sheep	Val		Ala

(*c*) H–Leu–Glu–Glu–Glu–Glu–Glu–Ala–Tyr(R)–Gly–Trp–Met–Asp–Phe–NH_2

Human minigastrin

Gastrin I, R = H
Gastrin II, R = SO_3H

Fig. 27.57 The chemically identified human gastrins and species variations. (*a*) Big gastrin [I, mol wt 3839 daltons] (456). Residues in the porcine molecule: 4 = Leu, 9 = Pro, 14 = Leu, 15 = Ala, 22 = Met. (*b*) Gastrin [I, mol wt 2098 daltons] equals sequence region 18–34 of big gastrin (460). (*c*) Minigastrin [I, mol wt 1647 daltons] equals sequence region 5–17 of gastrin (461).

of the released heptadecapeptide changes spontaneously to pyroglutamyl (457). The basic dipeptide connecting sequence preceding the COOH-terminal heptadecapeptide in big gastrin is analogous to the basic dipeptide connecting sequences in proinsulin (Section 8.1.4) and proparathyrine (Section 6.1.2). Although a direct biosynthetic precursor relationship remains to be demonstrated, big gastrin is probably the prohormone of gastrin. Minigastrin may be a metabolite. The nature and relationship of several other immunoreactive forms of gastrin in plasma, such as "big big gastrin", is still unclear (457).

Gastrin has the smallest highly active core of all known peptide hormones. The COOH-terminal tetrapeptide exhibits about 10% of the secretagogue activity of gastrin on a molar basis (464). This finding stimulated the most prolific synthetic analog program yet established in a single institution. Of about 600 synthetic tri- to heptapeptides (465), several were highly active agonists, but a desired potent inhibitor was not discovered. Of the potent small-size analogs, pentagastrin (Boc–β–Ala–Trp–Met–Asp–Phe–NH_2) is used clinically for the diagnosis of gastric acid secretion. Pentagastrin is inactivated by passage through the liver, but native gastrin is not (454), and it is possible that some compounds of potential clinical interest have escaped detection because most of the analog program has been confined to small COOH-terminus-related peptides.

9.1.2 SYNTHESIS AND STRUCTURE-ACTIVITY RELATIONSHIPS. Synthesis of gastrin I was announced (466) simultaneously with the disclosure of the molecule's structure. The carboxyl protected fragment 6–13 was condensed with fragment 1–5, and the ensuing tridecapeptide was coupled with the COOH-terminal tetrapeptide amide to complete the chain assembly. Removal of the protecting groups yielded a gastrin preparation possessing a potency 110% that of the native hormone. Big gastrin has very recently been synthesized from the intermediate fragments 1–19 and 20–34 (467).

Structure-activity relations have been most thoroughly studied at the carboxy-terminal pentapeptide region, which has all the biological activities of the whole gastrin molecule. Removal of the amide to form the free acid results in total loss of activity, but one of the hydrogens of the amide can be substituted by CH_3 or NH_2 with retention of all activity. The phenyl ring of Phe^{17} can be hydrogenated or substituted in the para position with retention of activity, but most changes of Asp^{16} cause total loss of activity. Oxidation of Met^{15} to sulfoxide causes complete loss, replacement by Leu or norleucine leads to enhancement of activity. With shorter gastrin fragments, potency is enhanced by blocking the NH_2-terminus (e.g., as in pentagastrin), which presumably increases resistance to enzymatic degradation (468).

9.2 Cholecystokinin (CCK)*

Cholecystokinin, identical with pancreozymin, once was thought to be a separate hormone. The 33 residue peptide (Fig. 27.58) has been isolated from extracts of porcine duodenum and purified by a series of chromatographic procedures. CCK exhibits dual effects on gall bladder contraction and pancreatic enzyme secretion (see Table 27.11). Tropic effects of CCK appear to be confined to growth stimulation of the exocrine pancreas, with no observable effects on gastrointestinal mucosa (445). Circulating levels of CCK in man fluctuate from 25 pg/ml before meals and 16 ng/ml afterwards. The half-life of circulation (454) of exogenously administered CCK is 2–3 min. Reviews are available (445, 452, 454, 463, 472).

The COOH-terminal (29–33)-pentapeptide amide is identical to that of gastrin.

* Synonym: pancreozymin.

H–Lys–Ala–Pro–Ser–Gly–Arg–Val–Ser–Met–Ile–Lys–Asn–Leu–Gln–Ser–Leu–Asp–Pro–Ser–His–

5 10 15 20

SO_3H

|

Arg–Ile–Ser–Asp–Arg–Asp–Tyr–Met–Gly–Trp–Met–Asp–Phe–NH_2

25 28 30 33

(*a*)

SO_3H

|

H–Asp–Arg–Asp–Tyr–Met–Gly–Trp–Met–Asp–Phe–NH_2

(*b*)

SO_3H

|

pGlu–Gln–Asp–Tyr–Thr–Gly–Trp–Met–Asp–Phe–NH_2

(*c*)

Fig. 27.58 The structures of porcine cholecystokinin and related peptides. (*a*) Porcine cholecystokinin (mol wt 3918 daltons) (469). (*b*) Synthetic cholecystokinin-(24–33)-decapeptide is the most potent fragment identified thus far (3–5 times as potent on a molar basis as native CCK) (470). (*c*) Caerulein (mol wt 1352 daltons) from frog skin (471).

This fragment is responsible for the biological actions of both hormones. The crucial difference is the location of the tyrosine residue. In gastrin it is six residues away from the COOH-terminus and in cholecystokinin seven residues away. Moreover, in CCK the tyrosine is always sulfated, since the sulfate group is important for high activity, in contrast to the nonessential role of this group for gastrin bioactivity. Thus the sulfated COOH-terminal heptapeptide is the smallest essential sequence in which the entire range of CCK bioactivity resides. The relative potency reaches a maximum with the COOH-terminal (24–33)-decapeptide (Fig. 27.58*b*), which is 3–5 times more potent on a molar basis than the parent 33 residue peptide. These investigations have gained impetus from the discovery of the potent effects of caerulein (Fig. 27.58*c*), a decapeptide from frog skin that exhibits 3–4 times higher CCK-like activity on a molar basis than native CCK. The COOH-terminal octapeptide of caerulein is identical with that of CCK except for the replacement of the 23-methionine residue by threonine. Desulfation of caerulein decreases its CCK-like effects and converts the molecule to a full agonist for gastric acid secretion.

A synthesis of the entire 33 peptide amide sequence of cholecystokinin has been reported recently (473). Since the synthetic product was the desulfated form, its CCK-like activity was low (0.25% of the standard native material) and synthesis of sulfated CCK has not yet been accomplished.

9.3 Secretin

Secretin is a 27 residue linear peptide of basic nature. It belongs to a family of peptides, including glucagon, GIP, and VIP, which show considerable sequence homology (Fig. 27.59). Secretin is difficult to isolate, and large amounts of porcine intestine are required—a typical yield is 1 mg of purified secretin from 1000 pigs (474). An instability recently traced to the acetate form is responsible for this low yield; the hydrochloride form is much more stable (475).

Secretin is the most potent known stimulant of pancreatic bicarbonate secretion. It also promotes pancreatic enzyme secretion (for reviews, see Refs. 452 and 476). The circulation half-life of secretin in

	1 5 10 15 20 25
Glucagon	His-Ser-Gln-Gly-Thr-Phe-Thr-Ser-Asp-Tyr-Ser-Lys-Tyr-Leu-Asp-Ser-Arg-Arg-Ala-Gln-Asp-Phe-Val-Gln-Trp-Leu- Met -Asn-Thr·NH_2
Secretin	His-Ser-*Asp*-Gly-Thr-Phe-Thr-Ser-Glu-Leu-Ser-*Arg-Leu-Arg*-Asp-Ser-Ala-Arg-Leu-Gln-Arg-Leu-*Leu*-Gln-Gly-Leu-Val·NH_2
VIP	His-Ser-*Asp*-Ala-Val-Phe-Thr-Asp-Asn-Tyr-Thr-*Arg-Leu-Arg*-Lys-Gln-Met-Ala-Val-Lys-Lys-Tyr-*Leu*-Asn-Ser- Ile - Leu -Asn·NH_2
GIP	Tyr-Ala-Glu-Gly-Thr-Phe-Ile-Ser-Asp-Tyr-Ser-Ile-Ala-Met-Asp-Lys-Ile-Arg-Gln-Gln-Asp-Phe-Val-Asn-Trp-Leu- Leu -Ala- Gln
	30 35 40 43
	-Gln-Lys-Gly-Lys-Lys-Ser-Asp-Trp-Lys-His-Asn-Ile-Thr-Gln

Fig. 27.59 Sequence homology between porcine glucagon, secretin, vasointestinal polypeptide (VIP), and gastric inhibitory polypeptide (GIP). Residues in identical positions to those in glucagon appear in boldface type. Additional residues in VIP identical to those in secretin are in italics. Number of identities: glucagon-GIP, 15; secretin-glucagon, 14; secretin-GIP, 9; VIP-secretin, 9; VIP-glucagon, 5; VIP-GIP, 4. From Butt (19). Reprinted with permission of Ellis Horwood, Ltd., Publ., Chichester.

dogs is 3.2 min; enzymatic degradation occurs in plasma and during liver passage. Similarities are observed in the actions of secretin and VIP, indicating that each hormone can interact with the other's receptor sites (477), but subject to species differences. Stimulation of pancreatic $HCO_3^{\ominus}$ secretion in dogs by VIP was 17% that of secretin. In birds, stimulation of pancreatic secretion by porcine secretin was weak (478). Conversely, porcine VIP showed potent activity in birds but was weak in mammals. Extracts of chicken or teleost intestine exhibited weak secretinlike effects on the mammalian pancreas, but strong effects on the pancreas of birds, suggesting a long evolutionary history of these hormones (478). The recent discovery that secretin stimulates insulin release from pancreatic islet cells opened up an active field of investigation (479). Other actions of secretin include stimulation of gastric pepsin secretion and increase in mesenteric blood flow. Secretin-induced mesenteric vasodilatation may be due partly to a direct effect of the hormone on vascular smooth muscle (480). Clinical use is made of secretin as a diagnostic aid for chronic pancreatitis or cancer of the pancreas, and in hypotonic duodenography (481).

Secretin was first synthesized by conventional methodology in two separate approaches: by stepwise addition of amino acids (482), and by segment condensation (482–484). Both syntheses provided products possessing the same potency (4000 IU/kg) and the same spectrum of biological activity as purified natural porcine secretin. Recent preparative scale syntheses of secretin have been carried out by advanced conventional methodology (484). Solid phase synthesis has only very recently been applied successfully (485) to the preparation of secretin with full biological activity (3.750–4.600 IU/mg). The benzhydrylamine resin support and coupling of symmetrical anhydrides of Boc-amino acids were used.

It has long been thought that the entire secretin molecule was required for biological activity and for assuming its partially helical folded conformation (486), since removal of even a single histidine residue at the NH_2-terminus caused inactivation. Surprisingly, however, the shorter synthetic secretin-(5–25)-tricosapeptide and its [Gln^9] and [Asn^{15}] analogs have recently been found to exhibit about 40% of the potency of native secretin in the rat and 5% in the guinea pig in stimulation of pancreatic enzyme secretion (487).

9.4 Gastric Inhibitory Polypeptide (GIP)

Gastric inhibitory polypeptide has been isolated from duodenal mucosa. The 43 residue straight chain peptide (Fig. 27.59) is the largest gastrointestinal hormone of known structure (488). Its sequence homology with glucagon, secretin, and VIP has been discussed (Fig. 27.59). GIP inhibits secretion of gastric acid and pepsin (445, 489). The second proved physiologic effect of GIP is its potent insulin-releasing activity (445), which was observed in dogs and in man at serum levels of 1 ng/ml (490).

The structure of GIP has been confirmed by solution synthesis (491). The synthetic product also displays the potent insulin-releasing activity observed with the native hormone. A synthetic intermediate, the COOH-terminal GIP-(15–43)-nonacosapeptide, exhibits approximately 25% of the activity of native GIP in the suppression of histamine-stimulated gastric acid secretion.

9.5 Vasointestinal Polypeptide (VIP)

Porcine vasointestinal polypeptide is a highly basic octacosapeptide (Fig. 27.59). Its structure (451, 492) has been confirmed by synthesis (493). The sequence of chicken VIP (494) differs in four positions: Ser^{11}, Phe^{13}, Val^{26}, and Thr^{28}. The entire molecule appears to be necessary for full biological activity. Smaller COOH-terminal fragments exhibit lower potency. VIP exhibits vasodilator and hypotensive actions in peripheral, splanchnic coronary, and pulmonary vascular beds. In the gastrointestinal tract, VIP inhibits gastric acid secretion. It stimulates pancreatic bicarbonate secretion and glycogenolysis (454, 492). Since the physiological role of VIP remains to be defined, this substance has been classified as a "candidate hormone" (453, 495). Recently the presence of VIP in neurons of the central and peripheral nervous systems and in human cerebrospinal fluid has been detected in immunocytochemical and radioimmunochemical studies (496).

9.6 Motilin

Motilin has been isolated from the mucosa of porcine small intestine. It is a linear 22 residue peptide (Fig. 27.60) whose structure (497) bears no similarity to any of the known gastrointestinal hormones. Motilin-secreting cells have been identified in human and animal duodenal and jejunal mucosa by immunofluorescent techniques (498). Motilin was discovered as a result of its motor stimulatory effect (at 100 ng/kg) on fundic and antral pouches of the dog stomach. The circulating half-life of exogenously administered motilin is 4–5 min (499). The peptide is released in response to alkalinization of the duodenum (500). However the physiological role of motilin remains to be determined, and presently it is to be considered as a "candidate hormone".

Motilin has been synthesized by conventional solution methods (501). The analogs [13-norleucine, 14-glutamic acid]motilin and [13-leucine]motilin have been similarly prepared (502). Their bioactivity compared well to that of native motilin.

10 CHORIONIC (PLACENTAL) HORMONES

When the female organism has been fertilized, the placenta begins to develop and to produce gonadotropic hormones.

H–Phe–Val–Pro–Ile–Phe–Thr–Tyr–Gly–Glu–Leu–Gln–Arg–Met–Gln–Glu–
1 5 10 15

Lys–Glu–Arg–Asn–Lys–Gly–Gln–OH
20 22

Fig. 27.60 The structure of porcine motilin (497).

Human *choriogonadotropin* (hCG)* is produced predominantly in early pregnancy; human *choriomammotropin* (hCS)† occurs in late pregnancy.

10.1 Choriogonadotropin (CG)

Human choriogonadotropin (hCG) is a glycoprotein that was discovered in the blood and urine of pregnant women. Its detection in the urine forms the basis of most tests for the early diagnosis of pregnancy. The major site of production in the placenta appears to be the syncytiotrophoblast. The role of hCG is to stimulate the corpus luteum into producing augmented amounts of estrogen and progesterone after fertilization. Its biological activity profile resembles that of pituitary lutropin (LH). Measurement of hCG levels by radioimmunoassay or a series of bioassays has been described in detail (503). For reviews, see Refs. 19, 504, and 505.

* Synonym: chorionic gonadotropin.

† Synonyms: chorionic somatomammotropin, placental lactogen (PL).

Most of the hCG that has been used for research purposes has been isolated from the urine of pregnant women and purified by ion exchange chromatography, gel filtration, and isoelectric focusing. Alternatively, hCG may be isolated from placental tissue. Highly purified hCG has a potency of about 15,000 IU/mg. Purification is complicated by heterogeneity because of variations in the sialic acid content of the hormone (504, 505).

Figure 27.61 presents the structure of hCG (mol wt *ca.* 35,000 daltons) (506,

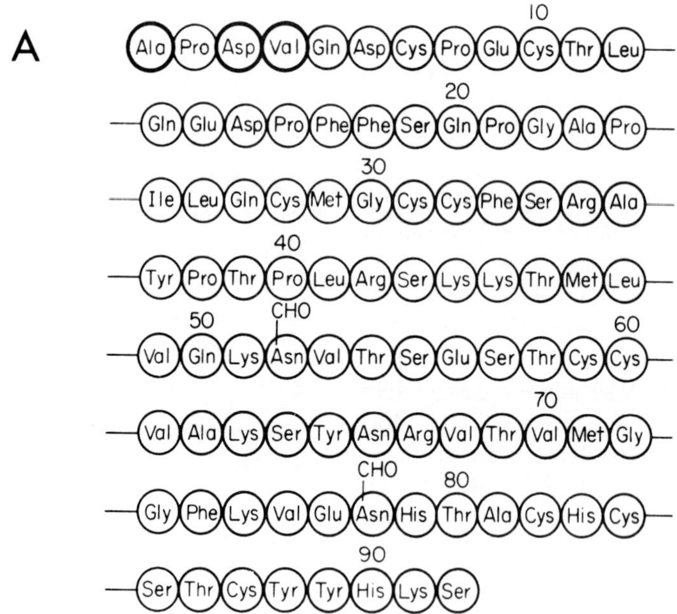

Fig. 27.61 Structure of human choriogonadotropin (hCG). (*a*) Amino acid sequence of the α-subunit. The residues appearing in heavy circles (1, 3, and 4) are found in varying proportions as the amino-terminus, indicating heterogeneity among the α-subunit peptide chains. The sites of carbohydrate attachment are indicated by CHO above the residues. From Canfield et al. (505). Reprinted with permission of Macmillan London and Basingstoke.

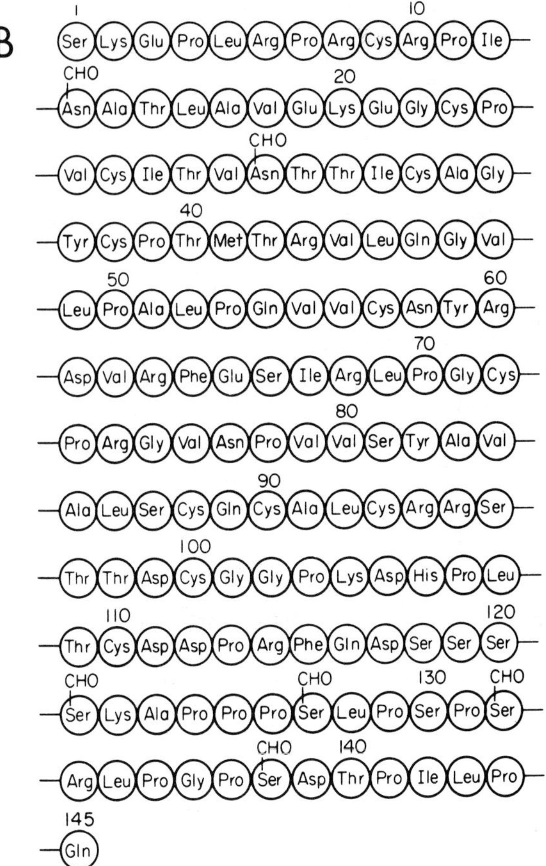

Fig. 27.61 (*Continued*) (*b*) Amino acid sequence of the β-subunit. From Canfield et al. (505). Reprinted with permission of Macmillan London and Basingstoke.

507). Like other glycoprotein hormones, hCG is composed of two dissimilar subunits, designated α and β in accordance with the nomenclature used for TSH, LH, and FSH. The α-subunit consists of 92 amino acid residues and exhibits an almost complete homology with the α-subunit of LH, which differs only in a two-residue inversion and a three-residue deletion at the NH_2-terminus (see Fig. 27.22). Indeed, the α-subunits of hCG, hLH, and hTSH are interchangeable, and the ensuing reconstituted hormones are indistinguishable from the native hormones in biologic, immunologic, and electrophoretic properties (504). The hCG β-subunit, which confers the hormonal specificity to the molecule, differs from hLH in 17 positions and contains a COOH-terminal sequence of 30 residues that does not occur in hLH. The structure of the carbohydrate units (Fig. 27.61*c*) has been studied by Bahl (504). Differing chains of repeated glucosamine-mannose units that are branched at mannose residues are attached to asparagine residues of the α- and β-subunits.

Therapeutically, hCG is used to induce ovulation in infertile women. The hCG-specific radioimmunoassay (508) has improved early detection of pregnancy and is very useful in the diagnosis of gestational choriocarcinoma, which produces massive

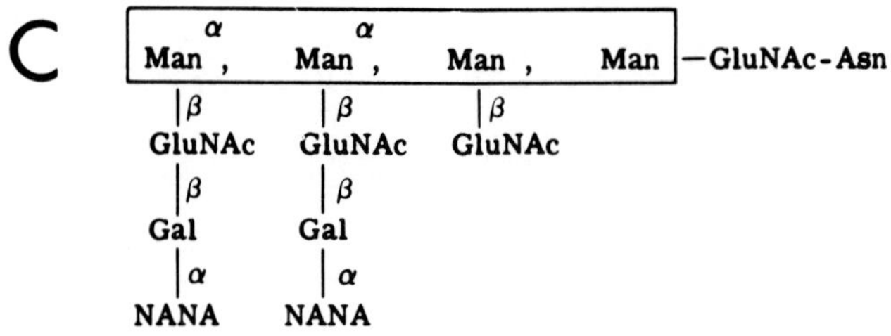

C

```
     α         α
  [ Man ,     Man ,     Man ,     Man ]—GluNAc-Asn
    |β        |β        |β
  GluNAc    GluNAc    GluNAc
    |β        |β
   Gal       Gal
    |α        |α
   NANA      NANA
```

Structure I

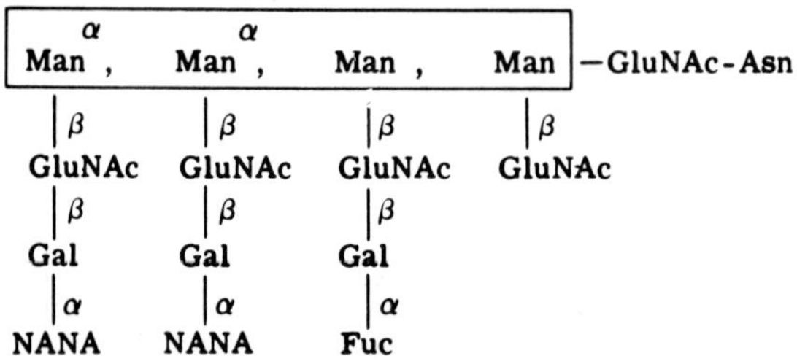

```
     α         α
  [ Man ,     Man ,     Man ,     Man ]—GluNAc-Asn
    |β        |β        |β        |β
  GluNAc    GluNAc    GluNAc    GluNAc
    |β        |β        |β
   Gal       Gal       Gal
    |α        |α        |α
   NANA      NANA      Fuc
```

Structure II

Fig. 27.61 (*Continued*) (*c*) Tentative structures of carbohydrate chains: I, sequence of monosaccharides in the carbohydrate units in HCG-α; II, sequence of monosaccharides in the carbohydrate units in HCG-β. NANA: *N*-Acetylneuraminic acid. From Bahl (504). Reprinted with permission of Academic Press, Inc.

amounts of hCG. The effectiveness of chemotherapy is monitored by measuring the decline of circulating hCG levels. To further improve the specificity of the radioimmunoassay for this purpose, it has been proposed to utilize the COOH-terminal sequence of 30 residues in the β-subunit of hCG (Fig. 27.61*b*) as an antigen. This sequence does not occur in hLH and offers the potential of developing highly hCG-specific antibodies. An eicosapeptide derivative related to the COOH-terminal hCG-(126–145) sequence region has been synthesized by conventional solution methods. It induced antibodies to hCG (509) and may become useful in the early detection of hCG-producing tumors.

10.2 Choriomammotropin (CS)

Human choriomammotropin (hCS) was discovered and isolated from aqueous placenta extracts (510). Radioimmunoassay is widely used for measuring blood levels of hCS during pregnancy, to test placental function. The half-life of circulation is 10–20 min. As in the case of hCG, the placental syncytiotrophoblast is the major site of hCS secretion. The hormone has a wide activity range, including somatotropic, mammotropic, lactotropic, and luteotropic effects. Its potency as a lactogen is considerable, and it seems likely that hCS contributes to breast development during pregnancy in humans. Thus the designation "placental lactogen" may best describe its function. It has been suggested that hCS, as well as hCG, exerts inhibitory effects on lymphocyte maturation. A suppression of cell-mediated immunity brought about in this manner might help to account for the failure of immunological rejection of the growing fetus by the mother (511). The biology and chemistry of choriomammotropin have been reviewed comprehensively (19, 512, 513).

Human choriomammotropin is a single-chain protein of 191 amino acid residues (mol wt 22,308 daltons) and contains two

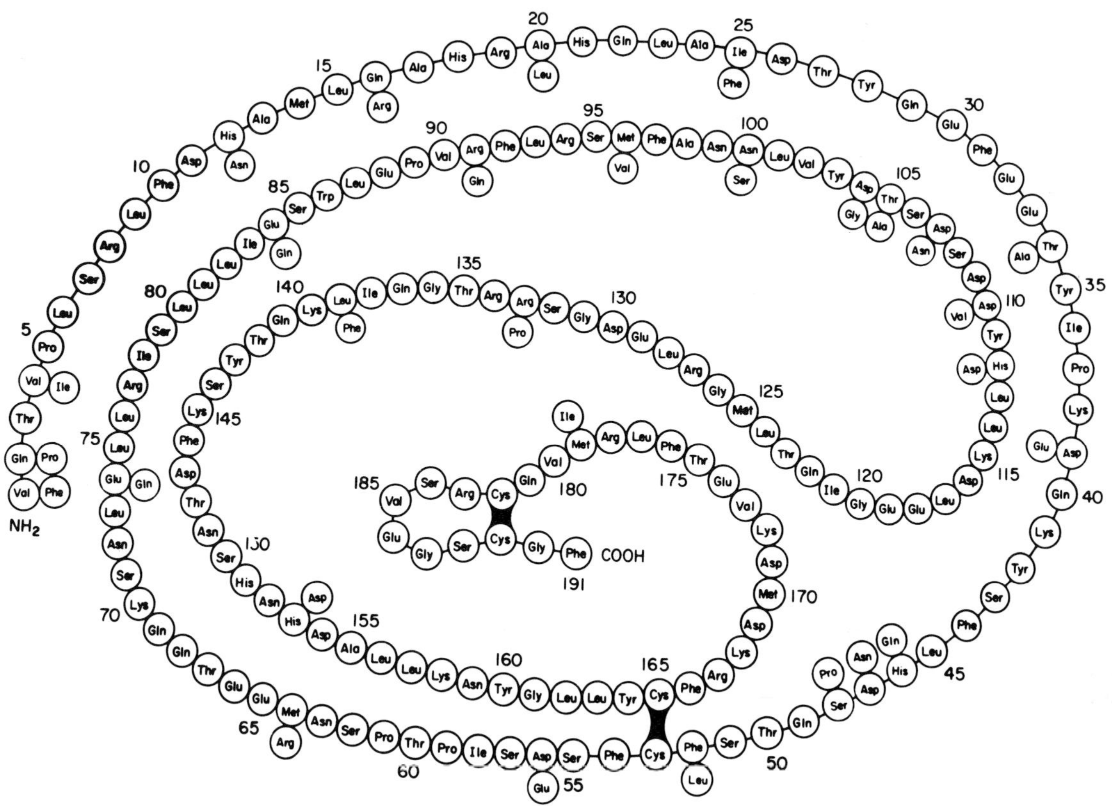

Fig. 27.62 The structure of human choriomammotropin (hCS, mol wt 22, 308 daltons) (514) as compared to human somatotropin (hGH, mol wt 22,005 daltons). The continuous chain is that of choriomammotropin. Residues that are different in hGH are shown alongside; others are common to both molecules. From Frantz (234). Reprinted with permission of Macmillan London and Basingstoke.

disulfide bridges (184, 514). As Fig. 27.62 suggests, hCS bears extensive (85%) structural homology to human somatotropin. About half the amino acid residues in hCs are in the α-helical conformation (515). CD studies show that there are considerable differences between the conformations of hCS and hGH (516).

Circulating big hCS (mol wt *ca.* 45,000 daltons) has been isolated and identified as consisting of two identical molecules of hCS, linked by a disulfide bond (517).

11 OVARIAN HORMONE: RELAXIN

In 1926 Hisaw (518) observed that the relaxation of the pubic symphysis during pregnancy in animals is controlled by a hormone that was subsequently isolated from aqueous extracts of porcine corpora lutea, and named relaxin. The hormone has since been detected in several animals. With the use of a specific radioimmunoassay for porcine relaxin (519), the hormone was discovered in the serum of pregnant women at term, when it is secreted by the pregnancy corpus luteum (520). Its secretion correlated with luteal progesterone secretion.

The porcine hormone has been purified by ion exchange chromatography. Relaxin is a basic peptide (pI *ca.* 10.7) having a molecular weight of about 5500 daltons. Disulfide bond reduction produces two peptide chains, a 22 residue A chain and a

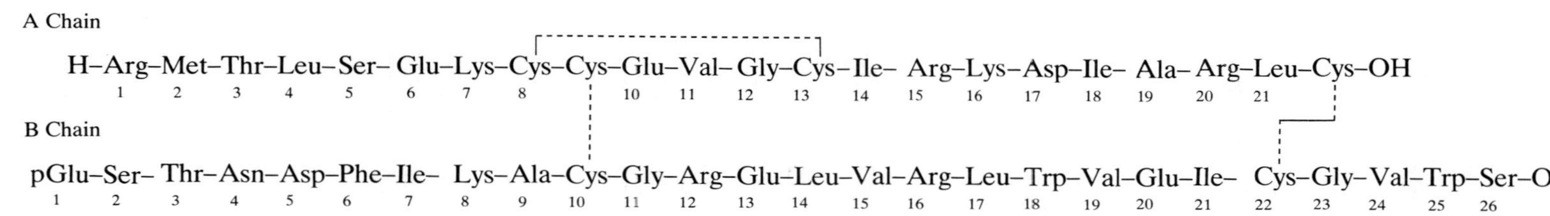

Fig. 27.63 The structure of porcine relaxin proposed by C. Schwabe et al. (522). The assignment of the disulfide bonds remains to be confirmed experimentally. The suggested disulfide bonds pattern shown is taken from that of insulin (see Fig. 27.41), assuming a "disulfide homology".

B chain consisting of 26–30 residues (521). Sequence analysis (522) revealed a structure (Fig. 27.63) that is surprisingly similar in overall molecular architecture to that of insulin (Fig. 27.41). The four half-cystine residues of the A chain and the two half-cystine residues of the B chain are spaced at exactly the same distances as in insulin. The disulfide positions still must be assigned, but very likely they will be found to correspond to those in insulin. This would then constitute the first case of a "disulfide homology" (522). Although only five other residues of relaxin are identical to those in equivalent positions of porcine insulin, model building, assisted by computer graphics, indicated that relaxin has also "conformational homology" with insulin (522a).

During pregnancy in women relaxin concentrations increase several-fold in the uterine cervix and bring about typical connective tissue changes. Relaxin has been used clinically to facilitate parturition (522b).

12 VASOACTIVE TISSUE HORMONES

The term "vasoactive tissue hormones" denotes biologically active polypeptides that are not secreted by a special gland or neuron but are released enzymatically from inactive precursors in blood plasma (angiotensinogen, bradykininogen), acting on smooth muscle and displaying vasoactive properties, i.e., hypo- or hypertensive action. Prominent among these is the family of angiotensin peptides, which exhibit a wide range of biologic and pharmacologic effects, and the kinins, which comprise a large number of vasoactive peptides originating from such diverse sources as human plasma and venoms of insects, amphibians, and molluscs. The vast amount of information gained from intensive studies of these peptides has been the subject of several authoritative treatises (523–526) and reviews (527–529). Here, a few selected highlights are discussed.

12.1 Angiotensin

When renin, an acid protease, is released from the kidney into the circulation, it reacts with a glycoprotein substrate (an α_2-globulin fraction) to produce the decapeptide angiotensin I by cleavage of a Leu-Leu bond (530). Human and other primate renins act on renin substrates of nearly every species, but nonprimate renins are inactive in man. Angiotensin I, which is biologically inactive, is rapidly converted into the octapeptide angiotensin II, (Fig. 27.64) by the action of "angiotensin-converting enzyme", a peptidyl dipeptidase that is present in large amounts in lung tissue or other vascular beds (528, 531). Angiotensin II is the most potent vasopressor agent known. Its short half-life of circulation (15 sec) indicates that it is quickly utilized by vascular smooth muscle. It is also attacked by a battery of enzymes, called angiotensinases, producing various metabolites (Fig. 27.64). One of the most exciting recent developments is the recognition of the strong agonist activity of one of the metabolites, the heptapeptide angiotensin III (des-Asp^1-angiotensin) (532). The physiologic importance of angiotensin III relative to angiotensin II remains to be determined (532a), as does the physiologic role of renin in hypertension (523).

The most important physiologic actions of angiotensin II are exerted on (1) the peripheral arterioles, to support and maintain arterial pressure, (2) the adrenal cortex, to stimulate release of aldosterone, a hormone that promotes sodium and fluid retention, and (3) the renal arterioles and juxtaglomerular cells of the kidney, to modulate renal hemodynamics and renin secretion, respectively.

Several hundred analogs have been synthesized, a large proportion of these with the use of Merrifield's solid phase

Angiotensinogen (Renin substrate)

H–Asp–Arg–Val–Tyr–Ile–His–Pro–Phe–His–Leu–Leu–Val–Tyr–Ser–Protein ⟵ liver

Renin ⟵ Kidney

H–Asp–Arg–Val–Tyr–Ile–His–Pro–Phe–His–Leu–OH
Angiotensin I

Converting enzyme ⟵ Lung Plasma Tissues

H–Asp–Arg–Val–Tyr–Ile–His–Pro–Phe–OH —angiotensinase B, C→ Inactive metabolites
Angiotensin II

angiotensinase A

H–Arg–Val–Tyr–Ile–His–Pro–Phe–OH
Angiotensin III

Fig. 27.64 Pathways of formation and degradation of angiotensin II.

method (8). Evaluation of their bioactivity and consideration of conformational data (534) have led to refined structure-activity relationships (535, 536) and permit predictive analog design. Several highly potent competitive inhibitors of the pressor and myotropic response to angiotensin II have been developed, e.g., [Phe^4, Tyr^8]angiotensin II (537, 538) and [Sar^1, Ile^8]angiotensin II (539). These antagonists suffered from initial transient agonist effects, but recently purer antagonists have been prepared (540), and of these [Sar^1, $Thr(Me)^8$]angiotensin II is thus far the most potent inhibitor.

Other approaches to suppression of angiotensin II levels in plasma encompass the use of synthetic competitive inhibitors of renin such as H–His–Pro–Phe–His–Leu–D-Leu–Val–Tyr–OH (541, 542) or inhibitors of angiotensin-converting enzyme, e.g., pGlu–Trp–Pro–Arg–Pro–Gln–Ile–Pro–Pro–OH (543). A proline derivative,

$$\begin{array}{c} CH_3 \\ | \\ HS–CH_2–CH–CO–Pro–OH, \end{array}$$

has recently been shown to be an orally effective inhibitor of angiotensin-converting enzyme (544).

Interesting new findings suggest a functional role for the angiotensin system in mammalian brain. Intraventricular administration of angiotensin II causes rise in blood pressure, thirst, and vasopressin release (545, 546). High affinity binding sites for angiotension II have been identified in certain areas of bovine and rat brain. The binding potency of angiotensin II and analogs to these receptor sites correlates with their *in vitro* potency and binding to adrenal cortex receptors (547). It will be fascinating to observe future studies on the suggestive role of angiotensin II peptides in the central nervous system.

12.2 Bradykinin and Other Kinins

There are more than 30 kinins of known structure, falling into two functional categories: (1) Physiologically significant mammalian tissue hormones (M1–6 in Table 27.12), and (2) inflammatory venoms

Table 27.12 Structures of Selected Kinins and Release of Mammalian Kinins from Precursor Plasma Protein

Homologies	Structure	Category	Kinin
	. . . Gly–Arg–Met–Lys–Arg–Pro–Pro–Gly–Phe–Ser–Pro–Phe–Arg. . .		Bradykininogen
	Plasma-kallikrein, trypsin	M-1	Bradykinin
	Glandular-kallikrein	M-2	Kallidin
	Plasmin	M-3	ML-bradykinin
	Pepsinlike protease	M-4	GAML-bradykinin
	H–Th–Ala–Thr(CH_2CH_2)–Thr–Arg–Arg–Arg–Gly–Arg–Pro–Pro–Gly–Phe–Ser–Pro–Phe–Arg–OH	V-1[a,b]	Vespulakinin 1
	H– Arg–Pro–Lys–Pro–Gln–Gln–Phe–Phe–Gly–Leu–Met–NH_2	M-5	Substance P
	pGlu–Ala–Asp–Pro–Asn–Lys–Phe–Tyr–Gly–Leu–Met–NH_2	V-2[c]	Physalaemin
	pGlu–Leu–Tyr–Glu–Asn–Lys–Pro–Arg–Arg–Pro–Tyr–Ile–Leu–OH	M-6	Neurotensin
	pGlu–Gly–Lys–Arg–Pro–Trp–Ile–Leu–OH	V-3	Xenopsin
	pGlu–Gln–Asp–Tyr(SO_3H)–Thr–Gly–Trp–Met–Asp–Phe–NH_2	V-4[d]	Caerulein
	pGlu–Val–Pro–Gln–Trp–Ala–Val–Gly–His–Phe–Met–NH_2	V-5	Ranatensin
	pGlu–Gln–Arg–Leu–Gly–Thr–Gln–Trp–Ala–Val–Gly–His–Leu–Met–NH_2	V-6	Alytesin
	pGlu–Gln–Arg–Leu–Gly–Asn–Gln–Trp–Ala–Val–Gly–His–Leu–Met–NH_2	V-7	Bombesin
	pGlu–Gln–Trp–Ala–Val–Gly–His–Phe–Met–NH_2	V-8	Litorin

[a] $CH_{1,2}$ = 1–3-*N*-Ac–galactosamine, 1–2 galactose.
[b] Related: polisteskinin, wasp kinin.
[c] Related: eledoisin, phyllomedusin.
[d] Compare with gastrin; related: phyllocaerulein.

of stinging insects, amphibians, and molluscs [V1–8]. Table 27.12 shows a few examples of kinin structures, many of which have been confirmed by synthesis (274, 526). Recent trends in mammalian kinin research (548) and in kinins of nonmammalian origin (549) have been reviewed.

Striking sequence homologies (Table 27.12) exist between bradykinin (M-1) and vespulakinin (V-1) (and also phyllokinins and other COOH-terminally extended kinins), between substance P (M-5) and physalaemin (V-2), between neurotensin (M-6) and xenopsin (V-3) (551), between gastrin and caerulein (V-4), and among the venoms ranatensin (V-5), alytesin (V-6), bombesin (V-7), and litorin (V-8) (552). Caerulein (V-4), with a COOH-terminal pentapeptide identical to that of both gastrin and CCK, is more potent than gastrin in stimulating gastric acid secretion in dogs (553). Physiologically, mammalian kinins may be involved in the regulation of blood pressure (554), capillary permeability, and blood clotting (548), and in anaphylactic and traumatic shock, in allergic and rheumatic disorders (525), and in the generation of pain. Neural control of kinin action has been suggested (525, 555). The clinical treatment of kinin-related disorders has been reviewed (525). Vespulakinins (V-1), recently isolated from the venom of the yellow jacket (550), are the first reported naturally occurring glycopeptide derivatives of bradykinin and the first reported vasoactive glycopeptides.

More than 200 analogs of the mammalian kinins have been synthesized. Analysis of structure-activity relations (274) show that the bradykinin molecule cannot be shortened without loss of activity and that the two arginine residues in the terminal positions are important for high bioactivity. Replacement of Phe^8 by D-Phe resulted in increased potency, presumably because of increased metabolic resistance (for a review, see Ref. 274).

13 GROWTH FACTORS

Serum contains a number of peptide or protein factors that promote cell growth. Some of these are at least partly regulated by somatotropin and are called somatomedins. All these growth-promoting factors seem to exert an anabolic action on their target tissue. Several growth hormone dependent factors have been described; viz; somatomedins A, B, and C, and NSILA-S.* Besides these, epidermal growth factor (EGF), urogastrone fibroblast growth factor (FGF), and nerve growth factor (NGF) have been isolated and purified. The complete structures of several of these have been determined. An entire volume of the *Advances in Metabolic Disorders* series reviews growth factors (556).

13.1 Somatomedins

Somatomedins are growth hormone dependent plasma factors of uncertain origin, found in man and in animals. High affinity binding sites have been noted in a variety of mammalian tissues, such as cartilage, liver, and muscle. Their physiological significance as growth-promoting agents has not yet been established. These factors (somatomedin A, B, and C, and NSILA-S) have weak insulinlike activity. However their ability to promote anabolic processes has been found recently to be 2 orders of magnitude greater than the insulinlike effects (557). NSILA is chemically best characterized and appears to be a single-chain peptide (mol wt *ca.* 6000 daltons), containing three disulfide bonds (558).

13.2 Epidermal Growth Factor and Urogastrone

Epidermal growth factor was discovered in 1962 by S. Cohen in extracts of the submaxillary gland of adult male mice. The

* NSILA, nonsuppressible insulinlike activity.

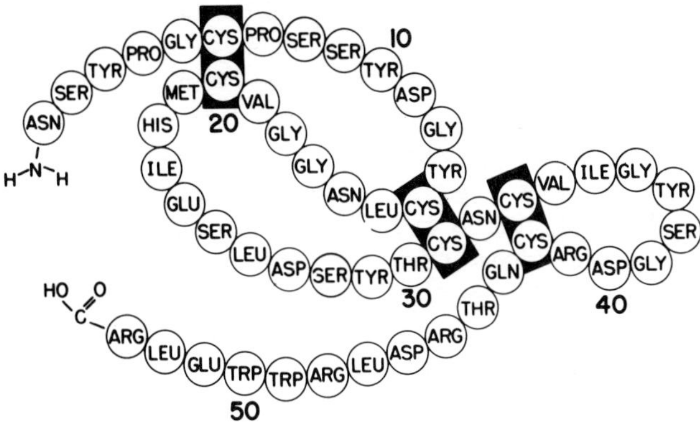

Fig. 27.65 The structure of murine epidermal growth factor. From Savage et al. (560). Reprinted with permission of the American Society of Biological Chemists.

peptide stimulates the proliferation and keratinization of various epidermal and epithelial tissues *in vivo* and *in vitro.* Among the major metabolic events in epidermal tissue, EFG affects the stimulation of protein and RNA synthesis, polysome formation, and ornithine decarboxylase formation. In human or mouse fibroblasts in culture, EGF is a potent mitogen. Inhibition of gastric acid secretion in dogs by EGF has been described (559). [Since this effect is observed at hundredfold lower doses (0.5 μg/kg in dogs) than those required for the gross anatomical changes in epidermal tissue (200 μg/kg s.c. per day in mice), the as yet unclear physiological role of EGF may be an involvement in the control of gastric acid secretion.

The structure of murine EGF (560) appears in Fig. 27.65. It is a single-chain peptide (mol wt 6045 daltons), with an isoelectric point at pH 4.60; it contains three disulfide bonds in 53 amino acid residues. The COOH-terminal pentapeptide sequence comprising both tryptophan residues is not required for bioactivity. These five residues can be removed with retention of full biological activity, while performic acid oxidation or disulfide bond reduction followed by *S*-aminoethylation results in loss of all activity.

A high molecular weight form of EGF (*ca.* 72,000 daltons) consists of 2 molecules of the peptide and 2 molecules of an arginine esteropeptidase (EGF-binding protein). It has been suggested that the arginine esteropeptidase might play a role in liberating EGF from a larger biosynthetic

H–Asn–Ser– Asp–Ser–Glu–Cys–Pro– Leu–Ser–His–Asp–Gly–Tyr–Cys–Leu–
1 5 10 15

His–Asp–Gly–Val–Cys–Met–Tyr–Ile– Glu–Ala– Asp–Lys–Tyr–Ala–
20 25 30

Cys–Asn–Cys–Val–Val–Gly–Tyr–Ile– Gly–Glu–Arg–Cys– Gln–Tyr–Arg–
35 40 45

Asp–Leu–Lys–Trp–Trp–Glu–Leu–Arg–OH
50

Fig. 27.66 The structure of human β-urogastrone. γ-Urogastrone lacks the 53-arginine residue. Extensive sequence homology (70%) exists with murine epidermal growth factor. From Gregory (563).

precursor (562). The chemistry and biology of EGF have been comprehensively reviewed (561).

An interesting possible relationship between EGF and *urogastrone* was recently suggested by Gregory (563). Two urogastrones (β-UG and γ-UG, differing in one COOH-terminal Arg residue) have been isolated from human urine. They possess potent specific inhibitory activity on gastric acid secretion in cats and dogs. Structure determination showed the urogastrons to be 53(52)-residue single-chain peptides with three disulfide bonds (Fig. 27.66). When this structure was compared to that of EGF, extensive homology of 37 common residues was evident. Subsequently, coincidence of biological activity was established, i.e., potent suppression of gastric acid secretion by EGF and stimulation of epidermal growth by urogastrone. It has been suggested, therefore, that β-urogastrone may be identical to human EGF (563).

13.3 Nerve Growth Factor

Nerve growth factors (NGF) are a group of proteins, distributed in many species, which

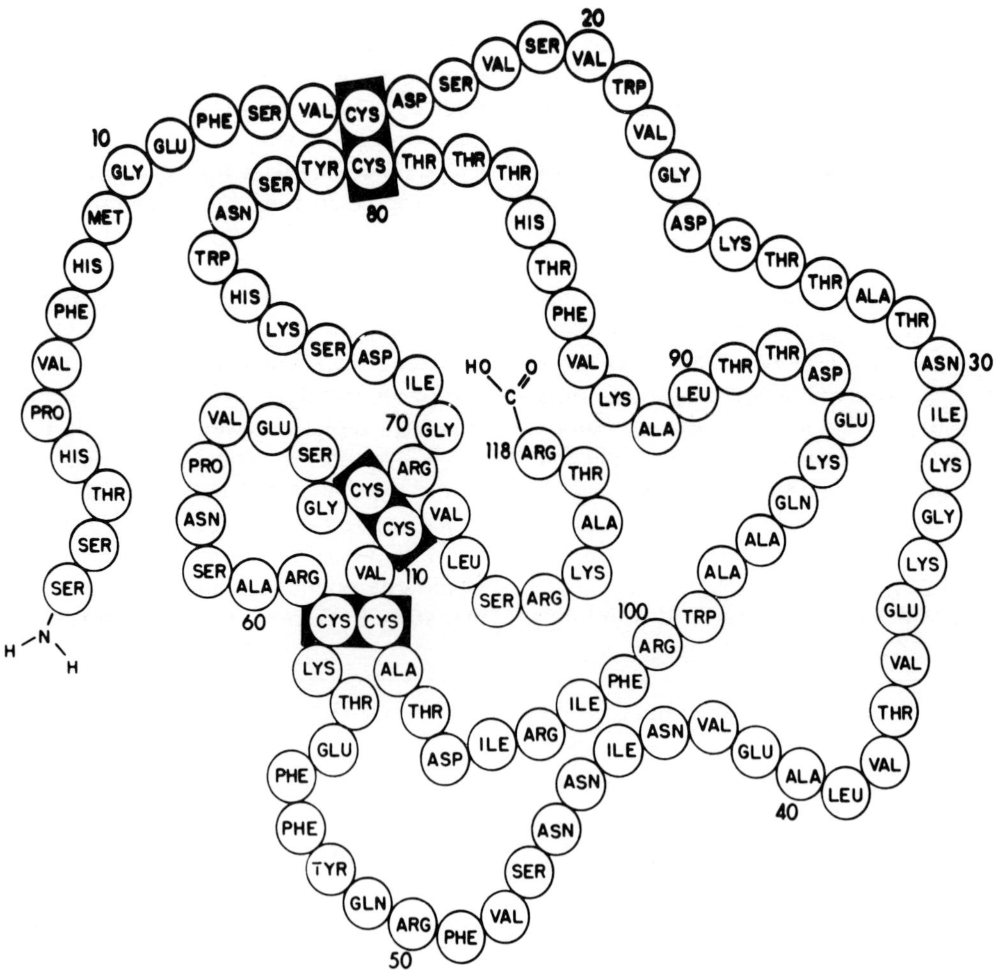

Fig. 27.67 The structure of murine nerve growth factor (monomer). From Angeletti and Bradshaw (568).

play a fundamental role in the embryonic development and the maintenance of the sympathetic nervous system. NGF was discovered in 1948 in two mouse tumors. Subsequently it was found in much larger amounts in the submandibular gland of male mice and in certain snake venoms (for reviews, see Refs. 564–566).

NGF has the remarkable ability of stimulating rapid neurite outgrowth from embryonic sensory and sympathetic ganglia *in vivo* and *in vitro*. The molecular mechanism of this effect is unknown, however binding of the protein to the surface of sensitive cells appears to be the initial event. The action of the growth factor may not be confined to the peripheral nervous system, since brain exhibits ^{121}I-NGF binding sites, and the regeneration of adrenergic neurons of the central nervous system can be stimulated by NGF. Studies on the origin and biosynthesis of NGF indicate that it is produced in a variety of different primary and transformed cells, including human cells. By immunologic and biologic criteria, NGF is present in human serum (567). The role of NGF in disease and its potential therapeutic uses are unknown.

The structure of murine NGF (568) is represented in Fig. 27.67. It consists of 118 amino acid residues (mol wt 13,250 daltons) and contains three disulfide bonds. The sequence of an NGF from the venom of the cobra *Naja naja* has been partially determined. Two molecules of NGF associate to form a dimer complex at 5–10 mg/ml concentration. However at the 1 ng/ml level it is to 99% monodisperse; i.e., the monomer seems to be the biologically active species. The biosynthesis of NGF may proceed by way of larger precursors (562).

Comparison of murine NGF with proinsulin showed certain similarities (21% identical residues), which led to the proposal that these proteins may be derived from a common, albeit distant, ancestral protein (564).

ACKNOWLEDGMENTS

For highly appreciated suggestions and manuscript corrections, I thank Drs. K. Gibson, A. L. Goldstein, C. H. Li, T. Mowles, C. Schwabe, C. W. Smith, S. Udenfriend, and R. Walter. Dr. P. Sorter and the Scientific Literature Department of Hoffman–La Roche, Inc., provided extensive literature information. Mrs. D. Dabaghian's expertise in preparing the manuscript is gratefully acknowledged.

REFERENCES

1. IUPAC–IUB Commission on Biochemical Nomenclature, Recommendations: (a) Peptide hormones; *J. Biol. Chem.*, **250,** 3215–3216 (1975). (*b*) *Ibid.*, **247,** 979–982 (1972); **242,** 555–557 (1967).
2. S. A. Berson and R. S. Yalow, Eds., *Peptide Hormones*, in *Methods in Investigative and Diagnostic Endocrinology*, Elsevier, New York, 1973. (a) Vol. 2A. (b) Vol. 2B.
3. S. Moore, in *Chemistry and Biology of Peptides*, J. Meienhofer, Ed., Ann Arbor Science Publishers, Ann Arbor, Mich., 1972, pp. 629–653.
4. K. A. Gruber, S. Stein, L. Brink, A. Radhakrishnan, and S. Udenfriend, *Proc. Nat. Acad. Sci., US*, **73,** 1314–1318 (1976).
5. (a) J. Bridgen, *Sci. Tools* (*LKB*), **24,** 1–6 (1977). (b) J. W. Jacobs and H. D. Niall, *J. Biol. Chem.*, **250,** 3629–3636 (1975). (c) D. J. McKean, E. H. Peters, J. I. Waldby, and O. Smithies, *Biochemistry*, **13,** 3048–3051 (1974). (d) J. Bridgen, *ibid.*, **15,** 3600–3604 (1976).
6. M. Bodanszky, Y. S. Klausner, and M. A. Ondetti, *Peptide Synthesis*, Wiley, New York, 1976.
7. F. M. Finn and K. Hofmann, in *The Proteins*, 3rd ed., Vol. 2, H. Neurath and R. L. Hill, Eds., Academic Press, New York, 1976, pp. 105–253.
8. B. W. Erickson and R. B. Merrifield, in *The Proteins*, 3rd ed., Vol. 2, H. Neurath and R. L. Hill, Eds., Academic Press, New York, 1976, pp. 255–527.
9. J. Meienhofer, in *Hormonal Proteins and Peptides*, Vol. 2, C. H. Li, Ed., Academic Press, New York, 1973, pp. 45–267
10. T. L. Blundell, G. G. Dodson, D. C. Hodgkin, and D. A. Mercola, *Advan. Protein Chem.*, **26,** 279–402 (1972).

11. V. J. Hruby, in *Chemistry and Biochemistry of Amino Acids, Peptides and Proteins*, Vol. 3, B. Weinstein, Ed., Dekker, New York, 1974, pp. 1–188. H. R. Wyssbrod and W. A. Gibbons, in *Survey of Progress in Chemistry*, Vol. 6, A. F. Scott, Ed., Academic Press, New York, 1973, pp. 210–326. Yu. A. Ovchinnikov and V. T. Ivanov, *Tetrahedron*, **31,** 2177–2209 (1975).
12. R. S. Yalow and S. A. Berson, *J. Clin. Invest.*, **39,** 1157–1175 (1960).
13. S. Spector, *Ann. Rev. Pharmacol*, **13,** 359–370 (1973); B. M. Jaffe and H. R. Behrman, Eds., *Methods of Hormone Radioimmunoassay*, Academic Press, New York, 1974.
14. K. Lübke, E. Schillinger, and M. Töpert, *Angew. chem. Int. Ed.*, **15,** 741–748 (1976).
15. G. S. Levey, Ed., *Hormone-Receptor Interaction, Molecular Aspects*, Modern Pharmacology-Toxicology Series, Vol. 9, Dekker, New York, 1976.
16. R. Acher, in *Polypeptide Hormones: Molecular and Cellular Aspects*, R. Porter and D. W. Fitzsimmons, Eds., Ciba Foundation Symposium No. 41, Excerpta Medica, New York, 1976, pp. 31–59.
17. M. O. Dayhoff, P. J. McLaughlin, W. C. Barker, and T. L. Hunt, *Naturwissenschaften*, **62,** 154–161 (1975).
18. J. A. Parsons, Ed., *Peptide Hormones*, University Park Press, Baltimore, 1976.
19. W. R. Butt, *Hormone Chemistry*, 2nd rev. ed., Vol. 1, Wiley, New York, 1975.
20. B. W. O'Malley and J. G. Hardman, Eds., *Peptide Hormones, Hormone Action*, Part B, *Methods in Enzymology*, Vol. 37, Academic Press, New York, 1975.
21. (a) F. Labrie, J. Meites, and G. Pelletier, Eds., *Hypothalamus and Endocrine Functions*, Plenum Press, New York, 1976 (b) H. Gainer, Ed., *Peptides in Neurobiology*, Plenum Press, New York, 1977. (c) L. L. Iversen, R. A. Nicoll, and W. Vale, Eds., *Neurobiology of Peptides*, Neurosciences Research Program Bulletin, Vol. 16, No. 2, MIT Press, Cambridge, MA, 1978.
22. R. O. Creep and E. B. Astwood, in *Handbook of Physiology*, Section 7, *Endocrinology*, American Physiological Society, Washington, D. C.. (a) Vol. 1, 1972. (b) Vol. 2, 1973. (c) Vol. 3, 1974. (d) Vol. 4, 1974. (e) Vol. 5, 1975. (f) Vol. 6, 1975. (g) Vol. 7, 1976.
23. R. Porter and D. W. Fitzsimmons, Eds., *Polypeptide Hormones; Molecular and Cellular Aspects*, Ciba Foundation Symposium No. 41, Excerpta Medica, New York, 1976.
24. O. Eichler et al., Eds., *Handbook of Experimental Pharmacology*, Springer, New York. (a) Vol. 23, 1968. (b) Vol. 25, 1970. (c) Vol. 32-I, 1971. (d) Vol. 34, 1973. (e) Vol. 37, 1974. (f) Vol. 32-II, 1975.
25. C. H. Li, Ed., *Hormonal Proteins and Peptides*, Academic Press, New York. (a) Vol. 1, 1973. (b) Vol. 2, 1973. (c) Vol. 3, 1975. (d) Vol. 4, 1977; Vol. 5, 1978; Vol. 6, 1978.
26. W. F. Ganong and L. Martini, Eds., *Frontiers in Neuroendocrinology*, Oxford University Press, New York. (a) Vol. 1, 1969. (b) Vol. 2, 1971. (c) Vol. 3, 1973. (d) Vol. 4, Raven Press, New York, 1976. (e) Vol. 5, Raven Press, New York, 1978.
27. K. Lübke, E. Schröder, and G. Kloss, *Chemie und Biochemie der Aminosäuren, Peptide und Proteine* (Thieme Taschenlehrbuch der Organischen Chemie, Vols. B2, B3). Thieme, Stuttgart, 1975.
28. J. Hughes, T. W. Smith, H. W. Kostcrlitz, L. A. Fothergill, B. A. Morgan, and H. R. Morris, *Nature* (London), **258,** 577–579 (1975).
29. (a) S. H. Snyder, *New Engl. J. Med.*, **269,** 266–271 (1977); *Sci. Am.*, **3,** 44–56 (1977). (b) A. Goldstein, *Science*, **193,** 1081–1086 (1976). (c) E. J. Simon, *Neurochem. Res.*, **1,** 3–28 (1976).
30. (a) C. H. Li, L. Barnafi, M. Chrétien, and D. Chung, *Nature* (London), **208,** 1093–1094 (1965). (b) C. H. Li and D. Chung, *ibid.*, **260,** 622–624 (1976).
31. (a) C. H. Li and D. Chung, *Proc. Nat. Acad. Sci., US*, **73,** 1145–1148 (1976). (b) A. F. Bradbury, D. G. Smyth, C. R. Snell, N. J. M. Birdsall, and E. C. Hulme, *Nature* (London), **260,** 793–795 (1976).
32. H. H. Loh, L. F. Tseng, E. Wei, and C. H. Li, *Proc. Nat. Acad. Sci., US*, **73,** 2895–2898 (1976).
33. (a) N. Ling, R. Burgus, and R. Guillemin, *Proc. Nat. Acad. Sci., US*, **73,** 3942–3946 (1976); R. Guillemin, N. Ling, R. Burgus, F. Bloom, and D. Segal, *Psychoneuroendocrinology*, **2,** 59–62 (1977). (b) A. Z. Ronai, L. Graf, J. I. Szekely, Z. Dumai-Kovacs, and S. Bajusz, *FEBS Lett.*, **74,** 182–184 (1977).
34. M. Rubinstein, S. Stein, L. D. Gerber, and S. Udenfriend, *Proc. Nat. Acad. Sci., US*, **74,** 3052–3055 (1977); M. Rubinstein, S. Stein, and S. Udenfriend, *ibid.*, **74,** 4969–4972 (1977).
35. (a) F. Bloom, D. Segal, N. Ling, and R. Guillemin, *Science*, **194,** 630–632 (1976). (b) Y. F. Jacquet and N. Marks, *ibid.*, **194,** 632–635 (1976). (c) W. H. Gispen, V. M. Wiegant, A. F. Bradbury, E. C. Hulme, D. G. Smyth, C. R. Snell, and D. DeWied, *Nature* (London), **264,** 794–795 (1976).

36. (a) H. W. Kosterlitz, Ed., *Opiates and Endogenous Opioid Peptides*, Elsevier/North Holland, Amsterdam, 1976. (b) W. A. Klee, in *Peptides in Neurobiology*, H. Gainer, Ed., Plenum Press, New York, 1977, pp. 375–396. (c) T. T. Chau-Pham, *Drug Metab. Rev.*, **7,** 255–294 (1978). (d) K. Verebey, J. Volavka, and D. Clouet, *Arch. Gen. Psych.*, **35,** 877-878 (1978). (e) G. R. Uhl, S. R. Childers, and S. H. Snyder, in *Frontiers in Neuroendocrinology*, Vol. 5, W. F. Ganong and L. Martini, Eds., Raven Press, New York, 1978, pp. 289–328. (f) E. Costa and M. Trabucchi, Eds., *The Endorphins, Advan. Biochem. Pharmacol.*, Vol. 18, Raven Press, New York, 1978. (g) S. H. Snyder, *Am. J. Psychiatry*, **135,** 645–652 (1978). (h) L. Terenius, *Annu. Rev. Pharmacol. Toxicol.*, **18,** 189–204 (1978).

37. R. C. A. Frederickson, *Life Sci.*, **21,** 23–42 (1977).

38. (a) C. H. Li, *Arch. Biochem. Biophys.*, **183,** 592–604 (1977). (b) C. H. Li, in *Hormonal Peptides and Proteins*, Vol. 5, C. H. Li, Ed., Academic Press, New York, 1978, pp. 35–73. (c) R. Guillemin, *Rec. Progr. Horm. Res.*, **33,** 1–28 (1977).

39. L. D. Gerber, S. Stein, M. Rubinstein, J. Wideman, and S. Udenfriend, *Brain Res.*, **151,** 117–126 (1978).

40. (a) J. D. Belluzzi, N. Grant, V. Garsky, D. Sarantakis, C. D. Wise, and L. Stein, *Nature* (London), **260,** 625–626 (1976). (b) H. H. Büscher, R. C. Hill, D. Römer, F. Cardinaux, A. Closse, D. Hauser, and J. Pless, *ibid.*, **261,** 423–425 (1976).

41. (a) W. L. Dewey, T. T. Chau-Pham, A. Day, M. Lujan, L. S. Harris, and R. J. Freer, in *Opiates and Endogenous Opioid Peptides*, H. W. Kosterlitz, Ed., Elsevier/North Holland, Amsterdam, 1976, pp. 103–110. (b) Y. Jacquet, N. Marks, and C. H. Li, *ibid.*, pp. 411–414.

42. (a) N. Marks, A. Grynbaum, and A. Neidle, *Biochem. Biophys. Res. Commun.*, **74,** 1552–1559 (1977). (b) J. M. Hambrook, B. A. Morgan, M. J. Rance, and C. F. C. Smith, *Nature* (London), **262,** 782–783 (1976). (c) N. Marks, in *Frontiers in Neuroendocrinology*, Vol. 5, W. F. Ganong and L. Martini, Eds., Raven Press, New York, 1978, pp. 329–377. (d) M. Knight and W. A. Klee, *J. Biol. Chem.*, **253,** 3843–3847 (1978).

43. (a) C. B. Pert, A. Pert, J. K. Chang, and B. T. W. Fong, *Science*, **194,** 330–332 (1976). (b) M. G. Baxter, D. Goff, A. A. Miller, and I. A. Saunders, *Proc. Brit. Pharm. Soc.*, 455P–456P (1977).

44. (a) S. Bajusz, A. Z. Rónai, J. I. Skékely, Z. Dunai-Kovács, I. Berzetai, and L. Gráf, *Acta Biochim. Biophys. Acad. Sci. Hung.*, **11,** 305–309 (1976); *FEBS Lett.*, **76,** 91–92 (1977). (b) D. Römer, H. H. Büscher, R. C. Hill, J. Pless, W. Bauer, F. Cardinaux, A. Closse, D. Hauser, and R. Huguenin, *Nature* (London), **268,** 547–549 (1977). (c) D. Yamashiro, L. F. Tseng, and C. H. Li, *Biochem. Biophys. Res. Commun.*, **78,** 1124–1129 (1977).

45. (a) L. Leybin, C. Pinsky, F. S. LaBella, V. Havlicek, and M. Rezek, *Nature* (London), **264,** 458–459 (1976). (b) J. M. Van Nueten, J. M. Van Ree, and P. M. Vanhoutte, *Eur. J. Pharmacol.*, **41,** 341–342 (1977).

46. (a) E. L. Lien, R. L. Fenichel, V. Garsky, D. Sarantakis, and N. H. Grant, *Life Sci.*, **19,** 837–840 (1976); E. L. Lien, D. E. Clark, and W. H. McGregor, *FEBS Lett.*, **88,** 208–210 (1978). (b) H. N. Bhargava, *Eur. J. Pharmacol.*, **41,** 81–84 (1977). (c) R. Schulz and A. Herz, *ibid.*, **39,** 429–432 (1976). (d) A. Pert and C. Sivit, *Nature* (London), **265,** 645–647 (1977). (e) R. Simantov and S. H. Snyder, *ibid.*, **262,** 505-507 (1976).

47. (a) N. P. Plotnikoff, A. J. Kastin, D. H. Coy, C. W. Christensen, A. V. Schally, and M. Spirtes, *Life Sci.*, **19,** 1283–1288 (1976). (b) A. J. Kastin, E. L. Scollan, M. G. King, A. V. Schally, and D. H. Coy, *Pharmacol. Biochem. Behav.*, **5,** 691–695 (1976). (c) J. D. Belluzzi and L. Stein, *Nature* (London), **266,** 556–558 (1977). (d) H. Frenk, G. Urca, and J. C. Liebeskind, *Brain Res.*, **147,** 327–337 (1978).

48. (a) J. Hughes, *Brain Res.*, **88,** 295–308 (1975). (b) R. Simantov, R. Goodman, D. Aposhian, and S. H. Snyder, *ibid.*, **111,** 204–211 (1976).

49. (a) T. Hokfelt, A. Ljungdahl, L. Terenius, R. Elde, G. Nilsson, *Proc. Nat. Acad. Sci., US*, **74,** 3081–3085 (1977). (b) G. R. Uhl, M. J. Kuhar, and H. S. Snyder, *ibid.*, **74,** 3081–3085 (1977). (c) S. J. Watson, H. Akil, S. Sullivan, and J. D. Barchas, *Life Sci.*, **21,** 733–738 (1977). (d) H.-Y. Yang, J. S. Hong, and E. Costa, *Neuropharmacology*, **16,** 303–307 (1977). (e) F. Bloom, E. Battenberg, J. Rossier, N. Ling, and R. Guillemin, *Proc. Nat. Acad. Sci., US*, **75,** 1591–1595 (1978).

50. (a) A. Wahlström, L. Johansson, and L. Terenius, in *Opiates and Endogenous Opioid Peptides*, H. W. Kosterlitz, Ed., Elsevier/North Holland, Amsterdam, 1976, pp. 49–56. (b) T. W. Smith, J. Hughes, H. W. Kosterlitz, and R. P. Sosa, *ibid.*, pp. 57–62. (c) J. Hughes, H. W. Kosterlitz, and T. W. Smith, *Brit. J. Pharmacol.*, **61,** 639–647 (1977).

51. J. D. Bower, K. B. Guest, and B. A. Morgan, *J. Chem. Soc., Perkin Trans. I*, 2488–2492 (1976).

52. (a) C. R. Beddell, R. B. Clark, G. W. Hardy, L. A. Lowe, F. B. Ubatuba, J. R. Vane, S. Wilkinson, K.-J. Chang, P. Cuatrecasas, and R. J. Miller, *Proc. Roy. Soc.*, London, **B198,** 249–265 (1977). (b) A. S. Dutta, J. J. Gormley, C. F. Hayward, J. S. Morley, J. S. Shaw, G. J. Stacey, and M. T. Turnbull, *Life Sci.*, **21,** 559–562. (1977). (c) D. H. Coy, P. Gill, A. J. Kastin, A. Dupont, L. Cusan, D. Britton, and R. Fertel, in *Peptides, Proceedings of the 5th American Peptide Symposium*, R. Walter and J. Meienhofer, Eds., Wiley, New York, 1977, pp. 107–110. (d) A. R. Day, R. J. Freer, and D. L. Marlborough, *ibid.*, pp. 114–116. (e) N. Ling, S. Minick, L. Lazarus, J. Rivier, and R. Guillemin, *ibid.*, pp. 96–99. (f) B. A. Morgan, J. D. Bower, K. P. Guest, B. K. Handa, G. Metcalf, and C. F. C. Smith, *ibid.*, pp. 111–113.

53. (a) D. H. Coy, A. J. Kastin, A. V. Schally, O. Morin, N. G. Caron, F. Labrie, J. M. Walker, R. Fertel, G. G. Berntson, and C. A. Sandman, *Biochem. Biophys. Res. Commun.*, **73,** 632–638 (1976). (b) L. Terenius, A. Wahlström, G. Lindeberg, S. Karlsson, and U. Ragnarsson, *ibid.*, **71,** 175–179 (1976). (c) J. K. Chang, T. W. Fong, A. Pert, and C. B. Pert, *Life Sci.*, **18,** 1473–1482 (1976). (d) N. Ling and R. Guillemin, *Proc. Nat. Acad. Sci., U.S.*, **73,** 3308–3310 (1976). (e) W. Feldberg and D. G. Smyth, *J. Physiol.*, **265,** 25P–27P (1977). (f) B. A. Morgan, C. F. C. Smith, A. A. Waterfield, J. Hughes, and H. W. Kosterlitz, *Commun. J. Pharm. Pharmac.*, **28,** 660–661 (1976).

54. B. von Graffenried, E. del Pozo, J. Roubicek, E. Krebs, W. Pöldinger, P. Burmeister, and L. Kerp, *Nature* (London), **272,** 729–730 (1978).

55. (a) C. H. Li and D. Chung, *Proc. Nat. Acad. Sci., US*, **73,** 1145–1148 (1976). (b) B. M. Cox, A. Goldstein, and C. H. Li, *ibid.*, **73,** 1821–1823 (1976). (c) L. Gráf, E. Barat, and A. Patthy, *Acta Biochim. Biophys. Acad. Sci. Hung.*, **11,** 121–122 (1976). (d) N. G. Saidah, N. Dragon, S. Benjannet, R. Routhier, and M. Chrétien, *Biochem. Biophys. Res. Commun.*, **72,** 1542–1547 (1976).

56. (a) C. H. Li, D. Chung, and B. A. Doneen, *Biochem. Biophys. Res. Commun.*, **72,** 1542–1547 (1976). (b) M. Chrétien, S. Benjannet, N. Dragon, N. G. Saidah, and M. Lis, *ibid.*, **72,** 472–478 (1976).

57. L. F. Tseng, H. H. Loh, and C. H. Li, *Nature* (London), **263,** 239–240 (1976).

58. (a) L. F. Tseng, H. H. Loh, and C. H. Li, *Biochem. Biophys. Res. Commun.*, **74,** 360–396 (1977). (b) L. F. Tseng, H. H. Loh, and C. H. Li, *Proc. Nat. Acad. Sci., US*, **73,** 4187–4189 (1976).

59. (a) A. Dupont, L. Cusan, M. Garon, F. Labrie, and C. H. Li, *Proc. Nat Acad. Sci., US*, **74,** 358–359 (1977). (b) C. Rivier, W. Vale, N. Ling, M. Brown, and R. Guillemin, *Endocrinology*, **100,** 238–241 (1977).

60. (a) B. J. Mayerson and L. Terenius, *J. Pharmacol.*, **42,** 191–192 (1977). (b) J. W. Holaday, H. H. Loh, and C. H. Li, *Life Sci.*, **22,** 1525–1536 (1978).

61. (a) R. E. Mains, B. A. Eipper, and N. Ling, *Proc. Nat. Acad. Sci., US*, **74,** 3014–3018 (1977). (b) J. L. Roberts and E. Herbert, *ibid.*, **74,** 4826–4830 (1977). (c) R. Guillemin, T. Vargo, J. Rossier, S. Minick, N. Ling, C. Rivier, W. Vale, and F. Bloom, *Science*, **197,** 1367–1369 (1977). (d) M. Rubinstein, S. Stein, and S. Udenfriend, *ibid.*, **75,** 669–671 (1978). (e) J. L. Roberts, M. Phillips, P. A. Rosa, and E. Herbert, *Biochemistry* 17, 3609–3618 (1978). (f) R. V. Lewis, S. Stein, L. D. Gerber, M. Rubinstein, and S. Udenfriend, *Proc. Nat. Acad. Sci., US*, **75,** 4021–4023 (1978).

62. (a) J. Rossier, T. Vargo, S. Minick, N. Ling, F. Bloom, and R. Guillemin, *Proc. Nat. Acad. Sci., US*, **74,** 5162–5165 (1977). (b) S. J. Watson, J. D. Barchas, and C. H. Li, *ibid.*, **74,** 5155–5158 (1977). (c) F. LaBella, G. Queen, J. Senyshyn, M. Lis, and M. Chrétien, *Biochem. Biophys. Res. Commun.*, **75,** 350–357 (1977).

63. C. H. Li, S. Lemaire, D. Yamashiro, and B. A. Doneen, *Biochem. Biophys. Res. Commun.*, **71,** 19–25 (1976).

64. (a) C. H. Li, D. Yamashiro, L. F. Tseng, and H. H. Loh, *J. Med. Chem.*, **20,** 325–328 (1977). (b) D. Yamashiro and C. H. Li, *Proc. Nat. Acad. Sci., US*, **71,** 4945–4949 (1974). (c) E. Atherton, M. Caviezel, H. Over, and R. C. Sheppard, *J. Chem. Soc. Chem. Commun.*, 819–821 (1977). (d) E. Atherton, H. Fox, C. J. Logan, and R. C. Sheppard, *ibid.*, 539–540 (1978). (e) D. H. Coy, P. Gill, A. J. Kastin, A. Dupont, L. Cusan, F. Labrie, D. Britton, and R. Fertel, in *Peptides, Proceedings of the Fifth American Peptide Symposium*, M. Goodman and J. Meienhofer, Eds., Wiley, New York, 1977, pp. 107–110. (f) D. S. Segal, R. G. Browne, F. Bloom, N. Ling, and R. Guillemin, *Science*, **198,** 411–414 (1977).

65. (a) C. Tzougraki, R. C. Makofske, T. F. Gabriel, S. S. Wang, R. Kutny, J. Meienhofer, and C. H. Li, *J. Am. Chem. Soc.*, **100,** 6248–6249 (1968). (b) M. Kubota, T. Hirayama, O. Nagase, and H. Yajima, *Chem. Pharm. Bull.*, **26,** 2139–2146 (1978).

66. D. Yamishiro, L. F. Tseng, B. A. Doneen, H. H.

Loh, and C. H. Li, *Int. J. Peptide Protein Res.*, **10,** 159–166 (1977).

67. C. H. Li, D. Yamashiro, L. F. Tseng, and H. H. Loh, *Int. J. Peptide Protein Res.*, **11,** 154–158 (1978).
68. D. Yamashiro, C. H. Li, L. F. Tseng, and H. H. Loh, *Int. J. Peptide Protein Res.*, **11,** 251–257 (1978).
69. J. Blake, L. F. Tseng, W. C. Chang, and C. H. Li, *Int. J. Peptide Protein Res.*, **11,** 323–328 (1978).
70. H. W. Yeung, D. Yamashiro, W. C. Chang, and C. H. Li, *Int. J. Peptide Protein Res.*, **12,** 42–46 (1978).
71. J. M. Walker, C. A. Sandman, G. G. Berntson, R. F. McGivern, D. H. Coy, and A. J. Kastin, *Pharmacol. Biochem. Behav.*, **7,** 543–548 (1977).
72. D. DeWied, G. L. Kovacs, B. Bohus, J. M. Van Ree, and H. M. Greven, *Eur. J. Pharmacol.*, **49,** 427–436 (1978).
73. N. S. Kline, C. H. Li, H. E. Lehmann, A. Lajtha, E. Laski, and T. Cooper, *Arch. Gen. Psychiatry*, **34,** 1111–1113 (1977); N. S. Kline and H. E. Lehmann, in *Endorphins in Mental Illness*, E. Usdin and W. E. Bunney, Jr., Eds., Macmillan Press, London, 1978.
74. C. Y. Su, S. H. Lin, Y. T. Wang, C. H. Li, L. H. Hung, C. S. Lin, and B. C. Lin, *J. Formosan Med. Assoc.*, **77,** 133–141 (1973).
75. D. H. Catlin, K. K. Hui, H. H. Loh, and C. H. Li, *Biochem. Psychopharm.*, **18,** 341–350 (1978).
76. Y. Hosabuchi and C. H. Li, *Commun. Psychopharm.*, **2,** 33–37 (1978).
77. K. M. Foley, R. F. Kaiko, C. E. Inturisi, J. B. Posner, C. H. Li, and R. W. Houde, Abstract, Int. Assoc. for the Study of Pain, 2nd Congress, Montreal, Canada, 1978.
78. W. M. A. Verhoeven, H. M. Van Praag, P. A. Botter, A. Sunier, J. M. Van Ree, and D. De-Wied, *Lancet*, 1046–1047 (1978).
79. W. Locke and A. V. Schally, Eds., *The Hypothalamus and Pituitary in Health and Disease*, Thomas, Springfield, Ill., 1972.
80. M. Motta, P. G. Crosignani, and L. Martini, Eds., *Hypothalamic Hormones, Chemistry, Physiology, Pharmacology and Clinical Uses*, Academic Press, New York, 1975.
81. R. Hall and A. Gomez-Pan, *Advan. Clin. Chem.*, **18,** 173–212 (1976).
82. S. Reichlin, R. Saperstein, I. M. D. Jackson, A. E. Boyd III, and Y. Patel, *Ann. Rev. Physiol.* **38,** 389–424 (1976); W. Vale, C. Rivier, and M. Brown, *ibid.*, **39,** 473–527 (1977).
83. A. W. Root, E. O. Reiter, and Y. Weisman, *Advan. Pediatr.*, **23,** 151–211 (1976).
84. A. Arimura and A. V. Schally, in *Hypothalamic Hormones, Chemistry, Physiology, Pharmacology and Clinical Uses*, M. Motta et al., Eds., Academic Press, New York, 1975, pp. 27–42. (a) S. M. McCann, Ed., *Localization of Hypophysiotropic Neurohormones* (Symposium), *Fed. Proc.*, **36,** 1952–1983 (1977); R. Guillemin, *Rec. Progr. Horm. Res.*, **33,** 1–28 (1977).
85. G. M. Besser and C. H. Mortimer, in *Frontiers in Neuroendocrinology*; W. F. Ganong and L. Martini, Eds., Vol. 4, Raven Press, New York, 1976, pp. 227–254; A. V. Schally, *Science*, **206,** 18–28 (1978).
86. A. V. Schally, A. Arimura, Y. Baba, R. M. G. Nair, H. Matsuo, T. W. Redding, L. Debeljuk, and W. F. White, *Biochem. Biophys. Res. Commun.*, **43,** 393–399 (1971).
87. R. Burgus, M. Butcher, N. Ling, M. Monahan, J. Rivier, R. Fellows, M. Amoss, R. Blackwell, W. Vale, and R. Guillemin, *C. R. Hebd. Seances Acad. Sci., Ser. D, Paris*, **273,** 1611–1613 (1971).
88. H. Matsuo, Y. Baba, R. M. G. Nair, A. Arimura, and A. V. Schally, *Biochem. Biophys. Res. Commun.*, **43,** 1334–1339 (1971); H. Matsuo, H. Arimura, R. M. G. Nair, and A. V. Schally, *ibid.*, **45,** 822–827 (1971).
89 A. V. Schally, A. Arimura, and A. J. Kastin, *Science*, **179,** 341–350 (1973).
90. W. Vale, G. Grant, and R. Guillemin, in *Frontiers in Neuroendocrinology*, Vol. 3, W. F. Ganong and L. Martini, Eds., Oxford University Press, New York, 1973, pp. 375–413.
91. E. C. Griffiths, *Hormone Res.*, **7,** 179–191 (1976); S. M. McCann, *New Engl. J. Med.*, **296,** 797–802 (1977).
92. J. F. Wilber, E. Montoya, N. P. Plotnikoff, W. F. White, R. Gendrich, L. Renaud, and J. B. Martin, *Rec. Progr. Hormone Res.*, **32,** 117–159 (1976).
93. A. J. Silverman, *Endocrinology*, **99,** 30–41 (1976); G. Pelletier, R. Leclerc, and D. Dübé, *J. Histochem. Cytochem.*, **24,** 864–871 (1976); J. S. Kizer, M. Palkovitz, M. Tappaz, J. Kebabian, and M. J. Brownstein, *Endocrinology*, **98,** 685–695 (1976).
94. F. A. Momany, *J. Am. Chem. Soc.*, **98,** 2990–2996 (1976); R. Deslauriers, R. A. Komoroski, G. C. Levy, J. H. Seely, and I. C. P. Smith, *Biochemistry*, **15,** 4672–4675 (1976); S. Mabrey and I. M. Klotz, *ibid.*, **15,** 234–242 (1976); P. Marche, T. Monteney-Garestier, P. Fromageot, and C. Helene, *ibid.*, **15,** 5738–5743 (1976).

95. K. Shigezane, S. Hatsuno, N. Takamura, T. Mizoguchi, and S. Sugasawa, *Chem. Pharm. Bull.* (Tokyo), **23,** 2696–2700 (1975).
96. H. Immer, V. R. Nelson, C. Revesz, K. Sestanj, and M. Götz, *J. Med. Chem.* **17,** 1060–1065 (1974).
97. R. Hirschmann and D. F. Veber, in *The Chemistry of Polypeptides*, P. G. Katsoyannis, Ed., Plenum Press, New York, 1973, pp. 125–142.
98. M. Fujino, S. Shinagawa, M. Obayashi, S. Kobayashi, T. Fukuda, I. Yamazaki, R. Nakayama, W. F. White, and R. H. Rippel, *J. Med. Chem.*, **16,** 1144–1147 (1973).
99. M. Fujino, I. Yamazaki, S. Kobayashi, T. Fukuda, S. Shinagawa, R. Nakayama, W. F. White, and R. H. Rippel, *Biochem. Biophys. Res. Commun.*, **57,** 1248–1256 (1974).
100. D. H. Coy, E. J. Coy, A. V. Schally, J. Vilchez-Martinez, Y. Hirotsu, and A. Arimura, *Biochem. Biophys. Res. Commun.*, **57,** 335–340 (1974).
101. M. W. Monahan, M. S. Amoss, H. A. Anderson, and W. Vale, *Biochemistry*, **12,** 4616–4620 (1973).
102. D. H. Coy, F. Labrie, M. Savary, E. J. Coy, and A. V. Schally, *Biochem. Biophys, Res. Commun.*, **67,** 576–582 (1975).
103. A. Arimura, J. A. Vilchez-Martinez, D. H. Coy, E. J. Coy, Y. Hirotsu, and A. V. Schally, *Endocrinology*, **95,** 1174–1177 (1974).
104. M. Fujino, T. Fukuda, S. Shinagawa, S. Kobayashi, I. Yamazaki, R. Nakayama, J. H. Seely, W. F. White, and R. H. Rippel, *Biochem. Biophys. Res. Commun.*, **60,** 406–413 (1974).
105. W. König, J. Sandow, and R. Geiger, in *Peptides: Chemistry, Structure and Biology*, R. Walter and J. Meienhofer, Eds., Ann Arbor Science Publishers, Ann Arbor, Mich., 1975, pp. 883–888.
106. W. Wiegelmann, H. G. Solbach, H. K. Kley, E. Nieschlag, K. H. Rudorff, and H. L. Krüskemper, *Hormone Res.*, **7,** 1–10 (1976).
107. W. Vale, G. Grant, J. Rivier, M. Monahan, M. Amoss, R. Blackwell, R. Burgus, and R. Guillemin, *Science*, **176,** 933–934 (1972).
108. D. H. Coy, E. J. Coy, A. V. Schally, J. A. Vilchez-Martinez, L. Debeljuk, W. H. Carter, and A. Arimura, *Biochemistry*, **13,** 323–326 (1974).
109. F. Labrie, M. Savary, D. H. Coy, E. J. Coy, and A. V. Schally, *Endocrinology*, **98,** 289–294 (1976).
110. R. W. A. Rees, T. J. Foell, S. Y. Chai, and N. Grant, *J. Med. Chem.* **17,** 1016–1019 (1974).
111. J. Rivier, N. Ling, M. Monahan, C. Rivier, M. Brown, and W. Vale, in *Peptides: Chemistry, Structure and Biology*, R. Walter and J. Meienhofer, Eds., Ann Arbor Science Publishers, Ann Arbor, Mich., 1975, pp. 863–870.
112. C. W. Beattie, A. Corbin, T. J. Foell, V. Garsky, W. A. McKinley, R. W. A. Rees, D. Sarantakis, and J. P. Yardley, *J. Med. Chem.*, **18,** 1247–1250 (1975); J. P. Yardley, T. J. Foell, C. W. Beattie, and N. H. Grant, *ibid.*, **18,** 1244–1247 (1975).
113. A. S. Dutta, B. J. A. Furr, and M. B. Giles, in *Peptides 1977, Proceedings of the 5th American Peptide Symposium*, M. Goodman and J. Meienhofer, Eds., Wiley, New York, 1977, pp. 189–192. (a) J. E. Rivier and W. Vale, *Life Sci.*, **23,** 869–876 (1978). (b) J. Humphries, Y.-P. Wan, K. Folkers, and C. Y. Bowers, *J. Med. Chem.*, **20,** 967–969; 1674–1677 (1977); A. V. Schally and D. Coy, in *Hypothalamic Peptide Hormones and Pituitary Regulation*, J. C. Porter, Ed., *Advances in Experimental Medicine and Biology*, Vol. 87, Plenum Press, New York, 1977, pp. 99–121; W. Vale, C. Rivier, M. Brown, and J. Rivier, *ibid.*, pp. 123–156.
114. R. Walter, in *Psychoneuroendocrinology*, N. Hatotani, Ed., Karger, New York, 1974, pp. 285–294; M. E. Celis, S. Taleisnik, and R. Walter, *Proc. Nat. Acad. Sci., US*, **68,** 1428–1433 (1971).
115. R. M. G. Nair, A. J. Kastin, and A. V. Schally, *Biochem. Biophys. Res. Commun.*, **43,** 1376–1381 (1971).
116. A. Vivas and M. E. Celis, in *Peptides: Chemistry, Structure and Biology*, R. Walter and J. Meienhofer, Eds., Ann Arbor Science Publishers, Ann Arbor, Mich., 1975, pp. 777–785; see also pp. 771–776.
117. N. P. Plotnikoff and A. J. Kastin, in *Peptides: Chemistry, Structure and Biology*, R. Walter and J. Meienhofer, Eds., Ann Arbor Science Publishers, Ann Arbor, Mich., 1975, pp. 645–649.
118. G. Pelletier, F. Labrie, A. J. Kastin, D. Coy, and A. V. Schally, *Pharmacol. Biochem. Behav.*, **3,** 675–679 (1975).
119. R. Greenberg, C. E. Whalley, F. Jourdikian, I. S. Mendelson, R. Walter, K. Nicolics, D. H. Coy, A. V. Schally, and A. J. Kastin, *Pharmacol. Biochem. Behav.*, **5,** Suppl. I, 151–158 (1976).
120. A. Dupont, F. Labrie, G. Pelletier, R. Puviani, D. H. Coy, A. V. Schally, and A. J. Kastin, *J. Endocrinol*, **64,** 243–248 (1975).
121. S. Björkman, S. Castensson, B. Lindeke, and H. Sievertsson, *Acta Pharm. Suec.*, **13,** 289–298 (1976).
122. W. Vale, P. Brazeau, G. Grant, A. Nussey, R.

Burgus, J. Rivier, N. Ling and R. Guillemin, *C. R. Acad. Sci. Paris, Ser. D*, **275,** 2913–2916 (1972); R. Burgus, N. Ling, M. Butcher, and R. Guillemin, *Proc. Nat. Acad. Sci., US*, **70,** 684–688 (1973).

123. W. Vale, P. Brazeau, C. Rivier, M. Brown, B. Boss, J. Rivier, R. Burgus, N. Ling, and R. Guillemin, *Rec. Progr. Horm. Res.*, **31,** 365–397 (1975).
124. R. Guillemin and J. E. Gerich. *Ann. Rev. Med.*, **27,** 379–388 (1976).
125. P. Brazeau, W. Vale, R. Burgus, N. Ling, M. Butcher, J. Rivier, and R. Guillemin, *Science*, **179,** 77–79 (1973).
126. A. Arimura, H. Sato, D. H. Coy, and A. V. Schally, *Proc. Soc. Exp. Biol. Med.*, **148,** 784–789 (1975).
127. C. Rufener, M. Amherdt, M. P. Dubois, and L. Orci, *J. Histochem. Cytochem.*, **23,** 966–969 (1975).
128. M. J. Brownstein, M. Palkovits, J. M. Saavedra, and J. S. Kizer, in *Frontiers in Neuroendocrinology*, Vol. 4, W. F. Ganong and L. Martini, Eds., Raven Press, New York, 1976, pp. 1–23; M. Brownstein, A. Arimura, H. Sato, A. V. Schally, and J. S. Kizer, *Endocrinology*, **96,** 1456–1461 (1975).
129. S. Efendic, T. Hokfelt, and R. Luft, *Rev. Invest. Clin.* (Mexico), **28,** 183–199 (1976).
130. E. A. Zimmerman, in *Frontiers in Neuroendocrinology*, Vol. 4, W. F. Ganong and L. Martini, Eds., Raven Press, New York, 1976, pp. 25–62; J. E. Gerich, S. Raptis, and J. Rosenthal, Eds., Somatostatin Symposium, *Metabolism*, **27,** Suppl. 1, 1129–1469 (1978).
131. N. Marks, F. Stern, and M. Benuck, *Nature* (London), **261,** 511–512 (1976); N. Marks and F. Stern, *FEBS Lett.*, **55,** 220–224 (1975); E. C. Griffiths, S. L. Jeffcoate, and D. T. Holland, *Neurosci. Lett.*, **4,** 33–37 (1977).
132. M. Benuck and N. Marks, *Life Sci.*, **19,** 1271–1276 (1976).
133. J. Rivier, M. Brown, and W. Vale, *Biochem. Biophys. Res. Commun.*, **65,** 746–751 (1975).
134. L. J. Deftos, M. Lorenzi, N. Bohanon, E. Tsalakian, V. Schneider, and J. E. Gerich, *J. Clin. Endocrinol. Metab.*, **43,** 205–207 (1976).
135. A. Gomez-Pan, J. D. Reed, M. Albinus, B. Shaw, R. Hall, G. M. Besser, D. H. Coy, A. J. Kastin, and A. V. Schally, *Lancet*, **1,** 888–890 (1975).
136. A. A. J. Barros D'sa, S. R. Bloom, and J. H. Baron, *Lancet*, **1,** 886–887 (1975).
137. R. M. Wilson, G. Boden, L. S. Shore, and N. Essa-Kumar, *Diabetes*, **26,** 7–10 (1977).
138. A. Prange-Hansen, K. Lundback, C. H. Mortimer, G. M. Besser, R. Hall, and A. V. Schally, in *Hypothalamic Hormones, Chemistry, Physiology, Pharmacology and Clinical Uses*, M. Motla et al., Eds., Academic Press, New York, 1975, pp. 337–345.
139. P. Mattes. S. Raptis, T. Heil, H. Rasche, and R. Scheck, *Hormone Metab. Res.*, **7,** 508–511 (1975).
140. H. C. Dollinger, S. Raptis, and E. F. Pfeiffer, *Hormone Metab. Res.*, **8,** 74–78 (1976).
141. N. Fujii and H. Yajima, *Chem. Pharm. Bull.* (Tokyo), **23,** 1596–1603 (1975).
142. A. M. Felix, M. H. Jimenez, T. Mowles, and J. Meienhofer, *Int. J. Peptide Protein Res.*, **11,** 329–339 (1978).
143. D. Sarantakis and W. A. McKinley, *Biochem. Biophys. Res. Commun.*, **54,** 234–238 (1973).
144. H. U. Immer, K. Sestanj, V. R. Nelson, and M. Götz, *Helv. Chim. Acta*, **57,** 730–734 (1974).
145. D. F. Veber, R. G. Strachan, S. J. Bergstrand, F. W. Holly, C. F. Homnick, R. Hirschmann, M. L. Torchiana, and R. Saperstein, *J. Am. Chem. Soc.*, **98,** 2367–2369 (1976).
146. M. Bodanszky and V. du Vigneaud, *J. Am. Chem. Soc.*, **81,** 5688–5691 (1959).
147. J. Meienhofer and K. Kuromizu, *Tetrahedron Lett.*, 3259–3262 (1974); *J. Am. Chem. Soc.*, **96,** 4978–4981 (1974).
148. N. Grant, D. Clark, V. Garsky, I. Jaunakais, W. McGregor, and D. Sarantakis, *Life Sci.*, **19,** 629–632 (1976).
149. S. Efendic, R. Luft, and H. Sievertsson, *FEBS Lett.*, **58,** 302–305 (1975).
150. D. Sarantakis, W. A. McKinley, I. Jaunakais, D. Clark, and N. H. Grant, *Clin. Endocrinol.*, **5,** 275–278 (1976).
151. M. Brown, J. Rivier, and W. Vale, in Glucagon Symposium, R. Unger, Ed., *Metabolism*, **25,** Suppl. 1, 1501–1503 (1976).
152. V. M. Garsky, D. E. Clark, and N. H. Grant, *Biochem. Biophys. Res. Commun.*, **73,** 911–916 (1976).
153. D. Sarantakis, J. Teichman, D. E. Clark, and E. L. Lien, *Biophys, Biochem. Res. Commun.*, **75,** 143–148 (1977).
154. C. Meyers, A. Arimura, A. Gordin, R. Fernandez-Durango, D. H. Coy, A. V. Schally, J. Dronin, L. Ferland, M. Beaulieu, and F. Labrie, *Biophys. Biochem. Res. Commun.*, **74,** 630–636 (1977).
155. J. Rivier, P. Brazeau, W. Vale, and R. Guillemin, *J. Med. Chem.*, **18,** 123–126 (1975).

156. J. E. Rivier, M. R. Brown, and W. Vale, *J. Med. Chem.*, **19,** 1010–1013 (1976).

157. D. Sarantakis, W. A. McKinley, and N. H. Grant, *Biochem. Biophys. Res. Commun.*, **55,** 538–542 (1973).

158. L. Ferland, F. Labrie, D. H. Coy, A. Arimura, and A. V. Schally, *Mol. Cell. Endocrinol.*, **4,** 79–88 (1976).

159. P. Brazeau, W. Vale, J. Rivier, and R. Guillemin, *Biochem. Biophys. Res. Commun.*, **60,** 1202–1207 (1974).

160. S. Ohashi, S. Sawano, T. Kokubu, M. Gondo, and K. Sakakibara, *Endocrinol. Japan*, **23,** 435–438 (1976).

161. R. Burgus, T. F. Dunn, D. M. Desiderio, D. N. Ward, W. Vale, R. Guillemin, A. M. Felix, D. Gillessen, and R. O. Studer, *Endocrinology*, **86,** 573–582 (1970).

162. J. Rivier, W. Vale, M. Monahan, N. Ling, and R. Burgus, *J. Med. Chem.*, **15,** 479–482 (1972).

163. H. H. Keller, G. Bartholini, and A. Pletscher, *Nature* (London), **248,** 528–529 (1974).

164. T. Hökfelt, K. Fuxe, O. Jahansson, S. Jeffcoate, and N. White, *Eur. J. Pharmacol.*, **34,** 389–392 (1975).

165. J. M. Cott, G. R. Breese, B. R. Cooper, T. S. Barlow, and A. J. Prange, Jr., *J. Pharmacol. Exp. Ther.*, **196,** 594–604 (1976). (a) B. J. Ormston, R. Garry, R. J. Cryer, G. M. Besser, and R. Hall, *Lancet*, **2,** 10–14 (1971).

166. C. Hatanaka, M. Obayashi, O. Nishimura, N. Toukai, and M. Fujino, *Biochem. Biophys. Res. Commun.*, **60,** 1345–1350 (1974). (a) S. Bajusz and I. Fauszt, *Acta Chim. Hung.*, **75,** 419–422 (1973).

167. G. Mattalia and O. Bucciarelli, *Experientia*, **31,** 874–875 (1975).

168. M. Monahan, J. Rivier, W. Vale, N. Ling, G. Grant, M. Amoss, R. Guillemin, R. Burgus, E. Nicolaides, and M. Rebstock, in *Chemistry and Biology of Peptides*, J. Meienhofer, Ed., Ann Arbor Science Publishers, Ann Arbor, Mich., 1972, pp. 601–608

169. B. Donzel, J. Rivier, and M. Goodman, *Biopolymers*, **13,** 2631–2647 (1974).

170. M. Montagut, B. Lemanceau, and A. M. Bellocq, *Biopolymers*, **13,** 2615–2629 (1974).

171. B. Donzel, M. Goodman, J. Rivier, N. Ling, and W. Vale, *Nature* (London), **256,** 750–751 (1975).

172. A. J. Prange, Jr., G. R. Breese, G. D. Jahuke, B. R. Martin, B. R. Cooper, J. M. Cott, I. C. Wilson, L. B. Alltop, M. A. Lipton, G. Bissette, C. B. Nemeroff, and P. T. Loosen, *Life Sci.*, **16,** 1907–1914 (1975).

173. G. Zetler, *Biochem. Pharmacol.*, **25,** 1817–1818 (1976).

174. C. Rivier, M. Brown, and W. Vale, *Endocrinology*, **100,** 751–754 (1977).

175. M. M. Chang, S. E. Leeman, and H. D. Niall, *Nature New Biol.*, **232,** 86–87 (1971); R. Carraway and S. E. Leeman, *J. Biol. Chem.*, **248,** 6854–6861 (1973); *ibid.*, **250,** 1907–1911; 1912–1918 (1975).

176. K. Kitagawa, T. Akita, T. Segawa, M. Nakano, N. Fujii, and H. Yajima, *Chem. Pharm. Bull.* (Tokyo), **24,** 2692–2698 (1976); H. Yajima, K. Kitagawa, T. Segawa, M. Nakano, and K. Katooka, *ibid.*, **24,** 544–546 (1976); **23,** 3299–3300 (1975).

177. F. Lembeck and G. Zetler, in *International Encyclopedia of Pharmacology and Therapeutics*, Sect. 72, Vol. 1, J. M. Walker, Ed., Pergamon Press, New York, 1972, pp. 29–71.

178. S. E. Leeman and E. A. Mroz, *Life Sci.*, **15,** 2033–2044 (1974); U. S. von Euler and B. Pernow, *Substance P*, Nobel Symposia, Vol. 37, Raven Press, New York, 1977; P. Skrabanek and D. Powell, *Substance P*, Annual Research Review, Eden Press, Montreal, Quebec, 1977.

179. P. Stern, S. Ćatović, and M. Stern, *Naunyn-Schmiedeberg's Arch. Pharmacol.*, **281,** 233–239 (1974).

180. T. Takahashi, S. Konishi, D. Powell, S. E. Leeman, and M. Otsuka, *Brain Res.*, **73,** 59–69 (1974).

181. G. R. Uhl and S. H. Snyder, *Eur. J. Pharmacol.*, **41,** 89–91 (1977); G. R. Uhl, J. P. Bennett, Jr., and S. Snyder, *Brain Res.*, **130,** 299–313 (1977).

182. G. Bissette, C. B. Nemeroff, P. T. Loosen, A. J. Prange, Jr., and M. A. Lipton, *Nature* (London), **262,** 607–609 (1976).

183. R. E. Carraway, L. M. Demers, and S. Leeman, *Endocrinology*, **99,** 1452–1462 (1976). (a) J. E. Rivier, L. H. Lazarus, M. H. Perrin, and M. R. Brown, *J. Med. Chem.*, **20,** 1409–1412 (1977).

184. C. H. Li, *Proc. Am. Phil. Soc.*, **116,** 365–382 (1972). (a) S. Udenfriend, M. Rubinstein, and S. Stein, in *Endorphins in Mental Health Research*, E. Usdin and W. E. Bunney, Eds., Macmillan Press, London, 1978, pp. 119–130.

185. C. H. Li, T. Hayashida, B. A. Doneen, and A. J. Rao, *Proc. Nat. Acad. Sci., US*, **73,** 3463–3465 (1976); C. H. Li and T. A. Bewley, *ibid.*, **73,** 1476–1479 (1976).

186. K. J. Catt and M. L. Dufau, *Ann. Rev. Physiol.*, **39,** 529–557 (1977).

187. F. M. Finn and K. Hofmann, *Acc. Chem. Res.*, **6,** 169–176 (1973); F. M. Finn, P. A. Johns, N.

Nishi, and K. Hofmann, *J. Biol. Chem.*, **251,** 3576–3585 (1976).

188. U. Lang, R. Schwyzer, D. Schulster, R. A. J. McIlhinney, and P. Cohen, in *Peptide Hormones*, J. A. Parsons, Ed., University Park Press, Baltimore, 1976, pp. 337–372.
189. R. Schwyzer and W. Rittel. *Helv. Chim. Acta*, **44,** 159–169 (1961); H. Kappeler and R. Schwyzer, *ibid.*, **44,** 1136–1141 (1961).
190. L. Graf, S. Bajusz, A. Patthy, E. Barat, and G. Cseh, *Acta Biochem. Biophys. Hung.*, **6,** 415–418 (1971).
191. A. Jöhl, B. Riniker, and L. Schenkel-Hulliger, *FEBS Lett.*, **45,** 172–174 (1974).
192. C. H. Li, *Advan. Protein Chem.*, **11,** 101–190 (1956).
193. J. Ramachandran, in *Hormonal Proteins and Peptides*, Vol. 2, C. H. Li, Ed., Academic Press, New York, 1973, pp. 1–28.
194. A. P. Scott, G. A. Bloomfield, P. J. Lowry, J. J. H. Gilkes, J. Landon, and L. H. Rees, in *Peptide Hormones*, J. A. Parsons, Ed., University Park Press, Baltimore, 1976, pp. 247–271.
195. T. H. Lee, D. Nelson, H. Matsuyama, A. Ruhmann-Wennhold, J. Kowal, H. E. Lebovitz, G. Sayers, N. D. Giordano, R. S. Yalow, S. A. Berson, R. J. Lefkowits, J. Roth, I. Pastan, C. Footier, F. Labrie, A. Brodish, and G. W. Little, in *Methods in Investigative and Diagnostic Endocrinology*, Vol. 2A, S. A. Berson and R. S. Yalow Eds., Elsevier, New York, 1973, pp. 331–404.
196. M. Löw, L. Kisfaludy, and S. Fermandjian, *Acta Biochem. Biophys. Hung.*, **10,** 229–231 (1975); D. Greff, F. Toma, S. Fermandjian, M. Löw, and L. Kisfaludy, *Biochim. Biophys. Acta*, **439,** 219–231 (1976).
197. R. Schwyzer and P. Sieber, *Nature* (London), **199,** 172–174 (1963).
198. K. Inouye, K. Watanabe, and H. Otsuka, *Bull. Chem. Soc. Japan*, **50,** 211–219 (1977).
199. K. Koyama, H. Watanabe, H. Kawatani, J. Iwai, and H. Yajima, *Chem. Pharm. Bull.* (Tokyo), **24,** 2558–2563 (1976).
200. F. Weygand, P. Huber, and K. Weiss, *Z. Naturforsch.*, **22b,** 1084–1085 (1967); T. Wieland, C. Birr, and F. Flor, *Angew. Chem. Int. Ed.*, **10,** 336; *Justus Liebigs Ann. Chem.*, 1595–1600; 1601–1605 (1973).
201. S. Lemaire, D. Yamashiro, C. Behrens, and C. H. Li., *J. Am. Chem. Soc.*, **99,** 1577–1580 (1977); D. Yamashiro and C. H. Li, *ibid.*, **95,** 1310–1315 (1973).
202. R. A. Boissonnas, S. Guttmann, and J. Pless, *Experientia*, **22,** 526 (1966).
203. P. A. Desaulles, B. Riniker, and W. Rittel, *Excerpta Medica, Int. Congr. Ser.*, No. 161, 489–491 (1968).
204. R. Geiger, *Justus Liebigs Ann. Chem.*, **750,** 165–170 (1971).
205. R. Schwyzer, P. Schiller, S. Seelig, and G. Sayers, *FEBS Lett.*, **19,** 229–231 (1971).
206. K. Hofmann, R. H. Andreatta, H. Bohn, and L. Moroder, *J. Med. Chem.*, **13,** 339–345 (1970).
207. R. Schwyzer, in *Peptides 1972*, H. Hanson and H. D. Jakubke, Eds., Elsevier, New York, 1973, pp. 424–436.
208. Y. Birk and C. H. Li, *J. Biol. Chem.*, **239,** 1048–1052 (1964); C. H. Li, L. Barnafi, M. Chretien, and D. Chung, *Nature* (London), **208,** 1093–1094 (1965).
209. M. Chretien, in *Methods in Investigative and Diagnostic Endocrinology*, Vol. 2A, S. A. Berson and R. S. Yalow, Eds., Elsevier, New York, 1973, pp. 617–632.
210. J. I. Harris, *Nature* (London), **184,** 167–169 (1959); H. B. F. Dixon, *Biochem. Biophys. Acta*, **37,** 38–42 (1960).
211. A. B. Lerner, T. H. Lee, D. P. Island, G. W. Liddle, A. J. Kastin, and A. V. Schally, in *Methods in Investigative and Diagnostic Endocrinology*, Vol. 2A, S. A. Berson and R. S. Yalow, Eds., Elsevier, New York, 1973, pp. 405-431; C. H. Li, in *Hormonal Proteins and Peptides*, Vol. 5, C. H. Li, Ed., Academic Press, New York, 1978, pp. 1–33.
212. H. Yajima and Y. Kiso, *Pharmacol. Ther. B*, **1,** 529–543 (1975).
213. A. Eberle, J. L. Fauchére, G. Tesser, and R. Schwyzer, *Helv. Chim. Acta*, **58,** 2106–2129 (1975); A. Eberle and R. Schwyzer, *ibid.*, **58,** 1528–1535 (1975).
214. A. P. Scott and P. J. Lowry, *Biochem. J.*, **139,** 593–602 (1974).
215. G. L. Dempsey, A. J. Kastin, and A. V. Schally, *Horm. Behav.*, **3,** 333–337 (1972); A. J. Kastin, C. Nissen, K. Nikolics, K. Medzihradszky, D. H. Coy, I. Teplan, and A. V. Schally, *Brain Res. Bull.*, **1,** 19–26 (1976); N. P. Plotnikoff and A. J. Kastin, *Life Sci.*, **18,** 1217–1222 (1976).
216. A. J. Kastin, L. H. Miller, D. Gonzalez-Barcena, W. D. Hawley, K. Dyster-Aas, A. V. Schally, M. L. Velasco De Parra, and M. Velasco, *Physiol. Behav.*, **7,** 893–896 (1971).
217. D. deWied, A. Witter, and H. M. Greven, *Biochem. Pharmacol.*, **24,** 1463–1468 (1975).
218. W. H. Bishop, A. Nureddin, and R. J. Ryan, in *Peptide Hormones*, J. A. Parsons, Ed., University Park Press, Baltimore, 1976, pp. 273–298.

219. E. Steinberger, *Pharmacol. Ther. B*, **2,** 771–786 (1976).

220. J. L. Vaitukaitis, G. T. Ross, G. D. Braunstein, and P. L. Rayford, *Rec. Progr. Horm. Res.*, **32,** 289–331 (1976).

221. N. R. Moudgal, Ed., *Gonadotropins and Gonadal Function*, Academic Press, New York, 1974.

222. M. R. Sairam and C. H. Li, in *Hormonal Proteins and Peptides*, Vol. 1, C. H. Li, Ed., Academic Press, New York, 1973, pp. 101–169.

223. H. Papkoff, in *Hormonal Proteins and Peptides*, Vol. 1, C. H. Li, Ed., Academic Press, New York, 1973, pp. 59–100; H. Papkoff, M. R. Sairam, S. W. Farmer, and C. H. Li., *Rec. Progr. Horm. Res.*, **29,** 563–590 (1973); D. N. Ward, L. E. Reichert, Jr., W. K. Liu, H. S. Nahm, J. Hsia, W. M. Lamkin, and N. S. Jones, *ibid.*, **29,** 533–561 (1973); N. R. Moudgal, A. Jagannadha, R. Maneckjee, K. Muralidhar, V. Mukku, and C. S. Sheela Rani, *ibid.*, **30,** 47–77 (1974).

224. L. E. Reichert, Jr., W. R. Butt, P. Franchimont, R. Guillemin, M. Amoss, R. Burgus, J. L. Gabrilove, N. Kase, and L. Sobrinho, in *Methods in Investigative and Diagnostic Endocrinology*, Vol. 2A, S. A. Berson and G. S. Yalow, Eds., Elsevier, New York, 1973, pp. 509–558.

225. M. R. Sairam and C. H. Li, *Arch. Biochem. Biophys.*, **165,** 709–714 (1974); J. G. Pierce, T. H. Liao, and R. B. Carlsen, in *Hormonal Proteins and Peptides*, Vol. 1, C. H. Li, Ed., Academic Press, New York, 1973, pp. 17–57.

226. J. G. Pierce, M. R. Faith, L. C. Guidice, and J. R. Reeve, in *Polypeptide Hormones: Molecular and Cellular Aspects*, R. Porter and P. W. Fitzsimmons, Eds., Ciba Foundation Symposium No. 41, Excerpta Medica, New York, 1976, pp. 225–250; J. G. Pierce, in *Methods in Investigative and Diagnostic Endocrinology*, Vol. 2A, S. A. Berson and G. S. Yalow, Eds., Elsevier, New York, 1973, pp. 433–445.

227. J. S. Cornell and J. G. Pierce, *J. Biol. Chem.*, **249,** 4166–4174 (1974); D. Chung, M. R. Sairam, and C. H. Li, *Arch. Biochem. Biophys.*, **159,** 678–682 (1973); Y. Combarnous and G. Hennen, *Biochem. Soc. Trans.*, **2,** 915–917 (1974). (a) P. G. Condliffe, J. L. Bakke, W. D. Odell, R. D. Utiger, J. M. Lowenstein, J. R. Hargadine, F. S. Greenspan, R. Guillemin, W. Vale, R. Burgus, J. Robbins, and J. E. Rall, in *Methods in Investigative and Diagnostic Endocrinology*, Vol. 2A, S. A. Berson and G. S. Yalow, Eds., Elsevier, New York, 1973, pp. 447–507. (b) M. R. Sairam and C. H. Li, *Biochem. Biophys. Res. Commun.*, **54,** 426–431 (1973). (c) B. R. Smith and R. Hall, in *Peptide Hormones*, J. A. Parsons, Ed., University Park Press, Baltimore, 1976, pp. 233–246. (d) M. R. Sairam and C. H. Li, *Can. J. Biochem.*, **55,** 755–760 (1977); in *Hormonal Proteins and Peptides*, Vol. 6, C. H. Li, Ed., Academic Press, New York, 1978,

228. C. S. Nicoll and H. A. Bern, in *Lactogenic Hormones*, G. E. W. Wolstenholme and J. Knight, Eds., Churchill-Livingston, London, 1972, pp. 299–317.

229. S. W. Farmer, H. Papkoff, T. A. Bewley, T. Hayashida, R. S. Nishioka, H. A. Bern, and C. H. Li, *Gen. Comp. Endocrinol.*, **31,** 60–71 (1977).

230. H. Papkoff, *Proc. Soc. Exp. Biol. Med.*, **153,** 498–500 (1976).

231. C. H. Li, *Int. J. Peptide Protein Res.*, **8,** 205–224 (1976). (a) B. Shome and A. F. Parlow, *J. Clin. Endocrinol. Metab.*, **45,** 1112–1115 (1977).

232. A. G. Frantz, in *Frontiers in Neuroendocrinology*, Vol. 3, W. F. Ganong and L. Martini, Eds., Oxford University Press, New York, 1973, pp. 337–374.

233. A. G. Frantz, *New Engl. J. Med.*, **298,** 201–207. (1978).

234. A. G. Frantz, in *Peptide Hormones*, J. A. Parsons, Ed., University Park Press, Baltimore, 1976, pp. 199–230.

235. C. H. Li, J. Meites, C. S. Nicoll, T. Hayashida, G. D. Bryant, F. C. Greenwood, H. Friesen, H. Guyda, and P. Hwang, in *Methods in Investigative and Diagnostic Endocrinology*, Vol. 2A, S. A. Berson and G. S. Yalow, Eds., Elsevier, New York, 1973, pp. 559–615; H.-D. Dellman, J. A. Johnson, and D. M. Klachko, Eds., *Comparative Endocrinology of Prolactin*, Plenum Publ. Corp., New York, 1977.

236. G. E. W. Wolstenholme and J. Knight, Eds., *Lactogenic Hormones*, Churchill-Livingston, London, 1972.

237. C. H. Li, M. S. Raben, J. N. Fain, M. P. Czech, R. Saperstein, H. M. Goodman, J. L. Kostyo, W. H. Daughaday, A. E. Wilhelmi, S. A. Berson, R. S. Yalow, S. M. Glick, A. V. Schally, and A. Arimura, in *Methods in Investigative and Diagnostic Endocrinology*, Vol. 2A, S. A. Berson and G. S. Yalow, Eds., Elsevier, New York, 1973, pp. 257–329.

238. A. Pecile and E. E. Müller, Eds., *Growth and Growth Hormone*, Excerpta Medica, Amsterdam, 1972. (a) L. L. Spielman and F. C. Bancroft, *Endocrinology*, **101,** 651–658 (1977).

239. C. H. Li, in *Hormonal Proteins and Peptides*, Vol. 3, C. H. Li., Ed., Academic Press, New York, 1975, pp. 1–40.

240. S. Raiti, Ed., *Advances in Human Growth Hormone Research*, US Department of Health, Education and Welfare Publication No. (NIH) 74–612, 1972.

241. C. H. Li and L. Gráf, *Proc. Nat. Acad. Sci., US*, **71,** 1197–1201 (1974). (a) C. H. Li and T. A. Bewley, *ibid.*, **73,** 1476–1479 (1976); C. H. Li, T. Hayashida, B. A. Doneen, and A. J. Rao, *ibid.*, **73,** 3463–3465 (1976).

242. F. M. Richards and P. J. Vithayathil, *J. Biol. Chem.*, **234,** 1459–1465 (1959).

243. H. Taniuchi and C. B. Anfinsen, *J. Biol. Chem.*, **243,** 4778–4786 (1968).

244. C. B. Anfinsen and H. A. Scheraga, *Adv. Protein Chem.*, **29,** 205–300 (1975).

245. A. W. Root, *Human Pituitary Growth Hormone*, C. Thomas, Springfield, IL., 1972.

246. J. M. Tanner, *Nature* (London), **237,** 433–439 (1972).

247. P. Vanamee, P. Sherlock, and S. J. Winawer, *Gastroenterology*, **62,** 824–825 (1972).

248. S. B. Chyatte, D. Rudman, J. H. Patterson, G. G. Gerron, I. F. O'Beirne, J. A. Barlow, P. Ahman, A. Jordan, and R. C. Mosteller, *Arch. Phys. Med. Rehabil.*, **53,** 470–475 (1972).

249. R. Walter, Ed., *Neurophysins, Carriers of Peptide Hormones, Ann. N.Y. Acad. Sci.*, **248** (1975).

250. B. T. Pickering and C. W. Jones, in *Hormonal Proteins and Peptides*, Vol. 5, C. H. Li, Ed., Academic Press, Inc., New York, 1978, pp. 103–185.

251. V. du Vigneaud, C. Ressler, J. M. Swan, C. W. Roberts, P. G. Katsoyannis, and S. Gordon, *J. Am. Chem. Soc.*, **75,** 4879–4880 (1953).

252. J. Rudinger, in *Drug Design*, Vol. 2, E. J. Ariëns, Ed., Academic Press, New York, 1971, pp. 319–419.

253. M. Manning, J. Lowbridge, J. Haldar, and W. H. Sawyer, *Fed. Proc.*, **36,** 1848–1852 (1977).

254. M. Zaoral, F. Brtnik, T. Barth, and A. Machova, *Endocrinol. Exp.*, **10,** 183–191 (1976).

255. R. Walter, C. W. Smith, P. K. Mehta, S. Boonjarern, J. A. L. Arruda, and N. A. Kurtzman, in *Disturbances in Body Fluid Osmolality*, T. E. Andreoli et al., Eds., American Physiological Society Publication, 1977, pp. 1–36; R. Walter, in *Endocrinology*, Vol. 2, V. H. T. James, Ed., *Excerpta Medica International Congress Series*, No. 403, Amsterdam, 1977, pp. 553–560.

256. B. M. Altura and B. T. Altura, *Fed. Proc.*, **36,** 1853–1860 (1977)

257. B. M. Altura, Ed., *Comparative Cellular and Pharmacological Actions of Neurohypophyseal Hormones on Smooth Muscle* (Symposium), *Fed. Proc.*, **36,** 1840–1878 (1977).

258. G. W. Bisset, in *Peptide Hormones*, J. A. Parsons, Ed., University Park Press, Baltimore, 1976, pp. 145–177.

259. R. Acher, in *Handbook of Physiology*, Section 7, *Endocrinology*, Part 1, American Physiological Society, Washington, D.C., 1974, pp. 119–130.

260. G. L. Robertson, *Ann. Rev. Med.*, **25,** 315–322 (1974).

261. E. A. Popenoe, C. Ressler, H. Sachs, A. Leaf, F. C. Bartter, L. Share, G. L. Robertson, J. Roth, C. Beardwell, L. A. Klein, M. J. Peterson, P. Gordon, S. M. Glick, R. J. Fitzpatrick, and F. Fuchs, in *Methods in Investigative and Diagnostic Endocrinology*, Vol. 2A, S. A. Berson and R. S. Yalow, Eds., Elsevier, New York, 1973, pp. 633–711.

262. W. H. Sawyer and M. Manning, *Annu. Rev. Pharmacol.*, **13,** 5–17 (1973).

263. W. H. Sawyer, *Fed. Proc.*, **36,** 1842–1847 (1977).

264. R. Acher, J. Chauvet, and M. T. Chauvet, *Nature New Biol.*, **244,** 124–126 (1973).

265. B. M. Altura, *Fed. Proc.*, **36,** 1840–1841 (1977).

266. R. Walter and C. W. Smith, private communication of latest bioassay data from literature card file, 1977. Cf. Ref. 280.

267. D. W. Urry and R. Walter, *Proc. Nat. Acad. Sci., US*, **68,** 956–958 (1971).

268. R. Walter, A. Ballardin, I. L. Schwartz, W. A. Gibbons, and H. R. Wyssbrod, *Proc. Nat. Acad. Sci., US*, **71,** 4528–4532 (1974).

269. R. Walter, *Fed. Proc.*, **36,** 1872–1878 (1977).

270. M. Bodanszky and V. du Vigneaud, *J. Am. Chem. Soc.*, **81,** 2504–2507 (1959).

271. J. Rudinger, J. Honzl, and M. Zaoral, *Coll. Czech. Chem. Commun.*, **21,** 202–210 (1956).

272. M. Wälti and D. B. Hope, *Experientia*, **29,** 389 (1973).

273. P. G. Pietta and G. R. Marshall, *J. Chem. Soc., D, Chem. Commun.*, 650–651 (1970).

274. E. Schröder and K. Lübke, *The Peptides*, Vol. 2, Academic Press, New York, 1966.

275. B. Berde and R. A. Boissonnas, in *Handbook of Experimental Pharmacology*, Vol. 23, O, Eichler et al., Eds., Springer, New York, 1968, pp. 802–870.

276. M. Manning, L. Balaspiri, M. Acosta, and W. H. Sawyer, *J. Med. Chem.*, **16,** 975–978 (1973); W. H. Sawyer, M. Acosta, L. Balaspiri, J. Judd, and M. Manning, *Endocrinology*, **94,** 1106–1115 (1974).

277. M. Zaoral and I. Blápa, *Coll. Czech. Chem. Commun.*, **42,** 3654–3657 (1977).

278. (a) H. Schulz and V. du Vigneaud, *J. Med. Chem.*, **9,** 647–650 (1966). (b) E. O. Lundell and M. F. Ferger, *J. Med. Chem.*, **18,** 1045–1047 (1975).

279. P. Marbach and J. Rudinger, *Experientia*, **30,** 696 (1974).

280. G. L. Stahl and R. Walter, *J. Med. Chem.*, **20,** 492–495 (1977).

281. J. Lowbridge, M. Manning, J. Haldar, and W. H. Sawyer, *J. Med. Chem.*, **20,** 120–123 (1977).

282. (a) C. W. Smith, C. R. Botos, and R. Walter, in *Peptides 1977, Proceedings of the Fifth American Peptide Symposium*, M. Goodman and J. Meienhofer, Eds., Wiley, New York, 1978, pp. 161–164. (b) C. W. Smith and R. Walter, *Science*, **199,** 297–299 (1978).

283. J. M. Beazley, *Sci. Basis Med., Ann. Rev.*, **80** (1973).

284. I. Vavra, A. Machova, V. Holecek, J. H. Cort, M. Zaoral, and F. Sorm, *Lancet*, **1,** 948–952 (1968).

285. J. T. Potts, Jr., D. H. Copp, P. F. Hirsch, C. W. Cooper P. L. Munson, R. S. Yalow, S. A. Berson, C. D. Arnaud, G. S. Gordan, B. S. Roof, A. H. Tashjian, Jr., A. D. Care, and G. A. Williams, in *Methods in Investigative and Diagnostic Endocrinology*, Vol. 2B, S. A. Berson and R. A. Yalow, Eds., Elsevier, New York, 1973, pp. 945–1026.

286. J. T. Potts, Jr., in *Peptide Hormones*, J. A. Parsons, Ed., University Park Press, Baltimore, 1976, pp. 119–142.

287. J. F. Habener, B. W. Kemper, A. Rich, and J. T. Potts, Jr., *Rec. Progr. Horm. Res.*, **33,** 249–308 (1977). (a) J. F. Habener, M. Rosenblatt, B. Kemper, H. M. Kronenberg, A. Rich, and J. T. Potts, Jr., *Proc. Nat. Acad. Sci., US*, **75,** 2616–2620 (1978).

288. H. Rasmussen and L. C. Craig, *J. Biol. Chem.*, **236,** 759–764 (1961).

289. H. T. Keutmann, G. D. Aurbach, B. F. Dawson, H. D. Niall, L. J. Deftos, and J. T. Potts, Jr., *Biochemistry*, **10,** 2779–2787 (1971).

290. H. T. Keutmann, M. M. Sauer, G. N. Hendy, J. L. H. O'Riordan, and J. T. Potts, Jr., *Biochemistry*, **17** (1978).

291. J. F. Habener and J. T. Potts, Jr., in *Handbook of Physiology*, Part VII, *Endocrinology*, American Physiological Society, Washington, D.C., 1976, pp. 313–342.

292. G. D. Aurbach, H. T. Keutmann, H. D. Niall, G. W. Tregear, J. L. H. O'Riordan, R. Marcus, S. J. Marx, and J. T. Potts, Jr., *Rec. Progr. Horm. Res.*, **28,** 353–398 (1972).

293. W. A. Peck, K. Messinger, G. Kimmich, and J. Carpenter, *Endocrinology*, **95,** 289–298 (1974).

294. J. F. Habener, J. T. Potts, Jr., and A. Rich, *J. Biol. Chem.*, **251,** 3893–3899 (1976).

295. G. W. Tregear, J. van Rietschoten, E. Green, H. D. Niall, H. T. Keutmann, J. A. Parsons, J. L. H. O'Riordan, and J. T. Potts, Jr., *Hoppe-Seyler's Z. Physiol. Chem.*, **355,** 415–421 (1974).

296. G. W. Tregear, in *Chemistry and Biology of Peptides*, J. Meienhofer, Ed., Ann Arbor Science Publishers, Ann Arbor, Mich., 1972, pp. 175–178.

297. N. H. Bell and P. H. Stern, *Am. J. Physiol.*, **218,** 64–68 (1970); G. L. Melson, L. R. Chase, and G. D. Aurbach, *Endocrinology*, **86,** 511–518 (1970).

298. T. K. Gray and P. L. Munson, *Science*, **166,** 512–513 (1969).

299. H. Rasmussen, M. Wong, D. Bikle, and D. B. P. Goodman, *J. Clin. Invest.*, **51,** 2502–2504 (1972).

300. A. H. Tashjian, Jr., B. G. Howland, K. E. W. Melvin, and C. S. Hill, Jr., *New Engl. J. Med.*, **283,** 890–895 (1970).

301. L. J. Deftos, *J. Am. Med. Assoc.*, **227,** 403–406 (1974).

302. F. R. Singer, *Postgrad. Med.*, **57** (3), 117–120 (1975).

303. S. F. Queener and N. H. Bell, *Metabolism*, **24,** 555–567 (1975).

304. H. Rasmussen and M. M. Pechet, *Sci. Am.*, **223** (4), 42–50 (1970).

305. S. Guttmann, J. Pless, R. L. Huguenin, E. Sandrin, H. Bossert, and K. Zehnder, *Helv. Chim. Acta*, **52,** 1789–1795 (1969).

306. P. Rivaille and G. Milhaud, *Helv. Chim. Acta*, **55,** 1617–1619 (1972); D. A. Ontjes, J. C. Roberts, J. F. Hennessy, H. J. Burford, and C. W. Cooper, *Endocrinology*, **92,** 1780–1785 (1973).

307. W. Rittel, R. Maier, M. Brugger, B. Kamber, B. Riniker, and P. Sieber, *Experientia*, **32,** 246–248 (1976).

308. R. Maier, B. Kamber, R. Riniker, and W. Rittel, *Horm. Metab. Res.*, **7,** 511–514 (1975).

309. R. Maier, B. Kamber, B. Riniker, and W. Rittel, *Clin. Endocrinol.*, **5,** Suppl., 327s–332s (1976).

310. J. F. A. P. Miller and D. Osoba, in *Nature and Origin of Immunologically Competent Cells*, G. E. W. Wolstenholme and J. Knight, Eds., Ciba Foundation Study Group, No. 16, Churchill, London, 1963, pp. 62–70.

311. D. H. Schlesinger and G. Goldstein, *Cell*, **5,** 361–366 (1975).

312. A. L. Goldstein, T. L. K. Low, M. McAdoo, J. McClure, G. B. Thurman, J. Rossio, C. Y. Lai, D. Chang, S. S. Wang, C. Harvey, A. H. Ramel, and J. Meienhofer, *Proc. Nat. Acad. Sci. US*, **74,** 725–729 (1977).

313. J.-F. Bach, M. Dardenne, J.-M. Pleau, and J. Rosa, *C.R. Acad. Sci. Paris*, **283,** 1605–1607 (1976); E. Bricas, J. Martinez, D. Blanot, G. Auger, M. Dardenne, J. M. Pleau, and J. F. Bach, in *Peptides 1977, Proceedings of the Fifth American Peptide Symposium*, M. Goodman and J. Meienhofer, Eds., Wiley, New York, 1978, pp. 564–567.

314. A. I. Kook, Y. Yakir, and N. Trainin, *Cell. Immunol.*, **19,** 151–157 (1975).

315. J.-F. Bach and C. Carnaud, *Progr. Allergy*, **21,** 342–408 (1976).

316. N. Trainin, *Physiol. Res.*, **54,** 272–315 (1974).

317. A. L. Goldstein and A. White, in *Contemporary Topics in Immunobiology*, Vol. 2, A. J. S. Davies and R. L. Carter, Eds., Plenum Press, New York, 1973, pp. 339–350.

318. T. D. Luckey, Ed., *Thymic Hormones*, University Park Press, Baltimore, 1973.

318a. G. Goldstein, *Nature* (London), **247,** 11–14 (1974); D. H. Schlesinger, G. Goldstein, and H. D. Niall, *Biochemistry*, **14,** 2214–2218 (1975).

319. A. L. Goldstein, F. D. Slater, and A. White, *Proc. Nat. Acad. Sci., US*, **56,** 1010–1017 (1966).

320. J. A. Hooper, M. C. McDaniel, G. B. Thurman, G. H. Cohen, R. S. Schulof, and A. L. Goldstein, *Ann. N.Y. Acad. Sci.*, **249,** 125–144 (1975).

321. A. L. Goldstein, J. A. Hooper, R. S. Schulof, G. H. Cohen, G. B. Thurman, M. C. McDaniel, A. White, and M. Dardenne, *Fed. Proc.*, **33,** 2053–2056 (1974).

322. (a) A. L. Goldstein, G. H. Cohen, J. L. Rossio, G. B. Thurman, C. N. Brown, and J. T. Ulrich, *Med. Clin. N. Am.*, **60,** 591–606 (1976). (b) M. H. Cohen, P. B. Chretien, D. C. Ihde, B. E. Fossieck, Jr., P. A. Bunn, D. E. Kenady, S. D. Lipson, and J. D. Minna, *Am. Assoc. Cancer Res., Abstracts*, No. 466, 1978.

323. G. Goldstein, *Nature* (London), **247,** 11–14 (1974).

324. K. Komuro and E. A. Boyse, *Lancet*, **1,** 740–743 (1973).

325. D. H. Schlesinger, G. Goldstein, M. P. Scheid, and E. A. Boyse, *Cell*, **5,** 367–370 (1975).

326. D. S. H. W. Nicol and L. F. Smith, *Nature* (London), **187,** 483–485 (1960).

327. J. Thomsen, K. Kristiansen, K. Brunfeldt, and F. Sundby, *FEBS Lett.*, **21,** 315–319 (1972).

328. L. Orci, in Glucagon Symposium, R. Unger, Ed., *Metabolism*, **25,** Suppl. 1, 1303–1313 (1976).

329. A. Marble, *Diabetes*, **21,** 632–636, (1972).

330. D. E. McMillan, *Diabetes*, **24,** 944–957 (1975); E. M. Kohner and N. W. Oakley, *Metabolism*, **24,** 1085–1102 (1975).

331. S. S. Fajans, *Diabetes*, **21,** 678–684 (1972).

332. A. Y. Chang, *Ann. Rep. Med. Chem.*, **11,** 170–179 (1976).

333. R. Unger, *Diabetes*, **25,** 136–151 (1976).

334. J. J. Abel, *Proc. Nat. Acad. Sci., US*, **12,** 132–136 (1926).

335. K. Freudenberg, W. Dirscherl, and H. Eyer, *Hoppe-Seyler's Z. Physiol. Chem.*, **202,** 128–158 (1931); **263,** 1–12 (1940); O. Wintersteiner, V. du Vigneaud, and H. Jensen, *J. Pharmacol. Exp. Ther.*, **32,** 367–385, 387–396, 397–411 (1928).

336. A. P. Ryle, F. Sanger, L. F. Smith, and R. Kitai, *Biochem. J.*, **60,** 541–556 (1955); H. Brown, F. Sanger, and R. Kitai, *ibid.*, **60,** 556–565 (1955); F. Sanger and E. O. P. Thompson, *ibid.*, **53,** 353–366, 366–374 (1953); F. Sanger and H. Tuppy, *ibid.*, **49,** 463–481, 481–490 (1951).

337. D. F. Steiner and P. E. Oyer, *Proc. Nat. Acad. Sci., US*, **57,** 473–480 (1967); D. F. Steiner, D. Cunningham, L. Spigelman, and B. Aten, *Science*, **157,** 697–700 (1967); C. Nolan, E. Margoliash, J. D. Peterson, and D. F. Steiner, *J. Biol. Chem.*, **246,** 2780–2795 (1971).

338. M. J. Adams, T. L. Blundell, E. J. Dodson, G. G. Dodson, M. Vijayan, E. N. Baker, M. M. Harding, D. C. Hodgkin, B. Rimmer, and S. Sheat, *Nature* (London), **224,** 491–495 (1969).

339. T. L. Blundell, J. F. Cutfield, S. M. Cutfield, E. J. Dodson, G. G. Dodson, D. C. Hodgkin, D. A. Mercola, and M. Vijayan, *Nature* (London), **231,** 506–511 (1971).

340. P. Sieber, B. Kamber, A. Hartmann, A. Jöhl, B. Riniker, and W. Rittel, *Helv. Chim. Acta*, **57,** 2617–2621 (1974); **60,** 27–37 (1977); B. Kamber, A. Hartmann, A. Jöhl, F. Märki, B. Riniker, W. Rittel, and P. Sieber, in *Peptides: Chemistry, Structure and Biology*, R. Walter and J. Meienhofer, Eds., Ann Arbor Science Publishers, Ann Arbor, Mich., 1975, pp. 477–485.

341. A. E. Renold et al., in *Hormones in Human Plasma*, H. N. Antoniades, Ed., Little, Brown, Boston, 1960, pp. 49–117.

342. G. F. Cahill, Jr., in *Peptide Hormones*, J. A. Parsons, Ed., University Park Press, Baltimore, 1976, pp. 85–100.

343. T. E. Prout, *J. Chronic Dis.*, **15,** 879–885 (1962).

344. M. A. Root, E. W. Shuey, W. R. Kirtley, and S. O. Waife, Eds., *Fiftieth Anniversary Insulin Symposium*, in *Diabetes*, Vol. **21** (2), 385–714 (1972).

345. J. Schlichtkrull, J. Brange, A. H. Christiansen, O. Hallund, L. G. Heding, and K. H. Jørgensen, in *Fiftieth Anniversary Insulin Symposium*, M. A. Root et al., Eds., in *Diabetes*, **21** (2), 649–656 (1972).

346. C. J. Epstein and C. B. Anfinsen, *Biochemistry*, **2,** 461–464 (1963).

347. C. Shipp and D. B. Stone, in *Diabetes Mellitus: Diagnosis and Treatment*, Vol. 3, S. S. Fajans and B. Sussman, Eds., 1971, pp. 173–179.

348. I. A. Mirsky, D. M. Kipnis, D. F. Steiner et al., in *Methods in Investigative and Diagnostic Endocrinology*, Vol. 2B, S. A. Berson and R. S. Yalow, Eds., Elsevier, New York, 1973, pp. 823–883.

349. J. E. Gerich, M. A. Charles, and G. M. Grodsky, *Ann. Rev. Physiol. Ser. II.*, **38,** 353–388 (1976).

350. S. J. Pilkis and C. R. Park, *Ann. Rev. Pharmacol.*, **14,** 365–388 (1974).

351. P. Cuatrecasas, *Biochem. Pharmacol.*, **23,** 2353–2361 (1974).

352. T. Fujita, Ed., *Endocrine, Gut, and Pancreas*, Elsevier, New York, 1976.

353. H. Klostermeyer and R. E. Humbel, *Angew. Chem. Int. Ed.*, **5,** 807–822 (1966).

354. A. C. Trakatellis and G. P. Schwartz, in *Progress in the Chemistry of Organic Natural Products*, Vol. 26, L. Zechmeister, Ed., Springer, New York, 1968, pp. 120–160.

355. R. Geiger, *Chem.-Ztg., Chem. App.*, **100,** 111–129 (1976).

356. D. F. Steiner, in *Peptide Hormones*, J. A. Parsons, Ed., University Park Press, Baltimore, 1976, pp. 49–64. (a) A. H. Rubenstein, D. F. Steiner, D. L. Horwitz, M. E. Mako, M. B. Block, J. I. Starr, H. Kuzuya, and F. Melani, *Rec. Progr. Horm. Res.*, **33,** 435–475 (1977).

357. P. E. Oyer, S. Cho, J. D. Peterson, and D. F. Steiner, *J. Biol. Chem.*, **246,** 1375–1386 (1971).

358. A. S. C. Ko, D. G. Smyth, J. Markussen, and F. Sundby, *Eur. J. Biochem.*, **20,** 190–199 (1971).

359. S. J. Chan, P. Keim, and D. F. Steiner, *Proc. Nat. Acad. Sci., US*, **73,** 1964–1968 (1976). (a) L. Villa-Komaroff, A. Efstratiadis, St. Broome, P. Lomedico, R. Tizard, S. P. Naber, W. L. Chick, and W. Gilbert, *Proc. Nat. Acad. Sci.*, **75,** 3727–3731 (1978).

360. R. A. Pullen, D. G. Lindsay, S. P. Wood, I. J. Tickle, T. L. Blundell, A. Wollmer, G. Krail, D. Brandenburg, H. Zahn, J. Gliemann, and S. Gammeltoft, *Nature* (London), **259,** 369–373 (1976).

361. R. A. Pullen, J. A. Jenkins, I. J. Tickle, S. P. Wood, and T. L. Blundell, *Mol. Cell. Biochem.*, **8,** 5–20 (1975).

362. F. H. Carpenter, *Am. J. Med.*, **40,** 750–758 (1966).

363. E. R. Arguilla, W. W. Bromer, and D. Mercola, *Diabetes*, **18,** 193–205 (1969).

364. The Conformational Study Group, Academia Sinica, *Sci. Sinica*, (Peking), **19,** 497–504 (1976).

365. F. K. Jansen, U. Kiesel, and D. Brandenburg, *Ann. Immunol.* (*Inst. Pasteur*), **128C,** 313–314 (1977).

366. G. Bentley, E. Dodson, G. Dodson, D. Hodgkin, and D. Mercola, *Nature* (London), **261,** 166–168 (1976).

367. D. A. Mercola, J. W. S. Morris, and E. R. Arguilla, *Biochemistry*, **11,** 3860–3874 (1972).

368. H. Lackner, *Angew. Chem., Int. Ed.*, **14,** 375–386 (1975).

369. J. Meienhofer and E. Atherton, "Structure-Activity Relations in the Actinomycins", in *Structure-Activity Relationships Among Semisynthetic Antibiotics*, D. Perlman, Ed., Academic Press, New York, 1977, pp. 427–529.

370. G. H. Dixon and H. C. Wardlaw, *Nature* (London), **188,** 721–724 (1960).

371. Y.-c. Du, Y.-s. Zhang, Z-x. Lu, and C.-l. Tsou, *Sci. Sinica* (Peking) **10,** 84–104 (1961).

372. J. Meienhofer, E. Schnabel, H. Bremer, O. Brinkhoff, R. Zabel, W. Sroka, H. Klostermeyer, D. Brandenburg, T. Okuda, and H. Zahn, *Z. Naturforsch*, **18b,** 1120–1121 (1963).

373. P. G. Katsoyannis, K. Fukuda, A. Tometsko, K. Suzuki, and M. Tilak, *J. Am. Chem. Soc.*, **86,** 930–932 (1964).

374. Y.-t. Kung et al., *Sci. Sinica* (Peking), **14,** 1710–1716 (1965).

375. K. Lübke and H. Klostermeyer, *Advan. Enzymol.*, **33,** 445–525 (1970).

376. D. F. Steiner and J. L. Clark, *Proc. Nat. Acad. Sci., US*, **60,** 622–629 (1968).

377. N. Yanaihara, T. Hashimoto, C. Yanaihara, and N. Sakura, *Chem. Pharm. Bull.* (Tokyo), **18,** 417–420 (1970); *J. Am. Chem. Soc.*, **94,** 8243–8244 (1972); N. Yanaihara, T. Hashimoto, C. Yanaihara, M. Sakagami, D. F. Steiner, and A. H. Rubenstein, *Biochem. Biophys. Res. Commun.*, **59,** 1124–1130 (1974).

378. V. K. Naithani, *Hoppe-Seyler's Z. Physiol. Chem.*, **354,** 141–146; 659–672 (1973); V. K. Naithani, M. Dechesne, J. Markussen, and L. G. Heding, *ibid.*, **356,** 997–1010 (1975).

379. R. Geiger, G. Jäger, and W. König, *Chem. Ber.*, **106,** 2347–2352 (1973).

380. D. Brandenburg and A. Wollmer, *Hoppe-Seyler's Z. Physiol. Chem.*, **354,** 613–627 (1973); D. Brandenburg, W. Schermutzki, and H. Zahn, *ibid.*, **354,** 1521–1524 (1973); A. Wollmer, D. Branderburg, H.-P. Vogt, and W. Schermutzki, *ibid.*, **355,** 1471–1476 (1974).

381. R. Geiger and R. Obermeier, *Biochem. Biophys. Res. Commun.*, **55,** 60–66 (1973); R. Obermeier and R. Geiger, *Hoppe-Seyler's Z. Physiol. Chem.*, **356,** 1631–1634 (1975).

382. W.-D. Busse and F. H. Carpenter, *J. Am. Chem. Soc.*, **96,** 5947–5949 (1974); W.-D. Busse, S. R. Hansen, and F. H. Carpenter, *ibid.*, **96,** 5949–5950 (1974).

383. H. Zahn and J. Meienhofer, *Makromol. Chem.*, **26,** 153–166 (1958).

384. L. Zervas and I. Photaki, *J. Am. Chem. Soc.*, **84,** 3887–3897 (1962); see review: I. Photaki, in The Chemistry of Polypeptides, P. G. Katsoyannis, Ed., Plenum Press, New York, 1973, pp. 59–85.

385. R. G. Hiskey, V. R. Rao, and W. G. Rhodes, in *Protective Groups in Organic Chemistry*, J. F. W. McOmie, Ed., Plenum Press, New York, 1973, pp. 235–308.

386. R. G. Hiskey, A. Wittinghofer, A. N. Goud, and R. R. Vunnam, in *Peptides: Chemistry, Structure and Biology*, R. Walter and J. Meienhofer, Eds., Ann Arbor Science Publishers, Ann Arbor, Mich., 1975, pp. 487–496.

387. D. F. Veber, J. D. Milkowski, R. G. Denkewalter, and R. Hirschmann, *Tetrahedron Lett.*, 3057–3058 (1968); *J. Am. Chem. Soc.*, **94,** 5456—5461 (1972).

388. P. G. Katsoyannis, A. Tometsko, and K. Fukuda, *J. Am. Chem. Soc.*, **85,** 2863–2865 (1963).

389. G. H. Dixon, *Excerpta Med. Found., Int. Congr. Ser.*, No. 58, 1207–1215 (1964).

390. The Shanghai Insulin Research Group, *Sci. Sinica* (Peking), **16,** 61–70 (1973).

391. G. Weitzel, F.-U. Bauer, and K. Eisele, *Hoppe-Seyler's Z. Physiol. Chem.*, **357,** 187–200 (1976).

392. R. Obermeier and R. Geiger, *Hoppe-Seyler's Z. Physiol. Chem.*, **357,** 759–767 (1976).

393. H.-G. Gattner, E. W. Smith, and V. K. Naithani, *Hoppe-Seyler's Z. Physiol. Chem.*, **356,** 1465–1467 (1975).

394. R. Geiger, K. Geisen, H. D. Summ, and D. Langer, *Hoppe-Seyler's Z. Physiol. Chem.*, **356,** 1635–1649 (1975).

395. H. J. Friesen, D. Brandenburg, C. Diaconescu, H.-G. Gattner, V. K. Naithani, J. Nowak, H. Zahn, S. Dockerill, S. P. Wood, and T. L. Blundell, in *Peptides 1977: Proceedings of the Fifth American Peptide Symposium*, M. Goodman and J. Meienhofer, Eds., Wiley, New York, 1978, pp. 136–140.

396. D. Brandenburg, W.-D. Busse, H.-G. Gattner, H. Zahn, A. Wollmer, J. Gliemann, and W. Puls, in *Peptides 1972*, H. Hanson and H. D. Jakubke, Eds., North-Holland/Elsevier, New York, 1973, pp. 270–283.

397. R. Geiger and D. Langner, in *Peptides 1974*, Y. Wolman, Ed., Wiley, New York, 1975, pp. 159–163.

398. E. L. Smith, R. L. Hill, and A. Bormann, *Biochem. Biophys. Acta*, **29,** 207–208 (1958).

399. P. G. Katsoyannis, C. Zalut, A. Harris, and R. J. Meyer, *Biochemistry*, **10,** 3884–3889 (1971).

400. L. I. Slobin and F. H. Carpenter, *Biochemistry*, **5,** 499–508 (1966).

401. P. G. Katsoyannis, J. Ginos, A. Cosmatos, and G. Schwartz, *J. Am. Chem. Soc.*, **95,** 6427–6434 (1973).

402. G. Weitzel, K. Eisele, H. Zollner, and U. Weber, *Hoppe-Seyler's Z. Physiol. Chem.*, **350,** 1480–1483 (1969).

403. H. G. Gattner, *Hoppe-Seyler's Z. Physiol. Chem.*, **356,** 1397–1404 (1975); Insulin Research Group, Shanghai, et al., *Sci. Sinica* (Peking), **19,** 351–357 (1976).

404. S. C. Chu, K. T. Li, C. P. Tson, Y. S. Chang, and T. H. Lu, *Sci. Sinica* (Peking), **16,** 71–78 (1973).

405. H. Berndt, H.-G. Gattner, and H. Zahn, *Hoppe-Seyler's Z. Physiol. Chem.*, **356,** 1469–1472 (1975).

406. U. Weber, F. Schneider, P. Köhler, and G. Weitzel, *Hoppe-Seyler's Z, Physiol, Chem.*, **348,** 947–949 (1967).

407. U. Weber, S. Hörnle, G. Grieser, K. H. Herzog, and G. Weitzel, *Hoppe-Seyler's Z. Physiol, Chem.*, **348,** 1715–1717 (1967).

408. G. Krail, D. Brandenburg, and H. Zahn, *Hoppe-Seyler's Z. Physiol. Chem.*, **356,** 981–996 (1975).

409. U. Weber, S. Hörnle, P. Köhler, G. Nagelschneider, K. Eisele, and G. Weitzel, *Hoppe-Seyler's Z. Physiol. Chem.*, **349,** 512–514 (1968).

410. Y. Okada and P. G. Katsoyannis, *J. Am. Chem. Soc.*, **97,** 4366–4372 (1975).

411. S. Hörnle, U. Weber, and G. Weitzel, *Hoppe-Seyler's Z. Physiol. Chem.*, **349,** 1428–1430 (1968).

412. A. Cosmatos, S. Johnson, B. Breier, and P. G. Katsoyannis, *J. Chem. Soc. Perkin Trans. I*, 2157–2163 (1975).

413. A. J. Moody, M. A. Stan, M. Stan, and J. Gliemann, *Horm. Metab. Res.*, **6,** 12–16 (1974).

414. D. Brandenburg, H.-G. Gattner, and A. Wollmer, *Hoppe-Seyler's Z. Physiol. Chem.*, **353,** 599–617 (1972).

415. D. G. Lindsay and S. Shall, *Eur. J. Biochem.*, **15,** 547–554 (1970); *Biochem. J.*, **121,** 737–745 (1971).

416. D. Levy and R. A. Paselk, *Biochim. Biophys. Acta*, **310,** 398–405 (1973).

417. G. Krail, Thesis, Technische Hochschule, Aachen, 1973.

418. D. Brandenburg, C. Diaconescu, I. Francis. H.-J. Friesen, H.-G. Gattner, V. K. Naithani, J. Novak, W. Schermutzki, E. Schmitt, A. Schüttler, and J. Weismann, Joint German-Russian Peptide Symposium, USSR, 1976.

419. A. Staub, L. G. Sinn, and O. K. Behrens, *Science*, **117,** 628–629 (1953).

420. W. W. Bromer, in *Progress in the Chemistry of Organic Natural Products*, Vol. 28, L. Zechmeister, Ed., Springer, New York, 1970, pp. 429–452.

421. F. Sundby, in Glucagon Symposium, R. Unger, Ed., *Metabolism*, **25,** Suppl. 1, 1319–1321 (1976).

422. L. G. Heding, E. K. Frandsen, and H. Jacobsen, in Glucagon Symposium, R. Unger, Ed., *Metabolism*, **25,** Suppl. 1, 1327–1329 (1976).

423. R. Unger, Ed., Glucagon Symposium, *Metabolism*, **25,** Suppl. 1, 1303–1533 (1976).

424. D. Baetens, C. Rufener, C. B. Srikent, R. Dobbs, R. H. Unger, and L. Orci, *J. Cell. Biol.*, **69,** 455–464 (1976).

425. L. Muñoz Barragan, C. Rufener, C. B. Srikant, R. E. Dobbs, W. A. Shannon, Jr., D. Beatens, and R. H. Unger, *Horm. Metab. Res.*, **9,** 37–39 (1977); R. H. Unger, P. Raskin, C. B. Srikant, and L. Orci, *Rec. Progr. Horm. Res.*, **33,** 477–517 (1977).

426. S. L. Pohl, L. Birnbaumer, and M. Rodbell, *Science*, **164,** 566–567 (1969).

427. R. Dobbs, H. Sakurai, H. Sasaki, G. Faloona, I. Valverde, D. Baetens, L. Orci, and R. Unger, *Science*, **187,** 544–547 (1975).

428. R. Sherwin, J. Wahren, and P. Felig, in Glucagon Metabolism, R. Unger, Ed., *Metabolism*, **25,** Suppl. 1, 1381–1383 (1976).

429. S. R. Bloom, A. J. Barnes, M. G. Bryant, and K. G. M. M. Alberti. in Glucagon Metabolism, R. Unger, Ed., *Metabolism*, **25,** Suppl. 1, 1481–1482 (1976).

430. P. J. Lefebvre and R. H. Unger, Eds., *Glucagon: Molecular Physiology, Clinical and Therapeutic Implications*, Pergamon Press, New York, 1972.

431. H. S. Tager and D. F. Steiner, *Proc. Nat. Acad. Sci., US*, **70,** 2321–2325 (1973).

432. A. C. Trakatellis, K. Tada, K. Yamaji, and P. Gardiki-Kouidou, *Biochemistry*, **14,** 1508–1512 (1975).

433. B. D. Noe, in Glucagon Metabolism, R. Unger, Ed., *Metabolism*, **25,** Suppl. 1, 1339–1341 (1976).

434. K. Sasaki, S. Dockerill, D. A. Adamiak, I. J. Tickle, and T. Blundell, *Nature* (London), **257,** 751–757 (1975).

435. T. L. Blundell, S. Dockerill, K. Sasaki, I. J. Tickle, and S. P. Wood, in Glucagon Metabolism, R. Unger, Ed., *Metabolism*, **25,** Suppl. 1, 1331–1336 (1976).

436. E. Wünsch, *Z. Naturforsch.*, **22B,** 1269–1276 (1967).

437. F. Weygand, D. Hoffmann. and E. Wünsch, *Z. Naturforsch.*, **21B,** 426–428 (1966).

438. W. W. Bromer, L. G. Sinn, A. Staub, and O. K. Behrens, *J. Am. Chem. Soc.*, **78,** 3858–3860 (1956).

439. Protein Synthesis Group. Shanghai, *Sci. Sinica* (Peking), **18,** 745–768 (1975).

440. V. J. Hruby, D. E. Wright, M. C. Lin, and M. Rodbell, in Glucagon Symposium, R. Unger, Ed., *Metabolism*, **25,** Suppl. 1, 1323–1325 (1976); *Biochemistry*, **14,** 1559–1563 (1975).

441. W. W. Bromer, in Glucagon Symposium, R. Unger, Ed., *Metabolism*, **25,** Suppl. 1, 1315–1316 (1976).

442. J. E. Gerich, in Glucagon Symposium, R. Unger, Ed., *Metabolism*, **25,** Suppl. 1, 1505–1507 (1976).

443. P. Felig and J. Wahren, in Glucagon Symposium, R. Unger, Ed., *Metabolism*, **25,** Suppl. 1, 1509–1510 (1976).

444. R. S. Sherwin, R. Hendler, R. DeFronzo, J. Wahren, and P. Felig, *Proc. Nat. Acad. Sci., US*, **74,** 348–352 (1977).

445. L. R. Johnson, *Ann. Rev. Physiol.*, **39,** 135–158 (1977).

446. A. G. E. Pearse, in *Endocrinology of the Gut*, W. Y. Chey and F. P. Brooks, Black, Thorofare, N.J., pp. 24–34.

447. S. R. Bloom, *Gut*, **15,** 502–510 (1974).

448. A. G. E. Pearse, in *Peptide Hormones*, J. A. Parsons, Ed., University Park Press, Baltimore, 1976, pp. 33–47; A. G. E. Pearse, J. M. Polak, and C. M. Heath, *Diabetologia*, **9,** 120–129 (1973); *Gut*, **12,** 783–788 (1971).

449. W. M. Bayliss and E. H. Starling, *J. Physiol.* (London), **28,** 325–353 (1902).

450. M. Bodanszky, Y. S. Klausner, and S. I. Said, *Proc. Nat. Acad. Sci., US,* **70,** 382–384 (1973).

451. V. Mutt and S. I. Said, *Eur. J. Biochem.*, **42,** 581–589 (1974).

452. J. Jorpes and V. Mutt, Eds., *Handbook Of Experimental Pharmacology,* O, Eichler et al. Eds., Vol. 7, *Secretin, Cholecystokinin, Pancreozymin, and Gastrin,* Springer, New York, 1973.

453. M. I. Grossman, in *Peptide Hormones,* J. A. Parsons, Ed., University Park Press, Baltimore, 1976, pp. 105–117.

454. P. L. Rayford, T. A. Miller, and J. C. Thompson, *New Engl. J. Med.*, **294,** 1093–1101; 1157–1164 (1976).

455. W. Y. Chey and F. P. Brooks, *Endocrinology of the Gut,* Black, Thorofare, N.J. 1974.

456. R. A. Gregory and H. J. Tracy, in *Gastrointestinal Hormones,* J. C. Thompson, Ed., University of Texas Press, Austin, 1975.

457. R. A. Gregory, in *Polypeptide Hormones: Molecular and Cellular Aspects,* R. Porter and D. W. Fitzsimmons, Eds., Ciba Foundation Symposium No. 41, Excerpta Medica, New York, 1976, pp. 251–265.

458. R. S. Yalow and S. A. Berson, *Gastroenterology,* **58,** 609–615 (1970).

459. H. Gregory, P. M. Hardy, D. S. Jones, G. W. Kenner, and R. C. Sheppard, *Nature* (London), **204,** 931–933 (1964).

460. P. H. Bentley, G. W. Kenner, and R. C. Sheppard, *Nature* (London), **209,** 583–585 (1966).

461. R. A. Gregory and H. J. Tracy, *Gut,* **15,** 683–685 (1974).

462. R. A. Gregory, M. I. Grossman, S. Emas, B. Uvnas, R. S. Yalow, S. A. Berson, and R. M. Zollinger, in *Methods of Investigative and Diagnostic Endocrinology,* Vol. 2B, S. A. Berson and R. S. Yalow, Eds., Elsevier, New York, 1973, pp. 1029–1058.

463. J. H. Walsh and M. I. Grossman, *New Engl. J. Med.*, **292,** 1324–1334, 1377–1384 (1975).

464. H. J. Tracy and R. A. Gregory, *Nature* (London), **204,** 935–938 (1964).

465. J. S. Morley, *Proc. Roy. Soc., Ser. B,* **170,** 97–111 (1968); *J. Chem. Soc.* (*C*), 809–813 (1969).

466. J. C. Anderson, M. A. Barton, R. A. Gregory, P. M. Hardy, G. W. Kenner, J. K. Macleod, J. K. Preston, and R. C. Sheppard, *Nature* (London), **204,** 933–934 (1964).

467. A. M. Choudhury, G. W. Kenner, S. Moore, R. Ramage, P. M. Richards, W. D. Thorpe, L. Moroder, G. Wendlberger, and E. Wünsch, in *Peptides 1976, Proceedings of the 14th European Peptide Symposium,* A. Loffet, Ed., Editions de l'Université de Bruxelles, Brussels, Belgium, 1976, pp. 257–261.

468. H. Wissmann, R. Schleyerbach, B. Schoelkeus, and R. Geiger, *Hoppe-Seyler's Z. Physiol. Chem.*, **354,** 1591–1598 (1973).

469. J. E. Jorpes, *Gastroenterology,* **55,** 157–164 (1968).

470. M. A. Ondetti, B. Rubin. S. L. Engel, J. Pluščec, and J. T. Sheehan, *Am. J. Dig. Dis.*, **15,** 149–156 (1970).

471. A. Anastasi, V. Erspamer, and E. Endean, *Arch. Biochem. Biophys.*, **125,** 57–68 (1968).

472. J. E. Jorpes, V. Mutt, M. I. Grossman, B. Rubin, S. L. Engel, J. D. Young, and H. D. Janowitz, in *Methods of Investigative and Diagnostic Endocrinology,* Vol. 2B, S. A. Berson and R. A. Yalow, Eds., Elsevier, New York, 1973, pp. 1075–1090.

473. H. Yajima, Y. Mori, K. Koyama, T. Tobe, M. Setoyama, H. Adachi, T. Kanno, and A. Saito, *Chem. Pharm. Bull.* (Tokyo), **24,** 2794–2802 (1976).

474. J. E. Jorpes and V. Mutt, *Acta Chem. Scand.*, **15,** 1790–1791 (1961).

475. W. König, M. Bickel, R. Geiger, R. Obermeier, V. Teetz, R. Uhman, and H. Wissmann, in *First International Symposium on Hormonal Receptors in Digestive Tract Physiology,* INSERM Symposium No. 3, Bonfits et al., Eds., Elsevier, New York, 1977, pp. 29–32.

476. V. Mutt, J. E. Jorpes, M. I. Grossman, L. J. Spingola, J. D. Young, and H. D. Janowitz, in *Methods of Investigative and Diagnostic Endocrinology,* Vol. 2B, S. A. Berson and R. A. Yalow, Eds., Elsevier, New York, 1973, pp. 1059–1074.

477. S. J. Konturek, P. Thor, A. Dembinski, and R. Krol, *Gastroenterology,* **68,** 1527–1535 (1975).

478. G. J. Dockray, *Gen. Comp. Endocrinol.*, **25,** 203–210 (1975).

479. J. A. Coddling, A. M. Rappaport, M. A. Ashworth, A. Kalnins, and R. E. Haist, *Horm. Metab. Res.*, **7,** 199–204 (1975); H. Stahlheber, M. Reiser, P. Lehnert, M. M. Forell, P. Botterman, and E. Jaeger, *Klin. Wochenschr.*, **53,** 339 (1975).

480. J. W. Fara, *Am. J. Dig. Dis.*, **20,** 346–353 (1975).

481. J. G. Gutiérrez, W. Y. Chey, A. Shah, and G. Holzwasser, *Radiology,* **113,** 563–566 (1974).

482. M. Bodanszky, in *Handbook of Experimental Pharmacology,* O. Eichler et al., Eds., Vol. 34, 1973, pp. 180–194.

483. E. Wünsch, in *The Chemistry of Polypeptides*, P. G. Katsoyannis, Ed., Plenum Press, New York, 1973, pp. 279–295.

484. G. Jäger, W. König, H. Wissmann, and R. Geiger, *Chem. Ber.*, **107,** 215–231 (1974).

485. B. Hemmasi and E. Bayer, *Int. J. Peptide Protein Res.*, **9,** 63–70 (1977).

486. M. Bodanszky and M. L. Fink, *Bioorganic Chem.*, **5,** 275–282 (1976); M. Bodanszky, M. L. Fink, K. W. Funk, and S. I. Said, *Clin. Endocrinol.*, **5,** Suppl., 195s–200s (1976).

487. M. Bodanszky, in *First International Symposium on Hormonal Regulators in Digestive Tract Physiology*, INSERM Symposium No. 3, Bonfils et al., Eds., Elsevier, New York, 1977, pp. 13–18; M. L. Fink and M. Bodanszky, *J. Am. Chem. Soc.*, **98,** 974–977 (1976).

488. J. C. Brown and J. R. Dryburgh, *Can. J. Biochem.*, **49,** 867–872 (1971).

489. J. C. Brown, J. R. Dryburgh, and R. A. Pederson, in *Endocrinology of the Gut*, W. Y. Chey and F. P. Brooks, Black, Thorofare, N. J., 1974, pp. 76–83.

490. J. Dupre, S. A. Ross, D. Watson, and J. C. Brown, *J. Clin. Endocrinol.*, **37,** 826–828 (1973).

491. H. Yajima, H. Ogawa, M. Kubota, T. Tobe, M. Fujimura, K. Henmi, K. Torizuka, H. Adachi, H. Imura, and T. Taminato, *J. Am. Chem. Soc.*, **97,** 5593–5594 (1975); *Chem. Pharm. Bull.* (Tokyo), **24,** 2447–2456 (1976).

492. S. I. Said and G. M. Makhlouf, in *Endocrinology of the Gut*, W. Y. Chey and F. P. Brooks, Black, Thorofare, N.J., 1974, pp. 83–87.

493. M. Bodanszky, Y. S. Klausner, C. Yang Lin, V. Mutt, and S. I. Said, *J. Am. Chem. Soc.*, **96,** 4973–4978 (1974).

494. A. Nilsson, *FEBS Lett.*, **60,** 322–326 (1975).

495. M. I. Grossman, *Gastroenterology*, **67,** 730–731 (1974).

496. J. Fahrenkrug, O. B. Schaffalitzky de Muckadell, and A. Fahrenkrug, *Brain Res.*, **124,** 581–584 (1977); M. G. Bryant, S. R. Bloom, J. M. Polak, R. H. Albuquerque, I. Modlin, and A. G. E. Pearse, *Lancet*, **1,** 991–993 (1976); A. Giachetti, S. I. Said, R. C. Reynolds, and F. C. Koniges, *Proc. Nat. Acad. Sci., US*, **74,** 3424–3428 (1977).

497. H. Schubert and J. C. Brown, *Can. J. Biochem.*, **52,** 7–8 (1974).

498. J. M. Polak, A. G. E. Pearse, and C. M. Heath, *Gut*, **16,** 225–229 (1975).

499. P. Mitznegg, S. R. Bloom, W. Domschke, S. Domschke, E. Wünsch, and L. Demling, *Gastroenterology*, **72,** 413–416 (1977).

500. J. R. Dryburgh and J. C. Brown, *Gastroenterology*, **68,** 1169–1176 (1975).

501. Y. Kai, H. Kawatani, H. Yajima, and Z. Itoh, *Chem. Pharm. Bull.* (Tokyo), **23,** 2346–2352 (1975); F. Shimizu, K. Imagawa, S. Mihara, and N. Yanaihara, *Bull. Chem. Soc. Japan*, **49,** 3594–3596 (1976).

502. E. Wünsch, E. Jaeger, S. Knof, R. Scharf, and P. Thamm, *Hoppe-Seyler's Z. Physiol Chem.*, **357,** 467–476 (1976).

503. R. E. Canfield, F. J. Morgan, J. L. Vaitukaitis, G. T. Ross, K. D. Bagshawe, and M. L. Taymor, in Glucagon Symposium, R. Unges, Ed., *Metabolism*, **25,** Suppl. 1, pp. 727–786.

504. O. P. Bahl, in Glucagon Symposium, R. Unger, Ed., *Metabolism*, **25,** Suppl. 1, pp. 171–199.

505. R. E. Canfield, S. Birken, J. H. Morse, and F. J. Morgan, in Endocrinology of the Gut, W. Y. Chey and F. P. Brooks, Black, Thorofare, N.J., pp. 299–315; S. Birken and R. E. Canfield, *J. Biol. Chem*; **252,** 5386–5392 (1977); *see also* H. T. Kentman and R. M. Williams, *ibid.*, **252,** 5393–5397 (1977).

506. R. Bellisario, R. B. Carlson, O. P. Bahl, and N. Swaminathan, *J. Biol. Chem.*, **248,** 6796–6809; 6810–6827 (1973).

507. F. J. Morgan, S. Birken, and R. E. Canfield, *Mol. Cell. Biochem.*, **2,** 97–99 (1973).

508. J. L. Vaitukaitis, *Ann. Clin. Lab. Sci.*, **4,** 276–280 (1974).

509. C. H. Schneider, K. Blaser, C. Pfeuti, and E. Gruden, *FEBS Lett.*, **50,** 272–275 (1975).

510. J. B. Josimovich and J. A. MacLaren, *Endocrinology*, **71,** 209–220 (1962).

511. S. F. Contractor and H. Davies, *Nature New Biol.*, **243,** 284–286 (1973).

512. B. N. Saxena, *Vitam. Horm.*, **29,** 95–151 (1971).

513. J. B. Josimovich, M. J. Levitt, M. M. Grumbach, S. L. Kaplan, and A. Vinik, in *Methods of Investigative and Diagnostic Endocrinology*, Vol. 2B, S. A. Berson and R. S. Yalow, Eds., Elsevier, New York, 1973, pp. 787–819.

514. C. H. Li, J. S. Dixon, and D. Chung, *Arch. Biochem. Biophys.*, **155,** 95–110 (1973).

515. S. Aloj and H. Edelhoch, *J. Biol. Chem.*, **246,** 5047–5052 (1971).

516. T. A. Bewley and C. H. Li, *Arch. Biochem. Biophys.*, **144,** 589–595 (1971).

517. A. B. Schneider, K. Kowalski, and L. M. Sherwood, *Biochem. Biophys. Res. Commun.*, **64,** 717–724 (1975).

518. F. L. Hisaw, *Proc. Soc. Exp. Biol. Med.*, **23,** 661–663 (1926); H. L. Fevold, F. L. Hisaw, and R. K. Meyer, *J. Am. Chem. Soc.*, **52,** 3340–3348 (1930).

519. O. D. Sherwood, K. R. Rosentreter, and M. L. Birkhimer, *Endocrinology*, **96,** 1106–1113 (1975).

520. G. Weiss, E. M. O'Byrne, and B. G. Steinetz, *Science*, **194,** 948–949 (1976).

521. C. D. Sherwood and E. M. O'Byrne, *Arch. Biochem. Biophys.*, **160,** 185–196 (1974).

522. C. Schwabe, J. K. McDonald, and B. Steinetz, *Biochem. Biophys. Res. Commun.*, **70,** 397–405 (1976); **75,** 503–510 (1977). (a) S. Bedarkar, W. G. Turnell, T. L. Blundell, and C. Schwabe, *Nature* (London), **270,** 449–451 (1977). (b) K. v. Maillot, M. Weiss, M. Nagelschmidt, and H. Struck, *Arch. Gynäk.*, **223,** 223–231 (1977).

523. I. H. Page and F. M. Bumpus, Eds., *Angiotensin*, Vol. 37 in *Handbook of Experimental Pharmacology*, O. Eichler et al., Eds., Springer, New York, 1974.

524. W. S. Peart, F. M. Bumpus, R. K. Türker, P. A. Khairallah, T. L. Goodfriend, and J. H. Laragh, in *Methods of Investigative and Diagnostic Endocrinology*, Vol. 2B, S. A. Berson and R. S. Yalow, Eds., Elsevier, New York, 1973, pp. 1145–1183.

525. J. V. Pierce, M. J. Reichgott, K. L. Melmon, M. E. Webster, R. C. Talamo, K. F. Austen, and E. Haber, in *Methods of Investigative and Diagnostic Endocrinology*, Vol. 2B, S. A. Berson and R. S. Yalow, Eds., Elsevier, New York, 1973, pp. 1185–1238.

526. E. G. Erdös and A. F. Wilde, Eds., *Bradykinin, Kallidin and Kallikrein*, Vol. 25, in *Handbook of Experimental Pharmacology*, O. Eichler et al., Eds., Springer, New York, 1970.

527. J. O. Davis, Chairman, Symposium on Advances in our knowledge of the Renin-Angiotensin System, *Fed. Proc.*, **36,** 1753–1787 (1977).

528. R. L. Soffer, *Ann. Rev. Biochem.*, **45,** 73–94 (1976).

529. P. Needleman and G. R. Marshall, Chairmen, Symposium on Angiotensin Antagonists: Overview and Projection, *Fed. Proc.*, **35,** 2486–2525 (1976).

530. L. T. Skeggs, M. Levine, K. W. Lentz, J. R. Kahn, and F. E. Dorer, *Fed. Proc.*, **36,** 1755–1759 (1977).

531. E. G. Erdös, *Fed, Proc.*, **36,** 1760–1765 (1977).

532. R. H. Freeman, J. O. Davis. T. E. Lohmeier, and W. S. Spielman, *Fed. Proc.*, **36,** 1766–1770 (1977). (a) F. M. Bumpus and M. C. Khosla, in *Hypertension, Physiopathology and Treatment*, J. Genest, E. Koiw, and O. Kuchel, Eds., McGraw-Hill, New York, 1977, pp. 183–201.

533. J. H. Laragh, D. B. Case, J. M. Wallace, and H. Keim, *Fed. Proc.*, **36,** 1781–1787 (1977).

534. R. Deslauriers, R. A. Komoroski, G. C. Levy, A. C. M. Paiva, and I. C. P. Smith, *FEBS Lett.*, **62,** 50–56 (1976).

535. M. C. Khosla, R. R. Smeby, and F. M. Bumpus, in *Angiotensin*, Vol. 37 in *Handbook of Experimental Pharmacology*, O. Eichler et al., Eds., Springer, New York, pp. 126–161, 1974.

536. G. R. Marshall, *Fed. Proc.*, **35,** 2494–2501 (1976).

537. G. R. Marshall, W. Vine, and P. Needleman, *Proc. Nat. Acad. Sci., US*, **67,** 1624–1630 (1970).

538. P. Needleman, J. R. Douglas, Jr., B. A. Jakschik, A. L. Blumberg, P. C. Isakson, and G. R. Marshall, *Fed. Proc.*, **35,** 2488–2493 (1976).

539. M. C. Khosla, R. R. Smeby, and F. M. Bumpus, in *Peptides: Chemistry, Structure and Biology*, R. Walter and J. Meienhofer, Eds., Ann Arbor Science Publishers, Ann Arbor, Mich., 1975, pp. 547–552.

540. M. C. Khosla, H. Mũnoz-Ramirez, M. M. Hall, R. R. Smeby, P. A. Khairallah, F. M. Bumpus, and M. J. Peach, *J. Med. Chem.*, **19,** 244–250 (1976).

541. K. Poulsen, J. Burton, and E. Haber, *Biochemistry*, **12,** 3877–3882 (1973).

542. A. I. Samuels, E. D. Miller, Jr., J. C. S. Fray, E. Haber, and A. C. Barger, *Fed. Proc.*, **35,** 2512–2520 (1976).

543. M. A. Ondetti, N. J. Williams, E. F. Sabo, J. Pluscec, E. R. Weaver, and O. Kocy, *Biochemistry*, **10,** 4033–4039 (1971).

544. M. A. Ondetti, B. Rubin, and D. W. Cushman, *Science*, **196,** 441–444 (1977).

545. J. P. Buckley, *Biochem. Pharmacol.*, **26,** 1–3 (1977).

546. W. B. Severs and A. E. Daniels-Severs, *Pharmacol. Rev.*, **25,** 415–449 (1973).

547. J. P. Bennett, Jr., and S. H. Snyder, *J. Biol. Chem.*, **251,** 7423–7430 (1976).

548. M. Rocha e Silva, *Life Sci.*, **15,** 7–22 (1974).

549. G. Bertaccini, *Pharmacol. Rev.*, **28,** 127–177 (1976).

550. H. Yoshida, R. G. Geller, and J. J. Pisano, *Biochemistry*, **15,** 61–64 (1976).

551. K. Araki, S. Tachibana, M. Uchiyama, T. Nakajima, and T. Yasuhara, *Chem. Pharm. Bull.* (Tokyo), **21,** 2801–2804 (1973).

552. F. Angelucci, R. de Castiglione, A. Anastasi, V.

Erspamer, and R. Endean, *Experientia*, **31,** 507–508, 510–511 (1975).

553. R. Faustini, C. Beretta, R. Cheli, and A. De Gresti, *Pharmacol. Res. Commun.*, **5,** 383–387 (1973).

554. J. C. McGiff, Chairman, Symposium on Kinin, Renal Function and Blood Pressure Regulation, *Fed. Proc.*, **35,** 172–206 (1976).

555. A. C. M. Camargo, F. J. Ramalho-Pinto, and L. J. Green, *J. Neurochem.*, **19,** 37–49 (1972).

556. R. Luft and K. Hall, Eds., *Somatomedins and Some Other Growth Factors*, in Advan. Metab. Disord., **8,** (1975).

557. K. Hall, K. Takano, L. Fryklund, and H. Sievertsson, *Advan. Metab. Disord.*, **8,** 19–46 (1975).

558. E. R. Froesch, U. Schlumpf, R. Heimann, J. Zapf, R. E. Humbel, and W. J. Ritschard, *Advan. Metab. Disord.*, **8,** 203–210 (1975).

559. J. M. Bower, R. Camble, H. Gregory, E. L. Gerring, and I. R. Willshire, *Experientia*, **31,** 825–826 (1975).

560. C. R. Savage, Jr., J. H. Hash, and S. Cohen, *J. Biol. Chem.*, **248,** 7669–7672 (1973).

561. S. Cohen, G. Carpenter, and K. J. Lembach, *Advan. Metab. Disord.*, **8,** 265–284 (1975); S. Cohen and J. M. Taylor, *Rec. Progr. Horm. Res.*, **30,** 533–550 (1974); S. Cohen and C. R. Savage, Jr., *ibid.*, **30,** 551–574 (1974).

562. A. C. Server and E. M. Shooter, *J. Biol. Chem.*, **251,** 165–173 (1976).

563. H. Gregory, *Nature* (London), **257,** 325–327 (1975); H. Gregory and B. M. Preston, *Int. J. Peptide Protein Res.*, **9,** 107–118 (1977).

564. R. A. Hogue-Angeletti, R. A. Bradshaw, and W. A. Frazier, *Advan. Metab. Disord.*, **8,** 285–299 (1975); A. C. Server and E. M. Shooter, *Adv. Protein Chem.*, **31,** 339–409 (1977); R. A. Bradshaw, *Ann. Rev. Biochem.*, **47,** 191–216 (1978).

565. R. A. Bradshaw and M. Young, *Biochem. Pharmacol.*, **25,** 1445–1449 (1976).

566. S. Varon, *Exp. Neurol.*, **48,** Part 2, 75–92 (1975).

567. J. D. Saide, R. A. Murphy, R. E. Canfield, J. Skinner, D. R. Robinson, B. G. W. Arnason, and M. Young, *J. Cell. Biol.*, **67,** Part 2, 376a (1975).

568. R. H. Angeletti and R. A. Bradshaw, *Proc. Nat. Acad. Sci., US*, **68,** 2417–2420 (1971).

CHAPTER TWENTY–EIGHT

The Male Sex Hormones and Analogs

R. E. COUNSELL

and

ROBERT BRUEGGEMEIER

Department of Pharmacology
University of Michigan Medical School
Ann Arbor, Michigan 48109, USA

CONTENTS

1 INTRODUCTION

Androgens are a class of steroids characterized by their biological effect on the primary and secondary sex characters of various male animals. In addition, androgens possess potent anabolic or growth-promoting properties. The search for substances that possess a preponderance of one or the other of these activities has been an ongoing concern of many investigators over the last 50 years. This chapter represents an attempt to mention all androgenic and anabolic steroids presently employed in clinical practice or animal husbandry in the United States and elsewhere. Modified androgens that have found use as biochemical or pharmacological tools also are included. The reader should consult several recently published books (1–4) for a more extensive treatment of the subject.

2 HISTORICAL

The first report of the isolation of a substance with androgenic activity was made by Butenandt (5, 6) in 1931. The material, isolated in very small quantities from human male urine (7), was named androsterone (28.**1**) (8). A second weakly androgenic steroid hormone was isolated

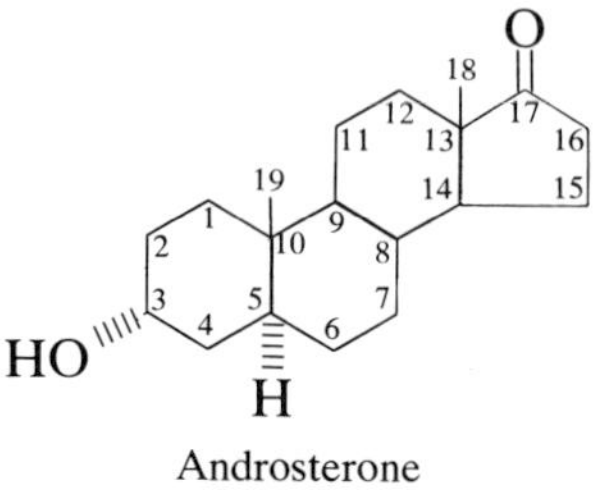

Androsterone

28.**1**

from male urine in 1934. This substance was named dehydroepiandrosterone (28.**2**)

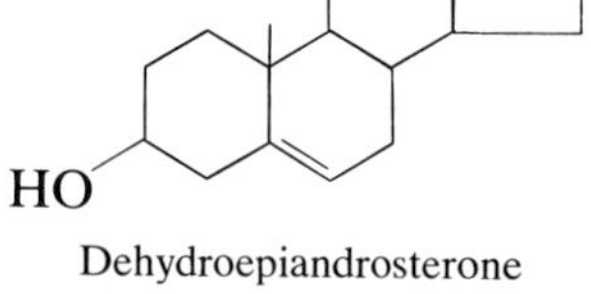

Dehydroepiandrosterone

28.**2**

because of its ready chemical transformation and structural similarity to androsterone (9). A year later Laqueur et al. (10, 11) reported the isolation of the testicular androgenic hormone, testosterone (28.**3**).

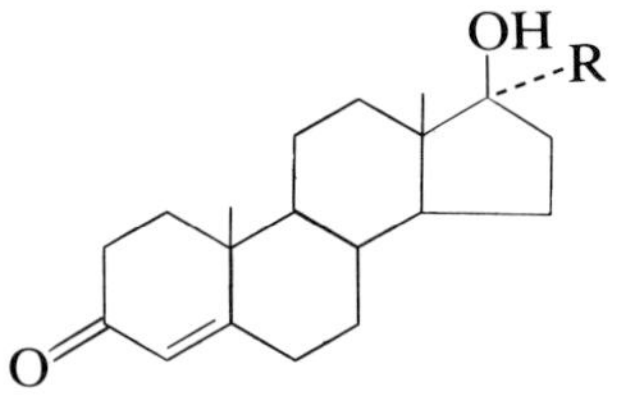

28.**3** R=H=testosterone
28.**4** $R=CH_3$ = 17α-methyltestosterone

This substance was nearly 10 times as potent as androsterone in promoting capon comb growth. Shortly after this discovery, the first chemical synthesis of testosterone was reported by Butenandt and Hanisch (12) and quickly confirmed by Ruzicka (13, 14).

For many years it was believed that testosterone was the active androgenic hormone in man. In 1968, however, research in two laboratories demonstrated that 5α-dihydrotestosterone (DHT, 28.**5**) was the

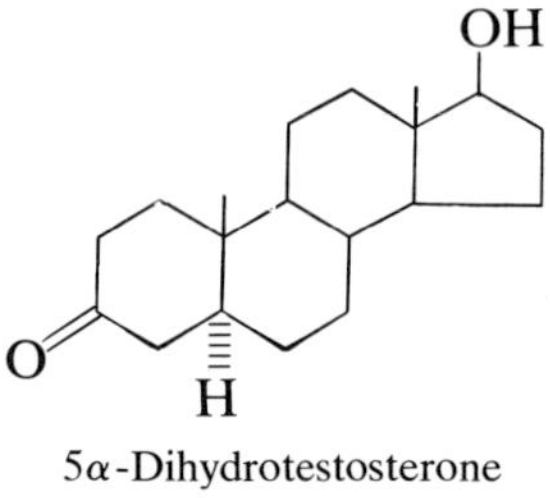

5α-Dihydrotestosterone

28.**5**

active androgen in target tissues, such as the prostate and seminal vesicles, and was formed from testosterone by a reductase present in these tissues (15, 16). Shortly thereafter a soluble receptor protein was isolated and demonstrated to be specific for DHT and related structures (17, 18).

The anabolic action of the androgens was first documented by Kochakian and Murlin in 1935 (19). In their experiments, extracts of male urine caused a marked retention of nitrogen when injected into dogs fed a constant diet. Soon afterward testosterone propionate was observed to produce a similar nitrogen-sparing effect in humans (20). Subsequent clinical studies demonstrated that testosterone was capable of causing a major acceleration of skeletal growth and a marked increase in muscle mass (21–23). This action on muscle tissue has been referred to more specifically as the myotrophic effect.

The first androgenic-like steroid used for its anabolic properties in humans was testosterone. Unfortunately, its use for this purpose was limited by the inherent androgenicity and the need for parenteral administration. 17α-Methyltestosterone (28.**4**) was the first androgen discovered to possess oral activity, but it too did not show any apparent separation of androgenic and anabolic activity. The promise of finding a useful, orally effective, anabolic agent free from androgenic side effects has prompted numerous clinical and biological studies over the past two decades.

3 OCCURRENCE AND BIOSYNTHESIS

The androgens are secreted not only by the testis, but also by the ovary and adrenal cortex. Testosterone is the principal circulating androgen and is formed by the Leydig cells of the testes. Other tissues, such as liver and human prostate, form testosterone from precursors, but this contribution to the androgen pool is minimal. Since dehydroepiandrosterone and androstenedione (see Fig. 28.3) are secreted by the adrenal cortex and ovary, they indirectly augment the testosterone pool because they can be rapidly converted to testosterone by peripheral tissues.

Plasma testosterone levels for men usually range between 0.61 and 1.1 μg/100 ml and are 5–100 times female values (24). The circulating level of DHT in normal adult men is about one-tenth the testosterone level (25). Daily testosterone production rates have been estimated to be 4–12 mg for young men and 0.5–2.9 mg for young women (26). Although attempts have been made to estimate the secretion rates for testosterone, these studies are hampered by the number of tissues capable of secreting androgens and the considerable interconversion of the steroids concerned (27, 28).

It is generally recognized that the synthesis of androgens in the testes is regulated by the trophic hormones, luteinizing hormone (LH) (also called interstitial cell-stimulating hormone, ICSH) and follicle-stimulating hormone (FSH). LH stimulates steroidogenesis in the Leydig cells, whereas FSH acts primarily on the germinal epithelium.

Our understanding of steroidogenesis in the endocrine organs has advanced considerably during the past decade. The current hypothesis, based largely on investigations with the adrenal cortex, appears to apply to the testis and ovary as well (29). Figure 28.1 outlines the following sequence of events known to be involved with steroidogenesis:

1. LH activates adenyl cyclase of the Leydig cells.
2. The intracellular concentration of cyclic AMP is increased.
3. Cyclic AMP activates certain protein kinases, which are involved with subsequent stages of the steroidogenesis pathway.
4. Cholesterol esters (storage form) are converted to free cholesterol, which is translocated to mitrochondria.
5. A cytochrome P-450 mixed-function oxidase system converts cholesterol to pregnenolone.
6. Nonmitochondrial enzymatic transformations convert pregnenolone to testosterone.

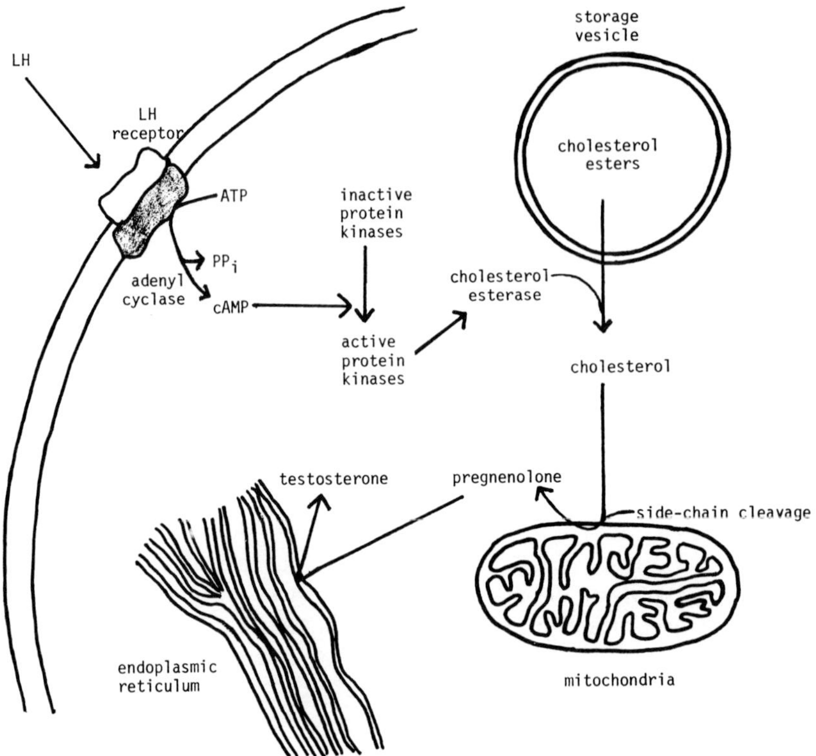

Fig. 28.1 Cellular events of steroidogenesis.

The conversion of cholesterol to pregnenolone has been termed the rate-limiting step in steroid hormone biosynthesis. The reaction requires NADPH and is catalyzed by cytochrome P-450. Although many of the details of this side chain cleavage reaction remain to be elucidated, the most widely held hypothesis proposes that the initial event involves hydroxylation at C-20 or C-22 followed by formation of the 20*R*,22*R*-diol (see Fig. 28.2). More recent studies, however, have served to cast doubt on this scheme. For example, Burstein and co-workers (30) found kinetic data to indicate that the 20*R*,22*R*-diol arises directly from cholesterol without the intermediacy of the monohydroxylated derivatives. Moreover, work in Lieberman's laboratory (31, 32) has shown that derivatives of cholesterol having a *t*-butyl or phenyl in addition to the hydroxyl group at C-20 (i.e., incapable of forming a C-20,22-dihydroxy derivative) could still give rise to pregnenolone. Lieberman's group postulates the formation of short-lived radicals or ionic species complexing with the enzyme system. The traditional side chain hydroxylated compounds would then be by-products of the reaction, arising from the transient, enzyme-bound radicals or ionic species (32).

Tracer studies have shown that two major pathways known as the "4-ene" and "5-ene" pathways are involved in the conversion of pregnenolone to testosterone. Both these pathways and the requisite enzymes are shown in Fig. 28.3. Earlier studies tended to favor the "4-ene" pathway, but more recent work has disputed this view and suggests that the "5-ene" pathway is quantitatively more important in man. The investigations of Vihko and

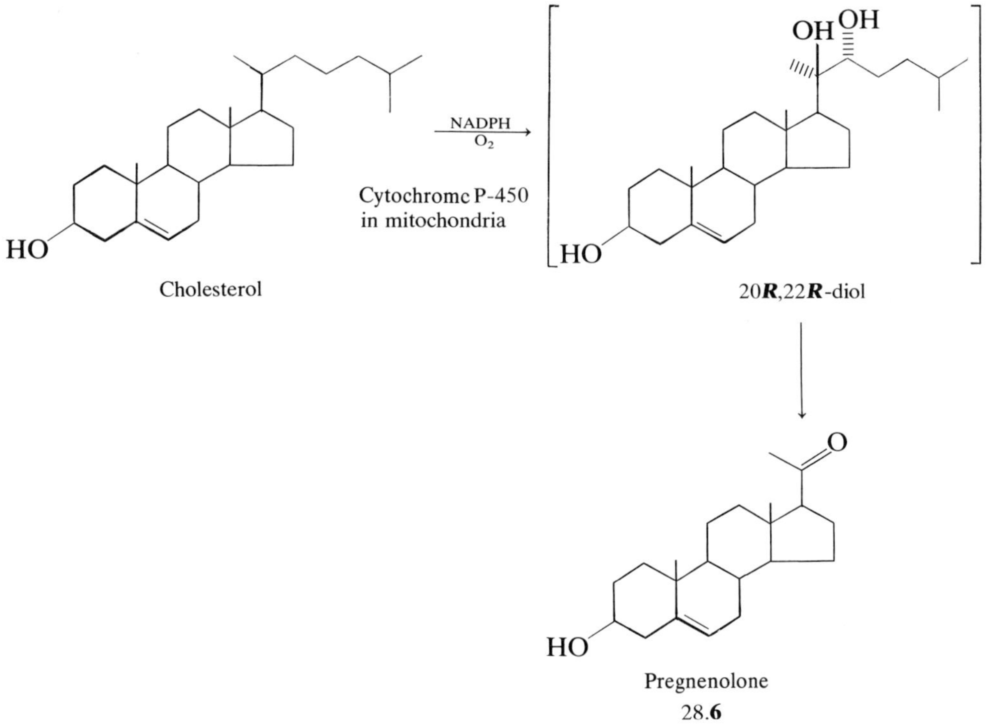

Fig. 28.2 Side-chain cleavage reaction.

Ruokonen (33) are particularly pertinent to this argument. These workers analyzed the spermatic venous plasma for free and conjugated steroids. The unconjugated steroids identified in normal males are listed in Table 28.1 along with the concentration in micrograms per 100 ml. All the intermediates of the "5-ene" pathway were identified, but progesterone (28.**7**), an important intermediate of the "4-ene" pathway, was not found. In addition, sulfate conjugates were present in significant quantities, especially androst-5-ene-3β,17β-diol 3-monosulfate. The data strongly suggest that this intermediate and its unconjugated form constitute an important precursor of testosterone in man. This view, however, was not supported by a kinetic analysis of the metabolism of androst-5-ene-3β,17β-diol (28.**11**) in man (34).

Table 28.1 Mean Concentration of Steroids in Spermatic Venous Plasma from Five Normal Males

Compound	Concentration (μg/100 ml)
5-Androstene-3β,17α-diol	4.0
5-Androstene-3β,17β-diol	18.5
Dehydroepiandrosterone	2.2
Androstenedione	2.5
Testosterone	74.0
Pregnenolone	4.8
17α-Hydroxypregnenolone	3.9
17α-Hydroxyprogesterone	6.2

Whichever pathway prevails, another important step is the conversion of the C-21 steroids to the C-19 androstene derivatives. Whereas the enzymes for side chain cleavage are localized in mitochondria, those responsible for cleavage of the C_{17}-C_{20} bond (C_{17}-C_{20} lyase) reside in the microsomes of the cell. Early studies implicated 17α-hydroxypregnenolone (28.**8**) or 17α-hydroxyprogesterone (28.**9**) as an obligatory intermediate in testosterone biosynthesis (35). Although such a sequence has

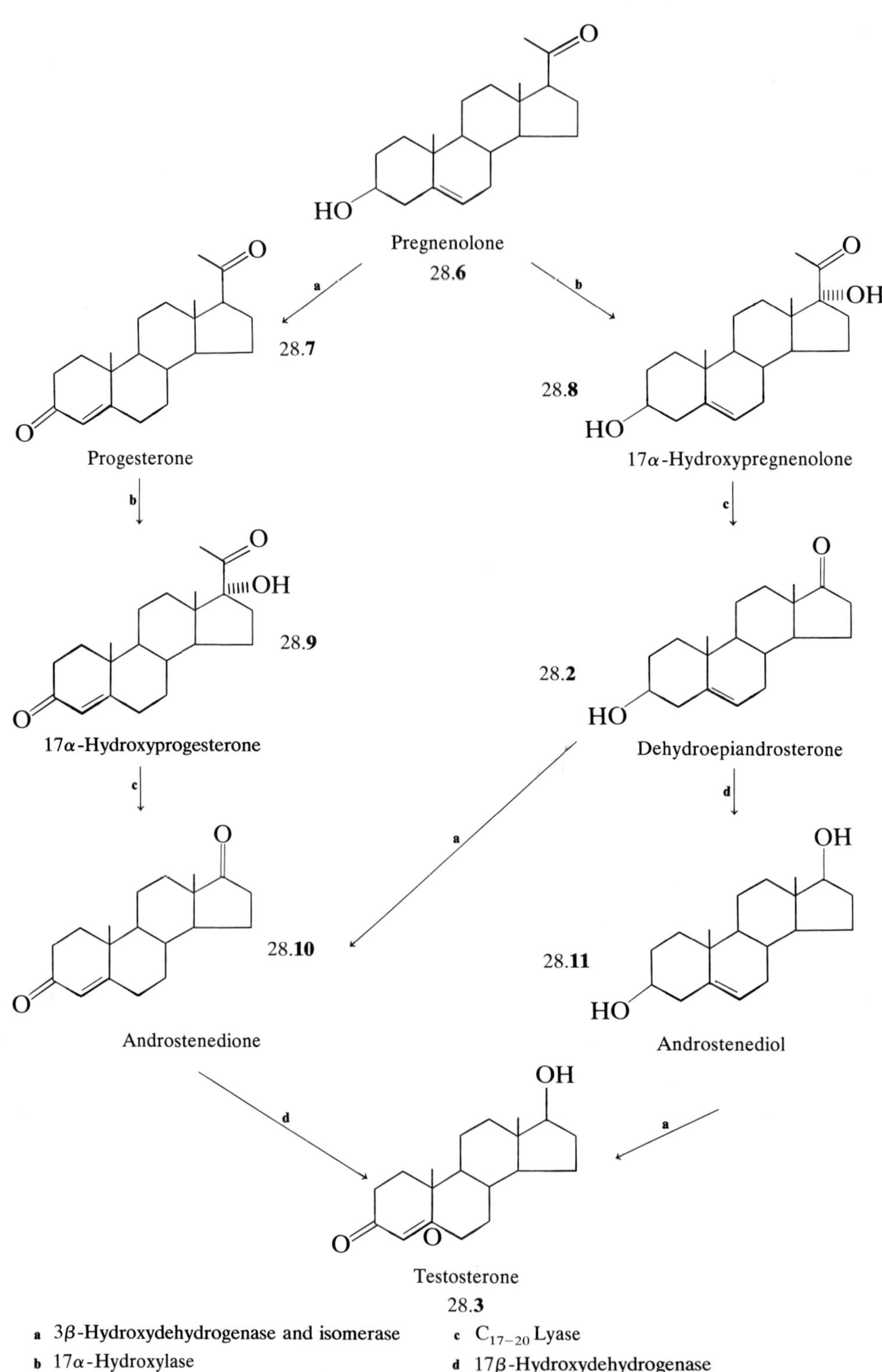
Pregnenolone
28.6
Progesterone
28.7
17α-Hydroxypregnenolone
28.8
17α-Hydroxyprogesterone
28.9
Dehydroepiandrosterone
28.2
Androstenedione
28.10
Androstenediol
28.11
Testosterone
28.3
a 3β-Hydroxydehydrogenase and isomerase
b 17α-Hydroxylase
c C_{17-20} Lyase
d 17β-Hydroxydehydrogenase

Fig. 28.3 Androgen biosynthesis.

been accepted dogma for the past quarter-century, the exact details of the lyase reaction are very much in doubt, especially when it can be shown that the C-20 deoxy analog of pregnenolone can also serve as a substrate for testosterone biosynthesis (36).

4 ABSORPTION AND DISTRIBUTION

Although considerable research has been devoted to the biochemical mechanism of action of the natural hormones and the synthesis of modified androgens, little is known about the absorption of these substances. It is well recognized that a steroid hormone might have high intrinsic activity but exert little or no biological effects because its physicochemical characteristics prevent it from reaching the site of action. This is particularly true in humans, where slow oral absorption or rapid inactivation may greatly reduce the efficacy of a drug. Even though steroids are commonly given by mouth, little is known of their intestinal absorption. One study in rats showed that androstenedione (28.**10**) was absorbed better than testosterone or 17α-methyltestosterone, and conversion of testosterone to its acetate enhanced absorption (37). Results with other steroids indicated that lipid solubility was an important factor for intestinal absorption. This may explain the oral activity of certain ethers and esters of testosterone.

Once in the circulatory system by either secretion from the testis or absorption of the administered drug, testosterone and other androgens will reversibly associate with certain plasma proteins, the unbound steroid being the biologically active form. The extent of this binding is dependent on the nature of the proteins and the structural features of the androgen.

The first protein to be studied was albumin, which exhibited a low association constant for testosterone and bound less polar androgens such as androstenedione to a greater extent (38–40). α-Acid glycoprotein (AAG) was shown to bind testosterone with a higher affinity than albumin (41, 42). A third plasma protein that binds testosterone is corticosteroid-binding α-globulin (CBG) (43). However under normal physiological conditions these plasma proteins are not responsible for extensive binding of androgens in plasma.

A specific protein termed sex steroid binding β-globulin (SBG) or testosterone-estradiol binding globulin (TEBG) was found in plasma that bound testosterone with a very high affinity (44, 45). The SBG–sex hormone complex serves several functions, such as transport or carrier system in the bloodstream, storage site or reservoir for the hormones, and protection of the hormone from metabolic transformations (46, 47). SBG has been purified and contains high affinity, low capacity binding sites for the sex hormones (48). Dissociation constants of approximately 1×10^{-9} M have been reported for the binding of testosterone and estradiol to SBG and are 2 orders of magnitude less than values reported for the binding of the hormone to the cytosolic receptor protein (49–51). The plasma levels of SBG are regulated by the thyroid hormones (52) and remain fairly constant throughout adult life in both the male and female (53). SBG is not present in the plasma of all animals (46, 53). For example, SBG-like activity is notably absent in the rat, and testosterone may be bound in the rat plasma to CBG.

Numerous studies have been performed on the specificity of the binding of steroids to human SBG (46, 47, 53–58). The presence of a 17β-hydroxyl group is essential for binding to SBG. In addition to testosterone, DHT, 5α-androstane-3β,17β-diol (28.**18**), and 5α-androstane-3α,17β-diol (28.**19**) bind with high affinity, and these steroids compete for a common binding site. Binding to SBG is decreased by 17α-substituents such as 17α-methyl and 17α-ethynyl moieties and by unsaturation at

C-1 or C-6. Also, 19-nortestosterone derivatives have lower affinity. SBG has been purified to homogeneity by affinity chromatography using a DHT-agarose adsorbant (59).

Another extracellular carrier protein exhibiting high affinity for testosterone, found in seminiferous fluid and the epididymis, originates in the testis and is called androgen binding protein (ABP) (60–62). This protein is produced by the Sertoli cells on stimulation by FSH (63, 64) and has very similar characteristics to those of plasma SBG produced in the liver (63). These proteins are distinctly separate from the intracellular cytoplasmic receptor protein (65), which is described in Section 7.

It is this cytoplasmic receptor protein and its high affinity for testosterone or DHT that accounts for the selective accumulation of these hormones in androgen target tissues. This selective uptake process is readily observed in rodents following administration of high specific activity tritiated androgens (66, 67).

The absorption of androgens and other steroids from the blood by target cells was usually assumed to occur by a passive diffusion of the molecule through the cell membrane. However studies in the early 1970s using tissue cultures or tissue slices suggested entry mechanisms for the steroids. Estrogens (68, 69) glucocorticoids (70, 71), and androgens (72–75) exhibit a temperature-dependent uptake into intact target cells, suggesting a protein-mediated process. Among the androgens, DHT exhibited a greater uptake than testosterone in human prostate tissue slices (72), and it was found that estradiol or androstenedione interfered with this uptake mechanism (73, 74). In addition, cyproterone (see Section 11) competitively inhibited androstenedione, testosterone, and DHT entry, whereas cyproterone acetate enhanced the uptake of these androgens (75). Little is known about the exit of steroids from target cells; the only reported research has dealt with an active transport of glucocorticoids out of cells (76, 77).

5 METABOLIC FATE

5.1 Reductive Metabolites

The metabolism of testosterone in a variety of *in vitro* and *in vivo* systems has been reviewed (35, 78, 79). The principal pathways for testosterone metabolism in man appear in Fig. 28.4. Human liver produces a number of metabolites, including androstenedione (28.**10**), androsta-4,16-dien-3-one, 5β-androstane-3α,17α-diol, 5α-androstane-3α,17β-diol (28.**19**), 5α-androstane-3β,17β-diol (28.**18**), and 3β-hydroxy-5α-androstan-17-one (28.**15**) (80, 81). In addition, cirrhotic liver was shown to produce more 17-ketosteroids than normal liver (82). Human adrenal preparations, on the other hand, gave 11β-hydroxytestosterone as the major metabolite (83). Intestinal metabolism of testosterone is similar to tranformations in the liver (79); the major metabolite in lung is androstenedione (84).

Studies on testosterone metabolism since the late 1960s have centered on steroid transformations by prostatic tissues. Normal prostate, benign prostatic hypertrophy (BPH), and prostatic carcinoma all contain 3α-, 3β-, and 17β-hydroxysteriod dehydrogenases, and 5α- and 5β-reductases, capable of converting testosterone to various metabolites. Prostatic carcinoma metabolizes testosterone more slowly than does BPH or normal prostate (85). In addition, increased levels of androgens are found in BPH (86). K. D. Voigt et al. (87–89) have extensively studied *in vivo* metabolic patterns of androgens in patients with BPH. Tritiated androgens were injected intravenously into these patients 30 min before prostatectomy, and prostatic tissue, tissue from surrounding skeletal muscle, and blood plasma were analyzed for

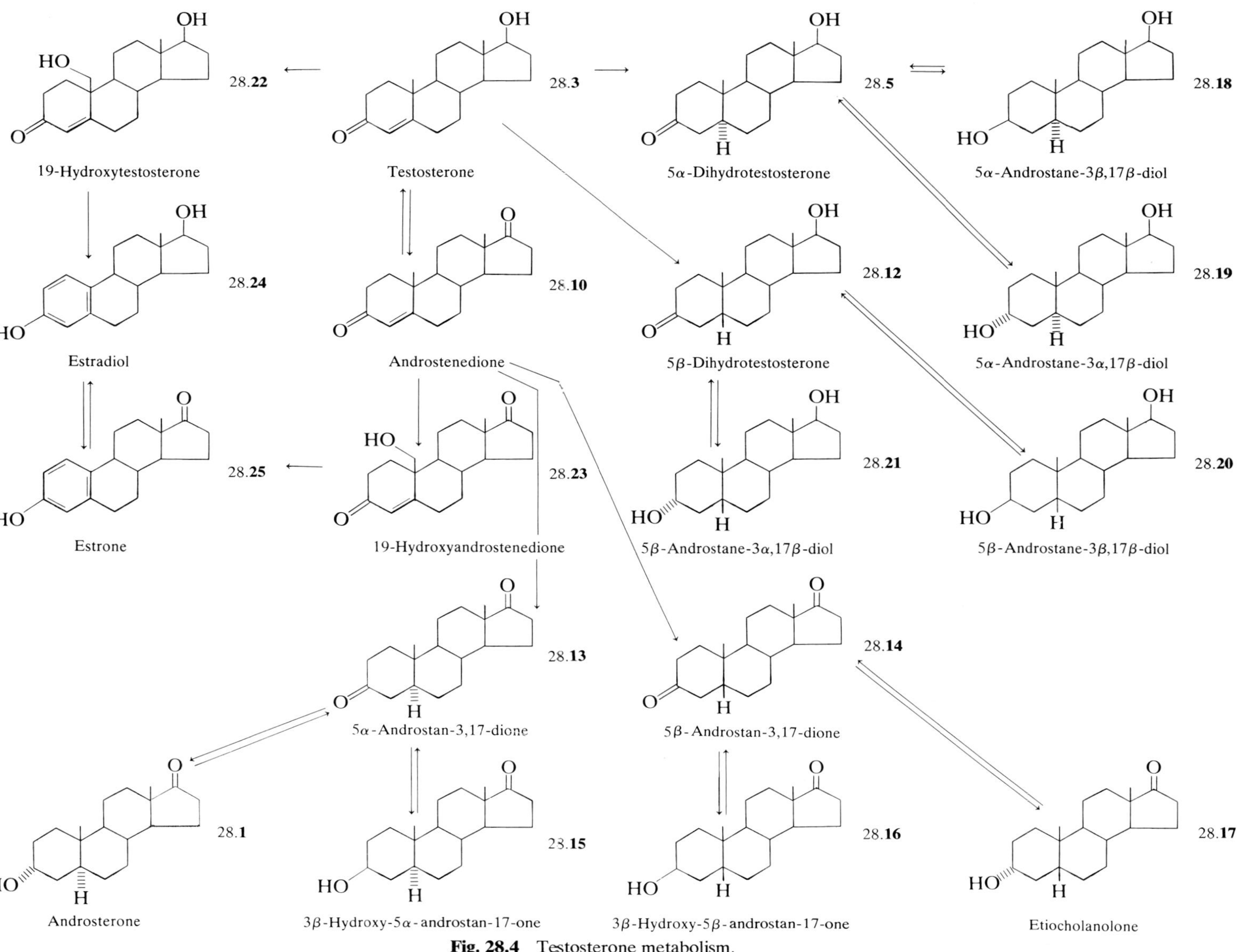
19-Hydroxytestosterone
28.22
Testosterone
28.3
5α-Dihydrotestosterone
28.5
5α-Androstane-3β,17β-diol
28.18
Estradiol
28.24
Androstenedione
28.10
5β-Dihydrotestosterone
28.12
5α-Androstane-3α,17β-diol
28.19
Estrone
28.25
19-Hydroxyandrostenedione
28.23
5β-Androstane-3α,17β-diol
28.21
5β-Androstane-3β,17β-diol
28.20
5α-Androstan-3,17-dione
28.13
5β-Androstan-3,17-dione
28.14
Androsterone
28.1
3β-Hydroxy-5α-androstan-17-one
23.15
3β-Hydroxy-5β-androstan-17-one
28.16
Etiocholanolone
28.17

Fig. 28.4 Testosterone metabolism.

metabolites. The major metabolite of testosterone found in BPH tissues was DHT, with minor amounts of diols isolated. Skeletal muscle and plasma contained primarily unchanged testosterone.

Table 28.2 lists the urinary metabolites that have been identified following the administration of testosterone to humans (see Fig. 28.4). These products are excreted as such or in the form of their glucuronide or sulfate conjugates. Androsterone (28.**1**) and etiocholanolone (28.**17**), the major urinary metabolites, are excreted predominantly as glucuronides, and only about 10% as sulfates (90). These conjugates are capable of undergoing further metabolism. Testosterone glucuronide, for example, is metabolized differently from testosterone in man, giving rise mainly to 5β-metabolites (91).

Table 28.2 Urinary Metabolites of Testosterone (cf. Ref. 92)

Metabolite	Approximate Conversion, %
Androsterone Etiocholanolone	25–50
5β-Androstane-3α,17β-diol	2
5α-Androstane-3α,17β-diol	1
5α-Androstan-3β-ol-17-one	1
Androst-16-en-3α-ol	0.4
3α,18-Dihydroxy-5β-androstan-17-one	0.3
3α,7β-Dihydroxy-5β-androstan-17-one	Trace
11β-Hydroxytestosterone	Trace
6α-, 6β-Hydroxytestosterone	Trace

It should also be pointed out that only a relatively small amount of the urinary 17-ketosteroids is derived from testosterone metabolism. In man at least 67% and in women about 80% or more of the urinary 17-ketosteroids are metabolites of adrenocortical steroids (93). This explains why a significant increase in testosterone secretion associated with various androgenic syndromes does not usually lead to elevated levels of 17-ketosteroid excretion.

Although androsterone and etiocholanolone are the major excretory products, the exact sequence whereby these 17-ketosteroids arise is still not clear. Studies with radiolabeled androst-4-ene-3β,17β-diol and the epimeric 3α-diol in humans showed that oxidation to testosterone was necessary before reduction of the A-ring (94). Moreover, in rats 5β-androstane-3α,17β-diol (28.**21**) was the major initial liver metabolite, but this decreased with time with the simultaneous increase of etiocholanolone (95). This formation of saturated diols agrees with studies using human liver (80) and provides evidence that the initial step in testosterone metabolism is reduction of the α,β-unsaturated ketone to a mixture of diols followed by oxidation to the 17-ketosteroids.

Until recently, it was generally thought that the excretory metabolites of testosterone were physiologically inert. Subsequent work has shown, however, that etiocholanolone has thermogenic effects when administered to man (96). Moreover, the hypocholesterolemic effects of parenterally administered androsterone have been described (97).

The metabolism of modified androgens or anabolic steroids is summarized in Table 28.3. As one would anticipate, many of the compounds are metabolized in a manner similar to testosterone. An important exception is 4-chlorotestosterone, which in humans gave rise to an allylic alcohol, 4-chloro-3α-hydroxyandrost-4-en-17-one (98). A number of other halogenated testosterone derivatives subsequently were found to take this abnormal reduction path *in vitro* (99). It was proposed that fluorine or chlorine substituents at the 2-, 4-, or 6-position in testosterone interfere with the usual α,β-unsaturated ketone resonance so that the C-3 carbonyl electronically resembles a saturated ketone.

Table 28.3 Metabolism of Modified Androgens

Substrate	Products	Test System	Species	References
17β-Hydroxyestra-4-en-3-one	5α-Estran-3α-ol-17-one 5β-Estran-3α-ol-17-one	*In vivo*	Human	100
	5α,5β-Estran-3α-ol-17-one plus 5α-Estran-3β-ol-17-one 5α-Estrane-3α,17β-diol 5α-Estrane-3β,17β-diol	Liver homogenate	Female rat	101
	Estra-4-ene-3,17-dione 5α-Estran-17β-ol-3-one 2-Methoxyestrone	Prostate slices	Human	102
1α-Methyl-17β-hydroxyestra-4-en-3-one acetate	1α-Methyl-5α-estran-3α-ol-17-one 1α-Methyl-5β-estran-3α-ol-17-one	*In vivo*	Human	103
17α-Methyl-17β-hydroxyestra-4-en-3-one	17α-Methyl-5α-estran-17β-ol-3-one 17α-Methyl-5α-estrane-3α,17β-diol	Liver homogenate	Female rat	104
17α-Methyltestosterone	17α-Methyl-5α-androstane-3α,17β-diol 17α-Methyl-5β-androstane-3α,17β-diol 17α-Methyl-5α-androstane-3β,17β-diol	*In vivo*	Human	105
17α-Methylandrost-5-ene-3β,17β-diol	17α-Methyltestosterone 11β-Hydroxy-17α-methyltestosterone	Adrenal	Male rat	106
17α-Methyl-17β-hydroxyandrosta-1,4-dien-3-one	17α-Methyl-6β,17β-dihydroxyandrosta-1,4-dien-3-one	*In vivo*	Human	107
1α-Methyl-17β-hydroxy-5α-androst-1-en-3-one acetate	1α-Methyl-5α-androstan-3α-ol-17-one	*In vivo*	Human	108
	1α-Methyl-5α-androst-1-ene-3,17-dione	*In vivo*	Human	109
	1α-methyl/compounds above plus: 1-Methylene-5α-androstan-3α-ol-17-one 1α-Methyl-5α-androstane-3,17-dione	*in vivo*	Human	110
4-Chloro-17β-hydroxyandrost-4-en-3-one acetate	4-Chloro-3α-hydroxyandrost-4-en-17-one	*In vivo*	Human	98
17β-Hydroxy-9β,10α-androst-4-en-3-one (retrotestosterone)	9β,10α-androst-4-ene-3,17-dione	Placenta	Human	111
D-Homo-17aβ-hydroxyandrost-4-en-3-one (D-homotestosterone)	D-Homo-5β-androstane-3α,17aβ-diol	*In vivo*	Human	112
1α-Methyl-5α-androstan-17β-ol-3-one	1α-Methyl-5α-androstan-3α-ol-17-one 1α-Methyl-5α-androstan-3α,17β-diol	*In vivo*	Human	113

The conversion of testosterone to DHT by 5α-reductase has major importance in the mechanism of action of the hormone. This enzymatic activity has been found in the microsomal fraction (114, 115) and in the nuclear membrane (116–122) of androgen-sensitive cells. In addition, the levels of 5α-reductase are under the control of testosterone and DHT (122); 5α-reductase activity decreases after castration and can be restored to normal levels of activity with testosterone or DHT administration (123).

5.2 Oxidative Metabolites

Another metabolic transformation of androgens leading to hormonally active compounds is their conversion to estrogens. Estrogens are biosynthesized in the ovaries and placenta and, to a lesser extent, in the testes, adrenals, and certain regions of the brain. This enzymatic activity was first identified by Ryan (124) in the microsomal fraction from human placental tissue. It is a cytochrome P-450 enzyme complex (125) and requires 3 moles of NADPH and 3 moles of oxygen per mole of substrate (126). The observation by Meyer (127) that 19-hydroxyandrostenedione (28.**23**) was a more active precursor of estrone (28.**25**) than the substrate androstenedione led to its postulated role in estrogen biosynthesis. This report and numerous studies that followed led to the currently accepted pathway for aromatization (128), as shown in Fig. 28.5.

The first two oxidations occur at the C_{19} position, producing the 19-alcohol (28.**23**) and then the 19-*gem*-diol (28.**27**), originally isolated as the 19-aldehyde (28.**26**) (129, 130). The final oxidation results in the stereospecific elimination of the 1β and 2β hydrogen atoms (131–133) and the concerted elimination of the oxidized C_{19} moiety as formic acid (130). 2β-Hydroxy-19-oxoandrostenedione (28.**28**) has been demonstrated to be the intermediate in this final oxidation, and this substance spontaneously aromatizes to estrone (128).

Incubation of a large number of testosterone analogs with human placental tissue (134–136) has provided some insight into the structural requirements for aromatization (see Table 28.4). Whereas androstenedione was converted rapidly to estrone, the 1-dehydro and 19-nor analogs were

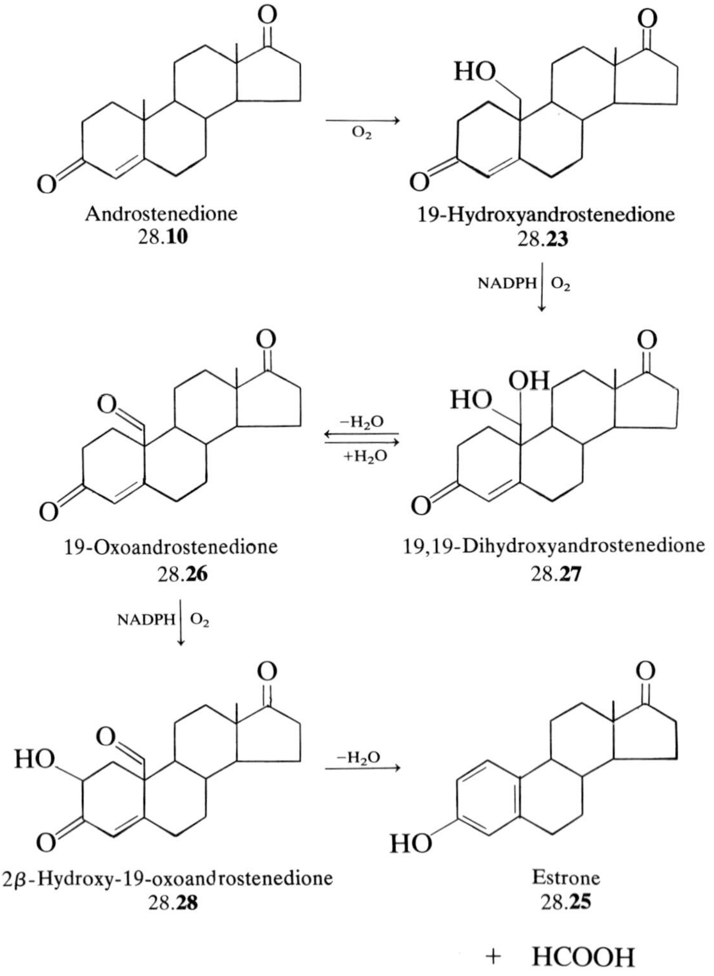

Androstenedione
28.**10**

O_2

19-Hydroxyandrostenedione
28.**23**

NADPH O_2

19-Oxoandrostenedione
28.**26**

$-H_2O$
$+H_2O$

19,19-Dihydroxyandrostenedione
28.**27**

NADPH O_2

2β-Hydroxy-19-oxoandrostenedione
28.**28**

$-H_2O$

Estrone
28.**25**

+ HCOOH

Fig. 28.5 Aromatization.

Table 28.4 Relative Substrate Activity in Aromatization[a]

Substrate	Activity, %
C_{19}-Steroids	
Androst-4-ene-3,17-dione	100
19-Hydroxyandrost-4-ene-3,17-dione	184, 133
17β-Hydroxyandrost-4-en-3-one	100
3β-Hydroxyandrost-5-en-17-one	66
5α-Androst-1-ene-3,17-dione	0
5α-Androstane-3,17-dione	0
1α-Hydroxyandrost-4-ene-3,17-dione	0
17β-Hydroxy-1α-methylandrost-4-ene-3-one	0
2β-Hydroxyandrost-4-ene-3,17-dione	15
2α-Hydroxyandrost-4-ene-3,17-dione	0
17β-Hydroxy-2β-methylandrost-4-en-3-one	0
11β-Hydroxyandrost-4-ene-3,17-dione	0
11α-Hydroxyandrost-4-ene-3,17-dione	100
17β-Hydroxy-17α-methylandrost-4-en-3-one	44
6β-Hydroxyandrost-4-ene-3,17-dione	21
6α-Fluoro-17β-hydroxyandrost-4-ene-3,17-dione	0
6β-Fluoro-17β-hydroxyandrost-4-ene-3,17-dione	0
9α-Fluoroandrosta-1,4-diene-3,17-dione	55
Androsta-1,4-diene-3,17-dione	22, 35
Androsta-4,6-diene-3,17-dione	0
Androsta-1,4,6-triene-3,17-dione	0
Androst-4-ene-3,11,17-trione	0
C_{18}-Steroids	
Estr-4-ene-3,17-dione	21
17β-Hydroxyestr-4-en-3-one	20
17β-Hydroxy-5α,10β-estr-3-one	0
C_{21}-Steroids	
Pregn-4-ene-3,20-dione	0
17α,19,21-Trihydroxypregn-4-ene-3,20-dione	0

[a] From Refs. 134–136.

metabolized slowly, and the 6-dehydro isomer and saturated 5α-androstane-3,17-dione remained unchanged. Hydroxyl and other substituents at 1α, 2β, and 11β interfered with aromatization, whereas similar substituents at 9α and 11α seemingly had no effect. Of the stereoisomers of testosterone, only the 8β,9β,10β-isomer aromatized, in addition to compounds having the normal configuration (8β, 9α, 10β). Thus the substrate specificity of aromatase appears to be limited to C_{19} steroids with the 4-en-3-one system. Inhibition studies with various steroids have provided additional insights into the structural requirements for the aromatase reaction (137–139). Such compounds as androsta-4,6-diene-3,17-dione and androsta-1,4,6-triene-3,17-dione with extended linear conjugation show increased inhibitory activity, and 5α-reduced C_{19}-steroids also inhibit aromatization. 4-Hydroxyandrostenedione (140) and various 7α-substituted androstenedione derivatives (141) are among the most potent inhibitors of aromatase *in vitro.*

The metabolism of androgens by the mammalian brain has also been investigated under *in vitro* conditions. Sholiton et al. (142) in 1966 first reported the metabolism of testosterone in rat brain, and later studies demonstrated the conversion of testosterone to DHT, androstenedione, 5α-androstane-3,17-dione and 5α-androstane-3β,17β-diol (143–147). The aromatization of androgens to estrogens was also found to occur in the hypothalamus and the pituitary gland (148–152). The full significance of these metabolites on various neuroendocrine functions, such as regulation of gonadotropin secretion and sexual behavior, is not yet fully understood (153).

6 PHYSIOLOGICAL ROLE AND METABOLIC EFFECTS

The natural androgen testosterone is responsible for the development and maintenance of the sexual characteristics of the male. The prostate, penis, seminal vesicles, and vas deferens are controlled by androgens; the development of these sex organs is evident during the stages of puberty. Secondary sex characteristics also develop under the influence of testosterone. Hair growth on the face, arms, legs, and trunk is stimulated by this hormone during younger years; in later years, testosterone is responsible for thinning of the hair and recession of the hairline. The growth of the larynx and the resultant deepening of the voice is dependent on testosterone. It also stimulates proliferation of the sebaceous glands, loss of subcutaneous fat, and an increase in the fructose content in human semen. The stimulation of male and female sexual behavior and changes in mood and aggressiveness are other characteristics associated with androgens.

In addition to these androgenic properties, testosterone also exhibits anabolic (myotropic) characteristics. This anabolic action is associated with a marked retention of nitrogen brought about by an increase of protein synthesis and a decrease of protein catabolism. The increase in nitrogen retention is manifested primarily by a decrease in urinary rather than fecal nitrogen excretion and results in a more positive nitrogen balance. For example, intramuscular administration of 25 mg of testosterone propionate twice daily can produce a nitrogen retention to appear within 1–3 days, reaching a maximum in about 5–8 days. This reduced level of nitrogen excretion may be maintained for at least a month and depends on the patient's nutritional status and diet (154).

Androgens and anabolic steroids influence skeletal maturation and mineralization, which is reflected in an increase in skeletal calcium and phosphorus (155). In various forms of osteoporosis, androgens decrease urinary calcium loss and improve the calcium balance in patients. This effect is not as noticeable in normal patients. Moreover the various androgen analogs differ markedly in their effects on calcium and phosphorus balance in man. 17α-Methyl-19-nortestosterone (28.**32**) is a very effective agent for increasing calcium balance in man, whereas fluoxymesterone (halotestin, 28.**53**) has essentially no effect on urinary or fecal calcium excretion (156).

Androgens and their 5β-metabolites (e.g., etiocholanolone) markedly stimulate erythropoiesis, presumably by increasing the production of erythropoietin and by enhancing the responsiveness of erythropoietic tissue to erythropoietin (157). This metabolic effect has prompted the evaluation of androgens and anabolic steroids in the treatment of various types of anemias.

The effects of androgens on carbohydrate metabolism appear to be minor and secondary to their primary protein anabolic property. The effects on lipid metabolism, on the other hand, seem to be unrelated to this anabolic property. As mentioned earlier, weakly androgenic metabolites such as androsterone have been found to lower serum cholesterol levels when administered parenterally. Among the anabolic steroids, oxandrolone (28.**56**) has been the most widely studied for its hypolipidemic effects. Since this agent has a more pronounced effect on triglycerides than cholesterol, it has been clinically evaluated for the treatment of types III, IV, and V hyperlipidemia (158).

Finally, testosterone exerts a major influence on the function of the central nervous system. Indeed, evidence now indicates that the development of gender identity as well as other aspects of behavior are under specific control of the male sex hormones. Moreover there appear to be distinct roles for the androgens, as suggested by the finding that testosterone but not DHT mediates the sex drive in rat (159).

7 MECHANISM OF ACTION

It would indeed be impossible to explain all the varied biological actions of testosterone by one biochemical mechanism. Over the last decade, the majority of investigations concerning the elucidation of the mechanisms of action of androgens have dealt with actions in androgen-dependent tissues and, in particular, the rat ventral prostate. The results of these studies indicate that androgens act in regulating protein synthesis by formation of a hormone-receptor complex, analogous to the mechanisms of action of estrogens and progestins. Numerous reviews have appeared on this subject (160–164).

Jensen and Jacobson (165), using radiolabeled 17β-estradiol (28.**24**), were the first to show that a steroid was selectively retained by its target tissues. Investigations of a selective uptake of androgens by target cells performed in the early 1960s were complicated by low specific activity of the radiolabeled hormones and the rapid metabolic transformations. Nonetheless, it was noted that target cells retained primarily unconjugated metabolites, whereas conjugated metabolites were present in nontarget cells such as blood and liver (166, 167). With the availability of steroids with high specific activity, later studies demonstrated the selective uptake and retention of androgens by target tissues (16, 17, 168–170). In addition, DHT was found to be the steroidal form selectively retained in the nucleus of the rat ventral prostate (16, 169). This discovery led to the current concept that testosterone is converted by 5α-reductase to DHT, which is the active form of cellular androgen in androgen-dependent tissues.

The rat prostate has been the most widely examined tissue, and current hypotheses on the mode of action of androgens are based largely on these studies (see Fig. 28.6). Present in the cytosol of prostate cells are proteins that bind DHT (17, 171). One particular protein receptor exhibits extremely high affinity and high specificity for DHT, with the steroid-receptor protein complex formed having a sedimentation coefficient of 3–3.5S in 0.4 M potassium chloride solutions. The binding of DHT with the receptor protein is a necessary step in the mechanism of action of the steroid in the prostate cell. Following this interaction, a conformational

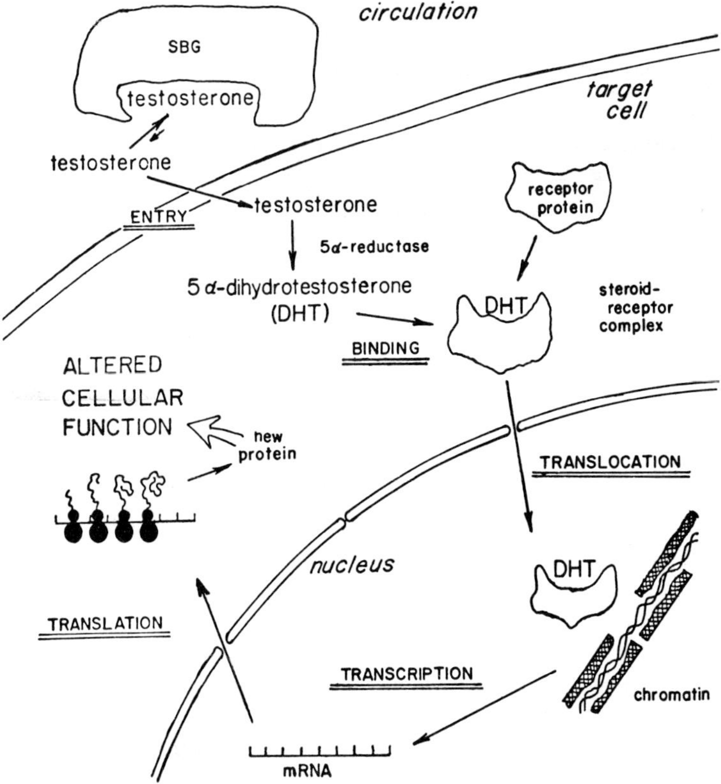

Fig. 28.6 A mechanism of action of testosterone.

change or activation of the steroid-receptor complex occurs. The activation process triggers the translocation of the steroid-receptor complex from the cytoplasm into the nucleus of the cell, where the complex acts to regulate protein synthesis. This nuclear complex formed by translocation has a sedimentation constant of 3*S*.

Studies of the interaction of the nuclear steroid-receptor complex with DNA have demonstrated that binding occurs, but not to specific sites on purified DNA (172, 173). Instead, the tissue specificity is regulated by nonhistone protein present in chromatin. These proteins, called "acceptor" proteins, are responsible for binding the steroid-receptor complex to specific sites on the chromatin. The effect of this binding in the nucleus is an increase in total cellular RNA. Recent experiments indicate that RNA is increased in response to androgens (174). In addition, the activities of DNA-dependent RNA polymerases are stimulated by testosterone treatment (175, 176). The exact nuclear events of gene transcription affected by androgens are poorly understood.

The ultimate action of androgens on target tissues is the stimulation of cellular growth and differentiation through regulation of protein synthesis. Numerous androgen-inducible proteins have been identified, such as a nerve-growth factor (177), an epidermal-growth factor (178), protease D (179), L-gulonolactonase (180), β-glucuronidase (180), and α_{2u}-globulin (181–183). Studies of these proteins suggest that the androgens act by enhancing transcription and/or translation of specific RNAs for the proteins.

Currently little is known concerning the release of steroid-receptor complexes from the nucleus. Liao and co-workers (184, 185) have isolated certain nuclear ribonucleoprotein (RNP) particles that bind the DHT-receptor complex. Liao has postulated that the steroid-receptor-bound RNP formed in the nucleus may enter the cytoplasm and participate in protein synthesis. The receptor protein and steroid may then be released and recycled in the cell. Future research will undoubtedly clarify this picture of hormone-receptor release from the nucleus.

While most biochemical studies focused on the rat ventral prostate, some researchers began to investigate the presence of cellular receptor proteins in other androgen-sensitive tissues. Table 28.5 lists tissues in which androgen receptors have been found. Although DHT is the active androgen in rat ventral prostate, it is not the only functioning form in other androgen-sensitive cells. In ventral prostate and seminal vesicles, DHT is readily formed. It is metabolized only slowly, however, and therefore can accumulate and bind to receptors. In other tissues such as brain or kidney, DHT is not readily formed and is metabolized quickly compared to testosterone. Species variations have also been demonstrated. The most striking example is the finding that 5α-androstane-3α,17α-diol interacts specifically with cytosolic receptor protein from dog prostate (209) and may be the active androgen in this species (210). Apparently the need for a 17β-hydroxyl is not essential in all species (see Section 10).

Thus current findings indicate that androgen receptor proteins vary in steroid specificity among different tissues from the same species as well as among different species. Nevertheless, the basic molecular mechanism of action of the androgens in androgen-sensitive tissues is consistent with the results of the studies on rat ventral prostate.

The manner whereby the androgens exert their anabolic effects has not been studied nearly as extensively. It has been reported that the conversion of testosterone to DHT is insignificant in skeletal and levator ani muscles, and suggests that the androgen-mediated growth of muscle is due to testosterone itself (211, 212). Muscle tissues display other differences, such as

Table 28.5 Tissues Containing Androgen Receptor Proteins

Tissue	Reference
Seminal vesicles	186, 187
Sebaceous gland	188–190
Testis	189, 191
Epididymis	189, 192, 193
Kidney	194
Submandibular gland	195, 196
Pituitary and hypothalamus	197–203
Bone marrow	204, 205
Liver	206
Androgen-sensitive tumors	207, 208

their inability to accumulate hormone and their lack of a cytoplasmic receptor protein typical of the androgen target organs (212, 213). Baulieu and co-workers (214, 215), on the other hand, have detected a typical steroid receptor for testosterone in the cytoplasm of the levator ani and quadriceps muscles of the rat. Unlike prostate receptor protein, DHT had a lower affinity than testosterone for this protein. Moreover, Powers and Florini (216) were able to demonstrate a direct effect of testosterone on muscle cells in tissue culture as measured by pulse-labeling of DNA with ^{3}H-thymidine. DHT failed to give a statistically significant stimulation of DNA synthesis. Thus although the exact mechanism for the anabolic action of testosterone is far from clear, there is some evidence for a direct action of testosterone and the involvement of specific receptor proteins.

The biochemical mechanism of action of androgens in human tissue appears to be similar in many aspects to the mechanisms described in numerous animal models. Again the majority of the studies on human tissues have concerned the role of androgens in the prostate gland. Similar characteristics for receptor proteins and for the enzymatic conversion of testosterone to DHT have been demonstrated. Despite the similarities of hormonal regulation in the prostate, considerable species differences exist concerning the structure and function of the prostate gland. In contrast to man, spontaneous prostatic tumors are rare in animals. The exception is benign prostatic hypertrophy in the dog; however this tumor is poorly comparable both histologically and therapeutically to that in man (217). Thus there is currently no ideal animal model for comparison of the action of androgens in humans.

8 METHODS OF BIOASSAY

8.1 Androgens

The various analytical methods used to establish the androgenic properties of steroidal substances have been reviewed by Dorfman (218). Traditionally, androgens have been assayed by the capon comb growth method and by the use of the seminal vesicles and prostate organs of the rodent. An increase in weight and/or growth of the capon comb have been used to denote androgenic activity following injection or topical application of a solution of the test compound in oil (219). A number of minor modifications of this test have been described (220–222). The increase in weight of the seminal vesicles and the ventral prostate of the immature castrated male rat has provided another measure of androgenic potency (223–226). The test compound is administered either intramuscularly or orally, and the weight of the target organs is compared with those of control animals.

8.2 Anabolic Agents

The methods employed to determine the anabolic or myotrophic properties of steroids have been reviewed (227). Generally, these are based on an increase in nitrogen retention and/or muscle mass in various laboratory animals. The castrated male rat is presently the most widely used and most sensitive laboratory animal for nitrogen balance studies (228). Dogs and ovariectomized monkeys have also been employed (229, 230). Although it is generally agreed that variations in urinary nitrogen excretion relate to an increase or decrease in protein synthesis, nitrogen balance assays are not without their limitations (231). This is partly because such studies fail to describe the shifts in organ protein and measure only the overall status of nitrogen retention in the animal (232).

The easily accessible levator ani muscle of the rat has provided a valuable index for measuring the myotrophic activity of steroidal hormones (224). By comparing the weight of levator ani muscle, seminal vesicles, and ventral prostate with controls, one can obtain a ratio of anabolic to androgenic activity (224, 226). There also appears to be some correlation between the levator ani response and urinary nitrogen retention (224). A modification of this muscle assay utilizes the parabiotic rat (233, 234) and allows for the simultaneous measurement of pituitary gonadotrophic inhibition and myotrophic activity. The suitability of the levator ani assay has been questioned on the possibility that its growth is more a result of androgenic sensitivity than of any steroid-induced myotrophic effect (235–237). Thus this assay is usually performed in conjunction with nitrogen balance studies or acceleration of body growth (238).

9 CLINICAL EVALUATION, UTILITY, AND SIDE EFFECTS

Relatively few methods are available for ascertaining androgenic and anabolic activity in humans. The most widely used tests involve measuring the change in nitrogen retention, sperm count suppression, and urinary testosterone levels following treatment. Since an increase in nitrogen retention is usually ascribed to the anabolic effects, this method serves only as an indirect measurement for androgenicity. Other clinical tests for androgenicity are much less quantitative and depend largely on the increased prominence of secondary sex characteristics. These effects are most readily observed in females, eunuchs, and prepubertal males, and are of limited practical value. Similarly, a high degree of individual variability was noted when testicular function and sperm count were used to measure androgenicity (239). An increase in viability and maturation of the sebaceous gland has also served as a criterion for androgenicity (240).

The main application of androgenic hormones is for replacement therapy in cases of testicular deficiency or decreased testosterone production such as is the case in hypogonadism in male children. In males, androgens are also used to treat abnormal testicular descent, impotency, pituitary dwarfism, benign prostatic hypertrophy, and certain types of cardiovascular disease (239). In females, they are used for the correction of menopausal symptoms, various forms of abnormal uterine bleeding, hypolibido, and other endocrine malfunctions. The masculinizing side effects, however, severely limit the use of androgens in treating female reproductive disorders. On the other hand, androgen analogs (e.g., calusterone, 28.**48**), which have minimal hormonal activity, produce beneficial results in the treatment of disseminated breast cancer (241).

Anabolic steroids have been used to enhance weight gain in underweight children (242) and adults (243, 244). They can also reverse the negative nitrogen balance associated with postoperative periods and glucocorticoid therapy (245, 246). Beneficial effects have also been noted in cases of bone decalcification associated with osteoporosis and the aging process (247, 248).

Moreover, the value of anabolic steroids for treating hyperlipidemia in individuals has been recognized (249–251). Oxandrolone (28.**56**) has been the compound most widely studied for its hypolipidemic effects. It has been found to lower triglyceride levels more consistently than cholesterol levels; therefore it has been investigated for the treatment of types III, IV, and V hyperlipoproteinemia (158).

The ability of anabolic steroids to stimulate erythropoiesis has led to their use in the treatment of various anemias. Particularly beneficial results have been demonstrated in the treatment of aplastic anemias when used alone or in combination with corticosteroid therapy (252).

Anabolic steroids have been widely used and abused by athletes in search of a shortcut to increase muscle mass and strength. Such results are not supported by clinical evidence, and the use of anabolic steroids or androgens for this purpose has been banned in international sports (253).

Unfortunately, the clinical use of androgens is limited by untoward side effects in humans. In addition to possible masculinization of females, both sexes may experience salt and subsequent water retention. Furthermore, certain 17α-alkylated androgens produce hepatic alterations as manifested by sulfobromophthalein (BSP) retention (254, 255) and in some instances by clinical jaundice (256). These hepatic changes appear to be transitory however, since normal function returns on cessation of therapy. Virilization (257) and premature acceleration of bone aging (epiphyseal closure) (258, 259) were noted in children who had received anabolic therapy.

10 STRUCTURALLY MODIFIED ANDROGENS

10.1 Early Modifications

Most of the early structure-activity relationship studies concerned minor modifications of testosterone and other naturally occurring androgens. Studies in animals (260) and humans (261) showed the 17β-hydroxyl function to be essential for androgenic and anabolic activity. In certain cases esterification of the 17β-hydroxyl group not only enhanced but also prolonged the anabolic and androgenic properties (262) (see Section 10.8). The early statement (263) that the 1-dehydro isomer of testosterone (28.**29**) was a weak androgen was subsequently disproved. This isomer and related compounds are potent androgenic and anabolic steroids (264).

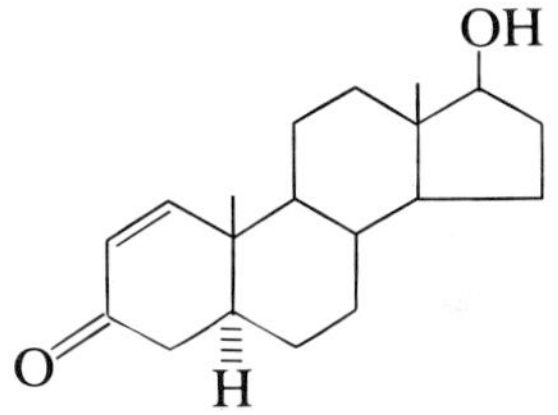

OH

O H

28.**29**

Reduction of the A-ring functional groups has variable effects on activity. For example, conversion of testosterone to DHT has little effect or may increase potency in a variety of bioassay systems (238, 265, 266). On the other hand, changing the A/B trans stereochemistry of known androgens such as androsterone (28.**1**) and DHT to the A/B *cis*-etiocholanolone (28.**17**) and 17β-hydroxy-5β-androstan-3-one (28.**12**), respectively, drastically reduces both the anabolic and androgenic properties (267–269). These observations established the importance of the A/B trans ring juncture for activity.

The discovery that C-17α methylation conferred oral activity on testosterone prompted the synthesis of additional *C*-17α-substituted analogs. Increasing the chain length beyond methyl invariably led to a decrease in activity (270). As a result of these studies, however, 17α-methylandrost-5-ene-3β,17β-diol (methandriol, 28.**30**) was widely evaluated in humans as an anabolic agent. Early biological studies with methandriol had shown a separation of anabolic and androgenic properties, but this was not confirmed by subsequent studies (225, 231). In addition, clinical studies showed no advantage of methandriol over 17α-methyltestosterone (28.**4**) (271).

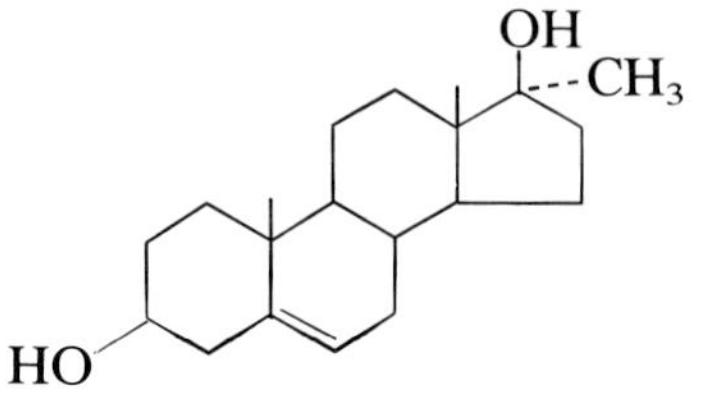

28.**30**

10.2 Nor and Homo Compounds

An important step toward developing an anabolic agent with minimal androgenicity was taken when Hershberger and associates (226), and later others (272, 273), found 19-nortestosterone (17β-hydroxyestr-4-en-3-one, nandrolone, 28.**31**) to be as myotrophic but only about 0.1 as androgenic as testosterone. This observation prompted the synthesis and evaluation of a variety of 19-norsteroids, including the 17α-methyl (normethandrone, 28.**32**) (274) and the 17α-cthyl (norethandrolone, 28.**33**) (275) homologs of 19-nortestosterone.

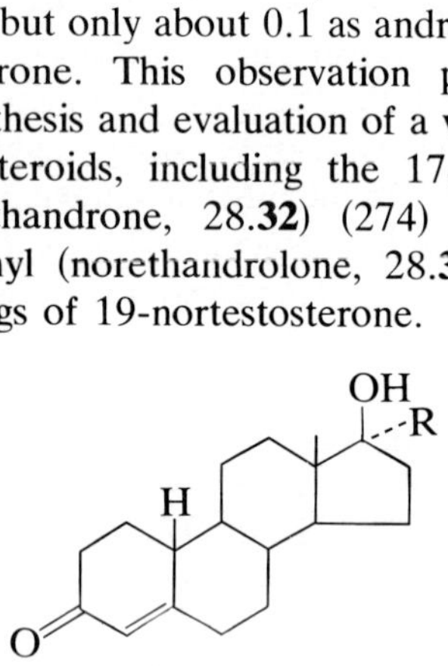

28.**31** R = H
28.**32** R = CH_3
28.**33** R = C_2H_5

Nandrolone in the form of a variety of esters (see Section 10.8) and norethandrolone have been widely used clinically. The latter, under the name Nilevar®, was the first agent to be marketed in the United States as an anabolic steroid. Androgenic (276) and progestational (277) side effects, however, led to its eventual replacement by other agents.

Nonetheless, these studies did stimulate the synthesis of other norsteroids. Interestingly, both 18-nortestosterone (278) and 18,19-bisnortestosterone (279) were essentially devoid of both androgenic and anabolic properties (280). Contraction of the B ring led to B-norsteroids, which were also lacking in androgenicity, but unlike the foregoing, this modification led to compounds with antiandrogenic activity (see Section 11).

Of the number of homoandrostane derivatives (those having one or more additional methylene groups included in normal tetracyclic ring system) that have been synthesized, only B-homo (281, 282) and D-homodihydrotestosterone (283, 284) have shown appreciable androgenic activity. A D-bishomo analog (28.**34**) was reported to be weakly androgenic (285).

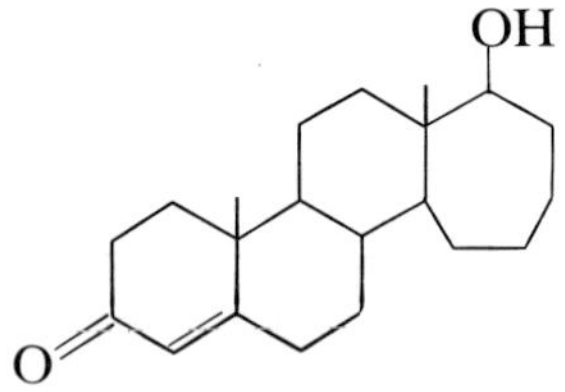

28.**34**

10.3 Dehydro Derivatives

The marked enhancement in biological activity afforded by introduction of a double bond at C_1 of cortisone and hydrocortisone prompted similar transformations in the androgens. The acetate of 17β-hydroxyandrosta-1,4-dien-3-one (28.**35**) (286) was as myotrophic as testosterone propionate but was much less androgenic. Furthermore, 17α-methyl-17β-hydroxyandrosta-1,4-dien-3-one (methandrostenolone, 28.**36**) had 1–2 times the oral potency of 17α-methyltestosterone in the rat nitrogen retention (287, 288) and levator ani muscle assays (289, 290). In clinical studies,

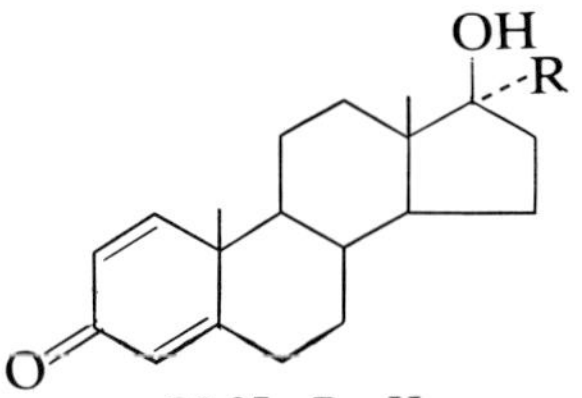

28.35 R = H
28.36 R = CH_3

methandrostenolone produced a marked anabolic effect when given orally at doses of 1.25–10 mg daily and was several times more potent than 17α-methyltestosterone (291).

In contrast with the 1-dehydro analogs, introduction of an additional double bond at the 6-position (28.**37**) markedly decreased both androgenic and myotrophic activity in the rat (286, 292). Moreover, removal of the C_{19}-methyl (293), inversion of the configuration at C_9 and C_{10} (294) and at C_8 and C_{10} (295), and reduction of the C_3-ketone failed to improve the biological properties (296).

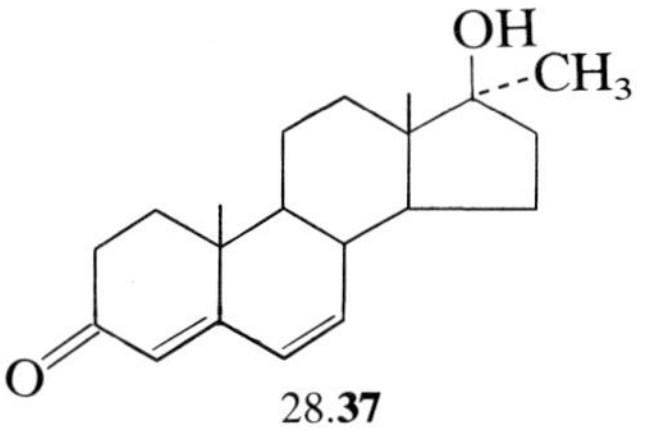

28.**37**

On the other hand, introduction of unsaturation into the B, C, and D rings has given rise to compounds with significant androgenic or anabolic activity. Ethyldienolone (28.**38**), for example, displayed an anabolic-to-androgenic ratio of 5 and was slightly more active than methyltestosterone when both were given orally (297).

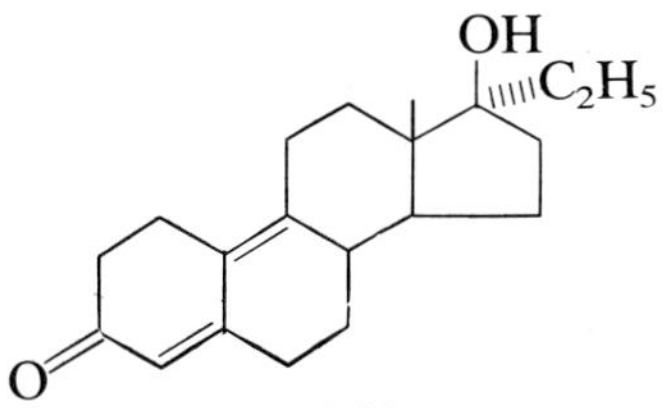

28.**38**

Segaloff and Gabbard (298) showed that introduction of a 14–15 double bond (28.**39**) increased androgenicity when compared with testosterone by local application in the chick comb assay. On the other hand, there was a 25% decrease in androgenicity when measured by the rat ventral prostate following subcutaneous administration. Conversion to the 19-nor analog (28.**40**) increased androgenicity, but the anabolic activity was significantly enhanced (299).

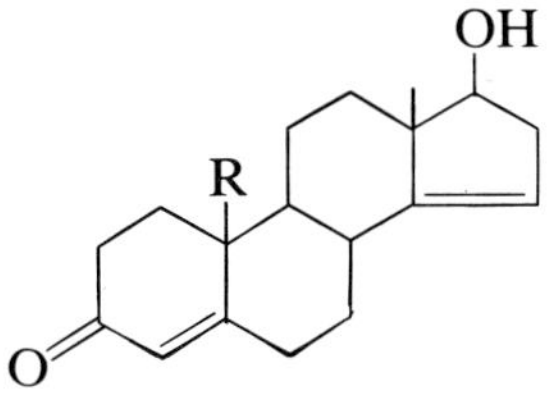

28.**39** R = CH_3
28.**40** R = H

Of a variety of triene analogs of testosterone that have been tested, only 17α-methyl-17β-hydroxyestra-4,9,11-trien-3-one (methyltrienolone, 28.**41**) showed significant activity in rats. Surprisingly, this compound had 300 times the anabolic and 60 times the androgenic potency of 17α-methyltestosterone when administered orally to castrated male rats (300). In this instance, however, the potent hormonal properties on rats did not correlate with later studies in humans (301–303). One study in patients with advanced breast cancer found methyltrienolone to have weak androgenicity and to produce severe hepatic dysfunction at very low doses (303).

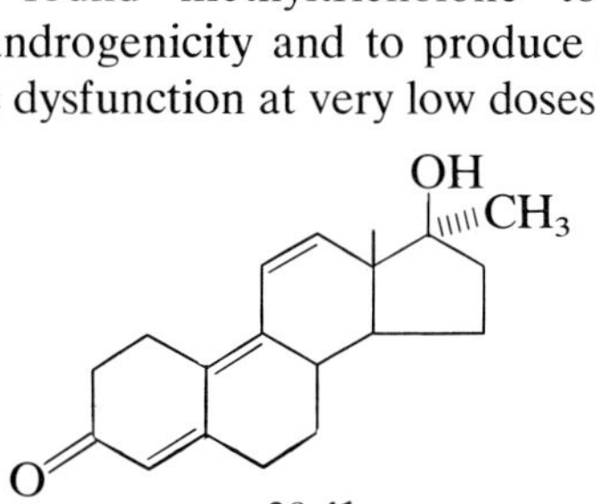

28.**41**

10.4 Alkylated Analogs

An extensive effort has been directed toward assessing the physiological effect of replacing hydrogen with alkyl groups at most positions of the steroid molecule. Although methyl substitution at C_3, C_4, C_5, C_6, C_{11}, and C_{16} has generally led to compounds with low anabolic and androgenic activity, similar substitution at C_1, C_2, C_7, and C_{18} has afforded derivatives of clinical significance.

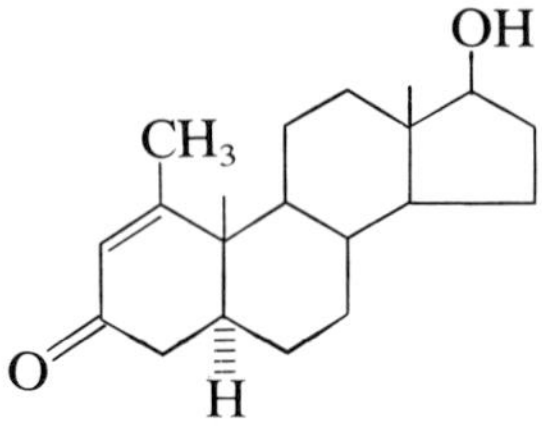

28.**42**

1-Methyl-17β-hydroxy-5α-androst-1-en-3-one (28.**42**) as the acetate (methenolone acetate) was about 5 times as myotrophic, but only 0.1 as androgenic, as testosterone propionate in animals (304). In addition, this compound or the free alcohol represented one of the few instances of a C_{17} nonalkylated steroid that possessed significant oral anabolic activity in animals (305) and in man (306). This effect may be related to the slow *in vivo* oxidation of the 17β-hydroxyl group when compared with testosterone (109). At a daily dose of 300 mg, methenolone acetate caused little virilization (307) or BSP retention (308). By contrast, the dihydro analog, 1α-methyl-17β-hydroxy-5α-androstan-3-one (mesterolone, 28.**43**), was found to possess significant oral androgenic activity in the cockscomb test (309) and in clinical assays (310).

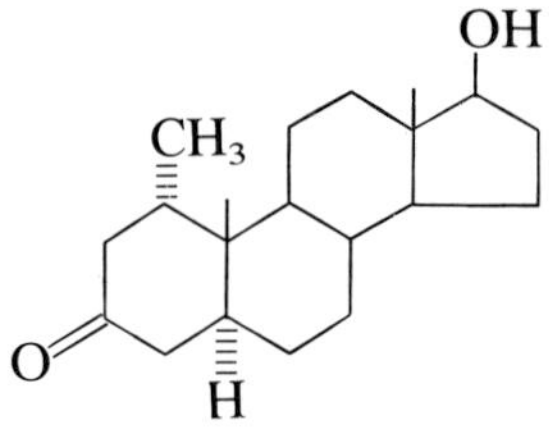

28.**43**

A comparison of the anabolic and androgenic activity of 28.**42** with its A-ring congeners revealed that the double bond was necessary at C_1 for anabolic activity. For example, 1α-methyl-17β-hydroxyandrost-4-en-3-one had a much lower activity (311). Furthermore, either reduction of the C_3 carbonyl group of 28.**43** (312) or removal of the C_{19} methyl group (313, 314) greatly reduced both anabolic and androgenic activity in this series.

Among the C_2-alkylated testosterone analogs, 2α-methyl-5α-androstan-17β-ol-3-one (drostanolone, 28.**44**) and its 17α-methylated homolog (28.**45**) have displayed anabolic activity both in animals (315) and in man (316). In contrast, 2,2-dimethyl and 2-methylenetestosterone or their derivatives showed only low anabolic or androgenic activity in animals (315, 317, 318). The most interest in drostanolone has been in relation to its potential as an antitumor agent with decreased masculinizing propensity.

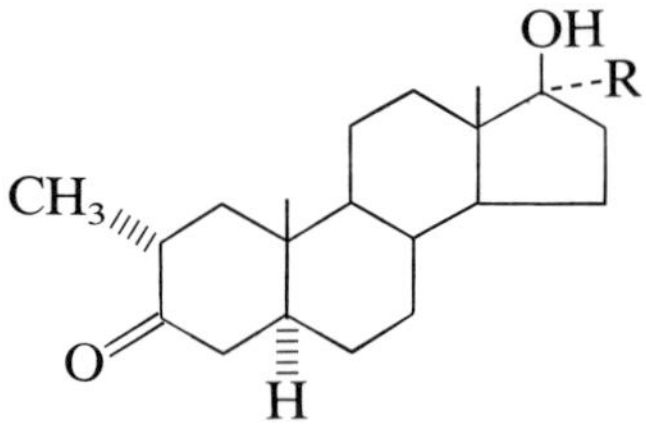

28.**44** R = H
28.**45** R = CH_3

7α,17α-Dimethyltestosterone (bolasterone, 28.**46**) had 6.6 times the oral anabolic potency of 17α-methyltestosterone in rats (319). Similar activity was observed in man at 1–2 mg/day without many of the usual side effects (320). Moreover, the corresponding 19-nor derivative was 41 times as active as 17α-methyltestosterone as an oral myotrophic agent in the rat (319).

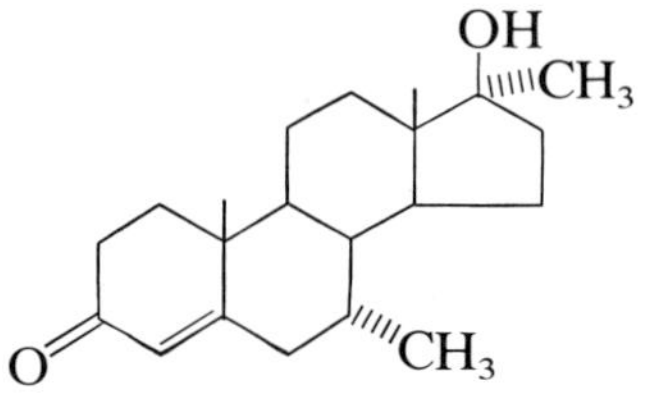

28.**46**

Segaloff and Gabbard (284) found 7α-methyl-14-dehydro-19-nortestosterone (28.**47**) to be approximately 1000 times as active as testosterone in the chick comb assay and about 100 times as active as testosterone in the ventral prostate assay.

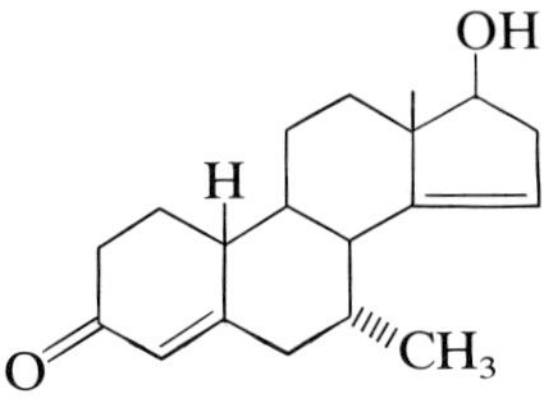

28.**47**

A fortuitious by-product in the synthesis of the 7α-methyltestosterone analogs was the 7β-methyl epimers (321, 322). Unlike 7α, the 7β-epimers have little androgenic activity. For this reason, 7β,17α-dimethyltestostosterone (calusterone, 28.**48**) was evaluated as a nonvirilizing agent for the treatment of advanced breast cancer and was shown to be a promising drug for this purposc (323, 324).

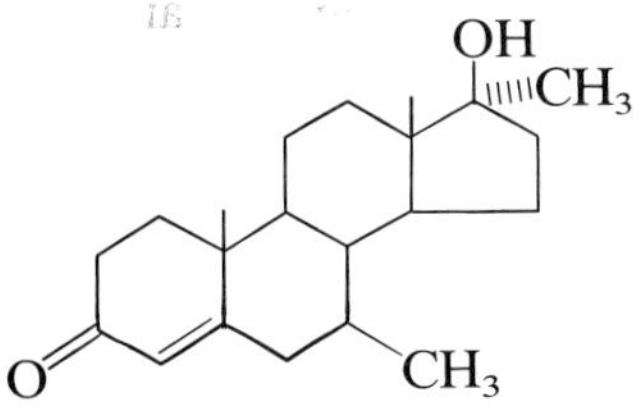

28.**48**

Certain totally synthetic 18-ethylgonane derivatives possessed pronounced anabolic activity. Similar to other 19-norsteroids, 13β,17α-diethyl-17β-hydroxygon-4-en-3-one (norbolethone, 28.**49**) was found to be a potent anabolic agent in animals and in man (325, 326). Since it is prepared by total synthesis, the product is isolated and marketed as the racemic DL-mixture. The hormonal activity resides in the D-enantiomer.

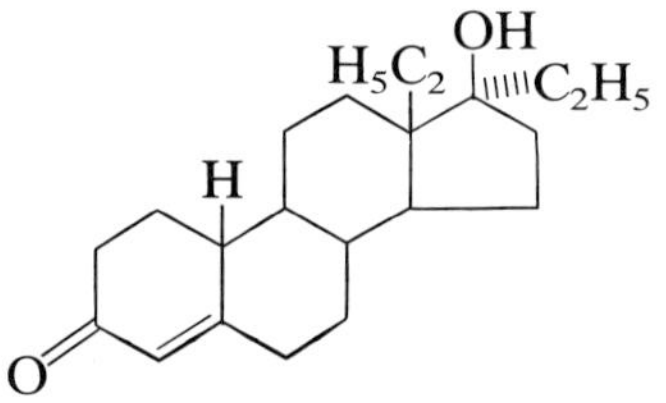

28.**49**

10.5 Halo, Hydroxy, and Mercapto Derivatives

In general, the preparation of halogenated testosterone derivatives has been therapeutically unrewarding. 4-Chloro-17β-hydroxyandrost-4-en-3-one (chlorotestosterone, 28.**50**) and its derivatives are the only chlorinated androgens that have been used clinically albeit sparingly (327).

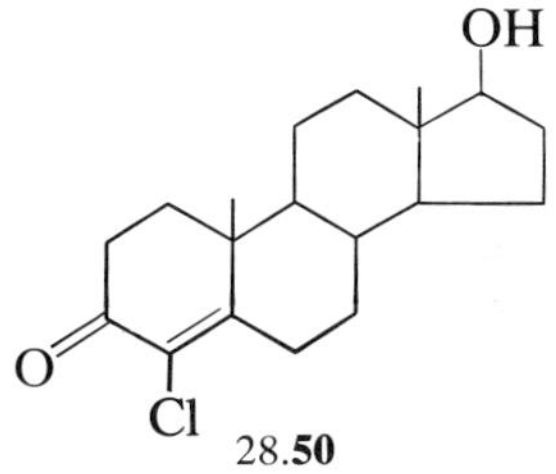

28.**50**

Testosteronc has been hydroxylated at virtually every position on the steroid nucleus. For the most part, nearly all these substances possess no more than weak myotrophic and androgenic properties. Two striking exceptions to this, however, are 4-hydroxy- and 11β-hydroxytestosterones. 4-Hydroxy-17α-methyltestosterone (oxymesterone, 28.**51**), for instance, had 3–5 times the myotrophic and 0.5 times the androgenic activity of 17α-methyltestosterone in the rat (328). In clinical studies, oxymesterone produced nitrogen retention in adults at a daily dose of 20–40 mg, and no adverse liver function was observed (329, 330).

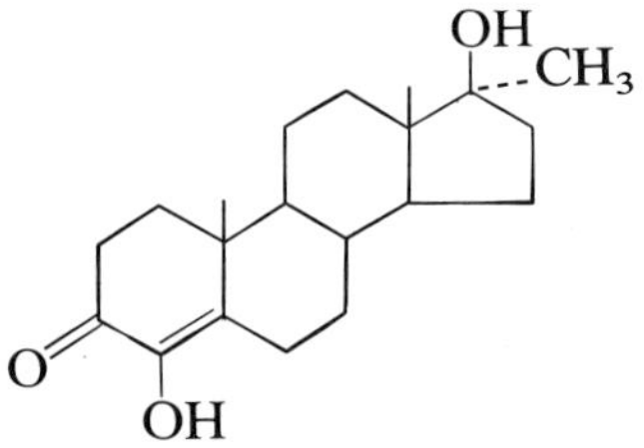

28.**51**

Introduction of an 11β-hydroxyl group in many instances resulted in a favorable effect on biological activity. 11β-Hydroxy-17α-methyltestosterone (28.**52**) was more anabolic in the rat than 17α-methyltestosterone (331), and 1.5 times as myotrophic in humans (332). This activity was enhanced by substitution of fluorine at the 9α-position. For example, 9α-fluoro-11β,17β-dihydroxy-17α-methylandrost-4-en-3-one (halotestin, 28.**53**) produced an oral anabolic effect 20 times and an androgenic response 9.5 times that of 17α-methyltestosterone in rats (333).

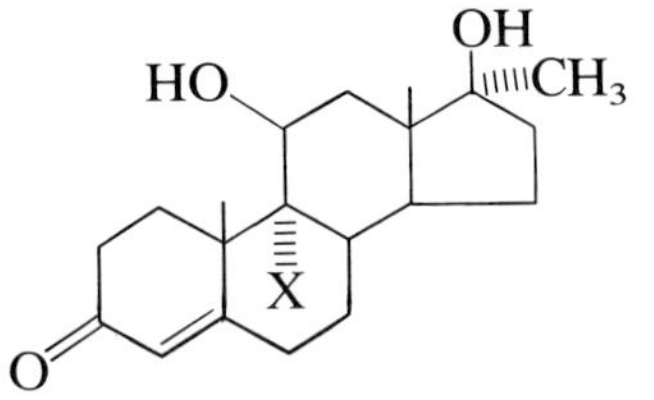

28.**52** X = H
28.**53** X = F

Early clinical studies with halotestin indicated an anabolic potency of 11 times that of the unhalogenated derivative (334, 335). Nitrogen balance studies, however, revealed an activity of only 3 times that of 17α-methyltestosterone (336). Because of the lack of any substantial separation of anabolic and androgenic activity, halotestin is used primarily as an orally effective androgen, particularly in the treatment of mammary carcinoma (337, 338).

One of the most widely studied anabolic steroids has been 2-hydroxymethylene-17α-methyl-5α-androstan-17β-ol-3-one (oxymetholone, 28.**54**). In animals it was found to be 3 times as anabolic and 0.5 times as androgenic as 17α-methyltestosterone (339, 340). Clinical studies confirmed these results (316, 339–341).

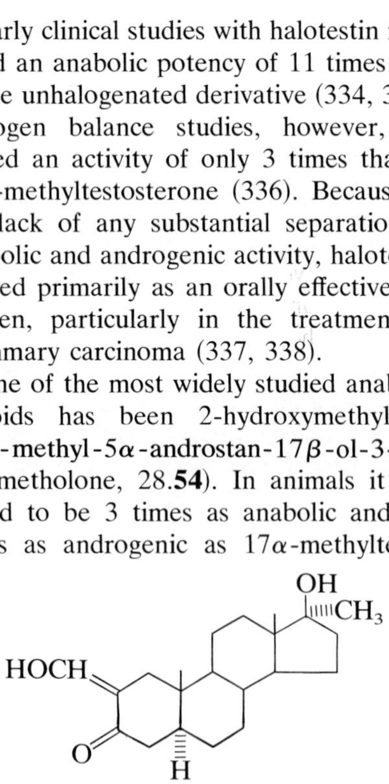

28.**54**

The substitution of a mercapto for a hydroxyl group has generally resulted in decreased activity. However the introduction of a thioacetyl group at C_1 and C_7 of 17α-methyltestosterone afforded 1α,7α-bis(acetylthio)-17α-methyl-17β-hydroxyandrost-4-en-3-one (thiomesterone, 28.**55**), a compound with significant activity. Thiomesterone was 4.5 times as myotrophic and 0.6 times as androgenic as 17α-methyltestosterone in the rat (342) and has been used clinically as an anabolic agent (343).

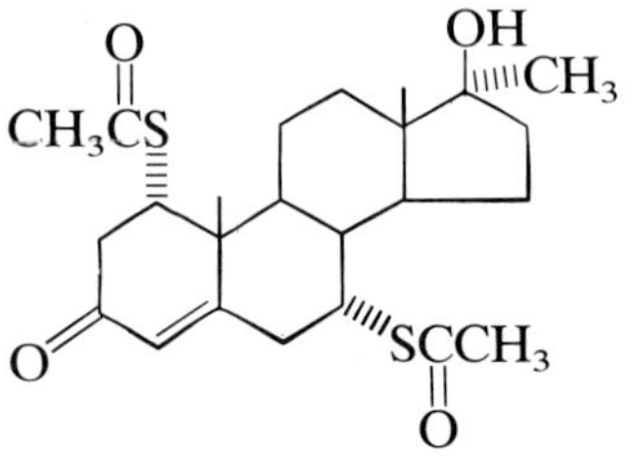

28.**55**

Moreover, numerous 7α-alkylthio androgens have exhibited anabolic-androgenic activity similar to that of testosterone propionate when administered subcutaneously (344, 345). Even though no clinically useful androgen resulted, similar 7α-substitutions were advantageous in the development of radioimmunoassays now employed in clinical laboratories (346). In addition, certain 7α-arylthioandrost-4-ene-3,17-diones were recently shown to be effective inhibitors of estrogen biosynthesis (141).

10.6 Oxa, Thia, and Aza Isosteres

A number of androgen analogs in which an oxygen atom replaces one of the methylene groups in the steroid nucleus have been synthesized and biologically evaluated. Of these derivatives, 17β-hydroxy-17α-methyl-2-oxa-5α-androstan-3-one (oxandrolone, 28.**56**) (347) was 3 times as anabolic and only 0.24 time as androgenic

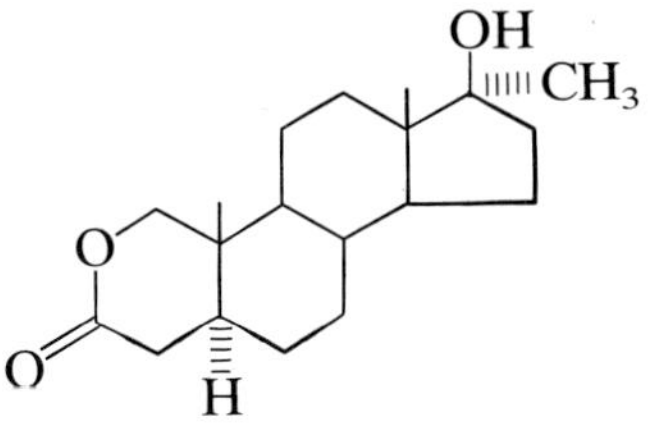

28.**56**

as 17α-methyltestosterone in the oral levator ani assay (348). By contrast, only minimal responses were obtained following intramuscular administration. The 2-thia (349) and 2-aza (350) analogs were essentially devoid of activity by both routes. The 3-aza-A-homoandrostene derivative 28.**57** displayed only 5% the anabolic-to-androgenic activity of methyltestosterone (351).

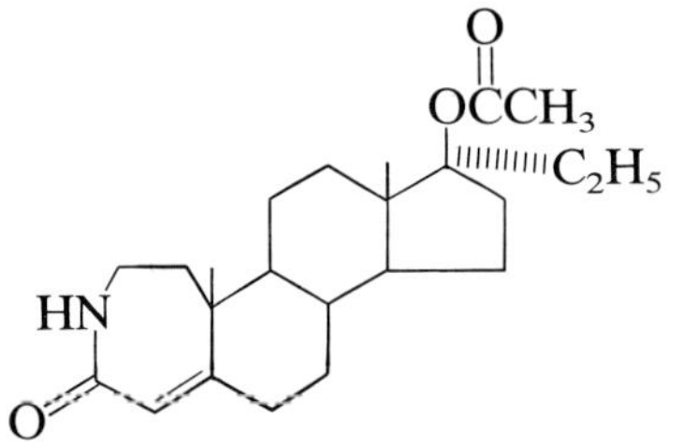

28.**57**

The clinical anabolic potency of oxandrolone was considerably more active than 17α-methyltestosterone and provided perceptible nitrogen sparing at a dose as low as 0.6 mg/day (352). Moreover, at dosages of 0.25–0.5 mg/kg, oxandrolone was effective as a growth-promoting agent without producing the androgenically induced bone maturation (353). Because of this favorable separation of anabolic from androgenic effects, oxandrolone has been one of the most widely studied anabolic steroids. Its potential utility in various clinical hyperlipidemias was discussed in Section 9.

The significant hormonal activity noted for estra-4,9-dien-3-ones such as 28.**38** (see Section 10.3) prompted the synthesis of the 2-oxa bioisosteres in this series. Despite the lack of a 17α-methyl group, 28.**58** had 93 times the oral anabolic activity of 17α-methyltestosterone. It was also 2.7 times as androgenic. As might be expected, the corresponding 17α-methyl derivative, 28.**59**, was the most active substance in this series. It had 550 times the myotrophic and 47 times the androgenic effect of 17α-methyltestosterone (354). These two compounds differed dramatically in progestational activity, however. The activity of 28.**58** was only 0.1 time, whereas the activity of 28.**59** was 100 times that of progesterone in the Clauberg assay (354). The pronounced oral activity of 28.**58** suggests that it is not a substrate for the 17β-alcohol dehydrogenase and represents an interesting finding.

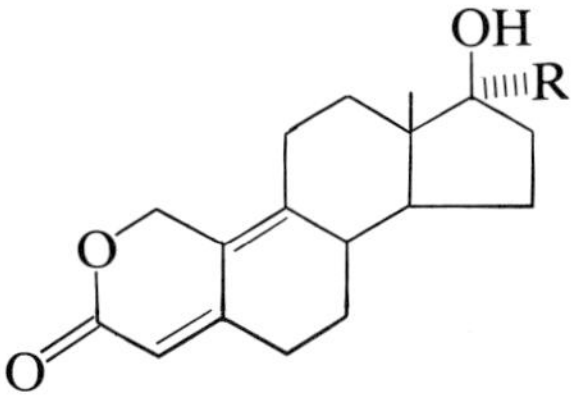

28.**58** R = H
28.**59** R = CH_3

10.7 3-Deoxy and Heterocyclic-Fused Analogs

Early studies by Kochakian (355) indicated that the 17β-hydroxyl group and the 3-keto group were essential for maximum androgenic activity. Based on this observation, the C_3 oxygen function was removed in the hope of decreasing the androgenic potency while maintaining anabolic activity (356). Unfortunately, the results failed to substantiate the rationale, and 17α-methyl-5α-androstan-17β-ol (28.**60**) was found to be a potent androgen in animals (357) and humans (358). However, Wolff and Kasuya

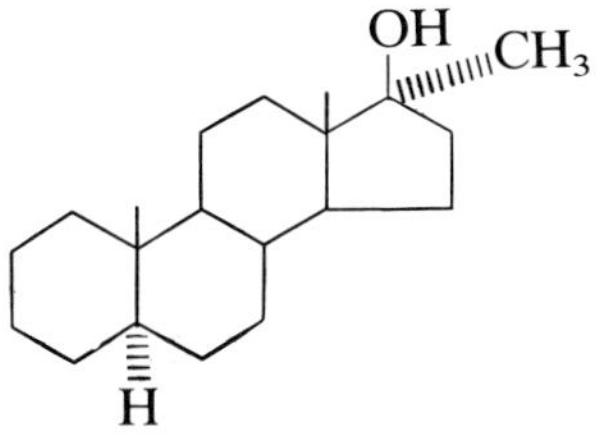

28.**60**

showed that this substance is extensively metabolized to the 3-keto derivative by rabbit liver homogenate (358a).

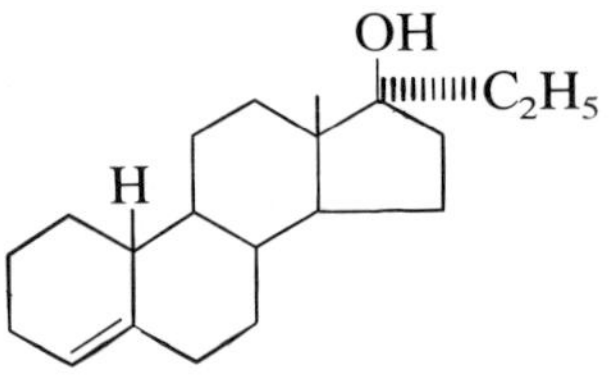

28.**61**

Other deoxy analogs of testosterone have been synthesized and tested. A 19-nor derivative, 17α-ethylestr-4-en-17β-ol (estrenol, 28.**61**) had at least 4 times the anabolic and 0.25 time the androgenic activity of 17α-methyltestosterone in animals (359) and was effective in humans at a daily dose of 3-5 mg (360–362). In addition, 17α-methyl-5α-androst-2-en-17β-ol (28.**62**) offered a good separation of anabolic from androgenic activity (357, 363).

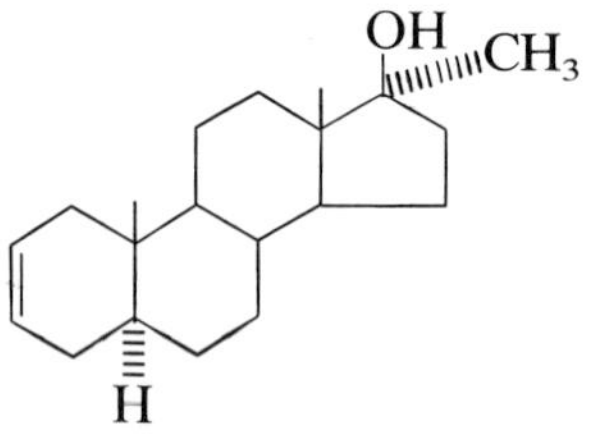

28.**62**

Since sulfur is considered to be isosteric with —CH=CH—, Wolff and Zanati (364) reasoned that 2-thia-A-nor-5α-androstane derivatives such as 28.**63** should have androgenic activity. Indeed, this compound possessed high androgenic and anabolic activity and served to verify that steric rather than electronic factors are inportant in connection with the structural requirements at C-2 and/or C-3 in androgens (365). Interestingly, the selenium and tellurium isosteres in the same series were found to have good androgenic activity (366, 367). Moreover experiments with a ^{75}Se-labeled analog have shown 28.**64** to selectively bind with the specific cytosol receptor for DHT in rat prostate (368).

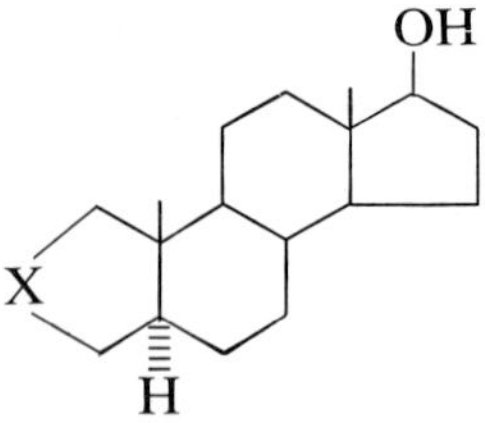

28.**63** X = S
28.**64** X = Se

The high biological activity noted for the 3-deoxy androstanes prompted numerous investigators to fuse various systems to the A-ring. The simplest such changes were 2,3-epoxy, 2,3-cyclopropano, and 2,3-epithioandrostanes. The 2α,3α-cyclopropano-5α-androstan-17β-ol was as active as testosterone propionate as an anabolic agent (368a). While the epoxides had little or no biological activity, certain of the episulfides possessed pronounced anabolic-androgenic activity (369). For example, 2,3α-epithio-17α-methyl-5α-androstan-17β-ol (28.**65**) was found to have approximately equal androgenic and 11 times the anabolic activity of methyltestosterone after oral administration to rats. The 2,3-β-episulfide, on the other hand, was much less active. 2,3α-Epithio-5α-androstan-17β-ol has been shown to have long-acting antiestrogenic activity, as well as some beneficial effects in the treatment of mammary carcinoma (370).

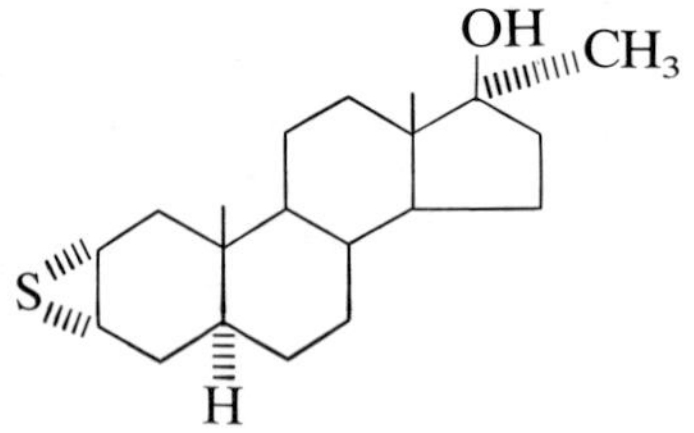

28.**65**

Other heterocyclic androstane derivatives have included the pyrazoles. Thus 17β-hydroxy-17α-methylandrostano-(3,2-*c*)-pyrazole (stanazolol, 28.**66**) was 10 times as active as 17α-methyltestosterone in improving nitrogen retention in rats (371). The myotrophic activity, however, was only twice that of 17α-methyltestosterone (372). Stanazolol at a dose of 6 mg/day produced an adequate anabolic response with no lasting adverse side effects (373, 374).

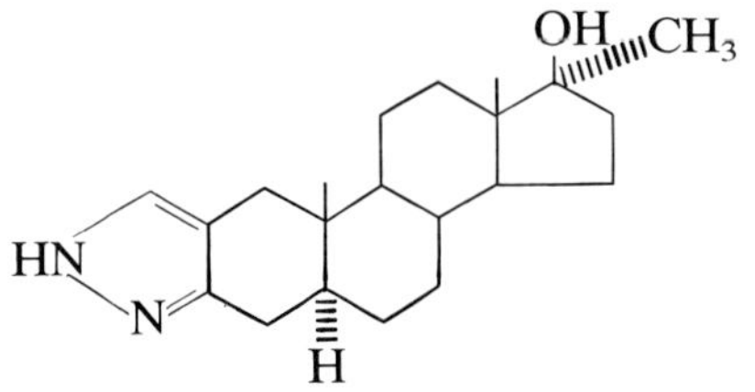

28.**66**

The high activity of the pyrazoles instigated the synthesis of other heterocyclic-fused androstane derivatives including isoxazoles, thiazoles, pyridines, pyrimidines, pteridines, oxadiazoles, pyrroles, indoles, and triazoles. One of the most potent was 17α-methylandrostan-17β-ol-(2,3-*d*)-isoxazole (androisoxazol, 28.**67**), which exhibited an oral anabolic-to-androgenic ratio of 40 (375). The corresponding 17α-ethynyl analog (danazol, 28.**68**) has been of most interest clinically. This compound has impeded androgenic activity and inhibits pituitary gonadotropin secretion (376). Since it depresses blood levels of androgens and gonadotropins, it has been studied as an antifertility agent in males (377). At doses of 200 or 600 mg daily, danazol lowered plasma testosterone and androstenedione levels, and this effect was dose related. In addition to an inhibition in gonadotropin release, a direct inhibition of Leydig cell androgen synthesis was observed. Other studies have shown danazol to be effective for the treatment of endometriosis, benign fibrocystic mastitis, and precocious puberty (378). Several reports have appeared relating to its disposition and metabolic fate (378, 379).

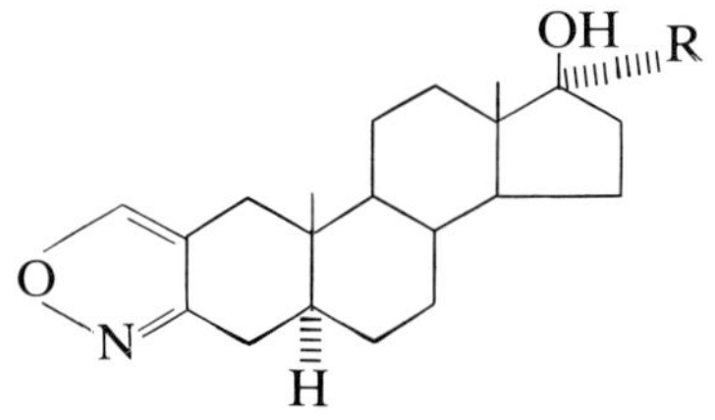

28.**67** $R = CH_3$
28.**68** $R = C{\equiv}CH$

10.8 Esters and Ethers

As early as 1936 it was known that esterification of testosterone markedly prolonged the activity of this androgen when it was administered parenterally (380). It was only natural that this approach to drug latentiation would be extended to the anabolic steroids. The acyl moiety is usually derived from a long chain aliphatic or arylaliphatic acid such as heptanoic (enanthoic), decanoic, cyclopentylpropionic, and β-phenylpropionic. For example, no less than 12 esters of 19-nortestosterone (nandrolone) have been used clinically as long-acting anabolic agents (381, 382).

In the case of nandrolone, the duration of action and thc anabolic-to-androgenic ratio increased with the chain length of the ester group (383, 384). The decanoate and laurate esters, for instance, were active 6 weeks after injection. Clinically, nandrolone decanoate appeared to be the most practical, since a dose of 25–100 mg/week produced marked nitrogen retention (385, 386).

Since the 17α-alkyl group has been implicated as the cause of the hepatotoxic side effects of oral preparations, the effect of esterification on oral efficacy has attracted attention. For example, esterification of dihydrotestosterone with short chain fatty acids resulted in oral anabolic and androgenic activity in rats (387). Moreover, esters of methenolone possessed appreciable oral anabolic activity (388). Unfortunately, follow-up studies in humans have not been reported.

The manner by which the steroid esters evoke their enhanced activity and increased duration of action has puzzled investigators for many years. The classical concept has been that esterification delays the absorption rate of the steroid from the site of injection, thus preventing its rapid destruction. Other factors must be involved, however, since the potency and prolongation of action vary markedly with the nature of the esterifying acid.

Recent studies by James and co-workers (389, 390) have shed the most light on this problem. They studied the effect of various aliphatic esters of testosterone on rat prostate and seminal vesicles and correlated androgenicity with lipophilicity and rate of ester hydrolysis by liver esterase. The peak androgenic response was observed with the butyrate ester, which was also the most readily hydrolyzed. The more lipophilic valerate ester was slightly less androgenic in a quantitative sense, but its action was longer lasting. It was concluded that the ease of hydrolysis controls the weight of the target organs, whereas lipophilicity was responsible for the duration of androgenic effect. These results explain the low androgenic activity previously noted for hindered trimethylacetate (pivalate) esters, which would be expected to be resistant to *in vivo* hydrolysis.

The effect of etherification on anabolic or androgenic activity has been studied less rigorously. Replacement of the 17β-OH with 17β-OCH_3 markedly reduced androgenic activity but did not affect greatly the ability to counteract cortisone-induced adrenal atrophy in male rats (391). A series of 17β-acetals (392, 393), alkyl ethers (394), and 3-enol ethers (395, 396), however, showed significant activity when given orally (397–399). The cyclohexyl enol ether of 17α-methyltestosterone, for example, was orally 5 times as myotrophic as 17α-methyltestosterone (399).

Other ethers such as the tetrahydropyranol (400, 401) and trimethylsilyl (402) have oral anabolic and androgenic activity in animals. The trimethylsilyl ether of testosterone (silandrone) had protracted activity following injection (403) and orally had twice the anabolic and androgenic activities of 17α-methyltestosterone (402). Solo et al. (404) evaluated a variety of ethers that would not be expected to be readily cleaved *in vivo* and found them to be almost devoid of anabolic and androgenic activity. This provides additional support for the necessity of a free 17β-hydroxyl for androgenic activity.

11 ANTIANDROGENS

Antiandrogens are substances that diminish the effectiveness of coadministered androgens on the various androgen-sensitive target organs. This action may be due to (1) modification of the entry of testosterone into the cell, (2) inhibition of the conversion of testosterone to DHT, or (3) competition with the natural hormone for binding to the cytoplasmic receptor protein. The antiandrogens most widely studied to date exert their action by the third mechanism.

A variety of modified progestins represent the most extensively investigated class of compounds. The best known is cyproterone acetate (28.**69**), a derivative of progesterone that competes with testosterone and DHT for the intracellular androgen receptor (17, 405, 406). As a consequence of this action, cyproterone acetate decreases the size and secretory function of the accessory sex organs in a variety of laboratory animals and man. Clinically it has been used with success in the treatment of pathological hypersexuality in men (407) and benign prostatic hypertrophy (408).

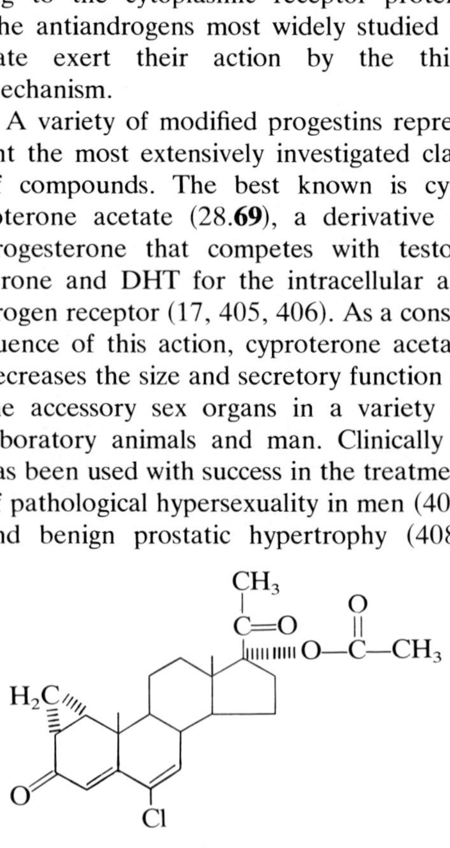

CH_3 C=O O—C(=O)—CH_3 H_2C O Cl

28.**69**

Another progestin, medrogesterone (28.**70**), has shown a similar profile of antiandrogenic effects in animals and man (409).

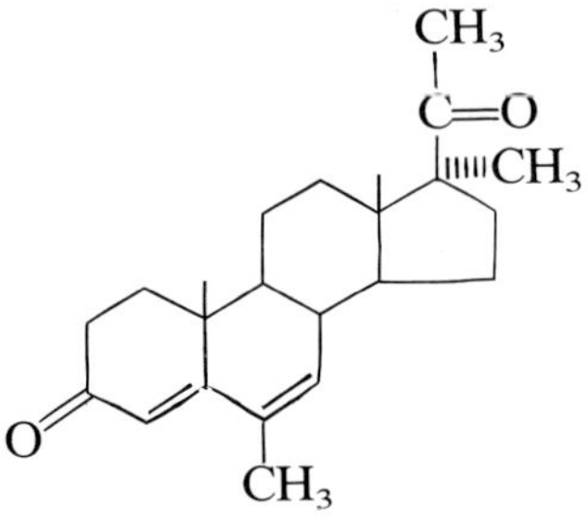

28.**70**

The antiandrogenic activity of 17α-methyl-B-nortestosterone (28.**71**) was reported by Saunders et al. (410) in 1964. Based on studies in experimental animals, they concluded that this B-norsteroid possessed neither androgenic, estrogenic, antiestrogenic, progestestational, antiprogestational, nor antigonadotropic activities. It was subsequently shown to inhibit receptor binding of DHT in rat prostate (411) and human prostatic hyperplasia (412). The compound has not been investigated widely in the clinic, but one study found it to have beneficial effects in acne and hirsutism (413).

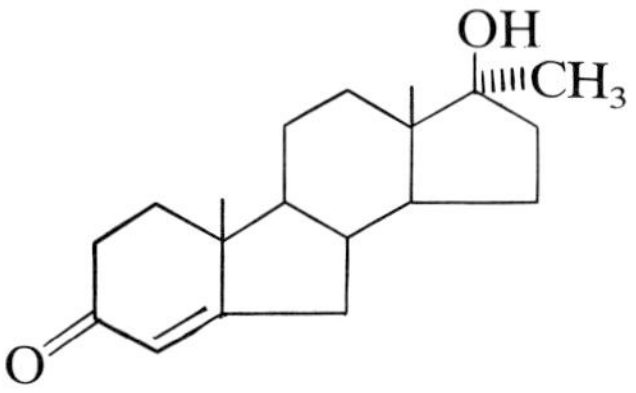

28.**71**

Several other antiandrogens, discovered since 1970, include 6α-bromo-17β-hydroxy-17α-methyl-4-oxa-5α-androstan-3-one (28.**72**, BOMT) (414, 415), 17-β-hydroxy-2α,2β,17α-trimethylestra-4,9,11-trien-3-one (28.**73**) (416), and 6α,7α-difluoromethylene-4′,5′-dihydro-1α,2α-methylene, 17(*R*)-spiro-[androst-4-ene-17,2′-(3′H)-furan]-3-one (28.**74**) (417, 418).

All the foregoing antiandrogens are steroid derivatives, and it is understandable

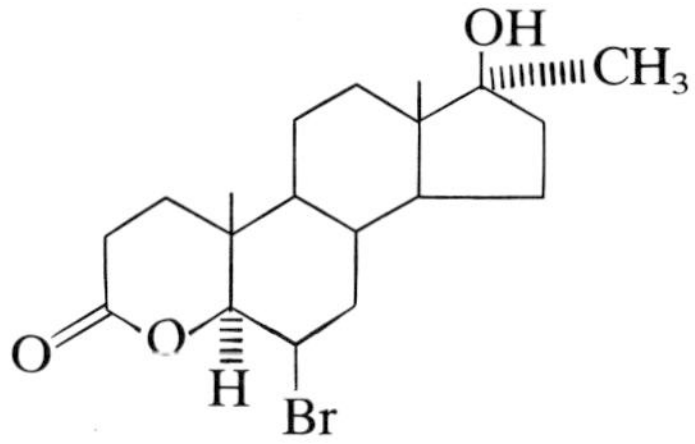

28.**72**

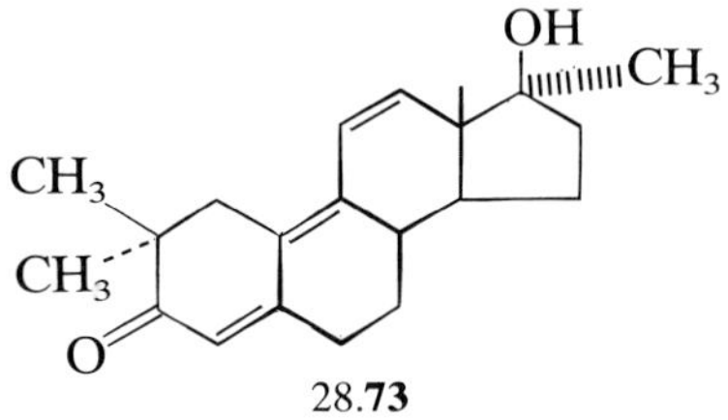

28.**73**

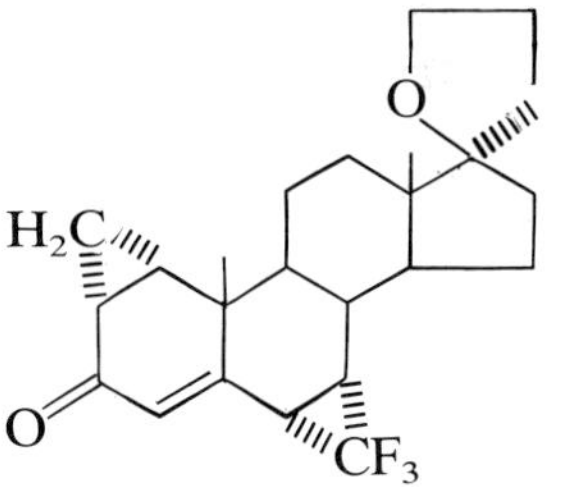

28.**74**

why they may compete with the natural hormone for receptor binding sites. Recently, however, a nonsteroidal antiandrogen known as flutamide (28.**75**) was also found to antagonize the binding of DHT to cytoplasmic and nuclear binding sites both *in vitro* and *in vivo* (419, 420). Flutamide and cyproterone acetate were about equipotent with antiandrogens *in vivo*, but the latter was about 10 times as active as flutamide in inhibiting the receptor binding of DHT *in vitro* (420). Unlike cyproterone acetate, however, flutamide is essentially devoid of hormonal effects. Acetanilide, a nonantiandrogen that has an acylanilide structure common to flutamide, had no effect on the receptor binding or nuclear retention of DHT. Whether flutamide is competing for the same receptor binding site as DHT remains to be established.

Moreover, a hydroxylated metabolite (28.**76**) has been identified and shown to have antiandrogenic action as well (421). The importance of this metabolite in the overall action of flutamide is still unclear. Initial clinical trials with flutamide in prostatic carcinoma have been encouraging, and trials in other hyperandrogenic syndromes are now in progress (422).

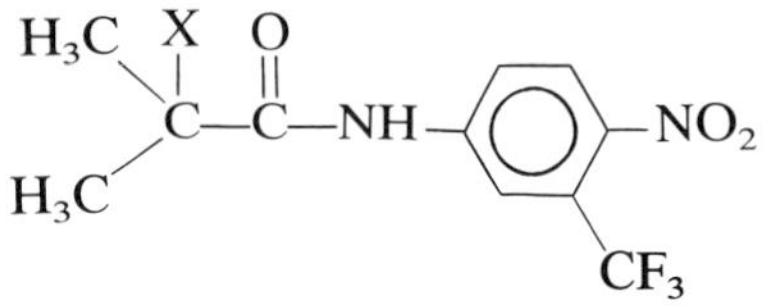

28.**75** X = H
28.**76** X = OH

12 STRUCTURE–ACTIVITY RELATIONSHIPS

As with other areas of medicinal chemistry, the desire to relate chemical structure to androgenic activity has attracted the attention of numerous investigators. Although it is often difficult to interrelate biological results from different laboratories, androgenicity data from the same laboratory afford useful information. In evaluating the data, one must be careful to note not only the animal model employed, but also the mode of administration. For example, marked differences in androgenic activity can be found when compounds are evaluated in the chick comb assay (local application) as opposed to the rat ventral prostate assay (subcutaneous or oral). The chick comb assay measures "local androgenicity" and is believed to minimize such factors as absorption, tissue distribution, and metabolism, which complicate the interpretation of *in vivo* data in terms of hormone-receptor interactions.

Furthermore, although the rat assays correlate well with what one eventually finds in humans, few studies of comparative pharmacology have been performed to date. Indeed, it is now realized that DHT may not be the principal mediator of androgenicity in all species. For example, a cytosol receptor protein has been found in normal and hyperplastic canine prostate that is specific for 5α-androstane-3α,17α-diol (209). Thus for the first time, even the sacrosanct position of the 17β-hydroxyl group is open to question!

Since the presence of the 17β-hydroxyl group was demonstrated very early to be an important feature for androgenic activity in rodents, most investigators interested in structure-activity relationships maintained this function and modified other parts of the testosterone molecule. Tables 28.6 and 28.7 compare the androgenic and anabolic activities of various A-ring modified derivatives of testosterone and DHT. The potencies, in percentage activity of testosterone propionate, were determined from the minimal levels at which significant increases in seminal vesicle and ventral prostate or levator ani muscle weights were obtained.

Three observations can be made based on these studies just mentioned.

1. The 1-dehydro isomer of testosterone is at least as active as testosterone.
2. The 1- and 4-keto isomers of testosterone and DHT have variable activity.
3. The 2-keto isomers of testosterone and DHT consistently lack appreciable activity.

The first attempt to ascertain the minimal structural requirements for androgenicity was by Segaloff and Gabbard (425). Whereas the oxygen function at position 3

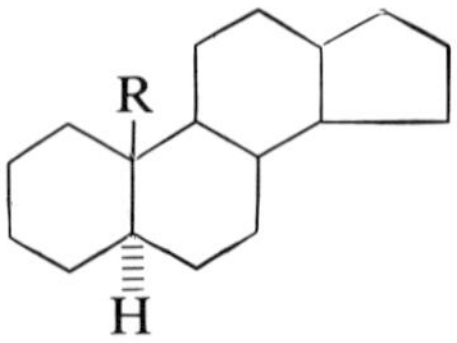

28.**77** R = CH_3
28.**78** R = H

Table 28.6 Androgenic and Myotrophic Activities of Testosterone Isomers Following Intramuscular Administration to Castrated Male Rats (423)

Steroid	Potency, % activity of testosterone propionate	
	Androgenic	Myotrophic
Testosterone propionate	100	100
Testosterone	35	26
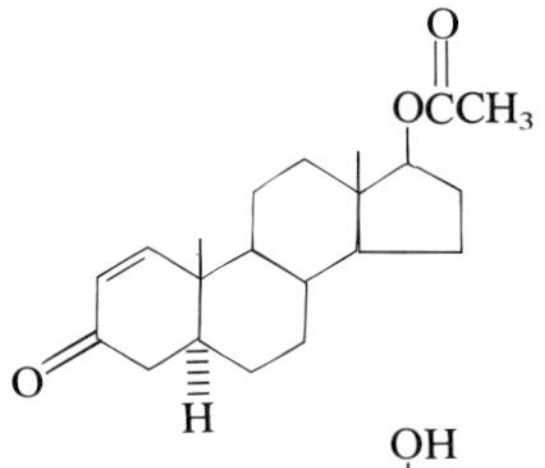 O, $OCCH_3$, O, H	100	400
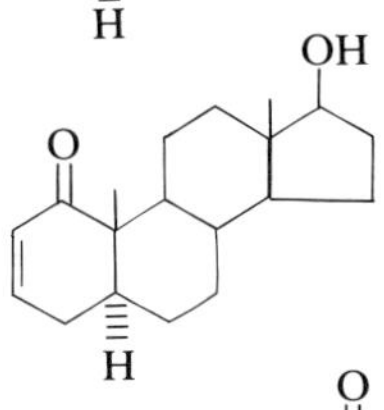 OH, O, H	1	5
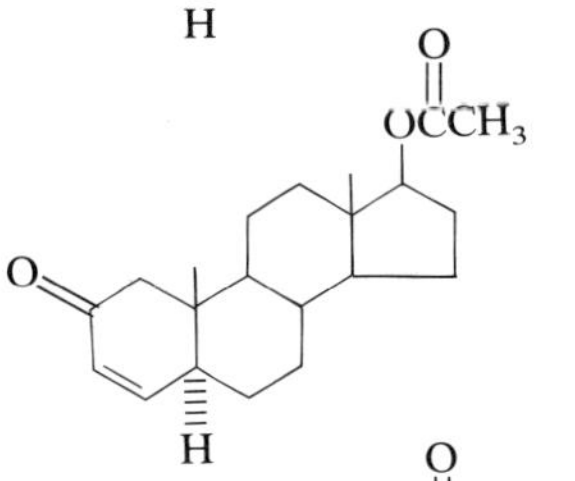 O, $OCCH_3$, O, H	1	4
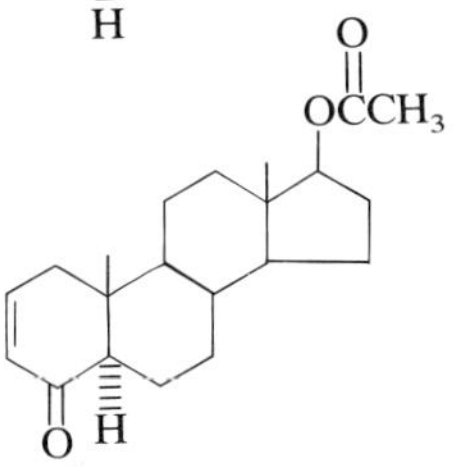 O, $OCCH_3$, O, H	25	200

could be removed from testosterone with little reduction in androgenic activity, removal of the hydroxyl group from position 17 sharply reduced the androgenicity. As a continuation of these studies, the hydrocarbon nucleus, 5α-androstane (28.**77**), was synthesized (425). It too was found to possess androgenicity when applied topically or given intramuscularly in the chick comb assay, albeit at high doses. On the other hand, it was learned later that the 19-nor analog, 5α-estrane (28.**78**), had less than 1% of the androgenic activity of testosterone propionate in castrated male rats (426).

Nonetheless, the work of Segaloff and Gabbard set the stage for a more thorough analysis of 3-deoxy testosterone analogs by Syntex scientists (427, 428). As shown in Table 28.8, the androgenicity of the

Table 28.7 Androgenic and Myotrophic Activities of DHT Isomers Following Intramuscular Administration to Castrated Male Rats (424)

	Potencies, % of activity of testosterone propionate	
Steroid	Androgenic	Myotrophic
Testosterone propionate	100	100
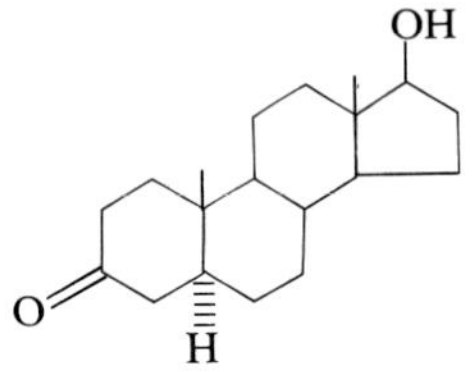	35	100
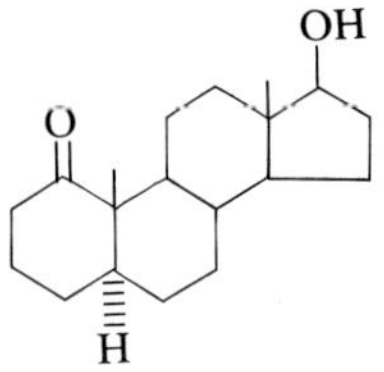	25	20
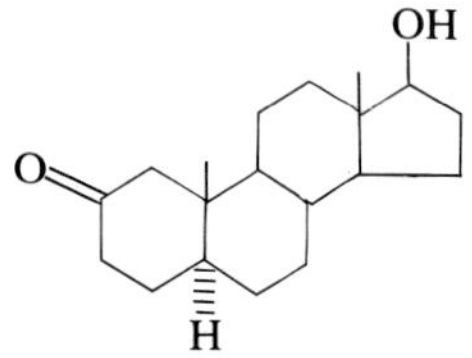	<1	<1
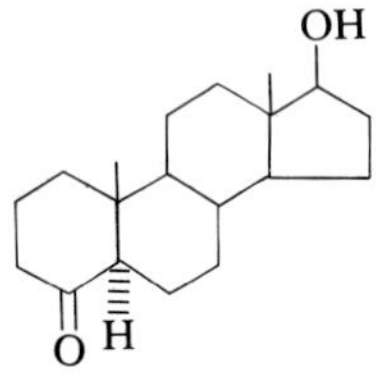	50	40

isomeric A-ring olefins was in the order $\Delta^1 > \Delta^2 > \Delta^3 > \Delta^4$. The Δ^2-isomer displayed the greatest anabolic activity and the best anabolic-to-androgenic ratio.

On the basis that sulfur is bioisosteric with CH═CH, Wolff and co-workers (364, 351) synthesized the thia, seleno, and tellurio androstanes represented by 28.**79**. All these analogs displayed androgenic activity. When the heteroatom was oxygen, however, the compound was essentially devoid of androgenicity (429). The oxygen analog was said to be inactive because oxygen is isosteric with CH_2 rather than $CH_2{=}CH_2$. Thus a minimum ring size was found to be required for activity. When the oxygen atom was introduced as part of a six-membered A-ring, an active androgen resulted (429).

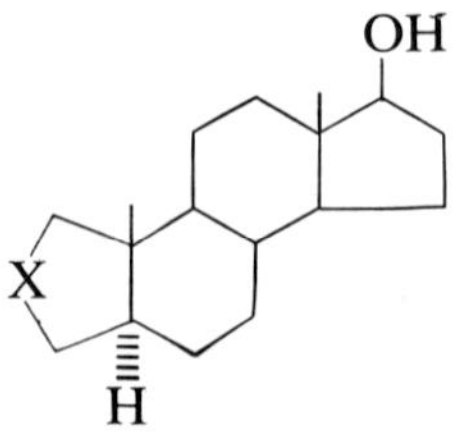

28.**79** X = O, S, Se, Te

Table 28.8 Relative Potency of Various 3-Deoxy Steroids Administered Subcutaneously to Castrated Male Rats (428)

Testosterone	Potency, % of activity of testosterone	
	Androgenic	Myotrophic
OH	100	100
OH	62	85
OH	42	69
O ‖ OCCH$_3$	20	18

As with the case of the double-bond isomers, the position of the oxygen atom was found to be important. The substitution of oxygen at C-2 gives rise to the most active compound, and the order of activity was 2 > 3 ≫ 4. As pointed out by Zanati and Wolff (429), these and earlier results are consistent with the concept that "the activity-engendering group in ring A is wholly steric and that, in principle, isosteric groups of any type could be used to construct an androgenic molecule." Further support for this idea has been obtained from X-ray crystallographic structure determinations (430). That even the full steroid nucleus is not essential for activity was shown by Zanati and Wolff (431) in the preparation of 7α-methyl 1,4-seco-2,3-bisnor-5α-androstan-17β-ol (28.**80**), having 50% of the anabolic activity of testosterone.

More recent studies by Segaloff and Gabbard (297) illustrated the marked enhancement of androgenicity achieved when

OH

CH_3 CH_3 H CH_3

28.**80**

a double bond was introduced at C-14. Both 14-dehydrotestosterone and the corresponding 19-nor analog were found to be potent androgens when applied topically. An extension of this series ascertained the effect of introducing a 7α-methyl (298). The results of this study are listed in Table 28.9, in terms of percentage increases in the weights of chick combs, rat ventral prostates, and rat levator ani induced by the test compounds as related to a similar dose of testosterone, the responses to the latter being described as 100%.

The effects of either 7α-methyl or 14-dehydro modification are more pronounced for 19-nortestosterone than for testosterone. The 14-dehydro modification had a greater effect on local androgenicity, whereas 7α-methylation had a more positive effect on systemic androgenicity. A marked synergism resulted when both the 14-dehydro and 7α-methyl modifications were present. The resultant compound, 7α-methyl-14-dehydro-19-nortestosterone, represents one of the most potent androgens reported to date.

The characterization of a specific receptor protein in androgen target tissues has made it possible to directly analyze the receptor affinity of various testosterone analogs. Liao and co-workers (432) were the first to employ this parameter for comparison with systemic androgenicity. Table 28.10 shows the receptor affinity and androgenic activity of a variety of androgens relative to DHT. The ability of the various steroids to be retained by prostate nuclei is also indicated.

Table 28.9 Comparison of the Androgenic and Myotrophic Activities of Testosterone Derivatives in the Chick Comb and Castrated Male Rat Assays Following Subcutaneous Administration

Testosterone Modification	Increase in Weight, % Chick Comb	Rat Ventral Prostate	Rat Levator Ani
None	100	100	100
19-Nor	81	42	90
7α-Methyl	11	97	135
7α-Methyl-19-nor	75	218	226
14-Dehydro	128	54	8
14-Dehydro-19-nor	320	69	133
14-Dehydro-7α-methyl-19-nor	435	352	330

As would be expected, the receptor affinity data did not necessarily correlate with the systemic androgenicity. In some cases, such as with 7α-methyl-19-nortestosterone, there was good agreement. Such was not the case, however, for 19-nortestosterone.

Receptor binding analysis of androgens has now been performed by other groups (433, 434). Shain and Boesel (431) measured the apparent binding constant for DHT and a number of steroidal and nonsteroidal compounds. Table 28.11 summarizes their findings.

Once again, no consistent relationship between receptor binding and *in vivo* androgenicity was apparent. Whereas the importance of the A/B trans ring fusion and 17β-hydroxyl prevailed, the data failed to demonstrate the potency previously noted for 7α-methyl-14-dehydro-19-nortestosterone. Moreover, 19-nortestosterone displayed a receptor affinity greater than that of DHT, yet its androgenicity is much less than DHT's.

Table 28.10 Relative Androgenicity and Receptor Binding Capacity of Various Androgens

Steroid	Androgenicity in Rat (s.c.)	Cytosol Receptor	Nuclear Retention
DHT	1.0	1.0	1.0
Testosterone (T)	0.4	<0.1	0.7
5α-Androstanedione	0.2	0.0	0.2
19-NorDHT	0.1	0.5	0.6
19-NorT	0.2	0.9	0.7
7α-CH_3-DHT	1.2	0.4	0.4
7α-CH_3-T	0.4	0.2	0.2
7β-CH_3-T	0.1	<0.1	<0.1
7α-CH_3-19-NorDHT	0.3	0.6	0.4
7α-CH_3-19-NorT	2.6	2.6	1.8

Table 28.11 Binding Affinity of Various Androgens for Rat Ventral Prostate Receptor Protein

Steroid	K_B, liters/mol
5α-DHT	6.9×10^8
5β-DHT	6.4×10^7
17β-Testosterone	4.2×10^8
17α-Testosterone	2.1×10^7
Androstenedione	1.3×10^7
5α-Androstanedione	3.5×10^7
19-Nortestosterone	8.6×10^8
14-Dehydrotestosterone	4.4×10^8
14-Dehydro-19-nortestosterone	5.9×10^8
7α-CH_3-14-Dehydro-19-nortestosterone	5.0×10^8

This lack of correlation between receptor assays and *in vivo* data should not cloud the importance of the receptor studies. The receptor assays measure affinity for the receptor protein, and this property is shared by androgens as well as antiandrogens. Moreover, such assays cannot predict the disposition and metabolic fate of an androgen following administration. Future more comprehensive studies should provide the basis for a more intelligent analysis of receptor studies and structure-activity relationships.

REFERENCES

1. J. A. Vida, *Androgens and Anabolic Agents. Chemistry and Pharmacology*, Academic Press, New York, 1969.
2. K. B. Eik-Nes, *The Androgens of the Testes*, Dekker, New York, 1970.
3. *Vitamins and Hormones*, Vol. 33, P. L. Munson, E. Diczfalusy, J. Glover, and R. E. Olsen, Eds., Academic Press, New York, 1975.
4. C. D. Kochakian, *Anabolic-Androgenic Steroids*, Springer-Verlag, New York, 1976.
5. A. Butenandt, *Angew. Chem.*, **44,** 905 (1931).
6. A. Butenandt and K. Tscherning, *Z. Physiol. Chem.*, **229**, 167 (1934).
7. T. F. Gallagher and F. C. Koch, *J. Biol. Chem.*, **84,** 495 (1929).
8. A. Butenandt, *Naturwiss.*, **21,** 49 (1933).
9. A. Butenandt and H. Dannenberg, *Z. Physiol. Chem.*, **229,** 192 (1934).
10. K. David, E. Dingemanse, J. Freud, and E. Laqueur, *Z. Physiol. Chem.*, **233,** 281 (1935).
11. K. David, *Acta Brevia Neerl. Physiol. Pharmacol. Microbiol.*, **5,** 85, 108 (1935).
12. A. Butenandt and G. Hanisch, *Berichte*, **68,** 1859 (1935); *Z. Physiol. Chem.*, **237,** 89 (1935).
13. L. Ruzicka, *J. Am. Chem. Soc.*, **57,** 2011 (1935).
14. L. Ruzicka, A. Wettstein, and H. Kagi, *Helv. Chim. Acta*, **18,** 1478 (1935).
15. N. Bruchovsky and J. D. Wilson, *J. Biol. Chem.*, **243,** 5953 (1968).
16. K. M. Anderson and S. Liao, *Nature (London)*, **219,** 277 (1968).
17. S. Fang, K. M. Anderson, and S. Liao, *J. Biol. Chem.*, **244,** 6584 (1969).
18. W. I. P. Mainwaring, *J. Endocrinol.*, **45,** 531 (1969).
19. C. D. Kochakian and J. R. Murlin, *J. Nutr.*, **10,** 437 (1935).
20. A. T. Kenyon, I. Sandiford, A. H. Bryan, K. Knowlton, and F. C. Koch, *Endocrinology*, **23,** 135 (1938).
21. R. K. Meyer and L. G. Hershberger, *Endocrinology*, **60,** 397 (1957).
22. S. L. Leonard, *Endocrinology*, **50,** 199 (1952).
23. J. M. Loring, J. M. Spencer, and C. A. Villee, *Endocrinology*, **68,** 501 (1961).
24. F. T. G. Prunty, *Brit. Med. J.*, **2,** 605 (1966).
25. A. Vermeulen, *Acta Endocrinol.* (Copenhagen), **83,** 651 (1976).
26. M. B. Lipsett and S. G. Korenman, *J. Am. Med. Assoc.*, **190,** 757 (1964).
27. A. Chapdelaine, P. C. MacDonald, O. Gonzalez, E. Gurpide, R. L. VandeWiele, and S. Lieberman, *J. Clin. Endocrinol. Metab.*, **25,** 1569 (1965).
28. J. F. Tait and R. Horton, *Steroids*, **4,** 365 (1964).
29. F. F. G. Rommerts, B. A. Cooke, and H. J. Van der Mulen, *J. Steroid Biochem.*, **5,** 279 (1974).
30. S. Burstein, H. L. Kimball, and M. Gut, *Steroids*, **15,** 808 (1970).
31. R. B. Hochberg, P. O. McDonald, S. Ladany, and S. Lieberman, *J. Steroid Biochem.*, **6,** 373 (1975).
32. R. B. Hochberg, P. O. McDonald, M. Feldman, and S. Lieberman, *J. Biol. Chem.*, **251,** 2087 (1976).
33. R. Vihko and A. Ruokonen, *J. Steroid Biochem.*, **5,** 843 (1974).

34. C. E. Bird, L. Morrow, Y. Fukumoto, S. Marcellus, and A. F. Clark, *J. Clin. Endocrinol. Metab.*, **43,** 1317 (1976).
35. R. I. Dorfman and F. Ungar, *Metabolism of Steroid Hormones*, Academic Press, New York, 1965.
36. R. B. Hochberg, S. Ladany, and S. Lieberman, *J. Biol. Chem.*, **251,** 3320 (1976).
37. H. P. Schedl and J. A. Clifton, *Gastroenterology*, **41,** 491 (1961).
38. K. B. Eik-Nes, J. Schellmann, A. R. Lumry, and L. T. Samuels, *J. Biol. Chem.*, **206,** 411 (1954).
39. B. H. Levedahl and H. Bernstein, *Arch. Biochem. Biophys.*, **52,** 353 (1954).
40. J. Schellmann, A. R. Lumry, and L. T. Samuels, *J. Am. Chem. Soc.*, **76,** 2808 (1954).
41. J. Kerkay and U. Westphal, *Biochim. Biophys. Acta*, **170,** 324 (1968).
42. J. Kerkay and U. Westphal, *Arch. Biochem. Biophys.*, **129,** 480 (1969).
43. P. I. Corvol, A. Chrambach, D. Rodbard, and C. W. Bardin, *J. Biol. Chem.*, **246,** 3435 (1971).
44. W. H. Pearlman and O. Crépy, *J. Biol. Chem.*, **242,** 182 (1967).
45. J. L. Guériguan and W. H. Pearlman, *Fed. Proc.*, **26,** 757 (1967).
46. B. E. P. Murphy, *Can. J. Biochem.*, **46,** 299 (1968).
47. O. Steeno, W. Heyus, H. Van Baelen, and P. De Moor, *Ann. Endocrinol.*, **29,** 141 (1968).
48. C. Mercier-Bodard, A. Alfsen, and E. E. Baulieu, *Acta Endocrinol.* (Copenhagen), **147,** 204 (1970).
49. M. C. Lebeau, C. Mercier-Bodard, J. Oldo, D. Bourguon, T. Brécy, J. P. Raynaud, and E. E. Baulieu, Ann. Endocrinol, 30, 183 (1969).
50. W. Rosner, N. P. Christy, and W. G. Kelley, *Biochemistry*, **8,** 3100 (1969).
51. W. H. Pearlman, I. F. F. Fong, and K. J. Tou, *J. Biol. Chem.*, **244,** 1373 (1969).
52. F. Dray, I. Mowezawicz, M. J. Ledru, O. Crépy,, G. Delzant, and J. Sebaoun, *Ann. Endocrinol.*, **30,** 223 (1969).
53. P. DeMoor, O. Steeno, W. Heyns, and H. Van Baelen, *Ann. Endocrinol.*, **30,** 233 (1969).
54. R. Horton, T. Kato, and R. Sherino, *Steroids*, **10,** 245 (1967).
55. A. Vermeulen and L. Verdonck, *Steroids*, **11,** 609 (1968).
56. T. Kato and R. Horton, *J. Clin. Endocrinol. Metab.*, **28,** 1160 (1968).
57. C. Mercier-Bodard and E. E. Baulieu, *Ann. Endocrinol.*, **29,** 159 (1968).
58. B. E. P. Murphy, *Steroids*, **16,** 791 (1970).
59. K. E. Mickelson and P. H. Petra, *Biochemistry*, **14,** 957 (1975).
60. E. M. Ritzen, S. N. Nayfeh, F. S. French, and M. C. Dobbins, *Endocrinology*, **89,** 143 (1971).
61. V. Hansson and O. Djoseland, *Acta Endocrinol.* (Copenhagen), **71,** 614 (1972).
62. F. S. French and E. M. Ritzén, *J. Reprod. Fertil.*, **32,** 479 (1973).
63. V. Hansson, O. Trygotad, F. S. French, W. S. McLean, A. A. Smith, D. J. Tindall, S. C. Weddington, P. Petruez, S. N. Nayfeh, and E. M. Ritzén, *Nature* (London), **250,** 387 (1974).
64. R. G. Vernon, B. Kopec, and I. B. Fritz, *Mol. Cell. Endocrinol.*, **1,** 167 (1974).
65. D. J. Tindall, V. Hansson, W. S. McLean, E. M. Ritzén, S. N. Nayfeh, and F. S. French, *Mol. Cell. Endocrinol.*, **3,** 83 (1975).
66. V. Hansson, K. J. Tveter, and A. Attramadal, *Acta Endocrinol.* (Copenhagen), **67,** 384 (1971).
67. L. E. Appelgren, *Steroids Lipids Res.*, **3,** 286 (1972).
68. D. Williams and J. Gorski, *Biochem. Biophys. Res. Commun.*, **45,** 258 (1971).
69. E. Milgrom, M. Atger, and E. E. Baulieu, *Biochim. Biophys. Acta*, **320,** 267 (1973).
70. R. W. Harrison, S. Fairfield, and D. N. Orth, *Biochemistry*, **14,** 1304 (1975).
71. R. W. Harrison, S. Fairfield, and D. N. Orth, *Biochem. Biophys. Res. Commun.*, **61,** 1262 (1974).
72. E. P. Gorgi, J. C. Stewart, J. K. Grant, and R. Scott, *Biochem. J.*, **122,** 125 (1971).
73. E. P. Gorgi, J. C. Stewart, J. K. Grant, and I. M. Shirley, *Biochem. J.*, **126,** 107 (1972).
74. E. P. Gorgi, J. K. Grant, J. C. Stewart, and J. Reid, *J. Endocrinol.*, **55,** 421 (1972).
75. E. P. Gorgi, I. M. Shirley, J. K. Grant, and J. C. Stewart, *Biochem. J.*, **132,** 465 (1973).
76. S. R. Gross, L. Aronow, and W. B. Pratt, *Biochem. Biophys. Res. Commun.*, **32,** 66 (1968).
77. S. R. Gross, L. Aronow, and W. B. Pratt, *J. Cell. Biol.*, **44,** 103 (1970).
78. P. Ofner, *Vitamins and Hormones*, Vol. 26, R. S. Harris, I. G. Wool and J. A. Lorraine, Eds., Academic Press, New York, 1968, p. 237.
79. K. Hartiala, *Physiol. Rev.*, **53,** 496 (1973).
80. M. Stylianou, E. Forchielli, M. Tummillo, and R. I. Dorfman, *J. Biol. Chem.*, **236,** 692 (1961).
81. D. Engelhardt, J. Eisenburg, P. Unterberger, and H. J. Karl, *Klin. Wochenschr.*, **49,** 439 (1971).

82. B. P. Lisboa, I. Drosse, and H. Breuer, *Z. Physiol. Chem.*, **342,** 123 (1965).
83. E. Chang, A. Mittelman, and T. L. Dao, *J. Biol. Chem.*, **238,** 913 (1963).
84. K. Hartiala and W. Nienstedt, *Int. J. Biochem.*, **7,** 317 (1976).
85. A. Vermeulen, R. Rubens, and L. Verdonck, *J. Clin. Endocrinol. Metab.*, **34,** 730 (1972).
86. P. K. Siiteri and J. D. Wilson, *J. Clin. Invest.*, **49,** 1737 (1970).
87. K. D. Voigt, H.-J. Horst, and M. Krieg, *Vitam. Horm.*, **33,** 417 (1975).
88. H. Becker, J. Kaufmann, H. Klosterhalfen, and K. D. Voigt, *Acta Endocrinol.* (Copenhagen), **71,** 589 (1972).
89. H. J. Horst, M. Dennis, J. Kaufmann, and K. D. Voigt, *Acta Endocrinol.* (Copenhagen), **79,** 394 (1975).
90. A. E. Kellie and E. R. Smith, *Biochem. J.*, **66,** 490 (1957).
91. P. Robel, R. Emiliozzi, and E. Baulieu, *J. Biol. Chem.*, **241,** 20 (1966).
92. F. T. G. Prunty, *Brit. Med. J.*, **2,** 605 (1966).
93. M. B. Lipsett and S. G. Korenman, *J. Am. Med. Assoc.*, **190,** 757 (1964).
94. N. Kundu, A. A. Sandberg, and W. R. Slaunwhite, Jr., *Steroids*, **6,** 543 (1965).
95. T. El Attar, W. Dirscherl, and K. O. Mosebach, *Acta Endocrinol.* (Copenhagen), **45,** 527 (1964).
96. A. Kappas and R. H. Palmer, in *Methods in Hormone Research*, Vol. 4, Part B, R. I. Dorfman, Ed., Academic Press, New York, 1965, p. 1.
97. L. Hellman, H. L. Bradlow, B. Zumoff, D. K. Fukushima, and T. F. Gallagher, *J. Clin. Endocrinol.*, **19,** 936 (1959).
98. E. Castegnaro and G. Sala, *Folia Endocrinol.*, **14,** 581 (1961).
99. H. J. Ringold, J. Graves, M. Hayano, and H. Lawrence, Jr., *Biochem. Biophys. Res. Commun.*, **13,** 162 (1963).
100. L. L. Engel, J. Alexander, and M. Wheeler, *J. Biol. Chem.*, **231,** 159 (1958).
101. D. Kupfer, E. Forchielli, and R. I. Dorfman, *J. Biol. Chem.*, **235,** 1968 (1960).
102. W. E. Farnsworth, *Steroids*, **8,** 825 (1966).
103. E. Caspi, A. Vermeulen, and H. B. Bhat, *Steroids*, Suppl. I, 141 (1965).
104. H. Okado, K. Matsuyoshi, and G. Tokuda, *Acta Endocrinol.* (Copenhagen), **46,** 40 (1964).
105. A. Segaloff, B. Gabbard, B. T. Carriere, and E. L. Rongone, *Steroids*, Suppl. I., 419 (1965).
106. R. Rembiesa, M. Holzbauer, P. C. M. Young, M. K. Birmingham, and M. Saffran, *Endocrinology*, **81,** 1278 (1967).
107. E. L. Rongone and A. Segaloff, *Steroids*, **1,** 179 (1963).
108. G. Lehnert and W. Mucke, *Arzneim.-Forsch.*, **16,** 603 (1966).
109. H. Langecker, *Arzneim.-Forsch.*, **12,** 231 (1962).
110. E. Gerhards, K. H. Kolb, and P. E. Schulze, *Z. Physiol. Chem.*, **342,** 40 (1965).
111. S. Dell'acqua, S. Manuso, G. Eriksson, and E. Diczfalusy, *Biochim. Biophys. Acta*, **130,** 241 (1966).
112. E. L. Rongone, A. Segaloff, B. Gabbard, A. C. Carter, and E. B. Feldman, *Steroids*, **1,** 664 (1963).
113. E. Gerhards, H. Gibian, and K. H. Kolb, *Arzneim.-Forsch.*, **16,** 458 (1966).
114. K. Nozu and B. I. Tamaski, *Biochim. Biophys. Acta*, **348,** 321 (1974).
115. K. Nozu and B. I. Tamaski, *Acta Endocrinol.* (Copenhagen), **76,** 608 (1974).
116. N. Bruchovsky and J. D. Wilson, *J. Biol. Chem.*, **243,** 2012 (1968).
117. N. Bruchovsky and J. D. Wilson, *J. Biol. Chem.*, **243,** 5953 (1968).
118. J. Shimazaki, N. Furuya, H. Yamanaka, and K. Shida, *Endocrinol. Jap.*, **16,** 163 (1969).
119. J. Shimazaki, I. Matsushita, N. Furuya, H. Yamanaka, and K. Shida, *Endocrinol. Jap.*, **16,** 453 (1969).
120. D. W. Frederiksen and J. D. Wilson, *J. Biol. Chem.*, **246,** 2584 (1971).
121. R. J. Moore and J. D. Wilson, *J. Biol. Chem.*, **247,** 958 (1972).
122. R. J. Moore and J. D. Wilson, *Endocrinology*, **93,** 581 (1973).
123. J. P. Karr, R. Y. Kirdani, G. P. Murphy, and A. A. Sandberg, *Life Sci.*, **15,** 501 (1974).
124. K. J. Ryan, *J. Biol. Chem.*, **234,** 268 (1959).
125. E. A. Thompson and P. K. Siiteri, *J. Biol. Chem.*, **249,** 5373 (1974).
126. E. A. Thompson and P. K. Siiteri, *J. Biol. Chem.*, **249,** 5364 (1974).
127. A. S. Meyer, *Biochim. Biophys. Acta*, **17,** 441 (1955).
128. J. Goto and J. Fishman, *Science*, **195,** 80 (1977).
129. M. Akhtar and S. J. M. Skinner, *Biochem. J.*, **109,** 318 (1968).
130. S. J. M. Skinner and M. Akhtar, *Biochem. J.*, **114,** 75 (1969).
131. J. D. Townsley and H. J. Brodie, *Biochem.*, **7,** 33 (1968).

132. H. J. Brodie, G. Possanza, and J. D. Townsley, *Biochim. Biophys. Acta*, **152,** 770 (1968).
133. Y. Osawa and D. G. Spaeth, *Biochem.*, **10,** 66 (1971).
134. K. J. Ryan, in *Proceedings of the First International Congress on Endocrinology*, Copenhagen, 350, (1960).
135. K. J. Ryan, in *Proceedings of the Fifth International Congress on Biochemistry*, Moscow, **7,** 381 (1963).
136. C. Gual, T. Morato, M. Hayano, M. Gut, and R. I. Dorfman, *Endocrinology*, **71,** 920 (1962).
137. W. C. Schwarzel, W. G. Kruggel, and H. J. Brodie, *Endocrinology*, **92,** 866 (1973).
138. P. K. Siiteri and E. A. Thompson, *J. Steroid Biochem.*, **6,** 317 (1975).
139. F. L. Bellino, S. S. H. Gilani, S. S. Eng, Y. Osawa, and W. L. Duax, *Biochemistry*, **15,** 4730 (1976).
140. A. M. H. Brodie, W. C. Schwarzel, A. A. Shaikh, and H. J. Brodie, *Endocrinology*, **100,** 1684 (1977).
141. R. W. Brueggemeier, E. E. Floyd, and R. E. Counsell, *J. Med. Chem.*, **21,** 1007 (1978).
142. L. S. Sholiton, R. T. Mornell, and E. E. Werk, *Steroids*, **8,** 265 (1966).
143. R. B. Jaffe, *Steroids*, **14,** 483 (1969).
144. L. S. Sholiton and E. E. Werk, *Acta Endocrinol.* (Copenhagen); **61,** 641 (1969).
145. L. S. Sholiton, I. L. Hall, and E. E. Werk, *Acta Endocrinol.* (Copenhagen), **63,** 512 (1970).
146. J. M. Stern and A. J. Eisenfeld, *Endocrinology* **88,** 1117 (1971).
147. R. Massa, E. Stupnicka, Z. Kniewald, and L. Martini, *J. Steroid Biochem.*, **3,** 385 (1972).
148. F. Naftolin, K. J. Ryan, and Z. Petro, *J. Clin. Endocrinol. Metab.*, **33,** 368 (1971).
149. F. Naftolin, K. J. Ryan, and Z. Petro, *Endocrinology*, **90,** 295 (1972).
150. F. Flores, F. Naftolin, and K. J. Ryan, *Neuroendocrinology*, **11,** 177 (1973).
151. F. Flores, F. Naftolin, K. J. Ryan, and R. J. White, *Science*, **180,** 1074 (1973).
152. J. A. Canick, D. E. Vaccaro, K. J. Ryan, and S. E. Leeman, *Endocrinology*, **100,** 250 (1977).
153. G. Perez-Palacios, K. Larsson, and C. Beyer, *J. Steroid Biochem.*, **6,** 999 (1975).
154. R. L. Landau, in *Anabolic-Androgenic Steroids*, C. D. Kochakian, Ed., Springer-Verlag, New York, 1967, p. 48.
155. H. Spencer, J. A. Friedland, and I. Lewin, in *Anabolic-Androgenic Steroids*, C. D. Kochakian, Ed., Springer-Verlag, New York, 1976, p. 419.
156. H. Spencer et al., in *Anabolic-Androgenic Steroids*, C. D. Kochakian, Ed., Springer-Verlag, New York, 1976, p. 433.
157. C. W. Gurney, in *Anabolic-Androgenic Steroids*, C. D. Kochakian, Ed., Springer-Verlag, New York, 1976, p. 483.
158. H. Kopera, in *Anabolic-Androgenic Steroids*, C. D. Kochakian, Ed., Springer-Verlag, New York, 1976, p. 573.
159. B. S. McEwen, *Sci. Am.*, **235** (1), 48 (1976).
160. B. W. O'Malley and A. R. Means, *Receptors for Reproductive Hormones*, Plenum Press, New York, 1974.
161. R. J. B. King and W. I. P. Mainwaring, *Steroid-Cell Interactions*, University Park Press, Baltimore, 1974.
162. S. Liao, *Int. Rev. Cytol.*, **41,** 87 (1975).
163. H. G. Williams-Ashman and A. H. Reddi, "Androgenic Regulation of Tissue Growth and Function" in *Biochemical Actions of Hormones*, Vol. 2, G. Litwack, Ed., Academic Press, New York, 1972, p. 257.
164. L. Chan and B. W. O'Malley, *New Engl. J. Med.*, **294,** 1322, 1372, 1430 (1976).
165. E. J. Jensen and H. I. Jacobson, *Rec. Progr. Hormone Res.*, **18,** 387 (1962).
166. W. H. Pearlman and M. R. I. Pearlman, *J. Biol. Chem.*, **236,** 1321 (1961).
167. B. W. Harding and L. T. Samuels, *Endocrinology*, **70,** 109 (1962).
168. K. J. Tveter and A. Attramadal, *Acta Endocrinol.* (Copenhagen), **59,** 218 (1968).
169. N. Bruchovsky and J. D. Wilson, *J. Biol. Chem.*, **243,** 2012 (1968).
170. W. I. P. Mainwaring, *J. Endocrinol.*, **44,** 323 (1969).
171. S. Fang and S. Liao, *J. Biol. Chem.*, **246,** 16 (1971).
172. W. I. P. Mainwaring and B. M. Peterken, *Biochem. J.*, **125,** 285 (1971).
173. J. L. Tymoezko and S. Liao, *Biochim. Biophys. Acta*, **252,** 607 (1971).
174. W. I. P. Mainwaring, P. A. Wilce, and A. E. Smith, *Biochem. J.*, **137,** 513 (1974).
175. W. I. P. Mainwaring, F. R. Mangan, and B. M. Peterken, *Biochem. J.*, **123,** 619 (1971).
176. P. Davies and K. Griffiths, *Biochem. J.*, **136,** 611 (1973).
177. I. Schenkein, M. Levy, and E. D. Bueker, *Endocrinology*, **94,** 840 (1974).
178. P. L. Barthe, L. P. Bullock, and I. Mowszowicz, *Endocrinology*, **95,** 1019 (1974).

179. M. F. Lyon, I. Hendry, and R. V. Short, *Endocrinology*, **58,** 357 (1973).

180. C. W. Bardin, L. P. Bullock, and R. J. Sherins, *Rec. Progr. Hormone Res.*, **29,** 65 (1973).

181. M. Kumar, A. K. Roy, and A. E. Axelrod, *Nature*, **223,** 399 (1969).

182. J. F. Irwin, S. E. Lane, and O. W. Neuhaus, *Biochim. Biophys. Acta*, **252,** 328 (1971).

183. A. K. Roy, *Endocrinology*, **92,** 957 (1973).

184. S. Liao, T. Liang, and J. L. Tymoczko, *Nature New Biol.*, **241,** 211 (1973).

185. S. Liao, T. Liang, T. C. Shao, and J. L. Tymoczko, *Advan. Exp. Med. Biol.*, **36,** 232 (1973).

186. K. J. Tveter and O. Unhjem, *Endocrinology*, **84,** 963 (1969).

187. J. M. Stern and A. J. Eisenfield, *Science*, **166,** 233 (1969).

188. K. Adachi and M. Kano, *Steroids*, **19,** 567 (1972).

189. W. I. P. Mainwaring and F. R. Mangan, *J. Endocrinol.*, **59,** 121 (1973).

190. S. Takayasu and K. Adachi, *Endocrinology*, **96,** 525 (1975).

191. V. Hansson et al., *Steroids*, **23,** 823 (1974).

192. D. J. Tindall, F. S. French, and S. N. Nayfeh, *Biochem. Biophys. Res. Commun.*, **49,** 1391 (1973).

193. J. A. Blaquier and R. S. Calandra, *Endocrinology*, **93,** 51 (1973).

194. E. M. Ritzén, S. N. Nayfeh, F. S. French, and P. A. Aronin, *Endocrinology*, **91,** 116 (1972).

195. J. F. Dunn, J. L. Goldstein, and J. D. Wilson, *J. Biol. Chem.*, **248,** 7819 (1973).

196. G. Verhoeven and J. D. Wilson, *Endocrinology*, **99,** 79 (1976).

197. P. Jouan, S. Samperez, M. L. Thieulant, and L. Mercier, *J. Steroid Biochem.*, **2,** 223 (1971).

198. P. Jouan, S. Samperez, and M. L. Thielant, *J. Steroid Biochem.*, **4,** 65 (1973).

199. M. Sar and W. E. Stumpf, *Endocrinology*, **92,** 251 (1973).

200. D. P. Cardinali, C. A. Nagle, and J. M. Rosner, *Endocrinology*, **95,** 179 (1974).

201. J. Kato, *J. Steroid Biochem.*, **6,** 979 (1975).

202. O. Naess, V. Hansson, O. Djoseland, and A. Attramadal, *Endocrinology*, **97,** 1355 (1975).

203. T. O. Fox, *Proc. Nat. Acad. Sci., USA*, **72,** 4303 (1975).

204. L. Valladares and J. Mingell, *Steroids*, **25,** 13 (1975).

205. J. Mingell and L. Valladares, *J. Steroid Biochem.*, **5,** 649 (1974).

206. A. K. Roy, B. S. Milin, and D. M. McMinn, *Biochim. Biophys. Acta*, **354,** 213 (1974).

207. N. Bruchovsky and J. W. Meakin, *Cancer Res.*, **33,** 1689 (1973).

208. N. Bruchovsky, D. J. A. Sutherland, J. W. Meakin, and T. Minesita, *Biochim. Biophys. Acta*, **381,** 61 (1975).

209. C. R. Evans and C. G. Pierrepoint, *J. Endocrinol.*, **64,** 539 (1975).

210. K. B. Eik-Nes, *Vitam. Horm.*, **33,** 193 (1975).

211. R. W. Gloyna and J. D. Wilson, *J. Clin. Endocrinol. Metab.*, **29,** 970 (1969).

212. V. Hansson, K. J. Tveter, O. Unhjem, and O. Djoseland, *J. Steroid Biochem.*, **3,** 427 (1972).

213. G. Giannopoulus, *J. Biol. Chem.*, **248,** 1004 (1973).

214. I. Jung and E. E. Baulieu, *Nature New Biol.*, **237,** 24 (1972).

215. M. G. Michel and E. E. Baulieu, *C.R. Acad. Sci. Paris*, **279,** 421 (1974).

216. M. L. Powers and J. R. Florini, *Endocrinology*, **97,** 1043 (1975).

217. F. Neumann, K. D. Richter, and T. Senge, *Vitam. Horm.* **33,** 103 (1975).

218. R. I. Dorfman, in *Methods in Hormone Research*, Vol. 2, A. Dorfman, Ed., Academic Press, New York, 1962, p. 275.

219. T. F. Gallagher and F. C. Koch, *J. Pharmacol. Exp. Ther.*, **55,** 97 (1935).

220. A. W. Greenwood, J. S. S. Blyth, and R. K. Callow, *Biochem. J.*, **29,** 1400 (1935).

221. C. W. Emmens, *Med. Res. Council, Spec. Rep. Ser.*, **234,** 1 (1939).

222. D. R. McCullagh and W. K. Cuyler, *J. Pharmacol. Exp. Ther.*, **66,** 379 (1939).

223. A. Segaloff, *Steroids*, **1,** 299 (1963).

224. E. Eisenberg and G. S. Gordan, *J. Pharmacol. Exp. Ther.*, **99,** 38 (1950).

225. F. J. Saunders and V. A. Drill, *Proc. Soc. Exp. Biol. Med.*, **94,** 646 (1957).

226. L. G. Hershberger, E. G. Shipley, and R. K. Meyer, *Proc. Soc. Exp. Biol. Med.*, **83,** 175 (1953).

227. F. A. Kincl, in *Methods in Hormone Research*, Vol. 4, R. I. Dorfman, Ed., Academic Press, New York, 1965, p. 21.

228. R. O. Stafford, B. J. Bowman, and K. J. Olson, *Proc. Soc. Exp. Biol. Med.*, **86,** 322 (1954).

229. E. Henderson and M. Weinberg, *J. Clin. Endocrinol.*, **11,** 641 (1951).

230. J. C. Stucki, A. D. Forbes, J. I. Northam, and J. J. Clark, *Endocrinology*, **66,** 585 (1960).

231. G. O. Potts, A. Arnold, and A. L. Beyler, *Endocrinology*, **67,** 849 (1960).

232. M. E. Nimni and E. Geiger, *Endocrinology*, **61,** 753 (1957).

233. J. N. Goldman, J. A. Epstein, and H. S. Kupperman, *Endocrinology*, **61,** 166 (1957).

234. F. A. Kincl, H. J. Ringold, and R. I. Dorfman, *Acta Endocrinol.*, **36,** 83 (1961).

235. M. E. Nimni and E. Geiger, *Proc. Soc. Exp. Biol. Med.*, **94,** 606 (1957),

236. R. O. Scow, *Endocrinology*, **51,** 42 (1952).

237. J. Leibetseder and K. Steininger, *Arzneim.-Forsch.* **15,** 474 (1965).

238. R. A. Edgren, *Acta Endocrinol.* (Copenhagen) Suppl., **87,** 3 (1963).

239. H. S. Kupperman, in *Encyclopedia of Sexual Behavior,* Albert Ellis, Ed., Hawthorn, Englewood Cliffs, N.J., 1961.

240. J. S. Strauss and P. E. Pochi, *Clin. Res.*, **13,** 233 (1965).

241. R. Rosso, G. Porcile, and F. Brema, *Cancer Chemother. Rep.*, **59,** 890 (1975).

242. W. A. Pacetti, *Curr. Ther. Res.*, **6,** 261 (1964).

243. R. C. Kory, R. N. Watson, M. H. Bradley, and B. J. Peters, *J. Clin. Invest.*, **36,** 907 (1957).

244. R. N. Watson, M. H. Bradley, R. Callahan, B. J. Peters, and R. C. Kory, *Am. J. Med.*, **26,** 238 (1959).

245. A. A. Renzi and J. J. Chart, *Proc. Soc. Exp. Biol. Med.*, **110,** 259 (1962).

246. A. A. Albanese, *J. New Drugs*, **5,** 208 (1965).

247. J. S. Bradshaw, W. E. Abbott, and S. Levey, *Am. J. Surg.*, **99,** 600 (1960).

248. G. S. Gordan and E. Eisenberg, *Proc. Roy. Soc. Med.*, **56,** 1027 (1963).

249. R. P. Howard and R. H. Furman, *J. Clin. Endocrinol.*, **22,** 43 (1962).

250. J. F. Dingman and W. H. Jenkins, *Metabolism*, **11,** 273 (1962).

251. S. Weisenfeld, S. Akgun, and S. Newhouse, *Diabetes*, **12,** 375 (1963).

252. D. W. Hughes, *Med. J. Aust.*, **2,** 361 (1973).

253. A. J. Ryan, in *Anabolic-Androgenic Steroids*, C. D. Kochakian, Ed., Springer-Verlag, New York, 1976, p. 515.

254. A. A. de Lorimier, G. S. Gordan, R. C. Lowe, and J. V. Carbone, *Arch. Intern. Med.*, **116,** 289 (1965).

255. I. M. Arias, in *Influence of Growth Hormone, Anabolic Steroids, and Nutrition in Health and Disease*, F. Gross, Ed., Springer-Verlag, Berlin, 1962, p. 434.

256. H. A. Kaupp and F. W. Preston, *J. Am. Med. Assoc.*, **180,** 411 (1962).

257. H. A. Plantier, *New Engl. J. Med.*, **270,** 141 (1964).

258. H. Hortling, K. Malmio, and L. Husi-Brummer, *Acta Endocrinol.* (Copenhagen) Suppl., **39,** 132 (1962).

259. A. Prader, *Acta Endocrinol.* (Copenhagen) Suppl., **63,** 78 (1962).

260. C. D. Kochakian, *Rec. Progr. Hormone Res.*, **1,** 177 (1948).

261. C. Huggins and E. V. Jensen, *J. Exp. Med.*, **100,** 241 (1954).

262. K. Junkmann, *Rec. Progr. Hormone Res.*, **13,** 389 (1957).

263. A. Butenandt and H. Dannenberg, *Berichte*, **73,** 206 (1940).

264. R. E. Counsell, P. D. Klimstra, and F. B. Colton, *J. Org. Chem.*, **27,** 248 (1962).

265. J. D. Wilson and R. E. Gloyna, *Rec. Progr. Hormone Res.*, **26,** 309 (1970).

266. F. J. Zeller, *J. Reprod. Fertil.*, **25,** 125 (1971).

267. L. H. Harris, *J. Clin. Endocrin. Metab.*, **21,** 1099 (1961).

268. C. Huggins, E. V. Jensen, and A. S. Cleveland, *J. Exp. Med.*, **100,** 225 (1954).

269. R. B. Gabbard and A. Segaloff, *J. Org. Chem.*, **27,** 655 (1962).

270. V. A. Drill and B. Riegel, *Rec. Progr. Hormone Res.*, **14,** 29 (1958).

271. J. W. Partridge, L. Boling, L. DeWind, S. Margen, and L. W. Kinsell, *J. Clin. Endocrinol. Metab.*, **13,** 189 (1953).

272. F. J. Saunders and V. A. Drill, *Endocrinology*, **58,** 567 (1956).

273. L. E. Barnes, R. O. Stafford, M. E. Guild, L. C. Thole, and K. J. Olson, *Endocrinology*, **55,** 77 (1954).

274. C. Djerassi, L. Miramontes, G. Rosenkranz, and F. Sondheimer, *J. Am. Chem. Soc.*, **76,** 4092 (1954).

275. F. B. Colton, L. N. Nysted, B. Reigel, and A. L. Raymond, *J. Am. Chem. Soc.*, **79,** 1123 (1957).

276. E. B. Feldman and A. C. Carter, *J. Clin. Endocrinol. Metab.*, **20,** 842 (1960).

277. J. Ferrin, *Acta Endocrinol.* (Copenhagen), **22,** 303 (1956).

278. K. V. Yorka, W. L. Truett, and W. S. Johnson, *J. Org. Chem.*, **27,** 4580 (1962).

279. W. F. Johns, *J. Am. Chem. Soc.*, **80,** 6456 (1958).

280. W. F. Johns, G. D. Searle & Co., private communication.

281. H. J. Ringold, *J. Am. Chem. Soc.*, **82,** 961 (1960).
282. A. Zaffaroni, *Acta Endocrinol.* (Copenhagen) Suppl., **50,** 139 (1960).
283. M. W. Goldberg, J. Sicé, H. Robert, and Pl. A. Plattner, *Helv. Chim. Acta*, **30,** 1441 (1947).
284. H. Heusser, P. T. Herzig, A. Furst, and Pl. A. Plattner, *Helv. Chim. Acta*, **33,** 1093 (1950).
285. G. Eadon and C. Djerassi, *J. Med. Chem.*, **15,** 89 (1972).
286. G. Sala, G. Baldratti, R. Ronchi, V. Clini, and C. Bertazzoli, *Sperimentale*, **106,** 490 (1956).
287. G. S. Gordan, *Arch. Intern. Med.*, **100,** 744 (1957).
288. A. Arnold, G. O. Potts, and A. L. Beyler, *Endocrinology*, **72,** 408 (1963).
289. P. A. Desaulles, *Helv. Med. Acta*, **27,** 479 (1960).
290. R. I. Dorfman and F. A. Kincl, *Endocrinology*, **72,** 259 (1963).
291. G. W. Liddle and H. A. Burke, Jr., *Helv. Med. Acta*, **27,** 504 (1960).
292. A. L. Beyler, G. O. Potts, and A. Arnold, *Endocrinology*, **68,** 987 (1961).
293. F. B. Colton, US Patent 2,874,170 (1959).
294. A. Smit and P. Westerhof, *Rec. Trav. Chim. Pays-Bas*, **82,** 1107 (1963).
295. R. Van Moorselaar, S. J. Halkes, and E. Havinga, *Rec. Trav. Chim. Pays-Bas*, **84,** 841 (1965).
296. J. S. Baran, *J. Med. Chem.*, **6,** 329 (1963).
297. R. A. Edgren, D. L. Peterson, R. C. Jones, C. L. Nagra, H. Smith, and G. A. Hughes, *Rec. Progr. Hormone Res.*, **22,** 305 (1966).
298. A. Segaloff and R. B. Gabbard, *Steroids*, **1,** 77 (1963).
299. A. Segaloff and R. B. Gabbard, *Steroids*, **22,** 99 (1973).
300. J. Tremolieres and E. Pequignot, *Presse Med.*, **73,** 2655 (1965).
301. H. L. Kruskemper and G. Noell, *Steroids*, **8,** 13 (1966).
302. H. L. Kruskemper, K. D. Morgner, and G. Noell, *Arzneim.-Forsch.*, **17,** 449 (1967).
303. A. Halden, R. M. Watter, and G. S. Gordan, *Cancer Chemother. Rep.*, **54,** 453 (1970).
304. G. K. Suchowsky and K. Junkmann, *Acta Endocrinol.* (Copenhagen), **39,** 68 (1962).
305. B. Pelc, *Collect. Czech. Chem. Commun.*, **29,** 3089 (1964).
306. O. Weller, *Endokrinologie*, **42,** 34 (1962).
307. O. Weller, *Endokrinologie*, **41,** 60 (1961).
308. H. L. Kruskemper and H. Breuer, *Excerpta Medica International Congress Series*, No. 51, 209 (1962).
309. F. Neumann, R. Wiechert, M. Kramer, and G. Raspe, *Arzneim.-Forsch.*, **16,** 455 (1966).
310. O. Weller, *Arzneim.-Forsch.*, **16,** 465 (1966).
311. B. Pelc and J. Jodkova, *Collect. Czech. Chem. Commun.*, **30,** 3575 (1965).
312. B. Pelc, *Collect. Czech. Chem. Commun.*, **30,** 3468 (1965).
313. C. Djerassi, R. Riniker, and B. Riniker, *J. Am. Chem. Soc.*, **78,** 6377 (1956).
314. A. Bowers, H. J. Ringold, and E. Denot, *J. Am. Chem. Soc.*, **80,** 6115 (1958).
315. O. Abe, H. Herraneu, and R. I. Dorfman, *Proc. Soc. Exp. Biol. Med.*, **111,** 706 (1962).
316. D. Berkowitz, *Clin. Res.*, **8,** 199 (1960).
317. R. E. Counsell and P. D. Klimstra, *J. Med. Chem.*, **6,** 736 (1963).
318. R. I. Dorfman and A. S. Dorfman, *Acta Endocrinol.* (Copenhagen), **42,** 245 (1963).
319. A. Arnold, G. O. Potts, and A. L. Beyler, *J. Endocrinol.*, **28,** 87 (1963).
320. D. R. Korst, C. Y. Bowers, J. H. Flokstra, and F. G. McMahon, *Clin. Pharmacol. Ther.*, **4,** 734 (1963).
321. J. A. Campbell, S. C. Lyster, G. W. Duncan, and J. C. Babcock, *Steroids*, **1,** 317 (1963).
322. J. A. Campbell and J. C. Babcock, *J. Am. Chem. Soc.*, **81,** 4069 (1959).
323. G. S. Gordan, S. Wessler, and L. V. Avioli, *J. Am. Med. Assoc.*, **219,** 483 (1972).
324. I. S. Goldenberg, N. Waters, R. S. Randin, F. J. Ansfield, and A. Segaloff, *J. Am. Med. Assoc.*, **223,** 1267 (1973).
325. R. A. Edgren, H. Smith, and G. A. Hughes, *Steroids*, **2,** 731 (1963).
326. R. B. Greenblatt, E. C. Jungck, and G. C. King, *Am. J. Med. Sci.*, **318,** 99 (1964).
327. G. Sala and G. Baldratti, *Proc. Soc. Exp. Biol. Med.*, **95,** 22 (1957).
328. G. Baldratti, G. Arcari, V. Clini, F. Tani, and G. Sala, *Sperimentale*, **109,** 383 (1959).
329. G. Sala, A. Cesana, and G. Fedriga, *Minerva Med.*, **51,** 1295 (1960).
330. A. A. Albanese, E. J. Lorenze, and L. A. Orto, *N.Y. State J. Med.*, **63,** 80 (1963).
331. S. C. Lyster, G. H. Lund, and R. O. Stafford, *Endocrinology*, **58,** 781 (1956).
332. H. A. Burke, Jr., and G. W. Liddle, *Abstr. Endocrine Society Meeting*, Atlantic City, N.J., 1959, p. 45.

333. S. C. Lyster, G. H. Lund, and R. O. Stafford, *Endocrinology*, **58,** 781 (1956).
334. R. M. Backle, *Brit. Med. J.*, **1,** 1378 (1959).
335. T. H. McGavack and W. Seegers, *Am. J. Med. Sci.*, **235,** 125 (1958).
336. G. H. Marquardt, C. I. Fisher, P. Levy, and R. M. Dowben, *J. Am. Med. Assoc.*, **175,** 851 (1961).
337. B. J. Kennedy, *New Engl. J. Med.*, **259,** 673 (1958).
338. H. Nowakowski, *Deut. Med. Wochenschr.*, **90,** 2291 (1965).
339. G. Sala, *Helv. Med. Acta*, **27,** 519 (1960).
340. R. M. Myerson, *Am. J. Med. Sci.*, **241,** 732 (1961).
341. W. W. Glas and E. H. Lansing, *J. Am. Geriatr. Soc.*, **10,** 509 (1962).
342. H. G. Kraft and H. Kieser, *Arzneim.-Forsch.*, **14,** 330 (1964).
343. H. L. Kruskemper, *Arzneim.-Forsch.*, **16,** 608 (1966).
344. R. E. Schaub and M. J. Weiss, *J. Org. Chem.*, **26,** 3915 (1961).
345. H. Kaneko, K. Nakamura, Y. Yamato, and M. Kurakawa, *Chem. Pharm. Bull.* (Tokyo), **17,** 11 (1969).
346. A. Weinstein, H. R. Lindner, A. Frielander, and S. Bauminger, *Steroids*, **20,** 789 (1972).
347. R. Pappo and C. J. Jung, *Tetrahedron Lett.*, 365 (1962).
348. H. D. Lennon and F. J. Saunders, *Steroids*, **4,** 689 (1964).
349. P. B. Sollman, G. D. Searle & Co., private communication.
350. R. Pappo, G. D. Searle & Co., private communication.
351. A. P. Shroff and C. H. Harper, *J. Med. Chem.*, **12,** 190 (1969).
352. M. Fox, A. S. Minot, and G. W. Liddle, *J. Clin. Endocrinol. Metab.*, **22,** 921 (1962).
353. C. G. Ray, J. F. Kirschvink, S. H. Waxman, and V. C. Kelley, *Am. J. Dis. Child.*, **110,** 618 (1965).
354. E. F. Nutting and D. W. Calhoun, *Endocrinology*, **84,** 441 (1969).
355. C. D. Kochakian, *Am. J. Physiol.*, **145,** 549 (1946).
356. C. D. Kochakian, *Proc. Soc. Exp. Biol. Med.*, **80,** 386 (1952).
357. E. F. Nutting, P. D. Klimstra, and R. E. Counsell, *Acta Endocrinol.* (Copenhagen), **53,** 627, 635 (1966).
358. I. A. Anderson, *Acta Endocrinol.* (Copenhagen) Suppl., **63,** 54 (1962).
358a. M. E. Wolff and Y. Kasuya, *J. Med. Chem.*, **15,** 87 (1972).
359. G. A. Overbeck, A. Delver, and J. deVisser, *Acta Endocrinol.* (Copenhagen) Suppl., **63,** 7 (1962).
360. J. L. Kalliomaki, A. M. Pirila, and I. Ruikka, *Acta Endocrinol.* (Copenhagen) Suppl., **63,** 124 (1962).
361. H. Kopera, *Excerpta Medica International Congress Series*, No. 51, 204 (1962).
362. A. Walser and G. Schoenenberger, *Schweiz. Med. Wochenschr.*, **92,** 897 (1962).
363. J. A. Edwards and A. Bowers, *Chem. Ind.* (London), 1962 (1961).
364. M. E. Wolff and G. Zanati, *J. Med. Chem.*, **12,** 629 (1969).
365. M. E. Wolff, G. Zanati, G. Shanmagasundarum, S. Gupte, and G. Aadahl, *J. Med. Chem.*, **13,** 531 (1970).
366. M. E. Wolff and G. Zanati, *Experientia*, **26,** 1115 (1970).
367. G. Zanati, G. Gaare, and M. E. Wolff, *J. Med. Chem.*, **17,** 561 (1974).
368. R. W. S. Skinner, R. V. Pozderac, R. E. Counsell, C. F. Hsu, and P. A. Weinhold, *Steroids*, **25,** 189 (1977).
368a. M. E. Wolff, W. Ho, and R. Kwok, *J. Med. Chem.*, **7,** 577 (1964).
369. P. D. Klimstra, E. F. Nutting, and R. E. Counsell, *J. Med. Chem.*, **9,** 693 (1966).
370. M. Fujimuri, *Cancer*, **31,** 789 (1973).
371. G. O. Potts, A. Arnold, and A. L. Beyler, *Excerpta Medica International Congress Series*, No. 51, 211 (1962).
372. G. O. Potts, A. L. Beyler, and D. F. Burnham, *Proc. Soc. Exp. Biol. Med.*, **103,** 383 (1960).
373. P. C. Burnett, *J. Am. Geriatr. Soc.*, **11,** 979 (1963).
374. W. G. Mullin and F. diPillo, *N.Y. State J. Med.*, **63,** 2795 (1963).
375. A. J. Manson, F. W. Stonner, H. C. Neumann, R. G. Christiansen, R. L. Clarke, J. H. Ackerman, D. F. Page, J. W. Dean, D. K. Phillips, G. O. Potts, A. Arnold, A. L. Beyler, and R. O. Clinton, *J. Med. Chem.*, **6,** 1 (1963).
376. G. O. Potts, A. Beyler, and H. P. Schane, *Fertil. Steril.*, **25,** 367 (1974).
377. R. J. Sherrins, H. M. Gandy, T. W. Thorsland, and C. A. Paulsen, *J. Clin. Endocrinol. Metab.*, **32,** 522 (1971).
378. D. Rosi, H. C. Neumann, R. G. Christiansen, H.

P. Schane, and G. O. Potts, *J. Med. Chem.*, **20,** 349 (1977).

379. C. Davison, W. Banks, and A. Fritz, *Arch. Int. Pharmacodyn. Ther.*, **221,** 294 (1976).

380. K. Miescher, E. Tschapp, and A. Wettstein, *Biochem. J.*, **30,** 1977 (1936).

381. G. A. Overbeck, *Anabole Steroide*, Springer-Verlag, Berlin, 1966.

382. H. L. Kruskemper, *Anabolic Steroids*, trans. by C. H. Doering, Academic Press, New York, 1968.

383. G. A. Overbeck, J. van der Vies, and J. de Visser, in *Protein Metabolism*, F. Gross, Ed., Springer-Verlag, Berlin, 1962, p. 185.

384. J. de Visser and G. A. Overbeck, *Acta Endocrinol.* (Copenhagen), **35,** 405 (1960).

385. G. A. Overbeck and J. de Visser, *Acta Endocrinol* (Copenhagen), **38,** 285 (1961).

386. H. Nowakowski, *Acta Endocrinol.* (Copenhagen) Suppl., **63,** 37 (1962).

387. A. Alibrandi, G. Bruni, A. Ercoli, R. Gardi, and A. Meli, *Endocrinology*, **66,** 13 (1960).

388. K. Junkmann and G. Suchowsky, *Arzneim.-Forsch.*, **12,** 214 (1962).

389. K. C. James, *Experientia*, **28,** 479 (1972).

390. K. C. James, P. J. Nicholl, and G. T. Richards, *Eur. J. Med. Chem.*, **10,** 55 (1975).

391. R. Gaunt, C. H. Tuthill, N. Antonchak, and J. H. Leathem, *Endocrinology*, **52,** 407 (1953).

392. P. Borrevang, *Acta Chem. Scand.*, **16,** 883 (1962).

393. R. Huttenrauch, *Arch. Pharm.*, **297,** 124 (1964).

394. F. B. Colton and R. E. Ray, US Patent 3,068,249 (1962).

395. A. Ercoli, R. Gardi, and R. Vitali, *Chem. Ind.* (London), 1284 (1962).

396. R. Vitali, R. Gardi, and A. Ercoli, *Excerpta Medica International Congress Series*, No. 51, 128 (1962).

397. R. I. Dorfman, A. S. Dorfman, and M. Gut, *Acta Endocrinol.* (Copenhagen), **40,** 565 (1962).

398. R. Vitali, R. Gardi, G. Falconi, and A. Ercoli, *Steroids*, **8,** 527 (1966).

399. A. Ercoli, G. Bruni, G. Falconi, F. Galletti, and R. Gardi, *Acta Endocrinol.* (Copenhagen) Suppl., **51,** 857 (1960).

400. A. D. Cross, I. T. Harrison, P. Crabbe, F. A. Kincl, and R. I. Dorfman, *Steroids*, **4,** 229 (1964).

401. A. D. Cross and I. T. Harrison, *Steroids*, **6,** 397 (1965).

402. R. R. Burtner, E. A. Brown, and R. A. Mikulec, *Excerpta Medica International Congress Series*, No. 111, 50 (1966).

403. F. J. Saunders, *Proc. Soc. Exp. Biol. Med.*, **123,** 303 (1966).

404. A. J. Solo, N. Bejba, P. Hebborn, and M. May, *J. Med. Chem.*, **18,** 165 (1975).

405. J. Stern and A. J. Eisenfeld, *Endocrinology*, **88,** 1117 (1971).

406. F. R. Mangan and W. I. P. Mainwaring, *Steroids*, **20,** 331 (1972).

407. F. Neumann, *Hormone Metab. Res.*, **9,** 1 (1977).

408. J. Geller, J. Fishman, and T. L. Cantor, *J. Steroid Biochem.*, **6,** 837 (1975).

409. N. Jagarinec and M. L. Givner, *Steroids*, **23,** 561 (1974).

410. H. L. Saunders, K. Holden, and J. F. Kerwin, *Steroids*, **3,** 687 (1964).

411. K. J. Tveter and A. Aakvaag, *Endocrinology*, **85,** 683 (1969).

412. V. Hansson and K. J. Tveter, *Acta Endocrinol.* (Copenhagen), **68,** 69 (1971).

413. A. Zarate, V. B. Mahesh, and R. B. Greenblatt, *J. Clin. Endocrinol. Metab.*, **26,** 1394 (1966).

414. A. Boris and M. Uskokovic, *Experientia*, **26,** 9 (1970).

415. A. Boris, L. DeMartino, and T. Trmal, *Endocrinology*, **88,** 1086 (1971).

416. E. E. Baulieu and I. Jung, *Biochem. Biophys. Res. Commun.*, **38,** 599 (1970).

417. G. H. Rasmusson, A. Chen. G. F. Reynolds, D. J. Patanelli, A. A. Patchett, and G. E. Arth, *J. Med. Chem.*, **15,** 1165 (1972).

418. J. R. Brooks, F. D. Busch, D. J. Patanelli, and S. L. Steelman, *Proc. Soc. Exp. Biol. Med.*, **143,** 647 (1973).

419. E. A. Peets, M. F. Jenson, and R. Neri, *Endocrinology*, **94,** 532 (1974).

420. S. Liao, D. K. Howell, and T. Chaug, *Endocrinology*, **94,** 1205 (1974).

421. R. Neri and E. A. Peets, *J. Steroid Biochem.*, **6,** 815 (1975).

422. W. W. Scott and D. S. Coffey, *Vitam. Horm.*, **33,** 455 (1975).

423. P. D. Klimstra and R. E. Counsell, *J. Med. Chem.*, **8,** 48 (1965).

424. P. D. Klimstra, R. Zigman, and R. E. Counsell, *J. Med. Chem.*, **9,** 924 (1966).

425. A. Segaloff and R. Bruce Gabbard, *Endocrinology*, **67,** 887 (1960).

426. R. E. Counsell, *J. Med. Chem.*, **9,** 263 (1966).

427. A. Bowers, A. D. Cross, J. A. Edwards, H. Carpio, M. C. Calzada, and E. Denot, *J. Med. Chem.*, **6,** 156 (1963).

428. F. A. Kincl and R. I. Dorfman, *Steroids*, **3,** 109 (1964).
429. G. Zanati and M. E. Wolff, *J. Med. Chem.*, **14,** 958 (1971).
430. W. L. Duax, M. G. Erman, J. F. Griffin, and M. E. Wolff, *Cryst. Struct. Comm.*, **5,** 775 (1976).
431. G. Zanati and M. E. Wolff, *J. Med. Chem.*, **16,** 90 (1973).
432. S. Liao, T. Liang, S. Fang, E. Casteneda, and T. Shao, *J. Biol. Chem.*, **248,** 6154 (1973).
433. S. A. Shain and R. W. Boesel, *J. Steroid Biochem.*, **6,** 43 (1975).
434. R. W. S. Skinner, R. V. Pozderac, R. E. Counsell, and P. A. Weinhold, *Steroids*, **25,** 189 (1975).

CHAPTER TWENTY–NINE

The Female Sex Hormones and Analogs

R. DEGHENGHI

and

M. L. GIVNER

Ayerst Research Laboratories,
Montreal, Quebec, Canada

CONTENTS

1 INTRODUCTION

The mammalian ovary is a source of steroid hormones whose influence on the reproductive processes was recognized long before their structure could be established. These physiological premises nursed the intense efforts of the chemists who successfully elucidated the structures of the estrogens and of progesterone. Many more years elapsed between the first isolation of these hormones in a pure state and their synthetic preparation in commercial quantities. Derivatives of greater potency were prepared and tested clinically. New drugs were developed for the treatment of hormonal insufficiency and disease states.

Without precedent, however, the most widespread use of these steroids is not a therapeutic one. As the ingredients of "the Pill", they were hailed as one of the most effective answers to one of mankind's many pressing problems (1); see also Chapter 30.

2 THE ESTROGENS

2.1 History

At the beginning of this century hormonal research was limited to the investigations performed by animal physiologists. More specifically, it was limited to the reporting of observations resulting from comparisons of different animal species and from the effects of organ removal or transplantation. These early investigations established that the ovaries secrete a hormone that maintains reproductive function. The role of the ovary as regulator of the genital organs was confirmed in 1900 by Knauer (2), who was able to prevent symptoms of gonadectomy by ovarian transplant.

In 1917 Stockard and Papanicolaou (3) reported that the type of cells in the vaginal smear could be correlated with the phases of the sexual cycle of the guinea pig. Subsequently, in 1923, Allen and Doisy (4) developed their well-known assay for the detection and quantitation of estrogen response. This test is based on the changes evoked by estrogen in the vaginal smear of the rat or mouse.

With a suitable assay available, chemists began to investigate the complex ovarian hormone. This research soon showed that the ovarian hormone was a mixture of chemically related substances. By 1927 the pioneering work of Aschheim and Zondek (5) established that urine of pregnant women was a rich source of estrogens. Soon after, in 1929, Doisy and co-workers (6) at the St. Louis University School of Medicine, and Butenandt (7) in Göttingen, Germany, independently isolated the first crystalline estrogen, estrone (E_1, 29.**1**), from this source.

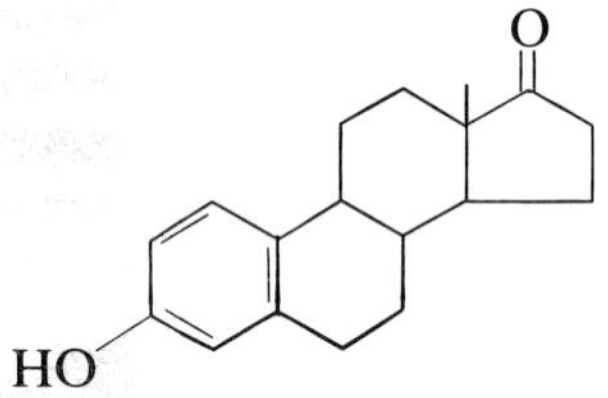

O
HO

29.**1**

In the following year Marrian (8) and Doisy et al. (9) announced almost simultaneously the isolation of estriol (E_3, 29.**2**)

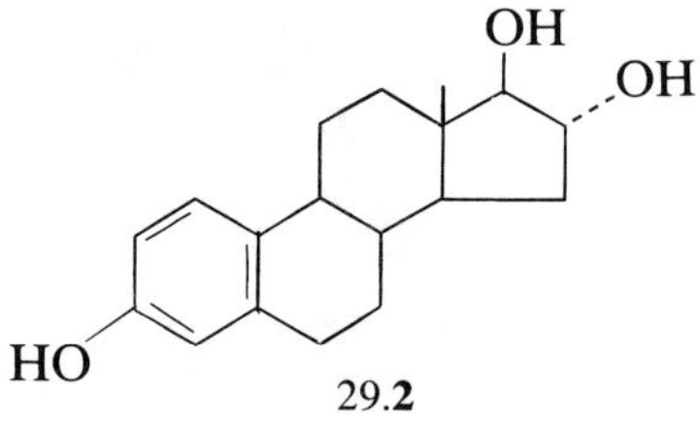

OH
OH
HO

29.**2**

from the same source. Ten years later, in 1940, 17β-estradiol (E_2, 29.**3**) was isolated

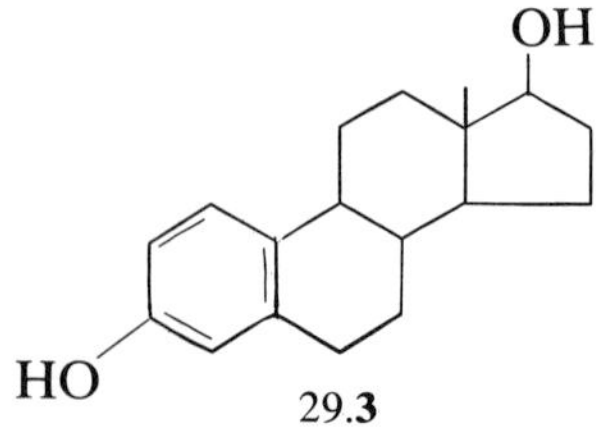

OH
HO

29.**3**

from the urine of pregnant women by the Doisy group (10). These three estrogens, the most abundant in human urine, are often called the "classical" estrogens.

Since the isolation of 17β-estradiol, evidence has accumulated for the existence of at least 15 other estrogens in human pregnancy urine. In addition to epimers and 16- or 17-keto derivatives of estriol, these urinary steroids include compounds with intriguing structures, such as 2-methoxyestrone (29.**4**) (11), 2-methoxyestriol (29.**5**)

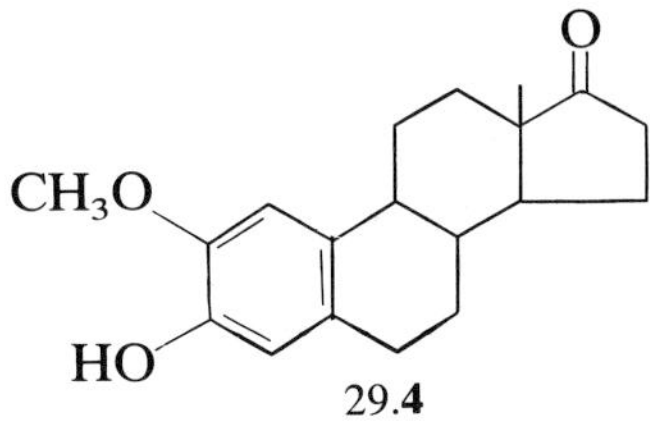

29.**4**

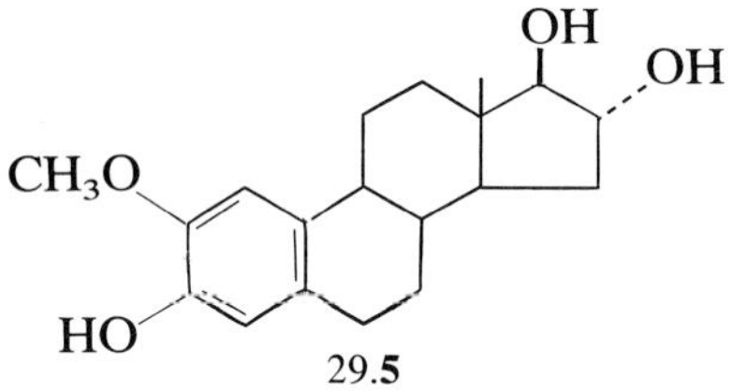

29.**5**

(12), 15α-hydroxyestriol (29.**6**) (13), and 18-hydroxyestrone (29.**7**) (14).

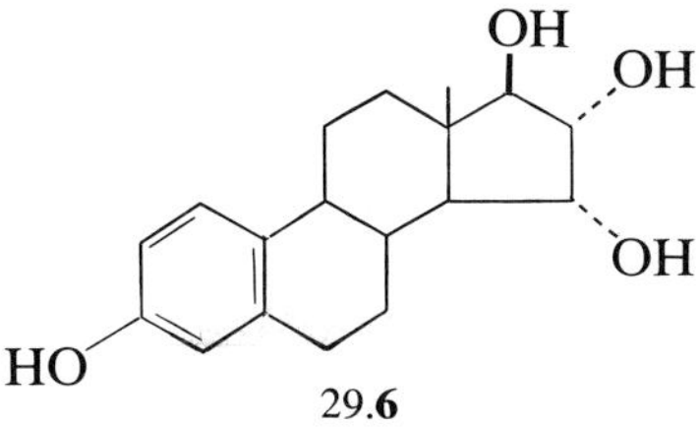

29.**6**

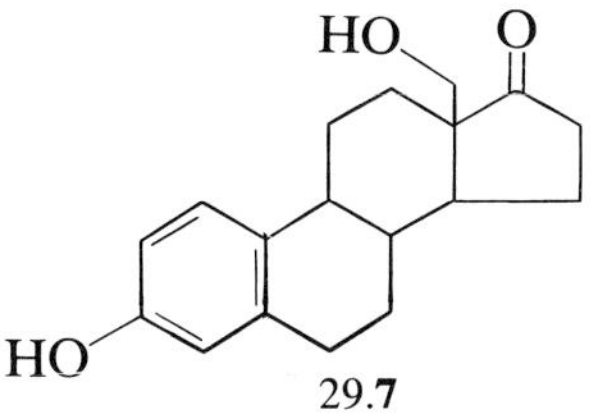

29.**7**

During these investigations of human pregnancy urine, evidence accumulated that correlated clinical signs of estrogenic activity with the amounts of estrogen excreted in the urine (15).

Investigations of another rich source of natural estrogens, the urine of pregnant mares (16), provided further evidence about the complexity of the "ovarian hormone". In 1930 Laqueur and collaborators (17) isolated estrone from pregnant mare's urine, and in 1932 Girard et al. (18) obtained three new estrogens from this source: equilin (29.**8**), equilenin (29.**9**), and

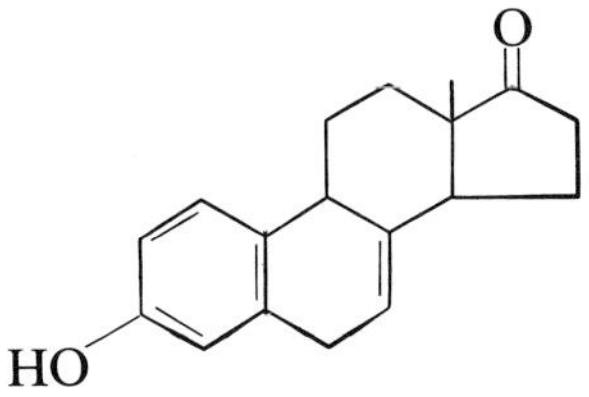

29.**8**

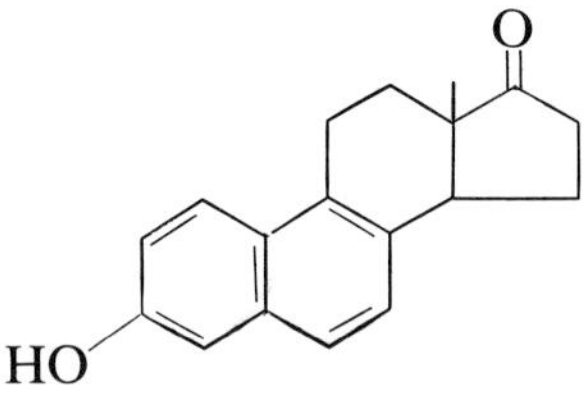

29.**9**

hippulin. The isolation of hippulin has never been confirmed; it has been suggested that it is 8-dehydro-14-isoestrone (19). The estrogens equilin and equilenin appear to be the unique property of the mare. Later investigations (20) showed that pregnant mare's urine is a rich source of estrone, equilin, and equilenin as well as the corresponding 17α-hydroxy derivatives of these three steroids.

In 1938 Inhoffen et al. made a significant contribution to the medicinal chemistry of estrogens (21). Estrone was treated with potassium acetylide in liquid ammonia to yield 17α-ethynylestradiol (29.**10**). When these investigators evaluated this synthetic estrogen in the Allen–Doisy rat assay, they discovered that it was 20 times more potent than estrone on oral administration. This surprising increase in oral activity was soon confirmed in humans (22). Today 17α-ethynylestradiol and its 3-methyl ether,

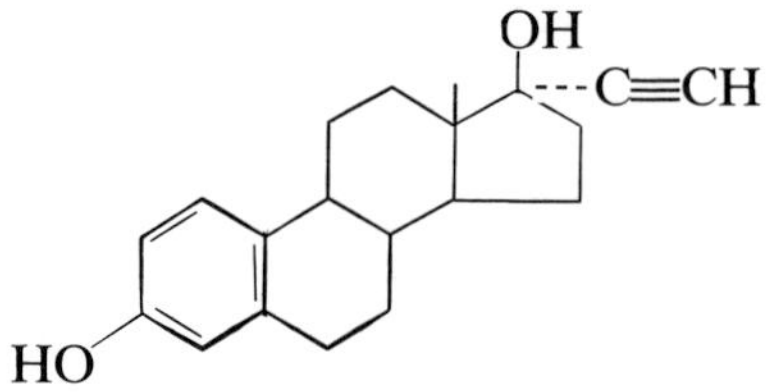

29.**10**

mestranol (29.**11**), are used widely as

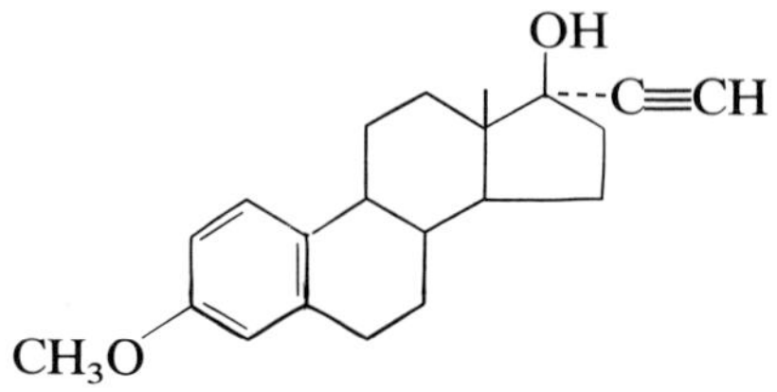

29.**11**

drugs, especially in the field of oral contraception. The realization that 17α-ethynylestradiol was a more potent orally active estrogen than the natural estrogens demonstrated that chemical alteration of the natural estrogens could be beneficial. Following this lead, the medicinal chemist has since produced several synthetic estrogens of therapeutic value.

2.2 Physiological Aspects of Estrogens

2.2.1 SOURCES. Estrogens are produced in the female by the ovary, placenta, and adrenal cortex, and in the male by the testis and the adrenal cortex. In the female, under normal physiological conditions, the ovary is the main site of estrogen production. During pregnancy, however, the placenta eventually becomes the main site, producing 100–1000 times more estrogen than the ovary toward the end of pregnancy. After menopause, small amounts of estrone are produced in the human female, at extraovarian sites. The mean concentration of ovarian steroids in serum under various physiological conditions is given in Table 29.1.

2.2.2 BIOGENESIS. The classical estrogens estrone, 17β-estradiol, and estriol are the three major estrogens in man and are frequently designated E_1, E_2, and E_3, respectively. 17β-Estradiol (29.**3**), the main secretory product of the ovary, is readily dehydrogenated *in vivo* to estrone (29.**1**), the major estrogen found in the blood. Estrone in turn is transformed into estriol (29.**2**), the most abundant estrogen excreted in the urine. These transformations take place mainly in the liver and have been summarized by Pincus and Zahl (23). However it was not until the 1950s that investigators began to unravel the many complexities of estrogen biosynthesis (24–26). Among the several investigations that have contributed to our present knowledge of the biogenetic pathway, the contributions of Engel and Ryan and their respective collaborators are

Table 29.1

	Concentration, pg/ml			
	E_1	E_2	E_3	Progesterone
Normal women				
Follicular phase	50	60	—	50
Midcycle	200	400	150	
Luteal phase	140	250	120	12,000
Postmenopausal	30	10	7	5
Pregnancy (3rd month)	1100	2600	970	35,000
Normal men	60	20	10	120

outstanding. Utilizing both *in vitro* and *in vivo* techniques, these groups demonstrated that the biogenesis of estrogens proceeds generally by the pathway shown in Fig. 29.1.

Alternative pathways for the biosynthesis of estrogens exist. During human pregnancy the placental-fetal unit is a source of increased amounts of estrogen, especially estriol. A considerable amount of this estriol is formed by pathways independent of estrone. For example, if labeled estrone or 17β-estradiol is administered to pregnant women, the specific activity of the urinary estriol is much lower than that of either the urinary estrone or 17β-estradiol (27, 28). 16α-Hydroxydehydroepiandrosterone (29.**12**) and androst-5-ene-3β, 16α,17β-triol (29.**13**) have been implicated as intermediates in these alternative pathways by *in vitro* experiments with placental preparations (29, 30) and by *in vivo* experiments (31). The exact nature of these alternative pathways awaits clarification (25).

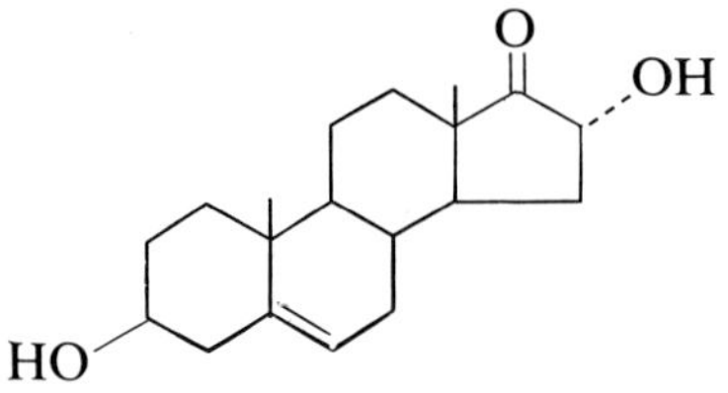

29.**12**

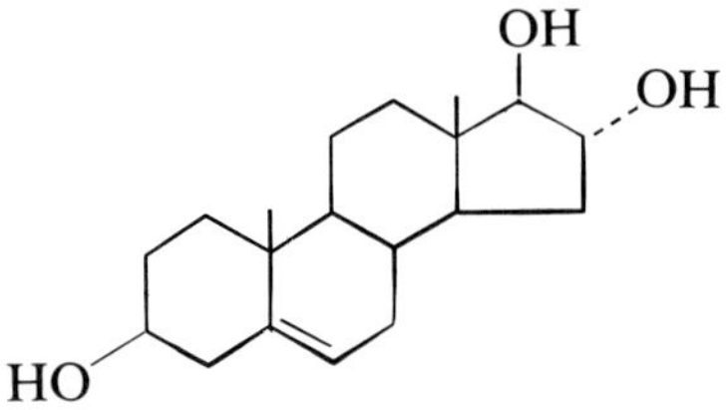

29.**13**

2.2.3 METABOLISM. Much of our knowledge concerning the metabolism of estrogens is due to the extensive investigations of Gallagher, Fishman, and their collaborators at the Sloan-Kettering Institute of Cancer Research, New York. Excellent reviews on this aspect of estrogens are available (15, 24, 32).

Our present view of the metabolic pathway of endogenous estrogens is based on a number of experiments in which ^{14}C-labelled estrone and 17β-estradiol were administered to healthy subjects and patients with cancer (33–37). According to these studies 17β-estradiol and estrone afford the same metabolic products; therefore the two are readily interconvertible in the body. This observation was confirmed (38) by administering a mixture of estrone-16-^{14}C and 17β-estradiol-6,7-^{3}H to patients. By comparing the isotope ratios of the metabolites, it was concluded that administered 17β-estradiol and, by inference, endogenous 17β-estradiol, are rapidly converted to estrone. Of the various routes of administration, the intravaginal one allows best the systemic absorption of estradiol without extensive conversion to estrone (39). All the other estrogen metabolites isolated represent further alterations of estrone. A most important alteration of estrone is its conversion to estriol, which occurs less rapidly than the conversion of 17β-estradiol to estrone. Another significant alteration of estrone is its conversion to 2-hydroxyestrone (29.**14**), which is further metabolized to 2-methoxyestrone (29.**4**). These reactions constitute the main processes for the metabolic pathway of 17β-estradiol, the principal secretory estrogen, as indicated by the study of urinary metabolites (Fig. 29.2).

In addition, small amounts of other metabolites of administered 17β-estradiol and estrone have been isolated from human pregnancy urine, indicating various other minor metabolic processes. Both the major and minor metabolites are listed in Table 29.2. This impressive list represents the culmination of many years of intensive research. It also reflects the progress achieved during this period in the techniques used for the isolation of natural products (e.g.,

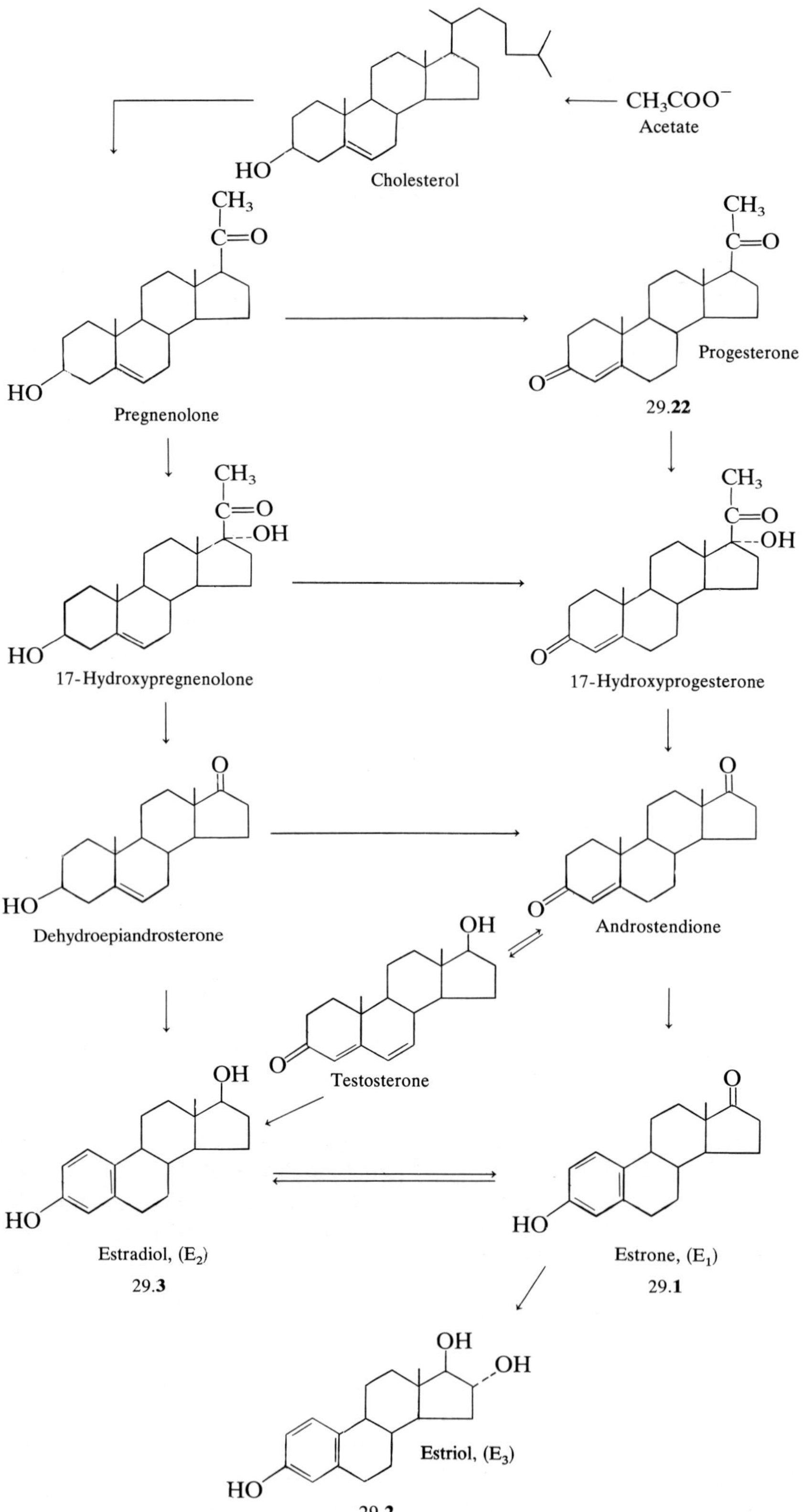

Fig. 29.1 Biogenetic pathway of the major urinary estrogens.

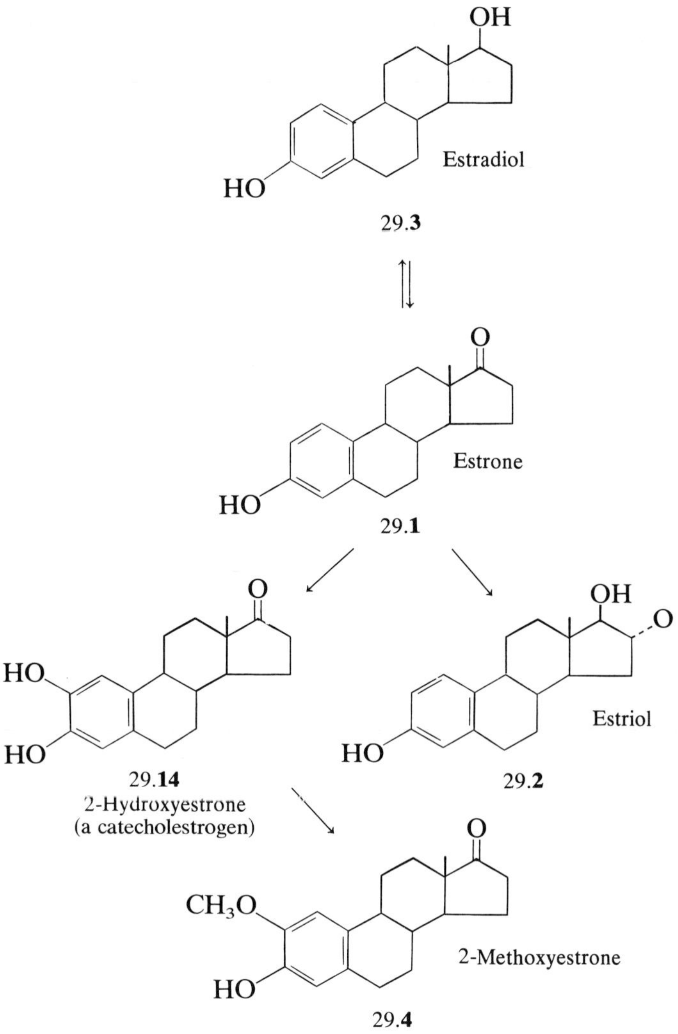

OH
HO
Estradiol
29.**3**

O
HO
Estrone
29.**1**

O
HO
HO
29.**14**
2-Hydroxyestrone
(a catecholestrogen)

OH
O
HO
Estriol
29.**2**

O
CH_3O
HO
2-Methoxyestrone
29.**4**

Fig. 29.2 Metabolic pathway of estradiol.

partition chromatography, isotopic techniques, and gas-liquid chromatography). It must be kept in mind, however, that the identification of some of the minor metabolites listed in Table 29.2 has been limited to chromatographic and partition properties, and in a few cases the lability of a certain precursor makes it difficult to discount the possibility that the new metabolite is an artifact.

The relative roles of the major pathways in the intermediary metabolisms of estrogens are illustrated in Fig. 29.3, which represents a collection of data on the relative amounts of known estrogens isolated from the urine of a number of patients treated with labeled 17β-estradiol (15). Also, from experiments similar to the ones just described, it has been possible to show that only about 50% of the administered 17β-estradiol is excreted in the urine within the first 24 hr. The remaining half of the administered estrogen appears in the bile during the first 24 hr. Because the bile normally empties into the gut, most of the biliary estrogen is reabsorbed from there

Table 29.2 Estrogens Isolated from Human Pregnancy Urine

Estrogen	Date of Isolation	Reference
Estrone	1929	6, 7
Estriol	1930	8, 9
17β-Estradiol	1940	10
16-Oxoestrone	1953	40
16β-Hydroxy-17β-estradiol	1955	41
18-Hydroxyestrone	1957	14a
2-Methoxyestrone	1957	11
16α-Hydroxyestrone	1957	42
16β-Hydroxyestrone	1958	43
16-Oxo-17β-estradiol	1958	43b, c
2-Methoxy-17β-estradiol	1959	44
16,17-Epiestriol	1959, 1960	45
17-Epiestriol	1960	46
2-Hydroxyestrone	1962	47, 88
2-Methoxyestriol 6α-Hydroxyestrone 6β-Hydroxyestrone 11β-Hydroxyestrone Δ^{16}-Estratrienol	1964	48
15α-Hydroxyestriol	1967	13

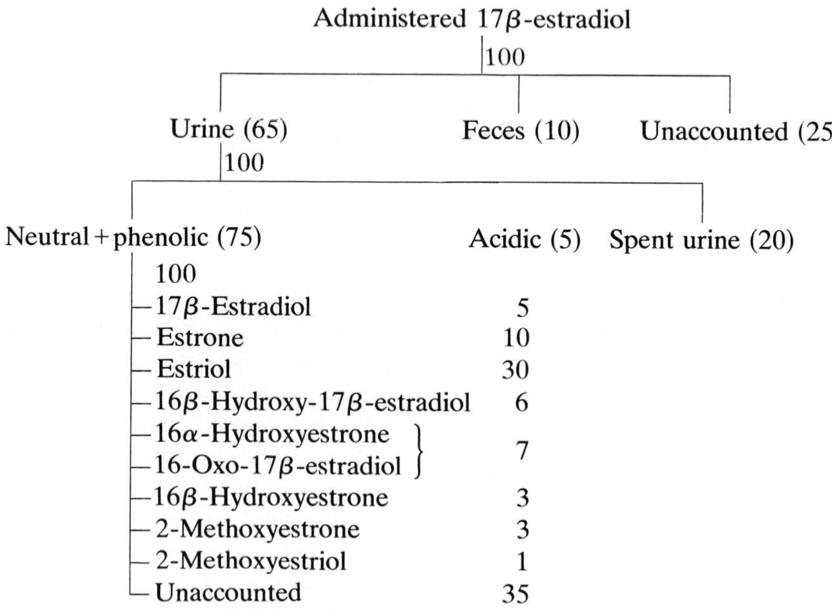

Fig. 29.3 The excretion of estrogen metabolites in the urine. All values shown are approximate percentages; they vary considerably from subject to subject. Data from Gallagher and co-workers (15).

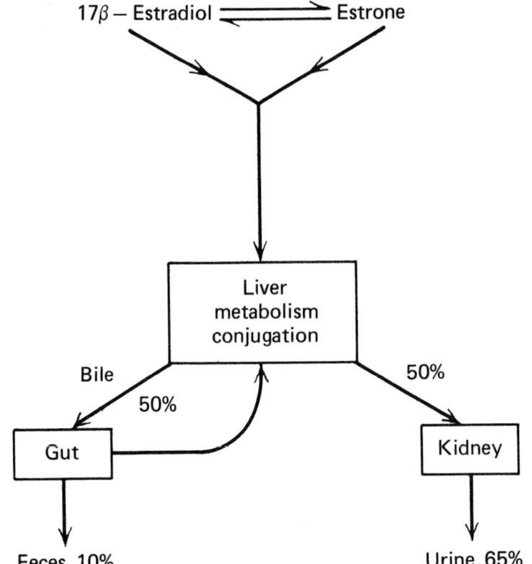

Fig. 29.4 The metabolism and excretion of 17-β estradiol and estrone.

and returned to the liver (see Fig. 29.4). This recirculation of the estrogen accounts for the relatively slow excretion of metabolites in the urine, in contrast to products derived from a hormone such as hydrocortisone. Eventually, after about 4–6 days, 50–80% of the administered estrogen is accounted for in the urine and about 1–18% is found in the feces. In these experiments approximately 30% of the radioactivity of the administered estrogen cannot be accounted for in the excretory products, and only about 40% of the radioactivity of the administered estrogen is contained in the metabolites that can be separated and analyzed from the excretory products.

To date, the determination of the relative amounts of estrogen metabolites in the urine not only has helped us to understand the nature of estrogen metabolism but also has proved useful for detecting a number of abnormal states related to hormone imbalance—for example, threatened abortion, cystic glandular hyperplasia, and various cancers and tumors (49).

2.2.4 CONJUGATION, TRANSPORT, AND EXCRETION. Estrogens act as regulators of various physiological processes in the body. In keeping with the dynamics of nature, any excess of these hormones, as well as their metabolites, must be eliminated from the body. Our present knowledge indicates that this prerequisite is met by either conjugation or degradation, or both. At times these two processes have been referred to collectively as "inactivation"; however this term is not appropriate when referring to the conjugation of estrogens, the most important process in the metabolism of these steroids. For example, Robson and Adler (50) found that estriol glucuronide was effective when administered intravaginally. Also, sodium estrone sulfate was twice as effective as the parent compound, estrone, when given orally to rats (51), and was effective in man as well (e.g., Ref. 52).

In reference to estrogens, the term "conjugation" is generally applied to a process whereby the estrogen becomes chemically bound to an acid by a natural process. This action renders the estrogen water soluble and facilitates its transport. The estrogens conjugate mainly with glucuronic acid or sulfuric acid. In the organs in which they originate, the greater portion of the estrogens are unconjugated, whereas in other parts of the body the estrogens appear to be predominantly in the conjugated form. On the other hand, from their work with doubly labelled dehydroepiandrosterone-7α-^{3}H sulfate-^{35}S, Oertel and co-workers (53, 54) have suggested that at least part of the estrogen sulfates may be biosynthesized directly from dehydroepiandrosterone sulfate.

The liver is considered to be the main site of estrogen conjugation. The kidney and intestine of rabbits (55), the bovine adrenal (56), and the human fetus (57, 58) are all capable of effecting conjugation. In humans, conjugation of estrogens with glucuronic acid occurs to a far greater extent than with sulfuric acid. Sodium estriol glucuronide (59), estrone sulfate (60, 61), estradiol sulfate (60, 61), estriol sulfate (61,

62), and estrone glucuronide (63) have been identified. Many investigators believe that the three classic estrogens occur as conjugates of both glucuronic and sulfuric acid. In addition, the estriol may be excreted in part as a mixed conjugate [i.e., estriol 3-sulfate 16(17?)-glucuronide] (64). Sodium estriol glucuronide (29.**15**) and sodium estrone sulfate (29.**16**) are examples of conjugates that have been isolated

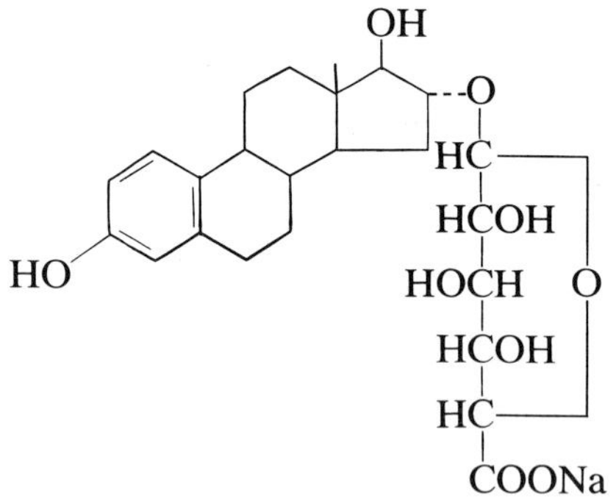

29.**15**

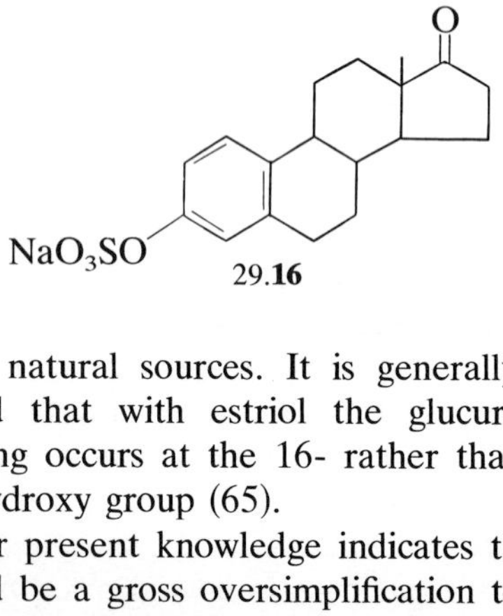

29.**16**

from natural sources. It is generally believed that with estriol the glucuronide binding occurs at the 16- rather than the 17-hydroxy group (65).

Our present knowledge indicates that it would be a gross oversimplification to describe the conjugation process of estrogens only as a means by which these hormones are solubilized for excretion by the kidney. Yet to be determined is the effect of the various conjugated forms on the distribution, action, and degradation of estrogens in the body.

2.2.5 MECHANISM OF ACTION. According to current concepts of the mechanism of action of steroid hormones (66–79), the interaction of the hormone with a protein receptor present in the cytoplasm of the "target" cell and the translocation of the complex formed into the nucleus are fundamental steps in eliciting a hormonal response, whatever the class of steroid hormone (estrogen, progestagen, androgen, gluco- and mineralocorticoids).

It is known that the gonadal sex steroids, 17β-estradiol, progesterone, and testosterone, regulate the expression of genes, control the synthesis of particular proteins, and are of basic importance in the metabolism of the cell and in growth and development.

Each of the steroid hormones affects only a few target tissues because only the cells of these tissues contain the appropriate receptor proteins. The estrogens form a complex with specific receptors in the uterus, vagina, breast, pituitary, and hypothalamus; progesterone interacts with its receptor proteins in the uterus, oviduct, ovary, pituitary, and hypothalamus, and testosterone (or its metabolite, 5α-dihydrotestosterone) interacts with androgen receptors in the seminal vesicles, prostate, testis, pituitary, and hypothalamus.

The hormones are recognized by their receptors on the basis of structure. The steroid hormones are small molecules with molecular weights of about 300, and they can diffuse into and out of most cells. However they selectively affect some cells, despite the very low concentrations in the blood (e.g., 10^{-9} mol/liter). The receptor molecule has a high affinity for its particular hormone but low affinity for other steroids with different biological activity. There are about 10,000 steroid receptor molecules per target cell. The receptor protein for 17β-estradiol has a molecular weight of about 200,000.

In nontarget cells, the hormone diffuses freely into the cell and out of it, and the concentration remains low. In a target cell, the hormone (e.g., progesterone) is sequestered by a receptor molecule. The receptor

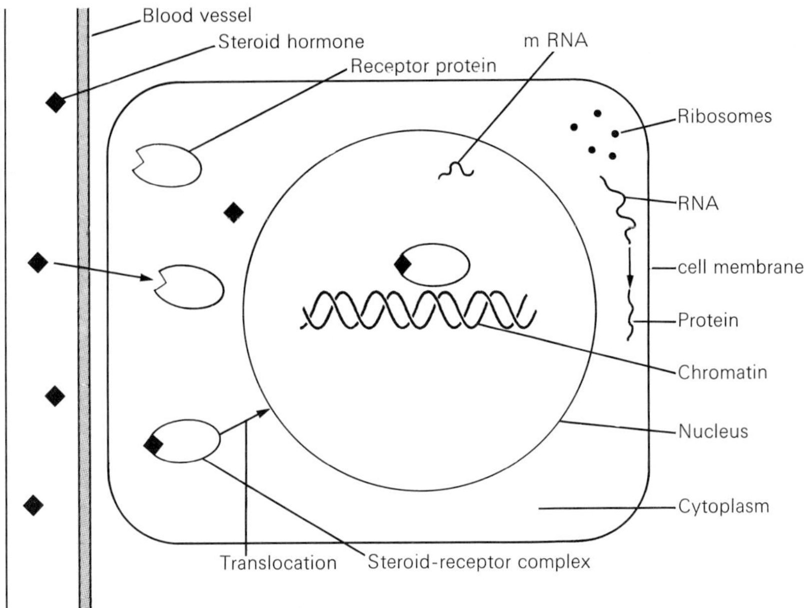

Fig. 29.5 A model of steroid hormone interactions on a target cell.

protein binds progesterone (72), forming a complex that enters the nucleus and becomes attached to the chromatin genetic material. Chromatin consists of DNA and two kinds of protein (histones and nonhistones). The progesterone-receptor complex stimulates the transcription of particular genes so that RNA encoding the information in those genes is synthesized (Fig. 29.5). On the organelles called ribosomes, the RNA is translated into proteins.

The magnitude of a cell's response appears to be related to the intracellular concentration of receptor proteins. Moreover, the concentration of receptors in a given tissue is not fixed; it can be altered by aging, by changes in the physiological state of development, and even by the presence of other hormones. It is known that estrogens stimulate the production of progesterone receptors and tissues treated with estrogens are more responsive to progesterone. Conversely, progesterone decreases the level of estrogen receptors and makes the tissue less responsive to estrogens.

It is possible to synthesize biologically inactive analogs of the natural steroid hormones that block the receptor binding sites and thereby suppress the hormonal response. Such "antihormones" have potential therapeutic value in the treatment of steroid-responsive benign and malignant growths.

The testing of these agents is accomplished by incubating them *in vitro* with a particular receptor protein (80, 82). The estrogen R-2828 (11β-methoxy-17-ethynyl-1,3,5(10)-estratriene-3,17β-diol) is much more uterotrophic than 17β-estradiol. Its 11α-isomer (Ru-16117) exhibits high antiestrogenic activity (80, 82) and is a potent inhibitor of chemically (DMBA)-induced rat mammary tumors (61). This antiestrogenic activity was attributed to the fast dissociation of this steroid-receptor complex (80). R-5020 (17,21-Dimethyl-19-nor-4,9-pregnadiene-3,20-dione, 29.**40**) is a potent synthetic progestagen (80, 81) that has great affinity for the progesterone receptor and is clinically effective as a progestagen. R-2323 (13-Ethyl-17-hydroxy-18,19-dinor-17α-4,9,11-pregnatrien-20-yn-3-0ne) interferes with the progesterone receptor and with gestation (82).

A significant proportion of breast cancers grow in response to estrogens circulating in the bloodstream and can be treated by the surgical removal of the estrogen-secreting organs. It has been shown that only human breast cancers that are rich with estrogen receptors are likely to respond to such ablative surgery (83, 84).

Reversible interference with specific receptor systems in target cells might provide a practical means of rendering reproductive tissues temporarily insensitive to the action of hormones normally responsible for their function, thus preventing at one of many possible stages the course of events leading to pregnancy. The specificity of receptor systems offers the possibility of controlling a limited group of tissues with few side effects on nontarget organs and without interfering with normal production and levels of hormones throughout the body. There are several possibilities in which receptor function might be modified, viz., influencing the synthesis or content of receptor in the target cell; inhibiting or modifying the binding of the hormone to receptor; interfering in some way with the subsequent result of hormone–hormone-receptor interaction in the nucleus, and limiting receptor function through immunologic means (86).

2.2.6 PHYSIOLOGICAL ACTION. The specific physiological effects of estrogens were first detailed by Pincus (89) and later by Diczfalusy and Lauritzen (32), as well as in several textbooks (90, 91). The more important effects on target organs are summarized in Table 29.3.

Table 29.3 Biological Effects of Estrogens on Various Target Organs

Organ	Effect
Ovary	Stimulate follicular growth; small doses cause weight increase of the ovary whereas large doses cause atrophy
Uterus	Endometrial growth
Vagina	Cornification of epithelial cells, accompanied by thickening and stratification of epithelium
Cervix	Increased amount of cervical mucus with a lowered viscosity, thus favoring sperm penetration and motility
Pituitary	Small doses promote secretion of pituitary gonadotropins (supportive effect): larger doses cause inhibition as well as general atrophy of this gland

2.2.7 ASSAYS

2.2.7.1 Chemical Methods. Comprehensive treatment of this subject has appeared in several reviews (15, 92, 93). Various methods are available for the estimation of estrogen levels in urine and blood. Frequently used techniques are colorimetric, fluorometric, and gas chromatographic methods. Isotopic (94) methods have also been used. The simpler techniques up to now have been colorimetric methods, which are based on a reaction originally described by Kober in 1931 (95). Gas-liquid chromatography is valuable for the separation and quantitation of pure estrogens (96–98). When used for the estimation of estrogens in body fluids, however, it is limited by the requirement for a high degree of purity of the final extract. This limitation is most critical when the amount of estrogen is relatively small, as in the case of blood or the urine from nonpregnant subjects. High pressure liquid chromatography (HPLC) and gas chromatography coupled with mass spectrometry are newer and promising methods of analysis of steroids in biological fluids (99, 100).

2.2.7.2 Bioassays. The estimation of estrogens by biological methods has been reviewed (92, 101). Only the two most extensively used assays, the vaginal cornification assay and the uterine weight assay, are discussed here. Less frequently used assays are based on the chick oviduct weight (102), vaginal mitosis and epithelial thickening (103), vaginal metabolic activity (104), and vaginal opening (105).

The vaginal cornification assay, or Allen–Doisy test, depends on the appearance of nucleated or cornified epithelial cells, but no leucocytes, in the vaginal smears from castrated female mice or rats (4). Numerous modifications of this test have occurred since its introduction in 1923 (106, 107). Because of the many variations (i.e., route and spacing of administration, different species of animals, different techniques for scoring smears) used in this test, it is imperative that a pure standard be assayed simultaneously, to obtain meaningful results. A reasonable degree of accuracy can be obtained for this test by employing two doses for both a standard and the test material, a 2+2 design (107). Each of the four groups should consist of 20 animals. Multiple doses must be given, and vaginal smears must be taken at intervals. Simpler modifications of this design are not reproducible.

The uterotropic assay uses the weight increase of the uterus of spayed or immature intact rats or mice as an end point. This test was developed by Dorfman and collaborators (108). Usually the animals are injected once or twice a day for 3 days; 24 hr after the last dose, the uteri are excised and weighed. Linear dose-response curves generally are obtained for the individual estrogens; however the curves for the various estrogens differ markedly from one another. Furthermore, giving progressively higher doses of estrogens eventually leads to a decrease in the uterine weight.

Table 29.4 Comparative Activity of Various Estrogens as Determined by the Allen–Doisy Test in Spayed Albino Rats (200–300 g)[a]

Compound	ED_{50} μg	
	p.o.	s.c.
Estrone	150	1.6
17β-Estradiol	60	0.1
Estriol	76	2.4
17α-Ethynylestradiol	33	0.12
17α-Ethynylestradiol 3-methyl ether	45	0.5

[a] Data from Ref. 81d.

Table 29.5 Relative Potency of Various Estrogens as Determined by Measurement of Their Uterotropic Activity in Swiss Albino Mice[a]

Compound	Relative Potency, %	
	p.o.	s.c.
Estrone	100	100
17β-Estradiol	300	280
17β-Estradiol benzoate		280
17α-Ethynylestradiol	2340	
17α-Ethynylestradiol 3-methyl ether	1120	25

[a] Data from Ref. 81e.

Comparative biological data for some of the estrogens of major importance are given in Tables 29.4 and 29.5.

2.2.7.3 Radioimmunoassays, Enzyme Immunoassays, and Metalloimmunoassays. Because of its high sensitivity and simplicity, radioimmunoassay has become quite popular in the determination of steroids, particularly in clinical laboratories (109–111). Chromatographic separations often are not needed because of the high specificity of most antisera. However there are problems of cross-reactivity between closely related steroids, as well as a general problem of handling and disposing of radioactive substances. To avoid the latter, enzyme immunoassays and metalloimmunoassays are currently under development (112, 113).

2.3 Chemistry

Estrogenic activity is one of the most common and nonspecific biological activities

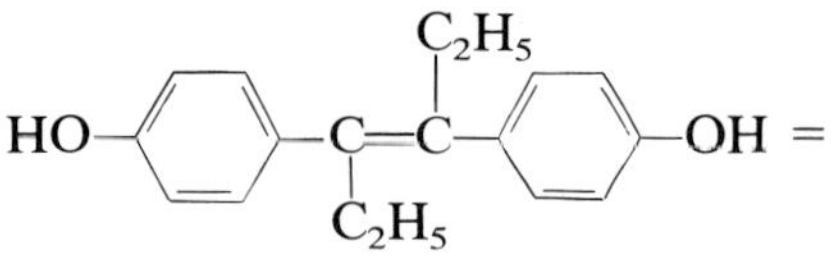

29.**17**

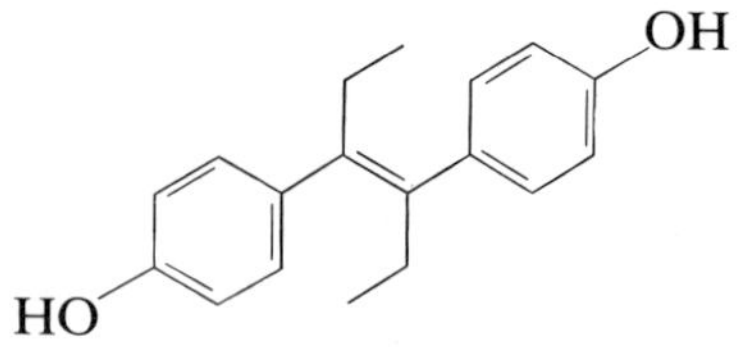

29.**17a**

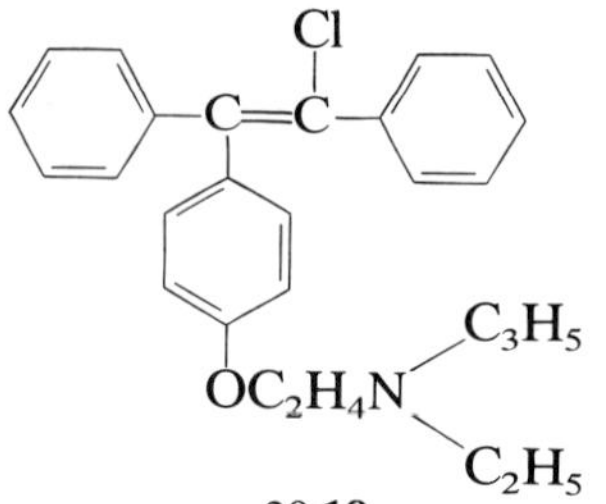

29.**18**

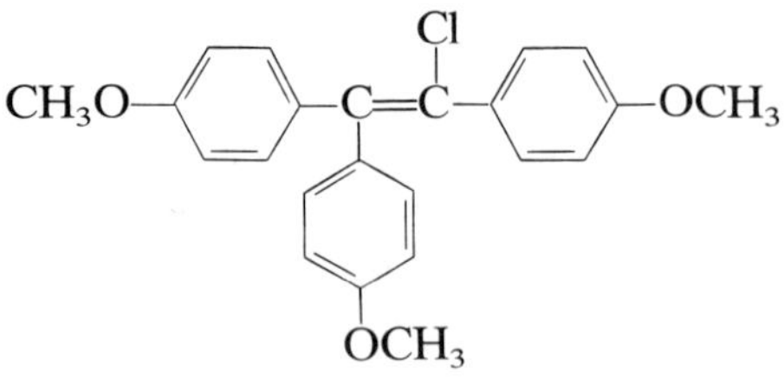

29.**19**

exhibited by chemical compounds. Hogg and Korman (106) listed many hundreds of compounds, in addition to the natural estrogens, that exhibit this activity, and classified them into 33 groups according to their main structural features—for example, diphenylethane, triphenylethane, naphthalene, and phenanthrene. Among the nonsteroidal estrogens, synthetic compounds of the diethylstilbestrol class have found wide application in medicine.

Diethylstilbestrol (DES, 29.**17**) was the first totally synthetic estrogen to be used therapeutically. It was synthesized by Dodds and colleagues in 1938 (121) and has become an important estrogen because of its high potency and low cost. On the other hand, a high incidence of side effects has been reported for this drug (see, e.g., Ref. 122).

Several detailed accounts of the discovery and ensuing investigations of related estrogens are available (123). It is interesting that Dodds and colleagues originally assigned the trans configuration to the most active isomer because it resembled more closely the spatial configuration of the natural estrogens (note formula 29.**17a**); subsequently this assignment proved to be correct.

In a related development, considerable interest has been focused on a number of compounds structurally similar to diethylstilbestrol. This group includes clomiphene (29.**18**) and chlorotrianisene (TACE, 29.**19**) (124). These compounds, though usually possessing weak estrogenic activity, are estrogen antagonists and interfere with implantation and development of ova in animals (125). Clomiphene, the most interesting compound in this group is therapeutically useful in humans for the induction of ovulation and the treatment of infertility (126).

In spite of the large number of synthetic compounds that possess estrogenic activity, however, only a few are used to any extent in medicine, probably because of the efficacy of the natural estrogens such as 17β-estradiol and conjugated equine estrogens. This situation is in contrast to the progestational field, in which potent synthetic progestins have almost entirely replaced the natural hormone, progesterone, as a drug.

17β-Estradiol, the most potent of the three classic estrogens when administered subcutaneously or intramuscularly, is relatively ineffective by the oral route at least in a nonmicronized formulation. Consequently it was most significant when, in 1938, Inhoffen et al. (21) reported the synthesis of ethynylestradiol, which soon

Table 29.6 Commercially Available Steroid Estrogens

Chemical Name	Available Preparations
17β-Estradiol	Pellets for implantation; suspension for injection; suppositories (vaginal); tablets for oral administration; tablets (buccal)
17β-Estradiol benzoate	Solution for injection
17β-Estradiol cyclopentylpropionate	Solution for injection
17β-Estradiol dipropionate	Solution for injection
17β-Estradiol valerate	Solution for intramuscular injection
Ethinylestradiol	Elixir for oral use; tablets for oral use
Estriol	Cream (topical and vaginal); lotion (topical); solution for injection; tablets for oral use
Estrogenic substances, conjugated	Cream for topical and vaginal application; lotion for topical application; powder for injection; solution for oral use; tablets for oral use
Estrone	Suspension for injection; pellets; suppositories (vaginal); tablets for oral use
Piperazine estrone sulfate	Elixir for oral use; tablets for oral use

was demonstrated to be a potent orally active estrogen in man (22). Later the 3-methyl ether of ethynylestradiol, although slightly less potent in humans, was shown to be equally effective.

In 1961 Ercoli and Gardi (127) found that the 3-cyclopentyl ether of 17α-ethynylestradiol was the most potent oral estrogen described thus far (45 times more potent than estrone by this route in mice).

Although only a few orally active estrogens have been developed by chemical modification of the natural hormones, this approach has produced a large number of long-acting estrogens for parenteral use, mainly through esterification of the oxygen functions. Table 29.6 lists the more commonly used estrogen drugs.

2.4 Therapeutic Applications

The principal use of estrogens in medicine is to control menopausal symptoms, such as hot flushes, headaches, nervousness, and depression. Other estrogen deficiency states for which estrogen therapy is recommended are menstrual irregularities such as dysmenorrhea and amenorrhea, the failure of ovarian development, vaginitis, and osteoporosis. Estrogens have also been applied beneficially in the treatment of prostatic carcinoma in men and breast cancer in postmenopausal women. The use of estrogens for the suppression of ovulation and the control of fertility is discussed in Chapter 30.

2.5 Effects of Estrogens on the Central Nervous System

Since the earliest therapeutic applications of estrogens, a definite, if ill-defined, effect on the central nervous system was noted. Only recently this "feeling of well-being" and in certain cases an antidepressant effect were studied and quantified (128). Improvements of estrogen-treated patients were noted in cases of anxiety, sleep disturbances, fatigue, restlessness, irritability, depression, and concentration and memory disturbances when compared to placebo treatment.

A similar double-blind controlled study (129) of the effect of estrone (piperazine) sulfate revealed only placebo effects on depression, anxiety, and hot flushes, but an objective decrease in the brokenness of sleep in perimenopausal women complaining of insomnia.

The existence of brain receptors sensitive to certain steroids and estrogens (similar to the opioid brain receptors) has been described (130).

2.6 Estrogens and Cancer

One of the physiologic mechanisms of action of estrogens is the regulation of gene expression, the synthesis of particular proteins, and the resulting growth and development of target tissues. Diethylstilbestrol (DES), taken during pregnancy, has been linked to neoplasias in the offspring. A number of reports have associated the clinical use of estrogens as replacement therapy in menopausal women with a higher incidence of endocrine (mainly uterine) cancers as determined by epidemiological criteria (131, 132).

Other studies have not shown a mutagenic effect of the naturally occurring estrogens by established criteria *in vitro*, nor any induction of chromosomal aberrations with human cell lines.

Additional investigations will help clarify this important issue.

3 PROGESTATIONAL AGENTS

Progesterone (29.**20**) is the least polar of all steroids of animal origin. An ovarian tissue,

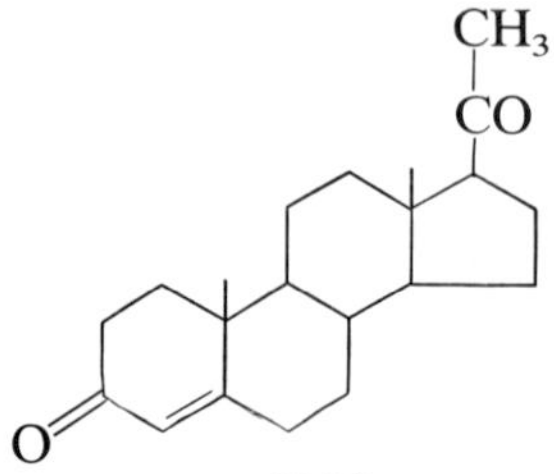

29.**20**

the corpus luteum, produces progesterone cyclically, as suggested by Fraenkel in 1903 and demonstrated by Corner and Allen 25 years later (133). Some of the physiological activities of this hormone are intimately connected with those of the estrogens and are believed to (1) modify uterine tissue, enabling transport, implantation, and development of the fertilized ovum, (2) suppress ovulation in a pregnant animal, (3) affect uterine motility, and (4) contribute to the development of mammary gland tissue. Progesterone is metabolized rapidly in the body and is excreted in the bile and urine, mainly as conjugates of pregnanediol (29.**21**). Loss of the pregnane side chain is

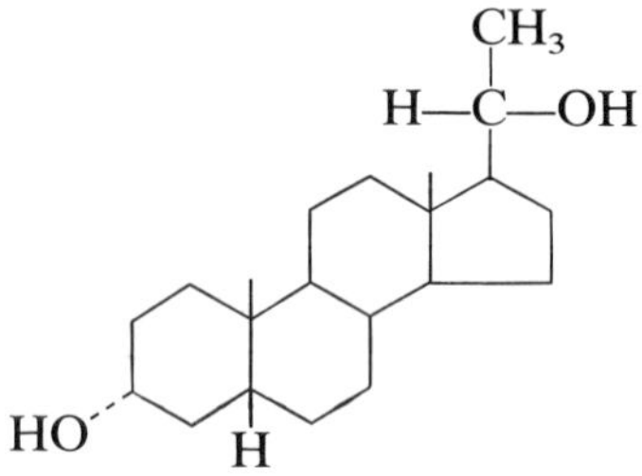

29.**21**

known to occur extensively. Metabolic hydroxylations of progesterone occur mainly in the liver; they diminish or destroy its progestational properties and account for its weak oral activity. Intranasal activity of progesterone in primates has been reported (134).

3.1 Oral Progestins

3.1.1 ANDROSTANE DERIVATIVES. Some androstane derivatives have progestational activity, and the early discovery of the oral activity of 17-alkylated testosterone led to the first oral progestational substance, ethisterone (29.**22**). Thus historically the way was paved for the development of progestational compounds not structurally related to progesterone. The modest potency of ethisterone was enhanced by

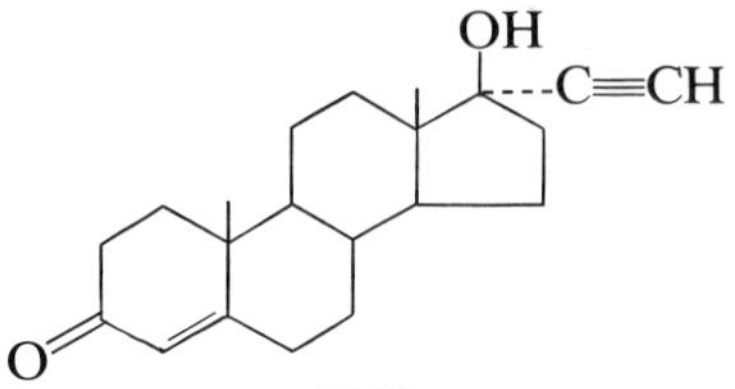

29.**22**

adding or eliminating appropriate methyl groups, as in dimethisterone (29.**23**), norethindrone (29.**24**), and norgestrel (29.**25**). Other manipulations include deconjugation of the double bond (norethynodrel, 29.**26**), esterification or etherification of the oxygen function in position 3 (ethynodiol diacetate, 29.**27**; quingestanol acetate, 29.**28**; norgestinate, 29.**29**), and even outright elimination of it (lynestrenol, 29.**30**; allylestrenol, 29.**31**; and tigestol, 29.**32**).

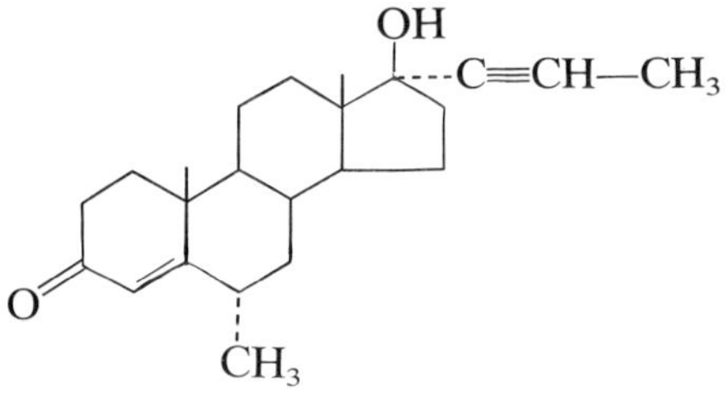

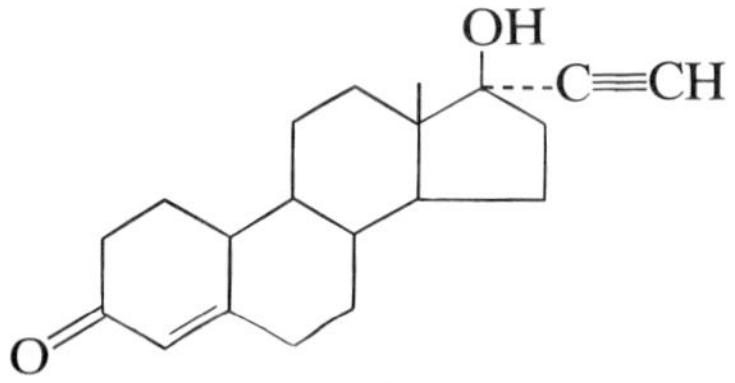

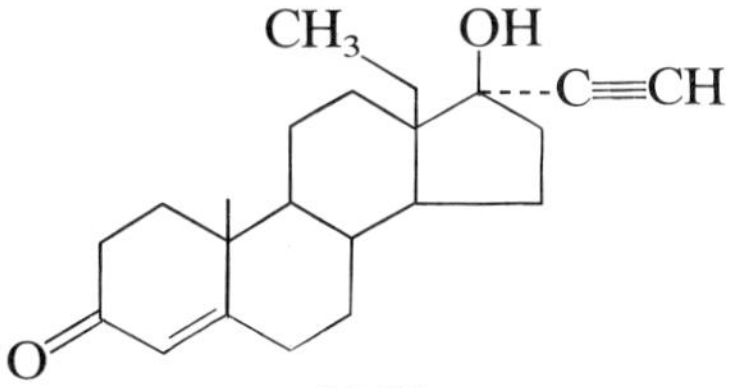

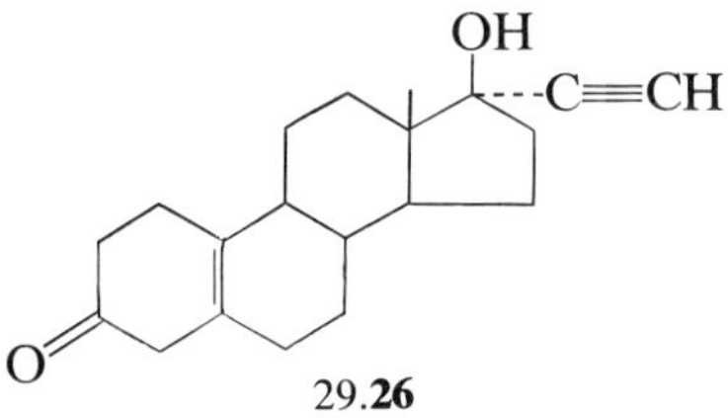

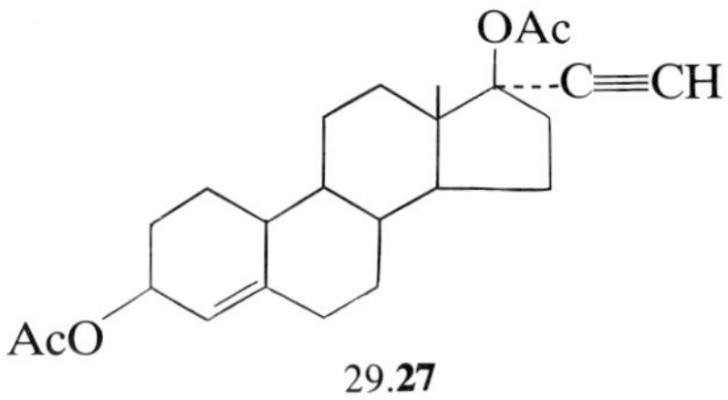

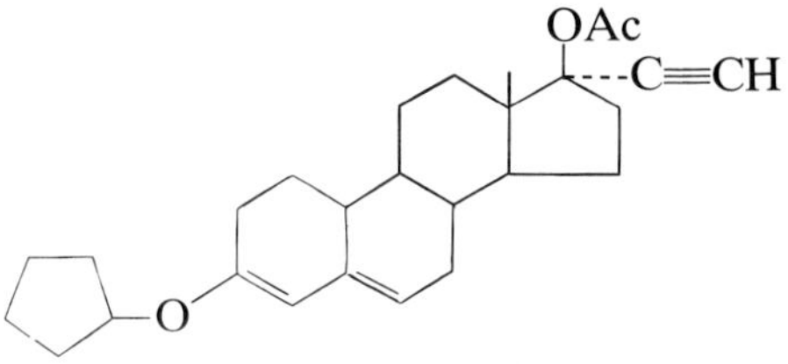

29.**23**

29.**24**

29.**25**

29.**26**

29.**27**

29.**28**

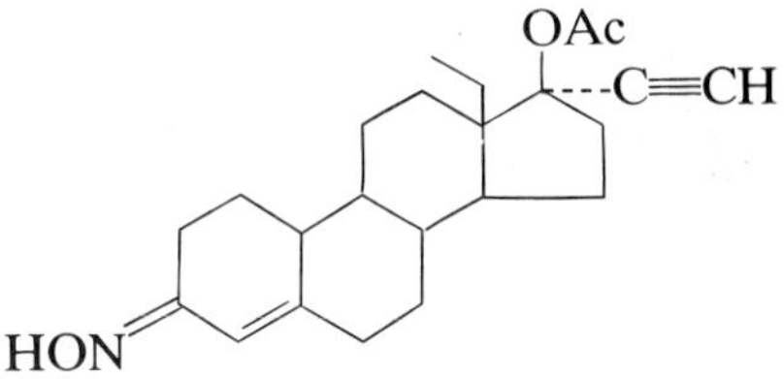

29.**29**

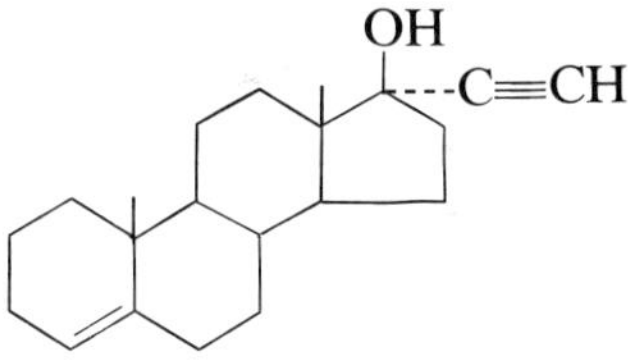

29.**30**

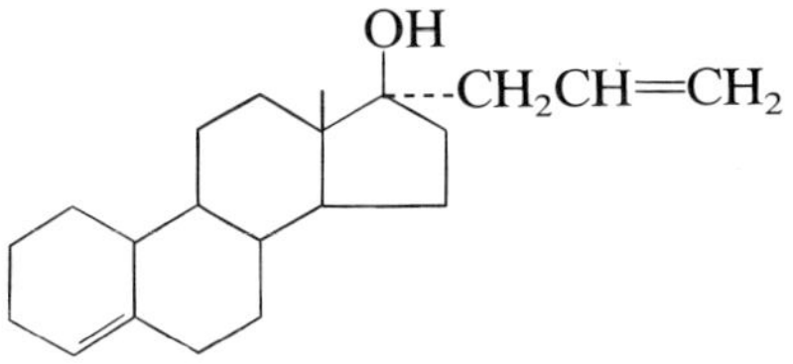

29.**31**

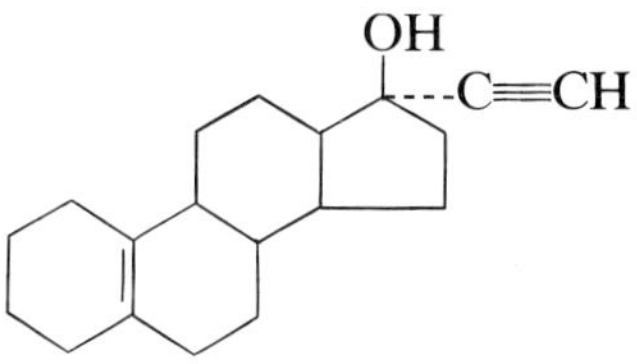

29.**32**

3.1.2 PREGNANE DERIVATIVES. The metabolic cleavage of the progesterone side chain can be impeded by appropriate 17α-substituents such as ester or alkyl groups. 17α-Acetoxyprogesterone (29.**33**) is mod-

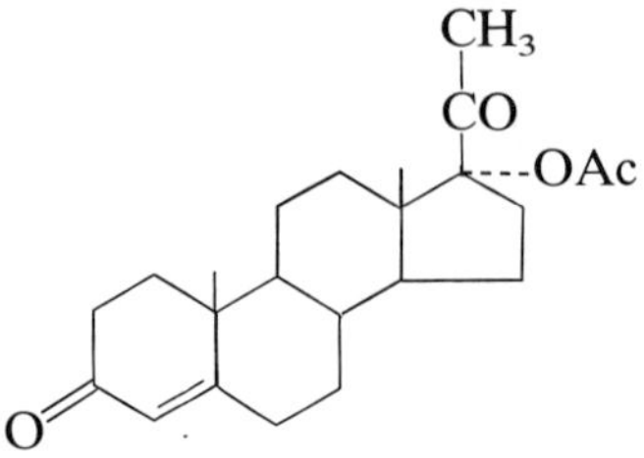

29.**33**

estly active by the oral route, and additional substituents are needed for greater oral potency. The 6α-methyl analog 29.**34**)

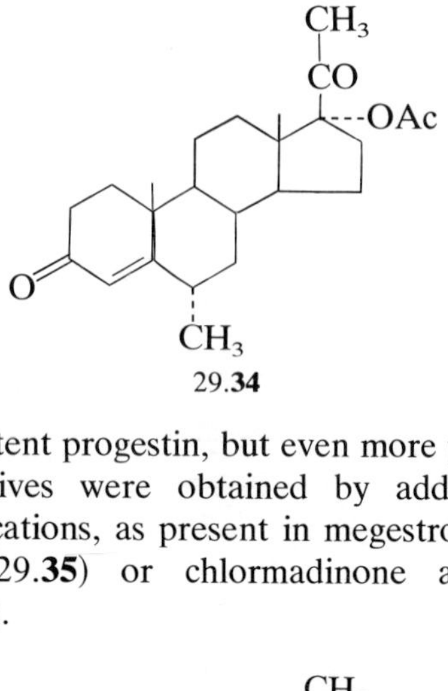

29.**34**

is a potent progestin, but even more potent derivatives were obtained by additional modifications, as present in megestrol acetate (29.**35**) or chlormadinone acetate (29.**36**).

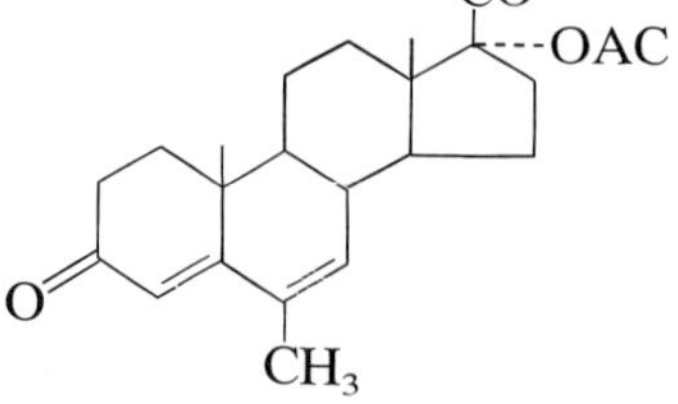

29.**35**

Medrogestone (29.**37**) is an example of a 17α-alkylated derivative. Dydrogesterone (9β, 10α-pregna-4,6-diene-3,20-dione

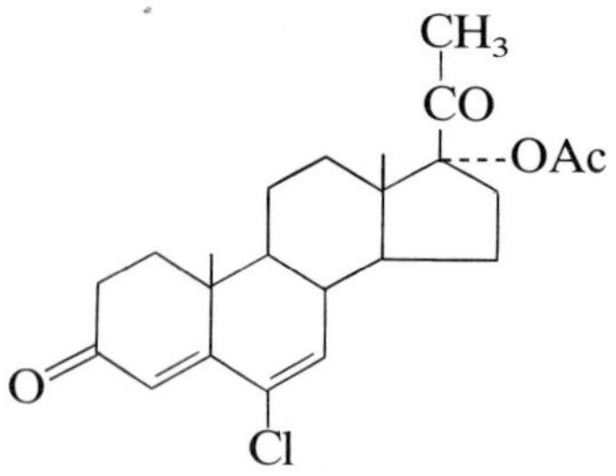

29.**36**

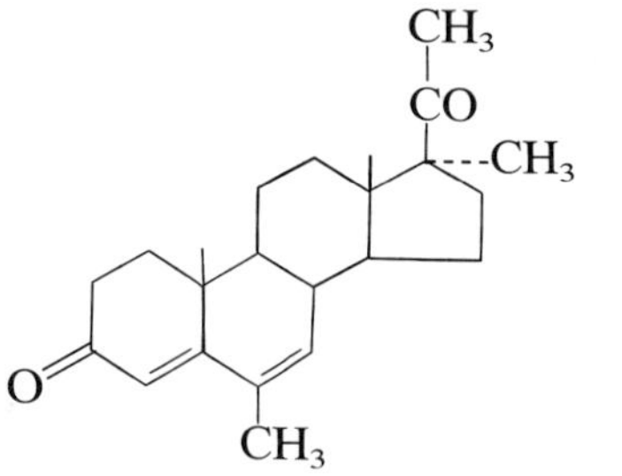

29.**37**

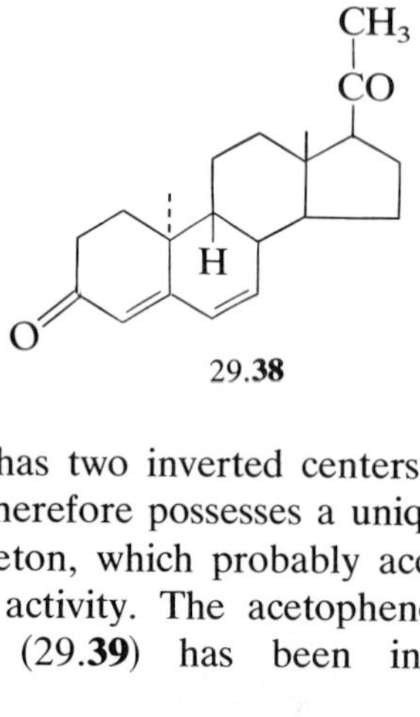

29.**38**

(29.**38**) has two inverted centers of asymmetry, therefore possesses a unique steroidal skeleton, which probably accounts for its oral activity. The acetophenonide derivative (29.**39**) has been investigated

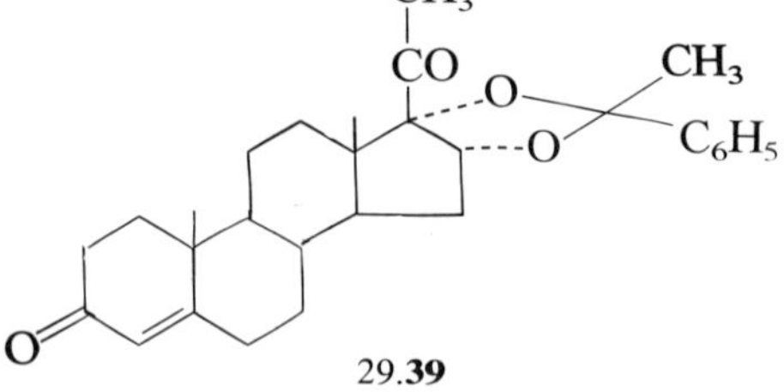

29.**39**

mainly for its long-acting properties when administered parenterally.

Promegestone (R-5020, 29.**40**) is a recent and interesting example with a hybrid

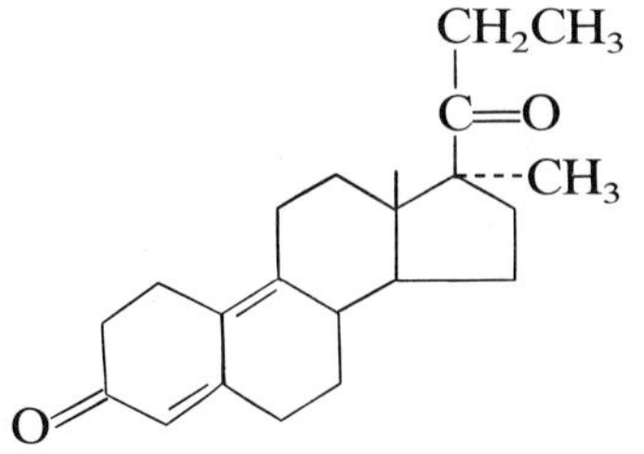

29.40

structure (a substituted pregnane side chain on an estradiene nucleus.

3.1.3. ASSAYS OF PROGESTINS. A battery of tests is available to determine the potency and biological profile of a progestational compound in animals. Some of the most frequently used are mentioned in Sections 3.1.3.1–3.1.3.8.

3.1.3.1 Endometrial Proliferation Test [*Clauberg–McPhail* (135)]. Immature female rabbits are primed with estrone for 6 days. From the seventh to the twelfth day of the experiment the test compound is given daily, either subcutaneously or orally. Then the animals are killed and sections are removed from the proximal, middle, and distal portions of each uterine horn. The stained sections are evaluated according to McPhail's grading system from +1 to +4 (1).

3.1.3.2 Local Test (136). This is similar to the Claubert–McPhail test, but the compound is injected directly into one uterine horn of the estrogen-primed rabbit.

3.1.3.3 Deciduoma Test (137, 138). This test measures the increase in weight of a uterine horn of ovariectomized rats primed with estrone and treated with the test compound. During treatment one uterine horn is traumatized chemically with histamine or mechanically with a burred needle. Under the influence of progestins, the rat uterus responds with rapid growth of stromal components to form a "deciduoma", which histologically resembles the maternal portion of the placenta.

3.1.3.4 Carbonic Anhydrase Test (139). This test measures *in vitro* the carbonic anhydrase content of an estrogen-primed rabbit uterus. A standard dose-response relation between progesterone and carbonic anhydrase concentration is obtained and measured.

3.1.3.5 Maintenance of Pregnancy Test in Rats (140). The test compound is given in a single dose on the ninth day or in multiple doses from the ninth to the twentieth day of pregnancy to ovariectomized rats. On the twenty-first day of pregnancy the number of implantations and the number of living and dead fetuses are recorded.

3.1.3.6 Antiovulatory Test (141). Ovulation is induced in rabbits by mating. The test compound is given, prior to mating, to adult female rabbits whose ovaries are subsequently inspected by laparotomy for ruptured points (ovulation). Effective doses inhibit such ovulation.

3.1.3.7 Gonadotropin-Inhibiting Activity (142). The test is performed on parabiotic rats (pairs of females attached surgically by the lateral skin and abdominal muscles), one of the partners being spayed, then given the test compound. The decrease in ovarian weight, measured at autopsy in the intact partner, reflects the inhibiting properties of the progestin. Serum LH and FSH levels can also be measured by radioimmunoassays.

3.1.3.8 Clinical Efficacy. Various parameters can be measured to determine the potency and efficacy of synthetic progestins in women. Endometrial biopsies, usually taken at the end of the menstrual cycle, provide an indication of endometrial proliferation. Progestational response can be detected by microscopic examination of vaginal smears. Plasma or urinary levels of gonadotropins might be affected, and urinary 17-ketosteroids are a measure of possible effect on the adrenals. Some synthetic progestins mimic progesterone in eliciting a characteristic thermogenic response. Delay of menses, pseudopregnancy, and withdrawal bleeding are also caused by synthetic progestins.

3.2 Therapeutic Applications

Progestational agents are used for the treatment of certain types of endocrine dysfunction such as amenorrhea, dysfunctional uterine bleedings (menorrhagia and methorrhagia), dysmenorrhea, and endometriosis. Other indications include therapy to avoid threatened abortion, endometrial carcinoma, resumption of menses in menopausal women and, to a lesser extent, as a test for pregnancy (143).

The major use of progestins is for contraception, as Chapter 30 discusses.

REFERENCES

1. R. Degheghi and A. J. Manson, in *Medicinal Chemistry*, 3rd Ed., A. Burger, Ed., Wiley-Interscience, New York, 1970, Ch. 35, pp. 900–922.
2. E. Knauer, *Arch. Gynäkol.*, **60,** 322 (1900).
3. C. R. Stockard and G. N. Papanicolaou, *Am. J. Anat.*, **22,** 225 (1917)
4. E. Allen and E. A. Doisy, *J. Am. Med. Assoc.*, **81,** 819 (1923).
5. S. Aschheim and B. Zondek, *Klin. Wochenschr.*, **6,** 1322 (1927).
6. E. A. Doisy, C. D. Veler, and S. A. Thayer, *Am. J. Physiol.*, **90,** 329 (1929).
7. A. Butenandt, *Naturwissenschaften*, **17,** 879 (1929).
8. G. F. Marrian, *J. Soc. Chem. Ind.* (London), **49,** 515 (1930); *Biochem. J.*, **24,** 435, 1021 (1930).
9. E. A. Doisy, S. A. Thayer, L. Levin, and J. M. Curtis, *Proc. Soc. Exp. Biol. Med.*, **28,** 288 (1930).
10. M. N. Huffman, D. W. MacCorquodale, S. A. Thayer, E. A. Doisy, G. V. Smith, and O. W. Smith, *J. Biol. Chem.*, **134,** 591 (1940).
11. (a) S. Kraychy and T. F. Gallagher, *J. Am. Chem. Soc.*, **79,** 754 (1957). (b) *J. Biol. Chem.*, **229,** 519 (1957). (c) J. Fishman, *J. Am. Chem. Soc.*, **80,** 1213 (1958). (d) K. H. Loke and G. F. Marrian, *Biochim. Biophys. Acta*, **27,** 213 (1958).
12. J. Fishman and T. F. Gallagher, *Arch. Biochem. Biophys.*, **77,** 511 (1958).
13. G. Zucconi, B. P. Lisboa, E. Simonitsch, L. Roth, A. A. Hagen, and E. Diczfalusy, *Acta Endocrinol.* (Copenhagen), **56,** 413 (1967).
14. (a) K. H. Loke, J. D. Watson, and G. F. Marrian, *Biochim. Biophys. Acta*, **26,** 230 (1957). (b) K. H. Loke, G. F. Marrian, W. S. Johnson, W. L. Meyer, and D. D. Cameron, *Biochim. Biophys. Acta*, **28,** 214 (1958).
15. J. B. Brown, *Advan. Clin. Chem.*, **3,** 157 (1960).
16. B. Zondek, *Klin. Wochenschr.*, **9,** 2285 (1930).
17. S. E. de Jongh, S. Kober, and E. Laqueur, *Biochem. Z.*, **240,** 247 (1931).
18. (a) A. Girard, G. Sandulesco, A. Fridenson, and J. J. Rutgers, *Compt. Rend.*, **194,** 909 (1932). (b) *Ibid.*, 981 (1932). (c) A. Girard, G. Sandulesco, A. Fridenson, C. Gaudefroy, and J. J. Rutgers, *ibid.*, **194,** 1020 (1932).
19. L. F. Fieser and M. Fieser, *Steroids*, Reinhold, New York, 1959, p. 463.
20. R. Gaudry and W. L. Glen, *Ind. Chem. Belg.*, Suppl. **2,** 435 (1959); *Chem. Abstr.*, **54,** 9030 (1960).
21. H. H. Inhoffen, W. Longemann, W. Hohlweg, and A. Serini, *Chem. Ber.*, **71,** 1024 (1938).
22. (a) C. Clauberg and Z. Ustum, *Zbl. Gynäkol.*, **62,** 1745 (1938). (b) V. J. Salmon, S. H. Geist, R. I. Walter, and N. Mintz, *J. Clin. Endocrinol. Metab.*, **1,** 556 (1941).
23. G. Pincus and P. A. Zahl, *J. Gen. Physiol.*, **20,** 879 (1937).
24. H. Breuer, *Vitam. Horm.*, **20,** 285 (1962).
25. E. Diczfalusy, *Fed. Proc.*, **23,** 791 (1964).
26. K. J. Ryan and O. W. Smith, *Rec. Progr. Hormone Res.*, **21,** 367 (1965).
27. J. Fishman, J. B. Brown, L. Hellman, B. Zumoff, and T. F. Gallagher, *J. Biol. Chem.*, **237,** 1489 (1962).
28. E. Gurpide, M. Angers, R. L. VandiWiele, and S. Lieberman, *J. Clin. Endocrinol. Metab.*, **22,** 935 (1962).
29. K. J. Ryan, *J. Biol. Chem.*, **234,** 268 (1959).
30. H. G. Magendantz and K. J. Ryan, *J. Clin. Endocrinol. Metab.*, **24,** 1155 (1964).
31. P. K. Suteri and P. C. MacDonald, *J. Clin. Endocrinol. Metab.*, **26,** 751 (1966).
32. E. Diczfalusy and C. Lauritzen, *Oestrogene beim Menschen*, Springer, Berlin, 1961.
33. C. T. Beer and T. F. Gallagher, *J. Biol. Chem.*, **214,** 335 (1955).

34. C. T. Beer and T. F. Gallagher, *J. Biol. Chem.*, **214,** 351 (1955).

35. A. A. Sandberg and W. R. Slaunwhite, *J. Clin. Invest.*, **36,** 1266 (1957).

36. B. T. Brown, J. Fishman, and T. F. Gallagher, *Nature* (London), **182,** 50 (1958).

37. C. J. Migeon, P. E. Wall, and J. Bertrand, *J. Clin. Invest.*, **38,** 619 (1959).

38. J. Fishman, H. L. Bradlow, and T. F. Gallagher, *J. Biol. Chem.*, **235,** 3104 (1960).

39. L. A. Rigg, B. Milanes, B. Villanueva, and S. S. C. Yen, *J. Clin. Endocrinol. Metab.*, **45,** 1261, (1977).

40. G. Serchi, *Chimica*, **8,** 9 (1953).

41. G. F. Marrian and W. S. Bauld, *Biochem. J.*, **59,** 136 (1955).

42. G. F. Marrian, E. J. D. Watson, and M. Panattoni, *Biochem. J.*, **65,** 12 (1957).

43. (a) B. T. Brown, J. Fishman, and T. F. Gallagher, *Nature* (London), **182,** 50 (1958). (b) D. S. Layne and G. F. Marrian, *ibid.*, p. 50. (c) D. S. Layne and G. F. Marrian, *Biochem. J.*, **70,** 244 (1958).

44. V. A. Frandsen, *Acta Endocrinol.* (Copenhagen), **31,** 603 (1959).

45. (a) H. Breuer and G. Pangels, *Biochim. Biophys. Acta*, **36,** 572 (1959). (b) *Z. Physiol. Chem.*, **322,** 177 (1960).

46. (a) H. Breuer, *Nature* (London), **185,** 613 (1960). (b) *Z. Physiol. Chem.*, **322,** 177 (1960).

47. V. Notchev and B. F. Stimmel, *Excerpta Medica International Congress Series*, No. 51, 175 (1962).

48. H. Breuer, in *Research on Steroids*, Vol. 1, C. Cassano, Ed., Pensiero Scientifico, Rome, 1964, p. 133.

49. J. B. Brown and G. D. Matthew, *Rec. Progr. Hormone Res.*, **18,** 337 (1962).

50. J. M. Robson and J. Adler, *Nature* (London), **146,** 60 (1940).

51. G. A. Grant and D. Beall, *Rec. Progr. Hormone Res.*, **5,** 307 (1950).

52. H. S. Kupperman, M. H. G. Blatt, H. Wiesbar, and W. Filler, *J. Clin. Endocrinol. Metab.*, **13,** 688 (1953).

53. G. W. Oertel, L. Treiber, and W. Rindt, *Experientia*, **23,** 97 (1967).

54. P. Knapstein, F. Wendlberger, and G. W. Oertel, *Experientia*, **23,** 97 (1967).

55. Y. Nose and F. Lipmann, *J. Biol. Chem.*, **233,** 1348 (1958).

56. A. Sneddon and G. F. Marrian, *Biochem. J.*, **86,** 385 (1963).

57. E. Diczfalusy, O. Cassmer, C. Alonso, and M. de Miquel, *Rec. Progr. Hormone Res.*, **17,** 147 (1961).

58. G. Mikhail, N. Wiqvist, and E. Diczfalusy, *Acta Endocrinol.* (Copenhagen), **42,** 519 (1963).

59. (a) S. L. Cohen and G. F. Marrian, *Biochem. J.*, **30,** 57 (1936). (b) S. L. Cohen and A. D. Odell, *ibid.*, **30,** 2250 (1936). (c) E. Menini and E. Diczfaluzy. *Endocrinology*, **67,** 500 (1960).

60. J. McKenna, E. Menini, and J. K. Norymberski, *Biochem. J.*, **79,** 11P. (1961).

61. J. C. Touchstone, J. W. Greene, Jr., R. C. McElroy, and T. Murawec, *Biochemistry*, **2,** 653 (1963).

62. E. Menini and E. Diczfalusy, *Endocrinology*, **68,** 492 (1961).

63. (a) I. B. Oneson and S. L. Cohen, *Endocrinology*, **51,** 173 (1952). (b) P. A. Katzman, R. F. Straw, H. J. Buchler, and E. A. Doisy, *Rec. Progr. Hormone Res.*, **9,** 45 (1954).

64. (a) R. F. Straw, P. A. Katzman, and E. A. Doisy, *Endocrinology*, **57,** 87 (1955). (b) P. Troen, B. Nilsson, N. Wiqvist, and E. Diczfalusy, *Acta Endocrinol.* (Copenhagen), **38,** 361 (1961). (c) J. C. Touchstone. J. W. Greene, Jr., R. C. McElroy, and T. Murawec, *Biochemistry*, **2,** 653 (1963). (d) R. Wilson, G. Ericksson, and E. Diczfalusy, *Acta Endocrinol.* (Copenhagen), **46,** 525 (1964). (e) E. Diczfalusy, M. Barr, and J. Lind, *ibid.*, **46,** 511 (1964). (f) M. Levitz, S. Shotsky, and G. H. Twombly, in *Estrogen Assays in Clinical Medicine*, C. A. Paulsen, Ed., University of Washington Press, Seattle, 1965, p. 155. (g) O. W. Smith and D. D. Hagerman, *J. Clin. Endocrinol. Metab.*, **25,** 732 (1965). (h) M. Levitz, *ibid.*, **26,** 773 (1966). (i) U. Goebelsmann, G. Eriksson, E. Diczfalusy, M. Levitz, and G. P. Condon, *Acta Endocrinol.* (Copenhagen), **53,** 391 (1966). (j) S. Emerman, G. H. Twombly, and M. Levitz, *J. Clin. Endocrinol. Metab.*, **27,** 539 (1967). (k) E. R. Smith and A. E. Kellie, *Biochem. J.*, **104,** 83 (1967).

65. M. Levitz, J. Katz, and G. H. Twombly, *Steroids*, **6,** 553 (1965).

66. E. V. Jensen, K. J. Catt, J. Gorski, and H. G. Williams–Ashman, in *Frontiers in Reproduction and Fertility Control*, R O. Greep and M. A. Koblinsky, Eds., MIT Press, Cambridge, Mass. 1977.

67. J. Gorski and F. Gannon, *Ann. Rev. Physiol.*, **38,** 425 (1976).

68. F. Gannon, B. Katzenellenbogen, G. Stancel, and G. Gorski, *The Molecular Biology of Hormone Action, 34th Symposium of the Society for*

Developmental Biology, Academic Press, New York, 1976, p. 137.

69. E. V. Jensen and E. R. De Sombre, *Science*, **182,** 126 (1973).
70. E. V. Jensen, S. Mohla, T. A. Gorell, and E. R. De Sombre, *Vitam. Horm.*, **32,** 89 (1974).
71. J. Gorski, R. A. Carlson, J. N. Harris, R. C. Manak, R. A. Maurier, W. L. Miller, and R. T. Stone, *Proceedings of the Fifth International Congress of Endocrinology, Hamburg*, Excerpta Medica, International Congress Series No. 402, *Endocrinology*, V. H. T. James, Ed., Excerpta Medica, Amsterdam, 1976, p. 7.
72. W. A. Coty, R. J. Schwartz, W. T. Schrader, and B. W. O'Malley, *Proceedings of the Fifth International Congress of Endocrinology, Hamburg*, Excerpta Medical Congress Series No. 402, *Endocrinology*, V. H. T. James, Ed., Excerpta Medica, Amsterdam, 1976 p. 526.
73. B. W. O'Malley and A. R. Means, *Science*, **183,** 610 (1974).
74. B. W. O'Malley and A. R. Means, Eds., *Receptors for Reproduction Hormones*, Plenum Press, New York, 1973.
75. R. J. B. King and W. I. P. Mainwaring, *Steroid-Cell Interactions*, University Park Press, Baltimore, 1974.
76. S. Liao, *Int. Rev. Cytol.*, **41,** 87 (1975).
77. E. E. Baulieu, *Mol. Cell Biochem.*, **7,** 157 (1975).
78. W. T. Schrader, W. A. Coty, R. G. Smith, and B. W. O'Malley, *Ann. N.Y. Acad. Sci.*, **286,** 64 (1977).
79. R. W. Kuhn, T. Schrader, W. A. Coty, P. M. Conn, and B. W. O'Malley, *J. Biol. Chem.*, **252,** 308 (1977).
80. J. P. Raynaud, *Med. Chem.* **5,** 451 (1977).
81. J. P. Raynaud, in *Progesterone Receptors in Normal and Neoplastic Tissues*, W. L. McGuire, J. P. Raynaud, and E. E. Baulieu, Eds., Raven Press, New York, 1977, p. 9.
82. J. P. Raynaud, C. Bonne, M. M. Bouton, M. Moguilewsky, D. Philibert, and G. Azadian–Boulanger, *J. Steroid Biochem.*, **6,** 615 (1975).
83. E. V. Jensen, S. Smith., and E. R. De Sombre, *J. Steroid Biochem.*, **7,** 911 (1976).
84. E. V. Jensen, *J. Am. Med. Assoc.*, **238,** 59 (1977).
85. P. A. Kelly, J. Asselin, M. G. Caron, F. Labrie, and J. P. Raynaud, *J. Nat. Cancer Inst.*, **58,** 623 (1977).
86. G. L. Greene, L. E. Closs, H. Fleming, E. R. De Sombre, and E. V. Jensen, *Proc. Nat. Acad. Sci., US*, **74,** 3681 (1977).
87. E. S. Shoemaker, J. P. Forney, and P. C. MacDonald, *J. Am. Med. Assoc.*, **238,** 1524 (1977).
88. J. Fishman, *Neuroendocrinology*, **24,** 367 (1977).
89. G. Pincus, in *The Hormones* Vol. 3, G. Pincus and K. V. Thimann, Eds., Academic Press, New York, 1955, p. 665.
90. P. Bard, *Medical Physiology*, 11th ed., Mosby, St. Louis, 1961.
91. C. H. Best and N. B. Taylor, *The Physiological Basis of Medical Practice*, 7th ed., Williams & Wilkins, Baltimore, 1961.
92. J. A. Loraine and E. T. Bell, in *Hormone Assays and Their Clinical Applications*, Williams & Wilkins. Baltimore, 1966, p. 225.
93. J. R. K. Preedy, *Methods Hormone Res.*, **1,** 1 (1962).
94. (a) C. T. Beer and T. F. Gallagher, *J. Biol. Chem.*, **214,** 335 (1955). (b) *Ibid.*, p. 351. (c) T. F. Gallagher, S. Kraychy, J. Fishman, J. B. Brown, and G. F. Marrian, *ibid.*, **233,** 1093 (1958).
95. S. Kober, *Biochem. Z.*, **239,** 209 (1931).
96. (a) W. J. A. Vanden–Heuvel, C. C. Sweeley, and E. C. Horning, *Biochem. Biophys. Res. Commun.*, **3,** 33 (1960). (b) W. J. A. Vanden–Heuvel, J. Sjovall, and E. C. Horning, *Biochim. Biophys. Acta*, **48,** 596 (1961).
97. T. Luukkainen, W. J. A. Vanden–Heuvel, E. O. A. Haahti, and E. C. Horning, *Biochim. Biophys. Acta*, **52,** 599 (1961).
98. H. H. Wotiz and H. F. Martin, *J. Biol. Chem.*, **236,** 1312 (1961).
99. G. J. Krol, C. A. Mannan, R. E. Pickering, D. V. Amato, B. T. Kho, and A. Sonnenschein, *Ann. Chem.* **49,** 1836 (1977).
100. H. Adlercrentz, F. Martin, O. Wahlroos, and E. Soini, *J. Steroid Biochem.*, **6,** 247 (1975).
101. C. W. Emment, *Methods Hormone Res.*, **2,** 59 (1962).
102. R. I. Dorfman and A. S. Dorfman, *Endocrinology*, **53,** 301 (1953).
103. L. Martin and P. J. Claringbold, *J. Endocrinol.*, **20,** 173 (1960).
104. L. Martin, *J. Endocrinol.*, **20,** 187 (1960).
105. (a) H. G. Lauson, C. H. Heller, J. B. Golden, and E. L. Severinghans, *Endocrinology*, **24,** 35 (1939). (b) J. L. Littrell, J. Tom, and C. J. Hartmann, *Fed. Proc.*, **5,** 65 (1946).
106. J. A. Hogg and J. Korman, in *Medicinal Chemistry*, Vol. 2, F. F. Blike and C. M. Suter, Eds., New York, 1956, p. 34.
107. C. W. Emmens, *Med. Res. Council (Brit.), Spec. Rep. Ser.*, 234 (1939).

108. (a) B. L. Rubin, A. S. Dorfman, L. Black, and R. I. Dorfman, *Endocrinology*, **49,** 429 (1951). (b) R. I. Dorfman, *Physiol. Rev.*, **34,** 138 (1954). (c) R. I. Dorfman and A. S. Dorfman, *Endocrinology*, **55,** 65 (1964). (d) C. Revesz, personal communication. (e) R. I. Dorfman and F. A. Kincl, *Acta Endocrinol.*, (Copenhagen), **52,** 619 (1966).
109. R. S. Yalow and S. A. Berson, *Nature*, **184,** 1648 (1959).
110. R. S. Yalow and S. A. Berson, *J. Clin. Invest.*, **39,** 1157 (1960)
111. R. P. Ekins, *Clin. Chim. Acta*, **5,** 453 (1960).
112. A. H. W. M. Schuurs and B. K. Van Weemen, *Clin. Chim. Acta*, **81,** 1 (1977).
113. M. Cais, S. Dani, Y. Eden, O. Gandolfi, M. Horn, E. E. Isaacs, Y. Josephy, Y. Saar, E. Slovin, and L. Snarsky, *Nature*, **270,** 534 (1977).
114. W. E. Bachmann, W. Cole, and A. L. Wilds, *J. Am. Chem. Soc.*, **61,** 974 (1939).
115. W. Klyne, *The Chemistry of the Steroids*, Wiley, New York, 1960.
116. T. B. Windholz and M. Windholz, *Angew. Chem.*, **76,** 249 (1964); *Angew. Chem., Int. Ed. Engl.*, **3,** 353 (1964).
117. P. Morand and J. Lyall, *Chem. Rev.*, **68,** 85 (1968).
118. (a) L. Velluz, G. Nominé, and J. Mathieu, *Angew. Chem.*, **72,** 725 (1960). (b) L. Velluz, G. Nominé, G. Amiard, V. Torelli, and J. Cérêde, *Compt. Rend.*, **257,** 3086 (1963).
119. G. H. Douglas, J. M. H. Graves, D. Hartley, G. A. Hughes, B. J. McLoughlin, J. Siddal, and H. Smith, *J. Chem. Soc.*, 5072 (1963).
120. H. Gibian, K. Kieslich, H.-J. Koch, H. Kosmol, C. Rufer, E. Schröder, and R. Vossing, *Tetrahedron Lett.*, 2321 (1966).
121. E. C. Dodds, L. Goldberg, W. Lawson, and R. Robinson, *Nature* (London), **141,** 247 (1938).
122. (a) R. Kurzrock, L. Wilson, and W. H. Perloff, *Endocrinology*, **26,** 581 (1940). (b) P. M. F. Bishop, G. C. Kennedy, and G. Wynn–Williams, *Lancet*, **255,** 764 (1948).
123. (a) F. von Wessely, *Angew. Chem.*, **53,** 197 (1940). (b) G. Masson, *Rev. Can. Biol.*, **3,** 491 (1944). (c) U. V. Solmssen, *Chem. Rev.*, **37,** 481 (1945).
124. A. L. Walpole, in *A Symposium on Agents Affecting Fertility*, C. R. Austin and J. S. Perry, Eds., Churchill, London, 1965, pp. 159–179.
125. J. M. Morris, G. von Wagenen, T. McCann, and D. Jacob, *Fertil. Steril.*, **18,** 18 (1967).
126. A. F. Goldfarb, A. Morales, A. E. Rakoff, and P. Protos, *Obstetr. Gynecol.*, **31,** 342 (1968).
127. A. Ercoli and R. Gardi. *Chem. Ind.* (London), 1037 (1961).
128. P. Fedor–Freybergh, *Acta Obstetr. Gynecol. Scand.*, Suppl. 64 (1977).
129. J. Thomson and I. Oswald, *Brit. Med. J.*, **2,** 1317 (1977).
130. F. LaBella, V. Havlicek, C. Pinsky, and L. Leybin, Neuroscience 111, Seventh Annual Meeting, Anaheim, Calif., November 6–10, 1977.
131. R. D. Gambrell, *J. Reprod. Med.*, **18,** 301 (1977).
132. A. R. Feinstein and R. I. Horwitz, *Brit. Med. J.*, **2,** 766 (1977).
133. L. Fieser and M. Fieser, *Steroids*, Reinhold, New York, 1959, Ch. 17.
134. T. C. Anand Kumar, G. F. X. David, and V. Puri, *Nature*, **270,** 532 (1977).
135. C. Clauberg, *Zbl. Gynekol.*, **54,** 7, 1154, 2757 (1930); modified by M. K. McPhail, *J. Physiol.* (London), **83,** 145 (1934).
136. D. A. McGinty, L. P. Anderson, and N. B. McCullough, *Endocrinology*, **24,** 829 (1939).
137. R. L. Elton and R. A. Edgren, *Endocrinology*, **63,** 464 (1958).
138. M. X. Zarrow, L. E. Peters, and L. A. Caldwell, *Ann. N.Y. Acad. Sci.*, **71,** 532 (1958).
139. Y. Ozawa and G. Pincus, *Endocrinology*, **68,** 680 (1961).
140. Z. Madjerek, J. DeVisser, J. Van der Vries, and G. A. Overbeck, *Acta Endocrinol.* (Copenhagen), **35,** 8 (1960).
141. G. Pincus and M. Chang, *Acta Physiol. Latino-Am.*, **3,** 177 (1953).
142. C. Biddulph, R. K. Meyer, and L. G. Gumbreck, *Endocrinology*, **26,** 280 (1940).
143. J. J. Gold, S. Bornsheck, L. Smith, and A. Scommegna, *Int. J. Fertil.*, **10,** 99 (1965).

CHAPTER THIRTY

Agents Affecting Fertility

RALPH I. DORFMAN

Department of Pharmacology
Stanford University
Stanford, California 94305, USA

CONTENTS

1 INTRODUCTION

This chapter discusses in detail the various agents affecting fertility in male and female mammals; compounds active in women and men are covered. The antifertility activity of plant materials has been summarized and discussed by Farnsworth et al. (1, 2) in considerable detail, and this material is not repeated here. The antifertility activity of steroid hormones and of related synthetic steroids that possess hormonal activity is discussed—the use of estrogens alone may be listed in this category. The unique antifertility activity of the combination of a progestogen plus estrogen is discussed for oral and injectable contraceptive treatment.

Progestogen and estrogen have been used for sequential contraceptive treatment. That is, estrogen alone is used for the first part of the menstrual cycle followed by a combination of progestogen plus estrogen to mimic the rise of progesterone during the second half of the normal menstrual cycle. The progestogens and estrogens used for these treatments are presented.

Contraceptive treatment by a progestogen alone (no estrogen) is discussed from the perspective of low dose continuous treatment. One study deals with low dose progestational treatment for 20 or 21 days plus 7 days with no active drug. Low dose continuous progestational therapy can be simulated with a single dosage by intramuscular injection. The data from these variants of continuous low dose progestogen treatment are presented.

Postcoital treatments with estrogens, estrogens plus progestogens, and progestogens alone are evaluated.

Data relating to various stages of abortion are discussed. Studies during the first and second trimesters of pregnancy show that prostaglandins are highly effective abortifacients and may be classified as agents affecting fertility. Nonprostaglandin abortifacients also are presented, mostly as applied in rodents. Nonhormonal, nonprostaglandin intravaginal spermicidal compounds are discussed.

LRF, the luteinizing hormone-releasing factor, plays an important role in ovulation. Inhibitors of LRF have been described which may be used to control the ovulation function and fertility as well. This possibility is analyzed.

Antifertility compounds effective in the

preimplantation phase of pregnancy are presented. These compounds have been studied in nonhuman female mammals and/or in women. Antifertility studies in men and in male nonhuman mammals are discussed. Results of antifertility studies in women are evaluated in terms of the Pearl Index, which is defined as the pregnancy rate per 100 woman-years of exposure (3). The Pearl Index is calculated as follows:

$$\text{Pearl Index} = \frac{\text{number of pregnancies} \times 1200}{\text{total months of exposure}}$$

The baseline or the control (at risk without any treatment) Pearl Index is about 40 (4).

The data are presented by a series of tables that cover the literature through 1976 with some 1977 reports included. A narrative is included for comments on the various agents affecting fertility. Finally, the structures of diverse antifertility compounds are represented in the figures, which are cross-referenced to the tables.

The data in this chapter deal essentially with thc efficacy of the agents affecting fertility in man and animals. The question of toxicity is mentioned only briefly. For complete discussions on toxicity and safety of these infertility agents the reader is referred to the following references:

1. H. W. Rudel, F. A. Kincl, and M. Henzl, *Birth Control*, Macmillan, New York, 1973.
2. J. P. Bennett, *Chemical Contraception*, Columbia University Press, New York, 1974.
3. C. R. Kay, *Oral Contraception Study*, Pitman Medical, New York, 1974.
4. *Population Reports, Oral Contraceptives*, Series A, No. 2, George Washington University Medical Center, Washington, D.C., March 1975.

2 ESTROGEN: ORAL, 20 DAYS' TREATMENT PER CYCLE (WOMEN)

Middleton (5) has studied (Table 30.1) the effect of 2 mg of diethylstilbestrol (Fig. 30.1) as a daily treatment for 20 days starting on day 5 of the menstrual cycle. Under these conditions, the Pearl Index was 3, a value significantly lower than 40, the Pearl Index considered as the control number.

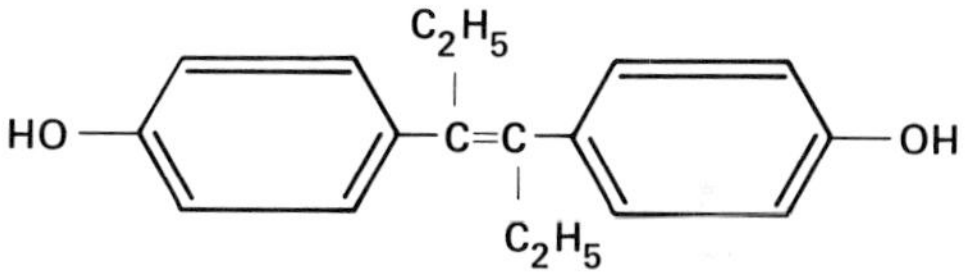

Fig. 30.1 Estrogen (diethylstilbestrol) used for antifertility studies (see Table 30.1).

3 COMBINATION OF PROGESTOGEN PLUS ESTROGEN (WOMEN)

Under normal conditions, ovulation occurs some 14 days before menstruation. The process of ovulation is dependent on the action of estrogens and progesterone from the ovary, follicle-stimulating hormone and

Table 30.1 Estrogen: Oral, 20 Days Treatment/Cycle (Women)

Compound	Number of Cycles or Months (Subjects)	Pregnancies, Pearl Index: Use	Reference
Diethylstilbestrol	1264 (86)	3	Middleton (5)

luteinizing hormone from the anterior pituitary, and releasing factors from the hypothalamus. Whether administered orally or by injection, estrogen and progestational agents in combination prevent ovulation from occurring by inhibiting the production of the required ovarian, anterior pituitary, and hypothalamic hormones. The menstrual cycle is preserved because the uterine endometrium is stimulated by the exogenous estrogens and progestogen and produces a menses-like bleeding on cessation of treatment. Thus the mechanism of action is severe decrease in hormone production and almost complete inhibition of ovulation.

3.1 Combination of Progestogen Plus Estrogen: Oral, 20–21 Days

The combination of a progestogen plus an estrogen administered orally for 20 to 21 days is the most effective of the hormonal contraceptive treatments on the basis of Pearl Index. Tables 30.2–30.11 indicate the various steroidal drugs that have been employed in effective combinations. The effective progestogens include norethindrone, norethindrone acetate, medroxyprogesterone acetate, norethynodrel, ethynodiol diacetate, lynestrenol, chlormadinone acetate, *dl*-norgestrel, *d*-norgestrel, and anagesterone; these progestogens are combined with ethynylestradiol or mestranol (see Figs. 30.2–30.6).

The Pearl Index by the combination method is well below 0.3, and many studies involving large numbers of cycles and subjects have resulted in values of zero, meaning no pregnancies. Over the last few years, less and less progestogen and estrogen have been used to produce highly efficacious treatments. In the case of norethindrone and mestranol, the first treatment schedule

Table 30.2 Combination of Norethindrone Plus Estrogen: Oral, 20 or 21 Days of Treatment, (Women)

Compounds		Number of Cycles or Months (Subjects)	Bleeding Interval Mean, days	Pregnancies, Pearl Index		Reference
Progestogen, mg/day	Estrogen, mg/day			Method	Use	
Norethindrone (0.5)	Ethynylestradiol (0.035)	8738 (613)	28.5[a] 27.9[b]	0	0.27	Pasquale and Yuliano (58)
Norethindrone (5)	Mestranol (0.075)	675 (113)	—	0	0	Swartz et al. (59)
Norethindrone (10)	Mestranol (0.06)	7194 (570)	—	0.16	0.8	Tyler et al. (60)
Norethindrone (10)	Mestranol (0.06)	6139 (210)	27	0	0	Goldzieher et al. (61)
Norethindrone (10)	Mestranol (0.06)	6062 (364)	27	0	0.6	Rice-Wray et al. (62)
Norethindrone (2)	Mestranol (0.1)	90 (32)	—	0	0	Andrews and Andrews (63)
Norethindrone (5)	Mestranol (0.075)	1249 (132)	—	0	0	Board (64)
Norethindrone (1)	Mestranol (0.08)	381 (50)	—	0	0	

[a] Before treatment.
[b] During treatment.

Table 30.3 Combination of Norethindrone Acetate Plus Ethynylestradiol: Oral, 20 or 21 Days of Treatment (Women)

Compounds		Number of Cycles or Months (Subjects)	Bleeding Interval Mean, days	Pregnancies, Pearl Index		Reference
Progestogen, mg/day	Estrogen, mg/day			Method	Use	
Norethindrone acetate (2.0)	Ethynylestradiol (0.04)	2810 (378)	—	0	0	Preston (65)
Norethindrone acetate (1.5)	Ethynylestradiol (0.03)	8979 (1102)	—	0.13	0.53	
Norethindrone acetate (0.6)	Ethynylestradiol (0.03)	7922 (1296)	—	0.15	0.91	
Norethindrone acetate (1.0)	Ethynylestradiol (0.02)	8284 (1218)	—	0.14	0.87	
Norethindrone acetate (4)	Ethynylestradiol (0.05)	156 (36)	—	0	0	Peeters et al. (66)
Norethindrone acetate (5)	Ethynylestradiol (0.05)	207 (22)	—	0	0	Bowman (67)
Norethindrone acetate (4)	Ethynylestradiol (0.05)	382 (53)	—	0	0	
Norethindrone acetate (4)	Ethynylestradiol (0.05)	1023 (166)	26–27	0	0	Mears and Grant (68)
Norethindrone acetate (4)	Ethynylestradiol (0.05)	1324	25–27	0	0	Bockner (69)

Table 30.4 Combination of Medroxyprogesterone Acetate Plus Ethynylestradiol: Oral, 20 or 21 Days of Treatment (Women)

Compounds		Number of Cycles or Months (Subjects)	Bleeding Interval Mean, days	Pregnancies, Pearl Index		Reference
Progestogen, mg/day	Estrogen, mg/day			Method	Use	
Medroxyprogesterone acetate (10)	Ethynylestradiol (0.05)	1188 (232)	—	0	0	Livingston (70)
Medroxyprogesterone acetate (10)	Ethynylestradiol (0.05)	1702 (268)	—	0	0	Moghissi et al. (71)
Medroxyprogesterone acetate (10)	Ethynylestradiol (0.05)	1100 (191)	26	0	0	Eichner (72)
Medroxyprogesterone acetate (10)	Ethynylestradiol (0.05)	481 (87)	28	0	0	Gold et al. (73)
Medroxyprogesterone acetate (10)	Ethynylestradiol (0.05)	692 (64)	—	0	0	Gould (74)
Medroxyprogesterone acetate (10)	Ethynylestradiol (0.05)	1009 (119)	—	0	0	Hass (75)

Table 30.5 Combination of Norethynodrel Plus Mestranol: Oral, 20 or 21 Days of Treatment (Women)

Compounds		Number of Cycles or Months (Subjects)	Bleeding Interval Mean, days	Pregnancies, Pearl Index		Reference
Progestogen, mg/day	Estrogen, mg/day			Method	Use	
Norethynodrel (5)	Mestranol (0.75)	3267 (216)	—	0	0.7	Mears (76)
Norethynodrel (2.5)	Mestranol (0.1)	2718 (262)	—	0	0.7	
Norethynodrel (9.85)	Mestranol (0.15)	8133 (830)	28.6	2.7	1.0	Pincus et al. (77) Rock et al. (78)
Norethynodrel (5)	Mestranol (0.75)	224	27.3	0	—	Pincus et al. (79)
Norethynodrel (2.5)	Mestranol (0.0375)	46	26.2	0	—	
Norethynodrel (2.5)	Mestranol (0.15)	589 (89)	—	2	—	Mears (80)
Norethynodrel (5.0)	Mestranol (0.75)	246 (49)	—	0	—	Pullen (81)
Norethynodrel (2.5)	Mestranol (0.1)	282 (34)	—	4.3	—	
Norethynodrel (2.3)	Mestranol (0.036)	129 (48)	35	130	—	Eckstein et al. (82)
Norethynodrel (2.5)	Mestranol (0.1)	1626 (238)	—	0.7	0.7	Chinnatamby (83)

Table 30.6 Combination of Ethynodiol Diacetate Plus Mestranol: Oral, 20 or 21 Days of Treatment (Women)

Compounds		Number of Cycles or Months (Subjects)	Bleeding Interval Mean, days	Pregnancies, Pearl Index		Reference
Progestogen, mg/day	Estrogen, mg/day			Method	Use	
Ethynodiol diacetate (0.5)	Mestranol (0.1)	354 (97)	27	0	0	Andrews et al. (84)
Ethynodiol diacetate (1.0)	Mestranol (0.1)	9,931 (410)	27	0	0	
Ethynodiol diacetate (2.0)	Mestranol (0.1)	2,833 (131)	27	0	0	
Ethynodiol diacetate (2)	Mestranol (0.1)	662 (124)	27.4	0	0	Pincus et al. (85)
Ethynodiol diacetate (2)	Mestranol (0.1)	981 (123)	—	0	0	Mears (86)
Ethynodiol diacetate (1)	Mestranol (0.1)	34,000 (4500)	—	0.04	0.2	Oldershaw (87)

Table 30.7 Combination of Lynestrenol Plus Ethynylestradiol: Oral 20 or 21 Days of Treatment (Women)

Compounds		Number of Cycles or Months (Subjects)	Bleeding Interval Mean, days	Pregnancies, Pearl Index		Reference
Progestogen, mg/day	Estrogen, mg/day			Method	Use	
Lynestrenol (0.75)	Ethynylestradiol (0.0375)	1,144 (134)	28	0	0	
		20,855	28	0.06	0.18	
Lynestrenol (5)	Ethynylestradiol (0.15)	794 (133)	—	0	7	Brehm (88)
Lynestrenol (5)	Ethynylestradiol (0.15)	567 (42)	26–34	0	0	Ferin (89)
Lynestrenol (2.5)	Ethynylestradiol (0.075)	180 (30)	—	0	0	Turpienen (90)
Lynestrenol (5)	Ethynylestradiol (0.15)	876 (120)	—	0	1.4	Hauser (91)
Lynestrenol (5)	Ethynylestradiol (0.15)	522 (100)	27	0	0	Hauser and Schubiger (92)
Lynestrenol (2.5)	Ethynylestradiol (0.075)	300 (87)	29.3	0	0	
Lynestrenol (0.75)	Ethynylestradiol (0.0375)	1,144 (134)	—	0 0	0 0	Altkemper et al. (93)
Lynestrenol (0.75)	Ethynylestradiol (0.0375)	4,857 (335)	96.2 28±3	0	0	Prsić and Kićović (94)

called for about 10 mg of the progestogen and 60 μg of the estrogen daily for 20 days. This prescription has been reduced to 1 mg of norethindrone and 50 μg of mestranol, with efficacy values as good as 0.1–0.3 (Pearl Index). In a second low dose combination, the daily steroid doses were 0.5 and 0.035 mg for norethindrone and ethynylestradiol, respectively. For 8738 cycles representing 613 subjects, the method Pearl Index was zero.

In the case of *d*-norgestrel in combination with ethynylestradiol, the dosage for active ingredients has been reduced without loss of efficacy as measured by the Pearl Index method. The low dose formula is

Table 30.8 Combination of Chlormadinone Acetate Plus Mestranol: Oral, 20 or 21 Days of Treatment (Women)

Compounds		Number of Cycles or Months (Subjects)	Bleeding Interval Mean, days	Pregnancies, Pearl Index		Reference
Progestogen, mg/day	Estrogen, mg/day			Method	Use	
Chlormadinone acetate (3)	Mestranol (0.1)	2525 (176)	27.5	0	0.4	Rice-Wray et al. (95)

Table 30.9 Combination of *dl*-Norgestrel Plus Ethynylestradiol: Oral, 20 or 21 Days of Treatment (Women)

Compounds		Number of Cycles or Months (Subjects)	Bleeding Interval Mean, days	Pregnancies, Pearl Index		Reference
Progestogen, mg/day	Estrogen, mg/day			Method	Use	
dl-Norgestrel (0.5)	Ethynylestradiol (0.05)	127,872 (6806)	28.2	0	0.19	Korba and Heil (96)
dl-Norgestrel (0.3)	Ethynylestradiol (0.03)	11,085 (852)	28.6 ± 3.5 (S.D.)	0.12	0.12	Woutersz (97)
dl-Norgestrel (0.750)	Ethynylestradiol (0.03)	5,231 (778)	—	0	0	Sartoretto and Moraes (98)
dl-Norgestrel (0.5)	Ethynylestradiol (0.05)	505 (63)	Normal	0	0	Apelo and Veloso (99)
dl-Norgestrel (0.5)	Ethynylestradiol (0.05)	14,486 (1929)	28	0	0.18	Andelman et al. (100)
dl-Norgestrel (0.5)	Ethynylestradiol (0.05)	3,175 (300)	28.2	0	0	Rice-Wray et al. (101)
dl-Norgestrel (0.3)	Ethynylestradiol (0.03)	754 (99)	28.6 ± 4.6 (S.D.)	0	1.6	Allen (102)

150 μg of *d*-norgestrel and 30 μg of ethynylestradiol (Table 30.10).

3.2 Combination of Progestogen Plus Estrogen: Oral

Table 30.12 summarizes the data indicating the antifertility efficacy according to the different progestogens and estrogen combinations used. A remarkably low Pearl Index value has been found for essentially all combinations. The data of Tietze's (6) composite analysis as well as the data summarized by Rutensköld (7) agree well with the summarized data presented in this chapter.

One must conclude from the mass of data now available that the combination of a progestational agent and estrogen administered daily for 20–21 days, starting with the fifth day of cycle, is a highly effective antifertility regimen. The combination of the progestogen plus estrogen inhibits the natural menstrual cycle, including ovulation, to the extent of better than 95%. The efficacy is better than 95%; perhaps closer to 100%. The additional efficacy from 95 to 100% occurs because the contraceptive mixture provides a hostile cervical secretion and a hostile uterine mucosa. This means that even if ovulation were to occur, the environment would provide an infertile rather than a fertile condition.

3.3 Combination: Oral, Alternate-Day Estrogen

To reduce estrogen intake to a minimum, a new regimen has been developed. The total estrogen per cycle has been reduced to 600 μg of ethynylestradiol. The estrogen dosage is 60 μg every other day. Efficacy is good, and the bleeding pattern is acceptable. The progestational agent is norethindrone at 0.5 mg daily (Table 30.13).

Table 30.10 Combination of *d*-Norgestrel Plus Ethynylestradiol: Oral, 20 or 21 Days of Treatment (Women)

Compounds		Number of Cycles or Months (Subjects)	Bleeding Interval Mean, days	Pregnancies Pearl Index		Reference
Progestogen, mg/day	Estrogen, mg/day			Method	Use	
d-Norgestrel (0.15)	Ethynylestradiol (0.03)	1,488	—	0	0	Apelo and Veloso (103)
d-Norgestrel (0.25)	Ethynylestradiol (0.05)	1,616 (220)	Normal	0	0	Apelo and Veloso (99)
d-Norgestrel (0.3)	Ethynylestradiol (0.03)	20,312 (1633)	28.5±5.6 (S.D.)	—	0.13	Woutersz (104)
d-Norgestrel (0.15)	Ethynylestradiol (0.03)	787 (120)	28.3±3	0	0	Altkemper et al. (93)
d-Norgestrel (0.15)	Ethynylestradiol (0.03)	1,076 (238)	28.4	1.2	1.2	Woutersz (105)
d-Norgestrel (0.15)	Ethynylestradiol (0.03)	423 (65)	28.3	0	0	Molina et al. (106)
d-Norgestrel (0.15)	Ethynylestradiol (0.03)	3,460 (590)	27.3	0	0	Moggia et al. (107)
d-Norgestrel (0.15)	Ethynylestradiol (0.03)	840 (75)	28.5±3.2	0	0	Briggs and Briggs (108)
d-Norgestrel (0.15)	Ethynylestradiol (0.03)	1,304 (132)	—	0	0	Fassa (109)
d-Norgestrel (0.15)	Ethynylestradiol (0.03)	754 (99)	28.6	0	0	Allen (102)
d-Norgestrel (0.15)	Ethynylestradiol (0.03)	11,980 (1320)	—	0.1	0.1	Rosenbaum (110)
d-Norgestrel (0.15)	Ethynylestradiol (0.03)	2,056 (150)	—	0.6	0.6	Bergstein et al. (111)
d-Norgestrel (0.15)	Ethynylestradiol (0.03)	767 (120)	28	0	0	Foss and Fotherby (112)

Table 30.11 Combination of Anagesterone Plus Mestranol: Oral, 20 or 21 Days of Treatment (Women)

Compounds		Number of Cycles or Months (Subjects)	Bleeding Interval Mean, days	Pregnancies, Pearl Index		Reference
Progestogen, mg/day	Estrogen, mg/day			Method	Use	
Anagesterone acetate (1);	Mestranol (0.08)	406 (35)	—	0	0	Board (64)
Anagesterone acetate	Mestranol (0.125)	71 (26)	—	0	0	Board (64)

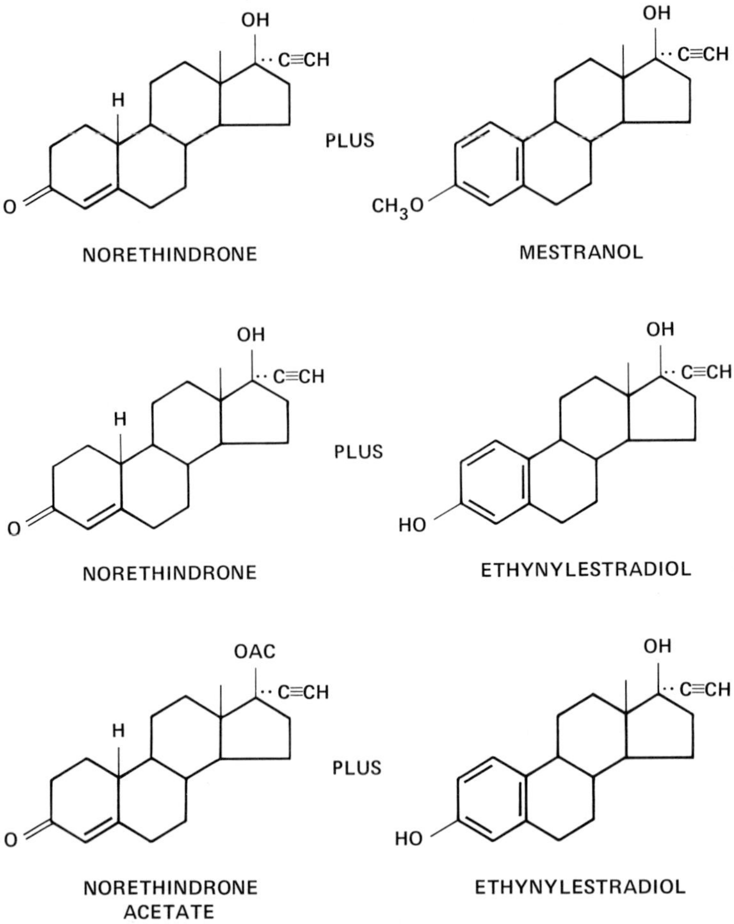

NORETHINDRONE PLUS MESTRANOL

NORETHINDRONE PLUS ETHYNYLESTRADIOL

NORETHINDRONE ACETATE PLUS ETHYNYLESTRADIOL

Fig. 30.2 Progestogen and estrogen combinations used for oral contraceptives (see Tables 30.2–30.14).

3.4 Combination of Progestogen Plus Estrogen: Oral, Every Other Day

Combination therapy is so highly effective that the accidentally missing of one day's tablet does not decrease the contraceptive effectiveness of the mixture. Table 30.14 indicates that the efficacy is unchanged, that is, zero pregnancies resulted, but that the bleeding pattern needs to be improved.

3.5 Combination of Progestogen Plus Estrogen: Oral, Once a Month

The long-acting steroids quingestanol acetate (progestogen) and quinestrol (estrogen) were synthesized with the objective of achieving efficacy and cycle control with a single combination treatment for the 28 day period. This has been accomplished. However the efficacy as judged by the Pearl Index was less favorable than the daily combination tablet for the 20 or 21 day therapy starting on day 5 of the cycle. (See Table 30.15, Fig. 30.7.)

3.6 Combination of Progestogen Plus Estrogen: Oral, Three Cycles (Tricycle)

On the basis of mechanism of action of combination therapy, it is known that the

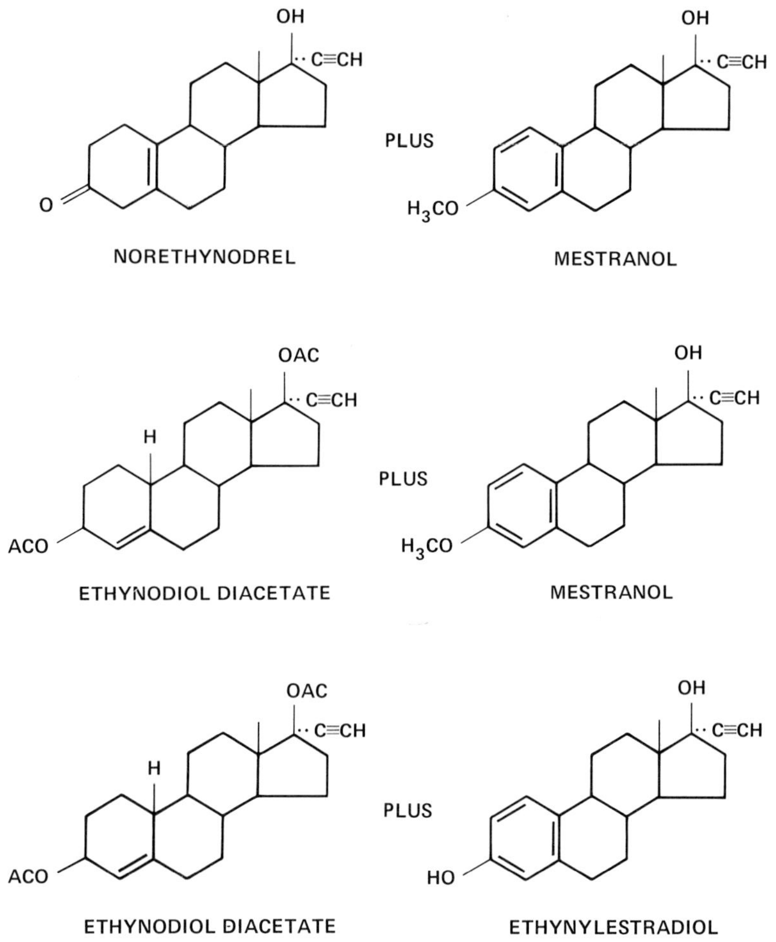

NORETHYNODREL PLUS MESTRANOL

ETHYNODIOL DIACETATE PLUS MESTRANOL

ETHYNODIOL DIACETATE PLUS ETHYNYLESTRADIOL

Fig. 30.3 Progestogen and estrogen combinations used for oral contraceptives (see Tables 30.2–30.14).

normal cycle including ovulation is essentially completely suppressed, and in its place an artificial cycle including withdrawal bleeding (menses) is instituted. Thus Loudon et al. (8) suggested that some women may not object to extending the cycle to 56 days, to 84 days, or even longer. Loudon et al. (8) have tested the acceptability of a reduced menstrual frequency when the subjects took lynestrenol (2.5 mg/day) plus ethynylestradiol (0.05 mg/day) daily for 84 days (Fig. 30.8). There were 202 subjects, and 53% completed a one year trial (Table 30.16). No pregnancies occurred. Of the subjects who completed a year's treatment, 82% liked having infrequent periods.

3.7 Combination of Progestogen Plus Estrogen: Single Injection, 28 Days

A combination of 150 mg of 16α,17α-dihydroxyprogesterone acetophenide (Fig. 30.9) and 10 mg of estradiol-17β-enanthate as a single injection will restrain fertility for 28 days. As Table 30.17 illustrates, a very low Pearl Index is attainable and cyclicity is good.

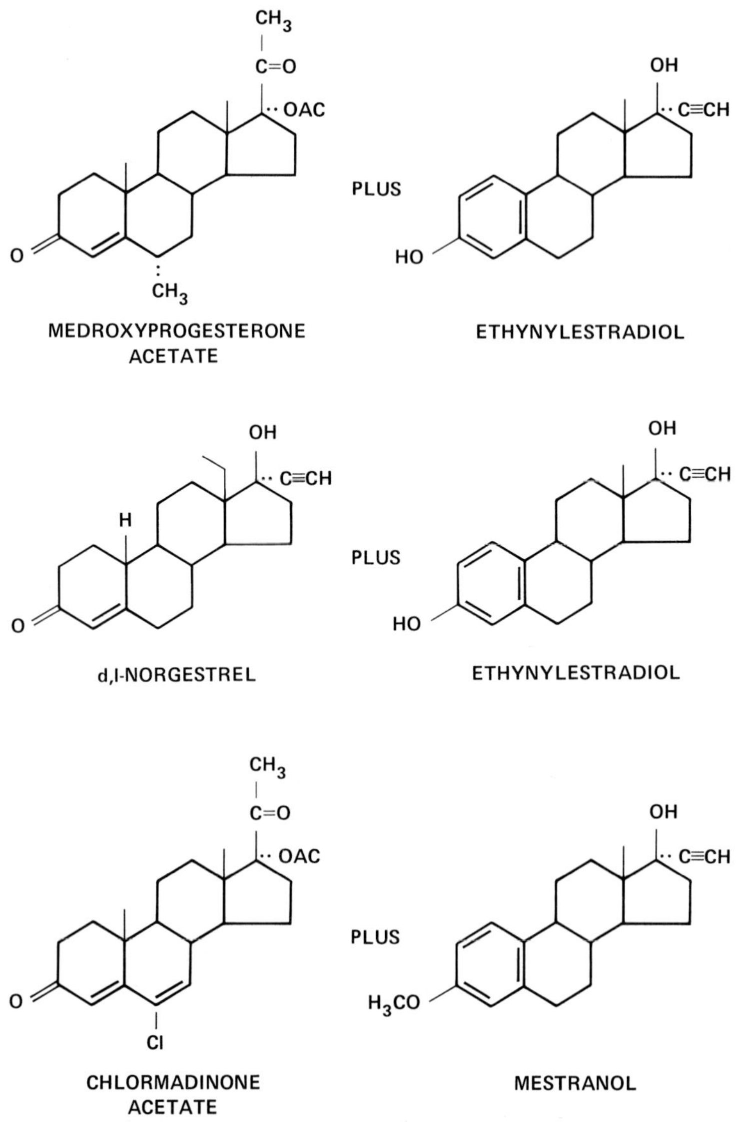

MEDROXYPROGESTERONE ACETATE PLUS ETHYNYLESTRADIOL

d,l-NORGESTREL PLUS ETHYNYLESTRADIOL

CHLORMADINONE ACETATE PLUS MESTRANOL

Fig. 30.4 Progestogen and estrogen combinations used for oral contraceptives (see Tables 30.2–30.14).

A combination of *dl*-norgestrel (25 mg) plus estradiol hexahydrobenzoate (5 mg) yielded zero pregnancies and good cycle control (Table 30.17).

Two concentrations of the combinations of norethindrone enanthate and estradiol-17β-unducelate have been studied (Table 30.17). No pregnancies occurred, and good cyclicity was reported. The estrogen is estradiol, therefore the 5 mg dose injected on the basis of 28 days means a low maximum mean dosage of 180 μg/day.

3.8 Combination of Progestogen Plus Estrogen: "Step Up"

The regimen outlined in Table 30.18 varies the progestogen *d*-norgestrel from 50 μg for the first 11 days of treatment to 125 μg

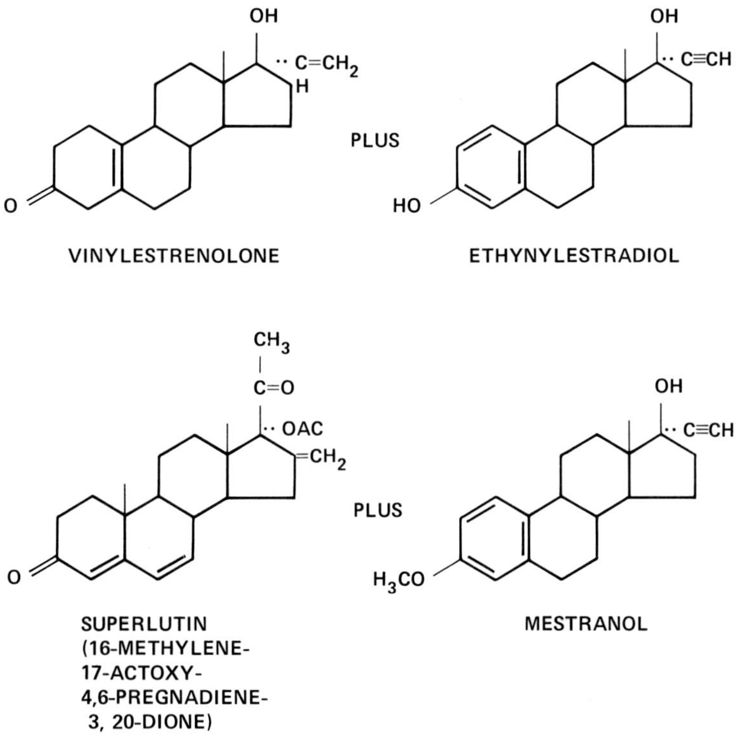
OH
C=CH2
H
O
PLUS
OH
C≡CH
HO
VINYLESTRENOLONE
ETHYNYLESTRADIOL
CH3
C=O
OAC
=CH2
O
PLUS
OH
C≡CH
H3CO
SUPERLUTIN
(16-METHYLENE-
17-ACTOXY-
4,6-PREGNADIENE-
3, 20-DIONE)
MESTRANOL

Fig. 30.5 Progestogen and estrogen combinations used for oral contraceptives (see Tables 30.2–30.14).

for the last 10 days; the estrogen ethynylestradiol remains constant at 50 μg for the total of 21 treatment days (Fig. 30.10). Under these conditions 1112 cycles for 178 subjects resulted in no pregnancies and a mean bleeding interval of 27.8 days.

3.9 Sequential: Oral Preparations

The combination contraceptive containing both estrogen and progestogen (Figs. 30.11–30.13) is administered from day 5 through day 25 or 26 of the cycle. In the normal menstrual cycle progesterone is essentially not present from days 5–15, and some investigators suggested that the combination tablet supplied an abnormal component, progestogen, in the first half of the cycle. To provide more natural hormonal conditions, a regimen was fashioned in which estrogen alone was administered from days 5–15 and a combination of estrogen plus progestogen treatment from days 15–25. A high efficacy rate is obtained with such a sequential treatment, and the mechanism by which this occurs is the same as already discussed under the mechanism of action of the combination treatment. Cyclicity is good, and cessation of treatment leads smoothly to endogenous hormone production and ovulation (Table 30.19).

3.10 Summaries: Sequential Oral Preparations

Summary Table 30.20 deals with the data collected by Tietze (6), as well as summaries of more recent studies. During a 5 year period, 1962–1967, Tietze calculated the Pearl Index of more than 70,000 cycles to be 0.5. This chapter contains data on

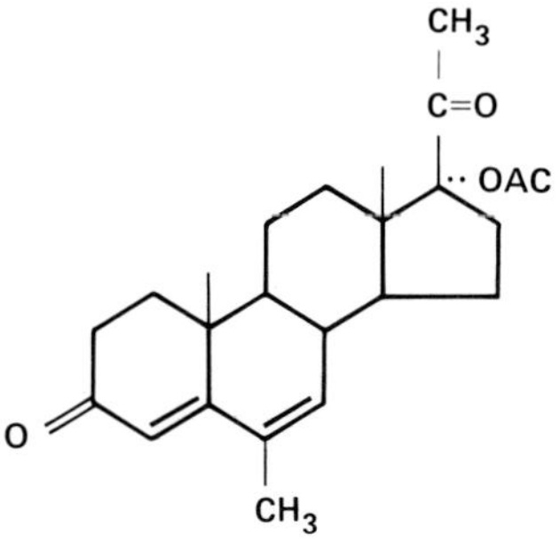

MEGESTROL ACETATE PLUS ETHYNYLESTRADIOL

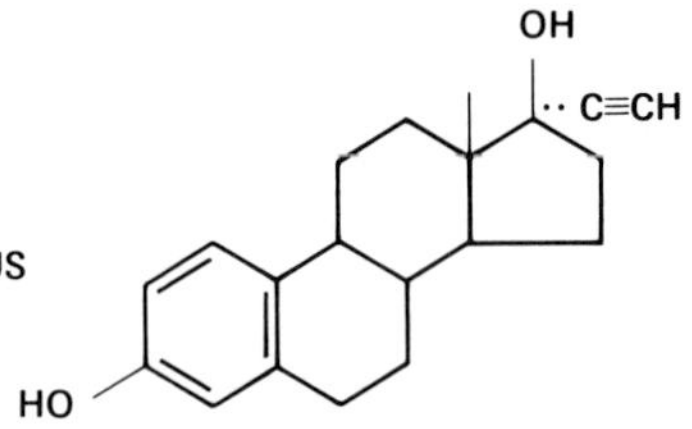

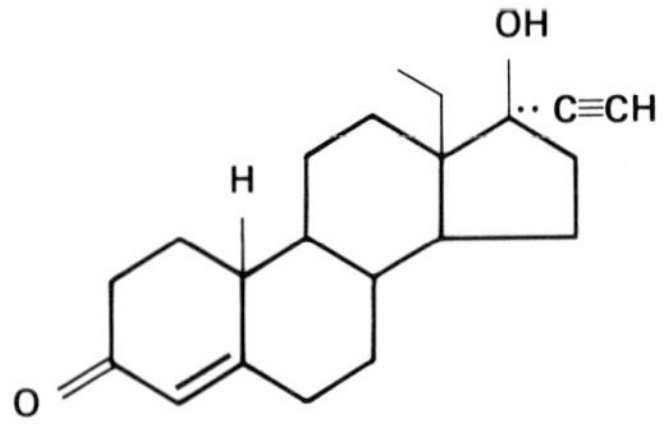

d-NORGESTREL PLUS ETHYNYLESTRADIOL

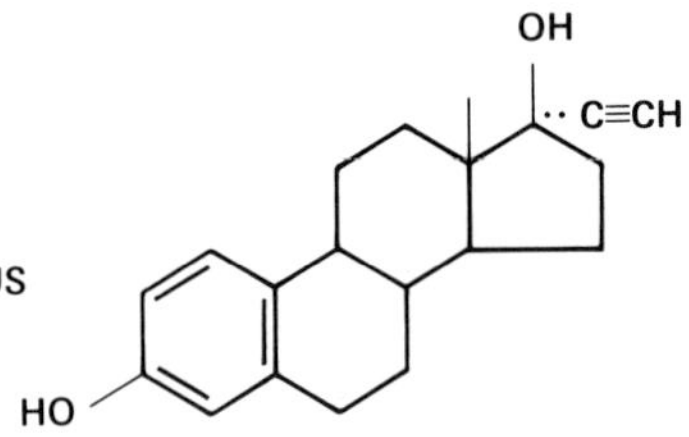

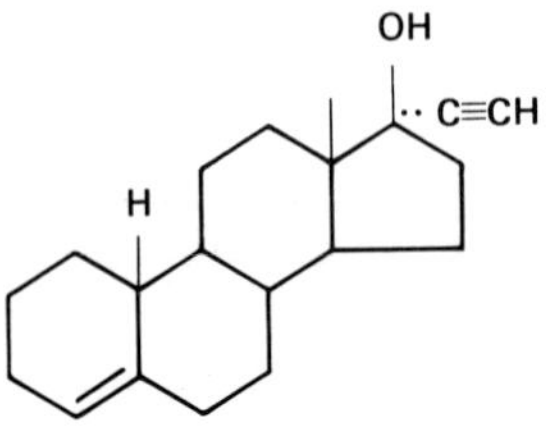

LYNESTRENOL PLUS MESTRANOL

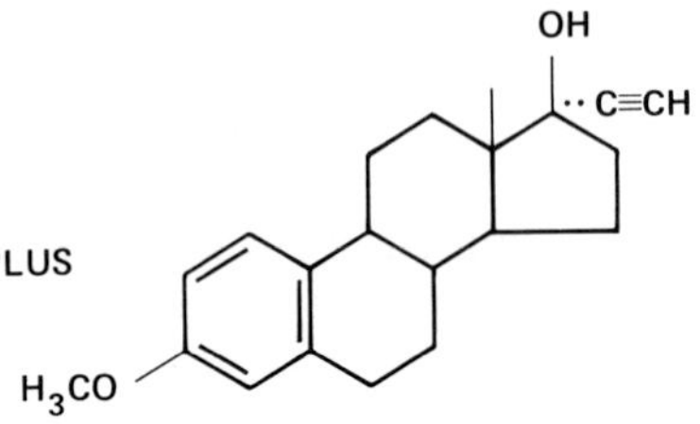

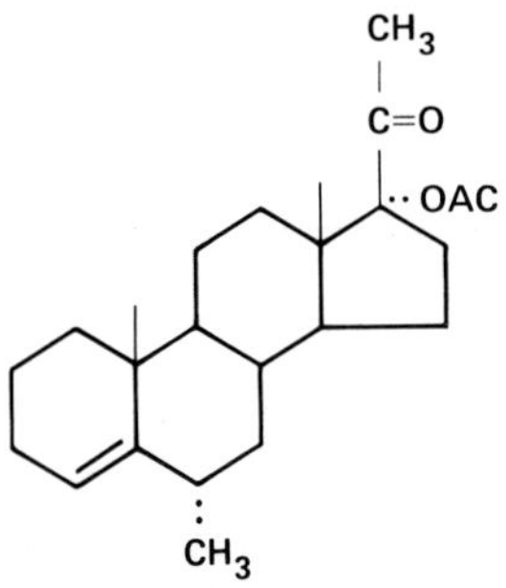

ANAGESTERONE PLUS MESTRANOL

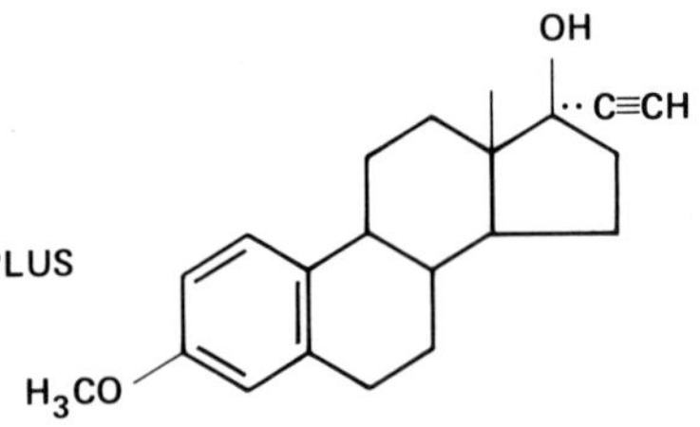

Fig. 30.6 Progestogen and estrogen combinations used for oral contraceptives (see Tables 30.2–30.14).

Table 30.12 Summaries: Combination of Progestogen Plus Estrogen: Oral (Women)

Compounds		Number of Cycles	Mean Pearl Index: Use	Reference
Progestogen	Estrogen			
14 Progestogens	Mestranol or ethynylestradiol	3,867,337 (combined studies)	0.005	Rutensköld (7)
Composite of various steroids, 1962–1967		200,000	0.1	Tietze (6)
Norethindrone	Mestranol or ethynylestradiol	30,527	0.21	This chapter
Norethindrone acetate	Ethynylestradiol (0.03 mg or less not included)	5,902	0	This chapter
Norethindrone acetate	Ethynylestradiol	6,172	0	This chapter
Medroxyprogesterone acetate	Ethynylestradiol	10,649	0	This chapter
Ethynodiol diacetate	Mestranol	14,761	0	This chapter
Lynestrenol	Ethynylestradiol	46,843	0.16	This chapter
d-Norgestrel	Ethynylestradiol	29,682	0.1	This chapter
Chlormadinone acetate	Mestranol	2,525	0.4	This chapter
dl-Norgestrel	Ethynylestradiol	162,354	0.15	This chapter
Anagesterone	Mestranol	477	0	This chapter

Table 30.13 Combination of Progestogen Plus Ethynylestradiol: Oral, Alternate-Day Estrogen, Progestogen Daily; 20 Days of Treatment (Women)

Compounds		Number of Cycles or Months (Subjects)	Bleeding Interval Mean, days	Pregnancies, Pearl Index		Reference
Progestogen, mg/day	Estrogen, mg/day			Method	Use	
Norethindrone (0.5)	Ethynylestradiol (0.060 every other day)	12,942 (1090)	—	0.18	0.73	Segre et al. (113)

Table 30.14 Combination of Progestogen and Estrogen: Oral, Every Other Day (Women)

Compounds		Number of Cycles or Months (Subjects)	Bleeding Interval, 24–33%	Pregnancies Pearl Index		Reference
Progestogen, mg every other day	Estrogen, mg every other day			Method	Use	
dl-Norgestrel (0.5)	Ethynylestradiol (0.05)	235 (51)	51.4[a]	0	0	Coutinho and De Souza (114)

[a] Amenorrhea, 12.7%, breakthrough bleeding, 35.6%.

Table 30.15 Combination Progestogen Plus Estrogen: Oral, Once a Month (Women)

Compounds		Number of Cycles or Months (Subjects)	Pregnancies, Pearl Index: Use	Reference
Progestogen, mg/4 weeks	Estrogen, mg/4 weeks			
Quingestanol acetate (norethindrone acetate 3-cyclopentyl enol ether) (5)	Quinestrol (ethynylestradiol cyclopentyl ether) (2)	16,000	Study in Mexico 1.5; study in Chile 4.0	Berman (115)
Quingestanol acetate (2.5)	Quinestrol (2)	36,000 (3600)	Various studies: 0, 1, 1.6, 4.2, 5.8	
Quingestanol acetate (2.5)	Quinestrol (2)	2,610 (256)	0	Rubio and Berman (116)
Quingestanol acetate (5)	Quinestrol (2)	2,420 (259)	1.5	Maqueo-Topete et al. (117)
Quingestanol acetate (2)	Quinestrol (2.5)	352 (55)	10.2	Nudemberg et al. (118)
Quingestanol acetate (2.5)	Quinestrol (2)	2,493 (503)	1.9	Larrañaga and Berman (119)
Quingestanol acetate (2.5)	Quinestrol (2)	3,130 (666)	5.1	Tejuja et al. (120)
Quingestanol acetate (2.5)	Quinestrol (2)	2,781 (212)	7.7	Mishell and Fried (121)
Quingestanol acetate (5)	Quinestrol (2)	7,441 (719)	4.0	Guiloff et al. (122)

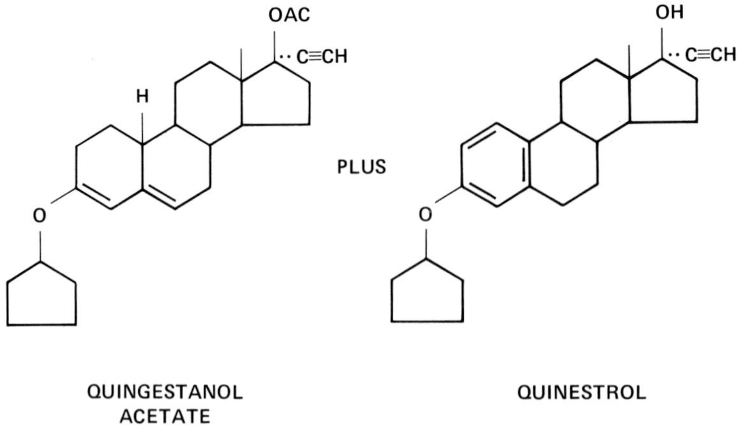

QUINGESTANOL ACETATE PLUS QUINESTROL

Fig. 30.7 Combination of progestogen and estrogen: once a month, oral (see Table 30.15).

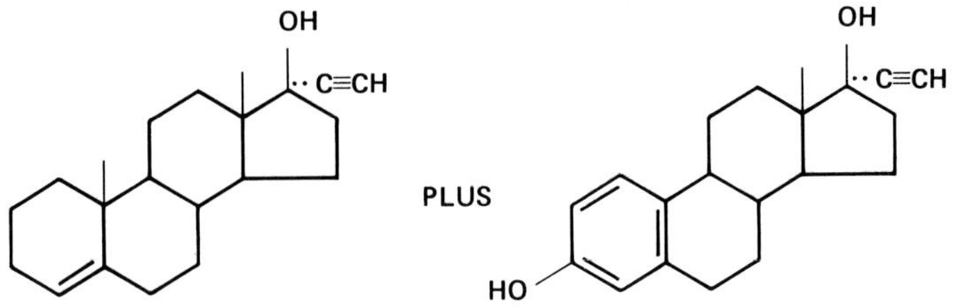

LYNESTRENOL PLUS ETHYNYLESTRADIOL

Fig. 30.8 Combination of lynestrenol plus ethynyl estradiol: daily tablet for 84 days (see Table 30.16).

Table 30.16 Combination of Progestogen Plus Estrogen: Oral, Three Cycles (Women)

Compounds		Subject		Pregnancies, Pearl Index		
Progestogen, mg/day	Estrogen, mg/day	Original Number	Completing One Year Trial, %	Method	Use	Reference
Lynestrenol (2.5)	Ethynylestradiol (0.05)	202	53	0	0	Loudon et al. (8)

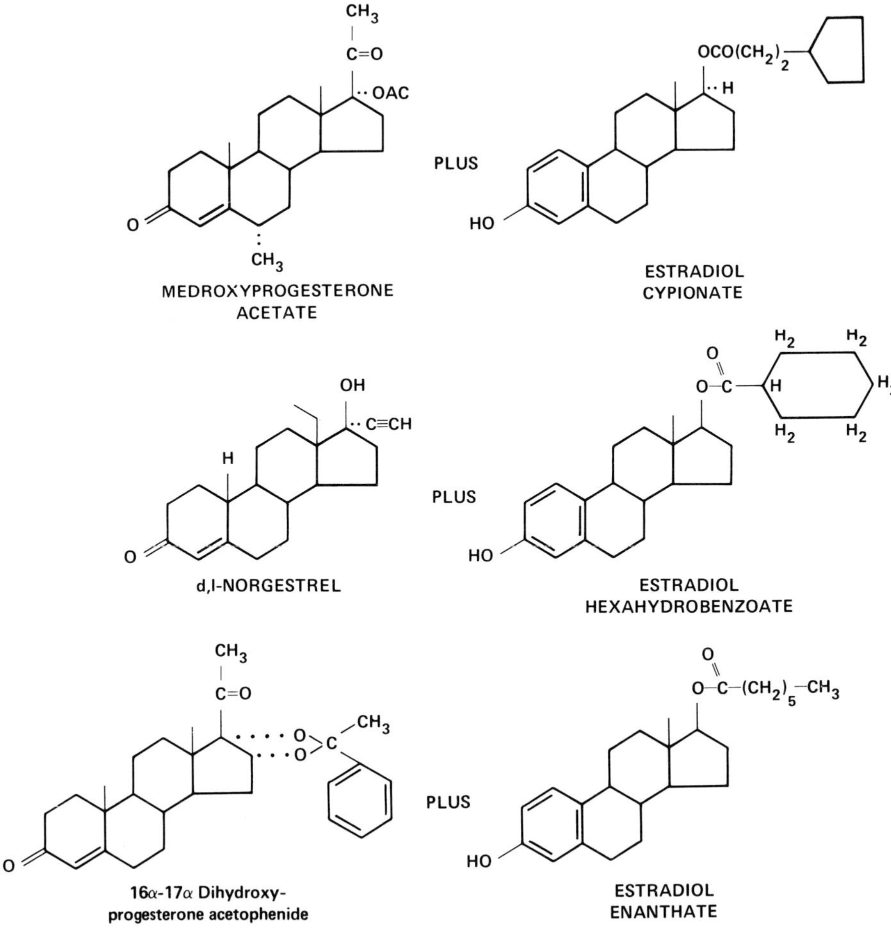

MEDROXYPROGESTERONE ACETATE PLUS ESTRADIOL CYPIONATE

d,l-NORGESTREL PLUS ESTRADIOL HEXAHYDROBENZOATE

16α-17α Dihydroxyprogesterone acetophenide PLUS ESTRADIOL ENANTHATE

Fig. 30.9 Combination of progestogen plus estrogen, once a month injection (see Table 30.17).

Table 30.17 Combination of Progestogen Plus Estrogen: Single Injection Every 28 Days (Women)

Compounds					
Progestogen, mg/month	Estrogen, mg/month	Cycle Lengths, 21–35 Days, %	Number of Cycles or Months (Subjects)	Pregnancies, Pearl Index: Use	Reference
Medroxyprogesterone acetate (25)	Estradiol cypionate (5)	85.1	623 (104)	0	Coutinho and De Souza (123)
dl-Norgestrel (25)	Estradiol hexahydrobenzoate (5)	75.0	550 (50)	0	De Souza and Coutinho (124)
16α,17α-Dihydroxyprogesterone acetophenide (150)	Estradiol enanthate (variable)	Mean cycle length, 26.8	4512 (385)	0	Wallach and Garcia (125)
16α,17α-Dihydroxyprogesterone acetophenide (variable)	Estradiol enanthate (variable)	88; mean cycle length, 24 days	590 (127)	0	Felton et al. (126)
16α,17α-Dihydroxyprogesterone acetophenide (150)	Estradiol enanthate (10)	74.2	198 (60)	0	Reifenstein et al. (127)
16α,17α-Dihydroxyprogesterone acetophenide (150)	Estradiol enanthate (10)	Mean cycle length, 26.3 days	511 (66)	0	James (128)
Medroxyprogesterone acetate (25)	Estradiol cypionate (5)	87	1108 (100)	0	Rubio et al. (129)
16α,17α-Dihydroxyprogesterone acetophenide (150)	Estradiol enanthate (10)	75	6197 (871)	0	Tyler et al. (130)
Norethindrone enanthate (50)	Estradiol unducelate (5)	88.8	431 (40)	0	Karim and El-Mahgoub
Norethindrone enanthate (70)	Estradiol unducelate (10)	85.9	392 (40)	0	(131)

additional 114,438 cycles of chlormadinone acetate calculated at 0.5 (Pearl Index), from 131,425 cycles of megestrol acetate calculated at 0.44, and from 57,492 cycles of dimethisterone calculated to be 0.77.

Thus the efficacy for oral sequentials is good, but the Pearl Index is somewhat greater than the Pearl Index of the combination regimen, calculated to be closer to 0.1–0.3.

Table 30.18 Combination of Progestogen Plus Estrogen: Oral, "Step Up" (Women)

d-Norgestrel (Progestogen) First 11 days, μg	Last 10 days, μg	Ethynyl-estradiol (Estrogen): 21 days, μg	Number of Cycles or Months (Subjects)	Bleeding Interval Mean, days	Pregnancies, Pearl Index Method	Use	Reference
50	125	50	1112 (178)	27.8	0	0	Brosens et al. (132)
50	125	50	570 (86)	27–28	0	0	Brosens et al. (133)

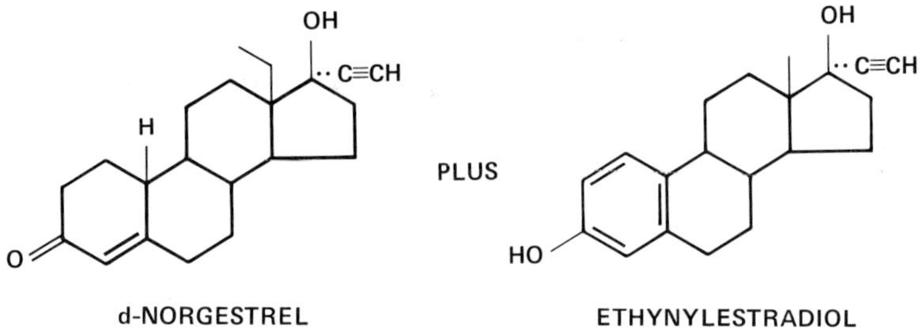

OH
C≡CH
H
O
PLUS
OH
C≡CH
HO
d-NORGESTREL
ETHYNYLESTRADIOL

Fig. 30.10 Combination of progestogen plus estrogen: "step-up," oral (see Table 30.18).

4 ETHYL NORGESTRIENONE

4.1 Single Compound: Oral, Dosage on Days 15, 16, and 17 of Cycle

R-2323 (Fig. 30.14) has been studied as a midcycle contraceptive administered at the level of 50 mg/day on days 15, 16, and 17 of the cycle. The treatment schedule is unique. Antifertility was demonstrated, with good cyclicity.* However use Pearl Indices of 9.5 and 10.1 are unacceptable values (Table 30.21). The method Pearl Indices of 5.0 and 4.6 are better but still excessive. The mean cycle length was 28±2 days in one study and 93% of the cycles were within the cycle lengths of 21–35 days.

* Good cyclicity occurs when treatment does not influence significantly the number of days between successive onsets of the menstrual flow, nor duration of flow.

4.2 Once a Week, Oral

Ethyl norgestrienone (R-2323) is the only compound that has been suggested as a once a week oral antifertility compound. The compound does have antifertility activity (Table 30.22); however the Pearl Index (use) of 8.7 (as one year) for the 5 mg weekly dosage is probably too high to warrant development of R-2323 as a practical contraceptive. The 2.5 mg/week dose was better, since at the lower dosage the Pearl Index (use) was 4.4 for 181 subjects studied for 2971 cycles.

5 PROGESTOGEN: LOW DOSE, CONTINUOUS

5.1 General Remarks

The use of a progestational agent at a low dose level on a continuous schedule has

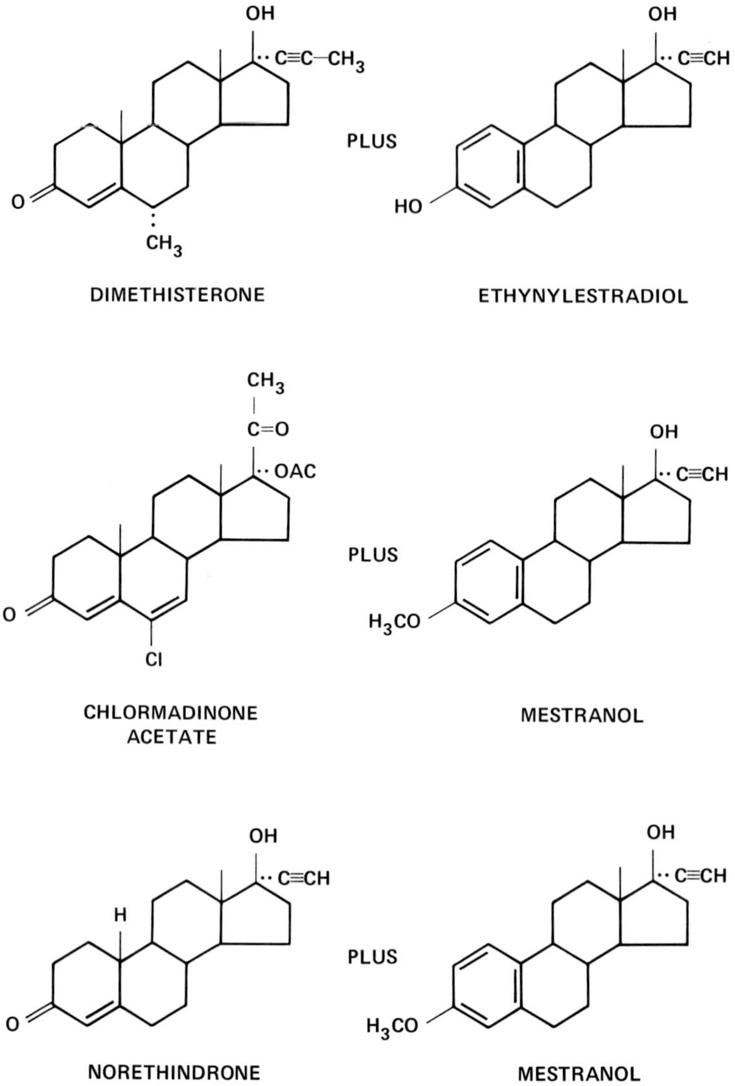

DIMETHISTERONE PLUS ETHYNYLESTRADIOL

CHLORMADINONE ACETATE PLUS MESTRANOL

NORETHINDRONE PLUS MESTRANOL

Fig. 30.11 Progestogen and estrogen for oral sequential treatment (see Tables 30.19, 30.20).

been developed as an effective contraceptive treatment.

The initial studies were done with chlormadinone acetate (9). This treatment affects the hypothalamic–anterior pituitary–ovarian axis minimally, in contrast to combination or sequential therapy, which depends on essentially total suppression of ovulation and endogenous hormone production. The contraceptive efficacy of the low dose continuous therapy appears to be due to a sperm barrier created by a viscous cervical mucus, a hostile endometrium for implantation, and abnormal transport rates for both sperm and ova.

Since the original discovery that 0.5 mg of chlormadinone acetate, on a continuous daily basis, is an effective antifertility agent, other progestogens have been employed with success.

Tables 30.23–30.30 document the data on the cyclicity and Pearl Index resulting

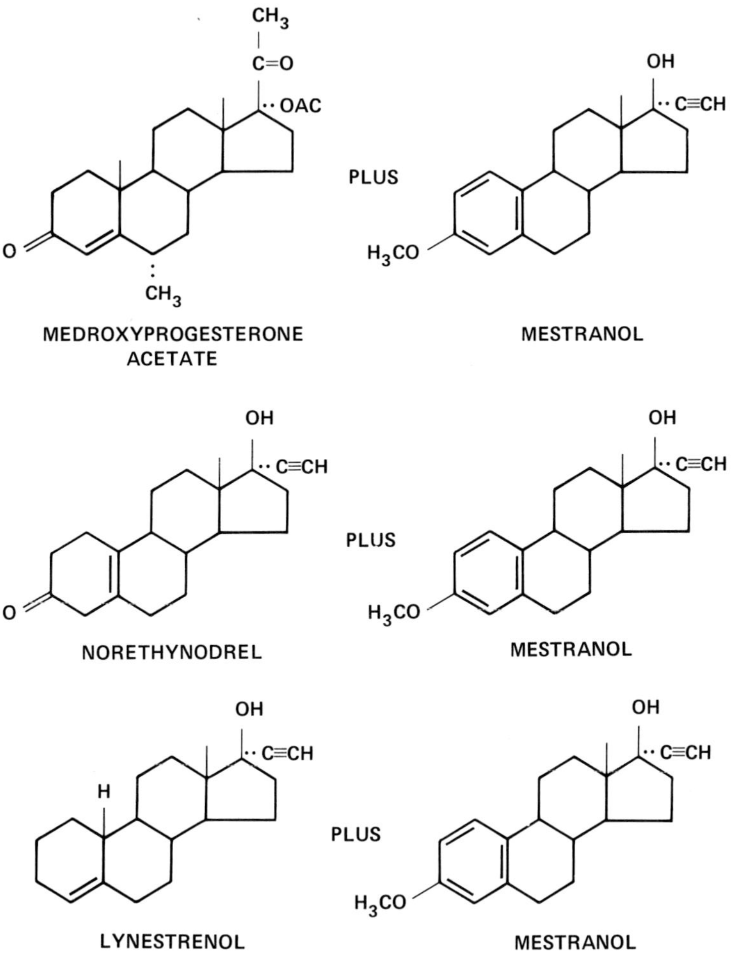

MEDROXYPROGESTERONE ACETATE PLUS MESTRANOL

NORETHYNODREL PLUS MESTRANOL

LYNESTRENOL PLUS MESTRANOL

Fig. 30.12 Progestogen and estrogen for oral sequential treatment (see Tables 30.19, 30.20).

from the use of eight progestational agents as low dose continuous contraceptive agents. These antifertility compounds are chlormadinone acetate, norethindrone, lynestrenol, ethynodiol diacetate, *dl*-norgestrel, *d*-norgestrel, quingestanol acetate, and megestrol acetate (Fig. 30.15).

5.2 Summaries: Low Progestogen Dose, Continuous Therapy

Table 30.31 summarizes the data on six agents. The data for two compounds were too limited for Pearl Index calculation. The overall Pearl Index varied from 0.9 for 55,837 cycles under the effects of lynestrenol to 4.0 for 85,594 cycles studied during administration of chlormadinone acetate. Norethindrone had an overall Pearl Index of 1.8 for 40,205 treated cycles.

At least eight progestational agents can function as antifertility agents at low doses when administered on a continuous basis (Table 30.31).

5.3 Progestogen: Low Dose, 21 Days Treatment-7 Days Off Treatment

Only a single study has been reported using the treatment schedule of 21 days on, 7 off,

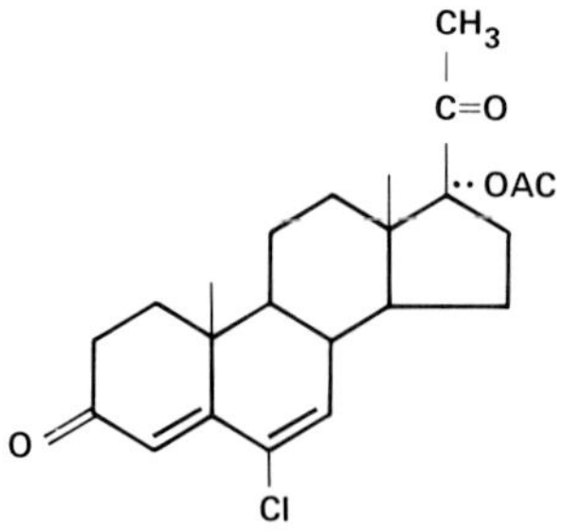

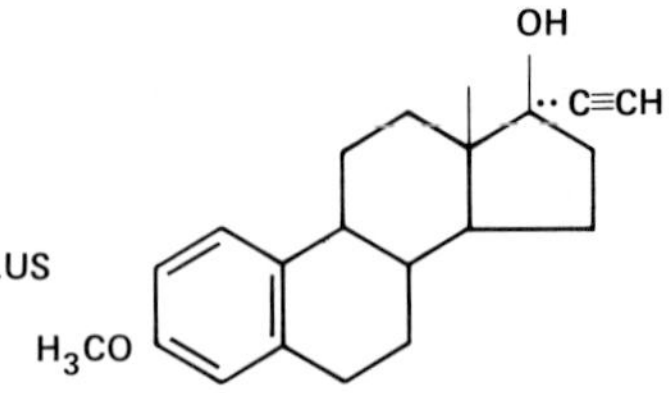

CHLORMADINONE ACETATE PLUS MESTRANOL

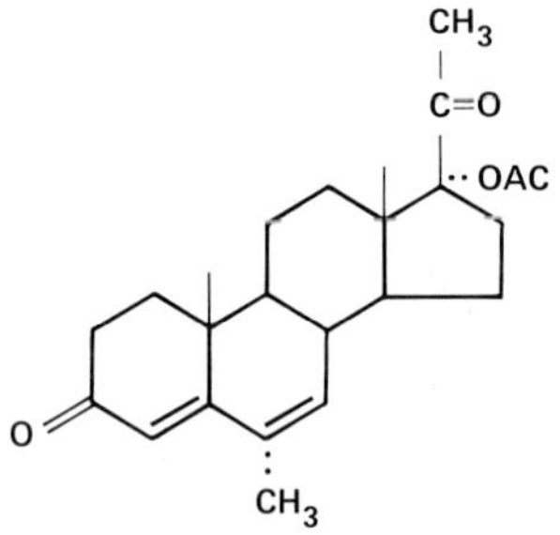

MEGESTROL ACETATE PLUS ETHYNYLESTRADIOL

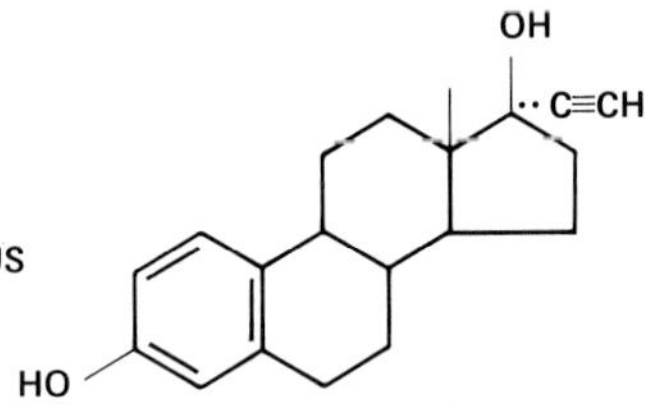

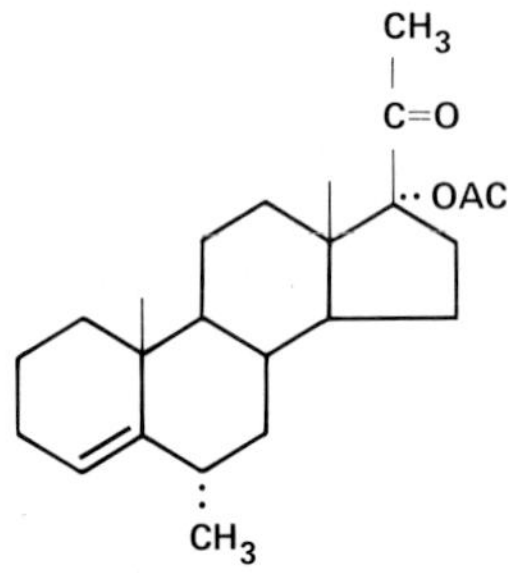

ANGESTERONE ACETATE PLUS MESTRANOL

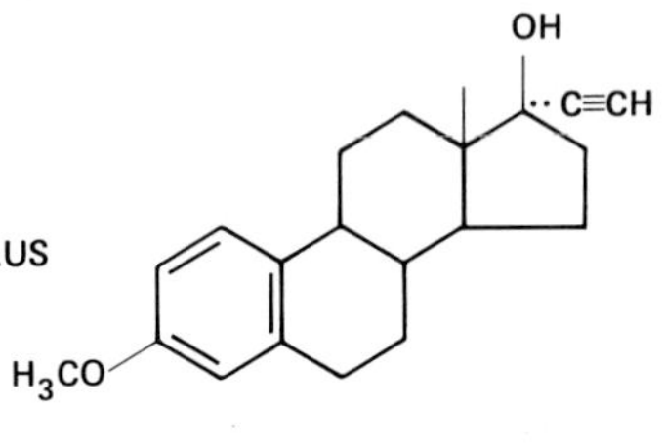

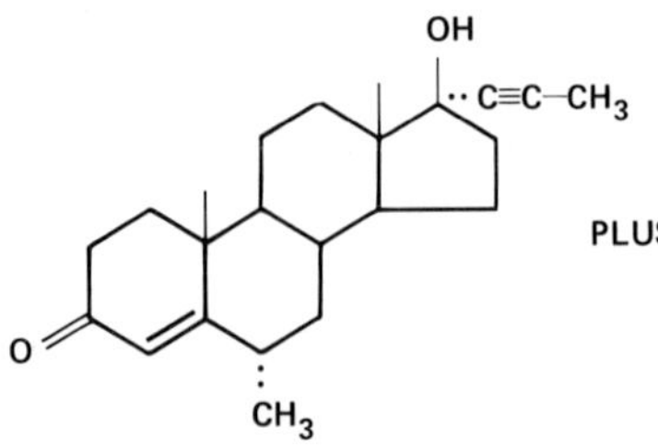

DIMETHISTERONE PLUS ETHYNYLESTRADIOL

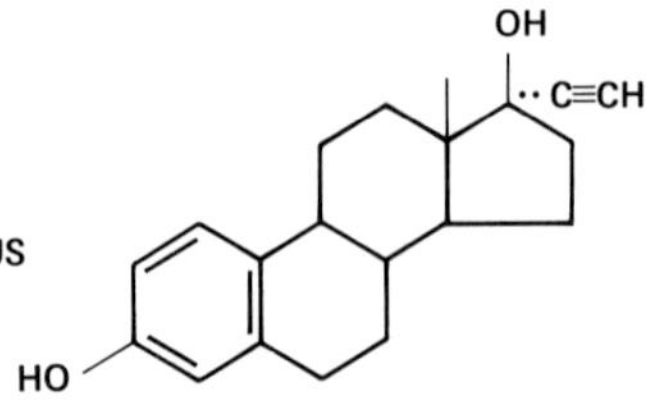

Fig. 30.13 Steroids used for oral sequential treatment (see Tables 30.19, 30.20).

Table 30.19 Sequential Oral Preparations (Women)

Phase I: Estrogen, mg	Phase II		Number of Cycles (Subjects)	I/II Phase, Days	Pregnancies, Pearl Index		Reference
	Estrogen, mg	Progestogen, mg			Method	Use	
Mestranol (0.08)	Mestranol (0.08)	Chlormadinone acetate (2)	11,730 (1191)	15/5	—	1.2	Goldzieher (134)
Mestranol (0.08)	Mestranol (0.08)	Chlormadinone acetate (2)	11,366 (500)	15/5	—	0.8	Rice-Wray (135)
Mestranol (0.08)	Mestranol (0.08)	Chlormadinone acetate (2)	1,513 (113)	15/5	—	3.3	Mears (76)
Mestranol (0.08)	Mestranol (0.08)	Chlormadinone acetate (2)	1,782 (122)	11/10	—	2.7	
Mestranol (0.1)	Mestranol (0.1)	Chlormadinone acetate (2)	534 (65)	11/10	0	0	
Mestranol (0.1)	Mestranol (0.1)	Chlormadinone acetate (2)	358 (97)	14/7	0	0.3	
Mestranol (0.08)	Mestranol (0.08)	Lynestrenol (2)	1,896 (144)	7/15	0	0	Rice-Wray et al. (136)
Mestranol (0.08)	Mestranol (0.08)	Lynestrenol (2)	1,500 (536)	7/15	0	0	Ijzerman (137)
Mestranol (0.08)	Mestranol (0.08)	Lynestrenol (2)	966 (106)	7/15	0	0	Persson et al. (138)
Ethynyl-estradiol (0.1)	Ethynyl-estradiol (0.1)	Megestrol acetate (4)	8,610 (600)	16/5	—	0.5	Mears (76)
Ethynyl-estradiol (0.1)	Ethynyl-estradiol (0.1)	Megestrol acetate (5)	1,006 (88)	16/5	1	0	
Ethynyl-estradiol (0.075)	Ethynyl-estradiol (0.05)	Megestrol acetate (4)	774 (80)	16/5	6	7.5	
Various steroids, 1962–1967			70,000	—	—	0.5	Tietze (6)
Mestranol (0.08)	Mestranol (0.08)	Chlormadinone acetate (2)	8,925 (550)	15/5	0.14	0.14	Tyler et al. (139)
Ethynyl-estradiol (0.05)	Ethynyl-estradiol (0.05)	Lynestrenol (1)	1,048 (125)	7/15	0	0	Brosens et al. (140)
Mestranol (0.08)	Mestranol (0.08)	Chlormadinone acetate (2)	62,343	15/5	—	0.64	Rutensköld (7)
Ethynyl-estradiol (0.1)	Ethynyl-estradiol (0.1)	Megestrol acetate (1)	121,045	—	—	0.40	
Mestranol (0.08)	Mestranol (0.08)	Chlormadinone acetate (2)	24,405 (1399)	15/5	0.10	0.49	Karrer and Smith (141)
Mestranol (0.08)	Mestranol (0.08)	Norethindrone (2)	2,091 (294)	14/6	0	0	Andrews et al. (84)

Table 30.19 (*continued*)

Phase I: Estrogen, mg	Phase II Estrogen, mg	Phase II Progestogen, mg	Number of Cycles (Subjects)	I/II Phase, Days	Pregnancies, Pearl Index Method	Pregnancies, Pearl Index Use	Reference
Ethynyl-estradiol (0.1)	Ethynyl-estradiol (0.1)	Dimethisterone (25)	57,492 (5952)	16/5	0.23	0.77	Sturtevant and Wait (142)
Mestranol (0.08)	Mestranol (0.08)	Norethindrone (2)	5,385 (184)	14/6 or 7	0.2	—	Board (64)
Mestranol (0.08)	Mestranol (0.08)	Anagesterone acetate (1)	405 (91)	14/6	3.0	—	
Mestranol (0.08)	Mestranol (0.08)	Anagesterone acetate (2)	6,721 (270)	14/6	1.2	—	
Mestranol (0.08)	Mestranol (0.08)	Chlormadinone acetate (2)	785 (116)	15/5	0	—	

Table 30.20: Summaries: Sequential Oral Preparations (Women)

Phase I: Estrogen	Phase II Estrogen	Phase II Progestogen	Number of Cycles	Pregnancies, Pearl Index: Use	Reference
Mestranol	Mestranol	Chlormadinone acetate	114,438	0.5	Summary, this chapter
Mestranol	Mestranol	Lynestrenol	5,410	0	Summary, this chapter
Ethynyl-estradiol	Ethynyl-estradiol	Megestrol acetate	131,425	0.44	Summary, this chapter
Ethynyl-estradiol	Ethynyl-estradiol	Dimethisterone	57,492	0.77	Summary, this chapter
Various steroids, 1962–1967			70,000	0.5	Tietze (6)
Mestranol	Mestranol	Angesterone acetate	7,126	1.2	Summary, this chapter

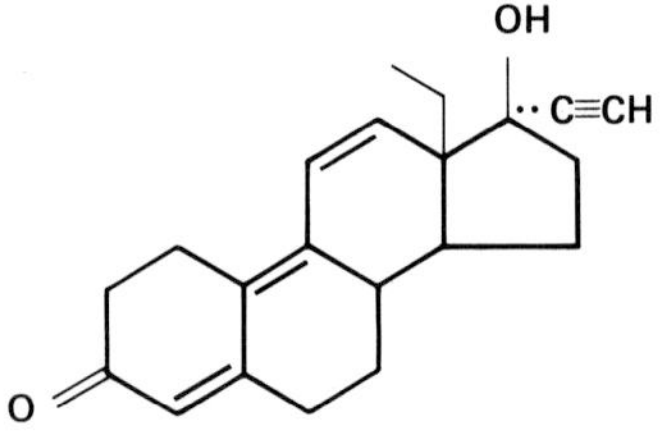

Fig. 30.14 Single compound (R-2323), dosage on days 15, 16, 17 of cycle (see Table 30.21) and single compound (R-2323), administered once a week, orally (see Table 30.22).

Table 30.21 Single Compound: Oral, Dosage on Days 15, 16, and 17 (Women)

Compound	Daily Dosage, mg	Number of Cycles (Subjects)	Cycle Length, days	Pregnancies, Pearl Index		Reference
				Method	Use	
RS-2323	50	2148 (160)	28±2	5	9.5	Azadian-Boulanger et al. (143)
RS-2323	50	1362 (140)	Normal 21–35 days, 93%	4.6	10.1	Sakiz et al. (14I)

Table 30.22 Single Compound: Oral, Once a Week (Women)

Compound	Dosage, mg/week	Number of Cycles or Months (Subjects)	Bleeding Interval, 21–35 days, %	Pregnancies, Pearl Index		Reference
				Method	Use	
R-2323 (13-Ethyl-17-hydroxy-18,19-dinor-17α-pregna-4,9,11-trien-20-yn-3-one); ethyl norgestrienone)	2.5	2971 (181)	56	2.8	4.4	Sakiz et al. (145)
R-2323	5	1944 (292)	51 (first 3 months); decreased to 36, 33, 37 in next 3 months	3.7 (at 1 yr)	8.7 (at 1 yr)	Mora et al. (146)

Table 30.23 Chlormadinone Acetate: Low Dose, Continuous Therapy (Women)

Chlormadinone Acetate: Daily Dose, mg	Number of Cycles or Months (Subjects)	Cycle Lengths, 21–35 Days, %	Pregnancies, Pearl Index		Reference
			Method	Use	
0.5	2,080 (260)	47	5.2	8.6	Howard et al. (147)
0.5	2,021 (194)	—	0.9	1.8	Jeppsson and Kullander (148)
0.5	1,600 (400)	—	0	0	Martinez-Manautou et al. (149)
0.5	771 (117)	—	6.2	9.3	Bergsjö and Koller (150)

Table 30.23 (*continued*)

Chlormadinone Acetate: Daily Dose, mg	Number of Cycles or Months (Subjects)	Cycle Lengths, 21–35 Days, %	Pregnancies, Pearl Index		Reference
			Method	Use	
0.5	7,002 (1328)	66	0.85	1.7	Christie (151)
0.5	3,199 (260)	21–24 weeks 69.2	3.7	4.5	Bernstein and Seward (152)
0.5	189 (40)	60	0	0	MacDonald et al. (153)
0.5	47,232 (2340)	65	—	4.2	Martinez-Manautou (154)
	4,100 Multicenter, UK	—	—	2.6	
	11,800 Multicenter, US (1639)	—	—	2.6	
0.5	5,600 (466)	—	—	4.0	Connell and Kelman (155)

Table 30.24 Norethindrone: Low Dose, Continuous Therapy (Women)

Norethindrone: Daily Dose, mg	Number of Cycles or Months, (Subjects)	Cycle Lengths, 21–35 Days, %	Pregnancies, Pearl Index		Reference
			Method	Use	
0.35	1,888 (154)	57	0.6	1.3	Board (156)
0.35	4,264 (168)	68	1.9	2.5	Board (157)
0.35	2,141 (151)	—	0.6	1.7	Keifer (158)
0.3	4,083 (221)	—	—	1.4	Larsson-Cohn (159)
0.35	3,453 (318)	—	2.1	2.4	McQuarrie (160)
0.35	12,000	—	0.68	1.75	Martinez-Manautou (154)

Table 30.25 Lynestrenol: Low Dose Continuous Therapy (Women)

Lynestrenol: Daily Dose, mg	Number of Cycles or Months (Subjects)	Cycle Lengths, 21–35 Days, %	Pregnancies, Pearl Index		Reference
			Method	Use	
0.5	7,039 (525)	—	0.7	1.2	Kićović et al. (161)
0.5	2,702 (274)	—	0.4	0.9	Prsić and Kićović (162)
0.5	2,442 (102)	—	0	0	Ravn (163)
0.5	3,553 (361)	—	0	0	Ravn (164)
0.5	37,405 (4731)	—	0.6	0.9	Voerman (165)
0.5	1,146 (50)	86	0	0	Rubio-Lotvin et al. (166)
0.5	1,550 (178)	58	1.0	3.1	Foley et al. (167)

Table 30.26 Ethynodiol Diacetate: Low Dose, Continuous Therapy (Women)

Ethynodiol diacetate: Daily Dose, mg	Number of Cycles or Months (Subjects)	Cycle Lengths, 21–35 Days, %	Pregnancies, Pearl Index		Reference
			Method	Use	
0.35	902 (112)	89	—	0	Ruiz-Velasco et al. (168)
0.5	811 (101)	76	—	2.95	
0.25	261 (86)	79	—	0	
0.5	1467 (34)	—	—	0.9	Postlethwaite (169)

Table 30.27 *dl*-Norgestrel: Low Dose, Continuous Therapy (Women)

dl-Norgestrel: Daily Dose, mg	Number of Cycles or Months (Subjects)	Cycle Lengths, 21–35 Days, %	Pregnancies, Pearl Index		Reference
			Method	Use	
0.075	29,006 (2202)	70 (21–45 days)	1.2	2.4	Korba and Paulson (170)
0.0375	770 (99)	46.6	1.6	1.6	Apelo and Veloso (171)
0.050–0.075	2,250 (188)	68 28 ± 5 days	2.0	3.0	Foss et al. (172)

Table 30.27 *(continued)*

dl-Norgestrel; Daily Dose, mg	Number of Cycles or Months (Subjects)	Cycle Lengths, 21–35 Days, %	Pregnancies, Pearl Index		Reference
			Method	Use	
0.075	1,887 (108)	66	1.3	2.0	Eckstein et al. (173)
0.05	2,288 (34)	—	0	0	Foss and Fotherby (174)
0.075	2,767 (290)	—	0.4	1.7	Hernandez-Torres (175)

Table 30.28 ***d*-Norgestrel: Low Dose, Continuous Therapy (Women)**

d-Norgestrel: Daily Dose, mg	Number of Cycles or Months (Subjects)	Cycle Lengths, 21–35 Days, %	Pregnancies, Pearl Index		Reference
			Method	Use	
0.0375	4,273 (565)	—	1.1	2.5	Ferrari et al. (176)
0.05	4,278 (242)	—	0.8	3.6	Foss (177)
0.03	15,393 (1969)	—	0.9	4.3	Scharff (178)
0.03	2,019 (167)	—	0	2.6	Rice-Wray et al. (179)
0.03	5,713 (643)	—	1.0	4.0	Kesserü et al. (180)

Table 30.29 **Quingestanol Acetate: Low Dose, Continuous Therapy (Women)**

Quingestanol Acetate: Daily Dose, mg	Number of Cycles or Months (Subjects)	Cycle Lengths, 21–35 Days, %	Pregnancies, Pearl Index		Reference
			Method	Use	
0.3	11,892 (1148)	—	1.5	4.3	Moggia et al. (181)
0.3	4,370 (400)	71	1.9	3.3	Maqueo et al. (182)
0.3	2,489 (181)	87	1.9	1.9	Rubio et al. (183)
0.3	3,208 (382)	—	0.9	2.9	Jubhari et al. (184)

Table 30.30 Megestrol Acetate: Low Dose, Continuous Therapy (Women)

Megestrol Acetate: Daily Dose, mg	Number of Cycles or Months (Subjects)	Cycle Lengths, 21–35 Days, %	Pregnancies, Pearl Index		Reference
			Method	Use	
0.25 mg Tablets	415 (131)	80	—	14.3	Avendaño et al. (185)
0.5 mg Tablets	1290 (238)	76	—	4.4	
0.25 mg Oil capsules	570 (146)	79	—	13.6	
0.5 mg Oil capsules	599 (152)	72	—	1.03	
0.5 mg Oil capsules	2938 (335)	69.9	1.2	6.1	Casavilla et al. (186)

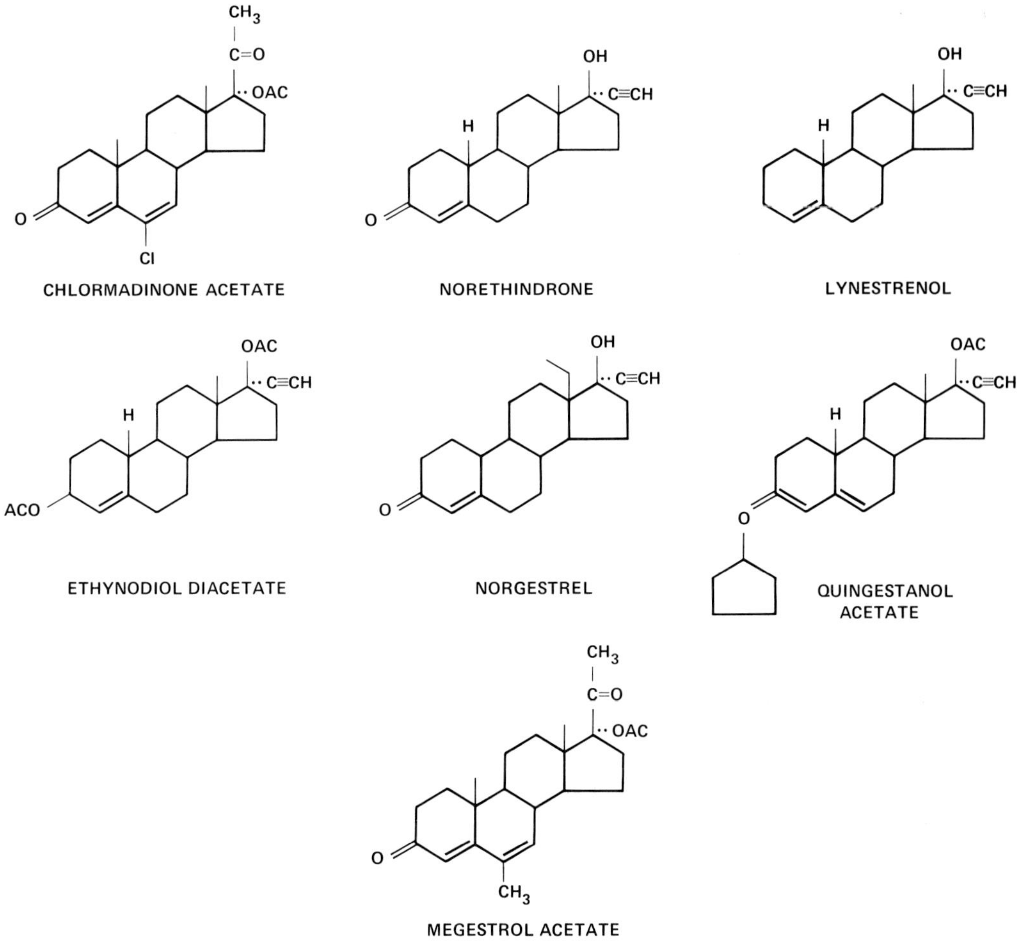

CHLORMADINONE ACETATE

NORETHINDRONE

LYNESTRENOL

ETHYNODIOL DIACETATE

NORGESTREL

QUINGESTANOL ACETATE

MEGESTROL ACETATE

Fig. 30.15 Progestogens used for low dose, continuous therapy (see Table 30.31).

Table 30.31 Summaries: Low Progestogen Dose, Continuous Therapy (Women)

Progestogen	Total Number of Cycles	Pearl Index, Use	Reference
Chlormadinone acetate	85,594	4.0	Summary, this chapter
Norethindrone	40,205	1.8	Summary, this chapter
Lynestrenol	55,837	0.9	Summary, this chapter
Ethynodiol diacetate	3,441	—[a]	
dl-Norgestrel	38,968	2.0	Summary, this chapter
d-Norgestrel	31,676	3.4	Summary, this chapter
Quingestanol	21,959	3.2	Summary, this chapter
Megestrol acetate only, use of 0.5 mg dose	4,827	—[a]	

[a] Number of cycles too small for calculation of Pearl Index.

Table 30.32 Progestogen, Low Dose: 21 Days on Treatment, 7 Days off Treatment (Women)

d-Norgestrel: Daily Dose, mg, for 21 Days Starting on Day 5 of Cycle	Number of Cycles (Subjects)	Cycle Lengths, 21–35 Days %	Cycle, Length days	Pearl Index: Use (Method)	Reference
0.5	218 (33)	63	33.5 ± 12.9	0 (0)	Roland et al. (187)
1.0	284 (55)	87	39.9 ± 9.5	0 (0)	
1.5	181 (28)	79	33.3 ± 13.5	0 (0)	
2.0	23 (9)	71	31.3 ± 6.8	0 (0)	

and Table 30.32 shows that Pearl Indices of zero were reported for all four concentrations of *d*-norgestrel used. Further studies employing this regimen are needed to test the possibility that the 7 day interruption is responsible for so dramatic an improvement in efficacy.

6 PROGESTOGEN ONLY: SINGLE INJECTION, LONG ACTING

6.1 Progestogen–Norigest (Norethindrone Enanthate): 84 days, 200 mg

Progestational agents, particularly medroxyprogesterone acetate and norethindrone enanthate (Table 30.33), may be used for fertility control by injection; the structures of these compounds appear in Fig. 30.16. For example, 150 mg of medroxyprogesterone acetate injected once every 3 months (Table 30.34) or 300 mg delivered at 6 month intervals (Table 30.35) and norethindrone enanthate injected every 84 days are highly effective contraceptive schedules. The mechanism of action is similar to that attributable to low dose continuous daily progestogen treatment.

El-Mahgoub and Karim (10) studied 171 women who received an injection of 200 mg of norethindrone enanthate every 84 days. No pregnancies were reported during 4329 months of the trial. Acceptable cycle control occurred in 46.4–71.4%

Table 30.33 Single Injection of Progestogen (Norethindrone Ethanate, 200 mg) Every 84 Days (Women)

Number of Cycles	Number of Subjects	Pearl Index	Reference
21,730	2177	0.88	Kesserü-Koss et al. (188)
4,391	520	2.3	Chinnatamby (11)
4,329	171	0	El-Mahgoub and Karim (10)

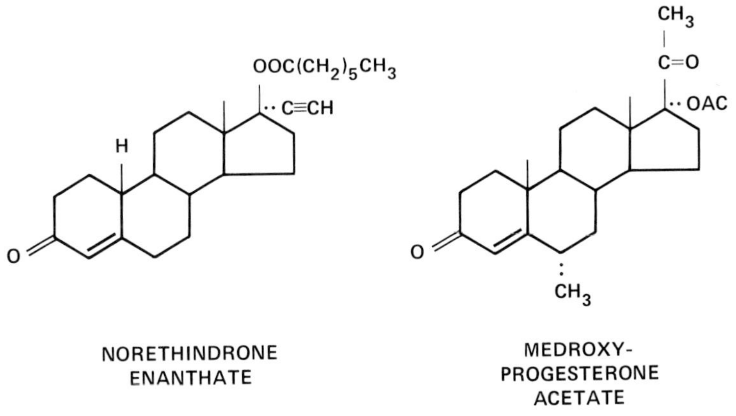

NORETHINDRONE ENANTHATE

MEDROXY-PROGESTERONE ACETATE

Fig. 30.16 Long-acting progestogens (see Tables 30.33–30.35).

of treatment months. Acceptability of cycle control increased with time. A relatively normal menstrual pattern was reestablished in 2–4 months, and normal cyclic endometrial pattern was regained within 3–6 months after treatment.

Another study deals with 21,730 cycles and gives an overall Pearl Index of 0.88; the highest Pearl Index (2.3 for 4391 cycles) was reported by Chinnatamby (11). The progestogen norethindrone enanthate is an effective antifertility agent when injected once every 84 days.

6.2 Progestogen–Medroxyprogesterone Acetate: 3 months, 150 mg

The data on the contraceptive use of medroxyprogesterone acetate, injected (150 mg) every 90 days, have been summarized (12). Fifteen pregnancies were reported for a total of 72,215 woman-months. The study involved 3857 women who were seen by 54 collaborating investigators. The overall efficacy was recorded as a Pearl Index of 0.25. Drug failures calculated by the life table method were 0.31 for 12 months, 0.37 for 18 months, 0.53 for 24 months, 0.53 for 30 months, and 0.90 for 36–70 months. On cessation of treatment, fertility returned (Table 30.34).

In addition to the summary report of Schwallie and Assenzo (12), more than 350,000 cycles of treatment every 3 months with 150 mg of medroxyprogesterone acetate per injection are reported in Table 30.34. The Pearl Indices are acceptable. In only one study of 24,399 cycles was a Pearl

Table 30.34 Single Injection of Progestogen (Medroxyprogesterone Acetate, 150 mg) Every 3 Months (Women)

Number of Cycles	Number of Subjects	Pearl Index	Reference
72,215	3,857	0.25	Schwallie and Assenzo (14)
750	90	0	Sajadi et al. (189)
30,734	1,883	0.04	Dodds (190)
2,490	250	0.48	Nunez (191)
5,009	690	0.72	Linthorst et al. (192)
24,399	886	1.2	Koetsawang et al. (13)
12,819	1,507	0.09	Leiman (193)
38,714	7,335	0.35	Bloch (194)
4,671	231	0	El-Mahgoub et al. (195)
18,261	1,000	0.02	Chinnatamby (196)
2,621	374	0	Tyler et al. (120)
10,110	752	0.12	Seymour and Powell (197)
14,001	1,123	0.09	Powell and Seymour (198)
9,109	226	0	Apelo et al. (199)
4,959	650	0.23	Scutchfield et al. (200)
5,067[a]	650	0.23	
4,677	584	0.77	Brat (201)
38,599	1,883	0.03	Dodds (202)
975	100	0	Mishell et al. (203)
4,128	298	0.29	Soichet (204)
2,514	214	0	Tyler (205)
22,000	561	0.25	Zañartu and Onetto (206)
4,528	480	0	Zartman (207)
132,000	13,523	0.1	Rall et al. (208)

[a] At 18th month.

Table 30.35 Single Injection of Medroxyprogesterone Acetate Every 6 Months (Women)

Number of Cycles (Dosage, mg)	Number of Subjects	Pregnancies, Pearl Index	References
21,470 (300)	991	1.73	Schwallie and Assenzo (12)
2,385 (300)	300	0.5	Nunez (209)
1,674 (300)	145	3.6	Khan et al. (210)
989 (300)	61	0	Mackay et al. (211)
904 (300)	92	0	El-Mahgoub et al. (212)
43,387 (250)	1099	1.4	Zañartu and Onetto (206)
88,530 (450)	6352	0.49	Rall et al. (208)
826 (400)	76	0	Ringrose (213)

Index greater than 1, and even in this report by Koetsawang et al. (13), the index was 1.2. A mean Pearl Index was calculated to be 0.21, a value that compares favorably with the Pearl Indices associated with the progestogen-estrogen combination for daily oral treatment.

6.3 Progestogen–Medroxyprogesterone Acetate: 6 months, 300 mg

The Pearl Index was 1.73 when 991 patients were treated for a total 21,470 months and the treatment was extended to 300 mg of medroxyprogesterone acetate every 6 months (Table 30.35) (14).

In addition to the study of Schwallie and Assenzo (14), four studies using a dose of 300 mg for 6 months are reported in Table 30.35. These reports total 5952 cycles; the mean Pearl Index is 1.0. The same table records additional studies indicating high efficacy when the dosage was 250, 400, and 450 mg per 6 month dose.

7 POSTCOITAL CONTRACEPTION

7.1 Postcoital Estrogens

Estrogens (see, e.g., Fig. 30.17) are effective postcoital compounds in rabbits (15), in monkeys, (16), and in women (17).

Morris and van Wagenen (16) have summarized their own postcoital studies and those documented in the literature. They conclude that administration of high dosages of estrogens in the postovulatory period appears to be effective, with a Pearl Index of the order of 0.03–0.3. Most of the studies concluded that diethylstilbestrol (DES) at the level of 25–50 mg/day for a minimum of 4 days afforded protection, since 5593 cumulative cycles of exposure resulted in about 0.5% failure.

Table 30.36 summarizes various studies involving diethylstilbestrol and other estrogens. The newer reports confirm the conclusions of the early studies that the therapy is effective and that all estrogens studied possess this type of antifertility activity. The mechanism of action is likely to be the prevention of implantation of a blastocyst.

7.2 Postcoital Progestogen: *d*-Norgestrel

Postcoital estrogens are effective for the prevention of unplanned pregnancies. For these purposes estrogens are useful on a one-time basis. However there exists a need for a postcoital contraceptive agent not involving estrogens but rather a compound that could be used after each sexual contact (i.e., one sexual contact, one postcoital tablet). Thus it was logical to search for a nonestrogen postcoital agent. Two progestogens have been so studied.

Postcoital studies using *d*-norgestrel are summarized in Table 30.37. The report by Kesserü et al. (18) involved a titration of *d*-norgestrel from 0.15–0.4 mg per dose. The highest dose level gave a method Pearl Index of 1.7 for the report on 25,558 cycles. Echeverry and Sarria (19) reported a Pearl Index of zero for 1185 cycles and a dosage of 1 mg of *d*-norgestrel. Moggia et al. (20), at the dosage level of 0.35 mg per contact and for 4282 cycles, reported a method Pearl Index of 0.8. Additional studies are included in Table 30.37. Although the data point to successful postcoital therapy, it should be noted that the number of sexual contacts per month was of the order of 8–10, and the quantity of *d*-norgestrel ingested could be equal to that of the low dose continuous progestogen therapy.

The study of López-Escobar et al. (21) showed a reasonable use Pearl Index of 4.9 at 0.4 mg per dose of *d*-norgestrel, with a mean of 3.2 sexual contacts per cycle. This finding appears to indicate a possible postcoital agent, but the Pearl Index needs improvement.

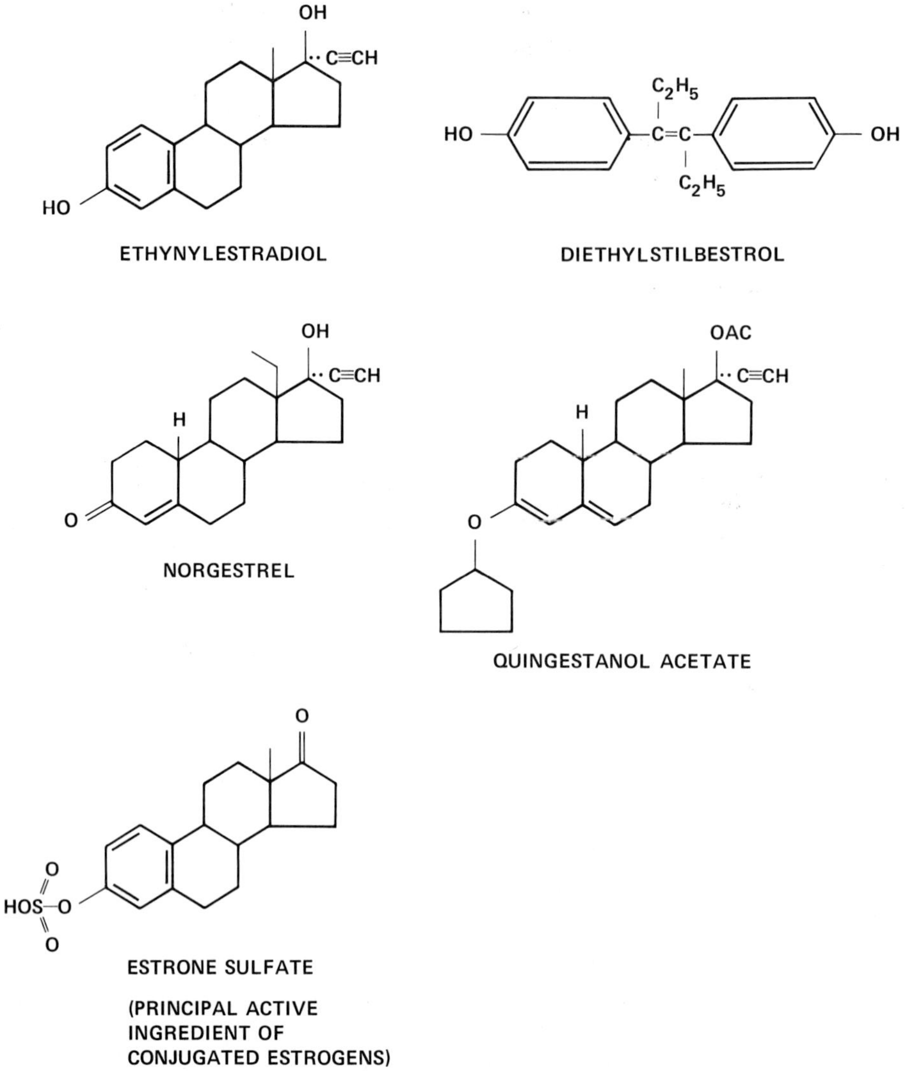

ETHYNYLESTRADIOL

DIETHYLSTILBESTROL

NORGESTREL

QUINGESTANOL ACETATE

ESTRONE SULFATE

(PRINCIPAL ACTIVE INGREDIENT OF CONJUGATED ESTROGENS)

Fig. 30.17 Compounds that appear to be active as postcoital compounds (see Tables 30.36–30.38).

7.3 Postcoital Progestogen: Quingestanol Acetate

Rubio et al. (22) have reported the use of the progestogen quingestanol acetate taken routinely in single doses within 24 hr of coitus as a successful postcoital contraceptive. The Pearl Index was zero for 1004 cycles at the 800 μg dose level. An average of 10.6 doses was taken per menstrual cycle. In view of the relatively large doses used by these workers, it is possible that the mechanism is not really postovulatory but equal to the low dose daily and continuous result (Table 30.38).

Moggia et al. (20) reported a method Pearl Index of 1.7 and a use index of 2.7 for a mean of 8 doses per cycle of quingestanol acetate (Table 30.38). Perhaps this good result is due to the ingestion of the antifertility agent within one hour of coitus.

Table 30.36 Postcoital Estrogens

Compound (Route)	Dosage	Number of Subjects	Pregnancies, Pearl Index	Reference
Ethynylestradiol (oral)	5 mg for 5 consecutive days	2336	2.0	Haspels (214)
Diethylstilbestrol (oral)	50 mg for 5 consecutive days	545		
Diethylstilbestrol (oral)	50 mg for 5 consecutive days	1298	0	Kuchera (215)
Conjugated estrogens (oral)	30 mg/day for 5 consecutive days	194 (follow-up 95%)	0	Crist, quoted by Blye (216)
Conjugated estrogens (oral)	50 mg/day on each of 2 consecutive days	200	0	Yussman, quoted by Blye (217)
Dienoestrol (oral)	2.5 mg 1st day 7.5 mg 2nd day	10	0	Szontagh and Kovacs (218)
Dienoestrol (D), ethynodioldiacetate (E) (oral)	1st day: 2.5 mg D+ 0.2 mg E 2nd day: 5 mg D+ 0.4 mg E	20	0	
Estradiol benzoate	12.5 mg			Haspels et al. (219)
Estradiol phenyl-propionate (injection)	10 mg	150	4 (pregnancies)	
Diethylstilbestrol (oral)	50 mg/day; 4–5 days	96 54	2.1 1.8	Coe (220)
Ethynylestradiol (oral)	1 mg/day for 5 days	32	0	Döring (221)
Diethylstilbestrol (oral)	25–50 mg/day for 5 days followed by 50 mg/day for 5 days	524	0.8	Haspels and Andriesse (222)
Ethynylestradiol (oral)	2.5 mg/day for 5 days followed by 5 mg/day for 5 days	1418	0.7	
Diethylstilbestrol (oral)	25 mg/day for 5 days	1217	0	Kuchera (223)
Ethynylestradiol (oral)	1. 6–10 mg over 3 days 2. 25 mg over 5 days	133	0	Lehfeldt (224)
Diethylstilbestrol (oral)	—	1100	0	Morris and Van Wagenen (16)
Diethylstilbestrol (DES); ethynylestradiol (EE)	25–50 mg DES or 0.5–2.0 mg EE for 5 days	100	0	Morris and Van Wagenen (17)
Diethylstilbestrol; diethylstilbestrol diphosphate; ethynylestradiol; conjugated estrogen	—	750	1.1	Morris and Van Wagenen (16)

Table 30.36 (*continued*)

Compound (Route)	Dosage	Number of Subjects	Pregnancies, Pearl Index	Reference
Diethylstilbestrol (oral)	50 mg/day for 5 days	124	2.4	Rosenfeld et al. (225)
Diethylstilbestrol (oral)	—	257	0	Morris and Van Wagenen (16)
Diethylstilbestrol (oral)	25 mg twice a day for 5 days	80	1.2	Sparrow (226)
Diethylstilbestrol (oral)	25 mg twice a day for 5 days	1000	0	Kuchera (215)

7.4 Postcoital Combination of Progestogen and Estrogen

The postcoital data on a combination of norgestrel and ethynylestradiol are presented in Table 30.39. The study of Yuzpe et al. (23) demonstrated no antifertility activity. This result may be due to the extended time, up to 5 days from coitus to start of steroid treatment. The second study looks more promising, with a Pearl Index of zero. Since the number of cycles was only 68, we must await confirmation.

Table 30.37 Postcoital Progestational Agents: *d*-Norgestrel

Dose, mg (Hours After Coitus)	Number of Cycles or Months	Doses per Cycle or Month	Pregnancies per 100 Woman-Years		Reference
			Method	Use	
0.15 (3)	239	—	30	45	Kesserü et al. (18)
0.25 (3)	8,762	—	3.8	6.2	
0.30 (3)	4,085	8.0	3.8	6.7	
0.35 (3)	3,158	8.0	3.0	3.0	
0.4 (3)	25,558	8.0	1.7	3.5	
1.0 (8)	1,185	—	0	0	Echeverry and Sarria (19)
0.35 (1)	4,282	8.0	0.8	2.2	Moggia et al. (20)
0.6	5,574	—	2.1	6.0	Schering A. G. (227)
0.8	3,688	—	1.6	5.8	
0.7	6,647	—	2.2	4.7	
1.0	3,528	—	0.7	3.4	
1.0	2,578	ca. 10[a]	2.8	6.5	Larrañaga et al. (228)
0.4 (1)	1,557	3.2[a]	—	4.9	López-Escobar et al. (21)

[a] Mean.

Table 30.38 Postcoital Progestational Agents: Quingestanol Acetate

Dose, mg (Hours After Coitus)	Number of Cycles or Months	Doses per Cycle or Month	Pregnancies per 100 Woman-Years		Reference
			Method	Use	
0.5 (24)	927	10.6	—	6.5	Rubio et al. (22)
0.8 (24)	1004	10.6	0	0	
1.5 (1)	4732	8.0	1.7	2.7	Moggia et al. (20)
0.5 (24)	514	11.7	—	11.7	Mischler et al. (229)
0.5 (24)	518	8.9	—	36.0	
0.75 (24)	2388	8.1	—	23.1	
0.75 (24)	1424	—	—	20.2	
1.5 (24)	3355	8.0	—	5.4	
1.5 (24)	1532	12.7	—	0.8	
2.0 (24)	861	7.8	—	1.2	

Table 30.39 Postcoital Combination of Progestogen and Estrogen

Daily Dose, mg (Hours After Coitus)		Number of Cycles	Doses per Cycle or Month	Pregnancies per 100 Woman-Years		Reference
Progestational Agent	Estrogen			Method	Use	
d-Norgestrel, 0.25 × 2	Ethynyl-estradiol, 0.05 × 2 (72)	68	—	0	0	Percival-Smith and Ross (229a)
dl-Norgestrel, (1.0)	Ethynyl-estradiol, 0.100 (120)	148 (143)	1	24	24	Yuzpe et al. (23)

8 PRECOITAL PROGESTOGENS: WOMEN

The study of Zañartu and Oberti (24) (Table 30.40) indicates that precoital oral treatment might be a possible contraceptive but that clogestone at the dose employed is not practical. The Pearl Index for the method was 6 and for use, 17. The report of Cox (25) indicates a reasonable Pearl Index, and on this basis one must consider megestrol acetate as a promising candidate for precoital antifertility development. Figure 30.18 shows the structure of clogestone and of megestrol acetate.

Table 30.40 Precoital Progestational Agents (Women)

Agent	Dose, mg (Hours Between Minimum and Maximum Hours Before Coitus)	Number of Cycles (Subjects)	Pregnancies, Pearl Index		Doses per Cycle	Reference
			Method	Use		
Megestrol acetate	0.5 (4 and 22)	667 (47)	—	5	9	Cos (25)
	0.5 (5 and 10)	468 (26)	0	1	9	
	0.5 (4 and 14)	187 (17)	0	0	9	
Clogestone (6-chloro-3β,17-dihydroxy-4,6-pregnadien-20-one-3,17-diacetate)	1.0 (5–6 hr before coitus)	649 (102)	6	17	Average 6 or more times per cycle	Zañartu and Oberti (24)

CLOGESTONE

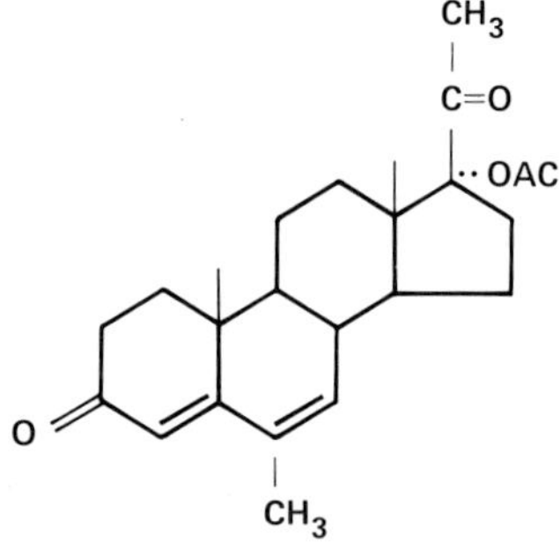

Fig. 30.18 Precoital treatment with progestogens (see Table 30.40).

9 PROSTAGLANDINS AND ABORTION

9.1 Prostaglandins and Abortion: $PGF_{2\alpha}$

Research in the field of abortifacients has accelerated dramatically as a result of changing social and legal attitudes. Scientific advances have occurred in the chemistry, pharmacology, and clinical application of prostaglandins, particularly as related to abortion research. These scientific efforts are aimed at the development of highly effective prostaglandin abortifacients possessing limited and acceptable side effects. The results of these efforts are presented in the Tables 30.41–30.47. The tables give the following information: gestation period, dose, route of administration, interval between induction and abortion, abortion of fetus with retention of placenta (incomplete abortion), abortion of fetus and placenta (complete abortion), vomiting episodes (side effect), and diarrhea (side effect). The compounds are diagrammed in Fig. 30.19.

Table 30.41 deals with the abortifacient activity of prostaglandin $F_{2\alpha}$ ($PGF_{2\alpha}$) and

Table 30.41 Prostaglandins and Abortion: Prostaglandin $F_{2\alpha}$

Gestation, weeks, or as noted	Dose (Route)	Results	Reference
8–20	15 mg in 20 min; the same dosage was repeated (intraamniotic)	1. Induction–abortion interval, 27.2 hr (7–48) 2. 16 of 20 aborted 3. Vomiting, 11 of 20	Brenner et al. (230)
14–19	Total dose varied from 10–124 mg and from 1–12 injections (intraamniotic)	1. Induction–abortion interval, 25 hr (12–51) 2. 9 of 9 aborted, 4 complete 3. Vomiting 2 subjects; 3 and 6 episodes	Bygdeman et al. (231)
16–22	*Group I:* 40 mg; booster of 20 mg at 6 hr, 40 mg at 24 hr p.r.n. (intraamniotic)	1. Induction–abortion interval, 18.1 ± 9.2 hr (S.D.) 2. 19–20 aborted in 36 hr; 14 complete 3. Vomiting, 9 of 20; diarrhea, 4 of 20	Corson and Bolognese (232)
	Group II: 40 mg repeated at 18–24 hr p.r.n. (intraamniotic)	1. Induction–abortion interval, 21.5 ± (10.1) hr (S.D.) 2. 20 of 20 aborted in 36 hr; 11 complete 3. Vomiting, 9 of 20; diarrhea, 2 of 20	
	Group III: 40 mg; 5 IU Pitocin/hr started at 6 hr (intraamniotic)	1. Induction–abortion interval, 15.9 ± 7.0 hr (S.D.) 2. 28 of 28 aborted in 36 hr; 21 complete 3. Vomiting, 9 of 28; diarrhea, 4 of 28	
	Group IV: 40 mg and laminaria tent; Pitocin, 10 IU/hr started at 6 hr (intraamniotic)	1. Induction–abortion interval, 16.1 ± 7.8 hr (S.D.) 2. 23 of 26 aborted in 36 hr 3. Vomiting, 8 of 26; diarrhea, 2 of 26	
16–21	Total dose 10–60 mg; 1–7 injections (intraamniotic)	1. Induction–abortion interval, 22.3 ± 8.7 hr (S.D.) 2. 35 of 35 aborted in 36 hr; 26 of 35 complete 3. Nausea, vomiting, and diarrhea "occurred in only 50% of the patients and were infrequent, late, and mild"	Anderson et al. (233)
11–14	Various (extra-amniotic, intra-amniotic, intravenous)	Serum progesterone and estradiol-17β decreased in a manner found during normal parturition or spontaneous abortion	Widholm et al. (234)

Table 30.41 (*continued*)

Gestation, weeks, or as noted	Dose (Route)	Results	Reference
Mean duration of amenorrhea, 40.2 days or 12 days after missed menstruation day	5 mg of $PGF_{2\alpha}$ over a 30 min period perfused into the uterine cavity; pretreatment with meperidine hydrochloride, atropine, and diazepam, i.m.	1. Mean onset of bleeding, 5.7 hr range 3–9 hr 2. All 100 patients aborted 3. 30% had 1 or more episodes of vomiting	Ragab and Edelman (235)
10–15	33–148 mg total dose (i.v. infusion)	1. Induction–abortion interval, 25 hr (8–31.5) 2. 10 of 10 aborted; 9 complete 3. Side effects in all patients; diarrhea, 5 of 10	Gillett et al. (236)
13–20	25 mg and 4–5 hr later 15 mg (intraamniotic)	1. Induction–abortion interval, 23 hr (6–83) 2. 46 of 50 aborted 3. Nausea, 26%; vomiting, 44%; diarrhea, 8%	Vaalamo and Tervilä (237)
	0.5 mg/dose given 5 times at 1–2 hr (extraamniotic)	1. Induction–abortion interval 40 hr (7–144) 2. 30 of 51 aborted 3. Nausea, 23%; vomiting, 33%; diarrhea, 2%	
14.7 ± 0.6 S.E. (12–16)	Up to 200 μg/min (i.v. infusion)	1. Abortion: 3 complete, 3 incomplete, 4 failures 2. All patients had nausea, vomiting, and diarrhea	Csapo et al. (238)
14–24	5–25 mg total dose (intraamniotic)	1. Induction–abortion interval, 28 hr (12–51) 2. 33 of 37 aborted; 16 complete 3. Vomiting, 1.4 episodes/patient; diarrhea, 0.8 episodes/patient	Toppozada et al. (239)
Pregnant; last period was 34–40 days prior to therapy	Total dose, 200–1100 mg (intravaginally)	1. Complete abortions, 3 of 9 2. Significant changes in steroid levels, 3 of 9 3. Time of onset of bleeding, 3.5–10 hr 4. Significant side effects such as vomiting and diarrhea, 7 of 9	Corlett et al. (240)
First trimester abortion; gestation 9.3 ± 0.4 weeks	10 mg (extraovular injection)	1. Decrease in plasma progesterone and estradiol-17β 2. 6 of 10 absorted completely in an average of 8 hr	Csapo et al. (241)

Table 30.41 *(continued)*

Gestation, weeks, or as noted	Dose (Route)	Results	Reference
11.9 ± 0.3	Total mean dose, 12.3 ± 0.9 mg (extraovular space)	1. Induction–abortion interval, 17.4 ± 1.6 hr 2. 19 of 20 aborted; 13 complete 3. Plasma progesterone decreased from 29.4 ± 2.5 to 12.8 ± 1.6 ng/ml	Csapo and Kivikoski (242)
Mean menstrual delay, 12 days	2.5 mg as a 7×2 mm pellet (intrauterine)	Uterine contractions started in few minutes; pregnancy test negative in 10 days	Csapo and Mocsary (243)
12–18	50 mg (intraamniotic injection)	1. Mean fall in progesterone, 55.7% 2. Mean fall in estradiol-17β, 46.6% 3. Highly significant correlation between decrease in both steroids and the instillation–abortion interval 4. Induction–abortion interval varied from 10.5 to 21.75 hr; mean 16.3 hr 5. 10 of 10 aborted in 24 hr	Tyack et al. (244)
16.2 ± 0.5	10 mg, then at 3 hr intervals 5 mg; total dose, 31.5 ± 3.2 mg (intraamniotic injection)	1. 7 of 10 aborted completely 2. Mean induction–abortion interval, 15.1 ± 1.8 hr	Csapo et al. (245)
12.3 ± 1.1	Initial dose, 8.1 ± 0.8 mg augmented by an average of 4 mg (extraamniotically injected)	1. 10 of 10 patients aborted; 7 completely 2. Mean induction–abortion interval, 10.9 ± 2 hr 3. Plasma estradiol-17β and progesterone decreased continuously	Csapo et al. (246)
16–19	75 mg (intraamniotic injections)	1. Induction–abortion interval, (6 hr, 58 min to 26 hr, 50 min); mean, 16 hr 2. 8 of 10 aborted in 24 hr	Craft et al. (247)

Plasma Steroid Levels

Hormone	Mean μg/100 ml (SE)	
	Preinjection	At 6 hr
Progesterone	3.1 ± 0.24	2.10 ± 0.30
17α-Hydroxy-progesterone	0.37 ± 0.05	0.30 ± 0.04
Estrone	0.46 ± 0.09	0.36 ± 0.07
Estradiol-17β	0.42 ± 0.08	0.31 ± 0.07
Estriol	0.21 ± 0.03	0.06 ± 0.02

Table 30.41 *(continued)*

Gestation, weeks, or as noted	Dose (Route)	Results	Reference
Early pregnancy: 12±1 (SE) after missed period	5 mg (intrauterine dose)	1. 20 of 22 aborted completely 2. Abortion score, 95 3. Side effects were infrequent, mild, and acceptable	Csapo et al. (248)
13–19	Initial dose of 500 μg followed by 2 mg at 15 min and 2 mg at 30 min; at 30 min $PGF_{2\alpha}$ was administered by pump at 67 μg/min; at 24 hr procedure stopped (continuous extra ovular)	1. Mean induction–abortion interval, 16.2 hr 2. 74 of 76 aborted; 82% in less than 24 hr; 72 were complete 3. Nausea, 6 of 76 (0.1 episodes/patient); vomiting, 17 of 76 (0.5 episodes/patient); diarrhea, 7 of 76 (0.3 episode/patient)	Lauersen and Wilson (249)
12–26	Varied: 25, 40, 50, 75 mg (single intra-amniotic)	1. Dose, mg — Success Within 48 hr, 25 — 64 40 — 89 50 — 97 75 — 93 2. Authors suggested dose, 40–50 mg 3. Side effects may be a problem at 70 mg; much less at 40–50 mg 4. Mean induction–abortion intervals, 17.4 and 20.4 hr, respectively, for nulliparous and multiparous	Hendricks et al. (250)
7 Volunteers, normal cycle	Total dose, 14–37.5 mg (i.v. infusion); duration, 5–7.5 hr	1. Progesterone fell markedly 2. Total estrogen declined slightly 3. Vaginal spotting occurred 2 days after the infusion 4. All had side effects, mostly GI	Hillier et al. (251)
8–12	Total 200 mg (vaginal pessaries)	1. Some degree of cervical dilatation in 8 of 10 patients, but useful only in multiparous patients 2. Side effects of uterine cramps, a flushed sensation, and the presence of diarrhea were relatively common	Craft (252)
14–22	25 mg (intraamniotic injection)	1. Mean induction–abortion interval, 40 hr (5–75) 2. 10 of 10 aborted; 5 complete in 75 hr	Symonds et al. (253)

Table 30.41 *(continued)*

Gestation, weeks, or as noted	Dose (Route)	Results	Reference
Early pregnancy, $n = 40$ Group 1, $n = 25$ Received 10 mg prochlorperazine on request; gestation, mean, 18.3 weeks Group 2, $n = 15$: Received 10 mg prochlorperazine 30 min before PG; gestation, mean, 17.4 hr	50 mg single dose (intraamniotically)	1. Incomplete abortion: group I, 24%; group II, 33% 2. Complete abortion, 68% 3. Induction–abortion interval, 19.1 hr 4. No serious complications	Brenner et al. (254)
10.8 ± 0.4	2–4 mg/hr; total dose 29.1 ± 3.9 mg (extraovular infusion)	1. 7 of 12 complete abortions; 2 incomplete 2. Induction–abortion interval, 9.4 ± 1.5 hr 3. Vomiting, 5 of 12 4. At the time of abortion, progesterone levels decreased to 14.6 ± 2.4 ng/ml; estradiol-17β to 0.4 ± 0.1 ml	Csapo et al. (255)
9–22	50 μg/min (i.v.)	1. Induction–abortion interval range, 4.3 ± 27.2 hr 2. 14 of 15 aborted in 28 hr; 13 complete 3. Vomiting, 3 of 15; diarrhea, 7 of 15	Karim and Filshie (256)
12–20	—	see subtable below	Aleem et al. (257)
6–11	100–2900 μg total dose (intrauterine)	1. Induction–abortion interval, 13 hr (8–17)	Roberts et al. (258)

Aleem et al. (257):

Abortion (Weeks)	n	Placental Progesterone, μg/g
Dilatation and suction	5	5.22 ± 0.31
Intraamniotic instillation of $PGF_{2\alpha}$ (12–14)	6	1.53 ± 0.14
(15–17)	3	1.50 ± 0.14
(18–20)	5	1.28 ± 0.21

Table 30.41 *(continued)*

Gestation, weeks, or as noted	Dose (Route)	Results	Reference
		2. 13 of 20 aborted in 24 hr; 0 of 20 complete 3. Vomiting, 1 of 20; Nausea, 4 of 20	
12–16	Total dosage, 0.75–42 mg over 12 hr period (i.v.)	1. Mean induction–abortion interval, 15.5 hr 2. 8 of 10 aborted; 4 complete 3. Nausea and vomiting, 10 of 10; diarrhea, 5 of 10	Cantor et al. (259)
10–23	25 mg repeated 6, 24, and 30 hr after first treatment (intraamniotic)	1. Mean induction–abortion interval, 18.9 hr 2. 21 of 22 aborted in 48 hr 3. Nausea and vomiting, 45%; diarrhea, 5%	Brenner et al. (260)
10–23	50 mg repeated after 24 hr (intraamniotic)	1. Mean induction–abortion interval, 23.8 hr 2. 23 of 24 aborted in 48 hr 3. Nausea and vomiting, 62%; diarrhea, 25%	
10–23	25 mg every 6 hr (intra-amniotic)	1. Mean induction–abortion interval, 21.5 hr 2. 24 of 25 aborted in 48 hr	
10–20	40 mg in a 5 min period (intraamniotic)	1. Mean induction–abortion intervals: 18.6 hr (multiparous); 32.2 hr (nulliparous) 2. 28 of 30 in 48 hr 3. Nausea and vomiting, 40%; diarrhea, 0%	Corlett and Ballard (261)
13–45	3 mg every 1–3 hr (extraovular)	1. Mean induction–abortion interval, 17.8 hr 2. 19 of 20 aborted in 48 hr 3. Nausea and vomiting, 45%	Shapiro (262)
14–20	40 mg in 5 min; 20 mg at 24 hr if needed (intra-amniotic)	1. Mean induction–abortion intervals: 21.6 hr (multi-parous), 24.3 hr (nulliparous) 2. 111 of 116 aborted in 48 hr	Duenhoelter et al. (263)
14–20	40 mg in 5 min; 20 mg after 24 hr if needed; laminaria tent and oxytocin (intraamniotic)	1. Mean induction–abortion interval, 16.2 hr 2. 99 of 100 aborted in 48 hr 3. Nausea and vomiting and diarrhea not clinically significant	Robins et al. (264)

Table 30.41 (*continued*)

Gestation, weeks, or as noted	Dose (Route)	Results	Reference
13–20	240 μg at start and 750 μg 2 hr later (extraovular)	1. Mean induction–abortion interval, 24 hr 2. 41 of 50 aborted in 48 hr 3. Nausea and vomiting, 18%; diarrhea, 0%	Himmelman et al. (265)
11–17	Dilute solution every 1 hr; total 0.5–1.2 g (intravaginally)	1. 1 of 5 aborted completely in 10.4 hr 2. Vomiting, 2 of 5; diarrhea, 1 of 5	Brenner et al. (266)
	Concentrated solution every 1 hr; total 0.3–1.2 g (intravaginally)	1. 6 of 9 aborted in 24 hr; 5 complete 2. Mean Induction-abortion interval, 11.5 hr (6–24) 3. Vomiting, 8 of 9; diarrhea, 5 of 9	
	Concentrated solution every 2 hr; total 0.55 g (intravaginally)	1. 3 of 8 aborted in 24 hr; all incomplete 2. Induction–abortion interval, 22.9 hr 3. Vomiting, 6 of 8; diarrhea 3 of 8	
	Vaginal tablets every hr; total dose (0.1–0.6 g) (intravaginally)	1. 4 of 6 aborted in 24 hr; 2 complete 2. Mean induction–abortion interval, 19.4 hr 3. Vomiting, 4 of 6; diarrhea, 2 of 6	
	Vaginal suppository every 2 hr; total dose (0.25–0.6 g)	1. 6 of 8 aborted in 24 hr; 3 complete 2. Mean induction–abortion interval, 13.6 hr 3. Vomiting, 10 of 10; diarrhea, 10 of 10	
7–13	Administration limited to 8 hr for 7–8 weeks gestation; total dose varied (2.5–5.7 mg, extraamniotic)	1. Induction–abortion interval, a. ca. 5–10 hr for patients 7–8 weeks b. 17.5 hr for 9–12 weeks c. 24.2 hr for 13 weeks 2. 55 of 60 aborted; 21 complete 12 hr 3. Vomiting, 1 episode	Wiqvist et al. (267)
6–8	Dose range 20–300 μg/min (i.v. infusion)	1. 6 of 6 completely aborted in 48 hr 2. Bleeding starting 4–7 hr 3. Vomiting, 2 of 7; diarrhea, 2 of 7	Wiqvist and Bygdeman (268)

Table 30.41 *(continued)*

Gestation, weeks, or as noted	Dose (Route)	Results	Reference
12–16	Dose range, 20–360 μg/min (i.v. infusion)	1. 4 of 6, complete inhibition 2. Bleeding starting 3–31 hr 3. Vomiting, 1 of 6	
15.7 ± 1.2 (S.E.)	40 mg (intraamniotic)	1. Mean induction–abortion interval, 20.1 ± 11.7 hr 2. 54 of 61 aborted; 10 complete 3. Nausea and vomiting, 19 of 61; diarrhea, 6 of 61	Elder (269)
Mainly 15–20; a few 13, 14, 21, and 22	25 mg at start and at 6 hr later (intra-amniotic)	1. Mean induction–abortion interval, 19.7 hr 2. 614 of 717 (86%) aborted within 48 hr; 439 of 717 (61%) aborted within 24 hr; 408 aborted completely in 48 hr 3. Diarrhea, 109 (15.2%), 0.4 episode/patient; vomiting, 384 (53.6%), 1.5 episodes/patient	WHO Study (270)
Mean of 11 days past expected menses; range, 5–17 days	Total dose, 300–700 mg in solution (intra-vaginally)	1. 6 of 8 aborted completely 2. vomiting, 1.1 episodes/patient; diarrhea, 0.6 episode/patient	Bolognese and Corson (271)
16–20	Range 40–180 mg; mean 88.8 ± 55.7 mg (S.D.) (intravaginally)	1. Mean induction–abortion interval, 12.7 ± 5.7 hr (S.D.) 2. 40 of 40 aborted in 36 hr; 21 complete 3. Vomiting and/or diarrhea, 30 of 40	Bolognese and Corson (272)
15.9 ± 0.6	Single dose 24.3 ± 1.1 mg (intraamniotic)	1. Induction–abortion interval, 16.5 ± 2.1 hr 2. 20 of 20 aborted completely (however 8 women had retained small placental residues) 3. Nausea, 3 of 20; vomiting, 4 of 20; diarrhea, 1 of 20	Saldana et al. (273)
16.8 ± 0.3 (13–20)	25 ± 1.13 mg (intra-amniotic)	1. Induction–abortion interval, 17.4 ± 1.22 hr 2. 47 of 50 aborted in 30 hr; 34 complete 3. Nausea and vomiting, 11; diarrhea, 5	Saldana et al. (274)
16–20	PGF_2: 15 mg (intra-amniotic); oxytocin (i.v. infusion); laminaria tent	1. Mean induction–abortion interval, 7 hr, 25 min (1 hr, 55 min–20 hr, 10 min) 2. 20 of 20 aborted in 24 hr	Engel et al. (275)

Table 30.41 (*continued*)

Gestation, weeks, or as noted	Dose (Route)	Results	Reference
		3. Vomiting, 13 episodes, 6 of 20 patients	
16–20	40 mg; single administrations over a 10 min period (intraamniotic)	1. Mean induction–abortion interval, 16.2 hr 2. 18 of 20 aborted in more than 24 hr; 17 complete 20 of 20 aborted; 17 complete 3. Nausea; 5 of 20 (7 episodes); vomiting, 11 of 20 (27 episodes); diarrhea 4 of 20 (8 episodes)	Lauersen and Wilson (276)
16 (14–19)	30 and 15 mg at 24 hr 15 mg at 42 hr if necessary (intra-amniotic infusion)	1. Induction–abortion interval, 24 ± 12 (S.D.) hr 2. 10 of 10 aborted in more than 24 hr 3. Estrone, estradiol-17β, and estriol levels fell to about half the preinfusion interval	Shutt et al. (277)
Group I, 11–16	25–200 μg/min (i.v.)	1. Mean induction–abortion interval, 10 hr 2. 2 of 5 aborted in 18 hr 3. Emesis, 5 of 5	Brenner (278)
Group II, 11–20	Progressive doses at specified times (i.v.)	1. Mean induction–abortion interval, 14 hr 2. 4 of 5 aborted in 18 hr 3. Emesis, 4 of 5	
Group III, 7–15	25 μg/min for 0.5 hr, maintained at 50 μg until abortion; maximum of 18 hr (i.v.)	1. Mean induction–abortion interval, 10 hr 2. 5 of 5 aborted 3. Emesis, 2 of 5	
14–20	5 + 35 mg repeated with 20 mg if needed (intraamniotic)	1. Induction–abortion intervals: multigravida, 25 hr; 51 min; primigravida, 29 hr, 31 min 2. 106 of 122 aborted in 48 hr 3. 70 uncomplicated 4. Nausea or vomiting, 29.5%	Duenhoelter and Gant (279)
10–26	80–100 μg/min until abortion (i.v.)	1. Average induction–abortion interval 10 hr 2. Progesterone levels in plasma did not respond in a uniform manner; Some patients showed decreases; in others drop occurred after abortion had taken place	Lehmann et al. (280)

Table 30.41 (*continued*)

Gestation, weeks, or as noted	Dose (Route)	Results	Reference
8–17	6 Patients 1. 25–250 μg/min over 12 hr 2. Rest 12 hr 3. Reinfuse if needed, or i.v. infusion 9 Patients 1. 50–100 μg/min over 24–33 hr 2. No reinfusion	1. 6 of 15, complete abortion 2. 3 of 15, incomplete abortion and required dilatation and curettage 3. 6 failed to abort in spite of strong uterine contraction and required dilatation and curettage 4. Nausea with vomiting and/or diarrhea, 11	Kirshen et al. (281)
12–22	0.5 mg at start, 0.5 mg at 5 min, 2.0 mg at 20 min, 2.0 mg at 50 min (extraovular)	1. Mean induction–abortion intervals; 13.4 hr (multiparous), 10.4 hr (nulliparous) 2. 55 of 60 aborted in 48 hr 3. Nausea and vomiting, 20%	Hodgson and Van Gorp (282)

cites many of the individual studies. These reports on $PGF_{2\alpha}$ are summarized in Table 30.42 on the basis of the percentage of treated patients that showed partial and complete abortion. Some reports do not separate the results with respect to partial and complete abortions.

Total abortions due to $PGF_{2\alpha}$, partial plus complete, accounted for 74–90% of the treated patients. This means that 10–26% of the patients did not abort, either partially or completely.

In each category of administration, the percentage of complete abortions was greater than the percentage of the partial abortions. Complete abortions varied from 47

Table 30.42 Summaries of Routes of Administration of Prostaglandins $F_{2\alpha}$ to Induce Abortion

Gestation, weeks	Route	Number of Patients	Number Aborted (%) Partial	Complete	Partial Plus Complete
10–24	Intraamniotic	1692	—	—	1525 (90)
10–24	Intraamniotic	1199	375 (31)	690 (58)	1065 (89)
11–20	Intravenous	72	—	—	60 (83)
10–16	Intravenous	42	8 (18)	26 (62)	34 (81)
7–22	Extraamniotic	212	—	—	185 (87)
7–20	Extraamniotic	92	42 (46)	47 (51)	89 (97)
6–14	Intrauterine	42	13 (31)	20 (48)	33 (79)
2–20	Intravaginal	93	25 (27)	44 (47)	69 (74)

Table 30.43 Prostaglandins and Abortion: Prostaglandin E_2

Gestation, weeks	Dose (Route)	Results	Reference
12–22	3.5–9.5 mg total; initial rate, 2.5 μg/min (i.v.); supplemented with oxytocin	1. Mean induction–abortion interval, 16 hr 2. 19 of 19 aborted in 24 hr; 13 complete 3. Vomiting, 13 of 14	Coltart and Coe (283)
9–28	260–6650 μg total dose over 21–24 to 60 hr (i.v. infusion)	1. Induction–abortion interval, 21.6 hr (6–60) 2. 28 of 30 aborted in 36 hr; 23 complete 3. Vomiting, 5 of 30	Embrey (284)
35–47 days since last menses	20 mg at 2 hr intervals; total dose, 80–120 mg (intravaginal)	1. Induction–abortion interval, 22 hr (7–54) 2. 7 of 10 aborted in 54 hr; 5 complete 3. Nausea, vomiting, and diarrhea were observed but not quantitated	Freid et al. (285)
16.7 ± 0.7 (S.E.)	Mean total dose, 57.3 ± 5.5 mg (intravaginal)	1. Induction–abortion interval, 12.6 ± 2.3 (S.E.) hr 2. 9 of 15 aborted 3. Vomiting, 11 of 15; diarrhea, 4 of 15	Schulman et al. (286)
16.0 ± 0.6 (S.E.)	Mean total dose 70.0 ± 6.1 mg (intravaginal) plus contraceptive diaphragm	1. Induction–abortion interval, 12.8 ± 2.3 (S.E.) hr 2. 16 of 16 aborted 3. Vomiting, 4 of 16; diarrhea, 2 of 16	
5–24	5–25 μg/min (i.v.)	1. Induction-abortion interval, 18 hr 2. 130 of 139 aborted in 48 hr; 105 complete 3. Nausea and/or vomiting, 50 of 139; diarrhea, 9 of 139	Karim and Filshie (287)
9–22	5 μg/min (i.v. infusion) until abortion was complete	1. Mean induction–abortion interval, 14.8 hr 2. 50 of 52 aborted in 48 hr; 43 complete 3. Nausea, 6 of 52; vomiting, 7 of 52; diarrhea, 3 of 52	Karim and Filshie (288)
8–27	10 mg suppository repeated after 1 hr, then 20 mg every 2 hr until abortion (intravaginal)	1. Mean induction–abortion intervals; 10.8 hr (multiparous), 13.2 hr (nulliparous) 2. 70 of 71 aborted in 48 hr 3. Nausea and vomiting, 50%; diarrhea, 18%	Lauersen et al. (289)

Table 30.43 *(continued)*

Gestation, weeks	Dose (Route)	Result	Reference
12–26	1.5 mg (extraovular)	1. Mean induction–abortion intervals: 11.3 hr (multiparous), 15.8 hr (nulliparous) 2. 24 of 24 aborted in 48 hr 3. Nausea and vomiting, 29%	Mackenzie et al. (290)

Table 30.44 Prostaglandins and Abortion: Comparisons

Compound	Gestation, weeks, or as noted	Dose (Route)	Results	Reference
PGE_2 $PGF_{2\alpha}$	Women who have passed their expected menstruation day by 2–7 days (intravaginal route) 8 of 12 had positive pregnancy test	PGE_2 total dose, 5–40 mg; 1–60 mg (intravaginally) $PGF_{2\alpha}$ total dose, 6–100 mg (intravaginally)	1. 1 of 6 aborted with infusion 2. One week later 5 of 6 had negative pregnancy tests 3. Bleeding started 1–6 hr after PG treatment 1. One week later, all 6 had negative pregnancy tests 2. Bleeding started 1–24 hr after PG treatment	Karim (291)
PGE_1 PGE_2	9–28	Total dose 2–5 mg (i.v. infusion) 2–5 μg/min	1. Mean induction–abortion interval, 19 hr (10–28) 2. 10 of 11 aborted; 8 complete 3. No side effects	Embrey (292)
PGE_2 $PGF_{2\alpha}$	7–23	*PGE_2*: 50 mg every 2 hr until labor was established (intravaginal) *$PGF_{2\alpha}$*: 50 mg every 2 hr until labor was established	1. Mean induction–abortion interval, 13.2 hr 2. 45 of 45 aborted in 24 hr? 40 completely 3. Vomiting, 6 of 45; diarrhea, 1 of 45	Karim and Sharma (293)
PGE_2 $PGF_{2\alpha}$	13–17	*Total dose PGE_2*: 2.5–7.5 mg (mean 4.6 mg) *Total dose $PGF_{2\alpha}$*: 15.0–22.5 (mean, 17.7 mg) (extraamniotic)	1. *PGE_2*: induction–abortion interval, 5 hr, 40 min, to 21 hr, 55 min (mean, 11 hr, 35 min). *$PGF_{2\alpha}$*: induction–abortion interval, 9 hr, 50 min, to 26 hr, 20 min (mean, 17 hr, 38 min)	Lippert and Modly (294)

Table 30.44 *(continued)*

Compound	Gestation, weeks, or as noted	Dose (Route)	Results	Reference
			2. 14 of 14 aborted completely in 24 hr (PGE_2); 6 of 6 aborted in 24 hr; 2 completely ($PGF_{2\alpha}$) 3. Vomiting, 5 of 14 (PGE_2); 0 of 6 ($PGF_{2\alpha}$)	
PGE_2	Mean delay in menstruation 10.5 (6–14) days, $n=2$	1 mg (intrauterine instillation)	Pregnancy Terminated 1. Mean uterine bleeding onset, 4.2 hr 2. Mean negative pregnancy test, 9.2 days (7–14)	Karim (295)
$PGF_{2\alpha}$	Mean delay in menstruation, 9.2 (7–14) days	4 mg (intrauterine instillation)	Pregnancy Terminated 1. Mean uterine bleeding onset, 4.1 hr 2. Mean negative pregnancy test, 7.3 days (5–10)	
$PGF_{2\alpha}$	Midtrimester abortion; composite of many studies, 2000 cases	First hr, 10 mg–50 (intraamniotic)	Efficacy, 91.4% in 30–36 hr; complete abortions, 80.2%; side effects: fleeting vomiting, 57.1%; diarrhea, 16.1%; infection, 0.5%	Southern and Gutknecht (296)
$PGF_{2\alpha}$	Midtrimester abortion; composite of many studies, 454 cases	doses 3.5–7.0 or more (extra-amniotic; between fetal membranes and uterine wall)	Efficacy, 82.8%; complete abortion, 72.6% with an initial dose of 3.5 mg and repeat at 2–4 hr. An efficacy of 98.2% can be anticipated. Incidence of vomiting and diarrhea lower than intraamniotic	
PGE_2	Midtrimester abortion; composite of many studies, 454 cases	Mean dose 96.1 mg (vaginal)	Mean time to abortion, 17.2 hr; efficacy, 82%; complete abortion, 52%; side effects: vomiting, 50%; diarrhea, 40%; headache, 20%	
PGE_2 $PGF_{2\alpha}$	1st and 2nd trimesters	*PGE_2*: 200 μg repeated at 1 or 2 hr; *$PGF_{2\alpha}$*: 750 μg repeated at 1 or 2 hr (extra-amniotic)	1. Mean induction–abortion interval, 22.4 hr 2. 94 aborted in 48 hr 3. Nausea, 4 of 94; vomiting, 25 of 94 (0.2 episode/patient); diarrhea, <0.01 episode	Embrey et al. (297)

Table 30.44 (*continued*)

Compound	Gestation, weeks, or as noted	Dose (Route)	Results	Reference
$PGF_{2\alpha}$	Midtrimester abortion	Suppositories, $PGF_{2\alpha}$-50 mg (intravaginally)	1 of 10 aborted in 10 hr	Béguin et al. (298)
PGF_2	Midtrimester abortion	Suppositories PGE_2-20 mg (intravaginally)	7 of 10 aborted in 10 hr	
16,16-Dimethyl-PGE_2-methyl ester	14–30	Mean total; 7.2 mg; 100 μg dose at 2 hr in-intervals (0.3–1.2) (oral)	1. Induction–abortion interval, 17 hr (12–28) 2. 7 of 11 aborted in 28 hr; 4 complete 3. Nausea, vomiting, and diarrhea, 11 of 11	Karim et al. (299)
16,16-Dimethyl-PGE_2	13–18	Mean total, 6.4 mg (0.2–1.8) 100 μg dose at 2 hr intervals (oral)	1. Induction–abortion interval, 16.7 hr (6–38) 2. 5 of 9 aborted in 38 hr; 2 complete 3. Nausea, 9 of 9; vomiting, 7 of 9; diarrhea, 7 of 9	
15-Methyl-$PGF_{2\alpha}$	8–24	350–500 μg at 2 hr intervals until abortion was achieved. Total drug varied from 0.9–8.4 mg (i.m.) All patients received prophylactic Lomotil® to reduce diarrhea. Prochlorperazine was used for severe and protracted bouts of vomiting; i.m. pentazocine for analgesia at patients' request.	1. Mean time to abortion 15.7 ± 6.5 (S.C.) hr 2. Complete abortion, 63% 3. Vomiting, 89% 4. Frequent GI side effects 5. Diarrhea, 89%	Bolognese and Corson (300)
15-Methyl-$PGF_{2\alpha}$ and 15-methyl PGE_1	Abortion	15-Methyl $PGF_{2\alpha}$: 350–500 mg at 2 hr intervals (i.m.)	Patients Receiving 15-Methyl-$PGF_{2\alpha}$	Patients Receiving 15-Methyl-PGE_1
		15-Methyl PGE_1: 20 mg at 4 hr	Induction–abortion interval: 15.7 ± 6.5	14.2 ± 6.3

Table 30.44 (*continued*)

Compound	Gestation, weeks, or as noted	Dose (Route)	Results			Reference
		intervals (vaginal suppositories)	(hr, ±S.D.)			
			Abortion			
			Complete	52	57	
			Incomplete	28	22	
			Failure	0	1	
			Side effects			
			Vomiting, (episodes)	89	74	
			Diarrhea (episodes)	89	23	
			Temperature ≥101.6°F	18	59	
$PGF_{2\alpha}$	13–16	250–750 μg every 2–4 hr (extra-ovular)	1. Mean induction–abortion interval, 21 hr 2. 36–40 aborted in 36 hr 3. Nausea and vomiting, 1.5 episodes/patient; diarrhea, 1.5 episodes/patient			Wiqvist et al. (301)
15-Methyl-$PGF_{2\alpha}$	13–16	500–850 μg, single instillation	1. Mean induction–abortion interval, 13.6 hr 2. 46 of 55 aborted in 36 hr 3. Nausea and vomiting, 1.5 episodes/patient; diarrhea, 1.5 episodes/patient			
$PGF_{2\alpha}$	10–14	3.5 and 3.8 mg total dose (intrauterine)	1. Induction–abortion intervals, 19 and 18 hr 2. 2 of 2 complete abortions 3. Diarrhea, 1 of 2			Embrey and Hillier (302)
PGE_2	6–20	1.2 mg total dose (intrauterine)	1. Induction–abortion interval, 18 hr (7.5–33) 2. 12 of 13 aborted in 34 hr; 9 complete 3. Vomiting, 0.17 episode; diarrhea, 0 episode			
$PGF_{2\alpha}$	13–16	37–158 mg total dose (i.v. infusion)	1. Induction–abortion interval, 11.6 hr (8.5–19.5) 2. 5 of 6 aborted in 24 hr 3. Vomiting, 5 of 6; diarrhea, 1 of 6			Kaufman et al. (309)
PGE_2	13–16	4.0–12.8 mg total dose (i.v. infusion)	1. Induction–abortion interval, 9.0–16.5 hr 2. 3 of 4 aborted in 24 hr; 1 of 4 complete 3. Vomiting, 2 of 4; diarrhea, 2 of 4			

Table 30.44 *(continued)*

Compound	Gestation, weeks, or as noted	Dose (Route)	Results	Reference
15(*S*)-15-Methyl-PGE_2-methyl ester	13–16	25 μg at 8 hr intervals (i.m.)	1. Induction–abortion interval, 10.5–18 hr 2. 3 of 3 aborted in 18 hr; all complete 3. Nausea and vomiting, 0 of 5; diarrhea, 0 of 5	Karim et al. (304)
	7–10	25 of 50 μg at 8 hr intervals (i.m.)	1. Induction–abortion interval, 6–14 hr 2. 5 of 5 aborted in 14 hr; 3 complete 3. Diarrhea, 1 of 5; nausea and vomiting, 0 of 5	
	?	50 μg every 8 hr until abortion (intravaginal)	1. Induction–abortion interval, 7–20 hr 2. 6 of 6 aborted in 20 hr; 5 complete 3. Vomiting, 1 of 6; diarrhea, 1 of 6	
15(S)-methyl-PGE_2	7–15	250 or 500 μg/dose, from 1 to 3 doses (i.m.)	1. Induction–abortion interval, 10–28 hr 2. 5 of 5 aborted in 28 hr; 3 complete 3. Vomiting, 3 of 5; diarrhea, 5 of 5	
	13–18	0.5 mg/dose, 1–3 doses (intravaginal)	1. Induction–abortion interval, 9–29 hr 2. 6 of 6 aborted; 5 complete 3. Vomiting, 3 of 6; diarrhea, 3 of 6	
	13–16	0.5 mg every 16 hr (intra-amniotic)	1. Induction–abortion interval, 8–32 hr 2. 6 of 6 aborted; 5 complete 3. Nausea and vomiting, 2 of 6; diarrhea, 0 of 6	
PGE_2	12–16	2.5–20 μg/min over 3.5 hr; if no abortion by 12 hr, additional PG treatment (i.v. infusion)	1. Induction–abortion interval, 20.9 (9–18) 2. 10 of 10 aborted in 38 hr; 7 complete 3. Vomiting, 10 of 10; diarrhea, 10 of 10	Hillier and Embrey (305)
$PGF_{2\alpha}$	15–16	25–200 μg/min over 3.5 hr; if no abortion by 12 hr, additional treatment (i.v. infusion)	1. Induction–abortion interval, 28.2 hr (10–49) 2. 10 of 10 aborted; 7 complete 3. Vomiting, 7 of 10; diarrhea, 5 of 10	

Table 30.44 (*continued*)

Compound	Gestation, weeks, or as noted	Dose (Route)	Results	Reference
15-Methyl-$PGF_{2\alpha}$	16.2	Single dose, 1.0 mg (intra-amniotic)	1. Induction–abortion interval, 20.1 hr 2. 6 of 13 aborted; 4 complete 3. Vomiting, 0.4 episode/patient; diarrhea, 0	Wiqvist et al. (306)
	16.7	Single dose, 2.5 mg (intra-amniotic)	1. Induction–abortion interval, 18.8 hr 2. 49 of 50 aborted; 25 complete 3. Vomiting, 1.5 episodes/patient; diarrhea, 0.1 episode/patient	
	17.7	Single dose, 5.0 mg (intra-amniotic)	1. Induction–abortion interval, 18.6 hr 2. 38 of 40 aborted; 25 complete 3. Vomiting, 2.0 episodes/patient; Diarrhea, 0.3 episode/patient	
$PGF_{2\alpha}$	16.6	Single dose, 40 mg (intraamniotic)	1. Induction–abortion interval, 18.5 hr 2. 25 of 33 aborted; 11 complete 3. Vomiting, 3.3 episodes/patient; diarrhea, 0.2 episode/patient	
15-Methyl-$PGF_{2\alpha}$	15.6	Mean, 6.1 mg; 1–2 mg every 6th hr until abortion (intravaginal)	1. Mean induction–abortion interval, 24.5 hr 2. 7 of 10 aborted in 24 hr; 3 complete 3. Vomiting, 1.9 episodes/patient; diarrhea, 1.3 episodes/patient	Bygdeman et al. (307)
15-Methyl-$PGF_{2\alpha}$-methyl ester	15.0	Mean 3.0 mg; 1.2 mg every 6th hr until abortion (intravaginal)	1. Mean induction–abortion interval, 18.4 hr 2. 9 of 10 aborted in 24 hr; 5 complete 3. Vomiting, 2.4 episodes/patient; diarrhea, 3.0 episodes/patient	
15-Methyl-$PGF_{2\alpha}$-methyl ester	15.7	Mean, 8.5 mg; 0.5 mg followed by 1 or 2 suppositories 1 mg every 3rd hr (intravaginal)	1. Induction–abortion interval, 16.4 hr 2. 9 of 13 aborted; 5 complete 3. Vomiting, 2.6 episodes/patient; diarrhea, 0.4 episode/patient	
15-Methyl-$PGF_{2\alpha}$	15.2	Mean, 2.007 mg/ 0.2–0.5 ng/ injection; mean of 5.5 injections (i.m.)	1. Mean induction–abortion interval, 16.1 hr 2. 30 of 30 aborted; 12 complete 3. Vomiting, 4.7 episodes/patient; diarrhea, 0.7 episode/patient	

Table 30.45 Summaries of Routes of Administration of Prostaglandins E_2 to Induce Abortion

Gestation, weeks	Route	Number of Patients	Number Aborted (%)		
			Partial	Complete	Total
3–27	Intravaginal	621	—	—	526 (85)
3–27	Intravaginal	509	143 (28)	281 (55)	424 (83)
1–28	Intravenous	260	48 (19)	193 (73)	241 (92)
12–26	Extraamniotic	38	—	—	38 (100)

Table 30.46 Prostaglandins and Abortion: 15-Methyl-PGF$_{2\alpha}$-Methyl Ester

Gestation, weeks, or as noted	Dose (Route)	Results	Reference
13–27 days (mean 20 days) menses delay	1 (Group I) to 1.5 (group II) mg suppository administered every 3rd hr (intravaginal)	1. *Complete abortion at* 1 *week:* group I, 3 of 20; group II, 2 of 20. *Complete abortion at* 2 *weeks:* group I, 14 of 20; group II, 16 of 20 2. Vomiting, mean 2.9 episodes, diarrhea, mean 5.6 episodes	Ylikorkala et al. (308)
Mean days since last menstrual period, 44.6	Long-acting vaginal device, 0.5% PG for 24 hr	1. 2.8 hr onset of bleeding; 13 days of bleeding 2. 5 of 5 aborted 3. Vomiting, mean 0.4 episode; diarrhea, mean 2.2 episodes	Bygdeman et al. (309)
Mean days since last menstrual, period 46.8	One-half of long-acting vaginal device, 0.5% PG for 24 hr	1. 5 hr onset of bleeding; 11.2 days of bleeding 2. 5 of 5 aborted 3. Vomiting, mean 1.8 episodes; diarrhea, 0	
Mean days since last menstrual period 41.5	Mean dose, 3.9 mg over 9–12 (intravaginal)	1. 4.4 hr onset of bleeding; 10.5 days of bleeding 2. 50 of 50 aborted 3. Vomiting, mean 0.7 episode; diarrhea, mean 0.7 episode	
12–21	*Group A* ($n = 35$): intravaginal silastic device, 0.5% PG, 24 hr	Gestation, weeks — Induction–Abortion interval, hr: 13–14 — 17.7±4.7 15–16 — 16.5±9.5 17–18 — 10.0±3.1 19–20 — 11.0±3.7 31 of 35 aborted in about 24 hr Nausea and vomiting, 27 episodes; diarrhea, 32 episodes	Lauersen and Wilson (310)

Table 30.46 (*continued*)

Gestation, weeks, or as noted	Dose (Route)	Results	Reference
	Group B ($n = 35$): intravaginal silastic device, 1.0% PG, 24 hr	Gestation, weeks / Induction–Abortion Interval, hr: 12 or less — 13.0±10.7 13–14 — 15.2±9.7 15–16 — 10.5±5.5 17–18 — 21.7±7.1 19–20 — 30 (one) 32 of 35 aborted in about 28 hr Nausea and vomiting, 74 episodes; diarrhea, 73 episodes	
10–20	Long-acting vaginal device, 0.5% PG, in place until aborted	1. Induction–abortion interval, 11.4±5.3 (S.D.) hr 2. 23 of 26 complete and incomplete abortions 3. Nausea and vomiting, 14 of 26; diarrhea, 14 of 26	Dillon et al. (311)
10–20	Long-acting vaginal device, 1.0% PG, in place until aborted	1. Induction–abortion interval, 13.5±7.5 (S.D.) hr 2. 24 of 24 complete and incomplete abortions 3. Nausea and vomiting, 17 of 24; diarrhea, 14 of 24	
Up to 3 weeks following 1st missed menstrual period (group I); $n = 45$, outpatient basis)	1 mg followed by either 1 or 1.5 mg every 3rd hr for a total of 3 or 4 mg administered over 12 hr (vaginal suppository); mean dose, 4.1 mg; range, (2.5±6.0 mg)	Terminated in 100% of early cases; 10 of 45 were not pregnant Bleeding (hr): Pregnant / Nonpregnant Onset — 6.2 / 5.2 Duration — 9.4 / 6.2 Vomiting, 0.5 episode/patient; diarrhea, 0.5 episode/patient	Bygdeman et al. (312)
Last menstrual period, 31-43 days	Total 2.5–5 mg (intravaginal)	1. Terminated 100% of pregnancies (10 of 10) 2. Bleeding of nonpregnant subjects, mean 6.5 days; of pregnant women, mean 8 days 3. Side effects were minimal and "Certainly clinically acceptable"	Bygdeman et al. (313)
12.5 (8–15)	Long-acting silastic vaginal device, 0.5% PG	1. Induction–abortion intervals, 19.6 hr (7–47) 2. 5 of 10 aborted in 48 hr 3. Vomiting, 1.8 mean episodes; diarrhea, 3.1 mean episodes	Hendricks et al. (314)

Table 30.46 *(continued)*

Gestation, weeks, or as noted	Dose (Route)	Results	Reference
12.4 (9–15)	Long-acting silastic vaginal device, 1.0% PG	1. Induction–abortion interval 14.1 hr (5–37) 2. 9 of 10 aborted in 48 hr 3. Vomiting, 2.3 mean episodes; diarrhea, 1.7 mean episodes	
Last menstrual period, 31–49 days	Long-acting silastic device, 0.5% PG; removed 24 hr after initiation of bleeding	1. Induction–abortion interval, 50 min–24 hr, 30 min 2. 9 of 9 aborted within 24 hr 3. Nausea and vomiting, 28 episodes; diarrhea, 24 episodes	Robins (315)
15.6 (9–20)	*Group I*: 250 μg every 2 hr for 24 hr, 500 μg for next 24 hr (i.m.)	1. Induction–abortion interval, 19.0 hr 2. 14 of 20 aborted in 24 hr 3. Vomiting, 5.2 episodes; diarrhea, 6.2 episodes	Gruber et al. (316)
12.9 (8–19)	*Group II:* PG same as group I plus prochlorperazine and Lomotil® (i.m.)	1. Induction–abortion interval, 15 hr 2. 17 of 20 aborted in 24 hr 3. Vomiting, 3.1 episodes; diarrhea, 0.6 episode	
15.1 (11–20)	*Group III:* same PG; same prochlorperazine plus Lomotil® plus laminaria tents (i.m.)	1. Induction–abortion interval, 17.5 hr 2. 14 of 20 aborted in 24 hr 3. Vomiting, 4.2 episodes; diarrhea, 1.2 episode	
10–21	Long-acting (0.5%) vaginal device left in place until aborted or 24 hr	1. Induction–abortion interval, 16.8 hr 2. 9 of 10 aborted in 24 hr 3. Vomiting, 0.7 mean episodes; diarrhea, 1.7 mean episodes	Bygdeman et al. (309)
13–20	Long-acting (1%) vaginal device left in place until aborted or 24 hr	1. Induction–abortion interval, 16.3 hr 2. 9 of 10 aborted in 24 hr 3. Vomiting, 2.4 mean episodes; diarrhea, 1.5 mean episodes	
13–20	Vaginal suppositories, mean, 7.8 mg, dosage every 3rd hr	1. Induction–abortion interval, 12.3 hr 2. 27 of 30 aborted in 24 hr 3. Vomiting, 1.5 mean episodes; diarrhea, 0.4 mean episodes	

Table 30.47 Summaries of Routes of Administration of Prostaglandin 15-Methyl-PGF$_{2\alpha}$ Methyl Ester in Inducing Abortion

Gestation, weeks	Route	Number of Patients	Abortions (%)		
			Partial	Complete	Total
Mean 14.5	Intramuscular	60	—	—	45 (75)
9–13	Intravaginal (device or suppository)	83	32 (39)	50 (60)	82 (99)
3–21	Intravaginal (device or suppository)	407	—	—	381 (94)

to 62% of the treated subjects, and partial abortions varied from 18 to 46% (Table 30.42).

9.2 Prostaglandins and Abortion: PGE$_2$

The antifertility activity of prostaglandin E$_2$ (PGE$_2$) is detailed in Table 30.43, and the comparative abortifacient activity of two or more prostaglandins studied simultaneously is contained in Table 30.44.

Summaries of PGE$_2$ administered by intravaginal, intravenous, and extraamniotic routes are considered in Table 30.45 from the viewpoint of partial and complete abortions attained. Again as for PGF$_{2\alpha}$, a higher percentage of complete than of partial abortions was reported. Complete abortions were 55% for the intravaginal route and 73% for the intravenous route. For partial abortions, the values of 28 and 19% were found for these routes, respectively.

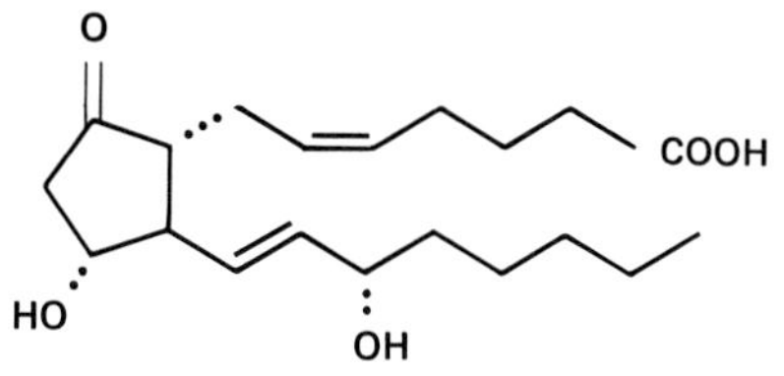

PGE$_2$

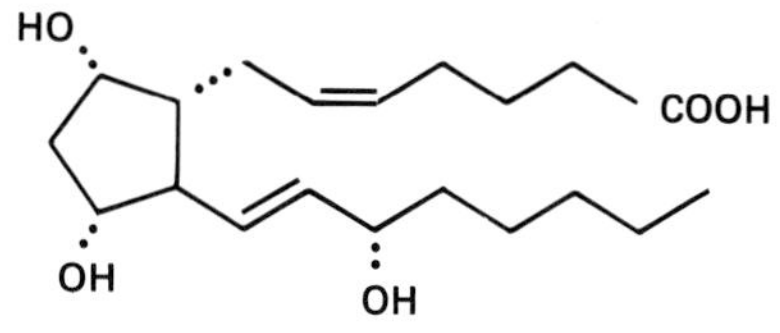

PGF$_{2\alpha}$

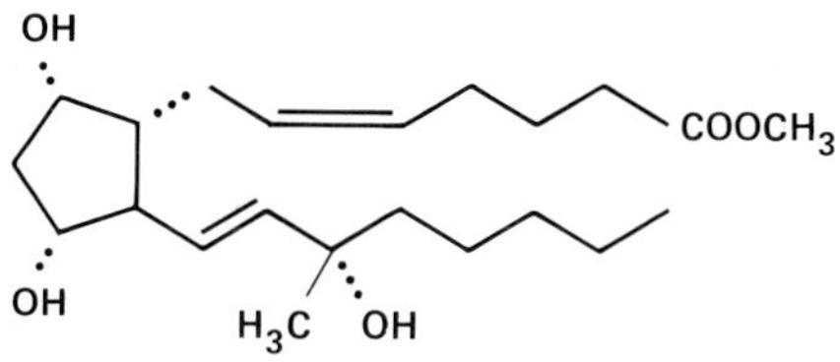

15-METHYL-PGF$_{2\alpha}$-METHYL ESTER

Fig. 30.19 Prostaglandins used to induce abortion in women (see Tables 30.41–30.47).

9.3 Prostaglandins and Abortion: 15-Methyl-$PGF_{2\alpha}$-Methyl Ester

The abortion data on the modified prostaglandin, 15-methyl-$PGF_{2\alpha}$-methyl ester, are recorded in Table 30.46, the summary information appears in Table 30.47. The intravaginal route gave a 99% abortion effectiveness, but only 60% were complete.

10 NONPROSTAGLANDIN ABORTIFACIENTS

Estrogens are abortifacient in various rodents and rabbits. Reports of these studies come from Greenwald (26, 27), from Dreisbach (28), and Selye et al. (29). Table 30.48 lists various nonprostaglandin abortifacients in addition to estrogens. The list

Table 30.48 Nonprostaglandin Abortifacients

Compound	Species (Route)	Results	Reference
Aminopterin	Rat (oral)	1. 0.2 mg/kg, one dose days 9–12 of pregnancy 2. Day 9 of 10, 100% effective; 0–30% effective on day 11 or 12	Murphy and Karnofsky (317)
Aminopterin	Women	1. 8–24 mg/day during 2–5 days to 3–8 weeks pregnancies 2. 10 of 12 women aborted	Thiersch (318)
N,N,N-Triethylenephosphoramide(TEPA)	Rat (i.m.)	1. 3 mg/kg 2. Abortifacient except placenta retained	Thiersch (319)
2,4-Diamino-5 *p*-chlorobenzyl-6-methylpyrimidine (antimalarial)	Rat (i.p., oral)	1. Day 7 treatment 2. Fetal death and resorption	Thiersch (320)
Chloropurine Thrioguanine	Rat (i.p.)	1. Treatment 7 and 8 days 2. 100% abortion	Thiersch (321)
6-Azauridine	Mouse (oral)	1. 0.5 mg/kg daily on days 8 and 9 of pregnancy 2. Abortifacient activity and low maternal toxicity	Sanders et al. (322)
Serotonin (5-HT)	Mouse (s.c.)	1. 2 mg on days 14, 15, or 16 2. Fetal death in 1 hr	Robson and Sullivan (323)
Sodium barbital	Rat (s.c.)	1. Injected days 8–9 of pregnancy 2. Complete resorption in 8 of 12 animals	Champakamalini and Rao (324)
Norethynodrel	Rat (oral)	1. Treatment days 9–13 of pregnancy 2. Terminates pregnancy	Davis (325)
MER-25 MRL-37 MRL-41	Rat (oral)	1. Treatment days 8–12 caused death of some embryos 2. Treatment days 13–17 had no harmful effects	Barnes and Meyer (326)
Clomiphene	Rat (oral)	Treatment from time of implantation had no significant effect on number of fetuses, but only small number delivered normally	Davidson et al. (327)

Table 30.48 *(continued)*

Compound	Species (Route)	Results	Reference
Norethynodrel	Rabbit (oral)	Treatment days 6–8 had no effect	Chang (328)
Oxymetholone; durabolin	Rat (?)	1. 1–5 mg/day starting on day 7 2. Oxymetholone abortifacient; durabolin activity may be due to conversion of durabolin to estrogen	Naqvi and Warren (329)
Chloropromazine	Rat (i.m.)	1. Every 8 hr on days 7 and 8 2. Produced abortion	Chambon (330)
Actinomycin D	Rabbit (i.p.)	1. Treatment between days 6 and 10 of pregnancy 2. Abortion and deformities	Tuchmann-Duplessis and Mercier-Parot (331)
Actinomycin D	Rat (i.p.)	1. Treatment on days 8 and 9 2. Resorbed teratological effects	
Bis(2-bromoethyl)-aminomethyl-4-methoxy-nitrobenzene; bis(2-hydroxyethyl)-aminomethyl-4-ethoxy-nitrobenzene	Rat (oral)	1. Active on treatment days 1–7 and days 1–3 2. Dose 1 mg/day 3. No estrogen data	Garg et al. (332)
Estradiol-17β; ethylestrenol	Rat (oral)	100% Abortion at days 9–13 and 5–19 at daily dose of 10 mg/100 g	Selye et al. (29)
2–(3-Methoxy-phenyl)-5,6-dihydro-*s*-triazole [5,1-*a*]; isoquinoline (L-10503)	Rat, mouse, hamster, rabbit, dog, monkey, baboon, rat	Resorption or expulsion of products of fertilization	Lerner et al. (333)
L-10503	Rat	1. Abortion 2. Primary effect at the utero-placentral level	Lerner and Carminati (334)

includes an antimetabolite (aminopterin), an antimalarial (2,4-diamino-5-*p*-chlorobenzyl-6-methylpyrimidine), serotonin, sodium barbital, weak estrogens (MER 25 and clomiphene), and androgen-anabolic compounds (testosterone, oxymetholone, durabolin); some of these are shown in Fig. 30.20.

Many compounds have antifertility-abortifacient activity, but these drugs usually have serious side effects and use in pregnant women is not possible (Table 30.48). Prostaglandins perhaps offer the most promise for providing for a smooth, minimum side effect interruption of a pregnancy in the first or second trimester.

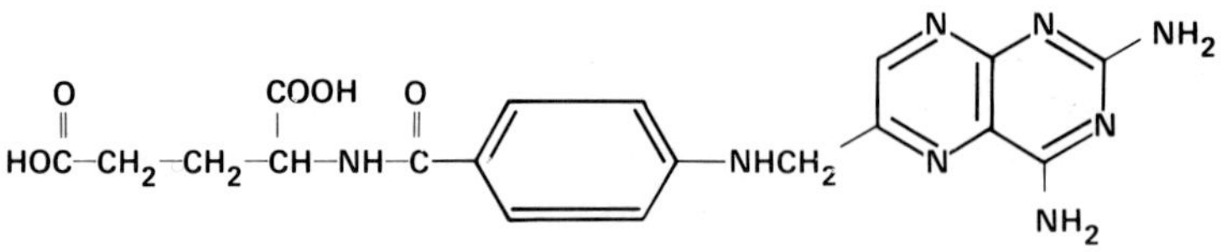

AMINOPTERIN

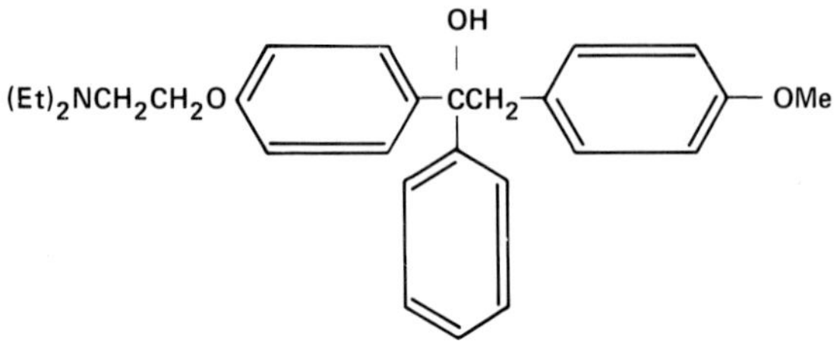

ETHAMOXYTRIPHETOL (MER-25)

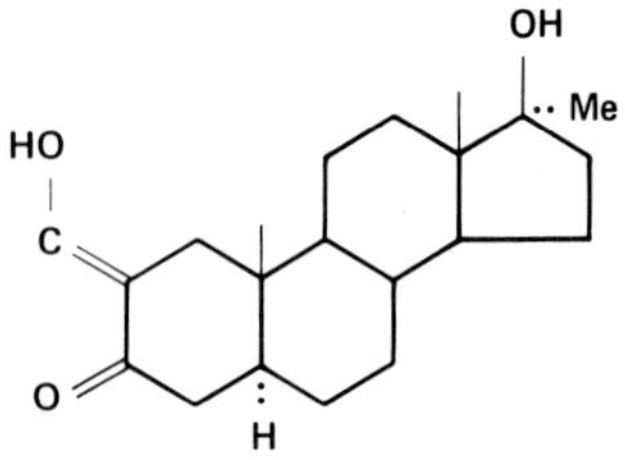

OXYMETHOLONE

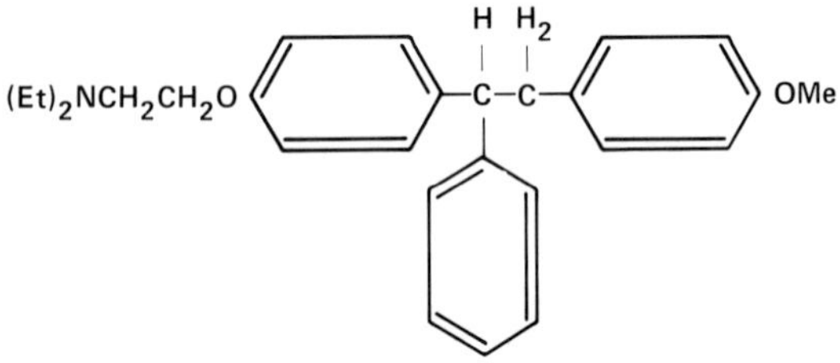

MRL-37

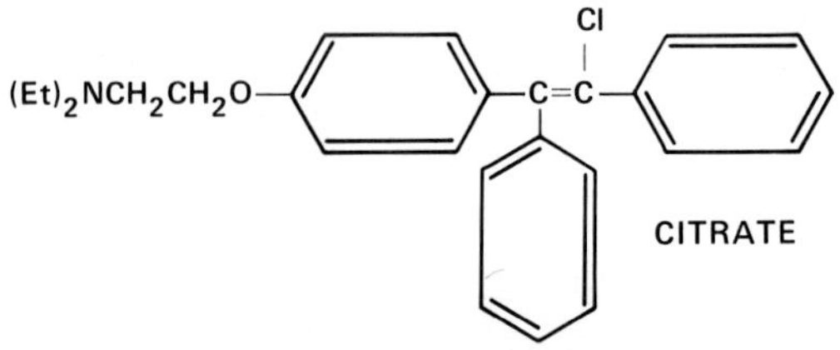

CITRATE

CLOMIPHENE (MRL-41)

Fig. 30.20 Some nonprostaglandin abortifacients (see Table 30.48).

11 NONHORMONAL SPERMICIDAL COMPOUNDS: INTRAVAGINAL

Data from studies using the sperimicidal compound nonoxynol-9 (Table 30.49) include results of five different formulations, of which the cream and C-Film yield reasonably good Pearl Indices. Five studies based on the cream formulations produced an overall mean Pearl Index of 6.5, for a total of 17,150 cycles. The mean Pearl Index for the C-Film formulation, for a total of 13,132 cycles, was 5.3. The Pearl Indices of the individual studies of the C-Film and cream formulations varied little from study to study. Specifically, the cream

Table 30.49 Nonhormonal Spermicidal Compounds: Intravaginal

Compound	Pharmaceutical Formulation	Number of Cycles or Months (Subjects or couples)	Pearl Index: Use	Reference
Nonoxynol-9	Foam	2,737 (130)	1.75	Bushnell (335)
Nonoxynol-9	Jelly	2,058 (195)	21	Kasabach (336)
Nonoxynol-9	Cream	2,915 (251)	9.06	Rovinsky (337)
Nonoxynol-9	Cream	6,783 (508)	6.19	Tyler (338)
Nonoxynol-9	Foam tablet	11,096 (1590)	14.4	
Nonoxynol-9	Foam tablet	1,749 (240)	22±3.8 (SEM)	Dingle and Tietze (339)
Nonoxynol-9	C-Film	5,194 (716)	5.31	Pariser (340)
Nonoxynol-9	C-Film	1,638 (91)	7.33	
Nonoxynol-9	Aerosol foam	1,116 (138)	7.53	Kleppinger (341)
Nonoxynol-9	Aerosol foam	5,572 (779)	28.3	Tietze and Lewit (342)
Nonoxynol-9	Aerosol foam	17,200 (1778)	3.14	Carpenter and Martin (343)
Nonoxynol-9	Aerosol foam	28,322 (1076)	3.98 (3.05)	Bernstein (344)
Nonoxynol-9	Aerosol foam	1,723 (142)	29.3	Paniagua et al. (345)
Nonoxynol-9	Foam tablets	1,809 (82)	11.9	Koya and Koya (346)
Nonoxynol-9	Gel Cream	3,728 (458) 633 (137)	8.0 7.6	Dubrow and Kuder (347)
Nonoxynol-9	C-Film	6,300 (720)	3.4	Hotay (348)
Dodecaethyleneglycol monolaurate (Immolin)	Jelly	5,103 (325)	10.8	Finkelstein et al. (349)
Diisobutylphenoxy-ethoxyethanol	Foam tablet	1,514 (147)	42.8	Finkelstein et al. (350)
Diisobutylphenoxypoly-ethoxy ethanol	Oil	3,280 (167)	9.5	Wulff and Jonas (351)
Fomos	Foam tablet	1,565 (166)	38	Tietze et al. (352)
7-Chloro-4-indanol; Lanesta-Gel	Gel	3,250 (259)	7.8	Margolis et al. (353)
Diisobutylphenoxy-polyethoxy	Jelly or cream	4,253 (291)	11.0	Finkelstein et al. (354)
Texofor FN11 (*p*-tri-isopropylphenoxy-polyethoxyethanol)	4% Coating on condom	(397 completed a questionnaire after 2 yr)	0.83	Potts and McDevitt (355)
TS-88 (*p*-methanyl-phenylpolyoxyethyl-ene ether)	Tablet	8,955 (475)	3.2	Ishihama and Inoue (356)

Table 30.49 *(continued)*

Compound	Pharmaceutical Formulation	Number of Cycles or Months (Subjects or couples)	Pearl Index: Use	Reference
Polysaccharide–polysulfuric acid ester	Suppository	1,344 (56)	1.79	Godts (357)
p-Methanylphenyl polyoxyethylene ether	Foam tablets	1,058 (124)	2.27	Population Report Series II (358)
p-Methanylphenyl polyoxyethylene ether	Foam	8,955 (5877)	3.22	IPPF Report to donors (359)

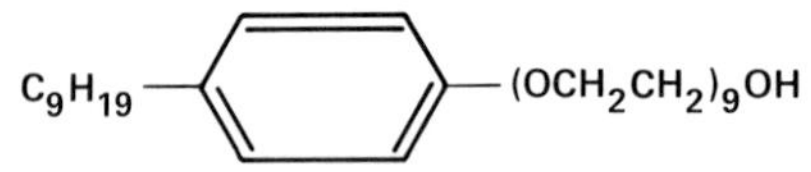

NONOXYNOL-9

p-METHANYLPHENYL
POLYOXYETHYLENE ETHER

$$HOCH_2CH_2O[CH_2CH_2O]_{10}\,CH_2CH_2O\overset{\displaystyle O}{\overset{\|}{C}}(CH_2)_{10}CH_3$$

(DODECAETHYLENEGLYCOL MONOLAURATE)

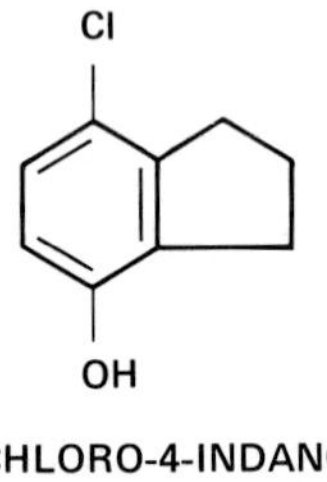

7-CHLORO-4-INDANOL

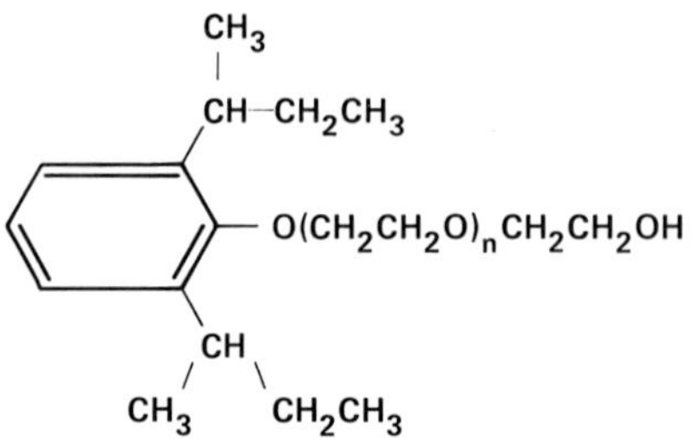

DIISOBUTYLPHENOXYPOLYEHTOXYETHANOL

Fig. 30.21 Structure of spermicidal compounds (see Table 30.49).

formulation had mean Pearl Indices variations from 3.9 to 9.1, and C-Film had variations of 3.4 to 7.3. These variations were reasonable compared to the wide variations of 1.8–22 for the foam, 10.8–21 for the jelly, and 3.1–29.3 for the aerosol foam. Some representative compounds appear in Fig. 30.21.

Table 30.49 contains a limited amount of contraceptive data using spermicidal compounds other than nonoxynol-9. However some quite acceptable Pearl Indices were reported. In three of the studies summarized, the effective agent is *p*-methanylphenylpolyoxyethylene ether, and the individual studies yielded Pearl Indices of 3.2 for 8955 cycles, 2.27 for 1058 cycles, and 3.22 for 8955 cycles. In a single limited study using polysaccharide polysulfuric acid ester in a suppository for 1344 cycles, the Pearl Index was 1.79.

12 INHIBITORS OF LRF (LUTEINIZING HORMONE–RELEASING FACTOR)

Theoretically, inhibitors of LRF (Table 30.50) may be considered to be antifertility agents. The specific use of these substances in women as contraceptive agents requires considerable development, but suggestions have been made that inhibitors be so employed. Schally et al. (30) speculated on the possible use of LH–RH inhibitors for fertility control. Coy et al. (31) synthesized the first peptide antagonists that are active *in vivo*.

By 1973 powerful antisera against LH–RH had been realized (32–34).

Table 30.50 Inhibitors of LRF (Luteinizing Hormone-Releasing Factor) in Women

Inhibitor Compound	Test (*in vivo* or *in vitro*)	Results	Reference
des-His^2-[D-Ala]-LRF	Method of Vale et al. (1972)	Antagonizes activity of LRF; more active inhibitor than des-H^2-LRF	Monahan et al. (360)
[D-Phe^2-D-Ala^6]-LH-RH ② [D-Phe^2-D-(Ph)-(Gly-]-LH-RH ⑥ [D-Phe^2-D-Phe^{62}]-LH-RH ⑦ [D-*p*-F-Phe^2-D-Ala^6]-LH-RH 9 [D-Phe^2-2-Me-Ala^6]-LH-RH ⑪	1. Rats, 200–250 g females 2. Peptides s.c. in corn oil; 1 mg/0.2 ml 3. Injections on half-hourly basis from 12:00 to 14:30 on day of proestrus (D_3) 4. Autopsied on morning of estrus (D_4)	Antiovulation test at 6 mg total dose produced 80% or greater inhibition	Beattie et al. (361)
LH-RH	*In vitro* rat pituitary	Inhibition of LH-RH at a 300,000 increase in dosage	Vale et al. (362)
[Gly^2]LRF	Rat anterior pituitary cell culture	1. Partial agonist 2. Decreased amount of LH secreted in response to LRF	
des-His^2-LRF	Rat anterior pituitary cell culture	1. Decreased amount of LH secreted in response to LRF 2. No agonist activity	

Table 30.50 *(continued)*

Inhibitor Compound	Test (*in vivo* or *in vitro*)	Results	Reference
des-His[2] peptide	Rat (*in vivo*)	Decreased amount of LH secreted in response to LRF	Coy et al. (363)
des-His-2-des-Gly-10-LH-RH-ethylamide	Rat (*in vivo*)	Blocked response to i.v. injection of LH-RH	Coy et al. (31)
D-[Phe]^2-D-[Ala]^6-LRH, WY-18,185	Preovulatory proestrus surge of serum LH and FSH in rats	Dampens response	Corbin and Beattie (364)
	Precoital effect in rats	Prevents pregnancy	
D-[Trp^2]-LH-RH D-[Phe^2]-LH-RH	Rat (*in vitro*)	Inhibit LH release by LH-RH	Rees et al. (365)

13 COMPOUNDS THAT AFFECT FERTILITY IN FEMALE NONHUMAN ANIMALS

This section deals with compounds that exert their action in nonhuman animals after fertilization and before implantation (Figs. 30.22–30.25; Table 30.51). The action of estrogens and progestogens as postcoital agents in women has already been presented.

As Table 30.51 indicates, estrogens are highly active anti-implantation compounds in the rabbit, the monkey, the rat, the mouse, the goat, the guinea pig, and women, as previously shown in postcoital

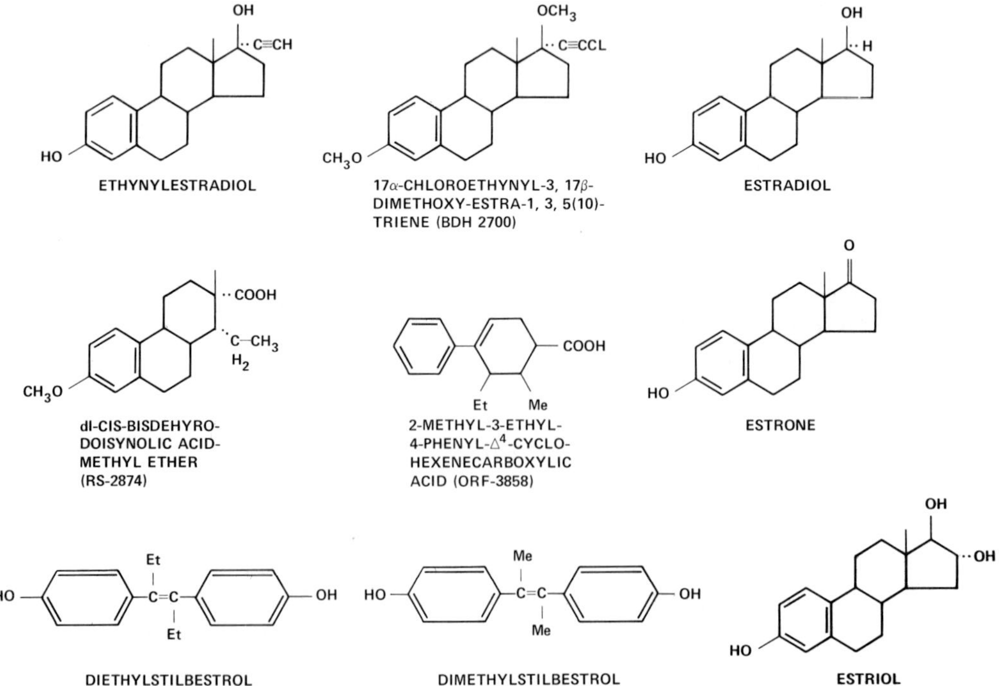

Fig. 30.22 Structures of estrogens that affect fertility in female nonhuman animals (see Table 30.51).

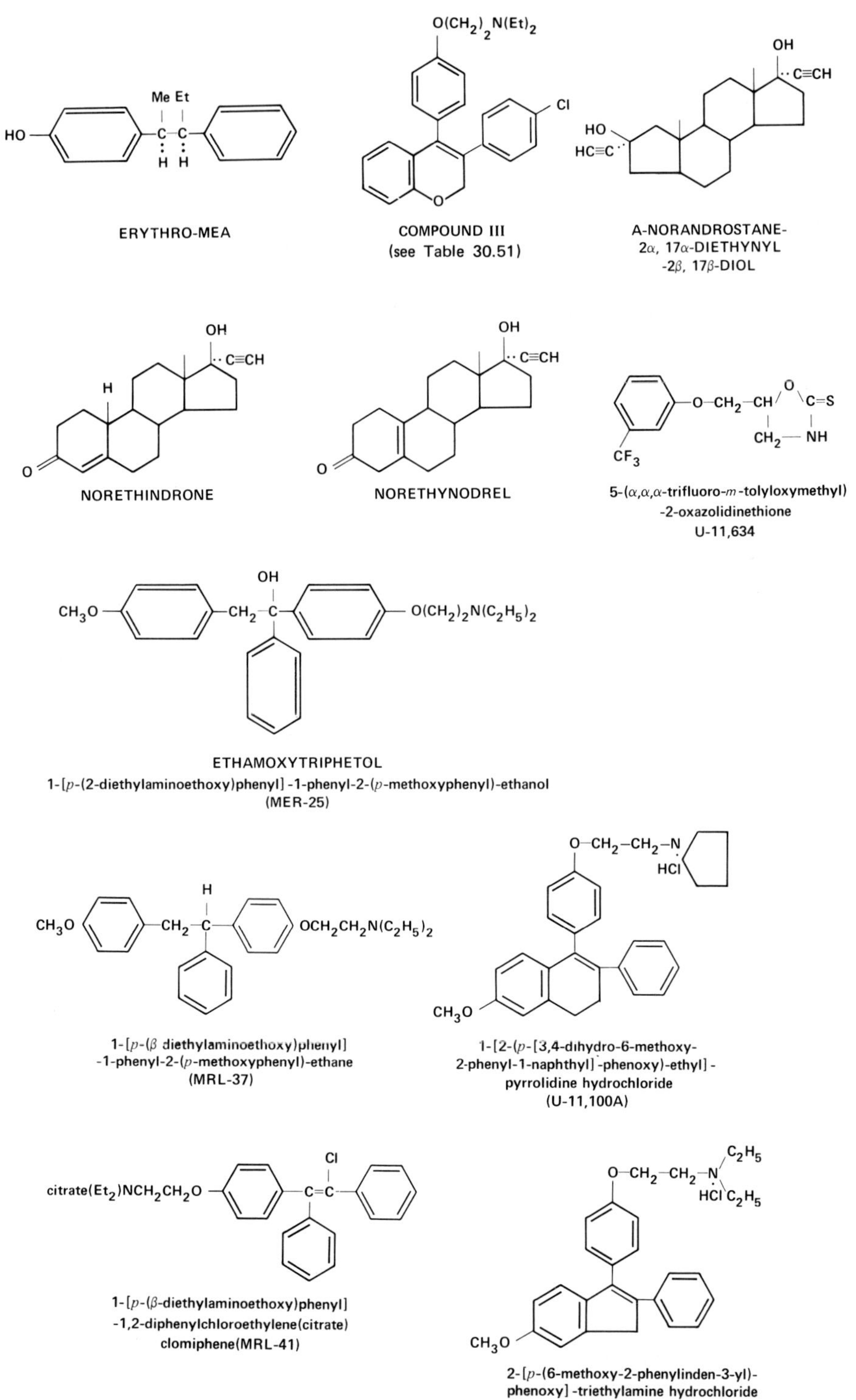

Fig. 30.23 Structures of compounds that affect fertility in female nonhuman animals (see Table 30.51).

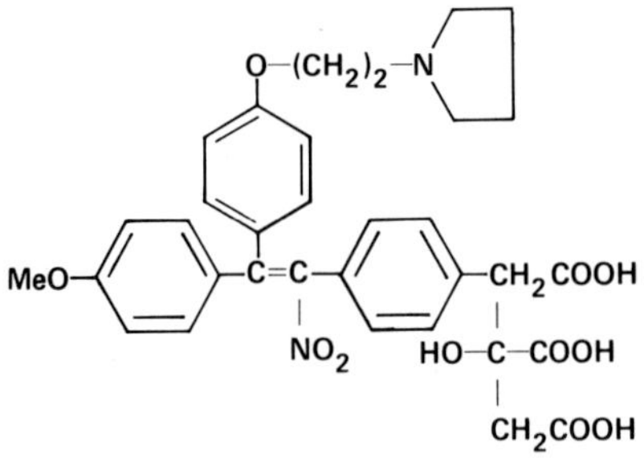

1-[2-(*p*-[α-(*p*-methoxy-phenyl)-β-nitrostyryl] phenoxy)ethyl] pyrrolidine monocitrate
CN-55,945-27

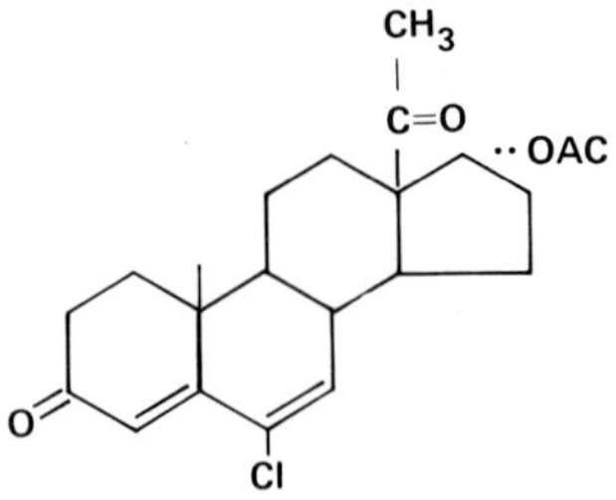

Chlormadinone Acetate

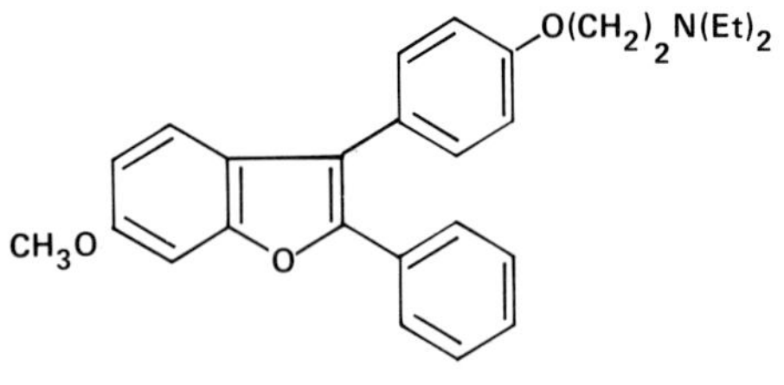

2-phenyl-3-diethylpyrol- indoethoxy-6-methoxy - benzofuran Hydrochloride

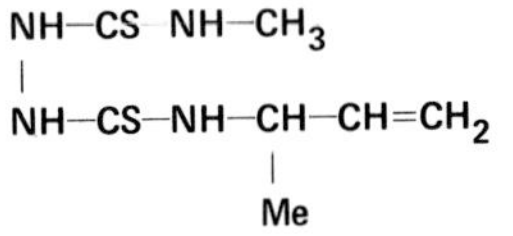

(1-(α-methylallylthiocarbamcyl)-2–(methylthiocarbamoyl)-hydrazine)
(ICI-33,828)

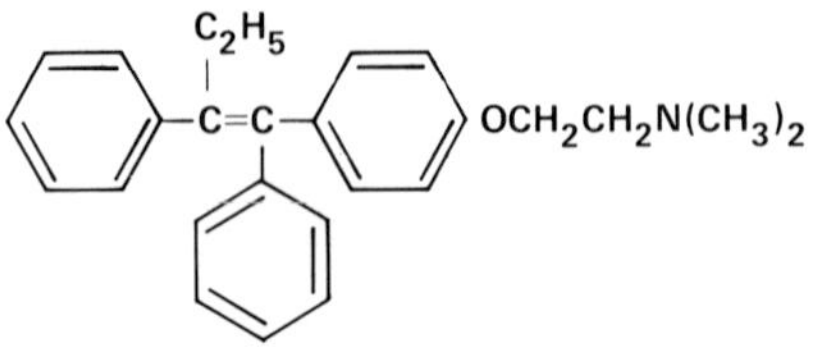

trans 1-(*p*-β-dimethylaminoethoxyphenyl)-1,2-diphenylbut-1-ene
(ICI-46,474)
(TAMOXIFEN)

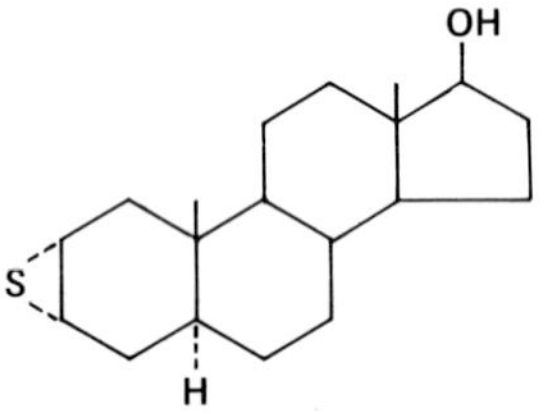

2α,3α-epithio-5-α androstan-17β-ol
(10275-S)

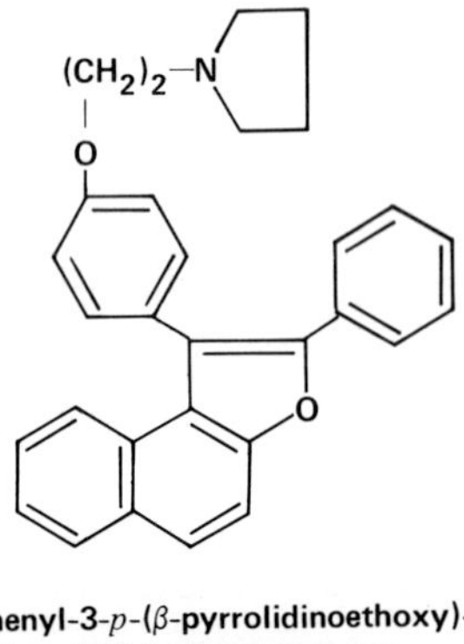

2-phenyl-3-*p*-(β-pyrrolidinoethoxy)-phenyl-(2:1,b)naphthofuran
(NF or 66/179)

Fig. 30.24 Structures of compounds that affect fertility in female nonhuman animals (see Table 30.51).

studies (Table 30.36). The mechanism of estrogen action as a postcoital agent is generally considered to be interference in the egg transport. Estrogen usually produces an acceleration of egg transport and in some species an arrest of egg movement—a phenomenon called "tube locking", usually due to excessive concentration of estrogens.

Norethindrone has postcoital anti-implantation activity produced by inhibition of speed of egg transfer (Table 30.51).

The group of antiestrogen compounds MER 25, MRL 37, and MRL 41 (clomiphene) has been studied in a variety of species to determine their preimplantation contraceptive activity. Depending on

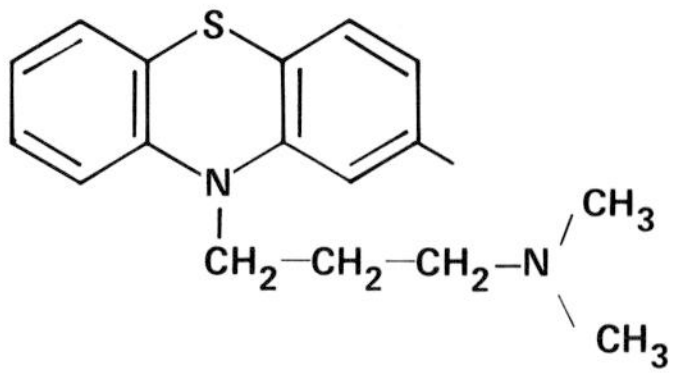

CHLORPROMAZINE

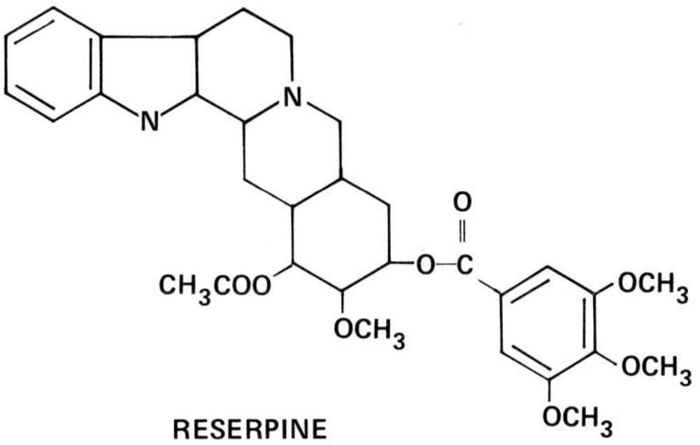

RESERPINE

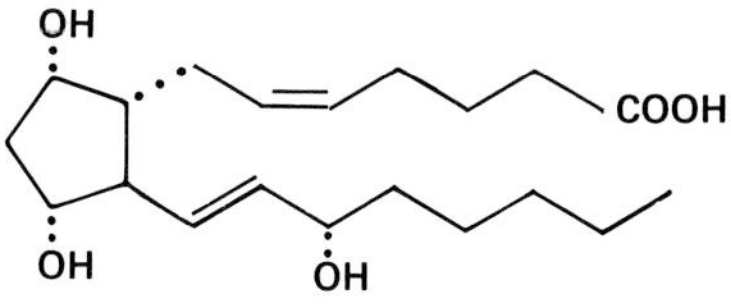

$PGF_{2\alpha}$

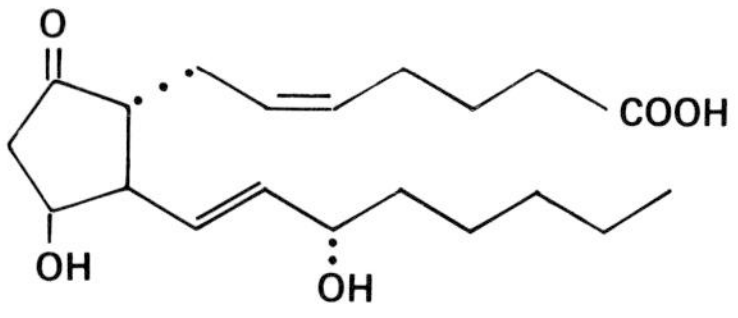

PGE_2

Fig. 30.25 Structures of compounds that affect fertility in female nonhuman animals (see Table 30.51).

Table 30.51 Compounds That Affect Fertility in Female Nonhuman Animals

Compound	Species (Route)	Results	Reference
dl-cis-Bisdehydro-doisynolic acid	Rabbit (s.c.)	1. Postcoital administration 2. Highly effective antifertility agent	Morris et al. (40)
dl-cis-Bisdehydro-doisynolic acid	Macaque monkey (oral)	1. Postcoital administration 2. Highly effective antifertility agent	
Estradiol-17β, mestranol, ethynylestradiol, diethylstilbestrol, *dl-cis*-bisdehydro-doisynolic acid, 2-methyl-3-ethyl-Δ^4-cyclohexene-carboxylic acid	Rabbit (s.c.)	1. Daily treatment for 1–3 days after coitus 2. Implantation inhibited	Morris and Van Wagenen (366)
Estrone	Rat (s.c.)	1. Treatment of 3, 4, 5, 6, or 7 days after mating 2. Prevents implantation	Dreisbach (28)
Estradiol-17β, diethylstilbestrol	Mouse (s.c.)	1. Treated 1, 2, 3 or 4, 5, 6 days after mating 2. Anti-implantation activity	Emmens and Martin (367)
Ethynylestradiol	Rabbit (oral)	1. Treatment 1 day after mating 2. Rate of egg transport time increased	Chang and Harper (15)

Table 30.51 *(continued)*

Compound	Species (Route)	Results	Reference
Diethylstilbestrol dipropionate	Angora goat doe (s.c.)	95% aborted, involving luteolytic process	Wentzel and Viljoen (368)
Diethylstilbestrol, dimethylstilbestrol, estradiol-17β	Mouse (oral)	Postcoital (days 1–6) antifertility activity	Martin et al. (369)
Estradiol cyclopentyl-propionate	Rat (s.c.), mouse (s.c.) rabbit (s.c.) guinea pig (s.c.), hamster (s.c.)	1. Postcoital-preimplantation 2. Accelerated rate of ovum transport	Greenwald (370)
Estriol-3-cyclo-pentylether	Rat (oral)	Postcoital contraceptive activity	Wotiz and Scublinsky (371)
Diphenyltetra-hydronaphthalene	Rat	Postcoital activity could be explained on basis of estrogenicity	Bencze et al. (372)
2-Methyl-3-ethyl-Δ4-cyclohexene-carboxylic acid	Rhesus monkey (oral)	1. Postcoital for 6 days at 2 ng/kg daily 2. No evidence of toxicity or teratogenicity 3. Highly active estrogen	Morris et al. (35)
Ethynylestradiol, BDH 2700	Rat (oral)	Estrogens increased significantly transport rate of fertilized eggs	Bennett et al. (373)
Diethylstilbestrol, dimethylstilbes-trol, estradiol	Mouse (oral)	Postcoital (days 1–6) antifertility activity	Martin et al. (369)
Erythro-MEA	Mouse	15 Times more potent as antifertility agent than would be expected based on antiestrogen activity	Emmens (374)
Dimethylstilbestrol, U-11, 100A	Mouse (s.c., i.v.)	Anti-implantation by estrogen and antiestrogen mechanism	
ORF 8511 1-Diphenylmethyl-enyl-2-methyl-3-ethyl-4-acetoxy-cyclohexane	Rat, mouse, hamster, (oral)	1. Suggests that postcoital anti-fertility activity and estro-genicity are related 2. Suggests that estrogens "may act as pharmaceutical agents only in species with low normal endogenous estrogen titers"	Hahn et al. (375)
A-Norandrostane-2α,17α-diethynyl-2β,17β-diol	Rat (s.c.)	1. Highly active preimplantation 2. Also estrogenic	Pincus et al. (376)
U-10,293 (2,8-Dichloro-6,12-diphenyldibenzo)	Rat (oral; s.c.)	1. Effective as single dose prior to implantation 2. Is estrogenic and antigonadotrophic 3. Low toxicity	Duncan et al. (377)

Table 30.51 *(continued)*

Compound	Species (Route)	Results	Reference
Norethindrone	Mouse (oral)	Postcoital (days 1–6) antifertility activity	Martin et al. (369)
Norethynodrel	Rat (s.c.)	Prevented nidation	Davis (325)
Norethynodrel, triethylamine	Rabbit (oral)	1. Postcoital treatment days 1, 2, and 3 2. Decrease number of normal blastocysts in uterus on day 6	Chang (328)
Norethindrone	Mouse (s.c.)	1. Treated days 1–3 2. Anti-implantation activity	Martin et al. (369)
Norethindrone	Rat (s.c.)	1. 0.9 mg single dose day 2 of pregnancy 2. Inhibits rate of egg transfer	Bennett and Vickery (378)
Norethindrone	Rabbit (s.c.)	1. 81 mg/kg on day 1 2. Inhibits rate of egg transfer	
MER-25, Clomiphene (MRL-41)	Rat, rabbit	Disturbed tubal transport	Pincus (379)
MRL-41, MER-25	Mouse	Disturbed tubal transport	Humphrey (380)
MRL-37, MRL-41, MER-25	Rat (oral)	1. Postcoital treatment 2. Anti-implantation activity	Barnes and Meyer (326)
Clomiphene MRL-41), U-11,555A	Mouse (oral)	1. Delayed tubal transport rate 2. Interference with implantation	Thomson (381)
Clomiphene	Rat (oral)	1. Postcoital treatment 2. Prevents implantation	Davidson et al. (382)
Clomiphene	Rat (oral)	1. Treatment on days 1–4 of pregnancy or single day treatment of day 1, 2, or 3 2. No implantation on day 10	Segal and Nelson (383)
Clomiphene	Mouse (oral)	1. Postcoital treatment 2. Arrested egg transport	Thomson (381)
Clomiphene	Rat (oral)	1. Postcoital treatment 2. Accelerated egg transport	Davidson et al. (382)
Clomiphene	Macaque monkey (s.c.)	1. Postcoital treatment 2. No antifertility effect	Morris et al. (35)
Clomiphene	Rabbit (oral)	1. Postcoital treatment, days 1–3 2. Decrease number of normal blastocysts in uterus on day 6	Chang (328)
MER-25	Rat	1. Prevents implantation 2. Antiestrogen mechanism	Lerner et al. (384)
MER-25	Rat (oral)	1. Postcoital treatment 2. Prevents implantation	Segal and Nelson (383)
MER-25	Rat (oral)	1. Postcoital treatment 2. Decrease in normal embryos	Chang (385)

Table 30.51 *(continued)*

Compound	Species (Route)	Results	Reference
		3. Increase in degenerating embryos before and after implantation	
MER-25	Mouse (oral)	Postcoital (days 1–6) antifertility activity	Martin et al. (369)
MER-25	Mouse (s.c.)	1. Postcoital treatment, days 1–3 2. Anti-implantation activity	
U-11,100A, A-Norandrostane-$2\alpha,17\alpha$-diethynyl-$2\beta,17\beta$-diol	Rabbit (oral)	1. Postcoital treatment, days 1–3 2. % Normal ova decreased significantly	Chang and Yanagimachi (386)
U-11,555A, U-11,100A	Rat (oral)	Antifertility effect produced by inhibiting progesterone (and possibly estradiol) production by ovary	Siddiqui et al. (387)
U-11,100A U-11,555A	Rat (oral)	Implantation reduction to about 40% of that of the controls was not due to an effect on egg transport or to delay of implantation	Siddiqui and Heald (388)
U-11,555A	Rat (oral)	1. Efficacy limited to period of tubal transport of zygote 2. Single doses, administered any time within 4 days of breeding, effectively inhibit pregnancy 3. After zygote had reached the uterus, compound was ineffective as a pregnancy inhibitor	Duncan et al. (389)
U-11,555A	Mouse (intravaginally or s.c.)	1. Weak estrogen and antiestrogen 2. Antifertility positive days 1–3 and 4–6 after mating	Emmens and Martin (367)
U-11,555A	Rat	1. Estrogenic activity does not explain the antifertility 2. Unstable 3. Photosensitizer	Morris et al. (35)
U-11,555A	Rat (oral)	Complete loss of blastocysts probably due to alteration in tubal and uterine mobility	Yoshida and Craig (390)
U-11,100A	Rat	Highly active when given for 7 days postcoitally	Lednicer et al. (391)
U-11,100A	Rhesus monkey	1. 6 Days treatment postcoitally 2. Inactive	Morris et al. (35)
U-11,100A	Rat, mouse	Rodent antifertility activity explained on basis of estrogenicity	Emmens et al. (392)
U-11,100A	Mouse (s.c.)	1. Postcoital treatment, 1–3 or 4–6 days 2. Anti-implantation activity	Emmens and Martin (367)

Table 30.51 (*continued*)

Compound	Species (Route)	Results	Reference
U-11,100A	Rabbit (oral), rat (oral), guinea pig (oral)	1. Postcoital treatment 2. Anti-implantation activity	Duncan et al. (393)
U-11,555A	Mouse (s.c.) Rat (s.c. or oral)	Antifertility activity days 1–3 or 4–6 Antifertility activity days 1–3 or 4–6	Emmens et al. (392)
U-11,634 (5[α,α,α-Trifluoro-*m*-tolyloxymethyl]-2-oxazolidinethione)	Rat (oral, s.c.)	1. Prevents implantation 2. Inactive as uterotropic and antiestrogenic agent 3. Nontoxic and not teratogenic at antifertility dose 4. At very high dose inhibits thyroid and causes hepatitis	Youngdale et al. (394)
2,3-Bis(4-methoxyphenyl)-pent-2-enenitrile (I); 3,4-bis(4-hydroxyphenyl)-hexan-2-one (II); 2,3-bis-(4-hydroxyphenyl)valeronitrile (IV)	Rat, hamster, rabbit (s.c.)	1. Compounds I, II, and IV had greater antifertility activity (preimplantation) than estrogenic activity compared to estrone 2. Accelerated rate of egg transport	Saunders and Rorig (37) Nutting and Sanders (38)
Bis(2-bromoethyl)aminomethylmethoxy-4-nitrobenzene (compound 5); bis(2-hydroxyethyl, aminomethyl-4-ethoxynitrobenzene (compound 8)	Rat (oral)	Compounds 5 and 8, administered at 1 mg/day from days 1–3 of pregnancy, produced 100% inhibition	Garg et al. (332)
Tamoxifen (ICI 46,474) [*trans*-1-(*p*-β-dimethylaminoethoxyphenyl)-1-2-diphenylbut-1-ene]	Rat (oral)	Administered on day 2 of pregnancy; the antifertility activity may be due to the "capacity to inhibit the synthesis of estradiol from progesterone"	Watson et al. (395)
Chlormadinone acetate	Rat (s.c.)	Infertility without marked impairment of sexual activity	Dörner et al. (396)
66/179, NP 2-phenyl-3-*p*-(β-pyrrolidinoethoxy)phenyl-(2:1,*b*)naphthofuran	Rat, rabbit, rhesus monkey (oral)	1. Postcoital treatment effective in all 3 species 2. Antiprogestational 3. Estrogenic activity in rat about $\frac{1}{4}$–$\frac{1}{3}$ estrone	Kamboj et al. (397)

Table 30.51 *(continued)*

Compound	Species (Route)	Results	Reference
H-1285	Mouse (oral)	1. Preimplantation activity at daily dose of 14 μg/kg (ED_{50}) 2. Vaginal smear estrogenic activity (ED_{50}) at 250 times antifertility dose	Emmens (398)
Tamoxifen (ICI 46,474)	Rat (oral)	1. When treated on day 2, the compound had a marginal effect on the transport of ova through the oviduct 2. Day 2 treatment is capable of affecting implantation without altering blastocyst transport through the oviduct 3. It is suggested that alteration of uterine metabolism is the main factor contributing to the antifertility activity	Major and Heald (399)
2-Phenyl-3-diethylpyrolidinoethoxy-6-methoxy-benzofuran hydrochloride	Rat, mouse, rabbit, monkey (oral)	1. When administered on days 1–5 or once on days 1–3, the antifertility activity was 100% and was reversible 2. "It appears to exert its antifertility effect by premature expulsion of ova from the fallopian tubes" (this may be due to estrogenicity)	Kar et al. (400)
Tamoxifen (ICI 46,474)	Rat (oral, i.v.)	Prevents implantation by counteracting the estrogen surge on day 4	Harper and Walpole (36)
ICI 33,828	Rat (oral)	Antifertility effects due to inhibiting effects on pituitary	Harper (401)
Metronidazole (Flagyl)	Rat (oral)	Antifertility effects may be due to action on zygote	Davidson and Davidson (402)
$2\alpha,3\alpha$-Epithio-5α-androstan-17β-ol	Rat (s.c.)	1. Treatment 1–6 days postcoitum effective 2. Treatment 8–13 days postcoitum no effect	Miyake and Takeda (39)
9α-Fluoro-11β,17-dihydroxy-3-oxo-4-androstene-17α-propionic acid (CS-1)	Rabbit (oral)	1. Prevents implantation 1st 8 days postcoitum 2. Not effective after 13th day of gestation 3. Antifertility effect abolished by progesterone or prolactin	Taché et al. (403)
CN-55,945-27	Rat (oral)	1. Treatment days 1–7 postcoitum 2. Antifertility activity by blocking	Callantine et al. (404)

Table 30.51 *(continued)*

Compound	Species (Route)	Results	Reference
		action of endogenous estrogen on uterus	
ICI 46,474 *Trans*-1-(*p*-β-dimethylamino-ethoxyphenyl)-1,2-diphenylbut-1-ene	Rat (oral)	1. Prevents implantation with single dose on day 1 or 2 2. Acclerated tubal transport 3. Suggests prevention of implantation by counteracting "estrogen surge on day 4"	Harper and Walpole (36)
Prostaglandin E_2, prostaglandin $F_{2\alpha}$	Rhesus monkey	Abortifacient	Kirton et al. (405, 406)
ICI 74205 (a C_{22} derivative of $PGF_{2\alpha}$)	Rat, hamster	4–5 Times more active than PGF_2 in terminating early pregnancy in hamsters and rats (s.c.) 20 times more potent in terminating early pregnancy in hamsters (oral)	Labhsetwar (407)
Tetrabenazine *p*-chlorophenyl-alanine	Mouse	Reduction in rate of egg transport in the oviduct	Kendle and Bennett (408)
Compound I 1-[2-[*p*-[α-(*p*-Methoxy-phenyl)-β-nitrostyryl]-phenoxy]ethyl]-pyrrolidine.	Prophylactic mouse test, 50 μg/kg daily (oral) Postcoital mouse test, 500 μg/kg (oral)	100% Effective	DeWald et al. (409)
	Anti-implantation rat test, 25 μg/kg daily (oral)	100% Effective	
	Dog, 250–500 μg/kg daily	ED_{100}	
Compound III (see Fig. 20 of Ref. 372)	Rat (oral)	Complete protection against pregnancy	Bencze et al. (372)
Reserpine, chlorpromazine	Mouse	Arrests egg transport	Bennett and Kendle (410)
Reserpine	Rhesus monkey	Antiovulatory	De Feo and Reynolds (411)
Dithiocarbamoyl-hydrozine	Rhesus monkey	Antiovulatory	McArthur and Ovadia (412)
Atropine, Dibenamine SKF-501, barbiturates, morphine	Rat, rabbit	Blocks ovulation primarily at central nervous system	Everett (413)

Table 30.51 (*continued*)

Compound	Species (Route)	Results	Reference
Chlorpromazine	Rat	Active at central nervous system plus other sites	
Reserpine, chlorpromazine	Rat	Interferes with implantation	Walpole (414)
Methallibure (ICI 33828)	Various species (oral)	Inhibition of LH and FSH leading to inhibition of ovulation	Walpole (414)
Reserpine	Mouse (i.p.)	Arrest of egg transport by single dose of 10 mg/kg on day 1 of pregnancy	Bennett and Kendle (410)

the species and the dose, these synthetic nonsteroidal compounds have accelerating or retarding effects on the transfer rate of eggs (Table 30.51).

Compounds U-11,555A and U-11,100A, which were found to be highly active postcoitally in the rat, are representative of the 2,3-diphenylindenes and dihydronaphthalene classes of compounds, respectively (Table 30.51). It has been suggested that the high oral activity in rats, guinea pigs, and rabbits may be due to inherent estrogenic and antiestrogenic activity. Although highly active in rodents, U-11,100A was inactive in the rhesus monkey at 25 and 250 mg daily dosages for 6 days postcoitally (35).

Tamoxifen (ICI 46, 474) (Table 30.51) is an antifertility compounds preventing implantation. Harper and Walpole (36) suggested that the mechanism involves the counteracting of the estrogen surge on day 4.

The objective of many of the studies reported in Table 30.51 was the identification of compounds high in antifertility activity and exceedingly low in hormonal activity. In studies of Saunders and Rorig (37) and Nutting and Sanders (38) three compounds (I, II, and IV) were synthesized; in the rat these had anti-implantation activity at a level significantly higher than would be expected on the basis of estrogenicity.

The antiestrogen $2\alpha,3\alpha$-epithio-5α-androstan-17β-ol was postcoitally active at 0.25 mg/day for treatment days 1–6 and inactive as an estrogen (Table 30.51).

dl-cis-Bisdehydrodoisynolic acid methyl ether proved to be a highly effective antifertility agent when administered postcoitally in the rabbit. Administration of 2 mg/day orally for 6 days following midcycle mating in the macaque monkey resulted in only one pregnancy in 98 positive matings. A positive mating involved sperm in the vagina. When given in a dose of 25 mg/day for 3 days starting on the 24–33 day of the cycle, there were two pregnancies out of 41 matings. These results represent significantly lower pregnancy rates than were encountered in untreated matings in the primate colony. Actually 18 pregnancies resulted from the same animals with 65 matings prior to the onset of the treatment periods (40).

14 MALE CONTRACEPTION IN HUMANS

By means of radioautography it has been found that one cycle of the seminiferous epithelium lasts 16 ± 1 days. Spermatogenesis in man extends over 4.6 cycles or a total of 74 days (41).

Male contraception may be accomplished by interfering with the process leading to mature ejaculated spermatozoa. The interfering may be affected by androgens, estrogens, progestogens, nonsteroidal compounds, or combinations thereof (Fig. 30.26; Table 30.52).

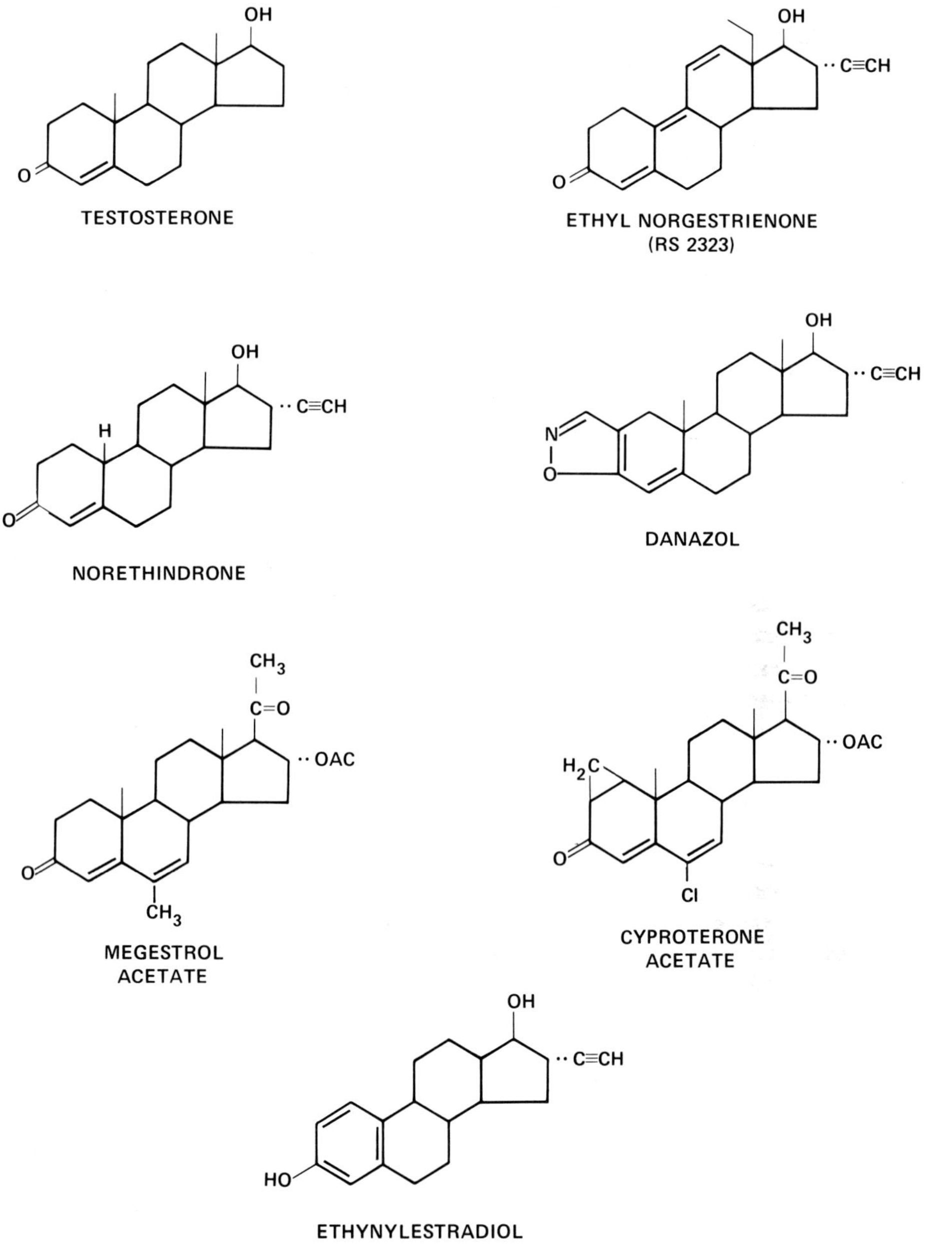
OH
O
TESTOSTERONE
OH
·· C≡CH
O
ETHYL NORGESTRIENONE
(RS 2323)
OH
·· C≡CH
H
O
NORETHINDRONE
OH
·· C≡CH
N
O
DANAZOL
CH3
C=O
·· OAC
O
CH3
MEGESTROL
ACETATE
CH3
C=O
·· OAC
H2C
O
Cl
CYPROTERONE
ACETATE
OH
·· C≡CH
HO
ETHYNYLESTRADIOL

Fig. 30.26 Some male antifertility compounds: human (see Table 30.52).

14.1 Androgens

Testosterone is a potentially valuable contraceptive agent. It reduces spermatogenesis, leading in time and in a high percentage of subjects to azoospermia. The action of testosterone does not affect libido or potency, and normal spermatogenesis returns on stopping the testosterone treatment.

Testosterone concentration in testis is many times higher than plasma level in various species, including man.

Steinberger et al. (42) demonstrated that

Table 30.52 Human Male Antifertility Compounds

Compound	Dose, mg (Route)	Effect on Spermatogenesis	Effect on Libido	Effect on Potency	Reference
Norethindrone	25 mg/day for 3 weeks, plus 25 mg/ week (oral)	Decreased sperm count	No change	No change	Johansson and Nygren (415)
Testosterine, norgestrienone	Silastic implant 50 mg twice/ week (implant and oral)	Marked decrease	No decrease	No decrease	Coutinho and Melo (416)
Testosterone, RS-2323	Silastic implant	Decrease	No decrease	No decrease	
Danazol (17α-pregn-4-en-20-yno-(2,3-*d*) isoxazol-17-ol) (D), testosterone propionate (TP)	200 mg, 3 times a day, oral, 4 months (D); 10 mg i.m. 3 times a week, 4 months (TP)	Decrease	No change	No change	Skoglund and Paulsen (49)
Danazol, testosterone enanthate	200 mg, 3 times a day, oral, 4 months; 200 mg, single monthly rate	Decrease	No change	No change	
Testosterone propionate	25 mg/day, 60 days	60 days of azoospermia	Normal	Normal	Reddy and Rao (417)
Testosterone implants	3 implants, 22 mg each	6–8 weeks of azo-ospermia (no change in testos-terone in plasma)	No change	—	Frick (418)
Megestrol acetate	30 mg daily for 3 weeks (oral)				
Testosterone implants	3 implants of 22 mg each	At 12 weeks 4 of 7 patients had azoospermia; 2 of 7 had $\frac{2}{3}$ re-duction (no change in test-osterone plasma)	No change	—	
Norethindrone	25 mg/day for 3 weeks				
Norethindrone implants	6				
Medroxypro-gesterone acetate	100 mg/ month s.c.	24 of 25 subjects had a marked drop in sperm count 1–3 months following 1st treatment	No change	No change	Melo and Coutinho (419)
Testosterone enanthate	250 mg/ month s.c.				

Table 30.52 *(continued)*

Compound	Dose, mg (Route)	Effect on Spermatogenesis	Effect on Libido	Effect on Potency	Reference
Cyproterone acetate	30 mg/day (oral)	1. Severe depression in 5 normal men after $7\frac{1}{2}$-$15\frac{1}{2}$ weeks of treatment 2. Complete restoration 4–5 months after stopping therapy	No complaints	No complaints	Petry et al. (46)
Methyltestosterone	20 mg/day (oral)	By week 18 all 5 subjects were	Normal	Normal	Briggs and Briggs (420)
Ethynylestradiol	40 μg/day (oral)	aspermic			
Ethynylestradiol	0.45 mg/day (oral)	1. Sperm count to zero in 4–6 weeks 2. Reversible	Decrease	Decrease	Patanelli (421)
Testosterone enanthate (TE)	(i.m.)	1. 250 mg weekly 2. In 70 days, loss of sperm	—	—	MacLeod and Tietze (45)
Medroxyprogesterone acetate	(i.m.)	1. 1 g weekly 2. Near aspermia in 70 days			
Medroxyprogesterone acetate	100 or 150 mg/month	Sperm production below 1 million	No change	—	Frick et al (422)
Testosterone	Various forms				
Testosterone enanthate	100 mg				
WIN 13,099 [*N,N'*-bis(dichloroacetyl)-*N,N'*-diethyl-1,4-xylylenediamine],	1. 2×500 mg daily (oral) 2. At 16th week increased to 2×1 g daily	1. Decreased 2. WIN 13,099 and WIN 18,446 decreased sperm count to 4×10^6 within 8 to 11 weeks	No change	No change	Heller et al. (47)
WIN 17,416 [*N,N'*-bis(dichloroacetyl)-*N,N'*-diethyl-1,6-hexanediamine],	3. At 22nd week increased to 2×1.5 g daily	3. Complete recovery on discontinuance			

Table 30.52 (*continued*)

Compound	Dose, mg (Route)	Effect on Spermatogenesis	Effect on Libido	Effect on Potency	Reference
WIN 18,446 [*N*,*N*′-bis(dichloroacetyl)-1,8-octanediamine]					
Clomiphene	100 mg/day (oral)	In 2–12 months produced oligospermia; azoospermia	—	—	Heller and Heller (423)
Cyproterone acetate	5–10 mg/day for 20 weeks	50–80% nonmotile; ability of sperm to penetrate cervical mucus decreased	No change	No change	Roy et al. (424)
Medroxyprogesterone acetate (MPA)	1 g MPA 1st injection, followed by 150 mg MPA injections monthly	11 of 12 sperm counts below 1 million	No change	—	Frick et al. (425)
Testosterone enanthate (TE)	TE, 250 mg/month				
WIN 13,099, WIN 17,416, WIN 18,446	—	1. Inhibition 2. Anomalies of both maturing spermatids and immature spermatids 3. No impairment of remainder of germinal epithelium or Leydig cells at minimal effective doses 4. No depression of hormonal secretion	—	—	Heller et al. (426)

1800 mg of testosterone enanthate administered over 9 weeks produced azoospermia in a 24-year-old man but did not increase the plasma testosterone.

Schoysman (43) lists as a disadvantage of the use of testosterone the inactivity of the hormone when administered by mouth. More recent studies indicate that testosterone undecanate given orally may be used to produce a suitable blood level of testosterone (44). Other disadvantages of testosterone administration mentioned by

Schoysman (43) are occasional aggressive behavior, acne, loss of hair, and delay in obtaining azoospermia. To these disadvantages may be possible added increased risk of prostatic cancer and possible increased incidence of atherosclerosis due to higher levels of plasma testosterone in treated subjects than in normal nontreated subjects.

14.2 Estrogens

Estrogens are highly effective inhibitors of spermatogenesis by means of hypothalamic–anterior pituitary inhibition. They cannot be considered to be useful contraceptive agents for men because of decrease in potency and libido. The possible side effect, gynecomastia, must be considered.

14.3 Progestogens

Progestogens alone, through their antigonadotrophic activity, produced degeneration of the germinal epithelium of the seminiferous tubules and a decrease in libido.

In the older preparations of the 19-nor type of progestogens, a significant concentration of estrogen was contained in the progestational preparation. For many years this has not been the case. New routes of synthesis of such progestogens as norethindrone have resulted in the preparation of essentially estrogen-free compounds.

A third type of progestogens includes 17α-acetoxy progesterone derivatives. These compounds are free of estrogen, and the antipituitary activity may be considered to be inhenent in the 17α-acetoxy compound.

It was reported by MacLeod and Tietze (45) that medroxyprogesterone acetate produced selective arrest of spermatogenesis even with a single injection of this progestogen. It was claimed that libido was not decreased and that the reduction in sperm count was reversible. In a study by Schoysman (43) on 30 subjects living a normal family life, diminished libido was found in five men. The Schoysman study also reported two of these subjects with gynecomastia.

Cyproterone acetate is a highly active progestational agent as well as an antiandrogen. When administered at a daily dose of 30 mg, spermatogenesis was strongly inhibited without any change in libido or potency (46).

Three compounds designated as WIN 13,099, WIN 17,416, and WIN 18,446 (Table 30.52) (Fig. 30.27) have high antispermatogenesis properties. WIN 13,099 and WIN 18,446 decreased the sperm count to 4 million within 8–11 weeks. Complete recovery of normal spermatogenesis following discontinuation of treatment was observed. During treatment, libido and potency remained unchanged. In spite of certain excellent properties, however, the compounds proved not to be valuable as male contraceptive pills because subjects who consumed alcohol reported becoming nauseated when they attempted to drink during treatment. WIN 18,446, when tested in men at 125–1000 mg dose levels, resulted in low sperm counts in 50 days and azoospermia after 80 days. On cessation of treatment, 100 days was required for spermatogenesis to be fully restored.

Compounds WIN 13,099, WIN 17,416, and WIN 18,446 did not inhibit the human pituitary and did not suppress Leydig cell synthesis of androgen, but they did influence spermatogenesis. Sperm output, and motility and sperm morphology, were adversely affected. Depression of spermatogenesis was reversible. The authors postulated that the effects resulted from "a direct action of the process of germinal-cell maturation at the site of the germinal epithelium" (47).

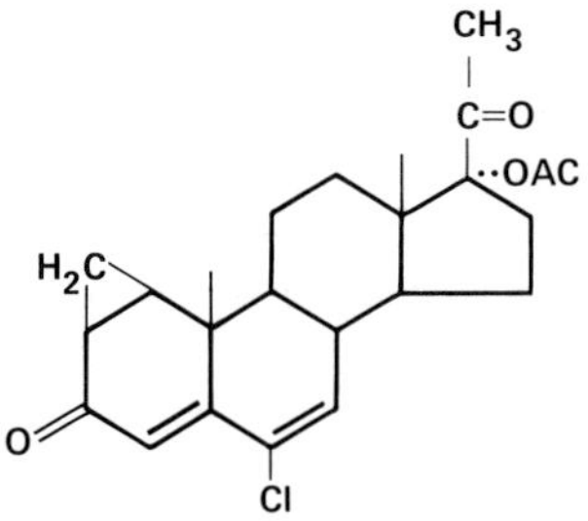

CYPROTERONE ACETATE

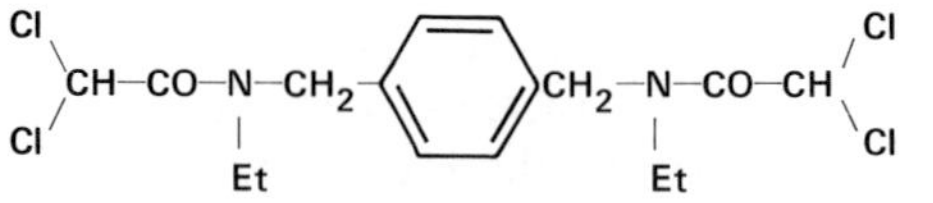

N,N′-bis(dichloroacetyl)-N,N′-diethyl-1,4-xylylenediamine
WIN-13,099

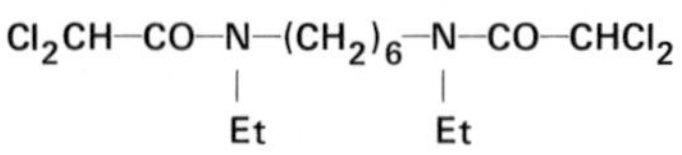

$Cl_2CH-CO-N(Et)-(CH_2)_6-N(Et)-CO-CHCl_2$

N,N′-bis(dichloroacetyl)-N,N′-diethyl-1,6-hexamethylenediamine
WIN-17,416

$Cl_2CH-CO-NH-(CH_2)_8-NH-CO-CHCl_2$

N,N′-bis(dichloroacetyl)-1.8-octamethylenediamine
WIN-18,446

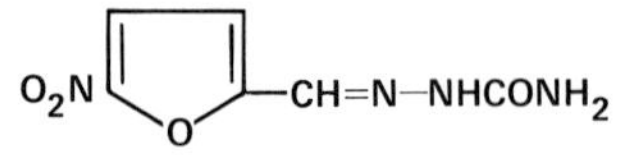

5-nitro-2-furaldehyde semicarbazone
(nitrofurazone)
(Furacin)

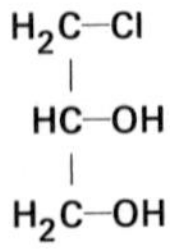

H_2C-Cl / $HC-OH$ / H_2C-OH

3-chloro-1,2-propanediol
(α-chlorohydrin)
(Y-5897)

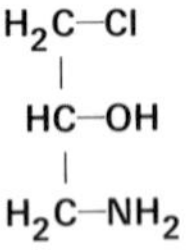

H_2C-Cl / $HC-OH$ / H_2C-NH_2

l-1-amino-3-chloro-
-2-propanol

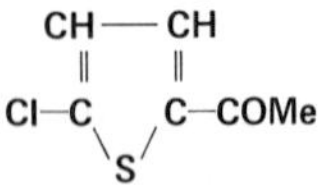

5-chloro-2-acetyl-thiophene
(Ba 11044)

Fig. 30.27 Male antifertility compounds: human and nonhuman (see Table 30.53).

14.4 Combinations

Sherins et al. (48) administered danazol at an oral daily dosage of 600 mg and found sperm counts of the order of 10–17 million per milliliter between the tenth and seventeenth weeks of treatment. Skoglund and Paulsen (49) modified the danazol treatment by incorporating testosterone in the schedule. The addition of testosterone in the form of the propionate or enanthate increased the antispermatogenic effects of danazol and improved the potency and libido of the subjects. The preliminary dosage as a contraceptive regimen is 600 mg of danazol by mouth per day and an intramuscular injection of 200 mg each month of testosterone enanthate.

When the most suitable danazol-testosterone dosage was employed, discontinuation of treatment permitted a return to pretreatment sperm count and sperm morphology. The return to normal occurred in 4 months (50). These workers concluded that danazol acts by inhibiting the spermatogenesis process at the spermatocyte-spermatid level.

The combination of testosterone as an implant and megestrol orally produced a promising treatment. At 6–8 weeks, azoospermia was observed without change in plasma testosterone and no change in libido (Table 30.52).

Methyltestosterone (20 mg/day, oral)

plus ethynylestradiol (40 μg/day, oral) produced aspermia in 18 weeks in all five subjects treated (Table 30.52).

Medroxyprogesterone acetate plus testosterone produced promising results on spermatogenesis without influencing libido or potency (Table 30.52).

14.5 Nitrofurans

The nitrofurans are heterocyclic compounds that are effective antispermatogenic agents in various species, including man (51, 52). At doses that suppress spermatogenesis, undesirable side effects were noted.

15 MALE CONTRACEPTION IN NONHUMAN ANIMALS

15.1 Steroids with Antispermatogenic Activity

Section 14 discussed the antispermatogenic activity of various steroids in men. As indicated in Table 30.53 and Figs. 30.27–30.29, antifertility activity in various nonhuman mammals shows similar responses to steroids. Estradiol benzoate, estradiol, estrone, and ethynylestradiol (Table 30.53) produce highly effective inhibition of spermatogenesis in the rat, through the decrease of LH and FSH, which means a decrease in testicular androgen production; a decrease in male accessories also occurs, as well as decreases in libido and potency.

Treatment of rodents with testosterone or methyltestosterone inhibits spermatogenesis through the hypothalamic–anterior pituitary–testicular axis. Two antiandrogens have been studied with respect to spermatogenesis. 17α-Methyl-B-nortestosterone was implanted in a hamster. The steroid appeared to impair an androgen-dependent epididymal function related to the fertilizing capacity of contained spermatozoa (Table 30.53) (53).

Cyproterone acetate has been implanted in rats, resulting in a male with defective spermatogenesis but no changes in mating behavior (54). This finding could be the basis of an elegant new method for male contraception, but first attempts to confirm it have failed (55).

Sperm taken directly from testis or vas deferens will not fertilize an ovum, but must first undergo capacitation. Jackson (56) reported that the monoesters of methanesulfonic acid prevent sperm from being capacitated and by this activity render the sperm infertile.

Various progestogens administered orally, by implant, and/or by injection, have been studied for antispermatogenetic activity. The progestogens previously discussed with respect to antipituitary activity in men (Table 30.52) include norethindrone, norgestrienone, danazol, megestrol, and medroxyprogesterone acetate. Nonhuman males also respond to progestogens with inhibition to the gonadotrophins. Table 30.53 presents such data. Cyproterone acetate is both a highly active progestogen and an inhibitor of spermatogenesis in rats. Other progestogens that show this type of activity in rats include norethindrone, norethynodrel, 17α-hydroxyprogesterone acetate, 17α-hydroxyprogesterone caproate, and deladroxone.

Steroid VI (57) was orally active in blocking of spermatogenesis but also caused decreases of weight in seminal vesicles, prostate, and epidydimus.

15.2 Nonsteroidal Gonadotrophin Inhibitors

Gonadotrophin inhibitor, ICI 33,828—methallibure—is an antifertility agent in rat, dogs, monkeys, and man but is inactive in mice, guinea pigs, rabbits, and horses.

Table 30.53 Antifertility Compounds for Nonhumans (Male)

Compound	Species (Route)	Results	Reference
l-1-Amino-3-chloro-2-propanol	Rat, mouse, hamster (oral)	Libido and coital performance unaffected; fertility returned 1–2 weeks, after compound was withdrawn	Coppola and Saldarini (427)
α-Chlorohydrin	Rat (oral)	1. Minimal effective daily dose, 5 mg/kg, for 14 days 2. Antifertility activity mediated by an effect on motility of vas deferens sperm stores 3. Antifertility effect reversible	Coppola (428)
5-Chloro-2-acetylthiophen (Ba 11044, Ciba)	Rat (oral)	1. After 20 days $\frac{2}{3}$ of tubules are damaged 2. Reduction of primary spermatocytes 3. Recovery of testis 25 days after cessation of treatment	Steinberger et al. (429)
2-*N*,*N*-Diethylaminoethanol (DEAE)	Rat, mouse (oral)	1. Treatment for days before mating 2. Reversible	Ketchel and Gresser (430)
Furacin	Rat	Most potent	Prior and Ferguson (431)
Furadroxyl, Furadantin	Rat spermatogenesis	1. Arrest of spermatogenesis at stage of primary spermatocytes 2. Reversible	Nelson and Steinberger (432)
5-Chloro-2-acetylthiophene	Rat	Arrest of spermatogenesis; an associated decrease in accessory organs	Steinberger et al. (433)
1-(*N*,*N*-Diethylcarbamylmethyl)-2,4-dinitropyrrole	Rat	Arrest of spermatogenesis	Patanelli and Nelson (434)
Progesterone Norethindrone Norethynodrel 17α-Hydroxyprogesterone acetate 17α-Hydroxyprogesterone caproate 6-Methyl-17α-hydroxyprogesterone acetate	Rat	Inhibition of spermatogenesis	Nelson (435)
WIN 17,416 [*N*,*N*′-bis(dichloroacetyl)-*N*,*N*′-diethyl-1,6-hexanediamine], WIN 18,446 [*N*,*N*′-bis(dichloroacetyl)-1,8-octanediamine],	Rat, dog, monkey (oral)	1. Relatively nontoxic 2. Testis effects: (*a*) reversible arrest of spermatogenesis; (*b*) normal Leydig, Sertoli, and spermatogonial cells	Coulston et al. (436)

Table 30.53 (*continued*)

Compound	Species (Route)	Results	Reference
WIN 13,099 [*N,N'*-bis(dichloro-acetyl)-*N,N'*-diethyl-1,4-xylylenediamine]			
WIN 17,416, WIN 18,446 WIN 18,099	Rat, monkey, dog (oral)	Inhibition and recovery of spermatogenesis	Drobeck and Coulston (437)
Cyproterone acetate	Rat (implant)	1. Caused reversible sterility 2. Mating behavior not affected 3. See Elger and von Berswordt-Wallrabe (56)	Prasad et al. (54)
α-Chlorohydrin (3-chloro-1,2-propanediol)	Rat	Damages the germinal epithelium and produces reversible sterility in male rats	Lubicz-Nawrocki and Glover (53)
17α-Methyl-B-nortestosterone	Hamster (implant)	Appears to impair an androgen-dependent epididymal function related to the fertilizing capacity of contained spermatozoa	
Furacin, Furadroxyl, Furadantin	Rat (oral)	1. Nontoxic at minimal effective antispermatogenesis doses 2. Complete recovery after 100 days of treatment	Nelson and Steinberger (432)
1-Amino-3-chloro-2-propanol hydro-chloride	Rat (oral)	Same activity as α-chlorohydrin on rat testis	Paul et al. (438)
dl-3-Chloro-1,2-propanediol (α-chlorohydrin)*dl*-1-Amino-3-chloro-2-propanol	Rat (oral)	1. Produce sterility by effect on epididymal spermatozoa 2. Negative to dominant lethal assay 3. Chloro derivative more active than amino derivative in single dose treatment	Jones and Jackson (439)
ICI 33,828, MRL 41, U-11,555	Rat (oral)	1. Spermatogenesis inhibited 2. Seminal vesicles, prostate, and epididymis decreased in size	Nelson and Patanelli (440)
WIN 18,446, Furacin, ORF-1616	Rat (oral)	1. Spermatogenesis inhibited 2. Seminal vesicles, prostate, and epididymis not affected	
Diethylstilbestrol, dienoestrol, triphenylethylene	Rat (implant crystals)	1. Testis decrease (inhibition of spermatogenesis) 2. Prostate and seminal vesicles decrease in size	Noble (441)
ICI 33,828	Rat (oral)	1. Testis decrease; antispermato-genesis 2. Prostate and seminal vesicles decrease in size	Walpole (442)

Table 30.53 *(continued)*

Compound	Species (Route)	Results	Reference
dl-α-Chlorohydrin	Rat (oral)	Single 50 mg/kg dose induced sterility in the 1st week and normal fertility in the 2nd week; by the 4th week there was permanent sterility condition due to bilateral obstructive lesions in the ductuli efferentes, which normally conduct sperm from testis to epididymis	Jackson and Robinson (443)
R-*l*-2-Chlorohydrin	Rat (oral)	Single 50 mg/kg did not induce sterility	
dl- or *l*-1-Amino-3-chloro-2-propanol	Rat (oral)	Ineffective in producing sterility	
Estradiol benzoate	Rat, immature (s.c.)	Severe testicular atropy; 50% decrease in testicular weight	Chemes et al. (444)
Estradiol benzoate + testosterone Estradiol benzoate + 5α-dihydro-testosterone Estradiol benzoate + 5α-androstane-3α,17β-diol	Rat, immature (s.c.)	Testicular decrease, 10–20%	
α-Chlorohydrin (U58,971), U15,646	Rat (oral s.c.)	1. Fertility lost in 1 week 2. Antifertility effect related to inability of sperm to fertilize ova	Ericsson and Baker (445)
U-5897, U-15,646, and others, including 25,352, 25,792, 27,045, 27,151, 27, 421, 27,574, 27,967	Rat (oral)	1. Treated for 8 days, starting on day 1 of pregnancy 2. Positive male antifertility test	Ericsson and Youngdale (446)
ICI 33,828, Methallibure	Rat (oral)	Antifertility due to reduced libido, arrest of spermatogenesis, and possibly induction of "lethal mutations" in developing germ cells	Hemsworth et al. (447)
Cyproterone acetate	Rat (implant)	Cannot confirm Prasad et al. (54)	Elger and von Berswordt-Wallrabe (55)
α-Chlorohydrin 4-Chloromethyl-2,2-methyl-1,3-dioxolane 4-Chloromethyl-2-penyl-1,3-dioxolane	Rat (oral)	Induced sterility	Banik et al. (448)

Table 30.53 *(continued)*

Compound	Species (Route)	Results	Reference
4-Chloromethyl-2-methyl-2-pentyl-1,3-dioxolane 1-Chloro-2,3-propanediol diacetate 1-Chloro-2,3-bis-tetrahydropyran-2-yloxy propane			
N,N'-Bis(dichloroacetyl)-*N,N'*-diethyl-1,4-xylylenediamine (I) *N,N'*-Bis(dichloroacetyl)-1,8-octamethylenediamine (II)	Rat (oral)	1. Testicular weight decrease 2. Atrophic seminiferous tubules 3. No change in Leydig cells 4. I and II showed no androgenic, estrogenic, progestational, or glycogenic activity	Beyler et al. (449)
Testosterone	Rabbit (implant)	1. Induced azoospermia 2. No change in plasma testosterone and accessory sex glands	Ewing et al. (450)
Bulsulfan (Myleran), Tretamine (TEM), isopropylmethanesulfonate (IMS)	Rabbit (i.v.)	1. Aspermia developed during weeks 10–11 after single administration of drugs 2. Toxic	Fox et al. (451)
Steroid VI (19-Norspiroxenone; oestr-4-en-3-one-spiro-17α-2'-tetrahydrofuran)	Rat (oral)	1. Blocked completion of spermatogenesis 2. Reduced number of fetuses 3. Diminished weight of seminal vesicle, prostate, testis, and epididymus 4. Suggest compound affects male fertility by antiestrogenic action in hypothalamus or testis	Goldman et al. (57)
Estradiol-17β, estrone, ethynylestradiol	Rat (s.c.)	Highly effective inhibition of spermatogenesis	Patanelli (421)
ICI 33,828 (Methallibure)	Rat	1. Inhibit spermatogenesis 2. Inhibit fertility 3. Loss of libido	Jackson and Schneider (452)
Deladroxone	Rat (i.m.)	1. In 48 days produced reversible arrest of spermatogenesis 2. Libido decreased	Setty and Kar (453)
	Rhesus monkey (i.m.)	No effect	
Testosterone, methyltestosterone	Rat (s.c.)	Arrest of spermatogenesis	Kincl et al. (454)

Table 30.53 *(continued)*

Compound	Species (Route)	Results	Reference
Cadmium chloride	Rhesus monkey	Antispermatogenic	Kar (455)
WIN 13,099 [*N,N*′-Bis(dichloro-acetyl)-*N,N*′-diethyl-1,4-xylylenediamine]	Rhesus monkey	Antispermatogenic	Coulston et al. (436)
Ciba 32,644-Ba [1-(5-Nitro-2-thiozolyl)-2-imidazolidione]	Rhesus monkey	Antispermatogenic	Sinari (456)
Busulfan (Myleran), Tretamine (TEM)	Rhesus monkey	Antispermatogenic	Kar et al. (457)
α-Chlorohydrin (U-5897)	Rhesus monkey	Functional sterility	Kirton et al. (405)
Myleran	Rat	1. Destruction of spermatogonia 2. Toxic	Jackson (458)
Tretamine	Rat	1. Destruction of spermatogonia 2. Sterilant effect on developing spermatids 3. Toxic	
ORF 1616 (adinitropyrrole)	Rat, mouse (oral)	1. Sterility in 6 weeks 2. Maintain sterility by once a month treatment	Nelson and Patanelli (440)
Hexamethylphos-phoramide (HMPA)	Rat (oral)	1. Sterilization 2. Toxic dose near effective dose	Jackson (458)
	Rabbit	Suppressant action on meiotic region of spermatogenesis	
Ethylenedimethan-sulfonate (EDS)	Rat (oral)	1. Sterilization in one week 2. Action on epididymal spermatozoa 3. Impairment of conversion of progesterone to testosterone	Jackson (458) BúLock and Jackson (459)
Trimethylphos-phate (TMP)	Rat, mouse (oral)	Infertility reversible	Jackson (458)
TMP (high doses), methyl methane-sulfonate, methylene dimethanesulfonate	Rat	1. Epididymal spermatozoa sterilized 2. Mechanism seems to involve donating of CH_3 groups	
α-Chlorhydrin	Rat (oral)	1. Effect is at the lower region of the epididymis 2. Prevents sperm from penetrating eggs 3. Animals become infertile within 48 hr 4. Reversible at low dose 5. Normal sex activity	

Table 30.53 *(continued)*

Compound	Species (Route)	Results	Reference
Thiotepa, Nitrofurazone, WIN-18,446 [*N*,*N*′-bis(dichloro-acetyl)-1,8-octanedi-amine]	Mouse (oral)	1. Serial mating method used 2. Thiotepa most active 3. Thiotepa active at 0.05 mg/day	Hershberger et al. (460)
ORF-1616	Rat (oral)	1. Pachytene spermatocytes VII–XIV most sensitive 2. Effect directly on testis; not mediated by pituitary gonadotropins 3. 6 month treatment maintains inhibition of spermatic development at stage VII	Patanelli and Nelson (461)

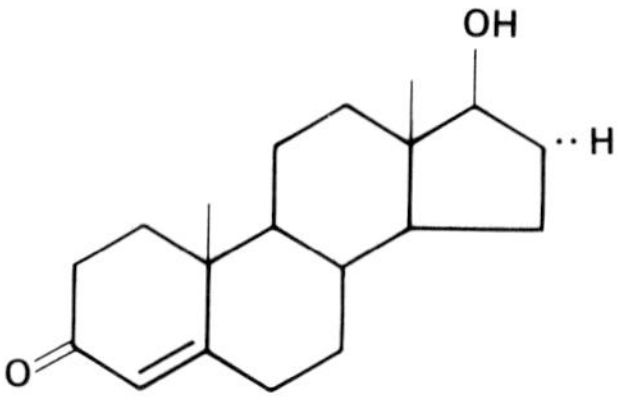

TESTOSTERONE

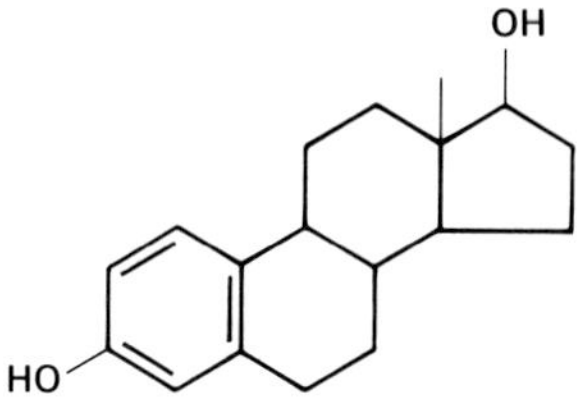

ESTRADIOL

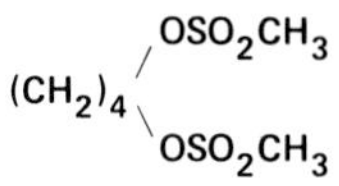

$(CH_2)_4(OSO_2CH_3)_2$

(MYLERAN, BUSULFAN)

O_2N–furan–$CH{=}N{-}N(CH_2CH_2OH)C(O)NH_2$

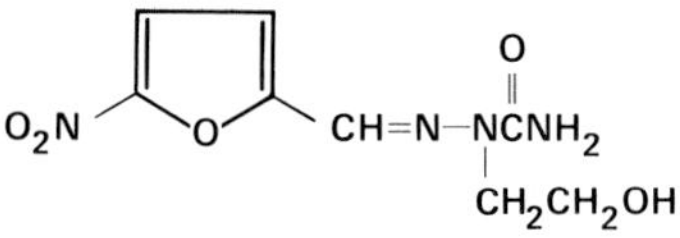

Furadroxyl [5-nitro-2-furfuraldehyde-2-(2-hydroxyethyl)-semicarbazone]

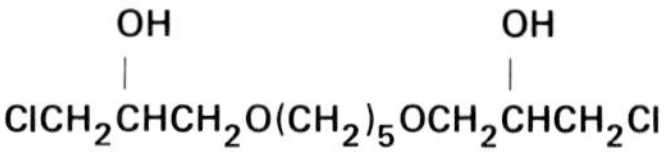

$ClCH_2CH(OH)CH_2O(CH_2)_5OCH_2CH(OH)CH_2Cl$

1,1′,-(pentamethylenedioxy)-bis(3-chloro-2-propanol) (U-15,646)

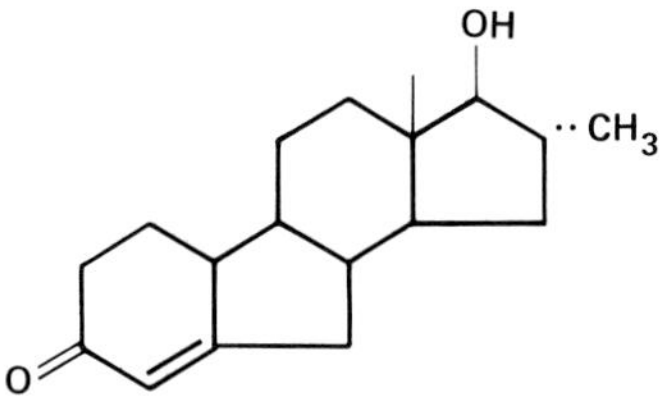

17α-methyl-B-nortestosterone

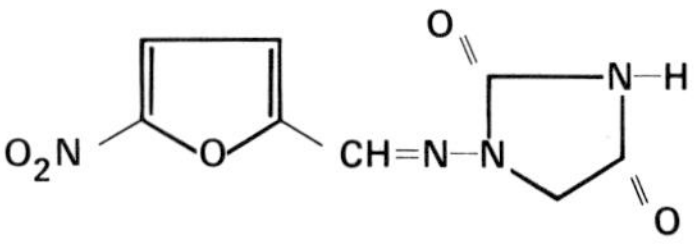

nitrofurantoin or furadantin [*n*-(5-nitro-2-furfurylidene) 1-amino-hydantoin]

Fig. 30.28 Male antifertility compounds: nonhuman (see Table 30.53).

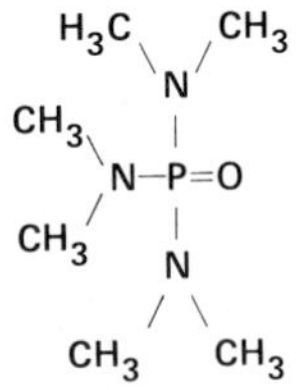

HMPA (Hexamethylphosphoramide)

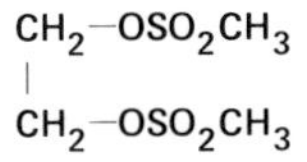

$CH_2{-}OSO_2CH_3$ / $CH_2{-}OSO_2CH_3$

EDS (Ethylenedimethanesulphanate)

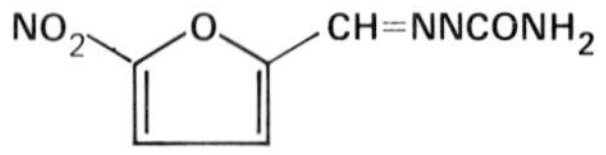

NO_2–furan–$CH{=}NNCONH_2$

NITROFURAZONE

$(CH_3O)_3PO$

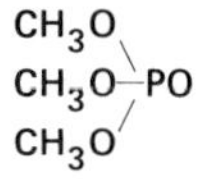

TMP (Trimethylphosphate)

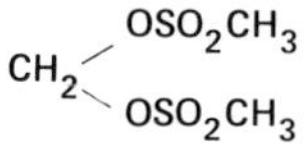

$CH_2(OSO_2CH_3)_2$

MDS (methylene dimethanesulphonate)

$CH_3 \cdot OSO_2CH_3$

MMS (methyl methanesulphonate)

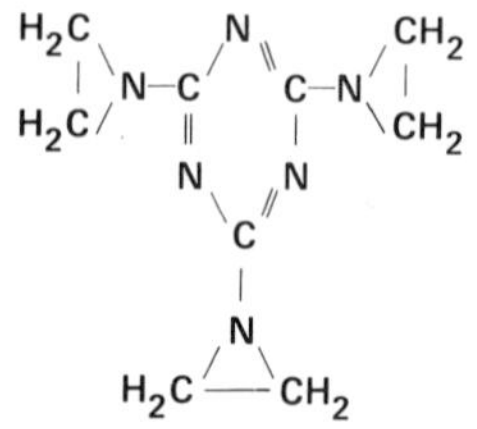

TRETAMINE (TEM)

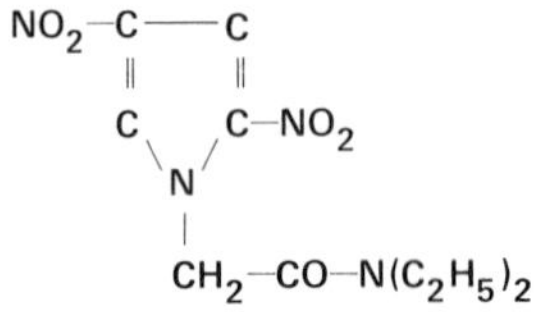

1-(*N*,*N*-diethylcarbamylmethyl) -2,4-dinitropyrrole

ORF-1616

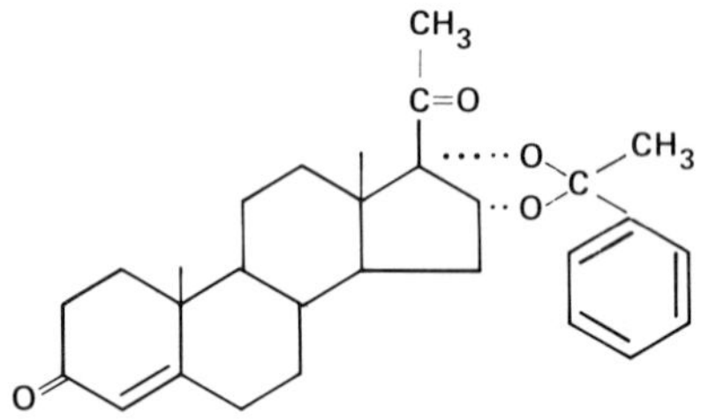

DELAROXONE

Fig. 30.29 Male antifertility compounds: nonhuman (see Table 30.53).

15.3 Dinitropyrroles

ORF-1616 is a highly active antispermatogenetic compound in rats. Complete infertility could be achieved in 3 weeks after a single oral administration. The antifertility effect continues for a total of 4 weeks. Cessation of treatment leads to restoration of fertility. Continuation of one treatment every 4 weeks causes complete infertility. ORF-1616 produces inhibition of spermatogenesis at the pachytene spermatocyte stage. The drug was abandoned because of "certain toxic effects seen in dogs."

15.4 Nitroimidazoles

The nitroimidazoles are best represented by 1-methyl-5-nitroimidazole, which has the highest activity. As indicated for other heterocyclic compounds, the action was in stopping sperm production at the primary spermatic stage. Side effects are unfavorable. High doses produce complete depopulation of the tubules.

15.5 Chlorohydrin

α-Chlorohydrin exerts its effect at high doses by damaging the germinal epithelium.

Also it adversely affects epididymal spermatozoa at low doses.

Epichlorohydrin and the 2,3-epoxypropanol produce infertility without spermatogenic damage.

16 SUMMARY AND CONCLUSION

This chapter has considered a variety of agents affecting fertility in females and males. The list of the rather large number of agents showing such activity is shortened when we consider only the compounds or combinations that are effective and/or promising contraceptive agents as judged by efficacy and toxicity studies in humans.

Table 30.54 summarizes the compounds and combinations that on the basis of efficacy data, indicate usefulness as contraceptives for women. A few compounds are included that are not now available for

Table 30.54 Summary of Agents Affecting Fertility in Women

Agents	Route	Available for Contraception on Basis of Scientific Data	In Development for Contraception
Combination Progestogen Plus Estrogen			
Norethindrone plus mestranol or ethynylestradiol	Oral	Available	—
Norethindrone acetate plus ethynylestradiol	Oral	Available	—
Medroxyprogesterone acetate plus ethynylestradiol	Oral	Available	—
Norethynodrel plus mestranol	Oral	Available	—
Ethynodiol diacetate plus mestranol	Oral	Available	—
Lynestrenol plus ethynylestradiol	Oral	Available	—
Chlormadinone acetate plus mestranol	Oral	Available	—
dl-Norgestrel plus ethynylestradiol	Oral	Available	—
d-Norgestrel plus ethynylestradiol	Oral	Available	—
Anagesterone plus mestranol	Oral	Available	—
Quingestanol plus quinestrol	Oral (once a cycle)	Available	—
Medroxyprogesterone acetate plus estradiol cypionate	Injection	Available	—
dl-Norgestrel plus estradiol hexahydrobenzoate	Injection	Available	—
16α,17α-Dihydroxyprogesterone acetophenide plus estradiol enanthate	Injection	Available	—
Norethindrone plus estradiol unducelate	Injection	Available	—
Sequential			
Chlormadinone acetate plus mestranol	Oral	Available	—
Megestrol acetate plus ethynylestradiol	Oral	Available	—
Lynestrenol plus ethynylestradiol	Oral	Available	—
Dimethisterone plus ethynylestradiol	Oral	Available	—
Anagesterone plus mestranol	Oral	Available	—
Norethindrone plus mestranol	Oral	Available	—

Table 30.54 (*continued*)

Agents	Route	Available for Contraception on Basis of Scientific Data	In Development for Contraception
Low Dose Continuous Progestogen			
Chlormadinone acetate	Oral	Available	—
Norethindrone	Oral	Available	—
Lynestrenol	Oral	Available	—
dl-Norgestrel	Oral	Available	—
d-Norgestrel	Oral	Available	—
Quingestanol	Oral	Available	—
Megestrol acetate	Oral	Available	—
Single Progestogen Injection for 84 Days or More			
Medroxyprogesterone acetate, 3 or 6 month	Injection	Available	—
Norethindrone enanthate, 84 days	Injection	Available	—
Postcoital Contraception			
Estrogens			
Diethylstilbestrol	Oral	Available	—
Ethynylestradiol	Oral	Available	—
Progestogens			
d-Norgestrel	Oral	—	In development
Quingestanol acetate	Oral	—	In development
Prostaglandins and Abortion: First and Second Trimester			
$PGF_{2\alpha}$	Injection	Available	—
PGE_2	Injection	Available	—
15-Methyl-$PGF_{2\alpha}$-methyl ester	Injection	—	In development
Spermicidal Compounds			
Nonoxynol	Intravaginal	Available	—
TS-88	Intravaginal	Available	—
p-Methanylphenol polyoxyethylene ether	Intravaginal	Available	—

contraceptive use but are undergoing development.

Fifteen combinations of progestogen plus estrogen are listed in Table 30.54. The greatest numbers of steroids are highly active contraceptive substances by the oral route. Six combinations have been effectively used as sequential therapy. Sequential therapy consists of estrogen treatment during the first half of the cycle followed by treatment with the combination of the progestogen and estrogen.

Seven progestogens have shown a relatively high efficacy in preventing pregnancy by using a low dose of the progestogen on a continuous basis.

Two agents, medroxyprogesterone acetate and norethindrone enanthate, have been used effectively as progestational agents to prevent fertility—by single injections whose effects last for 84 days in the case of norethindrone enanthate and for as long as 6 months in the case of medroxyprogesterone acetate.

Table 30.55 Agents Affecting Fertility in Men

Agents	Route	Available for Contraception on Basis of Scientific Data	In Development for Contraception
Norgestrienone plus testosterone	Silastic implant plus oral	Not available	In development
Danazol plus testosterone ester	Oral plus injection	Not available	In development
Medroxyprogesterone acetate, testosterone enanthate	Injection	Not available	In development
Norethindrone, testosterone	Implants and oral	Not available	In development
Cyproterone acetate	Oral	Not available	In development
Methyltestosterone, ethynylestradiol	Oral	Not available	In development

Diethylstilbestrol and ethynylestradiol have been developed as postcoital contraceptives for emergency use. The progestogens *d*-norgestrel and quingestanol acetate are being considered for postcoital contraceptives.

Prostaglandins are highly effective abortifacients in the first and second trimesters. $PGF_{2\alpha}$ and PGE_2 are available for use. 15-Methyl-$PGF_{2\alpha}$-methyl ester is being developed for this purpose. Three spermicidal compounds, nonoxynol, TS-88, and *p*-methanylphenol polyoxyethylene ether gave a reasonable Pearl Index.

Thus there are 37 compounds and/or combination of agents affecting fertility effectively enough and safely enough to be used as contraceptive agents for women. In addition, three agents are being developed as contraceptives for women.

Research on male contraceptives has been modest in quantity and far less successful than contraceptive research for women. Table 30.55 indicates some half-dozen male contraceptive regimens that are under study, but these still require considerable development.

REFERENCES

1. N. R. Farnsworth, A. S. Bingel, G. A. Cordell, F. A. Crane, and H. H. S. Fong, *J. Pharm. Sci.*, **64,** 535 (1975).
2. N. R. Farnsworth, A. S. Bingel, G. A. Cordell, F. A. Crane, and H. H. S. Fong, *J. Pharm. Sci.*, **64,** 717 (1975).
3. R. Pearl, *Human Biol.*, **4,** 363 (1932).
4. J. Peel and M. Potts, *Textbook of Contraceptive Practice*, Cambridge University Press, Cambridge, 1969, p. 40.
5. E. B. Middleton, *Obstetr. Gynecol.* **26,** 253 (1965).
6. C. Tietze, *Int. J. Fertil.*, **13,** 377 (1968).
7. M. Rutensköld, *Acta Obstetr. Gynecol. Scand.*, **50,** 203 (1971).
8. N. B. Loudon, S. R. N. M. Foxwell, D. M. Potts, A. L. Guild, and R. V. Short, *Brit. Med. J.*, **2,** 487 (1977).
9. J. Giner-Velazquez and J. Martinez-Manautou, *Control of Fertility, Hormonal Contraceptives*, (Proceedings of the Fourth Asian Congress on Obstetrics and Gynaecology, Singapore, 1968), p. 131.
10. S. El-Mahgoub and M. Karim, *Contraception*, **5,** 21 (1972).
11. S. Chinnatamby, *Aust. N.Z. J. Obstetr. Gynaecol.*, **11,** 2R3 (1971).

12. P. C. Schwallie and J. R. Assenzo, *Fertil. Steril.*, **24,** 331 (1973).
13. S. Koetsawang, S. Srisupandit, S. Srivanaboon, P. Bhiraleus, D. Rachawat, O. Kiriwat, and A. Koetsawang, *J. Med. Assoc. Thailand*, **57,** 396 (1974).
14. P. C. Schwallie and J. R. Assenzo, *Contraception*, **6,** 315 (1972).
15. M. C. Chang and M. J. K. Harper, *Endocrinology*, **78,** 860 (1966).
16. J. M. Morris and G. Van Wagenen, *Am. J. Obstetr. Gynecol.*, **115,** 101 (1973).
17. J. M. Morris and G. Van Wagenen, *Proceedings of the Eighth International Conference of the International Planned Parenthood Federation*, Santiago, April 1967, p. 256.
18. E. Kesserü, A. Larrañaga, and J. Parada, *Contraception*, **7,** 367 (1973).
19. G. Echeverry and C. Sarria, cited in *Population Reports*, J-149 (1976) (unpublished).
20. A. Moggia, A. Beauquis, F. Ferrari, M. L. Torrado, J. L. Alonso, E. Koremblit, and T. Mischler, *J. Reprod. Med.*, **13,** 58 (1974).
21. G. López-Escobar, H. Willomitzer, and J. D. Castillo, *Rev. Soc. Colomb. Endocrinol.*, **9,** 63 (1973).
22. B. Rubio, E. Berman, A. Larrañaga, E. Guiloff, and J. J. Aguirre, *Contraception*, **1,** 303 (1970).
23. A. A. Yuzpe, H. J. Thurlow, I. Ramzy, and J. I. Leyshon, *J. Reprod. Med.*, **13,** 53 (1974).
24. J. Zañartu and C. Oberti, in *Regulation of Human Fertility*, K. S. Moghissi and T. N. Evans, Eds., Wayne State University Press, Detroit, 1976, p. 101.
25. H. J. E. Cox, *J. Reprod. Fertil.*, Suppl. 5, 167 (1968).
26. G. S. Greenwald, *J. Exp. Zool.*, **135,** 461 (1957).
27. G. S. Greenwald, *Endocrinology*, **69,** 1068 (1961).
28. R. H. Dreisbach, *J. Endocrinol.*, **18,** 271 (1959).
29. H. Selye, F. Taché, and S. Szabo, *Fertil. Steril.*, **22,** 735 (1971).
30. A. V. Schally, A. J. Kastin, and A. Arimura, *Am. J. Obstetr. Gynecol.*, **114,** 423 (1972).
31. D. H. Coy, J. A. Vilchez-Martinez, E. J. Coy, A. Arimura, and A. V. Schally, *J. Clin. Endocrinol. Metab.*, **37,** 331 (1973).
32. A. Arimura and A. W. Schally, *Fed. Proc.*, **32,** 239A (1973).
33. A. Arimura, H. Sato, T. Kumasaka, R. B. Worobec, L. Debeljuk, J. Dunn, and A. V. Schally, *Endocrinology*, **93,** 1092 (1973).
34. A. Arimura, H. Sato, D. H. Coy, R. B. Worobec, A. V. Schally, N. Yanaihara, T. Hashimoto, C. Yanaihara, and N. Sukura, *Acta Endocrinol.* (Copenhagen), **78,** 222 (1975).
35. J. M. Morris, G. Van Wagenen, T. McCann, and D. Jacob, *Fertil. Steril.*, **18,** 18 (1967).
36. M. J. K. Harper and A. L. Walpole, *J. Endocrinol.*, **37,** 83 (1967).
37. F. J. Saunders and K. Rorig, *Fertil. Steril*, **15,** 202 (1964).
38. E. F. Nutting and F. J. Saunders, *Proc. Soc. Exp. Biol. Med.*, **131,** 1326 (1969).
39. R. M. Miyake and K. Takeda, in *Excerpta Medica International Congress Series* No.111, E. B. Romanoff and L. Martini, Eds., Amsterdam, 1966, p. 616.
40. J. M. Morris, G. Van Wagenen, and R. I. Dorfman, *Contraception*, **4,** 15 (1971).
41. C. G. Heller and Y. Clermont, in *Recent Progress in Hormone Research*, Vol. 20, G. Pincus, Ed., Academic Press, New York, 1964, p. 570.
42. E. Steinberger, in *Regulation of Human Fertility*, K. S. Moghissi and T. N. Evans, Eds., Wayne State University Press, Detroit, 1976, p. 291.
43. R. Schoysman, *Progr. Reprod. Biol.*, **1,** 294 (1976).
44. C. Hirschhäuser, C. R. N. Hopkinson, G. Stürm, and A. Coert, *Acta Endocrinol.* (Copenhagen), **80,** 179 (1975).
45. J. MacLeod and C. Tietze, in *Annual Review of Medicine*, Vol. 15, A. C. Degraff and W. P. Creger, Eds., Annual Reviews, Palo Alto, 1964, p. 299.
46. R. Petry, J. Mauss, J.-G. Rausch-Stroomann, and A. Vermeulen, *Horm. Metab. Res.*, **4,** 386 (1972).
47. C. G. Heller, D. J. Moore, and C. A. Paulsen, *Toxicol. Appl. Pharmacol.*, **3,** 1 (1961).
48. R. J. Sherins, H. M. Gandy, T. W. Thorslund, and C. A. Paulsen, *J. Clin. Endocrinol. Metab.*, **32,** 522 (1971).
49. R. D. Skoglund and C. A. Paulsen, *Contraception*, **7,** 357 (1973).
50. M. Ulstein, N. Netto, J. Leonard, and C. A. Paulsen, *Contraception*, **12,** 437 (1975).
51. E. Heinke and H. Jaeschke, *Therapiewoche*, **19,** 1664 (1969).
52. W. O. Nelson and R. G. Bunge, *J. Urol.*, **77,** 275 (1957).
53. C. Lubicz-Nawrocki and T. D. Glover, *J. Reprod. Fertil.*, **34,** 331 (1973).
54. M. R. N. Prasad, S. P. Singh, and M. Rajalakshmi, *Contraception*, **2,** 165 (1970).

55. W. Elger and R. von Berswordt-Wallrabe, *Acta Endocrinol.* (Copenhagen) Suppl., **173,** 120 (1973).
56. H. Jackson, B. W. Fox, and A. W. Craig, *J. Reprod. Fertil.*, **2,** 447 (1961).
57. A. S. Goldman, B. H. Shapiro, and A. W. Root, *J. Endocrinol.*, **69,** 11 (1976).
58. S. A. Pasquale and E. Yuliano, *Contraception,* **12,** 495 (1975).
59. D. P. Swartz, J. H. Walters, E. R. Plunkett, and R. A. H. Kinch, *Fertil. Steril.*, **14,** 320 (1963).
60. E. T. Tyler, H. J. Olson, L. Wolf, S. Finkelstein, J. Thayer, N. Kaplan, M. Levin, and J. Weintraub, *Obstretr. Gynecol.*, **18,** 363 (1961).
61. J. W. Goldzieher, L. E. Moses, and U. L. T. Ellis, *J. Am. Med. Assoc.*, **180,** 359 (1962).
62. E. Rice-Wray, M. Schulz-Contreras, I. Guerrero, and A. Aranda-Rosell, *J. Am. Med. Assoc.*, **180,** 355 (1962).
63. W. C. Andrews and M. C. Andrews, 19th Annual Meeting, American Society for the Study of Sterility, New York, 1963, p. 75.
64. J. A. Board, *Curr. Ther. Res.*, **13,** 1 (1971).
65. S. N. Preston, *Contraception,* **6,** 17 (1972).
66. F. Peeters, M. van Roy, and H. Oeyen, *Med. Klin.*, **56,** 1679 (1961).
67. R. Bowman, *Med. J. Aust.*, **1,** 715 (1962).
68. E. Mears and E. C. G. Grant, *Brit. Med. J.*, **2,** 75 (1962).
69. V. Bockner, *Med. J. Aust.*, **1,** 809 (1963).
70. N. B. Livingston, *Int. J. Fertil.*, **8,** 699 (1963).
71. K. S. Moghissi, A. Rosenthal, and N. Moss, *Int. J. Fertil.*, **8,** 703 (1963).
72. E. Eichner, *J. Ky. Med. Assoc.*, **62,** 195 (1964).
73. J. J. Gold, L. Smith, A. Scommegna, and S. Borushek, *Int. J. Fertil.*, **8,** 725 (1963).
74. J. Gould, *Int. J. Fertil.*, **8,** 737 (1963).
75. T. Hass, *Int. J. Fertil.*, **8,** 743 (1963).
76. E. Mears, in *Excerpta Medica International Congress Series* No. 111, E. B. Romanoff and L. Martin, Eds., Amsterdam, 1966, p. 196.
77. G. Pincus, D.-R. Garcia, J. Rock, M. Paniagua, A. Pendleton, F. Laraque, R. Nicolas, R. Borno, and V. Pean, *Science,* **130,** 81 (1959).
78. J. Rock, C.-R. Garcia, and G. Pincus, *Am. J. Obstetr. Gynecol.*, **79,** 758 (1960).
79. G. Pincus, J. Rock, and C.-R. Garcia, *Proceedings of the Sixth International Conference on Planned Parenthood,* New Delhi, 1959, p. 216.
80. E. Mears, *Brit. Med. J.*, **2,** 1179 (1961).
81. D. Pullen, *Brit. Med. J.*, **2,** 1016 (1962).
82. P. Eckstein, J. A. Waterhouse, G. M. Bond, W. G. Mills, D. M. Sandilands, and D. M. Shotton, *Brit. Med. J.*, **2,** 1172 (1961).
83. S. Chinnatamby, in *Excerpta Medica International Congress Series,* No. 72, G. W. Cadbury, H. D. Connolly, K. V. Earle, and A. S. Parkes, Eds., Amsterdam, 1964, p. 319.
84. M. C. Andrews, W. C. Andrews, and W. L. LeHew, *Am. J. Obstretr. Gynecol.*, **96,** 48 (1966).
85. G. Pincus, C.-R. Garcia, M. Paniagua, and J. Shepard, *Science,* **138,** 439 (1962).
86. E. Mears, *Fam. Plann. Perspect.*, **2,** 61 (1963).
87. K. L. Oldershaw, *Clin. Trials J.*, **13,** 131 (1968).
88. H. Brehm, *Int. J. Fertil.*, **9,** 45 (1964).
89. J. Ferin, *Int. J. Fertil.*, **9,** 29 (1964).
90. K. Turpienen, *Int. J. Fertil.*, **9,** 137 (1964).
91. G. A. Hauser, *Bib. Gynecol. Basel* **21,** 123 (1965).
92. G. A. Hauser and V. Schubiger, *Arch. Gynäkol.*, **202,** 175 (1965).
93. R. Altkemper, W. Prinz, and W. Soergel, *Curr. Med. Res. Opin.*, **4,** 353 (1976).
94. J. Prsić and P. M. Kićović, *Curr. Med. Res. Opin.*, **2,** 204 (1974).
95. E. Rice-Wray, S. A. deFerrer, I. Perez-Huerta, and J. Gorodovsky, *Contraception,* **1,** 389 (1970).
96. V. D. Korba and C. G. Heil, Jr., *Fertil. Steril.*, **26,** 973 (1975).
97. T. B. Woutersz, *J. Reprod. Med.*, **15,** 87 (1975).
98. J. N. Sartoretto and R. Moraes, *Contraception,* **10,** 127 (1974).
99. R. Apelo and I. Veloso, *Contraception,* **2,** 391 (1970).
100. M. B. Andelman, J. Zackler, and J. E. Walters, *J. Reprod. Fertil.*, **Suppl. 5,** 117 (1968).
101. E. Rice-Wray, C. Avila, and J. Gutierrez, *Obstetr. Gynecol.*, **31,** 368 (1968).
102. H. H. Allen, *Curr. Med. Res. Opin.*, **2,** 101 (1974).
103. R. Apelo and I. Veloso, *Fertil. Steril.*, **26,** 283 (1975).
104. T. B. Woutersz, *J. Reprod. Med.*, **16,** 338 (1976).
105. T. B. Woutersz, *Curr. Med. Res. Opin.*, **2,** 95 (1974).
106. R. Molina, R. Torres, and F. Boscan, *Invest. Clin.*, **14,** 159 (1973).
107. A. V. Moggia, E. Koremblit, and A. Beauquis, in *Excerpta Medica International Congress Series,* No. 344, D. V. I. Fairweather, Ed., Amsterdam, 1974, p. 87.

108. M. H. Briggs and M. Briggs, *Curr. Med. Res. Opin.*, **3,** 613 (1976).
109. I. Fassa, Paper read at 21st Meeting on Obstetrics and Gynecology, Brasilia, September 1974.
110. H. Rozenbaum, *Rev. Med. Ther.*, **27,** 1793 (1974).
111. N. A. M. Bergstein, A. A. Haspels, G. Linthorst, and U. Lachnit, *Med. Monatschr.*, **28,** 83 (1974).
112. G. L. Foss and K. Fotherby, *Curr. Med. Res. Opin.*, **3,** 72 (1975).
113. E. J. Segre, M. R. Henzl, J. Giner-V., C. Scheel, and S. Bessler, *Contraception*, **12,** 155 (1975).
114. E. M. Coutinho and J. C. DeSouza, *J. Reprod. Fertil.*, **16,** 137 (1968).
115. E. Berman, *J. Reprod. Med.*, **5,** 196 (1970).
116. B. Rubio Lotvin and E. Berman, *Obstetr. Gynecol.*, **35,** 933 (1970).
117. M. Maqueo-Topete, E. Berman, J. Soberon, and J. J. Calderon, *Fertil. Steril.*, **20,** 884 (1969).
118. F. Nudemberg, M. Kothari, K. Karam, and M. L. Taymor, *Fertil. Steril.*, **24,** 185 (1973).
119. A. Larrañaga and E. Berman, *Contraception*, **1,** 137 (1970).
120. S. Tejuja, S. D. Choudhury, N. C. Saxena, U. Malhotra, and G. Bhinder, *Contraception*, **10,** 375 (1974).
121. D. R. Mishell, Jr., and N. D. Freid, *Contraception*, **8,** 37 (1973).
122. E. Guiloff, E. Berman, A. Montiglio, R. Osorio, and C. W. Lloyd, *Fertil. Steril.*, **21,** 110, (1970).
123. E. M. Coutinho and J. C. DeSouza, *J. Reprod. Fertil.*, **15,** 209 (1968).
124. J. C. DeSouza and E. M. Coutinho, *Contraception*, **5,** 395 (1972).
125. E. E. Wallach and C.-R. Garcia, *Contraception*, **1,** 185 (1970).
126. H. T. Felton, E. W. Hoelscher, and D. P. Swartz, *Fertil. Steril.*, **16,** 665 (1965).
127. E. C. Reifenstein, Jr., T. E. Pratt, K. A. Hartzell, and W. B. Shafer, *Fertil. Steril.*, **16,** 652 (1965).
128. W. F. B. James, *J. Nat. Med. Assoc.*, **60,** 314 (1968).
129. B. Rubio Lotvin, J. A. Ruiz Moreno, R. Bolio Arista et al., *Prensa Med. Mex.*, **39,** 48 (1974). *Index Medicus* **16,** 1956 (1975).
130. E. T. Tyler, M. Levin, J. Elliot, and H. Dolman, *Fertil. Steril.*, **21,** 469 (1970).
131. M. Karim and S. E. El-Mahgoub, *Am. J. Obstetr. Gynecol.*, **110,** 740 (1971).
132. I. A. Brosens, F. A. Van Assche, and W. B. Robertson, in *Excerpta Medica International Congress Series*, No. 344, D. V. I. Fairweather, Ed., Amsterdam, 1974, p. 995.
133. I. A. Brosens, W. B. Robertson, and F. A. Van Assche, *Brit. Med. J.*, **4,** 643 (1974).
134. J. W. Goldzieher, C. Becerra, C. Gual, N. B. Livingston, Jr., M. Maqueo, L. E. Moses, and C. Tietze, *Am. J. Obstetr. Gynecol.*, **90,** 404 (1964).
135. E. Rice-Wray, *Rev. Fac. Med. Mex.*, **9,** 5 (1967).
136. E. Rice-Wray, J. Gorodovsky, and A. Peña, *Contraception*, **5,** 457 (1972).
137. G. L. Ijzerman, *J. Egypt. M.A.*, **51,** 975 (1968).
138. J. Persson and I. Rahbek, *Ugeskr. Laeg.*, **133,** 747 (1971).
139. E. T. Tyler, E. M. Matsner, and M. Gotlib, *Obstetr. Gynecol.*, **34,** 820 (1969).
140. I. Brosens, R. Rombaut, and A. Van Assche, *Pharmatheropeutica*, **1,** 96 (1976).
141. M. C. Karrer and E. R. Smith, *Am. J. Obstetr. Gynecol.*, **102,** 1029 (1968).
142. F. M. Sturtevant and R. B. Wait, *Contraception*, **2,** 187 (1970).
143. G. Azadian-Boulanger, J. Secchi, F. Laraque, J.-P. Raynaud, and E. Sakiz, *Am. J. Obstetr. Gynecol.*, **125,** 1049 (1976).
144. E. Sakiz, G. Azadian-Boulanger, F. Laraque, and J.-P. Raynaud, *Contraception*; **10,** 467 (1974).
145. E. Sakiz, G. Azadian-Boulanger, T. Ojasoo, and F. Laraque, *Contraception*, **14,** 275 (1976).
146. G. Mora, A. Faundes, and U. Pastore, *Contraception*, **10,** 145 (1974).
147. G. Howard, M. Blair, M. Elstein, and N. F. Morris, *Lancet*, **2,** 24 (1969).
148. S. Jeppson and S. Kullander, *Fertil. Steril.*, **21,** 307 (1970).
149. J. Martinez-Manautou, V. Cortez, J. Giner, R. Aznar, J. Casasola, and H. W. Rudel, *Fertil. Steril.*, **17,** 49 (1966).
150. P. Bergsjø and O. Koller, *Int. J. Fertil.*, **17,** 35 (1972).
151. G. A. Christie, *Med. J. Aust.*, **2,** 185 (1969).
152. G. S. Bernstein and P. Seward, *Contraception*, **5,** 369 (1972).
153. R. R. MacDonald, I. B. Lumley, A. Coulson, and S. R. Stitch, *J. Obstetr. Gynaecol. Brit. Commonw.*, **75,** 1123 (1968).
154. J. Martinez-Manautou, in *Control of Human Fertility*, E. Diczfalusy and V. Borell, Eds., Wiley, New York, 1971, p. 53.
155. E. B. Connell and C. D. Kelman, *Fertil. Steril.*, **20,** 67 (1969).
156. J. A. Board, *Am. J. Obstetr. Gynecol.*, **109,** 531 (1971).
157. J. A. Board, *South. Med. J.*, **69,** 49 (1976).

158. W. Keifer, in *A Clinical Symposium on Micronor (norethindrone 0.35 mg) Continuous Regimen Low-Dose Contraceptive*, Ortho Pharmacetical, Raritan, N.J., 1973, pp. 9–14. Cited in *Pop. Rep. Ser. A*, No. 3, A56 (1975).

159. U. Larsson-Cohn, in *A Clinical Symposium on Micronor (norethindrone 0.35 mg) Continuous Regimen Low-Dose Contraceptive*, Ortho Pharmaceutical, Raritan, N.J., 1973, pp. 4–8. Cited in *Pop. Rep. Ser. A*, No. 3, A56 (1975).

160. H. G. McQuarrie, in *A Clinical Symposium on Micronor (norethindrone 0.35 mg) Continuous Regimen Low-Dose Contraceptive*, Ortho Pharmaceutical, Raritan, N.J., 1973, pp. 15–18. Cited in *Pop. Rep. Ser. A*, No. 3, A56 (1975).

161. P. M. Kićović, S. Kovačevik, L. J. Djokic, S. Milojević, J. Janoskov, B. Behlilović, and N. Jeremić, *Int. J. Fertil.*, **19,** 171 (1974).

162. J. Prsić and P. M. Kićović, *Contraception*, **8,** 315 (1973).

163. J. Ravn, *Curr. Med. Res. Opin.*, **1,** 605 (1973).

164. J. Ravn, *Arzneim-Forsch.* (*Drug Res.*), **22,** 104 (1972).

165. J. Voerman, Abstract prepared by Organon Medical Information Service. Cited in *Pop. Rep. Ser. A*, No. 3, A56 (1975).

166. B. Rubio-Lotvin, J. A. Ruiz-Moreno, R. Bolio-Arista, E. Meza-y-Gutiérrez, and R. Gonzalez-Ansorena, *Curr. Med. Res. Opin.*, **3,** 431 (1975).

167. M. Foley, B. Law, J. Davies, and K. Fotherby, *Int. J. Fertil.*, **18,** 246 (1973).

168. V. Ruíz-Velasco, J. D. O. Mariscal, H. J. Salgado, G. R. Salinas, A. P. Zelaya, and J. B. Partida, *Fertil. Steril.*, **25,** 927 (1974).

169. D. L. Postlethwaite, *Practitioner*, **217,** 439 (1976).

170. V. D. Korba and S. R. Paulson, *J. Reprod. Med.*, **13,** 71 (1974).

171. R. Apelo and I. Veloso, *Fertil. Steril.*, **24,** 191 (1973).

172. G. L. Foss, E. K. Svendsen, K. Fotherby, and D. J. Richards, *Brit. Med. J.*, **4,** 489 (1968).

173. P. Eckstein, M. Whitby, K. Fotherby, T. K. Mukherjee, C. Butler, J. B. C. Burnett, D. J. Richards, and T. P. Whitehead, *Brit. Med. J.*, **3,** 195 (1972).

174. G. L. Foss and K. Fotherby, *J. Biosocial Sci.*, **7,** 269 (1975).

175. A. Hernandez-Torres, in *Advances in Planned Parenthood*, Vol. 5, A. J. Sobrero and C. McKee, Eds., *Excerpta Medica International Congress Series*, No. 207, Amsterdam, 1970, pp. 125–130.

176. A. Ferrari, J. C. Meyrelles, J. N. Sartoretto, and A. Soares Filho, *Int. J. Fertil.*, **18,** 133 (1973).

177. G. L. Foss, in *Current Problems in Fertility*, A. Ingelman-Sundberg and N.-O. Lunell, Eds., Plenum Press, New York, 1971, pp. 139–144.

178. H. J. Scharff, *Excerpta Medica International Congress Series*, No. 278, Amsterdam, 1973, p. 900.

179. E. Rice-Wray, I. I. Beristain, and A. Cervantes, *Contraception*, **5,** 279 (1972).

180. E. Kesserü, A. Larrañaga, H. Hurtado, and G. Benavides, *Int. J. Fertil.*, **17,** 17 (1972).

181. A. Moggia, T. Mischler, A. Beauquis, J. Zarate, M. Torrado, F. Ferrari, and E. Koremblit, *J. Reprod. Med.*, **10,** 186 (1973).

182. M. Maqueo, T. W. Mischler, and E. Berman, *Contraception*, **6,** 117 (1972).

183. B. Rubio, T. W. Mischler, and E. Berman, *Fertil. Steril.*, **23,** 668 (1972).

184. S. Jubhari, M. E. Lane, and A. J. Sobrero, *Contraception*, **9,** 213 (1974).

185. S. Avendaño, H. J. Tatum, H. W. Rudel, and O. Avendaño, *Am. J. Obstetr. Gynecol.*, **196,** 122 (1970).

186. F. Casavilla, J. Stubrin, C. Maruffo, B. Van Nynatten, and V. Pérez, *Contraception*, **6,** 361 (1972).

187. M. Roland, D. Leisten, and L. J. Caruso, *Obstetr. Gynecol.*, **41,** 595 (1973).

188. E. Kesseru-Koss, A. Larrañaga-Leguia, H. Hurtado-Koos, and H.-J. Scharff, *Acta Eur. Fertil.*, **4,** 203 (1973).

189. H. E. Sajadi, G. Borazjani, and M. S. Ardekany, *Int. J. Fertil.*, **17,** 217 (1972).

190. G. Dodds, in *Proceedings of the Fifth Asian Congress of Obstetrics and Gynecology*, Djakarta, Indonesia, October 8–15, 1971, S. T. Hudono, Ed., pp. 169–175.

191. J. A. Nunez, Paper presented at Sixth Latin-American Obstetrics and Gynecology Meeting, San Jose, Costa Rica, March 29–April 7, 1970, 13 pp.

192. G. Linthorst, F. P. Wibaut, and R. E. DeJongh, *Ned. Tijdschr. Gen.*, **116,** 1694 (1972).

193. G. Leiman, *Am. J. Obstetr. Gynecol.*, **144,** 97 (1972).

194. B. Bloch, *South Afr. Med. J.*, **45,** 777 (1971).

195. S. El-Mahgoub, Y. El-Gamal, M. Karim, A. Wishah, R. Hassan-Aly, and H. Madiha, *Int. J. Gynaecol. Obstetr.*, **10,** 48 (1972).

196. S. Chinnatamby, in *Proceedings of the Fifth Asian Congress of Obstetrics and Gynecology*, Djakarta, Indonesia, October 8–15, 1971, S. T. Hudono, Ed., p. 176.

197. R. J. Seymour and L. C. Powell, Jr., *Obstetr. Gynecol.*, **36,** 589 (1970).

198. L. C. Powell and R. J. Seymour, *Am. J. Obstetr. Gynecol.*, **110,** 36 (1971).

199. R. A. Apelo, J. R. De La Cruz, and F. C. Lopez, *IPPF Med. Bull.*, **8,** 1 (1974).

200. F. D. Scutchfield, W. N. Long, B. Corey, and W. Tyler, *Contraception*, **3,** 21 (1971).

201. T. M. Brat, in *Seventh World Congress on Fertility and Sterility*, October 1971, R. Kleinman and V. R. Pickles, Eds., *Excerpta Medica International Congress Series*, No. 234a, p. 85.

202. G. H. Dodds, *Contraception*, **11,** 15 (1975).

203. D. R. Mishell, Jr., M. A. El-Habashy, R. G. Good, and D. L. Moyer, *Am. J. Obstetr. Gynecol.*, **101,** 1046 (1968).

204. S. Soichet, *Int. J. Fertil.*, **14,** 33 (1969).

205. E. T. Tyler, in *Proceedings, Sixth World Congress on Fertility and Sterility, Tel Aviv, 1968*, Jerusalem, Israel Academy of Sciences and Humanities, 1970, p. 1.

206. J. Zañartu and E. Onetto, *Aust. N.Z. J. Obstetr., Gynaecol.*, **12,** 65 (1972).

207. E. R. Zartman, in *Advances in Planned Parenthood*, Vol. 2, A. J. Sobrero and S. Lewit, Eds., *Excerpta Medica International Congress Series* No. 138, Amsterdam, 1964, p. 116.

208. H. J. S. Rall. W. A. van Niekerk, B. H. J. Engelbrecht, and D. J. van Schalkwyk, *J. Reprod. Med.*, **18,** 55 (1977).

209. J. A. Nunez, in *Seventh World Congress on Fertility and Sterility, October 1971*, R. Kleinman and V. R. Pickles, Eds., *Excerpta Medica International Congress Series*, No. 234a, Amsterdam, 1971, p. 85.

210. T. Khan, A. Kazi, and B. Razu, in *Proceedings of the Seventh Biannual Seminar on Research in Population Planning*, Karachi, April 12–14, 1973. Karachi, National Research Institute of Fertility Control (1973), pp. 97–103.

211. E. V. Mackay, S. K. Khoo, and R. R. Adam, *Aust. N.Z. J. Obstetr. Gynaecol.*, **11,** 148 (1971).

212. S. El-Mahgoub, S. Karim, and R. Ammar, *Acta Obstetr. Gynecol. Scand.*, **51,** 251 (1972).

213. C. A. D. Ringrose, *J. Reprod. Med.*, **8,** 75 (1972).

214. A. A. Haspels, *Contraception*, **14,** 375 (1976).

215. L. K. Kuchera, *J. Am. Med. Assoc.*, **218,** 562 (1970).

216. T. Crist, quoted by R. P. Blye, *Am. J. Obstetr. Gynecol.*, **116,** 1044 (1973).

217. M. A. Yussman, quoted by R. P. Blye, *Am. J. Obstetr. Gynecol.*, **116,** 1044 (1973).

218. F. E. Szontagh and L. Kovacs, *Med. Gynaecol. Sociol.*, **4,** 36 (1969).

219. A. A. Haspels, G. A. Linthorst, and P. M. Kicovic, *Contraception*, **15,** 105 (1977).

220. B. B. Coe, *J. Am. Coll. Health Assoc.*, **20,** 286 (1972).

221. G. K. Döring, *Deuts. Arzteblatt.*, **35,** 2395 (1971).

222. A. A. Haspels and R. Andriesse, *Eur. J. Obstetr. Gynaec. Reprod. Biol.*, **3,** 113 (1973).

223. L. K. Kuchera, *Contraception*, **10,** 47 (1974).

224. H. Lehfeldt, *Am. J. Obstetr. Gynecol.*, **116,** 892 (1973).

225. D. L. Rosenfeld, G. R. Huggins, A. M. Jusczyk, C.-R. Garcia, and K. Rickels, in *Excerpta Medica International Congress Series*, No. 225, A. J. Sobrero and C. McKee, Eds., 1976, p. 19.

226. M. J. Sparrow, *N.Z. Med. J.* **79,** 862 (1974).

227. Schering A. G., Norigest Injectable Contraceptive, Symposium, Berlin, Schering A. G., October 1973, 121 pp. Cited in *Pop. Rep.*, J-149 (1976).

228. A. Larrañaga, M. Winterhaltel, and J. N. Sartoretto, *Int. J. Fertil.*, **20,** 156 (1975).

229. T. W. Mischler, E. Berman, B. Rubio, A. Larrañaga, E. Guiloff, and A. V. Moggia, *Contraception*, **9,** 221 (1974). (a) R. Percival-Smith and A. Ross, *B. C. Med. J.* **18,** 240 (1976).

230. W. E. Brenner, J. T. Braaksma, J. I. Fishburne, F. G. Kroncke, Jr., C. H. Hendricks, and L. G. Staurovsky, *Obstetr. Gynecol.*, **39,** 628 (1972).

231. M. Bygdeman, M. Toppozada, and N. Wiqvist, *Acta Physiol. Scand.*, **82,** 415 (1971).

232. S. L. Corson and R. J. Bolognese, *J. Reprod. Med.*, **14,** 47 (1975).

233. G. A. Anderson, J. C. Hobbins, V. Rajkovic, L. Speroff, and B. V. Caldwell, *Prostaglandins*, **1,** 147 (1972).

234. O. Widholm, P. Kajanoja, and E. D. B. Johansson, *Acta Obstetr. Gynecol. Scand.*, **54,** 135 (1975).

235. M. I. Ragab and D. A. Edelman, *Prostaglandins*, **11,** 275 (1976).

236. P. G. Gillett, R. A. H. Kinch, L. S. Wolfe, and C. Pace-Asciak, *Am. J. Obstetr. Gynecol.*, **112,** 330 (1972).

237. P. Vaalamo and L. Tervilä, *Ann. Chir. Gynaecol. Fenn.*, **63,** 483 (1974).

238. A. I. Csapo, J. P. Sauvage, and W. G. Wiest, *Am. J. Obstetr. Gynecol.*, **111,** 1059 (1971).

239. M. Toppozada, M. Bygdeman, and N. Wiqvist, *Contraception*, **4,** 293 (1971).

240. R. C. Corlett, B. Sribyatta, D. R. Mishell, Jr., C.

Ballard, R. M. Nakamura, and I. H. Thorneycroft, *Prostaglandins*, **2,** 453 (1972).

241. A. I. Csapo, B. Ruttner, and W. G. Wiest, *Prostaglandins*, **1,** 365 (1972).

242. A. I. Csapo and A. Kivikoski, *Prostaglandins*, **6,** 65 (1974).

243. A. I. Csapo and P. Mocsary, *Lancet*, **2,** 789 (1974).

244. A. J. Tyack, C. Lambadarios, R. J. Parsons, C. R. Stewart, and I. D. Cooke, *J. Obstetr. Gynaecol. Brit. Commonw.*, **81,** 52 (1974).

245. A. I. Csapo, A. Kivikoski, and W. G. Wiest, *Prostaglandins*, **1,** 305 (1972).

246. A. I. Csapo, A. Kivikoski, and W. G. Wiest, *Prostaglandins*, **2,** 125 (1972).

247. I. Craft, E. Carriere, and E. Youssefnejadian, *Obstetr. Gynecol.*, **44,** 135 (1974).

248. A. I. Csapo, P. Mocsary, T. Nagy, and H. L. Kaihola, *Prostaglandins*, **3,** 125 (1973).

249. N. H. Lauersen and K. H. Wilson, *Am. J. Obstetr. Gynecol.*, **120,** (1974).

250. C. H. Hendricks, W. E. Brenner, J. I. Fishburne, Jr., and J. T. Braaksma, *Prostaglandins*, **6,** 55 (1974).

251. K. Hillier, A. Dutton, C. S. Corker, A. Singer, and M. P. Embrey, *Brit. Med. J.*, **4,** 333 (1972).

252. I. Craft, *Prostaglandins*, **3,** 377 (1973).

253. E. M. Symonds, D. Fahmy, C. Morgan, G. Roberts, C. R. Gomersall, and A. C. Turnbull, *J. Obstetr. Gynaecol. Brit. Commonw.*, **79,** 976 (1972).

254. W. E. Brenner, J. R. Dingfelder, C. H. Hendricks, and L. Staurovsky, *Prostaglandins*, **4,** 485 (1973).

255. A. I. Csapo, A. Kivikosi, M. O. Pulkkinen, and W. G. Wiest, *Prostaglandins*, **1,** 295 (1972).

256. S. M. M. Karim and G. M. Filshie, *Lancet*, **1,** 157 (1970).

257. F. A. Aleem, H. Schulman, L. R. Saldana, and H. C. Hung, *Am. J. Obstetr., Gynecol.*, **123,** 202 (1975).

258. G. Roberts, R. Cassie, and A. C. Turnbull, *J. Obstetr. Gynaecol. Brit. Commonw.*, **78,** 834 (1971).

259. B. Cantor, R. Jewelewicz, M. Warren, I. Dyrenfurth, A. Patner, and R. L. Vande Wiele, *Am. J. Obstetr. Gynecol.*, **113,** 607 (1972).

260. W. E. Brenner, C. H. Hendricks, J. I. Fishburne, Jr., J. T. Braaksma, L. G. Staurovsky, and L. C. Harrell, *Am. J. Obstetr. Gynecol.*, **116,** 923 (1973).

261. R. C. Corlett, Jr., and C. Ballard, *Am. J. Obstetr. Gynecol.*, **118,** 353 (1974).

262. A. Shapiro, *Am. J. Obstetr. Gynecol.*, **121,** 333 (1975).

263. J. Duenhoelter, N. Gant, and J. Jimenez, *Obstetr. Gynecol.*, **47,** 469 (1976).

264. J. Robins, H. Nathanson, R. Fox, and L. Mann, in *Advances in Planned Parenthood*, Vol. 4, A. J. Sobrero and C. McKee, Eds., Excerpta Medica, Amsterdam, 1976, p. 12.

265. A. Himmelman, P. Myhrman, and S. G. Svanberg, *Contraception*, **12,** 645 (1975).

266. W. E. Brenner, C. H. Hendricks, J. T. Braaksma, J. I. Fishburne, Jr., and L. G. Staurovsky, *Prostaglandins*, **1,** 455 (1972).

267. N. Wiqvist, F. Béguin, M. Bygdeman, I. Fernström, and M. Toppozada, *Prostaglandins*, **1,** 37 (1972).

268. N. Wiqvist and M. Bygdeman, *Lancet*, **1,** 889 (1970).

269. M. G. Elder, *Contraception*, **10,** 607 (1974).

270. World Health Organization International Multicentre Study by the Task Force on the Use of Prostaglandins for the Regulation of Fertility and World Health Organization's Expanded Programme on Research, Development, and Research Training in Human Reproduction, *Brit. Med. J.*, **1,** 1373 (1976).

271. R. J. Bolognese and S. L. Corson, *Am. J. Obstetr. Gynecol.*, **117,** 246 (1973).

272. R. J. Bolognese and S. L. Corson, *Am. J. Obstetr. Gynecol.*, **120,** 281 (1974).

273. L. Saldana, H. Schulman, and W.-h. Yang, *Prostaglandins*, **3,** 847 (1973).

274. L. R. Saldana, H. Schulman, W.-h. Yang, M. A. Cunningham, and G. Randolph, *Obstetr. Gynecol.*, **44,** 579 (1974).

275. T. Engel, B. Greer, N. Kochenour, and W. Droegemueller, *Fertil. Steril.*, **24,** 565 (1973).

276. N. H. Lauersen and K. H. Wilson, *Am. J. Obstetr. Gynecol.*, **118,** 210 (1974).

277. D. A. Shutt, I. D. Smith, and R. P. Shearman, *Prostaglandins*, **4,** 291 (1973).

278. W. E. Brenner, *Am. J. Obstetr. Gynecol.*, **113,** 1037 (1972).

279. J. H. Duenhoelter and N. F. Gant, *Obstetr. Gynecol.*, **46,** 247 (1975).

280. F. Lehmann, F. Peters, M. Breckwoldt, and G. Bettendorf, *Acta Endocrinol.* (Copenhagen), *Suppl.*, **159,** 61 (1972).

281. E. J. Kirshen, F. Naftolin, and K. J. Ryan, *Am. J. Obstetr. Gynecol.*, **113,** 340 (1972).

282. J. Hodgson and P. Van Gorp. *Fertil. Steril.*, **27,** 1359 (1976).

Ramadan, S. Fotiou, and S. Bergström, *Prostaglandins*, **12** (Suppl.), 27 (1967).
283. T. M. Coltart and M. J. Coe, *Lancet*, **1,** 173 (1975).
284. M. P. Embrey, *J. Reprod. Med.*, **6,** 256 (1971).
285. N. D. Freid, D. R. Tredway, and D. R. Mishell, Jr., *Contraception*, **8,** 255 (1973).
286. H. Schulman, L. Saldana, T. Tsai, T. Leibman, M. Cunningham, and G. Randolph, *Prostaglandins*, **7,** 195 (1974).
287. S. M. M. Karim and G. M. Filshie, *J. Obstetr. Gynaecol. Brit. Commonw.*, **79,** 1 (1972).
288. S. M. M. Karim and G. M. Filshie, *Brit. Med. J.*, **3,** 198 (1970).
289. N. H. Lauersen, N. J. Secher, and K. H. Wilson, *Am. J. Obstetr. Gynecol.*, **122,** 947 (1975).
290. I. Z. Mackenzie, K. Hillier, and M. Embrey, *Brit. Med. J.*, **1,** 240 (1975).
291. S. M. M. Karim, *Contraception*, **3,** 173 (1971).
292. M. P. Embrey, *Brit. Med. J.*, **2,** 258 (1970).
293. S. M. M. Karim and S. D. Sharma, *J. Obstetr. Gynaecol. Brit. Commonw.*, **78,** 294 (1971).
294. T. H. Lippert and T. Modly, *J. Obstetr. Gynaecol. Brit. Commonw.*, **80,** 1025 (1973).
295. S. M. M. Karim, *Lancet*, **2,** 794 (1973).
296. E. M. Southern and G. D. Gutknecht, *J. Reprod. Med.*, **13,** 63 (1974).
297. M. P. Embrey, K. Hillier, and P. Mahendran, *Brit. Med. J.*, **3,** 146 (1972).
298. F. Béguin, M. Bygdeman, M. Toppozada, and N. Wiqvist, *Prostaglandins*, **1,** 397 (1972).
299. S. M. M. Karim, R. Sivasamboo, and S. S. Ratnam, *Prostaglandins*, **6,** 349 (1974).
300. R. J. Bolognese and S. L. Corson, *Fertil. Steril.*, **26,** 695 (1975).
301. N. Wiqvist, M. Bygdeman, C. Papageorgiou, and M. Toppozada, *Prostaglandins*, **6,** 193 (1974).
302. M. P. Embrey and K. Hillier, *Brit. Med. J.*, **1,** 588 (1971).
303. R. G. Kaufman, R. K. Freeman, and D. R. Mishell, Jr., *Contraception*, **3,** 121 (1971).
304. S. M. M. Karim, S. D. Sharma, and G. M. Filshie, *J. Reprod. Med.*, **9,** 383 (1972).
305. K. Hillier and M. P. Embrey, *J. Obstetr. Gynaecol. Brit. Commonw.*, **79,** 14 (1972).
306. N. Wiqvist, M. Bygdeman, and M. Toppozada, *Contraception*, **8,** 113 (1973).
307. M. Bygdeman, J. N. Martin, N. Wiqvist, K. Gréen, and S. Bergström, *Prostaglandins*, **8,** 157 (1974).
308. O. Ylikorkala, P. A. Järvinen, M. Puukka, and L. Viinikka, *Prostaglandins*, **12,** 609 (1976).
309. M. Bygdeman, K. Gréen, V. Lundström, M.
310. N. H. Lauersen and K. Wilson, *Prostaglandins*, **12** (Suppl.), 63 (1976).
311. T. F. Dillon, H. Mootabar, L. L. Phillips, and A. Risk, *Prostaglandins*, **12** (Suppl.), 81 (1976).
312. M. Bygdeman, U. Borell, A. Leader, V. Lundström, J. N. Martin, Jr., P. Eneroth, and K. Gréen, *Advan. Prostaglandins Thromboxane Res.*, **2,** 693 (1976).
313. M. Bygdeman, J. M. Martin, P. Eneroth, A. Leader, and V. Lundström, *Am. J. Obstetr., Gynecol.*, **124,** 495 (1976).
314. C. H. Hendricks, J. R. Dingfelder, and W. S. Gruber, *Prostaglandins*, **12** (Suppl.), 99 (1976).
315. J. Robins, *Prostaglandins*, **12** (Suppl.), 123 (1976).
316. W. Gruber, W. E. Brenner, L. G. Staurovsky, J. R. Dingfelder, and J. S. Wells, *Fertil. Steril.*, **27,** 1009 (1976).
317. M. L. Murphy and D. A. Karnofsky, *Cancer*, **9,** 955 (1956).
318. J. B. Thiersch, *Am. J. Obstetr. Gynecol.*, **63,** 1298 (1952).
319. J. B. Thiersch, *Proc. Soc. Exp. Biol. Med.*, **94,** 36 (1957).
320. J. B. Thiersch, in *Third International Congress on Chemotherapy*, Vol. 1, 1964, Hafner, New York, p. 367.
321. J. B. Thiersch, *Proc. Soc. Exp. Biol. Med.*, **94,** 40 (1957).
322. M. A. Sanders, B. P. Wiesner, and J. Yudkin, *Nature*, **189,** 1015 (1961).
323. J. M. Robson and F. M. Sullivan, *J. Physiol.*, **184,** 717 (1966).
324. A. V. Champakamalini and M. A. Rao, *Curr. Sci.*, **36,** 2 (1967).
325. B. K. Davis, *Nature*, **197,** 308 (1963).
326. L. E. Barnes and R. K. Meyer, *Fertil. Steril.*, **13,** 472 (1962).
327. O. W. Davidson, K. Wada, and S. J. Segal, *Fertil. Steril.*, **16,** 195 (1965).
328. M. C. Chang, *Fertil. Steril.*, **15,** 97 (1964).
329. R. H. Naqvi and J. C. Warren, *Steroids*, **18,** 731 (1971).
330. Y. Chambon, *Ann. Endocrinol.*, **18,** 80 (1957).
331. H. Tuchmann-Duplessis and L. Mercier-Parot, *C. R. Séances. Soc. Biol.*, **154,** 914 (1960).
332. S. K. Garg, V. J. Dhar, and K. A. N. Narendranath, *Indian J. Med. Res.*, **64,** 244 (1976).
333. L. J. Lerner, G. Galliani, M. C. Mosca, and A. Omodei-Solé, *Fed. Proc.*, **34,** 338 (1974).
334. L. J. Lerner and P. Carminati, *Advan. Prostaglandin Thromboxane Res.*, **2,** 645 (1976).

335. L. F. Bushnell, *Pacif. Med. Surg.*, **73,** 353 (1965).
336. H. Y. Kasabach, *Clin. Med.*, **69,** 894 (1962).
337. J. J. Rovinsky, *Obstetr. Gynecol.*, **23,** 125 (1964).
338. E. T. Tyler, *Pacif. Med. Surg.*, **73,** 79 (1965).
339. J. T. Dingle and C. Tietze, *Am. J. Obstetr., Gynecol.*, **85,** 1012 (1963).
340. G. Pariser, United States Vitamin Corporation, International Division, Paris, 1974.
341. R. K. A. Kleppinger, *Pa. Med. J.*, **68,** 31 (1965).
342. C. Tietze and S. Lewit, *J. Sex Res.*, **3,** 295 (1967).
343. G. Carpenter and J. E. Martin, in *Advances in Planned Parenthood*, Vol. 5, A. J. Sobrero and C. McKee, Eds., Excerpta Medica, Amsterdam, 1970, p. 170.
344. G. S. Bernstein, *Contraception*, **3,** 37 (1971).
345. M. E. Paniagua, H. W. Vaillant, and C. J. Gamble, *J. Am. Med. Assoc.*, **177,** 125 (1961).
346. Y. Koya and T. Koya, *Milbank Mem. Fund. Q. Biol.*, **38,** 167 (1960).
347. H. Dubrow and K. Kuder, *Obstetr. Gynecol.*, **11,** 586 (1958).
348. Hotay, *IPPF Med. Bull.*, **2,** 4 (1968).
349. R. Finkelstein, R. F. Guttmacher, and R. Goldberg, *Am. J. Obstetr. Gynecol.*, **63,** 664 (1952).
350. R. Finkelstein, E. W. Best, and F. S. Jaffe, *Simple Methods of Contraception*, Planned Parenthood Federation of America, New York, 1958, p. 12.
351. G. Wulff, Jr. and H. S. Jonas, *Am. J. Obstetr. Gynecol.*, **72,** 549 (1956).
352. C. Tietze, D. N. Pai, C. E. Taylor, and C. J. Gamble, *Am. J. Obstetr. Gynecol.*, **81,** 174 (1961).
353. A. J. Margolis, A. T. Cavanaugh, and M. Ems, *Fertil. Steril.*, **13,** 265 (1962).
354. R. Finkelstein, A. F. Guttmacher, and R. Goldberg, *Obstetr. Gynecol.*, **4,** 217 (1954).
355. M. Potts and J. McDevitt, *Contraception*, **11,** 701 (1975).
356. A. Ishihama and T. Inoue, *Contraception*, **6,** 401 (1972).
357. P. Godts, *Ars Med.*, **28,** 1055 (1973).
358. *Population Reports Series H*, No. 3, January 1975.
359. *International Planned Parenthood Federation Report to Donors: 1970–1972*, London, September 1971, 557 pp. Cited in Ref. 358.
360. M. W. Monahan, M. S. Amoss, H. A. Anderson, and W. Vale, *Biochemistry*, **12,** 4616 (1973).
361. C. W. Beattie, A. Corbin, T. J. Foell, V. Garsky, W. A. McKinley, R. W. A. Rees, D. Sarantakis, and J. P. Yardley, *J. Med. Chem.* **18,** 1247 (1975).
362. W. Vale, G. Grant, J. Rivier, M. Monahan, M. Amoss, R. Blackwell, and R. Guillemin, *Science*, **176,** 933 (1972).
363. D. H. Coy, E. J. Coy, A. V. Schally, J. A. Vilchez-Martinez, L. Debeljuk, W. H. Carter, and A. Arimura, *Biochemistry*, **13,** 323 (1974).
364. A. Corbin and C. W. Beattie, *Endocrinol. Res. Commun.*, **2,** 1 (1975).
365. R. W. A. Rees, T. J. Foell, S.-y. Chai, and N. Grant, *J. Med. Chem.*, **17,** 1016 (1974).
366. J. M. Morris and G. Van Wagenen, *Am. J. Obstetr. Gynecol.*, **96,** 804 (1966).
367. C. W. Emmens and L. Martin, *J. Reprod. Fertil.*, **9,** 269 (1965).
368. D. Wentzel and K. S. Viljoen, *Agroanimalia*, **7,** 41 (1975).
369. L. Martin, C. W. Emmens, and R. I. Cox, *J. Endocrinol.*, **20,** 299 (1960).
370. G. S. Greenwald, *Anat. Rec.*, **157,** 163 (1967).
371. H. H. Wotiz and A. Scublinsky, *Steroids*, **20,** 223 (1972).
372. W. L. Bencze, W. J. Carney, L. I. Barsky, A. A. Renzi, L. Dorfman, and G. de Stevens, *Experientia*, **21,** 261 (1965).
373. J. P. Bennett, K. E. Kendle, D. K. Vallance, and B. H. Vickery, *Acta Endocrinol.* (Copenhagen), **53,** 433 (1966).
374. C. W. Emmens, *Brit. Med. Bull.*, **26,** 45 (1970).
375. D. W. Hahn, G. Allen, J. L. McGuire, and J. P. Da Vanzo, *Contraception*, **9,** 393 (1974).
376. G. Pincus, U. K. Banik, and J. Jacques, *Steroids*, **4,** 657 (1964).
377. G. W. Duncan, S. C. Lyster, and J. B. Wright, *Proc. Soc. Exp. Biol. Med.*, **120,** 725 (1965).
378. J. P. Bennett and B. H. Vickery, unpublished; cited in *Chemical Contraception*, Columbia University Press, New York, 1974, p. 113.
379. G. Pincus, *The Control of Fertility*, Academic Press, New York, 1965.
380. K. W. Humphrey, *Proceedings of the Second Asia and Oceania Congress of Endocrinology*, Manila, 1968, p. 784.
381. J. L. Thompson, *J. Reprod. Fertil.*, **16,** 363 (1968).
382. O. W. Davidson, E. B. Schuchner, and K. Wada, *Fertil. Steril.*, **16,** 495 (1965).
383. S. J. Segal and W. O. Nelson, *Proc. Soc. Exp. Biol. Med.*, **98,** 431 (1961).
384. L. J. Lerner, F. J. Holthaus, Jr., and C. R. Thompson, *Endocrinology*, **63,** 295 (1958).

385. M. C. Chang, *Endocrinology*, **65,** 339 (1959).
386. M. C. Chang and R. Yanagimachi, *Fertil. Steril.*, **16,** 281 (1965).
387. U. Siddiqui, P. J. Heald, and J. Watson, *J. Endocrinol.*, **69,** 39P (1976).
388. U. A. Siddiqui and P. J. Heald, *J. Reprod. Fertil.*, **47,** 251 (1976).
389. G. W. Duncan, J. C. Stucki, S. C. Lyster, and D. Lednicer, *Proc. Soc. Exp. Biol. Med.*, **109,** 163 (1962).
390. K. Yoshida and J. M. Craig, *Fertil. Steril.*, **19,** 637 (1968).
391. D. Dednicer, S. C. Lyster, and G. W. Duncan, *J. Med. Chem.*, **10,** 78 (1967).
392. C. W. Emmens, B. G. Miller, and W. H. Ower, *J. Reprod. Fertil.*, **15,** 33 (1968).
393. G. W. Duncan, S. C. Lyster, J. J. Clark, and D. Lednicer, *Proc. Soc. Exp. Biol. Med.*, **112,** 439 (1963).
394. G. A. Youngdale, G. W. Duncan, D. E. Emmert, and D. Lednicer, *J. Med. Chem.*, **9,** 155 (1966).
395. J. Watson, F. B. Anderson, M. Adam, J. E. O'Grady, and P. J. Heald, *J. Endocrinol.*, **65,** 7 (1965).
396. G. Dörner, F. Gotz, and K. Mainz, *J. Endocrinol.*, **52,** 197 (1972).
397. V. P. Kamboj, H. Chandra, B. S. Setty, and A. B. Kar, *Contraception*, **1,** 29 (1970).
398. C. W. Emmens, *J. Reprod. Fertil.*, **34,** 23 (1973).
399. J. E. Major and P. J. Heald, *J. Reprod. Fertil.*, **36,** 117 (1974).
400. A. B. Kar, V. P. Kamboj, and B. S. Setty, *Indian J. Exp. Biol.*, **5,** 80 (1967).
401. M. J. K. Harper, *J. Reprod. Fertil.*, **7,** 211 (1964).
402. O. W. Davidson and J. R. Davidson, *Fertil. Steril.*, **27,** 211 (1976) (Abstr.).
403. Y. Taché, J. Taché, and H. Selye, *J. Reprod. Fertil.*, **37,** 257 (1974).
404. M. R. Callantine, R. R. Humphrey, S. L. Lee, B. L. Windsor, N. H. Schothin, and O. P. O'Brien, *Endocrinology*, **79,** 153 (1966).
405. K. T. Kirton, R. J. Ericsson, J. A. Ray, and A. D. Forbes, *J. Reprod. Fertil.*, **21,** 275 (1970).
406. K. I. Kirton, B. B. Pharriss, and A. D. Forbes, *Biol. Reprod.*, **3,** 163 (1970).
407. A. P. Labhsetwar, *Prostaglandins*, **2,** 375 (1972).
408. K. E. Kendle and J. P. Bennett, *J. Reprod. Fertil.*, **20,** 435 (1969).
409. H. A. De Wald, O. D. Bird, G. Rodney, D. H. Kaump, and M. L. Black, *Nature*, **211,** 538 (1966).
410. J. P. Bennett and K. E. Kendle, *J. Reprod. Fertil.*, **13,** 345 (1967).
411. V. G. De Feo and S. R. M. Reynolds, *Science*, **124,** 726 (1956).
412. J. W. McArthur and S. R. M. Reynolds, *Biol. Reprod.*, **5,** 183 (1971).
413. J. E. Everett, in *Agents Affecting Fertility*, C. R. Austin and J. S. Perry, Eds., Churchill, London, 1965, p. 244.
414. A. L. Walpole, *J. Reprod. Fertil. Suppl.*, **4,** 3 (1968).
415. E. D. B. Johansson and K.-G. Nygren, *Contraception*, **8,** 219 (1973).
416. E. M. Coutinho and J. F. Melo, *Contraception*, **8,** 207 (1973).
417. P. R. K. Reddy and J. M. Rao, *Contraception*, **5,** 295 (1972).
418. J. Frick, *Contraception*, **8,** 191 (1973).
419. J. F. Melo and E. M. Coutinho, *Contraception*, **15,** 627 (1977).
420. M. H. Briggs and M. Briggs, *Nature*, **252,** 585 (1974).
421. D. J. Patanelli, in *Handbook of Physiology* Section 7, Vol. 5, R. O. Greep and E. B. Astwood, Eds., American Physiology Society, Washington, D.C., 1975, p. 245.
422. J. Frick, G. Bartsch, and W.-H. Weiske, *Contraception*, **15,** 649 (1977).
423. G. V. Heller and C. G. Heller, *Clin. Res.*, **17,** 143 (1969).
424. S. Roy, S. Chatterjee, M. R. N. Prasad, A. K. Poddar, and D. C. Pandey, *Contraception*, **14,** 403 (1976).
425. J. Frick, G. Bartsch, and W.-H. Weiske, *Contraception*, **15,** 669 (1977).
426. C. G. Heller, B. Y. Flageolle, and L. J. Matson, *Exp. Mol. Pathol. (Suppl.)*, **2,** 107 (1963).
427. J. A. Coppola and R. J. Saldarini, *Contraception*, **9,** 459 (1974).
428. J. A. Coppola, *Life Sci.*, **8,** 43 (1969).
429. E. Steinberger, A. Boccabella, and W. O. Nelson, *Anat. Rec.*, **125,** 319 (1956).
430. M. Ketchel and J. D. Gresser, in *Advances in the Biosciences*, Vol. 10, G. Raspé and S. Bernhard, Eds., Pergamon Press, Oxford, 1972, p. 247.
431. J. T. Prior and J. H. Ferguson, *Cancer*, **3,** 1062 (1950).
432. W. O. Nelson and E. Steinberger, *Fed. Proc.*, **12,** 103 (1953).
433. E. Steinberger, A. Boccabella, and W. O. Nelson, *Anat. Rec.*, **125,** 312 (1956).
434. D. J. Patanelli and W. O. Nelson, *Arch. Anat. Micros. Morphol. Exp.* **48** (Suppl.), 199 (1959).

435. W. O. Nelson, *Proceedings of the Sixth International Congress of Planned Parenthood*, New Delhi, 1959, International Planned Parenthood Foundation, London, p. 143.

436. F. Coulston, A. L. Beyler, and H. P. Drobeck, *Toxicol. Appl. Pharmacol.*, **2,** 715 (1960).

437. H. P. Drobeck, and F. Coulston, *Exp. Mol. Pathol.*, **1,** 251 (1962).

438. R. Paul, R. P. Williams, and E. Cohen, *Contraception*, **9,** 451 (1974).

439. P. Jones and H. Jackson, *Contraception*, **13,** 639 (1976).

440. W. O. Nelson and D. J. Patanelli, in *Agents Affecting Fertility*, C. R. Austin and J. S. Perry, Eds., Churchill, London, 1965, p. 78.

441. R. L. Noble, *Lancet*, **2,** 192 (1938).

442. A. L. Walpole, in *Agents Affecting Fertility*, C. R. Austin and J. S. Perry, Eds., Churchill, London, 1965, p. 158.

443. H. Jackson and B. Robinson, *Chem. Biol. Interact.*, **13,** 193 (1976).

444. H. E. Chemes, E. Podesta, and M. A. Rivarola, *Biol. Reprod.*, **14,** 332 (1976).

445. R. J. Ericsson and V. F. Baker, *J. Reprod. Fertil.*, **21,** 267 (1970).

446. R. J. Ericsson and G. A. Youngdale, *J. Reprod. Fertil.*, **21,** 263 (1970).

447. B. N. Hemsworth, H. Jackson, and A. L. Walpole, *J. Endocrinol.*, **40,** 275, (1968).

448. U. K. Banik, T. Tanikella, and S. Rahkit, *J. Reprod. Fertil.*, **30,** 117 (1972).

449. A. L. Beyler, G. O. Potts, F. Coulson, and A. R. Surrey, *Endocrinology*, **68,** 819 (1961).

450. L. L. Ewing, L. G. Stratton, and C. Desjardins, *J. Reprod. Fertil.*, **35,** 245 (1973).

451. B. W. Fox, H. Jackson, A. W. Craig, and T. D. Glover, *J. Reprod. Fertil.*, **5,** 13 (1963).

452. H. Jackson and H. Schnieder, in *Annual Review of Pharmacology*, Vol. 8, H. W. Elliott, W. C. Cutting, and R. H. Dreisbach, Eds., Annual Reviews, Palo Alto, 1968, p. 467.

453. B. S. Setty and A. B. Kar, *Steroids*, **8,** 33 (1966).

454. F. A. Kincl, M. Maqueo, and R. I. Dorfman, *Acta Endocrinol.* (Copenhagen), **49,** 145 (1965).

455. A. B. Kar, *Endocrinology*, **69,** 1116 (1961).

456. V. S. P. Sinari, *Acta Tropica* (Basel) **Suppl. 9,** 289 (1966).

457. A. B. Kar, V. P. Kamboj, and H. Chandra, *J. Reprod. Fertil.*, **16,** 165 (1968).

458. H. Jackson, *Am. Sci.*, **61,** 188 (1973).

459. D. E. Bu'Lock and C. M. Jackson, *Gynecol. Invest.*, **2,** 305 (1971/2).

460. L. G. Hershberger, D. M. Hansen, and L. M. Hansen, *Proc. Soc. Exp. Biol. Med.*, **131,** 667 (1969).

461. D. J. Patanelli, and W. O. Nelson, in *Recent Progress in Hormone Research*, Vol. 20, G. Pincus, Ed., Academic Press, New York, 1964, p. 491.

CHAPTER THIRTY-ONE

Blood Glucose Regulation

BENJAMIN BLANK

Research and Development Laboratories
Smith Kline & French Laboratories
Philadelphia, Pennsylvania 19101, USA

Contents

1 INTRODUCTION

In the last 20 years most of the advances in the medicinal chemistry of diabetes have been medicinal rather than chemical. No new drug types have been added to the clinical arsenal in that time, although insight has been gained in several biological areas: (1) the etiology and diagnosis of diabetes, (2) the biochemical processes that are aberrant in diabetes and to some extent how they are modulated, (3) the mechanisms of insulin synthesis and secretion, and (4) insulin-receptor interactions. It is highly probable that as the body of biological data increases, the basis for rational new chemical studies will be developed, eventually leading to new and more effective drug therapy. A survey of diabetes makes evident the need for more effective diabetic therapy, as contrasted to better hypoglycemic therapy alone, and the existence of genuine concern about what is appropriate diabetic therapy and the ultimate value of such treatment in allowing the diabetic patient to lead a relatively normal life.

Diabetes is a disease that is becoming an increasingly important medical problem, not only in terms of growing patient population but also in terms of the effectiveness of modern therapy (1). There has been a steady increase in diabetes mortality with advancing age, with the number doubling in the age group 40–49 over that in the age group 30–39 (2). Counting deaths caused directly and indirectly by diabetes, the disease accounts for 2% of all deaths in the United States, making it this country's third largest killer (3–5), in addition to being the leading cause of blindness in adults. An estimated 4 million Americans have diabetes, and only about half of these cases are diagnosed (6). To some extent, the reported increase in diabetes reflects better diagnosis and health care. On the other hand, it is a reflection of greater affluency, more food, and less need for physical exertion. The tandem of obesity and diabetes is now a well-established fact (1).

This recent apparently greater incidence of diabetes probably can be blamed, in some measure, on the discovery and use of insulin. In 1921 Banting and Best isolated insulin and demonstrated its ability to lower blood glucose and to ameliorate the symptoms of diabetes (7). The advent of this therapy led to the assumption that the cause and cure for diabetes were at hand. This frame of mind produced a throttling down of research in the area. Only in the late 1940's and early 1950's when patients undergoing insulin therapy began to develop retinopathies and to suffer from strokes and renal and cardiac problems at a rate greater than the general population, did it become evident that insulin replacement alone was not the answer in the treatment of diabetes (8–12). Renewed interest and study revealed a host of new insights and problems, but we still are not certain of all the changes brought about by insulin, either in laboratory animals or man.

1.1 Diabetes Mellitus

Juvenile (brittle or unstable) diabetics are often lean, have an absolute requirement for insulin, and usually suffer with the disease from an early age. In addition to a hereditary basis, there is also epidemiologic evidence to suggest that a virus may act as a causative agent. Adult-onset or maturity-onset diabetics are often overweight, may not require any treatment except dietary restriction, and are usually older when the disease is discovered; the basis for the disease in these cases appears to be genetic.

Juvenile diabetics produce insignificant amounts of insulin. This, in turn, results in an inability to metabolize and utilize carbohydrate. Since this foodstuff serves as a major source of metabolic intermediates and energy, the body reverts to protein and lipid as alternatives. These changes are manifested by polyuria (loss of water and salts), polydipsia (insatiable thirst), and polyphasia (excessive hunger). Clinical tests show hyperglycemia and glucosuria (excess glucose in the blood and urine) and ketosis and ketonemia (ketones and fatty acids in the breath, blood, and urine).

Maturity-onset diabetes, on the other hand, can be more subtle and is really a continuum of disease states, ranging from the individual with overt, readily detectable hyperglycemia to the individual who is chemically diabetic or prediabetic. Chemical diabetes is unmasked when the subject is given a glucose tolerance test. Blood glucose values return to normal in 2 hr in nondiabetics; in diabetics the glucose peak is higher and of longer duration (6).

Subjects who are felt to be disposed toward diabetes (prediabetic or latent diabetic), on the basis of a familial history of diabetes, can be given cortisone (stress agent) before a glucose tolerance test. The diabetogenic properties of the steriod often lead individuals who are predisposed to diabetes to respond as overt diabetics (13–15). However there is now some question about the validity of this finding, and a number of studies have been and are being conducted to find a parameter that is associated consistently with the development of diabetes (16–21). A recent and still somewhat controversial assessment of prediabetes and diabetes is based on the premise that there is a defect in the binding of insulin to monocytes and lymphocytes from human diabetics and prediabetics (21, 22). Other studies measuring insulin binding to cultured human fibroblasts show that these cells develop an insulin "insensitivity" with just normal or precocious aging (23).

There is enough epidemiologic evidence to suggest that juvenile diabetes may have a viral origin (24–29). This etiology is supported by animal studies. It is felt that viral attack in genetically susceptible individuals triggers an autoimmune reaction that causes destruction of the pancreatic B-cells, the source of insulin (24, 30–32). It has also been shown in a small group of patients highly resistant to insulin that autoantibody formation has altered the binding capacity of their monocyte insulin receptors (33–35). If the viral etiology proves to be correct, treatment may ultimately depend on the development of a suitable vaccine. Although both juvenile and maturity-onset diabetes appear to be familial, the latter form of the disease seems to have more definite genetic and hereditary characteristics (1, 16, 17, 36).

The biochemical parameters that are altered prior to or concomitant with the symptomatology of diabetes are not always apparent. The most readily recognized action of insulin is its effect on carbohydrate metabolism. In this respect it promotes the active transport of glucose through the cell membrane in adipose and muscle tissue. In the former situation it promotes protein synthesis and inhibits the release of fatty acids and glycerol into the blood (37). Thus in light of this knowledge, the clinical findings noted in diabetes become understandable.

Insulin controls many of the enzymic steps in gluconeogenesis (the *de novo* synthesis of glucose) as well as the flow of gluconeogenic substrates and cofactors (fatty acids, amino acids, acetyl coenzyme A, NADH, ATP). Thus in diabetes with the lack of insulin, this control is lost, and despite the high circulating levels of blood glucose, glucose continues to be synthesized from lactate, pyruvate, and amino acids (38–40).

Gluconeogenesis is a normal process whose rate accelerates during periods of low carbohydrate intake. The initial response to fasting is glycogenolysis, the breakdown of glycogen, a polymeric storage form of glucose. Gluconeogenesis provides a longer term remedy to fasting and at the same time provides an outlet for the reutilization of lactate and glycerol produced during periods of increased physical and sympathetic nervous activity. This anabolic process also provides a "sink" for amino acids generated during protein catabolism (38).

A serious consequence of diabetes is alteration to the basement membranes of several tissues, particularly the kidney and vasculature (1, 8, 9, 41–45). This change does not seem to be controlled by hypoglycemic therapy (8, 9, 44–52), and it leads ultimately to serious cardiovascular problems. Much less is known about this complication of diabetes than about the effect of the disease on muscle, adipose tissue, and liver. It is known that there are alterations in the composition of glomerular basement membrane protein of the diabetic, especially the glycoprotein. Normal basement membrane contains two classes of glycoprotein. The level of one of these constituents, which has as its carbohydrate component a heteropolysaccharide, is unchanged in diabetes, but the second constituent may be increased. This second carbohydrate component is a disaccharide of galactose and glucose, and it is attached to hydroxylysine side chains in the protein backbone. In diabetes the number of hydroxylysine residues in the protein backbone is increased, and more disaccharide is incorporated than in either normal membrane or membrane from patients with other kidney diseases. Thus these changes seem to be a consequence of diabetes (9, 41–43). These membrane changes have also been associated with increases in the levels of an enzyme responsible for the attachment of the disaccharide unit to the protein backbone. The activity of the enzyme is controlled by insulin and is also influenced by the patient's age and the duration of the diabetes (9, 41–43, 53).

Glomerular basement membrane prepared differently has yielded different analytical data and has led to different conclusions. These studies disclosed a marked decrease in the cystine (54–56) and sialic acid content (56) of diabetic membranes, whereas glucose content was elevated (56) and hydroxylysine concentration was unchanged (54–56). It has also been shown that there are no free sulfhydryl groups in glomerular basement membrane (57). These data have been interpreted to indicate a decreased number of inter- and intrachain cross-links in the membrane. This provides a possible explanation for the increased glomerular capillary permeability to macromolecules often seen in diabetes.

Immunofluorescent studies were carried out using kidney tissue from diabetic patients. In more than half the samples, evidence was found for serum proteins in the membrane. The immunoglobulins so detected were not fixed as antibodies, and it was concluded that their presence is due to increased "trapping" of serum protein in the membrane (56).

The relationship between blood glucose levels carefully normalized with insulin and the development of microangiopathies has been the topic of much discussion in the recent literature. Apparently, both duration and severity of hyperglycemia are related to the severity of the microangiopathy seen in diabetes (52, 58–65). Earlier it was suggested that the glomerular membrane changes noted in diabetes did not necessarily reflect insulin insufficiency but could be the result of other genetic factors that became evident later than hyperglycemia (8). This view is supported somewhat by a recent review of Williamson and Kilo (66). Their conclusions are as follows: (1) capillary basement membrane changes associated with diabetes mellitus are a complication of insulin deficiency, (2) the pathogenesis of the membrane changes noted is multifactorial, and (3) the basement membrane changes seem to be the result of nonspecific reactions and are evidence of abnormal vascular function and/or injury. The changes do serve as a useful monitor of the deleterious effect(s) of diabetes on the vasculature. The cellular mechanism for the cause and effect is unknown. Despite contradictory reports, it is currently presumed that membrane changes are effected by a lack of insulin or an increase in growth hormone or both, and recommended therapy calls for lowering of elevated glucose levels (8, 9, 58, 59, 65).

In addition to overt differences between juvenile and maturity-onset diabetes, a number of biochemical differences seem to lie at the heart of the choice of therapy to be employed. It is known that circulating levels of insulin are greater than normal both in humans and experimental models of adult-onset diabetes (67–69). Immunoassays as well as biologic assay of blood confirm this and suggest that cells normally sensitive to insulin have become less sensitive (resistant). This, in turn, has led to the study of insulin receptors (21, 70–78).

There is recent evidence that insulin binding results in an interaction between binding sites, and it has been suggested that the binding site for cooperative interaction of insulin requires insulin dimers (79). Although there is evidence for the formation of higher molecular weight forms of insulin (80), and the ability of an insulin-sepharose complex ("super"-insulin) to evoke biological responses in tissue previously unresponsive to monomeric insulin (81), the physiological significance of these findings is still moot.

Insulin binding to its cell surface receptor is not a simple bimolecular phenomenon. On the basis of equilibrium and kinetic studies as well as other data, it has been proposed that the interactions are of the negative cooperative type and the receptor exists in both high and low affinity forms (76, 82, 83). The conversion of the receptor from the high affinity to the low affinity form can be induced by insulin, low pH, high temperature, urea, and antireceptor antibodies (83, 84). Models for negative cooperativity of surface receptors suggest subunit interactions (83, 85, 86) or movement of proteins within a "fluid mosaic" membrane (87–89). However results of work with solubilized insulin receptors suggest that a planar membrane is not required (90). Studies in which the insulin receptor size was measured using gel filtration indicated that insulin brought about a reversible change in the Stokes radius of the receptor from a larger form to a smaller form and led to the development of a model for the insulin receptor site.

This model proposes a tetrameric high affinity conformation, which, upon interaction with insulin at any of the sites, undergoes a small conformational change in all the subunits to produce a tetrameric receptor having decreased affinity for insulin (negative cooperativity). In the continued presence of insulin, this form converts to a monomeric low affinity form. This model is compatible with gel filtration binding data and a thermodynamic receptor model (82, 91).

There is considerable evidence that weight gain produces elevation of insulin blood levels (92–96), and preliminary findings indicate that high levels of insulin lead to a reduced number of receptors (21, 97, 98), possibly because of insulin's proteolytic activity (21). However there is a correlation between numbers of receptors (resistance) and the metabolic derangement of diabetes (19). Although this appears to be valid for lymphocytes, it does not appear to be true for adipocytes. The decrease in responsiveness of this cell type is not attributable either to the quantity of receptor cells or to their affinity for insulin (99, 100). The remarkable finding in all this work has been that a restriction of caloric intake is accompanied by a decrease in insulin concentration and an increase in the number of receptors, even though weight loss may be very modest (21, 101). This has an obvious implication for diabetic therapy.

These conclusions are modified somewhat by recent findings from a study with isolated adipocytes from fasted rats. It was shown that fasting increased insulin's overall binding affinity to this cell type, but the number of receptors per cell remained constant. Glucose oxidation was attenuated markedly, and there was a 40–50%

decrease in the apparent maximal transport capacity of 2-deoxyglucose with no change in K_m. The decrease in glucose oxidation is much greater than glucose transport, indicating impaired intracellular oxidation. It was concluded that fasting causes the adipocyte insulin receptors to undergo conformational changes that perhaps represent a regulatory mechanism whereby some metabolic change causes a change in receptor affinity (102).

Additional support for the concept that events distal to the binding of insulin to its receptor modulate subsequent sensitivity of the receptor for insulin is gleaned from studies with hepatic plasma membrane from streptozotocin-diabetic rats. It was suggested that the increased binding of insulin by hepatic membrane from the diabetic rats resulted from an enhanced binding capacity for insulin rather than from an increase in the affinity of the binding site. Insulin treatment decreased the binding capacity to normal and indicated that insulin controls its own binding (103). Similar findings with Chinese hamsters and diabetic mice confirm these results (104).

1.2 Insulin

Insulin is synthesized in the B-cells of the islets of Langerhans. The amino acid sequence of insulin from cattle was first determined by Sanger and co-workers (105, 106). Subsequently, the amino acid sequence of insulins from a variety of mammalian and nonmammalian sources has been determined (Fig. 31.1).

The discovery by Steiner and his colleagues of proinsulin in a human islet cell adenoma led to the delineation of the nature of insulin biosynthesis. The hormone is synthesized as a single chain with appropriate intramolecular disulfide bridges. Subsequently a portion of the center (the C chain) is removed enzymatically to give what appears to be two strands joined by intermolecular disulfide bonds (107, 108). When reduced natural insulin or the individual A and B chains of insulin are allowed to oxidize *in vitro*, they recombine poorly. This reluctance of insulin A and B chains to recombine efficiently is readily understandable in light of what is now known of insulin biosynthesis, although at one time a specific enzyme was invoked to carry out this recombination (37). Although there is great similarity between insulins from various mammalian sources the disparity between the C chains is much greater.

Katsoyannis and his co-workers, despite the difficulties of others, were successful in recombining the two chains of insulin in 60–80% yields (109). They have also continued to inspect the relationship between the chemical structure of insulin and its biological and immunological activity (110–112), while others have studied the relationship between the chemical structures of proinsulin and modified insulins and their binding capacities (113–127). For additional comment on the structure and synthesis of insulin and proinsulin, see Chapter 27.

1.3 Storage and Release of Insulin

Proinsulin is converted to insulin within the B-cell. The insulin is stored in secretory granules, which are translocated by way of a cytoskeleton composed of microtubules to the cell surface, where the cell membrane invaginates and expels the insulin (emiocytosis, exocytosis) (128, 129). In response to glucose and/or other stimuli, insulin is rapidly passed into the circulation. This rapid response is followed by a slower response, which can be modulated by inhibitors of protein synthesis and energy production or modifiers of microtubular translocation (108, 130–140). Thus the rapid response is probably due to the release of stored, preformed insulin, whereas the later, more sustained release results

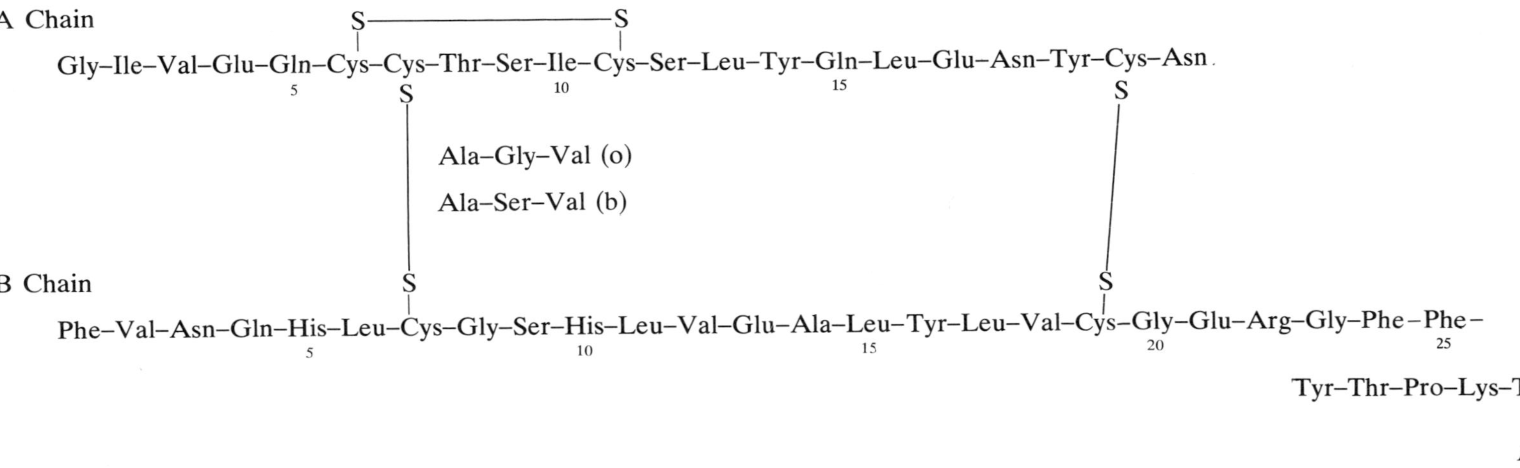

Fig. 31.1 Structure of human insulin. The structures of ovine (o), bovine (b), and porcine (p) insulins are also indicated with only the differences in amino acid sequence given between positions 8 and 10 in the A chain and at position 30 in the B chain.

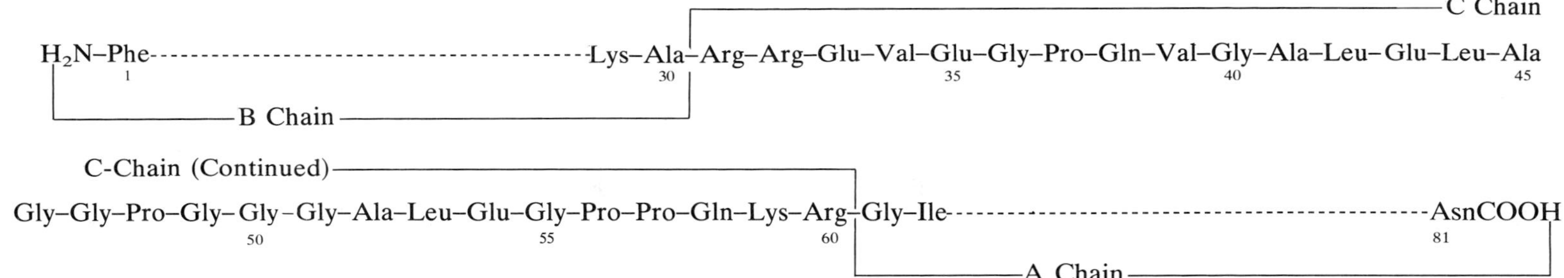

Fig. 31.2 Amino acid sequence of the bovine proinsulin connecting segment. Insulin B chain ends at residue 30, and insulin A chain begins at residue 61.

from new protein synthesis and translocation of the newly formed protein to the cell membrane (141).

The mechanism(s) by which glucose fosters the release of insulin is still the subject of intensive study. The initial step in this process may be the recognition by glucose of a receptor on the B-cell membrane. This, in turn, triggers subsequent events ("regulator site hypothesis") (142). Support for this hypothesis comes from the observation that the α-anomer of glucose is more effective than the β-anomer as a secretagogue (143–147) and as a protector against the necrotic action of alloxan (148, 149), but the two anomers are equally good as substrates in the islet cell in the early stages of glycolysis (150). However quite recent studies have produced data that conflict with the latter finding (151).

Alternatively, binding to the receptor may be followed by another reaction (metabolism) leading to the release of insulin by way of a glycolytic intermediate ("substrate-site hypothesis") (152–155). D-Glyceraldehyde and dihydroxyacetone have been implicated as key intermediates because of their potency in stimulating insulin release (154–156). These studies support a third possible mechanism for glucose-induced insulin release, namely, a "two-site" system made up of an "initiator" site sensitive to glucose and its metabolizable analogs, and a "potentiator" site that has much less specificity. Binding at the "potentiator" site effects insulin release only when the "initiator" site is also activated (153, 157). None of these hypotheses is yet generally accepted (129, 133, 158).

The insulin switch can be turned on or off by the dietary state of the animal (159, 160), as well as by a number of substances other than glucose (or its metabolites). These include phosphodiesterase inhibitors (161), glucagon, gastrointestinal hormones (secretin, pancreozymin, gastrin) (129, 133), modulators of α and β-adrenergic responses (129, 133, 162–165), other sugars (166–169), derivatives of cyclic AMP (170), nucleotides (171–174), prostaglandins (175), quinaldic acid (176), fatty acids (177–179), certain cations (158, 180–184), and sulfonylureas (129, 133, 158). These agents potentiate the release of insulin by stimulating adenyl cyclase, by substituting for cyclic AMP, or by inhibiting its degradation. These agents, however, fail to produce a large or sustained release of insulin except in the presence of glucose (129, 133). On the other hand, glucose, a primary stimulator of insulin release, has been reported either to increase (184, 185) or to have no effect (129) on cyclic AMP levels. Perhaps it would be more accurate to assign a modulating role to cyclic AMP in the glucose-induced process of insulin release (129, 133).

Agents that stimulate insulin release through the intermediacy of cyclic AMP also elicit an increase in the levels of both a protein kinase (186) and a phosphoprotein phosphatase in islet tissue. Either enzyme could control insulin secretion and, in either case, calcium ion is involved (129, 133). Despite certain contradictory data, cyclic AMP does increase the rate of insulin release.

Glucose-dependent release of insulin requires the presence of extracellular calcium ion. The accumulation of this cation intracellularly is an essential component of the insulin release mechanism. In fact, calcium ion can sustain insulin release in the absence of other stimulators as long as its transport into the cell is assured, as by the action of an ionophore (129, 158, 180–185, 187). It is still unclear where in the sequence of events calcium ion exerts its effects.

Somatostatin, a tetradecapeptide, of which more is said in the following section (and Chapter 27), directly affects the release of insulin. It inhibits the effects of all stimuli studied, and although its presence in pancreas has been demonstrated, its role in regulating insulin and glucagon release *in vivo* is unknown.

An interesting challenge has recently been extended to the commonly accepted theorem that the elevated glucose levels of diabetes are a consequence of an inadequate insulin supply. It has been suggested that the converse is true: that hyperglycemia is the stimulus that keeps insulin levels at the required minimal level for the anabolic processes needed for cell growth, and this is more important than nutrient regulation (188).

1.4 Glucagon and Somatostatin

In addition to the insulin-producing B-cells, pancreatic islet tissue contains A- and D-cells. The A-cells produce glucagon, a hormone that is antagonistic to insulin. The D-cells produce somatostatin (189, 190), a peptide that inhibits the release of both insulin and glucagon.

Glucagon (Fig. 31.3) is a peptide of 29 amino acids. There is some evidence that like insulin, it is derived from a prohormone, proglucagon (191). A peptide formed in the gut also has glucagonlike activity but is immunologically distinct from the pancreatic form (192–194). Recently a third source of glucagon has been established. Assay for glucagon in depancreatectomized dogs with a 30 K antiserum, specific for pancreatic glucagon, shows that this third source, which is comparable in its elicited physiological responses to pancreatic glucagon, is derived from the gastrointestinal tract (193, 195–198). Further information on the chemistry of glucagon is presented in Chapter 27.

The metabolic effects of glucagon, which are mediated by the liver through the action of cyclic AMP, result in glucose synthesis and glycogen breakdown. Glucagon has a profound stimulatory effect on phosphoenolpyruvate carboxykinase, a key enzyme in controlling the rate of gluconeogenesis. In addition, glucagon influences the rates of other gluconeogenic and glycolytic enzymes (38, 199–201). It is suggested that glucagon functions as a stimulator of gluconeogenesis in both fed and fasted animals (202). Suppression of glucagon release by somatostatin results in total shutdown of hepatic glucose synthesis.

The discovery, isolation, identification, and synthesis of a number of peptides released in the hypothalamus have brought new insight to our concepts of the release mechanisms of several hormones. These hypothalamic peptides control the release of humoral factors from the pituitary gland either by direct stimulation, as does thyroid release factor, or by inhibition, as does growth hormone release inhibitory factor [(GHRIF), somatotropin release inhibitory factor (SRIF), somatostatin]. The latter compound (Fig. 31.4) is a tetradecapeptide and exists naturally, with its two cysteine residues oxidized to form a disulfide bridge (203). It has now been shown using immunological techniques that this factor, in addition to its presence in the hypothalamus, is found in the D-cells of the pancreas, as well as being widely distributed elsewhere in the body (189, 190, 204–206). In some instances, the oxidized and reduced forms of somatostatin have been reported to have comparable activity (203, 207), but it has also been suggested the native or cyclic form suppresses basal insulin levels more effectively (208).

Somatostatin produces hypoglycemia

H–His–Ser–Gln–Gly–Thr–Phe–Thr–Ser–Asp–Tyr–Ser–Lys–Tyr–Leu–Asp–Ser–Arg–Arg–Ala–Gln–Asp–
5 10 15 20

Phe–Val–Gln–Trp–Leu–Met–Asn–Thr–OH
25

Fig. 31.3 Amino acid sequence of glucagon.

```
H–Ala–Gly–Cys–Lys–Asn–Phe–Phe–Trp–Lys–Thr–Phe–Thr–Ser–Cys–OH
          |         5                   10                |
          S-----------------------------------------------S
```

Fig. 31.4 Amino acid sequence of somatostatin.

when infused into normal, fasted baboons (209) and simultaneously blocks the release of the "glucostatic" hormones insulin and glucagon. Thus the hypoglycemia noted in these instances could not be attributed to any action of insulin. With the advent of an immunoassay for glucagon, it had been shown that hyperglucagonemia is a characteristic of naturally occurring or experimentally produced diabetes (193, 210). Hypoglycemia induced by somatostatin can be reversed by concomitant infusion of exogenous glucagon. Thus in recent years the role of elevated glucagon levels in producing the hyperglycemia attendant with diabetes has received considerable attention (193, 194, 210–221).

Perfusion of rat pancreas with somatostatin blocks glucagon and insulin release in the presence and absence of stimulators (222–225). Infusion of somatostatin into normal, fasted baboons and normal and diabetic dogs, with and without stimulation of glucagon release, causes simultaneous blockage of glucagon and insulin release and a lowering of circulating blood glucose (193, 209, 214, 218). Similar studies in humans with normal and diabetic volunteers have led to comparable findings (210, 213, 215, 216, 218, 221, 226–231).

Thus somatostatin has the unusual property of affecting simultaneously two substances with antithetical metabolic actions. It has been suggested that it is not the absolute amounts of insulin and glucagon, but their ratio, that controls carbohydrate metabolism, ketogenesis, and proteolysis (232). Varying a fixed glucagon-to-insulin ratio by factors of 100–1000 did not change the rates of gluconeogenesis, ketogenesis, urogenesis, glycogenolysis, or lactate production in perfused rat livers (226). The hepatic effects of somatostatin are not due to any direct action on the liver (209), nor is the action of somatostatin mediated by way of the action of growth hormone (213), or by an impairment of hepatic responsiveness to glycogenolytic stimulation (212). The data indicate that somatostatin inhibits insulin and glucagon secretion by a direct action on pancreatic A- and B-cells (223).

Somatostatin inhibits the release of growth hormone stimulated by barium or potassium ion (233) as well as the release of insulin (234–237) and glucagon (237) activated by calcium ion. Interestingly, cyproheptadine, 4-(5H-dibenzo [*a*, *d*] cyclohepten-5-ylidene)-1-methylpiperidine, an antagonist of histamine and serotonin, produces similar results (238). Increasing the concentrations of the above-named cations in the systems cited reverses the inhibition by somatostatin (233–236) and to some extent the effect of cyproheptadine (238). Thus it appears that somatostatin acts by blocking general cation-induced secretory processes (212).

In diabetes, glucagon release is no longer sensitive to hyperglycemia (213, 216). This supports the notion that diabetes is as much a disease of hyperglucagonemia as it is of hypoinsulinemia (193, 194, 210–221, 227). It is felt that somatostatin may facilitate the attainment and maintenance of euglycemia in insulin-dependent diabetic (210, 213, 217, 219) and in fact has been so used on an acute basis (215, 216, 228).

Conversely, a growing body of evidence suggests that the glucagon effects just listed occur only when there is a deficiency of insulin and that the lack of insulin is the key determinant for the observations noted. These conclusions are based in part on findings from pancreatectomized humans in which no measurable glucagon was detected (239–242). However it has also been reported that glucagon from extrapancreatic sources is available in such patients (197, 198). Despite these contradictory findings, it seems likely that insulin deficiency *per se*, rather than an alteration in a glucagon-to-insulin ratio, determines whether a diabetic symptomatology is present (240–245). In fact, when glucagon levels were maintained by infusion into maturity-onset diabetics on a constant diet and in juvenile diabetics treated with insulin, there was no change in glucose, urinary urea nitrogen, or total nitrogen. Thus the augmented gluconeogenesis and protein catabolism seen in ketoacidosis do not occur when adequate insulin is available and cannot be explained primarily as the result of hyperglucagonemia (246).

Although somatostatin has several desirable therapeutic characteristics for the treatment of diabetes—it lowers glucagon and glucose levels (193, 210, 212–214, 228), is rapidly reversible (209, 212), and produces no tachyphylaxis [infusions carried out for 7.5 and 24 hr in alloxan-diabetic dogs, (193, 214)]—it also has a number of disadvantages. It must be administered by intravenous infusion, and its action ceases as soon as infusion is halted. Moreover it inhibits insulin release, interferes with the secretion of TSH and gastrin, has a blunting effect on the secretion of prolactin and ACTH, interferes with the release of gastric acid as well as the secretion of the exocrine pancreas (secretin), and impairs platelet function (205, 206, 247, 248).

Despite the shortcomings of somatostatin, its ability to lower glucose levels in diabetics makes it an exciting candidate for structural modification, and some success has already been achieved. Removal of the *N*-terminal dipeptide of somatostatin, alone or in conjunction with *N*-acylation of the resulting dodecapeptide, produced compounds that inhibited growth hormone secretion for 24–72 hr after subcutaneous injection. These analogs did not require intravenous adminstration for activity and were reported to produce a prolonged response (207, 249, 250).

More recently, however, when the compounds were examined in a slightly different experimental model, the longevity of the response became suspect (251). On the other hand, two somatostatin-related peptides with no disulfide bridges suppressed growth hormone effects but were without action on the release of glucagon and insulin (Fig. 31.5). This was also true for a bicyclosomatostatin analog (254). In terms of specificity of action, this is an improvement on early modifications that inhibited growth hormone and insulin release without affecting glucagon levels significantly (255).

Evidence that neither a disulfide bridge nor the free thiol form of somatostatin is required for its activity was gleaned from the foregoing reports (253, 254), from a study of [Ala^{3,14}] somatostatin (251), and from cyclic analogs in which the sulfur atoms in the disulfide bridge were replaced with methylene groups (256). D-Trp^{8}-somatostatin proved to be 6–8 times more

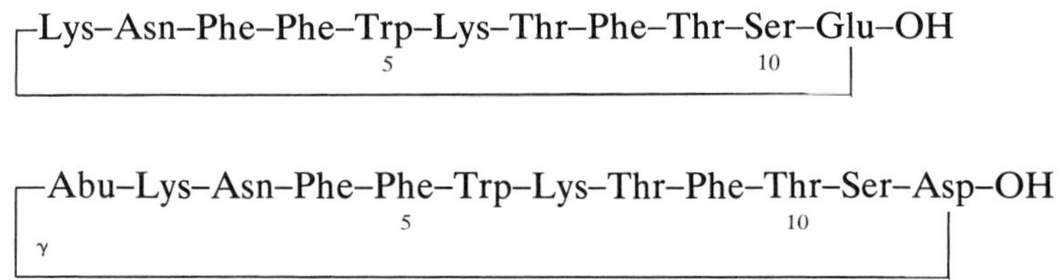

Fig. 31.5 Somatostatin analogs without disulfide bridges; these analogs were active in suppressing pentobarbital-stimulated release of growth hormone (252, 253).

potent than the native peptide in inhibiting arginine-induced release of insulin and glucagon in the rat (257). This is interpreted as the result of conformational changes in the molecule or resistance to enzymic degradation. In light of more recent studies, the former alternative appears to be the more likely (258).

Deletion of Ala^1–Gly^2 alone or concomitant with Asn^5 yielded analogs that inhibited arginine-stimulated release of insulin but had little or no effect on the associated release of glucagon (255, 259). A similar activity was noted for the des-Asn^5 and des-Asn^5-[D-Trp^8] analogs of somatostatin, with the latter compound having enhanced potency (260). This indicates that the structural changes produced are additive, in that a dissociation of activities has been coupled with enhanced potency (260).

Further elaboration of these findings has produced three somatostatin analogs, [D-Cys^{14}]-, [Ala^2, D-Cys^{14}]-, and [D-Trp^8, D-Cys^{14}]-somatostatin, which sharply suppressed the release of growth hormone *in vitro* and glucagon *in vivo*, but had less effect on insulin secretion *in vivo*. These analogs, particularly the [D-Trp^8-D-Cys^{14}]-somatostatin, are beginning to show the type of activity that could be useful in the treatment of diabetes (261).

The most serious challenge to the usefulness of somatostatin in the treatment of diabetes has come recently from the laboratory of Philip Felig. This investigator and his co-workers have shown that somatostatin behaves differently in oral and intravenous glucose tolerance tests carried out in insulin-dependent, juvenile-onset diabetics. In the oral test, somatostatin infusion brings about a 75–100% reduction in blood glucose. In the intravenous test no glucose lowering was noted. Similar studies with xylose and an observed 30% decrease in splanchnic blood flow in normals together with the glucose experiments indicate that somatostatin may act by decreasing and/or delaying carbohydrate absorption, possibly because of decreased splanchnic blood flow (245, 262, 263).

2 DIABETES THERAPY

2.1 Insulin

For the juvenile diabetic, there are no treatment alternatives to diet and exogenously administered insulin. The only consideration is the form of insulin to be used. Several insulin preparations are available in which insulin derived from either beef or pork is precipitated under varying conditions of pH and zinc ion concentration. These variables control the form of the insulins produced. Large crystals and high zinc content lead to insulin preparations with a slow onset and a long duration of activity. Amorphous insulin is rapid in onset of activity and short acting. Insulin preparations complexed with protamine and zinc (PZI insulin) act as a depot of the hormone after injection. The insulin is released slowly but provides glucose control over a number of hours, depending on the physical and dietary activity of the patient.

Insulin with an immediate onset of action is known as regular insulin, either acid or neutral. NPH or lente insulin has activity of intermediate duration. Mixtures of this form and the regular form have to be "customized" for each patient empirically, by analyzing frequently taken urine and/or blood samples for glucose. PZI insulin is also usually used together with regular insulin, and this combination also has to be individually titrated (6, 11).

The very recent availability of highly purified insulins has led to regular insulins, free of impurities, that are soluble only at acidic pH. This, allows the ready use of these new single peak or single component insulins with lente and complexed insulins. The occasional immunologic responses noted in insulin-dependent diabetics can be minimized, since the allergic responses are thought to be triggered by the protein impurities (insulin C chain) rather than by insulin *per se.* Though these problems statistically are not of great importance, to the individuals benefited they are lifesaving (264).

For insulin-dependent diabetics unable to administer insulin injections safely, a rectal form of the hormone (0.5–5.0 units/suppository) has recently become available. The preparations were studied in rabbits, and immunoreactive insulin and blood glucose levels were found to be affected as expected, demonstrating the effectiveness of the suppositories (265).

2.2 Oral Therapy

Drugs available to the clinician treating diabetic patients in the United States today have not changed in 10 years. They include several sulfonylureas and until recently phenethylbiguanide. The latter agent has been removed from the US market. If one includes hypoglycemic drugs used in Great Britain, four additional sulfonylureas and another biguanide can be added to the list (266–271). The US entries are 1-butyl-3-*p*-toluenesulfonylurea (tolbutamide, 31.**1**), 1-*p*-acetylbenzenesulfonyl-3-cyclohexylurea (acetohexamide, 31.**2**), 1-*p*-chlorobenzenesulfonyl-3-*n*-propylurea (chlorpropamide, 31.**3**), 1-(hexahydro-1*H*-azepin-1-yl)-3-(*p*-toluenesulfonyl)urea (tolazamide, 31.**4**),

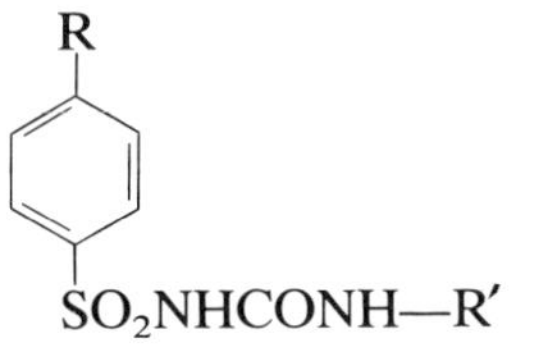

R

SO$_2$NHCONH—R′

31.**1** R = CH_3, R′ = *n*-C_4H_9 (tolbutamide)
31.**2** R = $COCH_3$, R′ = cyclohexyl (acetohexamide)
31.**3** R = Cl, R′ = *n*-C_3H_7 (chlorpropamide)

31.**4** R = CH_3, R′ = N (tolazamide)

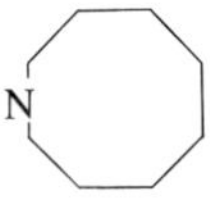

and *N*′-phenethylformamidinyliminourea (phenformin, DBI, 31.**5**). The British entries are *N*-[5-(2-methoxyethoxy)-2-pyrimidinyl)]-benzenesulfonamide (glymidine, 31.**6**), 1-{4-[2-(5-chloro-2-methoxybenzamido)-ethyl]phenylsulfonyl)-3-cyclohexylurea (glibenclamide, 31.**7**), [1-*S*(endo, endo)]-*N*-{[(3-hydroxy-4,7,7,-trimethylbicyclo-[2.2.1]hept-2-yl)amino]-carbonyl}-4-methylbenzenesulfonamide (glibornuride, 31.**8**), 1-cyclohexyl-3-{*p*-[2-(5-methylpyrazine-2-carboxamido)ethyl]phenylsulfonyl}urea (glipizide, 31.**9**), and 1,1-dimethylguanidine (metformin, 31.**10**). Although 31.**4** is actually a semicarbazide and 31.**6** is really a sulfonamide, they are usually grouped with the sulfonylureas because of their close resemblance.

31.**8** R = CH_3; R′ = (glibornuride)

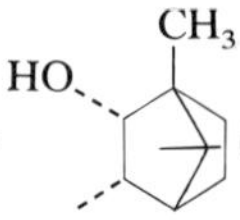

R—NH—C(=NH)—NH—C(=NH)—NH_2

31.**5** R = $C_6H_5(CH_2)_2$—(phenformin)
31.**10** R = $(CH_3)_2$ (metformin)

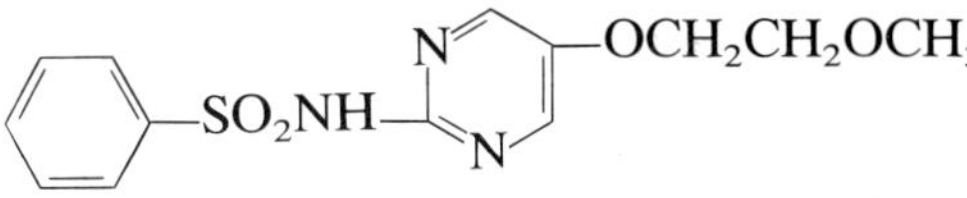

—SO$_2$NH— —$OCH_2CH_2OCH_3$

Glymidine

31.**6**

2.2.1 SULFONYLUREAS. The sulfonylureas arose from chance observations that certain antibacterial sulfonamides caused hypoglycemia (272). Development of that biological lead resulted in the discovery that certain nonantibacterial sulfonylureas also lowered blood glucose levels. This has produced a plethora of analogs, all of which do the same thing to a greater or lesser degree (273–278).

The sulfonylureas exert their hypoglycemic effect only in patients who still have the capacity to synthesize and secrete

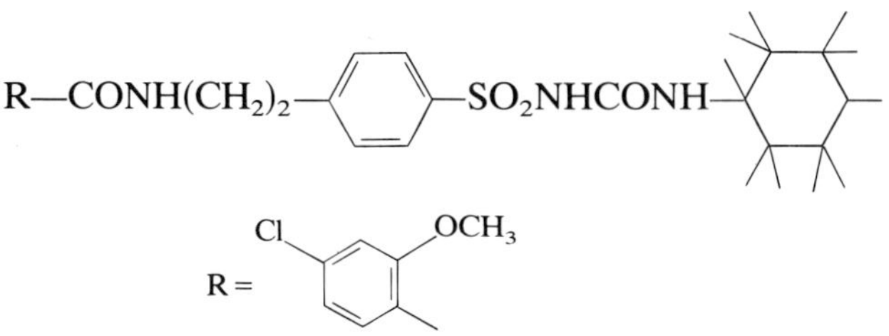

R—CONH$(CH_2)_2$—⟨C₆H₄⟩—SO_2NHCONH—⟨cyclohexyl⟩

R = (5-chloro-2-methoxyphenyl: Cl, OCH_3)

Glibenclamide
31.**7**

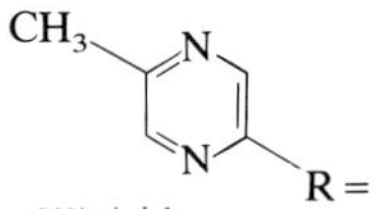

R = (CH_3-pyrazinyl)

Glipizide
31.**9**

insulin. It has been well established that these compounds function, for the main part, by stimulating the release of endogenous reserves of insulin from the pancreas (11, 266–271, 279). The differences between individual sulfonylureas are traceable to their potencies, which in turn are related to blood levels of the drugs. This property seems to be dependent on the drugs' metabolic half-lives (267), although this allegation has been questioned (269, 270). Tolbutamide (31,**1**) is converted to an inactive *p*-carboxy derivative and has a half-life of 4–5 hr; acetohexamide (31.**2**) is reduced to an active hydroxy metabolite and has a half-life of 6–8 hr, whereas chlorpropamide (31.**3**) is excreted unchanged and has a half-life of 35 hr. The metabolic pattern of these three drugs is reflected in their potencies and effective daily doses: 31.**1**, 0.5–3.0 g; 31.**2**, 0.25–1.5 g; 31.**3**, 0.1–0.5 g (267). Chlorpropamide is the most potent and longest acting, acetohexamide is intermediate in these respects, and tolbutamide is the least potent and shortest acting (267). Of great potential interest is the report that chlorpropamide enhances the ability of insulin receptors to bind the hormone in animals that are resistant or insensitive to insulin (21). Implications that drugs of this type are effective because of hepatic effects are dispelled somewhat by the finding that glibenclamide (31.**7**), a sulfonylurea approximately 100 times as potent as tolbutamide, inhibited two gluconeogenic enzymes *in vitro* but was devoid of this activity *in vivo* in rats that were unresponsive to insulin (280).

Because of their mechanism of action, the sulfonylureas are used primarily in maturity-onset patients over 40 years old with diabetes of less than 10 years' duration (270, 271). Some feel that the sulfonylureas should be used only in nonobese diabetics (268).

Recently it has been demonstrated that the antilipemic agent halofenate, 2-acetamidoethyl-(4-chloro-3-trifluoromethylphenoxy)acetate, reduces sulfonyl urea requirements or improves the control of hyperglycemia in diabetics with type IV hyperlipoproteinemia. These findings were not noted with clofibrate, 2-(*p*-chlorophenoxy)-2-methylpropionic acid ethyl ester, another hypolipemic agent (281). In an animal model of hyperlipemia, halofenate altered the insulin-to-glucagon ratio in favor of insulin (282). This has also been noted in humans during clofibrate treatment (283). The significance of these observations in the overall therapy of diabetes is uncertain.

The major problem with sulfonylurea therapy is failure of the patient to respond. There can be failure to respond from the onset of therapy (primary failure), or failure can occur after a period of effective treatment (secondary failure). In the first instance another agent must be tried. In the second, failure is often due to dietary indiscretion. If this can be ruled out, another agent must be tried (268–271).

2.2.2 BIGUANIDES. The use of phenformin (31.**5**) as a hypoglycemic agent is also the result of a chance observation. It was noted that a simple guanidine derivative lowered blood sugar levels in rabbits (284). Exploration of this finding led eventually to phenformin (285–290).

Unlike the sulfonylureas, this agent lowers blood glucose levels in pancreatectomized animals, thus it does not act by stimulating the release of insulin from the pancreas. In fact, although known and used for more than 20 years, its mode of action is still not clearly understood. In general, three schools of thought exist: (1) biguanides are effective by virtue of inhibiting intestinal transport and absorption of sugars (291–293), (2) they function at the level of the liver by inhibiting gluconeogenesis (294–299), or (3) these drugs affect metabolism in peripheral tissues by enhancing glucose uptake (300, 301) or inhibiting oxidative phosphorylation (295, 302). Regardless of whether any or all of these mechanisms are correct (303), they nonetheless provide a biochemical basis for the clinical findings, both beneficial and toxic. The US Food and Drug Administration ruled recently that the benefit to risk ratio of phenformin does not warrant its continued use and the drug is no longer used for the treatment of diabetes in the US.

A more current and speculative explanation proposes that phenformin and related structures are effective because of their interaction with biological membranes. The interactions are said to be nonspecific, and this would explain the diversity and multiplicity of the effects observed (304).

2.2.3 UGDP STUDY. For the maturity-onset diabetic, diet and weight loss currently are the treatments of choice (6, 267, 269, 270, 305). Where this regimen alone is not sufficient for maintenance of euglycemia, carefully titrated doses of insulin are recommended (58–64, 267, 269, 270, 305). This therapy results from the findings of a prospective study launched in 1961 at 12 diabetes centers in the United States—the University Group Diabetes Program (UGDP). The study was intended to determine whether control of blood glucose levels would prevent or delay the cardiovascular complications associated with long-term diabetes. Of particular interest was an assessment of the value of oral hypoglycemics which, to a considerable extent, have usurped the role played by diet and insulin in the handling of the mild, maturity-onset diabetic. The major design features of the program were a common study protocol for the collection of comparative data, random allocation of patients, double blind evaluation of the orally administered drugs, the incorporation of a placebo group; the long-term study of the patients, and central collection, editing, and monitoring of the acquired data.

The patients in the study were newly diagnosed diabetics willing to participate in the study, with a good prognosis for 5 year survival. Other clinical parameters assessed were a glucose tolerance test in the diabetic range and no evidence of ketosis over a 1 month period of dietary control. The patients were assigned to one of five groups (the fifth group was added about 18 months after the start of the study). The groups were: (1) variable insulin dose (insulin administered in sufficient quantity to maintain normal glucose levels); (2) standard dose of insulin (10–16 units/day, depending on the patient's estimated body surface); (3) tolbutamide (1.5 g/day); (4) placebo (dosage schedule similar to the oral hypoglycemics); and (5) phenformin (100 mg/day in two equal doses) (46, 47).

Although much controversy surrounds the conclusions drawn from the study and the actions taken (266–271, 305–308), there were in fact a greater number of cardiovascular incidents in the groups treated with a fixed dose of insulin and either of the two oral hypoglycemic agents. The group maintained on placebo and diet fared as well as the group on a variable dose of insulin in terms of cardiovascular effects, even though blood glucose control was attained in only 25% of these patients. However body weight control was best in the placebo-diet group. Thus the conclusion drawn was that none of the therapeutic regimens effectively delayed or prevented the degenerative vascular complications associated with diabetes of some standing (50).

A recent addition to earlier studies has been issued. This report deals more extensively with nonfatal events for patients treated with tolbutamide and diet compared with patients treated with diet alone and patients treated with diet plus insulin. These data were gathered at scheduled follow-up examinations at which tolbutamide treatment was discontinued. This review does nothing to change the earlier UGDP findings. Review of all the findings for fatal and nonfatal events provides no evidence of benefit associated with the long-term use of tolbutamide (309).

Though the UGDP study questions the value of regulating glycemic levels to preclude subsequent vascular complications, there has been much recent medical comment to suggest that very careful control of blood glucose is the preferred form of treatment (59–65). Since this approach has only recently been espoused, its worth must be evaluated in the future.

2.3 Miscellaneous Types of Hypoglycemic Agent

2.3.1 HYPOGLYCIN, METHYLENE CYCLOPROPANE ACETIC ACID, CYCLOPROPANE CARBOXYLIC ACID, PENTENOIC ACID. Hypoglycin (31.**11**), a natural product, has caused severe hypoglycemia in rats and humans (310). Its metabolite, methylene cyclopropaneacetic acid (31.**12**), was shown to be the active moiety (311).

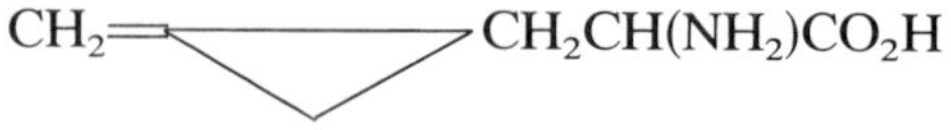

CH_2= (cyclopropane) $CH_2CH(NH_2)CO_2H$

31.**11**

CH_2= (cyclopropane) CH_2CO_2H

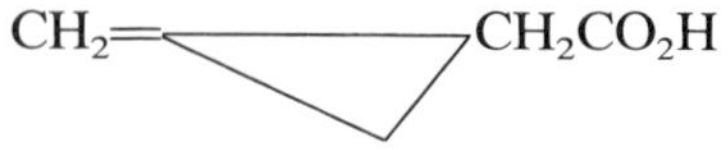

31.**12**

Studies with related structures led to the discovery that 4-pentenoic acid (31.**13**) was a potent hypoglycemic agent having a mechanism of action similar to that of hypoglycin and cyclopropanecarboxylic acid (31.**14**) (312–316).

$CH_2=CH(CH_2)_2CO_2H$

31.**13**

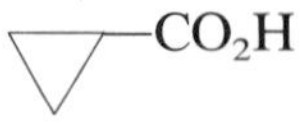

(cyclopropane)—CO_2H

31.**14**

These acids act by inhibiting fatty acid oxidation and as a result inhibit gluconeogenesis. The sites of action are the acylcarnitine transferase enzymes, which are involved in the transport of fatty acids across the mitochondrial membrane. It is assumed these compounds form "nonmetabolizable" forms of acyl coenzyme A and block the transport system (317–324). Unfortunately, formidable toxicity is associated with these compounds.

2.3.2 ISOXAZOLE AND PYRAZOLE CARBOXYLIC ACIDS. 3,5-Dimethylisoxazole (31.**15**) and pyrazole (31.**16**) are hypoglycemic in glucose-primed and diabetic rats because of their metabolism to the corresponding 5-carboxylic acids (31.**17** and 31.**18**).

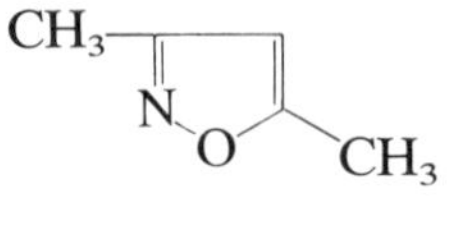

CH_3, N, O, CH_3

31.**15**

CH_3, N, N, H, CH_3

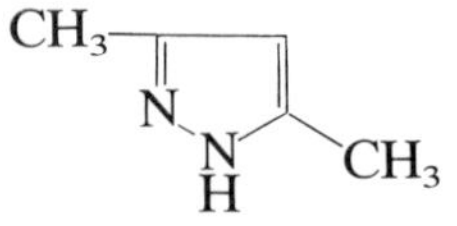

31.**16**

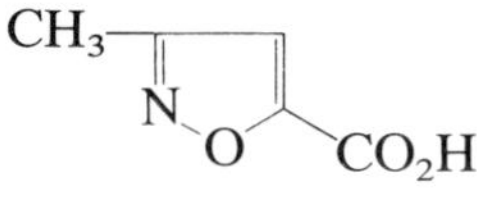

31.17

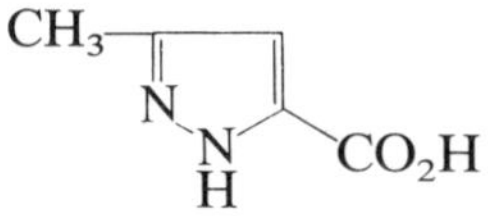

31.18

These compounds act primarily on adipose tissue by inhibiting lipolysis, promoting the conversion of glucose to triglyceride, and stimulating glycogenesis (325, 326).

The utility of the isoxazole has been demonstrated in human maturity-onset diabetics. Unfortunately, these patients became refractory to therapy after 12 days (327), confirming observations with both ring systems in rats (328–330).

2.3.3 OTHER SULFONYLUREAS. Innumerable examples of this class of drug have been prepared. Presented below are those for which hypoglycemic data are available from an appropriate screen.

The best in this series, 31.**19** (R = Cl), is similar to chlorpropamide in action. However there is also some evidence of a peripheral activity measured by an enhanced tissue uptake of glucose and by an inhibition of glycogenolysis (331, 332).

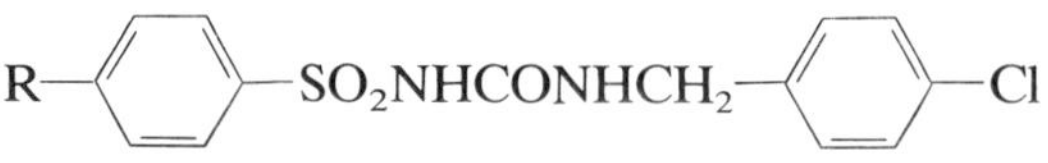

31.**19** R=H, Br, Cl, OCH_3, CH_3

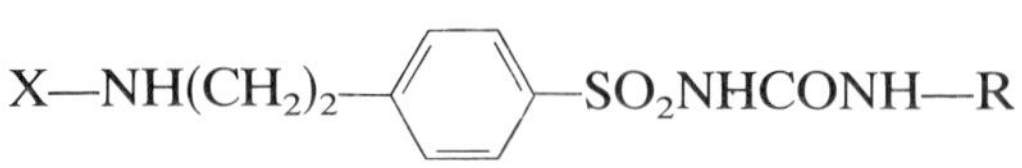

X = ..., R = cyclohexyl, ...

31.**20**

These compounds have good hypoglycemic activity in rats. The best, 31.**20** with X = 5-methylpyrazine-2-carbonyl and R = cyclohexyl (glydiazinamide), was 100 times as active as tolbutamide and glybenclamide in humans (333, 334).

When X in 31.**20** was a benzo analog of a five or six-membered heterocyclic ring containing an oxygen or one or two nitrogen atoms, the only reasonably active members were the quinoline, isoquinoline, and quinoxaline 2-carbonyl analogs (335, 336).

An extensive series of quinoline-8-acyl sulfonylureas (31.**21**) and semicarbazides and sulfonamido-2-pyrimidines showed good hypoglycemic activity in rabbits (337).

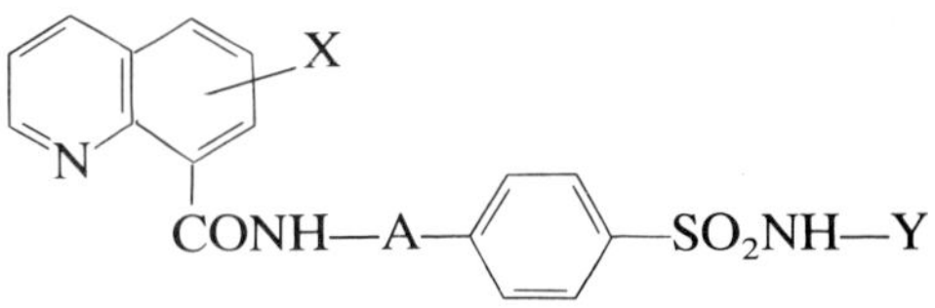

X = halogen
A = alkyl or branched alkyl
Y = 2-pyrimidinyl, CONH-cycloalkyl, CON

31.**21**

In a series of isoxazole, isothiazole, and pyrazole carbonylaminoalkylbenzenesulfonylureas, semicarbazides, and amides of aminopyrimidine, glisoxepid (31.**22**) was deemed best. It is about 300 times as potent as tolbutamide in normal, fasted humans (338, 339) and has been reported to

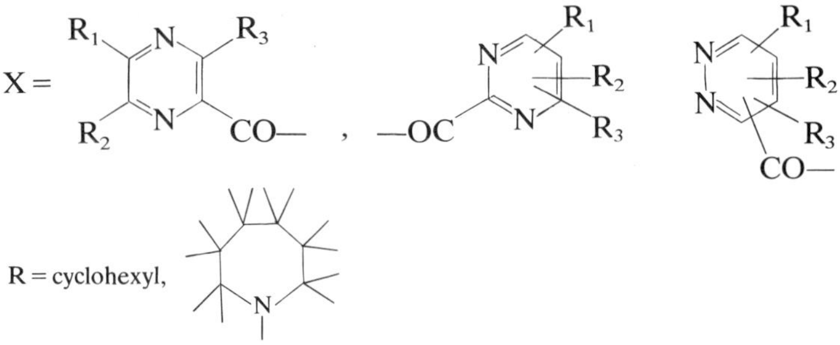

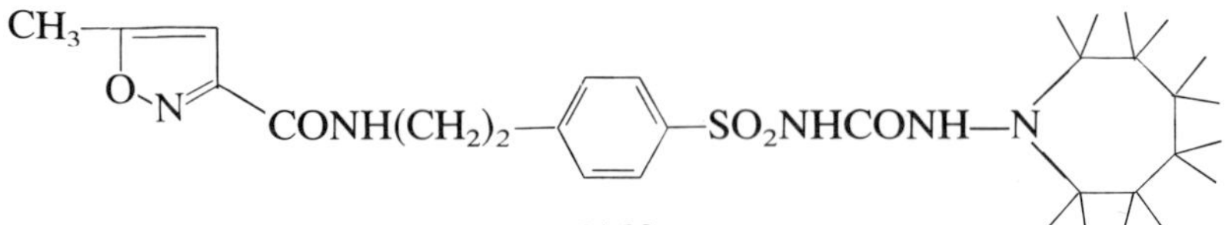

31.**22**

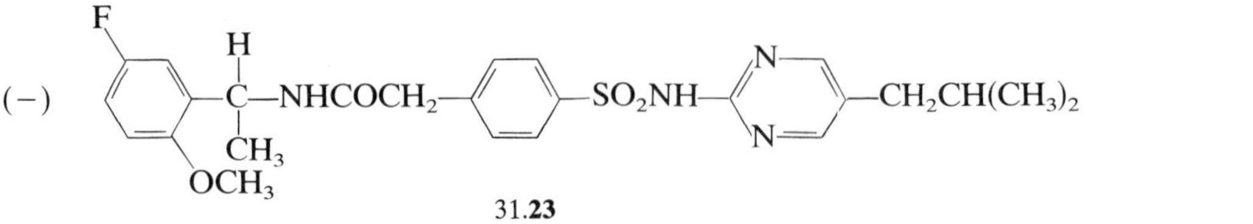

31.**23**

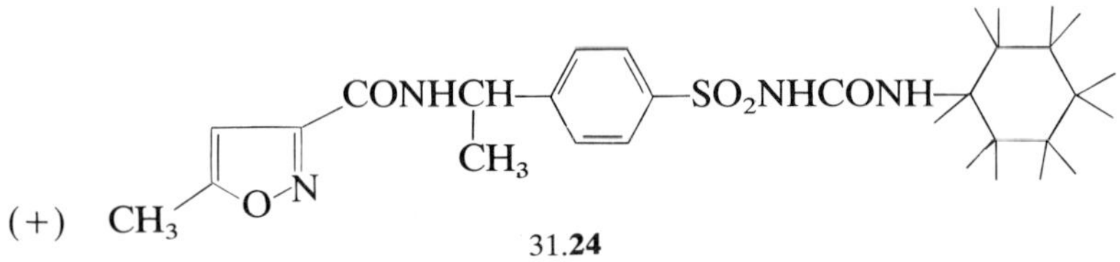

31.**24**

inhibit gluconeogenesis from lactate and alanine in rat liver (340).

Gliflumide (31.**23**) has activity similar to that of tolbutamide and glibenclamide in human maturity-onset diabetics but is more potent (341, 342).

The introduction of asymmetry into the alkyl side chain of these molecules markedly enhanced their hypoglycemic potency, with the activity residing primarily in the *S*-isomers. This lends credence to the belief that there is a second binding site for these compounds that the *S*-isomers fit better than the *R*-isomers. The effects noted with these compounds in rabbits have also been seen in other species, including man (343).

In a related but different series, the most potent members were the *R*-antipodes (31.**24**) (344).

Gliclazide (31.**25**) effectively lowers blood glucose levels in animals and humans. It is more potent and longer acting than tolbutamide (345). Of possible significance is the report that gliclazide reverses some of the microvascular abnormalities seen in diabetes (346). It is proposed that gliclazide accomplishes this by decreasing platelet stickiness or stimulating the disaggregation of these bodies. Alternatively, the effect might be achieved by fibrinolytic properties of 31.**25** (347).

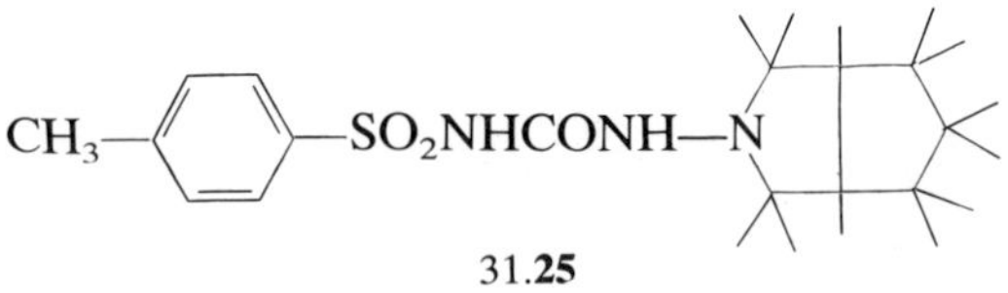

31.**25**

Glypentide (31.**26**) is reported to be long acting and 200–1000 times as active as tolbutamide (348).

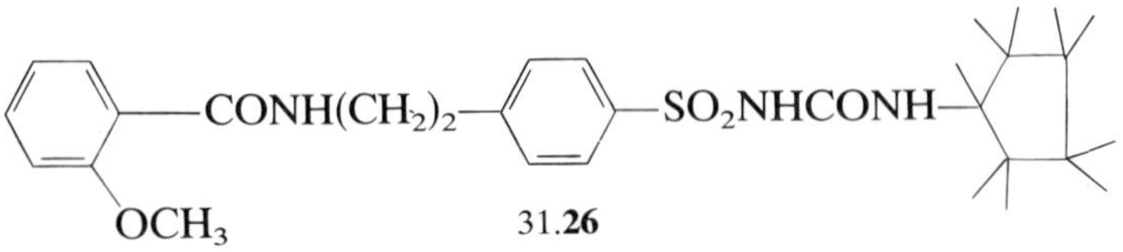

31.**26**

A new hypoglycemic sulfonylurea (31.**27**) is said to have an effect on gluconeogenesis (349).

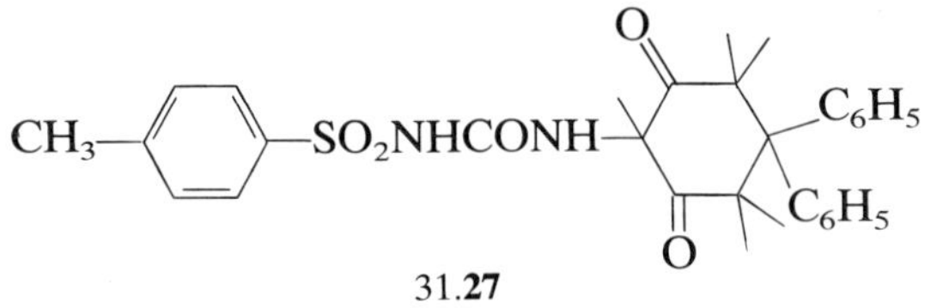

31.**27**

Other workers have claimed that the heterocyclic sulfonylurea 31.**28** is superior to tolbutamide and similar to glibenclamide (350, 351).

Sulfamylureas and semicarbazides have been studied as alternatives to the corresponding sulfonyl derivatives. Several have been found that have enhanced potency over earlier members in the series. They behave biologically as sulfonylureas. One, 31.**29**, has been chosen for clinical trials, but no reports have been issued (352–357).

2.3.4 COMPOUNDS WITH BIGUANIDELIKE ACTIVITY. A phosphorylated analog of phenformin was prepared and shown to have similar properties and potency. However this compound (31.**30**) was reported to have a greater separation between its hypoglycemic and hyperlacticacidemic properties and to cause fewer gastrointestinal problems (358).

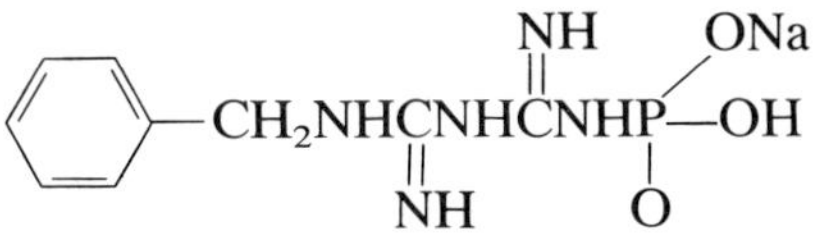

31.**30**

Morpholinobiguanides (31.**31**) were reported to have promising hypoglycemic activity (359).

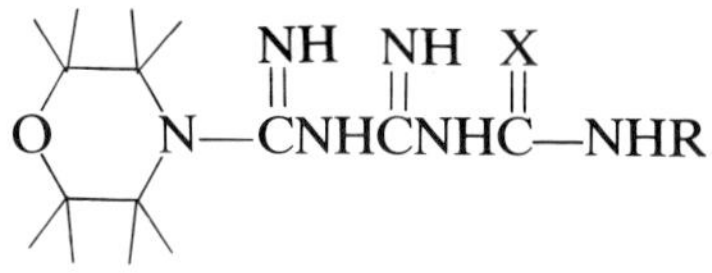

X = O or S R = alkyl, alkenyl, aralkyl, alicyclic

31.**31**

An extensive series of azolyl methylpyridinium quaternary salts (31.**32**) has been prepared and shown to be hypoglycemic in several animal models. These included pyrazolyl (360, 361), isoxazolyl (362–365), isothiazolyl (366), 1,2,4-oxadiazolyl (367), thiazolyl (368), oxazolyl (369), thienyl, furyl, and pyrrolyl (370), as well as some inactive azolyl derivatives (371).

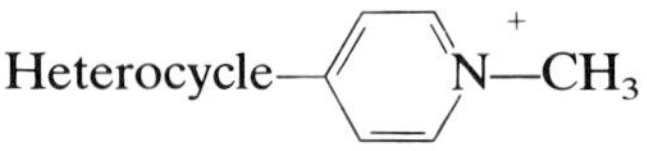

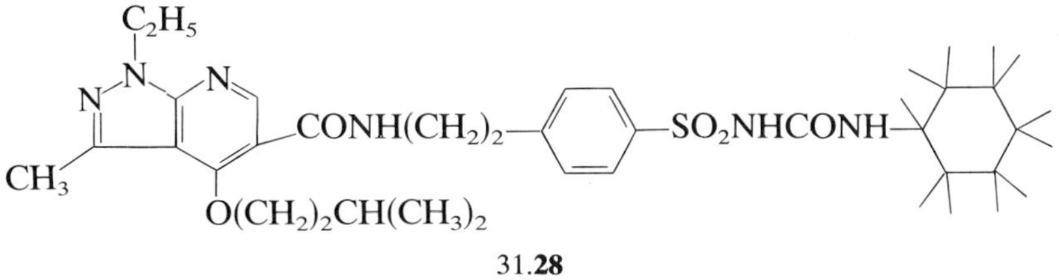

31.**32**

31.**28**

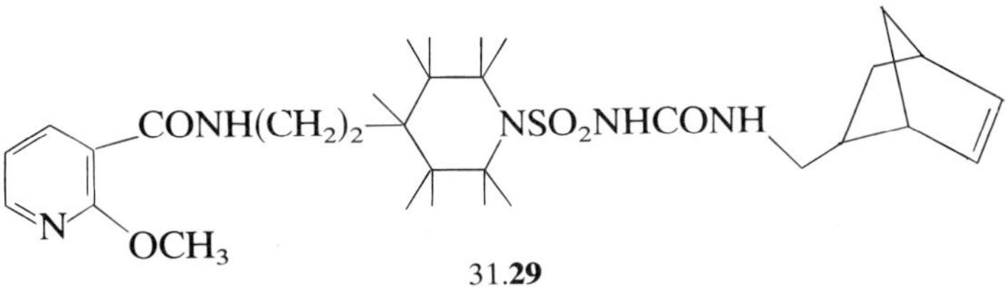

31.**29**

Replacing the five-membered rings with pyrimidine led to an inactive series (372), whereas replacement of the quaternized pyridine with a quaternized pyridazine (31.**33**) gave compounds that reduced blood sugar 23–62% in mice (373).

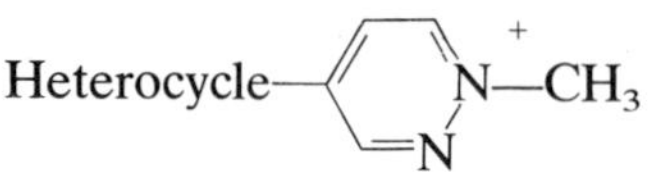

31.**33**

The 3-methyl-5-isoxazolylpyridinium salt of 31.**32** was reported to have an activity and a mechanism of action similar to those of phenformin in normal and diabetic models (374, 375).

4-Imino-1-(2-pyrimidinyl)-1,4-dihydropyridine (31.**34**) has a pattern of activity

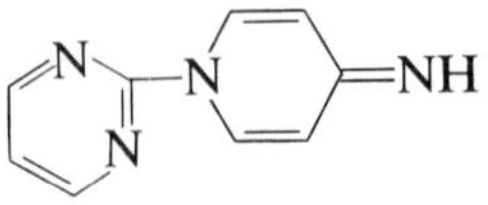

31.**34**

that mimics phenformin and isoxazolylpyridinium salts. The dihydropyridine causes a significant reduction of hyperglycemia in humans (376) and inhibits gluconeogenesis from lactate (377).

2.3.5 INHIBITORS OF GLUCONEOGENESIS. It has been demonstrated in a number of studies that tryptophan (31.**35**), as well as several of its metabolites (3-hydroxyanthranilic acid, 31.**36**, quinolinic acid, 31.**37**, quinaldic acid, 31.**38**), inhibit gluconeogenesis at one or more enzymatic sites, and in so doing lower glucose levels (378–386). Despite these findings, tryptophan, 3-hydroxyanthranilic acid, and

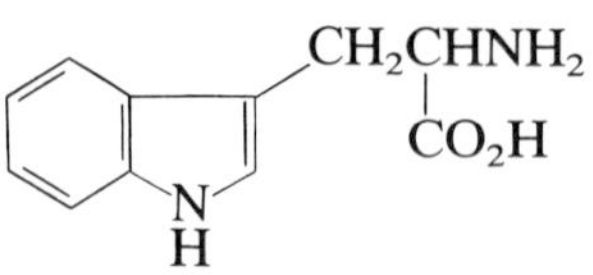

31.**35**

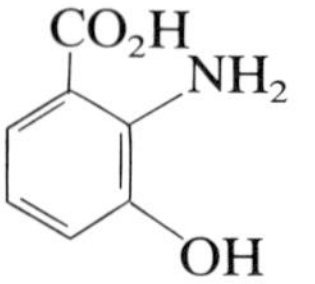

31.**36**

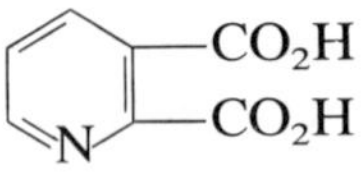

31.**37**

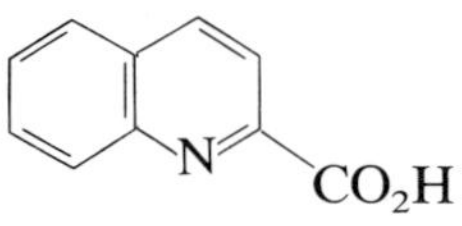

31.**38**

quinolinic acid were ineffective as inhibitors of gluconeogenesis in either alloxan- or streptozotocin-diabetic rats (387). In light of this report, the value of these compounds as lead structures in the search for better agents becomes suspect, although their ineffectiveness may be simply a matter of potency (*vide infra*).

An offshoot of the early work with tryptophan and its metabolites was the attempt to find potent agents that would control the hyperglycemia of diabetes by inhibiting gluconeogenesis. The tryptophan metabolite quinolinic acid served as the focal point for this study. A number of related structures were prepared, and of these 3-mercaptopicolinic acid (31.**39**) was shown

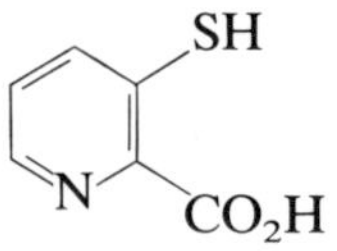

31.**39**

to be hypoglycemic in fasted rats, mice, guinea pigs (388, 389), and monkeys (390). Mercaptopicolinic acid was also active in alloxan-diabetic rats (389) and streptozotocin-diabetic guinea pigs (390).

In vitro experiments established that the glucose-lowering effect was accomplished by inhibiting gluconeogenesis. This was also suggested by the inactivity of mercaptopicolinic acid in fed animals, where the rate of gluconeogenesis is basal (389, 390). Cross-over studies (391) and studies with isolated systems confirmed the hypoglycemic activity of this agent and demonstrated that it interfered with gluconeogenesis primarily at the site of phosphoenolpyruvate carboxykinase (PEPCK) (389, 392–396). Mercaptopicolinate also inhibits ketogenesis in fasted and diabetic rats (393), as well as interfering with oxalacetate decarboxylation and the carboxylation activity of PEPCK during C_4 photosynthesis (397).

Structure-activity studies with isomers, derivatives, and analogs indicated that hypoglycemic activity was restricted to mercaptopicolinate (388, 398, 399). Using 3-mercaptopicolinic acid, an attempt was made in a limited clinical study to validate the hypothesis that inhibitors of gluconeogenesis would be beneficial in the treatment of diabetes. The results were inconclusive because the study was short-lived—the result of the compound's relative lack of potency and by the appearance of dermatitis in two of 10 patients (390).

5-Methoxyindole-2-carboxylic acid (MICA, 31.**40**) lowers blood sugar in mice

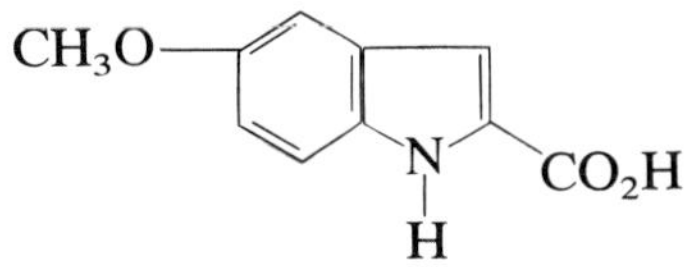

31.**40**

and rats by inhibiting gluconeogenesis. It does this by blocking pyruvate carboxylation and oxidation. The concomitant blockage of α-ketoglutarate metabolism and the attendant effects on the citric acid cycle are serious side effects, as is the accumulation of lactic acid resulting from the blockage of pyruvate oxidation (400–405).

Diphenyleneiodonium sulfate (31.**41**) is hypoglycemic in rats. It inhibits

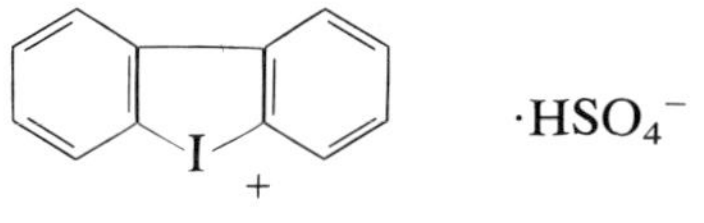

$\cdot HSO_4^-$

31.**41**

gluconeogenesis from lactate and aspartate but not from xylitol, dihydroxyacetone, or glycerol. This inhibition is associated with a deficiency of ATP resulting from inhibition of mitochondrial NADH-linked substrate oxidation (406). Similar studies were performed with this iodonium salt and derivatives in isolated hepatocytes (407).

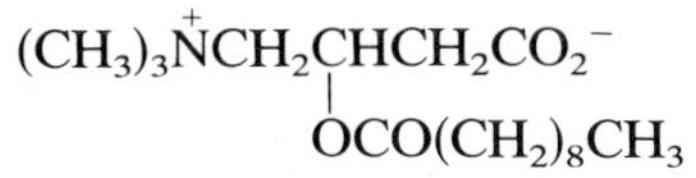

$$(CH_3)_3\overset{+}{N}CH_2CH(OCO(CH_2)_8CH_3)CH_2CO_2^-$$

31.**42**

In the absence of insulin, (+) decanoylcarnitine (31.**42**) reverses ketosis in diabetic rats and augments the action of insulin administered in this situation. Decanoylcarnitine also inhibits fatty acid stimulation of gluconeogenesis by preventing oxidation of these substrates. However without oleic acid stimulation of fatty acid oxidation, this carnitine derivative is ineffective. The action of decanoylcarnitine on fatty acid oxidation is rapidly reversible on removal of the inhibitor (408, 409).

α-Bromopalmitic acid, an irreversible inhibitor of fatty acid oxidation, is also hypoglycemic (410, 411). Other carnitine derivatives were found to be neither inhibitors of fatty acid oxidation nor hypoglycemic (412).

2.3.6 ALDOSE REDUCTASE INHIBITOR. Aldose reductase is a constituent of the sorbitol pathway for metabolizing aldoses. The enzyme catalyzes the conversion of glucose to sorbitol and is found in specific cells in the lens, nervous tissue, kidney, and islets of the pancreas. The sorbitol pathway is implicated in the changes noted in these tissues in diabetes.

Aldose reductase has low specificity for its substrates and is operative only at high aldose concentrations. The resulting polyols are difficult to metabolize and lead to increased hypertonicity and osmotic swelling. Such changes are felt to be involved in the mechanism of diabetic cataract formation and are associated with the demyelination seen in experimental diabetes in rats.

1,3-Dioxo-1*H*-benz[*d, e*]isoquinoline-2-(3*H*)-acetic acid (31.**43**) inhibits aldose reductase and reduces levels of sorbitol. This agent effectively suppresses cataract formation in galactosemic rats (413).

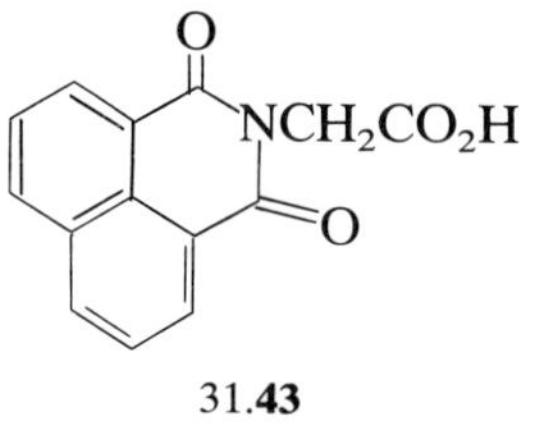

31.43

2.3.7 MISCELLANEOUS AGENTS. 5-Hydroxytryptophan (31.**44**) produces hypoglycemia in fed or fasted, normal mice treated with

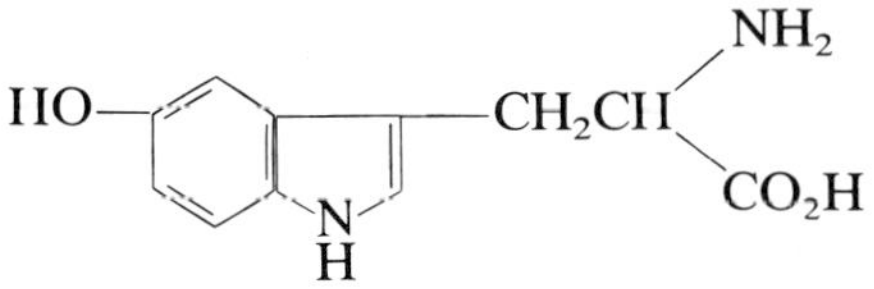

31.44

the monoamine oxidase inhibitor nialamide [(*N*-benzyl-*β*-(isonicotinoylhydrazine)propionamide)], with no concomitant increase in immunoreactive insulin. 5-Hydroxytryptophan is also effective in alloxan-diabetic mice. The hypoglycemic response is accompanied by a head-twitching response. Both responses can be abolished by pretreatment with serotonin antagonists and are augmented by antihistamines (414).

The anorectic agent fenfluramine (31.**45**) was shown to have a biphasic effect on

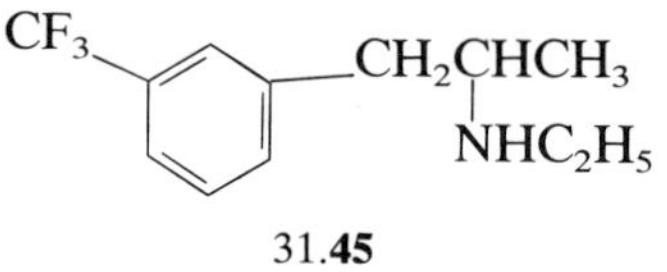

31.45

glucose uptake by skeletal muscle in a forearm perfusion model, lowering glucose levels in the initial phase and being without effect in the later phase. The compound is most effective when given just before eating, and it has been shown to lower blood glucose in maturity-onset diabetics who were both dependent and independent of insulin. It was more effective in the insulin-independent group. Since there was no evidence of lacticacidosis or changes in insulin secretion, it is suggested that fenfluramine increases glucose uptake and oxidation (415).

Among a series of *α*-alkoxybenzylamidoximes, amidines, and cycloamidines, 31.**46** had 60% of the hypoglycemic activity of tolbutamide and the greatest separation between hypoglycemic activity and toxicity. However there were species differences in the doses that caused death. This compound also produced a profound inhibitory effect on certain liver enzymes (416).

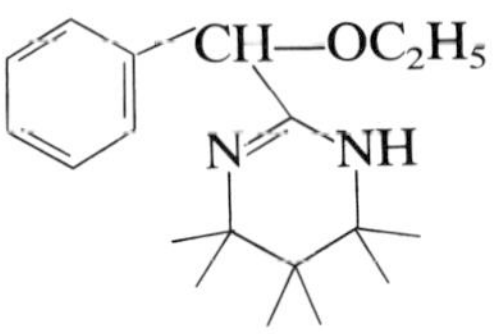

31.46

2.3.7.1 Lactamimides. An intensive study has been made of the relationship between hypoglycemic activity and the structure of lactamimides (417–419) and imidazo-[1,2-*a*]azacycloalkanes (420) derived from the lactamimides. Three of the most active members of these series are 31.**47**–31.**49**.

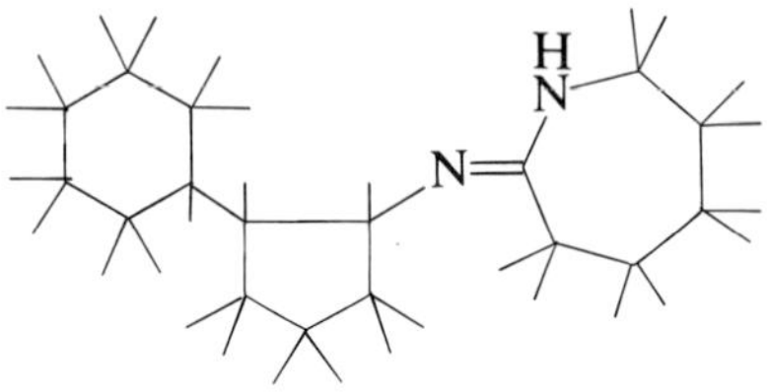

31.47

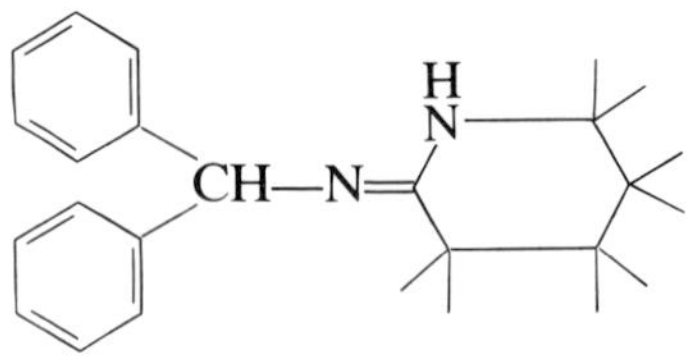

31.48

Two, 31.**48** and 31.**49**, are being evaluated for clinical trial (418).

The lactamimide 31.**47** is hypoglycemic in rats, dogs, and monkeys and lowers

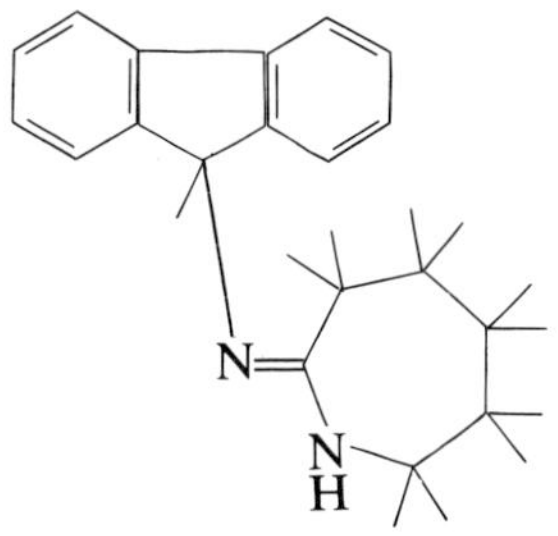

31.**49**

plasma free fatty acids, but not glucose, in alloxan-diabetic rats. It markedly stimulates insulin release from cultured islet cells (421). Some other members of this series that have activity are 31.**50**–31.**52**.

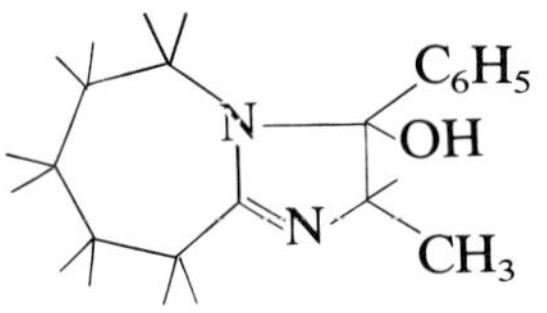

31.**50**

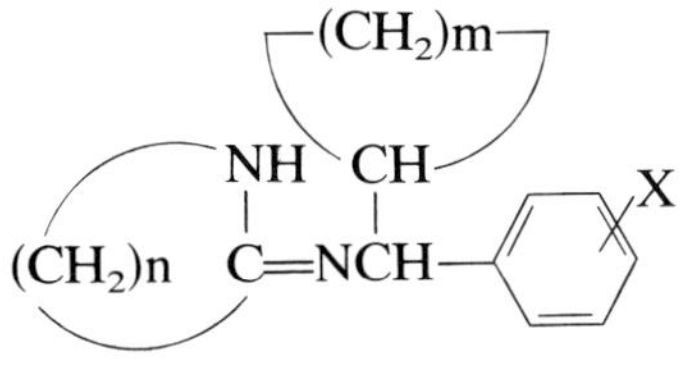

$m = 2$
$n = 7$
X = 2, 4-dimethyl

31.**51**

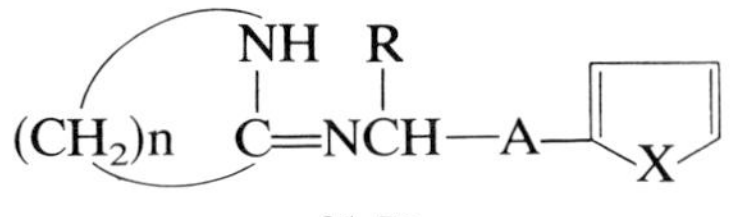

31.**52**

X	*n*	A	R
S	5	$CHCH_3$	CH_3
S	5	CH_2	Allyl
S	5	—	Cyclopropyl
O	6	—	Phenyl
S	6	—	Phenyl

In a series of *N*-substituted pyrroles, 31.**53** was the most active. It lowered blood glucose by stimulating its uptake. However, it had an undisclosed side effect (422, 423).

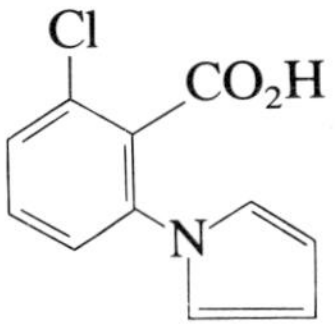

31.**53**

Diazirines with structures 31.**54** and 31.**55** produced 25–85% reductions in blood glucose values in normal mice (424).

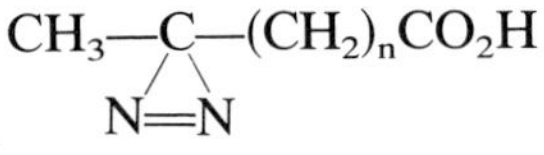

$n = 2$; methyl and 4-pyridylmethyl esters, amides, and hydrazides
$n = 3$; methyl ester

31.**54**

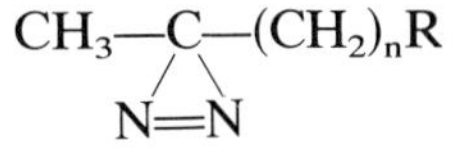

$n = 1$ and 2, $R = CH_2OH$
$n = 1$; $R = CH(OCH_3)_2$
$n = 1$; $R = CH_2NH_2$

31.**55**

Pyrazine-2-carboxamide (31.**56**), an antitubercular agent, is metabolized to the acid 31.**57**, which has hypoglycemic activity (425). Several amide (426), thiosemicarbazide, and thiadiazole derivatives also have moderate hypoglycemic activity (427).

In a series of indanes, the various members had highly variable hypoglycemic potency.

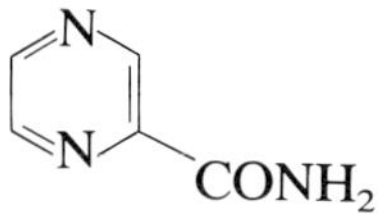

31.**56** 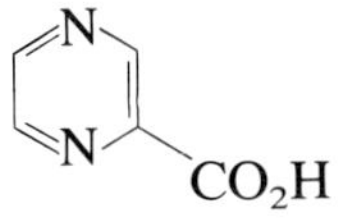 31.**57**

In compound 31.**58** the substituent X = OCH_3 gave compounds with more hypoglycemic activity than compounds with X = H. In general, series 31.**58** was more active than series 31.**59**. The nature of R and R′ markedly influences hypoglycemic activity (428–430). In the 31.**59** series, compounds

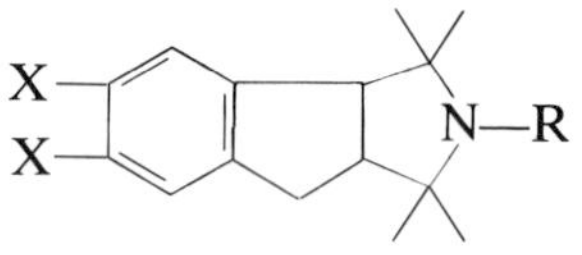

X = H or OCH_3
R = alkyl, cycloalkyl, or benzyl

31.**58**

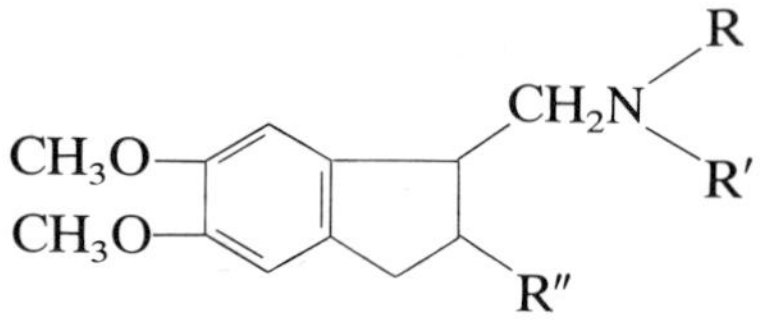

R and R′ = alkyl or H
R″ = H or CH_3

31.**59**

with R′ = R″ = n-C_3H_7, R = CH_3, R′ = n-butyl, and R″ = CH_3 had modest activity in normal and alloxan-diabetic rabbits.

Two thiadiazine sulfones (31.**60** and 31.**61**) are moderately hypoglycemic in mice (431).

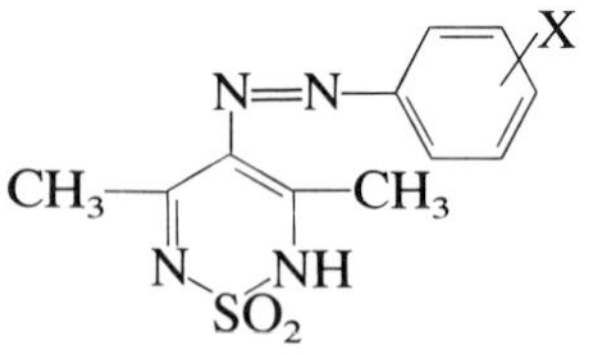

31.**60** X = 2,3-dimethyl
31.**61** X = 3,5-dichloro

2.3.7.2 Dichloroacetate. In fasted and diabetic rats, dichloroacetate (31.**62**) lowers

$Cl_2CHCO_2^-$ M^+
M = isopropylamine or monovalent cation

31.**62**

blood glucose and insulin levels after oral (432) and intraperitoneal administration (433–435). It has been suggested that dichloroacetate functions by inhibiting net release of gluconeogenic precursors from extrahepatic sites due to enhanced pyruvate oxidation and by inhibiting ketone body production in severe ketoacidosis (433, 436–438).

In rat hepatocytes dichloroacetate treatment did not block glucose production beyond glyceraldehyde-3-phosphate dehydrogenase, did not produce any consistent changes in the oxidation-reduction state of the cytosol, did not stimulate respiration, and did not alter the ATP/ADP ratio. The agent had no effect on the oxidation of pyruvate or lactate to carbon dioxide but did prevent the conversion to glucose of added lactate and pyruvate (439).

When administered to nonketotic, maturity-onset diabetics maintained on a constant diet, dichloroacetate caused plasma glucose, lactate, and free fatty acid levels to fall, but without an effect on insulin levels. These results support the proposed mechanism of action (440).

Several naphthylacetic acids (37.**63**) have been reported to have hypoglycemic activity comparable to that of chlorpropamide (441–445).

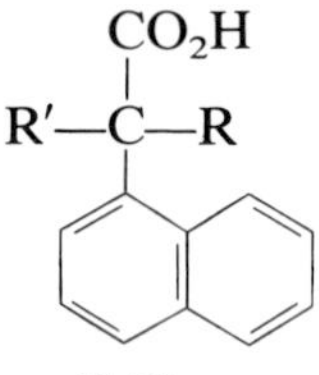

R = i-C_3H_7, R′ = $(CH_3)_2N(CH_2)_3$
R = R′ = $(CH_3)_2N(CH_2)_3$
R = i-C_3H_7, R′ = $(C_2H_5)_2N(CH_2)_2$

31.**63**

2-Piperazino-4-quinazolone (31.**64**) had hypoglycemic activity in some animal models but not others. No explanation was offered (446, 447). Currently it is believed 31.**64** stimulates insulin release from the pancreas (448).

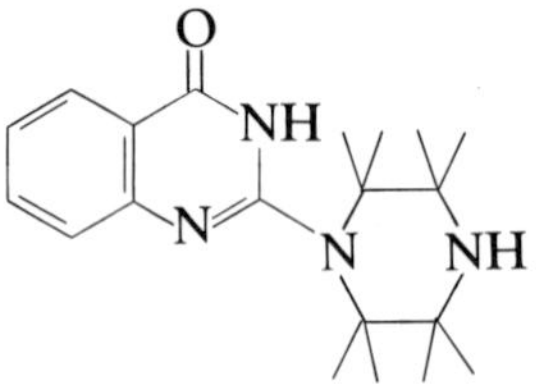

31.**64**

2-Aminonorbornane-2-carboxylic acid (31.**65**) has the property of enhancing tolbutamide-induced hypoglycemia. This

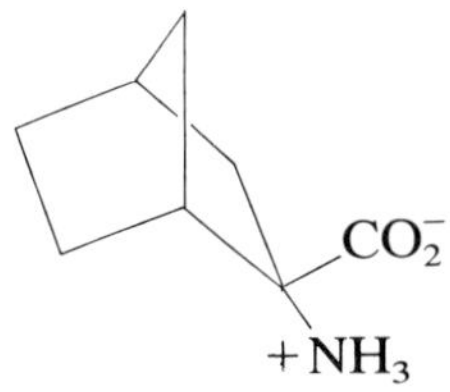

CO_2^-
$+NH_3$
31.**65**

property resides in the isomer with an exo-carboxylic acid function and the absolute configuration 1*R*, 2*S*, 4*S*. It provides information about the receptor site for the release of insulin stimulated by neutral amino acid (449).

A series of triphenylphenacylphosphoranes and phosphonium salts (31.**66** and 31.**67**) caused a marked depression in

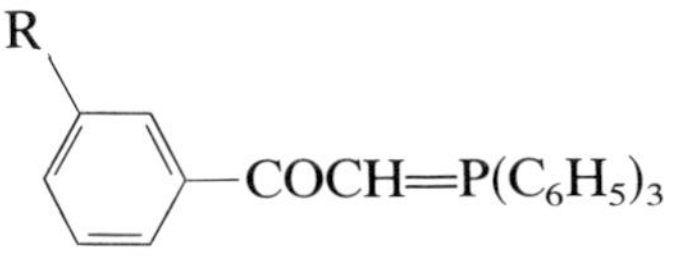

R
$-COCH{=}P(C_6H_5)_3$
31.**66**

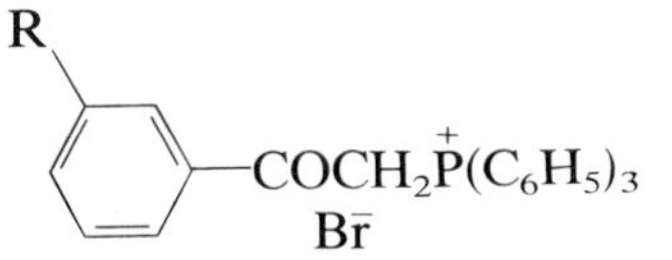

R
$-COCH_2\overset{+}{P}(C_6H_5)_3$
Br^-
31.**67**

blood glucose levels in fasted, fed, and diabetic rats. The activity was noted only in the parent and *m*-substituted phenacyl compounds. The biological activity could not be confirmed in rabbits, guinea pigs, or dogs. There was no explanation for this species specificity (450).

2.3.8 PEPTIDES. Insulin covalently bound to a polyacrylate polymer was prepared in a water-soluble form. After subcutaneous administration, this material was slowly released into the blood over an extended period. The polymer is degraded like the natural hormone. The biologic activity was attributed to the entire molecule, rather than to the result of *in vivo* splitting to insulin (451).

Liposomes containing insulin offer an attractive drug delivery system that possibly could circumvent some of the problems inherent in the oral administration of peptides. Insulin entrapped in dipalmitoylphosphatidylcholine/cholesterol liposomes and administered intragastrically lowered blood glucose levels for prolonged periods. The mechanism by which this type of insulin reaches the periphery is unknown (452).

A peptide isolated from human urine potentiates insulin activity in rabbits and rats, being much more active in the rat. This peptide has activity comparable to that seen with the human growth hormone peptide fragment sequence 6–13 (453). This peptide together with synthetic fragments of the amino-terminal sequence of human growth hormone were studied *in vitro* and *in vivo*. The abilities to enhance glucose uptake into diaphragm *in vitro* and to potentiate insulin activity *in vivo* were correlated with 31.**68**, the octapeptide cited previously (454).

3 FUTURE TRENDS

Earlier in this discussion it was suggested that the discovery of insulin acted as a deterrent to progress in diabetes research. To some extent this lack of drive and purpose has been perpetuated. Late in 1975 a National Commission on Diabetes reported on the state of the disease and its therapy. A review of the report states, "Problem Severe, Therapy Inadequate" (3). The disease now affects 5% of the population in the United States and it is projected that

H_2N--------------Leu–Ser–Arg–Leu–Phe–Asp–Asn–Ala
6 7 8 9 10 11 12 13
31.**68**

the number will double every 15 years. The average newborn American has a better than 20% chance of developing diabetes, and even with the best of current medical care, diabetic complications will develop.

On a more optimistic note, if the correlation between a viral etiology and juvenile diabetes can be firmly established, development of a vaccine may prevent development of the disease. New animal models for diabetes provide the researcher with systems closer to the human disease state (455). New insight into the disease and its complications has been acquired from the findings that certain biological systems coming into play during hyperglycemia lead to the activation of aldose reductase, the thickening of glomerular basement membrane, and the nonenzymatic addition of glucose to hemoglobin A_{1c} as a posttranslation transformation (456–460).

New surgical, cell culture, and bioengineering procedures offer the hope of long-lived, functioning surrogate pancreases (1, 52, 461, 462). The first of these approaches requires the surgical implantation of islet cells from an external source; the second would inject islet cells from cell cultures, ideally initiated by cells from the recipient himself. In this way host rejection would be obviated or greatly minimized. The third technique makes use of a glucose-sensing system attached to an external source of insulin. Glucose would be constantly monitored and insulin administered as needed. Finally, a valuable adjunct to the overall therapy of diabetes would be the development of diagnostic techniques that unambiguously determine whether a person has a predisposition toward diabetes (prediabetes), so that prophylactic measures, such as weight control and dieting, could be implemented as early as possible.

Surgical implantation of pancreatic tissue currently is the most promising and successful of the approaches just listed. For example, a complete reversal of streptozotocin-induced diabetes has been attained in the rat. This is accomplished with a single fetal pancreas, first grown in a normal syngenetic carrier before transplantation. The important feature seems to be allowing the fetal pancreas to develop for a time in a "normal glucose environment" before exposure to diabetic glucose levels (463–465).

Of a number of new biologic and medical insights that have been achieved in recent years, the discovery of an agent that inhibits aldose reductase has the potential to lead to a drug that could ameliorate the eye disturbances associated with diabetes (413). In fact, recently new and more potent inhibitors of aldose reductase have been discovered (flavonoids, and in particular quercitrin and its acetate, 31.**69**). These recent studies have shown for the first time in an intact, diabetic animal model, that onset of cataract formation is delayed when quercitrin is administered continually. Since the rat develops eye lesions over 3–4 months and the time of the appearance of opacity varies considerably from animal to animal, a new animal model was used, the degu, a rodent indigenous to the Andes of South America. Results indicate quercitrin does indeed delay the development of cataracts, although it does not prevent their formation or lower glucose levels in diabetic degus (466–468).

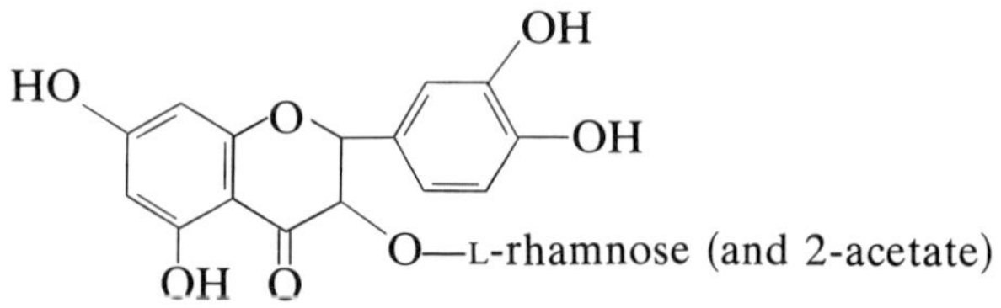

HO OH OH O
O—L-rhamnose (and 2-acetate)
OH O

31.**69**

If the observations marking the increased presence of hydroxylysine and disaccharide in diabetic glomerular basement membrane are valid (9, 41–43, 53), agents that interfere with some of the postribosomal steps of basement membrane synthesis, such as hydroxylation, glycosylation, export, and cross-link formation, might provide tools for dealing with this disorder (53). In addition, careful clinical and immunohistochemical examination of diabetic patients whose tissue shows evidence of increased "trapping" of serum proteins might help to determine whether this phenomenon is of prognostic or pathogenic consequence in the development of diabetic microangiopathy (56).

New knowledge about the basic happenings in glucose metabolism, in several systems affected in diabetes, has provided information that may allow the design of agents to effectively alter these systems and return them to their physiologic state. In so doing, it is hoped, that the overall diabetic state will be improved.

REFERENCES

1. G. F. Cahill, Jr., in *US News and World Report*, November 24, 1975, pp. 51–54.
2. G. Faludi, at the Annual Philadelphia Diabetes Forum, Philadelphia, November 7, 1975.
3. T. H. Maugh, II, *Science*, **191,** 272 (1976).
4. P. J. Palumbo, L. R. Elveback, C.-P. Chu, D. C. Connolly, and L. T. Kurland, *Diabetes*, **25,** 566 (1976).
5. D. L. Rimoin, *Calif. Med.*, **119,** 14 (1973).
6. M. A. Kimble, *J. Am. Pharm. Assoc., NS*, **14,** 80 (1974).
7. F. G. Banting and C. H. Best, *J. Lab. Clin. Med.*, **7,** 251 (1922).
8. G. F. Cahill, Jr., and J. S. Soeldner, *N. Engl. J. Med.*, **291,** 577 (1974).
9. R. G. Spiro, *Diabetologia*, **12,** 1 (1976).
10. E. P. Joslin, *Diabetes*, **5,** 67 (1956).
11. G. Sayers and R. H. Travis, "Insulin and Oral Hypoglycemic Drugs," in *The Pharmacological Basis of Therapeutics*, 3rd ed., L. S. Goodman and A. Gilman, Eds., Macmillan, New York, 1965, p. 1579.
12. T. H. Maugh, II, *Science*, **188,** 920 (1975).
13. S. S. Fajans and J. W. Conn, *Diabetes*, **3,** 296 (1954).
14. S. Berger, J. L. Downey, H. S. Traisman, and R. Metz, *N. Engl. J. Med.*, **274,** 1460 (1966).
15. S. Berger, J. L. Downey, and H. S. Traisman, *Ann. N.Y. Acad. Sci.*, **148,** 859 (1968).
16. R. V. Heinzelman, "Antidiabetics," in *Annual Reports in Medicinal Chemistry, 1967*, C. K. Kain, Ed., Academic Press, New York, 1968, p. 156.
17. K. Johansen, J. S. Soeldner, and R. E. Gleason, *Metabolism*, **23,** 1185 (1974).
18. J. L. Day and R. B. Tattersall, *Metabolism*, **24,** 145 (1975).
19. H. Ginsberg, J. M. Olefsky, and G. M. Reaven, *Diabetes*, **23,** 674 (1974).
20. J. L. Kyner, R. I. Levy, J. S. Soeldner, R. E. Gleason, and D. S. Fredrickson, *J. Lab. Clin. Med.*, **88,** 345 (1976).
21. T. H. Maugh, II, *Science*, **193,** 220 (1976).
22. S. Goldstein, M. Blecher, R. Binder, P. V. Perrino, and L. Recant, *Endocrinol. Res. Commun.*, **2,** 367 (1975).
23. A. L. Rosenbloom, S. Goldstein, and C. C. Yip, *Science*, **193,** 412 (1976).
24. A. A. Like and A. A. Rossini, *Science*, **193,** 415 (1976).
25. J. E. Craighead and M. F. McLane, *Sciene*, **162,** 913 (1968).
26. Editorial, *Lancet*, **2,** 804 (1971).
27. D. W. Boucher and A. L. Notkins, *J. Exp. Med.*, **137,** 1226 (1973).
28. T. H. Maugh, II, *Science*, **188,** 347 (1975).
29. T. H. Maugh, II, *Science*, **188,** 436 (1975).
30. A. A. F. Mahmoud and K. S. Warren, *Clin. Res.*, **23,** 565A (1974).
31. S. W. Huang and N. K. Maclaren, *Science*, **192,** 64 (1976).
32. A. A. F. Mahmoud, H. M. Rodman, M. A. Mandel, and K. S. Warren, *J. Clin. Invest.*, **57,** 362 (1976).
33. J. S. Flier, C. R. Kahn, J. Roth, and R. S. Bar, *Science*, **190,** 63 (1975).
34. C. R. Kahn, J. S. Flier, R. S. Bar, J. A. Archer, P. Gorden, M. M. Martin, and J. Roth, *N. Engl. J. Med.*, **294,** 739 (1976).
35. J. S. Flier, C. R. Kahn, D. B. Jarrett, and J. Roth, *J. Clin. Invest.*, **58,** 1442 (1976).

36. F. A. Grunwald, "Hypoglycemic Agents," in *Medicinal Chemistry*, Part 2, 3rd ed., A. Burger, Ed., Wiley-Interscience, New York, 1970, p. 1172.
37. H. Klostermeyer and R. E. Humbel, *Angew. Chem., Int. Ed. Engl.*, **5,** 807 (1966).
38. J. H. Exton, *Metabolism*, **21,** 945 (1972).
39. P. Felig and J. Wahren, *Israel J. Med. Sci.*, **11,** 528 (1975).
40. S. R. Wagle, W. R. Ingebretsen, Jr., and L. Sampson, *Diabetologia*, **11,** 411 (1975).
41. R. G. Spiro and M. J. Spiro, *Diabetes*, **20,** 641 (1971).
42. P. J. Beisswenger and R. G. Spiro, *Diabetes*, **22,** 180 (1973).
43. P. J. Beisswenger, *Diabetes*, **22,** 744 (1973).
44. F. I. R. Martin and G. L. Warne, *Metabolism*, **24,** 1 (1975).
45. J. T. Ireland, *Brit J. Clin. Pract.*, **30,** 149 (1976).
46. C. R. Klimt, G. L. Knatterud, C. L. Meinert, and T. E. Prout, *Diabetes*, **19** (Suppl. 2), 747 (1970).
47. C. L. Meinert, G. L. Knatterud, T. E. Prout, and C. R. Klimt, *Diabetes*, **19** (Suppl. 2), 789 (1970).
48. T. E. Prout, *Med. Clin. North Am.*, **55,** 1065 (1971).
49. G. L. Knatterud, C. L. Meinert, C. R. Klimt, R. K. Osborne, and D. B. Martin, *J. Am. Med. Assoc.*, **217,** 777 (1971).
50. M. G. Goldner, G. L. Knatterud, and T. E. Prout, *J. Am. Med. Assoc.*, **218,** 1400 (1971).
51. K. Prasannan and P. A. Kurup, *Atherosclerosis*, **18,** 459 (1973).
52. T. H. Maugh, II, *Science*, **190,** 1281 (1975).
53. R. G. Spiro, *Diabetes*, **25** (Suppl. 2), 909 (1976).
54. N. A. Kefalides, *J. Clin. Invest.*, **53,** 403 (1974).
55. T. Sato, H. Munakata, K. Yoshinaga, and Z. Yosizawa, *Clin. Chem. Acta*, **61,** 145 (1975).
56. N. G. Westberg, *Diabetes*, **25** (Suppl. 2), 920 (1976).
57. B. G. Hudson and R. G. Spiro, *J. Biol. Chem.*, **247,** 4229 (1972).
58. G. F. Cahill, Jr., D. D. Etzwiler, and N. Freinkel, *N. Engl. J. Med.*, **294,** 1004 (1975).
59. G. F. Cahill, Jr., D. D. Etzwiler, and N. Freinkel, *Diabetes*, **25,** 237 (1976).
60. W. W. Winternitz, *N. Engl. J. Med.*, **295,** 509 (1976).
61. D. A. Gorelick and N. Feldman, *N. Engl. J. Med.*, **295,** 510 (1976).
62. J. I. Malone and A. L. Rosenbloom, *N. Engl. J. Med.*, **295,** 510 (1976).
63. J. Jung and J. D. Cohen, *N. Engl. J. Med.*, **295,** 510 (1976).
64. M. Shoshkes, *N. Engl. J. Med.*, **295,** 511 (1976).
65. G. F. Cahill, Jr., *N. Engl. J. Med.*, **295,** 511 (1976).
66. J. R. Williamson and C. Kilo, *Diabetes*, **26,** 65 (1977).
67. A. Bloom, *Postgrad. Med. J.*, **47** (June Suppl.), 430 (1971).
68. H. Ginsberg, G. Kimmerling, J. M. Olefsky, and G. M. Reaven, *J. Clin. Invest.*, **55,** 454 (1975).
69. G. Kimmerling, W. C. Javorski, J. M. Olefsky, and G. M. Reaven, *Diabetes*, **25,** 673 (1976).
70. P. Cuatrecasas, *Proc. Nat. Acad. Sci., US*, **69,** 318 (1972).
71. J. A. Archer, P. Gorden, J. R. Gavin, III, M. A. Lesniak, and J. Roth, *J. Clin. Endocrinol. Metab.*, **36,** 627 (1973).
72. P. Cuatrecasas, *Biochem. Pharmacol.*, **23,** 2353 (1974).
73. M. D. Hollenberg and P. Cuatrecasas, *Fed. Proc.*, **34,** 1556 (1975).
74. P. Cuatrecasas, *J. Biol. Chem.*, **246,** 7265 (1971).
75. J. M. Hammond, L. Jarett, I. K. Mariz, and W. H. Daughaday, *Biochem. Biophys. Res. Commun.*, **49,** 1122 (1972).
76. P. DeMeyts, J. Roth, D. M. Neville, Jr., J. R. Gavin, III, and M. A. Lesniak, *Biochem. Biophys. Res. Commun.*, **55,** 154 (1973).
77. E. A. Siess, M. L. Nestorescu, and O. H. Wieland, *Diabetologia*, **10,** (1974).
78. P. Freychet, *Diabetologia*, **12,** 83 (1976).
79. E. J. M. Helmreich, *FEBS Lett.*, **61,** 1 (1976).
80. H. N. Antoniades, D. Stathakos, and J. D. Simon, *Endocrinology*, **95,** 1543 (1974).
81. T. Oka and Y. J. Topper, *Science*, **188,** 1317 (1975).
82. P. DeMeyts, *Endocrinology*, **98** (Suppl.), 68 (1976).
83. P. DeMeyts, A. R. Bianco, and J. Roth, *J. Biol. Chem.*, **251,** 1877 (1976).
84. J. S. Flier, C. R. Kahn, and J. Roth, *Clin. Res.*, **24,** 457A (1976).
85. A. Levitzki, *J. Theor. Biol.*, **44,** 367 (1974).
86. A. Colosimo, M. Brunori, and J. Wyman, *J. Mol. Biol.*, **100,** 47 (1976).
87. S. J. Singer and G. L. Nicolson, *Science*, **175,** 720 (1972).
88. S. Jacobs and P. Cuatrecasas, *Biochim. Biophys. Acta*, **433,** 482 (1976).
89. C. R. Kahn, *J. Cell Biol.*, **70,** 261 (1976).

90. B. H. Ginsberg, R. M. Cohen, and C. R. Kahn, *Diabetes*, **25** (Suppl. 1), 322 (1976).

91. B. H. Ginsberg, C. R. Kahn, J. Roth, and P. DeMeyts, *Biochem. Biophys. Res. Commun.*, **73,** 1068 (1976).

92 T. J. Merimee, *N. Engl. J. Med.*, **285,** 856 (1971).

93. J. D. Bagdade, E. L. Bierman, and D. Porte, Jr., *Diabetes*, **20,** 664 (1971).

94. G. D. Bompiani and E. Laudicina, *Israel J. Med. Sci.*, **8,** 823 (1972).

95. C. R. Kahn, D. M. Neville, Jr., P. Gorden, P. Freychet, and J. Roth, *Biochem. Biophys. Res. Commun.*, **48,** 135 (1972).

96. P. Freychet, M. H. Laudat, P. Laudat, G. Rosselin, C. R. Kahn, P. Gorden, and J. Roth, *FEBS Lett.*, **25,** 339 (1972).

97. J. A. Archer, P. Gorden, and J. Roth, *J. Clin. Invest.*, **55,** 166 (1975).

98. *Nutr. Rev.*, **34,** 145 (1976).

99. G. V. Bennett and P. Cuatrecasas, *Science*, **176,** 805 (1972).

100. J. M. Amatruda, J. N. Livingston, and D. H. Lockwood, *Science*, **188,** 264 (1975).

101. A. H. Soll, C. R. Kahn, D. M. Neville, Jr., and J. Roth, *J. Clin. Invest.*, **56,** 769 (1975).

102. J. M. Olefsky, *J. Clin. Invest.*, **58,** 1450 (1976).

103. M. B. Davidson and S. A. Kaplan, *J. Clin. Invest.*, **59,** 22 (1977).

104. R. Remer, H. J. von Funcke, and K. D. Hepp, *Diabetologia*, **12,** 416 (1976).

105. F. Sanger, *Chem. Ind.* (London), 104 (1959).

106. F. Sanger, *Science*, **129,** 1340 (1959).

107. D. F. Steiner, *Trans. N.Y. Acad. Sci.*, **30,** 60 (1967).

108. D. F. Steiner, *N. Engl. J. Med.*, **280,** 1106 (1969).

109. P. G. Katsoyannis, *Science*, **154,** 1509 (1966).

110. P. G. Katsoyannis, J. Ginos, A. Cosmatos, and G. P. Schwartz, *J. Chem. Soc. Perkins Trans.*, **I,** 464 (1975).

111. A. Cosmatos and P. G. Katsoyannis, *J. Biol. Chem.*, **250,** 5315 (1975).

112. A. Cosmatos, Y. Okada, and P. G. Katsoyannis, *Biochemistry*, **15,** 4076 (1976).

113. T. L. Blundell, G. G. Dodson, E. Dodson, D. C. Hodgkin, and M. Vijayan, *Rec. Progr. Hormone Res.*, **27,** 1 (1971).

114. P. Freychet, D. Brandenburg, and A. Wollmer, *Diabetologia*, **10,** 1 (1974).

115. J. Gliemann and S. Gammeltoft, *Diabetologia*, **10,** 105 (1974).

116. J. Gliemann and H. H. Sorensen, *Diabetologia*, **6,** 499 (1970).

117. D. Brandenburg, W. Busse, H. Gattner, H. Zahn, A. Wollmer, J. Gliemann, and W. Puls, "Structure-Function Studies with Chemically Modified Insulins. Peptides 72," in *Proceedings of the Twelfth European Peptide Symposium, Reinhardsbrunn Castle, German Democratic Republic, September 1972*, North-Holland, Amsterdam, 1973, pp. 270–283.

118, N. R. Lazarus, J. C. Penhos, T. Tanese, L. Michaels, R. Gutman, and L. Recant, *J. Clin. Invest.*, **49,** 487 (1970).

119. T. Blundell, G. Dodson, D. Hodgkin, and D. Mercola, *Advan. Protein Chem.*, **26,** 279 (1972).

120. D. Brandenburg, *Hoppe-Seylers Z. Physiol. Chem.*, **353,** 869 (1972).

121. D. Brandenburg, H. G. Gattner, and A. Wollmer, *Hoppe-Seylers Z. Physiol. Chem.*, **353,** 599 (1972).

122. C. V. Tompkins, P. H. Sonksen, and R. H. Jones, *J. Endocrinol.*, **65,** 59P (1975).

123. S. P. Wood, T. L. Blundell, A. Wollmer, N. R. Lazarus, and R. W. J. Neville, *Eur. J. Biochem.*, **55,** 531 (1975).

124. R. A. Pullen, D. G. Lindsay, S. P. Wood, I. J. Tickle, T. L. Blundell, A. Wollmer, G. Krail, D. Brandenburg, H. Zahn, J. Gliemann, and S. Gammeltoft, *Nature*, **259,** 369 (1976).

125. C. R. Snell and D. G. Smyth, *J. Biol. Chem.*, **250,** 6291 (1975).

126. P. Freychet, *J. Clin. Invest.*, **54,** 1020 (1974).

127. R. H. Jones, D. I. Dron, M. J. Ellis, P. H. Sonksen, and D. Brandenburg, *Diabetologia*, **12,** 601 (1976).

128. W. J. Malaisse, *Diabetologia*, **9,** 167 (1973).

129. G. W. G. Sharp, C. Wollheim, W. A. Muller, A. Gutzeit, P. A. Trueheart, B. Blondel, L. Orci, and A. E. Renold, *Fed. Proc.*, **34,** 1537 (1975).

130. D. L. Curry, L. L. Bennett, and G. M. Grodsky, *Endocrinology*, **83,** 572 (1968).

131. G. M. Grodsky, H. Sando, J. Gerich, J. Karam, and R. Fanska, "Synthesis and Secretion of Insulin in Dynamic Perfusion Systems," in *Advances in Metabolic Disorders*, Vol. 7, R. Levine and R. Luft, Eds., Academic Press, New York, 1974, p. 155.

132. G. M. Grodsky, *J. Clin. Invest.*, **51,** 2047 (1972).

133. J. E. Gerich, M. A. Charles, and G. M. Grodsky, *Ann. Rev. Physiol., Ser. II*, **38,** 353 (1976).

134. E. Van Obberghen, G. Somers, G. Devis, G. D. Vaughan, F. Malaisse-Lagae, L. Orci, and W. J. Malaisse, *J. Clin. Invest.*, **52,** 1041 (1973).

135. G. Devis, E. Van Obberghen, G. Somers, F. Malaisse-Lagae, L. Orci, and W. J. Malaisse, *Diabetologia*, **10,** 53 (1974).

136. G. Somers, E. Van Obberghen, G. Devis, M. Ravazzola, F. Malaisse-Lagae, and W. J. Malaisse, *Eur. J. Clin. Invest.*, **4,** 299 (1974).

137. E. Van Obberghen, G. Devis, G. Somers, M. Ravazzola, F. Malaisse-Lagae, and W. J. Malaisse, *Eur. J. Clin. Invest.*, **4,** 307 (1974).

138. W. J. Malaisse, E. Van Obberghen, G. Devis, G. Somers, and M. Ravazzola, *Eur. J. Clin. Invest.*, **4,** 313 (1974).

139. E. Van Obberghen, G. Somers, G. Devis, M. Ravazzola, F. Malaisse-Lagae, L. Orci, and W. J. Malaisse, *Endocrinology*, **95,** 1518 (1974).

140. M. McDaniel, C. Roth, J. Fink, G. Fyfe, and P. Lacy, *Biochem. Biophys. Res. Commun.*, **66,** 1089 (1975).

141. G. M. Grodsky, *Handb. Exp. Pharmakol.*, **32,** 1 (1975).

142. F. M. Matschinsky, R. Landgraf, J. Ellerman, and J. Kotler-Brajtburg, *Diabetes*, **21** (Suppl. 2), 555 (1972).

143. G. M. Grodsky, R. Fanska, L. West, and M. Manning, *Science*, **186,** 536 (1974).

144. A. Niki, H. Niki, I. Miwa, and J. Okuda, *Science*, **186,** 150 (1974).

145. A. A. Rossini, J. S. Soeldner, J. M. Hiebert, G. C. Weir, and R. E. Gleason, *Diabetologia*, **10,** 795 (1974).

146. G. M. Grodsky, R. Fanska, and I. Lundquist, *Endocrinology*, **97,** 573 (1975).

147. F. M. Matschinsky, A. S. Pagliara, B. A. Hover, M. W. Haymond, and S. N. Stillings, *Diabetes*, **24,** 369 (1975).

148. A. A. Rossini, M. Berger, J. Shadden, and G. F. Cahill, Jr., *Science*, **183,** 424 (1974).

149. A. A. Rossini, G. F. Cahill, Jr., D. A. Jeanloz, and R. W. Jeanloz, *Science*, **188,** 70 (1975).

150. L. A. Idahl, J. Sehling, and I. B. Taljedal, *Nature*, **254,** 75 (1975).

151. W. J. Malaisse, A. Sener, M. Koser, and A. Herchuelz, *FEBS Lett.*, **65,** 131 (1976).

152. P. J. Randle, S. J. H. Ashcroft, and J. R. Gill, in *Carbohydrate Metabolism and Its Disorders*, F. Dickens, P. J. Randle, and W. J. Whelan, Eds., Academic Press, London, 1968, p. 427.

153. S. J. H. Ashcroft, L. C. C. Weerasinghe, and P. J. Randle, *Biochem. J.*, **132,** 223 (1973).

154. B. Hellman, L. A. Idahl, A. Lernmark, J. Sehlin, and I. B. Taljedal, *Arch. Biochem. Biophys.*, **162,** 448 (1974).

155. W. J. Malaisse, G. Devis, D. G. Pipeleers, G. Somers, and E. Van Obberghen, *Diabetologia*, **10,** 379 (1974).

156. K. Jain, J. Logothetopoulos, and P. Zucker, *Biochim. Biophys. Acta*, **399,** 384 (1975).

157. S. J. H. Ashcroft and J. R. Crossley, *Diabetologia*, **11,** 279 (1975).

158. E. Cerasi, *Diabetologia*, **11,** 1 (1975).

159. E. A. Nikkila and M. R. Taskinen, *Postgrad. Med. J.*, **47** (June Suppl.), 412 (1971).

160. R. S. Bosboom, J. Zweens, and P. R. Bouman, *Diabetologia*, **9,** 243 (1973).

161. M. A. Charles, R. Fanska, F. G. Schmid, P. H. Forsham, and G. M. Grodsky, *Science*, **179,** 569 (1973).

162. R. Bressler, M. V. Cordon, and K. Brendel, *Arch. Intern. Med.*, **123,** 248 (1969).

163. H. Aleyassine and R. J. Gardiner, *Endocrinology*, **96,** 702 (1975).

164. B. J. Lin and R. E. Haist, *Endocrinology*, **96,** 1247 (1975).

165. K. E. Quickel, Jr., J. M. Feldman, and H. E. Lebovitz, *J. Clin. Endocrinol. Metab.*, **33,** 877 (1971).

166. P. E. Lacy, D. A. Young, and C. J. Fink, *Endocrinology*, **83,** 1155 (1968).

167. R. C. Turner, B. Schneeloch, and J. D. N. Nabarro, *J. Clin. Endocrinol. Metab.*, **33,** 301 (1971).

168. E. E. Muller, L. A. Frohman, and D. Cocchi, *Am. J. Physiol.*, **224,** 1210 (1973).

169. D. G. Pipeleers, M. Marichal, and W. J. Malaisse, *Endocrinology*, **93,** 1001 (1973).

170. J. M. Feldman and T. B. Jackson, *Endocrinology*, **94,** 388 (1974).

171. D. Watkins, S. J. Cooperstein, P. K. Dixit, and A. Lazarow, *Science*, **162,** 283 (1968).

172. D. Watkins, S. J. Cooperstein, and A. Lazarow, *Endocrinology*, **88,** 1380 (1971).

173. H. P. T. Ammon and J. Steinke, *Endocrinology*, **91,** 33 (1972).

174. H. P. T. Ammon and J. Steinke, *Diabetes*, **21,** 143 (1972).

175. S. Pek, T. Y. Tai, A. Elster, and S. S. Fajans, *Prostaglandins*, **10,** 493 (1975).

176. H. Okamoto, S. Miyamoto, H. Mabuchi, Y. Yoneyama, and R. Takeda, *Biochem. Biophys. Res. Commun.*, **53,** 1297 (1973).

177. N. J. Greenberger, M. Tzagournis, and T. M. Graves, *Metabolism*, **17,** 796 (1968).

178. I. Tamir, D. B. Grant, A. S. Fosbrooke, M. N. Segall, and J. K. Lloyd, *J. Lipid Res.*, **9,** 661 (1968).

179. W. Montague and K. W. Taylor, *Nature*, **217,** 853 (1968).

180. D. G. Pipeleers, M. Marichal, and W. J. Malaisse, *Endocrinology*, **93,** 1012 (1973).

181. B. Hellman, L. A. Idahl, A. Lernmark, J. Sehlin, and I. B. Taljedal, *Biochem. J.*, **138,** 33 (1974).

182. B. Hellman, *FEBS Lett.*, **54,** 343 (1975).

183. B. Hellman, *Biochim. Biophys. Acta*, **399,** 157 (1975).

184. M. A. Charles, J. Lawecki, R. Pictet, and G. M. Grodsky, *J. Biol. Chem.*, **250,** 6134 (1975).

185. V. Grill and E. Cerasi, *J. Biol. Chem.*, **249,** 4196 (1974).

186. K. J. Chang, N. A. Marcus, and P. Cuatrecasas, *J. Biol. Chem.*, **249,** 6854 (1974).

187. H. H. Conaway, M. A. Griffey, S. R. Marks, and J. E. Whitney, *Horm. Metab. Res.*, **8,** 351 (1976).

188. R. C. Turner and R. R. Holman, *Lancet*, **1** (7972), 1272 (1976).

189. L. Orci, D. Baetens, M. P. Dubois, and C. Rufener, *Hormone Metab. Res.*, **7,** 400 (1975).

190. T. Hokfelt, S. Efendic, C. Hellerstrom, O. Johansson, R. Luft, and A. Arimura, *Acta Endocrinol.* (Copenhagen), **80** (Suppl. 200), 5 (1975).

191. B. D. Noe and G. E. Bauer, *Endocrinology*, **97,** 868 (1975).

192. I. Valverde, D. Rigopoulou, J. Marco, G. R. Faloona, and R. H. Unger, *Diabetes*, **19,** 614 (1970).

193. R. Dobbs, H. Sakurai, H. Sasaki, G. Faloona, I. Valverde, D. Baetens, L. Orci, and R. Unger, *Science*, **187,** 544 (1975).

194. T. Matsuyama, W. H. Hoffman, J. C. Dunbar, N. L. Foa, and P. P. Foa, *Hormone Metab. Res.*, **7,** 452 (1975).

195. H. Sasaki, B. Rubalcava, D. Baetens, E. Blazquez, C. B. Srikant, L. Orci, and R. H. Unger, *J. Clin. Invest.*, **56,** 135 (1975).

196. D. Baetens, C. Rufener, B. C. Srikant, R. Dobbs, R. Unger, and L. Orci, *J. Cell Biol.*, **69,** 455 (1976).

197. J. P. Palmer, P. L. Werner, J. W. Benson, and J. W. Ensinck, *Lancet*, **1,** 1290 (1976).

198. J. L. Botha and A. I. Vinik, *Lancet*, **1,** 1290 (1976).

199. R. P. Eaton, D. M. Kipnis, I. Karl, and A. B. Eisenstein, *Am. J. Physiol.*, **227,** 101 (1974).

200. M. G. Clark, N. M. Kneer, A. L. Bosch, and H. A. Lardy, *J. Biol. Chem.*, **249,** 5695 (1974).

201. J. M. Wimhurst, K. L. Manchester, and E. J. Harris, *Biochim. Biophys. Acta*, **372,** 72 (1974).

202. S. R. Wagle, *Biochem. Biophys. Res. Commun.*, **59,** 1366 (1974).

203. P. Brazeau, W. Vale, R. Burgus, N. Ling, M. Butcher, J. Rivier, and R. Guillemin, *Science*, **179,** 77 (1973).

204. A. Arimura, H. Sato, A. Dupont, N. Nishi, and A. V. Schally, *Science*, **189,** 1007 (1975).

205. C. Lucke, H. J. Mitzkat, and A. von zur Muhlen, *Klin. Wochenschr.*, **54,** 293 (1976).

206. B. L. Pimstone, M. Berelowitz, and S. Kronheim, *South Afr. Med. J.*, **50,** 1471 (1976).

207. J. Rivier, P. Brazeau, W. Vale, and R. Guillemin, *J. Med. Chem.*, **18,** 123 (1975).

208. H. Leblanc and S. S. C. Yen, *J. Clin. Endocrinol. Metab.*, **40,** 906 (1975).

209. D. J. Koerker, W. Ruch, E. Chideckel, J. Palmer, C. J. Goodner, J. Ensinck, and C. C. Gale, *Science*, **184,** 482 (1974).

210. J. E. Gerich, M. Lorenzi, V. Schneider, C. W. Kwan, J. H. Karam, R. Guillemin, and P. H. Forsham, *Diabetes*, **23,** 876 (1974).

211. J. E. Gerich, M. Langlois, C. Naocco, J. H. Karam, and P. H. Forsham, *Science*, **182,** 171 (1973).

212. J. E. Gerich, M. Lorenzi, V. Schneider, and P. H. Forsham, *J. Clin. Endocrinol. Metab.*, **39,** 1057 (1974).

213. J. E. Gerich, M. Lorenzi, V. Schneider, J. H. Karam, J. Rivier, R. Guillemin, and P. H. Forsham, *N. Engl. J. Med.*, **291,** 544 (1974).

214. H. Sakurai, R. Dobbs, and R. H. Unger, *J. Clin. Invest.*, **54,** 1395 (1974).

215. F. R. Ward, H. Leblanc, and S. S. C. Yen. *J. Clin. Endocrinol., Metab.*, **41,** 527 (1975).

216. J. E. Gerich, M. Lorenzi, S. Hane, G. Gustafson, R. Guillemin, and P. H. Forsham, *Metabolism*, **24,** 175 (1975).

217. R. P. Eaton, *Diabetes*, **24,** 523 (1975).

218. H. Sakurai, R. E. Dobbs, and R. H. Unger, *Metabolism*, **24,** 1287 (1975).

219. R. H. Unger, *Diabetes*, **25,** 136 (1976).

220. G. C. Weir, S. D. Knowlton, R. F. Atkins, K. X. McKennan, and D. B. Martin, *Diabetes*, **25,** 275 (1976).

221. J. E. Gerich, M. Lorenzi, D. M. Bier, E. Tsalikian, V. Schneider, J. H. Karam, and P. H. Forsham, *J. Clin. Invest.*, **57,** 875 (1976).

222. G. C. Weir, S. D. Knowlton, and D. B. Martin, *Endocrinology*, **95,** 1744 (1974).

223. J. E. Gerich, R. Lovinger, and G. M. Grodsky, *Endocrinology*, **96,** 749 (1975).

224. S. Efendic and R. Luft, *Acta Endocrinol.* (Copenhagen), **78,** 510 (1975).

225. S. Efendic, A. Claro, and R. Luft, *Acta Endocrinol.* (Copenhagen), **81,** 753 (1976).

226. G. W. DeVane, T. M. Siler, and S. S. C. Yen, *J. Clin. Endocrinol., Metab.*, **38,** 913 (1974).

227. F. P. Alford, S. R. Bloom, J. D. N. Nabarro, R. Hall, G. M. Besser, D. H. Coy, A. J. Kastin, and A. V. Schally, *Lancet*, **2,** 974 (1974).

228. C. Meissner, C. Thum, W. Beischer, G. Winkler, K. E. Schroder, and E. F. Pfeiffer, *Diabetes*, **24,** 988 (1975).
229. S. Efendic and R. Luft, *Acta Endocrinol.* (Copenhagen), **78,** 516 (1975).
230. S. Efendic, P. E. Lins, G. Sigurdsson, B. Ivemark, P. O. Granberg, and R. Luft, *Acta Endocrinol.* (Copenhagen), **81,** 525 (1976).
231. S. Efendic, R. Luft, and A. Claro, *Acta Endocrinol.* (Copenhagen), **81,** 743 (1976).
232. S. R. Wagle, *Biochem. Biophys. Res. Commun.*, **67,** 1019 (1975).
233. R. Parilla, M. N. Goodman, and C. J. Toews, *Diabetes*, **23,** 725 (1974).
234. J. G. Schofield, F. Mira-Moser, M. Schorderet, and L. Orci, *FEBS Lett.*, **46,** 171 (1974).
235. W. Y. Fujimoto and J. Teague, *Endocrinology*, **97,** 1494 (1975).
236. T. Taminato, Y. Seino, Y. Goto, and H. Imura, *Biochem. Biophys. Res. Commun.*, **66,** 928 (1975).
237. W. Y. Fujimoto and J. W. Ensinck, *Endocrinology*, **98,** 259 (1976).
238. H. G. Joost, J. Beckmann, S. Holze, S. Lenzen, W. Poser, and A. Hasselblatt, *Diabetologia*, **12,** 201 (1976).
239. A. J. Barnes and S. R. Bloom, *Lancet*, **1,** 219 (1976).
240. J. E. Gerich, J. H. Karam, and M. Lorenzi, *Lancet*, **1,** 855 (1976).
241. M. Donowitz and P. Felig, *Lancet*, **1,** 855 (1976).
242. A. J. Barnes, S. R. Bloom, F. P. Alford, and R. C. G. Russell, *Lancet*, **1,** 967 (1976).
243. R. S. Sherwin, M. Fisher, R. Hendler, and P. Felig, *N. Engl. J. Med.*, **294,** 455 (1976).
244. R. Levine, *N. Engl. J. Med.*, **294,** 494 (1976).
245. P. Felig, J. Wahren, R. Sherwin, and R. Hendler, *Diabetes* **25,** 1091 (1976).
246. R. S. Sherwin, R. Hendler, and P. Felig, *Metabolism*, **26,** 53 (1977).
247. P. Robberecht, M. Deschodt-Lanckman, P. DeNeef, and J. Christophe, *Biochem. Biophys. Res. Commun.*, **67,** 315 (1975).
248. G. Boden, M. C. Sivitz, and O. E. Owen, *Science*, **190,** 163 (1975).
249. P. Brazeau, W. Vale, J. Rivier, and R. Guillemin, *Biochem. Biophys. Res. Commun.*, **60,** 1202 (1974).
250. M. Brown, J. Rivier, W. Vale, and R. Guillemin, *Biochem. Biophys. Res. Commun.*, **65,** 752 (1975).
251. L. Ferland, F. Labrie, D. H. Coy, A. Arimura, and A. V. Schally, *Mol. Cell. Endocrinol.*, **4,** 79 (1976).
252. N. Grant, D. Clark, V. Garsky, I. Jaunakais, W. McGregor, and D. Sarantakis, *Life Sci.*, **19,** 629 (1976).
253. V. M. Garsky, D. E. Clark, and N. H. Grant, *Biochem. Biophys. Res. Commun.*, **73,** 911 (1976).
254. D. Sarantakis, J. Teichman, D. E. Clark, and E. L. Lien, *Biochem. Biophys. Res. Commun.*, **75,** 143 (1977).
255. D. Sarantakis, W. A. McKinley, I. Jaunakais, D. Clark, and N. H. Grant, *Clin. Endocrinol.*, **5,** (Suppl.), 275s (1976).
256. D. F. Veber, R. G. Strachan, S. J. Bergstrand, F. W. Holly, C. F. Homnick, R. Hirschmann, M. Torchiana, and R. Saperstein, *J. Am. Chem. Soc.*, **98,** 2367 (1976).
257. J. Rivier, M. Brown, and W. Vale, *Biochem. Biophys. Res. Commun.*, **65,** 746 (1975).
258. N. Marks, F. Stern, and M. Benuck, *Nature*, **261,** 511 (1976).
259. S. Efendic, R. Luft, and H. Sievertsson, *FEBS Lett.*, **58,** 302 (1975).
260. M. Brown, J. Rivier, and W. Vale, *Fed. Proc.*, **35,** 782 (1976).
261. C. Meyers, A. Arimura, A. Gordin, R. Fernandez-Durango, D. H. Coy, A. V. Schally, J. Drouin, L. Ferland, M. Beaulieu, and F. Labrie, *Biochem. Biophys. Res. Commun.*, **74,** 630 (1977).
262. J. Wahren and P. Felig, *Lancet*, **2,** 1213 (1976).
263. P. Felig and J. Wahren, *Metabolism*, **25,** 1509 (1976).
264. A. B. Scoville, Jr., *South. Med. J.*, **69,** 1116 (1976).
265. S. Bakth, P. May, S. Akgun, and N. Etrel, *Clin. Res.*, **24,** 636A (1976).
266. R. J. Jarrett and H. Keen, *Brit. J. Hosp. Med.*, **11,** 265 (1974).
267. S. W. Shen and R. Bressler, *Dis. Mon.*, **22,** 3 (1976).
268. B. F. Clarke, *Brit. J. Clin. Pract.*, **30,** 136 (1976).
269. S. A. Hagg, *J. Maine Med. Assoc.*, **67,** 246 (1976).
270. S. A. Hagg, *Am. J. Hosp. Pharm.*, **33,** 943 (1976).
271. G. Faludi, *Geriatrics*, **31,** 67 (1976).
272. A. Loubatieres, *Ann. N.Y. Acad. Sci.*, **71,** 4 (1957).
273. W. J. H. Butterfield and W. V. Westering, Eds.,

Tolbutamide After Ten Years, Excerpta Medica, New York, 1967.

274. E. Haack, *Arzneim.-Forsch.*, **8,** 444 (1958).
275. H. Ruschig, G. Korger, W. Aumuller, H. Wagner, R. Weyer, A. Bander, and J. Scholz, *Arzneim.-Forsch.*, **8,** 448 (1958).
276. F. J. Marshall and M. V. Sigal, Jr., *J. Org. Chem.*, **23,** 927 (1958).
277. D. R. Cassady, C. Ainsworth, N. R. Easton, M. Livezey, M. V. Sigal, Jr., and E. Van Heyningen, *J. Org. Chem.*, **23,** 923 (1958).
278. B. Blank, F. A. Farina, J. F. Kerwin, and H. Saunders, *J. Org. Chem.*, **26,** 1551 (1961).
279. U. Krause, H. Puchinger, and A. Wacker, *Arzneim.-Forsch.*, **25,** 1231 (1975).
280. J. M. Foy and V. F. Standing, *Arzneim.-Forsch.*, **24,** 1279 (1974).
281. A. K. Jain, J. R. Ryan, and F. G. McMahon, *N. Engl. J. Med.*, **293,** 1283 (1975).
282. R. P. Eaton, R. Oase, and D. S. Schade, *Metabolism*, **25,** 245 (1976).
283. R. P. Eaton and D. S. Schade, *Metabolism*, **23,** 445 (1974).
284. E. Frank, M. Nothmann, and A. Wagner, *Klin. Wochenschr.*, **7,** 1996 (1928); *Chem. Abstr.*, **23,** 1684 (1929).
285. G. Ungar, L. Friedman, and S. L. Shapiro, *Proc. Soc. Exp. Biol. Med.*, **95,** 190 (1957).
286. S. L. Shapiro, V. A. Parrino, and L. Friedman, *J. Am. Chem. Soc.*, **81,** 2220 (1959).
287. S. L. Shapiro, V. A. Parrino, E. Rogow, and L. Friedman, *J. Am. Chem. Soc.*, **81,** 3725 (1959).
288. S. L. Shapiro, V. A. Parrino, and L. Friedman, *J. Am. Chem. Soc.*, **81,** 3728 (1959).
289. S. L. Shapiro, V. A. Parrino, and L. Friedman, *J. Am. Chem. Soc.*, **81,** 4635 (1959).
290. B. Elpern, *Ann. N.Y. Acad. Sci.*, **148,** 577 (1968).
291. W. Caspary and W. Creutzfeldt, *Diabetologia*, **7,** 379 (1971).
292. A. Czyzyk, J. Lawecki, J. Sadowski, I. Ponikowska, and Z. Szczepanik, *Diabetes*, **17,** 492 (1968).
293. F. A. Kruger, R. A. Altschuld, S. L. Hollobaugh, and B. Jewett, *Diabetes*, **19,** 50 (1970).
294. R. Haeckel, H. Haeckel, and M. Anderer, *Biochem. Pharmacol.*, **20,** 1053 (1971).
295. N. O. Jangaard, J. N. Pereira, and R. Pinson, *Diabetes*, **17,** 96 (1968).
296. J. M. Medina, F. Sanchez-Medina, and F. Mayor, *Rev. Esp. Fisiol.*, **27,** 253 (1971).
297. R. A. Altschuld and F. A. Kruger, *Ann. N.Y. Acad. Sci.*, **148,** 612 (1968).
298. G. A. O. Alleyne, H. S. Besterman, and H. Flores, *Clin. Sci.*, **40,** 107 (1971).
299. F. Meyer, M. Ipaktchi, and H. Clauser, *Nature*, **213,** 203 (1967).
300. R. Beckmann, W. Lintz, and J. Nijssen, *Experientia*, **27,** 127 (1971).
301. H. Daweke and I. Bach, *Metabolism*, **12,** 319 (1963).
302. R. A. Kreisberg, *Diabetes*, **17,** 481 (1968).
303. I. Polacek and J. Ouart, *Diabetes*, **23,** 25 (1974).
304. G. Schafer, *Biochem. Pharmacol.*; **25,** 2005 (1976).
305. P. L. Poffenbarger and F. A. White, *Conn. Med.*, **39,** 137 (1975).
306. G. R. Constam, *Diabetologia*, **7,** 237 (1971).
307. H. S. Seltzer, *Diabetes*, **21,** 976 (1972).
308. D. R. Hadden, *Ir. J. Med. Sci.* (May Suppl.), 11 (1973).
309. M. Miller, G. L. Knatterud, B. S. Hawkins, and W. B. Newberry, Jr., *Diabetes*, **25,** 1129 (1976).
310. D. B. Jellife and K. L. Stuart, *Brit. Med. J.*, **1,** 75 (1954).
311. C. von Holt, M. von Holt and H. Bohm, *Biochim. Biophys. Acta*, **125,** 11 (1966).
312. R. Bressler, C. Corredor, and K. Brendel, *Pharmacol. Rev.*, **21,** 105 (1969).
313. W. G. Duncombe and T. J. Rising, *Biochem. J.*, **109,** 449 (1968).
314. W. G. Duncombe and T. J. Rising, *Biochem. Pharmacol.*, **21,** 1075 (1972).
315. W. G. Duncombe and T. J. Rising, *Biochem. Pharmacol.*, **21,** 1089 (1972).
316. C. C. Guilbert and A. E. Chung, *J. Biol. Chem.*, **249,** 1026 (1974).
317. A. E. Senior and H. S. Sheratt, *Biochem. J.*, **108,** 46P (1968).
318. C. Corredor, K. Brendel, and R. Bressler, *Proc. Nat. Acad. Sci., US*, **58,** 2299 (1967).
319. N. Ruderman, E. Shafrir, and R. Bressler, *Life Sci.*, **7,** 1083 (1968).
320. M. Entman and R. Bressler, *Mol. Pharmacol.*, **3,** 333 (1967).
321. C. Corredor, K. Brendel, and R. Bressler, *Fed. Proc.*, **27,** 836 (1968).
322. P. Walter, V. Paetkau, and H. A. Lardy, *J. Biol. Chem.*, **241,** 2523 (1966).
323. K. Brendel, C. F. Corredor, and R. Bressler, *Biochem. Biophys. Res. Commun.*, **34,** 340 (1969).
324. N. B. Ruderman, C. J. Toews, C. Lowy, I. Vreeland, and E. Shafrir, *Am. J. Physiol.*, **219,** 51 (1970).

325. E. R. Froesch, M. Waldvogel, V. A. Meyer, A. Jakob, and A. Labhart, *Mol. Pharmacol.*, **3,** 429 (1967).

326. G. C. Gerritsen and W. E. Dulin, *J. Pharmacol. Exp. Ther.*, **150,** 491 (1965).

327. G. Geyer and B. Sokopp, *Acta Endocrinol. (Copenhagen)*; **72,** (Suppl. 173), 127 (1973).

328. G. C. Gerritsen and W. E. Dulin, *Proc. Soc. Exp. Biol. Med.*, **126,** 524 (1967).

329. J. N. Pereira and G. F. Holland, *J. Pharmacol. Exp. Ther.*, **157,** 381 (1967).

330. D. L. Smith, J. C. Wagner, and G. C. Gerritsen, *J. Pharm. Sci.*, **56,** 1150 (1967).

331. T. P. Gandhi and M. N. Jindal, *Arzneim.-Forsch.*, **21,** 961 (1971).

332. T. P. Gandhi and M. N. Jindal, *Arzneim.-Forsch.*, **21,** 968 (1971).

333. V. Ambrogi, K. Bloch, S. Daturi, P. Griggi, W. Logemann, M. A. Parenti, T. Rabini, and R. Tommasini, *Arzneim.-Forsch.*, **21,** 200 (1971).

334. F. Pedrazzi, A. Pisani Ceretti, S. Lose, F. Bommartini, D. Artini, and H. Emanueli, *Arzneim.-Forsch.*, **21,** 220 (1971).

335. V. Ambrogi, K. Bloch, P. Cozzi, S. Daturi, W. Logemann, M. A. Parenti, and R. Tommasini, *Arzneim.-Forsch.*, **21,** 204 (1971).

336. V. Ambrogi, K. Bloch, S. Daturi, W. Logemann, M. A. Parenti, and R. Tommasini, *Arzneim.-Forsch.*, **22,** 542 (1972).

337. R. Weyer, W. Aumuller, A. Bander, R. Heerdt, W. Pfaff, R. Schweitzer, and H. Weber, *Arzneim.-Forsch.*, **24,** 269 (1974).

338. H. Plumpe, H. Horstmann, and W. Puls, *Arzneim.-Forsch.*, **24,** 363 (1974).

339. W. Puls, W. Losert, O. Loge, E. Schillinger, U. Keup, and G. Kroneberg *Arzneim.-Forsch.*, **24,** 375 (1974).

340. H. D. Söling and A. Seck, *FEBS Lett.*, **51,** 52 (1975).

341. K. Gutsche, E. Schroder, C. Rufer, and O. Loge, *Arzneim.-Forsch.*, **24,** 1028 (1974).

342. L. Blumenbach, E. Gerhards, H. Gutsche, W. Kelin, O. Loge, W. Losert, E. Schillinger, U. Speck, H. Vetter, and H. Wendt, *Int. J. Clin. Pharmacol. Biopharm.*, **12,** 141 (1975).

343. C. Rufer, H. Biere, H. Ahrens, O. Loge, and E. Schroder, *J. Med. Chem.*, **17,** 708 (1974).

344. H. Biere, C. Rufer, H. Ahrens, O. Loge, and E. Schroder, *J. Med. Chem.*, **17,** 716 (1974).

345. J. Duhault, M. Boulanger, F. Tisserand, and L. Beregi, *Arzneim.-Forsch.*, **22,** 1682 (1972).

346. J. Duhault and F. Lebon, *Arzneim.-Forsch.*, **22,** 1686 (1972).

347. P. Desnoyers, J. Labaume, M. Anstett, M. Herrara, J. Pesquet, and J. Sebastien, *Arzneim.-Forsch.*, **22,** 1691 (1972).

348. J. Morell, *Biochem. Pharmacol.*, **23,** 2922 (1974).

349. R. J. Eberhard, R. Bressler, K. Brendel, and J. S. Hayes, *Pharmacologist*, **17,** 184 (1975).

350. I. Polacek, E. Schulze, H. Burg, and J. Ouart, *Arzneim.-Forsch.*, **24,** 1242 (1974).

351. H. Hohn, I. Polacek, and E. Schulze, *J. Med. Chem.*, **16,** 1340 (1973).

352. J. M. McManus, J. W. McFarland, C. F. Gerber, W. M. McLamore, and G. D. Laubach, *J. Med. Chem.*, **8,** 766 (1965).

353. J. W. McFarland, C. F. Gerber, and W. M. McLamore, *J. Med. Chem.*, **8,** 781 (1965).

354. J. M. McManus, and C. F. Gerber, *J. Med. Chem.*, **9,** 256 (1966).

355. J. M. McManus, *J. Med. Chem.*, **9,** 967 (1966).

356. J. R. Ryan, F. G. McMahon, and A. K. Jain, *Clin. Pharmacol. Ther.*, **17,** 243 (1975).

357. R. Sarges, D. E. Kuhla, H. E. Wiedermann, and D. A. Mayhew, *J. Med. Chem.*, **19,** 695 (1976).

358. G. Loiseau, R. Millischer, G. Berthe, A. M. Donadieu, P. Lohier, and J. P. Marquet, *Arzneim.-Forsch.*, **23,** 1571 (1973).

359. M. M. El-Kerdawy and H. A. Selim, *Pharmazie*, **30,** 768 (1975).

360. W. E. Dulin, G. H. Lund, and G. C. Gerritsen, *Proc. Soc. Exp. Biol. Med.*, **118,** 499 (1965).

361. V. J. Bauer, H. P. Dalalian, W. J. Fanshawe, S. R. Safir, E. C. Tocus, and C. R. Boshart, *J. Med. Chem.*, **11,** 981 (1968).

362. V. J. Bauer, W. J. Fanshawe, H. P. Dalalian, and S. R. Safir, *J. Med. Chem.*, **11,** 984 (1968).

363. S. J. Riggi, D. A. Blickens, and C. R. Boshart, *Diabetes*, **17,** 646 (1968).

364. D. A. Blickens and S. J. Riggi, *Toxicol. Appl. Pharmacol.*, **14,** 393 (1969).

365. D. A. Blickens and S. J. Riggi, *Diabetes*, **18,** 612 (1969).

366. G. E. Wiegand, V. J. Bauer, S. R. Safir, D. A. Blickens, and S. J. Riggi, *J. Med. Chem.*, **14,** 1015 (1971).

367. W. J. Fanshawe, V. J. Bauer, S. R. Safir, D. A. Blickens, and S. J. Riggi, *J. Med. Chem.*, **12,** 381 (1969).

368. G. E. Wiegand, V. J. Bauer, S. R. Safir, D. A. Blickens, and S. J. Riggi, *J. Med. Chem.*, **12,** 891 (1969).

369. G. E. Wiegand, V. J. Bauer, S. R. Safir, D. A. Blickens, and S. J. Riggi, *J. Med. Chem.*, **12,** 943 (1969).

370. G. E. Wiegand, V. J. Bauer, S. R. Safir, D. A. Blickens, and S. J. Riggi, *J. Med. Chem.*, **14,** 214 (1971).

371. V. J. Bauer, G. E. Wiegand, W. J. Fanshawe, and S. R. Safir, *J. Med. Chem.*, **12,** 944 (1969).
372. V. J. Bauer, H. P. Dalalian, and S. R. Safir, *J. Med. Chem.*, **11,** 1263 (1968).
373. G. E. Wiegand, V. J. Bauer, S. R. Safir, D. A. Blickens, and S. J. Riggi, *J. Med. Chem.*, **15,** 1326 (1972).
374. D. A. Blickens and S. J. Riggi, *J. Pharmacol. Exp. Ther.*, **177,** 536 (1971).
375. R. Haeckel, *Z. Klin. Chem, Klin, Biochem.*, **11,** 179 (1973).
376. J. R. Ryan, G. E. Maha, F. G. McMahon, and A. Kyriakopoulos, *Diabetes*, **20,** 734 (1971).
377. M. Oellerich and R. Haeckel, *Biochem. Pharmacol.*, **24,** 1085 (1975).
378. I. A. Mirsky, G. Perisutti, and D. Diengott, *Endocrinology*, **59,** 369 (1956).
379. I. A. Mirsky, G. Perisutti, R. Jinks, and M. Kaufman, *Endocrinology*, **60,** 318 (1957).
380. D. O. Foster, P. D. Ray, and H. A. Lardy, *Biochemistry*, **5,** 563 (1966).
381. P. D. Ray, D. O. Foster, and H. A. Lardy, *J. Biol. Chem.*, **241,** 3904 (1966).
382. C. M. Veneziale, P. Walter, N. Kneer, and H. A. Lardy, *Biochemistry*, **6,** 2129 (1967).
383. H. A. Lardy, "Site Specific Inhibitors of Gluconeogenesis," in *Inhibitors—Tools in Cell Research*, T. Bucher and H. Sies, Eds., Springer-Verlag, New York, 1969, p. 374.
384. H. G. McDaniel, W. J. Reddy, and B. R. Boshell, *Biochim. Biophys. Acta*, **276,** 543 (1972).
385. H. G. McDaniel, B. R. Boshell, and W. J. Reddy, *Diabetes*, **22,** 713 (1973).
386. H. Endou, E. Reuter, and H. J. Weber, *Nauyn-Schmiedeberg's, Arch. Pharmacol.*, **287,** 297 (1975).
387. F. L. Alvares and P. D. Ray, *J. Biol. Chem.*, **249,** 2058 (1974).
388. B. Blank, N. W. DiTullio, C. K. Miao, F. F. Owings, J. G. Gleason, S. T. Ross, C. E. Berkoff, H. L. Saunders, J. Delarge, and C. L. Lapiere, *J. Med. Chem.*, **17,** 1065 (1974).
389. N. W. DiTullio, C. E. Berkoff, B. Blank, V. Kostos, E. J. Stack, and H. L. Saunders, *Biochem. J.*, **138,** 387 (1974).
390. H. L. Saunders, private communication.
391. M. N. Goodman, *Biochem. J.*, **150,** 137 (1975).
392. V. Kostos, N. W. DiTullio, J. Rush, L. Cieslinski, and H. L. Saunders, *Arch. Biochem. Biophys.*, **171,** 459 (1975).
393. P. J. Blackshear, P. A. H. Holloway, and K. G. M. M. Alberti, *Biochem. J.*, **148,** 353 (1975).
394. B. H. Robinson and J. Oei, *FEBS Lett.*, **58,** 12 (1975).
395. M. Jomain-Baum, V. L. Schramm, and R. W. Hanson, *J. Biol. Chem.*, **251,** 37 (1976).
396. F. I. Bennett and G. A. O. Alleyne, *FEBS Lett.*, **65,** 215 (1976).
397. T. B. Ray and C. C. Black, *J. Biol. Chem.*, **251,** 5824 (1976).
398. B. Blank, N. W. DiTullio, L. Deviney, J. T. Roberts, and H. L. Saunders, *J. Med. Chem.*, **20,** 577 (1977).
399. B. Blank, N. W. DiTullio, F. F. Owings, L. Deviney, C. K. Miao, and H. L. Saunders, *J. Med. Chem.*, **20,** 572 (1977).
400. N. Baumann, B. Pease, and C. Hill, *Fed. Proc.*, **26,** 507 (1967).
401. N. Baumann and C. J. Hill, *Biochemistry*, **7,** 1322 (1968).
402. N. Baumann and B. S. Pease, *Biochem. Pharmacol.*, **18,** 1093 (1969).
403. N. Baumann, S. Gordon, and B. S. Pease, *Biochem. Pharmacol.*, **18,** 1241 (1969).
404. R. L. Hanson, P. D. Ray, P. Walter, and H. A. Lardy, *J. Biol. Chem.*, **244,** 4351 (1969).
405. J. Reed and H. A. Lardy, *J. Biol. Chem.*, **245,** 5297 (1970).
406. P. C. Holland, M. G. Clark, D. P. Bloxham, and H. A. Lardy, *J. Biol. Chem.*, **248,** 6050 (1973).
407. S. J. Gately, S. S. Al-Bassam, J. R. Taylor, and H. S. A. Sherratt, *Biochem. Chem. Trans.*, **3,** 333 (1975).
408. J. R. Williamson, E. T. Browning, R. Scholz, R. A. Kreisberg, and I. B. Fritz, *Diabetes*, **17,** 194 (1968).
409. J. D. McGarry and D. W. Foster, *J. Clin. Invest.*, **52,** 877 (1973).
410. R. A. Burges, W. D. Butt, and A. Baggaley, *Biochem. J.*, **109,** 38P (1968).
411. G. F. Tutwiler, *Experientia*, **29,** 1340 (1973).
412. S. G. Boots and M. R. Boots, *J. Pharm. Sci.*, **64,** 1949 (1975).
413. D. Dvornik, N. Simard-Duquesne, M. Krami, K. Sestanj, K. H. Gabbay, J. H. Kinoshita, S. D. Varma, and L. O. Merola, *Science.* **182,** 1146 (1973).
414. B. L. Furman, *Brit. J. Pharmacol.*, **50,** 575 (1974).
415. J. R. Turtle and J. A. Burgess, *Diabetes*, **22,** 858 (1973).
416. D. M. Bailey, C. G. DeGrazia, D. Wood, J. Siggins, H. R. Harding, G. O. Potts, and T. W. Skulan, *J. Med. Chem.*, **17,** 702 (1974).

417. J. M. Grisar, G. P. Claxton, A. A. Carr, and N. L. Wiech, *J. Med. Chem.*, **16,** 679 (1973).
418. J. M. Grisar, G. P. Claxton, N. L. Wiech, R. W. Lucas, R. D. MacKenzie, and S. Goldstein, *J. Med. Chem.*, **16,** 885 (1973).
419. J. M. Grisar, G. P. Claxton, and N. L. Wiech, *J. Med. Chem.*, **19,** 365 (1976).
420. G. P. Claxton, J. M. Grisar, and N. L. Wiech, *J. Med. Chem.*, **17,** 364 (1974).
421. B. W. Siegel, N. L. Wiech, and T. R. Blohm, *Fed. Proc.*, **34,** 754 (1975).
422. Y. Hamuro, K. Nishikawa, W. Watari, and Z. Suzuoki, *Biochem. Pharmacol.*, **23,** 3218 (1974).
423. H. Sugihara, N. Matsumoto, Y. Hamuro, and Y. Kawamatsu, *Arzneim.-Forsch.*, **24,** 1560 (1974).
424. R. F. R. Church, R. R. Maleike, and M. J. Weiss, *J. Med. Chem.*, **15,** 514 (1972).
425. V. S. Fang, *Arch. Int. Pharmacodyn. Ther.*, **176,** 193 (1968).
426. F. Uchimaru, S. Okada, A. Kosasayama, and T. Konno, *Chem. Pharm. Bull.* (Tokyo), **19,** 1337 (1971).
427. V. Ambrogi, K. Bloch, S. Daturi, W. Logemann, and M. A. Parenti, *J. Pharm. Sci.*, **61,** 1483 (1972).
428. S. C. Lahiri and B. Pathak, *J. Pharm. Sci.*, **57,** 1013 (1968).
429. S. C. Lahiri and N. C. De, *J. Med. Chem.*, **11,** 900 (1968).
430. S. C. Lahiri and B. Pathak, *J. Med. Chem.*, **14,** 888 (1971).
431. H. G. Garg and C. Prakash, *J. Med. Chem.*, **15,** 435 (1972).
432. H. L. Eichner, P. W. Stacpoole, and P. H. Forsham, *Diabetes*, **23,** 179 (1974).
433. M. Lorini and M. Ciman, *Biochem. Pharmacol.*, **11,** 823 (1962).
434. P. W. Stacpoole and J. M. Felts, *Metabolism*, **19,** 71 (1970).
435. P. W. Stacpoole and J. M. Felts, *Metabolism*, **20,** 830 (1971).
436. P. J. Blackshear, P. A. H. Holloway, and K. G. M. M. Alberti, *Biochem. J.*, **142,** 279 (1974).
437. P. J. Blackshear, P. A. H. Holloway, and K. G. M. M. Alberti, *Biochem. J.*, **146,** 447 (1975).
438. M. Goodman, T. T. Aoki, and N. Ruderman, *Diabetes*, **25** (Suppl. 1), 332 (1976).
439. P. W. Stacpoole, *Metabolism*, **26,** 107 (1977).
440. P. W. Stacpoole, D. M. Kornhauser, O. B. Crofford, D. Rabinowitz, and J. A. Oates, *Diabetes*, **25** (Suppl. 1), 328 (1976).
441. Ng. Ph. Buu-Hoi, *Compt. Rend.*, **247,** 2223 (1958).
442. G. Coppi, P. Fresia, and G. Bernardi, *Chim. Ther.*, 452 (1966).
443. G. Pala, T. Bruzzese, E. Marazzi-Uberti, and G. Coppi, *J. Med. Chem.*, **9,** 603 (1966).
444. S. Casadio, T. Bruzzese, G. Pala, G. Coppi, and C. Turba, *J. Med. Chem.*, **9,** 707 (1966).
445. G. Pala, S. Casadio, T. Bruzzese, and G. Coppi, *J. Med. Chem.*, **9,** 786 (1966).
446. C. M. Gupta, A. P. Bhaduri, N. M. Khanna, and S. K. Mukherjee, *Indian J. Chem.*, **9,** 201 (1971).
447. S. K. Mukherjee, *Biochem. Pharmacol.*, **22,** 1529 (1973).
448. S. S. Mukherjee, P. S. R. Murthi, and S. K. Mukherjee, *Acta Diabet. Lat.*, **13,** 8 (1976).
449. H. S. Tager and H. N. Christensen, *Biochem. Biophys. Res. Commun.*, **44,** 185 (1971).
450. B. Blank, N. W. DiTullio, L. Deviney, J. T. Roberts, and H. L. Saunders, *J. Med. Chem.*, **18,** 952 (1975).
451. D. M. Kramer and K. Lehmann, *FEBS Lett.*, **22,** 49 (1972).
452. G. Dapergolas and G. Gregoriadis, *Lancet*, **2,** 824 (1976).
453. F. M. Ng, P. Z. Zimmet, G. Seiler, P. Taft, and J. Bornstein, *Diabetes*, **23,** 950 (1974).
454. F. M. Ng, J. Bornstein, C. Welker, P. Z. Zimmet, and P. Taft, *Diabetes*, **23,** 943 (1974).
455. C. E. Hunt, J. R. Lindsey, and S. U. Walkley, *Fed. Proc.*, **35,** 1206 (1976).
456. S. Rahbar, *Clin. Chim. Acta*, **22,** 296 (1971).
457. L. A. Trivelli, H. M. Ranney, and H-T. Lai, *N. Engl. J. Med.*, **284,** 353 (1971).
458. E. P. Paulsen, *Metab. Clin. Exp.*, **22,** 269 (1973).
459. H. F. Bunn, D. N. Haney, K. H. Gabbay, and P. M. Gallop, *Biochem, Biophys. Res. Commun.*, **67,** 103 (1975).
460. H. F. Bunn, D. N. Haney, S. Kamin, K. H. Gabbay, and P. M. Gallop, *J. Clin. Invest.*, **57,** 1652 (1976).
461. J. Brown, I. G. Molnar, W. Clark, and Y. Mullen, *Science*, **184,** 1377 (1974).
462. F. C. Goetz, *Metabolism*, **23,** 875 (1974).
463. J. Brown, W. R. Clark, I. G. Molnar, and Y. S. Mullen, *Diabetes*, **25,** 56 (1976).
464. P. Mazur, J. A. Kemp, and R. H. Miller, *Proc. Nat. Acad. Sci., US*, **73.** 4105 (1976).
465. Y. S. Mullen, W. R. Clark, I. G. Molnar, and J. Brown, *Science*, **195,** 68 (1977).
466. S. D. Varma, I. Mikuni, and J. H. Kinoshita, *Science*, **188,** 1215 (1975).
467. S. D. Varma and J. H. Kinoshita, *Biochem. Pharmacol.*, **25,** 2505 (1976).
468. S. D. Varma, A. Mizuno, and J. H. Kinoshita, *Science*, **195,** 205 (1977).

CHAPTER THIRTY–TWO

Anticoagulants, Antithrombotics, and Hemostatics

K. N. VON KAULLA

University of Colorado Medical Center
Denver, Colorado 80262, USA

CONTENTS

1 FREQUENCY OF VARIOUS FORMS OF THROMBOEMBOLISM

Anticoagulants and antithrombotic agents are some of the most important drugs in existence, although there is considerable room for improvement. In humans these drugs prevent and/or treat intravascular clotting, a pathological process that in its various forms, primarily thrombosis and embolism, represents a major cause of disease and death.

In the United States, venous thromboembolism annually causes approximately 300,000 patients to be hospitalized, and of these more than 50,000 die (1). About 948,000 people annually suffer an acute myocardial infarction; of these patients, about 227,000 died (2). The reported incidence of coronary thrombosis in hearts with infarcts varies from 21% (3) to 100% (4). Among the white population of the United States, about 400,000 individuals per year were reported to undergo a cerebral infarct (5), and thromboembolic phenomena are involved in virtually all cases of cerebral infarction (6). Venous thromboembolism can also develop in childhood (7) and, as detected with ^{125}-I-fibrinogen leg scanning, occurs in 3% of childbirths (8). Thrombophlebitis leading to pulmonary embolism has been stated to cause as many as 9% of hospital deaths (9).

In the United States, pulmonary emboli are detected each year in an estimated 700,000 patients, and more than 90% can be traced to deep vein thrombosis (10). Thromboembolic disease was found to contribute to 12.5% of all postoperative deaths (11). This is not surprising because depending on the type of surgery, thrombosis was detected in 14%–74% of all cases (8). More than 5 million individuals in the United States over the age of 40 undergo major surgery (12). Of great importance is the observation that 20% of the thrombi formed during or after surgery continue to grow, thus requiring treatment, whereas the remainder of thrombi regress spontaneously (13). This regression clearly reflects the activity of the body's own defense mechanism, the fibrinolytic system. As discussed later, there are clear-cut potentials to activate this defense mechanism by drugs, an important challenge for the medicinal chemist, who can make very essential contributions to reduce human suffering.

Whereas thromboembolism is the most common form of intravascular clotting, other forms also have great clinical importance, and when not treated very early, these forms use up most of the clotting factors, resulting in the tendency to hemorrhage. Disseminated intravascular coagulation is the most common type of this pathological process (for review, see Ref. 14). In addition, certain drugs have a potential thrombogenic effect (15). Of these, the estrogen-containing oral contraceptives are of the greatest interest (16). There exists also hereditary thrombosis (17), a tendency that requires prophylactic anticoagulant treatment with quite a number of procedures. Finally, it is essential to point out that the anticoagulant heparin is required for the functioning of the heart-lung machine on which modern heart surgery is based, and only the use of heparin enables the dialysis machine (the artificial kidney) to function. Approximately 16,000 persons presently are subjected to renal dialysis in the United States (18).

2 PATHWAY OF APPROACHES

2.1 General Remarks

The literature concerning blood coagulation in both its clinical and biochemical aspects is enormous and increases rapidly. This also applies to the properties and functioning of anticoagulants and fibrinolytic agents. Very little, however, has been published in relation to attempts to develop better antithrombotic agents, research that would be very valuable and desirable from the clinical viewpoint. Also essential from the clinical point of view are the development and application of methods to discover, for instance, thrombosis tendency, thus permitting efficient prophylactic treatment. Methods have been developed (17, 19, 20) that reveal a pathologic tendency for intravascular clotting, that is, such individuals do not necessarily develop intravascular clots, but they have an increased tendency to do so in situations that might induce such a tendency (poor circulation in the lower extremities, certain types of surgery, other diseases that require long bed rest, etc.).

The detection of fibrin monomers or fibrin split products is now the center of interest, but finding these only provides confirmation that some intravascular clotting has already taken place, whereas the thrombin generation test (19) detects such a tendency mostly before any intravascular clotting has occurred. Various reasons for the triggering of intravascular clotting are known, although this is still a wide open field for clinical research.

2.2 Protective Mechanisms and Their Deficiencies

In the human blood there are two basic protective mechanisms against intravascular clotting; one, which deactivates activated clotting factors in the blood, is based on antithrombin III activity. The other mechanism, which at least partially dissolves intravascularly formed clots, is based on the fibrinolytic enzyme system. It has been proved that markedly reduced activity of each of these systems results in an increased potential for intravascular clotting. Hereditary thrombosis tendencies, based on a reduction of one of these two activities, have been described many times. Another condition that can cause localized intravascular clotting, mostly in the arterial side of the vascular system, is abnormally high aggregability of the thrombocytes.

2.3 The Value of Prior Coagulation Analysis

Before any treatment with anticoagulants is started, it should be determined whether abnormalities such as those just described exist, and if so, which type. Prothrombin-depressing agents are not very beneficial if there is markedly increased spontaneous aggregability of the platelets or hereditary antithrombin III deficiency, for example. Also, treatment of intravascular clotting with heparin might be less successful if the euglobulin lysis time indicates the absence of fibrinolytic potential in the blood (21). These introductory remarks are made to point out that it would be highly desirable clinically to analyze the clotting situation of the blood of a patient to ensure that the appropriate antithrombotic drug or combination of drugs is prescribed. It is realized that for technical reasons such an analysis is not always possible, particularly in smaller hospitals.

2.4 Desirability of Improvements of Anticoagulants and Antithrombotic Drugs

The anticoagulants and antithrombotic drugs are discussed in some detail in the sections that follow. Basically, these drugs are supposed to prevent intravascular clotting or to stop further intravascular clotting. Heparin is very efficient in this regard; prothrombin-depressing agents are less efficient. Certain agents prevent increased platelet aggregation, a property that contributes to thrombosis tendency. Fibrinolytic agents dissolve intravascular clots (thrombi, emboli). None of these drugs is highly effective in all clinical situations; they may induce side reactions, etc. Although the development of these drugs has very considerably increased the possibilities of preventing or treating all variations of thromboembolic disease, there is a good deal of room for further improvement. Here the medicinal chemist, in cooperation with clinicians who have the experimental interest and the experience, can be of decisive importance. For many years, no new and better anticoagulant drugs have been developed.

3 HEPARIN

3.1 History

Heparin, still the most effective anticoagulant, was discovered in 1916 by Jay McLean (22), a sophomore medical student, in Howell's laboratory at the John Hopkins University, Baltimore. Shortly afterward, Howell (23) reported that the preparation prevented blood coagulation *in vitro* and *in vivo* when injected intravenously into dogs. In 1918 Howell and Holt (24) named this anticoagulant heparin, to indicate its abundance in liver tissues. The first paper describing heparin treatment of patients was submitted for publication in February 1937 by Crafoord (25) in Stockholm, followed by Murray et al. (26) in March 1937 in Toronto. The number of publications relating to heparin is enormous. The earlier observations were well described in 1939 by Jorpes (27); further developments were covered by Engelberg in 1963 (28), whereas some of the latest biochemical and clinical results were published in a monograph by Kakkar and Thomas (29). Attempts to replace heparin by semisynthetic heparinlike compounds have been partially successful (see Section 4, on heparinoids).

3.2 Sources and Molecular Sizes

Jorpes (30) and Jorpes and Bergström (31) first showed that heparin contains glucuronic acid, hexosamine, and esterified sulfonic acids and is a mucopolysaccharide polysulfonic acid ester. Presently, there are more detailed insights into the heparin structure, although the correlation between structure and physiological activity remains largely unknown (32). Heparin for therapeutic use is obtained mostly from bovine lung tissue and from intestinal mucosa of pigs and cattle. In 1973 more than 35 million pounds of intestinal mucosa was used for production of heparin (33). Heparinlike substances have been isolated from whale lung and liver (34), fish scales (35), and common surf and ocean clam (36). Lately, heparin has been defined as a polydisperse, negatively charged, sulfated mucopolysaccharide with a molecular weight of 3000–57,500 (37). Opinions differ with regard to molecular weight (38, 39); for instance, ranges of 6000–25,000 (40) and 3000–37,000 (41) have been reported. Only fractions above a molecular weight of 7000 are said to have an anticoagulant action (41). However it has been claimed that special enzymatic degradation of heparin results in fragments possessing a molecular weight of approximately 5000 (42), which were designated λ-heparin. Studies have shown that after oral administration in mice, λ-heparin delays blood coagulation for up to 30 min. If this substance could be further developed as tablets for use in patients, it would represent great therapeutic progress.

3.3 Structure of Heparin

The presently recognized structural features of heparin (43) appear in Fig. 32.1. The polysaccharide is composed of alternating uronic acid (α-L-iduronic acid or β-D-glucuronic acid) and α-D-glucosamine

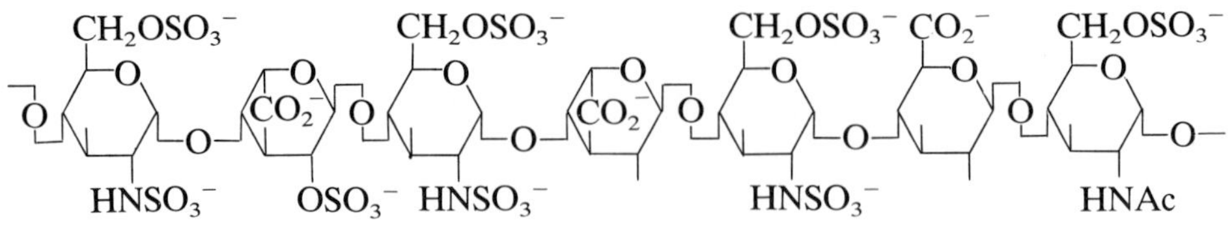

Fig. 32.1 Structure of heparin.

monosaccharide units, joined by 1→4 glycosidic linkages (for a recent review, see Ref. 44). The glucosamine residues have sulfated (major portion) or acetylated (minor portion) amino groups. Most of the glucosamine units carry —O—sulfate groups at C-6; in addition, most, but not all of the iduronic acid residues are sulfated at C-2. The glucuronic acid component invariably appears to be nonsulfonated (45). The structural specificity of heparin has also been summarized as follows: (1) presence of monosaccharide building stones: D-glucosamine, D-glucuronic acid, L-iduronic acid, all in pyranoside form; (2) structural and stereochemical requirements of 1→4 glycosidic conjugation, α-D- and α-L-anomeric linkage of the uronate residues, covalently linked sulfates in the amino and in the C-6 hydroxyl groups of the D-glucosamine residue, and conformation of hexopyranoside sugars in the heteropolysaccharide chain; and (3) heteropolysaccharide macromolecular character: polyanionic acid properties possessing high pK values (40). The heparins possess no branchings in the heteropolysaccharide chain. The requirement of a straight molecule for anticoagulant action has also been demonstrated for sulfonated polysaccharides with anticoagulant action: such compounds with identical molecular weights lose anticoagulant activity when they are branched and have none when they are globular (46).

3.4 Attempts at Synthesis

Attempts to synthetize heparin have not been completely successful; however there are some interesting approaches. For example, starting from an amylose derivative, the important 2-sulfonamido and 5-carboxyl groups in the α(1→4) linked polysaccharide chain were prepared by controlled chemical transformation. Heparinlike heteropolysaccharides were obtained that possessed appreciable anticoagulant activity (47).

3.5 Presence of Heparin in Blood

Although there has been some discussion of whether heparin is present in human blood, there is now abundant evidence that heparin normally occurs in the blood of man. Since it is protein bound, methods that detect free heparin only give false negative results. The material extracted from human plasma has the same biological activity as commercial heparin, and there is scant justification for any further doubt that the substance is indeed heparin (48). When heparin was extracted from human plasma it showed only the metachromatic reaction with toluidine blue after the precipitated heparin protein complex had been digested with tryptic enzymes. Heparin is stored in the mast cells, which are quite numerous in man and are located beneath the endothelium in most vessels (49).

3.6.1 THERAPEUTIC APPLICATIONS: METHODS. The therapeutic application of heparin as an anticoagulant in man is carried out in three ways depending on the clinical situation: intravenous infusion, intravenous injection, and subcutaneous injection; recently the latter route has been very widely used, particularly for prevention of intravascular clotting. Figure 32.2 shows how

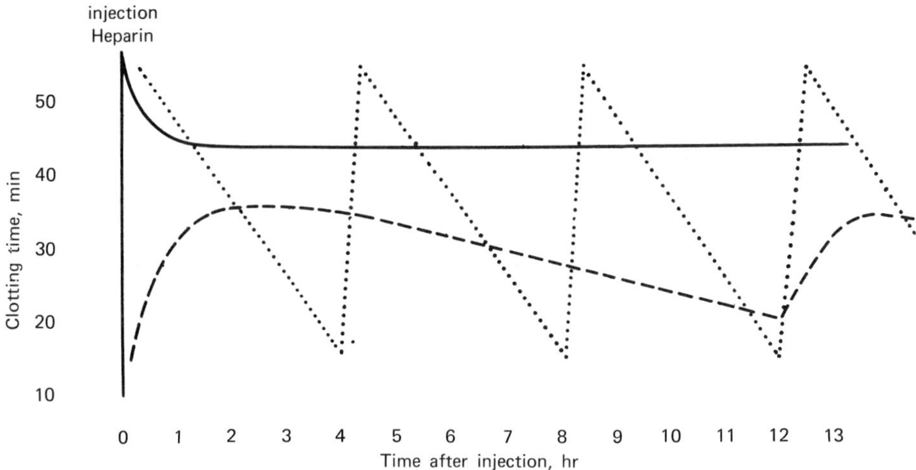

Fig. 32.2 Therapeutic application of heparin in man, showing different effects on blood clotting time: solid curve, i.e. loading dose followed by constant i.v. infusion; dotted curve, repeated i.v. injections; dashed curve, s.c. injection (every 12 hr).

these three applications affect or prolong, respectively, blood coagulation in man. The half-life of intravenous heparin (0.47–6 mg/kg) for man was found to be about $1\frac{1}{2}$ hr (50); a half-life of 60 min was also reported (51). As demonstrated with dogs, heparin applied *in vivo* not only reduces or prevents the coagulation of blood but, with some time delay, acts similarly on the lymph (52), an effect that might be quite valuable clinically.

3.6.2 THERAPEUTIC APPLICATIONS: CLINICAL RESULTS. The literature on the clinical use of heparin both as prophylactic agent and for treatment of thromboembolism is enormous. The use of low dose subcutaneous heparin as a prophylactic agent in patients undergoing elective general surgery is a more recent development. In regard to the incidence of thrombosis in these patients as assessed with ^{125}-I-fibrinogen leg scanning, an international trial with 1292 patients revealed occurrence of thrombosis in 25% of the untreated patients and in 8% of the patients who received heparin subcutaneously (53). The prophylaxis with low dose heparin was, however, ineffective after hip fractures and hip surgery. There are various other statistics reflecting similar results. Subcutaneous injections of 5000 units of heparin in normal subjects and in postoperative patients was also reported to decrease blood viscosity for 4–6 hr (54). Although subcutaneous heparin is not 100% effective as a prophylactic agent (and here are clear possibilities for further pharmaceutical developments), it is much more effective than other drugs used as antithrombotic agents. Thus in one study the thrombosis incidence of patients treated with coumarin was 18%, but only 2% in those treated with low dose subcutaneous heparin (55). In another study it was shown that the frequency of isotopically assessed deep vein thrombosis was 36% in untreated patients, 40.6% in a group treated with xantinol-nicotinate, 21.7% in the dextran-40 group, and only 12.8% in the heparin group. Occasional bleeding in the heparin group could not be completely avoided (56).

For the treatment of actual intravascular clotting with clear clinical symptoms (thromboses, embolism), generally much larger amounts of heparin are required, given as an infusion or as repeated intravenous injections. Heparin is also used in a variety of diseases involving fibrin deposition in very small vessels or capillaries, for instance, glomerulonephritis (for latest results and review of literature concerning heparin-treated glomerulonephritis, see Ref. 57). Labeled heparin applied topically was found to penetrate the human skin rapidly when lanolin was used as base; the effect on blood coagulation was not examined (58).

3.7 Assessment of the Effect of Heparin on the Coagulation System

There are numerous published methods for assessing the effect of heparin on blood (or plasma) coagulation *in vivo* and *in vitro*, or on components of the coagulation system. For a listing of various methods, see Ref. 59; five clotting methods used for heparin assay in plasma are compared in Ref. 60. From the clinical standpoint, the use of unstored whole blood is most desirable; however such a method, which was recently published, uses tubes containing diatomaceous earth (61), which provides an undesirable rough surface. It has also been found that some stored vacuum containers that are being utilized for sending drawn blood to the laboratory develop antiheparin activity (62).

A simple temperature-controlled bedside recording device has been developed in which whole blood from a patient can be used immediately after drawing without any additions; the machine produces coagulation curves revealing the dynamic action of heparin on the blood coagulation of the patient (63). It has been reported that assessment of clotting factor activities and coagulation screening tests can be carried out in heparinized blood when heparin is removed by chromatography (64).

3.8 Interaction with the Coagulation System

Figure 32.3 shows the interference of heparin with various components of the coagulation system. The drug exerts its anticoagulant effect only in the presence of a plasma cofactor, antithrombin III. Antithrombin III is a naturally occurring inhibitor of activated clotting factors that have a reactive serine residue at their enzymatically active center. These factors are IXa, Xa, XIa, thrombin, and probably XIIa. Antithrombin III combines with and inactivates these coagulation enzymes in a progressive and irreversible manner. Heparin binds to lysyl residues on the antithrombin III molecule, thus very markedly accelerates the inhibitory effect of antithrombin III (59).

Heparin appears to inactivate factor Xa more effectively than it does thrombin, which can also be inactivated by antithrombin alone (65). After subcutaneous injection of sodiumheparin it was found that heparin with a low molecular weight (9000) has a much more pronounced anti-Xa-potentiation effect than a preparation with a molecular weight of 22,000. Calcium-heparin (which is commercially used in Europe) was also less effective (66). Approximately one-third of heparin is bound to antithrombin III. This fraction accounts for 85% of the total heparin activity as measured in terms of thrombin inactivation (67). However previously it was found that antithrombin III is the main inactivator of thrombin even in the absence of heparin (68).

The requirements of antithrombin III for heparin anticoagulant activity have been shown in various ways. For instance, after heparin has been separated into two distinct fractions by antithrombin-substituted sepharose, only the fraction with high affinity to this sepharose exhibits anticoagulant activity. The two fractions do not have any structural dissimilarities. For structural requirements for the interaction of heparin with antithrombin III and the resulting structural changes, see Refs. 69 and 70. Antithrombin III activity is the most important human protective mechanism

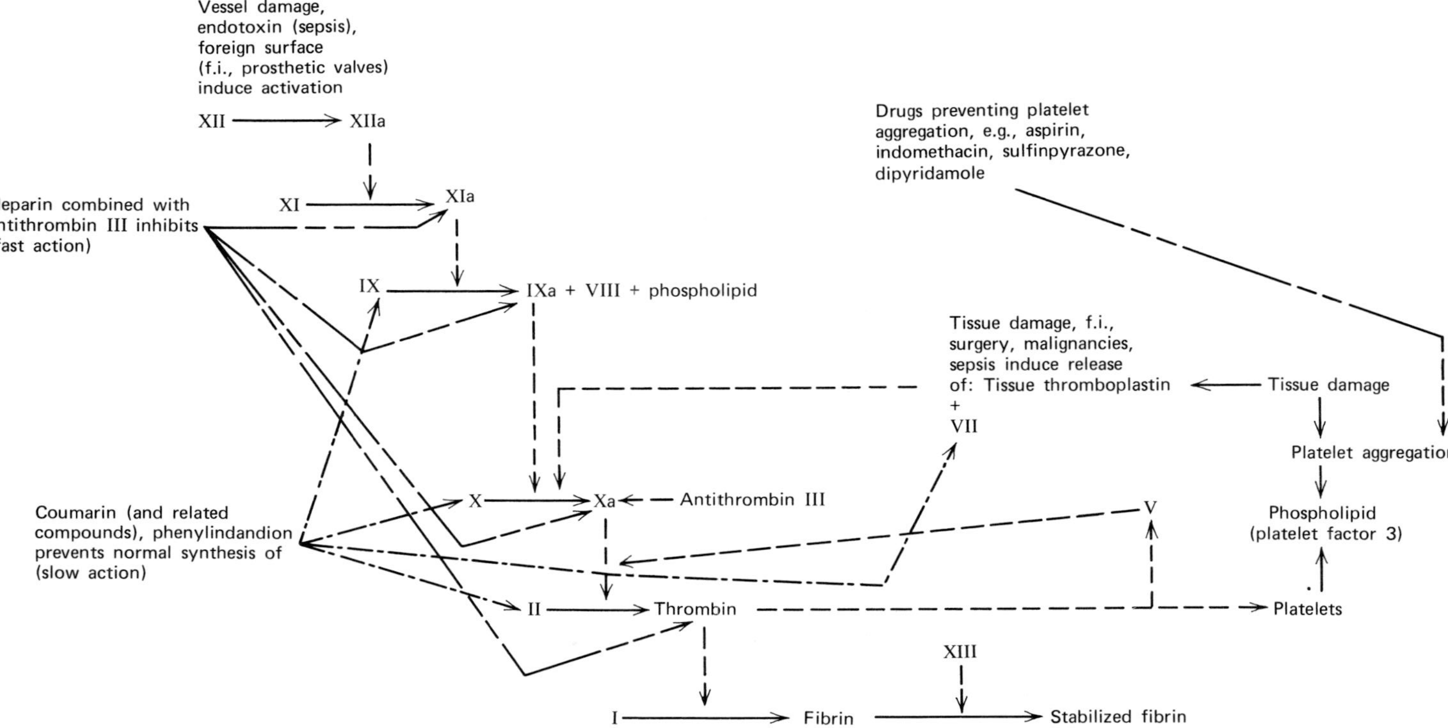

Fig. 32.3 The blood coagulation system. Pathways of action of anticoagulants: Solid lines, transformation; broken lines, action.

against intravascular clotting. Low hereditary antithrombin III activity results in hereditary tendency to thrombosis (17). This has been shown in many recent publications, and such reduced activity has also been found in normal persons who develop thrombosis tendency. Therefore it is important to realize that continuous intravenous infusion of large amounts of heparin (750–2000 U/hr) decreases antithrombin III activity in man, with a return to normal levels within 2 days after cessation of therapy. This finding was considered to represent a potential paradoxical thrombosis-inducing effect of heparin (71). Here is an open field for research on improvement of antithrombotic agents and therapy, respectively, particularly in regard to antithrombin III activity.

It has been demonstrated that coumadin and related drugs enhance antithrombin III activity in man and exert little protective antithrombotic action in patients in whom this little known effect does not occur, even if the prothrombin level is low (17). Recently a semisynthetic heparin analogue, a glycosamine polysulfate of bovine origin, having no anticoagulant effect *in vitro* yet increasing antithrombin III activity in man after intravenous injection, has been described. Based on this observation it was pointed out that an ideal drug for preventing thrombosis would selectively potentiate the action of antithrombin III without significantly delaying the clotting process (72).

3.9 Clearance of Heparin from Blood

The pathway of removing heparin from blood is not clearly understood. It has been claimed that the disappearance of heparin depends primarily on blood constituents, most specifically on platelets, not on clearance by kidney and other organs (73). However it has been demonstrated that patients with severely impaired kidney function show a significant but moderate decrease of heparin elimination (74). It was also found that platelets take up free heparin only, not heparin complexed with antithrombin III (75).

3.10 Heparin-Platelet Interaction

Whether heparin facilitates or prevents platelet aggregation is still an open question (76). For a review of this heparin function, see Ref. 77. Observations in patients with coronary artery disease also indicate that a heparin-neutralizing activity is released into the plasma after platelet aggregation (78). Occasionally heparin can also induce severe thrombocytopenia in patients (79), and it has been suggested that a causal relation, mediated by an immune mechanism, exists between heparin therapy and thrombocytopenia (80). One study even disclosed that thrombocytopenia occurred in 31% and disseminated intravascular clotting developed in 12% of patients receiving a standard dose of heparin therapy (81). However the reduced half-life of heparin and increased clearance rate with pulmonary embolism appear not to be related to binding of heparin on platelets (82). Heparin under experimental conditions is adsorbed onto human erythrocytes (83).

3.11 Lipid-Clearing Activity

Heparin is also a lipid-clearing agent. It activates a lipoprotein lipase normally present in plasma, an effect that appears particularly rapidly after intravenous injection in man. This effect is distinct from heparin's anticoagulant properties, and it may be of significance in protection against vascular atheroma and thrombosis (84). The lipoprotein lipase hydrolyzes complex lipids, releasing complex fatty acids to the plasma where they have a high affinity for albumin, displacing much of previously bound drugs.

Thus during postoperative therapy when a patient may be receiving heparin for 8–20 days, its administration can easily result in the activation of large amounts of the previously albumin-bound drugs (85). By blockade of the carboxyl groups of heparin, it is possible to separate the lipoprotein-clearing activity of this drug from its anticoagulant activity (86, 87).

3.12 Heparin and the Immunologic Mechanism

As mentioned earlier, heparin is stored in the mast cells, and from these sites it easily diffuses into the bloodstream. In the mast cells themselves, the metachromatic granules contain a histamine-heparin complex. Thus heparin functions these cells to bind and presumably inactivate histamine. This action of heparin plus its reversible binding and neutralization of complement, the inactivation of autoagglutinins in hemolytic anemia, the well-documented modification of a variety of allergic effects, and its antibody-increasing effect, all strongly suggest that endogenous heparin functions in the cellular immunologic mechanism (88).

3.13 Heparin and the Fibrinolytic System

The relation of heparin to the fibrinolytic system is a clinically important matter. In a purified system it has been observed that when plasmin is incubated together with antithrombin-heparin cofactor, a progressive inhibition of the proteolytic activity of the enzyme occurs and the presence of heparin dramatically accelerates the rate of interaction (89). Although such observations in a purified system do not necessarily reveal what might happen in the human blood, it appears that high heparin concentration can inhibit the functioning of the human fibrinolytic system, which is undesirable. We have observed in patients that the marked activation of the fibrinolytic system by intravenous pyrogen injections does not occur if, shortly before this injection, a large amount of heparin is given intravenously (90). This inhibiting effect, which has been mentioned in various publications, appears to be dose dependent, since after intravenous injection of 10,000 units of heparin in humans, activation of the fibrinolytic system occurs only after about 30–60 min, when the blood heparin concentration has already been reduced (91). Small amounts of heparin, however, activate the human fibrinolytic system both in *in vitro* (90, 92) and *in vivo* (93, 94). *In vitro* a fraction of one unit of heparin already enhanced fibrinolytic activity in various experimental arrangements (90), an observation that may explain the finding that less than one unit (0.4–0.6 U/ml) has an antithrombotic effect in experimental venous thrombosis (95). These investigations may help to explain the protective effect of low dose heparin in man (76).

Small amounts of heparin *in vitro* enhance the fibrinolytic activity in human blood induced by streptokinase (96), and in man the fibrinolysis-inducing capacity of nicotinic acid is similarly enhanced (97). These observations indicate the potential for development of anticoagulants with additional fibrinolytic activity. Indeed, recently a heparin-aspirin complex has been developed that *in vitro* exerts anticoagulant together with fibrinolytic activity and induces these two activities in rats after oral, intramuscular, and especially intravenous application (98). This combination is of great interest because it has been found that the proportions of cases of postsurgical vein thrombosis [as diagnosed with the ^{125}-I-labeled fibrinogen screening test (38)] are as follows: 30% in patients treated with acetylsalicylic acid, 19% with subcutaneous heparin, but only 9% with a combination of acetylsalicylic acid and low dose heparin

(39). Whether this effect is based on an increased fibrinolytic activity of this combination or the inhibition of platelet aggregation by aspirin is an open question.

3.14 Heparin-drug interactions

Heparin interactions with various drugs have been reported. Such interactions occur between heparin and monomycin, streptomycin, neomycin, polymycins B and M, gentamicin, erythromycin, thiazine derivatives, phenylbutazone, indomethacin, and many others. Antihistaminics and digitaloids antagonize the antithrombin activity of heparin. For a review of heparin-drug interaction, see Ref. 85.

4 HEPARINOIDS AND RELATED COMPOUNDS

4.1 General Remarks

There are many publications relating to the experimental and clinical use of heparinoids and most of them are published in European journals. A recent book on heparin (99) contains a chapter on heparinoids, but only dextran sulfates are mentioned. Heparinoids are sulfuric acid esters of high organic molecular compounds, such as polysaccharides, polyuronic acids, mucopolysaccharides, and synthetic polymers. Thus by reaction with chlorosulfonic acid, glycogen, starch, and chitin, chondroitin sulfuric acid, pectic acid, gum arabic (100), cellulose, and polyvinylalcohol (101) were transformed to sulfonic acid esters having anticoagulant activity *in vitro*.

4.2 Sulfonated Xylans (Pentosan)

The most interesting heparinoids in regard to therapeutic potential are sulfonated xylans (pentosans), with a sulfur content of about 17%, obtained from the wood of birch and beech trees (102). The heparinoid possesses very high anticoagulant activity, inhibits the heat coagulation of plasma, and exerts a higher anticomplement activity than heparin. It was also shown that the sulfonated molecule had to be chainlike to exert anticoagulant activity (103). Experiments with artificial thrombi revealed marked thrombus regression in the animals treated with sulfonated pentosans; a lower dosage (3×2 mg/kg) was clearly more effective than a higher dosage (3×1 mg/kg), and it is assumed that these results are primarily due to a fibrinolytic effect, not to the anticoagulant action, which is weaker than that of heparin (104). Figure 32.4 gives the structural formula of sulfonated pentosan.

4.2.1 THERAPEUTIC APPLICATIONS: ANTITHROMBOTIC EFFECT. The sulfonated pentosans (xylans) were the first heparinoids used in man for therapeutic purposes. A

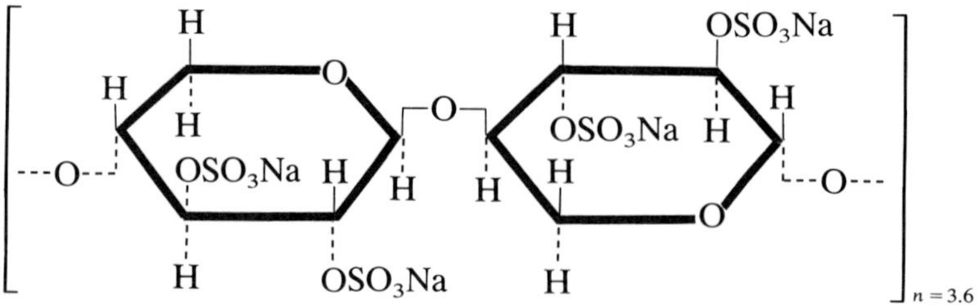

Fig. 32.4 Structure of pentosan polysulfonated ester.

thrombolytic effect was claimed in a number of publications (*vide infra*). Incorporated with some other components into an ointment and applied locally, the pentosan polysulfonate esters have been reported to be very effective clinically with superficial and deep thrombophlebitis, postthrombotic syndrome, and ulcus cruris (105). A smaller sulfonated pentosan compound with a molecular weight of about 2000 is presently the heparinoid most often used in the clinic. Much is being written on the effect of the pentosan polysulfonate ester as an antithrombotic agent. For example, postoperative venous thrombosis, as revealed by the ^{125}-I-fibrinogen test, bilateral venography and ultrasonic venography could be reduced from 51 to 15% ($p<0.005$) (106). This heparinoid, applied as intramuscular injection during the first week after apoplexy and as tablets during the following 3 weeks, also clearly enhanced the clinical improvement after this cerebral apoplexy due to thrombosis (107). Excellent results—namely, complete resolution when the occlusion was not older than 2 days—were also reported for thrombosis of the central vein of the retina (108). Since the anticoagulant activity of this pentosan polysulfonated with a molecular weight of about 2000 is very weak compared with the first used pentosan polysulfonated ester compound with a molecular weight of about 7000, its antithrombotic effect is considered to be caused by other activities. With a ^{35}S-marked preparation, it was shown that the compound is adsorbed through the skin and is found in the bloodstream when given orally or rectally.

4.2.2 THERAPEUTIC APPLICATIONS: LIPOLYTIC EFFECT. The anticoagulant activity of pentosan polysulfonated ester is a fraction of that of heparin, but it exerts other activities having clinical significance. The most important one is probably the claimed induction of fibrinolytic activity; the pentosan polysulfonated ester also induces marked lipolysis, and both activities are much more pronounced than those induced by heparin (109). Such an effect after intravenous injection in man was reported to be much more pronounced than the one obtained by heparin (110).

The lipolytic antilipemic effect is considered to be based on hydrolytic splitting of neutral fats in the circulation, accompanied by increased fibrinolytic activity that is more pronounced in arterial than in venous blood (111). Reduction of the lipoids of blood is more pronounced with abnormal high original values, an effect of great clinical importance with generalized arteriosclerosis. The lipoid values, however, are not reduced below normal values (112). The pentosansulfonate-induced activation of lipoprotein-lipase can be maintained for several months in patients with hyperlipemia by oral application of the heparinoid (113). The compound penetrates also into the cartilage, inhibits hyaluronidase there, and thus is seen to possess potential for inhibiting arthrotic changes of the cartilage (114).

4.2.3 EFFECT ON THE FIBRINOLYTIC SYSTEM. There are numerous reports that pentosan polysulfonated esters with a low molecular weight induce increased fibrinolytic activity *in vitro* and *in vivo* in experimental animals and in man (healthy persons and patients) as measured by various methods. Space does not permit citation of all publications concerning this subject. As examples, see Refs. 115 and 116, describing marked thrombolysis of artificial thrombi in mice, observed after oral application of the pentosan polysulfonated ester with the small molecule. It is assumed that the activation mechanism is based on a dissociation of an activator-inhibitor complex (117). The induction of fibrinolytic activity by various synthetic sulfated polysaccharides *in vitro* and *in vivo* has been considered lately as a "well-known phenomenon" probably based on a dissociation of plasminogen and inhibitors (118).

4.3 Effect of Natural Heparinoids on the Fibrinolytic and Coagulation Systems

Fibrinolytic activity is also induced by a natural heparinoid contained in the duodenal mucous membrane, an activity once thought to be due to the antilipemic effect induced by this compound in patients, because lipemia exerts an antiplasmin activity (119). This natural duodenal heparinoid served to obtain a persistent increase of fibrinolytic activity in patients, even after oral application with a daily dose of 60 mg for 6 months (120). The assessment of fibrinolysis-inducing capacity of heparinoids is essential for their evaluation as potential antithrombotic drugs. It can be very misleading to claim that heparinoids may not have such an effect, as was done in man for glucuronyl-glucose-amine-glycan sulfate, because in contrast to heparin they do not potentiate the factor Xa-inhibitor activity (121). The anticoagulant effect might also be concentration dependent, for it was shown that heparan-sulfate, a heparinoid prepared from the human aorta, like heparin, potentiates the inactivation of thrombin and of factor Xa by antithrombin III, but at a much lower concentration than is required by heparin (122). For the chemical similarities and differences between this heparinoid and heparin, see Ref. 123.

Recently it was reported that a heparinoid extracted from swine duodenal mucosa exerted in various animal test systems both plasma-clearing (lipoprotein lipase) and fibrinolysis and that a 1:5 heparin-heparinoid combination synergized these activities (124). It has been claimed that heparinoids mobilize heparin from depots in the tissues (125) and also, as tested *in vitro*, from protein complexes in human plasma, an effect that was demonstrated for polysulfuric acid esters of pentosan, dextran, pectins, and chondroitin (126), thus revealing a heparin-releasing effect.

4.4 Various Sulfonate Polysaccharides and Related Compounds

A sulfonated pectin derivative consisting of about 6–9 galacturonic acid units with an average molecular weight of 2500 ± 500 (127) incorporated into ointments is being used clinically for the local treatment of superficial thrombophlebitis, varicose veins, and hematoma (128), and inflammation of superficial veins (129). The transcutaneous adsorption of this heparinoid was proved with a ^{35}S-labeled preparation (130). On the pharmaceutical market, there are several other heparinoids incorporated into ointments with other mostly anti-inflammatory compounds. One such heparinoid was prepared by sulfatation of polysaccharides obtained from certain cellular membranes (131).

Another heparinoid was obtained from the lungs of young cattle and subsequently sulfated. This glycosaminglycanpolysulfate is being used primarily for arthrosis after intraarticular injection (but also after intramuscular injection). It diffuses into the cartilage, where by competitive inhibition it blocks the enzymes that degrade the mucopolysaccharides, thus interrupting the pathologic destruction of the cartilage (132). This heparinoid, for instance, inhibits the lysosomal enzymes β-glucuronidase and β-*N*-acetylglucosaminidase (133), which are particularly increased with joint inflammations. The good clinical results with this heparinoid in treating moderate arthrosis are quite remarkable (134). This heparinoid, and pentosan polysulfates, are the most potent inhibitors of neutral protease (down to $10^{-8}\,M$). Antirheumatic pyrazolone derivatives exert this action only at 10^{-5} *M*. Inhibition of neutral protease may be one way in which some antirheumatic drugs exert therapeutic effect in rheumatic disease (135).

4.5 Dextran Sulfate and Dextran

Dextran sulfate, a heparinoid prepared from dextran, which is a linear glucose polymer produced by bacteria growing on a sucrose substrate, also possesses anticoagulant activity. On a weight basis, this activity is 10–20 times less than that of heparin. At low concentrations dextran sulfate exerts a synergistic effect with the heparin anticoagulant activity. Dextran sulfate-25 accelerates *in vitro* the inhibition of factor Xa; however this occurs at higher concentration than is required by heparin. In clinical studies dextran sulfate-25 proved to be too toxic (99). For discussion of its potential fibrinolysis-inducing capacity *in vitro*, see Ref. 136.

Dextran itself has been used as an antithrombotic agent, as discussed in many publications. The preparations used have molecular weights of about 40,000 and 70,000. It was claimed that in venous thrombosis the desired clinical results can be accomplished more rapidly than with heparin (137). Its antithrombogenic effect, as shown in patients with acute stroke, was attributed, at least in this disease, to normalization of the hyperactivity of platelets. This suggestion supports the observations of inhibition of platelet aggregation as reported in the literature (138).

It has also been reported that dextran induces reversible changes of the structure and function of factor VIII, a property that may be responsible for its antithrombotic effect (139). The same paper showed that dextran reduces platelet adhesiveness and increases thrombus lysis *in vitro*. Studies in patients given ^{125}-I-labeled fibrinogen the day before surgery revealed that thrombi formed in Chandler tubes from the blood of these treated patients; then exposed to plasmin, lyse much more extensively after dextran treatment. From these results it was concluded that 500 ml of dextran infused into patients during surgery increases the lysability of thrombi formed during or after surgery. It is suggested that this finding at least partly explains the antithrombotic effect of dextran.

When dextran was given to patients, the maximum increase of lysability of the clots was found not at maximum dextran concentration, but when the concentration had decreased to about 6.4 mg/ml blood (140). The observed enhancement of thrombolysis is not quite compatible with the *in vitro* observation that dextran shortens clotting times and increases fibrin polymerization rates (141). However artificial systems *in vitro* do not always reflect what may happen in the living organism.

It has been suggested that dextran given intravenously can be recommended only for postoperative venous thrombosis (142). For side effects and further literature, see Ref. 142. Using the ^{125}I-fibrinogen isotopic test, deep vein thrombosis after surgery was found in 36% of the controls, in 12.8% of the heparin-treated group, and in 21.7% of the dextran group. Bleeding complications occurred in 8 out of 94 patients in the heparin group and only in 1 out of the 92 of the dextran group. In this patient group a reduced factor X activity was found (56). The persistence of dextran in the circulation may well be of clinical significance, since 50–75% of the postoperative thromboembolic complications begin during or in the first few days after surgery. In patients receiving 1000 ml of dextran-70 before surgery, the blood volume increased by dextran did not return to preoperative levels for 3–5 days, whereas in those receiving 500 ml, the preoperative blood volume was regained 1–2 days after surgery (143).

4.6 Hydroxychloroquine Sulfate

Hydroxychloroquine sulfate (7-chloro-4 4-[ethyl (2-hydroxyethyl) amino]-1-methyl-amino quinoline sulfate) is an antimalarial and anti-inflammatory agent that recently has been used successfully ($p < 0.005$) as tablets to prevent deep vein thrombosis in patients with fractures of hip, pelvis, or thoracolumbar spine, patients in whom subcutaneous heparin is not a very effective prophylactic agent. The drug does not interfere directly with the clotting process. Its mechanism of action is not yet clearly established (144).

5 DEFIBRINATING AGENTS

5.1 Mechanism of Action

A defibrinating agent is under investigation as an antithrombotic agent. It is a purified coagulant fraction, a glycoprotein (Ancrod) contained in the venom of the Malayan pit viper. This agent, having a molecular weight of about 30,000, converts fibrinogen to fibrin (145). It acts by removing fibrinopeptide A from fibrinogen (146). The fibrin thus formed is much more susceptible to fibrinolysis (147) than is fibrin formed by a normal clotting process because the former is not cross-linked (148).

It has also been suggested that a part of the antithrombotic effect of this defibrinating agent is a platelet-disaggregating action induced by fibrinolytic breakdown products deriving from the fibrin it forms (149). The main pathway of such antithrombotic action involves the lowering of the plasma fibrinogen concentration to a level at which formation or extension of thrombi through fibrin deposition is not supposed to occur. The degree of defibrination in patients can be regulated by varying the given dose. Slow intravenous infusion of 1 IU/kg body weight over 12 hr followed by further infusions of 0.5–1 IU/kg every 12 hr results in sustained hypofibrinogenemia of about 50 mg/100 ml (150).

The optimum level of hypofibrinogenemia for prevention or treatment of various thrombotic disorders is not yet known. After intravenous injection, Ancrod initially disappears from the circulation with a plasma half-life of 3–5 hr; but after 90% of the dose has been cleared, the remaining defibrinating agent is cleared more slowly, with a plasma half-life of 9–12 days (151). Spontaneous bleeding has been rare during Ancrod therapy, even when there is marked hypofibrinogenemia (152).

5.2 Clinical Application

Clinical studies have been limited and have concentrated mainly on venous thrombosis. Treatment with Ancrod prevented further extension of the thrombosis, but did not produce significant thrombolysis as assessed by repeated venography (153). The use of this defibrinating agent for the prevention of venous thrombosis after hip fracture did not reduce the incidence of postoperative thrombosis but appeared to reduce the frequency of pulmonary embolism (150). This defibrinating agent is considered to be an interesting alternative to heparin, but further well-controlled comparative studies are needed to define its role in practical patient management.

6 ORAL ANTICOAGULANTS (PROTHROMBIN–DEPRESSING AGENTS)

6.1 General Remarks

Oral anticoagulants, although beneficial for many patients, are certainly second-rate anticoagulants. For more than 20 years, my wife and I ran a central coagulation laboratory at a large medical center that did not as a rule perform routine tests such as determinations of the prothrombin time.

Instead, studies were carried out in patients, many from outside, who were referred to because of various problems with oral anticoagulants. It became quite obvious that oral anticoagulants do not provide the same protection against intravascular clotting as heparin does. In addition, there were side reactions, interactions with many drugs, and so on. The introductory comments do not imply that oral anticoagulants have no clinical value, for indeed they do.

6.2 Disadvantages of Oral Anticoagulants

However, one must be aware of the "weakness" of oral anticoagulants, as is discussed in this section, with a few examples. There exists, for instance, a hereditary resistance against the anticoagulant effect of warfarin (154). In many of the patients, we observed, despite a prothrombin activity distinctly within the therapeutic range, there was no protection against intravascular clotting. Although experience has led us to consider elevation of antithrombin III activity to be a necessary effect of oral coagulants (155–157), in many of these treated patients no such elevation was reported. This effect was also observed by other investigators (158). Hereditary antithrombin III deficiency has been shown to be the cause of a pronounced thrombosis tendency (153, 158).

In spite of identical prothrombin times, the test and its results (values) usually used to determine the effect of oral anticoagulants in performing the thrombin generation test (159) in human plasma, one can demonstrate that there are quite different dynamics of the coagulation (Fig. 32.5). The thrombin generation curve *N* reflects average normal values. A shift to the left and also down in relation to this control curve indicates hypercoagulability, a shift up and to the right, hypocoagulability. The more pronounced this shift, the more pronounced is the deviation from the normal average values. The upper thrombin generation curves obtained from patients with a prothrombin activity of 34–38% indicate that actually only one patient, B, is somewhat protected. The thrombin generation of patient J shows almost no protection, whereas patients R and W have distinct hypercoagulability, which indicates a potential thrombosis tendency. The lower thrombin generation curves obtained from patients with a prothrombin time on the "better side" of the therapeutic range reveal that the coagulation tendency is reduced in only two patients, whereas there is no effect on this tendency in the two others. Theoretically it could be claimed that preexisting relative hypercoagulability had been normalized in these patients, which may or may not indicate some protection. However, patients in whom thrombin generation is reduced by oral anticoagulants can develop hypercoagulability as measured with this test when walking on a treadmill band. The reduced prothrombin time, though, did not change in these patients, whereas antithrombin III decreased in many patients during this stress period.

One problem that has significantly complicated the use of oral anticoagulants is lack of uniformity of effect of a given dose. This has been attributed to individual variations among patients, speed of adsorption and action of the drug, genetic resistance, inaccuracies of assay, dietary variations, and the effect of alcohol and drugs (*vide infra*), as well as many other factors. For instance, simple mobilization of a patient previously at bedrest will significantly increase the anticoagulant requirement (160). These observations do not indicate that the oral anticoagulants have little clinical value, but they show that there is considerable room for improvement. The oral anticoagulants have clinical value, particularly as prophylactic agents, but the potential problems must be realized. Acute thrombi or emboli cannot be treated with these

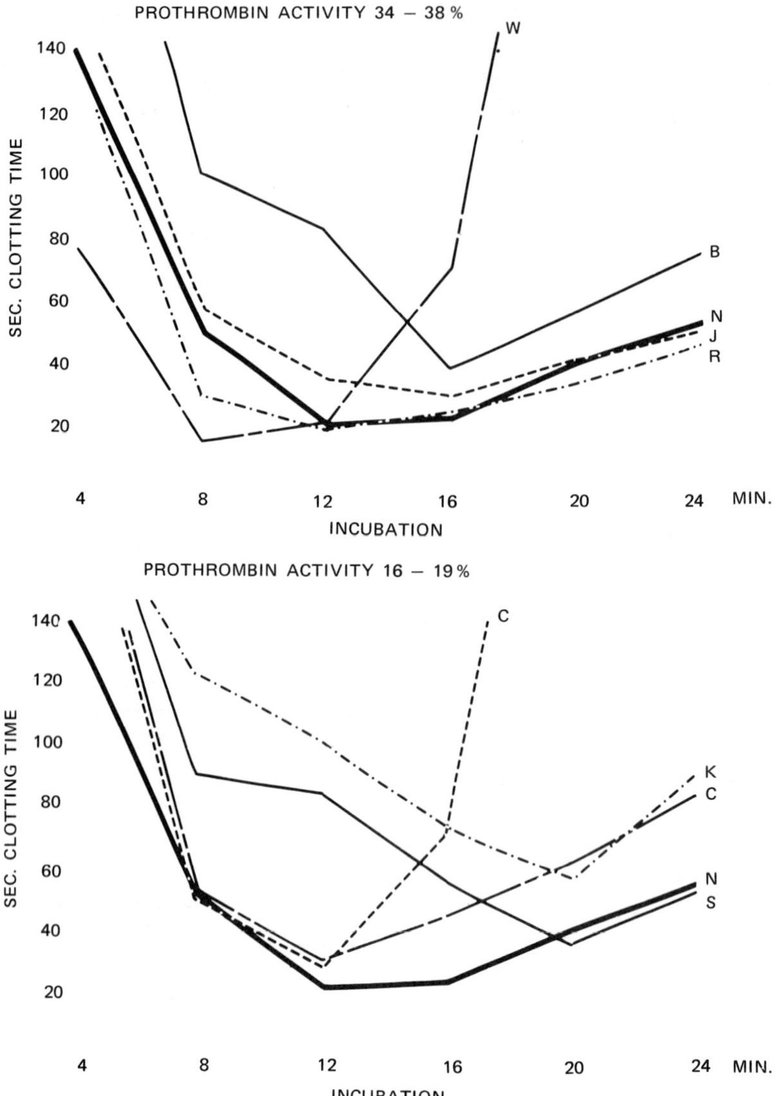

Fig. 32.5 Thrombin generation in patients receiving warfarin: note poor relationship of the dynamics of thrombin generation with prothrombin activity as measured with routine laboratory test.

drugs; here a heparin treatment for at least 7 days is indicated.

6.3 History

A serious disease plaguing the cattle of North Dakota and Canada was described by Schofield (161) in 1922 as "sweet clover disease". Its principal symptom was a severe bleeding tendency. The poisonous substance that caused it was identified in 1939 by Link as 3,3-methylene-bis(4-hydroxycoumarin), commonly known as the oral anticoagulant dicoumarol. In 1940 Link (162) synthesized this compound, although it had already been synthesized by Anschütz (163) in 1903. The first clinical application was made by Bingham and coworkers (164) in 1941.

Interestingly enough, another coumarin derivative also synthesized by Link (165), first used as a hemorrhagic rat poison, is now widely used clinically under the name warfarin. Bis(4-hydroxy-2-oxo-2*H*-1-benzopyran-3-yl)acetic ethyl ester or ethyldicoumarol acetate was the second oral anticoagulant introduced to clinical use (166, 167). It acts much faster but for a shorter time than dicoumarol. Together with dicoumarol, it was the first oral anticoagulant whose levels were determined in the blood. It was shown that the chemical level determination could not be used as a control of therapy (168). Later, several additional oral anticoagulants were developed, but they did not represent any improvements.

6.4 Chemical Structure

For discussion of synthesis and observations on the relationship of structure to anticoagulant activity, see Ref. 169. Figure 32.6 shows the basic structure and the substitutions of coumarin derivatives presently used as oral anticoagulants. Figure 32.7 gives the structure of phenylindandione, a compound that is related to coumarin derivatives phenindione (Hedulin), which was introduced in 1944 by Kabat (170), but produces clinically considerably more side effects than do coumarin derivatives.

OH, CH, R_1, R_2, O, O

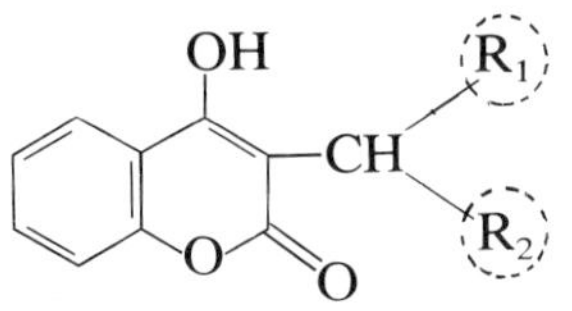

32.1 $R_1 = C_2H_5$ = marcumar
$R_2 = C_6H_5$
32.2 $R_1 = CH_2COCH_3$ = coumadin, warfarin
$R_2 = C_6H_5$
32.3 $R_1 = CH_2COCH_3$ = sintrom
$R_2 = C_6H_4NO_2$

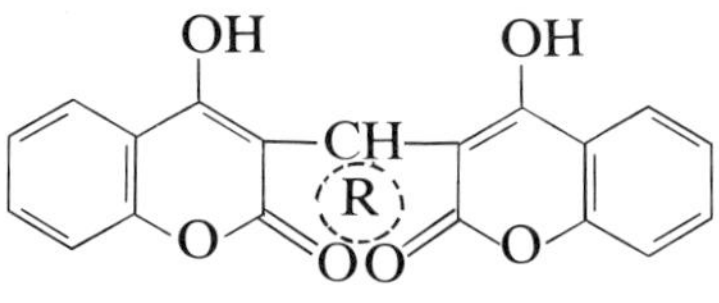

OH, OH, CH, R, O, O, O, O

32.**4** R = H = dicumarol
32.**5** R = $COOC_2H_5$ = tromexan

Fig. 32.6 Structures of coumadin derivatives presently used as oral anticoagulants.

O, O

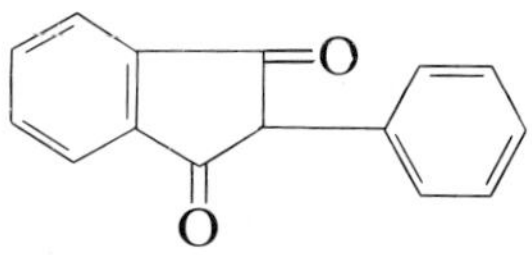

Phenylindandione

Fig. 32.7 Structure of phenylindandione.

6.5 Pathway of Action on the Coagulation System

Basically the anticoagulant activities of coumarin and related derivatives are induced by the same pathway. The drugs inhibit the effect of vitamin K in a postribosomal step in the hepatic synthesis of clotting factors II, VII, IX, and X (for a review of present knowledge, see Ref. 171), thus treatment with oral anticoagulants leads to the synthesis of biologically inactive, but immunologic detectable forms of these clotting proteins (172, 173). The modified proteins lack several carboxyl groups on glutamic acid side chains which are necessary for binding of calcium to the molecule. Since calcium form the link between these clotting proteins and phospholipid, the lack of calcium binding results in defective binding of the molecule to phospholipid, hence in failure of activation of these clotting factors (174).

The anticoagulant effect of the oral anticoagulants is delayed until the metabolic clearance of the clotting factors, whose normal synthesis has been blocked by these drugs, has them reduced to a "therapeutic" level. Thus peak plasma levels of sodium warfarin occur within 6 hr of oral administration, but the peak hypoprothrombinemic effect comes only 36–72 hr after drug administration (175). In other words, the prothrombin time cannot be reduced to the therapeutic level until much of the prothrombin and the clotting factors VII, IX, and X, present in the circulation, have been metabolized. However, there is some difference in speed and duration of their effects on the prothrombin time, the test method generally used to assess the effect of these drugs on the blood coagulation. The doubling of the pretreatment control values is reached by ethylbiscoumacetate within 18–30 hr; the effect is short lasting. Plasma half-life of this compound is $2\frac{1}{2}$ hr. With dicumarol, phenindione, warfarin, and phenprocouman, the doubling of the prothrombin time is obtained within 36–48 hr. The half-life in plasma is $24\frac{1}{2}$ and 42 hr for the first three compounds, but 160 hr for the last compound, which exerts the longest anticoagulant activity. After the last dose, 7–14 days is required for normalization of the prothrombin time with the last compound, whereas only about 2 days is required with ethylbiscoumacetate. The average required oral doses are as follows: phenprocouman, initial dose 24 mg, average maintenance dose 4 mg; warfarin, 20–40 and 8 mg; phenindione, 200 and 100 mg; dicumarol, 300 and 75 mg; ethylbiscoumacetate 900–1200 and 450 mg, respectively.

6.6 Binding to Albumin

With exception of dicumarol, the compounds are fast acting and are nearly completely adsorbed from the upper gastrointestinal tract. Once they have entered the circulation, they are extensively bound to plasma proteins, primarily to albumin, which binds 90–99%, depending on the compound. It has been claimed, as shown for warfarin, that the binding to albumin is different among individuals possessing different genetic forms of albumin (176). Moreover, there are drugs that bind more strongly to albumin the oral anticoagulants, thus replacing them, which may result in an "overdose" (*vide infra*).

6.7 Control of Action

The anticoagulant activity of the oral anticoagulants must be carefully controlled. With a weak reduction of the vitamin K-dependent clotting factors II, VII, IX, and X, there is absolutely insufficient protection against thromboses. If there is too much reduction, however, there exists considerable danger of bleeding. The control is carried out with the so-called prothrombin time (or thromboplastin time) determination. To plasma, thromboplastin is added together with calcium, resulting in a clotting time measured in seconds. This time is short because by adding thromboplastin a "short cut" is taken, excluding the first steps in the coagulation process. A prolongation of this prothrombin time into a certain range, which can be read from standard curves (mostly 15–25% of normal prothrombin activity) must be reached for good therapeutic effect. The best thromboplastin to be used is the one prepared from the grey substance of human brain, a thromboplastin that can not be used commercially. Commercial preparations react somewhat differently to the reduction of the clotting factors II, VII, and X. For comparison of commercial preparations, see Ref. 177. In many countries are now undertaking a standardization. There are many conditions that interfere with a correct test result—an incorrectly filled vacutainer, too long a storage of the blood sample, an injection of heparin given soon before the test, etc.

6.8 The Clinical Anticoagulant Effect

The oral anticoagulants are useful for long-term treatment, under certain conditions even life-long treatment, of certain pathologic conditions such as repeated episodes of thromboembolism, repeated heart infarcts, persisting tendency to arterial occlusion, morbus embolicus, and repeated transitory cerebral ischemias (178). Concerning other situations, there are contradictory reports. Thus it has been claimed that warfarin given prophylactically did not at all prevent venous thrombosis after hip surgery (179). However in another recent report it was shown that after total hip replacement, thromboembolic complications with warfarin prophylactic treatment were reduced from 31–50% of the controls to 5%. Low dose heparin did not exert a preventive effect (180).

Recent data indicate that drugs that prevent platelet aggregation (see next section) may under certain conditions be more effective than warfarin. A large multicenter European study showed that of patients who had suffered a heart infarct and had received antiaggregating agents, only 4% died from a secondary infarct or suddenly, whereas 7% of patients on warfarin and 8% of patients on placebo died from the same cause (181). These are a few examples taken from the numerous publications.

6.9 Other Therapeutic Effects

This section discusses some additional therapeutic effects of oral anticoagulants. For example, it has been claimed that with individual variations, dicumarol (bishydroxycoumarin) reduces the viscosity of the blood, and this effect is thought to explain the relief of angina pain in patients who suffer from coronary heart disease (182). Experimentally as well as on a clinical basis, oral anticoagulants have been shown to exert some anticarcinogenic action. In one controlled clinical trial, warfarin treatment as an adjuvant therapy to chemotherapy of cancer resulted in a 2-year survival of 40.6% for the warfarin group, compared with survival of the catotoxic therapy alone of 17.7% (183). For a review of this subject, see Refs. 184a and 183.

6.10 Clinical Side Effects

Side effects resulting from treatment with oral anticoagulants are relatively rare; nonspecific dermatitis (184b), skin necroses (185), and other conditions have been described. The use of phenindione which causes more side reactions than the coumarin derivatives, can be associated with agranulocytosis as well as liver and kidney damages. It also exerts antithyroid activity by affecting the organic binding of iodine (186), hence receives only limited clinical use compared to the coumarin drugs, which have few idiosyncratic side effects. For example, warfarin given to a pregnant woman may cross the placenta, consequently causing a variety of fetal abnormalities (187, 188).

6.11 Bleeding Tendencies

A tendency to bleed can develop under various conditions. Overdose and interaction with additional drugs are just two examples. The treatment of hemorrhage occurring under therapy with oral anticoagulants depends on the type of bleeding. Acute severe hemorrhage may require blood or plasma transfusion or, even better, factor concentrates followed by intravenous administration of vitamin K_1. In many cases vitamin K can be given orally. Two points must be considered: with a severe preexisting thrombosis tendency, fast and complete normalization of the clotting process may induce intravascular clotting, and the vitamin K treatment must be continued for a longer period with oral anticoagulants such as marcumar, which have a long half-life. Minor bleeding or bleeding that can be stopped by local treatment should not be treated with vitamin K. For a review of hemorrhagic complications, see Ref. 189.

6.12 Interaction of Oral Anticoagulants with Other Drugs

Many drugs interact in various ways with oral anticoagulants. Some drugs exert an additive hypoprothrombinemic effect: salicylates, propylthiouracil, quinidine, and others result in decreased prothrombin activity. Others have the same effect by decreasing vitamin K synthesis by the gut bacteria: chloramphenicol, kanamycin, neomycin, streptomycin, sulfonamides. The effect of the oral anticoagulants is also enhanced by their displacement from the albumin-binding plasma protein (by clofibrate, diphenylhydantoin, mefenamic acid, oxyphenbutazine, phenylbutazone) or by inhibition of their metabolism (phenyramidol and probably disulfiram). Other drugs reduce their anticoagulant effect by stimulating their metabolism (barbiturates, chloralhydrate, blutethimide, griseofulvin) or by reducing decrease absorption (probably barbiturates and cholestyramine). For further details, see Ref. 190.

Sudden discontinuation of barbiturate application with unchanged dose of the oral anticoagulant can result in hemorrhage (191). Occupational exposure to insecticides reduces the effect of warfarin (192), and the same effect has been reported for rifampicin. It was assumed that this effect is due to stimulation of the metabolism of the anticoagulant in the liver (193). The anticoagulant effect can also be reduced by stimulation of the synthesis of clotting factors by corticosteroids and oral contraceptives (194).

Metronidazole increases the warfarin level and the hypoprothrombinemia with the use of racemic $S(-)$-warfarin; none occurred with $R(+)$-warfarin. Thus the interaction of racemic warfarin and metronidazole is stereoselective and can be lessened and even avoided by use of $R(+)$-warfarin alone for long-term therapy (195). Oral anticoagulants can potentiate the effect of other drugs. Thus dicumarol administration results in the prolongation of the half-life time of the hypoglycemic drug tolbutamide (196). Dicumarol also increases the half-life of diphenylhydantoin. Phenprocoumon prolongs the half-life of diphenylhydantoin, too, but not tolbutamide, whereas warfarin and phenindione do not affect the half-life of those drugs (197). The foregoing are some characteristic examples of the interaction of oral anticoagulants with drugs; space does not permit coverage of the entire field.

7 INHIBITORS OF PLATELET AGGREGATION

7.1 Reviews

Drugs that inhibit platelet aggregation and function as antithrombotic prophylactic agents are being used with increasing frequency, despite many discussions relating to mechanism of action and the identity of the clinically the most advantageous drugs. For recent reviews, see Refs. 198–200. The difference of opinions is at times quite impressive: in their review, Steele et al. (206) did not mention dextran as an antiaggregating agent at all, which resulted in a protest by a physician (201) who had used dextrans successfully as antiaggregating agents; others also had recommended this drug, particularly for use after surgery to prevent thrombosis (202, 203).

7.2 Role of Aggregation of Thrombocytes in hemostasis and Thrombogenesis

Lesion of the vessel or slight endothelium damage immediately results in adhesion and, in particular, in aggregation of thrombocytes, an effect that leads to formation of a thrombus under certain circumstances. Thrombocytes adhere to collagen and other substituents of the vessel wall and release platelet components, including the important ADP, which induce the platelets to aggregate and to form an initially loose and unstable hemostatic plug. Blood coagulation is accelerated by a platelet phospholipid (platelet factor 3) that is made available on the surface of the platelet aggregate. This process results in thrombin generation, which induces further release of ADP from platelets. Thrombin converts fibrinogen to fibrin (204) (see Fig. 32.3).

The development and structure of a thrombus are similar in many ways to those of the hemostatic plug, but there are also differences. The hemostatic plug is largely extravascular, whereas the thrombus is intravascular. In addition, hemostatic plug formation is primarily initiated by tissue damage, whereas the initiation stimulus of thrombosis may involve damage to the vessel wall, stimulation of platelet adhesion, or aggregation (205). Adherence of the platelets to one another is called platelet aggregation. It is essentially the prevention of this aggregation that represents the preventive effect of certain antithrombotic drugs (*vide infra*).

7.3 Measurements of Thrombus-Related Platelet Function

To measure the antithrombotic potential of drugs, their preventive effects on adhesiveness or aggregability are being recorded. There are differences of opinion over whether increased adhesiveness (206) or aggregability (207) can be assessed to indicate a thrombosis tendency or an active venous thrombosis. For induction of *in vitro* aggregation of the platelets for the assessing of antiaggregating agents, both collagen and epinephrine are utilized. Collagen aggregates platelets by inducing release of endogenous ADP. Exogenous ADP and epinephrine both aggregate platelets directly (first phase aggregation) and induce release of endogenous ADP (second phase aggregation). Aspirin, for example, inhibits platelet aggregation by inhibiting the release reaction, whereas prostaglandin E inhibits aggregation directly, for instance, induced by exposing platelets to ADP.

The assessment of the aggregability of the platelets is carried out with various methods and also at different times after the drawing of blood. These differences explain the various results that have been obtained with almost identical groups of patients. Our own experiences make it quite clear that the blood of a patient (or that of a healthy individual, obtained for research purposes) must be drawn into siliconized equipment, and that this blood or the platelet-rich plasma obtained from it cannot be stored at all. Storage results in morphological changes of the thrombocytes which affect their functions. It is important to control the citrate-to-blood ratio in the clinical platelet aggregation studies and in the assessment of antiplatelet drugs (208). (For a critical review of platelet function tests and their interpretation, see Ref. 209.)

Furthermore, we found that stirring the platelets, which is being done before the addition of aggregation agents, must also be carried out in a control sample to which no aggregating agent has been added. We observed that such spontaneous aggregation occurs in transient blindness due to large platelet aggregates (210) among other diseases, as well as in many patients with thrombosis tendency. An increase of spontaneous platelet aggregation related to thrombosis tendency of various types was also observed by others (211). This aggregation tendency explains, at least in part, the antithrombotic effect of the various inhibitors of platelet aggregation.

7.4 Platelet Aggregation and Its Relation to Thromboembolism

The platelet aggregation mechanism is not completely understood. For instance, inactivation of complement components by cobra venom factor prevents aggregation of human platelets by collagen (212). This observation points to the possibility that pentosan polysulfonate ester (see Section 4) might function as an antiaggregation agent because of its high anticomplementary activity (213). The anticoagulant heparin (which at very small concentrations occurs normally in blood) interacts also with the platelets. It has been claimed that factor Xa inhibitor and heparin together comprise a potent blockade of platelet aggregation (214).

On the other hand, a platelet factor, a heat-stable protein with a low molecular weight, acts as a heparin-neutralizing substance. It is released from the platelets during the initial stages of blood coagulation. Recent reports indicate that increased platelet factor 4 activity is closely related to thromboembolic phenomena. In one study, for example, about 30% of the patients who suffered from a thromboembolic episode up to 4 weeks before the assessment had increased platelet factor 4 activity (215).

The increased aggregability is the most widely investigated function of the platelets. Among healthy persons this spontaneous aggregability is very low in younger people, but it increases with age. However in both age groups, somewhat more among the older segment, the aggregability of platelets is very much increased before the development of thromboembolic diseases, including myocardinal infarcts and venous or arterial thromboses (216). As assessed for the entire group, this increase was observed in 55–75% before appearance of symptoms of thromboembolic disease, clearly indicating the potential prophylactic value of antiaggregating agents. The aggregability of platelets was also reported in patients, particularly the younger ones, with transient ischemic attacks and strokes (217–219). It has been claimed that aspirin and dipyridamole fail to block the formation of platelet aggregates in acute cerebral ischemia, even though aggregation *in vitro* is inhibited (218). This opinion is not shared by others, who assign great value to antiaggregating (and antiadhesive) agents in the preventive and therapeutic management of ischemic stroke (for quotations, see Ref. 219).

In the acute stage of thrombosis, enhancement of adrenalin-induced platelet aggregation was observed (220), but spontaneous platelet aggregation, which we consider to be very significant clinically, was not measured. Thrombocythemia, a secondary feature of other diseases, particularly when combined with increased adhesiveness and/or spontaneous aggregation of the platelets, also predisposes an individual to thrombosis (221). Increased platelet aggregation, to give another example, has been observed in the myocardial microcirculation of patients with coronary disease who died suddenly (222). The rationale for administering antiplatelet drugs to patients with ischemic heart disease may be summarized as follows:

1. These agents may prevent the formation of a platelet-fibrin thrombus within one of the major epicardial vessels.
2. They may prevent the aggregation of platelets on these thrombi and their subsequent embolization.
3. They may prevent platelet aggregation in the myocardial microcirculation (223).

Platelet thrombi on prosthetic devices and vascular catheters have been described (224).

7.5 Prostaglandins and Their Effect on Platelet Aggregation

Recent research has revealed the important role of prostaglandins in relation to platelet function. The effects of these lipids, depending on the type, are opposite. Thus the prostaglandins E_2 and $E_{2\alpha}$ (PGE_2 and $PGE_{2\alpha}$) tend to stimulate platelet aggregation, in contrast to PGE_1, which inhibits aggregation (225).

It has been suggested that intermediates in the biosynthesis of prostaglandins, the prostaglandin endoperoxides, are produced by the platelets and induce platelet aggregation (226). Aspirin has been shown to inhibit the synthesis of prostaglandin endoperoxides by the platelets, as well as the formation of their products PGE_2 and $PGE_{2\alpha}$ (227, 228). In contrast to these prostaglandins, PGE_1 very markedly inhibits platelet aggregation. The immediate effect may represent direct competition with aggregation agents, and the observed additional slow effect may be mediated through stimulation of adenylcyclase (229).

Lately, a prostaglandin derivative has been synthesized that is 10–25 times more potent than PGE_1 in inhibiting platelet aggregation. Its biological half-life is only 1–2 min. A derivative, a thiaprostacycline, is stable, although it is 2–4 times less active than prostacycline (230). Here again are new possibilities for the synthesis of an inhibitor of platelet aggregation, so important clinically.

7.6 Aggregation Inhibitors Other than PGE and Related Compounds

7.6.1 ASPIRIN. There are numerous reports on aspirin (acetylsalicylic acid) as a preventive antithrombotic agent, and some of these reports are contradictory to others. For instance, a recent paper points out that aspirin cannot be recommended for the prevention of postoperative thromboembolic complications (231). Among the authors whose work is cited in this report, Harris et al. (232) are quoted as having said that aspirin has no prophylactic value in hip surgery. Harris himself, however, recently reported a clear reduction of venous thrombosis by aspirin after hip surgery (181). Reduction of postoperative thromboembolic complications by aspirin after hip surgery has been reported previously, as well (233).

After surgery in general, aspirin in combination with dipyridamole (persantin) was shown to have a preventive antithrombotic effect as assessed by the ^{125}-I-fibrinogen method (234). Yet recently it has been claimed that aspirin administered under these circumstances, and using the same method of leg scanning, is of little value (235). Clinical evidence published (for references, see Ref. 236) and results of double-blind studies suggest a preventive effect of aspirin in postoperative venous thrombosis and in embolism from artificial heart valves (236). Aspirin has been shown to reduce thrombus deposition on renal dialysis membranes (237).

The most impressive evidence for an antithrombotic effect comes from reports that aspirin prevents peripheral ischemia in patients with thrombocytosis and with spontaneous platelet aggregation (238). For a discussion of the values of aspirin in treating occlusive arterial disease, see Ref. 239. Aspirin has also been said to prevent secondary heart infarction better than warfarin does (181) and to prevent, thromboembolism in patients with Starr-Edwards valves, but only in combination with warfarin (181). For a review of intolerance to aspirin, see Ref. 240.

7.6.2 SULFINPYRAZONE. Sulfinpyrazone [1,2-diphenyl-3,5-dioxo-4-(2′-phenyl sulfinylethyl)pyrazolidine] lengthens the shortened survival time of platelets in patients with rheumatic disease, particularly those with a history of thromboembolism (241). It has also been shown to decrease the platelet clumping in both venous and arterial thromboses (242). Its mechanism is not completely established, but it was shown that collagen-induced serotonin release from platelets is reduced in platelet-rich plasma of patients who have taken sulfinpyrazone. Furthermore, platelet prostaglandin synthesis was strongly inhibited by the compound (243).

Sulfinpyrazone may exert its effect on platelet activity by inhibiting the surface sialyltranserase activity (244). The compound has been reported to reduce the incidence of transient ischemic attacks (245), to exert a protective effect in decreasing the platelet adhesion to atrioventricular shunts used for long-term renal dialysis (246), and to increase the platelet survival in patients with prosthetic mitral valves (247). Of particular interest is the observation that sulfinpyrazone normalizes reduced platelet survival in patients with recurring venous thrombosis resistant to anticoagulants (248). In contrast to aspirin, sulfinpyrazone is effective as an inhibitor of platelet function only as long as it is present in the circulation. Further studies are under way.

7.6.3 DIPYRIDAMOLE (PERSANTIN FORTE). Dipyridamole [2,6-bisdiethanolamino-4,8-dipiperidinopyrimido(5,4-*d*)-pyrimidin], a vasodilator, is also being used as an inhibitor of platelet aggregation. The reports on its mode of action are somewhat conflicting, as are the clinical results. Dipyridamole has been reported to inhibit cAMP phosphodiesterase activity in platelets, an effect shared by other pyrimido-pyrimidin compounds (RA-233, RA-433, VK 774), which are more important inhibitors *in vitro* than dipyridamole but have a less antithrombotic effect *in vivo* than this compound (249). Arterial thromboembolism involves platelet consumption, a process that is interrupted by dipyridamole but not by heparin. Acetylsalicylic acid exerts little activity for interruption of this process, but it potentiates the effect of dipyridamole (250). Dipyridamole in combination with oral anticoagulants reduced the incidence of embolism of aortic or prosthetic heart valves (251) and in combination with immunosuppressive agents; with heparin or warfarin, it improved the prognosis of patients with rapidly progressive glomerulonephritis (252). For a discussion of the mechanism of action of dipyridamole in regard to platelet function, see Ref. 253.

7.6.4 OTHER SYNTHETIC COMPOUNDS LESS WELL INVESTIGATED CLINICALLY. Bencyclan (*N*-[3-(benzylcycloheptyloxypropyl]*N*,*N*-dimethylamine), at very low concentrations, inhibits ADP-, epinephrine- and collagen-induced (254) or spontaneous platelet aggregation *in vitro* (255), but in humans such inhibition occurs only after intravenous injection (200–400 mg) and only for 1 hr (255).

Clofibrate {ethyl-[2-(*p*-chlorophenoxy)]-2-methylproprionate}, a hypolipidemic agent, appears to reduce platelet adhesiveness to glass (256). Its testing as an antithrombotic agent in various clinical studies did not provide convincing evidence for its effect in this regard (257). A lately developed derivative of clofibrate, 2⟨4-[2-(4-chlorobenzymido)ethyl]phenoxy⟩-2-methylproprionic acid, was found to inhibit collagen-induced aggregation of thrombocytes, to enhance the action of oral anticoagulants, and to reduce a pathologically prolonged euglobulin lysis time (258). Enhancement of fibrinolytic activity in man has also been observed for clofibrate (259).

Ibuprofen [α-(*p*-isobutylphenyl)-proprionic acid], an antirheumatic and antiphlogistic agent, has been reported to inhibit synthesis of prostaglandins, resulting in inhibition of aggregation of thrombocytes and erythrocytes (260).

Phenformin [1(β-phenylethyl)biguanid], together with anabolic steroids, given as a prolonged therapy, reduced significantly the number of platelet-leukocyte aggregates observed in patients with myocardial infarction, coronary insufficiency, venous thrombosis, and arteriosclerosis of the lower limbs (261).

7.6.5 AGGREGATING COMPOUNDS ASSESSED EXPERIMENTALLY ONLY. Suloctidil [1-(4-isopropylthiophenyl)-2n-octylaminopropanol], a new vascular antispasmodic agent, inhibits ADP-induced platelet aggregation by 70% and is about 10 times more potent than dipyridamole. It reduced the experimentally induced arterial thrombus formation in rats (262).

Flubiprofen, [2-(3′-fluor diphenyl-4yl)-proprionic acid] (263) and ditazole [4,5-diphenyl-2-bis(2-hydroxyethyl)aminoxacol] (264) were found to inhibit *in vitro* aggregation of human platelets induced by various other agents.

The synthesized dibutyryl-cAMP was observed to induce a (somewhat delayed) inhibition of platelet aggregation brought on by adenosinephosphate, epinephrine, and thrombin (229), an indication of a new therapeutic potential.

Carbenicillin has recently been reported to inhibit experimental formation of arterial thrombosis in dogs by marked impairment of platelet adhesiveness and aggregation (265).

7.6.6 HEPARIN. It has been claimed that platelets *in vitro* take up only free heparin, not heparin complexed with antithrombin III: 20% of the heparin was released by completed aggregation of the platelets (266a). Heparin was seen to inhibit to various degrees collagen-induced platelet aggregation, but also to potentiate adrenalin-induced aggregation (267a). Given intravenously to humans, heparin inhibited ristocetin-induced platelet aggregation in blood obtained after injection (268a), but had no effect on postoperative increased platelet retention on glass beads columns when applied in small doses subcutaneously (269a).

For the *in vitro* inhibition of collagen-induced aggregation of human platelets left in their plasma by synthetic fibrinolytic agents, see Section 9, on synthetic fibrinolytic agents.

8 ENZYMATIC FIBRINOLYTIC AGENTS

8.1 Negative Aspects of the Clinical Use of Streptokinase and Urokinase

Although there are many reports on useful thrombolytic effects obtained with streptokinase and urokinase (for review, see Ref. 266b), there are also various negative aspects indicating the need of safer, more effective, and less expensive thrombolytic agents. After intravenous injection of infusion into circulating blood, streptokinase and urokinase activate plasminogen to plasmin (for the streptokinase mechanism, see Section 8.2). This activation occurs not only within the thrombus to be lysed but primarily in the circulating blood, an effect that often results in a more or less severe tendency to bleed, for instance, from postoperative wounds (267b) or also from various parts of the body.

Some examples of the many reports include statistical data for streptokinase citing a tendency to bleed that developed in 37% of the treated patients and side reactions in 4% (268b). In another study, thrombolysis of venous occlusions was complicated by hemorrhage in 45%, by toxic allergic reactions in 40%, by pyrexia in 68%, by phlebitis at the infusion site in 26%, by pulmonary embolism in 6%, and by infections in 6%. Thrombolysis of arterial occlusion was accompanied by hemorrhage in 29%, by toxic allergic reactions in 55%, by pyrexia in 57%, by phlebitis at the infusion site in 10%, by arterial embolism in 10%, and by infections in 4% (269b). Although streptokinase treatment has been proved to be beneficial in several types of thromboembolic disease despite the side reactions, reports of its effectiveness as a therapeutic agent for fresh myocardial infarction have been contradictory (for quotations, see a negative report, Ref. 270).

Bleeding complications with urokinase occur also but are somewhat less frequent than with streptokinase (271) (streptokinase-urokinase embolism trial). In one report 45% of the patients treated with urokinase were found to have bleeding complications (272). Urokinase is extremely expensive; the amounts needed to treat one patient requires the volume of urine equivalent to the total output of one year from one single individual (272).

8.2 Streptokinase-Induced Activation of the Fibrinolytic System; Its Action on the Clotting System

Streptokinase, a product of β-hemolytic streptococci, is a single chain protein with a molecular weight of 48,000 (273). Streptokinase activates human plasminogen indirectly by first combining with plasminogen in equimolecular proportions to form an activator complex, which subsequently activates the remaining noncomplexed plasminogen to plasmin by cleaving a single arginyl-valine bond (274, 275). The plasmin generated by streptokinase reduces in the circulation the level of fibrinogen factors V and VIII (277). Streptokinase fails to induce lysis of retracted clots or does so very poorly (276), whereas synthetic fibrinolytic agents do exhibit a lysing effect (see Section 9).

The plasminogen in the blood of patients can be reduced considerably by streptokinase treatment. Therefore after cessation of therapy a new thrombosis may develop when plasminogen reaches its lowest point. For this reason, most treatment programs recommend the adminstration of heparin or dextran for a few days after treatment with the thrombolytic agent has ceased (278). Streptokinase was the first agent used for thrombolytic therapy. It certainly represents therapeutic progress—a progress, however, that leaves open a very wide field for improvements.

8.3.1 BIOLOGICAL ACTIVITIES OF UROKINASE. Urokinase is isolated from human urine. The first preparation, described in 1954 (279), had a molecular weight of 53,000 (280). Urokinase is clearly distinct from the circulating physiologic plasminogen activator (see Section 9). For details of the mechanism of the urokinase-catalyzed activation of human plasminogen, see Ref. 281. Urokinase is not antigenic to man, and its use is not complicated (as is the use of streptokinase) by the presence of neutralizing antibodies (282). After intravenous infusion, urokinase is cleared from the circulation with a plasma half-life of 10–15 min (283). Human urokinase excretion with the urine is reduced with certain diseases. This reduction is very pronounced with various types of carcinoma (284).

8.3.2 INTERFERENCE BY UROKINASE WITH THE COAGULATION SYSTEM. Urokinase infusion produces a plasma coagulation defect that is due to the action of the resulting plasmin on fibrinogen factors V and VIII. However it has been shown that urokinase treatment can also induce hypercoagulability during the first hours of application, and pretreatment with a small dose of intravenous heparin has been recommended (285).

8.3.3 THROMBOLYTIC TREATMENT WITH UROKINASE. Space does not permit the mention of all clinical papers, some of them published more than 10 years ago. With massive pulmonary embolism a 24 hr treatment with urokinase gave better results in reducing the emboli than did streptokinase treatment, but there was no difference in mortality (271). Urokinase has also been applied in ophthalmology—for instance, for the treatment of thrombi in retinal vessels (286).

8.3.4 SOURCES OF UROKINASE OTHER THAN URINE. Urokinase has been obtained from tissue cultures of human embryonic kidney cells (287) or organ cultures of human kidneys. The immunologic identity of this type of urokinase with urokinase from urine has been demonstrated (288).

8.4 Porcine Plasmin

Porcine plasmin was the first fibrinolytic enzyme with which a fibrinolytic activity was induced in experimental animals (289). This fibrinolytic enzyme, however, was clinically applied only recently. In a double-blind trial clinical and phlebographic evidence disclosed that with deep vein thrombosis, thrombolysis was obtained in 65% of the plasmin-treated group but improvements were achieved in only 15% of control patients (290). A combination of porcine plasmin with streptokinase resulted in a distinct thrombolytic effect, with deep vein thrombosis in 71.5% as compared with 55.8% with streptokinase alone (291). Plasmin is the active fibrinolytic enzyme, in contrast to streptokinase and urokinase, which activate plasminogen to plasmin.

8.5 Aspergillus Protease

Brinase, a protease from *Aspergillus oryzae*, was tested to a limited extent in patients with thrombotic disorders (294) but has not been properly evaluated. Brinase increases the negative charge of blood vessel walls and reduces platelets' adhesion (293). Brinase removes fibrin from lung vessels of rats in which intravascular clotting has been induced experimentally, and the fibrinolytic activity decreased (294).

8.6 Conclusions

Enzymatic fibrinolytic agents act, with some limitations, as thrombolytic drugs, but many aspects of this treatment require marked improvements both from biochemical and clinical viewpoints. Synthetic fibrinolytic agents, as described in the next section, offer clear potentials for such improvements.

9 SYNTHETIC FIBRINOLYTIC AGENTS: A LITTLE EXPLORED POTENTIAL FOR THE DEVELOPMENT OF BETTER ANTITHROMBOTIC DRUGS

9.1 General Remarks: The Fibrinolytic Potential of Human Blood

The value of streptokinase and urokinase has been summarized as follows: "... in order to decide on the risk versus the benefit for any particular patient, the physician will need to consider many factors before using these unique and potent agents" (295). As a better potential approach for the thrombolytic treatment, we discuss synthetic fibrinolytic agents.

That human blood possesses a high fibrinolytic potential can be proved by several methods, such as the regression of thrombi as demonstrated by various techniques, the very marked increase of fibrinolytic activity lasting for hours after intravenous injection of protein-free pyrogens (296), and highly increased fibrinolytic activity in several pathologic conditions.

9.2 Different Pathways of Fibrinolysis Induction Between Vascular Activator, Stimulated by Synthetic Fibrinolysis-Inducing Compounds, and Urokinase

The vascular plasminogen activator that triggers the fibrinolytic activity of the blood has properties quite different from those of the expensive urokinase. The biochemical analysis of these properties was carried out by a number of investigators after a method had been developed to extract large amounts of the vascular activator from human cadavers (297, 298).

The most important property of the vascular activator is its adsorption onto fibrin strands (299, 300). These strands adsorb also plasminogen from the blood, but antiactivator and antiplasmin are adsorbed in addition. If a human plasma clot is incubated with synthetic organic anions that inactivate these inhibitors (301, 302), strong fibrinolytic activity develops. The adsorption of activator and plasminogen to the fibrin strands is precisely demonstrated by using the "flat clots"—human plasma clots centrifuged free of serum at 36,000 g. These clots (Fig. 32.8) dissolve when exposed to a buffered solution of synthetic fibrinolytic compounds. Urokinase is completely inactive at any concentration with these flat clots. When after a certain exposure time such a flat clot is transferred to a compound-free buffered saline solution, it still dissolves. The adsorption of the fibrinolytic compounds to the fibrin strands has been proved by chemical analysis and by fluorescence (303).

Figure 32.9 shows the types of human clots we use for serial testing for potential synthetic fibrinolytic agents. With the plasma clots on the left, the substances are dissolved in citrated human plasma, which subsequently is clotted by recalcification. With the hanging clot on the right side, the preformed clot made from human plasma is incubated in the buffered compound solution. The important reasons for the difference in the required compound concentrations are discussed shortly.

Table 32.1 reveals that in contrast to the synthetic compounds, urokinase induces lysis in the plasma clot at relatively low concentrations, yet there is only partial lysis with the hanging clot at the same concentrations and, in contrast to synthetic compounds, no fibrinolysis at all with the flat clots. The adsorption of the compounds to the fibrin strands (in contrast to urokinase) is proved in Table 32.2. Fluorescent synthetic compounds that are added on a slide to

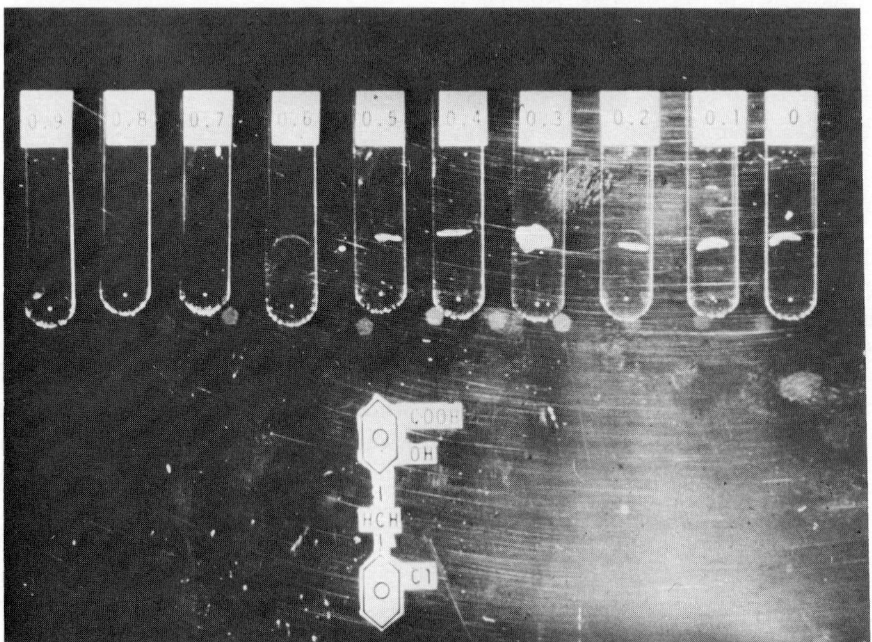

Fig. 32.8 Dissolution (left side) of human serum-free flat clots by a synthetic fibrinolytic compound concentrations expressed in millimoles).

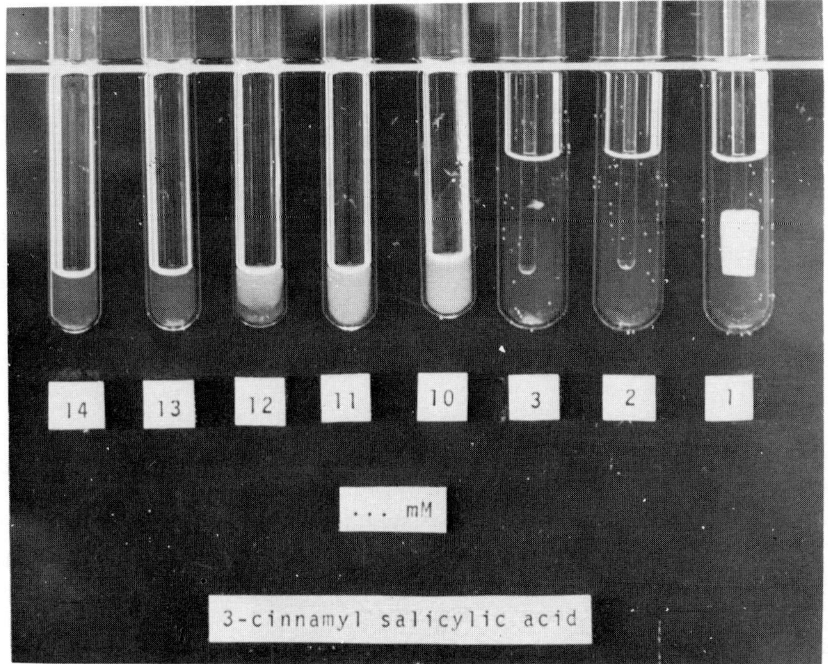

Fig. 32.9 Types of clot made from human citrated plasma for *in vitro* testing of synthetic organic compounds for their fibrinolysis-inducing potential. Plasma clots, left side (lysed at 14 and 13 mM), hanging clots, right side (lysed at 3 and 2 mM).

Table 32.1 Urokinase vs. Compound-Induced Fibrinolysis[a] of Various Types of Clots Originating from Human Plasma

Type of Clot	Urokinase (CTA units), ml																
	2000	1000	750	500	400	300	200	100	90	80	70	60	50	40	30	20	10
Plasma clot								+	+	+	+	+	+	+	(+)	−	−
Hanging clot		+	+	+	+	+	+	+	+	(+)	(+)	(+)	(+)	(+)	(+)	−	−
Serum-free clot	−	−	−	−	−	−	−	−	−	−	−	−	−	−	−	−	−

Type of Clot	*N*-(4-Isopropylphenyl)anthranilic acid, Concentration in mM																							
	20	19	18	17	16	15	14	13	12	11	10	9	8	7	6	5	4	3	2	1	0.9	0.8	0.7	0.6
Plasma clot			(+)	+	+	+	+	+	(+)	−														
Hanging clot											+	+	+	(+)	(+)	(+)	−	−						
Serum-free clot																		−	(+)	+	+	(+)	(+)	−

[a] +, Complete lysis within 24 hr; (+), partial lysis within 24 hr; −, no lysis.

Table 32.2 Evidence of Absorption onto Fibrin on Synthetic Fibrinolytic Compounds

Procedure	Evidence
Hanging clot incubated in B.S.[a]-containing compound, transferred into compound-free B.S. and incubated	Clot dissolves
Compound dissolved in human plasma, plasma clotted, centrifuged at 36,000 g., clot washed 3 times with B.S. and incubated in B.S.	Clot dissolves
Fluorescent compound added to plasma, clotted on slide, clot washed 3 times with B.S. and incubated	Fluorescent fibrin strands, which dissolve

[a] B.S. = Buffered Saline.

a plasma clot render the fibrin strands fluorescent because they diffuse into the strands and cannot be washed off. Such an exposed (to pamoic acid) and washed clot, which is already partially lysed, appears in Fig. 32.10.

9.3 Pathway of Fibrinolysis Induction by Synthetic Compounds: Difference Between Vascular Activator and Urokinase

The observations described indicate that the mechanism of the fibrinolysis of human clots induced by the synthetic compounds is as follows. The fibrin strands adsorb vascular activator, plasminogen, antiactivator, and antiplasmin. The fibrin strands adsorb

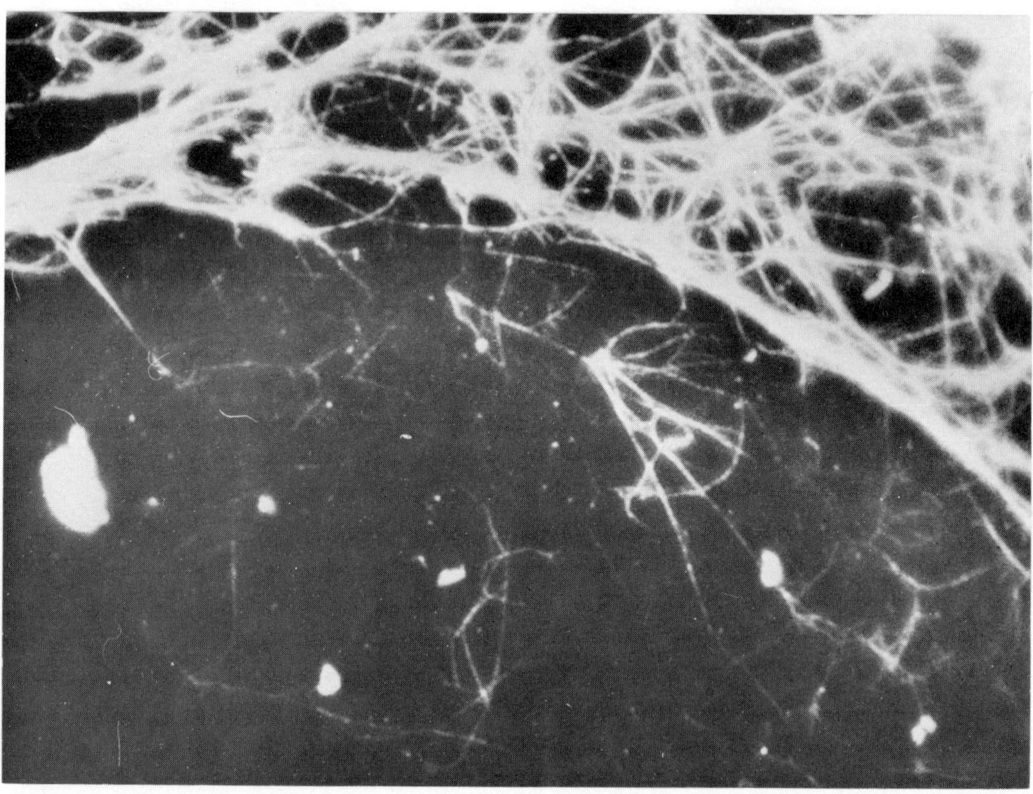

Fig. 32.10 Human plasma clot, made on a slide, exposed to the fluorescent fibrinolysis-inducing pamoic acid at 3 m*M*. After exposure, clot was washed several times with buffered saline; upon incubation, the clot dissolves. Photomicrograph taken with ultraviolet light.

Table 32.3 Parameters that Differentiate Vascular Activator from Urokinase

1. Differences in molecular weights
2. Antisera against urokinase do not react with vascular activator
3. Acetylglycyllysine methyl ester is hydrolyzed at different kinetics
4. Stability in salt solution is different
5. Vascular activator is much stronger bound to fibrin than is urokinase
6. Vascular activator induces clot lysis at lower CTA units than urokinase does
7. Vascular activator-induced fibrinolytic activity does not result in destruction of protein required for clotting, whereas urokinase-induced one does

very strongly synthetic fibrinolytic compounds. These compounds inactivate the adsorbed inhibitors, thus permitting the vascular activator to activate plasminogen to plasmin, which subsequently induces fibrinolysis. The vascular activator is different from urokinase, as various publications report (298, 299, 304). Table 32.3 gives the most essential differences. The fibrinolytic destruction by urokinase-induced fibrinolysis of proteins required for coagulation (item 7 in Table 32.3) results frequently in hemorrhages in patients treated with urokinase (or streptokinase). For statistical data on this subject, see Section 8.

9.4 Structure-Activity Relationships

Synthetic fibrinolytic compounds active *in vitro*, which induce fibrinolytic activity primarily on the fibrin strands, would be a desirable alternative to urokinase. It appears to be quite possible to develop these compounds for clinical use. After the discovery of such compounds by von Kaulla (305), numerous confirming reports were published (306–308). Some compounds discovered and/or studied at my laboratory, together with pathways for further developments, are described next. Fibrinolytic activity is induced in the test tube with clots made from human plasma by many synthetic organic anions. Figure 32.11 presents examples. Not shown, for instance, are various 2-phenethynylcyclopropane-carboxylates, which are active at about 15 m*M* (309) in the hanging clot system that is mostly used for serial testing. As a further example, in Fig. 32.12 indicates that the activity can be markedly increased by appropriate substitution.

9.5 Binding of the Compounds to Albumin

Figure 32.9 illustrates with 3-cinnamyl salicylic acid the differences in the compound concentration necessary for inducing fibrinolysis with the plasma clot and with the hanging clot. Because of the binding of the compounds to albumin, the plasma clots are lysed by 13 m*M*, in contrast to the hanging clots, which are lysed with only 2 m*M*. With the hanging clot, there is a surplus of compound solution (2.5 ml solution, 0.5 ml clot), and the binding of the compound to albumin does not reduce the compound concentration very much. This reduction, however, occurs with the plasma clot; here the compound is dissolved in the plasma before being clotted.

The binding of the fibrinolytic compounds to albumin is proved by the adsorption of labeled compounds to albumin and the reduction of the required compound concentration, when albumin is removed from plasma or when the binding sites of albumin are blocked by oxacillin. The suggested binding mechanism to albumin for the synthetic fibrinolytic agent flufenamic acid is the insertion of the aromatic portion of the drug into the hydrophobic crevice of this protein, while the

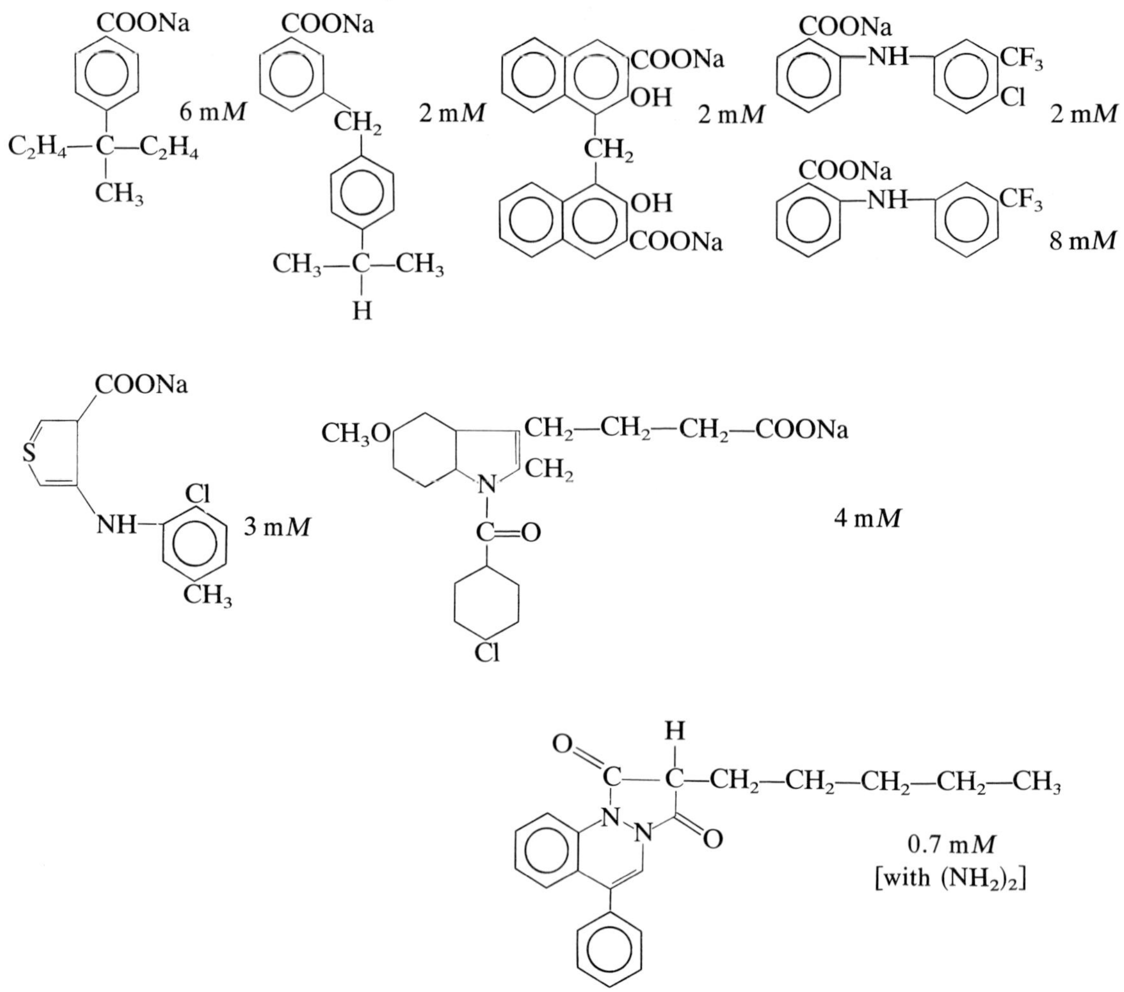

Fig. 32.11 Various structures of synthetic organic fibrinolysis-inducing compounds. Hanging clot method. Lowest active concentration (24 hr) given in italics to the right of each structure.

carboxylate group of the drug interacts with a cationic site of the protein surface (310).

The synthetic fibrinolytic agents are bound to albumin at quite different degrees. This can be concluded from the marked variations in the relation of the concentrations required for the lysis of plasma clots and hanging clots. Table 32.4 lists examples for these variations. In this table, compound 1 has a very high binding to albumin, in contrast to compound 4, which has a good relationship between molarities required for the lysis of clots of both types. This small difference gives a clear pointer for further developments of synthetic compounds. Niflumic acid [2-(3-trifluoromethylanilino)nicotinic acid] is also noteworthy from another stand point (see Section 9.7.) Compounds with little binding to albumin would be most useful. We discovered such a compound, with an activity relationship of 1 : 1 between plasma clot and hanging clot, indicating a minimal binding of the compound to albumin. The required molarity for the lysis of both types of clot was 14 m*M*. The structure of the

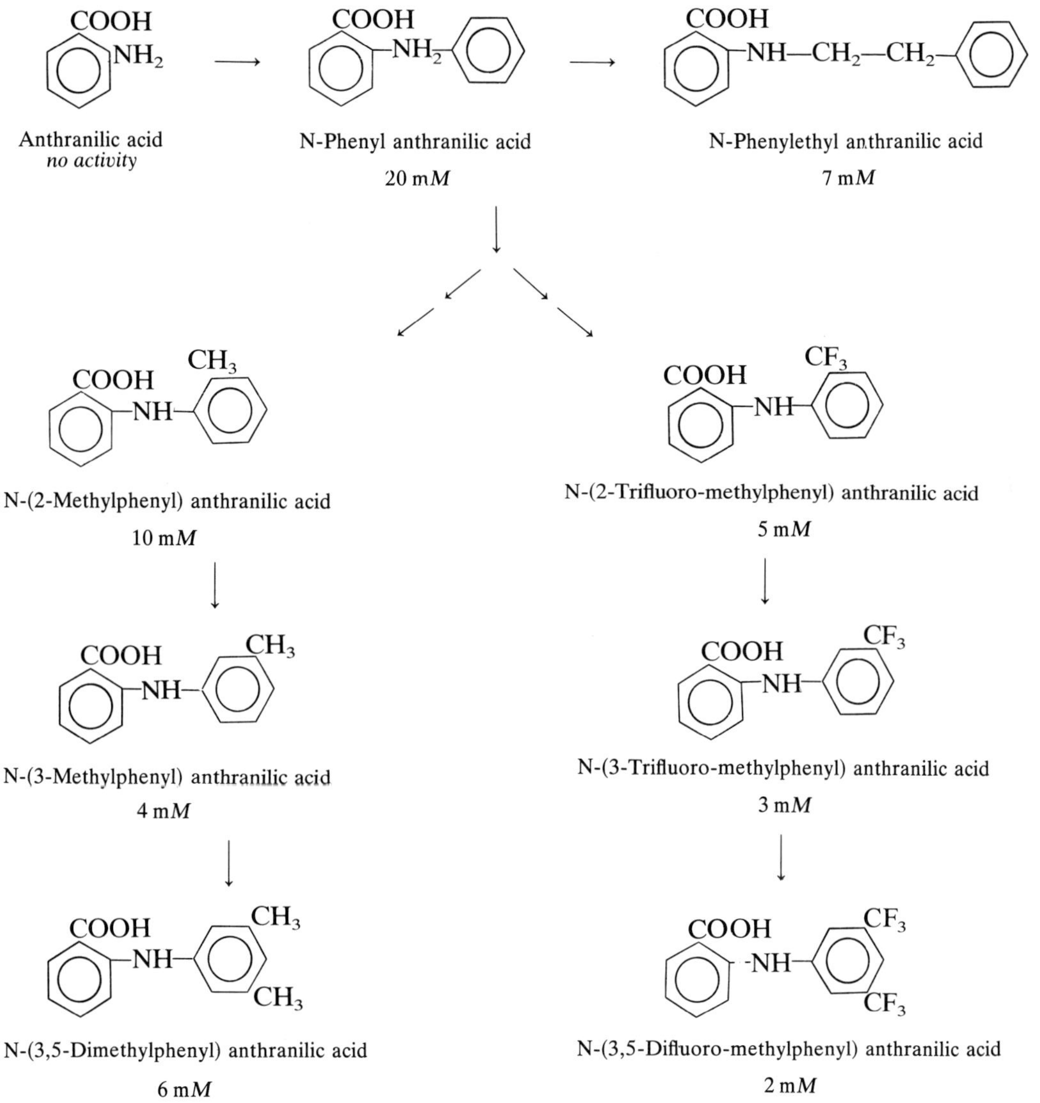
COOH
NH_2
Anthranilic acid
no activity
COOH
NH_2
N-Phenyl anthranilic acid
20 mM
COOH
$NH—CH_2—CH_2$
N-Phenylethyl anthranilic acid
7 mM
COOH
CH_3
NH
N-(2-Methylphenyl) anthranilic acid
10 mM
COOH
CF_3
NH
N-(2-Trifluoro-methylphenyl) anthranilic acid
5 mM
COOH
CH_3
NH
N-(3-Methylphenyl) anthranilic acid
4 mM
COOH
CF_3
NH
N-(3-Trifluoro-methylphenyl) anthranilic acid
3 mM
COOH
CH_3
NH
CH_3
N-(3,5-Dimethylphenyl) anthranilic acid
6 mM
COOH
CF_3
NH
CF_3
N-(3,5-Difluoro-methylphenyl) anthranilic acid
2 mM

Fig. 32.12 Enhancement of *in vitro* fibrinolysis-inducing capacity of anthranilic acid derivatives by various substitutions.

compound, Deriphat-160, is given in Fig. 32.13.

9.6 Enhancement of Fibrinolysis-Inducing Capacity of Synthetic Compounds

Hydrazine enhances the fibrinolysis-inducing capacity of the synthetic compounds both *in vitro* and *in vivo*, probably by further reducing the activity of antiplasmin (312). Table 32.5 gives examples of this enhancing effect *in vitro*. Here is yet another wide open field for further research.

9.7 Synthetic Compounds that Induce Fibrinolytic Activity *in vitro* and *in vivo*

Nicotinic acid induces fibrinolysis not only in the test tube, but also *in vivo* (in rats).

Table 32.4 Examples for the Relation Between Fibrinolytic Activity as Measured with Hanging Clot and with Plasma Clot

Fibrinolytic Compound	Concentration, m*M* Hanging Clot	Concentration, m*M* Plasma Clot	Ratio
1. 3-(4-Isopropylbenzoic)-salicylic acid	2	12	1:6
2. *N*-(3,5-Ditrifluoromethylphenyl)anthranilic acid	2	11	1:5.5
3. 3-(2-Methyl-3-chloroaniline)-4-thiophene carboxylic acid	3	11	1:3.7
4. Niflumic acid	8	11	1:1.5

Figure 32.14 plots the pronounced temporary shortening of the eugobulin lysis time in a rat after intravenous injection of 10 mg/kg of niflumic acid. Niflumic acid (311) induces fibrinolytic activity by two pathways: suppression of antiactivator and antiplasmin activity *in vitro*, and triggering of release of vascular activator *in vivo* (see Fig. 32.15). Search for compounds with these two types of fibrinolysis-inducing activity may well lead to more effective fibrinolytic drugs.

9.8 Synthetic Compounds That Induce Fibrinolytic Activity *in Vivo*

9.8.1 SHORT-ACTING COMPOUNDS. Oral application of certain agents has been

$$CH_3—(CH_2)_{10}—N\begin{cases} CH_2—CH_2—COONa \\ CH_2—CH_2—COOH \end{cases}$$

Fig. 32.13 Structure of Deriphat 160 C (*N*-lauryl-β-iminodipropionic acid monosodium salt), a synthetic fibrinolysis-inducing compound. Required concentration for plasma clot and hanging clot, 1:1.

Table 32.5 Enhancement of Fibrinolytic activity Induced by Synthetic Organic Compounds, Achieved by Preincubation (60 min) of Plasma with 2.5 m*M* Hydrazine

Compound	Concentration, m*M*[a] Without N_2H_4	Concentration, m*M*[a] With N_2H_4	Activity Increase %
Niflumic acid	12	8	66
3-(3,5-Ditrifluoromethyl-anilino)-4-thiophene carboxylic acid	8	5	75
3-(4-Isopropylbenzyl)salicylic acid	12	7	83
n-(3,5-Dimethylphenyl)anthranilic acid	11	6	91
4-(*n*-Decyl)benzenesulfonic acid	Not active	7	—
5-*n*-Nonyl salicylic acid	Not active	7	—
Lauryl sulfate	Not active	7	—

[a] Lowest molarity inducing complete clot lysis within 24 hr. Plasma clot method (human).

found to induce a mild but clear-cut fibrinolytic reaction in humans. Oral application of paraaminobenzoic acid (18 g: 2 g every 3 hr) induced a marked fibrinolytic reaction, i.e., lysis of diluted clots within 24 or 48 hr in 40 and 64% of treated patients (313). It was also claimed that injection of 1.8 g of aspirin increases fibrinolytic activity in human subjects as measured by the ^{125}-I-fibrinogen assay (314). Very shortly after ingestion, cayenne pepper (*Capsicum*) was found to induce a marked shortening of the euglobulin lysis time (315). It has also been reported that ingestion of onions enhanced fibrinolysis in man; cycloalliin, which shortens the euglobulin lysis time by 42%, has been identified as an active compound (316). In addition, xantinol nicotinate was shown to induce short-lived but intense fib-

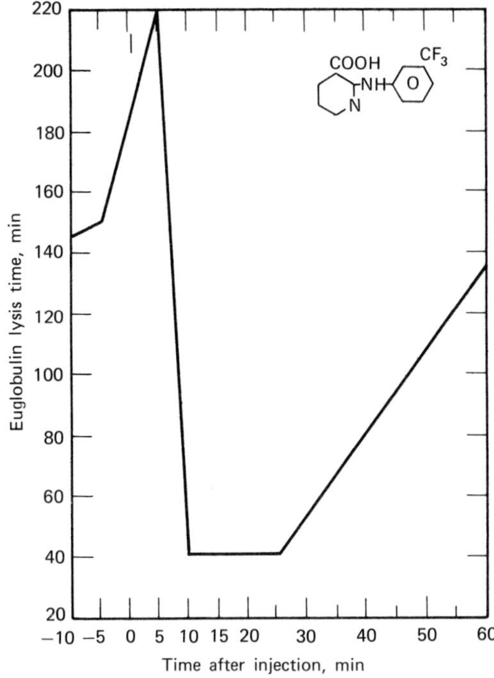

Fig. 32.14 Shortening of euglobulin lysis time after intravenous injection of 10 mg/kg of niflumic acid into a rat.

rinolytic activity in man, after oral application and also after intravenous infusion (317). Similar results after oral application were reported for a peripheral vasodilator hexanicit (*cis*-1,2,3,5-*trans*-4,6-cyclohexane) (318).

There are pharmacological compounds that induce short but very pronounced fibrinolytic activity, mainly after intravenous injection. Many years ago, adrenaline (319) and procaine hydrochloride (320) were observed to produce this action. Pitressin is another such compound (321). For a review of these compounds, including the more recently discovered ones exerting this activity, see Ref. 322.

This fibrinolysis-inducing effect of many drugs indicates a potential to develop compounds that very rapidly bring about a fibrinolytic, i.e. a thrombolytic, effect in humans. Obviously, a longer lasting effect is required for fibrinolytic therapy. Such an effect, lasting several hours after intravenous injection in man, was recently reported for furosemide (4-chloro-*N*-furfuryl-5-

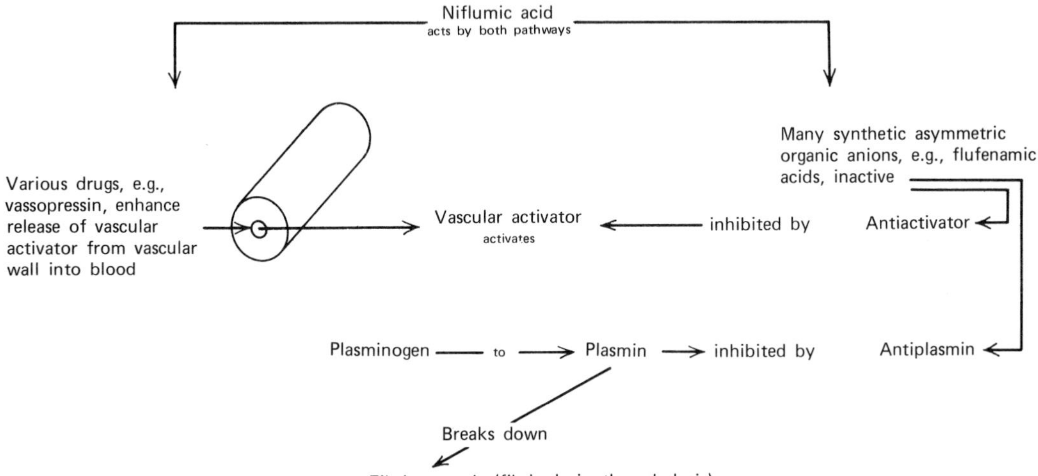

Fig. 32.15 The two pathways of the nonenzymatic activation of the fibrinolytic system. Niflumic acid acts in both pathways. The plasmin activators not occurring in the blood (i.e., urokinase and streptokinase) also activate plasminogen to plasmin, although urokinase and streptokinase use a somewhat different pathway.

sulfamonylanthranilic acid), and the enhancement of fibrinolytic activity could be repeated (323).

9.8.2 LONG-ACTING COMPOUNDS. A number of oral compounds increase the fibrinolytic activity of the blood on a long-term basis. Furazabol (17-methyl-5α-androstanol-[2,3-*c*]-furazan-17β-ol), an anabolic steroid, in doses of 0.04–1.0 mg daily per rat, increases the plasminogen activator activity in the blood and also of the lung of this animal. One month after cessation of treatment, these parameters returned to normal (324).

Other drugs normalize a reduced fibrinolytic activity and/or even increase the fibrinolytic activity of the blood in human beings. This is important because it has been shown that in many patients with recurrent venous thromboses the plasminogen activator content in the vein walls is decreased and/or the release of this vascular activator from the vein walls is defective (325, 326).

Several orally given drugs have been reported to activate fibrinolysis in these patients. Fearnley et al. (327) have found that phenformin (1-phenylbiguanide) and stanozolol (17β-hydroxy-17α-methyl-androstano[3,2-*C*]pyrazole), alone or in combination, evoke lasting fibrinolysis activation in the blood, as well as decreases in fibrinogen levels, platelet adhesiveness, and blood cholesterol level. However the increase of fibrinolytic activity is slow, and many days may be required to reach an effective level. Recently these findings were reconfirmed (328). Isacson and Nilsson (329) confirmed the same findings in regard to fibrinolytic activity and furthermore noted an increase of plasminogen activator content in the vein walls. Recently it was again observed that 100 mg of phenformin administered daily and/or 8 mg of ethylestrenol daily for 3–48 months increased the fibrinolytic activity of the blood and the level of fibrinolytic activity in the vein walls. This treatment normalized initially low fibrinolytic activity and decreased the frequency of thrombotic episodes (330).

Similar results were obtained in a 5 year study by Walker and Davidson (331). However phenformin has some undesirable side reactions (332). Therefore a phenformin-like substance, moroxydine chloride [N^1,N^1-anhydrobis(β-oxiethyl)biguanid HCl] was studied in patients having a defective fibrinolytic defense mechanism and a history of recurrent deep vein thromboses. This compound was quite effective; it increased the fibrinolytic release capacity of the vessel walls during the first 3 months of treatment and increased the fibrinolytic activity of the vessel walls (333).

9.9 Inhibition of Platelet Aggregation by Synthetic Fibrinolytic Compounds

Many of the compounds inducing fibrinolytic activity *in vitro* possess a second important antithrombotic potential, namely, the inhibition of the aggregation of human platelets by collagen (334). Table 32.6 indicates this for the derivative of phenyl-4-aminothiophene-3-carboxylic acid. The fibrinolytic activity is measured with the hanging clot system as well as the inhibition of aggregation of human thrombocytes in citrated plasma aggregated by collagen. This combined activity makes evident the possibility for development of antithrombotic drugs with a dual effect, that is, prevention and treatment of intravascular clotting. Some of the compounds prevent, too, the aggregation of platelets induced by foreign serum (335). The potential therapeutic value of this observation has not yet been investigated.

10 HEMOSTATIC AGENTS

10.1 General Remarks

Hemostatic agents can be divided into two general groups: agents that are applied in-

Table 32.6 Fibrinolytic Activity and Inhibition of Collagen-Induced Aggregation of Human Thrombocytes Left in the Plasma by Derivatives of Phenyl-4-Aminothiophene-3-Carboxylic Acid

	Lower Limits of	
Acid Derivatives	Fibrinolytic Activity, *M*	Aggregation Inhibiting (50%), *M*
[Thiophene-3-carboxylic acid	5×10^{-2}	4×10^{-3}]
N-2,6-Dimethyl-	5×10^{-3}	1×10^{-3}
N-2-Chloro-5-methyl-	3×10^{-3}	1×10^{-3}
N-2-Chloro-6-methyl-	4×10^{-3}	5×10^{-4}
N-2,3-Dimethyl-	7×10^{-3}	5×10^{-4}
N-2,4,6-Trichloro-	2×10^{-3}[a]	5×10^{-4}
N-2,4,6-Trichloro-3-methyl-	5×10^{-3}[a]	5×10^{-4}
N-2,4,6-Trimethyl-	3×10^{-3}	4×10^{-4}
N-3-Trifluoromethyl-	6×10^{-3}	4×10^{-4}
N-2-Chloro-3-methyl-	3×10^{-3}	5×10^{-5}

[a] Partial lysis.

travenously, intramuscularly, or orally, and agents that are applied locally. The ones applied "*in vivo*" are of different types depending on the clotting abnormality that must be treated to prevent a bleeding episode or to arrest an actual hemorrhage.

10.2 Replacement of Reduced Clotting Factors

The most common clotting abnormality due to a reduced clotting factor is hemophilia. There are about 20,000 hemophiliacs in the United States, and the vast majority suffer from a factor VIII deficiency; some are deficient in factor IX. In a severe hemophiliac the factor activity was found to be only a few percent of normal, sometimes even below 1%. The present treatment consists of infusion or intravenous injection of concentrates of the reduced factor prepared from human blood (mostly factor VIII). Its use varies from patient to patient. In some nonbleeding patients it is utilized to prevent bleeding, in others it is applied to stop an actual bleeding, to normalize the patient's clotting process before as well as during surgery, etc.

So far, no attempts have been made to replace factor VIII, the antihemophilic globulin, by a synthetic compound, although it was found that certain asymmetric organic anions exert factor VIII activity in the test tube in hemophilic plasma (336). Deficiencies, although some are rather rare, have been reported for almost all the clotting factors (for details, see Ref. 337).

10.3 Inactivation of Circulating Anticoagulants

Abnormal blood coagulation inhibitors of genetic origin (338) or inhibitors acquired during certain diseases [e.g., lupus erythematosus (339)] exist, though they are rare. There are also acquired inhibitors, which are directed against one individual clotting factor; they result principally from repeated transfusions. Thus it has been found that 16.5% of hemophilia A patients develop an inhibitor against factor VIII. In 30% of these patients the inhibitor titer is very low, so that its activity can be overcome by factor VIII infusions (340). If no active hemorrhage is in progress and requiring treatment, the titer may decrease spontaneously over a period of 3–6 months.

Cortisone has been used successfully to treat the abnormal circulating anticoagulant of some patients. In others, cortisone was without effect. Immune suppression with antimetabolites has similarly shown mixed effect (337). An unexplored therapeutic potential is the effect of the procoagulant fraction of human urine, which in the test tube normalizes the coagulation of a human plasma that contains a high titer circulating anticoagulant (341, 342).

10.4 Normalization of Abnormally High Fibrinolytic Activity

The (potential) fibrinolytic activity of the human blood is an important protective mechanism against intravascular clotting, i.e., formation of thrombi and emboli. However an abnormal increase of this activity can result in a bleeding tendency or even in severe hemorrhage because hemostatic clots are being dissolved. Such abnormal activation of the fibrinolytic system was observed during the early days of the heart-lung machine (343). This activation can be connected further with very severe liver damage, sudden shock, cancer of the prostate, and other diseases.

ε-Aminocaproic acid (EACA) reduces or normalizes pathologically increased fibrinolytic activity *in vivo*, primarily inactivating the activator of plasminogen (344). The use of EACA as an antifibrinolytic agent in primary fibrinolysis is indicated only in selected cases, because, to give one example, it has been reported that the competitive action of EACA for essential amino acids worsens hepatic coma, which as such may increase fibrinolytic activity very markedly (337). Patients with congenital cyanotic heart disease show significantly increased fibrinolytic activity and may require several days of treatment with EACA infusions before they are hemostatically safe for surgical intervention (345). The dosage is up to 20 g orally within 24 hr. If necessary, the treatment can be started with 1–2 g intravenously.

In Europe, the kallikrein inhibitor Trasylol, which is also a proteinase inhibitor given intravenously or as continuous infusion, is being used by various clinicians as an antifibrinolytic agent. Trasylol is a polypeptide of bovine origin. For structure, see Ref. 346; further details are given in Ref. 347.

10.5 Thrombocytopenia

Thrombocytopenia, i.e., low platelet count, generally occurs as an acquired disorder. However occasionally it is also seen with genetic anomalies such as the Wiskott-Aldrich syndrome and the May Hegglin disorder. There are several types of familial thrombocytopenia, too. Acquired thrombocytopenia can be divided into two basic types as caused by underproduction of thrombocytes or by overdestruction of the thrombocytes. The overdestruction can be on an immunological basis—one example being the neonatal purpura resulting from passive transfer of maternal autoantibodies—or from isologous incompatibility. The underproduction has many causes, including drug-induced bone marrow aplasia or metal intoxication. In these situations the treatment of the basic disease is indicated.

Thrombocytopenia has also been reported in association with heparin therapy (348) and in relation to alcohol consumption (349). Severe thrombocytopenia may also occur with various types of consumption coagulopathy. Under certain circumstances platelet concentrates can be transfused with good clinical results, but such a therapeutic approach must be very carefully evaluated. So far, no attempts have been made to develop synthetic compounds that exert at least some of the hemostatic platelet functions. Probably such compounds would not be affected by platelet antibodies.

10.6 Capillary Bleeding due to Increased Capillary Permeability

Bleeding of the capillaries that is attributable to increased capillary permeability can be controlled by carbazochrome salicylate (Adrenosemsalicylate, 3-hydro-1-methyl-5,6-indolinedion semicarbazone with sodium salicylate). It is administered orally (or intramuscularly) in doses of 1–5 mg. This dose can be repeated.

10.7 Neutralization of the Heparin Effect

Neutralization of the heparin effect in patients might become necessary for various reasons, for instance, emergency surgery in a patient who had been undergoing heparin treatment. The anticoagulant effect of heparin is (*in vitro*) immediately counteracted by numerous highly basic substances such as toluidine blue, protamine, and a synthetic quaternary ammonium polymer known as polybrene, an antiheparin agent too unstable for pharmaceutical distribution.

Protamine used as protamine sulfate and protamine chloride is presently the clinically applied antagonist of heparin. It is derived from testes and sperm of commercial fish. Its heparin-neutralizing effect was first described by Chargaff et al. (350). Protamine sulfate is a strongly basic substance that combines with and neutralizes heparin: 1 mg of protamine neutralizes approximately 1 mg of heparin. Because heparin clearance is rapid, however, only 50% of this dose needs to be given 60 min after heparin injection and only 25% after 2 hr. After subcutaneous heparin injection, protamine sulfate should be given in a dose equivalent to 50% of the last heparin dose. This may need to be repeated. Nevertheless, if clinically absolutely necessary, heparin should be neutralized *in vivo* only by protamine. The neutralization represents a potential danger of intravascular clotting. Heparin neutralization after use of the heart-lung machine to assure hemostasis is a distinct indication. "Heparin rebound", a new bleeding tendency that sometimes develops within a few hours of protamine injection (351), may require injection of additional protamine sulfate. For further information on protamine sulfate, see Bang (352).

10.8 Hypoprothrombinemia

All forms of hypoprothrombinemia can be treated with vitamin K. The most frequently used vitamin K is K_1 (2-methyl-3-phytyl-1,4-naphthoquinone), which was first isolated from alfalfa and was synthesized for commerce. It is used for treatment of many prothrombin complex (factors II, VII, IX, X) deficiencies occurring during liver disease. The synthesis of these factors is vitamin K dependent. These patients, however, should also be checked for primary fibrinolysis and for fibrinogen (factor I) deficiency. Vitamin K_1 (and other related compounds) is absorbed from the gastrointestinal tract only in the presence of bile salts. For therapeutic purposes it may also be applied intramuscularly or intravenously, a way of application that might be more efficient.

Vitamin K_1 is used primarily as an antidote for oral antithrombotic ("prothrombin-depressing") agents. In patients treated with these agents vitamin K rapidly normalizes factors VII and IX, whereas factors II and X return slowly. After intravenous vitamin K_1, the prothrombin time is normalized in 12–14 hr in these patients (353). With a high dose of vitamin K_1, a patient might become resistant to the anticoagulant effect of coumarin for about 2 weeks, an effect that is therapeutically undesirable (354). Because of side reactions, however, intravenous injection should not be given faster than 5 mg/min. When there is no drug-induced bleeding, yet the prothrombin time has been prolonged above safe levels, oral treatment with 2.5–10 mg of vitamin K_1 is usually sufficient (355). In patients treated with prothrombin-depressing agents, vitamin K_1 should be given only when absolutely necessary because an increase of the prothrombin activity above a certain level has the potential of inducing intravascular coagulation.

10.9 Topical Hemostatic Agents

Thrombin is a coagulant that is formed during blood coagulation (see Fig. 32.3) and rapidly converts fibrinogen into fibrin. This commercially available product (e.g., as Topostasin or Akrithrombin) is prepared from bovine plasma in a lyophilized sterilized form. It is being used to arrest oozing bleeding on superficial areas; a very firm clot, however, is not necessarily formed.

Oxydized cellulose is applied by means of a specially treated surgical gauze or cotton, whose hemostatic action depends on the formation of an artificial clot by cellulosic acid when used in surgery. It is valuable for control of moderate bleeding under conditions where suturing is not practical, such as in operations on the biliary tract, partial hepatectomy, or injuries of pancreas, spleen, or kidneys.

In a canine arterial bleeding model, it was lately found that microcrystalline collagen was more effective than oxydized cellulose. Microcrystalline collagen was also highly effective initially after large doses of heparin and in the presence of platelets with function rendered deficient by acetylsalicylate (356).

Human urine contains a very powerful procoagulant that clots even blood with circulating anticoagulants. From 1 ml of urine can be extracted enough procoagulant to normalize *in vitro* up to 10 ml of blood of a patient with severe hemophilia (357). We have purified this urinary procoagulant, which is also contained in urine of hemophiliacs; it is successful with tooth extractions and minor surgery in bleeders, primarily hemophiliacs, even if there is a circulating anticoagulant, thus avoiding transfusions.

A biochemist in India, interested in an investigation of this powerful procoagulant recently wrote me: "It is usual practice among many tribal people in our country to apply one's own urine on bleeding injuries and nothing else. It stops bleeding and it has amazing healing power" (358). The human urinary procoagulant is a very important but almost completely neglected hemostatic agent.

11 SUGGESTIONS FOR FURTHER RESEARCH FOR THE DEVELOPMENT OF BETTER ANTITHROMBOTIC–FIBRINOLYTIC AGENTS

11.1 General Remarks

Without the cooperation of the medicinal chemist, the development of more effective antithrombotic drugs cannot be achieved. Suggestions for such developments, which are extremely important for ill persons, might derive from various sides; those made by a physician who has much experimental experience might be the most realistic ones. Some proposals follow.

11.2 Fibrinolytic Activity

11.2.1 SPONTANEOUS FIBRINOLYSIS-THROMBOLYSIS. It has been distinctly demonstrated by many recent *in vivo* studies with ^{131}I-labeled fibrinogen that there exists, with great variations, a tendency of the thrombi to regress or dissolve completely. Enhancement of this process without application of enzymes would be very desirable. Treatment with the thrombolytic enzymes streptokinase or urokinase can very markedly enhance this process. As already mentioned, these two activators of the human fibrinolytic system do not occur in the blood; therefore their clinical utilization poses problems. The protective mechanism of the human fibrinolytic system is also revealed by the observation that a reduced fibrinolytic potential may result in increased tendency toward thrombosis (359).

11.2.2 LIVER AND THE FIBRINOLYTIC SYSTEM. The liver plays an important role in the regulation of the fibrinolytic activity of the blood. Complete exclusion of the liver from the circulation results within a very few minutes in an enormous increase of the fibrinolytic activity of the blood. This has been observed with the first human liver transplantation (360), with liver bypass in the rat (361), and in the pig (362). Reimplantation of a liver very quickly normalizes the increased fibrinolytic activity (363). Most likely, the liver removes plasminogen activator from the blood, thus suppressing increased plasminogen activation, an activation that can be highly desirable to prevent intravascular clotting under certain pathological conditions, or for the actual treatment of thromboembolism.

I know of no attempts to develop drugs that suppress specifically this particular liver function for the reduction of fibrinolytic activity, as the oral anticoagulants do with synthesis of the prothrombin complex. Such a drug would be extremely valuable, because activation of the body's own fibrinolytic activity by endogenous activators, as referred to in the discussions of fibrinolytic agents, is certainly less dangerous than the application of plasminogen activators that do not occur in the blood. There are, too, some indications, as demonstrated in the rat, that the spleen and the adrenal glands may also participate in the regulation of the fibrinolytic activity of the blood (364).

11.2.3 ORAL FIBRINOLYTIC AGENTS. Another possible means of activating the body's own fibrinolytic system are drugs that can be given orally. Such drugs exist, however treatment for several weeks is needed to obtain the desired effect, which thus far is not very pronounced (365). For half-synthetic heparinoids, given orally, a fast reduction of fibrinolytic activity has been reported (see Section 4, on heparinoids), and this effect would be worthy of further exploration. It was shown that orally given *p*-aminobenzoic acid induces a marked increase of fibrinolytic activity in the blood of patients. So does a certain pepper that grows in Thailand (see Section 9.8). The question arises whether the effect of the pepper contributes to the low thrombosis tendency of the Thai. These quoted observations certainly indicate a potential for further development of fibrinolytic-thrombolytic drugs.

11.2.4 COMBINED FIBRINOLYTIC AND ANTI-AGGREGATING EFFECTS. At very low *in vitro* concentrations, many synthetic fibrinolytic agents also exert an inhibitory effect on collagen-induced aggregation of human platelets left in fresh citrated human plasma (334). Here is an interesting avenue for the development of antithrombotic drugs with dual action.

11.3 Antithrombin III Activity

Antithrombin III is the most important natural protecting agent against intravascular clotting. Its reduced value reveals a thrombosis tendency, and very low values are connected with hereditary thrombophilia. In our experience, antithrombin III activity as measured by antithrombin III time, must be evaluated when using prothrombin-depressing agents so that these compounds give real protection against thromboembolism. When no increase occurs, there is no true protection by these agents. Compounds that considerably increase antithrombin III activity without affecting the prothrombin complex would be probably better and safer antithrombotic agents than the ones that reduce the prothrombin complex. Such possibilities exist. For instance, in all our patients who were being treated with prednisone we observed a very marked increase of antithrombin III activity (366). Prednisone, interestingly enough, moreover yet not immediately increases the fibrinolytic activity of the blood of treated patients (365). There are also compounds that increase antithrombin III activity *in vitro.* For example, *N*-(2-chloro-6-methylphenyl)-4-aminothiophene-3 carboxylic acid at 4 m*M* does so in human serum. Again we have little explored possibilities for the development of new antithrombotic drugs (366).

11.4 Variations of Heparin

Heparin with a lower molecular weight might be faster absorbed after subcutaneous injection at concentrations that might in addition increase the fibrinolytic activity of the blood. This possibility should be further explored, as well as the combination of heparin with aspirin, which in addition to exerting an anticoagulant effect might normalize pathologically increased of platelets aggregability, which contributes to a tendency toward thrombosis.

11.5 Synthetic Agents with Antihemophilic Globulin Activity

The possibility of developing synthetic compounds with factor VIII activity has been indicated by the property of certain organic anions to exert factor VIII activity in the test tube (367). This has not been investigated any further. Furthermore, although not a synthetic agent, the procoagulant of human urine, which proved to be very useful in man to arrest local bleeding in hemophiliacs even when a circulating anticoagulant was present (368), has not been really analyzed. Such analysis might reveal effective components that could be synthesized.

ACKNOWLEDGMENTS

The very helpful assistance of Mrs. Edith von Kaulla in preparing the manuscript is gratefully acknowledged.

REFERENCES

1. S. Wessler, *Fed. Proc.*, **36** (1), 66 (1977).
2. M. A. Ibrahim, D. L. Sakett, and W. Winkelstein, "Acute Myocardial Infarction: Magnitude of the Problem in Thrombosis, in *Thrombosis*, S. Sherry, K. M. Brinkhous, E. Genton, and J. M. Stengle, Eds., National Academy of Sciences, Washington, D.C., 1969, p. 106.
3. A. W. Branwood and G. L. Montgomery, *Scot. Med. J.*, **1**, 367 (1956).
4. W. B. Robertson, Coronary Thrombosis, M. D. thesis, St. Andrew University, 1960.
5. R. M. Acheson, "Strokes: An Estimate of the Magnitude of the Problem in the United States 1965," in *Thrombosis*, S. Sherry, K. M. Brinkhous, E. Genton, and J. M. Stengle, Eds., National Academy of Sciences, Washington, D.C. 1969, p. 136.
6. C. H. Millikan, "Incidence and Significance of Thromboemboli in Acute Cerebrovascular Occlusion," in *Thrombosis*, S. Sherry, K. M. Brinkhous, E. Genton, and J. M. Stengle, Eds., National Academy of Sciences, Washington, D.C., 1969, p. 155.
7. M. C. MacIntyre, D. R. B. Jones, and C. V. Ruckley, *Thromb. Diath. Haemorrh.* **34,** 563 (1975).
8. A. S. Gallus and J. Hirsh, *Drug*, **12,** 41 (1976).
9. R. H. Alexander, R. Folse, J. Pizzorno, and R. Conn, *Ann. Surg.* **180,** 883 (1974).
10. *Medi. World News*, February 7, 1977, p. 62.
11. J. V. H. Kemble, *Brit. J. Hosp. Med.*, **6,** 721 (1971).
12. Council on Thrombosis of the American Heart Association, Prevention of Venous Thromboembolism in Surgical Patients by Low-Dose Heparin," *Circulation*, **55,** 423A–425A (1977).

13. V. V. Kakkar, "Isotopic Detection of Deep Venous Thrombosis" in Thromboembolism: Diagnosis and Treatment, V. V. Kakkar, and A. J. Jouhar, Eds., Churchill Livingstone, Edinburgh, 1972.

14. R. W. Colman, St. J. Robby, and J. D. Minna, *Am. J. Med.*, **52,** 681 (1972).

15. G. Zbinden, *Ann. Rev. Pharmacol. Toxicol.* **16,** 177 (1976).

16. E. von Kaulla, W. Droegemueller, N. Aoki, and K. N. von Kaulla, *Am. J. Obstetr. Gynecol.*, **109,** 868 (1971).

17. E. von Kaulla and K. N. von Kaulla, *J. Med.* **3,** 349 (1972).

18. R. A. Ackerman, *Dialysis Transplant.*, **6** (3), 16 (1977).

19. K. N. von Kaulla and E. von Kaulla, *Circ. Res.*, **14,** 436 (1964).

20. E. von Kaulla and K. N. von Kaulla, *Am. J. Clin. Pathol.*, **61,** 810 (1974).

21. K. N. von Kaulla and R. L. Schultz, *Am. J. Clin. Pathol.*, **29,** 104 (1958).

22. J. MacLean, *Am. J. Physiol.*, **41,** 250 (1916).

23. W. H. Howell, Harvey Lectures, 1916–1917, Series XII.

24. W. H. Howell and E. Holt, *Am. J. Physiol.*, **47,** 328 (1918).

25. C. Crafoord, *Acta Chir. Scand.*, **74,** 407 (1937).

26. D. W. G. Murray, L. B. Jaques, T. S. Perrett, and C. H. Best, *Surgery*, **2,** 163 (1937).

27. E. J. Jorpes, *Heparin, Its Chemistry, Physiology and Application in Medicine*, Oxford University Press, Oxford, 1939.

28. H. Engelberg, *Heparin, Metabolism, Physiology and Clinical Application*, Thomas, Springfield, Ill., 1963.

29. V. V. Kakkar and D. P. Thomas edrs., *Heparin and Clinical Usage*, Academic Press, London, 1976.

30. E. Jorpes, *Biochem. J.* **29,** 1817 (1935).

31. E. Jorpes and S. Bergström, *Z. Physiol. Chem.*, **244,** 253 (1935).

32. J. Kiss, in *Heparin and Clinical Usage*, V. V. Kakkar and D. P. Thomas, Eds., Academic Press, London, 1976, p. 1.

33. *Chemical Marketing Reporter*, October 7, 1974.

34. Z. Yosizawa, *Biochem. Biophys. Res. Commun.* **16,** 336 (1964).

35. C. Veil and D. Quivy, *C. R. Séances Soc. Biol. Paris*, **144,** 14983 (1950).

36. L. H. Frommhagen, M. J. Fahrenbach, J. A. Brockmann, and E. L. R. Stockstead, *Proc. Soc. Exp. Biol. Med.*, **82,** 280 (1953).

37. A. S. Gallus and J. Hirsh, *Drugs*, **12,** 41 (1976).

38. G. J. H. Den Ottolander, A. P. C. van der Maas, and W. Schopman, *Thromb. Diath. Haemorrh.*, **32,** 277 (1974).

39. D. Loew, P. Brücke, W. Simma, H. Vinazzer, E. Dienstl, and K. Boehme, *Thromb. Res.* **11,** 81 (1977).

40. J. Kiss, *Thromb. Diath. Haemorrh*, **33,** 20 (1974).

41. B. H. Nader, N. M. McDuffie, and C. P. Dietrich, *Biochem. Biophys. Res. Commun.*, **57,** 488 (1974).

42. S. E. Lasker, US Patent 3,766,167, October 16, 1973.

43. U. Lindahl, M. Höök, G. Bäckström, J. Jacobsson, J. Riesenfeld, A. Malström, L. Rodén, and D. S. Feingold, *Fed. Proc.*, **31** (1), 19 (1977).

44. U. Lindahl, in *Carbohydrates*, Vol. 7 in International Reviews of Science: Organic Chemistry, Series 2, G. O. Aspinall, Ed. Butterworths, London, 1976, p. 283.

45. U. Lindahl and O. Axelsson, *J. Biol. Chem.*, **246,** 74 (1971).

46. K. N. von Kaulla and E. Husemann, *Experientia*, **2** (6), 1 (1946).

47. D. Horton and E. K. Just, *Carbohyd. Res.*, **30,** 349 (1973).

48. H. Engelberg, *Fed. Proc.*, **36** (1), 70 (1977).

49. H. Engelberg, A. Dudley, and L. Freeman, *J. Lab. Clin. Med.*, **46,** 653 (1955).

50. W. J. Estes and P. F. Poulin, *Throm. Diath. Haemorrh.*, **33,** 17 (1974).

51. A. S. Gallus and J. Hirsh, *Drugs*, **12,** 54 (1976).

52. K. N. von Kaulla and E. B. Pratt, *Am. J. Physiol.*, **187,** 89–93 (1956).

53. International Multicentre Trial, *Lancet*, **2,** 45 (1975).

54. A. Erdi, V. V. Kakkar, D. P. Thomas, D. A. Lane, and J. A. Dormandy, *Lancet*, **2,** 342 (1976).

55. T. J. M. V. van Vroonhoven, J. van Zijl, and H. Milier, *Lancet*, **1,** 375 (1974).

56. V. F. Gruber, F. Duckert, R. Fridrich, J. Rothorst, and J. Rem, *Lancet*, **1,** 207 (1977).

57. E. Quellhorst, W. Reichel, E. Fernandez-Redo, and F. Scheler, *Med. Klin.*, **72** (22), 981 (1977).

58. H. Schaefer and A. Zesch, *Pharmazie*, **31** (4), 251 (1976).

59. A. S. Gallus and J. Hirsh, *Drug*, **12,** 46 (1976).

60. A. N. Teien and M. Lie, *Thromb. Res.* **7,** 777 (1975).

61. P. G. Hattersley, *Am. J. Clin. Pathol.*, **66,** 899 (1976).

62. J. Hirsh, J. Bishop, M. Johnson, and C. Walker, *Blood*, **48** (6), 1004 (1976).
63. K. N. von Kaulla, P. Ostendorf, and E. von Kaulla, *J. Med.*, **6,** 73 (1975).
64. A. R. Thompson and R. B. Counts, *J. Lab. Clin. Med.*, **88,** 922 (1976).
65. E. T. Yin, *Thromb. Diathes. Haemorrh.*, **33,** 43 (1974).
66. E. A. Johnson, T. B. L. Kirkwood, Y. Stirling, J. Perez-Requejo, G. I. C. Ingram, D. R. Baugham, and M. Brozovic, *Thromb. Haemostas.*, **35** (3), 586 (1976).
67. L. O. Andersson, T. W. Barrowcliffe, E. Holmer, E. A. Johnson, and G. E. C. Sims, *Thromb. Res.* **9,** 575 (1976).
68. U. Abildgaard, *Scand. J. Clin. Lab. Invest.* **19,** 190 (1967).
69. J. Riesenfeld, M. Hook, I. Bjork, U. Lindahl, and B. Ajaxon, *Fed. Proc.*, **36** (1), 39 (1977).
70. G. Villanueva and I. Danishefky, *Fed. Proc.*, **36** (3), 645 (1977).
71. E. Marciniak and J. P. Gockerman, *Clin. Res.*, **25** (3), 478 (1977).
72. D. P. Thomas, D. A. Lane, R. Michalski, E. A. Johnson, and V. V. Kakkar, *Lancet*, **1,** 120 (1977).
73. J. M. Ramstack, L. Zuckerman, J. A. Caprini, and L. F. Mockros, *Proc. Ann. Conf. Eng. Med. Biol.*, **17,** 222 (1975).
74. A. N. Teien and J. Bjoernson, *Scand. J. Haematol.*, **17** (1), 29 (1976).
75. J. N. Shanberge, J. Kambayashi, and M. Nakagawa, *Thromb. Res.*, **9,** 595 (1976).
76. S. Wessler, *Fed. Proc.*, **36** (1), 66 (1977).
77. M. B. Zucker, *Thromb. Diath. Haemorrh.*, **33,** 63 (1974).
78. B. Dana, L. Ellman, N. Carvalho, W. M. Daggett, and A. M. Hutter, *Am. J. Cardiol.*, **38,** 9 (1976).
79. D. Green, M. Roberts, N. Reynolds, and R. Patterson, *Clin. Res.*, **25** (3), 476A (1977).
80. R. B. Babcock, C. W. Domper, and W. B. Scharfman, *New Engl. J. Med.*, **295,** 237 (1976).
81. W. R. Bell, P. A. Tomasulo, and B. M. Alving, *Ann. Intern. Med.*, **85,** 755 (1976).
82. H. K. Chiu, W. G. van Aken, J. Hirsh, E. Regoeczi, and A. A. Horner, *J. Lab. Clin. Med.*, **90** (1), 204 (1977).
83. K. N. von Kaulla and W. Henkel, *Schweiz. Med. Wochensch.*, **82,** 1128 (1952).
84. J. L. Tullis, *Clot*, Thomas, Springfield, Ill., 1976, p. 495.
85. W. A. Colburn, *Drug Metab. Rev.*, **5** (2), 281 (1976).
86. I. Danishefsky, *Advan. Exp. Biol. Med.*, **52,** 105 (1975).
87. C. Ehnholm, D. J. Neaf, L. Kaijser, P. K. J. Kinnunen, and L. A. Carlson, *Atherosclerosis*, **27,** 35 (1977).
88. H. Engelberg, *Fed. Proc.*, **36** (1), 70 (1977).
89. R. D. Rosenberg, *Fed. Proc.*, **36,** 10 (1977).
90. K. N. von Kaulla and T. S. McDonald, *Blood*, **13,** 811 (1958).
91. H. Lackner and C. Merskey, *Brit. J. Haematol.*, **6,** 402 (1960).
92. M. Schmidhauser-Kopp and E. Eichenberger, *Experientia*, **8,** 354 (1952).
93. H. Vinazzer, *Wien. Z. Inn. Med.*, **32,** 167 (1951).
94. H. B. W. Greig, *Lancet*, **2,** 16 (1956).
95. H. M. Chiu, J. Hirsh, W. L. Yung, E. Regoeczi, and M. Gent, *Blood*, **49,** 171 (1977).
96. Y. Konttinen, *Scand. J. Clin. Lab. Invest.*, **14,** 15 (1962).
97. F. K. Beller and D. Sellin, *Arzneim.-Forsch.*, **10,** 758 (1960).
98. B. A. Kudryashov and L. A. Lyapina, *Vopr. Med. Khim.*, **23,** 44 (1977), *Chem. Abstr. Biochem. Sect.*, **86,** p. 28, Abstr. 150, 444 (1977).
99. E. T. Yin and O. Tangen. "Heparin, Heparinoids and Blood Coagulation," in *Heparin, Chemistry and Clinical Usage*, V. V. Kakkar and D. P. Thomas, Eds., Academic Press, London, 1976, p. 121.
100. S. Bergström, *Z. Physiol. Chem.*, **238,** k63 (1936).
101. E. Chargaff, F. W. Bancroft, and M. Stanley-Brown, *J. Biol. Chem.*, **115,** 155 (1936).
102. E. Husemann, *J. Prakt. Chem.*, **155,** 13 (1940).
103. E. Husemann, K. N. von Kaulla, and R. Kappesser, *Z. Naturforsch.*, **1,** 584 (1946).
104. W. Sandritter, M. Huppert, and G. Schlüter, *Klin. Wochenschr.*, **36,** 651 (1958).
105. H. J. Dauer, *Z. Allgemeinmed.*, **47,** 1816 (1971).
106. S. N. Joffee, E. J. Immelman, and J. H. Louw, *South Afr. J. Surg.*, **2** (3), 108 (1973).
107. R. Bokonjic, *Ärztl. Prax.*, **23,** 2033 (1971).
108. R. Stelzer, *Klin. Mitteilungsbl. Augenheilkd.*, **143** (4), 519 (1966).
109. R. Taugner and K.-P. Karsunky, unpublished expertise, 1968.
110. H. Schön and M. Sauer, *Arzneim.-Forsch.* (*Drug Res.*), **13** (8), 718 (1963).
111. A. C. Asmal, W. P. Leary, J. Carboni, and C. J. Lockett, *South Afr. Med. J.* **49,** 1091 (1975).

112. H. Felix and P. Canal, *Vie Méd. M. T.*, **4,** 141 (1962).

113. G. Frandoli and P. L. Spreafico, *Farmaco*, **27,** 514 (1972).

114. D. Platt, *Med. Welt*, **23,** 1767 (1972).

115. W. Henk and G. Nebosis, *Wien. Klin. Wochenschr.*, **10,** 191 (1968).

116. H. Köstering, F. König, S. Weber, E. Warmann, and M. Guerrero, *Med. Welt*, **24,** 139 (1973).

117. E. S. Oleson, *Activation of the Blood Fibrinolytic System*, Munksgaard, Copenhagen, 1965.

118. S. Coccheri and V. de Rosa, in *Proceedings of the Third International Conference on Synthetic Fibrinolytic Agents, Glasgow*, 1976, Raven Press, New York, 1978.

119. Y. Konttinen, *Scand. J. Clin. Lab. Invest.*, **14** (1), 72 (1962).

120. G. Cultrera, C. Pasotti, A. Gibelli, P. Giarola, A. E. Tammaro, and P. De Nicola, *Arzneim.-Forsch.* (*Drug Res.*), **19,** 372 (1969).

121. P. M. Mannucci, C. di Santo, and F. Franchi, *Experientia*, **33,** 1478 (1976).

122. A. N. Teien, U. Abildgaard, and M. Höök, *Thromb. Res.* **8,** 859 (1976).

123. M. Höök, U. Lindahl, and P.-H. Iverius, *Biochem. J.*, **137,** 33 (1974).

124. E. Marmo, E. Lampa, C. Vacca, F. Rossi, R. Spadaro, and A. Sannino, *Arch. Sci. Med.*, **132,** 83 (1975). *Chem. Abstr.* **86** (37478), 11 (1977).

125. R. Pulver, *Arzneim.-Forsch.* (*Drug-Res.*), **12,** 528 (1962).

126. R. Pulver, *Arzneim.-Forsch.* (*Drug-Res.*), **15,** 1320 (1965).

127. R. Pulver, C. Montigel, and B. Herrmann, *Arzneim.-Forsch.* (*Drug Res.*), **13,** 194 (1963).

128. F. Gycha, G. Osterheld, and A. Taller, *Med. Welt*, **23,** 310 (1972).

129. M. Erlac, *Med. Welt*, **22,** 2067 (1971).

130. W. Burkl, *Arzneim.-Forsch.* (*Drug Res.*), **15** (3), 253 (1965).

131. E. Marmo and A. Matera, *Arzneim.-Forsch.* (*Drug Res.*), **23,** 846 (1973).

132. A. C. Enislidis, *Med. Welt*, **23,** 733 (1972).

133. H. Greiling and M. Kaneko, *Arzneim.-Forsch.* (*Drug Res.*), **23,** 593 (1973).

134. J. Schoch, *Fortschr. Med.* **93,** 133 (1975).

135. D. Kruze, K. Fehr, H. Menninger, and A. Böni, *Z. Rheumatol.*, **35,** 377 (1976).

136. S. Okamoto, "Mode of Action of Nonenzymatic Activators of Fibrinolysis: With Reference to an Antitumor Agent and to Dextran Sulfate, in *Synthetic Fibrinolytic Thrombolytic Agents*, K. N. von Kaulla and J. F. Davidson, Eds., Thomas, Springfield, Ill., 1975, p. 118.

137. J. A. Moncrief, "Specificity of Sharply Cut Dextran Fraction to Inhibit Thrombosis Propagation," in *Dextrans, Current Concepts of Basic Actions and Chemical Applications*, J. R. Derrick and M. M. Guest, Eds., Thomas, Springfield, Ill., 1971, p. 77.

138. M. I. Barnhart, J. Gilroy, and J. S. Meyer, "Platelet Function in Acute Stroke. Patients Treated with Rheomacrodex," in *Dextrans, Current Concepts of Basic Actions and Chemical Applications*, J. R. Derrick and M. M. Guest, Eds., Thomas, Springfield, Ill., 1971, p. 162.

139. S. E. Bergentz, *Anesth. Analg. Reanim.* **33** (9), 573 (1976).

140. M. Åberg, S. E. Bergentz, and U. Hedner, *Ann. Surg.*, **181** (3), 342 (1975).

141. M. W. Rampling, D. A. Lane, and V. V. Kakkar, *Thromb. Res.*, **9,** 379 (1976).

142. A. S. Gallus and J. Hirsh, *Drugs*, **12,** 134 (1976).

143. J. W. Walkley, J. Tillman, and J. Bonnar, *J. Pharm. Pharmacol.*, **28,** 29 (1976).

144. E. H. Hansen, P. Jessing, H. Lindewald, P. Ostergaard, T. Olesen, and E. I. Malver, *J. Bone Joint Surg.* **58-A** (8), 1089 (1976).

145. W. R. Bell, G. Bolton, and W. R. Pitney, *Brit. J. Haematol.*, **13,** 581 (1967).

146. M. R. Ewart, M. W. C. Hatton, J. M. Basford, and K. S. Dodgson, *Biochem. J.*, **118,** 603 (1970).

147. S. V. Pizzo, M. L. Schwartz, R. L. Hill, and P. A. McKee, *J. Clin. Invest.*, **51,** 2841 (1972).

148. G. H. Barlow, W. R. Hollemann, and L. Lorand, *Res. Commun. Chem. Pathol. Pharmacol.*, **1,** 39 (1970).

149. G. R. M. Prentice, A. G. G. Turpie, and A. A. Hassanein, *Lancet*, **1,** 644 (1969).

150. W. W. Barrie, E. H. Wood, P. Crumlish, C. D. Forbes, and G. R. M. Prentice, *Brit. Med. J.*, **4,** 130 (1974).

151. E. Regoeczi and W. R. Bell, *Brit. J. Haematol.*, **16,** 573 (1969).

152. A. A. Sharp, B. A. Warren, A. M. Paxton, and M. J. Allington, *Lancet*, **1,** 493 (1968).

153. D. A. Tibbutt, E. W. Williams, M. W. Walker, C. N. Chectermann, J. M. Holt, and A. A. Sharp, *Brit. J. Haematol.* **27,** 407 (1974).

154. R. A. O'Reilly, *N. Engl. J. Med.*, **282,** 1448 (1970).

155. E. von Kaulla and K. N. von Kaulla, *Münch. Med. Wochenschr.* **116,** 1387 (1974).

156. E. von Kaulla and K. N. von Kaulla, *Am. J. Clin. Pathol.*, **48,** 69 (1967).

157. E. von Kaulla and K. N. von Kaulla. *Proceedings of the Ninth Congress of the International Society of Haematology, Mexico 1962,* Karger, Basel, 1964, pp. 133–139.
158. E. Marciniak, C. H. Farley, and D. E. De-Simone, *Blood,* **43,** 219 (1974).
159. K. N. von Kaulla and E. von Kaulla, *Circ. Res.,* **14,** 436 (1964).
160. P. Wahlberg and D. Nyman, *N. Engl. J. Med.,* **286,** 46 (1972).
161. F. W. Schofield, *Can. Vet. Rec.,* **3,** 74 (1932).
162. K. P. Link, *Harvey Lect.,* **39,** 162 (1943–1944).
163. R. Anschütz, *Ber. Chem. Ges.,* **36,** 465 (1903).
164. J. B. Bingham. O. O. Meyer, and F. J. Pohle, *Am. J. Med. Sci.* **202,** 563 (1941).
165. K. P. Link, *Circulation,* **19,** 97 (1949).
166. E. Petraček, *Čas. Lék. Čes.,* **83,** 1204 (1944).
167. K. N. von Kaulla and R. Pulver, *Schweiz. Med. Wochenschr.,* **78,** 806 (1948).
168. R. Pulver and K. N. von Kaulla, *Schweiz. Med. Wochenschr.,* **78,** 956 (1948).
169. S. Divald and M. M. Joullié, in *Medicinal Chemistry,* 3rd ed., Part II, A. Burger, Ed., Wiley-Interscience, New York, 1970, Ch. 41, pp. 1092–1122.
170. H. Kabat, E. F. Stohlman, and M. I. Smith, *J. Pharmacol. Exp. Ther.,* **80,** 160 (1944).
171. J. W. Suttie, G. A. Grant, C. H. T. Esmon, and D. V. Shah, *Mayo Clin. Proc.,* **49,** 933 (1974).
172. S. H. Goodnight, D. I. Feinstein, B. Østerud, and S. I. Rapaport, *Blood,* **38** (1), 1 (1971).
173. M. J. Larrieu and D. Meyer, *Lancet,* **2,** 1085 (1970).
174. C. T. Esmon, J. W. Suttie, and C. M. Jackson, *J. Biol. Chem.,* **250,** 4095 (1975).
175. A. S. Gallus and J. Hirsh, *Drugs,* **12,** 47 (1976).
176. G. Wilding, B. S. Blumberg, and E. S. Vesell, *Science,* **195** (4282), 991 (1977).
177. L. Poller, *Proc. Roy. Soc. Med.,* **68** (10), 629 (1975).
178. L. Biland, O. Rüst, D. Nyman, and F. Duckert, *Schweiz. Rundsch. Med.* **63** (52), 1568 (1974).
179. D. J. Pinto, *Brit. J. Surg.,* **57,** 349 (1970).
180. M. A. Ritter and C. W. Hamilton, *Ann. Surg.,* **181,** 896 (1975).
181. *Med. World News,* August 22, 1977, p. 36.
182. G. A. Mayer, *Am. J. Clin. Pathol.,* **65,** 402 (1974).
183. R. D. Thornes, *J. Ir. Coll. Phys. Surg.,* **2,** 41 (1972).
184. (a) P. Hilgard and R. D. Thornes, *Eu. J. Cancer,* **12,** 755 (1976). (b) R. M. Nalbandian, I. J. Mader, J. L. Barret, and J. F. Pearce, *J. Am. Med. Assoc.,* **192,** 603 (1965).
185. H. Schneider and F. K. Beller, *Med. Welt,* **28,** 432 (1977).
186. E. D. Williams and I. Doniach, *Endocrinology,* **21,** 421 (1961).
187. M. Carson and M. Reid, *Lancet,* **1,** 1356 (1976).
188. *J. Am. Med. Assoc.* (*Med. News*), **234,** 1015 (1975).
189. W. W. Coon and P. K. Willis, *Arch. Intern. Med.,* **133,** 386 (1974).
190. P. D. Hansten, *Drug Interactions,* Lea & Febiger, Philadelphia, 1973, pp. 17ff.
191. F. Koller, *Schweiz. Rundsch. Med.* **66** (2), 37 (1977).
192. W. H. Jeffery, T. A. Ahlin, C. Goren, and W. R. Hardy, *J. Am. Med. Assoc.* **236** (25), 2881 (1976).
193. D. Bethge, *Deut. Med. Wochenschr.,* **102,** 590 (1977).
194. J. J. Schrogie, H. M. Solomon, and P. D. Zieve, *Clin. Pharmacol. Ther.,* **8,** 670 (1970).
195. R. A. O'Reilly, *New Engl. J. Med.* **295,** 354 (1976).
196. M. Kristensen and J. Moelholm-Hansen, *Diabetes,* **16** (4), 211 (1967).
197. L. Skovsted, M. Kristensen, J. Mølholm-Hansen, and K. Siersback-Nielsen, *Acta Med. Scand.,* **199,** 513 (1976).
198. H. J. Weiss, *Am. Heart J.,* **92,** 86 (1976).
199. A. S. Gallus and J. Hirsh, *Drugs,* **12,** 132 (1976).
200. E. Genton, M. Gent, J. Hirsh, and L. Harker, *New Engl. J. Med.,* **293,** 1174–1178, 1296 (1973).
201. M. Atik, Letter to the Editor, *New Engl. J. Med.* **294,** 1122 (1976).
202. J. M. Lambie, *Brit. Med. J.,* **2,** 144 (1970).
203. J. Bonnar, J. J. Walsh, and M. Haddon, *Abstract* 243, 4th International Congress on Thrombosis and Haemostasis, Vienna, June 1973, p. 278.
204. J. Hirsh, E. F. O'Sullivan, and A. S. M. Martin, *Blood,* **32,** 726 (1968).
205. J. F. Mustard and M. A. Packham, *Circulation,* **42,** 1 (1970).
206. P. P. Steele, H. S. Weily, and E. Genton, *N. Engl. J. Med.,* **288,** 1149 (1973).
207. T. Sano, M. G. J. Boxer, L. A. Boxer, and M. Yokoyama, *Thromb. Diath. Haemorrh.,* **25,** 524 (1971).
208. C.-H. Ts'ao, R. Lo, and J. Raymond, *Am. J. Clin. Pathol.,* **65** (4), 518 (1976).
209. J. H. Weiss, *J. Lab. Clin. Med.,* **87** (6), 909 (1976).

210. J. Mundall, P. Quintero, K. N. von Kaulla, B. Harmon, and J. Austin, *Neurology*, **22,** 280 (1972).
211. K. Breddin, H. J. Krywanek, and M. Ziemen, *Acta Clin. Belg.*, **30,** 3 (1975).
212. B. V. Chater, *Brit. J. Haematol.*, **32,** 513 (1976).
213. F. C. Berthoux, A. M. Freyria, and J. Traeger, *Pathol. Biol.*, **25** (3), 179 (1977).
214. E. T. Yin, L. C. Guidice, and S. Wessler, *J. Lab. Clin. Pathol.*, **82,** 390 (1973).
215. T. Okuno and D. Crockatt, *Am. J. Clin. Pathol.*, **67,** 351 (1977).
216. K. Breddin, H. J. Krzywanek, and M. Ziemen, in *XVIII Hamburger Symposion über Blutgerinnung 1975*, R. Marx and H. A. Thies, Eds., Roche, Grenzach-Wyhlen p. 109.
217. J. R. Couch and R. S. Hassanein, *Neurology*, **26,** 888 (1976).
218. J. H. Dougherty, D. E. Levy, and B. B. Weksler, *Lancet*, **1,** 821 (1977).
219. S. C. Sharma, G. P. Vijayan, M. L. Suri, and H. N. Seth, *J. Clin. Pathol.*, **30** (7), 649 (1977).
220. H. Yamazaki, T. Sano, T. Asano, and H. Hidaka, *Thromb. Res.*, Suppl. II, **8,** 217 (1976).
221. J. Vreeken, *Lancet*, **1,** 774 (1977).
222. J. W. Haerem, *Atherosclerosis*, **15,** 199 (1972).
223. J. F. Mustard and M. A. Packham, *Circulation Suppl.*, **39,** 40 (1969).
224. S. Berger and E. D. Salzmann, "Thromboembolic Complications of Prosthetis Devices," in *Progress in Haemostasis and Thrombosis*, Vol. 2, T. H. Spaet, Ed., Grune & Stratton, New York, 1974, p. 273.
225. J. B. Smith, C. Ingerman, J. J. Kocsis, and M. J. Silver, *J. Clin. Invest.*, **52,** 965 (1973).
226. A. L. Willis, *Prostaglandins*, **5,** 1 (1974).
227. J. B. Smith, C. Ingerman, and J. J. Kocsis, *J. Clin. Invest.*, **53,** 1468 (1974).
228. G. J. Roth and P. W. Majerns, *J. Clin. Invest.*, **56,** 624 (1975).
229. T. Y. Wang, C. V. Hussey, and J. C. Garancis, *Am. J. Clin. Pathol.*, **67** (4), 362 (1977).
230. *Chem. Eng. News*, September 5, 1977, p. 19.
231. M. Pfenninger and U. F. Gruber, *Schweiz. Med. Wochenschr.*, **107** (28), 1335 (1977).
232. W. H. Harris, E. W. Salzman, C. Athanasoulis, A. C. Waltman, S. Baum, and R. W. DeSanctis, *J. Bone Joint Surg.*, **56A,** 1522 (1974).
233. E. W. Salzman, W. H. Harris, and R. W. DeSanctis, *New Engl. J. Med.*, **284,** 1287 (1971).
234. J. T. G. Renney, E. F. O'Sullivan, and J. G. Lynch, 16.*Arbeitstagung der D.A.B., Bonn*, 1972, Schattauer Verlag, Stuttgart, 1973.
235. C. P. Clagett, D. F. Brier, C. B. Rosoff, P. B. Schneider, and E. W. Salzman, *Surg. Forum*, **25,** 473 (1974).
236. K. Breddin and I. Scharrer, *Folia Angiol.*, **23,** 187 (1973).
237. J. H. Stewart, P. C. Farrell, and M. Dixon, *Aust. N.Z. J. Med.* **5,** 117 (1975).
238. F. E. Preston, I. G. Emmanuel, D. A. Winfield, and R. G. Malia, *Brit. Med. J.* **3,** 548 (1974).
239. Colfarit Symposion III, Acetylsalicylsäure bei arterieller Verschlusskrankheit, Bayer, Cologne, 1975.
240. M. A. Abrishami and J. Thomas, *Ann. Allerg.*, **39** (1), 28 (1977).
241. P. Steele, J. Rainwater, and E. Genton, *Clin. Res.*, **25** (2), 145A (1977).
242. J. A. Blakely, N. Seth, and N. Varik, *Abstract* 130, Fourth International Congress on Thrombosis and Haemostasis, Vienna, June 1973, p. 164.
243. M. Ali and W. D. McDonald, *J. Lab. Clin. Med.*, **89** (4), 868 (1977).
244. K. K. Wu and C. S. L. Ku, *Fed. Proc.*, **36** (2), 380 (1977).
245. G. E. Evans, *Surg. Forum*, **23,** 239 (1972).
246. A. Kaegi, G. Pineo, and A. Shimizu, *N. Engl. J. Med.*, **290,** 304 (1974).
247. H. S. Weily and E. Genton, *Circulation*, **42,** 967 (1970).
248. P. P. Steele, H. S. Weily, and E. Genton, *New Engl. J. Med.*, **288,** 1148 (1973).
249. M. P. Cucuiano, E. E. Nishizawa, and J. F. Mustard, *J. Lab. Clin. Med.*, **77,** 958 (1971).
250. L. A. Harker and S. J. Schlichter, *Thromb. Diath. Haemorrh.*, **31,** 188 (1974).
251. J. E. Arrants and P. Hairston, *Am. Surg.*, **38,** 432 (1972).
252. J. S. Cameron, D. Gill, D. R. Turner, C. Chantler, C. S. Ogg, G. Vosnides, and D. G. Williams, *Lancet*, **2,** 923 (1975).
253. S. Niewiarowski, H. Lukasiewicz, N. Nath, and A. T. Sha, *J. Lab. Clin. Med.*, **86,** 64 (1975).
254. O. Ponari, E. Civardi, A. G. Detori, A. Megha, R. Poti and G. Bulleti, *Arzneim.-Forsch.* (*Drug Res.*), **26** (8), 1532 (1976).
255. W. Jäger, I. Scharrer, U. Satkowski, and K. Breddin, *Arzneim.-Forsch.* (*Drug Res.*), **25** (12), 1938 (1975).
256. R. L. Kinlough-Rathbone, "The Effects of Some Other Drugs on Platelet Function, in *Platelets, Drugs and Thrombosis*, J. Hirsh, J. F. Cade, A. S. Gallus, and E. Schonbaum, Eds., Karger, Basel 1975, p. 124.

257. Coronary Drug Project Research Group, *J. Am. Med. Assoc.*, **231,** 360 (1975).

258. R. Zimmermann, A. Hoffrichter, E. Walter, W. Ehlers, K. Andrassy, P. D. Lang, G. Schlierf, E. Weber, and P. Barth. *Deut. Med. Wochenschr.*, **102,** 509 (1977).

259. C. M. Ogston, D. Ogston and G. M. MacAndrew, *Curr. Ther. Res.*, **7,** 437 (1965).

260. C. D. Brooks, *Curr. Ther. Res.*, **15,** 180 (1973).

261. M. I. Kusin, I. N. Bokarew, A. J. Smoljanizki, I. P. Ljubezow, and I. C. Ippolitow, *Folia Haematol.* (Leipzig), **102,** 230 (1975).

262. J. Roba, R. Bourgain, R. Andries, M. Claeys, W. van Opstal, and G. Lambelin, *Thromb. Res.*, **9,** 585 (1976).

262. E. E. Nishizawa, D. J. Wynalda, and D. E. Svydam, *Thromb. Diath. Haemorrh.*, Suppl., **60,** 415 (1974).

264. G. de Gaetano, M. C. Tonolli, M. P. Bertoni, and M. C. Roncaglioni, *Haemostasis*, **6,** 127 (1977).

265. B. T. Lyman and G. J. Johnson, *Fed. Proc.*, **36** (3), 380 (1977), abstract.

266. (a) J. N. Shanberge, J. Kambayashi, and M. Nakagawa, *Thromb. Res.*, **9,** 595 (1976). (b) A. S. Gallus and J. Hirsh, *Drugs*, **12,** 132 (1976).

267. (a) S. Bygdeman and O. Tangen, *Thromb. Res.*, **11,** 141 (1977). (b) J. F. Cade, D. Basu, T. J. Muckle, and J. Hirsh, *Thromb. Diath. Haemorrh.*, **32,** 592 (1974).

268. (a) Y. Pekcelen and S. Inceman, *Thromb. Haemostas.*, **35** (2), 485 (1976). (b) E. Johannson, *Läkartidningen*, **71,** 2687 (1974).

269. (a) T. C. Economopoulos, A. G. Papayannis, N. E. Stathakis, G. Arapakis, and C. Gardikas, *Acta Haematol.*, **57,** 266 (1977). (b) P. Six, G. A. Marbet, M. Walter, D. Nyman, F. Duckert, G. Mader, A. da Silva, and L. K. Widmer, in *Blutgerinnung und Antikoagulantien*, K. Neuhaus and F. Duckert, Eds., Schattauer-Verlag, Stuttgart, 1976, p. 111.

270. H. Poliwoda, R. Schneider, and H. J. Avenarius, *Med. Klin.*, **72,** 451 (1977).

271. Urokinase-Streptokinase Embolism Trial, Phase 2, Results, *J. Am. Med. Assoc.*, **229,** 1606 (1974).

272. S. S. Shapiro, in *Drugs and Hematologic Reactions*, N. V. Dimitrov and J. H. Nadine, Eds., Grune & Stratton, New York, 1974, p. 311.

273. E. C. DeRenzo, P. K. Siiteri, B. L. Hutchings, and P. H. Bell, *Biol. Chem.* **242,** 533 (1967).

274. K. N. N. Reddy and G. Markus, *J. Biol. Chem.*, **247,** 1683 (1972).

275. H. Trobisch, *Postgrad. Med. J.*, **49** (suppl. 5), 17 (1973).

276. R. Gottlob, E. B. Nashef, P. Donas, F. Piza, and R. Kolb, *Thromb. Diath. Haemorrh.*, **29,** 393 (1973).

277. R. Schmutzler and F. Koller, "Thrombolytic Therapy," in *Recent Advantages in Blood Coagulation*, L. Poller, Ed., Churchill, London, 1969, p. 299.

278. J. L. Tullis, *Clot*, Thomas, Springfield, Ill. 1976, p. 474.

279. K. N. von Kaulla, *J. Lab. Clin. Med.*, **44,** 944 (1954).

280. A. Lesuk, L. Terminello, and J. H. Travez, *Science*, **147,** 880 (1965).

281. B. N. Violand and F. J. Castellino, *J. Biol. Chem.*, **251** (1), 3906 (1976).

282. E. Genton and H. N. Claman, *J. Lab. Clin. Mech.*, **75,** 619 (1970).

283. A. P. Fletcher, N. Alkjaersig, S. Sherry, E. Genton, J. Hirsh, and F. Bachmann, *J. Lab. Clin. Med.*, **65,** 713 (1965).

284. N. Riggenbach and K. N. von Kaulla, *Cancer*, **14,** 889 (1961).

285. B. Bizzi, G. Leone, and F. Accorrà, *Haemostasis*, **5,** 147 (1976).

286. G. Coscas, *Med. Trib.*, **49,** 4 (1974).

287. G. H. Barlow and L. Lazer, *Thromb. Res.*, **1,** 201 (1972).

288. B. Astedt, B. Bladh, and L. Holmberg, *Experientia*, **33** (5), 589 (1977).

289. K. N. von Kaulla, *Klin. Wochenschr.*, **29,** 422 (1951).

290. O. Storm, P. Ollendorff, E. Drewsen, and P. Tang, *Thromb. Diath. Haemorrh.*, **32,** 468 (1974).

291. G. A. Marbet, M. Walter, P. Six, D. Nyman, O. Rüst, L. Biland, F. Duchert, G. Madar, A. da Silva, L. K. Widmer, H. E. Schmitt, and J. Vokal, in *Blurgerinnung und Antikoagulantien*, K. Neuhaus and F. Duckert, Eds., Schattauer-Verlag, Stuttgart, 1976, p. 87.

292. D. E. Fitzgerald, E. P. Frisch, and R. D. Thornes, *J. Ir. Coll. Phys. Surg.*, **1,** 123 (1972).

293. P. N. Sawyer, *Thromb. Res.*, **10,** 531 (1977).

294. C. Diffong and T. Saldeen, *Thromb. Res.*, **9** (6), 611 (1976).

295. J. C. Frantantoni, *Am. Heart J.*, **93,** 271 (1977).

296. K. N. von Kaulla, *Circulation*, **17,** 187 (1958).

297. N. Aoki and K. N. von Kaulla, *Am. J. Clin. Pathol.*, **55,** 171 (1971).

298. N. Aoki, *J. Biochem.*, **75,** 731 (1974).

299. S. Thorsen, P. Glas-Greenwalt, and T. Astrup, *Thromb. Diath. Haemorrh.*, **28,** 65 (1972).
300. V. Gurewich, E. Hyde, and B. Lipinski, *Blood,* **46,** 555 (1975).
301. N. Aoki and K. N. von Kaulla, *Thromb. Diath. Haemorrh.*, **22,** 251 (1969).
302. K. N. von Kaulla, *Thromb. Diath. Haemorrh.*, **9,** 220 (1963).
303. K. N. von Kaulla, D. Fogleman, and H. Mueller, "Clot Penetration and Fibrin Adsorption of Synthetic Fibrinolytic Compounds," in *Progress in Chemical Fibrinolysis and Thrombolysis*, Vol. 1, J. F. Davidson, M. M. Samama, and P. C. Desnoyer, Eds., Raven Press, New York, 1975, p. 45.
304. N. Aoki and K. N. von Kaulla, *J. Lab. Clin. Med.*, **78,** 354 (1971).
305. K. N. von Kaulla, *Arch. Biochem. Biophys.*, **96,** 4 (1962).
306. K. N. von Kaulla, in *Chemical Control of Fibrinolysis-Thrombolysis*, J. E. Shor, Ed., Wiley-Interscience, New York, 1970, p. 1.
307. K. N. von Kaulla and J. F. Davidson, Eds., *Synthetic Fibrinolytic Thrombolytic Agents. Chemical, Biochemical, Pharmacological and Clinical Aspects*, Thomas, Springfield Ill., 1975.
308. J. F. Davidson, M. M. Samama, and P. C. Desnoyers, Eds., *Progress in Chemical Fibrinolysis and Thrombolysis*, Vol. 1, Raven Press, New York, 1975.
309. M. Yoshimito, K. N. von Kaulla, and C. Hansch, *J. Med. Chem.*, **10,** 276 (1975).
310. C. F. Chignell, *Mol. Pharmacol.*, **5,** 455 (1969).
311. K. N. von Kaulla, *Experientia*, **30,** 959 (1974).
312. K. N. von Kaulla, in K. N. von Kaulla and J. F. Davidson, Eds., *Synthetic Fibrinolytic Thrombolytic Agents*, Thomas, Springfield, Ill., 1975, p. 166.
313. K. N. von Kaulla, *Wien. Z. Inn. Med.*, **8** (33), 329 (1952).
314. L. A. Moroz, *New Engl. J. Med.*, **296,** 525 (1977).
315. S. Visudhiphan, personal communication.
316. K. T. Augusti, M. E. Benaim, H. A. Bevur, and R. Virden, *Atherosclerosis*, **21,** 409 (1975).
317. C. A. Bouvier, and S. Berthoud, *Helv. Med. Acta*, **34,** 170 (1968).
318. G. Schulze, H. Polivoda, and H. Köstering, *Münch. Med. Wochenschr.*, **105,** 1692 (1963).
319. R. Biggs, R. G. Macfarlane, and J. Pilling, *Lancet*, **1,** 402 (1947).
320. K. N. von Kaulla, *Schweiz. Med. Wochenschr.*, **77,** 313 (1947).
321. S. A. Schneck and K. N. von Kaulla, *Neurology*, **11,** 959 (1961).
322. J. D. Cash, in *Progress in Chemical Fibrinolysis and Thrombolysis*, Vol. 1, J. F. Davidson, M. M. Samama, and P. Desnoyers, Eds., Raven Press, New York, 1975, p. 97.
323. I. S. Chohan, I. Singh, J. Vermylen, and M. Verstraete, *Exp. Haematol.*, **5,** 153 (1977).
324. T. Kumada and A. Yasushi, *Thromb. Haemostas.*, **36** (2), 451 (1976).
325. M. Pandolfi, M. S. Isacson, and I. M. Nilsson, *Acta Med. Scand.*, **186,** 1 (1969).
326. S. Isacson and I. M. Nilsson, *Acta Chir. Scand.*, **138,** 313 (1972).
327. G. R. Fearnley, G. V. Chakrabarti, and E. Hocking, *Lancet*, **2,** 1008 (1967).
328. A. Perzanowski, M. Bielawiec, and M. Myśliwiec, *Folia Haematol.* (Leipzig), **103,** 381 (1976).
329. S. Isacson and I. M. Nilsson, *Scand. J. Haematol.*, **7,** 404 (1970).
330. U. Hedner, I. M. Nilsson, and S. Isacsson, *Folia Haematol.* (Leipzig), **103,** 372 (1976).
331. J. D. Walker and J. F. Davidson, in *Proceedings of the Third International Conference on Synthetic Fibrinolytic-Thrombolytic Agents, Glasgow 1976*, Raven Press, New York, 1978.
332. P. H. Wise, M. Chapman, D. W. Thomas, A. R. Clarkson, P. E. Harding, and J. B. Edwards, *Brit. Med.*, **1,** 70 (1976).
333. U. Hedner and I. M. Nilsson, in *Proceedings of the Third International Conference on Synthetic Fibrinolytic-Thrombolytic Agents, Glasgow 1976*, Raven Press, New York, 1978.
334. D. Thilo and K. N. von Kaulla, *J. Med. Chem.*, **13,** 503 (1970).
335. J. Gerloff and K. N. von Kaulla, *Proc. Soc. Exp. Biol. Med.*, **141,** 298 (1972).
336. E. von Kaulla and K. N. von Kaulla, *Nature New Biol.* **240,** 144 (1975).
337. J. L. Tullis, *Clot*, Thomas, Springfield, Ill., 1976, p. 163.
338. J. Robinson, P. M. Aggeler, G. P. Nicol, and A. S. Douglas, *Brit. J. Haematol.*, **13,** 510 (1967).
339. E. Bidwell, *Ann. Rev. Med.*, **20,** 63 (1969).
340. *Med. World News*, July 25, 1977, p. 41.
341. K. N. von Kaulla and T. Matsumura, *Klin. Wochenschr.*, **46,** 26 (1968).
342. K. N. von Kaulla and E. von Kaulla, *Acta Haematol.*, **30,** 25 (1963).
343. K. N. von Kaulla and H. Swan, *J. Thorac. Surg.*, **36,** 519 (1958).
344. N. Alkjaersig, A. P. Fletcher, and S. Sherry, *J. Biol. Chem.*, **234,** 832 (1959).

345. D. Green, *Lancet*, **2,** 486 (1971).
346. F. A. Anderer, *Z. Naturforsch.*, **20b,** 462 (1965).
347. N. U. Bang, F. K. Beller, E. Deutsch, and E. F. Mammen, *Thrombosis and Bleeding Disorders: Theory and Methods*, Thieme, Stuttgart, Academic Press, New York, 1971, p. 311.
348. M. M. Stevenson and V. Anido, Abstract 271, American Society of Hematologists, December 1970.
349. R. Ryback and J. F. Desforges, *Arch. Intern. Med.*, **125,** 475 (1970).
350. G. Chargaff and K. B. Olson, *J. Biol. Chem.*, **122,** 1953 (1938).
351. B. H. Hyun, R. E. Pence, J. C. Davila, J. Butcher, and R. P. Custer, *Surg. Gynecol., Obstetr.*, **115,** 191 (1962).
352. N. U. Bang, F. K. Beller, E. Deutsch, and E. F. Mammen, *Thrombosis and Bleeding Disorders: Theory and Methods*, Thieme, Stuttgart; Academic Press, New York, 1971, pp. 280–281.
353. *U.S. Dispensatory*, 26th ed., Lippincott, Philadelphia, 1967, p. 904.
354. J. L. Tullis, *Clot*, Thomas, Springfield, Ill., 1976, p. 469.
355. A. S. Douglas, *Anticoagulant Therapy*, Blackwell, Oxford, 1962, p. 333.
356. W. B. Abott and W. Austen, *Surgery*, **78** (6), 723 (1975).
357. N. Aoki and K. N. von Kaulla, *Thromb. Diath. Haemorrh.*, **16,** 586 (1966).
358. K. K. Nagda, personal communication, 1976.
359. S. Isacson and I. M. Nilsson, in *Synthetic Fibrinolytic Thrombolytic Agents*, K. N. von Kaulla and J. F. Davidson, Eds., Thomas, Springfield, Ill. 1975, p. 312.
360. T. E. Starzl, T. L. Marchioro, K. N. von Kaulla, G. Herman, R. S. Brittain, and W. R. Waddell, *Surg. Gynecol. Obstetr.*, **117,** 657 (1963).
361. S. Wasantapruek and K. N. von Kaulla, *Thromb. Diath. Haemorrh.*, **15,** 284 (1966).
362. K. N. von Kaulla, P. Ostendorf, and L. Leppke, "*In Vitro* Synergism of Endogenously Increased Fibrinolysis with Compound-Induced Fibrinolysis," in *Progress in Chemical Fibrinolysis and Thrombolysis*, Vol. 1, J. F. Davidson, M. M. Samama, and P. C. Desnoyers, Eds., Raven Press, New York, 1975, p. 385.
363. J. Homatas, S. Wasantapruek, E. von Kaulla, K. N. von Kaulla, and B. Eiseman, *Acta Hepato-Splenol.*, **18** (1), 14 (1971).
364. K. N. von Kaulla, E. von Kaulla, S. Wasantapruek, *Acta-Hepato-gastroentrol*, **28,** 1978, in press.
365. R. Chakrabarti, G. R. Fearnley, and E. D. Hocking, *Brit. Med. J.*, **1,** 534 (1964).
366. E. von Kaulla, unpublished results.
367. E. von Kaulla and K. N. von Kaulla, *Klin. Wochensch.*, **51,** 706 (1973).
368. K. N. von Kaulla and E. von Kaulla, *Acta Haematol.*, **30,** 25 (1963).

CHAPTER THIRTY–THREE

Prostaglandins

ROBERT T. BUCKLER
and
DAVID L. GARLING

Chemistry Department
Miles Laboratories, Inc.
Elkhart, Indiana 46514, USA

CONTENTS

1 INTRODUCTION

In the previous edition of this work, the field of prostaglandin research was not deemed extensive enough to merit a chapter of its own. Indeed, the stereochemistry and the absolute configuration of the first few prostaglandins were established conclusively only in 1968. But between 1968 and the end of 1976, prostaglandin research became one of the major areas of interdisciplinary research in the biological sciences. The phenomenal upswing in interest in prostaglandins can best be grasped by an appreciation of the raw statistics of the growth of prostaglandin literature. Through 1970 some 2000 scientific publications appeared, dealing with the chemical, physiological, pharmacological, and other aspects of prostaglandins (1). The yearly rate of issue of scientific publications and patents for 1971–1976 is detailed in Table 33.1 (2). Although returns for 1976 are incomplete, the rate of issue of scientific articles having to do with prostaglandins appears to have leveled off at about 3 per day.

Table 33.1 Yearly Appearance of Prostaglandin Literature Since 1970

Year of Publication	Articles and Monographs	Patents
1976	1053	201
1975	1104	226
1974	1047	138
1973	943	96
1972	604	41
1971	362	21
	5113	723

Thus more than 7000 scientific publications represent, to the end of 1976, the body of scientific knowledge concerning prostaglandins. Clearly it is beyond the scope of this chapter to present anything like a critical, comprehensive summary of the field. Instead this work focuses on areas of prostaglandin research that are relevant to medicinal chemists, namely, areas where prostaglandins are thought to be involved in the etiology of disease states.

Prostaglandins have been implicated, if not always convincingly, not only in major diseases like hypertension, inflammation, and gastrointestinal disturbances, but in such seemingly unrelated disorders as male sterility, asthma (3), psoriasis (4), migraine (5), cystic fibrosis (6), sunburn (7), and simple itch (8).

Many of these diseases seem to offer the opportunity for treatment by replacement therapy with a PG analog if the disease is due to lack of prostaglandins, or with prostaglandin inhibitors if overproduction of prostaglandins is the cause. Just such reasoning has stimulated the synthesis of some 10,000 prostaglandin analogs (our estimate), and many of them appearing in print are taken up in the final section of this chapter. That so many PG analogs have been synthesized is a tribute to the development of many elegant synthetic routes to the prostaglandin system. The overall synthetic chemistry of prostaglandins is not considered here, but it is well discussed in Refs. 1 and 9–12.

Listed for 1975 are 149 review articles on prostaglandins, of which 107 are in English (2). Although this figure is exaggerated by the loose definition of what constitutes a review article, there are still many thorough, recent treatments of almost every aspect of prostaglandin research. The best overall review up to 1973 is Ref. 1. The most up-to-date critical summary of the pharmacology, biochemistry, and physiology of prostaglandins is a three volume series edited by S. M. M. Karim (12–14).

The end of 1976 is not the best time to be reviewing the field of prostaglandin research. Evidence now accumulating suggests that the primary prostaglandins, PGEs and PGFs, may not always be the principal effectors of physiological activity. With the discovery and characterization of the thromboxanes and PGI_2 has come the realization that these substances and the prostaglandin endoperoxides, with their short *in vivo* half-lives, might be the real primary species and, in some cases, the PGEs and PGF's, only intermediates in their catabolic deactivation. This apparently is the case in regard to platelet aggregation. Whether it is generally true has yet to be determined, but the next few years will undoubtedly see a reinterpretation of the importance of the primary prostaglandins, PGE and PGF.

1.1 History of the Discovery of Prostaglandins

During the 1920s and 1930s the realization that many of the body's processes were controlled or affected by small molecules and peptides led to the examination of extracts of a number of tissues and organs for the presence of physiologically active substances. Important discoveries resulted, such as Loewi's identification of the cardiac depressor substance *vagusstoffe* as acetylcholine and Abel's isolation of oxytocin and vasopressin from the posterior lobe of the pituitary gland.

In 1930 Kurzrok and Leib found that human semen both relaxed and contracted human uterine muscle strips (15). From this, they inferred the presence in semen of two substances, one contractile, the other a relaxant (15, 16). A few years later, Goldblatt isolated a depressorlike substance from human seminal plasma that contracted isolated rabbit intestine and isolated guinea pig uterus (17). The active principle could be extracted from seminal plasma with alcohol and, when given intravenously to cats, caused a large fall in blood pressure lasting 30–45 min. The active substance was unstable to alkali and heat, but not to weak acids, behavior that clearly differentiated it from acetylcholine, histamine, and adenosine (18).

At about the same time, von Euler found that similar activity was displayed by extracts of prostate glands and seminal vesicles of several animal species (19, 20). In 1935 he coined the name "prostaglandin" for the substance, by this time known to be an acidic lipid, and a year later he published an extensive description of its pharmacological properties (21, 22). von Euler reported that intravenous administration of prostaglandin caused peripheral vasodilation and lowered blood pressure. It contracted intestinal smooth muscle and stimulated the isolated uterus of many species and was distinct from other lipids such as substance P and vesiglandin.

Interest in prostaglandins declined during World War II but was revived in the late 1940s and early 1950s by Bergström and associates at the Karolinska Institute. In 1947, using a concentrated extract of sheep vesicular glands, they showed that prostaglandin activity was associated with several unsaturated, hydroxy, lipidlike acids. Not until 1956, however, when a program was developed for the large-scale collection and processing of sheep vesicular glands, was enough extract obtained to allow purification and structure determination of the active components (23). By 1960, monitoring their chromotographies with a bioassay based on the ability of prostaglandins to stimulate the rabbit duodenum, Bergström and Sjovall isolated, in crystalline form, the first two prostaglandins: PGE_1 (33.**1**) and $PGF_{1\alpha}$ (33.**2**) (24). Both substances stimulated the rabbit duodenum at concentrations of 10^{-9} g/ml, although PGE_1 was the more active of the two in lowering blood pressure (25, 26). Elemental analysis and mass spectrometry showed both to contain 20 carbon atoms and to have the empirical formulas $C_{20}H_{34}O_5$ (PGE_1) and $C_{20}H_{36}O_5$ ($PGF_{1\alpha}$) (24). Prostaglandin E_1 was determined to be ketonic, and the frequency of the infrared carbonyl stretching absorption (*ca.* 1730 cm^{-1}) indicated a five-membered cyclic ketone (27, 28). Reduction of the ketone function of PGE_1 with sodium borohydride gave two isomeric trihydroxy compounds, one identical to $PGF_{1\alpha}$.

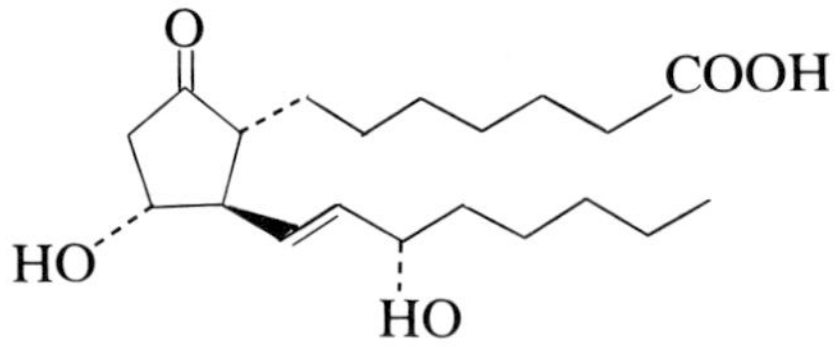

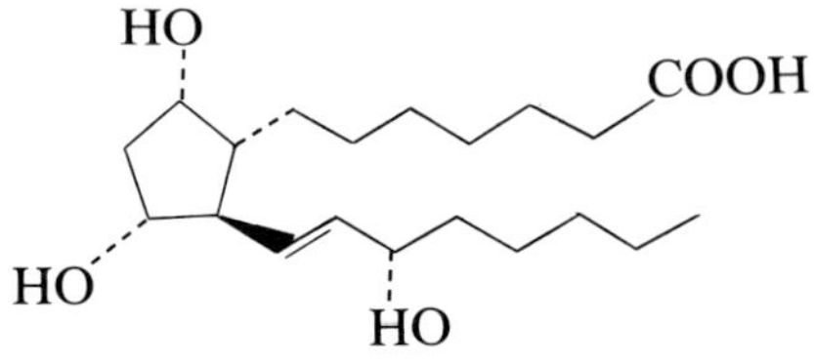

33.**1**

33.**2**

Treatment of PGE_1 with dilute alkali gave a new prostaglandin, named PGA_1 (33.**3**), whose UV absorption at 217 nm indicated it to be a conjugated cyclopentenone. More vigorous treatment with alkali produced an isomer of PGA_1, labeled PGB_1 (33.**4**). Its UV absorption at 278 nm indicated a doubly conjugated structure arising from migration of the ring double bond of PGA_1 (24). This base-catalyzed transformation to PGAs and then to PGBs is characteristic of all E-type prostaglandins and accounts for their instability at high pH.

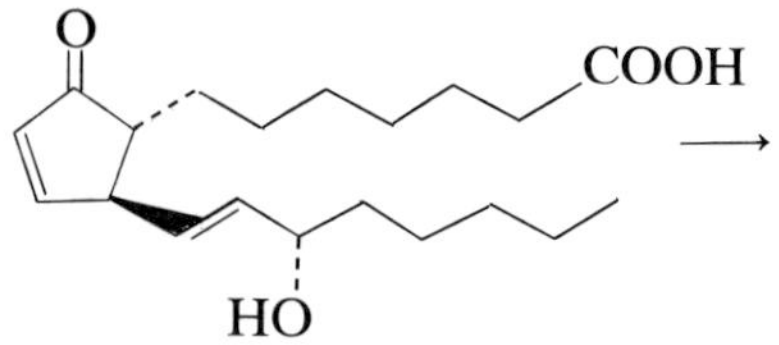

33.**3**

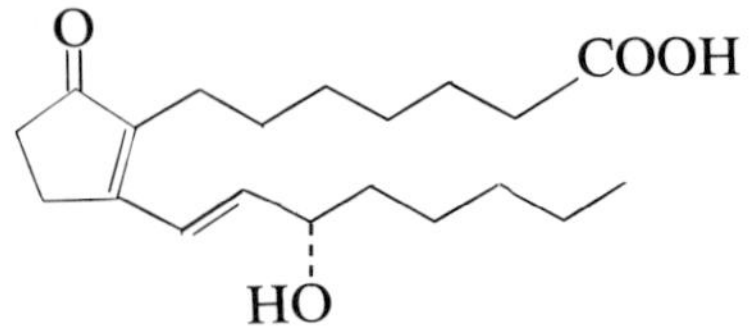

33.**4**

Oxidation of PGE_1 and $PGF_{1\alpha}$ with chromic acid produced suberic acid, showing that both possessed six methylene groups in a linear chain (23). The base-catalyzed elimination of water from PGE_1 to give an $\alpha\beta$-unsaturated ketone placed one of its two hydroxyl groups β to the ketone function. The other hydroxyl group was placed by oxidative ozonolysis of the 15-acetate of PGA_1, which gave, after deacetylation, L-2-hydroxyheptanoic acid of known absolute configuration (29). Further degradation studies located the trans double bond in the lower arm.

These and other studies suggested structures 33.**1** and 33.**2** for PGE_1 and $PGF_{1\alpha}$. X-Ray analysis confirmed these structures and completed the assignment of the absolute stereochemistry and configuration of the chiral centers (29–31).

Two more prostaglandins, PGE_2 (33.**5**) and PGE_3 (33.**6**), were later isolated from sheep vesicular glands. PGE_2 was found to differ from PGE_1 by the presence of a cis double bond at C_5–C_6. PGE_3 also possesses the $\Delta^{5,6}$ cis double bond, as well as a second cis double bond at C_{17}–C_{18} (32).

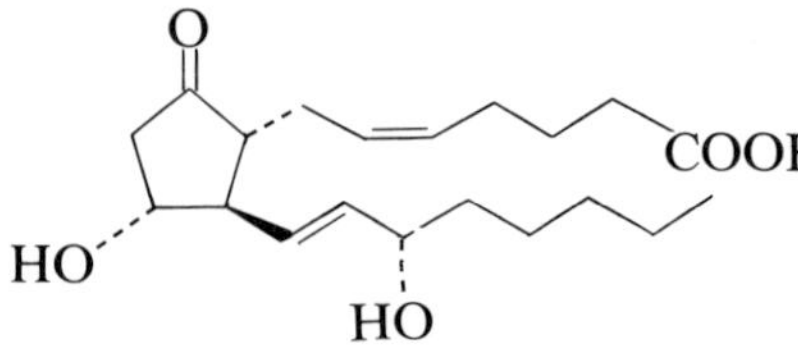

33.**5**

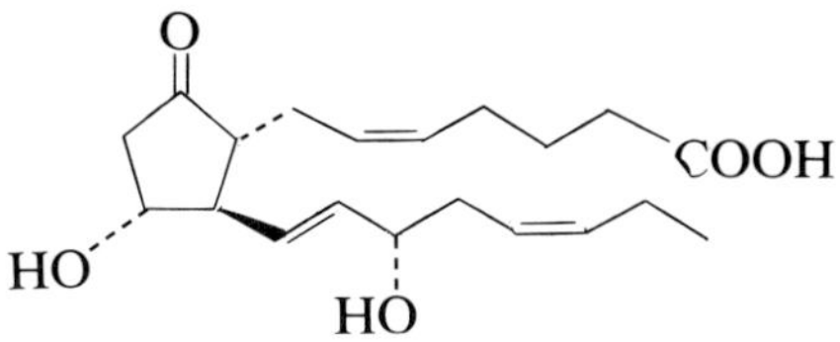

33.6

The corresponding $PGF_{2\alpha}$ (33.**7**) and $PGF_{3\alpha}$ (33.**8**) were later isolated from sheep and bovine lung tissues, respectively (23, 33).

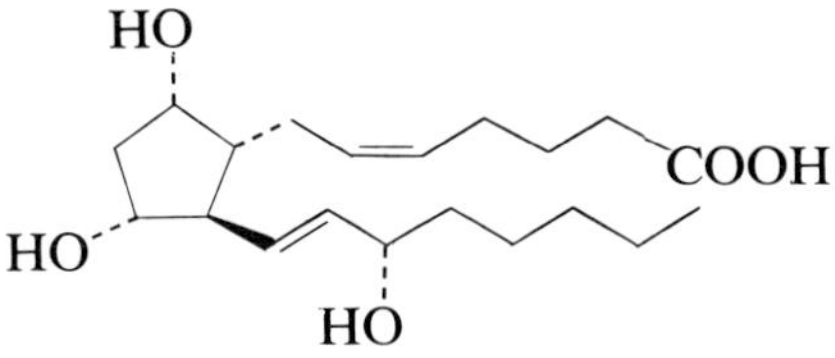

33.7

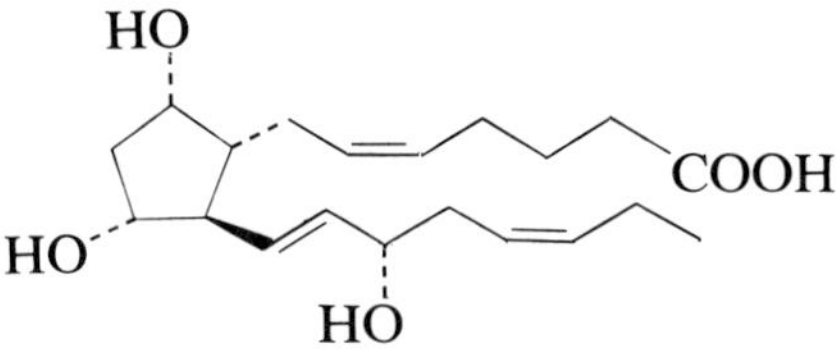

33.8

In addition to the primary prostaglandins, PGE_1, E_2, and E_3 and their A_1, A_2, A_3, B_1, B_2, B_3, and $F_{2\alpha}$ and $F_{1\alpha}$ counterparts, human semen (but not sheep semen) also contains 19-hydroxy prostaglandins (23). Early workers detected 19-hydroxy PGA_1, A_2, B_1, and B_2 there in relatively large quantities. However recent workers, using human semen frozen immediately after ejaculation, converted the prostaglandins present to their heat-stable O-methyl oximes–methyl esters–silyl ethers. When this mixture was analyzed by combined gas chromatography–mass spectrometry, only small amounts of 19-hydroxy PGAs or PGBs were detected. Instead, large amounts of the previously unknown 19-hydroxy PGE_1 (33.**9**) and 19-hydroxy PGE_2 (33.**10**) were found. These two PGs are now known to be the preponderant prostaglandins of human semen, together present at levels up to 100 μg/ml (34, 35).

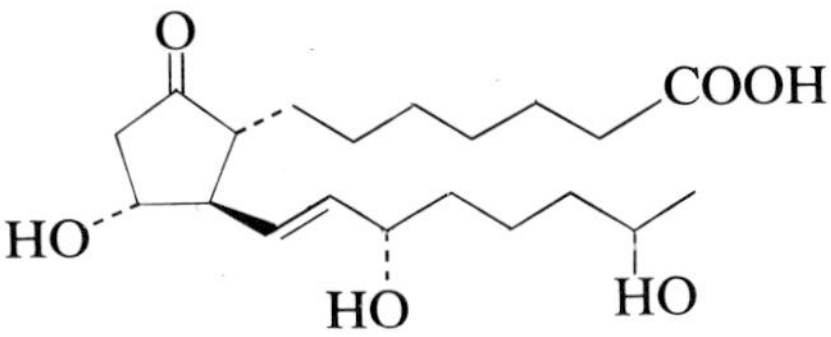

33.9

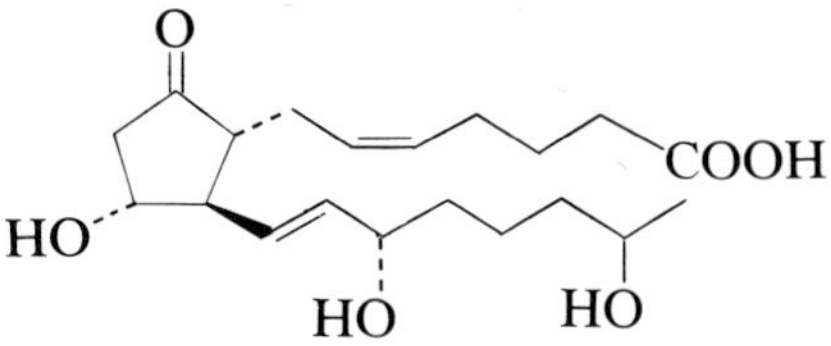

33.10

This finding suggests that the 19-hydroxy As and Bs found in semen are largely artifacts of the isolation process.

The expected intermediates in the rearrangement of prostaglandins A_1 and A_2 to B_1 and B_2 have been characterized and named PGC_1 (33.**11**) and PGC_2 (33.**12**). Although the conversion PGA→C→B is chemically facile and undoubtedly occurs to some degree during isolation, at least some PGC_1 is produced from PGA_1 by enzymatic action. An isomerase able to catalyze the reaction has been detected in the blood of several mammals, including man (36–38). And there is evidence that in humans the conversion $PGC_1 \rightarrow B_1$ may also be enzymatically controlled (38, 39). Although not isolated so far from biological sources,

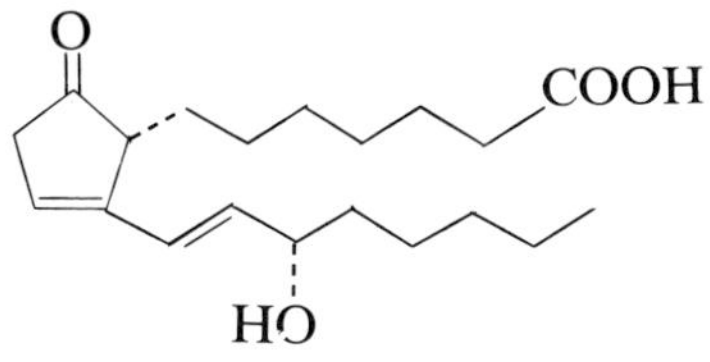

33.11

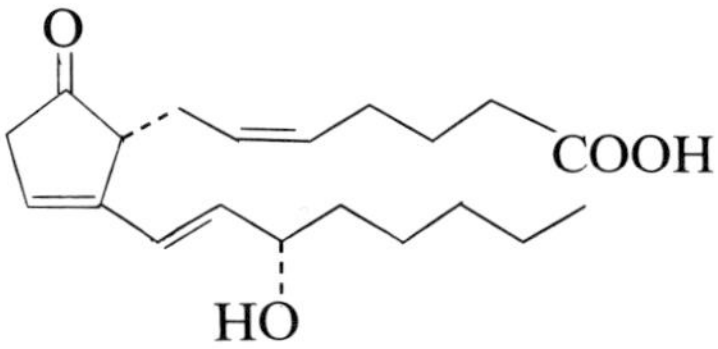

33.12

PGC_2 and 15-epi PGC_2 have been prepared by incubating PGA_2 and 15-epi PGA_2 with a PGA isomerase obtained from cat serum (40).

Prostaglandin C_1 is more potent than PGA_1 in lowering blood pressure (37). Nevertheless, the great ease of converting PGCs to inactive PGBs suggests that the sequence PGE→A→C→B is a route of metabolic inactivation of PGEs in which the Cs are simply intermediates, playing no role themselves in physiological processes.

In 1968 a new type of prostaglandin, PGD_1 (33.**13**), was isolated from the mixture produced by incubating 8,11,14-eicosatrienoic acid (33.**21**) with homogenates of sheep vesicular glands (40). Both PGD_1 and PGD_2 (33.**14**), derived from arachidonic acid, are formed in minor amounts by the endoperoxide isomerase that normally catalyzes the formation of PGE_1 and PGE_2. Although the enzyme seems to be present in most tissues, minor amounts of both PGDs are also produced by the nonenzymatic breakdown of the endoperoxides (41, 42). However much higher yields of PGDs can be obtained by the enzymatic process when serotonin is added to the incubation mixture accompanying the bovine seminal vesicle preparation (43). This suggests that the ratio of PGE to PGD can be controlled by tissues, perhaps in response to hormonal mediation. But though PGD_2 has a pressor effect in sheep, the PGDs are much less active than the substances from which they are derived and may be only intermediates in the biological inactivation of the endoperoxides (44).

HO COOH O HO

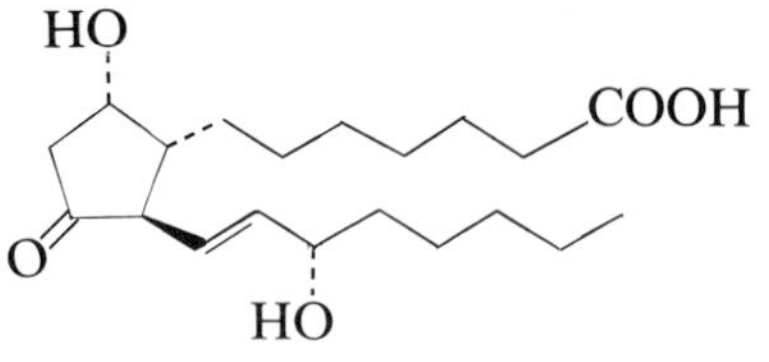

33.**13**

HO COOH O HO

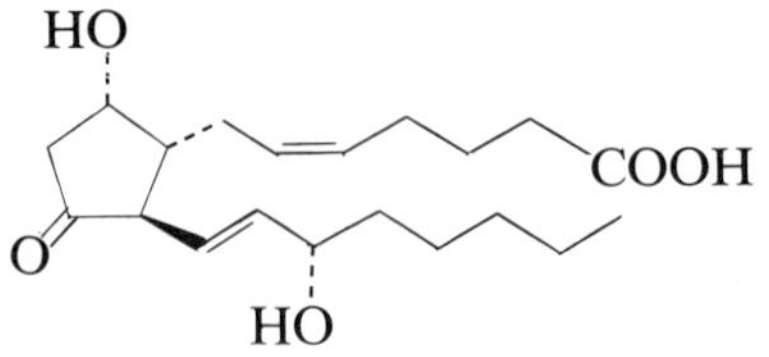

33.**14**

Table 33.2 Prostaglandins Isolated from Mammalian Sources

PGE_1	PGE_2	PGE_3	19 HO-PGE_1	19 HO-PGE_2
$PGF_{1\alpha}$	$F_{2\alpha}$	$F_{3\alpha}$		
PGA_1	A_2		19 HO-A_1	19 HO-A_2
PGC_1				
PGB_1	B_2		19 HO-B_1	19 HO-B_2
PGD_1	D_2			

Thus the family of prostaglandins isolated from biological sources has grown to more than 20 members (Table 33.2). However the compounds listed in this table are not the only prostaglandinlike materials produced in organs and tissues by catabolism of the essential fatty acids. The other substances are discussed in Section 2, Biosynthesis.

Prostaglandins are considered by convention to be derivatives of the completely unsubstituted acid, given the trivial name prostanoic acid (33.**15**), and are numbered as shown for the parent (45).

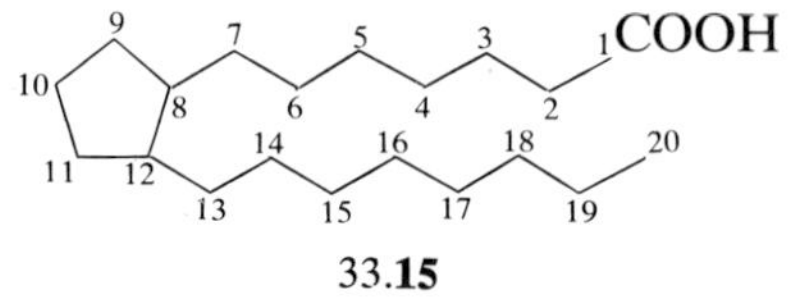

9 7 5 3 1COOH 10 8 6 4 2 14 16 18 20 11 12 13 15 17 19

33.**15**

As indicated earlier, the letter E designates the prostaglandins having a β-hydroxy cyclopentanone ring and the letter F those that possess a dihydroxy cyclopentane ring. The subscript numeral refers to the number of carbon-carbon double bonds in the molecule. The subscripts α and β are taken from steroid nomenclature. An α-substitutent is one projecting down from the plane of the molecule when the molecule is displayed with the ring to the left; a β-substitutent is one projecting above the plane. Thus $PGF_{2\alpha}$ is the isomer derived from PGE_2 by reduction of the 9-ketone function to give a 9α-hydroxyl group. In $PGF_{2\beta}$, the 9-hydroxyl group projects above the plane of the ring. In the naturally occurring prostaglandins the two "arms" are trans to each other. The carboxyl-bearing "upper arm" is attached in the α-configuration. Mirror images of the natural prostaglandins are designated *enantiomeric* or *ent* prostaglandins. The "arms" are still trans to each other but the upper arm is now β and the lower is α (46).

The chiral center at C-15 is designated by the Cahn-Ingold-Prelog notation. It is *S* in the natural prostaglandins (47). The absolute configuration at C-19 has been determined to be *R* for 19-hydroxy PGB_1 isolated from human semen (48). It is likely that other 19-hydroxy PGs are also *R* at C-19.

The hydroxyl group at C-11 in the E series has the α-configuration in the natural substance. However, compounds having the unnatural configuration at C-11 or C-15 are not always designated as 11β or 15 (*R*) but occasionally as 11-epi or 15-epi, particularly in the older literature. Thus 33.**16** is 11-epi PGE_1 and 33.**17** is 11-epi, 15-epi, ent PGE_2, or simply ent-11,15-epi-PGE_2 (49).

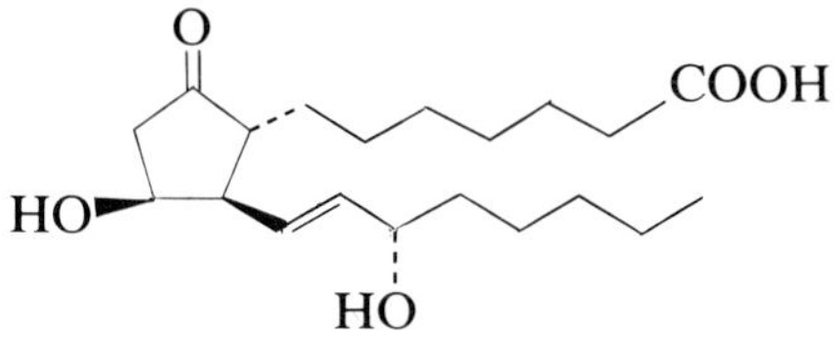

O, COOH, HO, HO

33.**16**

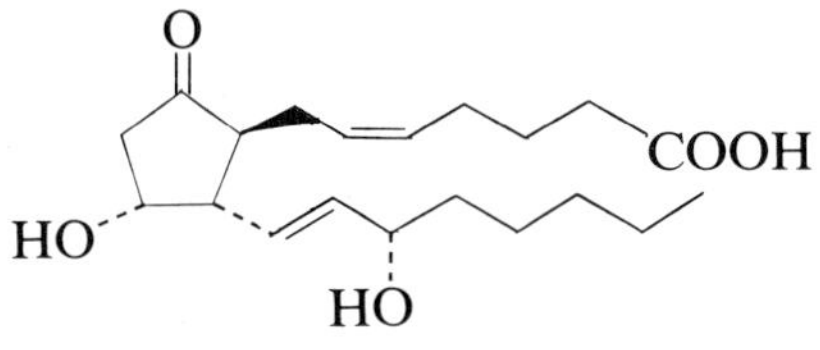

O, COOH, HO, HO

33.**17**

Prostaglandins having the arms fused cis to each other are named isoprostaglandins, e.g., 8-isoprostaglandin E_1 (33.**18**).

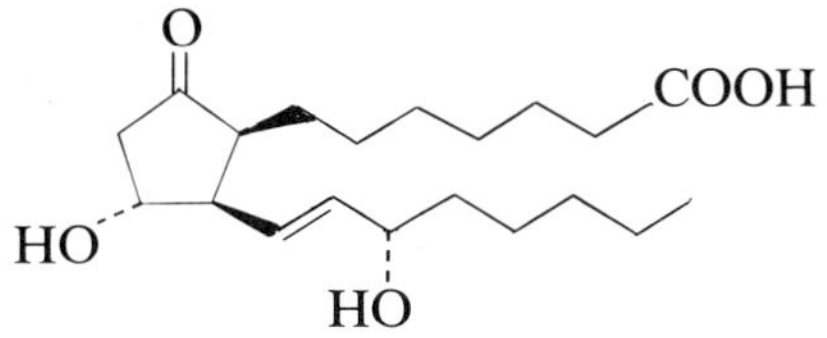

O, COOH, HO, HO

33.**18**

Prostaglandins of the E and F families have been termed the primary prostaglandins, since they are the primary products of the PG synthetase systems (other types being artifacts, metabolites, or minor products), as well as the chief effectors of the physiological activity of prostaglandins. Although very recent work suggests that in some cases the endoperoxides (*vide infra*) are the real effectors of PG activity and the Es and Fs themselves only metabolites, use of the term "primary" in reference to PGEs and PGFs is well entrenched.

1.2 Occurrence

Although human seminal plasma is the richest mammalian source of prostaglandins, containing up to 300 μg/ml of a mixture of a least 15 of them, prostaglandins are also found in significant amounts in reproductive tissues of both male and female, the developing fetus and decidua, umbilical cord, amniotic fluid, endometrium, menstrual fluid, kidneys, lungs, eyes, stomach mucosa, epidermis, thymus, thyroid, nerves, and probably many other tissues as well (1). Except in genital tissue, most of the prostaglandin is present as PGE_2 and $PGF_{2\alpha}$. In the adrenal medulla, for example, levels of E_2 are as high as 45 ng/g. Substantial amounts of $PGF_{2\alpha}$, as much as 50 ng/g, are also found in lung tissue, and up to 100 ng/g occurs in thyroid tissue. Very little is detected in the pancreas, parotid gland, and adrenal medulla (50, 51).

Only the semen of primates and sheep contains prostaglandins. However, many other organs of higher mammals contain prostaglandins, and again PGE_2 and $PGF_{2\alpha}$

predominate (50). There is no obvious significance in the pattern of PG distribution among organs and tissues of a species. For example, high levels of PGEs and PGFs can be detected in the thyroids of rats, guinea pigs, rabbits, and chickens, low levels in the cat, and none in the dog (52). Nevertheless, in higher species, prostaglandins are generally found in the principal organs, glands, and skeletal muscles.

Prostaglandin E-like activity has also been found in the gastrointestinal tracts of lower vertebrates such as sheatfish, carp, and leopard shark, in amounts proportional to those found in mammals. Smaller amounts have been detected in the mussel, scallop, crawfish, blue crab, sea anemone, and several species of annelids (53). The small amount present in the sea anemone contrasts with the high level of 15-epi PGA_2 found in the gorgonian coral *Plexaura homomalla* (54).

1.3 Release

Even though relatively large amounts of prostaglandins can be detected in only a few tissues, the capacity for prostaglandin biosynthesis can be demonstrated in almost all tissues. Prostaglandins are rarely stored in tissues; usually they are synthesized rapidly, in response to local stimulation, from tissue stores of their fatty acid precursors (55). Stimulation can be mechanical (stretch or distension), chemical (catecholamines, serotonin, histamine, acetylcholine, glucagon), or neural (56). Probably anything that disrupts or disturbs cell membranes provokes some degree of prostaglandin release. Because of this, many estimates of prostaglandin levels in organs and tissues are likely too high because of the cell disruption that necessarily occurs during isolation. The ability of tissues to synthesize prostaglandins is determined by incubating tissue homogenates with tritium-labeled arachidonic acid and measuring the amount of labeled PGE_2 produced (57).

The precursors of prostaglandins are fatty acids: arachidonic acid (33.**22**) (5,8,11,14-eicosatetraenoic acid) for the PG_2 series, and dihomo-γ-linolenic acid (8,11,14-eicosatrienoic acid 33.**21**) for the PG_1 series. Both are derived from the dietary essential fatty acid, linoleic acid (33.**19**) (56). Tissue concentrations of arachidonic and dihomo-γ-linolenic acids are no higher than those of prostaglandins themselves. These lipids are not pooled as such but are stored in cell membranes as phospholipids. They are liberated from these stores when PG biosynthesis is required by the action of the enzyme phospholipase A (55, 58, 59). The availability of these fatty acid substrates appears to be the controlling step in prostaglandin synthesis.

1.4 Prostaglandins and Essential Fatty Acids

In 1930 it was discovered that linoleic acid (33.**19**) is a necessary element in the diet of healthy rats (60). Lack of it causes poor growth, skin lesions, kidney damage, and sterility (60, 61). This finding was later extended to other species, including humans. When it was recognized that many tissues are able to convert linoleic acid to γ-linolenic acid (33.**20**), and this intermediate to the prostaglandin precursors dihomo-γ-linolenic acid (33.**21**) and arachidonic acid (33.**22** see Fig. 33.1), it was theorized that these fatty acids are essential because they are the necessary precursors of prostaglandins (62–64).

There are many fatty acids in the normal diet, and their essential fatty acid (EFA) potencies relative to linoleic acid are known (65). Subsequent experiments have demonstrated that only fatty acids capable of yielding biologically active prostaglandins display appreciable EFA activities. And the degree of EFA activity of these

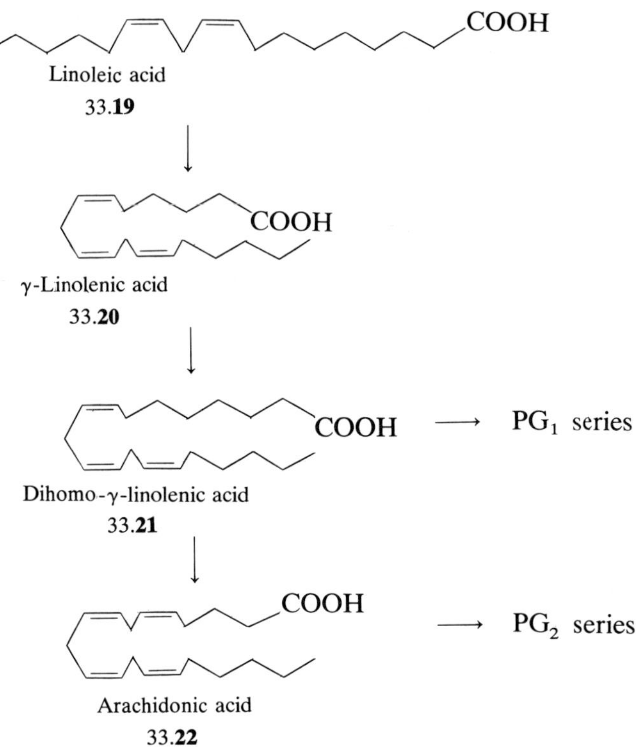

Fig. 33.1 Bioconversion of linoleic acid to prostaglandins.

acids is proportional to their rates of conversion into prostaglandins by rat liver mitochondria (66).

Although dihomo-γ-linolenic acid and arachidonic acid are more active than linoleic acid in curing symptoms of fatty acid deficiency in rats, prostaglandins are not active at all (67). This may be due, however, to the instability of prostaglandins or to the lack of a specific uptake mechanism for them in the affected tissues. Prostaglandins do not readily penetrate membranes except those of tissues such as lung, liver, and kidneys, which possess specific transport systems for them (68, 69).

2 BIOSYNTHESIS

Efforts to discover the pathways and mechanisms of prostaglandin biosynthesis have been underway since the discovery of PGs in human seminal fluid in the 1930s. Current understanding of these transformations has been developed largely through the study of urinary metabolites and the products obtained by incubating prostaglandins and their precursors with tissue homogenates. Prior to 1960 most experiments were performed using precursors labeled with tritium or ^{14}C, followed by chromatographic separation and bioassay of the labeled products for substances exhibiting prostaglandinlike activity (70). The recent advent of sophisticated analytical techniques such as gas-liquid chromatography using electron capture detectors (61), radioimmunoassay, high pressure liquid chromatography, and quantitative gas chromatography–mass spectrometry employing multiple ion detection has brought about rapid progress in this area (71–74). In 1975 and 1976 such methods revealed the existence of the endoperoxides, thromboxanes, and PGI_2. These substances had heretofore gone undetected, and their physiological effects had been attributed to the primary prostaglandins or to unidentified factors.

Prostaglandins are biosynthesized from the essential polyunsaturated fatty acids and can be found in nearly every tissue, although the amounts vary from organ to organ and from species to species. Prostaglandins of the "1" series arise from 18,11,14-eicosatrienoic acid (33.**21**), whereas the PG_3s originate from 5,8,11,14,17-eicosapentaenoic acid (33.**23**). For purposes of brevity, this discussion focuses chiefly on the biosynthesis of PGE_2 (33.**5**) and $PGF_{2\alpha}$ (33.**7**) and other substances from arachidonic acid (33.**22**). These are the prostaglandins of greatest significance in man and are the ones most thoroughly studied. The biochemical transformations of 33.**21** and 33.**23** leading to the PG_1 and PG_3 series have been less studied, but they appear to be similar to arachidonic acid pathways.

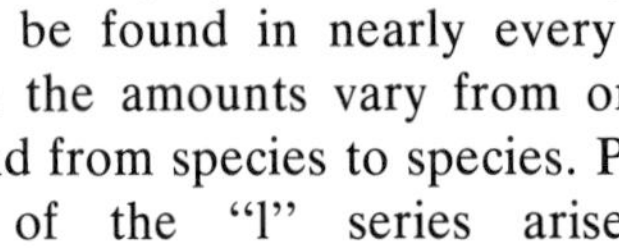

COOH

33.**23**

Biosynthesis of prostaglandins in man can be stimulated by oral administration of arachidonate esters, as shown by increases of up to 47% in amounts of urinary metabolites excreted (75). Analysis of urinary metabolite production has also demonstrated that endogenous prostaglandin synthesis increases in response to cold stress in the rat (76), scalding in the guinea pig and dog (77, 78), guinea pig anaphylaxis (79), and human pregnancy (80).

2.1 The Cyclooxygenase Pathway

Tritiated arachidonic acid can be converted to tritiated PGE_2 in 20–32% yield by incubating it with a homogenate of sheep vesicular glands. When only the supernatant fraction from the vesicular gland homogenate is employed, all the arachidonic acid is consumed during a 1 hr period (63, 64). The catabolism of arachidonic acid is initiated by the action of the enzyme phospholipase A, which liberates it from membrane-bound phospholipids. It is then converted to the primary prostaglandins by the prostaglandin synthetase system. The latter transformation can be inhibited by indomethacin and other nonsteroidal anti-inflammatory agents, as well as by 5,8,11,14-eicosatetraynoic acid, the acetylenic analog of arachidonic acid (78, 81–83). Although prostaglandin synthetase can be prepared as an acetone-pentane powder, it is not a homogeneous enzyme but a complex of enzymes and cofactors (84). It acts on arachidonic acid to produce not only PGE_2 and $PGF_{2\alpha}$ but other prostaglandins and nonprostaglandin products as well, as shown in Fig. 33.2 (85, 86).

The efficiency of the prostaglandin synthetase system depends on the amount of substrate available (87). The addition of arachidonic acid or phospholipase A to perfused frog intestines results in the rapid appearance of PGE_2 in the perfusate (58, 88). Phospholipase A appears to control the availability of the substrate by virtue of its ability to free the fatty acid from its storage sites (55, 89). The rate of formation of prostaglandins in bovine seminal vesicles has been found to be a function of phospholipase activity (90). And incubation of phospholipids with prostaglandin synthetase preparations has confirmed that phospholipids are able to function as a source of arachidonic acid. Furthermore, the yields of prostaglandins obtained are markedly increased following pretreatment of the phospholipids with a phospholipase A obtained from snake venom (91, 92). The participation of phospholipase A_2 in the biosynthesis of

PGs by the thyroid gland has recently been demonstrated. In the thyroid gland, arachidonic acid appears to be liberated from two sources, the most important of which is phosphatidylinositol. This process is dependent on calcium ions, is independent of cyclic AMP, and is stimulated by large amounts of thyrotropin (TSH). A less significant source of arachidonate is triglycerides, from which it is released by a cyclic AMP-dependent lipase (93).

A key step in the conversion of arachidonic acid to prostaglandins is the incorporation of the oxygen atoms at positions C-9, C-11, and C-15 to produce the endoperoxide PGG_2 (33.**24**). To explore the mechanism of this process C-14 labeled 8,11,14-eicosatrienoic acid (33.**21**) was incubated in an atmosphere of $^{18}O_2$ with sheep vesicular gland homogenates to produce doubly labeled PGE_1. It was possible to demonstrate that not only did all the incorporated oxygen arise from molecular oxygen, but that the oxygen atoms at C-9 and C-11 were derived from the same molecule of oxygen (94). Although as early as 1965 an endoperoxide was proposed as the logical type of intermediate to account for this observation, it was eight years before endoperoxides (33.**24**) and (33.**25**) were finally isolated and characterized.

Indirect evidence for the existence of the endoperoxides was provided earlier by the finding that PGE and PGF arise independently from a common intermediate. Several experiments in which homogenates of guinea pig lung of sheep vesicular glands transformed labeled fatty acids simultaneously into PGE, PGF and PGD showed that PGE and PGF do not interconvert under physiological conditions, as might have been expected on the basis of their

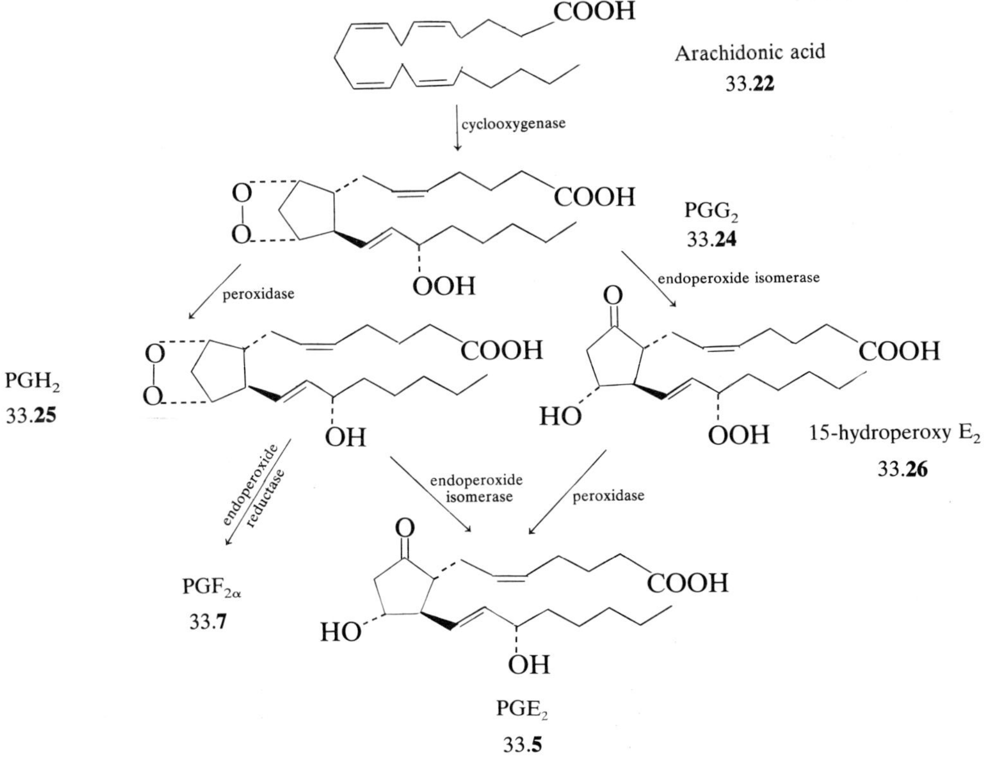

Fig. 33.2 Biosynthesis of the "primary" prostaglandins.

close chemical resemblance (42, 95, 96, 97, 98). In addition, in the oxygenation of 8,11,14-eicosatrienoic acid (33.**21**) and arachidonic acid by sheep vesicular glands, small amounts of malonaldehyde and 12-hydroxy-8,10-heptadecadienoic acid were obtained. This formation was also rationalized by assuming the involvement of an endoperoxide as the precursor (42, 98, 99).

It was subsequently determined that arachidonic acid is converted into two endoperoxides, PGG_2 (33.**24**) and PGH_2 (33.**25**), by a fatty acid cyclooxygenase. In 1973, short-term incubations of arachidonic acid with the microsmal fractions of sheep vesicular gland homogenates provided the first direct evidence for the intermediacy of endoperoxides in PG biosynthesis (81). When the incubation was carried out in the presence of 4-chloromercuribenzoate, both PGG_2 and PGH_2 were detected (41, 100). In addition, the partial purification of an endoperoxide isomerase, which is almost entirely associated with the microsomal fraction of the homogenate, has been reported (101). This enzyme is at least partially responsible for directing the breakdown of the endoperoxides. Its activity is increased by reduced glutathione (GSH) and inhibited by 4-chloromercuribenzoate. The activity of the peroxidase present in the PG synthetase system is also increased by GSH.

The structural assignments of PGG_2 and PGH_2 were based mainly on chemical evidence. Both endoperoxides can be reduced to $PGF_{2\alpha}$ by either stannous chloride or triphenylphosphine. The presence of the 15-hydroperoxy group in PGG_2 was inferred by its conversion to a 15-keto endoperoxide with lead tetraacetate, and reduction of this to 15-keto $PGF_{2\alpha}$.

The endoperoxides are unstable in aqueous media. PGG_2 breaks down to give 15-hydroperoxy PGE_2 (33.**26**) as the major product, and PGH_2 decomposes to PGE_2 and PGD_2 (33.**14**) in a ratio of 4 : 1. PGH_2 has a half-life of 4–5 min in an aqueous buffer, pH 7.4, at 37°.

The endoperoxides display considerable activity in stimulating respiratory and other smooth muscles (102, 103). They also induce irreversible platelet aggregation.

The biological fate of the endoperoxides seems to vary depending on the tissues studied. When PGG_2 and PGH_2 are incubated with sheep vesicular gland homogenates, PGE_2 is the major product, accompanied by a fourth as much PGD_2 (41). When PGH_2 is incubated with bovine serum albumin, however, PGD_2 becomes the predominant product and PGE_2 the minor, the ratio now being 4 : 1 in favor of PGD_2 (104). This conversion does not proceed by way of PGE_2, for PGE_2 is unchanged under these conditions. Boiling the serum albumin before the incubation destroys part of the factor responsible for conversion to PGD_2 and causes $PGF_{2\alpha}$ to become the major product. The conversion of PGH_2 to PGD_2 is not inhibited by the sulfhydryl scavenger *N*-ethylmaleimide or PGE_2, but it is inhibited by preincubation with the completely saturated eicosanoic acid. This implies that the sulfhydryl group of serum albumin is not involved in this transformation and that PGH_2 must bind to fatty acid binding sites in serum albumin before the conversion to PGD_2 can occur. It has been suggested that a hydrophobic binding site could provide the environment necessary to shift the product distribution in favor of PGD_2. There is some precedent for this: PGH_2 is known to rearrange spontaneously to PGD_2 on silica gel (81).

When the experiment was repeated using serum albumin from other genera, differences were observed that could not be explained on the basis of differential inhibition of PGH_2 binding by competition with other fatty acids. The incubation of bovine and guinea pig serum albumin with PGH_2 gave PGD_2 to PGE_2 in a ratio of 4 : 1, horse and human serum albumin gave a ratio of 1 : 1, and rabbit and rat albumin gave a ratio of

0.3 : 1. This compares with a ratio of formation in aqueous solution of 0.25 : 1, PGD_2 to PGE_2. Moreover, when egg albumin and PGH_2 were simultaneously added to the incubation mixture, the major products became $PGF_{2\alpha}$ and HHT (33.**29**), with PGE_2 and PGD_2 present in lesser amounts (85). The significance of these findings is hard to determine. They suggest that endogenous serum factors might be able to control the product distribution in the breakdown of the endoperoxides, thus acting as some kind of physiological control mechanism. If so, the mechanism has yet to be established (105).

2.2 The Lipoxygenase Pathway

Evidence for a second pathway of arachidonate bioconversion was first suggested in 1971, when the participation of a hydroperoxidation step was proposed to account for the inhibition of arachidonate catabolism by the enzyme glutathione peroxidase (106, 107). Glutathione peroxidase, in the presence of reduced glutathione, inhibits all product formation during the incubation of arachidonic acid with preparations of sheep vesicular glands. It was later found that incubation of arachidonic acid with human platelets led to several substances that could not be products of the cyclooxygenase pathway, namely, 12-hydroperoxy-5,8,10,14-eicosatetraenoic acid (HPETE) (33.**27**) and 12-hydroxy-5,8,10,14-eicosatetraenoic acid (HETE, 33.**28**) (85, 86). see Fig. 33.3.

Both the cyclooxygenase and the lipoxygenase pathways contribute to the catabolism of arachidonic acid. Subsequently, it was found that aspirin and indomethacin specifically inhibit the cyclooxygenase pathway, but have, at the most, a slight stimulating effect on the lipoxygenase route; a finding that explains the known ability of aspirin to block platelet aggregation (86). 5,8,10,14-Eicosatetraynoic acid blocks both routes.

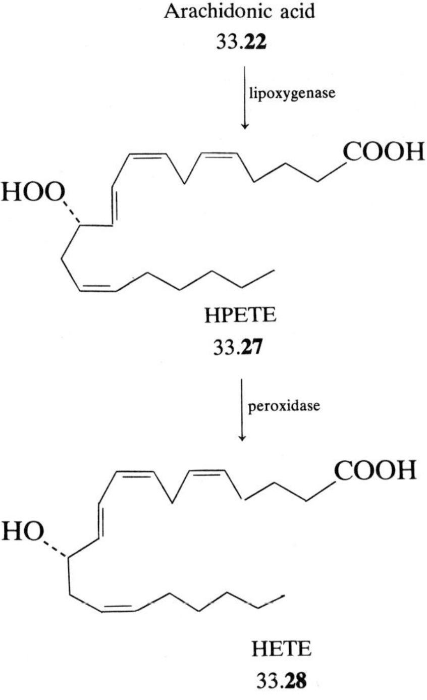

Fig. 33.3 The lipoxygenase pathway of arachidonate catabolism.

To examine the lipoxygenase pathway more closely, investigators turned to a simpler but analogous enzyme, soybean fatty acid oxygenase (lipoxygenase), which could be obtained in a more highly purified form than could prostaglandin synthetase. Earlier work with this enzyme had established its substrate requirements and had demonstrated that hydrogen removal was the initial step in its mechanism of action (108, 109).

The activity of soybean lipoxygenase is also inhibited by glutathione peroxidase in the presence of glutathione (110). The addition of *N*-ethylmaleimide (which combines with the sulfhydryl group of glutathione), restores the activity of the lipoxygenase to the levels existing before glutathione peroxidase treatment. This suggests that a lipid hydroperoxide is required to activate the enzyme, a suggestion confirmed by finding a lag phase at the start of the oxygenation step that can be overcome by the addition of organic hydroperoxides (110). Self-destruction of the enzyme also occurs at a rate depending on the particular fatty acids acting as substrate, and its action is inhibited by large concentrations of substrate. (These probably displace the hydroperoxide activator from its binding sites.)

The physiological significance of the lipoxygenase route and its exact relationship to the cyclooxygenase mechanism is not clear at this time. It may be that the products of this pathway exert some type of feedback inhibition on the rate or control the direction of breakdown of the endoperoxides.

2.3 Biosynthesis in Platelets

During aggregation, platelets transform arachidonic acid into a number of substances, at least some of which can affect the further progress of aggregation. The role of platelets in hemostasis and the part played by prostaglandins in platelet aggregation are discussed more fully in Section 4. As Fig. 33.4 indicates, platelets convert arachidonic acid into HPETE and HETE by the lipoxygenase pathway present in other tissues. And, as in other tissues, the cyclooxygenase pathway produces the endoperoxides PGG_2 and PGH_2. In platelets,

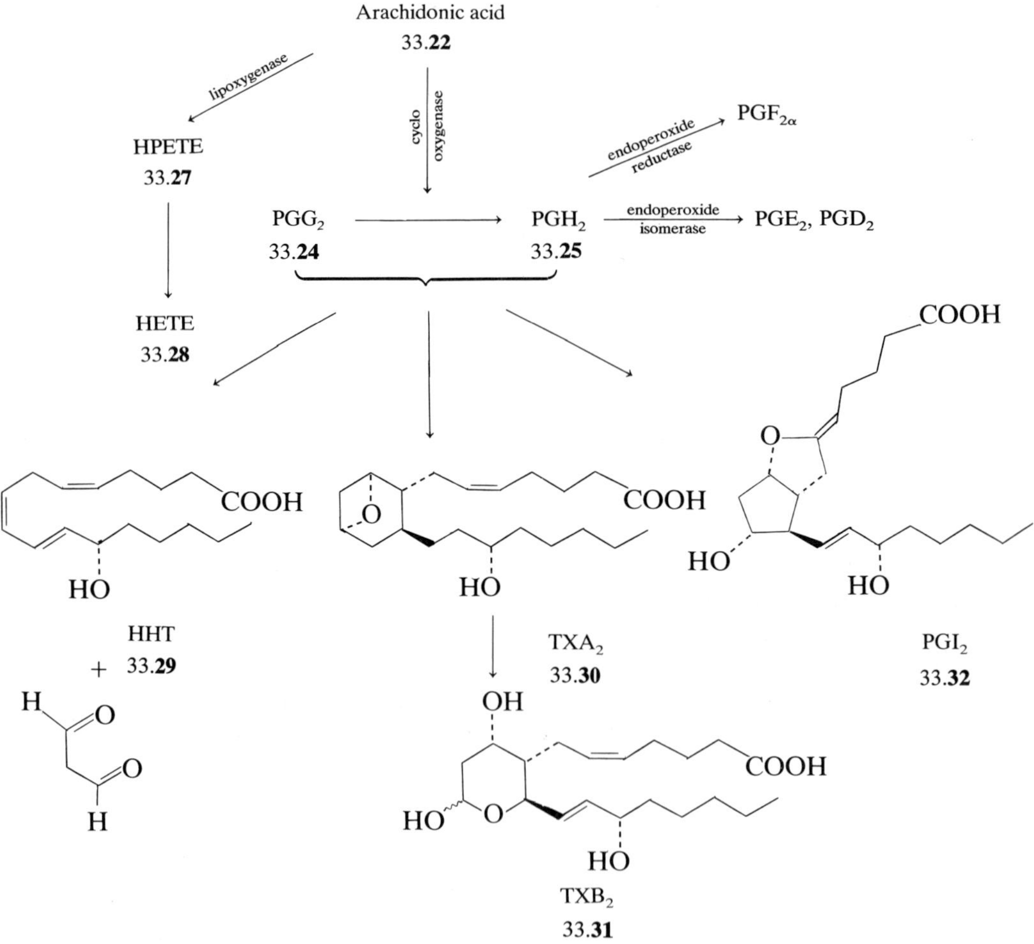

Fig. 33.4 Products of arachidonate bioconversion in platelets.

however, only small amounts of the endoperoxides are converted to the primary prostaglandins, PGE_2 and $PGF_{2\alpha}$, and PGD_2 (33.**14**). This finding was the first indication that substances other than the primary prostaglandins could be direct participants in the regulation of cell functions (85, 86, 107).

The incubation of labeled arachidonic acid with human platelets gives rise to four nonprostaglandin oxygenated lipids. The first of these was characterized as 12-hydroxy-5-*cis*, 8-*trans*, 10-*trans*-heptadecatrienoic acid (HHT, 33.**29**). This substance is likely to be produced by fragmentation of the endoperoxide with expulsion of malonaldehyde (98). As already mentioned, its 5,6-dihydro analog, 12-hydroxy-8-*trans*,10-*trans*-heptadecadienoic acid is produced when 8,11,14-eicosatrienoic acid (33.**21**) is incubated with preparations of sheep vesicular glands (42, 99). The formation of HHT can be suppressed by the addition to the incubation mixture of glutathione and an antioxidant such as hydroquinone. Also isolated from platelets was a new substance, first called PHD but later renamed thromboxane B_2 (TXB_2, 33.**31**) (106). Thromboxane B_2 was identified as a six-membered, cyclic hemiacetal by mass spectrometry and chemical degradation. Incubation of human platelets with arachidonic acid in an atmosphere of $^{18}O_2$ showed that TXB_2 arises from PGG_2 by rearrangement and incorporation of one water molecule (85). Attempts to trap the intermediate in this transformation provided evidence of a highly unstable substance named thromboxane A_2 (TXA_2, 33.**30**). It has a half-life of 32 sec in plasma and is a potent stimulator of platelet aggregation and smooth muscle (111–113). It is TXA_2 that is responsible for the platelet-aggregating activity of arachidonic acid and probably of the endoperoxides as well (114–118).

Before all the postulated products of arachidonate catabolism in platelets had been identified, another material called rabbit aorta contracting substance (RCS) was isolated along with PGE_2, $PGF_{2\alpha}$, SRS-A (slow reacting substance in anaphylaxis), and histamine during anaphylaxis induced in guinea pig lungs (119). As the name implies, RCS is a powerful contractor of arterial smooth muscle. It was later found to be released along with PGE_2 during stimulation of perfused rabbit spleens (118). When the perfusate was held at 37° for 3 min, the RCS activity disappeared, and the loss in RCS activity appeared to be balanced by an increase in PGE_2 activity. At the same time, the biosynthesis of RCS was found to be antagonized by nonsteroidal anti-inflammatory drugs, the same drugs known to inhibit prostaglandin synthetase (118). Thus for a while it seemed that RCS might be either the long postulated endoperoxide or some other PGE_2 precursor (118). When the endoperoxides were characterized, however, their half-lives were found to be longer than that of RCS. The subsequent discovery of TXA_2 and characterization of its physiological properties showed it to be the factor mainly responsible for the activity of RCS (119, 120).

Recently an enzyme has been isolated from the arterial walls of several species that transforms the endoperoxides into yet another substance first called PGX, later given the trivial name prostacyclin (121–124), and now called prostaglandin I_2 (125). Substantial amounts of PGI_2 have been obtained by incubating PGG_2 or PGH_2 with microsomes of rabbit or pig aorta, and its structure has been determined to be 5-*Z*-9-deoxy-6,9α-epoxy-$\Delta^5PGF_{1\alpha}$ (33.**32**). PGI_2 has a short half-life under biological conditions, presumably because of its chemical instability: it is rapidly hydrolyzed to 6-keto $PGF_{1\alpha}$ (33.**33**) (126, 127).

The structure of prostaglandin I_2 resembles that of the bicyclic acid (33.**34**) isolated as a major product from the incubation of tritiated arachidonic acid with

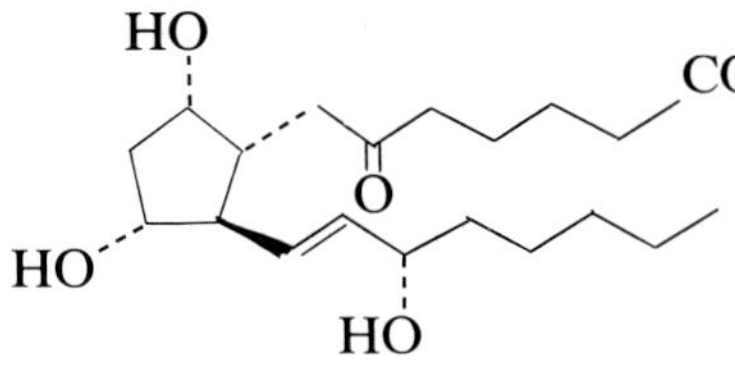

HO COOH O HO HO

33.**33**

COOH O HO HO

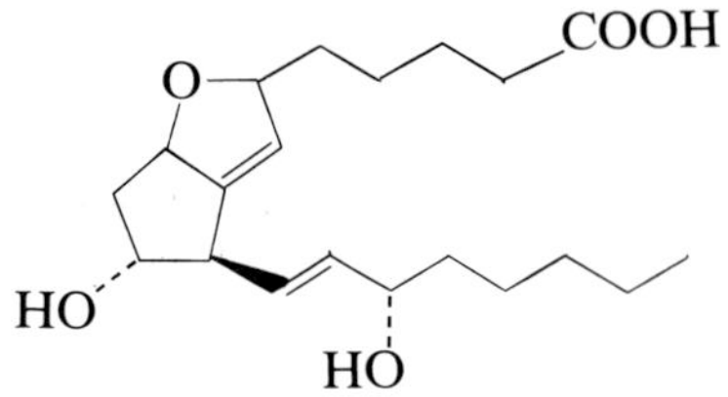

33.**34**

homogenized rat stomachs or seminal vesicle powders (128, 129). [Along with 33.**34** were detected a tetrahydrofuran derivative, 33.**35**, and a pyran derivative, 33.**36** (129).]

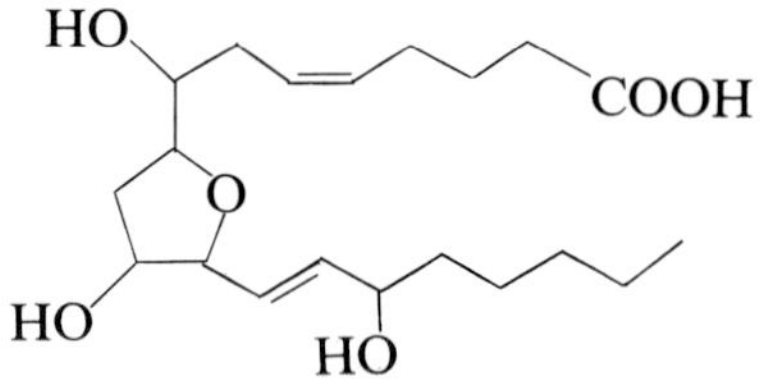

HO COOH O HO HO

33.**35**

HO COOH O HO HO

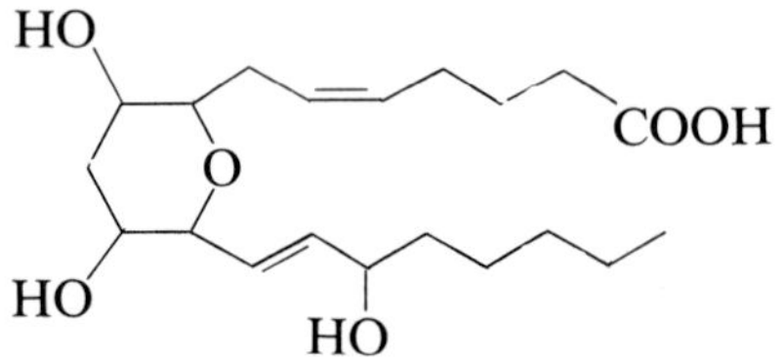

33.**36**

2.4 Summary

Platelets are highly specialized cells, and it now appears that some of their functions in hemostasis are affected by thromboxanes and PGI_2. Nevertheless, thromboxanes occur in other tissues too. Incubation of arachidonate with guinea pig lung homogenates, or perfusion in guinea pig lungs, gives TXB_2 (and HHT) as the major products (130). TXB_2 has also been found in carrageenin-induced granulomas in rats (111). It is not clear what role thromboxanes fulfill in cells other than platelets, although their presence in lungs might be related to their ability to stimulate smooth muscle. And it is not certain that thromboxanes and endoperoxides are the chief products of the action of prostaglandin synthetase in all tissues. In other tissues, PGEs and PGFs may still be the primary products and effectors of PG-like activity. Not all tissues transform arachidonic acid the same way. In the case of primary prostaglandins, mostly $PGF_{2\alpha}$ is produced in lungs, whereas mostly Es are produced in reproductive tissue (131).

Nor is it clear what part, if any, is played by oxygenated lipids like HETE (33.**28**), HHT (33.**29**), and 33.**34** to 33.**36** in physiological processes. It may be that these substances are simply by-products of the free radical pathways leading to the endoperoxides and thromboxanes. Free radical reactions are high energy processes, and their intermediates are prone to a certain amount of fragmentation.

3 METABOLISM

Although the metabolism of prostaglandins has been studied in nearly every organ in which these substances occur, the major metabolizing organs (lung, liver, and kidney) have been most thoroughly investigated. In the circulation prostaglandins are quickly destroyed, chiefly by the lungs. When infused into pulmonary arteries of guinea pigs, PGE_2 loses 92% of its activity in one pass. $PGF_{2\alpha}$ loses 90% of its activity, and PGA_2 loses 64% (132, 133). These PGs are chiefly deactivated by the enzyme 15-hydroxyprostaglandin dehydrogenase, which is found in all tissues examined to date, although its activity varies from organ to organ and species to species (118–120).

This enzyme exhibits two types of activity, one depending on NAD+ and the other on NADP+ as cofactors (134, 135). Its substrate requirements are stereospecific with respect to prostaglandin configuration at C-15; it requires the *S*-configuration, and it is inhibited in noncompetitive fashion by 15*R* PGEs (134). The activity of the enzyme is unaffected by variations in the carboxylic acid side chain of the substrate but it is inhibited by PGBs (136).

As Fig. 33.5 illustrates for PGE_2, the second step in prostaglandin metabolism is the reduction of the C_{13}-C_{14} double bond of the 15-keto metabolite (33.**37**) to give the 13,14-dihydro-15-keto prostaglandin 33.**38** (71). Some of this metabolite undergoes further stereospecific reduction of the 15-keto group to give back the 15*S* alcohol 33.**39** (121). Thus the primary products of PGE_2 metabolism are 33.**38** and 33.**39** (137–139). This is the general route of physiological deactivation of most prostaglandins in most tissues (140).

Studies of urinary and liver metabolites have revealed further metabolic transformations that involve β-and ω-oxidations. Incubation of PGs E_1, B_1, $F_{1\alpha}$, and $F_{1\beta}$ with enzymes derived from rat liver mitochondria give the corresponding homologs in which the upper arm has been shortened by two carbon atoms (141). The incubation of PGE_2 with the guinea pig liver homogenates gives 15-keto PGE_2 (33.**37**) and 13,14-dihydro PGE_2 (33.**39**) as major products. They are accompanied by significant amounts of the corresponding $PGF_{2\alpha}$ metabolites, suggesting the additional participation of a 9-keto reductase (142). Subcutaneous administration of $PGF_{1\alpha}$ in the rat gives dinor $PGF_{1\alpha}$ as the major product (143). (Nor = the one-carbon atom lower homolog formed by removal of a methylene group from the upper arm; dinor = the two-carbon lower homolog, etc.)

The metabolism of prostaglandins E_2 and $F_{2\alpha}$ has been thoroughly studied in intact animals by Krister Gréen and others. In the guinea pig, $PGF_{2\alpha}$ is metabolized chiefly to 5,7-dihydroxy-11-keto-tetranorprostanoic acid (33.**40**) (144). In the rat, the intravenous administration of labeled $PGF_{2\alpha}$ has led to the detection of nine different metabolites (Fig. 33.6). Most of them are excreted in the urine (144–146).

There appear to be three separate pathways of $F_{2\alpha}$ metabolism in the rat. $PGF_{2\alpha}$ can simultaneously undergo reduction of the C_5-C_6 cis double bond and successive β-oxidations to give dinor $PGF_{1\alpha}$ (33.**41**) and tetranor $PGF_{1\alpha}$ (33.**42**). Dinor $PGF_{1\alpha}$ (33.**41**) can be hydroxylated to give 5,7,11,15-tetrahydroxy tetranorprost-9-enoic acid (33.**43**) and 5,7,11,16-tetrahydroxy tetranorprost-9-enoic acid

PGE_2 $\xrightarrow{\text{dehydrogenase}}$ 33.**37** $\xrightarrow{\text{reductase}}$ 33.**38** $\longrightarrow$ 33.**39**

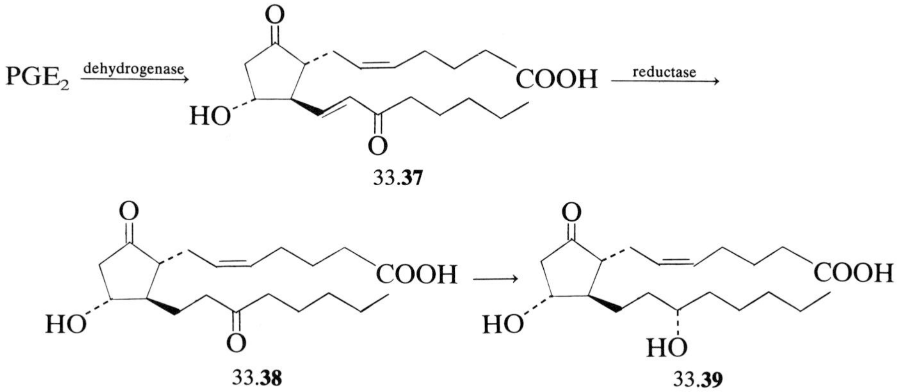

Fig. 33.5 Metabolic inactivation of PGE_2

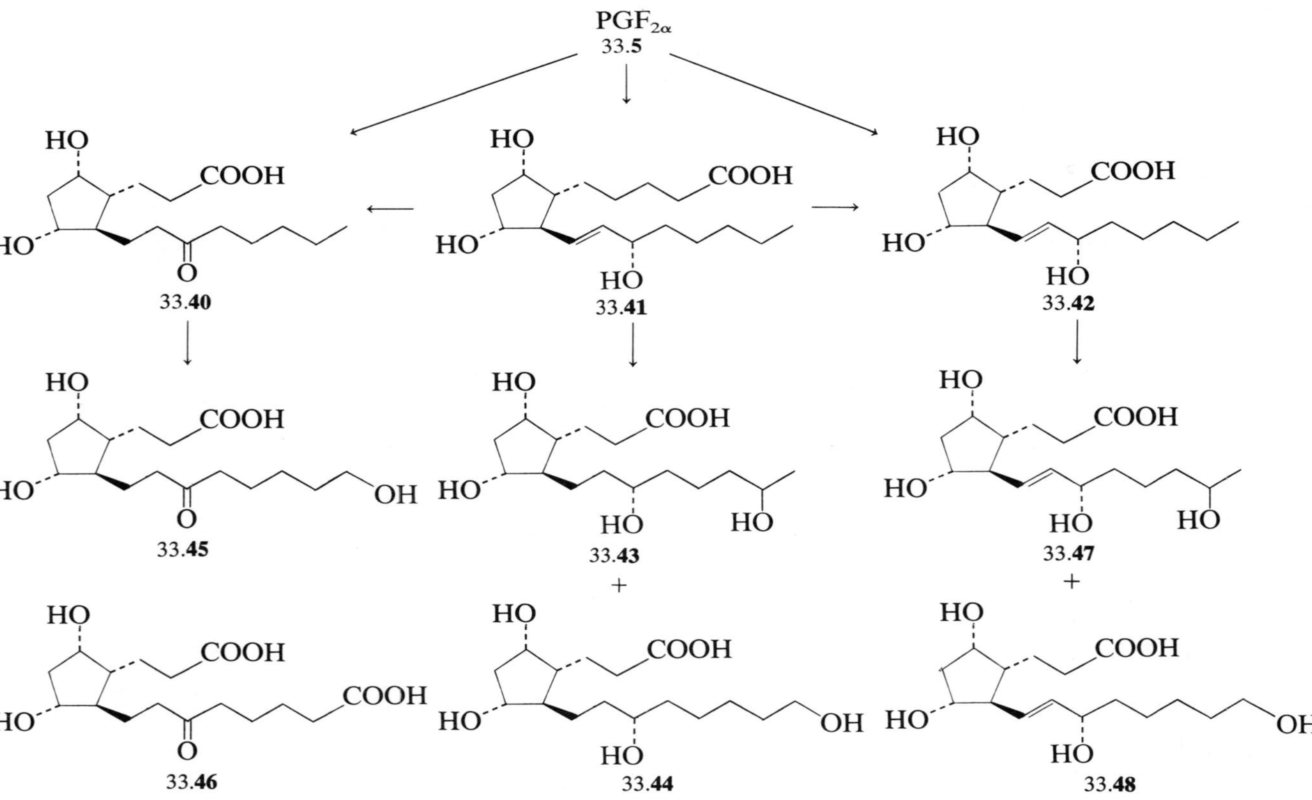

Fig. 33.6 Metabolism of prostaglandin $F_{2\alpha}$ in the rat.

(33.**44**). $PGF_{2\alpha}$ and dinor $PGF_{1\alpha}$ can also be converted in several steps to 5,7-dihydroxy-11-keto-tetranorprostanoic acid (33.**40**), which can undergo further oxidation to give 5,7,16-trihydroxy-11-keto-tetranorprostanoic acid (33.**45**) and 5,7-dihydroxy-11-keto-tetranorprosta-1,16-dioic acid (33.**46**). Finally, both $PGF_{2\alpha}$ and dinor $PGF_{1\alpha}$ can be transformed into 5,7,11,15- and 5,7,11,16-tetrahydroxy tetranorprostanoic acids (33.**47**, 33.**48**) by a combination or reduction of the C_{13}-C_{14} double bond and β-and ω-oxidations (146).

Prostaglandin E_2 is metabolized in rats much the same way as $PGF_{2\alpha}$. The metabolite 33.**40** is common to both pathways, and E_2 gives rise to metabolites that are analogs of 33.**40**, 33.**42**, 33.**45**, and 33.**46**, containing a 9-keto function in place of the 9α-hydroxy group (147, 148). In addition to these, the rat converts PGE_2 into four isomers formally derived from PGB_2, the product of dehydration and rearrangement of PGE_2 (Fig. 33.7). They are tetranor PGB_1 (33.**49**), 11,16-dihydroxy-5-keto-tetranorprosta-4(8),9-dienoic acid (33.**50**), 11-15-dihydroxy-5-keto-tetranorprosta-4(8),9-dienoic acid (33.**51**), and 11-hydroxy-5-keto-tetranorprosta-4(8),9-diene-1,16-dioic acid (33.**52**) (148).

In man the principal urinary metabolites of $PGF_{2\alpha}$ and PGE_2 are the dicarboxylic acid 33.**46** and its 9-keto counterpart. These are the final products of at least five metabolic steps: dehydrogenation of the 15-hydroxyl group, reduction of the trans double bond at C_{13}-C_{14}, two β-oxidation steps, and an ω-oxidation step (149, 150). The basal levels of these metabolites have been established in humans and could prove to be useful for monitoring endogenous prostaglandin concentrations in disease states (151).

Recent studies of prostaglandin metabolism as a function of age have revealed variations in metabolism during animal development in both the products formed and the activities of the enzymes involved. In general, the 15-hydroxyprostaglandin dehydrogenase and the 13,14-reductase enzymes are most active in the immature animal, whereas the 9-prostaglandin dehydrogenase and β-oxidases become more active in the adult. In early fetal organs, only the 15-dehydrogenase can be found (152).

4 SOME BIOLOGICAL PROCESSES INVOLVING PROSTAGLANDINS

4.1 The Renal-Cardiovascular System

It has long been known that the kidney

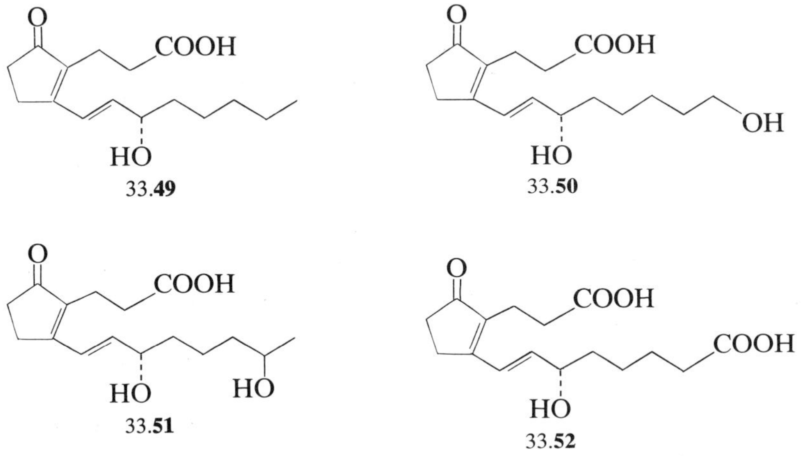

O COOH HO 33.**49**

O COOH OH HO 33.**50**

O COOH HO HO 33.**51**

O COOH COOH HO 33.**52**

Fig. 33.7 Some metabolites of PGE_2 in the rat.

contributes to the regulation of systemic blood pressure in addition to controlling sodium excretion and urine formation. It possesses the potential for elevating blood pressure by means of the renal renin-angiotensin system and renal sympathetic enervation. Thus infusion of norepinephrine or angiotensin II into the renal artery causes renal vasoconstriction, hence reduced renal blood flow. But the kidney possesses a potential antihypertensive mechanism as well. In a series of experiments beginning in the late 1930s, it was discovered that experimental renoprival hypertension caused by manipulation of one kidney (by constriction of the renal arteriole or cellophane wrapping) was much less effective if the other kidney remained intact (153, 154). Removal of the intact kidney produced a much more marked hypertension. Experimental hypertension due to removal of both kidneys was reversed almost completely by implantation of a normal kidney (155, 156). Thus normal kidneys exert a protective action against the development of hypertension.

This led to the suggestion by a number of investigators, principally J. B. Lee (157, 158), E. E. Muirhead (159), and J. C. McGiff (160) that the kidney secretes a humoral antihypertensive substance able to lower blood pressure in response to various hypertensive stimuli. This hypothesis was supported by the finding that the development of experimental renoprival hypertension could be prevented by administration of extracts of renal medulla or kidney homogenates, or by transplantation of renal medullary tissue (161, 163). However such an antihypertensive function of the kidney could be manifested in several ways: by secretion of a vasodilator substance able to act either systemically or intrarenally, or by increased sodium excretion.

Systemic arterial blood pressure is determined chiefly by the pumping action of the heart and the total peripheral resistance to blood flow. The degree of resistance is a function of the elasticity and diameter of the small blood vessels, mainly the arterioles, but also the capillaries. All the various vascular beds of the circulation, including the renal bed, contribute to this resistance. In the resting condition, normal renal blood flow accounts for about 20% of total cardiac output. Within the kidney, the rate of blood flow varies in each portion, being much greater in the cortex than in the medulla. When systemic blood pressure rises, the renal cortical vasculature constricts, to maintain unchanged blood flow to the cortex. However blood flow to the renal medulla does increase.

In 1965 Lee reported the discovery of medullin, extracted from the renal medulla of rabbits, which seemed to fulfill the criteria of a renal antihypertensive hormone (164). Medullin, a potent vasodilator, was quickly found to be identical with prostaglandin A_2; later PGE_2 and $PGF_{2\alpha}$ were also detected in renal medulla (165).

Both PGE_1 and E_2 are powerful vasodilators when given intraarterially, causing a fall in blood pressure that is accompanied by a reflex increase in heart rate due to a direct dilation of the vascular smooth muscle. The effect is not inhibited by α- or β-adrenergic blocking agents, antihistamines, LSD, ganglionic blocking agents, or vagotomy (166, 167). Prostaglandins A_1 and A_2 are about one-tenth as active as the corresponding E compounds, and though lacking any stimulatory effects on nonvascular smooth muscle, they possess roughly the same pharmacological profile of activity on the renal-cardiovascular system (168–170). In human hypertension, infusion of PGA at rates varying from 0.3 to 5 μg/(kg)(min) substantially reduces blood pressure, and the reduction is accompanied by increased natriuresis (171, 172). The response occurs in two stages. An initial rise in sodium excretion and urine flow is quickly followed by a fall in systemic blood pressure resulting from decreased peripheral resistance due to peripheral arteriolar vasodilation. After 30 min, urinary flow returns to near-normal levels (173). When infusion is halted, blood pressure returns to hypertensive levels.

Injection of 25 μg of prostaglandin A_1 in normotensive individuals produces a transient drop in mean arterial blood pressure associated with increased subclavian and femoral blood flow (174). Prolonged infusion of PGA seems to have no effect beyond this initial, transient fall in blood pressure. This suggests the existence of a pressor mechanism that is able to prevent PGA_1 from lowering the blood pressure below normal levels (157).

Thus prostaglandins A_1, A_2, E_1, and E_2 are potent lowerers of systemic blood pressure in human hypertensive subjects, but do not evoke significant side effects when given in a manner that permits sufficient blood levels to be achieved. This would make them ideal candidates for antihypertensive drug therapy, were it not for their rapid removal from the circulation by lung and kidney. Effective blood levels can be maintained only by continuous infusion of the PGs.

Prostaglandin $F_{2\alpha}$ is also present in the kidney in substantial quantity. And although it shares the potent smooth muscle stimulating property of E_1 and E_2, its effects on the renal-cardiovascular system are completely different. Infusion of $PGF_{2\alpha}$ in man in doses ranging from 0.01 to 2.0 μg/(kg)(min) for 60 min produces no effect on blood pressure, heart rate, or respiration (175). In dogs, $PGF_{2\alpha}$ has some pressor effects due to increased venoconstriction that leads to increased cardiac output (176).

Prostaglandins C_1 and C_2 possess about half the arterial blood pressure lowering ability of the corresponding PGEs. The PGBs are about one-hundredth as active as the PGEs (177).

As is usual in other tissues of the body, prostaglandins are not stored as such in the kidney. There is continuous low level synthesis of PGE_2 and $F_{2\alpha}$ that is thought to contribute, by way of the vasodilator actions of E_2, to the maintenance of basal intrarenal blood flow (178). When angiotensin II (A II) is infused into the renal artery, there is an immediate drop in renal blood flow and urine flow. Within 5 min, however, blood and urine flows return to normal levels in spite of continued infusion of A II. But when the PG synthetase inhibitor indomethacin is given, the hypertensive effect of A II persists (179). This suggests that at least one prostaglandin is synthesized on demand by a synthetase system that is not evenly distributed throughout the kidney but is located chiefly in the renal papilla, at its junction with the outer medulla (180, 181). This synthetase system is almost completely absent from the renal cortex.

A great deal of controversy exists as to how much prostaglandin A_2 is present in the kidney and whether it is synthesized enzymatically or by adventitious dehydration of PGE_2 (157, 182, 183). The weight of evidence accumulated so far suggests that prostaglandins of the A type are not primary prostaglandins but rather are artifacts of the corresponding E types, produced by dehydration during the procedure used to extract them from tissue. This point has not been conclusively established, however, and there is reasonable evidence that PGAs are not artifacts and do play a definite role in physiological regulation (184, 185). The future development of more sensitive prostaglandin bioassays will be needed to resolve the question.

Recently prostaglandin D_2 (33.**14**) was found to be a major product of a synthetase system isolated from rabbit renal medulla, suggesting that it may have a significant role in renal physiology (186). Or it may be the endoperoxide precursor to E_2, $F_{2\alpha}$, and D_2 that is responsible for the observed activities.

Prostaglandins of the 1-series are not observed in the kidney.

4.1.1 PROSTAGLANDINS AS RENAL HORMONES. Recognition of the important biological effects of prostaglandins in the kidney has led to the development of a general theory of the role of the kidney in regulating blood pressure and the volume of body fluids. According to this theory, arterial blood pressure is regulated by a balance of the actions of renin-angiotensin, norepinephrine, and prostaglandin E_2 on the arterioles. Elevations in blood pressure stimulate renal cortical vasoconstriction that tends to maintain a constant rate of blood flow through the renal cortex. This is the "autoregulatory" function of the kidney. However blood flow through the medulla is not autoregulated. Increases in systemic arterial blood pressure produce increased blood flow to the medulla that is sensed by the interstitial cells. These cells respond by increasing the synthesis and release of PGE_2, which acts on the outer medulla and cortex to reduce the tone of the cortical vasculature, increase blood flow, and so lower blood pressure. PGE_2 also blocks sodium resorption in the proximal tubules, leading to natriuresis and consequent plasma volume reduction. Although volume reduction can be as high as 10%, it cannot be the sole cause of blood pressure reduction (172).

It has also been suggested that some of the prostaglandin E_2 or A_2 synthesized intrarenally escapes into the general circulation and produces a systemic antihypertensive effect by way of peripheral vasodilation (157, 182, 183). However it is hard to see how this is likely to contribute greatly to the blood pressure lowering process. The amounts of PGE_2 released by the kidneys are smaller than those required to demonstrate a systemic effect when given by intraarterial infusion. Also, PGE_2 is rapidly destroyed in the lungs and liver.

4.1.2 PROSTAGLANDINS AS NATRIURETIC HORMONES. The observations that infusion of PGAs and PGEs increases urine flow and sodium excretion led to the suggestion that E_2 is a natriuretic hormone (157, 160, 182, 183). When PGA_2 or PGE_2 is administered into the renal artery, sodium and water excretion increases while the glomerular filtration rate (GFR) remains the same. The same pattern is seen when saline is administered, which suggests that elevated sodium levels stimulate release of a factor capable of causing the excretion of sodium ions without significantly increasing GFR. In experimental animals maintained on low sodium diets, the concentration of PGA in the renal papilla was found to be high—3600 pg/mg, falling to 500 pg/mg in the outer medulla, and very low in the cortex. When a high sodium diet was administered, the concentration of prostaglandin A in the papilla fell by half, but it rose to about 1300 pg/mg in the outer medulla (157). When indomethacin, a PG synthetase inhibitor, was given to salt-loaded animals, sodium excretion dropped sharply, and this was mirrored by greatly reduced levels of PGA in the medulla and cortex. All of which implicates PGA_2 or PGE_2 as an endogenous natriuretic hormone. The mechanism of natriuresis has been suggested to proceed by way of inhibition of salt and water resorption in the proximal tubules (187). A number of specific biochemical mechanisms have been proposed for this inhibition but none have been definitely established (188).

The theory that renal prostaglandins contribute to the regulation of systemic blood pressure appears to be correct overall. However the weight of evidence so far accumulated suggests that this homeostatic function is mediated almost exclusively by PGE_2 and that PGA_2, originally suspected to fulfill the role of renal antihypertensive hormone, is present in the kidney in at best negligible quantities. And although both PGEs and PGAs, by causing peripheral arterial vasodilation, reduce systemic blood pressure in human and experimental hypertension when given intraarterially, they do not normally act as circulating hormones. Rather, they act intrarenally to lower elevated blood pressure by a combination of increased renal blood flow, reduced blood volume, and increased sodium excretion and diuresis.

Prostaglandin $F_{2\alpha}$ is present in the kidneys in quantity, but it has been assigned no definite role in intrarenal physiology. It has been suggested that $F_{2\alpha}$ could contribute to the renal control of blood pressure by acting as a "venous hormone." That is, its release into the venous circulation by the kidney might serve to increase cardiac output (160).

4.2 Inflammation

The term "inflammation" broadly describes the body's normal defense reactions to injury or tissue insult. The stimulus may be external as with a burn, chemical irritation, or mechanical trauma; or internal, such as a neoplasm, or viruses, or bacteria. Depending on the nature of the stimulus, the inflammatory response can be either acute or chronic. In the case of tissue damage due to an acute event—a burn, for example—inflammation takes the form of a transient, reparative response that ceases when normal tissue function is restored. Tissue damage due to a more or less ongoing stimulus, such as an infection, produces a chronic inflammatory response that seeks to destroy the source of the irritation or to wall it off from the rest of the organism, as in the case of granuloma formation in pulmonary tuberculosis.

The inflammatory response is a complex process that varies slightly depending on the stimulus that evokes it. It is a combination of many kinds of biological and chemical events that begins with the recognition of the injurious stimulus, continues with mobilization of natural defense mechanisms, and culminates in tissue repair or the sealing off of the offending body. This inflammation-repair process is accomplished chiefly by the elements present in the circulation—circulating antibodies, white blood cells, and complement factors—which are mainly responsible for the recognition and destruction steps.

The early stage of inflammation is marked by dilation of the peripheral vasculature, the venules and capillaries, in the affected area. Fluid and proteins leak into the interstitial spaces and produce edema. The vessels become more permeable and "sticky" toward leukocytes, particularly polymorphonuclear leukocytes (PMNs), which adhere to the vasculature, migrate through the walls, and accumulate locally (183, 190, 191). These white blood cells engulf and digest the offending agents and tissue debris in a process accompanied by the release of proteolytic enzymes (called lysozymes) from their lysosomes. Pain, reddening of the skin, and locally elevated temperature also occur. PMNs derive their name from the many granules they contain in which are located digestive and hydrolytic enzymes, including phosphatases, needed to digest bacteria, dead tissue, etc. It is the nonspecific action of these enzymes that appears to be responsible for damage to healthy tissue. The PMNs are the actual effectors of inflammation and are present as several cell types, e.g., basophils, neutrophils, and eosinophils. Neutrophils are end cells, incapable of division. About 1% are present in the circulation, where their lifetime is about 6 hr. The rest are held in reserve in the bone marrow. Eosinophils are similar to the neutrophils in genesis and life span. They are found in large numbers (up to $500\times$blood) in some tissues, particularly in organs, such as lung, intestines, and skin, which are in contact with the environment. They also contain lysosomal granules similar to those of neutrophils except for having a basic protein that is responsible for the eosin stain reaction. Eosinophils are able to release substances that antagonize histamine, bradykinin, and serotonin, suggesting that at least part of their participation in the inflammatory response might be to restore the damaged area to normal (192).

Monocytes and macrophages are other kinds of leukocytes that play a role in inflammation. Monocytes are the largest of blood cells. They take up foreign elements in the circulation by both pinocytosis and phagocytosis. In inflammation monocytes leave the blood and move into the perivascular area where they give rise to macrophages. Macrophages are giant cells, 5 times the size of the monocytes from which they are derived. The richest sources of these cells are lung, liver, and connective tissue. Their life span is much longer than that of PMNs, and their chief function appears to be the engulfment and removal of larger debris left behind by the action of PMNs and other agents on damaged tissue, bacteria, etc. (191, 192).

Perhaps the last cell to arrive at the site of inflammation is the platelet. Platelets are white blood cells involved in the clotting mechanism. They also seem to be responsible for returning vascular permeability to normal after it has been increased, as in inflammation. The platelets aggregate to form a plug that seals off leaks in injured small blood vessels. They first adhere to the damaged vessels by a mechanism qualitatively similar to other leukocyte adhesions, then to one another to form a clump. It may be that platelets are simply specialized white blood cells that service damaged blood vessels just as PMNs and macrophages service damaged tissues, except that they do not appear to be phagocytic. It is interesting to note that platelets release $PGF_{2\alpha}$, which may counter some of the inflammatory actions of PGEs. This, and the ability of platelets to restore normal vascular permeability and circulation, can be thought of as an anti-inflammatory response that helps terminate the inflammatory response. However some investigators have described the platelet itself as an inflammatory cell, at least potentially, although conclusive evidence for this in clinical inflammation is lacking (193, 194). Figure 33.8 outlines the basic processes and time course of the inflammatory response, with the reservation that the latter phases are not distinct but rather tend to overlap to varying degrees (195).

There are at least 10 substances able to act as mediators of the various stages of inflammation depicted in Fig. 33.8: histamine, serotonin, slow reacting substance of anaphylaxis (SRS-A), kinins, plasmin, activated Hageman factor, complement, lysosomal enzymes, lymphokines, and prostaglandins (189). Vasodilating substances such as histamine, serotonin, and kinins are thought to be mainly responsible for the exudative stage, the "initial burst" of inflammation caused by increased capillary permeability. Prostaglandins appear to modulate the latter stages of inflammation involving PMN emigration into the affected area (195). In one model of experimental inflammation, the carrageenin-induced rat foot edema, inhibitors of histamine, serotonin, and kinins delay by several hours the onset, but not the peak, of edema formation (196–198). Prostaglandin E_2 appears at the site of carrageenin inflammation at about 3 hr and reaches a peak between 12

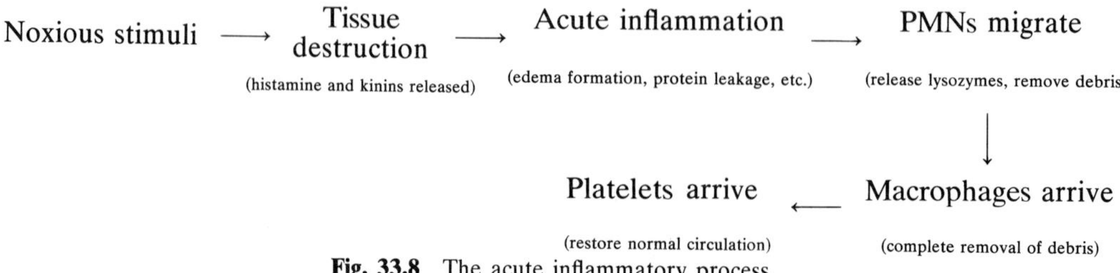

Fig. 33.8 The acute inflammatory process.

and 24 hr, approximately at the time PMNs begin to appear (198).

It has been suggested that prostaglandins are responsible for the transition from the acute exudative phase of inflammation to the chronic, ongoing state (199). Support for this idea comes from the finding that prostaglandin E_1 is chemotactic for PMNs, even though PGE_1 elevates intracellular levels of cyclic AMP and such elevated cyclic AMP levels are known to reduce PMN motility (200, 201). This is an apparent contradiction unless it can be thought of as a "trapping mechanism." Perhaps freely circulating PMNs flow into the inflamed area, absorb PGE_1, and lose their motility, thus remaining in the area to begin the process of phagocytosis of foreign and damaged tissue. This process in turn liberates phosphoesterases, which release prostaglandin precursors from their phospholipid storage sites. The ubiquitous synthetase system then makes more prostaglandins, which trap more PMNs at the site. Once the noxious stimulus and the damaged tissue have been removed by hydrolysis and phagocytosis, local production of prostaglandins decreases and the inflammatory response diminishes. This theory fits in nicely with the well-known ability of nonsteroidal anti-inflammatory drugs, which inhibit PG synthetase, to inhibit chemotaxis (202). However prostaglandins are not chemotactic for leukocytes in all systems studied, and a quantitative relationship between cyclic AMP stimulation and inhibition of chemotaxis has not been established (203, 204). Prostaglandins E_1, E_2, $F_{1\alpha}$, and $F_{2\alpha}$ also increase vascular permeability, a property that could contribute to the maintenance of edema during later stages of inflammation (205).

Most of the evidence linking prostaglandins to inflammation is based on finding them in exudates of experimental inflammation (195, 206) and in human inflammation (207). Furthermore, rats deficient in essential fatty acids (leading to decreased ability to synthesize prostaglandins) resist developing carrageenin-induced inflammation, as do rats that have been immunized against prostaglandins (208, 209).

The most important of the inflammatory diseases is rheumatoid arthritis. Although it takes many forms, the most debilitating and most common symptom is impaired joint function (210). Opposing surfaces of bones are covered with cartilage, and opposition of two bones is maintained by the fibrous joint capsule and the muscles that span the joint. The space between the joint capsule and the articulating cartilage is occupied by the synovial membrane. This membrane secretes synovial fluid, which lubricates and supplies nutrients to the avascular cartilage (210). Inflammation of this synovial membrane (synovitis) is characterized by the presence of cells releasing hydrolytic enzymes into the synovial fluid. These begin to digest the cartilage, causing it to lose resilience and slipperiness. In chronic inflammation the synovial membrane becomes overgrown with inflammatory cells, hypertrophies, and eventually destroys the joint (210). Clearly, a drug able to interrupt the crucial "prostaglandin phase" or leukocyte migration process would be extremely beneficial in treating many forms of inflammation, particularly chronic varieties.

Of the many drugs used to treat arthritis, aspirin stands out as having been used most and longest, even though how it acts was only recently elucidated. In reviewing the pharmacology of aspirin in 1969, Collier suggested that its diverse effects on many physiological events could have a common cause. He proposed that aspirin acts to depress some local humoral process involved in a natural defense mechanism (211). The inference for arthritis was that the aspirin owed its therapeutic properties to its ability to inhibit the particular natural defense mechanism of inflammation.

Since prostaglandins had recently been established as important mediators of a crucial phase of inflammation, their antagonism by aspirin would have offered a convenient explanation of aspirin's anti-inflammatory activity. But it was well known that aspirin has no inhibitory effect on responses evoked by the administration of prostaglandins in several experimental models. The explanation was finally provided in 1971 by the simultaneous publication of three articles demonstrating that therapeutic doses of aspirin and the potent anti-inflammatory drug indomethacin were able to block the enzymatic synthesis of PGE_2 and $PGF_{2\alpha}$ in guinea pig lung (212), dog spleen (213), and human platelets (214). Additional studies confirmed that aspirin and other nonsteroidal anti-inflammatory agents do not act *directly* to inhibit the actions of prostaglandins but rather act *indirectly* by preventing their synthesis. Their inhibitory potencies against PG synthetase are of the same degree and rank order as their clinical potencies (215, 216). However there are many prostaglandin synthetase systems, and their susceptibility to anti-inflammatory drugs varies depending on species and organ. The relative activities of indomethacin (33.**53**) and aspirin on rabbit brain synthetase, for example, is 19 : 1, whereas on the synthetase system from bovine seminal vesicles the ratio is 2140 : 1 (217).

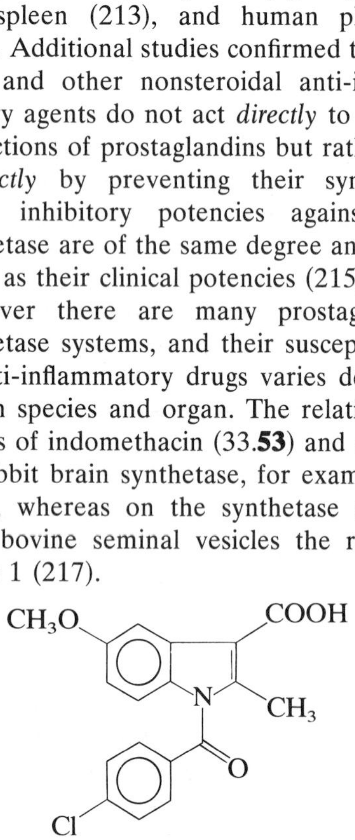

Indomethacin
33.**53**

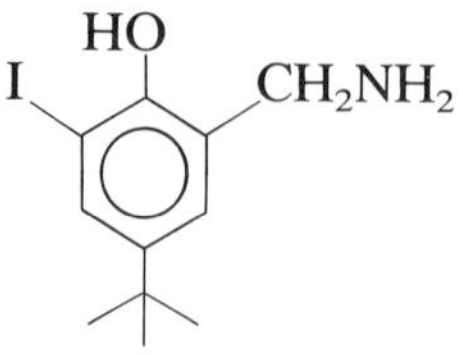

33.**54**

The varying sensitivity of synthetase systems may explain why not all kinds of inflammation respond to the same degree to various anti-inflammatory drugs. For example, although elevated levels of prostaglandins are present in many inflammatory conditions of the human skin, such inflammations are not sensitive to treatment by aspirin and other potent nonsteroidal anti-inflammatory drugs. Recently, however, the prostaglandin synthetase system present in human skin was found to be unaffected by such drugs but was greatly inhibited by the anti-inflammatory steroid fluocinolone acetonide (218, 219). This seems to explain, at least partially, the inactivity of aspirin and the success of lipophilic corticosteroids in treating dermal inflammations.

Systemic anti-inflammatory steroids, on the other hand, appear to act by stabilizing cell membranes, thus preventing the release of arachidonic acid, the prostaglandin precursor, from its storage sites (220).

Studies of several models of experimental inflammation in the rat have further substantiated both the role of prostaglandins in inflammation and the physiological consequences of the inhibition of their synthesis by aspirinlike drugs. Such anti-inflammatory drugs were found to inhibit consistently the delayed phase of inflammation by preventing the migration of mononuclear cells, and perhaps also PMNs, into the inflamed area. The degree of inhibition paralleled the extent of reduction of prostaglandins in the inflammatory exudate (221–223). In addition, evidence now indicates that such drugs can block the transport of prostaglandins across cell membranes and thereby prevent them from acting as inflammatory mediators (224).

Recently it has been found that both PGD_2 (33.**14**) and the endoperoxide PGG_2 (33.**24**) can act as mediators of inflammation (225, 226). In acute inflammation at least, the endoperoxide appears to be all important. The inhibition of its formation by the cyclooxygenase pathway accounts for the efficacy of acidic, nonsteroidal anti-inflammatory agents such as aspirin and indomethacin (33.**53**), but at least one other nonsteroidal anti-inflammatory drug, 2-aminomethyl-4-*t*-butyl-6-iodophenol (MK-447 33.**54**), actually stimulates the synthesis of the primary prostaglandins. This finding has led to the proposal that PGEs are not primarily responsible for inflammation but are merely artifacts of PGG_2, which is. And that compound MK-447 acts by speeding the conversion of PGG_2 to PGH_2, and so to the primary prostaglandins (226). Whether this explanation can be substantiated and extended to other nonacidic, nonsteroidal anti-inflammatory agents that are not prostaglandin synthetase inhibitors, remains to be seen.

4.3 Human Reproduction

4.3.1 THE MENSTRUAL CYCLE. In no other area of mammalian physiology are there so many control mechanisms as exist in the human female for regulation of reproduction. And at least some of these control mechanisms now appear to involve prostaglandins. In women, reproductive ability is governed by the reproductive or menstrual cycle. The events of the menstrual cycle are designed to facilitate conception; they occur chiefly in the ovaries and are reflected by changes in the endometrium—the mucous lining of the uterus. The pituitary gland, located at the base of the brain and connected to the central nervous system (CNS), regulates the activities of the ovaries and coordinates the timing of various aspects of the cycle in response to both internal and external stimuli (227). The pituitary gland accomplishes this by secreting into the general circulation two glycoprotein gonadotropins: follicle-stimulating hormone (FSH) and luteinizing hormone (LH).

The ovary is a flattened ellipsoid, about 2 in. at its greatest length. It contains tens of thousands of ova, which are located in cystlike bodies called graafian follicles. Under the influence of FSH, several follicles begin to develop and enlarge toward the surface of the ovary. Normally, during one menstrual cycle, only a single follicle completes the process of development, ruptures, and discharges its ovum into the peritoneal cavity. This is called ovulation. The egg is released in the vicinity of the ciliary processes surrounding the opening (ostium) of the fallopian tubes. The fallopian tubes, or oviducts, are 4–5 in. long and connect the ovaries to the uterus. The rapid beat of the cilia at the mouth of the tube provides a current that, together with the muscle activity of the duct, carries the liberated ovum through the oviduct toward the uterus. During this 3–4 day journey, the egg is nourished by the secretions of cells lining the oviduct. If the egg encounters sperm along the way, conception occurs and the fertilized ovum is swept along toward the uterus (228).

The uterus is a hollow, pear-shaped, muscular organ with walls about $\frac{1}{2}$ in. thick, consisting of a lower, narrow neck, the cervix, projecting down into the vagina and an upper, larger body called the fundus. The entire organ is held in place in the pelvic cavity by several types of ligament. The cavity of the upper uterus is triangular, and from the two upper, lateral apices, the fallopian tubes extend to the ovaries. The hollow interior (lumen) of each fallopian tube is continuous with the uterine cavity.

As the follicle develops prior to ovulation, it secretes increasing amounts of estrogen and smaller amounts of progesterone. Estrogen acts to increase the spontaneous muscle activity of the fallopian tubes, to facilitate movement of the egg toward the uterus. It also causes the endometrial lining of the uterus to proliferate, increasing its thickness two-to-threefold, and readying it to receive the fertilized egg, the blastocyst. If conception does not occur, the egg dies and the thickened endometrium becomes hemorrhagic, sloughs off, and is discharged through the cervix and vagina in about 5 days of menstrual flow. The endometrium then returns to the inactive state until again stimulated by ovulation.

As soon as ovulation occurs, the cells of the now-empty follicle are stimulated by LH to organize and form a structure known from its color as the corpus luteum. The corpus luteum exists to secrete the steroid hormone progesterone. Under the influence of increased levels of progesterone, the endometrium develops a secretory function, which assists it in accepting and nourishing the fertilized ovum. If pregnancy does not occur, the corpus luteum regresses within 2 weeks and circulating levels of progesterone decline sharply. It is this decrease in progesterone secretion by the corpus luteum that is mainly responsible for loss of the endometrium. If pregnancy does occur, cells of the developing placenta secrete another hormone, human chorionic gonadotropin (HCG). This hormone acts to prolong the lifetime of the corpus luteum with its needed production of progesterone until the placenta develops sufficiently to produce its own. This occurs by the end of the first trimester of pregnancy, after which the corpus luteum becomes nonfunctional and regresses.

The lifetime of the corpus luteum in nonpregnancy is controlled by the uterus. In many nonprimate species, this endocrine function of the uterus is mediated at least partially by prostaglandin $F_{2\alpha}$, now generally accepted to be identical with "luteolysin," the long sought uterine luteolytic hormone (229). Administration of indomethacin greatly prolongs estrus in the guinea pig. Immunization of sheep and guinea pigs against prostaglandin $F_{2\alpha}$ accomplishes the same thing, and the increase in length of the estrous cycle and persistence of the corpus luteum is proportional to the titer of antibodies to $PGF_{2\alpha}$ (229). In cattle, sheep, and swine, $PGF_{2\alpha}$ is produced by the uterus and reaches the ovary by diffusing directly from the uteroovarian vein to the adjacent ovarian artery (229, 230). Neither the oviduct nor the lymphatic channels are involved. No such local pathway from uterus to ovary exists in other species. In the horse, for example, $PGF_{2\alpha}$ secreted by the uterus is returned to the ovary by the general circulation. Luteolysin acts directly on the ovary to limit corpus luteum function, not indirectly by inhibiting gonadotropin release from the pituitary gland (231, 232). It appears to inhibit the actions of gonadotropins on the ovary by competing directly with them for receptor sites (233). In the rat, $PGF_{2\alpha}$ and LH are mutual antagonists of their opposite effects on progesterone secretion. There is some evidence that the decrease in progesterone synthesis is accomplished by the ability of $PGF_{2\alpha}$ to inhibit the enzyme cholesterol esterase. This enzyme releases cholesterol, the necessary substrate for progesterone biosynthesis, from its intercellular storage sites (229).

The regression of the corpus luteum is attributed to the influence of $PGF_{2\alpha}$ on local blood flow. Although it was originally postulated that total blood flow to the ovary was diminished, it now appears that total ovarian blood flow is relatively unchanged. Instead, $PGF_{2\alpha}$ acts to redistribute blood flow within the ovary away from the corpus luteum, causing it to atrophy and regress (234). There is a degree of similarity between this mechanism and the postulated role of PGE_2 in redistributing blood flow in the kidney in response to hypertensive stimuli.

In primates, the influence of prostaglandin $F_{2\alpha}$ on luteolysis is much less marked. In one study, infusion of $PGF_{2\alpha}$ reduced plasma progesterone levels late in the luteal phase of the cycle but did not shorten the cycle (235). In women, infusion of $PGF_{2\alpha}$ in doses up to 50 μg/min for as long as 8 hr early in the luteal phase shortened the phase in only about one-third of the patients studied. And luteolysis could not be induced by intravaginal administration of prostaglandins (235). Thus in spite of the existence of specific ovarian binding sites for $PGF_{2\alpha}$ that suggest for it a specific controlling function of the corpus luteum, $F_{2\alpha}$ does not seem to be responsible for luteolysis in the human, at least not by a mechanism similar to the one found in subprimates (236). Nevertheless, intrauterine administration of $PGF_{2\alpha}$ will terminate early human pregnancy (within a few weeks of delayed menstruation), a time during which maintenance of pregnancy entirely depends on progesterone secreted by the corpus luteum. However this does not seem to be due to a luteolytic effect; rather, it appears to be the result of sustained uterine contraction and vasoconstriction that dislocate the developing blastocyst (237, 238).

Prostaglandins do mediate at least some of the ovulatory actions of LH in humans: local production of $PGF_{2\alpha}$ is elevated in the follicles and ovaries in response to LH. In rats, pharmacological blockade of this preovulatory elevation of prostaglandin blocks ovulation as well (239). Prostaglandin $F_{2\alpha}$ stimulates oocyte maturation, and the $PGF_{2\alpha}$ responsible for the rupture of the follicle is produced by the follicle itself (240, 241).

Prostaglandins may affect the reproductive cycle by yet another mechanism, by acting directly on the pituitary gland. Exogenous prostaglandins stimulate LH secretion from the pituitary in rats, and this stimulation is followed by fresh ovulation (242). However this effect may be due simply to potentiation of adrenergic transmission, which is necessary for the secretion of LH. The extent to which PGs affect LH release in humans has not been definitely established (243).

Prostaglandin $F_{2\alpha}$ also induces muscle activity in the oviducts and may act there to facilitate egg transport (244). Prostaglandin E induces contractions in the proximal quarter of the oviduct but relaxes the distal portions. Since there is much PGE in sperm, this action may facilitate conception by aiding egg transport through the oviduct (245).

Prostaglandins increase the motility of the nonpregnant uterus at about the time of ovulation but not at other times of the menstrual cycle, and this too may facilitate conception by aiding sperm transport (246).

4.3.2 PARTURITION. The pregnant uterus is sensitive at all times to the presence of prostaglandins; they are among the most potent stimulants known, with the PGEs being about 10 times more potent than $PGF_{2\alpha}$. Intravenous infusion of 0.6–9.0 μg/ml of PGE_1 increases both the amplitude and frequency of uterine contractions and, if continued, can result in expulsion of the fetus (247). Prostaglandins stimulate uterine smooth muscle directly by acting on discrete prostaglandin receptors in the myometrium, the smooth muscle coat of the uterus (248). They act at all stages of gestation and are active whether administered parenterally or locally.

Much evidence has been collected during the last 10 years suggesting that prostaglandins play a major role in labor and parturition, and numerous efforts have been made to determine exactly the levels of prostaglandins in peripheral and uterine blood during pregnancy. Although estimates vary greatly depending on the analytical technique used, a clear pattern presents itself. Compared to nonpregnant females, peripheral blood levels of $PGF_{2\alpha}$ are elevated in the first and third trimesters of pregnancy but decreased in the second. Levels are also high in umbilical blood, and during labor a peak of $PGF_{2\alpha}$ appears 45–60 sec after a contraction.

Both prostaglandins E_2 and $F_{2\alpha}$ appear in the amniotic fluid. Concentrations are low during the first 36 weeks but later rise sharply to above 300 pg/ml and to above 1000 pg/ml as labor commences (249, 250).

This increase parallels estrogen increase during gestation and may be the result of it.

The amount of prostaglandins present in the amniotic fluid during labor is directly proportional to the degree of cervical dilation (251–253). They seem to arise from the decidua and may be produced and released by these tissues in response to the stretching and contraction that occur during labor. And their release causes more stretch and contraction that contribute to the accelerating cyclic process that leads to parturition. Nonsteroidal anti-inflammatory drugs, which block prostaglandin synthesis, prolong parturition in the rat, and there is some evidence that prolonged ingestion of aspirin in humans has a similar effect (235).

Labor at term can be induced by prostaglandins and is identical with spontaneous labor or labor induced by oxytocin. In a study of 100 patients, $PGF_{2\alpha}$ and oxytocin gave almost equivalent results in inducing labor. Side effects, principally uterine hypertonus, were slightly greater with $F_{2\alpha}$. However the prostaglandin was able to induce contractions at any stage of pregnancy, whereas oxytocin is usually effective only at term (243).

4.3.3 MALE FERTILITY. Only humans, monkeys, and sheep have prostaglandins in their semen, and there is not much in the sheep. However, lower animals reproduce themselves ably enough, suggesting that perhaps prostaglandins in semen are a consequence of higher evolution. The total amount present in human semen has been estimated to be as high as 300 μg/ml. Some 15 different PGs have been detected, but the relative concentrations are hard to determine. With seminal plasma, as with blood, the manner of isolation allows a substantial amount of the PGEs to dehydrate to As and rearrange to Bs. Even so, concentrations of the labile PGE_1 and PGE_2 are high, above 25 μg/ml, and are accompanied by one-fifth as much PGE_3. Prostaglandins $F_{1\alpha}$ and $F_{2\alpha}$, stable under the conditions of isolation, are present in only small concentrations, roughly 5 μg/ml (254).

Since human semen contains such large amounts of prostaglandins, it is almost certain that they play a definite role in reproduction. However there is no correlation between the prostaglandin content of human seminal fluid and the number or motility of spermatozoa present (235). On the other hand, samples of seminal fluid from men in infertile marriages contain less PGEs than from men with children (255). A number of studies have shown that aspirin, a prostaglandin synthetase inhibitor, can reduce levels of PGs in seminal fluid by 30–80%, but this has yet to be linked to male infertility (256, 257).

Not much is definitely known about the physiological effects of prostaglandins on male reproductive tissues, although they do stimulate the corpus cavernosa muscle of the penis (258). This, along with their other smooth muscle stimulating actions, may contribute to the maintenance of the peristalsis involved in ejaculation. Local vasodilation caused by PG release may also contribute to erection (235).

It has already been pointed out that prostaglandins provided by semen affect smooth muscle activity in the vagina and oviducts, possibly facilitating egg and sperm transport. Thus it may be that prostaglandins in semen have no effect on fertility in the male, but only in the female after semen has been deposited.

4.4 The Gastrointestinal Tract

4.4.1 GASTROINTESTINAL MOTILITY. Prostaglandins are present in all portions of the human alimentary canal and affect many of the physiological processes that take place there, especially gastric acid secretion, intestinal and pancreatic secretion, ion transport, and smooth muscle activities.

The musculature of the stomach consists of three layers of fibers: inner circular ones distributed over the entire organ, outer longitudinal fibers concentrated along the curvature of the stomach, and oblique fibers concentrated toward the upper end of the stomach. Superimposed on the resting tone of these muscles is the muscle activity known as peristalsis, coupled waves of up to four different kinds of muscle activity that, in man, originate in the longitudinal fibers but are the product of rhythmic contractions and relaxations of all three. Gastric peristalsis assists digestion by breaking up the stomach contents and moving them toward the intestines. Peristaltic waves continue through the duodenum, the foot-long upper portion of the small intestine, and become somewhat irregular and of lower frequency in the lower portions of the small intestine, the jejunum and ileum. Movement is slower still and less regular in the lower intestines, the cecum and colon, although it still originates in longitudinal fibers.

Prostaglandins E_2 and $F_{2\alpha}$ are present in gastric tissue and gastric juice chiefly as E_2, less so as $F_{2\alpha}$. There is about 1 μg of PGE_2 per gram of wet mucosa and about 2 ng/ml of gastric juice (259, 260). It is not clear whether the amount present in gastric juice is actively secreted or arises adventitiously through cell turnover. However there is a circadian variation of PGE levels in human gastric juice that is reciprocal to gastric acid output; PGE levels are higher during the day than during the night. This circadian rhythm is disturbed in peptic ulcer patients; in normal subjects it can be abolished and PGE levels lowered by therapeutic doses of aspirin (261, 262). This suggests that PGE_2 actually is present in gastric juice under normal conditions. PGE is located chiefly in the mucosal and submucosal regions of the stomach, with less in muscle layers (263). The gastric mucosa releases prostaglandin upon vagal stimulation, or stimulation by histamine or pentagastrin (264).

Prostaglandins are among the most potent stimulators of gastric smooth muscle known, although sensitivity varies from species to species and from place to place in the alimentary canal of each species. In man and guinea pig, PGEs relax circular smooth muscle but contract longitudinal muscles in both stomach and small intestines. In the rat, both muscles are contracted. Prostaglandins appear to act directly on gut muscle, although there is also some stimulation of intestinal cholinergic nerves (260). In man, administration of 0.8–3.2 mg of PGE is known to cause pain and increased gut motility, secretions, and some bile reflux into the stomach (265, 266). However the motility of the sigmoid colon was significantly reduced by the infusion of 0.08 μg/(kg)(min) of PGE_2. $PGF_{2\alpha}$ at 0.8 μg/(kg)(min) was without effect (267). In man, PGE_2 reduces sphincter pressure and peristalsis in the lower esophagus but has no effect on the upper esophagus (268).

The extreme sensitivity of gastric and intestinal smooth muscles to PGs, their presence in the alimentary canal, and their rapid metabolic inactivation in the gut wall, suggest that PGE_2 is at least partly responsible for both basal tone and peristalsis. This idea is supported by the finding that aspirin and indomethacin, which block prostaglandin synthesis, inhibit peristalsis in the ileum and colon of the guinea pig (269).

Of perhaps even greater physiological significance is the effect of prostaglandins on gastric and intestinal secretions.

4.4.2 GASTROINTESTINAL SECRETIONS. To prepare the contents of the stomach for digestion, the stomach produces gastric juice, comprised mainly of hydrochloric acid (HCl) secreted by the parietal cells, mucus secreted by the mucous cells, and the pepsin precursor, pepsinogen, secreted by the chief cells of the fundus. The mechanism of HCl secretion is not completely understood, but it is an ATP-dependent process under the control of cyclic AMP and involves the enzyme *carbonic anhydrase.* Water is separated at the parietal cell membrane; the hydroxide ion is neutralized by bicarbonate ion enzymatically formed from carbon dioxide, and the hydrogen ion is excreted into the stomach. Chloride ion is actively secreted as the counterion, and water is passively transported as an accompaniment of solute movement. To help protect the cells of the stomach lining from being themselves digested by the acidic milieu, mucoprotein is secreted by the mucous cells. This gel-like mucus adheres strongly to the surface epithelium, lubricating it, and at the same time forming a physical barrier to acid penetration. Its constant erosion by stomach acid is balanced by its constant synthesis. Although mucus secretion is stimulated by gastric acid among other things, prolonged hyperacidity is associated with the development of various ulcers (270).

Most of the work of digesting and absorbing nutrients takes place in the small intestine. Aside from mucus, the small intestine secretes electrolytes and water to dilute the products of digestion to isotonicity, to facilitate absorption. The major digestive enzymes, amylase, lipase, trypsin, chymotrypsin, are secreted into the duodenum by the adjacent pancreas. This large multilobed gland also secretes bicarbonate to raise the pH of the incoming gastric chyme to that necessary for the efficient workings of the intestinal digestive enzymes.

Gastric, intestinal, and pancreatic secretions are subject to extremely close control by neural and humoral mediators as well as by stimulatory and inhibitory hormones.

Although the role of prostaglandins in the stomach is still unknown, gastric acid secretion is inhibited by PGEs in many species. PGAs have no effect on gastric smooth muscle, but they too reduce acid secretion when given orally (271). Since the Es are more active in man when given intravenously, the oral activity of PGA might be a reflection of the relative gastric stabilities of the two types. Prostaglandin $F_{2\alpha}$ has no effect on gastric secretion. In man, PGs inhibit basal acid secretion as well as secretion induced by histamine and pentagastrin, and the degree of inhibition is dose dependent. In rats, an oral dose of 2 mg/kg of PGE_2 reduces acid output by 50% (272, 273). Pepsin output and mucus synthesis do not seem to be greatly affected by the natural prostaglandins (263, 274). The prostaglandins appear to act directly on the acid-producing cells, perhaps by a local elevation of cyclic AMP levels rather than by reducing blood flow to the gastric mucosa (275). Prostaglandins E_1 and E_2, together with cyclic AMP, are known to inhibit the membrane-bound Na^+, K^+-dependent ATPase responsible for cation transport across the parietal cell membrane (276). It may be that in the stomach, PGE_2 participates in a negative feedback mechanism limiting acid secretion induced by food or pentagastrin (260).

In contrast to their different actions on gastric acid secretion, both E-type prostaglandins and $F_{2\alpha}$ stimulate secretions of water, electrolytes, and perhaps mucus by the small intestine. In man, infusion of 0.4 or 0.8 μg/(kg)(min) of $PGF_{2\alpha}$ increases ileal secretion up to 25-fold. Absorption of electrolytes by the jejunum is inhibited, but water resorption in the colon is unaffected (263, 277–279). PGE_2 is similarly active, and again this activity may be related to elevations in cyclic AMP levels.

Prostaglandin Es and $F_{2\alpha}$ are potent inducers of vomiting and diarrhea in humans, to a degree that limits their usefulness in labor induction and other therapeutic applications. The diarrhea appears to be the double consequence of enhanced fluid secretion by the ileum that overwhelms the resorptive capacity of the colon (279), and reduced motility of the sigmoid colon that facilitates the onward propulsion of the more fluid contents (267). The diarrhea associated with a number of disease states (ulcerative colitis, cholera, etc.) has been attributed to elevated levels of intestinal prostaglandins (263, 280, 281).

4.4.3 ANTISECRETORY PROSTAGLANDIN ANALOGS. The ability of some prostaglandins to reduce gastric acid secretion has led to a search for orally active antisecretory PGE analogs that lack the side effects leading to diarrhea. The 16,16-dimethyl analog 33.**55** of PGE_2, together with 15(*S*) and 15(*R*)-methyl PGE_2 (33.**56**, 33.**57**) and their respective methyl esters, are all potent oral inhibitors of both basal and stimulated gastric acid secretion in humans. The free acid 33.**55** possesses an ED_{50} of 40 μg, with an effect lasting longer than that of PGE_2 methyl ester. Similar potency is seen in the free acid 33.**56** and its methyl ester. Some abdominal cramping occurs at higher doses, possibly because intestinal motility is reduced (282). One study reported that pepsin output was reduced and there was some incidence of diarrhea at doses of 2 μg/kg (283, 284). On oral administration in humans, the unnatural 15(*R*)-isomer 33.**57** and its methyl ester are roughly equivalent to 33.**55** and 33.**56**, and are better tolerated, but both are inactive when given intravenously (285).

In the rat, 33.**55** and 33.**56** are 40 times as active as PGE_2 in inhibiting pentagastrin-induced gastric acid secretion when given orally and 100 times as active when administered subcutaneously. The unnatural isomer 33.**57** is inactive when given parenterally but is active when first incubated at pH 2 (286), conditions that favor epimerization of 33.**57** to a mixture of 33.**56** and 33.**57**.

In dogs, the methyl ester of 33.**55** not only inhibits acid secretion but strongly inhibits bicarbonate and fluid secretion by the pancreas (287).

The methyl ester 33.**58** of 16-methylene PGE_2 was equipotent to 33.**55** and an order of magnitude superior to PGE_2 on infusion in the rat. It also protected the rat against indomethacin-induced ulcers (288).

Moving the 15-hydroxyl group of PGE_1 methyl ester to the adjacent methylene gave 33.**59**, equipotent with but longer acting in the rat than PGE_1 methyl ester itself. Compound 33.**60**, with the hydroxyl group at C-17, was without gastric antisecretory activity (289).

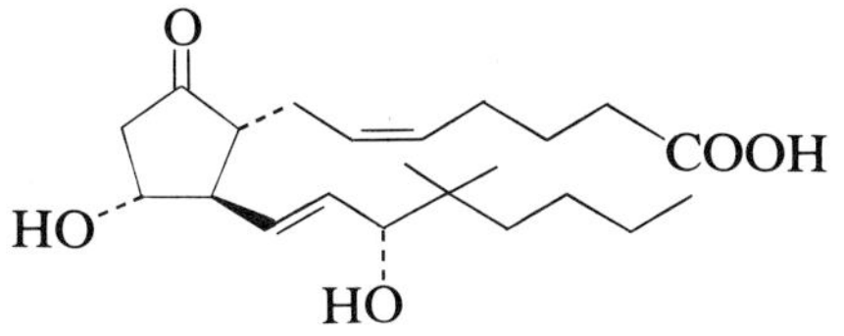

33.**55**

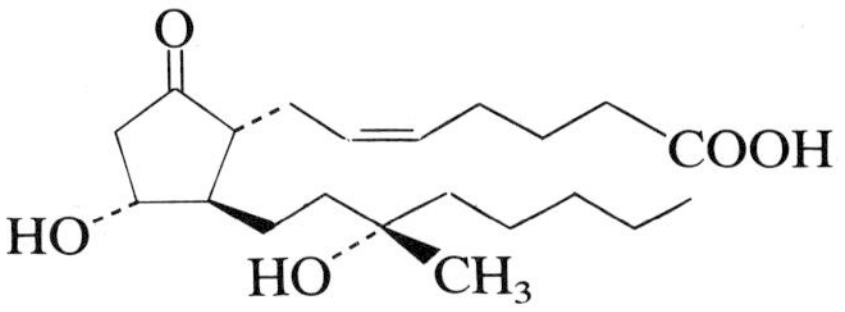

33.**56**

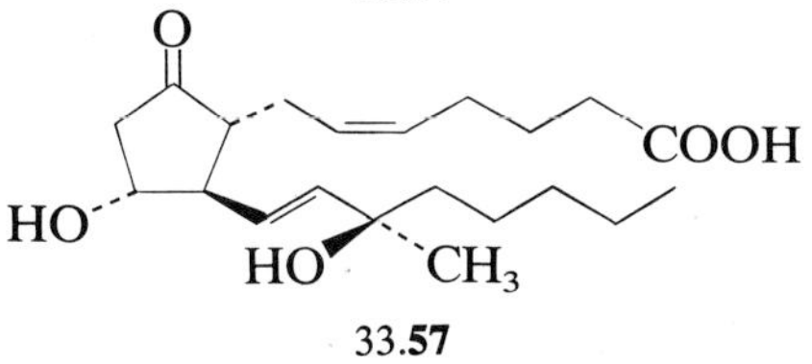

33.**57**

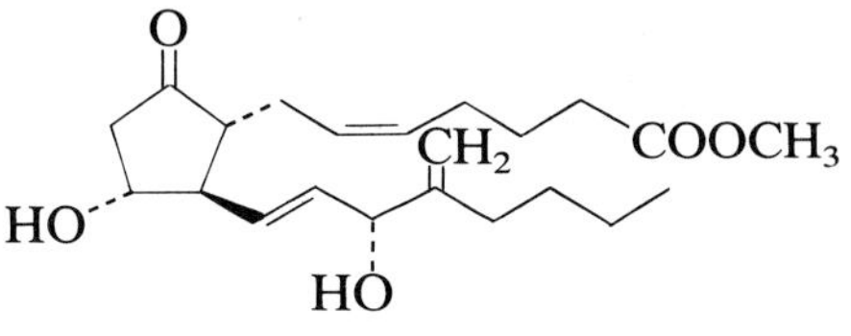

33.**58**

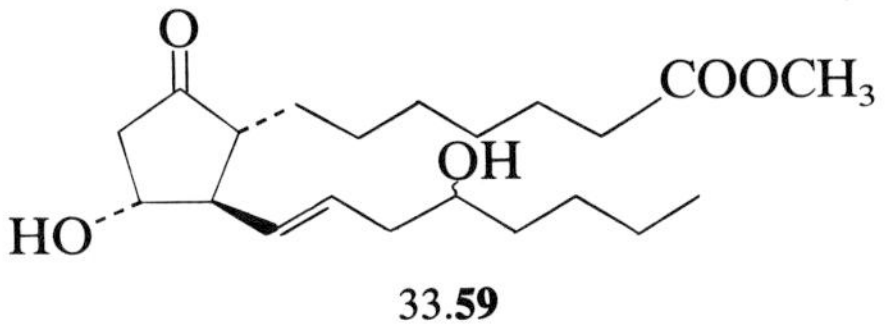

33.**59**

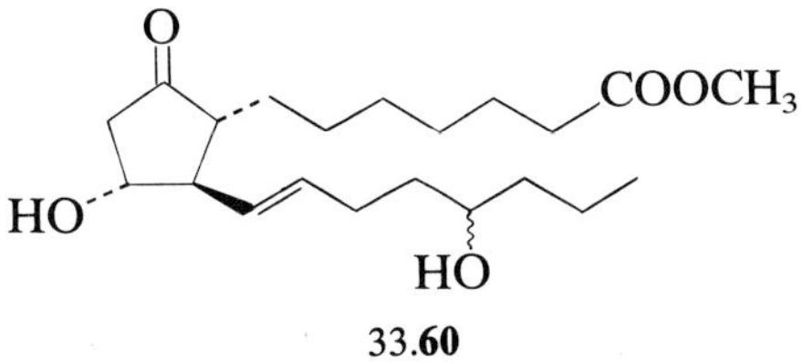

33.**60**

The finding that analogs like 33.**55** and 33.**56** reduce gastric acid secretion in man, produce little diarrhea, and inhibit experimental ulcer production in rats offers hope that a clinically useful antiulcer drug of this type will be available for human use soon.

The increase in antisecretory potency of 15- and 16-substituted prostaglandins is the consequence of steric crowding around the 15-hydroxyl group that renders it insensitive to the 15-dehydrogenase enzyme, the chief PG-deactivating enzyme in the human gut wall (136, 290).

The 11-desoxy analogs of 33.**55** and 33.**56** also reduce gastric acidity, but not gastric volume, in the pentagastrin-stimulated rat (291). Some gastric antisecretory activity in the rat has also been claimed for 11-desoxy-15(*S*),-15-methyl prostaglandin E_1 (292).

The 1-carbinol analog 33.**61** of PGE_1 is a potent inhibitor of acid secretion in several animal models. The cyclohexyl analog 33.**62** is equipotent to 33.**61** in this regard but lacks some of the prostaglandinlike side effects of 33.**61** (293).

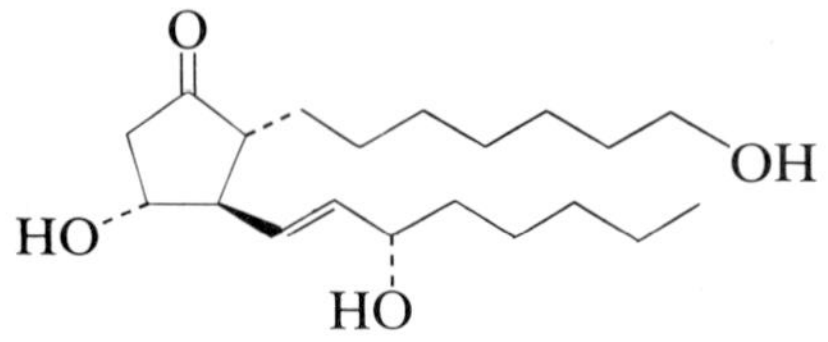

33.**61**

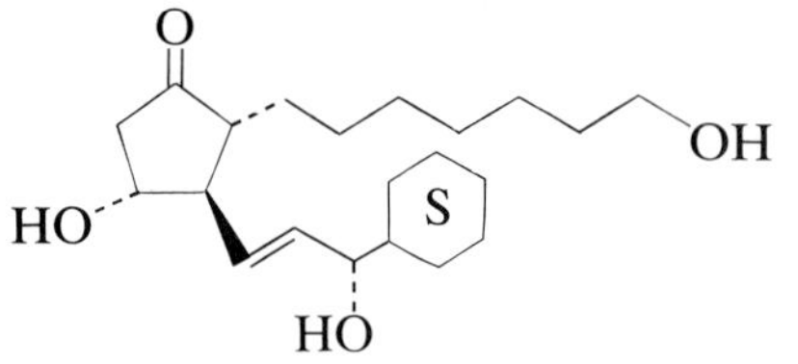

33.**62**

4.5 Fever

Fever is the rise in whole body temperature associated with infection and inflammation, as opposed to the hyperthermia associated with exercise or exposure to a hot environment. Fever may be induced either by exogenous pyrogens—stimuli arising outside the body from sources like bacteria, viruses, fungi, yeasts, and protozoa—or it may be caused by internal stimuli—pyrogens produced within the body by inflammation, antigen-antibody reactions, etc. (294). Endogenous pyrogen is produced by leukocytes and other defensive cells of the reticuloendothelial system upon stimulation by exogenous pyrogens such as endotoxins derived from gram-negative bacteria. Endogenous pyrogen is a protein with a molecular weight between 10,000 and 20,000 (295). It is this substance, when released into the general circulation, that is the common mediator of fever. Its actions on the anterior hypothalamus of the CNS result in metabolic changes that decrease heat loss and increase heat gain, resulting in a hyperthermic state.

Although both endogenous pyrogen and endotoxin cause fever when injected directly into the brains of experimental animals, they do not act directly on the CNS in the intact animal; they are too hydrophilic to penetrate the blood-brain barrier. How they produce fever was unknown until it was discovered that prostaglandins E_1 and E_2, when injected intracerebrally in the cat, produce fevers of short duration but similar in all other respects to fever induced by endotoxin (296–298). And levels of PGE_2, normally low in the cerebrospinal fluid of the cat, were found to be elevated considerably during pyrogen-induced fever (299). Furthermore, fevers caused by endotoxin in the cat, or arachidonic acid in the rat, were suppressed by the antipyretic drug 4-acetamidophenol, but fever caused by PGE_1 was not (300). These findings led to the suggestion that bacterial pyrogens produce fever by stimulating in the CNS the synthesis and release of E-prostaglandins, probably PGE_2, and that antipyretic drugs act by blocking this synthesis. Subsequently, indomethacin, aspirin, and 4-acetamidophenol were found to inhibit rabbit brain prostaglandin synthetase in about the same order and degree as their clinical effectiveness as antipyretics (301, 302).

The fever-producing effect of PGE, at least in rabbits, is due to a norepinephrine-mediated increase in levels of cyclic AMP in hypothalamic neurones (303, 304).

Prostaglandins do not seem to be concerned with heat production or conservation in nonfebrile states, at least in experimental animals (305, 306).

4.6 Prostaglandins, Bronchoconstriction, and Asthma

There is a dynamic equilibrium in mammals that governs and balances normal bronchial airway capacity. Acetylcholine, bradykinin, histamine, and prostaglandin $F_{2\alpha}$ are bronchoconstrictors; catecholamines and PGE_2 are bronchondilators. In most species, both prostaglandin $F_{2\alpha}$ and prostaglandin E_2 are present in tissues of the respiratory tract: $PGF_{2\alpha}$, the constrictor, is synthesized in the lung; the dilator PGE_2 in the bronchial wall (307). Both are rapidly inactivated by conversion to their respective inactive 13,14-dihydro-15-keto metabolites by the joint action of the 15-dehydrogenase and 13,14-reductase enzymes also present in these tissues (308, 309)

In experimental animals, prostaglandins display diverse effects depending on the species and type of respiratory muscle studied. PGEs relax tracheal smooth muscle only in species such as guinea pig, ferret, sheep, and pig, where there is a natural state of constriction or tone. They are not active in monkeys, cats, and rabbits, where tone must be induced by histamine or acetylcholine (308). They produce bronchodilation in the cat, guinea pig, and monkey, but not in the dog. Prostaglandins are most active when inhaled as aerosols, a route of administration that avoids the extensive metabolic inactivation consequent to systemic adminstration (310). PGE_1, when given by aerosol, is 30 times as active as isoprenaline in antagonizing acetylcholine-induced bronchoconstriction in the cat. In the guinea pig, it is 100 times as potent as isoprenaline (311).

When given by aerosol to normal humans, 55 μg of PGE_1 lowers airway resistance 10–20% and lowers it up to 40% in asthmatics (312). Some bronchial and pharyngeal irritation is observed.

Prostaglandin $F_{2\alpha}$ is a potent bronchoconstrictor. In man, inhalation produces decreased airway conductance, cough, and occasional wheezing (313). The bronchoconstriction can be inhibited by isoprenaline and PGE_2 but not by disodium cromoglycate or inhibitors of prostglandin synthesis (314, 315). Unlike E_2, $F_{2\alpha}$ retains its bronchoconstrictor properties when given intravenously, leading to some respiratory side effects when used for termination of pregnancy (316).

Unlike $PGF_{2\alpha}$, its 9β-isomer $PGF_{2\beta}$ is a potent bronchodilator (317). Prostaglandin As display some bronchoconstriction in the dog, and PGBs exhibit about one-fiftieth the relaxant activity of PGE_2. However on human circular smooth muscle, PGB_2 is more active as a stimulant than $PGF_{2\alpha}$ (318). Some bronchodilating activity has been reported for 11-desoxy PGE_1 and its 15-methyl analog (319).

In dogs, prostaglandin D_2 displays a bronchoconstrictor potency 4–6 times that of $PGF_{2\alpha}$, suggesting that a portion of the bronchial tone ascribed to $F_{2\alpha}$ could be due to PGD_2 (320).

Prostaglandins affect respiratory smooth muscle directly, not by acting through ganglionic or β-adrenergic pathways. Their influence on resting tone appears to be mediated by cyclic nucleotides (308, 321).

That the disease of asthma stemmed from an imbalance in respiratory prostaglandin production was suggested by finding asthmatics to be several hundred times more sensitive to $PGF_{2\alpha}$ than normal subjects, and blood levels of $PGF_{2\alpha}$ in asthmatics that were twice the normal values (318). In addition, prostaglandins, along with histamine and SRS-A, are known to be released from the sensitized lungs of many animals, including man, on exposure to a variety of antigens (313). However aspirin and indomethacin evoke a protective response in only a small fraction of asthmatics, which argues against overproduction of $PGF_{2\alpha}$ being a cause of the disease (321). However, two intermediate metabolites of $PGF_{2\alpha}$, 15-keto $PGF_{2\alpha}$ and 13,14-dihydro $PGF_{2\alpha}$. are equipotent to $PGF_{2\alpha}$ itself as a bronchoconstrictor. Thus asthma could be due not to overproduction of $PGF_{2\alpha}$, but to a disorder in its metabolism that permits the buildup of a bronchoconstrictive metabolite (322). Since the cause of bronchial asthma is still unknown, it is not yet possible to rule out a role for prostaglandins. In any case, a bronchodilating prostaglandin that lacks the local irritation side effects of PGEs and the adrenergic side effects of isoproterenol would be a useful drug in the treatment of asthma.

4.7 Lipolysis

An important source of fuel for the body is fatty acids, liberated by the hydrolysis of triglycerides stored in cells of adipose tissue. The rate of mobilization of triglycerides in adipocytes is controlled by numerous hormones including epinephrine, norepinephrine, glucagon, ACTH, and TSH, all of which appear to act by the common mechanism of elevating intracellular levels of cyclic AMP.

Some time ago, it was observed that low levels of prostaglandin E_1 inhibit fat mobilization *in vitro* by rat epididymal tissue and by human adipose tissue when elicited by catecholamines, glucagon, and TSH. PGE_1 also inhibits lipolysis in canine adipose tissue induced by sympathetic nerve stimulation (323–326). The high blood levels of glycerol and free fatty acids produced in unanesthetized dogs by injecting 10 $\mu g/kg$ of epinephrine can be lowered by injecting 30 $\mu g/kg$ of PGE_1 (326). At lower doses, however, PGE_1 itself induces lipolysis in dogs and humans. This stimulation can be abolished by ganglionic blocking agents, which suggests that it is mediated by the sympathetic nervous system. The PGAs and PGFs have little effect on lipolysis, but PGE_2 is 3 times as potent as PGE_1 in rat adipose tissue (327).

Nevertheless, the ability of PGEs to inhibit lipolysis is well established and is correlated with decreased levels of cyclic AMP in adipocytes. The adipocyte is unusual in that prostaglandins depress rather than increase the intracellular cyclic AMP content of these cells, even though the same E-receptor is present here as in other tissues (328, 329). Specifically, PGE is thought to inhibit lipolysis by interfering with the binding of ATP to adenylate cyclase, resulting in decreased production of cyclic AMP, which is needed to activate triglyceride lipase (329).

The evidence that PGEs inhibit hormone-induced lipolysis, together with the finding that both nervous and hormonal stimulation of adipose tissue releases PG-like substances (330), led to the concept that when released in adipose tissue, prostaglandins act as negative feedback inhibitors of lipolysis. Although much evidence has been accumulated in support of the theory, the argument is compromised by the finding that in the dog, the prostaglandin synthetase inhibitor indomethacin does not enhance lipolysis induced either basally or by norepinephrine (331). But total inhibition of PG synthesis is hard to accomplish, and even a little E_2 may be sufficient to inhibit lipolysis.

4.8 Platelets

The role of platelets in hemostasis was discussed earlier in connection with changes in vascular permeability during inflammation. Although normal blood vessels offer no attraction to these thrombocytes, injury to blood vessels exposes collagen in underlying connective tissues. Platelets adhere strongly to injured blood vessels and release a clot-forming factor and ADP. These agents stimulate other platelets to accumulate in the area of injury and form a plug or thrombus.

The prostaglandin synthetase system is present in platelets, and its products both augment and inhibit their hemostatic functions. Although PGE_2 and $PGF_{2\alpha}$ are released from platelets during aggregation, they are now known not to be the cause of platelet aggregation, even though PGE_2 has a stimulating effect on ADP-induced aggregation (332–334). Prostaglandin $F_{2\alpha}$ is inactive, but the methylated analogs of PGE_2 are equiactive with PGE_2 (335). On the other hand, PGE_1, which does not appear in human platelets in concentrations as low as 10 ng/ml, is a potent inhibitor of *in vitro* platelet aggregation induced by ADP, ATP, norepinephrine and serotonin, collagen, and thrombin, as well as of platelet-to-glass adhesiveness in whole blood (333). PGBs are inactive and PBAs are about one-tenth as active as PGE_1 as inhibitors (336, 337). The ability of PGE_1 to inhibit aggregation has been correlated with its ability to increase cyclic AMP in platelets (338).

Prostaglandin D_2 (33.**14**) has been found to be a potent inhibitor of human platelet aggregation induced by PGG_2, ADP, or collagen (339). Since it too is a product of endoperoxide breakdown and since the ratio PGE_2 to PGD_2 can be affected by endogenous factors, the possibility exists that PGD_2 might be formed to act as a feedback inhibitor of aggregation (340, 341).

Recently the endoperoxides PGG_2 and PGH_2 were discovered to be much more potent than PGE_2 in causing rapid platelet aggregation (332, 342). Thromboxane A_2 is also able to aggregate platelets (343, 344).

In 1976 it was discovered that microsomes from the inner lining of normal blood vessels contain enzymes that convert the endoperoxides, not to the platelet-aggregating thromboxanes, but to a new substance, prostaglandin I_2 (PGX, prostacyclin). Prostaglandin I_2 is the most potent *inhibitor* of platelet aggregation yet discovered, possessing 30 times the activity of PGE_1 (123). It is capable of destroying platelet clumps even after they have formed in the test tube. Thus the endoperoxides produce PGI_2, an inhibitor of platelet aggregation, when in contact with normal blood vessels, and thromboxanes, stimulators of aggregation, in the presence of the products of blood vessel damage. Though it is attractive to see in this a homeostatic mechanism of controlling platelet function, not enough is known at this time to allow more than speculation.

4.9 The Autonomic Nervous System

Prostaglandins affect sympathetic transmission in the autonomic nervous system in various ways and degrees, depending on the concentration and kind of prostaglandin considered, the species of animal studied, and the organ or vascular bed examined. Generally, PGEs depress synaptic transmission at sympathetic neuroeffector junctions. They can act prejunctionally by blocking the release of the adrenergic transmitter norepinephrine, and postjunctionally by reducing effector responses to what norepinephrine is released (345, 346). For example, stimulation of the guinea pig vas deferens by way of the hypogastric nerve can be blocked by subnanogram amounts of PGE, and this inhibition can be abolished by a PG-synthesis inhibitor (347). In the isolated cat spleen, infusion of PGE_2 does not affect basal output of norepinephrine. However, it does reduce the effect of electrical stimulation on this organ in a dose-dependent manner that is also proportional to the ability of PGE_2 to inhibit the stimulated release of norepinephrine (348). And contraction of the spleen induced by nerve stimulation or norepinephrine leads to the local release of prostaglandin E_2.

Prostaglandin As are less active than Es, as are PGG_2 and PGH_2, whereas 16,16-dimethyl PGE_2 is an order of magnitude more potent than E_2 itself on the guinea pig vas deferens (349).

The concept that prostaglandins modulate sympathetic autonomic transmission by feedback inhibition of transmitter release was a result of the observations that PGEs are released in the region of the neuroeffector junction in a number of tissues and organs by adrenergic stimulation, and that they in turn inhibit the local release of norepinephrine (346, 350). This theory accounts for the actions of PGEs in a number of tissues, but it does not appear to be universally applicable, since PGEs actually facilitate responses to norepinephrine in accessory reproductive tissues of several species.

E-Type prostaglandins appear to have no effect on cholinergic neuroeffector transmission. Their role in ganglionic transmission in the autonomic nervous system has been little studied (347, 349).

Although less studied than the Es, prostaglandin $F_{2\alpha}$ has the opposite effect of facilitating sympathetic autonomic transmission, particularly in vascular smooth muscle. It appears to act by facilitating the release of transmitter on sympathetic stimulation (346, 351).

4.10 The Central Nervous System

The central actions of prostaglandins having to do with fever were discussed in a previous section. However prostaglandins occur throughout the CNS—not just in neurones concerned with thermoregulation. Although only small amounts of PGs are present in the CNS under resting conditions (as with most other tissues), the capacity exists to synthesize them in large amounts. Nevertheless, the CNS differs from most other tissues in two important ways: stimulation releases more $PGF_{2\alpha}$ than PGE_2 (up to 4 times as much), and once released, prostaglandins are metabolized less extensively in adult brains than elsewhere (352–354). Rather than limiting their central actions by converting them to inactive metabolites, the CNS excretes prostaglandins into the general circulation, from which they are removed by the lung, liver, and kidneys.

There were early suggestions that prostaglandins, particularly the Es, functioned as central neurotransmitters, since iono-phoretic administration of prostaglandins to brain stem cells or direct application to exposed spinal cords of cats increases the rate of firing of the stimulated neurons (254). And administration of PGEs to intact animals produces symptoms of depression and sedation that are short-lived when the PGs are given by the parenteral route, but increase in duration and intensity when they are given intraventricularly (354). This central depressant action of prostaglandin Es enhances the sedative action of barbiturates and inhibits the analeptic activity of strychnine and pentylenetetrazole (351). The mechanism by which PGEs produce this central sedation is unknown. They do not cross the blood-brain barrier, and even when given intraventricularly, only small amounts are taken up by nerve tissue (354, 355). But endogenous pyrogen, which cannot cross the blood-brain barrier either, causes fever nonetheless. Perhaps both substances interact first with the glial cells lining the blood vessels of the CNS to release a factor able to act directly on neurones.

Many agents cause the release of prostaglandins within the CNS: nerve stimulation, analeptics, low blood flow states, trauma, and serotonin; and the rate of PG release correlates with changes in neuronal activity.

Nevertheless, prostaglandins are no longer considered to act as transmitters in the CNS. Here, as in the autonomic nervous system and in many other tissues, prostaglandins are released postsynaptically by the action of transmitter, where they act to increase local levels of cyclic AMP, which are responsible for the response of the cell. The action of transmitter, cyclic AMP, or both, may stimulate the formation of PGE to act as a negative feedback inhibitor of adenylate cyclase as a way of modulating synaptic transmission (356, 357). However, this theory seems to be at variance with the fact that mostly $PGF_{2\alpha}$ is formed in the CNS (or detected anyway). Two possible explanations exist. The enzyme PGE 9-keto-α-reductase has been identified in the brains of several species (358, 359), suggesting that $PGF_{2\alpha}$ may be simply a product of the metabolic inactivation of PGE_2 in the CNS. [$PGF_{2\alpha}$ has no effect on the adenylate cyclase system (354).] On the other hand, prostaglandin $F_{2\alpha}$ has the ability to elevate cyclic GMP levels, and in many biological systems cyclic GMP antagonizes the actions of cyclic AMP (360), a subject discussed more fully in the next section.

5 HOW PROSTAGLANDINS ACT

Before asking "What is the mechanism of action of a substance"? one must know what response is the consequence of the action. If the substance in the question is a drug, the ultimate response will be a clinical improvement in a patient, such as lowered blood pressure. This is a pharmacological result of some physiological event like peripheral vasodilation. The vasodilation is itself the physiological expression of some biochemical event that reduces tone in arterioles. This biochemical response is the consequence of some chemical interaction of the drug with a particular subunit of a protein or membrane. And, in many cases, even the chemical interaction may be the sum of several submolecular perturbations (Fig. 33.9). Furthermore, some responses may result from more than one physiological process, or the processes depicted in Fig. 33.9 may be subdivided into several steps. So when asking how prostaglandins act, one must first specify the level of organization at which the action is taking place.

Much is known of the pharmacological and physiological mechanisms by which prostaglandins act. Various prostaglandins lower blood pressure, alter capillary permeability, inhibit gastric acid secretions, inhibit lipolysis, etc. Less is known about their biochemical mechanisms of action: mostly that they alter intracellular levels of cyclic nucleotides and affect Ca^{2+} turnover. But almost nothing is known about the chemical mechanisms of action that give rise to these effects.

5.1 As Systemic Hormones

Prostaglandins are ubiquitous and affect nearly all physiological processes. Trying to place them in their proper perspective in mammalian physiology has led various investigators to propose that they act as "autocoids" (361), "modulators" (362), "intracellular messengers" (363), and hormones.

One definition of a "classical" hormone is some substance that on stimulation of a

Submolecular perturbation ⟶ Chemical interaction ⟶ Biochemical effect
↓
Clinical manifestation ⟵ Pharmacological consequence ⟵ Physiological response

Fig. 33.9 Cause-effect relationships in drug responses.

gland or organ is released into the general circulation to act on distant tissues. Although $PGF_{2\alpha}$ may act as a circulating luteolytic hormone in horses, it is unlikely that prostaglandins as a family act this way in humans. The "venous hormone" hypothesis, devised to account for all the $PGF_{2\alpha}$ present in the human kidney, may be an exception, but it requires further substantiation (160). And convincing proof is lacking that prostaglandins A or E are released into the general circulation by the kidneys to lower systemic blood pressure (364). Prostaglandins are removed so quickly from the circulation by lungs, liver, and kidneys that significant blood levels are not achieved under normal circumstances.

It is less easy to rule out the possibility that prostaglandins act as intracellular messengers. Since most cells synthesize prostaglandins in response to hormones and other stimuli, the newly synthesized PGs could function inside cells as regulators of cyclic nucleotide and Ca^{2+} levels, or by directly affecting enzyme activity (363). In the adipocyte, PGEs contribute to the regulation of lipolysis by negative feedback inhibition of cyclic AMP, but the adipocyte may be an isolated example (365). Calcium ion is a necessary component of many of the biological actions of cyclic AMP, and it is well known that prostaglandins affect Ca^{2+} turnover in several systems by stimulating its release from subcellular binding sites (366, 367). In platelets, added Ca^{2+} counteracts the inhibition of PGE_1 on aggregation (368). It is possible that in some cases, prostaglandins act as intracellular messengers by altering cyclic AMP levels by way of intracellular regulation of Ca^{2+} transport.

In contrast to this picture, Bito has assembled a convincing argument that prostaglandins are not intracellular messengers. He argues that the prostaglandin synthetase enzyme complex is embedded in cellular membranes in such a fashion as to release newly synthesized prostaglandins only into blood or extracellular fluid (361). Thus prostaglandins would not accumulate within cells unless they are actively transported there by specific carrier systems, such as are present in the ovaries and major metabolizing organs. Otherwise PGs act only at cell membrane surfaces as local extracellular hormones (361).

5.2 As Local Hormones

Since prostaglandin biosynthesis can be virtually abolished by nonlethal doses of aspirin and indomethacin, their formation cannot be essential for the continued existence of the organism (362). This inescapable fact, and most of what is known about prostaglandins, is compatible with the concept that these substances are secreted into extracellular space, or the local circulation, to affect nearby cells. This concept may not be strictly applicable to prostaglandin actions in all tissues, e.g., the autonomic or central nervous systems, but there is abundant evidence that this is their physiological mechanism of action in reproductive tissues, platelets, kidneys, and lungs, in inflammation, and in other systems. The biochemical mechanism by which prostaglandins accomplish this often, perhaps always, requires the mediation of cyclic nucleotides.

5.3 Prostaglandins and Cyclic AMP

It should be clear from the preceding discussions that the physiological consequences of prostaglandin actions are frequently linked to alterations in intracellular concentrations of cyclic AMP. Progress in the field of cyclic AMP research in the last 10 years has led to the development of the concept that cyclic AMP is a "second messenger", that is, the agent of intracellular information transfer between extracellular hormones and intracellular enzymes

(369). A large number of tissues respond to their relevant hormones with increased intracellular levels of cyclic AMP. Cyclic AMP is produced by a hormone-sensitive enzyme, adenylate cyclase, which resides in the plasma membrane and makes cyclic AMP from ATP (369–371). According to the second messenger concept, basal levels of a cellular response are due to a steady state output of cyclic AMP, and increases or decreases in the response are due to increases or decreases in cellular cyclic AMP concentrations.

In the early 1970s, the proposal was made that many of the actions of prostaglandins were mediated by cyclic AMP (372, 373). Except for the adipocyte, where PGEs lower cyclic AMP levels in the stimulated cell, E-type prostaglandins generally elevate intracellular levels of the cyclic nucleotide in a dose-dependent manner. They act by stimulating its synthesis, not inhibiting its destruction by phosphodiesterase (372, 374). Specific binding proteins have been shown to exist for E-type prostaglandins in mouse ovary, lipocyte, rat stomach, thyroid, and other tissues (370, 372, 373). The receptor has the characteristics of a sulfhydryl containing protein and is located on the cell membrane (1). The receptor appears to be specific for PGEs and may be associated with adenylate cyclase. F-Type prostaglandins are able to stimulate the synthesis of cyclic AMP only at high concentrations—concentrations so high that the PGE receptor(s) probably fails to distinguish it from PGE.

5.4 Prostaglandins and the Yin-Yang Theory of Cyclic Nucleotide Control

The consistent inability to demonstrate that prostaglandin $F_{2\alpha}$ altered intracellular cyclic AMP levels was the first evidence that this cyclic nucleotide does not act alone as a "second messenger" of hormone activity (372). A second clue was the finding that the metabolic effects of insulin (which are antagonized by glucagon and epinephrine—hormones that elevate cyclic AMP) are manifested without a reduction of cyclic AMP levels (375). This led to a search for a cellular component able to promote cellular events in opposite fashion to cyclic AMP.

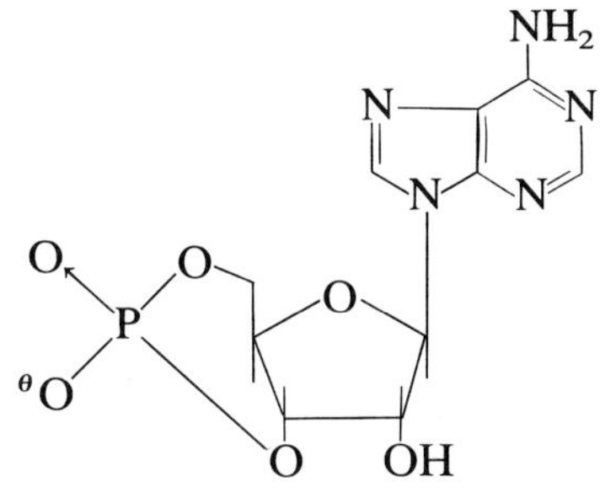

Cyclic AMP

Recent research has shown that 3′,5′-cyclic guanosine monophosphate (cyclic GMP) is a naturally occurring component of mammalian and other animal tissues, perhaps as widely distributed as cyclic AMP, although its concentration in most cells and tissues is generally one-tenth to one-fiftieth that of cyclic AMP (376). This has, in turn, led to the finding that altered intracellular concentrations of cyclic GMP are frequently linked with agents that produce effects opposite to cyclic AMP (377).

Rather than unidirectional control by cyclic AMP, N. D. Goldberg has proposed that many biological systems are subject to bidirectional control by a balance of the contrasting actions of cyclic AMP and cyclic GMP (378). Recalling that the *yin* and

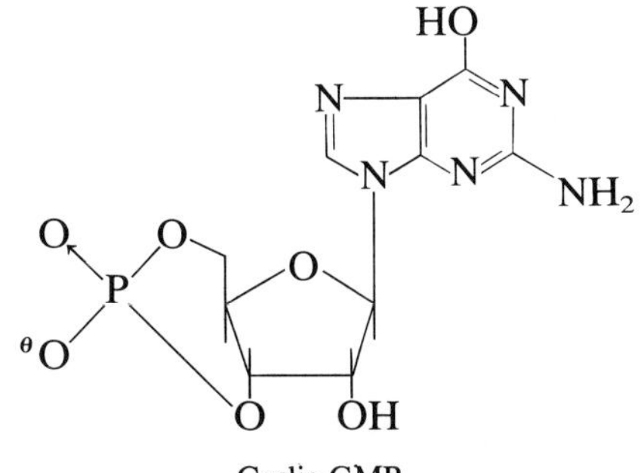

Cyclic GMP

the *yang* are the positive and negative principles, respectively, of Confucian cosmology, Goldberg suggested the term "yin-yang" to describe the phenomenon. Thus "yin-yang" symbolizes a dualism between two natural forces and also allows for the possibility that the two forces may also enter into a mutual interaction that results in a synthesis (377–380).

Actually, two kinds of bidirectionally controlled systems are proposed: A-type systems that are facilitated by cyclic AMP and suppressed by cyclic GMP, and B-types that are promoted by cyclic GMP and inhibited by cyclic AMP (379, 380). Cardiac muscle contraction is one example of an A-type system; contraction of vascular and uterine smooth muscles, cell proliferation, and leukotaxis are B-type systems (379). B-Type systems appear to be more common: release of lysosomal enzymes from stimulated PMNs is enhanced by cyclic GMP and inhibited by cyclic AMP (381). A similar pattern is seen in the rat cerebral cortex: cyclic GMP excites pyramidal tract neurons, cyclic AMP depresses them (360).

To complete the picture, evidence has begun to accumulate that F-type prostaglandins act by way of stimulation of intracellular cyclic GMP levels and that the often opposing actions of PGEs and PGFs can be explained by extending Goldberg's yin-yang hypothesis to prostaglandins (382). However, there are cases of PGEs and PGFs that have qualitatively the same actions (e.g., in luteolysis in rodents and on some smooth muscles). Here the prostaglandin–cyclic nucleotide relationship is less well established. In these systems, the presence of both cyclic nucleotides may be required to produce a response (a synthesis in terms of the yin-yang theory).

Nevertheless, in spite of its attractiveness, the concept that the many actions of E- and F-prostaglandins are mediated by the contrasting action of cyclic AMP and cyclic GMP is solidly at variance with the idea expressed earlier that the primary prostaglandins themselves are not the effectors of biological activity but rather, the endoperoxides, thromboxanes, and PGI_2 fulfill this function. These two new and so far separate lines of research will no doubt collide in the near future and resolve themselves into one unified concept of mediator control of biological processes.

6 STRUCTURE–ACTIVITY RELATIONSHIPS

The natural prostaglandins exhibit several kinds of activity that would be useful therapeutically if side effects could be eliminated. The potential development of PGs as antihypertensives, inhibitors of gastric acid secretion, and bronchodilators, and for use in labor induction is limited chiefly by their stimulation of gastrointestinal smooth muscle, which results in diarrhea and gastric distress when the PGs are administered systemically. Although the rapid metabolic inactivation of prostaglandins by 15-dehydrogenase can be overcome in many instances by placing small alkyl or fluoro groups in the vicinity of the 15-hydroxyl function, rendering the PGs insensitive to the enzyme (383), and in spite of the synthesis of thousands of prostaglandin analogs, as of 1977 not one has yet achieved significant therapeutic usage. This is due almost entirely to the failure to make potent analogs that are lacking in side effects.

Generally, a substance that exhibits more than one kind of biological activity does so by one of two mechanisms. It may act on identical receptors attached to cells of different effector tissues. Acetylcholine, for example, has an inhibitory effect on cardiac muscle but a stimulatory effect on ileal smooth muscle, even though the two receptors are identical as judged by structure-activity studies of agonists and antagonists (384). In such cases, achieving a separation of activities by design and synthesis of structural analogs is a practical impossibility. Since prostaglandins are thought to act as intracellular messengers, the receptors for them must be located on the surface of the cells of the responding tissues. Thus, as depicted in Fig. 33.10, PGE could possibly evoke three dissimilar responses by binding to three identical E-receptors located on the cell membrane and coupled to adenylate cyclase.

Actually, identical receptors are rarely found on dissimilar tissues. More commonly, a substance evokes different responses by interacting with receptors of different kinds. The receptors "recognize" different structural patterns in the same molecule. Adrenal steroids, for example, possess both glucocorticoid and mineralocorticoid activity—and these activities are differentiated by the 11- and 17-hydroxyl functions. PG receptors appear to fall in this category. And although similar tissues probably bear similar receptors, giving some overlap, Andersen and Ramwell have grouped prostaglandin activities (and by inference their receptors) into four general classes (385):

Class I. Receptors that respond about equally to PGAs and PGEs but not to $PGF_{2\alpha}$. Important responses are natriuresis, lowered blood pressure, and perhaps inhibition of gastric acid secretion.

Class II. Responses almost exclusively associated with PGEs and frequently associated with elevations of intracellular cyclic AMP; this may be the largest category.

Class III. Receptors interacting with both E- and F-prostaglandins and producing responses of gastric, intestinal, and uterine smooth muscle stimulation.

Class IV. F-Specific responses of bronchoconstriction, luteolysis, and perhaps other processes associated with elevations of intracellular cyclic GMP levels.

If this division of responses is accurate, it should be possible to prepare prostaglandin analogs whose activities are specific at least for the tissues bearing the receptors of a particular class.

When discussing structure-activity patterns within a family of related molecules, it is convenient to examine separately the

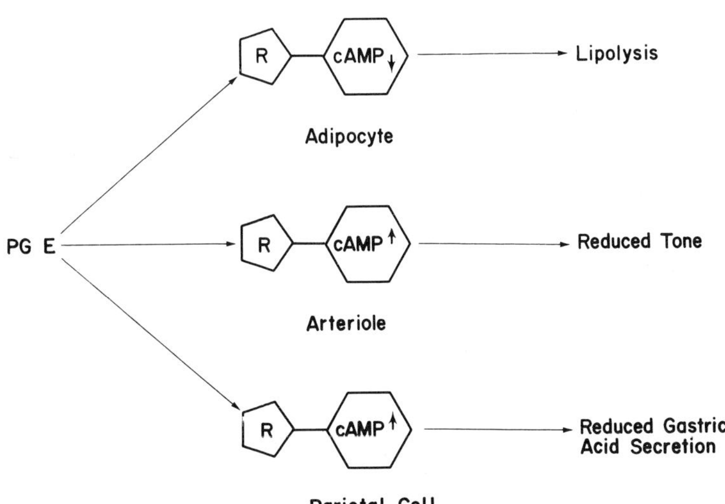

Fig. 33.10 A possible mode of PG–cell interaction.

three ways in which changes in structure can cause changes in biological activity. Namely, the effect of changes in constitution (what functional groups are varied), the effect of changes in geometrical or optical configuration, and the effect of changes in conformation (how the functional groups are displayed in space relative to one another).

6.1 Constitution

It is an accepted strategem in drug development to eliminate an unwanted activity from a drug by removing its structural determinants from the lead molecule. In the prostaglandin family, the activity determinants are the oxygen functions at C-1, C-9, C-11, and C-15, and the double bonds. In spite of all the PG analogs made and tested, only a few general statements can be made concerning what specific biological activities are determined by what functional groups.

Removal of the 11α-hydroxyl function of PGEs and PGFs eliminates most of the diarrhea potential and irritation of gastric smooth muscle. Saturation of the *trans* double bond at C_{13}-C_{14} has a similar result. The potency of 13,14-dihydro PGs is also decreased in other assays, but this may be due to loss of rigidity in the lower arm. Thus these two structural features appear to be determinants for some types of smooth muscle stimulation (385, 386). Generally, the 11-desoxy PGEs resemble the PGEs in their profile of activity but are less potent.

The oxygen function at C-9 is also a determinant of smooth muscle activity. It must be present as a ketone or as the α-alcohol; the 9β-isomer is usually weaker in activity or relaxes smooth muscle. Obviously the oxygen function at C-9 also serves to distinguish E-prostaglandins from the Fs in the majority of tissues that respond differently to the two types.

Oxidation of the 15*S* alcohol to a ketone usually inactivates the molecule, as does alkylating the alcohol function.

Reduction of the carboxyl function of PGs to a primary alcohol has been accomplished, but the pharmacological profile of the resulting prostaglandin 1-carbinols has not been reported. The prostaglandin 1-aldehydes appear to resemble the corresponding carboxylic acids in their spectrum of activity (386).

Reduction of the *cis* double bond at C_5-C_6 has no qualitative effect on PG activity except in platelet aggregation. Isomers of prostaglandins having a *trans* double bond at C_5-C_6 have been synthesized and appear to be less active than the natural *cis* isomers (388). Prostaglandins having a *cis* instead of a *trans* double bond at C_{13}-C_{14} have been prepared but apparently are not active (389).

Thus considering constitution alone, there are no clear structure-activity relationships among prostaglandins.

6.2 Configuration

There are five chiral centers in the PGF family and four in the PGE family. Of the 32 and 16 possible isomers of each, biological activity is almost exclusively associated with the isomer having the all-"natural" configuration. The inversion or elimination of any one of these chiral centers reduces the activity of the molecule drastically. However, there are reports that prostaglandins having unnatural configuration at two or more chiral centers are more potent than their all "natural" counterparts. Although 15-*epi* PGE_1 and A_1 are inactive, *ent* 15-*epi* PGE_1 (33.**63**) and *ent* 15-*epi* PGA_1 (33.**64**) are more active than PGs E_1 and A_1 on several isolated smooth muscle preparations (390, 391). *Ent* 11,15-*epi* PGE_1 (33.**65**) is several times more active than PGE_1 on the rat uterus and rabbit jejunum (390). The methyl ester of *ent*

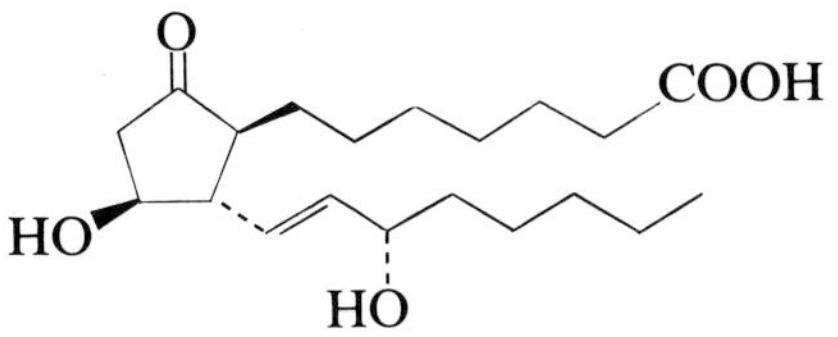

33.**63**

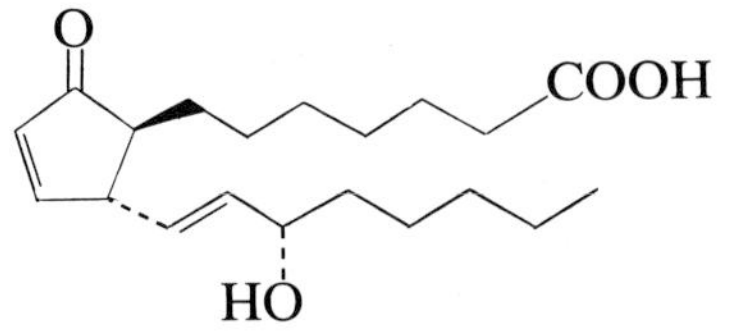

33.**64**

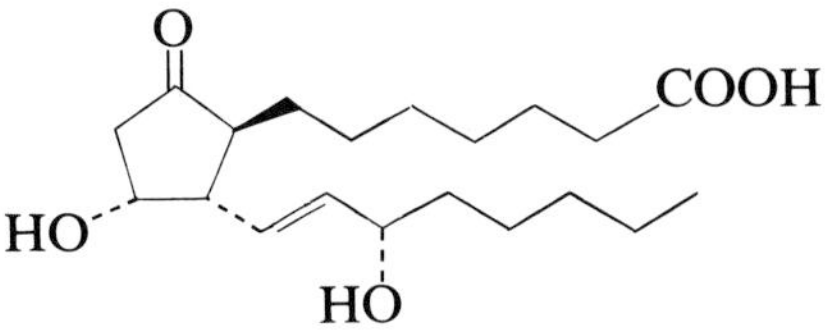

33.**65**

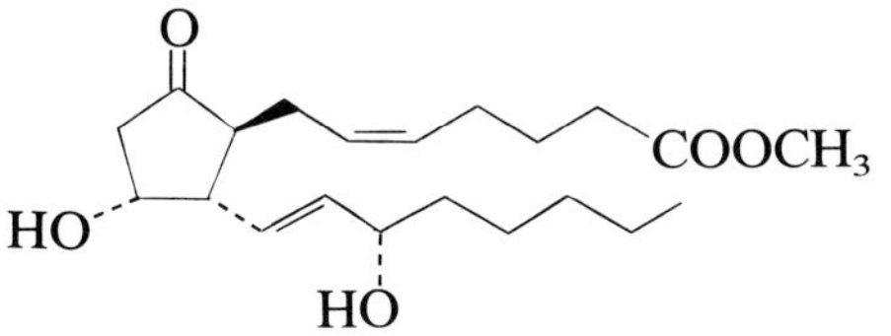

33.**66**

11,15-*epi* prostaglandin E_2 (33.**66**) is much more active than PGE_2 in several assays (392).

These diastereoisomers still retain the natural *S*-configuration at C-15, the one feature essential to prostaglandin activity in every system. And although the backbone of the prostaglandin skeleton has been reversed by these transformations, the oxygen functions largely remain in the same spatial relationship as in the natural prostaglandins. The increase in activity may be because the inverted skeleton makes a better interaction with the receptors involved. However, these isomers are also poorer substrates for the chief prostaglandin-deactivating enzyme, PG 15-dehydrogenase (393). Some of their enhanced activity may be due to their much longer biological half-lives.

6.3 Conformation

The confusing pattern of structure-activity relationships among prostaglandins may be due partially to their lack of structural rigidity. There are many possible degrees of rotational freedom in the two prostaglandin side chains, giving rise to hundreds of potential rotational isomers, each displaying the activity-determining oxygen atoms in a slightly different spatial arrangement. Two different receptors might be able to produce two different responses by undergoing the same chemical interaction with exactly the same PG structural elements displayed in two different conformations. This is an often-encountered phenomenon when dealing with endogenous substances. The nicotinic and muscarinic receptors of acetylcholine are known to respond to different conformations (rotomers) of the transmitter (394). Histamine contracts smooth muscles by acting on H1-receptors responsive to the staggered conformation of its side chain, and stimulates gastric acid secretion by way of H2-receptors responsive to the gauche conformation (395). This kind of multiple activity is characteristic of many small molecules produced by the body to control biological processes. It is economical. One molecule can do the work of several simply by having more than one way in which its functional groups can be presented to different receptors. The flexibility of the side chains makes it likely that some prostaglandin receptors are also capable of distinguishing different prostaglandin conformations.

The preferred conformation of most primary prostaglandins has been determined in the crystalline state. Prostaglandins E_1 and $F_{1\beta}$ adopt conformations with their side chains fully extended and in close contact, resembling the interactions found in long chain fatty acids (396). The dispersion interaction between the two chains amounts to several kilocalories per mole of stabilization. In the PG_1 family, the interchain interaction decreases in the order $E_1 > F_{1\alpha} > A_1 > B_1$, a trend that parallels their activity in the rat uterus preparation. In PGA_1, the Δ^{10} double bond tends to flatten the ring and move the two arms apart, decreasing their interaction. PGA_1 has been crystallized in two forms that differ slightly in the arrangement of the side chains (397, 398). PGE_2 also crystallizes in a fully extended conformation. In its crystalline state, energies of lattice packing and hydrogen bonding seem to be more important than the lipophilic interaction between chains, probably because the *cis* double bond at C_5-C_6 creates an impediment to close packing of the chains (399).

Molecular orbital calculations on prostaglandins E_1 and $F_{1\beta}$ confirm the extended conformations as the most stable (in the absence of outside influences), and suggest 2 kcal/mol for the interaction stabilization between chains (400, 401). The calculations also predict an extremely large number of available conformations for these prostaglandins, of which a significant number are energetically favorable enough to be appreciably populated at room temperature.

The relaxation times in aqueous solution of the 20 carbon atoms of PGs E_1 and $F_{2\alpha}$ have been measured with ^{13}C NMR (402, 403). These values give some idea of the rigidity or flexibility of the carbon skeleton under approximate biological conditions. In PGE_1, relaxation times are slower toward the middle of the chains and in the ring, with the exception of C-10. In solution, prostaglandin E_1 displays little segmental motion from C-5 to C-15; it is fairly rigid, again suggesting an interaction between the two chains (403). Prostaglandin $F_{2\alpha}$ presents nearly the same picture. It is rigid from C-5 to C-15 and flexible at the ends of each chain. The relaxation times for $PGF_{2\beta}$ indicate it to be even more rigid than $F_{2\alpha}$. Overall, the prostaglandin molecule may be viewed as possessing the rigidity of a bicyclic structure from C-5 to C-15 to which a butyric acid and an *n*-pentyl side chain are attached (403).

The CD spectrum of $PGF_{2\alpha}$ also shows the two side chains of $PGF_{2\alpha}$ to be in close proximity in solution and the interaction between them to be diminished in the less potent stereoisomers $PGF_{2\beta}$ and 11-*epi* $PGF_{2\alpha}$ (404, 405).

The overall picture that emerges from these studies is that prostaglandins exist as distorted elongated ellipsoids with a lipophilic core and the polar oxygen atoms directed out and away from the center of the molecule. Although the central portion of the moleucle is rigid (except for C-10), considerable segmental rotation can occur at the ends of both chains. This "tertiary" structure is probably further stabilized under physiological conditions. The two chains, being lipophilic structures in a hydrophilic environment, would tend to be shoved together, allowing greater hydrogen bonding to occur at the oxygen atoms. Although this description suggests a kind of "internal" micelle (and prostaglandins are known to form micelles above concentrations of 0.1 *M*), prostaglandins do not form true micelles at physiological concentrations (406, 407). There is evidence that even small changes in the structure of the primary prostaglandins result in significant perturbation of this "tertiary" structure that can alter the spatial pattern of the oxygen atoms, hence altering or lowering the biological response. This presupposes that the prostaglandin receptors are themselves quite rigid and unable to interact with prostaglandin conformations even slightly perturbed from what the receptor usually sees. All the spectra and physicochemical measurements of prostaglandins agree that their structures are conformationally well defined between C-5 and C-15. It may be no accident that most changes in prostaglandin structure between C-5 and C-15 tend to lower activity remarkably.

6.4 Prostaglandin Analogs

Despite the synthesis of thousands of prostaglandin analogs, only a fraction have appeared in publications, and then mostly in the patent literature. Biological data are often sketchy or absent, or given in general terms that make comparisons of related structures difficult. Nevertheless, a comprehensive discussion of the structure-activity relationships of even the analogs that are known would be beyond the space available for this chapter. What follows, instead, is a brief summary of some of the simpler structural variations that have been made in the prostaglandin skeleton (see also Ref. 408).

6.4.1 VARIATIONS IN THE UPPER CHAIN. Analogs of PGE_2 (33.**67**), $PGF_{2\alpha}$, and PGE_1 have been prepared having a 5-tetrazolyl group in place of the carboxyl function. The 5-alkyl tetrazole moiety is about as acidic as the carboxyl, and the activities of analogs like 33.**67** in the rat blood pressure assay and on the gerbil colon are roughly equivalent to those of the natural prostaglandins (409). Analogs of PGE_2 (33.**68**), PGE_1, PGA_2, and $PGF_{2\alpha}$ having a sulfonic acid function in place of the carboxyl have been synthesized, but do not appear to be active (410). Simple esters of prostaglandins are rapidly hydrolyzed to the free acids by

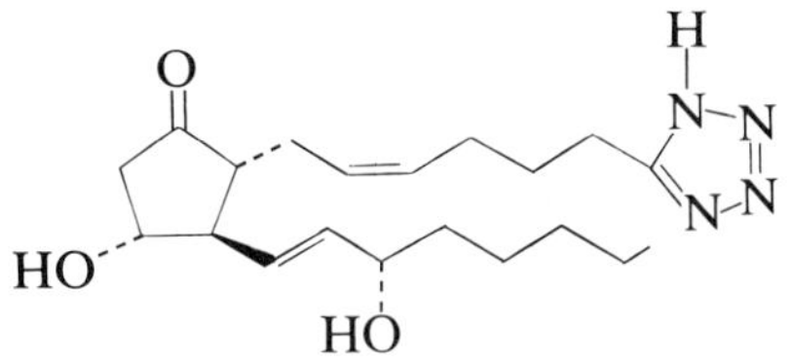

33.**67**

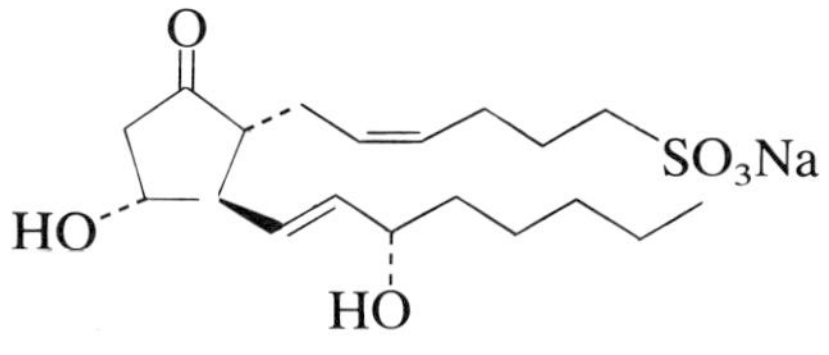

33.**68**

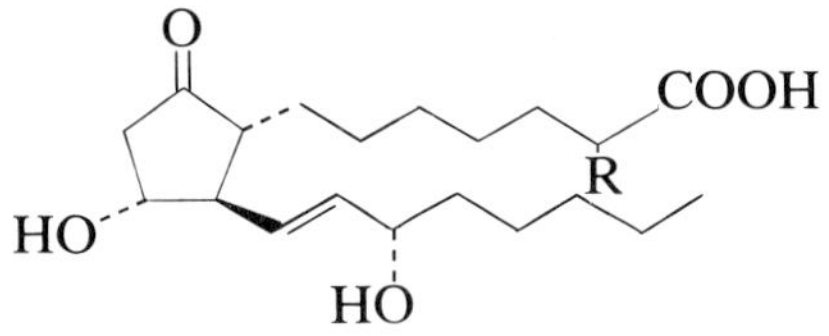

33.**69**

R = CH_3, n-C_4H_9, CH_2OH, C_6H_5, Br, F, CN, OCH_3, CH_2OCH_3, COOH, $COOCH_3$

serum esterases; such esters might be useful in developing formulations of improved stability. PGE_1 and PGE_2 have been couped to the amine group of phosphatidylethanolamine to give prostaglandin amides that are as active as the free acids but with a slower onset of action. These amides are converted to free prostaglandins by enzymes present in tissues but are not hydrolyzed in the blood (411).

Many 2-substituted prostaglandin E_1s (33,**69**), A_1s, and $F_{1\alpha}$s bearing small alkyl groups, substituted alkyl groups, halogen groups, and conjugating groups have been made by incubating the corresponding eicosatrienoic acids with a sheep vesicular gland preparation (412–414). Conversions were lower than with eicostrienoic acid 33.**21** itself. Although biological activities were generally much less than the natural PGs, 2-fluoro PGE_1 (33.**69**: R = F), was more active than PGE_1 in increasing coronary blood flow in the rat heart, and 2-cyano PGE_1 (33.**69**: R = CN) was half as active as E_1 in lowering rat arterial blood pressure.

3-Methyl PGE_1 (33.**70**) and 3-methoxy $PGF_{1\alpha}$ (33.**71**) have been reported but do not appear to be active (412, 415). The synthesis of 7-ketoprostaglandin E_1 (33.**72**) and its 11-desoxy counterpart has been accomplished but no activity was reported (416), which is unfortunate in view of the coronary vasodilating activity recently reported for 6-keto $PGF_{1\alpha}$ (33.**33**) (417).

The 7-oxa analog of PGE_1 33.**73**, is much less active than prostaglandin E_1; 7-oxa $PGF_{1\alpha}$ (33.**74**: X = O) possesses some

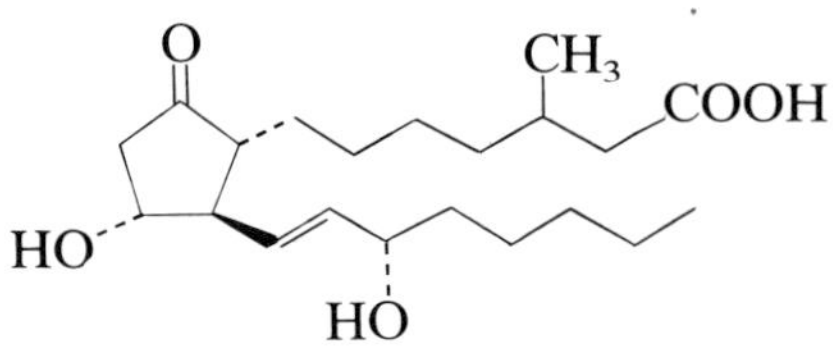

33.70

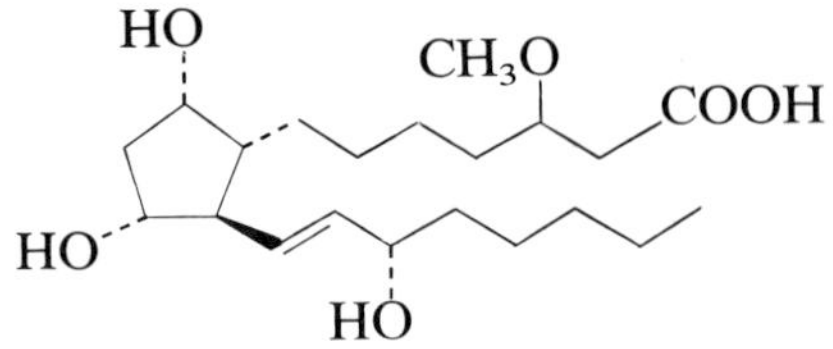

33.71

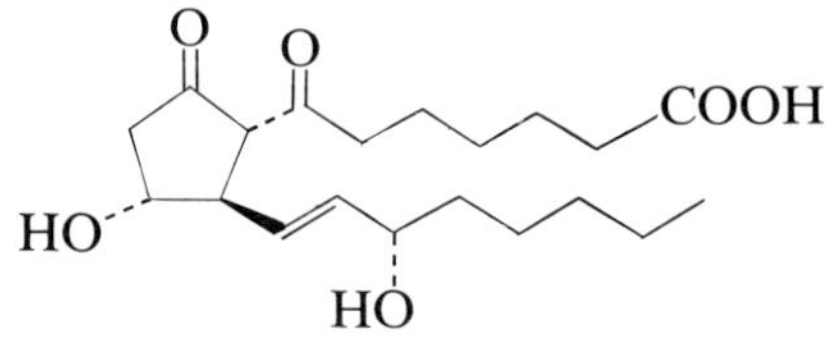

33.72

stimulatory action on the gerbil colon (418, 419). However, the 9,11,15-tridesoxy analog 33.**75** antagonizes the activity of both E_1 and $F_{1\alpha}$ on the gerbil colon (420). The 7-thia analog 33.**74** (X = S) displays weak agonist activity in stimulating cyclic AMP in the mouse ovary and in binding to the bovine corpus luteum receptor, but it inhibits placental 15-dehydrogenase (421).

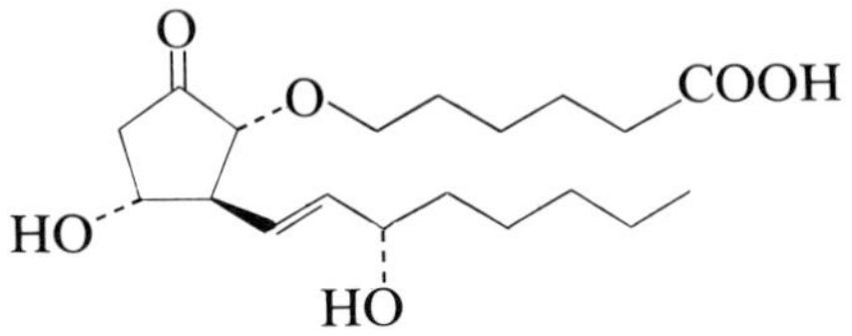

33.73

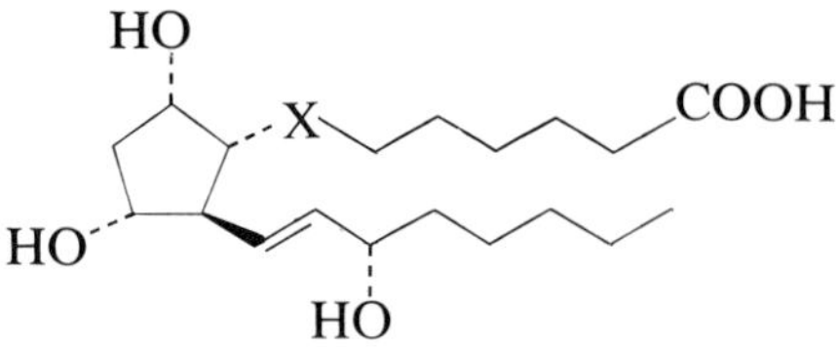

33.74 X = O, S

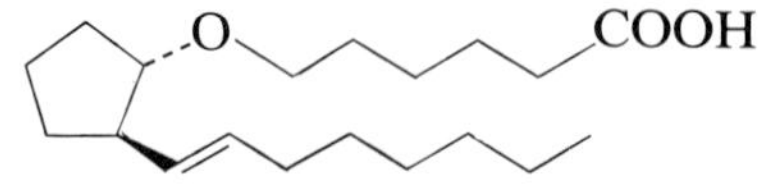

33.75

The ethyl ester of 3-oxaprostaglandin E_1 (33.**76**) was prepared to prevent metabolic deactivation by β-oxidation, but it is much less active than E_1 on isolated smooth muscle preparations (422). The 4-oxa and 5-oxa analogs of prostaglandins of the 1-family have been disclosed in the patent literature and appear to possess weak agonist activity (423, 424). However the methyl ester of the phenyl analog 33.**77**, although weakly active on isolated smooth muscle, is 10 times as potent as PGE_1 in inhibiting human platelet aggregation (425).

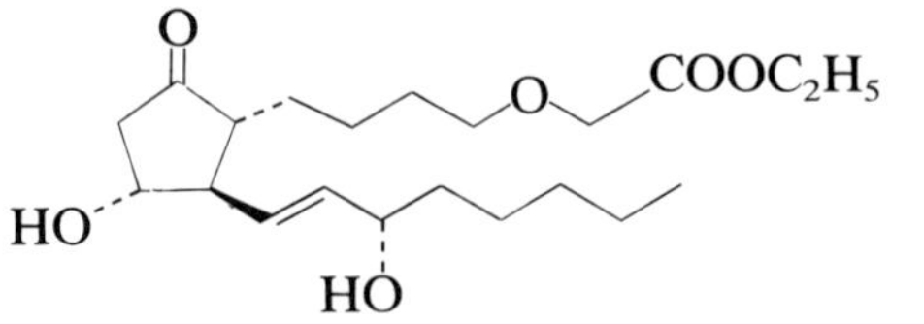

33.76

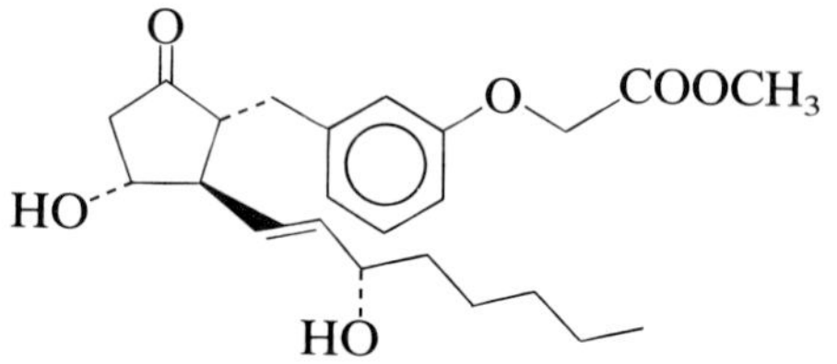

33.77

The synthesis of *trans*-Δ^2-prostaglandins E_1 (33.**78**), A_1, and $F_{1\alpha}$ has been accomplished by two groups (415, 426). The PGE_1 analog is a potent inhibitor of platelet aggregation but is weaker than PGE_1 in stimulating the guinea pig ileum. The *trans*-Δ^3- and *trans*-Δ^5-PGE_1 analogs lack both activities, as does *cis*-Δ^4-PGE_1 (426). Both the cis and trans isomers of 2,3-methylene PGE_1 (33.**79**) show some stimulation of the gerbil colon; 3,3-dimethyl PGE_1 is inactive (412). Δ^4-$PGF_{1\alpha}$ has been prepared and found to be more resistant to β-oxidation and 15-dehydrogenation then $PGF_{2\alpha}$, but no pharmacological activity has been reported for it (427).

The *cis* 5,6-double bond of the PG_2 series has been replaced by an allene function as in Δ^4-PGE_2 (33.**80**) and an

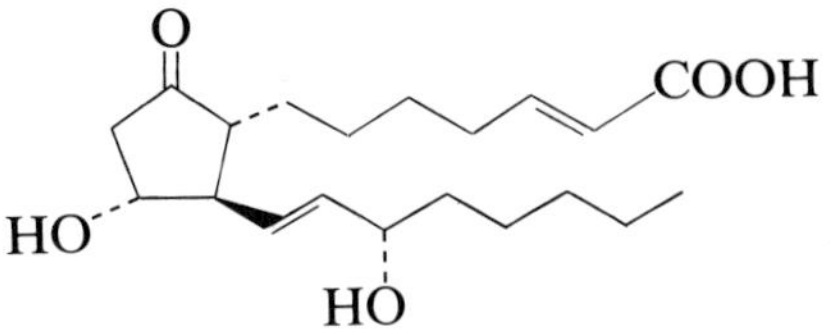

33.**78**

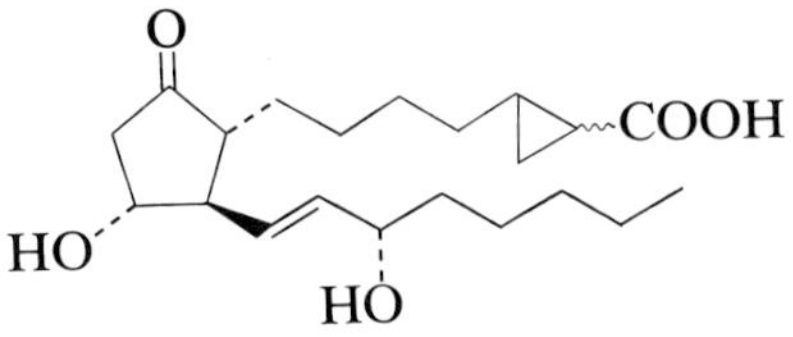

33.**79**

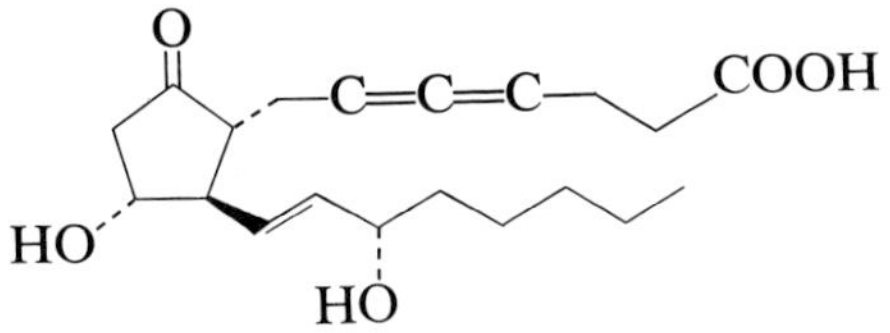

33.**80**

acetylene function as in 5,6-dehydroprostaglandin E_2 (33.**81**) (428–431). They do not appear to possess prostaglandinlike activity.

Analogs of the primary prostaglandins have been made containing eight carbon atoms in the upper arm, e.g., α-homo PGE_1 (33.**82**), and six carbon atoms in the upper arm, e.g., α-nor-ω-homo PGE_1 (33.**83**) (141, 432, 433). They appear to possess negligible PG activity, although some of them are substrates for PG 15-dehydrogenase (432).

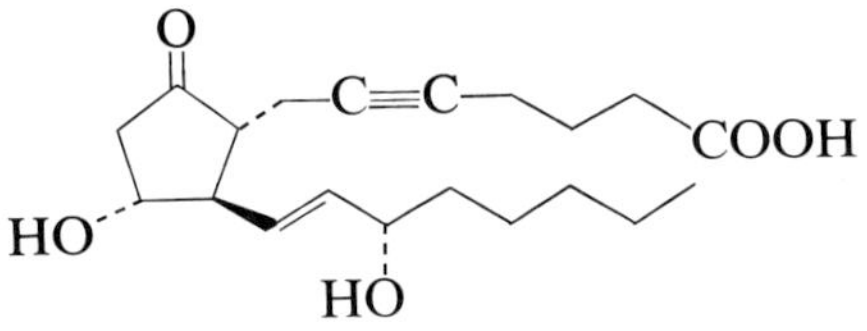

33.**81**

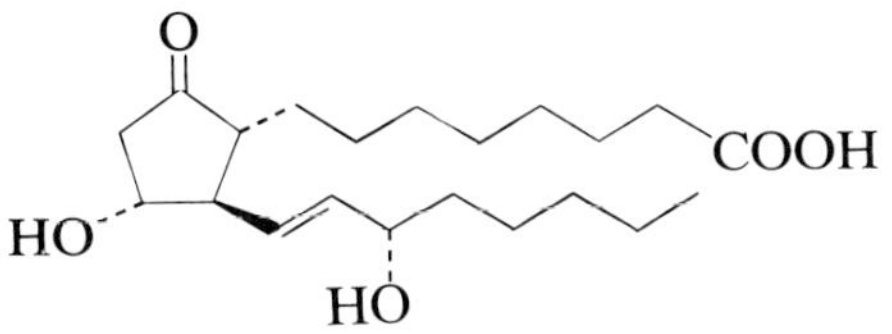

33.**82**

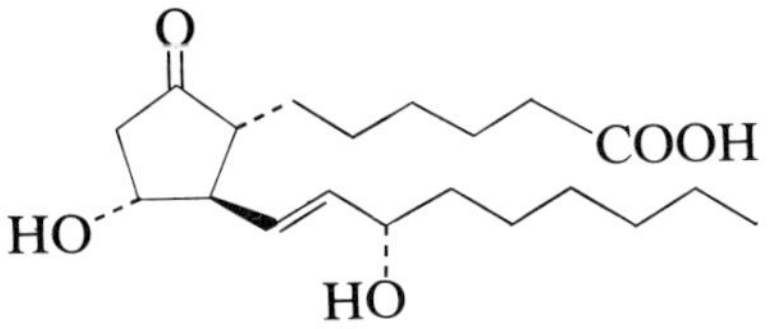

33.**83**

Benzo-[5,6]prostaglandins E_2 (33.**84**), A_2, and $F_{2\alpha}$, having the cis-$\Delta^{5,6}$ double bond incorporated into a phenyl ring, are devoid of significant activity (434).

Considering structures 33,**80**–33.**83**, it is clear that the distance separating the carboxyl group on the upper chain from the cyclopentane ring is critical for PG activity. Departing from this distance by altering the length of the chain or by changing the geometry by varying the unsaturation drastically, reduces activity. Even the substitution of small groups on the upper chain produces steric effects that must perturb the spatial arrangement of the two chains. Replacing carbon atoms in the chain by heteroatoms does not alter geometry much, but it diminishes the lipophilic character of the chains, which in turn will affect the chain-chain interaction.

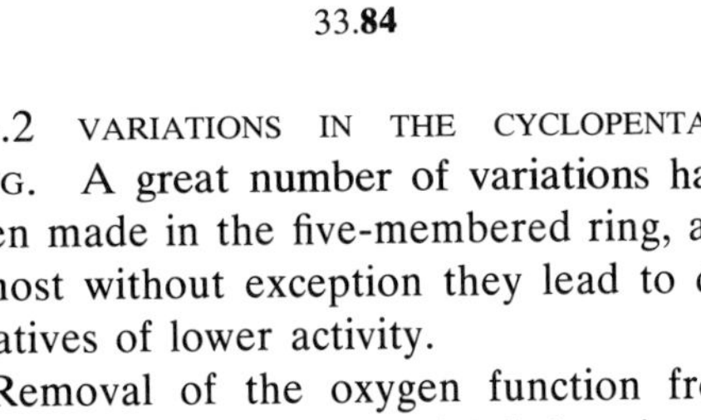

33.**84**

6.4.2 VARIATIONS IN THE CYCLOPENTANE RING. A great number of variations have been made in the five-membered ring, and almost without exception they lead to derivatives of lower activity.

Removal of the oxygen function from position 9 gives 33.**85**, which is inactive, as is its PG_2 counterpart (435, 436). Some 8-substituted 11-desoxy PGE_1s (33.**86**) and E_2s have been prepared, but no activities were reported (437–439).

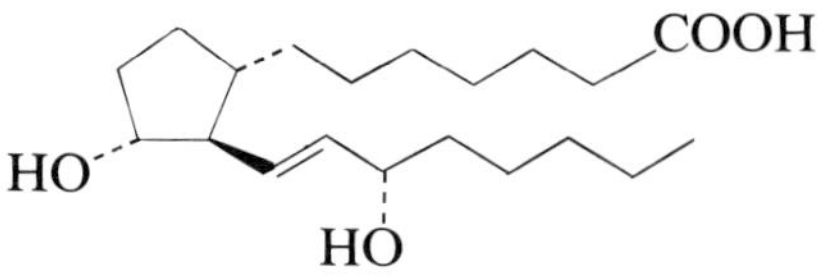

33.**85**

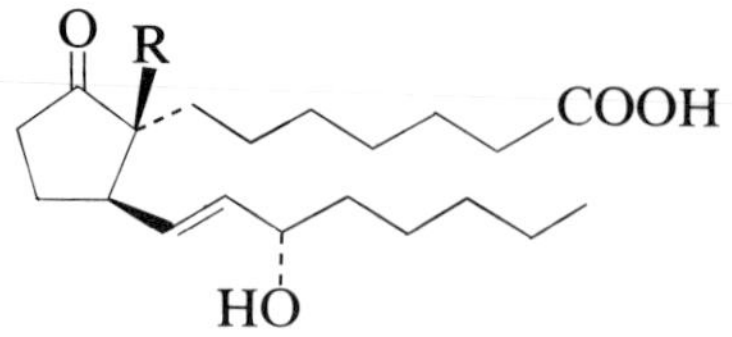

33.**86** R = CH_3, SC_6H_5, $COOCH_3$

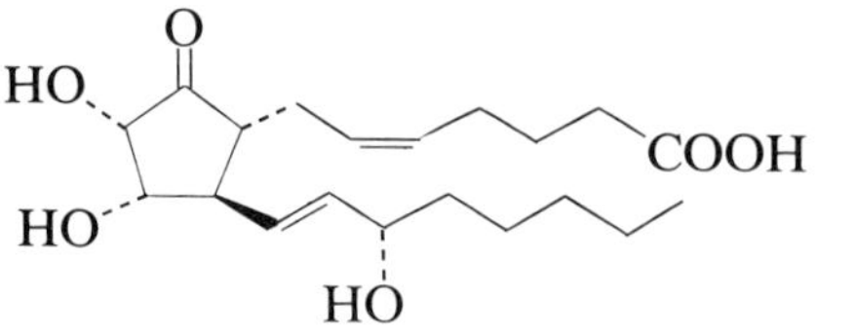

33.**87**

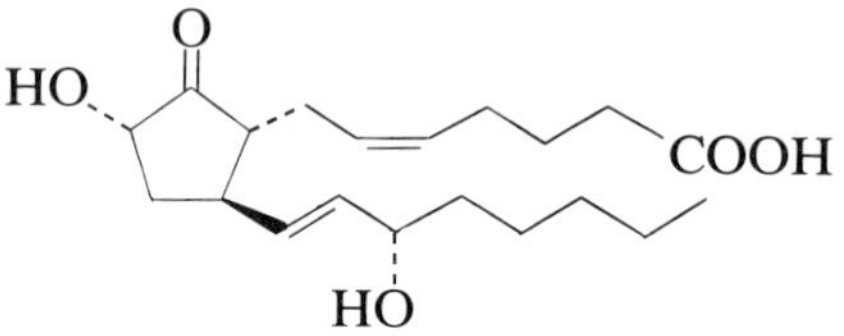

33.**88**

10α-Hydroxyprostaglandin E_2 (33.**87**) and $F_{2\alpha}$ have been prepared (440), as have 10α-hydroxy-11-desoxyprostaglandin E_2 (33.**88**), $F_{2\alpha}$ and their 10β-epimers, but no activities have been reported for them (441, 442).

Analogs of prostaglandin $F_{2\alpha}$ have been synthesized in which the 9α-hydroxy and the 11α-hydroxyl groups were replaced with hydroxymethyl groups, giving 33.**89** and 33.**90** (443, 444). No activities were reported, but the 9-keto analog of 33.**90**, 11α-hydroxymethyl-11-desoxy

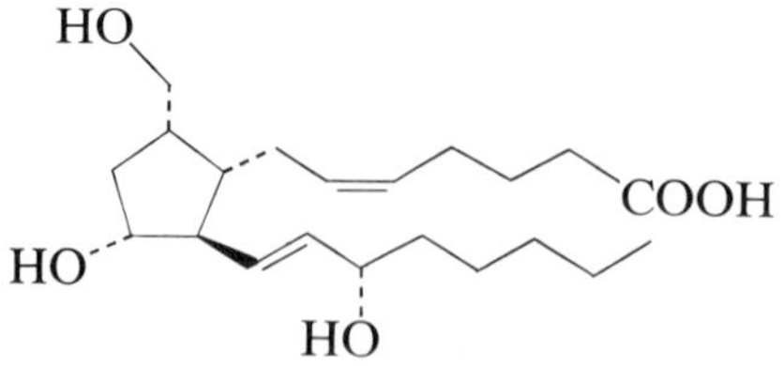

33.**89**

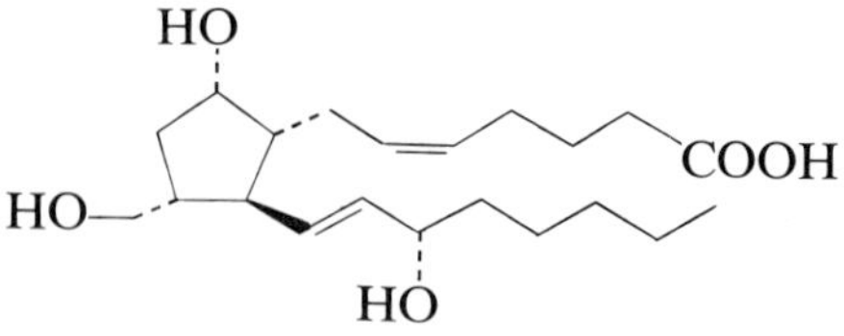

33.**90**

PGE_2, is said to exhibit the specific activity of uterine contraction (445, 446). The doubly homologated *bis*-9α,11α-hydroxymethyl-9,11-desoxy $PGF_{2\alpha}$ (33.**91**) has been made (447), but no activity was reported for it or for 12α-hydroxymethyl $PGF_{2\alpha}$ methyl ester (448)

Both the α- and β-isomers of 10,11-methylene-11-deoxy PGE_2 (33.**92**) and the α-isomer (33.**93**) of 11,12-difluoromethylene PGE_2 have been prepared but were not reported to be active (449–451).

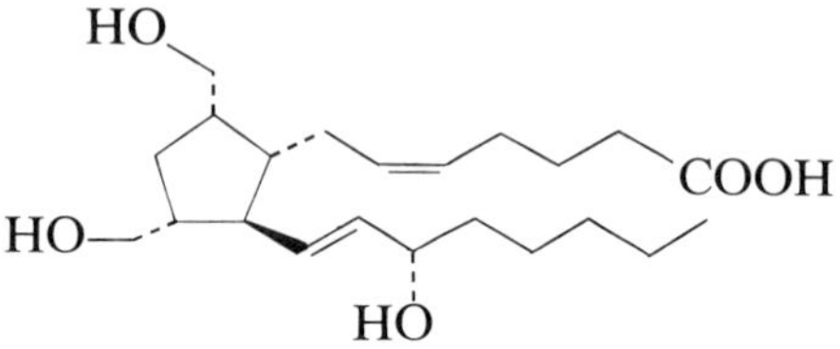

33.**91**

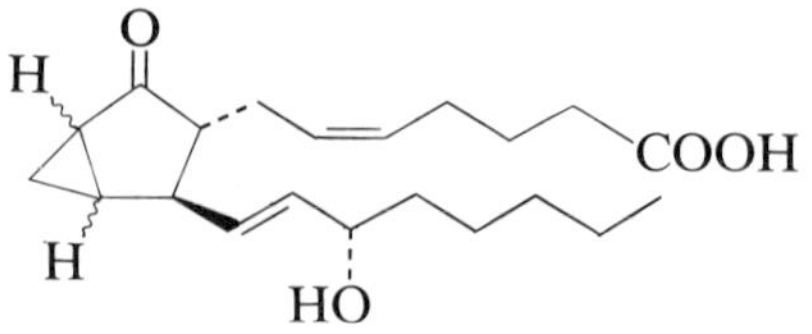

33.**92**

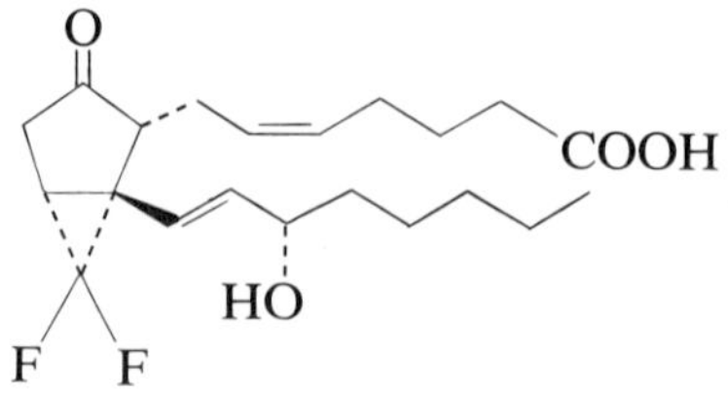

33.**93**

10,10-Dimethyl prostaglandin E_2 (33.**94**) and other similarly substituted PGs of the 1- and 2-series have been prepared but are inactive (452). No activity has been reported for the methyl ester of 11-methyl prostaglandin E_2 (33.**95**), A_2, or $F_{2\beta}$ (449, 453, 454), or for 11α-methyl-11-desoxy

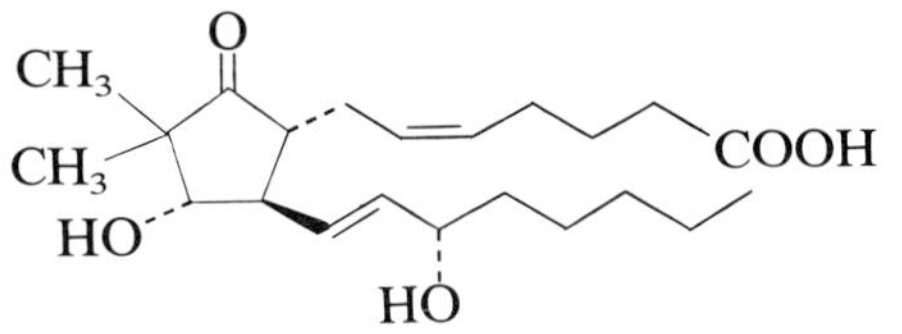

33.**94**

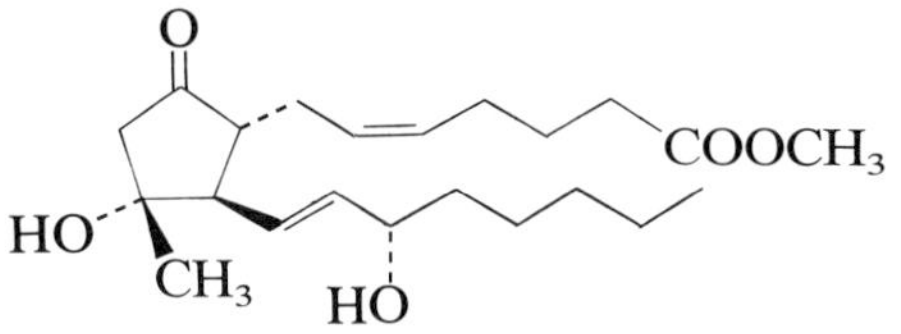

33.**95**

PGE_2 methyl ester (455). Other 11-desoxy prostaglandins have been prepared with small functional groups substituted at position 11 (CHO, CH_2NO_2, $CONH_2$, SCH_3, $CH{=}CH_2$, etc.), but none appears to be active (444, 455, 456).

A number of 12α-methyl substituted prostaglandins have been made in an effort to block the metabolic transformation PGA → PGB that occurs in the blood and is an important systemic means of inactivating PGEs and PGAs. However 12α-methyl PGA_2 (33.**96**) is without effect on dog blood pressure or gastric acid secretion in rats (457). No activity has been reported for the E_2 and $F_{2\alpha}$ analogs of 33.**96** (458, 459), or for 12α-methyl-11-desoxy PGE_2 methyl ester (33.**97**) (460). 12α-Fluoro $PGF_{2\alpha}$ methyl ester (33.**98**) has recently been made, but no activity was reported for it (461).

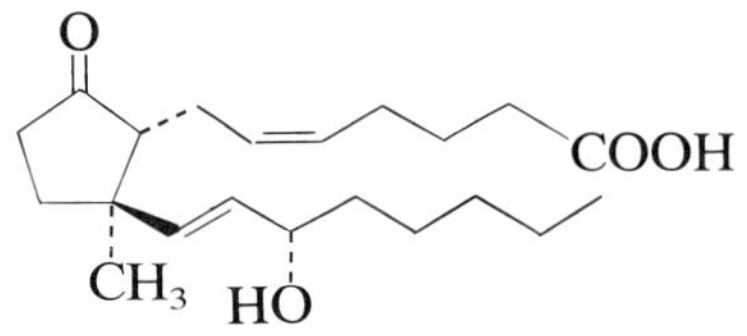

33.**96**

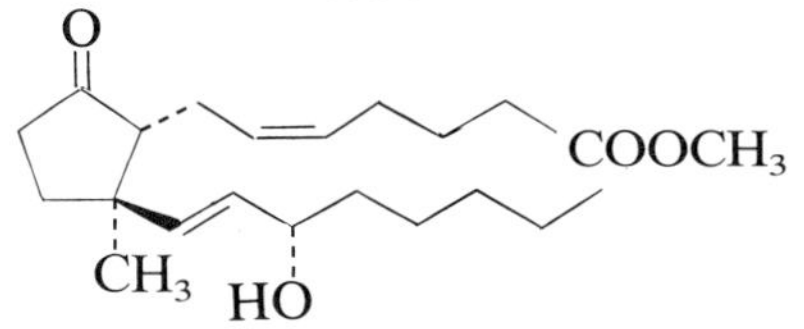

33.**97**

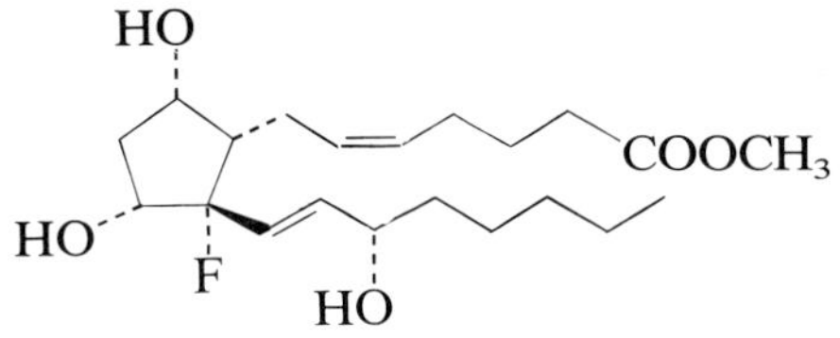

33.**98**

The cyclohexyl analog 33.**99** of prostaglandin $F_{2\alpha}$ has been described as less potent than the natural substance (462), and the fluorinated analog 33.**100** is at least 2 orders of magnitude less active than prostaglandin $F_{2\alpha}$ (463). The cyclobutanone analog 11-nor PGE_2 (33.**101**) has recently been synthesized, but its activity has not been reported (464). This is one of the few PG analogs in which the cyclic portion of the molecule has been transformed into a structural unit smaller than that occurring in the natural prostaglandins. The 9-desoxy-9-carboxy analog of 33.**101** exhibited one-tenth the potency of prostaglandin $F_{2\alpha}$ in the hamster antifertility assay (465). 11-Nor $PGF_{2\alpha}$ has been prepared, but no activity was reported (466).

The photolytic 2+2 cycloaddition of ethylene to a PGA_2 precursor was the key

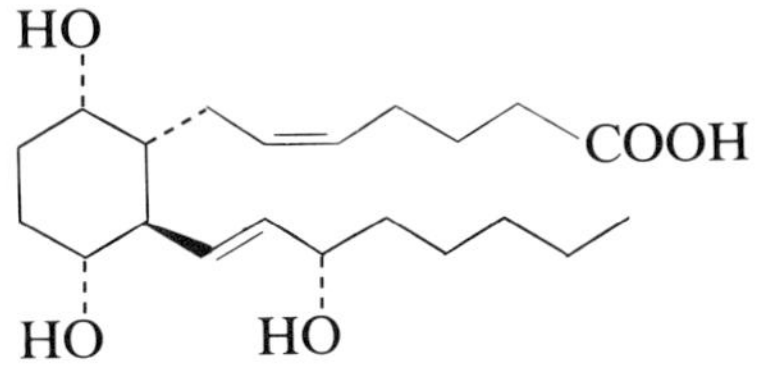

33.**99**

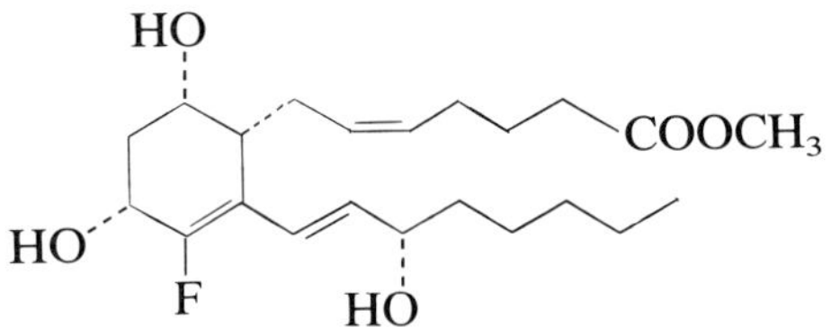

33.**100**

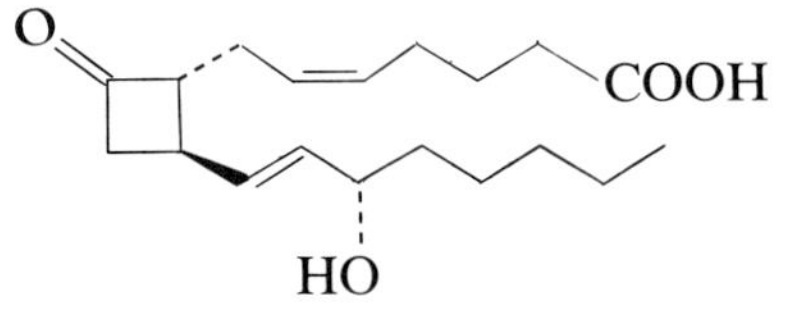

33.**101**

step in the synthesis of the bicyclic analog 33.**102** (467). No activity has been reported for it or for the photoaddition products of allene and PGA_2.

The prostaglandin structure has also been varied by replacing certain carbon atoms of the cyclopentane ring by oxygen, sulfur, and nitrogen atoms. Both 9-oxa and 9-thia analogs (33.**103**) of the PG_1 series have been made (468, 469). No activity was reported for these compounds, for the sulfoxide analog of 33.**103** (X = S), or for the 13,14-dihydro analog of 33.**103** (X = O) (470). 10-Oxa-11-desoxy PGE_1 methyl ester (33.**104**) has been made, but no activity was reported (471). The 11-oxa and 11-thia analogs (33.**105**) of prostaglandin E_1 are weakly active in the gerbil colon assay,

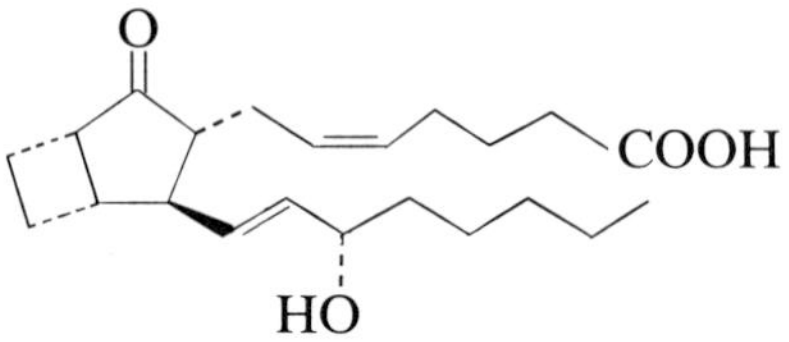

33.**102**

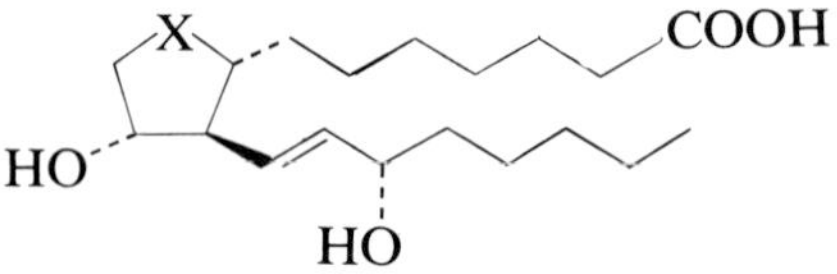

33.**103** X = O, S

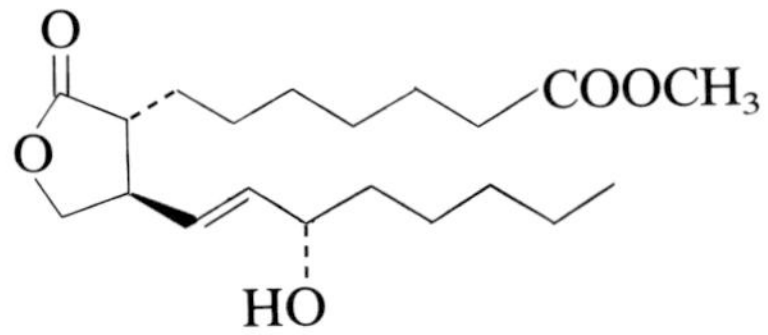

33.**104**

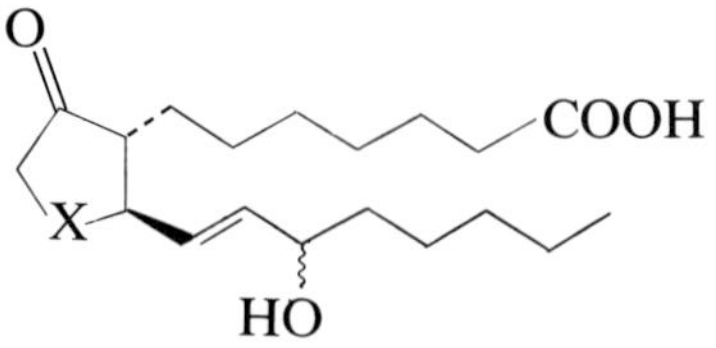

33.**105** X = O, S, $>S^+—O^-$

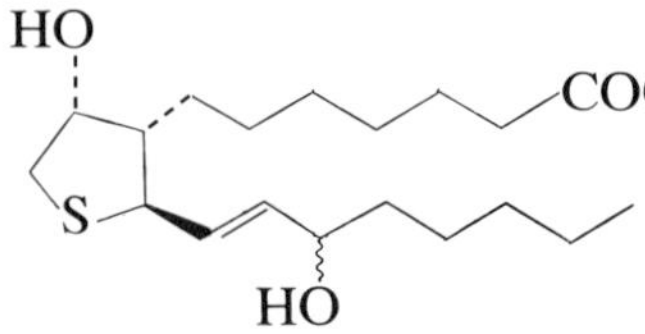

33.**106**

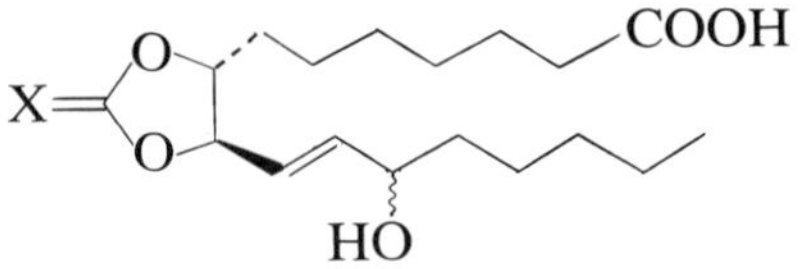

33.**107**; X = H_2, O

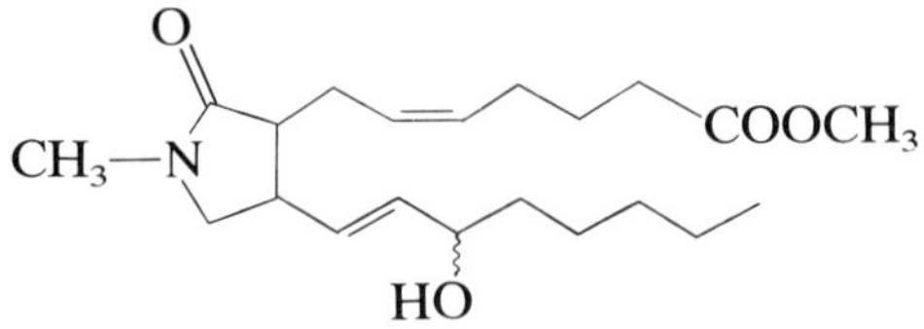

33.**108**

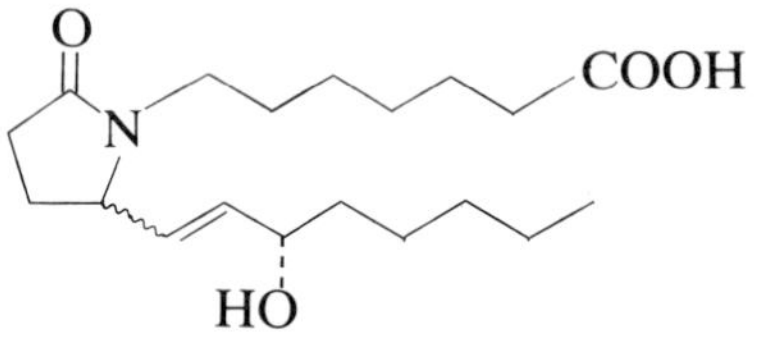

33.**109**

but the sulfoxide 33.**105** (X = $>S^+—O^-$) is inactive (472, 473). No activity was reported for 11-oxa PGE_2 (474), or 11-thia $PGF_{1\alpha}$ (33.**106**) (472). Replacement of both carbon atoms at positions 9 and 11 gave 9,11-*bis*-oxa PGE_1 and its 10-keto derivative 33.**107**, both weakly active in the gerbil colon assay (475). *N*-Methyl-10-aza-11-desoxy PGE_2 methyl ester (33.**108**) has been reported to possess spasmolytic and broncholytic activity (476, 477). 8-Aza-11-desoxy PGs E_2 and E_1 (33.**109**) have been synthesized (478, 479); the methyl ester of 33.**109** exhibits gastric antisecretory and antihypertensive activity (479). 11-Desoxy-12-aza PGE_1 (33.**110**) displays substantial activity on rat fundus and rat uterus smooth muscles (480); but no activity was reported for the 9-desoxy-$\Delta^{9,10}$ analog of (481).

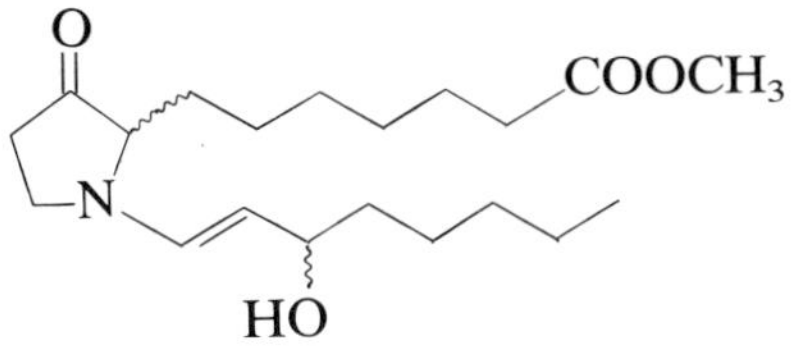

HO

33.**110**

Some oxazole and thiazole analogs of PGE_1 have been made; the most potent is 33.**111**, which displays one-twentieth the activity of prostaglandin $F_{2\alpha}$ on the rat uterus preparation (482).

The realization that the endoperoxides PGG_2 (33.**24**) and PGH_2 (33.**25**) are responsible for many of the actions originally attributed to the primary prostaglandins has led to a search for stable analogs that might act as mimics or inhibitors of the natural substances. The all-carbon analog 33.**112** of PGH_1 specifically inhibits the aspect of PG synthetase activity that leads to PGE_1, but it increases slightly the production of $PGF_{1\alpha}$ (483). The bicyclic analogs 33.**113** and 33.**114** of PGH_2 strongly inhibit the production of PGE_2 by ram seminal vesicle preparation. However when epinephrine is used as cofactor, $PGF_{2\alpha}$ production is suppressed more than is E_2 production (484). And the methyl ester of 33.**113** actually stimulates the production of PGE_2. There is no obvious explanation for these remarkable observations. Compound 33.**113** is one-tenth as potent as prostaglandin G_2 in aggregating human platelets (485, 486).

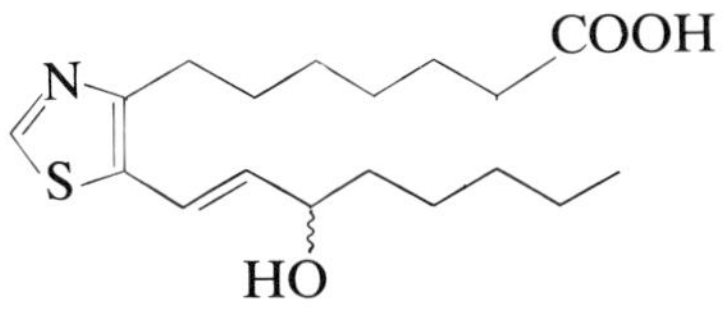

HO

33.**111**

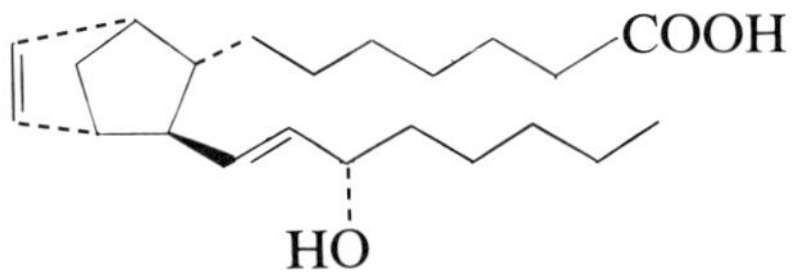

HO

33.**112**

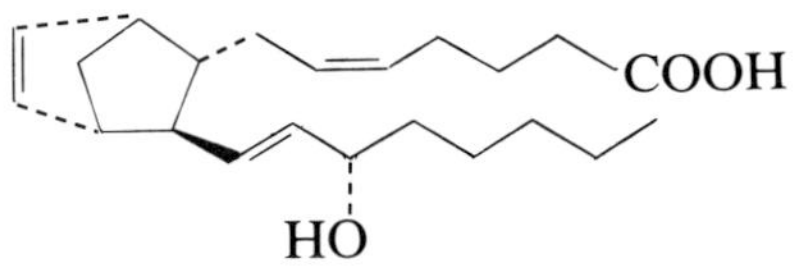

HO

33.**113**

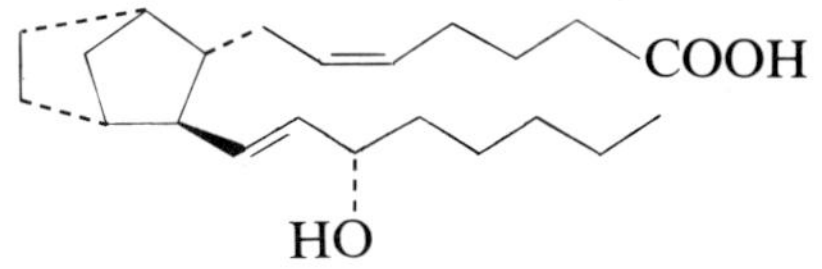

HO

33.**114**

HO

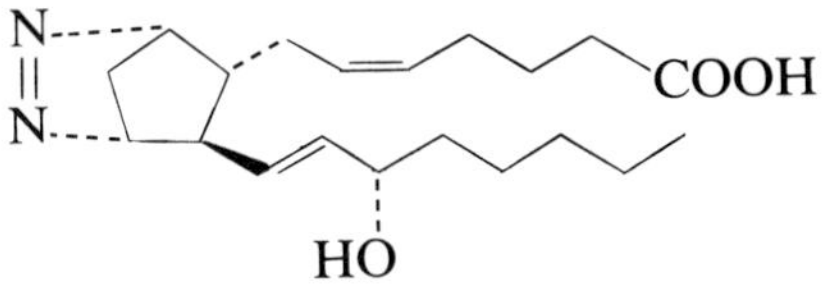

33.**115**

9,11-Aza PGE_2 (33.**115**) is a stable endoperoxide analog that is 8 times as potent as PGG_2 in aggregating human platelets and 7 times as potent as PGH_2 in the rabbit aorta strip assay (487, 488). Both monocarbon analogs of PGH_2 (33.**116**, 33.**117**) are potent bronchoconstrictors. They are more active than G_2 in aggregating platelets and are several times more potent than H_2 in causing contractions of rabbit aorta strips (489, 490).

The dithia analog (33.**118**) of PGH_2 methyl ester appears to be without effect on prostaglandin biosynthesis (491). The $PGF_{2\alpha}$ acetal (33.**119**) of acetaldehyde resembles the endoperoxides in structure and

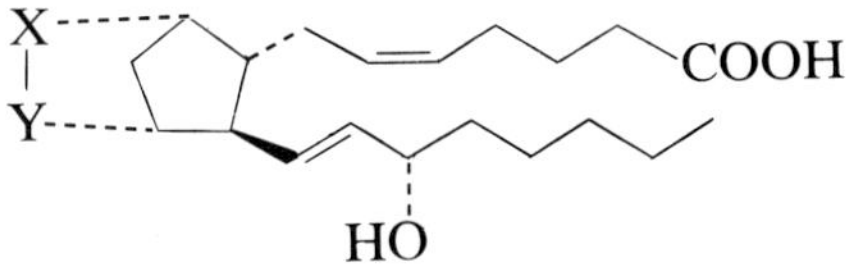

HO

33.**116** X = O, Y = CH_2
33.**117** X = CH_2, Y = O

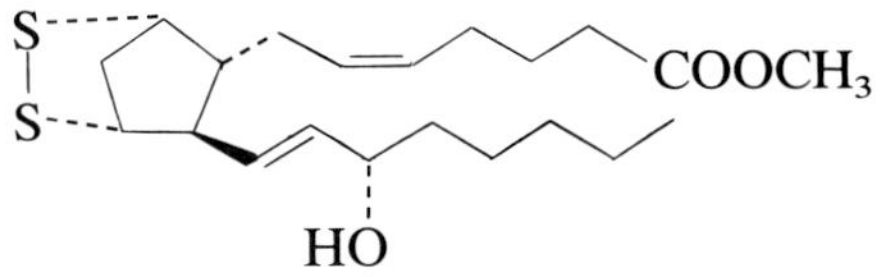

HO

33.**118**

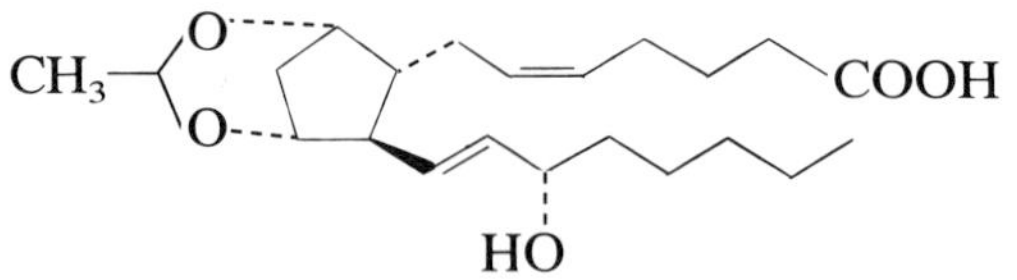

33.**119**

profile of activity. It has one-fiftieth the potency of PGG_2 in the platelet aggregation test and is slightly less potent in the gerbil colon and rabbit aorta assays (492).

Although relatively few endoperoxide analogs have been tested, they seem to be much less sensitive to variation in the heteroatom bridge than the primary prostaglandins are to variations in the cyclopentane ring. If endoperoxides truly are the principal effectors of activity, the prospect of obtaining analogs of improved therapeutic utility would seem to be better for them than for the primary prostaglandins.

6.4.3 VARIATIONS IN THE LOWER CHAIN. This type of structural variation contains the largest number of prostaglandin analogs; they are more accessible synthetically, and variations between C-15 and C-20 have produced analogs with narrower activity profiles. The effects on activity of reducing the C_{13}-C_{14} double bond and oxidizing the 15*S*-hydroxyl group are discussed in Section 6.

The acetylenic analog 33.**120** of prostaglandin $F_{2\alpha}$ displays enhanced luteolytic activity in the hamster, decreased activity in the gerbil colon assay, and inhibits placental 15-dehydrogenase (493, 494). The PGE_2 methyl ester analog of 33.**120** is about one-fifth as active as PGE_1 in binding to rat lipocytes and stimulating cyclic AMP production in mouse ovaries (493).

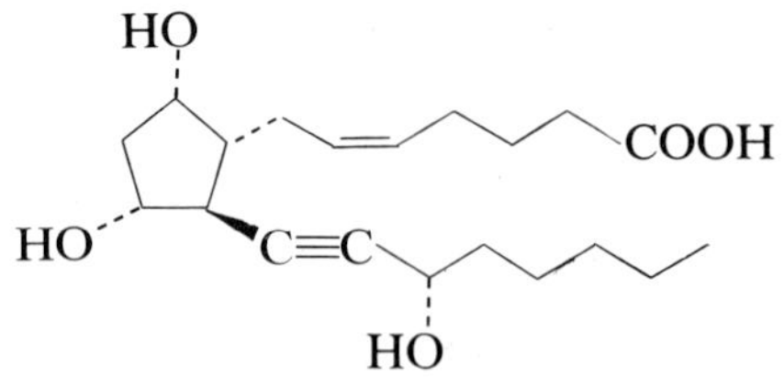

33.**120**

The syntheses of 13,14-dihydro-13,14-methylene PGE_2 (33.**121**) and $F_{2\alpha}$ have been reported but without any mention of activity (495). The formic acid catalyzed allylic rearrangement of 15-*epi* PGA_2 methyl ester gave the 13-hydroxy-Δ^{14}-isomer 33.**122**; it possesses slight pressor activity in the rat (496, 497).

The 14-chloro and 14-phenyl analogs (33.**123**, 33.**124**) of $PGF_{2\alpha}$ are largely inactive, as are the corresponding PGEs (494, 498). 14-Alkyl prostaglandins have been reported only in the patent literature: 14-methyl PGE_1 is about one-twentieth as active as prostaglandin E_2 in inhibiting gastric acid secretion and in lowering dog blood pressure. Both 14-methyl PGE_1 and PGE_2 do retain the potent bronchodilator activity of the PGEs (499).

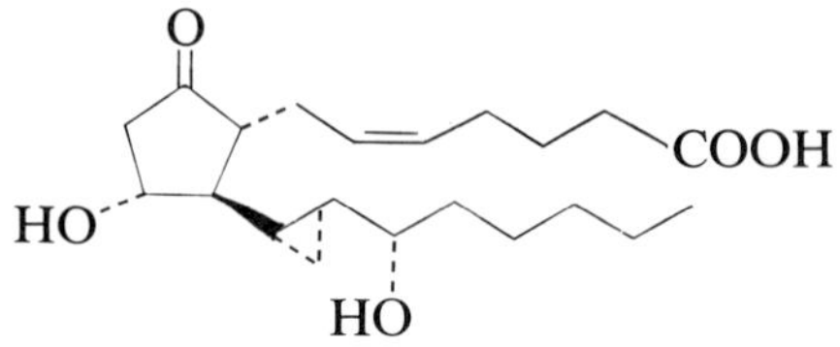

33.**121**

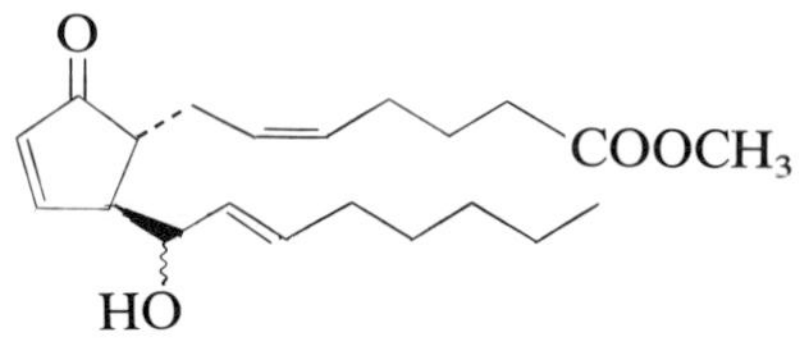

33.**122**

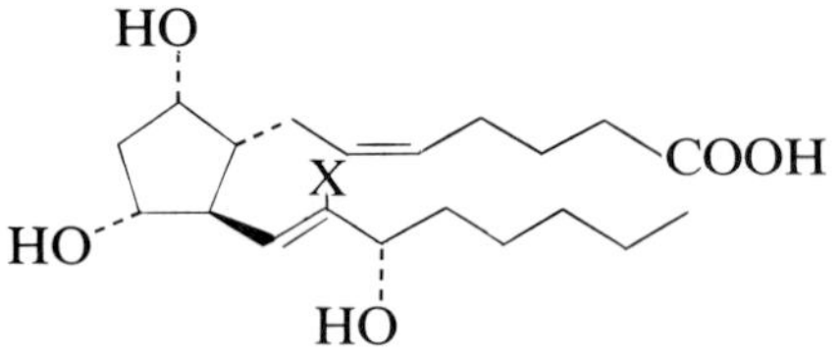

33.**123** X = Cl
33.**124** X = C_6H_5

Shortening the lower chain by one methylene gives ω-norprostaglandins, comparable in activity to the natural substances. Higher ω-homologs of PGE_1 have recently been prepared, and they display interesting patterns of activity (500). ω-Homo PGE_1 (33.**125**: R = n-C_6H_{13}) is half as active as PGE_1 in the gerbil colon assay, but the ω-ethyl and ω-propyl homologs (33.**125**: R = n-C_7H_{15} and n-C_8H_{17}) are only one-twentieth and one two-hundredth as active. The hypotensive potencies in the anesthetized rat fall off less rapidly: the potency of ω-methyl PGE_1 is 0.68 that of PGE_1, ω-ethyl PGE_1 is 0.84 that of PGE_1; ω-propyl is 0.42 as potent and ω-butyl (33.**125**: R = n-C_8H_{19}) is less than one-tenth as potent (500). In the dog, ω-methyl PGE_1 is equipotent to prostaglandin E_1 in inhibiting gastric acid secretion, but the higher homologs are inactive.

ω-Dihomoprostaglandin $F_{2\alpha}$ (33.**126**) is reported to be 20 times as potent as $PGF_{2\alpha}$ in the hamster antifertility test, but with less than one-third the smooth muscle stimulating activity (501).

11-Desoxy-ω-dihomo PGE_2 and $PGF_{1\alpha}$ have also been reported (502, 503); the activity of the latter in stimulating smooth muscle is less than that of 11-desoxy $PGF_{1\alpha}$ (503).

A series of alkoxy-substituted analogs of prostaglandin $F_{2\alpha}$ was prepared and several of the analogs were found to be potent luteolytic agents in hamsters (504, 505). 20-Methoxy $PGF_{2\alpha}$ (33.**127**) is equipotent to $F_{2\alpha}$, and 17-n-butoxytri-ω-nor $PGF_{2\alpha}$ (33.**128**) and 18-n-propoxy-di-ω-nor $PGF_{2\alpha}$ (33.**129**)—these are the 18-oxa and 19-oxa analogs of 33.**126**—are 4–5 times

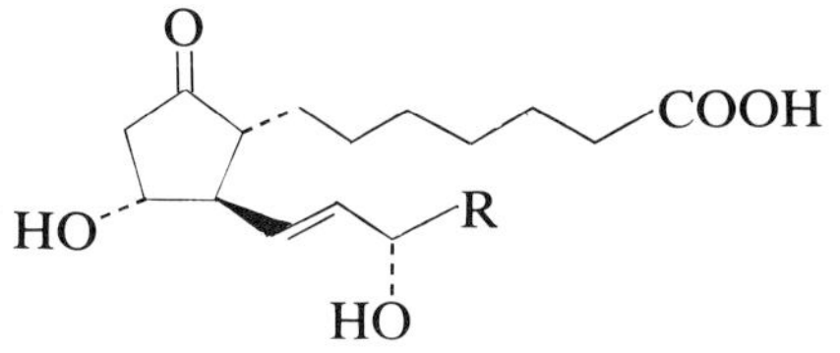

33.**125**

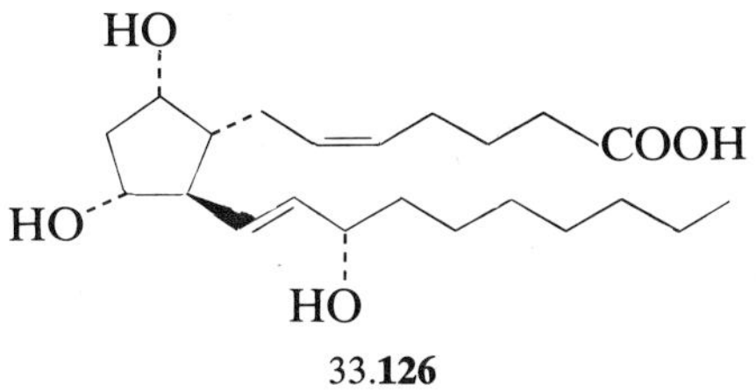

33.**126**

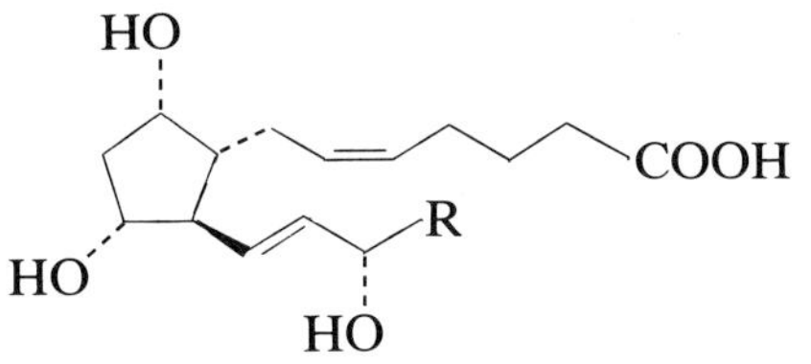

33.**127** R =

33.**128** R =

33.**129** R =

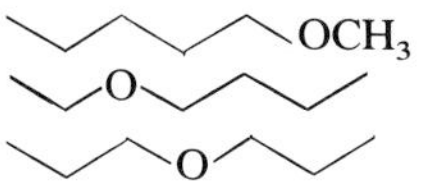

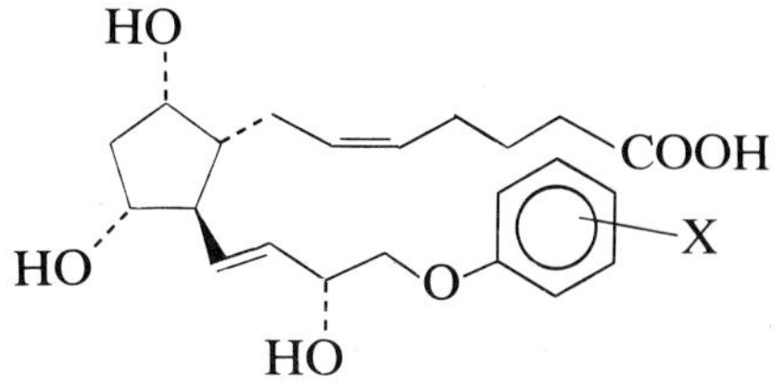

33.**130**

more luteolytic than $F_{2\alpha}$. Further investigations led to the discovery of substituted 16-phenoxy-tetra-ω-nor $PGF_{2\alpha}$ analogs (33.**130**) of even greater luteolytic potency. Activity is highest when X is an electron-withdrawing substituent. The chloro, trifluoromethyl, 4-fluoro derivatives 33.**130** (X = 3-Cl, X = 3-CF_3 and X = 4-F) are several hundred times more potent than $PGF_{2\alpha}$ in inducing luteolysis (504). The mechanism of action of these compounds is not known, but they may suppress uterine microcirculation. They are not substrates for the 15-dehydrogenase but are metabolized chiefly by β-oxidation. In spite of their potent luteolytic actions, these compounds are less active than $F_{2\alpha}$ in stimulating uterine smooth muscle. The PGE_2 analog of 33,**130** (X = 4-Cl) is also a potent luteolytic agent, but in the E_2-series increased luteolytic potency is accompanied by enhanced uterine smooth muscle stimulation (505, 506).

A series of 17-phenyl-ω-trinorprostaglandins has been made and evaluated in a number of assays (507–509). The pressor potency of the $F_{2\alpha}$ analog 33.**131** was 5 times that of $F_{2\alpha}$ itself and 90 times that of $F_{2\alpha}$ as a luteolytic agent in the hamster antifertility test. The PGE_1 and E_2 analogs

HO HO COOH C_6H_5 HO

33.**131**

O COOCH$_3$ HO HO

33.**132**

of 33.**131** were almost equal to PGE_1 in inhibiting gastric acid secretion in dogs (509).

The cyclooctylidine derivative 33.**132** of PGE_1 methyl ester has recently been synthesized. This conformationally constrained prostaglandin lacks smooth muscle activity but displays significant peripheral vasodilator activity in the dog (510).

REFERENCES

1. J. S. Bindra and R. Bindra, *Prog. Drug Res.*, **17,** 410 (1973).
2. *Chemical Abstracts*, Chemcon Data Base.
3. R. B. Zurier, *Arch. Intern. Med.*, **133,** 101 (1974).
4. K. F. Jacobs and M. M. Jacobs, *Rocky Mt. Med.*, **71,** 507 (1974).
5. *Med. News*, September 9, 1974.
6. H. P. Chase, *Pediatrics*, **57,** 441 (1976).
7. D. S. Snyder and W. H. Eaglstein, *J. Invest. Dermatol.*, **60,** 110 (1973).
8. M. W. Greaves and W. McDonald-Gibson, *Brit. Med. J.*, **73,** 608 (1973).
9. N. M. Weinshenker and N. H. Andersen, in *The Prostaglandins*, Vol. 1, P. W. Ramwell, Ed., Plenum Press, New York, 1973, p. 5.
10. E. J. Corey, in *Selected Organic Synthesis*, Ian Fleming, Ed., Wiley, London, 1973, p. 208.
11. U. Axen, J. E. Pike, and W. P. Schneider, in *The Total Synthesis of Natural Products*, Vol. 1, John ApSimon, Ed., Wiley-Interscience, New York, 1973, p. 81.
12. *Prostaglandins: Chemical and Biochemical Aspects*, S. M. M. Karim, Ed., University Press, Baltimore, 1976.
13. *Prostaglandins: Physiological, Pharmacological and Pathological Aspects*, S. M. M. Karim, Ed., University Park Press, Baltimore, 1976.
14. *Prostaglandins and Reproduction*, S. M. M. Karim, Ed., University Park Press, Baltimore, 1976.
15. R. Kurzrok and C. C. Leib, *Proc. Soc. Exp. Biol. Med.*, **28,** 268 (1930).
16. J. R. Cockrill, E. G. Miller, Jr., and R. Kurzrok, *Am. J. Physiol.*, **112,** 577 (1935).
17. M. W. Goldblatt, *Chem. Ind.* (London), **11,** 1056 (1933).
18. M. W. Goldblatt, *J. Physiol.*, **84,** 208 (1935).
19. U. S. von Euler, *Arch. Exp. Path. Pharmacol.*, **175,** 78 (1934).
20. U. S. von Euler, *Skand. Arch. Physiol.*, **81,** 65 (1939); *Chem. Abstr.* **33,** 29642 (1939).
21. U. S. von Euler, *Klin. Wochensch.*, **14,** 1182 (1935); *Chem. Abstr.* **30,** 30403 (1936).
22. U. S. von Euler, *J. Physiol.*, **88,** 213 (1936).
23. S. Bergström, *Science*, **157,** 382 (1967).
24. (a)–(c) S. Bergström and J. Sjövall, *Acta Chem. Scand.*, **14,** 1693, 1701, 1706 (1960).
25. S. Bergström, R. Eliasson, U. S. von Euler, and J. Sjövall, *Acta Physiol. Scand.*, **45,** 133 (1959).
26. S. Bergström, H. Dunér, U. S. von Euler, B. Pernow, and J. Sjövall, *Acta Physiol. Scand.*, **45,** 145 (1959).
27. S. Bergström, L. Krabisch, B. Samuelsson, and J. Sjövall, *Acta Chem. Scand.*, **16,** 969 (1962).
28. S. Bergström, R. Ryhage, B. Samuelsson, and J. Sjövall, *Acta Chem. Scand.*, **16,** 501 (1962).
29. D. H. Nugteren, D. A. van Dorp, S. Bergström, M. Hamberg, and B. Samuelsson, *Nature*, **212,** 38 (1966).
30. S. Abrahamsson, *Acta Crystallograp.*, **16,** 409 (1963).
31. S. Abrahamsson, S. Bergström, and B. Samuelsson, *Proc. Chem. Soc.*, 332 (1962).
32. B. Samuelsson, *J. Am. Chem. Soc.*, **85,** 1878 (1963).
33. B. Samuelsson, *Biochim. Biophys. Acta*, **84,** 707 (1964).
34. P. L. Taylor and R. W. Kelly, *Nature*, **250,** 665 (1974).
35. H. T. Jonsson, Jr., B. S. Middleditch, and D. M. Desiderio, *Science*, **187,** 1093 (1975).
36. R. L. Jones, *J. Lipid Res.*, **13,** 511 (1972).

37. R. L. Jones and S. Cammock, *Advan. Biosci.*, **9,** 61 (1973).
38. H. Polet and L. Levine, *J. Biol. Chem.*, **250,** 351 (1975).
39. E. Horton, R. Jones, C. Thompson, and N. Poyser, *Ann. N.Y. Acad. Sci.*, **180,** 351 (1971).
40. R. L. Jones, *Prostaglandins*, **5,** 283 (1974).
41. D. H. Nugteren and E. Hazelhof, *Biochem. Biophys. Acta*, **326,** 448 (1973).
42. D. H. Nugteren, R. K. Beerthuis, and D. A. van Dorp, *Rec. Trav. Chim. Pays-Bas*, **85,** 405 (1966).
43. C. J. Sih, C. Takeguchi, and P. Foss, *J. Am. Chem. Soc.*, **92,** 6670 (1970).
44. R. L. Jones, in *Advances in Prostaglandin and Thromboxane Research* Vol. 1, B. Samuelsson and R. Paoletti, Eds., Raven Press, New York, 1976, p. 221.
45. B. Samuelsson and G. Stallberg, *Acta Chem. Scand.*, **17,** 810 (1963).
46. N. H. Andersen, *Ann. N.Y. Acad. Sci.*, **180,** 14 (1971).
47. E. L. Eliel, *Stereochemistry of Carbon Compounds*, McGraw-Hill, New York, 1962, p. 92.
48. M. Hamburg, *Eur. J. Biochem.*, **6,** 147 (1968).
49. C. Gandolfi, G. Doria, and P. Gaio, *Tetrahedron Lett.*, 4303 (1972).
50. E. J. Christ and D. A. van Dorp, *Biochim. Biophys. Acta*, **270,** 537 (1972).
51. S. M. M. Karim, M. Sandler, and E. D. Williams, *Brit. J. Pharmacol. Chemother.*, **31,** 340 (1967).
52. S. M. M. Karim, K. Hillier, and J. Devlin, *J. Pharm. Pharmacol.*, **20,** 749 (1968).
53. T. Nomura and H. Ogata, *Biochim. Biophys. Acta*, **431,** 127 (1976).
54. A. J. Weinheimer and R. L. Spraggins, *Tetrahedron Lett.* **59,** 5185 (1969).
55. H. Kunze and W. Vogt, *Ann. N.Y. Acad. Sci.*, **180,** 123 (1971).
56. W. O. Lundberg, *Chem. Ind.* (London), 572 (1965).
57. P. Piper and J. Vane, *Ann. N.Y. Acad. Sci.*, **180,** 363 (1971).
58. J. H. Bartels, H. Kunze, W. Vogt, and G. Wille, *Arch. Pharmakol.*, **266,** 199 (1970).
59. W. Vogt, U. Meyer, H. Kunze, E. Lufft, and S. Babilli, *Arch. Pharmakol.*, **262,** 124 (1969).
60. G. O. Burr and M. M. Burr, *J. Biol. Chem.*, **86,** 587 (1930).
61. G. H. Jouvenaz, D. H. Nugteren, R. K. Beerthuis, and D. A. Van Dorp, *Biochim. Biophys. Acta*, **202,** 231 (1970).
62. D. R. Howton and J. F. Mead, *J. Biol. Chem.*, **235,** 3386 (1960).
63. D. A. Van Dorp, R. K. Beerthuis, D. H. Nugteren, and H. Vonkeman, *Biochim. Biophys. Acta*, **90,** 204 (1964).
64. S. Bergström, H. Danielsson, and B. Samuelsson, *Biochim. Biophys. Acta*, **90,** 207 (1964).
65. H. J. Thomasson, *Nature*, **194,** 973 (1962).
66. R. K. Beerthuis, D. H. Nugteren, H. J. J. Pabon, and D. A. Van Dorp, *Rec. Trav. Chem. Pays-Bas*, **87,** 461 (1968).
67. F. P. Kupiecki and J. R. Weeks, *Fed. Proc.*, **25,** 719 (1966).
68. L. Z. Bito, H. Davson, and E. V. Salvador, *J. Physiol.*, **256,** 257 (1976).
69. L. Z. Bito, M. Wallenstein, and R. Baroody, in *Advances in Prostaglandin and Thromboxane Research*, Vol. 1, B. Samuelsson and R. Paoletti, Eds., Raven Press, New York, 1976, p. 297.
70. M. P. L. Caton, *Prog. Med. Chem.*, **8,** 317 (1971).
71. B. Samuelsson, E. Granström, K. Gréen, M. Hamberg, and S. Hammarström, *Ann. Rev. Biochem.*, **44,** 669 (1975).
72. C. G. Hammar, B. Holmstedt, and R. Ryhage, *Anal. Biochem.*, **25,** 532 (1968).
73. C. C. Sweeley, W. H. Elliott, I. Fries, and R. Ryhage, *Ann. Chem.*, **38,** 1549 (1966).
74. K. Gréen, *Chem. Phys. Lipids*, **3,** 254 (1969).
75. H. W. Seyberth, O. Oelz, T. Kennedy, B. J. Sweetman, A. Danon, J. C. Frölich, M. Heimberg, and J. A. Oates, *Clin. Pharmacol. Ther.*, **18,** 521 (1975).
76. K. Gréen and B. Samuelsson, *Eur. J. Biochem.*, **22,** 391 (1971).
77. E. Änggård and C. E. Jonsson, *Acta Physiol. Scand.*, **81,** 440 (1971).
78. M. Hamberg and C. E. Jonsson, *Acta Physiol. Scand.*, **87,** 240 (1973).
79. K. Strandberg and M. Hamberg, *Prostaglandins*, **6,** 159 (1974).
80. M. Hamberg, *Life Sci.* **14,** 247 (1974).
81. M. Hamberg and B. Samuelsson, *Proc. Nat. Acad. Sci. US*, **70,** 899 (1973).
82. M. Hamberg and B. Samuelsson, *J. Biol. Chem.*, **247,** 3495 (1972).
83. M. Hamberg, *Biochem. Biophys. Res. Commun.*, **49,** 726 (1972).
84. D. P. Wallach and E. G. Daniels, *Biochim. Biophys. Acta*, **231,** 445 (1971).
85. M. Hamberg and B. Samuelsson, *Proc. Nat. Acad. Sci., US*, **71,** 3400 (1974).

86. M. Hamberg, J. Svensson, and B. Samuelsson, *Proc. Nat. Acad. Sci., US,* **71,** 3824 (1974).
87. C. Pace-Asciak and L. S. Wolfe, *Biochim. Biophys. Acta,* **218,** 539 (1970).
88. H. Kunze, *Biochim. Biophys. Acta,* **202,** 180 (1970).
89. W. Vogt, R. Suzuki, and S. Babilli, *Mem. Soc. Endocrinol.,* **14,** 137 (1966).
90. H. Kunze and R. Bohn, *Arch. Pharmakol.,* **264,** 263 (1969).
91. W. E. M. Lands and B. Samuelsson, *Biochim. Biophys. Acta,* **164,** 426 (1968).
92. H. Vonkeman and D. A. Van Dorp. *Biochim. Biophys. Acta,* **164,** 430 (1968).
93. B. Haye, S. Champion, and C. Jacquemin, in *Advances in Prostaglandin and Thromboxane Research* Vol. 1, B. Samuelsson and R. Paoletti, Eds., Raven Press, New York, 1976, p. 29.
94. B. Samuelsson, *J. Am. Chem. Soc.,* **87,** 3011 (1965).
95. E. Änggård and B. Samuelsson, *J. Biol. Chem.,* **246,** 3518 (1965).
96. M. Hamberg and B. Samuelsson, *J. Biol. Chem.,* **242,** 5336 (1967).
97. E. Granström, W. E. M. Lands, and B. Samuelsson, *J. Biol. Chem.,* **243,** 4104 (1968).
98. P. Wlodower and B. Samuelsson, *J. Biol. Chem.,* **248,** 5673 (1973).
99. M. Hamberg and B. Samuelsson, *J. Biol. Chem.,* **242,** 5344 (1967).
100. M. Hamberg, J. Svensson, T. Wakabayashi, and B. Samuelsson, *Proc. Nat. Acad. Sci., US,* **71,** 345 (1974).
101. T. Miyamoto, S. Yamamoto, and O. Hayaishi, *Proc. Nat. Acad. Sci., US,* **71,** 3645 (1974).
102. B. Samuelsson and M. Hamberg, in *Prostaglandin Synthetase Inhibitors,* H. J. Robinson and J. R. Vane, Eds., Raven Press, New York, 1974, p. 107.
103. M. Hamberg, P. Hedqvist, K. Strandberg, J. Svensson, and B. Samuelsson, *Life Sci.,* **16,** 451 (1975).
104. M. Hamberg and B. Samuelsson, *Biochim. Biophys. Acta,* **431,** 189 (1976).
105. E. Christ–Hazelhof, D. H. Nugteren, and D. A. Van Dorp, *Biochim. Biophys. Acta,* **450,** 450 (1976).
106. W. E. M. Lands, H. W. Cook, and L. H. Rome, in *Advances in Prostaglandin and Thromboxane Research,* Vol. 1, B. Samuelsson and R. Paoletti, Eds., Raven Press, New York, 1976, p. 7.
107. W. Lands, R. Lee, and W. Smith, *Ann. N.Y. Acad. Sci.,* **186,** 107 (1971).
108. K. Gréen, M. Hamberg, and B. Samuelsson, in *Advances in Prostaglandin and Thromboxane Research,* Vol. 1, B. Samuelsson and R. Paoletti, Eds., Raven Press, New York, p. 47.
109. M. Hamberg and B. Samuelsson, *J. Biol. Chem.,* **242,** 5329 (1967).
110. W. L. Smith and W. E. M. Lands, *J. Biol. Chem.,* **247,** 1038 (1972).
111. E. F. Ellis, *Science,* **193,** 1135 (1976).
112. W.-c. Chang, S.-i. Murota, and S. Tsurufuji, *Prostaglandins,* **13,** 17 (1977).
113. P. P. K. Ho, C. P. Walters, and H. R. Sullivan, *Prostaglandins,* **12,** 951 (1976).
114. J. Svensson and M. Hamberg, *Prostaglandins,* **12,** 943 (1976).
115. P. Needleman, S. Moncada, S. Bunting, J. R. Vane, M. Hamberg, and B. Samuelsson, *Nature,* **261,** 558 (1976).
116. M. Hamberg, J. Svensson, and B. Samuelsson, *Proc. Nat. Acad. Sci., US,* **72,** 2994 (1975).
117. S. Moncada, P. Gryglewski, and S. Bunting, *Nature,* **263,** 663 (1976).
118. P. Needleman, P. S. Kulkarni, and A. Raz, *Science,* **195,** 409 (1977).
119. P. J. Piper and J. R. Vane, *Nature,* **223,** 29 (1969).
120. R. Gryglewski and J. R. Vane, *Brit. J. Pharmacol.,* **43,** 37 (1972).
121. J. R. Vane, *Nature New Biol.,* **231,** 232 (1971).
122. *Chem. Eng. News,* December 20, 1976, p. 17.
123. R. A. Johnson, D. R. Morton, J. H. Kinner, R. R. Gorman, J. C. McGuire, and F. F. Sun, *Prostaglandins,* **12,** 915 (1976).
124. G. J. Dusting, S. Moncada, and J. R. Vane, *Prostaglandins,* **13,** 3 (1977).
125. *Science,* **196,** 1072 (1977).
126. P. C. Isakson, A. Raz, S. E. Denny, E. Pure, and P. Needleman, *Proc. Nat. Acad. Sci. US,* **74,** 101 (1977).
127. W.-c. Chang and S.-i. Murota, *Biochim. Biophys. Acta,* **486,** 136 (1977).
128. C. Pace–Asciak and L. S. Wolfe, *Chem. Commun.,* 1234 (1970).
129. C. Pace–Asciak and L. S. Wolfe, *Chem. Commun.,* 1235 (1970).
130. M. Hamberg and B. Samuelsson, *Biochem. Biophys. Res. Commun.,* **61,** 942 (1974).
131. E. Änggård and B. Samuelsson, *J. Biol. Chem.,* **240,** 3518 (1965).
132. E. Änggård and C. Larsson, *Eur. J. Pharmacol.,* **14,** 66 (1971).
133. P. J. Piper, J. R. Vane, and J. H. Wyllie, *Nature,* **225,** 600 (1970).

134. S. C. Lee, S. S. Pong, D. Katzen, K. Y. Wu, and L. Levine, *Biochemistry*, **14,** 142 (1975).

135. E. Änggård, F. M. Matschinsky, and B. Samuelsson, *Science*, **163,** 479 (1969).

136. J. Nakano, E. Änggård, and B. Samuelsson, *Eur. J. Biochem.*, **11,** 386 (1969).

137. E. Änggård and B. Samuelsson, *J. Biol., Chem.*, **239,** 4097 (1964).

138. E. Änggård, K. Gréen, and B. Samuelsson, *J. Biol. Chem.*, **264,** 1932 (1965).

139. E. Änggård and B. Samuelsson, *Biochemistry*, **4,** 1864 (1965).

140. E. Anggård and E. Oliev, *Agents Actions*, **6,** 498 (1976).

141. M. Hamberg, *Eur. J. Biochem.*, **6,** 135 (1968).

142. M. Hamberg and V. Israelsson, *J. Biol. Chem.*, **245,** 5107 (1970).

143. E. Granström, V. Inger, and B. Samuelsson, *J. Biol. Chem.*, **240,** 457 (1965).

144. E. Granström and B. Samuelsson, *Eur. J. Biochem.*, **10,** 411 (1969).

145. K. Gréen, *Acta Chem. Scand.*, **23,** 1453 (1969).

146. K. Gréen, *Biochim. Biophys. Acta*, **231,** 419 (1971).

147. M. Hamberg and B. Samuelsson, *Biochem. Biophys. Res. Commun.*, **34,** 22 (1969).

148. K. Gréen, *Biochemistry*, **10,** 1072 (1971).

149. M. Hamberg and B. Samuelsson, *J. Am. Chem. Soc.*, **91,** 2177 (1969).

150. E. Granström and B. Samuelsson, *J. Am. Chem. Soc.*, **91,** 3398 (1969).

151. K. Gréen and B. Samuelsson, *Biochem. Med.*, **11,** 298 (1974).

152. C. R. Pace-Asciak, in *Advances in Prostaglandin and Thromboxane Research*, Vol. 1, B. Samuelsson and R. Paoletti, Eds., Raven Press, New York, 1976, p. 35.

153. J. D. Fasciolo, B. A. Houssay, and A. C. Taquini, *J. Physiol.*, **94,** 281 (1938).

154. H. Goldblatt, J. Lynch, R. F. Hanzal, and W. W. Summerville, *J. Exp. Med.*, **59,** 347 (1934).

155. W. J. Kolff and I. H. Page, *Am. J. Physiol.*, **178,** 75 (1954).

156. E. E. Muirhead, G. B. Brown, G. S. Germain, and B. E. Leach, *J. Lab. Clin. Med.*, **76,** 641 (1970).

157. J. B. Lee, *Arch. Intern. Med.*, **133,** 56 (1974).

158. J. B. Lee, *Am. J. Med.*, **61,** 681 (1976).

159. E. E. Muirhead, in *The Prostaglandins: Pharmacological and Therapeutic Advances*, M. F. Cuthbert, Ed., Heinemann, London, 1973, p. 201.

160. J. C. McGiff, in *Prostaglandins and Cyclic AMP*, R. H. Kahn and W. E. M. Lands, Eds., Academic Press, New York, 1973, p. 119.

161. E. E. Muirhead, F. Jones, and J. A. Stirman, *J. Lab. Clin. Med.*, **56,** 167 (1960).

162. E. E. Muirhead, E. G. Daniels, E. Booth, W. A. Freyburger, and J. W. Hinman, *Arch. Pathol.*, **80,** 43 (1965).

163. J. B. Lee, R. B. Hickler, C. A. Saravis, and G. W. Thorn, *Circ. Res.*, **13,** 359 (1963).

164. J. B. Lee, B. G. Covino, B. H. Takman, and E. R. Smith, *Circ. Res.*, **17,** 57 (1965).

165. J. B. Lee, K. Crowshaw, and B. H. Takman, *Biochem. J.*, **105,** 1251 (1967).

166. S. Bergström, L. A. Carlson, and L. Orö, *Acta Physiol. Scand.*, **60,** 170 (1964).

167. C. G. Strong and D. F. Bohr, *Am. J. Physiol.*, **213,** 725 (1967).

168. K. V. Malik and J. C. McGiff, in *Prostaglandins: Physiological, Pharmacological and Pathological Aspects*, S. M. M. Karim, Ed., University Park Press, Baltimore, 1976, p. 103.

169. H. Kannegiesser and J. B. Lee, *Nature*, **229,** 498 (1971).

170. J. B. Lee, J. Z. Gougoutas, B. H. Takman, E. G. Daniels, M. F. Grostic, J. E. Pike, J. W. Hinman, and E. E. Muirhead, *J. Clin. Invest.*, **45,** 1036 (1966).

171. A. R. Chrislieb, S. J. Dobrzinsky, C. J. Lyons, and R. B. Hickler, *Clin. Res.*, **17,** 234 (1969).

172. A. A. Carr, *Am. J. Med. Sci.*, **259,** 21 (1970).

173. E. E. Westura, H. Kannegiesser, J. D. O'Toole, and J. B. Lee, *Circ. Res.*, **27,** (Suppl. 1), I-131 (1970).

174. H. B. Barner, G. C. Kaiser, M. Jellinck, and J. B. Lee, *Am. Heart J.*, **85,** 584 (1973).

175. S. M. M. Karim, K. Somers, and K. Hillier, *Eur. J. Pharmacol.*, **5,** 117 (1969).

176. D. W. Du Charme, J. R. Weeks, and R. G. Montgomery, *J. Pharmacol., Exp. Ther.*, **160,** 1 (1968).

177. R. L. Jones, *Brit. J. Pharmacol.*, **45,** 144P (1972).

178. J. W. Aiken and J. R. Vane, *J.* … *l. Exp. Ther.*, **184,** 678 (1973).

179. J. C. McGiff, K. Crowsha… J. Lonigro, *Circ. Res.* … (1970).

180. P. T. Schnatz, J. B … Vance, *Clin. Re* …

181. A. Prezyna, … man, and J …

182. J. B. Le … (1975 …

183. J. B. Lee, in *The Prostaglandins*, P. Ramwell, Ed., Plenum Press, New York, 1973, p. 133.
184. J. C. Frolich, W. M. Williams, B. J. Sweetman, M. Smigel, K. Carr, J. W. Hollifield, S. Fleisher, A. S. Nies, M. Frish–Holmberg, and J. A. Oates, in *Advances in Prostaglandin and Thromboxane Research*, Vol. 1, B. Samuelsson and R. Paoletti, Eds., Raven Press, New York, 1976, p. 65.
185. A. Attallah, W. Payakkapan, J. Lee, A. Carr, and E. Brazelton, *Prostaglandins*, **5,** 69 (1974).
186. C. J. Blackwell, R. J. Flowers, and J. R. Vane, *Biochim. Biophys. Acta*, **398,** 178 (1975).
187. M. Martinez–Maldonado, N. Tsaparas, G. Eknoyan, and W. W. Suki, *Am. J. Physiol*; **222,** 1147 (1972).
188. G. R. Zins, *Am. J. Med.*, **58,** 14 (1975).
189. G. Weissman, in *Mediators of Inflammation*, G. Weismann, Ed., Plenum Press, New York, 1974, p. 2.
190. J. L. Marx, *Science*, **177,** 780 (1972).
191. G. Kaley and R. Weiner, *Ann. N.Y. Acad. Sci.*, **180,** 338 (1971).
192. H. R. Schumacher and C. A. Agudelo, *Science*, **175,** 1139 (1972).
193. R. L. Nachman and B. Weksler, *Ann. N.Y. Acad. Sci.*, **201,** 131 (1972).
194. M. A. Packham, E. E. Anderson, and J. F. Mustard, *Biochem. Pharmacol.*, **17,** 171 (1968).
195. A. L. Willis, *J. Pharm. Pharmacol.*, **21,** 126 (1969).
196. M. DiRosa, J. P. Giraud, and D. A. Willoughby, *J. Pathol.*, **104,** 15 (1971).
197. M. DiRosa and L. Sorrentino, *Brit. J. Pharmacol.*, **38,** 214 (1970).
198. A. L. Willis, in *Prostaglandins, Peptides and Amines*, P. Mantegazza and E. W. Horton, Eds., Academic Press, London, 1969, p. 31.
199. R. B. Zurier, *Arch. Intern. Med.*, **133,** 101 (1974).
200. G. Weissmann, S. Hoffstein, S. Kammerman, and H. H. Tai, *J. Clin Invest*, **53,** 297 (1974).
201. G. Weissmann, R. B. Zurier, and S. Hoffstein, *Adv. Biosci.*, **9,** 435 (1973).
202. I. Rivkin, G. V. Foschi, and C. H. Rosen, *Proc. Soc. Exp. Biol. Med.*, **153,** 236 (1976).
203. I. Rivkin, J. Rosenblatt, and E. L. Becker, *J. Immunol.*, **115,** 1126 (1976).
204. J. L. Diaz–Perez, M. E. Goldyne, and R. K. Winkelmann, *J. Invest. Dermatol.*, **66,** 149 (1976).
205. T. J. Williams and J. Morley, *Nature*, **246,** 215 (1973).
206. C. J. Whelan, *J. Pharm. Pharmacol.*, **26,** 356 (1974).
207. M. W. Greaves, J. Søndergaard, and W. McDonald-Gibson, *Brit. Med. J.*, **2,** 258 (1971).
208. S. H. Ferreira, R. J. Flower, M. F. Parsons, and J. R. Vane, *Prostaglandins*, **8,** 433 (1974).
209. I. L. Bonta, H. Chrispyn, J. Noordhoek, and J. E. Vincent, *Prostaglandins*, **5,** 495 (1974).
210. H. E. Paulus, in *Antiinflammatory Agents: Chemistry and Pharmacology*, Vol. 1, R. A. Scherer and M. W. Whitehouse, Eds., Academic Press, New York, 1974, p. 3.
211. H. O. J. Collier, in *Advances in Pharmacology and Chemotherapy*, Vol. 7, S. Garattini, A. Goldoni, F. Hawking, and I. J. Kopin, Eds., Academic Press, New York, 1969, p. 382.
212. J. R. Vane, *Nature New Biol.*, **231,** 232 (1971).
213. S. H. Ferreira, S. Moncada, and J. R. Vane, *Nature New Biol.*, **231,** 237 (1971).
214. J. B. Smith and A. L. Willis, *Nature New Biol.*, **231,** 235 (1971).
215. H. O. J. Collier, *Nature New Biol.*, **232,** 17 (1971).
216. R. Flower, R. Gryglewski, K. Herbaczýnska-Cedro, and J. R. Vane, *Nature New Biol.* **238,** 104 (1972).
217. S. H. Ferreira and J. R. Vane, *Ann. Rev. Pharmacol.*, **14,** 57 (1974).
218. M. W. Greaves and W. McDonald-Gibson, *J. Invest. Dermatol.*, **61,** 127 (1973).
219. M. W. Greaves and W. McDonald-Gibson, *Brit. Med. J.*, 527 (1972).
220. Y. Floman, N. Floman, and V. Zor, *Prostaglandins*, **11,** 591 (1976).
221. R. Vinegar, J. F. Traux, and J. L. Selph, *Proc. Soc. Exp. Biol. Med.*, **143,** 711 (1973).
222. A. Blackham and R. T. Owen, *J. Pharm. Pharmacol.*, **27,** 201 (1975).
223. M. Di Rosa, *Pol. J. Pharm. Pharmacol.*, **26,** 25 (1974).
224. L. Z. Bito and E. Salvador, *J. Pharmacol. Exp. Ther.*, **198,** 481 (1976).
225. R. J. Flower, E. A. Harvey, and W. P. Kingston, *Brit. J. Pharmacol.*, **56,** 229 (1976).
226. F. A. Kuehl, Jr., J. L. Humes, R. W. Egan, E. A. Ham, G. C. Beveridge, and C. G. Van Arman, *Nature*, **265,** 170 (1977).
227. H. M. Goodman, in *Medical Physiology*, 13th ed., Vol. 2, V. B. Mountcastle, Ed., Mosley, St. Louis, 1974, p. 1741.
228. C. W. Bardin and H. E. Morgan, in *Best and Taylor's Physiological Basis of Medical Practice*, 9th ed., J. R. Brobeck, Ed., Williams & Wilkins, Baltimore, 1973, pp. 7–95.

229. E. W. Horton and N. L. Poyser, *Physiol. Rev.*, **56,** 595 (1976).

230. J. A. McCracken, J. C. Carlson, M. E. Glew, J. R. Goding, D. T. Blaird, K. Gréen, and B. Samuelsson, *Nature New Biol.*, **238,** 129 (1972).

231. T. M. Nett and A. M. Akbor, *Biol. Reprod.*, **9,** 87 (1973).

232. J. C. Carlson, B. Barcikowski, and J. A. McCracken, *J. Reprod. Fertil.*, **34,** 357 (1973).

233. H. R. Behrman, T. S. Ng, and G. R. Orczyk, in *Gonadotropins and Gonadal Function*, N. R. Moudgal, Ed., Academic Press, New York, 1974, p. 332.

234. L. L. Anderson, K. P. Bland, and R. M. Melampey, *Rec. Prog. Hormone Res.*, **25,** 57 (1969).

235. S. M. M. Karim and K. Hillier, in *Prostaglandins and Reproduction*, S. M. M. Karim, Ed., University Park Press, Baltimore, 1975, p. 37.

236. W. S. Powell, S. Hammarström, and B. Samuelsson, *Lancet*, 1120 (1974).

237. A. I. Csapo, M. O. Pulkkinen, and H. L. Kaihola, *Am. J. Obstet. Gynecol.*, **112,** 1061 (1974).

238. S. M. M. Karim and J.-J. Amy, in *Prostaglandins and Reproduction*, S. M. M. Karim, Ed., University Park Press, Baltimore, 1975, p. 78.

239. D. T. Armstrong, Y. S. Moon, and J. Zamecnik, in *Gonadotropins and Gonadal Function*, N. R. Moudgal, Ed., Academic Press, New York, 1973, p. 345.

240. C. V. Rao, in *Advances in Prostaglandin and Thromboxane Research*, Vol. 1, B. Samuelsson and R. Paoletti, Eds., Raven Press, New York, 1976, p. 247.

241. J. M. Marsh, N. S. T. Yang, and W. J. LeMaire, *Prostaglandins*, **7,** 269 (1974).

242. H. R. Behrman and G. G. Anderson, *Arch. Intern. Med.*, **133,** 77 (1974).

243. A. C. Wentz and G. S. Jones, *Obstet Gynecol.*, **42,** 172 (1973).

244. F. Sandberg, A. Ingelman-Sundberg, and G. Ryden, *Acta Obstetr. Gynecol. Scand.*, **44,** 585 (1965); *Chem. Abstr.*, **65,** 2590 (1966).

245. F. Sandberg, A. Ingelman-Sundberg, and G. Ryden, *Acta Obstetr. Gynecol. Scand.*, **43,** 95 (1964), *Chem. Abstr.*, **63,** 2092*b* (1965).

246. E. M. Coutinho and H. S. Maia, *Fertil. Steril.*, **22,** 539 (1971).

247. W. E. Brenner, *Am. J. Obstetr. Gynecol.*, **123,** 306 (1975).

248. S. Hammarström, W. S. Powell, V. Kyldén, and B. Samuelsson, in *Advances in Prostaglandin and Thromboxane Research*, Vol. 1, B. Samuelsson and R. Paoletti, Eds., Raven Press, New York, 1976, p. 235.

249. J. A. Salmon and J.-J. Amy, *Prostaglandins*, **4,** 523 (1973).

250. B. M. Hibbard, S. C. Sharma, R. J. Fitpatrick, and J. D. Hamlett, *J. Obstetr. Gynaecol. Brit. Commonw.*, **81,** 35 (1974); *Chem. Abstr.*, **81,** 36092t (1974).

251. M. J. N. C. Keirse and A. C. Turnbull, *Prostaglandins*, **4,** 263 (1973).

252. M. J. N. C. Keirse, A. P. C. Flint, and A. C. Turnbull, *J. Obstetr. Gynaecol. Brit. Commonw.*, **81,** 131 (1974); *Chem. Abstr.*, **81,** 36088w (1974).

253. S. M. M. Karim and J. J. Amy, in *Amnionic Fluid*, D. V. I. Fairweather and T. K. A. B. Eskes, Eds., Excerpta Medica, Amsterdam, 1973, p. 287.

254. E. W. Horton, *Physiol. Rev.*, **49,** 122 (1969).

255. M. Bygdeman, B. Fredericsson, K. Swanback, and B. Samuelsson, *Fertil. Steril.*, **21,** 622 (1970).

256. H. O. J. Collier and R. J. Flower, *Lancet*, **11,** 852 (1971).

257. E. W. Horton, R. L. Jones, and C. G. Marr, *J. Reprod. Fertil.*, **33,** 385 (1973).

258. S. M. M. Karim and P. G. Adaikan, quoted in *Prostaglandins and Reproduction*, S. M. M. Karim, Ed., University Park Press, Baltimore, 1976, p. 26.

259. A. Bennett, in *Topics in Gastroenterology*, S. C. Truelove and D. P. Jewell, Eds., Blackwell, Oxford, 1973, p. 285.

260. A. Bennett and B. Fleshler, *Gastroenterology*, **59,** 790 (1970).

261. M. G. Tonnesen, W. Jubiz, J. G. Moore, and J. Frailey, *Am. J. Digest. Dis.*, **19,** 644 (1974).

262. C. Child, W. Jubiz, and J. G. Moore, *Gut*, **17,** 54 (1976).

263. A. Bennett, in *Prostaglandins: Physiological, Pharmacological and Pathological Aspects*, S. M. M. Karim, Ed., University Park Press, Baltimore, 1976, p. 247.

264. F. Coceani, C. Pace–Asciak, F. Volta, and L. S. Wolfe, *Am. J. Physiol.*, **213,** 1056 (1967).

265. E. W. Horton and I. H. M. Main, *Gut*, **9,** 655 (1968).

266. J. J. Misiewicz, S. L. Waller, and M. Kiley, *Lancet*, **1,** 648 (1969).

267. R. L. Hunt, J. B. Dilawari, and J. J. Misiewicz, *Gut*, **16,** 47 (1975).

268. A. Mukhopadhyay, S. Rattan, and R. K. Goyal, *J. Appl. Physiol.*, **39,** 479 (1975).

269. A. Bennett, K. G. Eley, and H. L. Stockley, *Brit. J. Pharmacol.*, **57,** 335 (1976).

270. H. W. Davenport, *Gut,* **6,** 513 (1965).
271. C. H. Spilman and R. T. Duby, *Prostaglandins,* **2,** 159 (1972).
272. A. Robert, in *Advances in Prostaglandin and Thromboxane Research,* Vol. 2, B. Samuelsson and R. Paoletti, Eds., Raven Press, New York, 1976, p. 507.
273. D. Bhana, S. M. M. Karim, D. C. Carter, and P. A. Ganesan, *Prostaglandins,* **3,** 307 (1973).
274. J. Lukaszewska, L. Wilson, and W. Hansel, *Proc. Soc. Exp. Biol. Med.,* **140,** 1302 (1972).
275. L. Way and R. P. Durbin, *Nature,* **221,** 874 (1969).
276. G. Mózsik, J. Kutas, L. Nagy, and G. Németh, *Eur. J. Pharmacol.,* **29,** 133 (1974).
277. C. Matuchansky and J. J. Bernier, *Gastroenterology,* **64,** 1111 (1973).
278. J. H. Cummings, A. Newman, J. J. Misiewicz, G. J. Milton–Thompson, and J. A. Billings, *Nature,* **243,** 169 (1973).
279. G. J. Milton–Thompson, J. H. Cummings, A. Newman, J. A. Billings, and J. J. Misiewicz, *Gut,* **16,** 42 (1975).
280. A. Tothill, *Prostaglandins,* **11,** 925 (1976).
281. A. Bennett, in *Advances in Prostaglandin and Thromboxane Research,* Vol. 2, B. Samuelsson and R. Paoletti, Eds., Raven Press, New York, 1976, p. 547.
282. B. Nylander and S. Andersson, in *Advances in Prostaglandin and Thromboxane Research,* Vol. 2, B. Samuelsson and R. Paoletti, Eds., Raven Press, New York, 1976, p. 521.
283. S. J. Konturek, J. Olesky, J. Biernat, E. Sito, and N. Kwiecién, *Am. J. Digest, Dis.,* **21,** 291 (1976).
284. S. J. Konturek, N. Keviecién, J. Swierczek, J. Olesky, E. Sito, and A. Robert, *Gastroenterology,* **70,** 683 (1976).
285. S. M. M. Karim and W. P. Fung, in *Advances in Prostaglandin and Thromboxane Research,* Vol. 2, B. Samuelsson and R. Paoletti, Eds., Raven Press, New York, 1976, p. 529.
286. I. H. M. Main and B. J. R. Whittle, *Brit. J. Pharmacol.,* **54,** 309 (1975).
287. V. Rosenberg, D. Biezunski, M. Gonda, D. A. Dreiling, J. Rudick, and A. Robert, *Surgery,* **79,** 509 (1976).
288. H. Miyake *et al., Chem. Lett.,* 211 (1976).
289. E. Z. Dajani, D. R. Driskill, R. G. Bianchi, P. W. Collins, and R. Pappo, *Prostaglandins,* **10,** 733 (1975).
290. B. M. Peskar and B. A. Peskar, *Biochim. Biophys. Acta,* **424,** 430 (1976).
291. W. Lippmann, *Prostaglandins,* **7,** 231 (1974).
292. W. Lippmann, *Prostaglandins,* **7,** 223 (1974).
293. H. C. Kluender and G. P. Peruzzotti, *Tetrahedron Lett.,* 2063 (1977).
294. A. S. Milton, *J. Pharm. Pharmacol.,* **28,** 393 (1976).
295. E. Atkins and P. Bodel, in *The Inflammatory Process,* 2nd ed., Vol. 3, L. Grant and R. T. McClusky, Eds., New York, Academic Press, 1974, p. 467.
296. A. S. Milton and S. Wendlandt, *J. Physiol.,* **207,** 76P (1970).
297. A. S. Milton and S. Wendlandt, *J. Physiol.,* **217,** 33P (1971).
298. W. Feldberg and P. N. Sazena, *J. Physiol.,* **217,** 547 (1971).
299. W. Feldberg and K. P. Gupta, *J. Physiol.,* **228,** 41 (1973).
300. J. A. Splawinski, K. Reichenberg, J. Vetulani, J. Marchaj, and J. Kaluza, *Pol. J. Pharmacol.,* **26,** 101 (1974).
301. J. Stitt, *J. Physiol.,* **232,** 163 (1973).
302. R. J. Flower and J. R. Vane, *Nature,* **240,** 410 (1972).
303. H. P. Laburn, C. Rosendorff, G. Willies, and C. Woolf, *J. Physiol.,* **240,** 49P (1974).
304. C. J. Woolf, G. H. Willies, H. Laburn, and C. Rosendorff, *Neuropharmacology,* **14,** 397 (1975).
305. Q. J. Pittman, W. L. Veale, and K. E. Cooper, *Can. J. Pharmacol. Physiol.,* **54,** 101 (1976).
306. W. I. Cranston, R. F. Hellon, and D. Mitchell, *J. Physiol.,* **249,** 425 (1975).
307. S. M. M. Karim, M. Sandler, and E. D. Williams, *Brit. J. Pharmacol.,* **31,** 340 (1967).
308. M. E. Rosenthale, *NY State J. Med.,* 374 (1975).
309. A. P. Smith, in *Prostaglandins: Physiological, Pharmacological and Pathological Aspects,* S. M. M. Karim, Ed., University Park Press, Baltimore, 1976, p. 83.
310. M. E. Rosenthale, A. Dervinis, and J. Kassarich, *J. Pharmacol. Exp. Ther.,* **178,** 541 (1971).
311. B. J. Large, P. F. Leswell, and D. R. Maxwell, *Nature,* **224,** 78 (1969).
312. A. P. Smith, M. F. Cuthbert, and L. S. Dunlop, *Clin. Sci.,* **48,** 421 (1975).
313. A. P. Smith, *Clin. Sci.,* **44,** 17 (1973).
314. A. P. Smith and M. F. Cuthbert, *Brit. Med. J.,* **2,** 212 (1972).
315. P. Hedquist, A. Holmgren, and A. A. Mathé, *Acta Physiol. Scand.,* **82,** 29a (1971).
316. A. P. Smith, *Clin. Sci.,* **44,** 17 (1973).

317. M. E. Rosenthale, A. Dervinis, J. Kassarich, A. Blumenthal, and M. I. Gluckman, in *Prostaglandins and Cyclic AMP*, R. H. Kahn and W. E. M. Lands, Eds., Academic Press, New York, 1973, p. 53.

318. P. Y. Lo, P. G. Adaikan, and S. M. M. Karim, *Prostaglandins*, **11**, 531 (1976).

319. R. Greenberg, K. Smorong, and J. F. Bagli, *Prostaglandins*, **11**, 961 (1976).

320. M. A. Wasserman, D. W. DuCharme, R. L. Griffin, G. L. DeGraaf, and F. G. Robinson, *Prostaglandins*, **13**, 255 (1977).

321. C. W. Parker and D. E. Snider, *Arch. Intern. Med.*, **8**, 963 (1973).

322. W. Dawson, R. L. Lewis, R. E. McMahon, and W. J. F. Sweatman, *Nature*, **250**, 331 (1974); W. Dawson and W. J. F. Sweatman, *Int. Arch. Appl. Immunol.*, **49**, 213 (1975).

323. B. B. Fredholm and P. Hedqvist, *Acta Physiol. Scand.*, **80**, 450 (1970).

324. D. Steinberg, M. Vaughan, P. Nestel, and S. Bergström, *Biochem. Pharmacol.*, **12**, 764 (1963).

325. S. Bergström and L. A. Carlson, *Acta Physiol. Scand.*, **63**, 195 (1965).

326. D. Steinberg and R. Pittman, *Proc. Soc. Exp. Biol. Med.*, **123**, 192 (1966).

327. S. Bergström, L. A. Carlson, and L. Orö, *Acta Physiol. Scand.*, **67**, 185 (1966).

328. F. A. Kuehl, Jr., and J. L. Humes, *Proc. Nat. Acad. Sci., US*, **69**, 480 (1972).

329. F. A. Kuehl, Jr., V. J. Cirillo, and H. G. Oien, in *Prostaglandins: Chemical and Biochemical Aspects*, S. M. M. Karim, Ed., University Park Press, Baltimore, 1976, p. 191.

330. J. E. Shaw, *Fed. Proc.*, **25**, 770 (1066).

331. B. B. Fredholm and P. Hedqvist, *Biochem. Pharmacol.*, **24**, 61 (1975).

332. C. Malmsten, M. Hamberg, J. Svensson, and B. Samuelsson, *Proc. Nat. Acad. Sci., US*, **72**, 1446 (1975).

333. J. W. D. McDonald and R. K. Stuart, *J. Lab. Clin. Invest.*, **84**, 111 (1974).

334. J. F. Mustard and M. A. Packham, *Pharmacol. Rev.*, **22**, 97 (1970).

335. J. L. Gordon and D. E. MacIntyre, *Brit. J. Pharmacol.*, **58**, 298P (1976).

336. J. R. Weeks, N. C. Sekhar, and D. W. DuCharme, *J. Pharm. Pharmacol.*, **21**, 103 (1969).

337. J. Kloeze, *Biochim. Biophys. Acta*, **187**, 285 (1969).

338. N. R. Marquis, R. L. Vigdahl and P. A. Tavormina, *Biochim. Biophys. Res. Commun.*, **36**, 965 (1969).

339. E. E. Nishizawa, W. L. Miller, R. R. Gorman, G. L. Bundy, J. Svensson, and M. Hamburg, *Prostaglandins*, **9**, 109 (1975).

340. O. Oelz, R. Oelz, B. J. Sweetman, and J. A. Oates, *Prostaglandins*, **11**, 469 (1976).

341. O. Oelz, R. Oelz, H. R. Knapp, B. J. Sweetman, and J. A. Oates, *Prostaglandins*, **13**, 225 (1977).

342. B. Samuelsson and M. Hamberg, in *Prostaglandin Synthetase Inhibitors*, H. J. Robinson and J. R. Vane, Eds., Raven Press, New York, 1974, p. 107.

343. B. Samuelsson, M. Hamberg, C. Malmsten, and J. Svensson, in *Advances in Prostaglandin and Thromboxane Research*, Vol. 2, B. Samuelsson and R. Paoletti, Eds., Raven Press, New York, 1976, p. 737.

344. E. W. Salzman, in *Advances in Prostaglandin and Thromboxane Research*, Vol. 2, B. Samuelsson and R. Paoletti, Eds., Raven Press, New York, 1976, p. 767.

345. P. J. Kadowitz, P. D. Joiner, and A. L. Hyman, *Ann. Rev. Pharmacol.*, **15**, 285 (1975).

346. M. J. Brody and P. J. Kadowitz, *Fed. Proc.*, **33**, 48 (1974).

347. G. Swedin, *J. Pharm. Pharmacol.*, **23**, 994 (1971).

348. P. Hedqvist, *Life Sci.*, **9**, 269 (1970).

349. P. Hedqvist, in *Advances in Prostaglandin and Thromboxane Research*, Vol. 1, B. Samuelsson and R. Paoletti, Eds., Raven Press, New York, 1976, p. 357.

350. P. Hedqvist, in *Prostaglandins*, Vol. 1, P. Ramwell, Ed., Plenum Press, New York, 1973, p. 101.

351. P. J. Kadowitz, C. S. Sweet, and M. J. Brody, *Eur. J. Pharmacol.*, **18**, 189 (1972).

352. F. Coceani, L. Puglisi, and B. Lavers, *Ann. NY Acad. Sci.*, **180**, 289 (1971).

353. S. W. Holmes and E. W. Horton, *J. Physiol.*, **195**, 731 (1968).

354. F. Coceani and C. R. Pace–Asiak, in *Prostaglandins: Physiological Pharmacological and Pathological Aspects*, S. M. M. Karim, Ed., University Park Press, Baltimore, 1976, p. 1.

355. S. W. Holmes and E. W. Horton, *Brit. J. Pharmacol.*, **34**, 32 (1968).

356. G. R. Siggins, E. F. Battenberg, B. J. Hoffer, F. E. Bloom, and A. L. Steiner, *Science*, **179**, 585 (1973).

357. B. J. Hoffer, G. R. Siggins, A. P. Oliver, and F.

E. Bloom, *J. Pharmacol. Exp. Ther.*, **184,** 553 (1973).

358. S. C. Lee and L. Levine, *J. Biol. Chem.*, **249,** 1369 (1974).
359. C. A. Leslie and L. Levine, *Biochem. Biophys. Res. Commun.*, **52,** 717 (1973).
360. T. W. Stone, D. A. Taylor, and F. E. Bloom, *Science,* **187,** 845 (1975).
361. L. Z. Bito, *Prostaglandins,* **9,** 851 (1975).
362. E. W. Horton, *J. Pharm. Pharmacol.*, **28,** 389 (1976).
363. M. J. Silver and J. B. Smith, *Life Sci.*, **16,** 1635 (1975).
364. J. B. Lee, R. V. Patak, and B. K. Mookerjee, *Am. J. Med.*, **60,** 798 (1976).
365. G. Burke, L. L. Chang, and M. Szabo, *Science,* **180,** 875 (1973).
366. S. Greenberg, J. P. Long, and F. P. J. Diecke, *Arch. Int. Pharmacodyn.*, **204,** 373 (1973).
367. F. Villani, A. Chiarra, S. Cristalli, and F. Piccinini, *Experientia,* **30,** 532 (1974).
368. P. R. Emmons, J. R. Hampton, M. J. G. Harrison, A. J. Honour, and J. R. A. Mitchell, *Brit. J. Med.*, **2,** 468 (1967).
369. K. J. Hittelman and R. W. Butcher, in *The Prostaglandins: Pharmacological and Therapeutic Advances,* M. F. Cuthbert, Ed., Heinemann, London, 1973, p. 151.
370. F. A. Kuehl, Jr., *Prostaglandins,* **5,** 325 (1974).
371. F. A. Kuehl, Jr., V. J. Cirillo, E. A. Ham, and J. L. Humes, *Advan. Biosci.*, **9,** 155 (1973).
372. F. A. Kuehl, Jr., J. L. Humes, V. J. Cirillo, and E. A. Ham, in *Advances in Cyclic Nucleotide Research,* Vol. 1, P. Greengard, R. Paoletti, and G. A. Robinson, Eds., Raven Press, New York, 1972, p. 493.
373. F. A. Kuehl, Jr., in *Prostaglandins and Cyclic AMP,* R. H. Kahn and W. E. M. Lands, Eds., Academic Press, New York, 1973, p. 223.
374. F. A. Kuehl, Jr., and J. L. Humes, *Proc. Nat. Acad. Sci., US,* **69,** 480 (1972).
375. N. D. Goldberg, C. Villar–Palaski, H. Sasko, and J. Larner, *Biochim. Biophys. Acta,* **148,** 665 (1967).
376. N. D. Goldberg, S. B. Dietz, and A. G. O'Toole, *J. Biol. Chem.*, **244,** 4458 (1969).
377. N. D. Goldberg, M. K. Haddox, E. Dunham, C. Lopez, and J. W. Hadden, in *Cold Spring Harbor Symposium on the Regulation of Proliferation in Animal Cells,* B. Clark and R. Baserga, Eds., Cold Spring Harbor Laboratory, New York, 1974, p. 609.
378. C. B. Kauffman, R. D. Meyers, and J. Koob, *Chemistry,* **49,** 12 (1976).
379. N. D. Goldberg, M. K. Haddox, S. E. Nichol, D. B. Glass, C. H. Sanford, F. A. Kuehl, Jr., and R. Estensen, in *Advances in Cyclic Nucleotide Research,* Vol. 5, G. I. Drummond, P. Greengard, and G. A. Robison, Eds., Raven Press, New York, 1975, p. 307.
380. N. D. Goldberg, M. K. Haddox, C. E. Zeilig, S. E. Nichol, T. S. Acott, and D. B. Glass, *J. Invest. Dermatol.*, **67,** 641 (1976).
381. G. Weissmann, I. Goldstein, S. Hoffstein, G. Chauvet, and R. Robineaux, *Ann. NY Acad. Sci.*, **256,** 222 (1975).
382. F. A. Kuehl, Jr., V. R. Cirillo, M. E. Zanetti, G. C. Beveridge, and E. A. Ham, in *Future Trends in Inflammation,* Vol. 2, J. P. Giroud, D. A. Willoughby, and G. P. Velo, Eds., Birkhäuser-Verlag, Basel, 1975, p. 165.
383. E. W. Yankee, D. E. Ayer, G. L. Bundy, F. H. Lincoln, E. L. Miller, Jr., and G. A. Youngdale, in *Advances in Prostaglandin and Thromboxane Research,* Vol. 1, B. Samuelsson and R. Paoletti, Eds., Raven Press, New York, 1976, p. 195.
384. A. S. V. Burgen and J. F. Mitchell, *Gaddum's Pharmacology,* Oxford University Press, Oxford, 1972, p. 8.
385. N. H. Andersen and P. W. Ramwell, *Arch. Intern. Med.*, **133,** 30 (1974).
386. J. Nakano, *Proc. Soc. Exp. Biol. Med.*, **136,** 1265 (1971).
387. M. Hayashi, S. Kori, and H. Endo, German Patent 2,400,451; *Chem. Abstr.*, **84,** 43440v (1976).
388. L. G. Brooke and R. C. Marschall, *J. Pharm. Pharmacol.* **26,** (Suppl.), 80P (1974).
389. A F. Kluge, K. G. Untch, and J. H. Fried, *J. Am. Chem. Soc.*, **94,** 9256 (1972).
390. P. W. Ramwell, J. E. Shaw, E. J. Corey, and N. Andersen, *Nature,* **221,** 1251 (1969).
391. E. J. Corey, *J. Org. Chem.*, **37,** 3039 (1972).
392. E. L. Cooper and E. W. Yankee, *J. Am. Chem. Soc.*, **96,** 5876 (1974).
393. H. Shio, P. W. Ramwell, N. H. Andersen, and E. J. Corey, *Experientia,* **26,** 355 (1970).
394. L. B. Kier, in *Fundamental Concepts of Drug-Receptor Interactions,* J. F. Danielli, J. F. Moran, and D. J. Triggle, Eds., Academic Press, New York, 1970, p. 15.
395. C. R. Ganellin *et al., J. Med. Chem.*, **16,** 610, 616, 620 (1973).
396. I. Rabinowitz, P. Ramwell, and P. Davison, *Nature New Biol.*, **233,** 88 (1971).

397. W. L. Duax and J. W. Edmonds, *Prostaglandins*, **3,** 201 (1973).

398. G. T. DeTitta, J. W. Edmonds, and W. L. Duax, *Prostaglandins*, **9,** 659 (1975).

399. J. W. Edmonds and W. L. Daux, *Prostaglandins*, **5,** 275 (1974).

400. J. R. Hoyland and L. B. Kier, *J. Med. Chem.*, **15,** 84 (1972).

401. A. Murakami and Y. Akahori, *Chem. Pharm. Bull.* (Tokyo), **22,** 1133 (1974).

402. C. Chachaty, Z. Wolkowski, F. Piriou, and G. Lukacs, *Chem. Commun.*, 951 (1973).

403. W. W. Conover and J. Fried, *Proc. Nat. Acad. Sci., US*, **71,** 2157 (1974).

404. E. M. K. Leovey and N. H. Andersen, *J. Am. Chem. Soc.*, **97,** 4148 (1975).

405. N. H. Andersen, P. W. Ramwell, E. M. K. Leovey, and M. Johnson, in *Advances in Prostaglandin and Thromboxane Research*, Vol. 1, B. Samuelsson and R. Paoletti, Eds., Raven Press, New York, 1976, p. 271.

406. T. J. Roseman and S. H. Yalkowsky, *J. Pharm. Sci.*, **62,** 1680 (1973).

407. M. C. R. Johnson and L. Saunders, *Biochim. Biophys. Acta*, **218,** 543 (1970).

408. T. K. Schaaf, *Ann. Rep. Med. Chem.*, **11,** 80 (1976).

409. N. A. Nelson, R. W. Jackson, and A. T. Au, *Prostaglandins*, **10,** 303 (1975).

410. Y. Iguchi, S. Kori, and M. Hayashi, *J. Org. Chem.*, **40,** 521 (1975).

411. H. Kunze, R. B. Ghooi, E. Bohn, and D. Le–Kim, *Prostaglandins*, **12,** 1005 (1976).

412. D. A. van Dorp and E. J. Christ, *Rec. Trav. Chim. Pays-Bas*, **94,** 247 (1975).

413. J. Buo and O. Kower, *Rec. Trav. Chim. Pays-Bas*, **94,** 232 (1975).

414. H. Miyake and M. Hayashi, *Prostaglandins*, **4,** 577 (1973).

415. H. Wakatsuka, S. Kori, and M. Hayashi, *Prostaglandins*, **8,** 341 (1974).

416. T. Tanaka, S. Kurozumi, T. Toru, M. Kobayashi, S. Miura, and S. Ishimoto, *Tetrahedron Lett.*, 1535 (1975).

417. A. Raz, P. C. Isakson, M. S. Minkes, and P. Needleman, *J. Biol. Chem.*, **252,** 1123 (1977).

418. J. Fried, M. M. Mehra, W. L. Kao, and C. H. Lin, *Tetrahedron Lett.*, 2695 (1970).

419. J. Fried, M. M. Mehra, and W. L. Kao, *J. Am. Chem. Soc.*, **93,** 5594 (1971).

420. J. Fried, C. H. Lin, M. M. Mehra, W. L. Kao, and P. Dalven, *Ann. N.Y. Acad. Sci.*, **180,** 38 (1971).

421. J. Fried, M. M. Mehra, and Y. Y. Chan, *J. Am. Chem. Soc.*, **96,** 6759 (1974).

422. G. Bundy, F. Lincoln, N. Nelson, J. Pike, and W. Schneider, *Ann. N.Y. Acad. Sci.*, **180,** 76 (1971).

423. N. A. Nelson, German Patent 2,423,155; 2,423,156; *Chem. Abstr.*, **83,** 9299a, 9300u (1975).

424. N. A. Nelson, *US Patent* 3,920,723; *Chem. Abstr.*, **84,** 105087w (1976).

425. N. A. Nelson, R. W. Jackson, A. T. Au, D. J. Wynalda, and E. E. Nishizawa, *Prostaglandins*, **10,** 795 (1975).

426. D. Van Dorp, *Ann. N.Y. Acad. Sci.*, **180,** 181 (1971).

427. K. Gréen, B. Samuelsson, and B. J. Magerlain, *Eur. J. Biochem.*, **62,** 527 (1976).

428. P. Crabbé and H. Carpio, *Chem. Commun.*, 904 (1972).

429. J. W. Patterson, Jr., and J. H. Fried, *J. Org. Chem.*, **39,** 2506 (1974).

430. C. H. Lin, S. J. Stien, and J. E. Pike, *Prostaglandins*, **11,** 377 (1976).

431. W. P. Schneider, German Patent, 2,011,969; *Chem. Abstr.*, **74,** P87486n (1971).

432. J. Kloeze, *Biochim. Biophys. Acta*, **187,** 285 (1969).

433. C. B. Struijk, R. K. Beerthuis, H. J. J. Pabon, and D. A. Van Dorp, *Rec. Trav. Chem. Pays-Bas*, **85**, 1233 (1966).

434. R. T. Buckler, H. E. Hartzler, F. E. Ward, and E. Kurchacova, *Eur. J. Med. Chem.*, **12,** 463 (1977).

435. N. Finch, J. J. Fitt, and I. H. S. Hsu, *J. Org. Chem.*, **40,** 206 (1975).

436. A. Guzman and P. Crabbé, *Chem. Lett.*, 1073 (1973).

437. S. Kurozumi, T. Toru, and T. Tanaka, *Tetrahedron Lett.*, 4091 (1976).

438. E. J. Corey and H. S. Sachdev, *J. Am. Chem. Soc.*, **95,** 8483 (1973).

439. T. Toru, S. Kurozumi, T. Tanaka, S. Miura, M. Kobayashi, and S. Ishimoto, *Tetrahedron Lett.*, 4087 (1976).

440. P. Crabbé, A. Guzmán, and E. Verlarde, *Chem. Commun.*, 1126 (1972).

441. G. Doria and C. Gandolfi, *Farmaco, Ed. Sci.*, **29,** 327 (1974).

442. P. Crabbé, A. Cervantes, and M. C. Meana, *Chem. Commun.*, 119 (1973).

443. K. Kojima and K. Sakai, *Tetrahedron Lett.*, 101 (1976).

444. A. Guzmán and J. M. Muchowski, *Tetrahedron Lett.*, 2053 (1975).

445. K. Sakai, J. Ide, and O. Oda, *Tetrahedron Lett.*, 3021 (1975).

446. J. Ide and K. Sakai, *Tetrahedron Lett.*, 1367 (1976).

447. I. T. Harrison, R. Grayshan, T. Williams, A. Semenovski, and J. H. Fried, *Tetrahedron Lett.*, 5151 (1972).

448. P. A. Grieco, C.-l. J. Wang, and F. J. Okuniewicz, *Chem. Commun.*, 939 (1976).

449. O. Vogel and P. Crabbé, *Helv. Chim. Acta*, **56,** 557 (1973).

450. A. Guzmán and J. M. Muchowski, *Chem. Ind.* (London), 790 (1975).

451. P. Crabbé and A. Cervantes, *Tetrahedron Lett.*, 1319 (1973).

452. O. G. Plantema, H. de Koning, and H. O. Huisman, in *Advances in Prostaglandin and Thromboxane Research*, Vol. 2, B. Samuelsson and R. Paoletti, Eds., Raven Press, New York, 1976, p. 875.

453. A. Guzmán, M. Vera, and P. Crabbé, *Prostaglandins*, **8,** 85 (1974).

454. C. H. Lin, *Chem. Ind.* (London), 994 (1976).

455. C. V. Grudzinskas and M. J. Weiss, *Tetrahedron Lett.*, 141 (1973).

456. A. Guzmán and P. Crabbé, *Chem. Ind.* (London), 635 (1973).

457. E. J. Corey, C. S. Shiner, R. P. Volante, and C. R. Cyr, *Tetrahedron Lett.*, 1161 (1975).

458. P. A. Grieco, C. S. Pogonowski, M. Nishizawa, and C.-l. J. Wang, *Tetrahedron Lett.*, 2541 (1975).

459. P. A. Grieco, N. Fukamiya, and M. Miyashita, *Chem. Commun.*, 573 (1976).

460. L. Godoy, A. Guzmán, and J. M. Muchowski, *Chem. Lett.*, 327 (1975).

461. C.-l. J. Wang, P. A. Greico, and F. J. Okuniewicz, *Chem. Commun.*, 468 (1976).

462. N. S. Crossley, *Tetrahedron Lett.*, 3327 (1971).

463. J. M. Muchowski and E. Velarde, *Prostaglandins*, **10,** 297 (1975).

464. A. E. Greene, J. P. Deprés, M. C. Meana, and P. Crabbé, *Tetrahedron Lett.*, 3755 (1976).

465. A. Guzmán, J. M. Muchowski, and M. A. Very, *Chem. Ind.* (London), 884 (1975).

466. D. Reuschling, K. Küblein, and A. Linkies, *Tetrahedron Lett.*, 17 (1977).

467. P. Crabbé, G. A. Garcia, and C. Rius, *Tetrahedron Lett.*, 2951 (1972).

468. I. Vlattas and L. Della Vecchia, *Tetrahedron Lett.*, 4455 (1974).

469. I. Vlattas and L. Della Vecchia, *Tetrahedron Lett.*, 4459 (1974).

470. D. K. Dikshit, R. S. Kapil, and N. Anand, *Indian J. Chem.*, **13,** 1353, 1359 (1975).

471. F. M. Hauser and R. C. Huffman, *Tetrahedron Lett.*, 905 (1974).

472. I. T. Harrison, R. J. K. Taylor, and J. H. Fried, *Tetrahedron Lett.*, 1165 (1975).

473. I. T. Harrison, V. R. Fletcher, and J. H. Fried, *Tetrahedron Lett.*, 2733 (1974).

474. I. Vlattas and A. O. Lee, *Tetrahedron Lett.*, 4451 (1974).

475. I. T. Harrison and V. R. Fletcher, *Tetrahedron Lett.*, 2729 (1974).

476. K. Kühlein, A. Linkies, and D. Reuschling, *Tetrahedron Lett.*, 4463 (1976).

477. D. Reuschling, M. Mitzlaff, and K. Kühlein, *Tetrahedron Lett.*, 4467 (1976).

478. G. Bollinger and J. M. Muchowski, *Tetrahedron Lett.*, 2931 (1975).

479. J. W. Bruin, H. de Koning, and H. O. Huisman, *Tetrahedron Lett.*, 4599 (1975).

480. R. M. Schribner, *Tetrahedron Lett.*, 3853 (1976).

481. J. C. Lapierre and U. K. Pandit, *Tetrahedron Lett.*, 897 (1977).

482. G. Ambrus and I. Barta, *Prostaglandins*, **10,** 661 (1975).

483. P. Wlodawer, B. Samuelsson, S. M. Albonico, and E. J. Corey, *J. Am. Chem. Soc.*, **93,** 2816 (1971).

484. T. J. Leeney, P. R. Marsham, G. A. F. Ritchie, and M. W. Senior, *Prostaglandins*, **11,** 953 (1976).

485. E. J. Corey, M. Shibasaki, K. C. Nicolaou, C. L. Malmsten, and B. Samuelsson, *Tetrahedron Lett.*, 737 (1976).

486. H. Shimomura, A. Sugie, J. Katsube, and H. Yamamoto, *Tetrahedron Lett.*, 4099 (1976).

487. E. J. Corey, K. C. Nicolaou, Y. Machida, C. L. Malmsten, and B. Samuelsson, *Proc. Nat. Acad. Sci., US*, **72,** 3355 (1975).

488. E. J. Corey, K. Narasaka, and M. Shibasaki, *J. Am. Chem. Soc.*, **98,** 6417 (1976).

489. G. L. Bundy, *Tetrahedron Lett.*, 1957 (1975).

490. C. Malmsten, *Life Sci.*, **18,** 169 (1976).

491. S. Ohki, N. Ogino, S. Yamamoto, O. Hayaishi, H. Yumamoto, H. Miyake, and M. Hayaski, *Proc. Nat. Acad. Sci., US*, **74,** 144 (1977).

492. P. S. Portoghese, D. L. Larson, A. G. Abatjoghou, E. W. Dunham, J. M. Gerrard, and J. G. White, *J. Med. Chem.*, **20,** 321 (1977).

493. J. Fried and C. H. Lin, *J. Med. Chem.*, **16,** 429 (1973).

494. C. Gandolfi, G. Doria, and P. Gaio, *Farmaco, Ed. Sci.*, **27,** 1125 (1972).

495. B. Radüchel, V. Mende, G. Cleve, G.-A. Hoyer, and H. Vorbrüggan, *Tetrahedron Lett.*, 633 (1975).
496. R. L. Spraggins, *Tetrahedron Lett.*, 4343 (1972).
497. J. A. Noguez and L. A. Maldonado, *Synth. Commun.*, **6,** 39 (1976).
498. R. T. Buckler and D. L. Garling, *Tetrahedron Lett.*, 2257 (1978).
499. M. Hayashi *et al.*, German Patent 2,221,301; British Patent 1,398,838.
500. E. Z. Dajani, L. F. Rozek, J. H. Sanner, and M. Miyano, *J. Med. Chem.*, **19,** 1007 (1976).
501. A. P. Labhsetwar, *Nature*, **238,** 400 (1972).
502. W. Bartmann, G. Beck, and U. Lerch, *Tetrahedron Lett.*, 2441 (1974).
503. D. W. R. Hall and K. D. Jaitly, *Prostaglandins*, **11,** 573 (1976).
504. N. S. Crossley, *Prostaglandins*, **10,** 5 (1975).
505. J. Bowler, N. S. Crossley, and R. I. Dowell, *Prostaglandins*, **9,** 391 (1975).
506. D. Binder, J. Bowler, E. D. Brown, N. S. Crossley, J. Hutton, M. Senior, L. Slater, P. Wilkinson, and N. C. A. Wright, *Prostaglandins*, **6,** 87 (1974).
507. G. L. Bundy and F. H. Lincoln, *Prostaglandins*, **9,** 1 (1975).
508. B. J. Magerlein, G. L. Bundy, F. H. Lincoln, and G. A. Youngdale, *Prostaglandins*, **9,** 5 (1975).
509. W. L. Miller, J. R. Weeks, J. W. Lauderdale, and K. T. Kirton, *Prostaglandins*, **9,** 9 (1975).
510. H. C. Arndt, W. G. Biddlecom, G. P. Peruzzotti, and W. D. Woessner, *Prostaglandins*, **11,** 569 (1976).

CHAPTER THIRTY–FOUR

Analogs of Cyclic Nucleotides

RICH B. MEYER, JR.

Department of Pharmaceutical Chemistry
School of Pharmacy
University of California
San Francisco, California 94143, USA

CONTENTS

1 INTRODUCTION

1.1 History

The discovery in 1957 of a heat-stable nucleotide that mediates the glycolytic action of the peptide hormone glucagon (1) must be recorded as the beginning of a field of research that has since branched into almost every classical subdivision of the biological sciences. That nucleotide, the "second messenger" of hormone action, proved to be adenosine cyclic 3′,5′-(hydrogen) phosphate (2) (cyclic AMP or cAMP, 34.**1**), and its

34.**1**

discoverer, Earl W. Sutherland, received the Nobel Prize in 1971 for his substantial contributions toward our understanding of its actions. As of 1977 this compound (together with one and possibly two other cyclic nucleotides that mediate cellular function) are the subject of one journal, several annual conferences, and a series of reviews. It seems, indeed, that research directed specifically toward elucidating the role of cAMP and other cyclic nucleotides in various biological processes has been a major factor in the advancement of understanding in these fields, which must include the functions of almost every tissue in the body.

It is beyond the scope of this chapter to review the involvement of cAMP in all biological functions. Attention is directed instead to studies that have been conducted using analogs of cAMP and on the relationship of the structure of the analog to the nature of the biological response elicited. It is hoped that the data presented here will serve as a guide for the possible use of cyclic nucleotide analogs as therapeutic agents.

1.2 Cyclic Nucleotide Action and Metabolism

In higher animal tissue, the formation, action, and degradation of cAMP is remarkably straightforward (3). As Fig. 34.1 illustrates, the enzyme that synthesizes cAMP, adenylate cyclase, is usually a membrane-bound enzyme. According to the usual scenario, the hormone ("first messenger") binds to a receptor on the outside of the cell membrane. This binding activates, possibly through a coupling

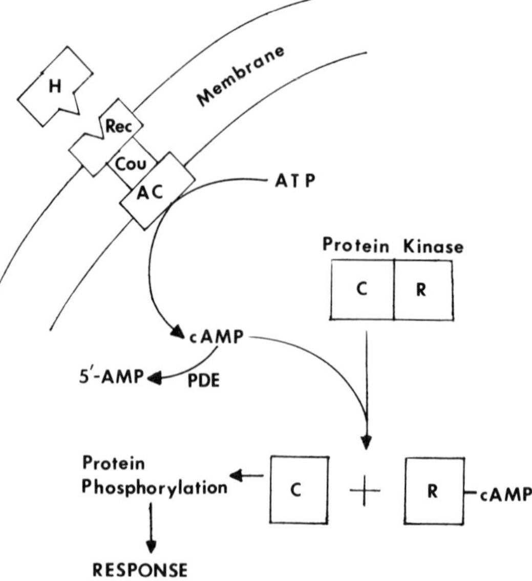

Fig. 34.1 Cellular mechanism of cAMP action: H, extracellular hormone; Rec, receptor; Cou, coupling protein; AC, adenylate cyclase; PDE, phosphodiesterase; C, catalytic subunit; R, regulatory subunit.

protein (4), the adenylate cyclase on the inside of the membrane, which then converts ATP to cAMP. There are only two enzyme systems in higher organisms with which cAMP then may interact. Cyclic nucleotide phosphodiesterase regulates cAMP levels by hydrolyzing the 3′-*O*→P bond to give adenosine 5′-phosphate (5′-AMP). Phosphodiesterase has been found in every tissue that has been examined to determine its presence, and it may exist in several forms (5). The action of cAMP, however, is mediated by another enzyme, protein kinase (6). Although the situation may be more complex, protein kinase can be thought of as being an inactive holoenzyme that upon binding cAMP, dissociates into the regulatory subunit (with cAMP bound) and the catalytic subunit. The sole role of the catalytic subunit is to catalyze phosphorylation of a target protein, whose identity and function would vary from tissue to tissue. It has been postulated that in higher organisms activation of protein kinase is the sole means by which cAMP exerts its actions (7).

There are at least two other naturally occurring nucleotides. In 1963 guanosine cyclic 3′,5′-phosphate (cGMP, 34.**2**) was

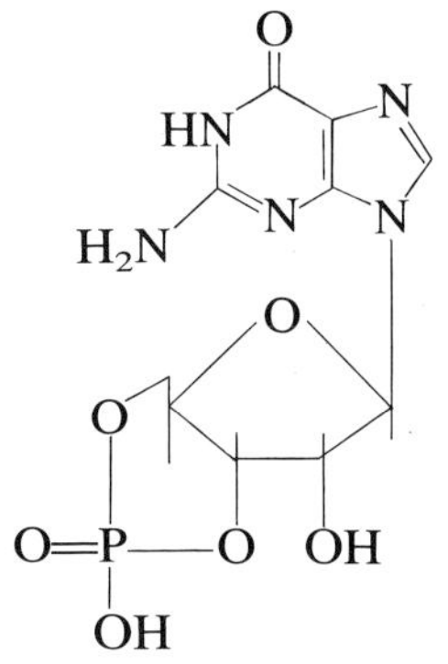

34.**2**

isolated from rat urine (8) and was subsequently identified in virtually all tissue (9). The formation, metabolism, and action of cGMP parallel almost exactly those of cAMP: it is formed from GTP by guanylate cyclase, its levels are regulated by cleavage to GMP by phosphodiesterase, and it is able to stimulate a cGMP-specific protein kinase (10). The ultimate effects of the latter action are not as well understood at this time as are those for cAMP. Possibly the most tantalizing prospect is the proposal by N. D. Goldberg of the yin-yang hypothesis (11): the effects of elevated levels of cAMP and cGMP are diametrically opposed, and most life processes are regulated by way of this dichotomy. (See also Chapter 33, Section 5.4.)

Another cyclic nucleotide, cytidine cyclic 3′,5′-phosphate (cCMP), has been isolated from natural sources only recently (12). Thus far all that is known about cCMP is that it induces growth of rodent leukemia cells in culture (13a) and that it has been positively identified in the urine of human cancer patients (13b).

Table 34.1 presents a few of the physiological responses known to be associated with changes in levels of cAMP.

Table 34.1 A Few of the Hormones that Exert Their Activity by way of cAMP[a]

Hormone	Tissue	Response
Glucagon	Liver	Glucose release
Vasopressin	Kidney	Increased water permeability
TSH	Thyroid	Thyroid hormone release
Catecholamines	Postsynaptic neurons	Membrane hyperpolarization[b]
Catecholamines	Cardiac muscle	Contraction[c]
ACTH	Adrenal cortex	Steroidogenesis
TRH	Anterior pituitary	TSH release

[a] Ref. 3, unless otherwise indicated.
[b] Ref. 14.
[c] Ref. 15.

1.3 Why Make Cyclic Nucleotide Analogs?

Given the amazing diversity of physiological functions in which cAMP and probably cGMP are involved, the synthesis of analogs must be looked on as something of a bonanza to the medicinal chemist. There is great potential in the utilization of these compounds in the control of proliferative diseases (psoriasis, cancer), cardiovascular abnormalities (hypertension, cardiac shock), hormonal disorders, respiratory ailments, nervous disorders, and many others. These and other possible uses of cyclic nucleotide analogs and other agents that act by way of systems that utilize cyclic nucleotides have been reviewed recently by Amer and coworkers (16–18). Further guides for the study of possible therapeutic uses of such analogs may be found in a series of reviews on cyclic nucleotides in disease states (19) and on clinical cyclic nucleotide research (20, 21).

Appropriate substitution of the cyclic nucleotide molecule might reasonably be expected to achieve one or more of the following goals:

1. *Resistance to Phosphodiesterase.* Agents that show selective resistance to phosphodiesterase from particular tissue would be especially interesting.
2. *Stimulation of Protein Kinase.* Again, the possibility of selectively stimulating protein kinase from given tissues is enticing.
3. *Inhibition of Phosphodiesterase.* Endogenous cyclic nucleotide levels might be raised.
4. *Tissue and Enzyme Selectivity.* The nature of the substituents might determine uptake of the analogs into certain types of tissue, in addition to the potential for enzyme specificity as mentioned in items 1 and 2.
5. *Nucleotide Prodrugs.* The cyclic nucleotides have only one negative charge, thus might penetrate tissues more readily than a 5′-nucleotide, to which they would be cleaved by phosphodiesterase.

As of this writing, no cyclic nucleotide has found use as an approved drug in this country, although there are many promising leads. The most straightforward method of evaluating new compounds is direct assay as activators of protein kinase (either cAMP or cGMP dependent) and as substrates and inhibitors of phosphodiesterase, since these are the only two enzymes involved in cyclic nucleotide action.

An alternate approach to development of therapeutic agents that interact with cyclic nucleotide utilizing systems is investigation of drugs that inhibit phosphodiesterase (see 3 and 4, above). Indeed, theophylline and papaverine, drugs that probably work by way of this mechanism, have been in clinical use for some time. There seem to be substantial differences in the affinity of phosphodiesterases from different tissue for given inhibitors, a condition that lends itself to the development of drugs with minimal side effects. Excellent comprehensive reviews on phosphodiesterase inhibitors are available (22, 23).

1.4 Chemistry and Nomenclature

This chapter describes the relationship of substitution on the cyclic nucleotides to their activity in the two key enzyme systems, and to activity in tissue culture and whole animals. Although the chemistry is of secondary importance here, it obviously dictated the direction of the analog investigation. By far the largest number of analogs have been prepared from either cAMP or cGMP for reasons of simplicity. In their pioneering work on the chemistry of cyclic nucleotides, Smith, Drummond, and Khorana showed that nucleoside 5′-phosphates could be cyclized to the cyclic 3′,5′-phosphates in refluxing pyridine solution using *N,N′*-dicyclohexylcarbodiimide as dehydrating agent to form the new phosphate ester bond (24, 25), a technique that Khorana's group had brilliantly exploited in the synthesis of phosphodiesters. For the intranucleoside linkage of the cyclic phosphates, however, it was necessary to carry out the reaction under very high dilution, and this did not lend itself to large-scale preparation of derivatives. Other methods of synthesis of cyclic nucleotides from derivatives of 5′-nucleotides also require high dilution (26, 27). All aspects of the chemistry of cyclic nucleotides have been recently reviewed (28–30).

The *Chemical Abstracts* name for cAMP is adenosine cyclic 3′,5′-(hydrogen) phosphate. For the number of compounds covered here, however, abbreviations are much more useful, and these are used according to the IUPAC Biochemical Nomenclature conventions. The cyclic 3′,5′-phosphates of adenosine, guanosine, inosine, xanthosine, cytidine, and uridine are abbreviated cAMP, cGMP, cIMP, cXMP, cCMP, and cUMP, respectively. The appropriate substituents are denoted by prefixes. Derivatives of 9-β-D-ribofuranosylpurine 3′,5′-phosphate that are not related to the preceding natural bases are denoted by cRMP with the appropriate prefix.

1.5 The Enzyme Systems

1.5.1 PROTEIN KINASE. A cyclic nucleotide analog would have little potential therapeutic benefit (except for use as a prodrug) if it could not mimic cAMP or cGMP by activating the appropriate protein kinase. The alternate type of activity, inhibition of cAMP or cGMP activation of the kinases by the analog, has not been rigorously investigated.

By and large, 6-aminopurine cyclic nucleotides are specific activators of cAMP-dependent protein kinases, and 2-aminopurin-6-one cyclic nucleotides are specific for cGMP-dependent protein kinases. The ability of a compound to stimulate the kinase will be expressed as K'_a, defined in equation 34.1.

$$K'_a = \frac{K_a \text{ (parent cyclic nucleotide)}}{K_a \text{ (analog)}} \tag{34.1}$$

where K_a is the kinetically determined activation constant, or ability of the nucleotide to half-maximally activate the kinase (31, 32). The use of K'_a eliminates tissue-to-tissue differences in the affinity of protein kinases for their respective cyclic nucleotides and gives a ready point of reference for the efficacy of the analogs with respect to the naturally occurring compounds. When analogs are tested as activators of the cAMP-dependent kinase, K'_a(cAMP) is reported; K'_a(cGMP) likewise is used for values determined with the cGMP-dependent protein kinase relative to the K_a of cGMP.

1.5.2 PHOSPHODIESTERASE. Cyclic nucleotide phosphodiesterase appears to be more than one protein and possesses two, three, or more catalytic activities (5). We are interested, however, in determining to what extent a new analog is cleaved in the biological environment. To this end the hydrolysis assay is customarily performed on a crude fraction at relatively high (*ca.* 1 m*M*) substrate concentration. Since there are usually high K_m and low K_m activities in the enzyme preparations (5), the hydrolysis by the high K_m fraction is normally measured, although probably the low K_m activity would be more significant at achievable cellular concentrations of exogenously administered analog.

The ability of the analog to be a phosphodiesterase substrate is expressed by the value *S*, defined in equation 34.2.

$$S = \frac{\text{rate of hydrolysis of analog}}{\text{rate of hydrolysis of cAMP}} \tag{34.2}$$

Rates of hydrolysis less than 0.05 that of cAMP are very difficult to measure, and compounds with *S* values less than 0.05 may be considered to be substantially resistant to phosphodiesterase.

Most cyclic nucleotide analogs have also been examined as inhibitors of phosphodiesterase. In the most comprehensive study, a large series of 8-substituted derivatives of cAMP, cGMP, cIMP, and cXMP were examined as inhibitors of cAMP and cGMP hydrolysis by enzyme preparations from two different tissues (33). For virtually none of the analogs yet examined was the I_{50} obtained as low as the K_m of the substrate, indicating that this inhibition is probably not an important factor in the pharmacological action of these drugs.

2 EFFECTS OF STRUCTURAL MODIFICATIONS ON ENZYMIC ACTIVITY

2.1 8-Substituted Derivatives

2.1.1 8-SUBSTITUTED CYCLIC AMP ANALOGS. Most of the 8-substituted analogs of cAMP and cGMP were prepared from 8-Br-cAMP or 8-Br-cGMP, which in turn were readily prepared by direct bromination of the parent compound (32, 33). The ease of this reaction has contributed to the preparation of a large number of these derivatives.

The placement of the 8-substituent on either cAMP or cGMP produces at least two of the results initially sought in investigations into cyclic nucleotide analogs: the new derivatives are resistant to phosphodiesterase yet largely retain the ability to stimulate protein kinases. Table 34.2 shows the ability of these compounds to activate a cAMP-dependent protein kinase: most compounds are good kinase activators, and some are better than cAMP itself. Only the 8-benzylamino and the 8-carboxymethylthio (which carries a negative charge) derivatives show reduced ability to mimic cAMP. The presence of a positive charge on the 8-substituent, as in the 8-(ε-aminoalkyl)amino-cAMP's, does not impair binding to any great extent. This class of compounds was prepared for use in affinity chromatography of cAMP binding protein (38). The 8-HO-cAMP and 8-HS-cAMP derivatives, which exist as the oxo and thioxo tautomers, respectively, are better activators of kinase than is cAMP. This indicates that the 7-position of the purine ring may not be specifically involved in binding, as further substantiated below. Generally 8-(alkyl or aryl)thio-substitution is most reliable in yielding compounds that are good kinase activators.

Table 34.2 Activation of cAMP-Dependent Protein Tissue by 8-Substituted cAMP Derivatives

R_8	K'_a (cAMP)	References
Cl	3.1	34
Br	2.9	32
I	2.1	34
CH_3	0.22	35
NH_2	1.5	32
N_3	0.68	32
$NHCH_3$	0.38	32
$N(CH_3)_2$	0.59	32
$NH(CH_2)_2NH_2$	0.34	38
$NH(CH_2)_8NH_2$	0.93	36
$NHCH_2C_6H_5$	0.02	32
OH	2.8	32
OC_6H_4Cl-*p*	0.87	33
SH	3.8	32
SCH_3	2.4	32
SC_2H_5	2.0	32
SCH_2COOH	0.004	32
$SCH_2C_6H_5$	2.1	32
SC_6H_5	3.0	37
SC_6H_4Cl-*p*	18.0	33
SC_6H_4Br-*p*	1.6	37

8-Substituted cAMP derivatives are less readily hydrolyzed by phosphodiesterase than any class of substituted analogs. Most analogs have very low rates of hydrolysis ($S = 0.05$) (32, 33, 39). Only 8-H_2N-cAMP ($S = 0.2$–0.8) (32, 39) and 8-H_3C-cAMP ($S = 0.3$) (35) show the slightest tendency to serve as a substrate for phosphodiesterase from various sources. These data have been correlated with the 8-substituent covalent radius (NH_2 has the smallest radius of examined substituents) and interpreted to infer that the cyclic nucleotide must be in the anti conformation for enzymic binding and substrate activity; the syn conformation forced by large 8-substituents is very inhibitory to proper binding for substrate activity (39). Conversely, this syn conformation must be preferred by protein kinase, since the analogs with large 8-substituents are the best activators (Table 34.2).

2.1.2 8-SUBSTITUTED CYCLIC GMP ANALOGS. These compounds were prepared either by treatment of 8-Br-cGMP with the appropriate nucleophile (33), or by free radical alkylation or acylation (40).

Even though the cGMP-dependent protein kinase (isolated from lobster muscle) (10) used for these assays is an enzyme completely different from the cAMP-dependent enzymes above, its specificity for an 8-substituent on cGMP is similar to the specificity of the cAMP-dependent enzyme for an 8-substituent on cAMP. Table 34.3 lists selected compounds.

The 8-Br and 8-(substituted thio)-cGMP analogs are the best activators of lobster muscle cGMP-dependent protein kinase, and the 8-(substituted amino) compounds show the poorest activity. The carbon substituents on the 8-position are also beneficial to activity. Interestingly, the 8-methyl substituent is far less active than its isosteric 8-bromo counterpart, and this was also found to be the case when comparing 8-Me-cAMP and 8-Br-cAMP.

It is important to point out that the protein kinases were highly specific for their respective cyclic nucleotides. Of all the 8-substituted derivatives examined, no 8-R-cAMP possessed a K'_a (cGMP) greater than 0.1, and no 8-R-cGMP possessed a K'_a (cAMP) greater than 0.06 (33). In most cases, these "crossover" K'_a values were substantially lower.

A bulky 8-substituent confers the same resistance to phosphodiesterase cleavage on cGMP as it does to cAMP. This parallelism is extended by the report that only 8-H_2N-cGMP ($S = 0.22$) and 8-H_3C-cGMP ($S = 0.25$) (40) were reliably efficient substrates.

Table 34.3 Activation of cGMP-Dependent Protein Kinase from Lobster Muscle by 8-Substituted cGMP's

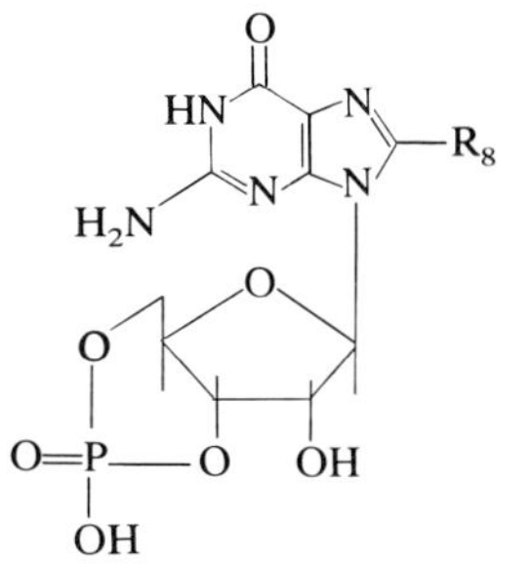

R_8	K'_a (cGMP)	Reference
Br	4	33
OH	2.5	33
$NHCH_3$	0.3	33
$NHCH_2C_6H_5$	0.005	33
SCH_3	4.9	33
$SCH_2C_6H_5$	4.5	33
SC_6H_4Cl-*p*	5.2	33
CH_3	0.07	40
$CH(CH_3)_2$	0.7	40
$COCH_3$	0.56	40
$CHOHCH_3$	1.8	40
COC_6H_5	0.7	40
$CHOHC_6H_5$	2.3	40

2.2 6-Substituted Derivatives of Cyclic RMP

2.2.1 AS CYCLIC AMP ANALOGS. Derivatives of cRMP that bear only a substituent in the 6-position might be expected to be closely analogous to cAMP, and this proves to be the case. As Table 34.4 indicates, all compounds with one or two alkyl or alkoxy groups on N^6 are approximately as good as cAMP itself in their ability to activate the cAMP-dependent protein kinases. The N^6-acyl, alkoxycarbonyl, and carbamoyl groups listed in Table

Table 34.4 Activation of cAMP-Dependent Protein Kinase by and Phosphodiesterase Hydrolysis of 6-Substituted cRMP

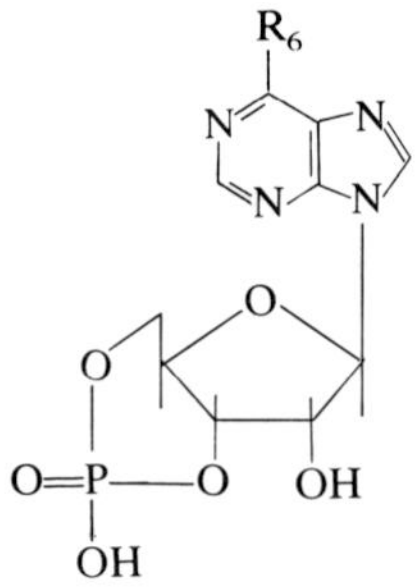

R_6	K_a' (cAMP)	S	Reference
N^6-Alkyl and alkoxysubstituents			
$NHCH_3$	1.3	0.22	36, 42
NHC_2H_5	0.8	0.20	41
NHC_4H_9-*n*	1.8	0.21	36, 42
$NHCH_2C_6H_5$	0.8	0.30	36
$N(C_2H_5)_2$	1.4	<0.09	41
NHOH	1.0	0.44	43
$NHOCH_3$	0.65	0.42	43
N^6-Acyl substituents			
$NHCOC_3H_7$-*n*	0.84	<0.05	44-46
$NHCO_2C_2H_5$	0.29	0.08	44
$NHCONHCH_3$	0.72	<0.05	44
$NHCONHC_3H_7$-*n*	1.1	<0.05	44
$NHCONHC_6H_5$	4.4	<0.05	44
Other 6-substituents			
SH	0.2	1.1	41
SCH_3	0.9	0.42	41
$SCH_2C_6H_5$	1.9	0.54	41
OH	0.59	0.46	41
OCH_3	0.62	0.53	41
Cl	1.4	1.2	41, 45

34.4 show that these groups also allow effective kinase stimulation by these analogs, and the more highly lipophilic substituents seem to contribute somewhat to binding (*vis,*N^6-CH_3NHCO-cAMP vs. N^6-C_6H_5NHCO-cAMP).

Good kinase activation is also obtained by 6-HO-cRMP (inosine cyclic 3′,5′-phosphate, cIMP), and by the 6-Cl, 6-CH_3O, and 6-alkylthio-cRMP derivatives. Similar results were obtained with other 6-substituted-cRMP derivatives when these were tested for their ability to influence the phosphorylation of phosphorylase *b* kinase by protein kinase (45). Thus the specificity for the cAMP-dependent protein kinase does not seem to lie in the 6-position, and a great many functional groups are tolerated. In particular, cIMP, which is tautomerically similar to cGMP at positions 1 and 6, is an effective stimulator of the cAMP-dependent kinase, whereas cGMP is not (*vide infra*).

The long-standing success of N^6-2′-*O*-dibutyryladenosine cyclic 3′,5′-phosphate (Bt_2cAMP) as an exogenously administered cAMP derivative that can elicit cAMP-mediated effects (47–49) is based on its hydrolysis, intra- or extracellularly, to N^6-Bt-cAMP which, as Table 34.4 shows, is a good stimulator of protein kinase (44–46). This compound, however, is a very poor phosphodiesterase substrate [see the review by Miller (50) for a discussion], and this is undoubtedly the basis of its success. As Table 34.4 reveals, other N^6-acyl, carbamoyl, or alkoxycarbonyl derivatives are also substantially resistant to phosphodiesterase. Among the N^6-alkyl derivatives, however, only N^6,N^6-Et_2cAMP shows similar resistance. All other monoalkyl derivatives are better substrates.

2.2.2 AS CYCLIC GMP ANALOGS. The K_a' (cGMP) of cAMP for the cGMP-dependent protein kinase from lobster muscle is very small (0.025–0.015) (33). The 6-substituted derivatives of cRMP, however, represent the only class of compounds that are not close cGMP analogs that show any substantial ability to activate the cGMP-dependent kinase (41).

2.3 2-Substituted Derivatives

A substantial number of cAMP analogs with varying 2-substituents were prepared from 5-amino-1-β-D-ribofuranosylimidazole-4-carboxamidine cyclic 3′,5′-phosphate (51, 52). Those compounds give a clear picture of the binding requirements of the bovine brain protein kinase at the 2-position of cAMP (52).

Table 34.5 2-Substituted Derivatives of cAMP as Activators of cAMP-Dependent Protein Kinase[a]

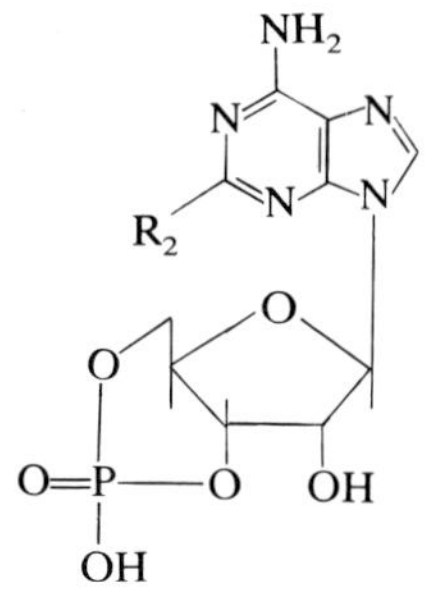

R_2	K_a' (cAMP)	S[b]
Cl	0.39	0.85
Br	*ca.* 1.0[c]	
CH_3	0.16	0.83
CF_3	0.43	0.43
C_2H_5	0.25	0.40
C_4H_9-*n*	0.46	0.64
C_4H_9-*i*	0.05	0.86
C_6H_{13}-*n*	0.91	0.76
C_8H_{17}-*n*	1.6	0.41
$C_{10}H_{21}$-*n*	0.28	0.28
C_6H_5	0.024	0.32
Pyridin-2-yl	0.009	0.76
C_6H_4Cl-*o*	0.09	0.71
NH_2	0.12	0.93
$N(CH_3)_2$	0.07	0.24
OH	0.06	0.66
SH	0.001	0.15
SCH_3	0.2	0.55
SC_2H_5	0.18	1.0
SC_3H_7	0.3	0.74
$SC_{10}H_{21}$-*n*	0.16	0.40
$SCH_2C_6H_5$	0.52	0.63

[a] Data from Ref. 52 unless otherwise specified.
[b] Data from Ref. 52 with a rabbit lung phosphodiesterase preparation.
[c] Data from Ref. 53.

Table 34.5 lists the results for selected compounds.

The data support the existence of some steric interference to kinase binding for a group in the 2-position of cAMP. It would be reasonable to expect this if the cAMP-dependent kinase were to "discriminate" against the 2-amino group of cGMP. Thus 2-H_2N-cAMP and 2-H_3C-cAMP have poor K_a' values. Interestingly, as a linear alkyl (or alkylthio) chain is extended from the 2-position to a maximum of eight atoms, increased binding is experienced, supporting the possibility of a hydrophobic pocket in the binding locale of the 2-position. Branching of the 2-substituent, as seen in the case of 2-Ph-cAMP and 2-*i*-C_4H_9-cAMP, is very detrimental to binding. The 2-mercapto and 2-hydroxy analogs gave very poor K_a' values, most likely because these compounds exist in the keto or thione tautomers, with a proton on N-3, and do not have the same electronic character as the other compounds.

The rates of hydrolysis of the 2-substituted cAMP derivatives by phosphodiesterase were all quite high, indicating not only that this region is not a binding point to the enzyme, but that there is substantial bulk tolerance in this region of the binding site. A wide variety of substituents were accommodated.

2.4 2′-*O*-Modified Cyclic Nucleotides

A free hydroxy group in the ribo configuration at the 2′-position of cAMP is essential for binding to and activation of protein kinase by cAMP analogs (46). Acylation or alkylation of the 2′-hydroxy of cAMP yields analogs (34.**3**) that have K_a' (cAMP) values less than 0.006 when assayed with cAMP-dependent protein kinase from either bovine heart or brain. The sole exception thus far reported is 2′-*O*-$ClCH_2CO$-cAMP, which gave a K_a' (cAMP) of 0.083 with porcine brain histone kinase (54). It should be noted that 2-*O*-acyl derivatives are relatively unstable, and even a very small amount of deacylated cyclic nucleotide will give rise to higher K_a' values.

Two other possible modifications at the 2′-position, inversion or removal of the hydroxyl, give relatively inactive compounds.

Both 9-β-D-arabinofuranosyladenine cyclic 3′,5′-phosphate (ara-cAMP, 34.**4**) and 2′-deoxyadenosine cyclic 3′,5′-phosphate (cdAMP 34.**5**) gave a K_a' (cAMP) less than 0.005 (46).

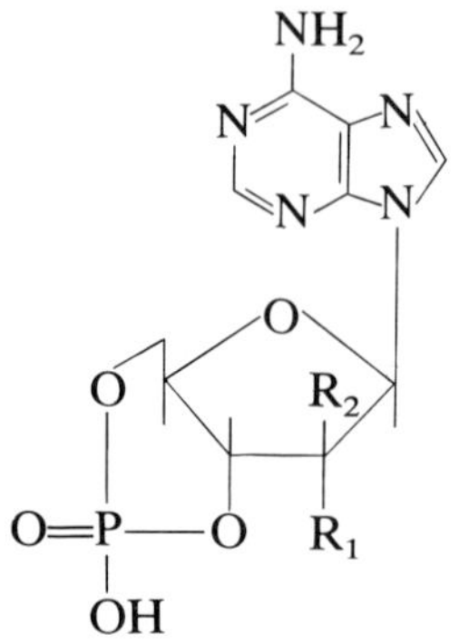

34.**3** R_1 = O-acyl or O-alkyl; R_2 = H
34.**4** R_1 = H; R_2 = OH
34.**5** R_1 = R_2 = H

In light of the parallel specificities of the cAMP- and cGMP-dependent protein kinases for 8-substituents on the respective parent cyclic nucleotides, it is interesting to note that a similar parallelism is found with 2′-*O*-substituents. Either acylation, inversion, or removal of the 2′-hydroxyl groups gave a derivative of cGMP that possessed a K_a' (cGMP) less than 0.009 with the lobster muscle protein kinase (55).

In sharp contrast to the deleterious effect of 2′-*O*-modification on protein kinase activity, only a minor decrease in phosphodiesterase substrate activity is noted with these compounds. A series of 2′-*O*-acyl-cAMP derivatives was hydrolyzed at approximately 0.3–0.7 times the rate of cAMP splitting (39, 46). Several 2′-*O*-acyl-cGMP analogs were substrates also, giving *S* values of 0.1–0.3 (55). The arabinosyl analogs of cAMP ($S = 0.17$) and cGMP ($S = 0.53$), as well as the 2′-deoxy derivatives of cAMP ($S = 0.67$) and cGMP ($S = 0.21$), were also substrates (46, 55).

2.5 Other Single Changes in the Purine Ring

2.5.1 THE 1-POSITION. A free nitrogen at the 1-position of cAMP is important for effective activation of protein kinase. 1-Me-cAMP gave a K_a' (cAMP) of 0.01, and 1-MeO-cAMP gave a K_a' (cAMP) of 0.094 (43). The aglycone of both of these compounds is a strong base, however, and probably protonated at physiological pH.

Among substituents that did not change the electronic character of the ring as drastically, cAMP-1-oxide (34.**6**) had a K_a' (cAMP) of 0.23 (43, 53) and 1-deaza-cAMP (34.**7**) had a K_a' (cAMP) of 1.0 (56).

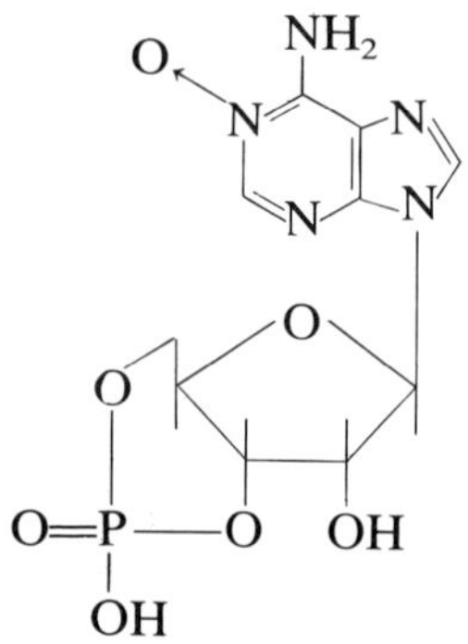

34.**6**

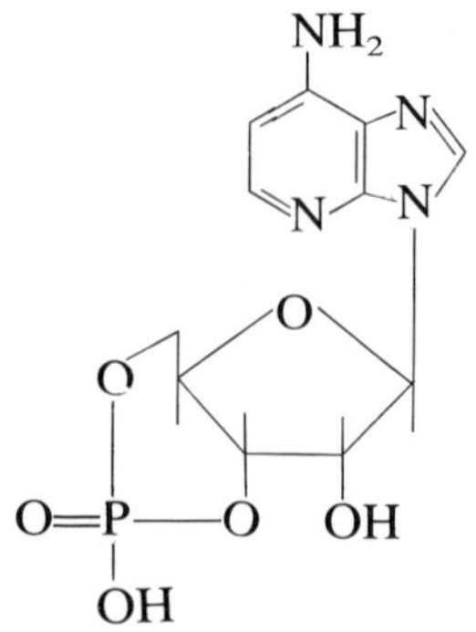

34.**7**

Among cGMP analogs, 1-Me-cGMP had a K_a' (cGMP) of 0.034 (36). None of the changes above substantially affected phosphodiesterase substrate activity.

2.5.2 THE 3-POSITION. The only compound with a modification in this position, 3-deaza-cAMP (34.**8**), had a K_a' (cAMP) of 0.04, indicating that the nitrogen in the 3-position is important for protein kinase binding (56).

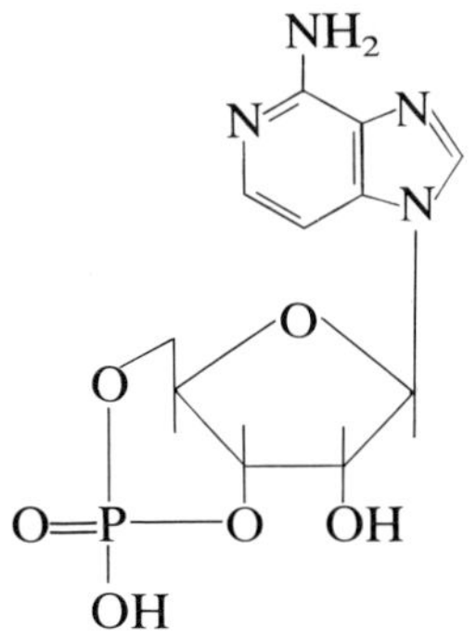

34.**8**

2.5.3 THE 7-POSITION. The nitrogen in the 7-position is apparently unimportant in kinase activation by cAMP, as already mentioned. Tubercidin cyclic 3′,5′-phosphate (7-deaza-cAMP, 34.**9**) had a K_a' (cAMP) of 1.5 (57, 58). Toyocamycin cyclic 3′,5′-phosphate (34.**10**) and sangivimycin cyclic 3′,5′-phosphate (34.**11**) had K_a' (cAMP) values of 0.52 and 0.23, respectively (57). All these compounds were phosphodiesterase substrates.

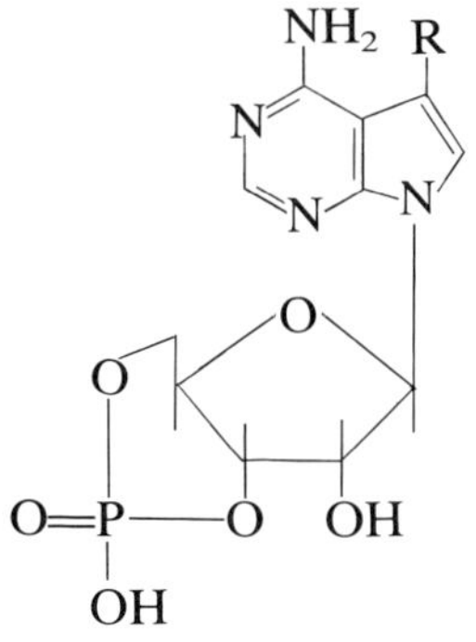

34.**9** R = H
34.**10** R = CN
34.**11** R = $CONH_2$

2.5.4 OTHER CHANGES IN THE RING. The purine ring carbon atoms at positions 2 and 8 have also been replaced with nitrogen. 2-Aza-cAMP (34.**12**) gave K_a' (cAMP) values of 0.06–0.10 in three different systems, and 8-Aza-cAMP (34.**13**) gave a K_a' (cAMP) range of 0.53–0.85 (56). The electronic effect of these changes on the calculated electron density at the 3-position was found to correlate with K_a' (56). The K_a' values given

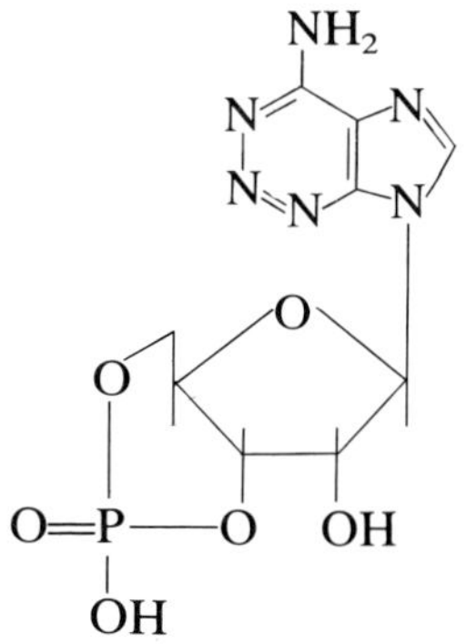

34.**12**

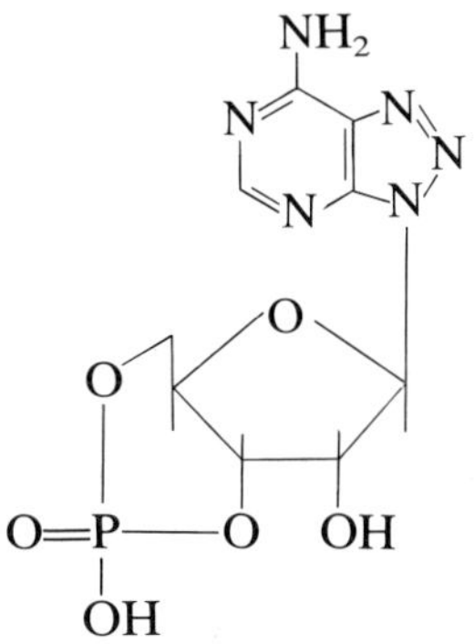

34.**13**

previously for 1-, 3-, and 7-deaza-cAMP agreed with this correlation.

2.6 Two Different Substituents on Cyclic RMP

Since cIMP may be considered to be an altered analog of either cAMP or 2-desamino-cGMP, it is useful to consider the activity of cIMP analogs on both cAMP- and cGMP-dependent kinases. As Table 34.6 shows, cIMP itself has a good K_a' (cAMP) and a poor K_a' (cGMP). Addition to the 8-position of substituents that increase the activity of cAMP itself (8-Br, 8-OH, 8-SC_6H_4Cl-*p*) does not have the same effect on cIMP. Both 8-HO-cIMP and 8-*p*-ClC_6H_4S-cIMP show marked improvements in their K_a' (cGMP), however (33). As expected (*vide supra*), the 8-substituted cIMP analogs are very poor phosphodiesterase substrates (33).

Table 34.6 Activity of 8-Substituted cIMP Derivatives as Activators of cAMP and cGMP-Dependent Protein Kinase[a]

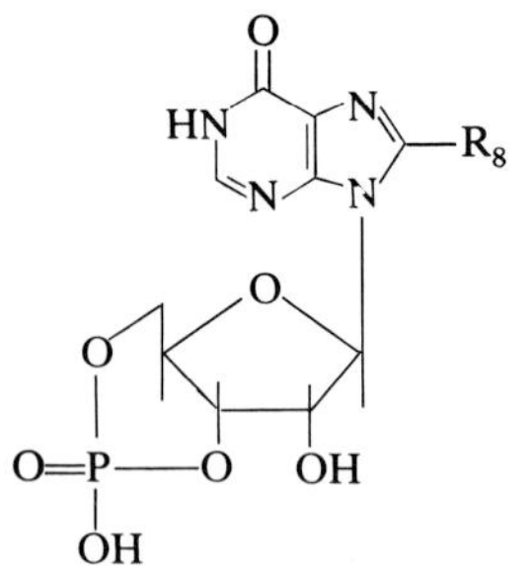

R_8	K_a' cAMP	K_a' cGMP
H	0.59	0.085
Br	0.14	0.02
OH	0.85	0.71
SCH_3	0.16	0.11
SC_6H_4Cl-*p*	1.0	0.84
NH_2	0.02	0.01

[a] Data from Ref. 33.

Table 34.7 considers the effect of addition of an 8-substituent to a 2-substituted cAMP. In all cases except one, the K_a' (cAMP) values lie midway between the values of the two corresponding singly substituted cAMP analogs (Table 34.2). Only 8-Br-2-Me-cAMP has an unusually high K_a'.

A large number of 6,8-disubstituted derivatives of cRMP have been prepared (59), and a few of these are abstracted in Table 34.8. By and large, the K_a' (cAMP) values are averages of the values obtained from the respective 8-substituted-cAMP (Table 34.2) and 6-substituted-cRMP (Table 34.4). This indicates that the contribution or detraction of the substituents to binding to kinase is additive to some extent.

Although 6-HS-cRMP gave a K_a' (cAMP) of 0.2 (see Table 34.4), the corresponding 2-amino analog was one hundredfold less active. The latter compound (the 6-mercapto analog of cGMP) was much better in its ability

Table 34.7 Stimulation of cAMP-Dependent Protein Kinase by Some 2,8-Disubstituted cAMP Analogs[a]

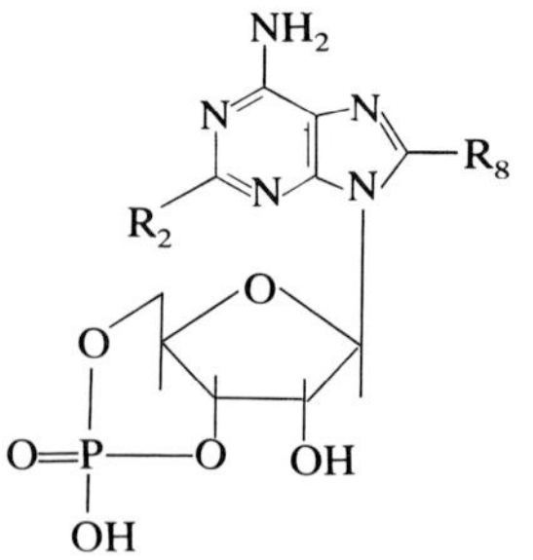

R_2	R_8	K_a' (cAMP)
CH_3	H	0.16
CH_3	Br	3.4
CH_3	$SCH_2C_6H_5$	0.95
CH_3	SC_6H_4Cl-*p*	2.3
C_4H_9-*n*	H	0.46
C_4H_9-*n*	Br	0.66
C_4H_9-*n*	$SCH_2C_6H_5$	1.1
C_4H_9-*n*	SC_6H_4Cl-*p*	2.2

[a] Data from Ref. 60.

Table 34.8 Stimulation of cAMP-Dependent Protein Kinase by Some 6,8-Disubstituted Derivatives of cRMP[a]

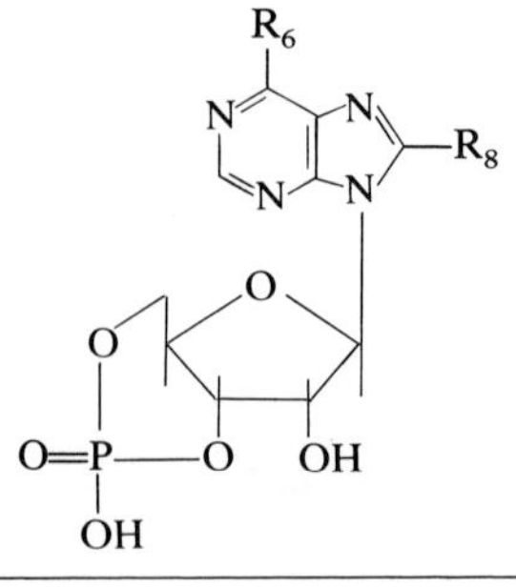

R_6	R_8	K_a' (cAMP)
NH-C_1 to C_6-Alkyl	$SCH_2C_6H_5$	1.8–5.0
$N(C_2H_5)_2$	$SCH_2C_6H_5$	1.1
$N(C_2H_5)_2$	SC_6H_4Cl-*p*	4.0
Pyrrolidino	$SCH_2C_6H_5$	16
SCH_3	SCH_3	1.7
Cl	OH	1.0
Cl	$N(C_2H_5)_2$	0.12

[a] Data from Ref. 37.

to stimulate cGMP-dependent protein kinase, giving a K_a' (cGMP) of 0.2 (59a).

The widespread acceptance of N^6,2'-O-Bt_2-cAMP as a cAMP analog with *in vivo* and cell culture activity has prompted the use of N^2,2'-O-Bt_2-cGMP as an exogenous cGMP source. It should be pointed out that although the hypothetical "active" metabolite, N^2-Bt-cGMP, is moderately resistant to phosphodiesterase ($S = 0.08$), it is a poor stimulator of lobster muscle cGMP-dependent protein kinase [K_a' (cGMP) = 0.029] (55). It is therefore advisable for those wishing to investigate elevated cGMP effects by an exogenously added analog to use one of the more active 8-substituted derivatives.

2.7 Changes in the Sugar and Cyclic Phosphate

Ara-cAMP and cdAMP have been mentioned: any change at 2' results in loss of kinase activation activity. The 4'-position is not as important; both 4'-thio-cAMP (34.**14**) and the carbocyclic analog 34.**15** had K_a'

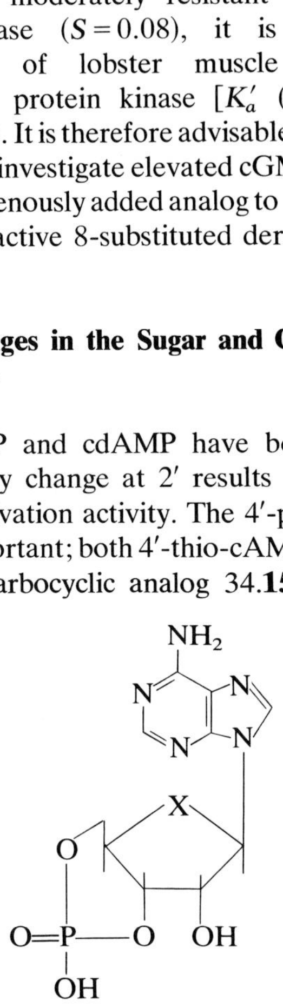

34.**14** X = S
34.**15** X = CH_2

(cAMP) values 0.2–0.5 (50). Compound 34.**14** was a good phosphodiesterase substrate, however (61). Inversion of the cAMP configuration at the 3'-position gives 9-β-D-xylofuranosyladenine cyclic 3',5'-phosphate (xylo-cAMP, 34.**16**). This compound was not effective in stimulating rabbit muscle protein kinase (50, 62).

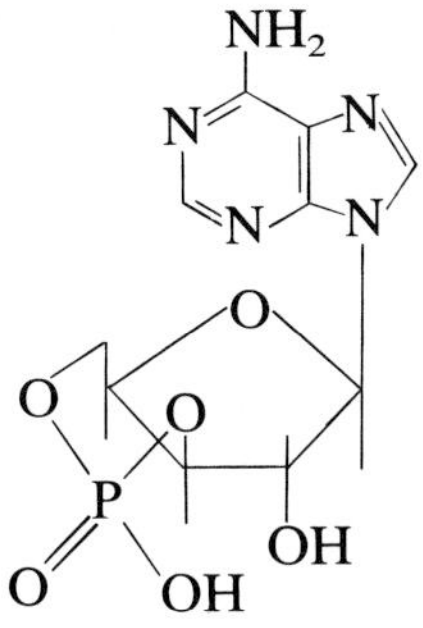

34.**16**

Table 34.9 Stimulation of cAMP-Dependent Protein Kinase by cAMP Analogs with Cyclic Phosphate Modifications

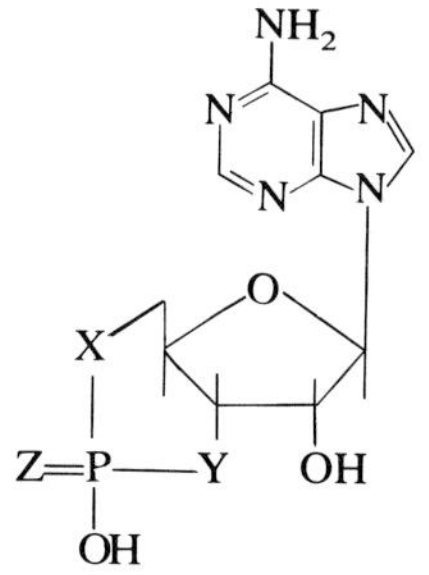

X	Y	Z	K_a' (cAMP)	Reference
O	CH_2	O	0.01	50, 58, 62, 63
CH_2	O	O	0.01	50, 58, 62, 63
O	NH	O	0.01	65
S	NH	O	0.001	64
NH	O	O	0.04	66
NH	O	S	0.04	66
$N(C_4H_9)$	O	O	0.01	66
$N(C_8H_{17})$	O	O	0.51	67
O	O	S	0.5	68

Table 34.9 gives the results of protein kinase activation by various cAMP derivatives in which one of the atoms attached to phosphorus has been changed to carbon, nitrogen, or sulfur. Clearly, the phosphate is very critical for binding to kinase. Only 5'-deoxy-5'-thioadenosine cyclic 3',5'-phosphorothiolate and adenosine cyclic 3',5'-phosphorothionate were effective stimulators of cAMP-dependent protein kinase.

The 5′-amino-5′-deoxyadenosine cyclic 3′,5′-phosphothionate in Table 34.9 gave an interesting result when tested for phosphodiesterase susceptibility: one of the epimers was a substrate and one was not (66).

The negative charge has been removed from cAMP by its conversion to esters (68–70) and amides (71), as shown in structure 34.**17**. These compounds are totally ineffective in activation of protein kinase.

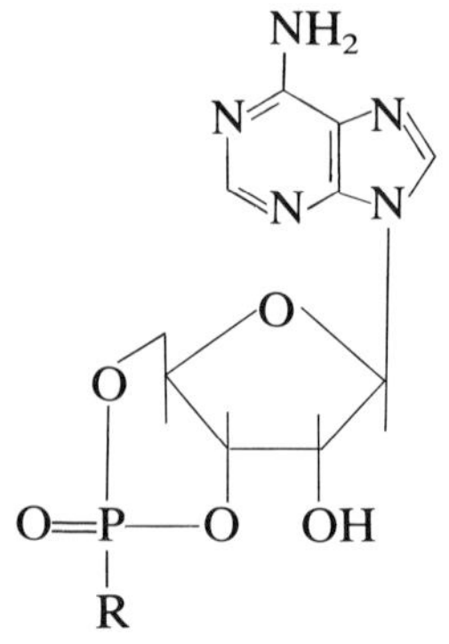

34.**17a** R = $—OCH_3$, $—OC_2H_5$, $—OC_3H_7$-*n*, $—OC_4H_9$-*n*, $—OC_{10}H_{21}$-*n*, $—OCH_2C_6H_5$
34.**17b** R = $—N(CH_3)_2$

The two possible 5′-*C*-methyl analogs of cAMP have been prepared: 9-(6-deoxy-β-D-allofuranosyl)adenine cyclic 3′,5′-phosphate (34.**18**) and its isomer 34.**19** in the talo configuration (72). The alloisomer has a K_a' (cAMP) of 0.6, and the taloisomer and the 5′,5′-di-*C*-methyl analog (34.**20**) (72) were much less active (50).

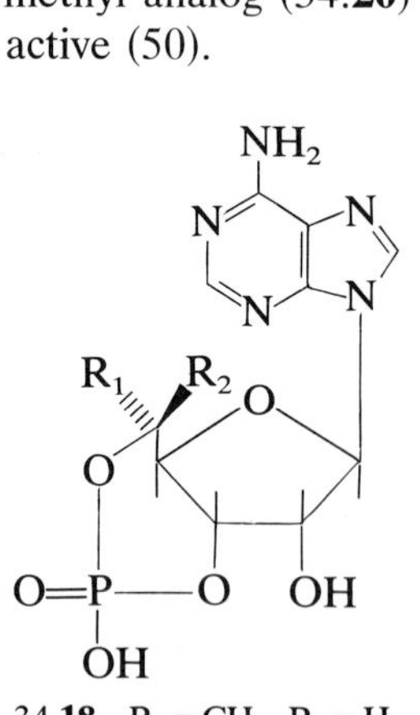

34.**18** $R_1 = CH_3$, $R_2 = H$
34.**19** $R_1 = H$, $R_2 = CH_3$
34.**20** $R_1 = R_2 = CH_3$

2.8 Imidazole Cyclic Nucleotides

Derivatives of 5-amino-1-β-D-ribofuranosylimidazole cyclic 3′,5′-phosphate of the type illustrated by structure 34.**21** are very poor activators of cAMP-dependent protein kinase (43).

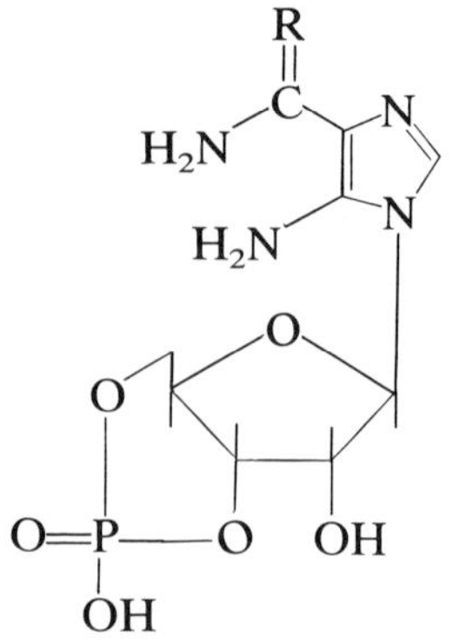

34.**21** R = O, S, NH, $NOCH_3$

2.9 Structure-Activity Relationship Summary

2.9.1 PROTEIN KINASE. The abilities of substituents in the indicated positions on cAMP to effect the stimulation of cAMP-dependent protein kinase are summarized below.

1. *The 2-Position.* Small substituents cause some decrease in activity, which is regained as a straight alkyl chain increases in length. Branched substituents are not allowed.
2. *The 6-Position.* Many substituted nitrogen, sulfur, and oxygen functions are allowed.
3. *The 8-Position.* Substituents with large atomic radii (—Br, —Cl, —S—R) often give better activity than cAMP; substituted amino functions are poor.
4. *The 2′-Position.* Any change destroys activity.
5. *The Cyclic Phosphate.* The only changes accommodated in the six-membered cyclic phosphate ring were the replacement of

either the 5′-oxygen or an exocyclic phosphate oxygen with sulfur.

2.9.2 PHOSPHODIESTERASE. Almost all 8-substituents eliminated phosphodiesterase substrate activity by the analogs. Acylation of N^6 of cAMP eliminated substrate activity in most cases. No other changes were predictable in eliminating phosphodiesterase cleavage of the analogs.

3 ACTIVITY OF CYCLIC NUCLEOTIDE ANALOGS IN TISSUE CULTURE OR ANIMAL SYSTEMS

The evaluation of cyclic nucleotide analogs for activity in whole cell or animal systems must take into account the intrinsic affinity of the analog for its target receptor (e.g., protein kinase), the degradation rate of the analog by phosphodiesterase, and the ability of the compound to penetrate the intact cells. Many studies have been performed using various analogs of cAMP and cGMP; this section concentrates on studies in which the comparative activity of several analogs allows the definition of structure-activity relationships.

3.1 Glucose Release from Liver Slices

The first analogs of cAMP were a series of N^6, 2′-*O*-diacyl, N^6-monoacyl, and 2′-*O*-monoacyl analogs prepared by Posternak (47, 48). These compounds were assayed first for activation of phosphorylase in the presence of dog liver and heart extracts (47). All derivatives were found to be less active than cAMP. The compounds were later tested for the amount of phosphorylase activation (as judged by glucose release) achieved by 1×10^{-5} *M* analog when incubated with dog liver slices. In this assay, N^6-Bt-cAMP, N^6,2′-*O*-Bt_2cAMP, and N^6-acyl derivatives showed good activity. It was in this work that the superiority of Bt_2cAMP to other acylated analogs was demonstrated, and two possibilities for this activity were presented: the nucleotide could gain greater cell penetration by virtue of its greater lipophilicity, or it could be more potent simply because its active metabolite, N^6-Bt-cAMP, was phosphodiesterase resistant (the negative effect of a 2′-*O*-acyl group on intrinsic activity had already been demonstrated). This matter is still in question, although one report has shown that Bt_2cAMP does not penetrate intact cells in culture better than cAMP (73).

Bauer and co-workers investigated the effect of several 8-substituted derivatives on glucose release from rat liver slices (74). The data are summarized in Table 34.10. The K_a values obtained for the compounds from bovine liver cAMP-dependent protein kinase are also given for comparison. The 8-substituted analogs display a close correspondence in rank between their ability to stimulate kinase and to release glucose; these compounds are all phosphodiesterase resistant. cAMP itself is almost inactive in the glucose release system, and Bt_2cAMP is quite active, although not as active as several of the 8-substituted analogs.

3.2 Steroidogenesis and Lipolysis

cAMP mediates the action of ACTH in the stimulation of lipolysis in adipocytes (75) and in the stimulation of steroidogenesis in adrenal cells (76). A variety of 8-substituted cAMP derivatives are capable of stimulating these responses in isolated adipocytes and adrenal cells (77). As Table 34.10 indicates, these analogs are, in general, much more potent than cAMP itself. The relationship of structure to activity, furthermore, parallels the ability of the compounds to stimulate protein kinase from bovine liver and brain (28), although the kinase from the cells in these assays was not tested.

3.3 Cell Growth and Differentiation

The possibility that the relative levels of cAMP and cGMP determine whether a cell is

Table 34.10 Comparison of Protein Kinase Activation with the Ability of cAMP Analogs to Activate Glucolysis, Steroidogenesis, and Lipolysis

R_8	$K_a \times 10^8$, M^a	Glucolysis A_{50}, μM^b	Adrenal A_{50}, μM^c	Lipocyte A_{50}, μM^d
H	2.5	100	330	8,500
SH	1.2	1.0	380	250
OH	1.7	1.3	90	260
$SCH_2C_6H_5$	1.1	2.7	190	1,400
SCH_3	3.9[e]	2.8	65	180
NH_2	4.9	4.6	150	1,200
$NHCH_2CH_2OH$	16.4	15.8	Inactive	14,000
Bt_2cAMP	—	5.0	95	500

[a] Activation constant of bovine liver protein kinase (74).
[b] Concentration for half-maximal stimulation of glucose release from rat liver slices (74).
[c] Concentration for half-maximal activation of steroidogenesis by isolated rat adrenal cells (77).
[d] Concentration for half-maximal stimulation of lipolysis in rat epididymal lipocytes (77).
[e] Activation of bovine brain protein kinase (32).

to grow or to differentiate is a tantalizingly simple hypothesis for the understanding of cell processes. This has been formulated by Goldberg and co-workers in the "yin-yang" hypothesis—the two cyclic nucleotides produce opposing results and their relative levels determine whether the cell will grow or differentiate (11). Tomkins and Kram have formulated a similar concept of pleiotypic control (78). To this end, the effect of cyclic nucleotide analogs on cell growth and differentiation-related processes has been examined.

A number of studies have shown that cAMP analogs inhibit growth, cause loss of viability, or kill cells in culture. By and large, the analogs giving the most pronounced effects are those that are able to stimulate protein kinase at relatively low concentrations and are somewhat phosphodiesterase resistant. Thus some 8-substituted cAMP derivatives, in addition to Bt_2cAMP, inhibited the growth of Reuber H35 hepatoma cells in a reversible manner (79). Several N^6-substituted cAMP derivatives decreased the viability of three tumor cell lines in culture (80), while in some cases neither the corresponding nucleoside nor 5′-phosphate showed cytostatic activity. Some cyclic nucleotides become cytotoxic after phosphodiesterase hydrolysis to their respective 5′-phosphates; these are a special case dealt with below. The ready reversibility of the cytostatic action found with the foregoing analogs, however, is most likely ascribable to some event mediated by cAMP receptor (most likely protein kinase). The mediary role of protein kinase in the cytotoxicity of cAMP and analogs toward S49 mouse lymphosarcoma cells has been elegantly demonstrated by Coffino, Bourne, Tomkins, and co-workers (81, 82).

Direct unequivocal evidence for promotion of cell growth by cGMP is much rarer. Mitogenic activity, however, has been observed for 8-Br-cGMP and other cGMP derivatives in B lymphocytes (83, 84). Bt_2cAMP was shown to be antimitotic in the same assay (85, 86).

If cAMP and analogs inhibit cell growth, is there a chance of using them to arrest growth of rapidly dividing tissue? Cho-chung has found that Bt_2cAMP, 8-Br-cAMP, and 8-MeS-cAMP reversibly arrested growth of some rat tumors while having no effect against others (87). The use of cAMP analogs that act solely on the cAMP receptors of the cells would seem to be limited, however, by the failure to produce a decisive cytotoxic event.

3.4 Enzyme Induction

In connection with the role of cAMP in promotion of differentiation, there is evidence that cAMP plays an intermediary role in the induction of the synthesis of certain enzymes. In particular, Wicks and co-workers found tyrosine transaminase and phosphoenolpyruvate carboxykinase levels to be markedly elevated after administration of Bt_2cAMP to rat hepatoma cells in culture (88). Furthermore, a series of 6- and 8-substituted cAMP analogs induced the synthesis of these two enzymes in the hepatoma culture system, and the activity of the compounds in this assay was closely parallel to the ability of the analogs to stimulate protein kinase.

A series of 23 cyclic nucleotide analogs has been examined for ability to induce tyrosine transaminase synthesis in adrenalectomized rats (89). These results, expressed as Ind_{50} (the concentration necessary, in micromoles per kilogram, for half-maximal induction of transaminase activity), were compared to the ability of the compounds to stimulate rat liver protein kinase (expressed as K_a, nM) and their relative rate of hydrolysis by rat liver phosphodiesterase (expressed as S). The results appear in Table 34.11. When log Ind_{50} was correlated with log K_a and log S, a very good fit was obtained:

$$\log(\mathrm{Ind}_{50}) = 0.90 + 0.47\log(S) + 0.80\log(K_a) \quad (34.3)$$
$$n = 20,\ s = 0.27,\ r = 0.92$$

Given the wide range of substitution types on the analogs, these data are strongly suggestive of the involvement of protein kinase in induction of this enzyme. The K_a and S values from rat liver were very close to those from other sources reported earlier in this chapter and, as might be expected, 8-p-ClPhS-cAMP was the most potent inducer of tyrosine transaminase, having an Ind_{50} more than twentyfold lower than that of Bt_2cAMP.

3.5 Stimulation of Pituitary Hormone Release

cAMP mediates the release of a number of hormones from a secretory glands (90). In a series of experiments on isolated rat pituitary glands, Cehovic, Posternak, and co-workers demonstrated that several analogs could mediate the release of several pituitary hormones. Several N^6- and 8-substituted cAMP derivatives were effective in stimulating the release of prolactin (91, 93), growth hormone (91, 92), and thyroid-stimulating hormone (TSH) (94).

The TSH-induced release of thyroxine and triiodothyronine from thyroid is also

Table 34.11 Correlation of the Ability of Cyclic Nucleotide Analogs to Induce Tyrosine Aminotransferase in Rats, with Their Rates of Hydrolysis by Phosphodiesterase and Their Ability to Activate Protein Kinase[a]

			Ind_{50}[d], μM/kg	
Compound	K_a[b], nM	S[c]	Experimental	Calculated[e]
8-Substituent on cAMP				
NH_2	12	0.9	168	56
$NHCH_2Ph$	240	0.06	368	174
OH	9.6	0.09	11	16
OCH_3	84	0.06	158	74
SH	5.4	0.1	5.8	10
SCH_3	10	0.08	7.4	15.3
SC_6H_4Cl-*p*	0.22	0.05	0.95	0.57
Br	7	0.11	3.9	13
N^6-Substituents on cAMP				
COC_3H_7	26	0.06	30	29
C_2H_5	30	0.29	36	68
$(C_2H_5)_2$	13	0.14	36	25
CH_2Ph	19	0.40	52	55
OC_2H_5	42	0.46	123	112
OCH_2Ph	17	0.55	57	59
$CO_2C_2H_5$	100	0.12	145	119
6-Substituent on cRMP				
SH	70	1.2	136	265
SCH_3	1.2	0.6	15	7
SCH_2Ph	10	0.72	37	43
OH (cIMP)	43	0.63	121	132
OCH_3	47	0.68	145	147

[a] Data recalculated from Ref. 89.
[b] Activation constant for rat liver protein kinase.
[c] Hydrolysis rate (relative to cAMP) by rat liver phosphodiesterase.
[d] Concentration to give half-maximal induction of tyrosine aminotransferase in adrenalectomized rats.
[e] Calculated from equation 34.3.

mediated by cAMP (90). A series of N^6,2′-*O*-dibutyryl-8-substituted-cAMP analogs has been shown to duplicate this effect in mice (95). In this experiment, a dose of 15–30 mg/kg of 8-MeS-cAMP, 8-H_2N-cAMP, or 8-N_3-cAMP (i.v.) was found to stimulate radioiodine release equivalent to that caused by 0.6–1.2 mU of TSH per mouse (i.v.). The corresponding butyrylated analogs were less active in this test, as were other 8-substituted analogs.

3.6 Activity on Cardiac and Smooth Muscle

cAMP mediates smooth muscle function, with high cAMP levels giving relaxation of this tissue. Rubin and co-workers investigated the response of guinea pig trachea and rat portal vein to a series of 8-substituted cAMP analogs (96). As might be expected from knowledge of the K_a' of these compounds (Section 2.1.1) 8-$PhCH_2$S-, 8-MeS-,

8-N_3-, and 8-HS-cAMP were the most potent analogs in causing smooth muscle relaxation. Theophylline, a cyclic nucleotide phosphodiesterase inhibitor, was more potent than any of the cyclic nucleotides in this assay, however, and cAMP itself was inactive.

In cardiac muscle, contraction is mediated by cAMP. Kukovetz and co-workers have shown excellent correlations between the ability of a series of compounds to inhibit phosphodiesterase and their potency in stimulating the positive inotropic response (97), and Bt_2cAMP has been shown to have inotropic activity (98). No detailed study of the effect of a greater variety of cAMP derivatives on cardiac contractility has been published, but one analog that emerged from a series screened had superior inotropic properties. That compound, 8-(benzylthio)-*N*-butyladenosine cyclic 3′,5′-phosphate (34.**22**) produced a noticeable increase in

NHC_4H_9-*n* $SCH_2C_6H_5$

34.**22**

peak developed tension of excised cat papillary muscle at 2×10^{-6} *M* (99).

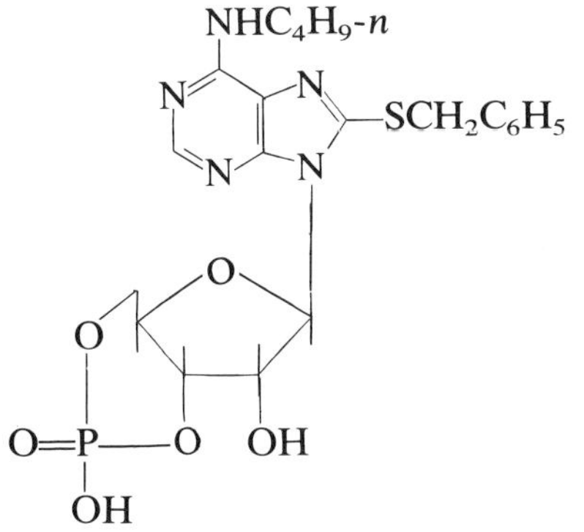

4 PYRIMIDINE CYCLIC NUCLEOTIDES

Recently Bloch has found that cytidine cyclic 3′,5′-phosphate (cCMP, 34.**23**) is capable of eliminating the characteristic time lag observed before a chilled leukemia L1210 culture, which has been brought to incubation temperature, starts to grow (13a). Furthermore, cCMP is itself produced by these cells (12), and it is found in the urine of human

NH_2

34.**23**

leukemia patients but not otherwise normal patients (13b). cAMP and cGMP do not affect this growth lag, but cUMP, which Bloch has isolated from rat liver extracts (13c), delays the growth lag considerably. This exciting discovery may lead to the elucidation of yet another "yin-yang" mechanism by which cell processes are controlled. Cytidylate cyclase activity has recently been found in normal and tumor cells (99a).

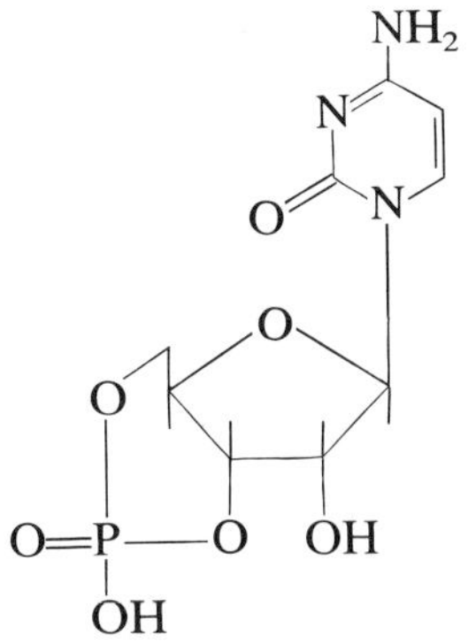

5 CYCLIC NUCLEOTIDES AS PRODRUGS

With the exception of psicofuranine and decoyinine (see Chapter 24), virtually all analogs of purines, pyrimidines, and their nucleosides that show carcinostatic activity must be intracellularly converted to their respective 5′-phosphates. These bioactive nucleotides are of little use in chemotherapy because they do not penetrate cells intact, presumably because of the two negative charges they carry. The cyclic nucleotides carry only one negative charge and are readily converted, in many cases, to the respective 5′-nucleotides by phosphodiesterase. Acylation of the 2′-hydroxyl yields cyclic nucleotides that may still be phosphodiesterase substrates. After the cyclic phosphate ring is opened, the 2′-*O*-acyl group becomes very labile. Thus cyclic nucleotides of bioactive nucleosides are potential prodrugs for the corresponding 5′-nucleotides.

phosphodiesterase and deacylation

34.**24**

The antileukemia drug 6-mercaptopurine must be converted to 6-thioinosine acid (34.**24**) by hypoxanthine–guanine phosphoribosyl transferase (HGPRT) to begin a chain of events terminating in cell death. Lack of this enzyme leads to resistance to 6-mercaptopurine. A series of 2′-*O*-acyl-9-β-D-ribofuranosyl-6-mercaptopurine derivatives (34.**25**) was examined for cytotoxicity to S49 mouse lymphosarcoma cells lacking HGPRT. The parent compound (34.**25**, R = H) and the derivatives with short acyl groups on the 2′-OH were active only at high concentrations (~1 m*M*). When the acyl group was lengthened to 16 carbons (34.**25**, $R = COC_{15}H_{31}$), the compound gave a 50% inhibition of cell growth at 65 μM (100). It is reasonable to conclude that the drug is penetrating the cells intact and being converted to 34.**24** as opposed to extracellular breakdown to cytotoxic products, since 6-mercaptopurine, its ribonucleoside, and the appropriate fatty acid control gave negative results with these cells.

Removal of the negative charge altogether would, of course, give a neutral molecule. An appropriately designed neutral compound might be a prodrug, therefore, for cAMP or an analog, or for one of the cyclic nucleotides of carcinostatic agents as discussed earlier. Nagyvary and co-workers have prepared some alkyl esters of cAMP (34.**17a**), and weak inhibition of tumor growth has been observed (101). Some substituted benzyl esters of cAMP were shown to raise cAMP levels in glioma cells, probably by serving as cAMP prodrugs (70). This class of esters apparently has a half-life in biological fluids that is short enough to furnish detectable quantities of cAMP inside the cells, but long enough to prevent total extracellular hydrolysis (70). Again, cAMP itself gave no effect at the concentrations tested.

Adenosine cyclic *N,N*-dimethylphosphoramidate (34.**17b**), which yields cAMP when incubated at acid pH, is too stable to act as a cAMP prodrug under neutral conditions (71).

6 CYCLIC AMP IN BACTERIA

There are some functions of cAMP in bacteria for which there are no established analogies in higher organisms. In *Escherichia coli* cAMP mediates the synthesis of inducible enzymes by binding to a specific protein (the cAMP receptor, or CRP, protein) that apparently binds to the promoter region of the operon and increases the frequency of initiation.

A number of analogs of cAMP were tested for their ability to inhibit the cAMP-CRP-stimulated transcription and for their ability to inhibit cAMP binding to CRP (103). Tubercidin cyclic 3′,5′-phosphate (34.**9**) 8-Br-, 8-HS-, N^6-Bt-cAMP, and cGMP were the most effective binding inhibitors, and 5′-deoxy-5′-octylaminoadenosine cyclic 3′,5′-phosphoramidate (see Table 34.9) was the most potent transcription inhibitor. The only analog that was able to replace cAMP as a transcription stimulant in the presence of CRP in this system was tubercidin cyclic 3′,5′-phosphate (34.**9**).

7 AFFINITY CHROMATOGRAPHY AND AFFINITY LABELING

After the structural requirements of a protein (phosphodiesterase, protein kinase) for binding cAMP have been determined, an appropriate spacer arm for attachment of the ligand to an immobilized support may be placed, and affinity chromatography of cAMP-binding proteins may be conducted. The most thorough study of the effect of point of attachment and length of spacer arm on the efficiency of affinity column chromatography has been done by Dills and co-workers (104). They prepared N^6-H_2N-$(CH_2)_n$-cAMP analogs ($n = 2, 4, 6, 9, 12$), 2-$H_2N(CH_2)_2NH$-cAMP, and 8-$H_2N(CH_2)_2NH$-cAMP. These derivatives were covalently attached to cyanogen bromide-activated Sepharose 4B and used to separate the regulatory subunit (which binds cAMP) from the catalytic subunit of rabbit muscle protein kinase. The 6- and 8-substituted ligands were the most effective in binding to protein kinase (see Tables 34.2, 34.4, 34.5). Little steric hindrance was experienced with different spacer arm length, since no difference was seen in the apparent affinity of the holoenzyme for the series of N^6-substituted ligands. The regulatory subunit was successfully eluted from the column with cAMP.

Analogs of cAMP capable of generating highly reactive carbenes or nitrenes under photolytic conditions have been used for photoaffinity labeling of the active sites of cAMP-binding proteins. The analogs used to date are the 2′-*O*- and N^6-ethoxycarbonyldiazoacetyl-cAMP (105–107) and 8-N_3-cAMP (108, 109).

In summary, cyclic nucleotides seem to be involved as a second messenger in so many of the essential processes of life that it is difficult to believe that some of the types of compounds described herein will not reach clinical utility in the near future. The rational design and testing of these compounds must be based on an understanding of the interactions between the nucleotides and their primary receptors, and it is hoped that this chapter contributes to that understanding.

REFERENCES

1. T. W. Rall, E. W. Sutherland, and J. Berthet, *J. Biol. Chem.*, **224,** 463 (1957).
2. E. W. Sutherland and T. W. Rall, *J. Am. Chem. Soc.*, **79,** 3608 (1957).
3. G. A. Robison, R. W. Butcher, and E. W. Sutherland, *Cyclic AMP*, Academic Press, New York, 1971.
4. M. E. Maguire, E. M. Ross, and A. G. Gilman, *Advan. Cyclic Nucleotide Res.*, **8,** 1 (1977).
5. M. M. Appleman, W. J. Thompson, and T. R. Russell, *Advan. Cyclic Nucleotide Res.*, **3,** 65 (1973).
6. T. A. Langan, *Advan. Cyclic Nucleotide Res.*, **3,** 99 (1973).
7. J. F. Kuo and P. Greengard, *Proc. Nat. Acad. Sci., US*, **64,** 1349 (1969).
8. D. F. Ashman, R. Lipton, M. M. Melicow, and T. D. Price, *Biochem. Biophys. Res. Commun.*, **11,** 330 (1963).
9. N. D. Goldberg, R. F. O'Dea, and M. K. Haddox, *Advan. Cyclic Nucleotide Res.*, **3,** 155 (1973).
10. J. F. Kuo and P. Greengard, *J. Biol. Chem.*, **245,** 2493 (1970).
11. N. D. Goldberg, M. K. Haddox, S. E. Nicol, D. B. Glass, C. H. Sanford, F. A. Kuehl, Jr., and R. Estensen, *Advan. Cyclic Nucleotide Res.*, **5,** 307 (1975).
12. A. Bloch, *Biochem. Biophys. Res. Commun.*, **58,** 652 (1974).
13. (a) A. Bloch, G. Dutschman, and R. Maue, *Biochem. Biophys. Res. Commun.*, **59,** 955 (1974). (b) A. Bloch, R. Hromchak, and E. S. Henderson, *Proc. Am. Assoc. Cancer Res.*, **16,** 191 (1975), (c) A. Bloch and R. J. Leonard, *Proc. Am. Assoc. Cancer Res.*, **17,** 203 (1976).
14. P. Greengard, D. A. McAfee, and J. W. Kebabian, *Advan. Cyclic Nucleotide Res.*, **1,** 337 (1972).
15. W. R. Kukovetz and G. Pöch, *Advan. Cyclic Nucleotide Res.*, **1,** 261 (1972).
16. M. S. Amer and G. R. McKinney, *Life Sci.*, **13,** 753 (1973).

17. M. S. Amer and G. R. McKinney, *Ann. Rep. Med. Chem.*, **9,** 203 (1974).
18. M. S. Amer and G. R. McKinney, *Ann. Rep. Med. Chem.*, **10,** 192 (1975).
19. *Cyclic Nucleotides and Disease*, B. Weiss, Ed., University Park Press, Baltimore, 1975.
20. F. Murad, *Advan. Cyclic Nucleotide Res.*, **3,** 355 (1977).
21. A. E. Broadus, *Advan. Cyclic Nucleotide Res.*, **8,** 509 (1977).
22. M. S. Amer and W. E. Kreighbaum, *J. Pharm. Sci.*, **64,** 1 (1975).
23. M. Chasin and D. N. Harris, *Advan. Cyclic Nucleotide Res.*, **7,** 225 (1976).
24. M. Smith, G. I. Drummond, and H. G. Khorana, *J. Am. Chem. Soc.*, **83,** 698 (1961).
25. G. I. Drummond, M. W. Gilgan, E. J. Reiner, and M. Smith, *J. Am. Chem. Soc.*, **86,** 1626 (1964).
26. R. K. Borden and M. Smith, *J. Org. Chem.*, **31,** 3247 (1966).
27. R. Marumoto, T. Nishimura, and M. Honjo, *Chem. Pharm. Bull. (Tokyo)*, **23,** 2295 (1975).
28. L. N. Simon, D. A. Shuman, and R. K. Robins, *Advan. Cyclic Nucleotide Res.*, **3,** 225 (1973).
29. R. B. Meyer, Jr., and J. P. Miller, *Life Sci.*, **14,** 1019 (1974).
30. J. P. Miller and R. K. Robins, *Ann. Rep. Med. Chem.*, **11,** 291 (1976).
31. E. Miyamoto, J. F. Kuo, and P. Greengard, *J. Biol. Chem.*, **244,** 6395 (1969).
32. K. Muneyama, R. J. Bauer, D. A. Shuman, R. K. Robins, and L. N. Simon, *Biochemistry*, **10,** 2390 (1971).
33. J. P. Miller, K. H. Boswell, K. Muneyama, L. N. Simon, R. K. Robins, and D. A. Shuman, *Biochemistry*, **12,** 5310 (1973).
34. K. Muneyama, D. A. Shuman, K. H. Boswell, R. K. Robins, L. N. Simon, and J. P. Miller, *J. Carbohydr. Nucleosides Nucleotides*, **1,** 55 (1974).
35. L. F. Christensen, R. B. Meyer, Jr., R. K. Robins, and J. P. Miller, unpublished results.
36. R. B. Meyer, Jr., R. K. Robins, and J. P. Miller, unpublished results.
37. K. H. Boswell, R. K. Robins, and J. P. Miller, unpublished results.
38. W. L. Dills, J. A. Beavo, P. J. Bechtel, and E. G. Krebs, *Biochem. Biophys. Res. Commun.*, **62,** 70 (1975).
39. G. Michal, K. Mühlegger, M. Nelboeck, C. Thiessen, and G. Weimann, *Pharmacol. Res. Commun.*, **6,** 203 (1974).
40. L. F. Christensen, R. B. Meyer, Jr., J. P. Miller, L. N. Simon, and R. K. Robins, *Biochemistry*, **14,** 1490 (1975).
41. R. B. Meyer, Jr., D. A. Shuman, R. K. Robins, R. J. Bauer, M. K. Dimmitt, and L. N. Simon, *Biochemistry*, **11,** 2704 (1972).
42. T. Posternak, I. Marcus, A. Baggai, and G. Cehovic, *C.R. Acad. Sci. Paris*, **269,** 2409 (1969).
43. R. B. Meyer, Jr., D. A. Shuman, R. K. Robins, J. P. Miller, and L. N. Simon, *J. Med. Chem.*, **16,** 1319 (1973).
44. K. H. Boswell, J. P. Miller, D. A. Shuman, R. W. Sidwell, L. N. Simon, and R. K. Robins, *J. Med. Chem.*, **16,** 1075 (1973).
45. M. Du Plooy, G. Michal, G. Weimann, M. Nelboeck, and R. Paoletti, *Biochim. Biophys. Acta*, **230,** 30 (1971).
46. J. P. Miller, D. A. Shuman, M. B. Scholten, M. K. Dimmitt, C. M. Stewart, T. A. Khwaja, R. K. Robins, and L. N. Simon, *Biochemistry*, **12,** 1010 (1973).
47. T. Posternak, E. W. Sutherland, and W. F. Henion, *Biochim. Biophys. Acta*, **65,** 558 (1962).
48. J. G. Falbriard, T. Posternak, and E. W. Sutherland, *Biochim. Biophys. Acta*, **148,** 99 (1967).
49. W. F. Henion, E. W. Sutherland, and T. Posternak, *Biochim. Biophys. Acta*, **148,** 106 (1967).
50. J. P. Miller, in *Cyclic Nucleotides: Mechanism of Action*, H. Cramer and J. Schultz, Eds., Wiley, London, 1977, p. 77.
51. R. B. Meyer, Jr., D. A. Shuman, and R. K. Robins, *J. Am. Chem. Soc.*, **96,** 4962 (1974).
52. R. B. Meyer, Jr., H. Uno, R. K. Robins, L. N. Simon, and J. P. Miller, *Biochemistry*, **14,** 3315 (1975).
53. B. Jastorff and W. Freist, *Bioorg. Chem.*, **3,** 103 (1974).
54. E. S. Severin, M. V. Nesterova, L. P. Sashchenko, V. V. Rasumova, V. L. Tunitskaya, S. N. Kochetkov, and N. N. Gulyaev, *Biochim. Biophys. Acta*, **384,** 413 (1975).
55. J. P. Miller, K. H. Boswell, A. M. Mian, R. B. Meyer, Jr., R. K. Robins, and T. A. Khwaja, *Biochemistry*, **15,** 217 (1976).
56. J. P. Miller, L. F. Christensen, T. A. Andrea, R. B. Meyer, Jr., S. Kitano, and Y. Mizuno, *J. Cyclic Nucleotide Res.*, **4,** 133 (1978).
57. J. P. Miller, K. H. Boswell, K. Muneyama, R. L. Tolman, M. B. Scholten, R. K. Robins, L. N. Simon, and D. A. Shuman, *Biochem. Biophys. Res. Commun.*, **55,** 843 (1973).
58. J. F. Kuo and P. Greengard, *Biochem. Biophys. Res. Commun.*, **40,** 1032 (1970).
59. K. H. Boswell, L. F. Christensen, D. A. Shuman,

and R. K. Robins, *J. Heterocycl. Chem.*, **12,** 1 (1975). (a) R. B. Meyer, Jr., H. Uno, D. A. Shuman, R. K. Robins, L. N. Simon, and J. P. Miller, *J. Cyclic Nucleotide Res.*, **1,** 159 (1975).

60. H. Uno, R. B. Meyer, Jr., D. A. Shuman, R. K. Robins, L. N. Simon, and J. P. Miller, *J. Med. Chem.*, **19,** 419 (1976).
61. A. K. M. Anisuzzaman, W. C. Lake, and R. L. Whistler, *Biochemistry*, **12,** 2041 (1973).
62. G. I. Drummond and C. A. Powell, *Mol. Pharmacol.*, **6,** 24 (1970).
63. G. H. Jones, H. P. Albrecht, N. P. Damordaran, and J. G. Moffatt, *J. Am. Chem. Soc.*, **92,** 5510 (1970).
64. M. Morr, *Tetrahedron Lett.*, 2127 (1976).
65. N. Panitiz, E. Rieke, M. Morr, K. G. Wagner, G. Roesler, and B. Jastorff, *Eur. J. Biochem.*, **55,** 415 (1975).
66. B. Jastorff and H. P. Bär, *Eur. J. Biochem.*, **37,** 497 (1973).
67. D. A. Shuman, J. P. Miller, M. B. Scholten, L. N. Simon, and R. K. Robins, *Biochemistry*, **12,** 2781 (1973).
68. R. N. Gohil, R. G. Gillen, and J. Nagyvary, *Nucleic Acids Res.*, **1,** 1691 (1974).
69. R. G. Gillen and J. Nagyvary, *Biochem. Biophys. Res. Commun.*, **68,** 836 (1976).
70. J. Engels and E. J. Schlaeger, *J. Med. Chem.*, **20,** 907 (1977).
71. R. B. Meyer, Jr., D. A. Shuman, and R. K. Robins, *Tetrahedron Lett.*, 269 (1973).
72. R. S. Ranganathan, G. H. Jones, and J. G. Moffatt, *J. Org. Chem.*, **39,** 290 (1974).
73. W. L. Ryan and M. A. Durick, *Science*, **177,** 1002 (1972).
74. R. J. Bauer, K. R. Swiatek, R. K. Robins, and L. N. Simon, *Biochem. Biophys. Res. Commun.*, **45,** 526 (1971).
75. G. A. Robison, R. W. Butcher, and E. W. Sutherland, *Cyclic AMP*, Academic Press, New York, 1971, p. 286.
76. G. A. Robison, R. W. Butcher, and E. W. Sutherland, *Cyclic AMP*, Academic Press, New York, 1971, p. 317.
77. C. A. Free, M. Chasin, V. S. Paik and S. M. Hess, *Biochemistry*, **10,** 3785 (1971).
78. R. Kram and G. M. Tomkins, *Proc. Nat. Acad. Sci., US*, **70,** 1659 (1973).
79. R. Van Wijk, W. D. Wicks, and K. Clay, *Cancer Res.*, **32,** 1905 (1972).
80. C. I. Hong, G. L. Tritsch, A. Mittelman, P. Hebborn, and G. B. Chheda, *J. Med. Chem.*, **18,** 465 (1975).
81. H. R. Bourne, P. Coffino, and G. M. Tomkins, *Science*, **187,** 750 (1975).
82. P. A. Insel, H. R. Bourne, P. Coffino, and G. M. Tomkins, *Science*, **190,** 896 (1975).
83. D. A. Chambers, D. W. Martin, Jr., and Y. Weinstein, *Cell*, **3,** 373 (1974).
84. Y. Weinstein, S. Segal, and K. L. Melmon, *J. Immunol.*, **115,** 112 (1975).
85. J. Watson, R. Epstein, and M. Cohn, *Nature*, **246,** 405 (1973).
86. Y. Weinstein, D. A. Chambers, H. R. Bourne, and K. L. Melmon, *Nature*, **251,** 352 (1974).
87. Y. S. Cho-chung, *Cancer Res.*, **34,** 3492 (1974).
88. K. Wagner, M. D. Roper, B. H. Leichtling, J. Wimalasena, and W. D. Wicks, *J. Biol. Chem.*, **250,** 231 (1975).
89. J. P. Miller, A. H. Beck, L. N. Simon, and R. B. Meyer, Jr., *J. Biol. Chem.*, **250,** 426 (1975).
90. G. A. Robison, R. W. Butcher, and E. W. Sutherland, *Cyclic AMP*, Academic Press, New York, 1971, pp. 353 ff.
91. G. Cehovic, I. Marcus, A. Gabbai, and T. Posternak, *C.R. Acad. Sci. Paris*, **271,** 1399 (1970).
92. T. Posternak, I. Marcus, and G. Cehovic, *C.R. Acad. Sci. Paris*, **272,** 622 (1971).
93. N.-b. Giao, G. Cehovic, M. Bayer, H. Gergeley, and T. Posternak, *C.R. Acad. Sci. Paris*, **279,** 1705 (1974).
94. T. Posternak and G. Cehovic, *Ann. N.Y. Acad. Sci.*, **185,** 42 (1971).
95. G. Cehovic, M. Bayer, and N.-b. Giao, *J. Med. Chem.*, **19,** 899 (1976).
96. B. Rubin, E. H. O'Keefe, M. H. Waugh, D. G. Kotler, D. A. DeMaio, and Z. P. Horowitz, *Proc. Soc. Exp. Biol. Med.*, **137,** 1245 (1971).
97. W. R. Kukovetz, G. Pöch, and A. Wurm, *Advan. Cyclic Nucleotide Res.*, **5,** 395 (1975).
98. T. Meinertz, H. Nawrath, and H. Scholz, *Arch. Pharmacol.*, **277,** 107 (1972).
99. D. B. Evans, C. S. Parham, M. T. Schenck, and R. J. Laffan, *J. Cyclic Nucleotide Res.*, **2,** 307 (1976).
100. R. B. Meyer, Jr., T. E. Stone, B. Ullman, and D. W. Martin, Jr., unpublished results.
101. F. A. Cotton, R. G. Gillen, R. N. Gohil, E. E. Hazen, Jr., C. R. Kirchner, J. Nagyvary, J. P. Rouse, A. G. Stanislowski, J. D. Stevens, and P. W. Tucker, *Proc. Nat. Acad. Sci., US*, **72,** 1335 (1975).
102. I. Pastan and R. Perlman, *Science*, **169,** 339 (1970).
103. W. B. Anderson, R. L. Perlman, and I. Pastan, *J. Biol. Chem.*, **247,** 2717 (1972).
104. W. L. Dills, Jr., J. A. Beavo, P. J. Bechtel, K. R.

Myers, L. J. Sakai, and E. G. Krebs, *Biochemistry*, **15**, 3724 (1976).

105. D. J. Brunswick and B. S. Cooperman, *Biochemistry*, **12**, 4074 (1973).
106. B. S. Cooperman and D. J. Brunswick, *Biochemistry*, **12**, 4079 (1973).
107. C. E. Guthrow, H. Rasmussen, D. J. Brunswick and B. S. Cooperman, *Proc. Nat. Acad. Sci., US*, **70**, 3344 (1973).
108. B. E. Haley, *Biochemistry*, **14**, 3852 (1975).
109. A. H. Pomerantz, S. A. Rudolph, B. E. Haley, and P. Greengard, *Biochemistry*, **14**, 3858 (1975).

CHAPTER THIRTY–FIVE

Antihyperlipidemic Agents

GERALD F. HOLLAND

Central Research
Pfizer Inc.,
Groton, Connecticut 06340, USA

CONTENTS

1 INTRODUCTION

Cardiovascular diseases—diseases of the heart and blood vessels—are the most serious health problems of contemporary society. In the United States some 28 million people are affected (1), and although the rising mortality rate for cardiovascular diseases observed since the beginning of the century appears to have leveled off (2), they still account for 51% or about 1 million, of all deaths each year (3). The chances for developing a cardiovascular disease by age 65 are 37% for a man and 18% for a woman (4). Ischemic (coronary) heart disease (IHD), an irregular thickening of the inner layer of the walls of the arteries, accounts for 66% of all cardiovascular deaths and for 34% of all deaths overall (3); it kills more Americans (643,000) each year than automobile accidents, and any other disease (including cancer) as well. Similar observations have been reported in other countries. Finland, for example, has a rate of IHD in middle-aged men that is even higher than the rate in United States (5). In England and Wales about 40% of deaths that occur in middle-aged men are due to IHD (6); it is the cause of more than a quarter of all deaths in the United Kingdom (7) and in the Soviet Union (8).

Worldwide epidemiological studies have shown the incidence of IHD is related to a number of *independent* risk factors, particularly high concentrations of serum lipids, high blood pressure, and cigarette smoking (1, 9–20). The Seven Countries Study (10) showed that serum cholesterol and blood pressure tend to be elevated in men living in countries where IHD is more common. Although high blood pressure was found to be the most reliable predictor in the Framingham prospective study (12, 13, 20), elevated serum cholesterol and cigarette smoking were also clearly identified as risk factors. In Japan, where serum cholesterol concentrations are low, risk factors such as diabetes and hypertension do not play the important role that they do in Western countries, suggesting that hypercholesterolemia is a major, and perhaps a principal, risk factor (21). Elevated levels of systolic blood pressure, cigarette smoking, and fasting triglyceride levels were the most notable risk factors in a random selection of men aged 40 in Edinburgh and Stockholm (17) who were at equal risk of heart disease as judged by serum cholesterol levels. Thus the current emphasis toward finding agents that lower plasma lipid levels (antihyperlipidemic agents) is based on the association between hyperlipidemia and an increased risk to IHD.

Ischemic heart disease usually involves a slow, subtle formation of atherosclerotic plaques leading to blockage of coronary arteries. The plaques develop gradually over a period of many years and contain an accumulation of smooth muscle cells from the arterial wall, lipids, especially cholesterol, and calcium (22–25). Epidemiological studies have shown that hypercholesterolemia is an independent risk factor; for example, data from the Framingham, Albany, and Minnesota studies show that the heart attack rate in men aged 35–44 was 5 times greater when the serum cholesterol exceeded 265 mg-% than when serum cholesterol was under 200 mg-% (26). Both the Framingham (27) and Minnesota (28) studies showed that the risk is an exponential function of the serum cholesterol levels, the incidence of the disease being proportional to the 2.66th (27) to the 3.4th (28) power of serum cholesterol level.

The significance of elevated triglyceride levels (hypertriglyceridemia) in IHD is still the subject of controversy in spite of the time that has elapsed since the association was first reported (29–31). Raised triglyceride levels were interpreted to be an independent risk factor in Stockholm men of all ages (32), in the retrospective Seattle survey (33), and for women over 50 but not for men in the Framingham study (13). However in a number of other studies (34–38), such as the 8.5 year Western Collaborative Group Study (36) and the Hawaii-Japanese Study (37), no independent effect of triglycerides could be detected. The consensus is that hypertriglyceridemia is not firmly established as an independent risk factor, mainly because of the problem in population studies in correcting for the degree of hypercholesterolemia that accompanies endogenous hypertriglyceridemia. The latter appears to be a risk factor in IHD only when accompanied by high cholesterol values.

Lipids, by definition, are insoluble in aqueous media, and a number of different natural systems exist that solubilize them in aqueous compartments, such as bile, intestinal contents, and plasma. Except for the unesterified fatty acids, virtually all the plasma lipids, including cholesterol, cholesterol esters, triglycerides, and phospholipids, interact with protein to form soluble lipoproteins, and it is in this form that they circulate (39–44). These lipoproteins are complex macromolecules composed of lipid noncovalently bound with protein and carbohydrate. The combination serves not only to solubilize but also to stabilize the lipid moiety in its transport through the plasma. The plasma lipoproteins are classified on the basis of their flotation in salt solutions in the ultracentrifuge and their electrophoretic mobilities. The four major fractions are the chylomicrons, the very low density (VLDL or pre-β), the low density (LDL or β) and the high density (HDL or α) lipoproteins. Elevations in plasma cholesterol are usually associated with increased concentrations of LDL, the lipoprotein particularly rich in cholesterol, elevations of endogenously derived plasma triglycerides are usually due to an increase in VLDL. A number of reviews have defined the various clinical hyperlipoproteinemias, types I–V (40, 45, 46).

2 TREATMENT

Diet and drug therapy are the usual methods employed to reduce plasma lipid levels. For patients who either are refractory or find an altered diet or drug therapy of limited value, such as patients with heterozygous or homozygous familial hypercholesterolemia, more heroic and drastic intervention procedures have been used. Such procedures include partial ileal bypass (47), terminal portacaval shunt (48), intravenous hyperalimentation (49), plasma exchange (50), extracorporeal affinity chromatography using agarose beads (51), and complete biliary diversion (52). Reduction of LDL cholesterol with the plasma exchange and affinity chromatography techniques is thought to be best achieved when these procedures are used in conjunction with drug treatment.

3 DIET THERAPY

Worldwide opinion leaders agree that there is a connection between diet and the development of IHD and that there is sufficient evidence to recommend a moderate change in the diet of the general population (53). In fact diet therapy is the basic treatment for hyperlipoproteinemia (54–57). Since hyperlipidemic patients tend to be overweight, the primary objectives of diet therapy are to reduce weight and to lower plasma lipids. Specific diets for each type of hyperlipoproteinemia are now available (56, 58, 59). The major dietary changes that are indicated for hyperlipoproteinemic patients are weight reduction, and restriction of dietary cholesterol, saturated fat, and carbohydrate, concomitant with an increased consumption of polyunsaturated fat. Which of these changes is emphasized for an individual patient depends on the lipid abnormality involved. A number of clinical dietary trials (1, 47, 60–65) carried out over the last decade have shown that diet therapy can reduce both plasma cholesterol and triglycerides by 10–20% and 30–40%, respectively. Dietary management under rigorous experimental design, such as metabolic ward studies using orally administered liquid-formula feeding, is capable of lowering plasma lipids by even greater amounts (66). Experience has shown, however, that maintaining lowered lipid levels by dietary measures alone is difficult because of poor adherence to diets over a period of years.

4 DRUG THERAPY

Antihyperlipidemic drugs are indicated when lipid abnormalities have failed to respond to adequate diet treatment, or when the patient cannot faithfully adhere to the particular diet regimen. In clinical practice drugs and diet are used simultaneously (54, 57, 67). That none of the current antihyperlipidemic agents is useful in all types of hyperlipidemia is not surprising, since hyperlipidemia is a manifestation of a number of heterogeneous dysfunctions, all differing in clinical profiles, prognosis, and responsiveness to therapy. Antihyperlipidemic agents have been reviewed extensively (57, 68–99), mainly from the viewpoint of clinical medicine.

5 CLOFIBRATE

Clofibrate (35.**1**), the ethyl ester of an aryloxyalkanoic acid, is the most widely used antihyperlipidemic agent. Its discovery in 1962 (100) followed from the observation in 1953 (101) that derivatives of

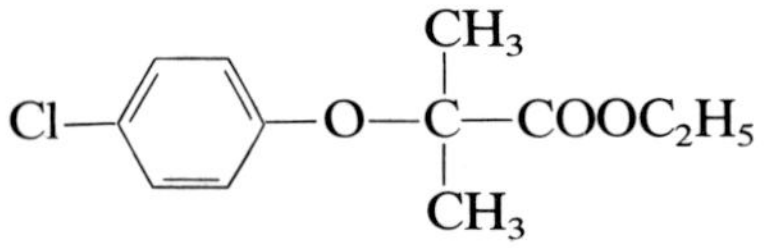

$$Cl-C_6H_4-O-C(CH_3)_2-COOC_2H_5$$

35.**1**

phenylacetic acid produced plasma cholesterol depressions both in the rat and in man. The structure-activity relationship studies of the phenyl- and phenoxyacetic acids that led to clofibrate have been reviewed (68, 69). Despite extensive studies in animals and man, the antihyperlipidemic mode of action of clofibrate is still not completely understood (57, 81–83, 86, 88, 92–95, 97, 98). Clinically it is mainly effective in reducing endogenous triglycerides of VLDL, with much less effect on plasma cholesterol and LDL levels. Because clofibrate is primarily a *hypotriglyceridemic agent*, any proposed mechanism of action should attempt to explain that relative specificity of action. One view is that the primary effect of clofibrate is to cause a net inhibition of hepatic triglyceride synthesis, leading to reduced hepatic triglyceride output. It has been suggested (102) that this follows from the increased rate of synthesis of hepatic mitochondrial α-glycerophosphate dehydrogenase. The enhancement of this enzyme leads to a reduction in the availability of precursor α-glycerophosphate for the synthesis of triglyceride. Another view is that clofibrate increases the removal rate of triglyceride-rich serum lipoproteins by increasing lipoprotein lipase activity (102).

5.1 Derivatives of Clofibrate

Clinical reports have appeared on other esters and derivatives of clofibric acid, the free acid and active agent of clofibrate. These include *alufibrate* (35.**2**) (103) the aluminum salt, and two esters, *simfibrate* (CLY-503, 35.**3**) (104), and *clofibride* (MG. 46, 35.**4**) (105). These derivatives appear to have the same clinical profile as clofibrate; their main effect is to reduce

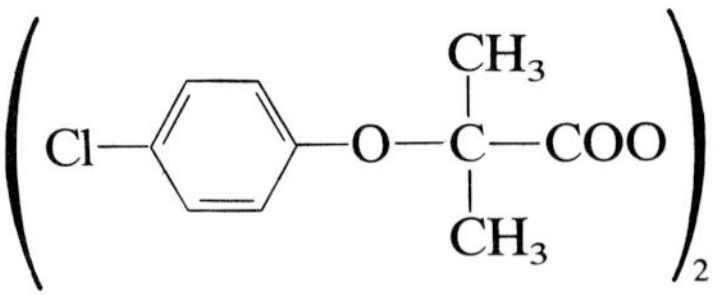

	R
35.2	AlOH
35.3	$CH_2CH_2CH_2$

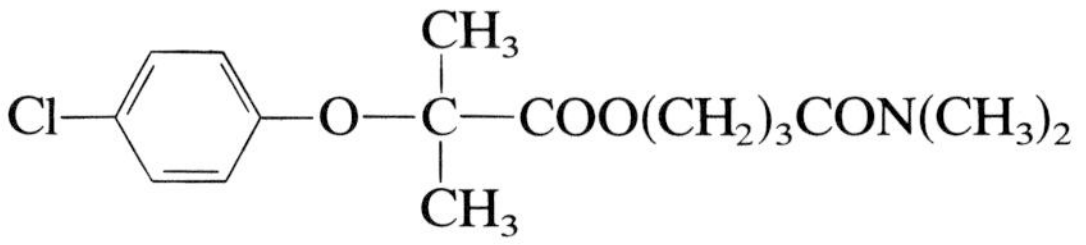

35.4

plasma triglycerides rather than cholesterol levels. Alufibrate and simfibrate give lower plasma levels of clofibric acid than either clofibrate or clofibride (104, 106).

5.2 Analogs of Clofibrate

Since the discovery of clofibrate, an almost endless array of analogs, some structurally quite similar and others quite novel, has been prepared. This worldwide effort to develop more potent and effective agents is logical in view of the relative safety and good toleration of clofibrate in more than a decade of clinical experience. These analogs appear to be qualitatively quite similar to clofibrate with regard to their antihyperlipidemic activity and also their ability to cause liver enlargement (hepatomegaly) in rats. Although a number of them showed high promise in early clinical studies in reducing LDL-cholesterol, unfortunately none has yet passed the current demands of a superior safety profile in animals and man, as well as having clinical advantages over clofibrate. Hepatotoxicity in animals and man has been a frequent finding among these compounds and appears to have been at least partially responsible for the failure of many otherwise attractive agents.

Clofibrate analogs are discussed in two categories: those that have been subjected to clinical evaluation, and those that have not.

5.2.1 CLOFIBRATE ANALOGS CLINICALLY EVALUATED. Clinical reports have appeared on a number of analogs of clofibrate; these compounds, listed in Table 35.1, include *nafenopin* (Su-13,437, 35.**5**), SaH 42-348, (35.**6**), *methyl clofenapate* (ICI-55, 695, 35.**7**), *halofenate* (MK-185, 35.**8**), GP-45,699 (35.**9**), HCG-004 (35.**10**), *procetofene* (LF-178, 35.**11**), *bezafibrate* (BM-15,075, 35.**12**), *gemfibrozil* (CI-719, 35.**13**), ICI-55,897 (35.**14**), ST-9067, (OGP, 35.**15**), and BL-J433 (35.**16**).

Nafenopin (Su-13,437, 35.**5**) is more potent than clofibrate in lowering cholesterol levels in rats (107). It has been reported (108–110) to have a greater cholesterol lowering effect than clofibrate in man, but others have been unable to confirm this (111, 112). The main effect of nafenopin is to reduce plasma triglyceride levels (76, 83, 85, 92). But long-term hepatotoxicity in man has been reported (113), and the development of liver pathology in long-term

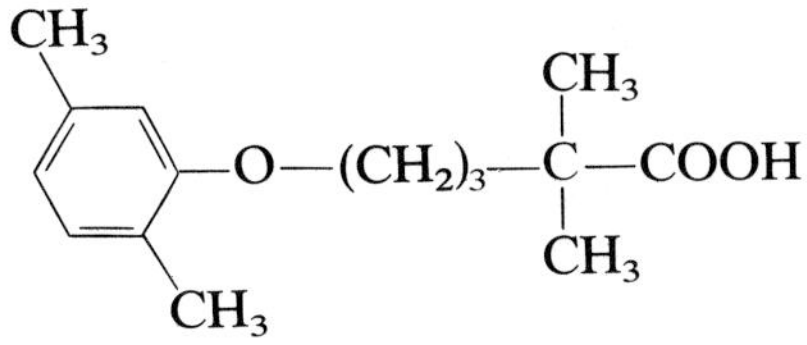

35.**13**

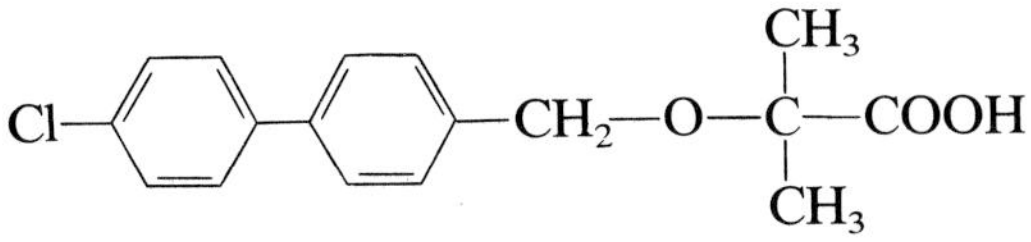

35.**14**

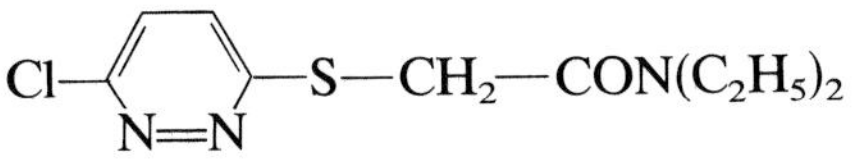

35.**15**

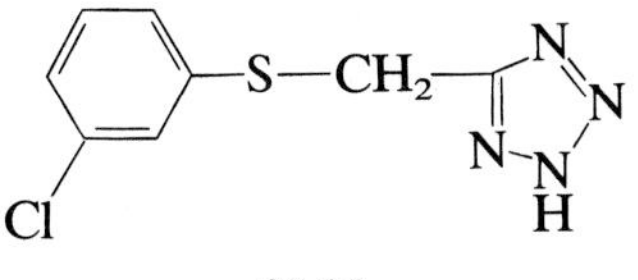

35.**16**

Table 35.1 Clofibrate Analogs That Have Been Clinically Evaluated

$$A-C_6H_4-O-C(R_1)(R_2)-COOB$$

Compound Number	NAME	*A*	R_1	R_2	*B*
35.**1**	Clofibrate	Cl	CH_3	CH_3	CH_2CH_3
35.**5**	Nafenopin, Su-13,437	(tetrahydronaphthyl)—	CH_3	CH_3	H
35.**6**	SaH 42-348	Cl	$Cl-C_6H_4-O$	H	—(piperidyl)NCH_3
35.**7**	Methyl clofenapate	$Cl-C_6H_4-$	CH_3	CH_3	CH_3
35.**8**	Halofenate, MK-185	3-CF_3	$Cl-C_6H_4-$	H	$CH_2CH_2NHCOCH_3$
35.**9**	GP-45,699	C_6H_5	C_5H_{11}	H	H
35.**10**	HCG-004	$Cl-C_6H_4-O$	CH_3	H	H
35.**11**	Procetofene, LF 178	$Cl-C_6H_4-C(=O)$	CH_3	CH_3	$CH(CH_3)_2$
35.**12**	Bezafibrate, BM 15,075	$Cl-C_6H_4-C(=O)NHCH_2CH_2$	CH_3	CH_3	H

animal studies prompted the withdrawal of this agent from clinical studies (114–116). Like clofibrate, nafenopin causes liver enlargement in rodents, which is accompanied by an increased proliferation of peroxisomes (microbodies) in liver cells. It has been suggested that peroxisome proliferation and hepatomegaly may be related to the mechanism by which these agents induce lipid lowering effects (115), although on short-term administration clofibrate has been shown to reduce plasma lipid levels in rats without affecting liver size (102).

SaH 42-348 (35.**6**) was found to be more active than clofibrate in the rat (117) and was reported to be more effective than clofibrate in reducing cholesterol levels in man (109). It has a plasma half-life of about 3 weeks (118). Elevations in lactic dehydrogenase (LDH) and glutamic oxalacetic transaminase (SGOT) have been observed with SaH 42-348 (119).

Methyl clofenapate (ICI-55,695, 35.**7**) appeared to satisfy the objective of developing a more potent analog, since it produces greater depressions of LDL and VLDL levels in man than does clofibrate (120–122). However, it was withdrawn from clinical studies because of hepatotoxicity in mice and rats during long-term studies (121, 122). The free acid, clofenapic acid, has an exceptionally long half-life in man of 30–40 days compared to 12 hr in the case of clofibric acid (120).

Halofenate (MK-185, 35.**8**) is a more potent clofibrate analog (123) that has been characterized by many reports (76, 83, 88, 92, 93, 124–128) as a clinically effective triglyceride lowering agent with little effect on cholesterol levels. However in one study it did lower cholesterol in a substantially higher proportion of patients than expected (129). In addition, it is significantly more effective than clofibrate in lowering serum uric acid levels (127, 130). It is distinguished from the other aryloxyalkanoic acids in being effective for both hypertriglyceridemia and hyperuricemia. Halofenate is highly protein bound and displaces thyroxine from thyroid binding globulin and other plasma proteins in man.

In one clinical study *GP-45,699* (35.**9**) reduced both cholesterol and triglycerides; in two other studies, however, cholesterol levels fell but triglyceride levels were elevated (131–133). This rebound phenomenon, whereby triglyceride levels tend to surpass starting values, is associated with an increase in plasma triglyceride turnover (131), however plasma triglycerides do return to normal after discontinuing therapy. GP-45,699 was temporarily withdrawn from clinical trials because of a fall in circulating leucocytes and impairment in liver function tests (131, 133).

HCG-004 (35.**10**) reduces serum cholesterol and triglyceride levels in normal and hyperlipidemic rats. As with clofibrate, liver enlargement is observed after high doses have been administered for several days. Liver cholesterol and triglyceride concentrations are also depressed. HCG-004 is more effective in reducing lipid levels than nafenopin in obese mice and clofibrate in fructose- or triton-induced hyperlipidemic rats. In normal rats it is 10.5 times more potent than clofibrate in lowering cholesterol and 26 times more in lowering triglyceride levels (134). Clinical trials indicate that it is less effective than clofibrate in reducing cholesterol levels, with its main effect on HDL cholesterol and only moderate influence on LDL cholesterol (133). Reducing HDL levels is probably a less than desirable effect in view of the recent evidence that HDL exerts a protective effect against the development of IHD (37, 135, 136). HCG-004 was withdrawn from clinical trials because of allergic skin reactions (133).

The structure-activity relationships leading to *procetofene* (LF-178, 35.**11**) reveal that replacement of the 4-chloro substituent of clofibrate by the 4-chlorobenzoyl moiety greatly enhances antihyperlipidemic activity in normal and triton-treated rats (137). Other acyl groups, aliphatic and alicyclic, as well as benzoyl substituted by 3-chloro or by dichloro, abolish activity. At 100 mg/kg, procetofene produces total lipid depressions twice those seen with clofibrate at 300 mg/kg. It is active, whereas clofibrate is not, in the senescent, dietary, and triton-hyperlipidemic rat, possibly indicating a somewhat different lipid lowering profile (138). However procetofene produces the increase in liver weight in rats that is typical of the aryloxyalkanoic lipid lowering agents. Procetofene is more potent than clofibrate in man in reducing LDL cholesterol and VLDL triglycerides at doses ranging from 200–400 mg/day. It was well tolerated and effective in a multicenter trial in which a mixed hyperlipidemic population was treated up to 12 months (139), suggesting potential value in treating diet-resistant hypercholesterolemic and hypertriglyceridemic patients. An unexpected and unwanted elevation in placelet count was observed in another study (140).

Bezafibrate (BM-15,075, 35.**12**) is 20 times more potent than clofibric acid in male rats in lowering cholesterol and triglyceride levels. Fructose-induced hypertriglyceridemia and triton-induced hypercholesterolemia are suppressed by 35.**12**. In human studies it is most effective in decreasing VLDL triglyceride and cholesterol levels, and it is effective in all types of hyperlipoproteinemia. This compound is somewhat more active than clofibrate as a hypotriglyceridemic agent. Bezafibrate decreases LDL levels in patients with elevated cholesterol to the same degree as clofibrate (141).

Gemfibrozil (CI-719, 35.**13**) is not a phenoxyacetic acid but a phenoxyvaleric acid. It is 10 times more effective than clofibrate in reducing serum triglyceride values in animals but has little effect on serum cholesterol levels (142). In hypertriglyceridemic patients it depresses levels of VLDL, leading to lowered plasma triglyceride and cholesterol. It decreases triglyceride turnover, free fatty acid (FFA) flux, and VLDL β-apoprotein turnover (143). In hypercholesterolemic patients it reduces cholesterol levels by 14% (142). The metabolism of gemfibrozil in laboratory animals has been described (144). A symposium has detailed the structure activity relationships, animal evaluation, and clinical studies with 35.**13** (145). In man gemfibrozil is effective particularly in lowering triglycerides, and in this respect it appears to be equal to clofibrate (142, 145).

ICI-55,897 (35.**14**), a benzyloxyalkanoic acid, resembles clofibrate and methyl clofenapate (35.**7**), both aryloxyalkanoic acids, in structure. Surprisingly, however, ICI-55,897 elevates cholesterol levels by 15% and LDL levels by 20%, producing only a 9% lowering of VLDL concentrations (146). These anomalous effects point out the difference in biological activity that sometimes arises from a seemingly subtle structural change.

ST-9067 (OGP 35.**15**) is a heterocyclic thioalkanoic amide that bears a structural resemblance to clofibrate. This choleretic agent (147) produces significant reductions in plasma cholesterol and triglyceride levels in man (148). No serious side effects have been noted during clinical evaluation of the choleretic and antihyperlipidemic effects of ST-9067 (148, 149).

BL-J433 (35.**16**) is the most active in a series of 5-aryloxyalkyl-, 5-arylthioalkyl-, and 5-anilinoalkyltetrazole analogs of clofibrate (150). Although it is comparable to clofibrate in rats, BL-J433 was not effective in lowering either serum cholesterol or triglyceride levels in two clinical studies (151).

5.2.2 CLOFIBRATE ANALOGS LIMITED TO ANIMAL EVALUATION. Despite reports that a number of other clofibrate analogs are quite effective antihyperlipidemic agents in laboratory animals, clinical evaluation of lipid lowering effects has not been described.

Somewhat akin structurally to SaH 42-348 (35.**6**) but cyclized by a methylene bridge, *treloxinate* (35.**17**), has a dioxocin ring structure. In rats it is 8 times more potent than clofibrate in reducing plasma cholesterol and 30 times as potent in reducing triglycerides. It affects only triglycerides in Sprague-Dawley rats but both triglycerides and cholesterol in Wistar rats. In rats, treloxinate and its analogs have a greater hypotriglyceridemic than hypocholesterolemic effect. Hepatomegaly similar to that observed with clofibrate occurs in treloxinate-treated rats. Treloxinate also reduces LDL-cholesterol in hypothyroid dogs (152, 153).

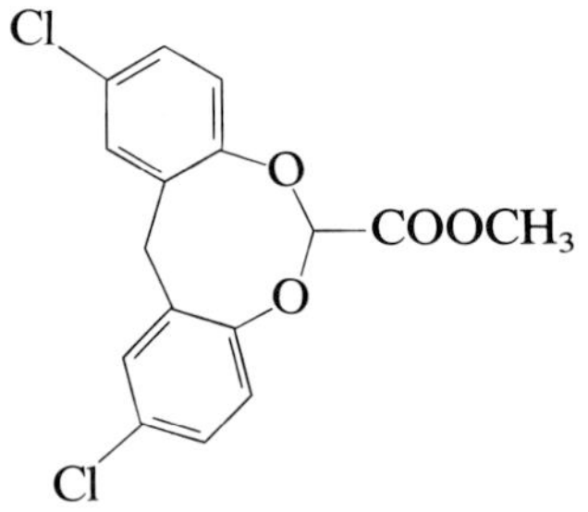

35.**17**

S-8527 (35.**18**) is 20–30 times as potent as clofibrate in reducing serum cholesterol and triglyceride levels in the rat (154, 155). At higher but not at lower doses it induces hepatomegaly, as well as histological and electron microscopic changes similar to

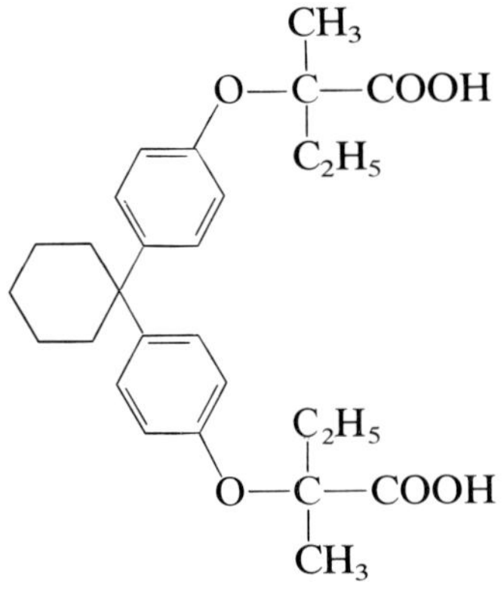

35.**18**

those observed with clofibrate (156). It has been suggested that 35.**18** lowers triglycerides (157) by inhibiting triglyceride synthesis in the liver and lowers cholesterol (158) by inhibiting hepatic lipoprotein synthesis and/or secretion.

WY-14,643 (35.**19**), a heterocyclic thioalkanoic acid (159) structurally related to ST-9067 (35.**15**), is 60 times as potent as clofibrate in lowering cholesterol in hypercholesterolemic rats (160). This agent has only a slight effect on serum cholesterol of

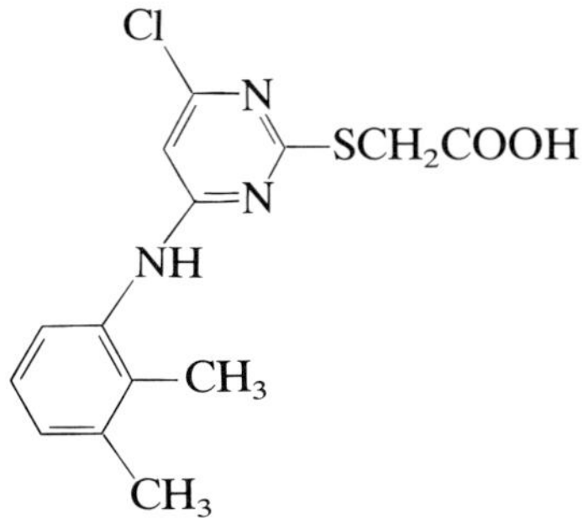

35.**19**

normal rats. Like clofibrate, it induces liver enlargement and peroxisome proliferation in liver cells. Members of a series of analogs that show no antihyperlipidemic activity fail to induce hepatomegaly and peroxisome proliferation (160), further supporting a mechanistic link between lipid lowering and hepatomegaly and peroxisome proliferation. WY-14,643 increases plasma cholesterol in female monkeys (161).

AT-308 (35.**20**) was found to be the most active (162, 163) agent from a series of heterocyclic 1,2,4-oxadiazole analogs of

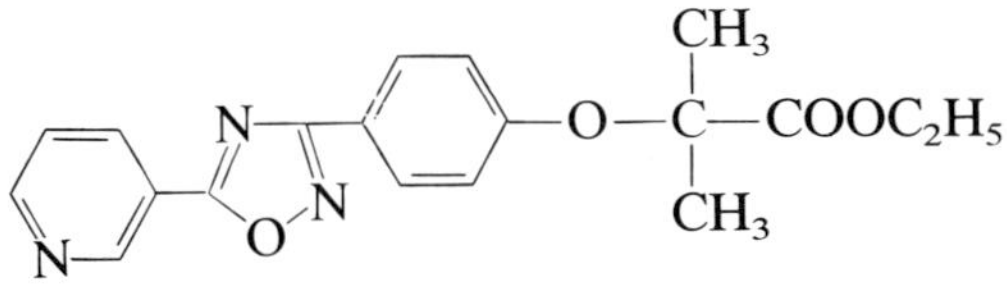

35.**20**

methyl clofenapate (35.**7**). It reduces cholesterol levels in normal and hypercholesterolemic rats (164); but unlike clofibrate it has no effect on plasma triglycerides, suggesting that this agent reduces plasma cholesterol selectively (165). AT-308 increases liver weight (164).

The absorption and disposition of the antihyperlipidemic agent *ciprofibrate* (WIN-35,833, 35.**21**) in rats, monkeys, and man

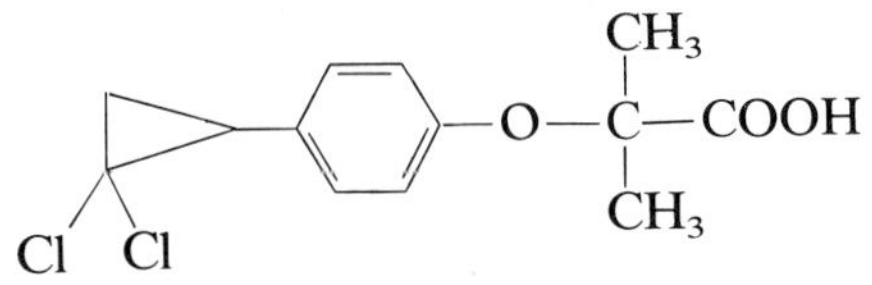

35.**21**

indicate that it is rapidly absorbed and extensively bound to human plasma protein (166).

Structure-activity relationships of cyclic aryloxy acids related to clofibrate including various chromans, chromanones, chromones, 1,4-benzodioxanes, 1,3-benzodiaxoles, various benzo-, dihydrobenzo-, and tricyclic benzofurans, as well as a number of non-oxygen-containing heterocyclic systems, have been extensively studied. Some compounds selectively reduce either cholesterol or triglyceride levels, others reduce both.

In the triton-induced hyperlipidemic rat model, 6-chlorochroman-2- (35.**22**) and 6-phenylchromone-2- (35.**23**) carboxylic acid ethyl esters compare favorably with clofibrate (167, 168) in hypocholesterolemic and hypotriglyceridemic activity, whereas 1,4-benzodioxane-2-carboxylic acid ethyl ester

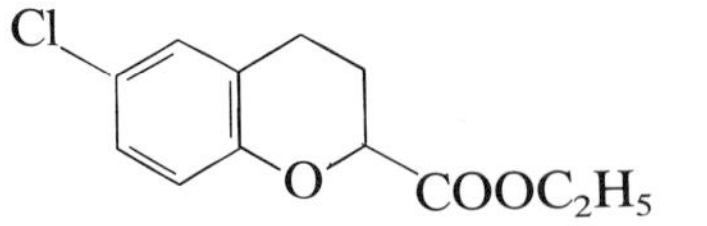

35.**22**

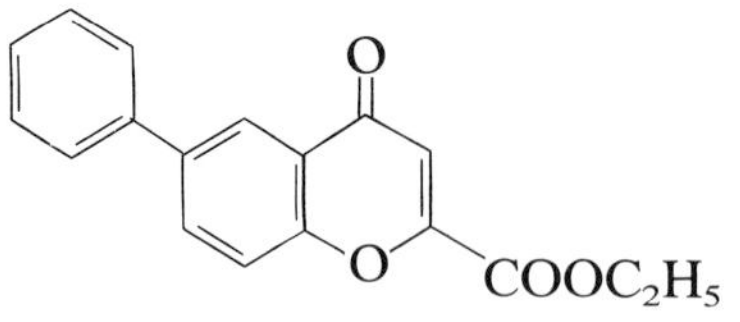

35.**23**

(35.**24**) mainly depresses elevated triglyceride levels (167). A series of 1,3-benzodioxole-2-carboxylates, such as 35.**25**, bearing structural resemblance to SaH 42-348 (35.**6**) and treloxinate (35.**17**), also possess antihyperlipidemic activity

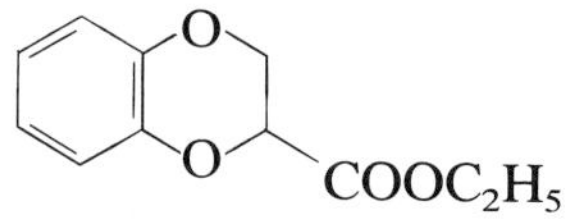

35.**24**

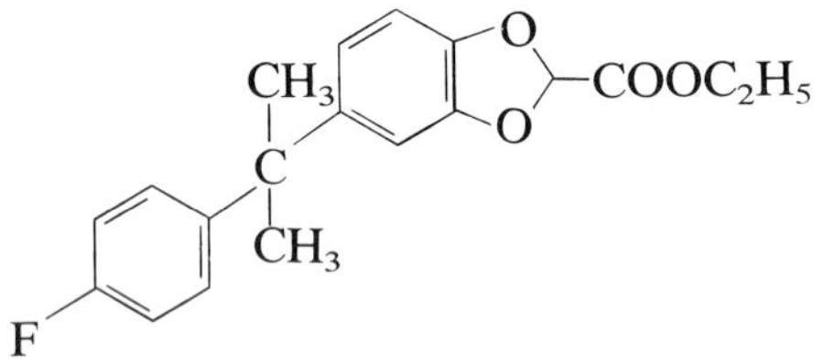

35.**25**

(169). Although 35.**25** is more effective than clofibrate in lowering both plasma cholesterol and triglyceride levels in normal rats, unfortunately the desired separation from hepatomegaly is not achieved (169). In the benzofuran, 2,3-dihydrobenzofuran, and 3(2*H*)-benzofuranone-2-carboxylates, hypocholesterolemic, hypotriglyceridemic, or both activities are observed (170, 171).

The dihydrobenzofurans (35.**26**, 35.**27**) show selective hypocholesterolemic activity (170) in the hyperlipidemic rat, whereas the benzofuran- (35.**28**–35.**31**) and 3(2*H*)-benzofuranone-2-carboxylates (35.**32**, 35.**33**) loose this selectivity (170, 171); see Table 35.2. Indeed both 35.**29** and 35.**32** are

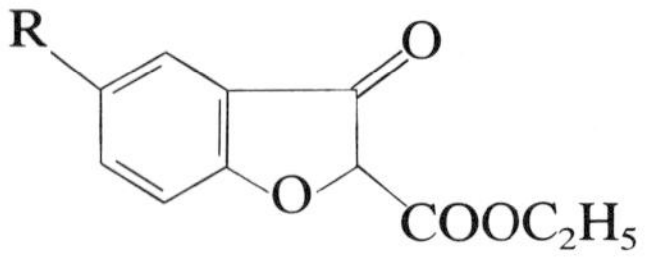

35.**32** R = Cl
35.**33** R = C_6H_5

selective against elevated triglyceride levels.

A number of tricyclic benzofurans have also been prepared and evaluated in hyperlipidemic rats. Ethyl-2-(4-dibenzofuranyloxy)-2-methylpropionate (35.**34**) is the

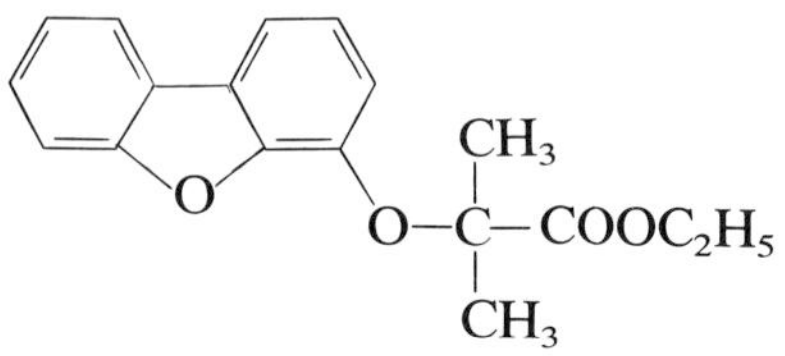

35.**34**

most effective in lowering cholesterol and triglyceride levels from a series of dibenzofuranyloxy and dibenzofuranylmethoxy compounds (172). Both tricyclic lactones 35.**35** (173) and 35.**36** (174) lower elevated triglyceride levels, however, only 35.**35** is effective in reducing

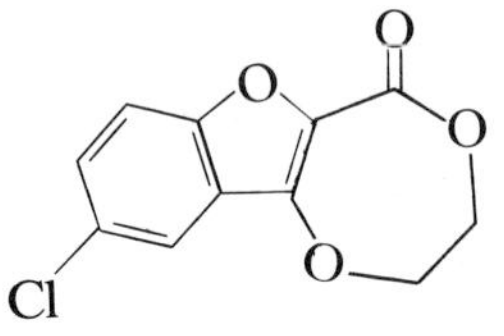

35.**35**

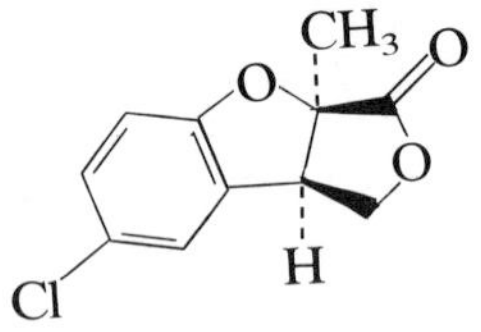

35.**36**

elevated cholesterol. A different testing model can lead to contrary findings—35.**35** in normolipidemic rats, as opposed to hyperlipidemic rats, is ineffective in lowering serum cholesterol levels (173).

Table 35.2 Benzofurans and Dihydrobenzofurans

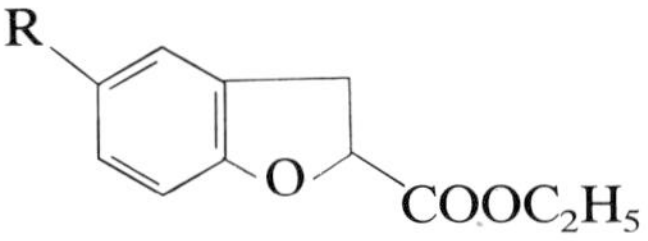

35.26 R = Cl
35.27 R = C_6H_5

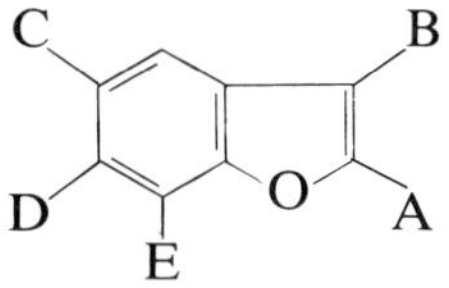

Compound Number	A	B	C	D	E
35.**28**	$COOC_2H_5$	H	Cl	H	H
35.**29**	$COOC_2H_5$	H	C_6H_5	H	H
35.**30**	C_6H_5	H	H	H	$O-C(CH_3)_2-COOC_2H_5$
35.**31**	H	C_6H_5	H	$O-C(CH_3)_2-COOC_2H_5$	H

Other acids containing certain structural features of clofibrate but in cyclized form have also been examined, including coumarilic acid (35.**37**) and such non-oxygen heterocyclic systems as

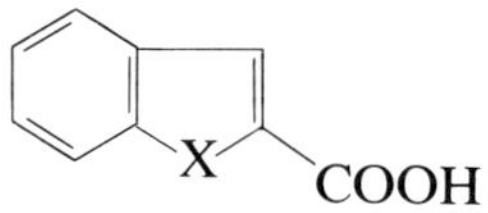

35.**37** X = O
35.**38** X = S
35.**39** X = NH

benzo[*b*]thiophen- (35.**38**) and indole- (35.**39**) 2-carboxylic acids (175). The 5-chloro analog of 35.**39** lowers plasma cholesterol in normal rats but differs from clofibrate in neither lowering triglycerides in normal rats nor reversing triton-induced hyperlipidemia. A tetrahydrocarbazole-2-carboxylic acid (35.**40**), an analog of 35.**39**, lowers serum cholesterol and triglycerides

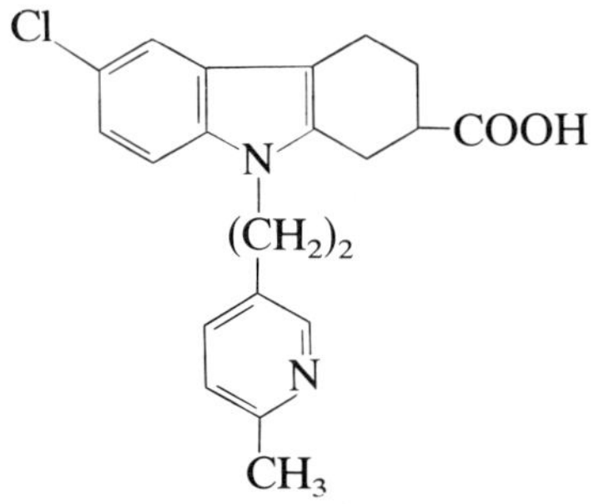

35.**40**

in normal and hyperlipidemic rats (176). At effective doses it also produces slight

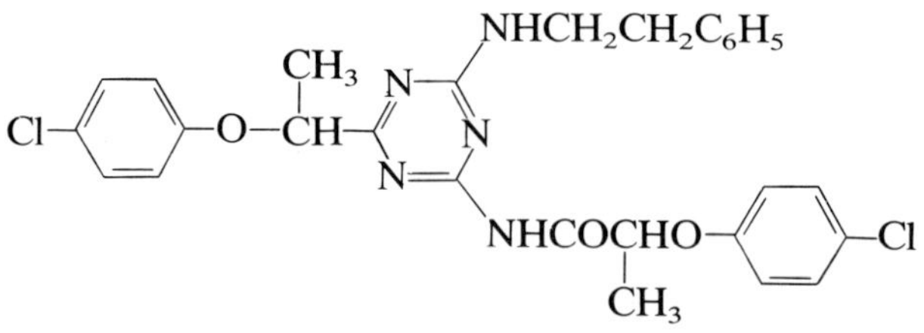

35.**41**

hepatomegaly; the agent 35.**40** is also claimed to have a mechanism of action similar to that of clofibrate. From a series of substituted aryloxy aminotriazines, 35.**41** shows moderate lipid-lowering activity (177).

A broad structural range of other aryloxyalkanoic acid structures related to clofibrate have also reported to exhibit antihyperlipidemic actiity in animals. These agents include aryloxymethyltetrazole analogs (178) of SaH 42-348 (35.**6**) and methyl clofenapate (35.**7**); heterocyclic analogs (179, 180) of methyl clofenapate and AT-308 (35.**20**); a variety of arylsubstituted derivatives (177, 180–182), including halogen, alkoxy, alkyl, aralkyl, alkene, styryl, benzyloxy, and benzoyl substitution; various α-substituted analogs (183); *urefibrate* (EGYT-1299, M-451) (184), a urea derivative of SaH 42-348; arylthio derivatives (185, 186) of clofibrate, and nafenopin (35.**5**). In addition, a wide variety of esters, amides, and salts have also been prepared (177, 181, 187, 188).

1-(Theophyllin-7-yl)-ethyl-2-(2-*p*-chlorophenoxy)-2-methylpropionate, ML-1024, an oxyalkyltheophylline ester of clofibric acid, shows favorable acute and chronic antihyperlipidemic activity as well as low toxicity in rats and minipigs (177).

The intense research effort to develop an acceptable and superior clofibrate analog that has taken place since the 1963 Buxton Symposium on Atromid (189) has so far been unsuccessful. The outcome of the clofibrate analogs still undergoing clinical evaluation is awaited with keen interest.

6 AGENTS STRUCTURALLY DISTINCT FROM CLOFIBRATE BUT HAVING MECHANISTIC OR CLINICAL SIMILARITIES

Since the discovery of clofibrate a number of antihyperlipidemic agents have been reported that are structurally dissimilar but do resemble it from either a mechanistic or a clinical viewpoint.

6.1 Tibric Acid

Tibric acid (2-chloro-5-(*cis*-3,5-dimethylpiperidinosulfonyl)benzoic acid, 35.**42**) proved to be the most potent member of a

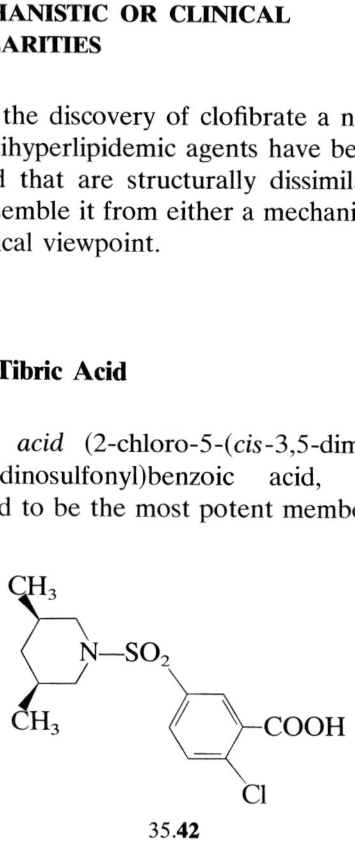

35.**42**

new structural class of antihyperlipidemic agents, the sulfamylbenzoic acids (190, 191). It is 10 times as potent as clofibrate in lowering plasma cholesterol levels in the rat, and it also lowers fasting plasma cholesterol and triglyceride levels in the dog. The lipid reductions produced by tibric acid have been tentatively attributed to increased synthesis of hepatic mitochondrial α-glycerophosphate dehydrogenase, which results in reduced concentrations of α-glycerophosphate and reduced triglyceride synthesis and secretion (192). A similar mode of action had been proposed previously for clofibrate (102). As expected, the lipid responses of tibric acid in man are quite similar to clofibrate: tibric acid is most effective in patients with elevated triglycerides, but the effect on total cholesterol is less pronounced (193–195).

The relationships of structure to antihyperlipidemic activity of other benzoic acid series have also been reported. These are the 4-alkoxy-, 4-benzyloxy- and the 4-aminobenzoates; although no mechanistic or clinical data are available for either of these series, they are included in this section because of their structural resemblance to tibric acid (35.**42**). The 4-alkoxybenzoates were prepared in an effort to circumvent the undesirable central nervous system side effects that were observed in dogs with 4-hexadecyloxybenzoic acid (35.**43**). Maximum cholesterol lowering activity in rats is seen when the 4-alkoxy

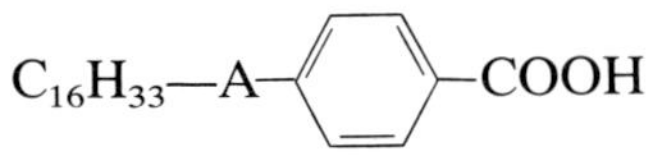

$C_{16}H_{33}$—A—C_6H_4—COOH

35.**43** A=O
35.**44** A=NH

chain contains 12–20 carbons. Alkyl chains with a chloro group enhance activity, whereas a number of other chain substituents, as well as aryl substitution, abolish activity (196). 4-Benzyloxybenzoic acid has also been shown to effectively lower cholesterol levels in male rats (197). 4-Aryloxy- and 4-benzyloxyphenylacetic acids also show antihyperlipidemic activity in rats (197). In the analogous series of 4-aminobenzoates (35.**44**), the hexadecyl substitution is the most favorable for lowering serum sterols in normal rats. Structure 35.**44** also shows antiatherogenic activity in cholesterol-fed rabbits (198).

6.2 Tiadenol

Tiadenol (fonlipol, LL-1558, 35.**45**) is a structurally unique antihyperlipidemic agent that lowers cholesterol levels in cholesterol-fed rats (199). In man 35.**45**

$HOCH_2CH_2$—S—$(CH_2)_{10}$—S—CH_2CH_2OH

35.**45**

has its most prominent effects on plasma triglyceride levels, with a considerably smaller depression on plasma cholesterol concentrations (200). It does show some effectiveness in lowering plasma cholesterol levels in patients with essential hypercholesterolemia (201, 202). Although little is known of the mechanism of action of tiadenol, it bears a number of biological and clinical similarities to clofibrate and tibric acid. The agent produces hepatomegaly and an increase in liver microbodies in rats. Furthermore, its clinical profile is similar both with respect to the type of hyperlipoproteinemic patient in which it is most effective, and to the magnitude of plasma triglyceride and cholesterol depression observed.

6.3 Gemcadiol

Gemcadiol (CI-720, 35.**46**) is a decanediol analog of tiadenol. It reduces plasma triglycerides at low doses and plasma cholesterol levels at higher doses in rats, mice, and rhesus monkeys (203). It is 10 times more effective than clofibrate in reducing triglycerides in normal rats. Like clofibrate and tiadenol, 35.**46** produces hepatomegaly in rats (203). It is effective in reducing elevated levels of cholesterol and triglycerides in hyperlipoproteinemic patients of various types (204, 205).

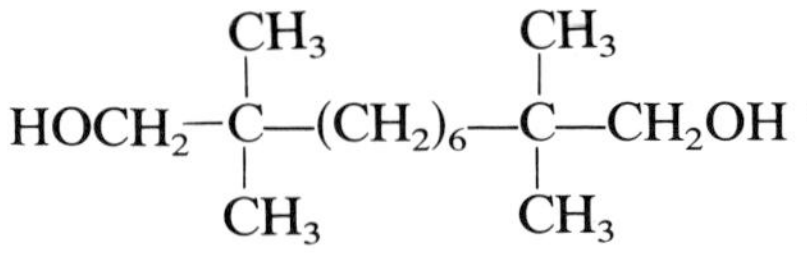

$HOCH_2$—$C(CH_3)_2$—$(CH_2)_6$—$C(CH_3)_2$—CH_2OH

35.**46**

7 AGENTS THAT INHIBIT LIPID ABSORPTION

Structurally diverse agents have been reported to decrease sterol lipid levels by inhibiting intestinal absorption of bile acids and/or cholesterol.

7.1 Bile Acid Binding Agents

An important development in antihyperlipidemic drug therapy has been the introduction of the anion exchange resins cholestyramine, colestipol, and polidexide. These resins reduce plasma cholesterol levels by binding bile acids in the small intestine, resulting in the interruption of the normal enterohepatic circulation of bile acids and enhancing their fecal excretion. In turn, the conversion of cholesterol to bile acids is enhanced and plasma cholesterol levels decrease. These agents are very effective in subjects with elevated LDL-cholesterol (type II hyperlipidemia).

7.1.1 CHOLESTYRAMINE. *Cholestyramine* (47, 57, 75, 81, 82, 86, 94, 95, 206, 207) is a high molecular weight copolymer of styrene and divinylbenzene with trimethylbenzyl ammonium groups as the ion exchange sites. The resin is hydrophilic but insoluble in water, remains unchanged in the intestinal tract, and is not absorbed. In the small intestine, the cholestyramine resin exchanges chloride ion for bile acids, forming an insoluble complex that results in an increased loss of fecal bile acids. To compensate for the interruption and diversion of the normal enterohepatic circulation of bile acids, cholesterol conversion to bile acids is enhanced. This increased rate of cholesterol catabolism is reflected in increased catabolism of LDL as the concentration of both cholesterol and LDL in serum is diminished. The action of cholestyramine resembles ileal bypass from the point of view of its effect on cholesterol metabolism (208). Increases in fecal excretion of neutral sterols are also observed (82, 87, 207). The agent is thus effective for lowering total plasma cholesterol and LDL-cholesterol levels. Reductions in cholesterol levels of the order of 15–25% have been consistently reported in various groups of type II patients (82). Cholestyramine has its main effect on LDL levels, while HDL lipids are unchanged; it is ineffective for type III, IV, and V patients, and in fact is contraindicated for such patients because it may actually elevate triglyceride levels (82, 209, 210). In type II patients a concomitant rise in VLDL can also lead to triglyceride elevations (209).

7.1.2 COLESTIPOL. An insoluble copolymer of diethylenetriamine and epichlorhydrin containing secondary and tertiary amine functionalities (211), *colestipol* appears to be quite similar to cholestyramine in mechanism of action, potency in reducing cholesterol levels, and toleration (57, 89, 206, 207, 211–219). As with cholestyramine, the decreased plasma LDL and cholesterol levels are sometimes accompanied by reciprocal increases in VLDL levels, resulting in the observed elevation in serum triglycerides (213–218). In one study thc level of VLDL returned to pretreatment levels during continued administration of the drug (217).

7.1.3 POLIDEXIDE. *Polidexide* (Secholex, DEAE-Sephadex), a nonabsorbable diethylaminoethyl derivative of a cross-linked dextran (206, 207, 220), is as effective as cholestyramine in reducing the serum cholesterol and LDL levels of patients with severe hypercholesterolemia (221–223). It significantly increases bile acid output, with only slight change in the excretion of neutral sterols, indicating slight, if any, effect on intestinal cholesterol absorption. In some studies VLDL and triglyceride levels were found to be moderately decreased (221, 224); in others, triglyceride levels were slightly elevated (222, 225) by polidexide.

7.2 Other Sterol Binding Agents

A number of other structurally different hypocholesterolemic agents have also been suggested to have a mechanism of action based on their ability to interfere with cholesterol and/or bile acid absorption in the intestine.

7.2.1 NEOMYCIN. *Neomycin*, an antibiotic that is poorly absorbed (226), appears to be as effective as cholestyramine in hypercholesterolemic (type II) patients (227). There is no significant effect on plasma triglyceride values. There is still controversy on its mechanism of action; some have suggested an alteration in the intestinal flora (228), a change in intestinal mobility (229), and formation of insoluble lipid complexes in the intestine (230, 231). Cholesterol-lowering activity in germfree animals and with nonantibiotic analogs indicates that the sterol effect observed is not dependent on changes in the intestinal flora. The failure to find a consistent increase in fecal acidic sterols in man suggests that neomycin is not a bile acid sequestering agent (229, 231). Sterol balance studies show a marked increase in fecal neutral sterol excretion, which could result from decreased cholesterol absorption. Animal studies also indicate that neomycin is not a bile acid sequestrant but affects cholesterol levels perhaps by increasing fecal excretion of neutral sterols (232).

7.2.2 SITOSTEROLS. *Sitosterols* are plant sterols that lower plasma cholesterol and LDL levels by about 10% without affecting triglycerides (57, 95). *β-Sitosterol* (35.**47**), the predominant member of this series, differs structurally from cholesterol in having a C-24 ethyl group. The sitosterols are thought to lower plasma levels of cholesterol by interfering with its absorption. The usual clinical dose of 10–20 g/day might be too high: a dose of 3 g/day reduced cholesterol absorption by 50%, and raising the dose to 9–12 g/day gave no further improvement (233). The sitosterols have always been considered to be poorly absorbed (<5%) and not to be present in the blood, but a number of cases of β-sitosterolemia have now been identified. Significant amounts of sitosterols—approximately 30%—are indeed absorbed and carried in the blood in the LDL fraction (234, 235). The development of β-sitosterolemia occurs regardless of whether plasma cholesterol levels are elevated. The C-24 methylene analog (35.**48**) decreases serum lipid levels in rats (236).

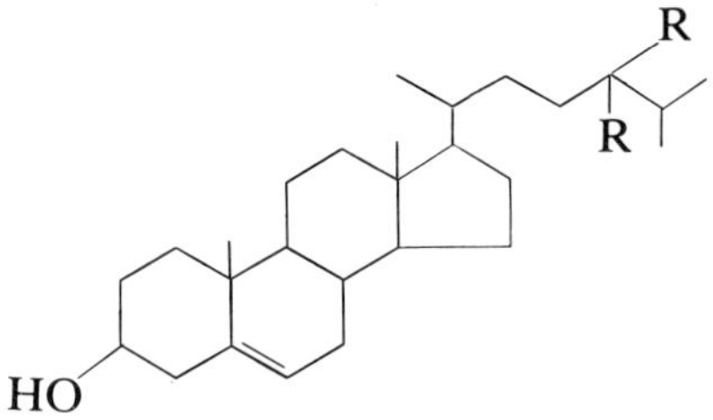

35.**47** R, R = H, C_2H_5
35.**48** R, R = CH_2

7.2.3 CHOLESTANE-3β, 5α, 6β-TRIOL. This compound (C-3-T, 35.**49**) was shown to be effective in preventing hypercholesterolemia in cholesterol-fed rabbits and chickens, and in triton-induced hyperlipidemic rats (237). Administration of 35.**49** to rats leads to an increased fecal excretion of sterols (238), whereas in pigeons an increased fecal excretion of both neutral sterols and bile acids accompanies the reduction of serum cholesterol (239). This agent inhibits cholesterol absorption through the intestinal mucosa, possibly by competing for sites of cholesterol esterification (240). A series of oxy analogs, esters

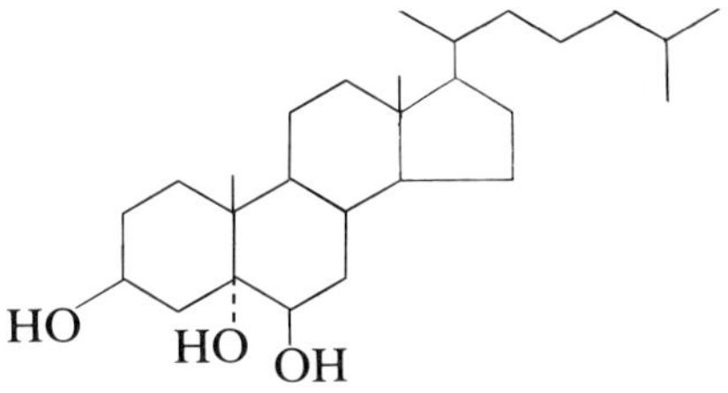

35.**49**

(241), and amino (242) derivatives has been prepared. The formation of aortic lesions in C-3-T-dosed rabbits has lessened clinical interest in the compound, however (243).

7.2.4 LINOLEIC ACID AMIDES. A series of amides of linoleic acid appears to lower lipid levels in a number of species and to prevent atherosclerosis in animals. Structure-activity studies indicate the superior activity of the *N*-cyclohexyl amide, *linolexamide* (35.**50**), and substituted *N*-phenyl analogs over the *N*-isopropyl, *N,N*-diphenyl, and the pyrrolidine derivatives (244). Structure-activity relationship delineation of compounds related to 35.**50** led

$$C_4H_9(CH_2CH{=}CH)_2{-}(CH_2)_7{-}\overset{O}{\overset{\|}{C}}NH{-}R$$

35.**50** R = cyclohexyl (linolexamide)

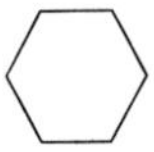

35.**51** R = $-\underset{C_6H_5}{\underset{|}{C}}HCH_3$ (AC-223)

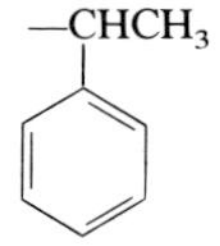

35.**52** R = $-\underset{C_6H_5}{\underset{|}{C}}HCH_2{-}C_6H_4{-}CH_3$ (moctamide, AC-485)

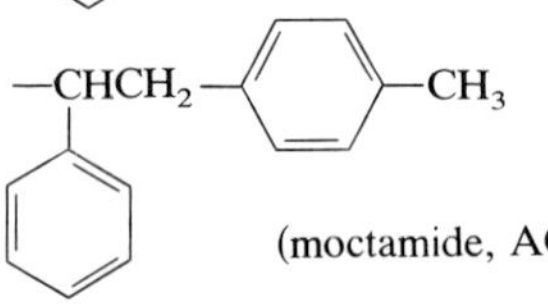

first to *N*-α-methylbenzyl linoleamide (AC-223, 35.**51**), which is more effective than 35.**50** in lowering both serum and liver cholesterol levels in cholesterol-fed rabbits. Resolution of 35.**51** shows that the (+)-isomer is superior to the DL-compound as a hypocholesterolemic agent (245). A further improvement in activity is found with *moctamide*, the (−)-*N*-α-phenyl-β-(*p*-tolyl)-ethyl amide (AC-485, (35.**52**), which is more than 5 times as potent as 35.**51** (246).

Mechanism studies with the linoleamides indicate that they inhibit cholesterol absorption (247). These agents have been extensively evaluated and found to be active in a number of different atherosclerotic animal models. They have been shown to be more effective than β-sitosterol, linoleic acid, ethyl linoleate, and safflower oil against cholesterol-induced atherosclerosis in rabbits (244). Both 35.**51** and 35.**52** have been tested in man (244, 248). At a dose of 1.5 g/day (0.5 g, t.i.d.), 35.**51** in a one year study produced a 19% reduction in plasma cholesterol levels (244). At a daily dose of 300 mg, moctamide (35.**52**) was found to be effective in inhibiting the elevation of serum cholesterol due to egg-yolk feeding (248). The absorption, excretion, and metabolism of both 35.**51** and 35.**52** have been described in animals and in man (249). More than 50% of 35.**51** and more than 75% of 35.**52** are excreted in human feces as unchanged drug.

AHR-6168, the linoleic acid amide of norfenfluramine, decreases serum cholesterol and LDL levels but increases HDL levels in a dose-dependent fashion in hypercholesterolemic rats. It does not affect triglycerides. In normal rats lipoprotein levels are not altered, but hepatic sterol synthesis is reduced (250).

7.2.5 SULFAGUANIDINE. *Sulfaguanidine* (35.**53**), a poorly absorbed sulfonamide, depresses plasma cholesterol in cholesterol-fed rats (251) and inhibits cholesterol absorption in mice and rats without affecting bile salt excretion (252). That the cholesterol lowering properties of 35.**53** are not general for sulfonamides was borne out by the inactivity of sulfanilylurea, sulfacetamide, sulfathiazole, sulfadiazine, sulfanilamide, and sulfadimethoxine. Furthermore, the effect of sulfaguanidine on cholesterol absorption is quite specific, since even minor structural modifications result in almost complete loss of hypocholesterolemic activity (253). The lipid

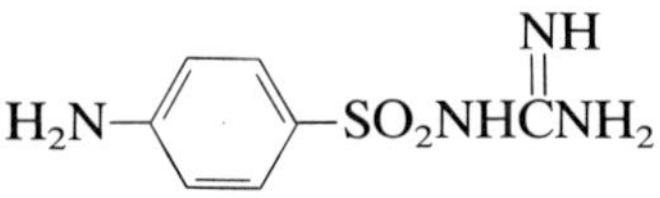

$$H_2N{-}C_6H_4{-}SO_2NH\overset{NH}{\overset{\|}{C}}NH_2$$

35.**53**

effect of 35.**53** is independent of any antimicrobial activity because inhibition of cholesterol absorption by 35.**53** occurs under germfree conditions (254).

7.2.6 POLYENE MACROLIDES. Polyene macrolide antibiotics are known to interact and produce complexes with cholesterol (255) and plasma lipoproteins (256). A number of them have been shown to lower plasma cholesterol levels in a variety of species. The original report (257) that the aromatic heptaene *candicidin*, the nonaromatic heptaene *amphotericin B*, and the nonaromatic pentaene *filipin* are effective after oral administration to dogs, was followed up by similar reports in cholesterol-fed chickens (258) and rats (259). Candicidin also was shown to produce a lower incidence of atherosclerosis in cockerels on either a cholesterol-rich or a cholesterol-free diet (260). In chickens candicidin increases the fecal excretion of cholesterol and bile acids, suggesting that the polyene macrolides lower plasma cholesterol by decreasing the intestinal absorption of both neutral and acidic sterols (261).

Candicidin also significantly reduces cholesterol absorption in other laboratory animals, including the mouse, rat, rabbit, hamster, and guinea pig (262). Low intravenous doses of amphotericin B in rats depress plasma cholesterol levels; this suggests another hypocholesterolemic mechanism (inhibition of *de novo* cholesterol synthesis has been proposed) that could be superimposed on and independent of inhibition of sterol absorption (259, 263), *Hamycin*, a heptaene macrolide antibiotic, was shown to be more effective than amphotericin B in lowering serum cholesterol levels in rats by either oral or intravenous routes (264).

7.2.7 CALCIUM. *Calcium*, administered as calcium carbonate, decreases serum cholesterol levels in both hypercholesterolemic and hypertriglyceridemic patients but is without effect on triglyceride levels. It has been suggested that calcium acts in the intestine by either binding bile acids or inhibiting cholesterol absorption (265). Calcium has also been proposed as the hypocholesterolemic factor in milk (266).

7.2.8 FIBER AND OTHER HIGH MOLECULAR WEIGHT AGENTS. A wide variety of high molecular weight materials either isolated or derived from natural sources have received wide publicity over the last few years because of their claimed usefulness as hypocholesterolemic and possibly as antiatherosclerotic agents (267). These include different dietary fibers such as lignin, wheat fiber (bran), cellulose, hemicelluloses, pectins, various gums, colloids, waxes, and a variety of other oligo- and polysaccharides. For the most part, unfortunately, the nature of the substance responsible for the cholesterol lowering effects is not known.

Some dietary fibers [i.e., remnants of plant cells that are resistant to the alimentary enzymes of man (267)] have the properties of sequestering bile acids and/or neutral sterols in the intestinal tract, thus interfering with their reabsorption and increasing their fecal excretion. It has been demonstrated that the dietary fibers with the greatest bile acid sequestering or cholesterol binding capacities are the most effective hypocholesterolemic agents. For example, cholestyramine is superior to either lignin or alfalfa as a sequestering agent (268) and is a superior cholesterol lowering agent. Wheat fiber (bran) and cellulose have very limited binding capacities and have little, if any, effect on plasma lipid levels.

There are conflicting clinical reports on the lipid-lowering efficacy of *lignin*, a polymer that originates from three phenylpropanoid monomers (269, 270); different preparations might account for these discrepant results. The preparation that is effective in man is also effective in rats, reducing serum cholesterol and increasing fecal neutral sterols without causing appreciable changes in fecal bile acids (271). *Wheat fiber* (bran), which has been evaluated in some 10 clinical studies, does not reduce plasma lipids substantially (272–274). Bran, also, was found to be ineffective in lowering cholesterol levels in animals (274).

Pectin, a complex carbohydrate polymer composed of repeating galacturonic acid units, originates primarily in the cell walls and fibrous portions of fruits, vegetables, and land plants. It reduces plasma cholesterol in man by some 12–15% and increases fecal neutral sterol and bile acid secretion (272, 275, 276). A reduction in serum LDL-cholesterol is correlated with a reduction in serum apolipoprotein-B, the main protein particle of LDL (273). *Guar gum*, a galactomannan, is slightly more effective than pectin in lowering serum cholesterol and increasing fecal bile acid output in normal individuals (272). It is also effective in hypercholesterolemic patients (277). A number of other gums have also been studied in animals and man (274, 278). In man, *psyllium seed gum*, a hydrophilic colloidal polysaccharide composed of arabinose and galacturonic acid units, produces a significant fall in serum cholesterol levels and increases fecal bile acid excretion (274, 279). *Locust bean gum*, *Konjac mannan* (280), and *carrageenan* lower plasma cholesterol levels in animals (274).

Of a variety of different legumes that have been studied, only *Bengal gram* and *blackgram* are hypocholesterolemic in man and in animals, respectively (281, 282). *Cellulose*, the linear polymer of repeating 1–4 linked D-glucose units, is the most abundant cell wall component of higher plants. It is ineffective in lowering cholesterol levels in animals and man unless very high doses are used (274). *Alfalfa* has a high saponin content and binds well with bile acids and cholesterol. The cholesterol lowering property of alfalfa in animals (283–285) has been correlated with its ability to form unabsorbable complexes with cholesterol in the intestinal lumen (286). The contrast of alfalfa and cellulose (287) can be accounted for by their respective lipid binding capacities (268). *Dextran*, a D-glucose polysaccharide, administered to man intravenously (288, 289), but not orally (289), lowers plasma cholesterol, triglycerides, and LDL.

Sucrose polyester is a noncaloric, nonabsorbable fat. These sucrose esters consist of a mixture of hexa-, hepta-, and octa- long chain fatty acids (290), and they decrease cholesterol absorption in the rat (290) and reduce total and LDL cholesterol in normal human subjects by 14 and 17%, respectively (291). The polyester appears to be less effective in hypercholesterolemic patients in one limited study (291).

The hypocholesterolemic effect of *soybean protein* (textured vegetable protein), in which vegetable protein is substituted for animal protein, is greater than that of a low cholesterol, low saturated fat diet containing an equal amount of animal protein. Significant decreases in both serum cholesterol and triglycerides were noted in type IIa and IIb patients, including some with familial hypercholesterolemia (292).

8 OTHER AGENTS CLINICALLY EVALUATED

8.1 Nicotinic Acid

The lipid-lowering activity of *nicotinic acid* was described more than 20 years ago. Since then many studies have shown it to be an effective agent for lowering triglyceride, cholesterol, VLDL, and LDL levels (47, 57, 86, 94, 95). It depresses plasma triglyceride levels within hours of administration by reducing VLDL synthesis, which precedes cholesterol and LDL depressions. Inhibition of adipose tissue lipolysis has been proposed as its mechanism of action. This effect on adipose tissue reduces the flux of free fatty acids to the liver and reduces the rate of triglyceride synthesis and decreases VLDL synthesis and secretion. This sequence explains the early fall in triglyceride and VLDL levels, but not the subsequent and delayed cholesterol and LDL depressions. Perhaps the longer half-life and slower turnover of LDL accounts for the latter observations.

A number of other mechanisms have also been proposed to explain the antihyperlipidemic activity of nicotinic acid. These include direct inhibition of hepatic VLDL synthesis, inhibition of hepatic cholesterol synthesis, increased cholesterol and/or VLDL catabolism, and activation of lipoprotein lipase leading to an enhanced clearance of chylomicrons and VLDL.

The renaissance of research on nicotinic acid as an antihyperlipidemic agent took place some 10 years ago (68, 69, 85, 92). The search for a superior analog with greater lipid lowering activity and better toleration led to several interesting compounds, the most promising being those in which the carboxyl group of nicotinic acid is altered, such as 3-pyridyltetrazole and 3-pyridylacetic acid, as well as variations of the heterocyclic nucleus, such as pyrazole and isoxazole carboxylic acids. The extensive structure-activity effort, however, failed to provide a replacement for nicotinic acid. The rapid metabolism of nicotinic acid and excretion of metabolites, and rebound in free fatty acids observed during therapy, limit its clinical usefulness. To circumvent these effects and prolong lipid lowering activity, a series of derivatives, including a polymer, a variety of esters, alcohols, ethers, and salts of nicotinic acid, was prepared and evaluated. One polymer containing about 25% nicotinic acid residues with a polysaccharide (starch) backbone, shows prolonged oral antilipolytic activity in the rat—about 6 times that of nicotinic acid (293). There is no rebound of free fatty acids.

A number of nicotinic acid esters have been prepared as prodrugs. These include pentaerythritoltetranicotinate (35.**54**), tetranicotinoylfructose (35.**55**), myoinositol

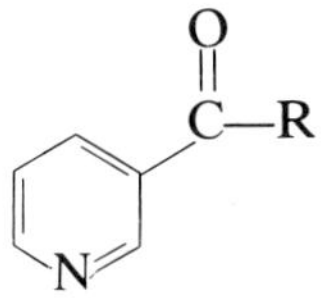

O
||
C—R
N

35.**54** R = pentaerythritol

35.**55** R = fructose

35.**56** R = myoinositol

35.**57** R = D-glucitol

(35.**56**) and D-glucitol (35.**57**) hexanicotinate, 2,2,6,6-tetra(nicotinoyloxymethyl)-cyclohexanol (35.**58**), and tocopherol-nicotinate. Administration of pentaerythritoltetranicotinate to hyperlipoproteinemic

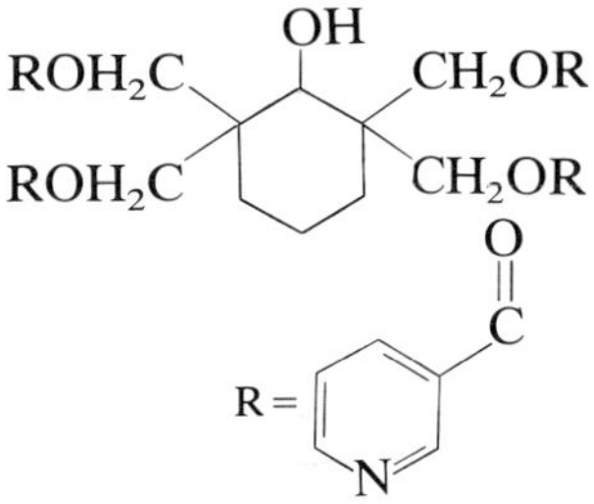

OH
ROH_2C CH_2OR
ROH_2C CH_2OR
O
||
C
R =
N

35.**58**

patients effectively reduces both cholesterol and triglyceride levels (294). The agent was claimed to cause less flushing than nicotinic acid, and there are conflicting reports on whether it produces fewer gastrointestinal side effects (295, 296). It has also been observed that 35.**54** produces elevated and prolonged blood levels (for up to 3 hr) of nicotinic acid. In 24 hr, 30% of 35.**54** was excreted in the form of nicotinic acid and nicotinic acid derivatives (297). Tetranicotinoylfructose (35.**55**) lowers free fatty acid concentration and flux, as well as triglyceride levels, in hypertriglyceridemic patients (298). It also lowers cholesterol levels (299). Myoinositol (35.**56**) and D-glucitol (35.**57**) hexanicotinate have been found to be effective in reducing both cholesterol and triglyceride levels in hypercholesterolemic and hypertriglyceridemic subjects (300, 301). Blood levels of nicotinic acid are raised for up to 24 hr after administration of 35.**56** to patients (300). 2,2,6,5-Tetra(nicotinoyloxymethyl)cyclohexanol (35.**58**) suppresses elevated levels of cholesterol and triglycerides in cholesterol-fed rabbits (302).

β-Pyridylcarbinol (35.**59**), which is oxidized to nicotinic acid *in vivo*, depresses serum cholesterol levels in hypercholesterolemic and hypertriglyceridemic subjects (303–305). It is equal to clofibrate in decreasing cholesterol levels (304), but much less consistent in affecting elevated triglycerides (303, 304). The 5-fluoro analog of 35.**59**, 5-fluoro-3-hydroxymethylpyridine (35.**60**), has been shown to

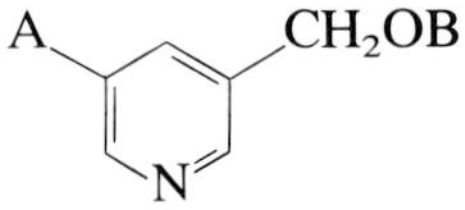

35.**59** A = H, B = H
35.**60** A = F, B = H
35.**61** A = H, B = CH_3

lower plasma free fatty acids. A significant reduction in ventricular arrhythmias of myocardial infarction patients is correlated with the fall in plasma free fatty acids, provided treatment with 35.**60** is initiated within 5 hr of onset of symptoms (306). The drug produces little skin flushing.

Structure 35.**61** is the most effective of a series of pyridylmethyl ethers in lowering both cholesterol and triglyceride levels in hyperlipidemic rats, and it is more potent than nicotinic acid. Unfortunately, however, 35.**61** is ulcerogenic (307). In a series of acetals of nicotinaldehyde, 35.**62** was

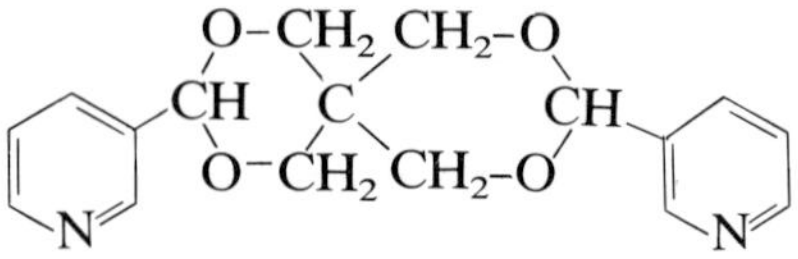

35.**62**

found to be superior to nicotinic acid in rats in lowering both elevated cholesterol and triglyceride levels, but it produces testicular degeneration in rats (308).

A wide variety of other pyridyl acids, esters, amides, and alcohols have also been tested for antilipolytic activity, but none is superior to nicotinic acid (309). Xanthinol nicotinate (35.**63**), a 7-[2-hydroxy-3-[(2-hydroxyethyl)methylamino]propyl] theophylline salt of nicotinic acid, reduces both cholesterol and triglyceride values in patients (310). Flushing and gastrointestinal intolerance is observed in only a small number of individuals. Blood levels of nicotinic acid lasting for more than 8 hr are attained in a slow release preparation (311).

8.2 Dextrothyroxine

Dextrothyroxine (35.**64**) is most effective in lowering plasma LDL and LDL-cholesterol levels (57, 94, 95). It increases cholesterol synthesis and catabolism and probably also LDL release and removal. The increased

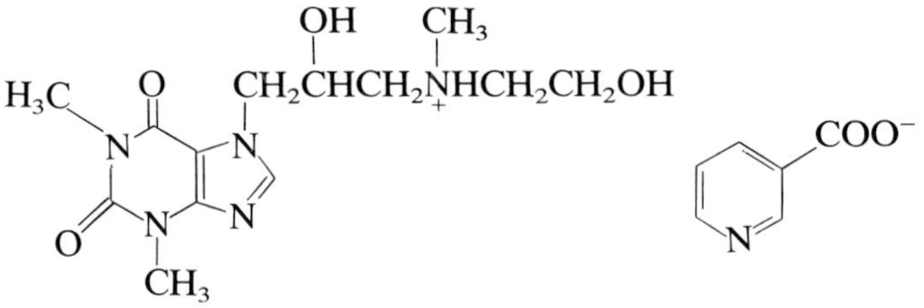

35.**63**

catabolism and removal rates are apparently greater than hepatic cholesterol synthesis and LDL release, for both neutral and acidic sterols are excreted and serum cholesterol levels are reduced. It is less effective in reducing serum triglyceride levels. Dextrothyroxine is limited in value as an antihyperlipidemic agent because of cardiac side effects, principally angina and arrhythmias (82, 94, 95). The sodium salt of 35.**64** was withdrawn from the Coronary Drug Project because of excess mortality and morbidity in patients with symptoms of cardiovascular disease (312).

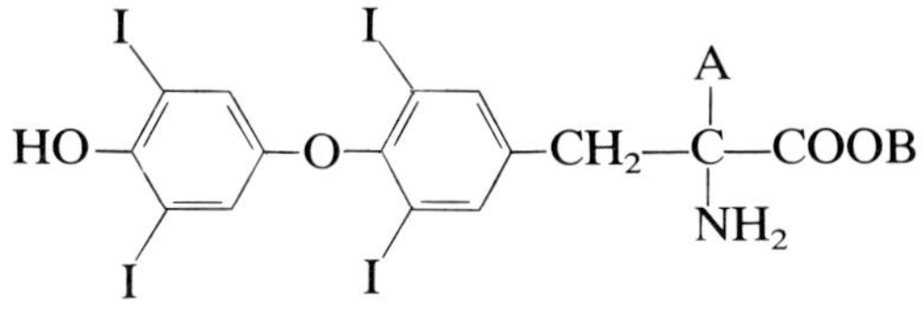

35.**64** A = H, B = H
35.**65** A = CH_3, B = CH_2CH_3

Etiroxate (CG 635, 35.**65**), the ethyl ester of α-methyl-DL-thyroxine, was prepared in an effort to dissociate the calorigenic activity from the antihyperlipidemic activity of dextrothyroxine (85). Studies in rats claim pronounced cholesterol lowering activity without corresponding effects on basal metabolic rate, heart, and thyroid gland (313). Similar claims have also been made in man. In two studies, 35.**65** reduced cholesterol levels in hypercholesterolemic patients by about 20% and it is reported that there is no significant incidence of angina (314) or changes in metabolic rate (315). Unfortunately neither study compared 35.**65** against placebo or dextrothyroxine. In another evaluation (316), however, there was no statistical difference in cardiac side effects between 35.**64**, 35.**65**, and placebo. Additional clinical studies will be required to determine whether α-methyl-DL-thyroxine ethyl ester does indeed have a more favorable side effect profile than dextrothyroxine.

8.3 Hormones and Analogs

Estrogens are no longer considered generally useful antihyperlipidemic agents, in spite of the early encouraging reports that they lower serum cholesterol and LDL levels (86, 95). Both the 2.5 and 5.0 mg/day doses were removed from the Coronary Drug Project because of lack of therapeutic effect and a suggestion of increased morbidity and mortality (317). In addition, they tend to increase the VLDL concentration, especially in hypertriglyceridemic patients. Estrogen therapy appears to have unique applicability to type III hyperlipoproteinemia, which is characterized by the presence of VLDL with abnormally high cholesterol content and abnormal electrophoretic mobility. In type III subjects the agent reduces both cholesterol and triglyceride concentrations, normalizes lipoprotein composition, and increases the catabolism of VLDL to LDL (318).

The progestational agent *norethindrone acetate* (35.**66**), used mainly in females,

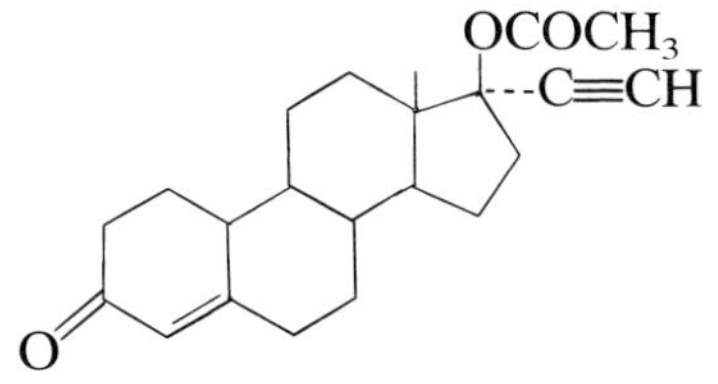

35.**66**

decreases triglyceride, VLDL, and chylomicron levels in normal and hypertriglyceridemic patients (319, 320). These lipid reductions are associated with an increase in postheparin lipolytic and triglyceride lipase activity, suggesting that 35.**66** lowers endogenous and exogenous triglycerides by increasing the activity of triglyceride lipases and improving the clearance of triglycerides from the plasma.

The anabolic steroid *oxandrolone* (35.**67**) has also been shown to be effective in lowering triglyceride levels in hypertriglyceridemic patients (320); it decreases both the chylomicron and VLDL fractions in a manner similar to that of 35.**66**. The estrogens, and

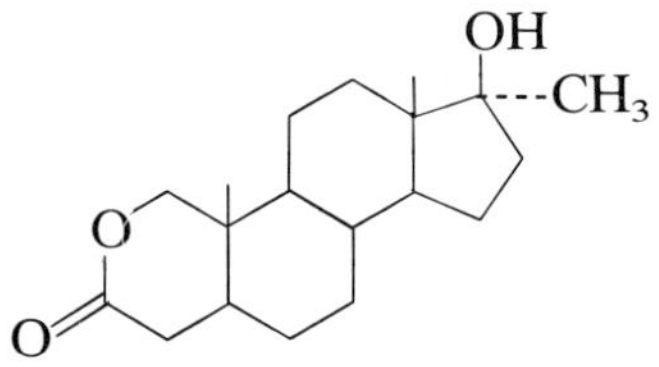

35.67

the progestational and anabolic agents cause a variety of disturbing endocrine side effects, as well as cardiac and thromboembolic problems. The antihyperlipidemic and side effect profiles of these agents have been thoroughly reviewed (57, 92, 95).

Glucagon has potent antihyperlipidemic activity in man, dog, fowl, and the rat (321, 322). Daily dosing for 10 days lowers cholesterol levels in hypercholesterolemic patients (323). It has been suggested that glucagon treatment might be attractive therapy in familial hypercholesterolemia, particularly for heterozygotes (324). *Insulin* decreases serum triglycerides in hypertriglyceridemic patients (325). In one study, administration of *human growth hormone* to hyper- and normocholesterolemic patients resulted in a decrease of serum cholesterol and an elevation of serum triglyceride and VLDL levels. In another study, no significant effect on cholesterol or triglyceride levels was observed (326). These conflicting results may be due to differences with regard to sex, age, dosage, and treatment duration among the investigations cited. *Somatostatin* reduces triglycerides in hypertriglyceridemic patients and alloxan-diabetic dogs, and, when combined with insulin, serum lipids in rats (327).

8.4 Salicylic Acids

A number of salicylic acids have antihyperlipidemic activity in clinical studies. *para-Aminosalicylic acid* (PAS, 35.**68**) was originally shown to have hypocholesterolemic activity in some patients who were under treatment for tuberculosis, and this observation was confirmed in a number of additional studies (57, 82, 95). PAS lowers serum cholesterol, triglyceride, and LDL levels in hypercholesterolemic patients (328, 329) and cholesterol, triglyceride, and VLDL levels in hypertriglyceridemic patients (330). Its mode of action has not been studied extensively, but inhibition of cholesterol absorption (328) and cholesterol and triglyceride synthesis (329) have been suggested for the action of PAS in hypocholesterolemic patients, and inhibition of VLDL production in the case of hypertriglyceridemia (330).

Salicylic acid and other salicyates are well-known inhibitors of free fatty acid mobilization. 3-Methylsalicylic acid (35.**69**)

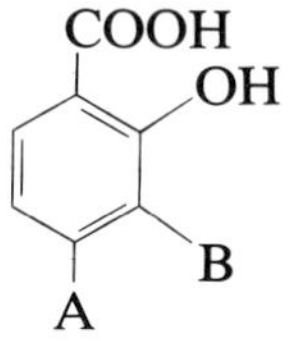

35.**68** A = NH_2, B = H
35.**69** A = H, B = CH_3

was studied because it has a longer half-life in man than salicylic acid. In rats and rabbits it decreases plasma free fatty acids, and in baboons, plasma cholesterol levels. Similarly, in man, 35.**69** decreases free fatty acids and is effective in lowering cholesterol levels in hypercholesterolemic patients (331).

5-Bromosalicylhydroxamic acid (35.**70**) reduces plasma cholesterol in man (332); of a

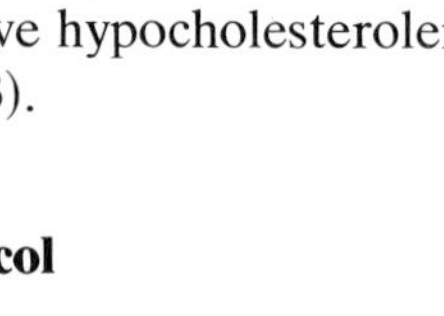

35.**70**

series of salicylhydroxamic acids, 35.**70** is the most effective hypocholesterolemic agent in rabbits (333).

8.5 Probucol

Probucol (DH-581, 35.**71**) is the most potent cholesterol lowering agent of a series of alkylidenedithiobisphenols (334). Substitution of a methyl or an isopropyl group for a *t*-butyl group on the phenolic ring, or higher substitution on the isopropylidene group, decreases hypocholesterolemic activity in mice. Clinical evaluation shows that 35.**71**

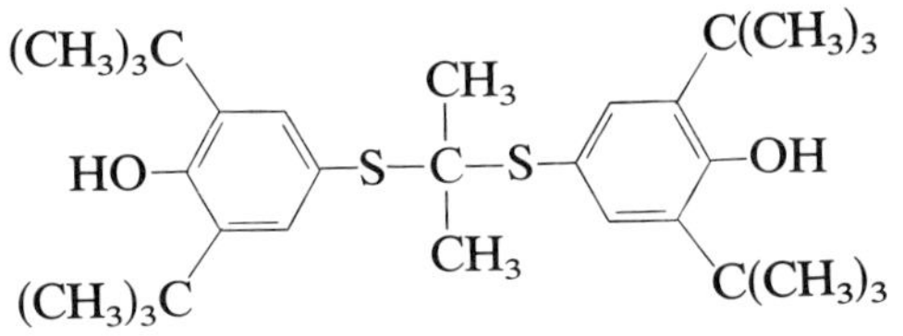

35.**71**

depresses cholesterol levels by some 15–20% in hypercholesterolemic subjects (88, 93, 335). Although a few studies with probucol have reported some plasma triglyceride reductions (336–338), for the most part the triglyceride effect has been erratic. The clinical indication for this agent is for use in hypercholesterolemic patients. It has been well tolerated in studies ranging from 2 to 7 years (339, 340). Probucol's plasma half-life in man is approximately 2 days (341); its mode of action is not known. Inhibition of cholesterol synthesis (342, 343), inhibition of cholesterol or lipoprotein transport (344, 345), inhibition of free fatty acid release from adipose tissue (345), and inhibition of cholesterol and bile acid absorption leading to an increased excretion of fecal cholesterol and bile acids (343, 346) have all been suggested as components of its mode of action.

DH-990, 2[(3,5-di-*t*-butyl-4-hydroxyphenyl)thio]hexanoic acid (35.**72**), which combines structural features of probucol (35.**71**) and clofibrate, was developed from a series of arylthioalkanoic acids. It lowers serum cholesterol levels in normal mice, rats,

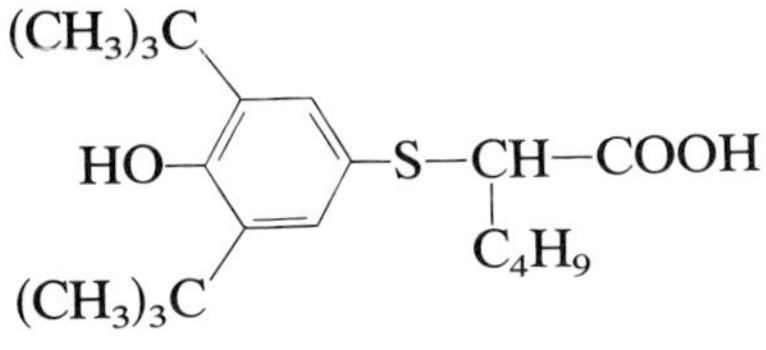

35.**72**

and monkeys (347). DH-990 differs from probucol in significantly reducing serum triglyceride levels in rats (344, 347). In one study it slightly increased liver weight in rats (347); in another it was reported to have no hepatomegalic effect (348). Structure-activity research in the arylthioalkanoic acids indicates that it is important that the thioether group be adjacent to the carboxyl and attached to a phenyl ring. A four-carbon aliphatic chain on the α-carbon is most favorable for both antihyperlipidemic activity and low toxicity. Removal of the phenolic hydroxyl or replacement of the sulfur by oxygen led to less desirable agents.

8.6 Hypoglycemic Agents

The biguanide hypoglycemic agents are effective in clinical hyperlipidemia, particularly in hypertriglyceridemia. *Metformin* (35.**73**) decreases plasma triglyceride and cholesterol

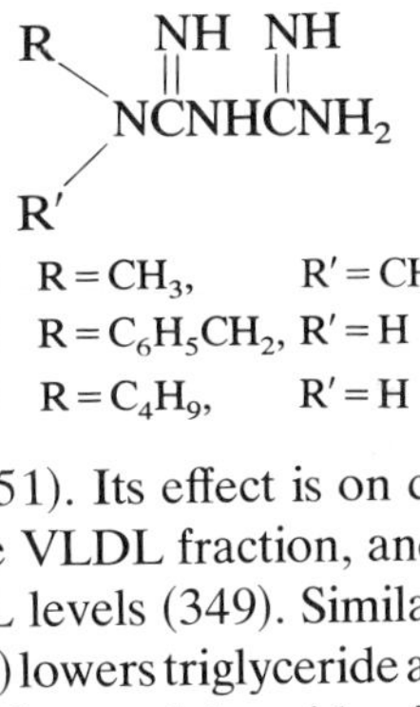

35.**73** $R = CH_3$, $R' = CH_3$
35.**74** $R = C_6H_5CH_2$, $R' = H$
35.**75** $R = C_4H_9$, $R' = H$

levels (349–351). Its effect is on cholesterol content of the VLDL fraction, and it has no effect on LDL levels (349). Similarly, *phenformin* (35.**74**) lowers triglyceride and cholesterol levels of hypertriglyceridemic patients, and its predominant effect is on VLDL (352, 353). *Buformin* (35.**75**) is less active than either metformin or phenformin in reducing elevated triglyceride levels (351). The biguanides act predominantly on VLDL metabolism by inhibiting its synthesis and/or release. In most studies the lipid effects appear to be unrelated to its hypoglycemic action and independent of changes in glucose tolerance, insulin secretion, or insulin concentration (349–351, 353). To the contrary, one study reported that basal insulin, fasting glucose, and free fatty acids are reduced after phenformin administration, and it is claimed that these effects contribute to the lowering of plasma triglyceride levels by reducing endogenous triglyceride production (352). The clinical usefulness of the biguanides, especially phenformin, is limited because of the increased incidence of lactic acidosis that is associated with this therapy (354).

There have been conflicting reports on the cholesterol and triglyceride lowering effects of the sulfonylurea hypoglycemic agents (354, 355). In some studies a small effect on plasma triglyceride levels has been noted. *Tolazamide* (35.**76**) reduces serum cholesterol in maturity-onset diabetics, independent of effects on blood glucose (354, 356).

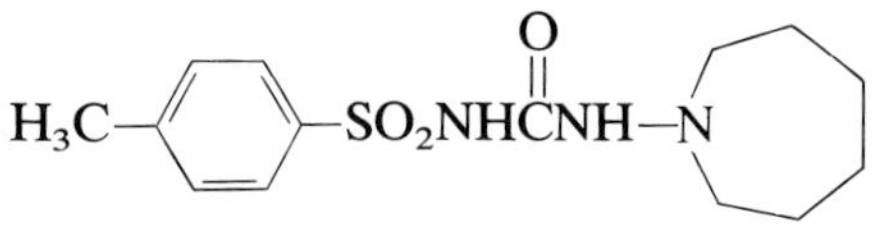

$H_3C-C_6H_4-SO_2NHC(=O)NH-N$ (azepane)

35.**76**

Sulfonylureas also depress plasma free fatty acids (357).

The hypoglycemic agent *dichloroacetate* lowers plasma free fatty acids, cholesterol, and triglycerides in nonketotic, adult-onset diabetics (358). The changes in triglycerides and cholesterol are primarily in the VLDL and LDL fractions, respectively.

8.7 Miscellaneous Agents

Chenic (*chenodeoxycholic*) *acid* (35.**77**), an effective agent for inducing dissolution of cholesterol gallstones, has been reported in a number of clinical studies to reduce significantly plasma triglyceride levels in normal and hyperlipidemic patients (359–362). The fall in triglycerides mainly reflects a fall in the triglyceride content of VLDL and is independent of the type of hyperlipoproteinemia. The magnitude of the reduction appears to correlate with the baseline triglyceride concentration. Patients with the initial highest values show the greatest response. It has been suggested that a decreased secretion of VLDL into plasma accounts for this effect (360, 362). Serum cholesterol was slightly depressed in one of these studies (360), but not in the others (359, 361). In a number of other trials no change in serum triglycerides was observed (363–365).

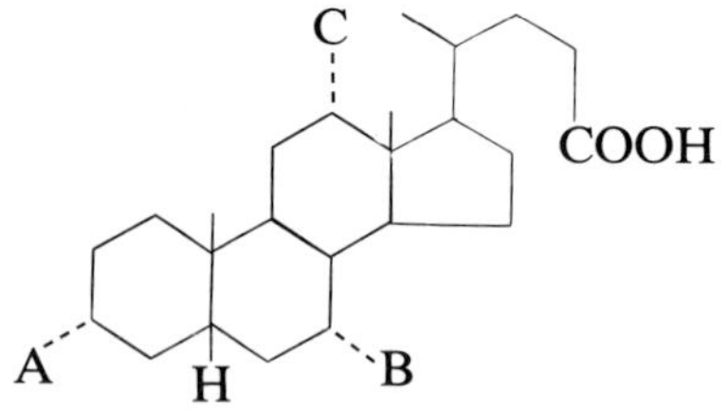

(Steroid skeleton with substituents A, B, C, H and side chain COOH)

35.**77** A, B = OH, C = H

35.**78** A, B, C = OH

35.**79** A, C = OH, B = H

Cholic and *deoxycholic acid*, two bile acids structurally related to chenic acid, have also been evaluated in human trials. In one study, cholic acid (35.**78**) reduced serum cholesterol in hypercholesterolemic patients. The hypertriglyceridemic subjects showed no cholesterol reduction and only a slight but insignificant fall in triglyceride values (366). In another study, chronic administration of cholic acid had no effect on serum cholesterol levels (367). Deoxycholic acid (35.**79**) decreased serum cholesterol levels in both normo- and hyperlipidemic patients (368, 369). The triglyceride levels were unchanged after deoxycholic acid treatment.

Eritadenine (35.**80**), earlier referred to as lentinacin or lentysine, and isolated from the edible mushroom *Lentinus*

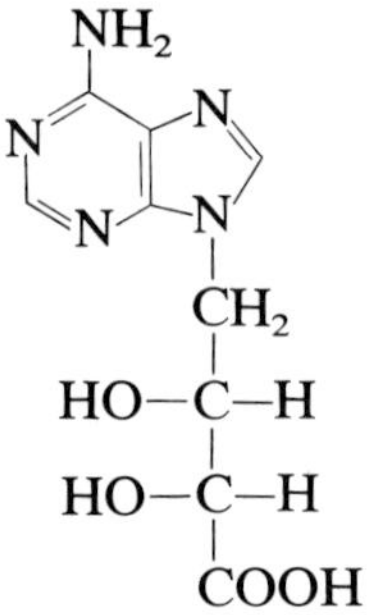

(Adenine-9-yl)–CH_2–CH(OH)–CH(OH)–COOH

35.**80**

edodes (370), is 2(*R*),3(*R*)-dihydroxy-4-(9-adenyl)butyric acid (371, 372). It is more than 10 times as active as clofibrate in lowering serum cholesterol and triglycerides in rats (373). It is less effective in the triton-induced hyperlipidemic rat. Eritadenine does not affect liver size (374), but liver lipids tend to increase (373). The agent causes a limited but significant enhancement in the rate of removal of cholesterol from the plasma compartment (375). Analog analysis has shown the importance of the side chain carboxyl and hydroxy functions, and an intact adenine nucleus (376–378). The most active analogs are monohydroxy esters, and some are 50 times as potent as 35.**80**. In a limited group of hyperlipidemic patients, eritadenine reduced both blood cholesterol and triglyceride levels (379).

Ascorbic acid (vitamin C, 35.**81**) has been a

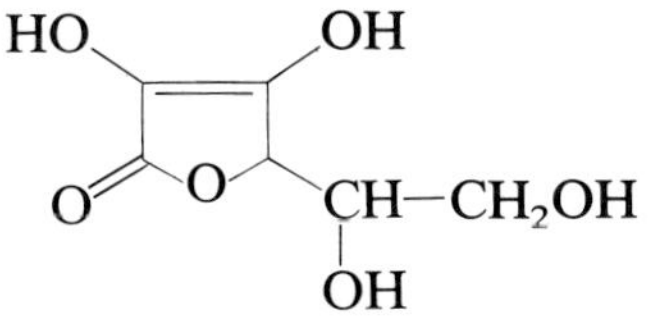

HO OH

O O $CH-CH_2OH$

OH

35.**81**

center of controversy ever since it was reported to lower serum cholesterol concentrations in hypercholesterolemic patients, some 30 years ago. Subsequently there has been little agreement on the effects of ascorbic acid in hypercholesterolemic patients; it is active in some studies but not in others (380). For example, in one study, ascorbic acid produced no significant change in plasma cholesterol, triglyceride, or lipoprotein levels in nine hypercholesterolemic subjects (381); in a second study, both serum cholesterol and triglycerides were depressed (382).

In still another study the age of the patient appeared to be important: ascorbic acid depressed cholesterol levels in young subjects, apparently free of atherosclerosis, but elevated the levels in older, atherosclerotic individuals. It was suggested that the latter observation was due to the mobilization of cholesterol from arterial tissues and would be of long-term benefit to atherosclerotic patients (383). This conclusion has been criticized because an elevation in plasma cholesterol levels is more likely to aggravate existing atherosclerosis than to be a benefit (384). It is generally agreed that ascorbic acid has no effect in subjects having normal cholesterol values (380, 385). Most of the clinical studies have been carried out with a limited number of patients, and it is unfortunate that a large controlled study in hypercholesterolemic subjects has not been reported.

Result of research on animals have also been ambiguous. There is disagreement on the effect of ascorbic acid in rabbits (386). It depresses serum cholesterol levels in hypercholesterolemic and hypothyroid rats (386, 387) but has no significant effect in primates (386). The hypocholesterolemic activity observed in some studies has been attributed to the formation of ascorbic acid-2-sulfate, claimed to be a requisite intermediate for cholesterol excretion (388). Others have suggested that the concentration of ascorbic acid in the liver, which is correlated with the oxidation of cholesterol to bile acids, is of greater importance (389, 390).

780SE (35.**82**) bears structural resemblance to the anorexigenic agent fenfluramine; it has a more pronounced effect on serum triglycerides in hyperlipidemic and obese hyperlipidemic rats than either clofibrate (35.**1**) or tiadenol (35.**45**). Furthermore,

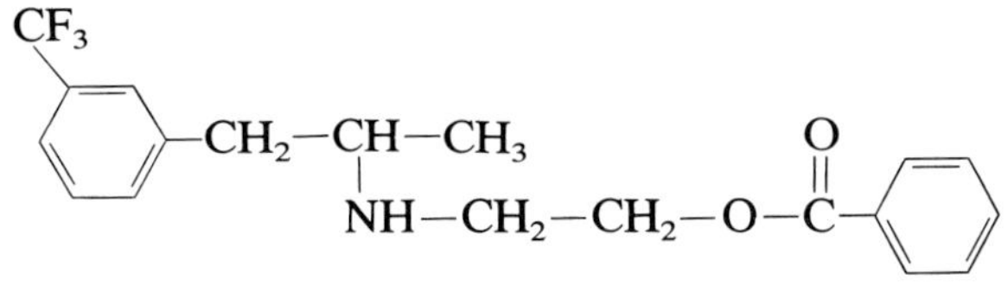

CF_3

$CH_2-CH-CH_3$ O

$NH-CH_2-CH_2-O-C$

35.**82**

unlike 35.**1** and 35.**45**, 35.**82** has no effect on rat serum cholesterol levels and does not increase liver weight (391). In man it lowers elevated cholesterol and/or triglyceride levels, with a range of activity similar to that of clofibrate. The agent also improves glucose tolerance in diabetic patients. *Fenfluramine* was also found to decrease serum cholesterol levels in man (392).

3-Hydroxy-3-methylglutaric acid (HMG, 35.**83**), a natural metabolite formed *in vivo* by deacylation of HMG–coenzyme A, lowers

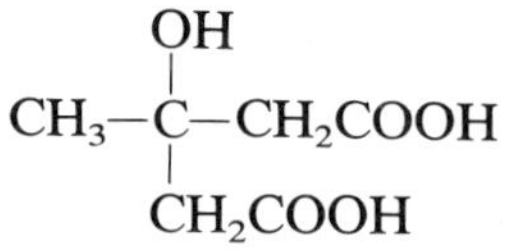

$$CH_3{-}\underset{\displaystyle CH_2COOH}{\overset{\displaystyle OH}{\underset{|}{\overset{|}{C}}}}{-}CH_2COOH$$

35.**83**

cholesterol and triglyceride levels in hyperlipidemic rats, rabbits, and men (393). In rats, it is 4 times as potent as nicotinic acid as an antihyperlipidemic agent and inhibits both hepatic and intestinal cholesterol biosynthesis. High drug levels have been shown to persist in the liver and intestine, the main sites of cholesterol biosynthesis (394). In a small group of familial hypercholesterolemic patients, 35.**83** lowered elevated levels of cholesterol and triglycerides (395). Serum triglycerides rose during the initial phase of therapy in patients who entered the study with normal triglyceride levels. Judging from toxicity and teratogenicity studies, 35.**83** is safe (396). HMG has been proposed as the hypocholesterolemic factor in yogurt (397) and milk (398). *Glutamic acid*, another five-carbon dicarboxylic acid, has also been reported to have hypocholesterolemic effects in man and animals (399, 400). Cholesterol levels in hypercholesterolemic rats are reduced by 1-(4-biphenyl)pentyl half-ester of 35.**83**, as well as the same half-ester of succinic, fumaric, and maleic acids (393).

Cynarin (35.**84**), the active hypocholesterolemic principle of the artichoke, decreases liver cholesterol synthesis and serum cholesterol levels in the rat. It also reduces serum and hepatic concentrations of triglycerides in the ethanol-induced hypertriglyceridemic rat (401). In a mixed population of hyperlipidemic patients, it was found to reduce serum cholesterol, triglyceride, and VLDL levels (402), with its most pronounced effect in moderately hypercholesterolemic subjects (403, 404). Cynarin is not effective in severe and familial hypercholesterolemia (404, 405).

Disodium ethane-1-hydroxy-1,1-diphosphonate (disodium etidronate, EHDP, 35.**85**), a bone-calcium regulator, has lipid

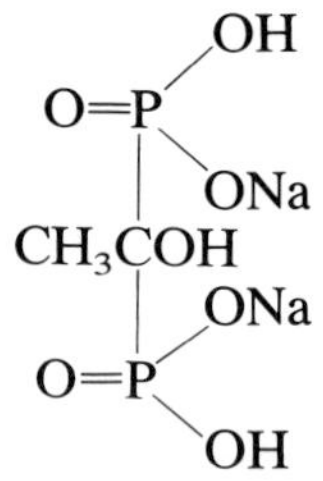

$$O{=}P(OH)(ONa){-}C(CH_3)(OH){-}P(ONa)(OH){=}O$$

35.**85**

lowering properties (406). In hypercholesterolemic and hypertriglyceridemic patients, 35.**85** produces a rapid decrease in total lipid, triglyceride, free, and esterified cholesterol, and VLDL levels. A parallel increase in LDL levels is noted. In the rabbit, this agent inhibits calcification, plaque formation, and lipid accumulation in arteries (407).

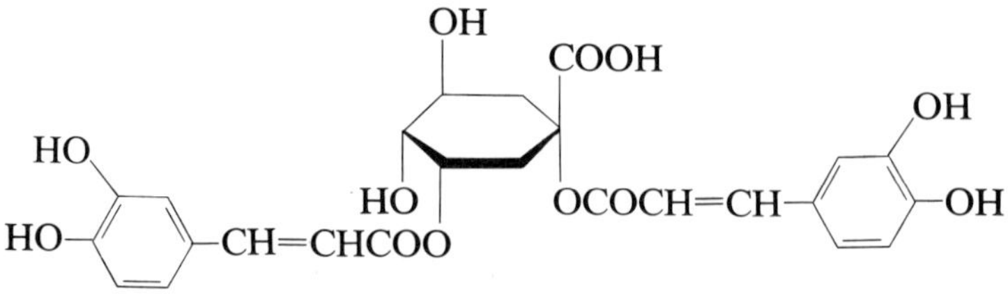

OH, COOH, OH, HO, HO, OCOCH=CH—, —OH, HO—, —CH=CHCOO

35.**84**

Polyunsaturated phosphatidylcholine (polyunsaturated lecithin) has been extensively evaluated in animals and in man. Antihyperlipidemic activity has been observed in some animal models but not in others. For example, in rats, chicks, and minipigs (408), but not in rabbits, baboons, and Japanese quail (409), reductions in elevated lipid levels are observed. Similar inconsistencies have also been reported in man. In a number of clinical studies either oral or intravenous administration resulted in an antihyperlipidemic effect. In one study (410) intravenous dosing resulted in depressions of cholesterol, triglyceride, and LDL levels. In studies with hypercholesterolemic and hypertriglyceridemic subjects, intravenous dosing lowered cholesterol and LDL levels, but triglycerides remained unaltered (409). Lowered lipid levels were maintained after switching to oral administration. Other results are less encouraging—some investigators observed no significant change in any lipid parameters after lecithin treatment (411).

9 OTHER AGENTS LIMITED TO ANIMAL EVALUATION

U-41,792 (35.**86**), a potent antihyperlipidemic agent in a number of animal species,

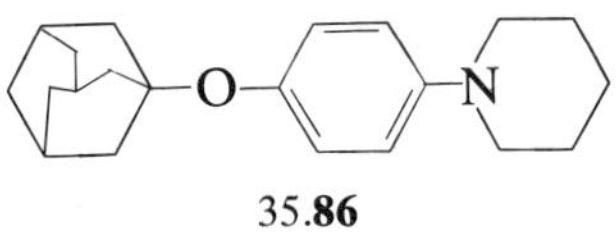

35.**86**

was selected from among a series of bicyclic and tricyclic oxyanilines (412, 413). The agent was examined in a system in which the atherogenic lipoproteins LDL and VLDL are precipitated from the serum by heparin; it produces a marked, specific reductions in the levels of LDL and VLDL, and an elevation in HDL in cholesterol–cholic acid-induced hypercholesterolemic rats. Analogs lacking the bicyclic or tricyclic ether functionality are inactive. Liver cholesterol and lipid levels decrease during chronic administration. Liver enlargement is observed both after single and multiple-day dosing. *U-25,030* (35.**87**), a sulfamyloxyaniline sharing structural features with 35.**86**, also produces

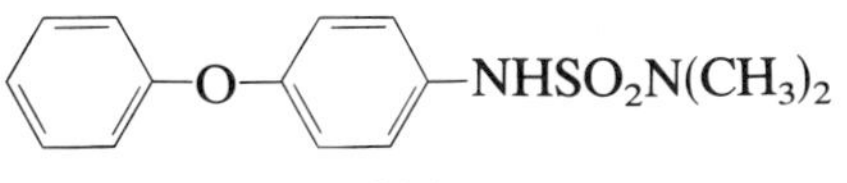

$-NHSO_2N(CH_3)_2$

35.**87**

marked reductions in cholesterol levels in hypercholesterolemic rats (414).

RMI-14514 (35.**88**) is a tetradecyloxyfurancarboxylic acid. The finding that a variety of 4-alkoxybenzoylacetates lower serum

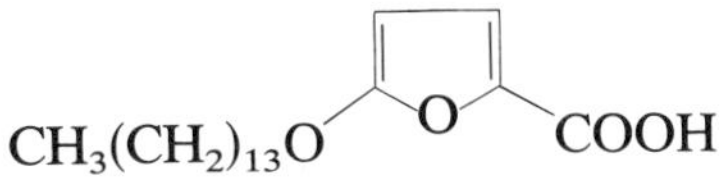

$CH_3(CH_2)_{13}O$ COOH

35.**88**

cholesterol and triglyceride levels, and the subsequent observation that the β-keto esters are metabolized to benzoic acids, led to an extended search of alkoxybenzoic and heterocyclic acids (415). Replacement of the benzene ring by either a furan or thiophene system improvcs antihyperlipidemic potency. A chain length of 12–18 carbon atoms in the alkoxy substituent is required for activity, with the tetradecyl as the most favorable chain length. The 5-tetradecyloxyfuran and thiophene-2-carboxylic acids are comparable in lipid lowering effects. The agent reduces cholesterol and triglyceride levels in rats, and plasma cholesterol in rhesus monkeys. Compound 35.**88** does not inhibit hepatic biosynthesis of cholesterol *in vivo*, but does so *in vitro*, and reduces fatty acid biosynthesis *in vivo* to one-third that of controls (416). Hepatomegaly is observed with this agent, but it is less than that seen after clofibrate. Its effect on hepatic lipogenesis appears to distinguish 35.**88** from clofibrate. A number of sulfamylthiophene-3-carboxylic acids reduce triglyceride, but not cholesterol, levels in rats (417).

A number of long chain aliphatic ketones such as *2-octanone* (35.**89**) and *2-hexadecanone* (35.**90**) demonstrate antihyperlipidemic activity (418, 419). The first

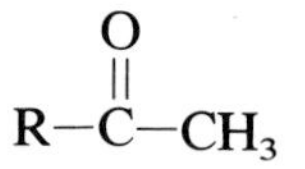

$$R-\overset{\overset{\displaystyle O}{\|}}{C}-CH_3$$

35.**89** $R=C_6H_{13}$
35.**90** $R=C_{14}H_{29}$

of these lowers both serum cholesterol and triglycerides (418), whereas 35.**90** only lowers cholesterol levels (419) in rats. Highest cholesterol lowering activity is found when the ketone group is at the 2-position of the carbon chain. The active members from this series inhibit HMG–coenzyme A reductase, the rate-limiting enzyme for cholesterol biosynthesis, in mice *in vivo*, and in mouse and rat liver *in vitro*. 2-Octanone (35.**89**) is the most potent inhibitor, and folding the aliphatic ketone into a cyclooctanone configuration decreases HMG–coenzyme A reductase inhibitory activity. Serum lipase activity is significantly elevated in rats after treatment with 35.**89**. It has been postulated that 2-octanone lowers serum cholesterol by inhibiting cholesterol synthesis and accelerating fecal sterol excretion, and lowers serum triglycerides by increasing catabolism by serum lipase and excretion (418). 2-Octanone (35.**89**) has advantages over some earlier long chain cyclic ketones, such as 2,8-dibenzylcyclooctanone (35.**91**), in not having

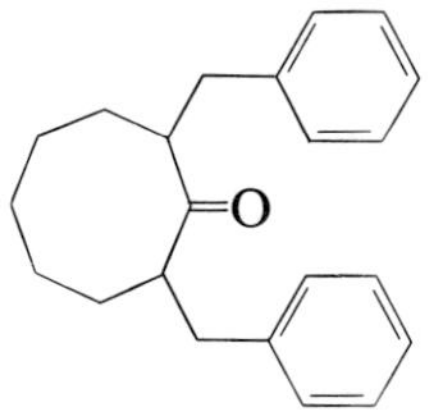

35.**91**

estrogenic activity in rats or antifertility activity in mice. Compound 35.**91** was found to be the most potent cholesterol lowering agent in rats from among a series of cycloalkanones (420), but its lipid lowering effects appear to parallel its estrogenic activity (421). A series of *1,5-diphenyl-3-pentanones* exhibits hypocholesterolemic, estrogenic, and antifertility activities similar to those of 35.**91**. Replacement of the benzylic carbon by oxygen gives the 1,5-diphenoxy-2-propanones. Two from this series, 35.**92** and 35.**93** appear to be quite similar to 2-octanone (35.**89**) in lowering serum cholesterol levels without displaying estrogenic or antifertility activities (422).

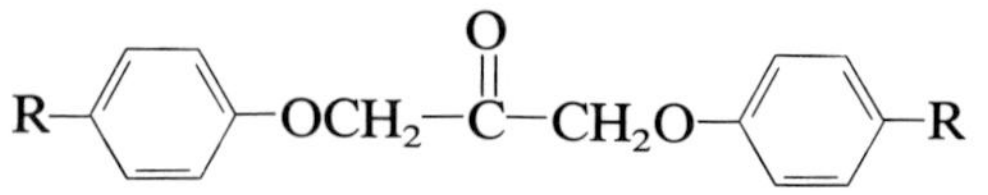

35.**92** $R=CH_3$
35.**93** $R=Cl$

A number of *N-alkylimidazoles* have been shown to inhibit cholesterol biosynthesis and depress lipid levels in animals (423, 424). *N*-substitution by *N*-decyl (35.**94**), *N*-dodecyl (35.**95**), geranyl (35.**96**), and farnesyl (35.**97**) are the most favorable for inhibiting

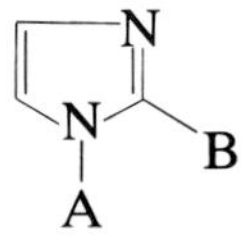

35.**94** A = decyl, $B=CH_3$
35.**95** A = dodecyl, B = H
35.**96** A = geranyl, B = H
35.**97** A = farnesyl, B = H

cholesterol biosynthesis. One of these, 35.**95**, inhibits the conversion of 2,3-oxidosqualene to lanosterol both *in vitro* and *in vivo*. Extension of the *N*-alkylimidazoles to *N*-benzyl substitution led to a number of compounds that effectively reduce both plasma cholesterol and triglyceride levels in mice. The most active *N*-benzylimidazoles are those with methoxy (35.**98**, 35.**99**) and methyl (35.**100**) substitution on the benzyl nucleus (424). Further substitution on the

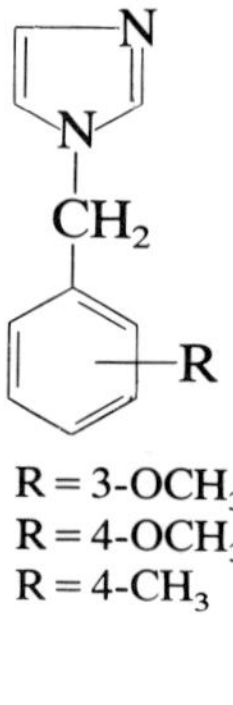

35.**98** $R=3\text{-}OCH_3$
35.**99** $R=4\text{-}OCH_3$
35.**100** $R=4\text{-}CH_3$

imidazole ring results in loss of activity. Unfortunately, the most potent *N*-alkyl- and *N*-benzylimidazole antihyperlipidemic agents tend to increase liver lipids; furthermore, those with the greatest hypocholesterolemic effects depress normal body weight gain and produce fatty livers in rats.

Beloxamide (*N*-γ-phenylpropyl-*N*-benzyloxyacetamide, W-1372, 35.**101**) lowers

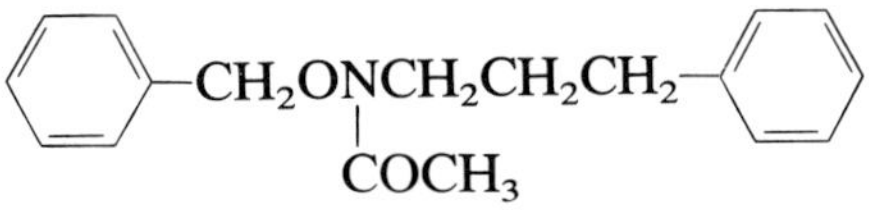

$C_6H_5CH_2ONCH_2CH_2CH_2C_6H_5$ ($COCH_3$ on N)

35.**101**

serum cholesterol levels in hypercholesterolemic rats and rabbits. It also lowers cholesterol and triglyceride levels in squirrel monkeys on normal as well as on a high cholesterol diet. In rats and monkeys, 35.**101** reduces LDL lipids without affecting hepatic cholesterol or triglyceride synthesis. It does, however, increase the triglyceride and cholesterol content of the liver. The accumulation of liver lipids and the decrease of serum lipids suggests that 35.**101** acts by preventing the release of lipoproteins from the liver (425). Although it inhibits the development of atheromata in rat, rabbits, and monkeys (92, 426), it unfortunately induces hepatic lesions similar to those induced by carbon tetrachloride, ethionine, or orotic acid (427).

3-Methyl-4-phenyl-3-butenoic acid (BBA, 35.**102**) inhibits cholesterol biosynthesis and is a hypocholesterolemic agent in

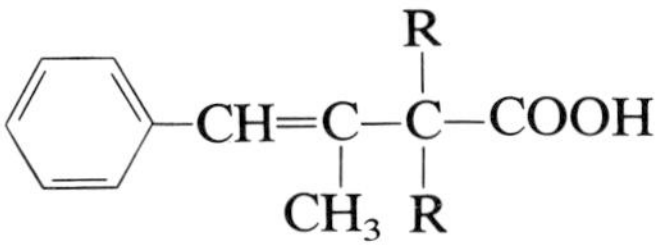

$C_6H_5CH{=}C(CH_3){-}CR_2{-}COOH$

35.**102** R = H, H
35.**103** R = CH_3, CH_3

animals (428). The diethylamide of 35.**102** reduces plasma free fatty acid levels and is an effective hypotriglyceridemic agent in fructose- and ethanol-induced hypertriglyceridemia (429). The *gem*-dimethyl analog (35.**103**) of 35.**102** also inhibits cholesterol biosynthesis (430), but a number of 2-butenoic acids (35.**104**) do not (431).

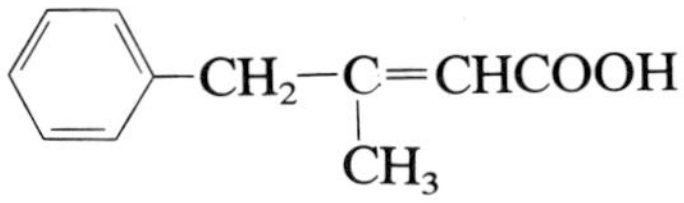

$C_6H_5CH_2{-}C(CH_3){=}CHCOOH$

35.**104**

The most effective antihyperlipidemic agents in a series of *dodecane*- and *cyclopentenecarboxylic acids* are 2-chloro-3,7,11-trimethyldodecanoic acid (35.**105**)

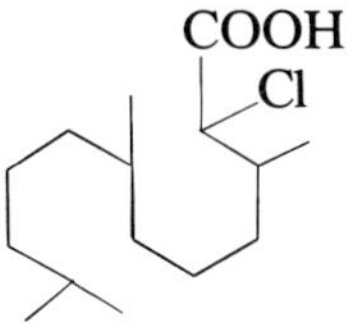

COOH, Cl

35.**105**

and 3-hydroxy-3-methyl-6-(2,2,3-trimethyl-3-cyclopentenyl)hex-4-enoic acid (35.**106**). They significantly depress elevated levels of cholesterol, triglycerides, and free fatty acids in hyperlipidemic rats (432).

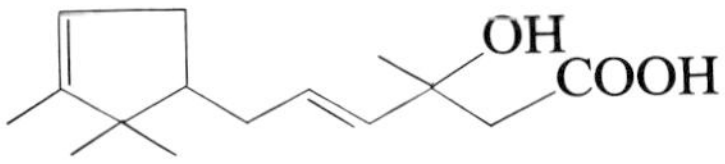

OH, COOH

35.**106**

Certain central nervous system drugs have antihyperlipidemic effects. Oral administration of a number of benzodiazepines to cholesterol-fed rabbits and triton-induced hyperlipidemic rats produces reduction in lipid levels. *Chlordiazepoxide* (35.**107**),

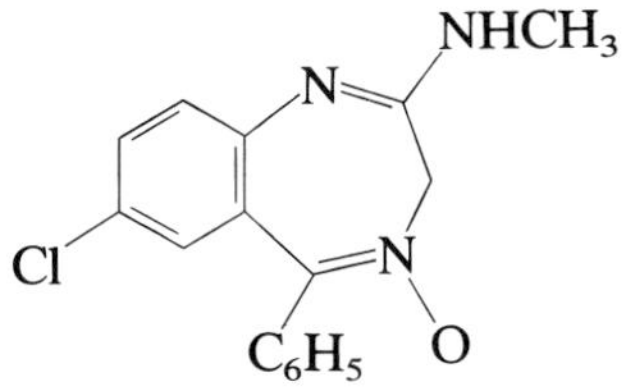

$NHCH_3$, N, Cl, N, C_6H_5, O

35.**107**

diazepam (35.**108**), and *lorazepam* (35.**109**) are the most effective in decreasing serum total lipids, cholesterol, and triglyceride levels; *oxazepam* (35.**110**), *medazepam* (35.**111**), and *nitrazepam* (35.**112**) are less

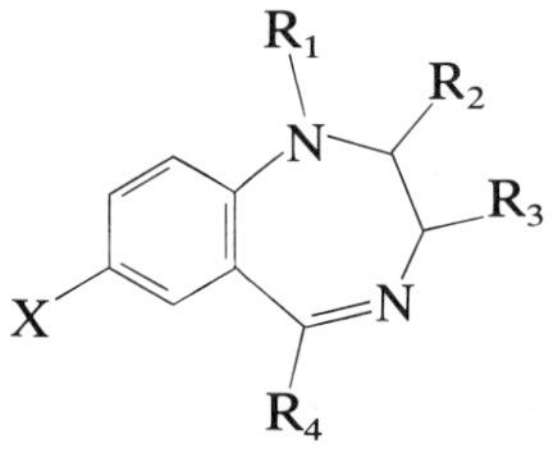

	X	R_1	R_2	R_3	R_4
35.**108**	Cl	CH_3	O	H	C_6H_5
35.**109**	Cl	H	O	OH	2-ClC_6H_4
35.**110**	Cl	H	O	OH	C_6H_5
35.**111**	Cl	CH_3	H,H	H	C_6H_5
35.**112**	NO_2	H	O	H	C_6H_5

effective. Compounds 35.**108** and 35.**109** produce changes in serum lipid content in rats similar to those due to clofibrate, but at approximately one-twentieth the dose (433). Diazepam (35.**108**) was found to increase hepatic cholesterol synthesis in normal man, a result not predicted from animal studies. This effect correlates with a significant increase of hepatocyte smooth endoplasmic reticulum (434). Antihistamines such as *chlorcyclizine* and *cinnarizine* have lipid lowering properties. Chlorcyclizine and a variety of other diarylalkylpiperazines lower serum cholesterol and triglycerides in rats and mice (435). Cinnarizine is effective in hyperlipidemic patients, especially those with hypertriglyceridemia (436).

RMI-12436A (35.**113**) is the most active cholesterol lowering agent in rats from a

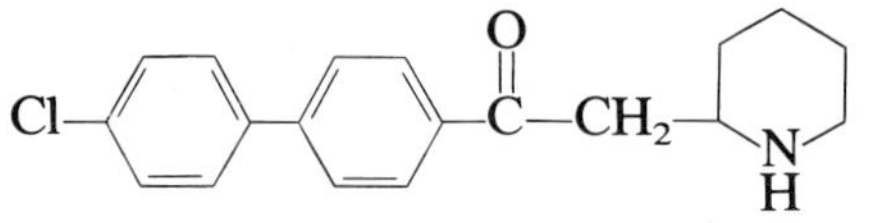

35.**113**

series of piperidine and pyrrolidine ethanones and ethanols (437). It was suggested that 35.**113** acts by inhibiting 7-dehydrocholesterol Δ^7-reductase. A wide variety of other amine derivatives, such as azasteroids and branched chain amines, also lower plasma cholesterol levels in animals by inhibiting either sterol Δ^7- or Δ^{24}-reductase (68, 92, 437).

1-(3-Chlorophenyl)-1-methyl-2-phenyl-2-(2-pyridine)ethanol (35.**114**) and its 2-(4-hydroxyphenyl) metabolite (35.**115**) lower

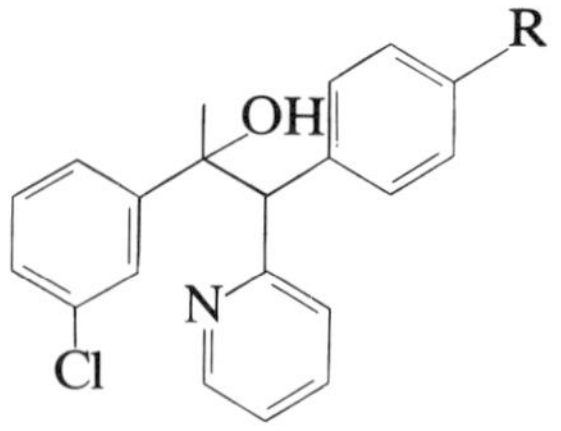

35.**114** R = H
35.**115** R = OH

cholesterol levels in normal rats. Compound 35.**114**, selected from a series of 2-(2-pyridine)-1,1-diarylalkanols, has no hypocholesterolemic activity in monkeys or man The unsaturated isomers of 35.**114** and 35.**115**, the isomers of 35.**115** are minor metabolites in the rat, also show hypocholesterolemic activity, some are of special interest because of their relatively low estrogenicity (438).

Sch 9122 (35.**116**), structurally related to diethylstilbestrol, lowers serum cholesterol in

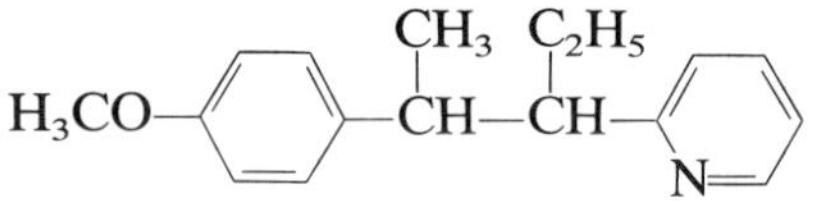

35.**116**

rats. At oral doses that lower serum cholesterol by 30%, 35.**116** does not produce estrogenic effects on secondary sex structures, stimulate mammary tissue, or have adverse fertility or mating behavior, and in these respects is unlike standard estrogenic agents (439).

Hypocholesterolemic effects of *phenolic* compounds, such as guaiacol, hydroquinone, quinhydrone, pyrocatechol, and gallic acid, have been reported. As a follow-up to these findings and in an effort to improve on their therapeutic index, a series of esters and sulfones of 2,5-dihydroxybenzene sulfonic acids was evaluated (440). A number of these phenols, such as 35.**117**, depress both plasma cholesterol and triglyceride levels to the same

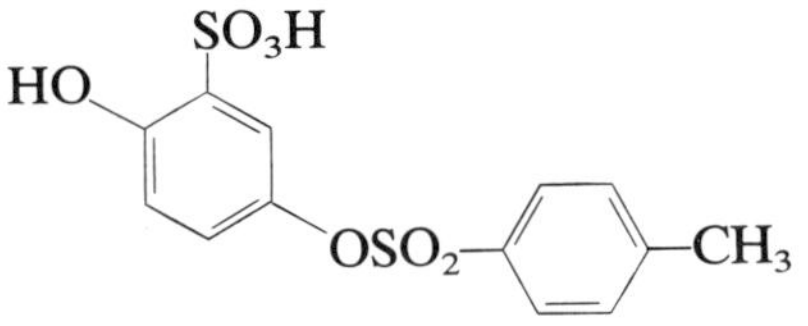

35.**117**

degree as clofibrate after oral administration to hyperlipidemic rats.

4-Biphenylyl-substituted acids are known to reduce plasma cholesterol levels in both animals and man. The structure-activity relationships around 5-(4-biphenylyl)-3-methylvaleric acid (35.**118**), the most potent member from the original series, has been further extended, and it was found that a number of other ring systems can replace the biphenyl group without loss of antihyperlipidemic activity. Most notable is 5-(4-phenylsulfonylphenyl)-3-methylvaleric acid (35.**119**), which depresses both cholesterol

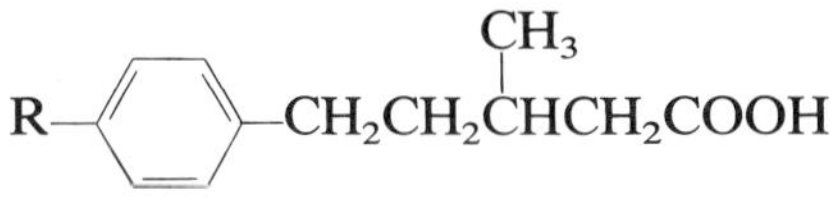

35.**118** $R = C_6H_5$
35.**119** $R = C_6H_5SO_2$

and triglyceride values in rats; its most pronounced effect is on lowering serum triglyceride levels. Compound 35.**119** is more potent than 35.**118** (441).

A number of members from the *Tetronic* (35.**120**) series of surface-active agents demonstrate hypocholesterolemic activity. They are prepared by the sequential addition of ethylene oxide and propylene oxide to ethylenediamine. Tetronic 701, which contains about 10% by weight of polyoxyethylene, is the most interesting member and lowers serum and liver cholesterol in normo- and hypercholesterolemic rats. Hypocholesterolemic effects are also observed in chicks and rabbits on hypercholesterolemic diets. This agent inhibits the uptake of cholesterol into liver and serum, suggesting inhibition of cholesterol absorption as its mechanism of action. Tetronic 701 in rats produces a dose-related growth depression. The tetrabenzoate ester of Tetronic 701 also lowers cholesterol levels but has a significantly smaller effect on growth depression. Hydrophobic detergents also lower serum levels of cholesterol and triglycerides in rats (442).

Bis(2-ethylhexyl)phthalate (35.**121**) produces in rats and mice a reduction in serum

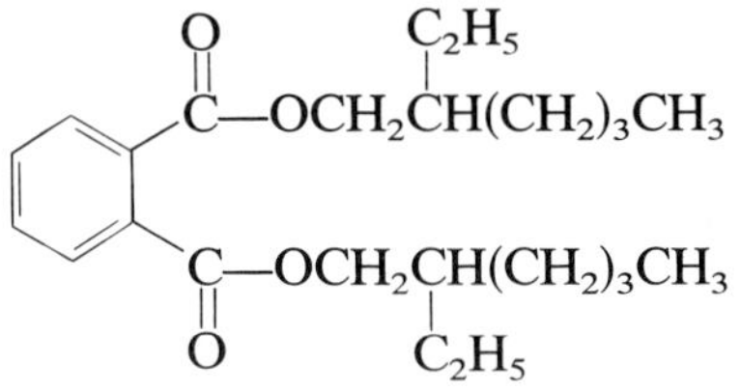

35.**121**

cholesterol and triglyceride levels. In rat liver slices it inhibits both sterol and squalene biosynthesis from acetate and mevalonate (443). In both rats and mice 35.**121** causes hepatomegaly that is attributed to the observed increase in liver peroxisomes. Elevations in hepatic catalase and carnitine acetyltransferase activity are observed, which parallel the peroxisome proliferation. It has been suggested that a relationship exists between the lipid lowering properties of 35.**121** and the induction of peroxisomal enzymes (444).

RU15350 (35.**122**), a 5-thiazolecarboxylic

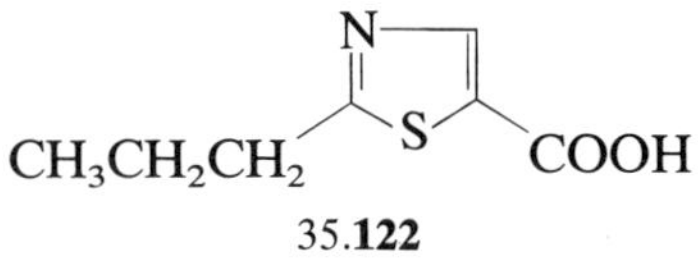

35.**122**

acid, is an antilipolytic and hypotriglyceridemic agent in rats. It is claimed to be superior to nicotinic acid with regard to its

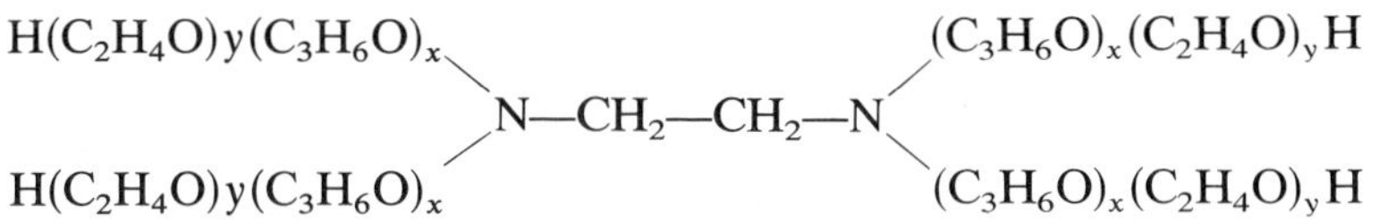

$$[H(C_2H_4O)_y(C_3H_6O)_x]_2N—CH_2—CH_2—N[(C_3H_6O)_x(C_2H_4O)_yH]_2$$

35.**120**

antilipolytic properties, which are not associated with rebound. Furthermore, 35.**122** exhibits less cutaneous vasodilator activity than nicotinic acid (445).

2-(o-Chlorophenyl)-3,4-diphenylisoxazolin-5-one (SC-27504) reduces serum cholesterol levels in rats. Triglyceride levels are not consistently affected. Cholesterol biosynthesis is inhibited at a step prior to mevalonate formation, but only at high doses. An increase in liver cholesterol is observed, suggesting an increased hepatic uptake of cholesterol from serum. *Ethyl 2-(4-chorophenyl)-5-ethoxy-4-oxazoleacetate* (Y-9738) is 7 times as potent as clofibrate in lowering cholesterol levels in both normal and cholesterol-fed rats. Y-9738 differs from clofibrate in lowering cholesterol in the rat fed cholesterol-propylthiouracil and also in not producing hepatomegaly (446).

5α-Cholest-8(14)-en-3β-ol-15-one has hypocholesterolemic activity in rats. There is no accumulation of other sterols in the serum. Administration also results in significantly depressed incorporation into hepatic sterols of acetate, but not mevalonate, indicating inhibition of cholesterol synthesis at the level of HMG–coenzyme A reductase. The 3β-palmitate and 3β-hemisuccinate esters are also effective in reducing serum cholesterol levels in rats (447).

3-Hydroxy-17,17-dimethylgona-1,3,5(10),8,11,13-hexaene and 3-alkoxy derivatives depress cholesterol levels in hypercholesterolemic rats rendered hypothyroid by administration of propylthiouracil. The 2-methylpropionic acid derivative is also effective in normal rats (448).

Antihyperlipidemic activity of two *isoindoline* series has been reported. The α,1-diphenylisoindoline-1-ethanols depress serum cholesterol and triglycerides in rats and cholesterol levels in dogs. Some bridged isoindoline derivatives show hypocholesterolemic effects in rats (449).

(−)Hydroxycitrate significantly reduces serum levels of cholesterol and triglycerides in rats. In two hypertriglyceridemic models—the genetically obese Zucker rat and in fructose-treated rats—elevated triglyceride levels, as well as hyperlipogenesis, were depressed. The agent reduces the biosynthesis of triglycerides, cholesterol, cholesterol esters, and free fatty acids *in vitro. In vivo*, (—)hydroxycitrate suppresses the hepatic rates of cholesterol and fatty acid synthesis (450).

2-Aminoethanol reduces both cholesterol and triglycerides in hyperlipidemic rats. The most potent hypotriglyceridemic agents are the *N*-monosubstituted derivatives, and 2-aminoethanol is the most effective hypocholesterolemic agent. It was suggested that the amino alcohols interfere with phospholipid metabolism (451). *Suloctidil*, 1-4(isopropylthiophenyl)-2-*n*-octylaminopropanol, a potent vasoactive agent reduces plasma cholesterol and LDL levels in hypercholesterolemic monkeys. It inhibits cholesterol biosynthesis and displays antilipolytic activity *in vitro* (452).

A number of *amino acids* lower plasma lipids. Glutamic acid is hypocholesterolemic both in animals and man (399, 400). In rats L-lysine decreases serum cholesterol, and administration of a mixture of L-lysine and L-tryptophan lowers both serum cholesterol and triglyceride levels in animals and man (453). *S*-Adenosyl-L-methionine reduces serum triglycerides, but not cholesterol, in hyperlipidemic patients (454).

Linoleyl (35.**123**) and *oleyl* (35.**124**) *esters* of *4-toluenesulfonic acid* depress plasma cholesterol levels of cholesterol-fed rats.

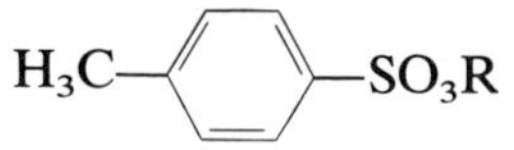

H_3C—⟨benzene⟩—SO_3R

35.**123** R = linoleyl
35.**124** R = oleyl

Both are more effective than ethyl linoleate, itself. Neither 35.**123** nor 35.**124** affects plasma cholesterol levels of normocholesterolemic rats. Whereas both agents also depress hepatic cholesterol levels, ethyl linoleate is without a similar effect. Since neither sodium 4-toluenesulfonate nor linoleyl methanesulfonate lowers cholesterol levels, it appears that the effects observed are due to both the alcohol and sulfonic moieties. Mechanism studies suggest that these agents inhibit intestinal cholesterol absorption (455).

Antihyperlipidemic activity has been claimed for a variety of other structurally distinct agents including vitamin A (456), heparin, chondroitin polysulfate and other mucopolysaccarides (457–459), 5β-cholanic acid (460), dipyridamole (461), and coenzyme A (462).

A number of other *natural products* exhibit antihyperlipidemic activity: *citrinin* (35.**125**),

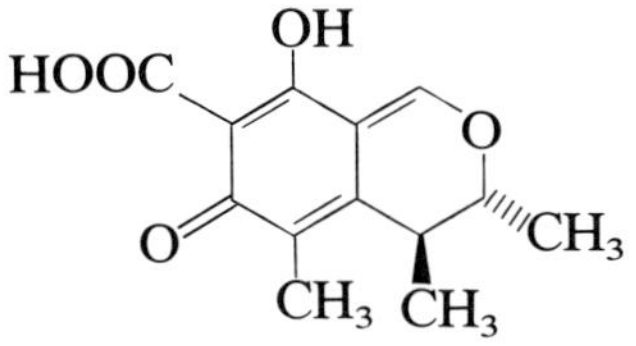

35.**125**

ML-236 *A* (35.**126**), *ML*-236 *B* (35.**127**), and *ML*-236 *C* (35.**128**) are fungal metabolites that lower serum cholesterol in rats after oral administration. Of these, 35.**125** and 35.**127** are the most effective, being approximately 20 times as potent as clofibrate. Chronic dosing of 35.**125** in rats results in lowered serum and liver cholesterol and triglyceride levels. These agents inhibit cholesterol biosynthesis *in vitro*, with 35.**127** being the most potent (463, 464). In addition, 35.**126** and 35.**127** inhibit hepatic cholesterol

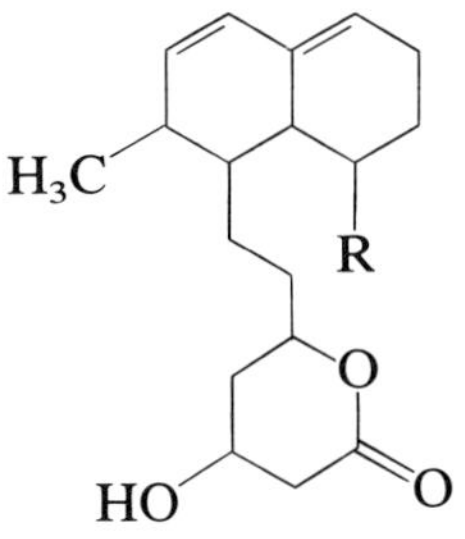

35.**126** R = OH
35.**127** R = $OCOCH(CH_3)(CH_2CH_3)$
35.**128** R = H

synthesis *in vivo* (464). Acetate but not mevalonate incorporation is inhibited, indicating that the site of inhibition is between acetate and mevalonate. It has been demonstrated that 35.**125** inhibits both HMG–coenzyme A reductase and acetoacetyl–coenzyme A thiolase, whereas 35.**126**–35.**128** inhibit HMG-coenzyme A reductase. The inhibition of HMG–coenzyme A reductase by 35.**125** is time dependent and irreversible. The acid forms of 35.**126** and 35.**127** are more effective reductase inhibitors than are their respective lactone forms. The cholesterol lowering properties of these four agents are attributed to their inhibitory effects on cholesterol biosynthesis (465, 466).

Ascofuranone (35.**129**) is another fungal metabolite that depresses serum lipids after single and chronic doses in normolipidemic

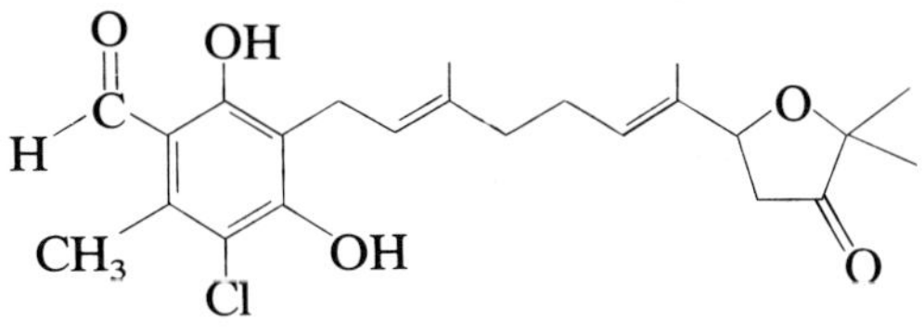

35.**129**

rats. It reduces serum free fatty acids, triglycerides, and cholesterol in cholesterol-fed rats—yet clofibrate, under the same conditions, depresses free fatty acid and triglyceride levels but is without effect on cholesterol levels. Ascofuranone increases liver weight but to a lesser extent than clofibrate, and it differs from clofibrate in reducing liver and cardiac cholesterol levels in cholesterol-fed rats. In addition, 35.**129** stimulates the excretion of bile acid (467).

The essential oils of *onion* and *garlic* have been reported to decrease serum cholesterol, triglyceride, and LDL levels, and also prevent a decrease in HDL levels, in cholesterol-fed rabbits (468–470). It was suggested that these effects account for the antiatherosclerotic properties in animals of both onion and garlic. A second study in rabbits confirmed the cholesterol lowering and antiatherosclerotic properties of garlic, but did not confirm similar findings after administration of onions (471).

The active principle of garlic is reported to be a mixture of sulfur compounds, one of which is *allicin* (35.**130**), which reduces serum

$$CH_2{=}CHCH_2{-}S{-}\overset{\overset{\displaystyle O}{|}}{S}{-}CH_2CH{=}CH_2$$

35.**130**

and liver lipid levels in rats, exerting its most pronounced effect on liver triglycerides and cholesterol (472). Freshly extracted garlic juice protects human subjects from fat-induced increases in serum cholesterol (473). As with the controversy in rabbits, there are conflicting reports on whether onions produce similar effects (473, 474).

S-Methyl-L-cysteine sulfoxide (35.**131**) is distributed abundantly in cabbage and depresses serum cholesterol levels of hyperlipidemic rats (475).

$$CH_3\overset{\overset{\displaystyle O}{|}}{S}{-}CH_2\underset{\underset{\displaystyle NH_2}{|}}{CH}{-}COOH$$

35.**131**

Crocetin, the aglycone of the principle pigment of saffron (from the stamens of crocus blossoms), reduces serum cholesterol and triglyceride levels and prevents atherosclerosis in rabbits (476).

A variety of *terpenes* have hypocholesterolemic activity. The tricyclic diterpenoid derivatives of totarol, abietane, and pimarane reduce serum cholesterol levels in hypercholesterolemic rats. Some, such as totarol and abietic acid, are as active as clofibrate, and more active than β-sitosterol, cholestyramine, nicotinic acid, or pectin. *THD-341* (35.**132**), a Δ^8-dihydroabietamide derivative of abietic acid, is the most effective in reducing serum cholesterol levels in hypercholesterolemic rats and rabbits; it is comparable to dextrothyroxine, more potent than estradiol, and far more potent than clofibrate. THD-341, totarol, and abietic acid are inactive in

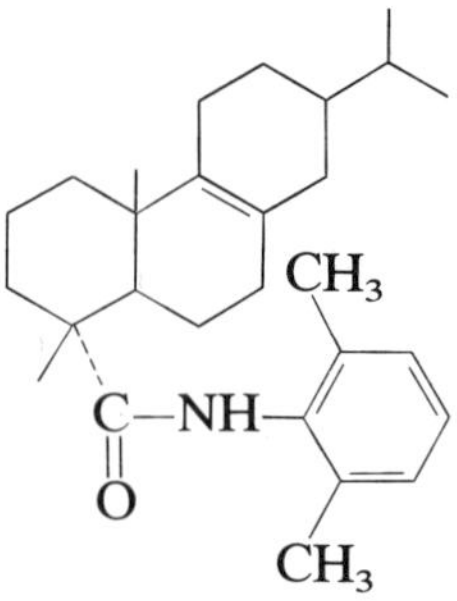

[Structure 35.132: tricyclic abietane skeleton bearing C(=O)–NH– linked to a 2,6-dimethylphenyl ring; labels: CH_3, C—NH—, O, CH_3]

35.**132**

normocholesterolemic rats on a normal diet. Mechanism studies suggest that THD-341, abietic acid and totarol, and possibly the other hypocholesterolemic tricyclic diterpenoids, exert their cholesterol lowering activity by inhibiting intestinal cholesterol absorption (477). Alisol A-24-monoacetate, a triterpene, also reduces cholesterol levels in rats on an atherogenic diet (478).

Various *saponins* have antihyperlipidemic activity. Saikosaponins, isolated from the root of *Bupleurum falcatum* L., reduces the elevated levels of plasma cholesterol and triglycerides in rats after cholesterol feeding (479). It increases hepatic cholesterol synthesis, plasma cholesterol turnover, and fecal excretion of neutral sterols and bile acids. A number of the saponins from an extract of ginseng reduce serum lipid levels in rats (480).

Breynins A and B, sulfur-containing *glycosides* extracted from *Breynia officinalis* Hemsl, possess significant hypocholesterolemic activity in rats (481).

10 COMBINATION THERAPY

The inadequacies of the available antihyperlipidemic agents has prompted the use of combination therapy (47, 57, 86, 94, 95). Combining lipid lowering agents that act by different mechanisms has been especially useful in refractory patients, such as those with heterozygous or homozygous familial hypercholesterolemia (50, 51, 94). In responsive subjects, lipid depressions greater than that anticipated from single-agent therapy have been observed. The combination of cholestyramine and nicotinic acid appears to function synergistically and is quite effective in reducing extremely high levels of LDL in both homozygotic and heterozygotic hypercholesterolemic subjects. The combination of clofibrate and a bile acid sequestering resin has been found useful not only in reducing plasma cholesterol and triglycerides, but also in producing maximum mobilization of body cholesterol (482). Other combinations that have been used are clofibrate and polidexide, clofibrate and neomycin, clofibrate and nicotinic acid, and neomycin and β-sitosterol. Lipid lowering agents such as colestipol, phytosterols, *para*-aminosalicylic acid, β-pyridylcarbinol, pentaerythritoltetranicotinate, myoinositol hexanicotinate, phenformin, butylbiguanide, and essential phospholipids have also been combined with either clofibrate, cholestyramine, or nicotinic acid.

Chemical combinations have also been found attractive. Clofibrate has been combined by an ester linkage with nicotinic acid and β-pyridylcarbinol. *Etofibrate*, a nicotinic acid ester of clofibrate, and *nicofibrate*, the β-pyridylcarbinol ester of clofibrate, lower both plasma cholesterol and triglyceride levels in patients (483, 484).

The popular use, and the wide variety of combinations that have been employed, attest to the need for more effective lipid lowering agents.

11 HIGH DENSITY LIPOPROTEINS (HDL)

A number of recent epidemiologic studies such as those in Honolulu (37), Framingham (485), Tromso (486), New Zealand (487), and London (488) have shown that HDL cholesterol level is an important indicator of ischemic heart disease and should be added to the other known cardiovascular risk factors. It was observed that the risk of developing ischemic heart disease correlates with decreased plasma concentrations of HDL cholesterol. At all levels of LDL cholesterol, considered to be the most "atherogenic" of all the lipoprotein fractions, persons with low levels of HDL have a higher rate of heart disease than subjects with moderate or high levels of HDL cholesterol. The studies show that low HDL level precedes heart disease and plays a critical role in the development of clinically evident atherosclerosis.

These findings have a number of important implications. For example, the assumption that total plasma cholesterol can effect heart disease is no longer valid or sufficient; rather, it is the *distribution* of cholesterol between the HDL and the combined LDL and VLDL fractions that is important. One must also question the validity and appropriateness of the routine plasma cholesterol test in evaluating heart-risk factors, for elevated cholesterol could be an indication of high HDL levels and could have a protective value, rather than acting as a risk factor.

Furthermore, the rationale of cholesterol lowering therapy must also be challenged, since agents that lower HDL-cholesterol could be harmful. Based on current evidence, it seems that therapeutic intervention should be targeted at favorably altering the distribution of cholesterol between HDL and the combined LDL and VLDL fractions, with the objective of increasing HDL levels. It would be appropriate for future clinical studies routinely to measure HDL cholesterol levels, especially in evaluations of morbidity and mortality. One should probably also question conclusions drawn from the long-term antihyperlipidemic studies that have evaluated morbidity and mortality, since HDL cholesterol levels, which could have been lowered, were not measured.

Although the mechanism for the protective action of elevated cholesterol in the HDL fraction is not known, it has been suggested that it plays a role in the transportation of cholesterol from tissue such as the arteries to the liver for disposal, as well as partially blocking the uptake of LDL by tissues. In either case HDL would reduce cholesterol concentrations in the arteries (489).

The value of elevating HDL cholesterol levels has not gone unnoticed as a diverse group of agents, including chlorinated hydrocarbons (490), such as lindane (491), phenytoin (492), estrogens and progestational agents (95, 493), ethyl alcohol (494), and bicyclic- and tricyclicoxyanilines, such as 35.**86** (412, 413), have been reported to elevate HDL levels in man and animals. Although clofibrate has been reported to produce a slight increase in plasma HDL, none of the established antihyperlipidemic agents is therapeutically effective in this respect. Some preliminary findings on the clofibrate analogs procetofene (35.**11**), bezafibrate (35.**12**), and gemfibrozil (35.**13**) indicate that they might favorably affect HDL levels (495).

12 STATUS OF ANTIHYPERLIPIDEMIC THERAPY

Two decades of the extensive and combined efforts of chemists, biologists, and clinicians has yielded a wide structural and mechanistic variety of antihyperlipidemic agents that are effective in man and animals. Unfortunately the availability of these agents has not allowed a definitive answer on the lipid hypothesis—namely, whether a reduction in plasma lipids will reduce the incidence of coronary heart disease. The lipid hypothesis has been tested in secondary and primary prevention trials by both diet and drug therapy.

Three secondary prevention trials with clofibrate failed to show a significant decrease in the incidence of deaths due to new coronary events. In the US Coronary Drug Project clofibrate did not statistically alter the incidence of either cardiovascular disease mortality or nonfatal myocardial infarctions in patients who were only moderately hyperlipidemic (mean baseline plasma cholesterol level, 251 mg-%; plasma triglyceride level, 165–170 mg-%) (496). Although the Newcastle-upon-Tyne study (497) showed that the clofibrate group had a lower rate of cardiovascular death than the placebo group, and both the Newcastle-upon-Tyne and Scottish (498) secondary prevention studies show a reduction in the incidence of definite, nonfatal myocardial infarction, these improvements were not statistically significant. In the Newcastle and Scottish studies, but not in the Coronary Drug Project, only a subgroup of patients with a history of angina pectoris showed a reduction in mortality and myocardial infarction. Nicotinic acid was also evaluated in the Coronary Drug Project, and although there was no evidence of a beneficial effect on mortality either in the entire treated group or in any subgroup, it did decrease the incidence of nonfatal myocardial infarction.

Similarly, the use of dietary intervention has been evaluated in a number of secondary and primary prevention trials in different parts of the world without any better success (47, 60, 65, 66). The diet studies in general suffer from serious shortcomings in study design, including size and age of the population, lack of randomization and double-blind protocols, and doubtful statistical procedures and analyses.

To date, the secondary and primary intervention studies have yielded negative or at best equivocal results in demonstrating the benefits of lowering plasma lipids (66, 499).

Two primary drug prevention studies are in progress: the World Health Organization (WHO) Cooperative Trial with clofibrate (500), and the National Heart and Lung Institute's Lipid Research Clinic (LRC) Primary Prevention Trial with cholestyramine (501). It is hoped that the cholesterol depressions in the LRC study with cholestyramine will be on the order of 25%, thus greater than those observed in the trials of secondary and primary drug and diet intervention. The poor cholesterol responses in those studies represent a serious shortcoming in attempts to adequately test the lipid hypothesis. The results of the WHO and LRC intervention trials will be anxiously awaited, since these studies could very well be the last trials of major antihyperlipidemic therapy to be funded (502).

If the drug intervention trials fail, it need not be the end of the era as some have predicted (503); it could very well be that the antihyperlipidemic agents of the future must be more specific. Is it not too much to expect that a single agent be effective in a large and varied population? Current information, such as that on HDL, as well as genetic studies on monogenic forms of hyperlipidemia, strongly suggest that the blanket approach in which all patients are treated in a homogeneous fashion is incorrect. It would seem to be more prudent to treat those at risk with therapies specifically designed to ameliorate that risk.

Rather than being pessimistic with regard to the lipid approach for the treatment of ischemic heart disease, it seems that one has every reason to be optimistic. There have been new insights in understanding the complex mechanisms whereby hyperlipidemia causes progressive atherosclerosis. Chronic hyperlipidemia has been shown to deposit lipids in the atheromatous lesions and perhaps to initiate the primary endothelial injury that predisposes to atherosclerosis (23, 24). There has also been good progress in understanding the mechanism of the transfer of lipoproteins into the arterial intima leading to plaque formation (504). And last and most important, the first demonstration of regression of human atherosclerosis by antihyperlipidemic drug therapy has been reported (505).

The time for renewed efforts to develop superior lipid regulating agents is now.

REFERENCES

1. G. B. Kolata and J. L. Marx, *Science*, **194,** 509 (1976).
2. Medical News, *J. Am. Med. Assoc.*, **231,** 691 (1975); W. J. Walker, *New Engl. J. Med.*, **297,** 163 (1977).
3. *Vital Statistics Report of the United States*, Vol. 25, No. 11, National Center for Health Statistics, Washington, D.C., 1977, p. 18.
4. W. B. Kannel, D. McGee, and T. Gordon, *Am. J. Cardiol.*, **38,** 46 (1976).
5. Editorial, *Brit. Med. J.*, **1,** 1105 (1976).
6. T. Khosla, R. G. Newcombe, and H. Campbell, *Brit. Med. J.*, **1,** 341 (1977).
7. Editorial, *Brit. Med. J.*, **4,** 765 (1971).
8. A. N. Klimov, *Atheroscler. Rev.*, **1,** 229 (1976).
9. Report of Intersociety Commission for Heart Disease Resources: "Primary Prevention of the Atherosclerotic Disease," *Circulation*, **42,** A-55 (1970).
10. A. Keys, Ed., "Coronary Heart Disease in Seven Countries," *Circulation*, **41** (Suppl. I), 1 (1970).
11. D. W. Simborg, *J. Chronic. Dis.*, **22,** 515 (1970).
12. T. Gordon, P. Sorlie, and W. B. Kannel, *The Framingham Study: An Epidemiological Investigation of Cardiovascular Disease*, Section 27, Government Printing Office, Washington, DC, 1971.
13. W. B. Kannel, W. P. Castelli, T. Gordon, and P. M. McNamara, *Ann. Intern. Med.*, **74,** 1 (1971).
14. A. Keys, C. Aravanis, H. Blackburn, F. S. P. van Buchem, R. Buzina, B. S. Djordjevic, F. Fidanza, M. J. Karvonen, A. Menotti, V. Puddu, and H. L. Taylor, *Circulation*, **45,** 815 (1972).
15. J. Stamler and F. H. Epstein, *Prevent. Med.*, **1,** 27 (1972).
16. Editorial, *Brit. Med. J.*, **2,** 375 (1973).
17. M. F. Oliver, I. A. Nimmo, M. Cooke, L. A. Carlson, and A. G. Olsson, *Eur. J. Clin. Invest.*, **5,** 507 (1975)
18. A. Keys, *Atherosclerosis*, **22,** 149 (1975).
19. Editorial, *Lancet*, **1,** 402 (1976).
20. L. Werko, *Am. Heart J.*, **91,** 87 (1976).
21. Editorial, *Brit. Med. J.*, **1,** 789 (1977).
22. *Arteriosclerosis, A Report by the National Heart and Lung Institute Task Force on Arteriosclerosis*, Vol. 1, 1971 [US Department of Health, Education and Welfare Publication No. (NIH) 72–137], Vol. 2, 1971 [US Department of Health, Education and Welfare Publication No. (NIH) 72–219], Government Printing Office, Washington, DC.
23. R. Ross and J. A. Glomset, *New Engl. J. Med.*, **295,** 369, 420 (1976).
24. R. Ross and L. Harker, *Science*, **193,** 1094 (1976).
25. G. B. Kolata, *Science*, **194,** 592 (1976).
26. W. E. Connor and S. L. Connor, *Prevent. Med.*, **1,** 49 (1972).
27. J. Cornfield, *Fed. Proc.*, **21** (Suppl. II), 58 (1962).
28. A. Keyes, H. L. Taylor, H. Blackburn, J. Brozek, J. T. Anderson, and E. Simonson, *Arch. Intern. Med.*, **128,** 201 (1971).

29. M. J. Albrink and E. B. Man, *Arch. Intern. Med.*, **103,** 4 (1959).
30. L. A. Carlson, *Acta Med. Scand.*, **167,** 399 (1960).
31. A. Antonis and I. Bersohn, *Lancet*, **1,** 998 (1960).
32. L. A. Carlson and L. E. Böttiger, *Lancet*, **1,** 865 (1972).
33. J. L. Goldstein, W. R. Hazzard, H. G. Schrott, E. L. Bierman, A. G. Motulsky, M. J. Levinski, and E. D. Campbell, *J. Clin. Invest.*, **52,** 1533 (1973).
34. D. F. Brown, S. H. Kinch, and J. T. Doyle, *New Engl. J. Med.*, **273,** 947 (1965).
35. L. Wilhelmsen, H. Wedel, and G. Tibblin, *Circulation*, **48,** 950 (1973).
36. R. H. Roseman, R. J. Brand, R. I. Sholtz, and M. Friedman, *Am. J. Cardiol.*, **37,** 903 (1976).
37. G. G. Rhoades, G. L. Gulbrandsen, and A. Kagan, *New Engl. J. Med.*, **294,** 293 (1976).
38. T. Gordon, W. P. Castelli, M. C. Hjortland, W. B. Kannel, and T. R. Dawber, *J. Am. Med. Assoc.*, **238,** 497 (1977).
39 S. Eisenberg and R. I. Levy, *Advan. Lipid Res.*, **13,** 1 (1975).
40. S. Eisenberg and R. I. Levy, *Handb. Exp. Pharmacol.*, **41,** 191 (1975).
41. J. D. Morrisett, R. L. Jackson, and A. M. Gotto, Jr., *Ann. Rev. Biochem.*, **44,** 183 (1975); *Biochim. Biophys. Acta*, **472,** 93 (1977).
42. C. B. Blum and R. I. Levy, *Ann. Rev. Med.*, **26,** 365 (1975).
43. R. L. Jackson, J. D. Morrisett, and A. M. Gotto, Jr., *Physiol. Rev.*, **56,** 259 (1976).
44. S. Eisenberg, *Atheroscler. Rev.*, **1,** 23 (1976).
45. D. S. Fredrickson, R. I. Levy, and R. S. Lees, *New Engl. J. Med.*, **276,** 34, 94, 148, 215, 273 (1967).
46. D. S. Fredrickson and R. I. Levy, in *Metabolic Basis of Inherited Diseases*, J. B. Stanbury, J. B. Wyngaarden, and D. S. Fredrickson, Eds., McGraw-Hill, New York, 1972, pp. 545–614.
47. H. Buchwald, R. B. Moore, and R. L. Varco, *Circulation*, **49** (Suppl. I), 1, 13, 22 (1974).
48. T. E. Starzl, H. P. Chase, C. W. Putnam, and K. A. Porter, *Lancet*, **2,** 940 (1973).
49. H. Torsvik, H. A. Feldman, J. E. Fischer, and R. S. Lees, *Lancet*, **1,** 601 (1975).
50. G. R. Thompson, R. Lowenthal, and N. B. Myant, *Lancet*, **1,** 1208 (1975).
51. P. J. Lupien, S. Moorjani, and J. Awad, *Lancet*, **1,** 1261 (1976); J. A. Awad, P. Lupien, S. Moorjani, and R. Cloutier, *Curr. Ther. Res. Clin. Exp.*, **21,** 525 (1977).
52. R. J. Deckelbaum, R. S. Lees, D. M. Small, S. E. Hedberg, and S. M. Grundy, *New Engl. J. Med.*, **296,** 465 (1977).
53. K. R. Norum, *Nutr. Metab.*, **22,** 1 (1978).
54. R. S. Lees and A. M. Lees, *Postgrad. Med.*, **60,** 99 (1976).
55. Report on Prevention of Coronary Heart Disease, *Atherosclerosis*, **24,** 591 (1976).
56. A. G. Shaper and J. W. Marr, *Brit. Med. J.*, **1,** 867 (1977).
57. J. Morganroth and R. I. Levy, in *Current Cardiovascular Topics*, Vol. 1, *Drugs in Cardiology*, E. Donoso, Ed., Stratton Intercontinental Medical Book Corp., New York, 1975, pp. 127–156.
58. D. S. Fredrickson, R. I. Levy, M. Bonnell, and N. Ernst, *The Dietary Management of Hyperlipoproteinemia: A Handbook for Physicians and Dietitians; Type I Diet; Type IIa Diet; Type IIb or III Diet; Type IV Diet; Type V Diet*, National Heart and Lung Institute, National Institutes of Health, Bethesda, Md., US Department of Health, Education, and Welfare Publication Nos. (NIH) 75–110, 76–111, 77–112, 76–113, 77–114, 73–115.
59. A. M. Gotto, Jr., M. E. DeBakey, J. P. Foreyt, L. W. Scott, and J. I. Thornby, *J. Am. Med. Assoc.*, **237,** 1212 (1977).
60. J. Cornfield and S. Mitchell, *Arch. Environ. Health*, **19,** 382 (1969).
61. S. Dayton, *Fed. Proc.*, **30,** 849 (1971).
62. P. J. Scott, *Drugs*, **6,** 1 (1973).
63. M. Albrink, *Postgrad. Med.*, **55,** 87 (1974).
64. A. K. Rider, *J. Am. Med. Assoc.*, **233,** 275 (1975).
65. I. D. Frantz, *Handb. Exp. Pharmacol.*, **41,** 409 (1975).
66. E. H. Ahrens, Jr., *Ann. Intern. Med.*, **85,** 87 (1976).
67. L. K. Smith, R. V. Luepker, S. S. Rothchild, A. Gillis, L. Kochman, and J. R. Warbasse, *Ann. Intern. Med.*, **84,** 22 (1976).
68. W. L. Bencze, R. Hess, and G. de Stevens, in *Progress in Drug Research*, Vol. 13, E. Jucker, Ed., Birkhäuser-Verlag, Basel, 1969, pp. 217–292.
69. F. L. Bach, in *Medicinal Chemistry*, 3rd ed., A. Burger, Ed., Wiley-Interscience, New York, 1970, pp. 1123–1171.
70. J. F. Douglas, *Ann. Rep. Med. Chem.*, **6,** 150 (1970).
71. E. H. Strisower, G. Adamson, and B. Strisower, *Med. Clin. North Am.*, **54,** 1599 (1970).
72. J. N. Moss and E. Z. Dajani, in *Screening Methods in Pharmacology*, Vol. 2, R. A. Turner and P. Hebborn, Eds., Academic Press, New York, 1971, pp. 121–143.
73. D. Kritchevsky, *Fed. Proc.*, **30,** 835 (1971).
74. R. S. Lees and D. E. Wilson, *New Engl. J. Med.*, **284,** 186 (1971).
75. R. I. Levy, D. S. Fredrickson, R. Shulman, D. W.

Bilheimer, J. L. Breslow, N. J. Stone, S. E. Lux, H. R. Sloan, R. M. Krauss, and P. N. Herbert, *Ann. Intern. Med.*, **77,** 267 (1972).

76. T. R. Blohm, *Ann. Rep. Med. Chem.*, **7,** 169 (1972).
77. D. Kritchevsky, in *Search for New Drugs*, A. A. Rubin, Ed., Dekker, New York, 1972, pp. 261–289.
78. D. Kritchevsky, *Lipids*, **9,** 97 (1974).
79. G. Crepaldi, R. Fellin, and G. Briani, *Advan. Exp. Med. Biol.*, **38,** 199 (1973).
80. C. Sirtori, R. Fumagalli, and R. Paoletti, *Advan. Exp. Med. Biol.*, **38,** 171 (1973).
81. R. J. Havel and J. P. Kane, *Ann. Rev. Pharmacol.*, **13,** 287 (1973).
82. R. I. Levy and B. M. Rifkind, *Drugs*, **6,** 12 (1973).
83. T. R. Blohm, *Ann. Rep. Med. Chem.*, **8,** 183 (1973).
84. A. S. Truswell, *Proc. Nutr. Soc.*, **33,** 215 (1974).
85. R. Howe, *Advan. Drug Res.*, **9,** 7 (1974).
86. R. I. Levy, J. Morganroth, and B. M. Rifkind, *New Engl. J. Med.*, **290,** 1295 (1974).
87. B. Murphy, *J. Am. Med. Assoc.*, **230,** 1683 (1974).
88. G. F. Holland and J. N. Pereira, *Ann. Rep. Med. Chem.*, **9,** 172 (1974).
89. D. Kritchevsky, *Advan. Exp. Med. Biol.*, **63,** 135 (1975).
90. C. R. Sirtori, *Pharmacol. Res. Commun.*, **7,** 103 (1975).
91. *Med. Lett.*, **17**(12), issue 428 (1975).
92. W. L. Bencze, *Handb. Exp. Pharmacol.*, **41,** 349 (1975).
93. J. N. Pereira and G. F. Holland, *Ann. Rep. Med. Chem.*, **10,** 182 (1975).
94. R. I. Levy, *J. Am. Med. Assoc.*, **235,** 2334 (1976); S. Margolis, *ibid.*, **239,** 2696 (1978).
95. D. Yeshurun and A. M. Gotto, Jr., *Am. J. Med.*, **60,** 379 (1976).
96. B. Morgan, *Biochem. Soc. Trans.*, **4,** 589 (1976).
97. J. G. Hamilton, L. Cheng, and A. C. Sullivan, *Ann. Rep. Med. Chem.*, **11,** 180 (1976).
98. A. C. Sullivan, L. Cheng, and J. G. Hamilton, *Ann. Rep. Med. Chem.*, **12,** 191 (1977).
99. C. R. Sirtori, A. Catapano and R. Paoletti, *Atheroscler. Rev.*, **2,** 113 (1977).
100. J. M. Thorp and W. S. Waring, *Nature*, **194,** 948 (1962).
101. J. Redel and J. Cottet, *C.R. Acad. Sci. Paris*, **236,** 2553 (1953).
102. J. N. Pereira and G. F. Holland, in *Atherosclerosis, Proceedings of the Second International Symposium*, R. J. Jones, Ed., Springer-Verlag, New York, 1970, pp. 549–554; J. Boberg, M. Boberg, R. Gross, S. Grundy, J. Augustin, and V. Brown, *Atherosclerosis*, **27,** 499 (1977).
103. H. B. Stahelin, J. T. Locher, and R. Maier, *Clin. Chim. Acta*, **54,** 115 (1974).
104. C. Harvengt and J. P. Desager, *Curr. Ther. Res. Clin. Exp.*, **19,** 145 (1976); P. Saba, F. Galeone, F. Salvadorini, and M. Guarguaglini, *Curr. Ther. Res. Clin. Exp.*, **22,** 741 (1977).
105. M. Leutenegger, H. Choisy, J. Caron, and H. Paris, *Therapie*, **29,** 599 (1974).
106. C. Harvengt and J. P. Desager, *Int. J. Clin. Pharmacol.*, **15,** 1 (1977).
107. R. Hess and W. L. Bencze, *Experientia*, **24,** 418 (1968).
108. G. Hartmann and G. Forster, *J. Atheroscler. Res.*, **10,** 235 (1969).
109. D. Berkowitz, *Circulation*, **40** (Suppl. III), 44 (1969).
110. D. Berkowitz, *Circulation*, **42** (Suppl. III), 12 (1970).
111. C. H. Duncan and M. M. Best, *Circulation*, **42,** 859 (1970).
112. C. A. Dujovne, P. Weiss, and J. R. Bianchine, *Clin. Pharmacol. Ther.*, **12,** 117 (1971).
113. R. Kattermann, R. Arnold, and W. Creutzfeldt, *Arzneim.-Forsch.*, **22,** 616 (1972).
114. J. K. Reddy, *Am. J. Pathol.*, **82,** 37a (1976).
115. J. K. Reddy, M. S. Rao, and D. E. Moody, *Cancer Res.*, **36,** 1211 (1976).
116. C. Russo and M. Mendlowitz, *Clin. Pharmacol. Ther.*, **12,** 676 (1971).
117. A. R. Timms, L. A. Kelly, R. S. Ho, and J. H. Trapold, *Biochem. Pharmacol.*, **18,** 1861 (1969).
118. D. Berkowitz, E. DeFelice, and P. Arcese, *Circulation*, **38** (Suppl. VI), 41 (1968).
119. F. Bochner, B. E. Cham, M. J. Eadie, W. D. Hooper, B. R. Knowles, J. M. Sutherland, and J. H. Tyrer, *Toxicol. Appl. Pharmacol.*, **24,** 653 (1973).
120. J. M. Thorp, in *Atherosclerosis, Proceedings of the Second International Symposium*, R. J. Jones, Ed., Springer-Verlag, New York, 1970, pp. 541–544.
121. G. M. Craig and K. W. Walton, *Atherosclerosis*, **15,** 189 (1972).
122. G. M. Craig, *Atherosclerosis*, **15,** 265 (1972).
123. J. L. Gilfillan, V. M. Hunt, and J. W. Huff, *Proc. Soc. Exp. Biol. Med.*, **136,** 1274 (1971).
124. C. Sirtori, A. Hurwitz, K. Sabih, and D. L. Azarnoff, *Lipids*, **7,** 96 (1972).
125. J. P. Morgan, J. R. Bianchine, T. H. Hsu, and S. Margolis, *Clin. Pharmacol. Ther.*, **12,** 517 (1971).
126. W. S. Aronow, M. del Vicario, K. Moorthy, J. King, M. Vawter, and N. P. Papageorges, *Curr. Ther. Res. Clin. Exp.*, **18,** 855 (1975).

127. C. A. Dujovne, D. L. Azarnoff, D. H. Huffman, P. Pentikainen, A. Hurwitz, and D. W. Shoeman, *Clin. Pharmacol. Ther.*, **19,** 352 (1976).
128. L. R. Mandel, *Lipids*, **12,** 34 (1977).
129. E. D. Rees, R. D. Hamilton, I. F. Kanner, S. Wasson, and T. Hearn, *Atherosclerosis*, **24,** 537 (1976).
130. E. M. Jepson, E. Small, M. F. Grayson, G. Bance, and J. D. Billimoria, *Atherosclerosis*, **16,** 9 (1972).
131. A. Gustafson and R. Sannerstedt, *Eur. J. Clin. Pharmacol.*, **5,** 259 (1973).
132. V. Beaumont, J. C. Buxtorf, B. Jacotot, and J. L. Beamont, *Atherosclerosis*, **20,** 141 (1974).
133. A. Gustafson, *Postgrad. Med. J.*, **51** (Suppl. 8), 66 (1975).
134. E. Granzer and H. Nahm, *Arzneim-Forsch.*, **23,** 1353 (1973).
135. Editorial, *Lancet*, **2,** 131 (1976).
136. E. A. Nikkila, *Lancet*, **2,** 320 (1976).
137. R. Sornay, J. Gurrieri, C. Tourne, F. J. Renson, B. Majoie, and E. Wulfert, *Arzneim.-Forsch.*, **26,** 885 (1976).
138. J. Gurrieri, M. Le Lous, F. J. Renson, C. Tourne, H. Voegelin, B. Majoie, and E. Wulfert, *Arzneim.-Forsch.*, **26,** 889 (1976).
139. J. Rouffy, C. Dreux, Y. Goussault, R. Dakkak, and F. J. Renson, *Arzneim-Forsch.*, **26,** 901 (1976); E. Wulfert, B. Majoie, and A. de Ceaurriz, *ibid.*, 906 (1976).
140. M. Afschrift, T. Mets, and G. Verdonk, *Lancet*, **2,** 311 (1977).
141. H. Stork and P. D. Lang, *Advan. Exp. Med. Biol.*, **63,** 485 (1975); A. G. Olsson, S. Rössner, G. Walldius, L. A. Carlson, and P. D. Lang, *Atherosclerosis*, **27,** 279 (1977).
142. D. H. Jones, R. H. Greenwood, R. F. Mahler, M. Thomas, and R. Couch, *Clin. Trials*, **13,** 42 (1976).
143. A. H. Kissebah, S. Alfarsi, P. W. Adams, M. Seed, J. Folkard, and V. Wynn, *Atherosclerosis*, **24,** 199 (1976).
144. R. A. Okerholm, F. J. Keeley, F. E. Peterson, and A. J. Glazko, *Fed. Proc.*, **35,** 327 (1976).
145. "Gemfibrozil: A New Lipid Lowering Agent," *Proc. Roy. Soc. Med.*, **69** (Suppl. 2), 1 (1976).
146. M. C. Stone, J. M. Thorp, and J. S. Wain, *Advan. Exp. Med. Biol.*, **63,** 151 (1975).
147. E. Kloimstein, R. Schönbeck, and H. Stormann, *Arzneim.-Forsch.*, **14,** 261 (1964).
148. H. Hammerl, C. Kränzl, G. Nebosis, O. Pichler, and M. Studlar, *Wien. Med. Wochenschr.*, **124,** 518 (1974).
149. G. Hitzenberger, *Arzneim.-Forsch.*, **14,** 279 (1964).
150. R. L. Buchanan, V. Sprancmanis, and R. A. Partyka, *J. Med. Chem.*, **12,** 1001 (1969).
151. D. T. Nash, L. Gross, W. Haw, and K. Agre, *J. Clin. Pharmacol.*, **8,** 377 (1968).
152. T. Kariya, T. R. Blohm, J. M. Grisar, R. A. Parker, and J. R. Martin, *Advan. Exp. Med. Biol.* **26,** 302 (1972).
153. J. M. Grisar, R. A. Parker, T. Kariya, T. R. Blohm, R. W. Fleming, V. Petrow, D. L. Wenstrup, and R. G. Johnson, *J. Med. Chem.*, **15,** 1273 (1972).
154. K. Toki, Y. Nakamura, K. Agatsuma, H. Nakatani, and S. Aono, *Atherosclerosis*, **18,** 101 (1973).
155. K. Suzuki, S. Aono, and H. Nakatani, *Jap. J. Pharmacol.*, **24,** 407 (1974).
156. S. Sakamoto, K. Yamada, T. Anzai, and T. Wada, *Atherosclerosis*, **18,** 109 (1973).
157. K. Suzuki, *Biochem. Pharmacol.*, **24,** 1203 (1975).
158. K. Suzuki, *Biochem. Pharmacol.*, **25,** 325 (1976).
159. A. A. Santilli, A. C. Scotese, and R. M. Tomarelli, *Experientia*, **30,** 1110 (1974).
160. R. M. Tomarelli, L. Bauman, and A. A. Santilli, *Abstr. Pap., Am. Chem. Soc.*, 170 Meeting MEDI 24 (1975); J. K. Reddy, D. E. Moody, D. L. Azarnoff, and R. M. Tomarelli, *Arch. Int. Pharmacodyn. Ther.*, **225,** 51 (1977).
161. M. R. Malinow, P. McLaughlin, and L. Papworth, *Clin. Res.*, **24,** 86A (1976).
162. S. Yurugi, A. Miyake, T. Fushimi, E. Imamiya, H. Matsumura, and Y. Imai, *Chem. Phar. Bull.* (Tokyo), **21,** 1641 (1973).
163. S. Yurugi, A. Miyake, M. Tomimoto, H. Matsumura, and Y. Imai, *Chem. Pharm. Bull.* (Tokyo), **21,** 1885 (1973).
164. Y. Imai and K. Shimamoto, *Atherosclerosis*, **17,** 121 (1973); M. Arakawa, H. Miyajima, H. Matsumura, M. Izukawa, and Y. Imai, *Biochem. Pharmacol.*, **27,** 167 (1978).
165. Y. Imai, H. Matsumura, S. Tamura, and K. Shimamoto, *Atherosclerosis*, **17,** 131 (1973).
166. C. Daveson, D. Benziger, A. Fritz, and J. Edelson, *Drug Metab. Dispos.*, **3,** 520 (1975).
167. H. A. I. Newman, W. P. Heilman, and D. T. Witiak, *Lipids*, **8,** 378 (1973).
168. D. T. Witiak, W. P. Heilman, S. K. Sankarappa, R. C. Cavestri, and H. A. I. Newman, *J. Med. Chem.*, **18,** 934 (1975).
169. J. M. Grisar, G. P. Claxton, R. A. Parker, F. P. Palopoli, and T. Kariya, *J. Med. Chem.*, **17,** 721 (1974).
170. D. T. Witiak, H. A. I. Newman, G. K. Poochikian, W. Loh, and S. K. Sankarappa, *Lipids*, **11,** 384 (1976).

171. G. Bondesson, T. Högberg, A. Misiorny, and N. E. Stjernström, *Acta Pharm. Suec.*, **13,** 97 (1976).

172. G. Bondesson, C. Hedbom, T. Högberg, O. Magnusson, N. E. Stjernström, and L. A. Carlson, *J. Med. Chem.*, **17,** 108 (1974); T. Högberg, G. Bondesson, and N. E. Stjernström, *Acta Pharm. Suec.*, **14,** 149 (1977).

173. D. T. Witiak, G. K. Poochikian, D. R. Feller, N. A. Kenfield, and H. A. I. Newman, *J. Med. Chem.*, **18,** 992 (1975); A. P. Goldberg, W. S. Mellon, D. T. Witiak, and D. R. Feller, *Atherosclerosis*, **27,** 15 (1977).

174. D. T. Witiak, E. Kuwano, D. R. Feller, J. R. Baldwin, H. A. I. Newman, and S. K. Sankarappa, *J. Med. Chem.*, **19,** 1214 (1976).

175. T. Kariya, J. M. Grisar, N. L. Wiech, and T. R. Blohm, *J. Med. Chem.*, **15,** 659 (1972).

176. C. Dalton and W. R. Pool, *J. Pharm. Sci.*, **66,** 348 (1977).

177. G. Metz and M. Specker, *Arzneim.-Forsch.*, **25,** 1686 (1975); G. Metz, M. Specker, W. Sterner, E. Heisler, and G. Grawuit, *ibid.*, **27,** 1173 (1977); G. Metz and M. Specker, *ibid.*, 1421 (1977).

178. R. L. Buchanan and V. Sprancmanis, *J. Med. Chem.*, **16,** 174 (1973).

179. S. Gronowitz, R. Svenson, G. Bondesson, O. Magnusson, and N. E. Stjernström, *Acta Pharm. Suec.*, **11,** 211 (1974).

180. F. Miyoshi and K. Nagao, *J. Pharm. Soc. Japan*, **94,** 1028 (1974); F. Miyoshi, H. Fukami and Y. Sako, *J. Pharm. Soc. Japan*, **94,** 1061 (1974).

181. M. Nakanishi, T. Kobayakawa, T. Okada, and T. Tsumagari, *J. Pharm. Soc. Japan*, **90,** 921 (1970).

182. T. Högberg, G. Bondesson, A. Misiorny, and N. E. Stjernstöm, *Acta Pharm. Suec.*, **13,** 427 (1976).

183. T. Högberg, G. Bondesson, A. Misiorny, and N. E. Stjernström, *Acta Pharm. Suec.*, **14,** 137 (1977).

184. A. Maderspach, J. Borsy, S. Elek, and I. Polgari, *Artery*, **2,** 360 (1976).

185. B. B. Chaudhari, *J. Pharm. Sci.*, **58,** 366 (1969).

186. F. Andreani, R. Andrisano, and A. Andreani, *Farmaco, Ed. Sci.*, **30,** 847 (1975).

187. J. Nordmann, G. Mattioda, and G. Loiseau, *Chem. Ther.*, **8,** 342 (1973).

188. F. Miyoshi, H. Kuroda, K. Hiraoka, H. Fukami, K. Onishi, M. Mori, K. Nagao, M. Shiga, and E. Sakakibara, *J. Pharm. Soc. Japan*, **94,** 387 (1974); F. Miyoshi, K. Hiraoka, M. Hirohashi, K. Nagao, and E. Sakakibara, *ibid.*, 397 (1974).

189. "Symposium on Atromid," *J. Atheroscler. Res.*, **3,** 347 (1963).

190. G. F. Holland and J. N. Pereira, *Abstr. Pap., Am. Chem. Soc.*, 168 Meeting MEDI 30, 1974.

191. J. N. Pereira and G. F. Holland, *Advan. Exp. Med. Biol.*, **63,** 474 (1975).

192. J. N. Pereira, G. A. Mears, and G. F. Holland, *Fed Proc.*, **34,** 789 (1975).

193. C. R. Sirtori, S. Zoppi, B. Quarisa, and E. Agradi, *Pharmacol. Res. Commun.*, **6,** 445 (1974).

194. J. B. Enticknap, R. S. Winwood, and P. L. Wright, *Artery*, **3,** 164 (1977).

195. P. Bielman, D. Brun, S. Morrjani, M. A. Gagnon, L. Tetreault, and P. J. Lupien, *Int. J. Clin. Pharmacol.*, **15,** 166 (1977); H. J. Lisch, S. Sailer, and H. Braunsteiner, *Arzneim.-Forsch.*, **27,** 2017 (1977).

196. V. G. de Vries, D. B. Moran, G. R. Allen, and S. J. Riggi, *J. Med. Chem.*, **19,** 946 (1976).

197. K. H. Baggaley, R. Fears, R. M. Hindley, B. Morgan, E. Murrell, and D. E. Thorne, *J. Med. Chem.*, **20,** 1388 (1977); R. I. Trust, F. J. McEvoy, and J. D. Albright, *Abstr. Pap., Am. Chem. Soc.*, JOINT Conference 40 (1977).

198. E. E. Largis, A. S. Katocs, Jr., L. Will, D. K. McClintock, and S. A. Schaffer, *J. Am. Oil Chem. Soc.*, **53,** 140A (1976); A. S. Katocs, Jr., and S. A. Schaffer, *Fed. Proc.*, **36,** 1160 (1977).

199. E. Assous, M. Pouget, J. Nadaud, G. Tartary, M. Henry, and J. Duteil, *Therapie*, **27,** 395 (1972).

200. J. Rouffy and M. J. Loeper, *Therapie*, **27,** 433 (1972).

201. J. Rouffy, *Therapie*, **30,** 815 (1975).

202. J. L. de Gennes, J. Truffert, and J. M. LeQuere, *Therapie*, **31,** 455 (1976).

203. G. Rodney, R. E. Maxwell, and P. Uhlendorf, *Fed. Proc.*, **35,** 598 (1976).

204. H. P. Blumenthal, J. R. Ryan, and F. G. McMahon, *Clin. Pharmacol. Ther.*, **17,** 229 (1975).

205. H. P. Blumenthal, J. R. Ryan, A. K. Jain, and F. G. McMahon, *Lipids*, **12,** 44 (1977).

206. K. Gundersen, in *Cardiovascular Drugs*, F. G. McMahon, Ed., Futura Publishing, Mount Kisco, New York, 1974, pp. 87–103.

207. H. R. Casdorph, *Lipid Pharmacology*, Vol. 2, R. Paoletti and C. J. Glueck, Eds., Academic Press, New York, 1976, pp. 221–256.

208. S. M. Grundy, E. H. Aherns, Jr., and G. Salen, *J. Lab. Clin. Med.*, **78,** 94 (1971).

209. R. J. Jones and L. Dobrilovic, *J. Lab. Clin. Med.*, **75,** 953 (1970).

210. B. J. Kudchodkar, H. S. Sodhi, L. Horlick, and D. J. Nazir, *Proc. Soc. Exp. Biol. Med.*, **148,** 393 (1975).

211. T. M. Parkinson, K. Gundersen, and N. A. Nelson, *Atherosclerosis*, **11,** 531 (1970).

212. C. J. Glueck, S. Ford, Jr., D. Scheel, and P. Steiner, *J. Am. Med. Assoc.*, **222,** 676 (1972).

213. J. R. Ryan, A. K. Jain, and F. G. McMahon, *Clin. Pharmacol. Ther.*, **17,** 83 (1975).

214. J. R. Ryan, A. K. Jain, and F. G. McMahon, *Clin. Pharmacol. Ther.*, **21,** 116 (1977).
215. P. Clifton-Bligh, N. E. Miller, and P. J. Nestel, *Clin. Sci. Mol. Med.*, **47,** 547 (1974).
216. N. E. Miller and P. J. Nestel, *Eur. J. Clin. Invest.*, **5,** 241 (1975).
217. J. L. Witztum, G. Schonfeld, and S. W. Weidman, *J. Lab. Clin. Med.*, **88,** 1008 (1976).
218. A. M. Lees, M. A. McCluskey, and R. S. Lees, *Atherosclerosis*, **24,** 129 (1976).
219. K. Gundersen, E. E. Cooper, G. Ruoff, T. Nikolai, and J. R. Assenzo, *Atherosclerosis*, **25,** 303 (1976).
220. L. A. Simons, *Clin. Exp. Pharmacol. Physiol.*, **3,** 99 (1976).
221. E. A. Nikkilä, T. A. Miettinen, and A. Lanner, *Atherosclerosis*, **24,** 407 (1976).
222. L. A. Simons and N. B. Myant, *Artery*, **2,** 129 (1976).
223. A. N. Howard and R. J. C. Evans, *Atherosclerosis*, **20,** 105 (1974).
224. A. Gustafson and A. Lanner, *Eur. J. Clin. Pharmacol.*, **7,** 65 (1974).
225. S. Ritland, A. Lanner, O. Fousa, J. P. Blomhoff, and E. Gjone, *Advan. Exp. Med. Biol.*, **63,** 479 (1975).
226. K. J. Breen, R. E. Bryant, J. D. Levinson, and S. Schenker, *Ann. Intern. Med.*, **76,** 211 (1972).
227. R. W. B. Schade, A. van't Laar, C. L. H. Majoor, and A. P. Jansen, *Acta Med. Scand.*, **199,** 175 (1976).
228. P. Samuel, C. M. Holtzman, E. Meilman, and W. Perl, *J. Clin. Invest.*, **47,** 1806 (1968).
229. A. Sedaghat, P. Samuel, J. R. Crouse, and E. H. Ahrens, Jr., *J. Clin. Invest.*, **55,** 12 (1975).
230. G. R. Thompson, M. MacMahon, and P. Claes, *Eur. J. Clin. Invest.*, **1,** 40 (1970).
231. T. A. Miettinen, *Eur. J. Clin. Invest*, **3,** 256 (1973).
232. W. A. Phillips and G. L. Elfring, *Lipids*, **12,** 10 (1977).
233. S. M. Grundy and H. Y. I. Mok, *J. Lipid Res.*, **18,** 263 (1977); A. M. Lees, H. Y. I. Yok, R. S. Lees, M. A. McCluskey, and S. M. Grundy, *Atherosclerosis*, **28,** 325 (1977).
234. A. K. Bhattacharyya and W. E. Connor, *J. Clin. Invest.*, **53,** 1033 (1974).
235. R. S. Shulman, A. K. Bhattacharyya, W. E. Connor, and D. S. Fredrickson, *N. Engl. J. Med.*, **294,** 482 (1976).
236. S. Teshima, A. Kanazawa, M. Yoshioka, and K. Kitahara, *J. Steroid Biochem.*, **5,** 69 (1974).
237. Y. Aramaki, T. Kobayashi, Y. Imai, S. Kikuchi, T. Matsukawa, and K. Kanazawa, *J. Atheroscler. Res.*, **7,** 653 (1967).
238. Y. Imai, S. Kikuchi, T. Matsuo, Z. Suzuoki, and K. Nishikawa, *J. Atheroscler. Res.*, **7,** 671 (1967).
239. A. M. Wartman and W. E. Connor, *J. Lab. Clin. Med.*, **82,** 793 (1973).
240. M. Ito, W. E. Connor, E. J. Blanchette, C. R. Treadwell, and G. V. Vahouny, *J. Lipid Res.*, **10,** 694 (1969).
241. D. T. Witiak, R. A. Parker, D. R. Brann, M. E. Dempsey, M. C. Ritter, W. E. Connor, and D. M. Brahmankar, *J. Med. Chem.*, **14,** 216 (1971).
242. D. T. Witiak, R. A. Parker, M. E. Dempsey, and M. E. Ritter, *J. Med. Chem.*, **14,** 684 (1971).
243. R. P. Cook and J. D. B. MacDougall, *Brit. J. Exp. Pathol.*, **49,** 265 (1968).
244. D. Kritchevsky, S. A. Tepper, and J. A. Story, *Lipids*, **12,** 16 (1977); Y. Suzuki, *J. Pharm. Soc. Japan*, **97,** 5 (1977).
245. H. Fukushima and H. Nakatani, *J. Atheroscler. Res.*, **9,** 65 (1969).
246. H. Nakatani, S. Aono, Y. Suzuki, H. Fukushima, Y. Nakamura, and K. Toki, *Atherosclerosis*, **12,** 307 (1970).
247. A. Nagata, H. Nakatani, and K. Toki, *Lipids*, **11,** 163 (1976).
248. N. Takeuchi and Y. Yamamura, *Clin. Pharmacol. Ther.*, **16,** 368 (1974).
249. A. Hirohashi, A. Nagata, H. Miyawaki, H. Nakatani, and K. Toki, *Xenobiotica*, **6,** 329 (1976); A. Nagata, *ibid.*, 339 (1976).
250. W. N. Dannenburg, M. S. Kearney, and R. T. Ruckart, *Fed. Proc.*, **36,** 1104 (1977).
251. G. A. Leveille and K. Chakrabarty, *J. Nutr.*, **95,** 88 (1968).
252. H. J. Eyssen, J. F. Van den Bosch, and G. A. Janssen, *Advan. Exp. Med. Biol.*, **4,** 549 (1969).
253. J. F. Van den Bosch, G. A. Janssen, H. Eyssen, and H. Vanderhaeghe, *J. Nutr.*, **101,** 1515 (1971).
254. H. Eyssen, H. Vanderhaeghe, and P. de Somer, *Fed. Proc.*, **30,** 1803 (1971).
255. A. W. Norman, A. M. Spielvogel, and R. C. Wong, *Advan. Lipid Res.*, **14,** 127 (1976).
256. A. N. Klimov, A. A. Nikiforova, and A. M. Tchistiakova, *Biochim. Biophys. Acta*, **380,** 76 (1975).
257. C. P. Schaffner and H. W. Gordon, *Proc. Nat. Acad. Sci., US*, **61,** 36 (1968).
258. H. Fisher, P. Griminger, and C. P. Schaffner, *Proc. Soc. Exp. Biol. Med.*, **132,** 253 (1969).
259. A. C. Parekh, R. J. Creno, and C. V. Dave, *Res. Commun. Chem. Pathol. Pharmacol.*, **9,** 307 (1974).
260. H. Fisher, P. Griminger, and W. Siller, *Proc. Soc. Exp. Biol. Med.*, **145,** 836 (1974).

261. I. Kwon and H. Fisher, *Fed. Proc.*, **33,** 690 (1974).

262. P. F. Micklewright and D. J. Trigger, *J. Pharm. Pharmacol.*, **26** (Suppl.), 108P (1974).

263. A. C. Parekh, R. K. Mathur, and C. V. Dave, *Res. Commun. Chem. Pathol. Pharmacol.*, **16,** 535 (1977).

264. C. V. Dave and A. C. Parekh, *Proc. Soc. Exp. Biol. Med.*, **149,** 299 (1975).

265. L. A. Carlson, A. G. Olsson, L. Orö, and S. Rössner, *Atherosclerosis*, **14,** 391 (1971); M. L. Bierenbaum, A. I. Fleischman, and R. I. Raichelson, *Lipids*, **7,** 202 (1972).

266. A. N. Howard, *Atherosclerosis*, **27,** 383 (1977).

267. H. Trowell and D. Burkitt, *Artery*, **3,** 107 (1977); D. Kritchevsky, *Am. J. Clin. Nutr.*, **30,** 979 (1977); *Nutr. Rev.*, **35,** 183 (1977); *Am. J. Clin. Nutr.*, **31,** S190 (1978).

268. J. A. Storey and D. Kritchevsky, *J. Nutr.*, **106,** 1292 (1976).

269. C. Thiffault, M. Belanger, and M. Pouliot, *Can. Med. Assoc. J.*, **103,** 165 (1970).

270. P. Lindner and B. Moller, *Lancet*, **2,** 1259 (1973).

271. P. A. Judd, R. M. Kay, and A. S. Truswell, *Proc. Nutr. Soc.*, **35,** 71A (1976).

272. D. J. A. Jenkins, A. R. Leeds, C. Newton, and J. H. Cummings, *Lancet*, **1,** 1116 (1975).

273. P. N. Durrington, A. P. Manning, C. H. Bolton, and M. Hartog, *Lancet*, **2,** 394 (1976).

274. A. S. Truswell, *Nutr. Rev.*, **35,** 51 (1977); C. Arvanitakis, C. L. Stamnes, J. Folscroft, and P. Beyer, *Proc. Soc. Exp. Biol. Med.*, **154,** 550 (1977).

275. T. A. Miettinen and S. Tarpila, *Clin. Chim. Acta*, **79,** 471 (1977).

276. R. M. Kay and A. S. Truswell, *Am. J. Clin. Nutr.*, **30,** 171 (1977).

277. D. J. A. Jenkins, A. R. Leeds, B. Slavin, and E. M. Jepson, *Lancet*, **2,** 1351 (1976).

278. G. A. Spiller and R. J. Amen, *CRC Crit. Rev. Food Sci. Nutr.*, **7,** 39 (1975).

279. M. M. Lieberthal and R. A. Martens, *Am. J. Dig. Dis.*, **20,** 469 (1975).

280. S. Kiriyama, A. Enishi, and K. Yura, *J. Nutr.*, **104,** 69 (1974).

281. K. S. Mathur, M. A. Khan, and R. D. Sharma, *Brit. Med. J.*, **1,** 30 (1968).

282. P. V. G. Menon and P. A. Kurup, *Biomedicine*, **24,** 248 (1976).

283. M. R. Malinow, P. McLaughlin, G. O. Kohler, and A. L. Livingston, *Steroids*, **29,** 105 (1977); M. R. Malinow, P. McLaughlin, L. Papworth, C. Stafford, G. O. Kohler, A. L. Livingston, and P. R. Cheeke, *Am. J. Clin. Nutr.*, **30,** 2061 (1977).

284. L. Horlick and S. Fedoroff, *Lancet*, **2,** 361 (1975).

285. R. M. G. Hamilton and K. K. Carroll, *Atherosclerosis*, **24,** 47 (1976).

286. A. W. Barichello and S. Fedoroff, *Brit. J. Exp. Pathol.*, **52,** 81 (1971).

287. D. Kritchevesky, *Lipids*, **12,** 49 (1977).

288. T. P. Whitehead, P. W. Dykes, J. Gloster, and P. Harris, *Clin. Sci.*, **38,** 233 (1970).

289. G. Blohme, J. Kerstell, and A. Svanborg, *Acta Med. Scand.*, **183,** 481 (1968).

290. F. H. Mattson, R. J. Jandacek, and M. R. Webb, *J. Nutr.*, **106,** 747 (1976).

291. R. W. Fallat, C. J. Glueck, R. Lutmer, and F. H. Mattson, *Am. J. Clin. Nutr.*, **29,** 1204 (1976).

292. C. R. Sirtori, E. Agradi, F. Conti, O. Mantero, and E. Gatti, *Lancet*, **1,** 275 (1977).

293. L. Puglishi, V. Caruso, R. Paoletti, P. Ferruti, and M. C. Tanzi, *Pharmacol. Res. Commun.*, **8,** 379 (1976).

294. S. Rössner, A. G. Olsson, and L. Orö, *Acta Med. Scand.*, **200,** 269 (1976).

295. L. Harthon and N. Svedmyr, *Atherosclerosis*, **20,** 65 (1974).

296. A. G. Olsson, L. Orö, and S. Rössner, *Atherosclerosis*, **19,** 407 (1974).

297. L. Harthon and K. Sigroth, *Arzneim.-Forsch.*, **24,** 1688 (1974).

298. A. H. Kissebah, P. W. Adams, P. Harrigan, and V. Wynn, *Eur. J. Clin. Invest.*, **4,** 163 (1974).

299. C. Boroda, *J. Int. Med. Res.*, **3,** 10 (1975).

300. H. Hammerl, C. Kränzl, O. Pichler, and M. Studlar, *Münch. Med. Wochenschr.*, **111,** 1912 (1969); H. Sommer, *Arzneim.-Forsch.*, **15,** 1337 (1965).

301. P. Avogaro, G. Bittolo-Bon, M. Pais, and G. C. Taroni, *Pharmacol. Res. Commun.*, **9,** 599 (1977).

302. Y. Aso, Y. Abe, K. Higo, T. Naruke, and T. Irikura, *J. Atheroscler. Res.*, **10,** 391 (1969).

303. U. H. Klemens and P. V. Löwis, *Deut. Med. Wochenschr.*, **98,** 1197 (1973).

304. G. Wolfram, C. Keller, S. Kilani, and N. Zöllner, *Deut. Med. Wochenschr.*, **101,** 76 (1976).

305. N. Zöllner, C. Keller, and G. Wolfram, *Atherosclerosis*, **26,** 611 (1977).

306. M. J. Rowe, J. M. M. Neilson, and M. F. Oliver, *Lancet*, **1,** 295 (1975).

307. G. Bondesson, C. Hedbom, O. Magnusson, and N. E. Stjernström, *Acta Pharm. Suec.*, **12,** 445 (1975).

308. G. Bondesson, C. Hedbom, O. Magnusson, and N. E. Stjernström, *Acta Pharm. Suec.*, **13,** 1 (1976).

309. L. A. Carlson, C. Hedbom, E. Helgstrand, A. Misiorny, B. Sjöberg, N. E. Stjernström, and G. Westin, *Acta Pharm. Suec.*, **9,** 411 (1972); D. M. Bailey, D. Wood, R. E. Johnson, J. P. McAuliff, J.

C. Bradford, and A. Arnold, *J. Med. Chem.*, **15,** 344 (1972).
310. J. Schneider and M. Palm, *Therapiewoche*, **25,** 7704 (1975).
311. G. Brenner, *Arzneim.-Forsch.*, **25,** 237 (1975).
312. Coronary Drug Project Research Group, *J. Am. Med. Assoc.*, **220,** 996 (1972).
313. J. Kuwashima, T. Tsuboi, B. Fujitani, K. Ishikawa, K. Nakamura, Y. Ohsawa, H. Kaneko, K. Yoshida, and M. Shimizu, *J. Pharm. Soc. Japan*, **94,** 1541 (1974).
314. W. Schwartzkopff and E. Russ, *Deut. Med. Wochenschr.*, **100,** 815 (1975).
315. H. Lageder and K. Irsigler, *Atherosclerosis*, **22,** 473 (1975).
316. W. Schwartzkopff and E. Russ, *Münch. Med. Wochenschr.*, **117,** 827 (1975).
317. Coronary Drug Project Research Group, *J. Am. Med. Assoc.*, **214,** 1303 (1970); **226,** 652 (1973).
318. A. Chait, J. J. Albers, J. D. Brunzell, and W. R. Hazzard, *Lancet*, **1,** 1176 (1977).
319. C. J. Glueck, R. I. Levy, and D. S. Fredrickson, *Ann. Intern. Med.*, **75,** 345 (1971).
320. C. J. Glueck, D. Scheel, J. Fishback, and P. Steiner, *Lipids*, **7,** 110 (1972); C. L. Malmendier, C. J. van den Bergen, G. Emplit, and C. Delcroix, *J. Clin. Pharmacol.*, **18,** 42 (1978).
321. B. Rothfeld, S. Margolis, A. Varady, Jr., and A. Karmen, *Biochem. Med.*, **10,** 122 (1974); R. P. Eaton, D. S. Schade, and M. Conway, *Lancet*, **2,** 1545 (1974).
322. S. O. Byers, M. Friedman, and S. R. Elek, *Proc. Soc. Exp. Biol. Med.*, **149,** 151 (1975).
323. F. Aubry, Y. L. Marcel, and J. Davignon, *Metab. Clin. Exp.*, **23,** 225 (1974).
324. Editorial, *Lancet*, **2,** 444 (1974).
325. R. C. Turner, R. R. Holman, and P. A. Harding, *Clin. Sci. Mol. Med.*, **53,** 3p (1977).
326. M. Friedman, S. O. Byers, R. H. Rosenman, C. H. Li, and R. Neuman, *Metab. Clin. Exp.*, **23,** 905 (1974); J. F. Aloia, I. Zanzi, and S. H. Cohn, *Metab. Clin. Exp.*, **24,** 795 (1975).
327. P. Micossi, J. C. Dunbar, A. E. Pontiroli, B. A. Baker, F. Lengel, M. F. Walsh, and P. P. Foa, *Diabetes*, **25** (Suppl. I), 377 (1976); H. Pointer, G. Hengl, P. M. Bayer, and U. Flegel, *Wien. Klin. Wochenschr.*, **89,** 224 (1977); V. Schusdziarra, M. Brown, J. Rivier, W. Vale, R. Dobbs, P. Raskin, and R. H. Unger, *FEBS Lett.*, **79,** 133 (1977).
328. P. J. Barter, W. E. Connor, A. A. Spectro, M. Armstrong, S. L. Connor, and M. A. Newman, *Ann. Intern. Med.*, **81,** 619 (1974).
329. P. T. Kuo, W. C. Fan, J. B. Kostis, and K. Hayase, *Circulation*, **53,** 338 (1976).
330. A. Goldberg, M. Chen, J. Brunzell, E. Bierman, and D. Porte, Jr., *Circulation*, **52** (Suppl. II), 4 (1975).
331. A. N. Howard, D. E. Hyams, W. Everett, I. W. Jennings, G. A. Gresham, A. Bizzi, S. Garattini, E. Veneroni, and T. A. Miettinen, *Eur. J. Pharmacol.*, **13,** 244 (1971).
332. A. Czyzyk and T. Urbanski, *Nature*, **197,** 381 (1963).
333. A. Czyzyk, A. Ostaszynski, H. Plenkiewicz, Z. Szczepanik, and T. Urbanski, *Arzneim.-Forsch.*, **22,** 465 (1972).
334. M. B. Neuworth, R. J. Laufer, J. W. Barnhart, J. A. Sefranka, and D. D. McIntosh, *J. Med. Chem.*, **13,** 722 (1970).
335. A. F. Salel, R. Zelis, H. S. Sodhi, J. Price, and D. T. Mason, *Clin. Pharmacol. Ther.*, **20,** 690 (1976).
336. H. B. Brown and V. G. deWolfe, *Clin. Pharmacol. Ther.*, **16,** 44 (1974).
337. R. S. Harris, Jr., H. R. Gilmore III, L. A. Bricker, I. M. Kiem, and E. Rubin, *J. Am. Geriatr. Soc.*, **22,** 167 (1974).
338. D. T. Nash, *J. Med.*, **6,** 305 (1975).
339. F. L. Canosa, A. M. Aparicio, and E. Boyle, Jr., *Clin. Pharmacol. Ther.*, **17,** 230 (1975).
340. D. McCaughan, *J. Am. Oil Chem. Soc.*, **53,** 144A (1976); H. L. Taylor, R. B. Nolan, R. E. Tedeschi, and C. J. Maurath, *Clin. Pharmacol. Ther.*, **23,** 131 (1978); W. B. Parsons, *Am. Heart J.*, **96,** 213 (1978).
341. J. A. Arnold, D. Martin, H. L. Taylor, D. R. Christian, and J. F. Heeg, *Fed. Proc.*, **29,** 356 (1970).
342. W. B. Parsons, Jr., *Circulation*, **46** (Suppl. II), 16 (1972).
343. T. A. Miettinen, *Atherosclerosis*, **15,** 163 (1972).
344. J. W. Barnhart, J. A. Sefranka, and D. D. McIntosh, *Am. J. Clin. Nutr.*, **23,** 1229 (1970).
345. J. W. Barnhart, J. D. Johnson, D. J. Rytter, and R. B. Failey, *Advan. Exp. Med. Biol.*, **26,** 275 (1972).
346. J. W. Barnhart, D. J. Rytter, and J. A. Molello, *Lipids*, **12,** 29 (1977); R. C. Heel, R. N. Brogden, T. M. Speight, and G. S. Avery, *Drugs*, **15,** 409 (1978).
347. A. A. Renzi, D. J. Rytter, E. R. Wagner, and H. K. Goersch, *Advan. Exp. Med. Biol.*, **63,** 477 (1975); E. R. Wagner, R. G. Dull, L. G. Mueller, B. J. Allen, A. A. Renzi, D. J. Rytter, J. W. Barnhart, and C. Byers, *J. Med. Chem.*, **20,** 1007 (1977).
348. D. Kritchevsky, S. A. Tepper, and J. A. Story, *Arzneim.-Forsch.*, **26,** 862 (1976).
349. C. R. Sirtori, E. Tremoli, M. Sirtori, F. Conti, and R. Paoletti, *Atherosclerosis*, **26,** 583 (1977).

350. D. Fedele, A. Tiengo, R. Nosadini, E. Marchiori, G. Briani, M. C. Garotti, and M. Muggeo, *Diabete Metab.* (Paris), **2,** 127 (1976).

351. P. Weisweiler and P. Schwandt, *Klin. Wochenschr.*, **54,** 283 (1976).

352. R. W. Stout, J. D. Brunzell, D. Porte, Jr., and E. L. Bierman, *Metab. Clin. Exp.*, **23,** 815 (1974).

353. P. D. Lang, J. Vollmar, U. H. Klemens, P. V. Löwis, F. A. Gries, T. Koschinsky, K. Huth, E. Pilz, G. Schlierf, G. J. Kremer, P. Lenhart, P. Schwandt, H. Hammerl, and M. Studlar, *Deut. Med. Wochenschr.*, **98,** 2280 (1973).

354. S. W. Shen and R. Bressler, *New Engl. J. Med.*, **296,** 493 (1977), M. H. Tan, C. A. Graham, R. F. Bradley, R. E. Gleason, and J. S. Soeldner, *Diabetes*, **26,** 561 (1977); R. Paisey, R. S. Elkeles, J. Hambley, and P. Magill, *Clin. Sci. Mol. Med.*, **54,** 37P (1978).

355. J. A. Moorhouse, *Can. Med. Assoc. J.*, **96,** 536 (1967).

356. G. Düntsch, *Arzneim.-Forsch.*, **20,** 577 (1970).

357. F. K. Gurgis, M. H. Ghanem, and M. M. Abdel-Hay, *Arzneim.-Forsch.*, **26,** 435 (1976).

358. P. W. Stacpoole, D. M. Kornhauser, O. B. Crofford, D. Rabinowitz, and J. A. Oates, *Diabetes*, **25** (Suppl. I), 328 (1976).

359. G. D. Bell, B. Lewis, A. Petrie, and R. H. Dowling, *Brit. Med. J.*, **3,** 520 (1973).

360. N. E. Miller and P. J. Nestel, *Lancet*, **2,** 929 (1974).

361. M. Kallner, *J. Lab. Clin. Med.*, **86,** 595 (1975).

362. F. Begemann, *Digestion*, **12,** 262 (1975).

363. M. J. Coyne, G. G. Bonorris, A. Chung, L. I. Goldstein, D. Lahana, and L. J. Schoenfield, *New Engl. J. Med.*, **292,** 604 (1975).

364. G. Schlierf, A. Stiehl, C. C. Heuck, P. D. Lang, P. Oster, and B. Schellenberg, *Eur. J. Clin. Pharmacol.*, **10,** 147 (1976).

365. U. Leuschner, E. Reber, and W. Erb, *Deut. Med. Wochenschr.*, **102,** 156 (1977).

366. K. Einarsson, K. Hellström, and M. Kallner, *Metab. Clin. Exp.*, **23,** 863 (1974).

367. N. F. LaRusso, N. E. Hoffman, A. F. Hofmann, T. C. Northfield, and J. L. Thistle, *Gastroenterology*, **69,** 1301 (1975).

368. N. F. LaRusso, P. A. Szczepanik, and A. F. Hofmann, *Gastroenterology*, **72,** 132 (1977).

369. J. Ahlberg, B. Angelin, K. Einarsson, K. Hellström, and B. Leijd, *Clin. Sci. Mol. Med.*, **53,** 249 (1977).

370. T. Kaneda and S. Tokuda, *J. Nutr.*, **90,** 371 (1966).

371. T. Kamiya, Y. Saito, M. Hashimoto, and H. Seki, *Tetrahedron Lett.*, 1969, 4729.

372. I. Chibata, K. Okumura, S. Takeyama, and K. Kodera, *Experientia*, **25,** 1237 (1969).

373. K. Takashima, K. Izumi, H. Iwai, and S. Takeyama, *Atherosclerosis*, **17,** 491 (1973).

374. T. Rokujo, H. Kikuchi, A. Tensho, Y. Tsukitani, T. Takenawa, K. Yoshida, and T. Kamiya, *Life Sci.*, **9,** 379 (1970).

375. K. Takashima, C. Sato, Y. Sasaki, T. Morita, and S. Takeyama, *Biochem. Pharmacol.*, **23,** 433 (1974).

376. M. Hashimoto, Y. Saito, H. Seki, and T. Kamiya, *Chem. Pharm. Bull.* (Tokyo), **20,** 1374 (1972).

377. A. Tensho, I. Shimizu, T. Takenawa, H. Kiruchi, T. Rokujo, and T. Kamiya, *J. Pharm. Soc. Japan*, **94,** 708 (1974).

378. K. Okumura, K. Matsumoto, M. Fukamizu, H. Yasuo, Y. Taguchi, Y. Sugihara, I. Inoue, M. Seto, Y. Sato, N. Takamura, T. Kanno, M. Kawazu, T. Mizoguchi, S. Saito, K. Takashima, and S. Takeyama, *J. Med. Chem.*, **17,** 846 (1974).

379. M. Matsuo and K. Hashimoto, *Nippon Yakurigaku Zasshi*, **67,** 11p (1971).

380. S. D. Turley, C. E. West, and B. J. Horton, *Atherosclerosis*, **24,** 1 (1976).

381. V. E. Peterson, P. A. Crapo, J. Weininger, H. Ginsberg, and J. Olefsky, *Am. J. Clin. Nutr.*, **28,** 584 (1975).

382. E. Ginter, *New Engl. J. Med.*, **294,** 559 (1976); E. Ginter, O. Cerna, J. Budlovsky, V. Balaz, F. Hruba, V. Roch, and E. Sasko, *Int. J. Vitam. Nutr. Res.*, **47,** 123 (1977).

383. C. R. Spittle, *Lancet*, **2,** 1280 (1971).

384. R. J. Morin, *Lancet*, **1,** 594 (1972).

385. G. P. M. Crawford, C. P. Warlow, B. Bennett, A. A. Dawson, A. S. Douglas, D. F. Kerridge, and D. Ogston, *Atherosclerosis*, **21,** 451 (1975).

386. J. P. Kotze, *South Afr. Med. J.*, **49,** 1651 (1975); B. Sokoloff, M. Hori, C. Saelhof, B. McConnell, and T. Imai, *J. Nutr.*, **91,** 107 (1967).

387. A. Scholz, *Klin. Wochenschr.*, **51,** 518 (1973).

388. A. J. Verlangieri and R. O. Mumma, *Atherosclerosis*, **17,** 37 (1973).

389. D. Hornig, F. Weber, and O. Wiss, *Z. Klin. Chem. Klin. Biochem.*, **12,** 62 (1974).

390. D. Hornig and H. Weiser, *Experientia*, **32,** 687 (1976).

391. J. Duhault, M. Boulanger, L. Beregi, N. Sicot, and F. Bouvier, *Atherosclerosis*, **23,** 63 (1976).

392. B. Riveline, *Postgrad. Med. J.*, **51** (Suppl. I), 162 (1975); M. S. Sian and A. J. Harding Rains, *Gut*, **18,** A951 (1977).

393. S. Y. K. Yousufzai and M. Siddiqi, *Lipids*, **12,** 258 (1977); K. E. Guyer, S. G. Boots, and M. R. Boots, *Biochem. Pharmacol.*, **26,** 2449 (1977).

394. L. L. Savoie and P. J. Lupien, *Can. J. Physiol. Pharmacol.*, **53,** 638 (1975).

395. P. J. Lupien, D. Brun, and S. Moorjani, *Lancet*, **1,** 1256 (1973); *Lancet*, **1,** 283 (1978).
396. L. L. Savoie and P. J. Lupien, *Arzneim.-Forsch.*, **25,** 1284 (1975).
397. G. V. Mann, *Atherosclerosis*, **26,** 335 (1977).
398. C. R. Nair and G. V. Mann, *Atherosclerosis*, **26,** 363 (1977).
399. R. E. Olson, G. Bazzano, and J. A. D'Elia, *Trans. Assoc. Am. Phys.*, **83,** 196 (1970).
400. J. D'Elia, G. S. Bazzano, and G. Bazzano, *Lipids*, **7,** 394 (1972).
401. J. Wojcicki, *Arzneim.-Forsch.*, **26,** 2047 (1976).
402. M. Montini, P. Levoni, A. Ongaro, and G. Pagani, *Arzneim.-Forsch.*, **25,** 1311 (1975).
403. H. Hammerl, K. Kindler, C. Kraenzl, G. Nebosis, O. Pichler, and M. Studlar, *Wien. Med. Wochenschr.*, **123,** 688 (1973).
404. H. Pristantz, *Wien. Med. Wochenschr.*, **125,** 705 (1975).
405. H. Heckers, K. Dittmar, F. W. Schmahl, and K. Huth, *Atherosclerosis*, **26,** 249 (1977).
406. A. Caniggia and C. Gennari, *Artery*, **3,** 188 (1977).
407. I. Y. Rosenblum, L. Flora, and R. Eisenstein, *Atherosclerosis*, **22,** 411 (1975).
408. F. Leuschner, H. H. Wagener, and B. Neumann, *Arzneim.-Forsch.*, **26,** 1743 (1976).
409. V. Blaton, F. Soetewey, D. Vandamme, B. Declercq, and H. Peeters, *Artery*, **2,** 309 (1976); P. Avogaro, G. Cazzolato, B. G. Bittolo, G. B. Quinci, F. Belussi, O. Mantero, and F. E. Conti, *Pharmacol. Res. Commun.*, **9,** 885 (1977).
410. L. Campanacci, G. Guarnieri, L. Faccini, and G. Bellini, *Arzneim.-Forsch.*, **25,** 1306 (1975).
411. H. F. ter Welle, C. M. van Gent, W. Dekker, and A. F. Willebrands, *Acta Med. Scand.*, **195,** 267 (1974).
412. C. E. Day, P. E. Schurr, D. E. Emmert, R. E. TenBrink, and D. Lednicer, *J. Med. Chem.*, **18,** 1065 (1975).
413. P. E. Schurr and C. E. Day, *Lipids*, **12,** 22 (1977).
414. W. A. Phillips, P. E. Schurr, and N. A. Nelson, *Fed. Proc.*, **29,** 385 (1970).
415. R. A. Parker, T. Kariya, J. M. Grisar, and V. Petrow, *J. Med. Chem.*, **20,** 781 (1977).
416. T. Kariya, R. A. Parker, J. M. Grisar, J. Martin, and L. J. Wille, *Fed. Proc.*, **34,** 789 (1975); E. Panek, G. A. Cook, and N. W. Cornell, *Lipids*, **12,** 814 (1977).
417. B. Dafgärd, S. Gronowitz, G. Bondesson, O. Magnusson, and N. E. Stjernström, *Acta Pharm. Suec.*, **11,** 309 (1974).
418. I. H. Hall and G. L. Carlson, *J. Med. Chem.*, **19,** 1257 (1976).
419. S. D. Wyrick, I. H. Hall, C. Piantadosi, and C. R. Fenske, *J. Med. Chem.*, **19,** 219 (1976).
420. G. L. Carlson, I. H. Hall, G. S. Abernethy, and C. Piantadosi, *J. Med. Chem.*, **17,** 154 (1974).
421. M. N. Cayen, J. Dubuc, and D. Dvornik, *Biochem. Pharmacol.*, **25,** 1537 (1976).
422. C. Piantadosi, I. H. Hall, S. D. Wyrick, and K. S. Ishaq, *J. Med. Chem.*, **19,** 222 (1976).
423. K. H. Baggaley, S. D. Atkin, P. D. English, R. M. Hindley, B. Morgan, and J. Green, *Biochem. Pharmacol.*, **24,** 1902 (1975).
424. K. H. Baggaley, M. Heald, R. M. Hindley, B. Morgan, J. L. Tee, and J. Green, *J. Med. Chem.*, **18,** 833 (1975).
425. P. Hill, W. G. Martin, and J. F. Douglas, *Proc. Soc. Exp. Biol. Med.*, **148,** 41 (1975).
426. F. M. Berger, J. F. Douglas, B. J. Ludwig, and S. Margolin, *J. Pharmacol. Exp. Ther.*, **170,** 371 (1969).
427. J. D. Khandekar, B. D. Garg, and K. Kovacs, *Arch. Pathol.*, **92,** 221 (1971).
428. M. L. Speranza, A. Gaiti, G. E. De Medio, I. Montanini, and G. Porcellati, *Biochem. Pharmacol.*, **19,** 2737 (1970).
429. R. Fumagalli, S. Gorini, C. Pezzini, C. Sirtori, and U. Valcavi, *Advan. Exp. Med. Biol.*, **63,** 450, 476 (1975); P. Avogara, G. Cazzolato, and C. Capri, *Artery*, **3,** 219 (1977).
430. E. S. Stratford, *J. Med. Chem.*, **18,** 242 (1975).
431. S. G. Boots, M. R. Boots, and K. E. Guyer, *J. Pharm. Sci.*, **60,** 614 (1971).
432. A. Plech, H. I. Trzeciak, A. Sokola, Z. S. Herman, and T. Zawisza, *Pol. J. Pharmacol. Pharm.*, **27,** 399 (1975).
433. J. Horak, B. Cuparencu, M. Cucuianu, A. Opincaru, E. Seusan, and I. Vincze, *Atherosclerosis*, **24,** 81 (1976).
434. F. Orlandi, F. Bamonti, M. Dini, M. Koch, and A. M. Jezequel, *Eur. J. Clin. Invest.*, **5,** 139 (1975).
435. R. A. Salvador, C. Atkins, S. Haber, C. Kozma, and A. H. Conney, *Biochem. Pharmacol.*, **19,** 1975 (1970); J. W. Barnhart, *Toxicol. Appl. Pharmacol.*, **27,** 449 (1974).
436. P. Saba, F. Galeone, F. Salvadorini, M. Guarguaglini, and J. L. Houben, *Artery*, **3,** 250 (1977).
437. J. M. Grisar, G. P. Claxton, K. T. Stewart, R. D. MacKenzie, and T. Kariya, *J. Med. Chem.*, **19,** 1195 (1976); J. A. Svoboda, T. R. Wrenn, M. J. Thompson, J. R. Weyant, D. L. Wood, and J. Bitman, *Lipids*, **12,** 691 (1977).
438. J. E. Sinsheimer, E. Van den Eeckhout, L. E. Hewitt, Y. Kido, D. R. Wade, D. W. Hansen, Jr., J. C. Drach, and J. H. Burckhalter, *J. Med. Chem.*, **19,**

647 (1976); J. M. Kokosa, J. E. Sinsheimer, D. R. Wade, J. C. Drach, and J. H. Burckhalter, *ibid.*, **21,** 225 (1978).

439. M. Steinberg and A. S. Watnick, *Proc. Soc. Exp. Biol. Med.*, **134,** 696 (1970).

440. J. Esteve, J. Pares, A. Colombo, I. Demestre, L. Rodriguez, R. Sagarra, and R. Roser, *Eur. J. Med. Chem.-Chim. Ther.*, **11,** 43 (1976).

441. J. H. Dygos, C. M. Jett, L. J. Chinn, and J. E. Miller, *J. Med. Chem.*, **20,** 1705 (1977).

442. J. Green, M. Heald, K. H. Baggaley, R. M. Hindley, and B. Morgan, *Atherosclerosis*, **23,** 549 (1976); W. J. Bochenek and J. B. Rodgers, *Biochim. Biophys. Acta*, **489,** 503 (1977).

443. F. P. Bell, *Lipids*, **11,** 769 (1976).

444. J. K. Reddy, D. E. Moody, D. L. Azarnoff, and M. S. Rao, *Life Sci.*, **18,** 941 (1976).

445. F. Clemence, O. Le Martret, R. Fournex, M. Dagnaux, and G. Plassard, *Eur. J. Med. Chem.-Chim. Ther.*, **11,** 567 (1976).

446. J. E. Miller and J. B. Hill, *J. Am. Oil Chem. Soc.*, **53,** 140A (1976); T. Kobayakawa, K. Osuga, H. Yasuda, and H. Imamura, *Jap. J. Pharmacol.*, **27,** 97P (1977).

447. D. L. Raulston, C. O. Mishaw, E. J. Parish, and G. J. Schroepfer, Jr., *Biochem. Biophys. Res. Commun.*, **71,** 984 (1976); A. Kisic, D. Monger, E. J. Parish, S. Satterfield, D. L. Raulston, and G. J. Schroepfer, Jr., *Artery*, **3,** 421 (1977).

448. L. J. Chinn and K. W. Salamon, *J. Med. Chem.*, **20,** 229 (1977).

449. L. Brzechffa, M. Eberle, R. Engstrom, L. Kelly, and S. Talati, *Abstr. Pap., Am. Chem. Soc.*, 172nd Meeting MEDI 47 (1976); J. W. H. Watthey, B. Henrici, S. Lausten, and M. Miller, *ibid.*, 173rd Meeting MEDI 12 (1977).

450. A. C. Sullivan, J. Triscari, J. G. Hamilton, and J. A. Ontko, *Lipids*, **12,** 1 (1977).

451. G. Bondesson, C. Hedbom, D. Magnusson, and N. E. Stjernström, *Acta Pharm. Suec.*, **11,** 417 (1974).

452. H. Peeters, V. Blaton, B. Declercq, D. Vandamme, J. Roba, R. Roncucci, and G. Lambelin, *Arzneim.-Forsch.*, **27,** 1964 (1977).

453. C. I. Jarowski and R. Pytelewski, *J. Pharm. Sci.*, **64,** 690 (1975); P. K. Raja and C. I. Jarowski, *J. Pharm. Sci.*, **64,** 691 (1975).

454. F. Consolo, F. Arrigo, G. Di Tommaso, and A. Trifiro, *Curr. Ther. Res. Clin. Exp.*, **22,** 751 (1977).

455. F. W. Quackenbush, P. G. Rand, and J. E. MacNintch, *Lipids*, **12,** 686 (1977); J. E. MacNintch, R. A. Harris, W. Grogan, C. L. Villemez, Jr., and F. W. Quackenbush, *Lipids*, **12,** 819 (1977).

456. J. W. Erdman, Jr., and P. A. Lachance, *Nutr. Rep. Int.*, **10,** 277 (1974).

457. D. Porte, Jr., and E. L. Bierman, *J. Lab. Clin. Med.*, **73,** 631 (1969).

458. T. Kobayakawa, *J. Pharm. Soc. Japan*, **92,** 919 (1972).

459. K. Nakazawa and K. Murata, *Advan. Exp. Med. Biol.*, **63,** 468 (1975); P. Rubba, A. Rivellese, S. Griffo, and M. Mancini, *Pharmacol. Res. Commun.*, **9,** 675 (1977); R. Turpini, *Artery*, **3,** 282 (1977); P. Avogaro, G. Bittolo-Bon, G. C. Taroni, G. Cazzolato, and F. Belussi, *Pharmacol. Res. Commun.*, **9,** 977 (1977).

460. E. E. Howe, D. K. Bosshardt, J. Gilfillan, V. M. Hunt, and J. W. Huff, *Arch. Biochem. Biophys.*, **129,** 264 (1969).

461. C. Bibracher, K. Krueger, and J. Roehren, *Ther. Gegenw.*, **114,** 1107 (1975).

462. F. Consolo, G. Di Tommaso, F. Arrigo, and A. Trifiro, *Boll. Soc. Ital. Biol. Sper.*, **51,** 1920 (1975).

463. A. Endo and M. Kuroda, *J. Antibiot.* (Tokyo), **29,** 841 (1976).

464. A. Endo, M. Kuroda, and Y. Tsujita, *J. Antibiot.* (Tokyo), **29,** 1346 (1976); A. Endo, Y. Tsujita, M. Kuroda, and K. Tanzawa, *Eur. J. Biochem.*, **77,** 31 (1977).

465. M. Koroda, Y. Hazama-Shimada, and A. Endo, *Biochem. Biophys. Acta*, **486,** 254 (1977); K. Tanzawa, M. Kuroda, and A. Endo, *ibid.*, **488,** 97 (1977).

466. A. Endo, M. Kuroda, and K. Tanzawa, *FEBS Lett.*, **72,** 323 (1976).

467. T. Hosokawa, K. Suzuki, T. Okutomi, M. Sawada, and K. Ando, *Jap. J. Pharmacol.*, **25,** 35 (1975).

468. A. Bordia, S. K. Verma, A. K. Vyas, B. L. Khabya, A. S. Rathore, N. Bhu, and H. K. Bedi, *Atherosclerosis*, **26,** 379 (1977).

469. R. C. Jain and D. B. Konar, *Lancet*, **1,** 918 (1976).

470. The Herbs and the Heart, *Nutr. Rev.*, **34,** 43 (1976).

471. R. C. Jain, *Lancet*, **1,** 1240 (1975).

472. K. T. Augusti and P. T. Mathew, *Experientia*, **30,** 468 (1974).

473. A. Bordia, H. C. Bansal, S. K. Arora, and S. V. Singh, *Atherosclerosis*, **21,** 15 (1975).

474. K. I. Baghurst, M. J. Raj, and A. S. Truswell, *Lancet*, **1,** 101 (1977).

475. M. Fujiwara, Y. Itokawa, H. Uchino, and K. Inoue, *Experientia*, **28,** 254 (1972).

476. J. L. Gainer and J. R. Jones, *Experientia*, **31,** 548 (1975).

477. H. Enomoto, Y. Yoshikuni, Y. Yasutomi, K. Ohata, K. Sempuku, K. Kitaguchi, Y. Fujita, and T. Mori, *Chem. Pharm. Bull.* (Tokyo), **25,** 507 (1977); H. Enomoto, Y. Yoshikuni, T. Ozaki, R. Zschocke, and K. Ohata, *Atherosclerosis*, **28,** 205 (1977).

478. Y. Imai, H. Matsumura and Y. Aramaki, *Jap. J. Pharmacol.*, **20,** 222 (1970).
479. M. Yamamoto, A. Kumagi, and Y. Yamamura, *Arzneim.-Forsch.*, **25,** 1240 (1975).
480. K. Sakakibara, Y. Shibata, T. Higashi, S. Sanada, and J. Shoji, *Chem. Pharm. Bull.* (Tokyo), **23,** 1009 (1975).
481. H. Koshiyama, M. Hatori, H. Ohkuma, F. Sakai, H. Imanishi, M. Ohbayashi, and H. Kawaguchi, *Chem. Pharm. Bull.* (Tokyo), **24,** 169 (1976).
482. S. M. Grundy and H. Y. I. Mok, *J. Lab. Clin. Med.*, **89,** 354 (1977).
483. H. Kaffarnik, J. Schneider, and W. Haase, *Deut. Med. Wochenschr.*, **100,** 2486 (1975).
484. G. Gragnoli, G. Postorino, I. Tanganelli, and L. Brandi, *Minerva Med.*, **68,** 1281 (1977).
485. T. Gordon, W. P. Castelli, M. C. Hjortland, W. B. Kannel, and T. R. Dawber, *Am. J. Med.*, **62,** 707 (1977).
486. N. E. Miller, D. S. Thelle, O. H. Forde, and O. D. Mjos, *Lancet*, **1,** 965 (1977).
487. J. M. Stanhope, V. M. Sampson, and P. M. Clarkson, *Lancet*, **1,** 968 (1977).
488. I. C. Ononogbu, *Experientia*, **33,** 1063 (1977).
489. S. M. Grundy, *Am. J. Clin. Nutr.*, **30,** 985 (1977).
490. T. T. Ishikawa, S. McNeely, P. M. Steiner, C. J. Glueck, M. Mellies, P. S. Gartside, and C. M. McMillin, *Metab. Clin. Exp.*, **27,** 89 (1978).
491. L. A. Carlson and B. Kolmodin-Hedman, *Acta Med. Scand.*, **201,** 375 (1977).
492. E. Nikkilä, M. Kaste, C. Ehnholm and J. Viikari, *Brit. Med. J.*, **2,** 99 (1978).
493. R. M. Krauss, F. T. Lindgren, A. Silvers, R. Jutagir, and D. D. Bradley, *Clin. Chim. Acta*, **80,** 465 (1977).
494. W. P. Castelli, T. Gordon, M. C. Hjortland, A. Kagan, J. T. Doyle, C. G. Hames, S. B. Hulley, and W. J. Zukel, *Lancet*, **2,** 153 (1977); K. Yano, G. G. Rhoads, and A. Kagan, *New Engl. J. Med.*, **297,** 405 (1977).
495. O. D. Mjos, *Scand. J. Clin. Lab. Invest.*, **37,** 191 (1977); *Abstracts Sixth International Symposium on Drugs Affecting Lipid Metabolism*, Philadelphia, Pa., 75, 68, and 38 (1977).
496. Coronary Drug Project Research Group, *J. Am. Med. Assoc.*, **231,** 360 (1975).
497. Physicians of the Newcastle-upon-Tyne Region, *Brit. Med. J.*, **4,** 767 (1971).
498. Research Committee of the Scottish Society of Physicians, *Brit. Med. J.*, **4,** 775 (1971).
499. N. O. Borhani, *Am. J. Cardiol.*, **40,** 251 (1977).
500. J. A. Heady, *Bull. W.H.O.*, **48,** 243 (1973); B. M. Rifkind, *Atheroscler. Rev.*, **2,** 67 (1977).
501. G. B. Kolata, *Science*, **190,** 764 (1975).
502. M. J. Finkel, *Lipids*, **12,** 64 (1977).
503. G. V. Mann, *New Engl. J. Med.*, **297,** 644 (1977).
504. C. E. Niehaus, R. Wootton, J. Lewis, A. Nicoll, B. Williams, D. J. Coltart, and B. Lewis, *Lancet*, **2,** 469 (1977).
505. D. H. Blankenhorn, S. H. Brooks, R. H. Selzer, and R. Barndt, Jr., *Circulation*, **57,** 355 (1978).

Index